PROPERTY OF
NATIONAL UNIVERSITY
LIBRARY.

CIRCULATING

HISPANIC MENTAL HEALTH RESEARCH:

A REFERENCE GUIDE

HISPANIC MENTAL HEALTH RESEARCH: A REFERENCE GUIDE

Frank Newton

Esteban L. Olmedo

Amado M. Padilla

NATIONAL UNIVERSITY
LIBRARY   SAN DIEGO

UNIVERSITY OF CALIFORNIA PRESS
Berkeley • Los Angeles • London

University of California Press
Berkeley and Los Angeles, California
University of California Press, Ltd.
London, England
Copyright © 1982 by The Regents of the University of California
ISBN 0–520–04166–6
Library of Congress Catalog Card Number: 81–52880
Printed in the United States of America
1   2   3   4   5   6   7   8   9

CONTENTS

ACKNOWLEDGMENTS

There are always countless numbers of people to thank in a project such as this. Perhaps the greatest debt is owed to Dr. James Ralph, Chief, Center for Minority Group Mental Health Programs and Dr. Juan Ramos, Director, Division of Special Mental Health Programs, National Institute of Mental Health. With their encouragement and assistance the authors were able to complete the bibliography presented here. Our sincere appreciation extends as well to the National Institute of Mental Health for its generous financial support of the project, through Research Grants MH 30276 and MH 24854 to the Spanish Speaking Mental Health Research Center at the University of California, Los Angeles. Finally, we must express our profound gratitude to our excellent staff, without whose diligence and devotion this project could not have succeeded. They served as abstractors, library workers, data entry operators on the computer, and in a variety of other capacities. These individuals, in alphabetical order, include: Diane Bloom, Cathy Bruno, Elizabeth Cooney, Maria Hewitt, Steve Lopez, Marcia Luna, Robert Perez, Arturo Romero, Cecilia Torres, Bruce Williams, Mary Williams, and Autumn VanOrd. Certainly, the quality of this bibliography, more than any words of appreciation we could express, is a tribute to the outstanding quality of all their efforts.

Amado M. Padilla
University of California, Los Angeles
September, 1981

INTRODUCTION

Interest in Hispanic Americans has accelerated since the mid-nineteen sixties. The major reason for this is the rise of ethnic awareness and interest in self-enhancement shown by Hispanics, most notably Mexican Americans, Puerto Ricans, and Cubans. This increased awareness has reached beyond the Hispanic community and is reflected in a number of aspects of our daily life. For example, people commonly speak of "salsa" and doing the "Latin hustle" or of the fact that bilingual education should be available to children from homes where Spanish is spoken. Today we recognize the first as a cultural evolution of music and dance. Similarly, in the case of bilingual education, the arguments pro and con are aired in the press and at educational conferences whereas a decade ago, although in existence, bilingual education did not carry the same significance that it does today.

This interest in things cultural has also had an effect in the behavioral and social sciences. There has in the past decade been an explosion of literature on Hispanics. Our interest at the Spanish Speaking Mental Health Research Center (SSMHRC) has been to collect and systematize into bibliographic form the literature that pertains to the mental health of the Hispanic American. This was obviously a large task and requires some definition of terms. Since mental health does not have an absolutely agreed upon definition by professionals in the field, we did not attempt a definition, other than to conceive of mental health in the broadest possible terms. For our purposes, mental health-related literature referred to any article—be it psychiatric, psychological, sociologial, educational or anthropological in nature—that was connected in some way with the mental well-being of the target population. This almost circular defintion meant that articles on "susto" (a condition of "magical fright") were as likely to be included in the bibliograpy as articles on the success of a particular psychotheraputic technique; and articles dealing with such topics as the cognitive development of Hispanic children were also eligible for citation, as were articles concerned with the training of students in social welfare or psychology. Moreover, our concern was to cite not only those studies which included Hispanic Americans in the subject population, but also those articles in the non-Hispanic American literature which further our understanding of Hispanic Americans—especially for areas in which little or no research exists on Hispanic Americans.

A second matter in need of clarification is the term "Hispanic American." In our usage of the term we are referring to all people of Spanish Speaking/Surname origin residing in the United States or Puerto Rico. Accordingly, Hispanic is a generic term which includes Cuban Americans, Mexican Americans, Puerto Ricans, and other Central or South American origin groups. A quick scanning of the entries in the bibliography will reveal that the majority of articles pertain either to Mexican Americans or Puerto Ricans. This is due to the fact that, until recently, literature on Hispanic groups other than these two was virtually non-existent. For example, a few years ago there was little information available on Cuban Americans and, with the exception of a few articles, there is still no body of literature on Hispanics from the Dominican Republic, other Caribbean islands, or other Central or South American countries. However, this situation is changing rapidly— evidenced by the fact that research on Cuban Americans has increased dramatically. We therefore fully expect that over the decade of the eighties, we will see the emergence of literature pertaining to all Hispanic American communities.

Finally, it is important to note that our bibliography only cites references to Hispanic groups residing in the United States. Users who are interested in transcultural work with inhabitants of Central or South American countries are referred to two recent volumes that may facilitate their search: (1) Ardila and Finley (1975) who, in a special issue of the Interamerican Journal of Psychology/Revista Interamericana de Psicologia, compiled a bibliography on psychology in Latin America; and (2) Favazza and Oman (1977) who recently published "Anthropological and Cross Cultural Themes in Mental Health: An Annotated Bibliography, 1925-1975" which contains a very large number of articles pertaining to Latin America.

Our purpose in compiling this bibliography was to make available to researchers, practitioners, and students a volume which they could easily consult for information about Hispanics and mental health-related issues. The need for such a bibliography became apparent in 1971 when one of the authors (A.M. Padilla) began a search of the Hispanic mental health literature. Since no readily apparent reference source existed in this field, work on the compilation of such a bibliography was begun in 1972. Because of the limited size of the literature, that first bibliography (Padilla and Aranda, 1974) appeared in annotated form containing only 497 citations from the early 1920s through 1972. Building upon this pioneering work, a second bibliography was published four years later (Padilla, Olmedo, Lopez, and Perez, 1978). It contained the original 497 citations in Padilla and Aranda's work plus approximately 1,300 new citations. That startling increase in size was not merely due to the more thorough search procedure employed in compiling the new bibliography, but clearly reflected the explosion of literature in the Hispanic mental health field in the 1970s.

The second bibliography differed from the first in the notable absence of article annotations. But it also improved upon that earlier volume by the inclusion of index terms to help users rapidly locate articles by subject matter. That change reflected our evolution as bibliographers and, in particular, our realization that the adequate storage and retrieval of the rapidly growing literature required a new, more efficient cataloging system. We therefore developed a computerized bibliographic retrieval system which allowed us to quickly add new citations to the bibliography and, by means of index terms, to immediately access the literature according to subject matter. As part of this effort to expand and improve our bibliographic project, we decided that reinstituting annotations (or abstracts) to the articles would be an invaluable aid to users. This new bibliography represents the culmination of our three years of work to make these changes in our bibliographic system. The 2,000 citations with abstracts presented in this volume include material contained in the two previous bibliographies plus several hundred new citations. Improvements in this new bibliography include more concise abstracts than those appearing in the first bibliography plus a larger set of index terms than that found in the second bibliography. This new bibliography contains all of the Hispanic mental health literature through 1977 and the more important citations for the years 1978-79. Obviously, our task as bibliographers is far from over. In subsequent work, we will complete abstracts on material from 1978-79 not included here, and we will add new material appearing in the early-1980s.

It should also be mentioned that since the bibliography is computerized for easy access and since it is constantly being updated, users can communicate with the staff at the Spanish Speaking Mental Health Research Center to learn whether new entries have been added to the bibliography on a particular topic following the publication of this volume. This requires a computer search of our files which can be done in a brief period of time for a very nominal charge.

SOURCES

No beginning date was established in our search procedure, although our searches of bibliographic data bases generally went back only to the late-1960s or early-1970s because of the time limitations of each data base. Therefore, the majority of our citations are from the past two decades, while some date back to the 1920s. Regarding the specifics of our searches of bibliographic data bases, we began with the National Clearinghouse for Mental Health Informtion (NCMHI). In addition, we obtained searches from the following data bases (listed by their commonly known acronyms, with their full names in parentheses):

PASAR (Psychological Abstracts Search and Retrieval)
ERIC (Educational Resources Information Center)
DISSERTATION ABSTRACTS
NTIS (National Technical Information Service)
SOCIOLOGICAL ABSTRACTS
SOCIOSEARCH (Social Science Citation Index)
NCAI (National Clearinghouse for Alcohol Information)
CAAAL (Classified Abstract Archive of the Alcohol Literature)

MEDLINE (National Library of Medicine's Medical Analysis and Retrieval System)

The tables of contents of a large number of journals were also searched during the period in which this bibliography was compiled. This resulted in the location of many relevant entries, especially of material published prior to 1960.

A number of conference resports and upublished manuscripts are included in the bibliography. These entries pose a particular problem because they are often difficult to obtain. They are included here because of their relevance and not necessarily because they are readily available in conference proceedings, from the authors themselves, or from the SSMHRC Clearinghouse. Moreover, it is not our contention that we have included all conference reports in compiling this bibliography since we were at times unable to locate relevant sources or complete citations. Many of the conference reports that are included here were forwarded by the authors directly to SSMHRC for inclusion in the bibliography. Accordingly, this has resulted in some unevenness in the inclusion of conference reports and unpublished papers. For example, only one report delivered at a professional meeting may be listed when, in fact, there may have been several other papers on an Hispanic theme that we did not know about or have access to.

A final point is that a large number of individuals were contacted and informed about the bibliographic project and asked to send relevant materials to SSMHRC—such as reprints, conference papers, technical reports, etc. This resulted, fortunately, in our inclusion of a number of valuable citations which might otherwise have gone unnoticed. Technical consultation was also obtained from experts in the field of information science who advised us on a variety of commercial bibliographic sources and on ways to maximize our search strategies.

IDENTIFYING ARTICLES

Bibliographic work is always problematic. A very large number of articles, chapters and books may, because of historical developments, be peripherally relevant or touch on a topic of interest in the development of a new line of inquiry and then move on to a totally different problem, thus creating headaches for the bibliographer. Trying to be too limiting in the compilation of a bibliography can be a mistake since important historical citations may be omitted, while trying to be too encompassing can result in a project that appears to have no central theme. Another problem in this kind of work is that the bibliographer always finds that it is necessary to add one more citation or that there is one more source that must be checked before completion. Still another difficulty is that relevant sources cannot always be identified from the title alone. For example, an article by Abad, Ramos, and Boyce (1974) is clearly identifiable as relevant to the field of Hispanic mental health by its title "A model for delivery of mental health services to Spanish-speaking minorities," while an article by Allinsmith and Goethals (1956) entitled

"Cultural factors in mental health: An anthropological perspective" is not at all identifiable by its title alone. Then there are titles that hint at relevance but which must be examined carefully, as in the case of the article by Aiello and Jones (1971) entitled "Field study of the proxemic behavior of young school children in three subcultural groups." In this case, the curious bibliographer must determine whether one of the subcultural groups in the study is Hispanic.

Our procedure for locating relevant articles began by searching for titles which appeared to deal with Hispanic Americans (or at least with ethnic/minority groups) and fell within our broad definition of mental health. Once these were identified, the articles were examined to determine whether they met our criteria for inclusion in the bibliography. The next step was to examine the author's reference list for titles of other potentially relevant citations. This procedure allowed us to add references which, by an examination of title alone, would probably not have been searched. Moreover, the branching out process of moving from one article's reference list to another's allowed us to gradually build up our body of citations in the bibliography.

Articles appearing in psychological, psychiatric, and social work-related journals were the most easily identifiable by title as relevant for our search. This was not true of the anthropological, educational, and sociological literature where articles could not always be identified by title and where some restrictions had to be imposed as to what articles would or would not be included in the bibliography. For instance, there are a large number of articles on family and kin structure among various Latin American groups in the anthropological literature. Further, it is clear from current work on Hispanic mental health (cf. Keefe, Padilla, & Carlos, 1979) that family and kin structure is an important consideration for a total understanding of how Hispanics resolve emotional problems. However, to include all relevant literature would obviously have taken us far beyond our goal of compiling a bibliography on Hispanics residing in the United States only. Accordingly, when review articles were available on important topics, we opted to include the review article rather than all of the possibly relevant literature. Thus, Carlos and Seller's (1972) important review of family and kin structure is included here. Similar problems occurred in the educational and sociological literature. In education we have included, for example, Hernandez's (1973) review of variables affecting achievement of middle school Mexican American students. Unfortunately, such systematic reviews do not yet exist in the sociological literature.

In conclusion, we have tried to be as encompassing as possible in the material that we have selected for inclusion. We have tried to use as broad a definition of mental health as possible so as not to exclude disciplines or areas of inquiry in our search. The core disciplines have been anthropology, education, psychology, psychiatry, sociology, and social work; nonetheless, work in public health, medicine and nursing has been added when appropriate. It is important to note that economic and political science-related journals were also searched from time to time to determine whether works of relevance could be located. A perusal of the bibliography will reveal that few articles could be located in these fields (e.g., Weaver, 1971). It is our belief that the absence of literature in these two disciplines should be corrected since it is clear that economics and politics enter directly into the determination of mental health policy. The role that Hispanics can and should play in the field of mental health cannot be achieved in the absence of a solid understanding of the impact of economics and politics on the profession.

CITATION FORMAT

In the computerized bibliographic format used, there are six fields which contain information about an article. The first field (AUTH) lists the last name and initials of the author(s). In the second field (TITL), the complete title of the article is given. The third field, source (SRCE), provides the user with the exact information necessary to be able to locate the article. For instance, the article by Abad et al. (1974) is available in the American Journal of Orthopsychiatry, was published in 1974, and can be found in volume 44, issue number 4, pages 584 to 595. In those cases where the article is not available in a journal or book, other important information is given in the source field to help the user obtain the desired article. For example, an unpublished manuscript by Acosta (1975) can be obtained by writing the author at the Department of Psychiatry, School of Medicine, University of Southern California. Similarly, a working paper by Anderson and Evans (1973) can be obtained from the Institute for the Study of Social Change at Purdue University or from the ERIC Document Reproduction Service No. ED 077 813.

The fourth field requires greater amplification. The index (INDX) field contains a listing of the most important descriptor terms. These descriptor terms have been employed to help users determine whether the article is appropriate for their needs. Following this introduction, the user will find the "Dictionary of Descriptor Terms" which was employed in carrying out the indexing of all citations. For example, a user who wants to know what is implied by the index term ACCULTURATION will see in the dictionary that it refers to: (1) a process of change or adaptation from one culture to another; and (2) studies measuring, manipulating, or making reference to the process of acculturation. Then turning to the "Inverted Index" further back, the user will see that ACCULTURATION is a term that has been used as a descriptor term for a large number of citations, beginning numerically with entry number 1 by Abad, Ramos, and Boyce (1977).

In addition to topical information, the index field conveys information on Hispanic subgroups. For instance, if an article pertains to Mexican Americans, this term is keyed in the index field of that article and appears as well in the Inverted Index of the bibliography. Other Hispanic subgroups indexed include Caribbean, Cuban, Puerto Rican, Mexican, and Spanish Surnamed. The latter term is used when the particular subgroup in a study or report is not specified.

The index field also contains information as to whether the author(s) reports findings from an empirical study, a survey, a case study, or whether the article is a review of literature, an essay, or a book. Each of these types of reports are defined in the bibliography's Dictionary of Descriptor Terms. Finally, where appropriate, the index field contains information about the age of the subject population in question. The term is broken down into five categories: infancy (up to age 2); children (2 to 12 years); adolescents (13 to 18 years); adults (19 to 59 years); and gerontology (age 60 and over).

It was felt that these added descriptor terms would assist users in determining whether or not a particular article meets their needs. They should serve the user well in alleviating the problem of spending time searching for studies that ultimately are not of direct interest. An example may help. Suppose that a user is interested in work of an empirical nature with children of Mexican American origin which bears on the general topic of intelligence. The user has several alternatives. One could begin with all of the articles on intelligence and intelligence testing, and then systematically eliminate all references which do not seem appropriate from the other descriptor terms listed. Another strategy would be to begin with children and eliminate all inappropriate citations. Either strategy will get the user to the same point, that is, to all references of an empirical nature with Mexican American children on intelligence and intelligence testing.

In discussing the INDX field, it is important to say a few words about the strategy employed to assign descriptor terms. Prior to assigning any descriptor terms, the article, chapter, or book was read by an abstractor. Titles alone were not used for making decisions about descriptor terms. Further, it was felt that since the INDX field is crucial to the use of the bibliography, we did not set a limit on the number of descriptors assigned to any reference. Accordingly, as many descriptor terms as the abstractor felt necessary to fully cover an entry were used.

The fifth field, abstract (ABST), also requires some explanation. Each entry is accompanied by an abstract of approximately 200 words. The abstracts were prepared in such a way as to accurately describe the entry in terms of the problem, subject population, method of study, results, and conclusions. No value judgments were made by the abstractors or editors concerning the subject matter, methodology, analysis, or conclusions derived by the author(s) of any entry. These judgments are left to the user. A second point, as users will note, is that some abstracts are followed by JOURNAL ABSTRACT, AUTHOR ABSTRACT, PASAR ABSTRACT, etc. These designations inform the user of the source of the abstract. The additional designation of MODIFIED (e.g., JOURNAL ABSTRACT MODIFIED) indicates that the abstract was edited by SSMHRC staff so as to conform to our criteria for completeness of information in abstracts. If an abstract is not followed by a source designation, this means that the abstract was written by our staff. Finally, each abstract is followed by the number of references cited by the article. This information is meant to help those users who wish to know if an article will aid them in an expanded search for relevant literature in their area of interest.

The sixth and final field, accession number (ACCN), presents a six-digit number assigned by our staff to the entry. This number is essentially an arbitrary designation for the convenience of our staff's record keeping. Specifically, in SSMHRC's offices there is a copy of each article cited in the bibliography, and this file is arranged by accession number. It should therefore be noted that if a user needs to contact SSMHRC regarding any reference in the bibliography, it would facilitate our staff's response if the reference's accession number is included in the user's inquiry.

Regarding format, the articles are generally in alphabetical order according to the primary author's last name. However, there are a few cases where this order is not strictly adhered to, due to limitations of the computer program used to develop the bibliography. The computer program interprets the ampersand in multiple author citations to precede all letters. Consequently, citations with three or more authors will be presented before the double author citations. For example, FABREGA, H., Jr., Swartz, J.D., & WALLACE, C.A. precedes FABREGA, H., Jr., & METZGER, D. Although there are these minor variations from a strictly alphabetized bibliography, the user should have no difficulty in locating the desired articles.

CONCLUDING COMMENT

Bibliographic work may not seem as challenging as conducting empirical research nor as intellectually stimulating as preparing an exhaustive review of literature. Yet it is a very gratifying endeavor. What motivates a bibliographer is more than knowing that a valuable service is being provided. One important point is that each abstract is an interesting challenge which requires the cobined talents of a scientist who can accurately discern the most essential elements of a research report and a writer who can clearly and completely describe the contents of a 5-page report or a 500-page book in a few hundred words. Moreover, it can be fascinating to uncover references which have lain forgotten for years and yet were important for the development of current interests, or to locate references which depict earlier stereotypes and prejudices of presumably unbiased social scientists. In the first case, the bibliographer may be motivated by a sense of history in seeing in print what earlier writers thought about a problem. A good example would be the early work of Sanchez (1932a, b; 1934a, b) on the intelligence testing of Hispanic children. Many of his observations are as current as if they had been written yesterday, yet they are largely ignored by mainstream psychometricians. In the second case, imagine finding three early articles entitled "Musical talent of Mexicans," A comparison of the intelligence of Mexican and mixed- and full-blood Indian children," and "Racial differences in bi-manual dexterity of Latin and American children." These studies demonstrate, in sum, that Mexican children are musical, good with their hands, and superior to full-blooded Indians because of elements of Caucasian blood in Mexicans, but not equal to whites. An examination of these articles reveals that their "scientific" conclusions were arrived at by established and well known psychologists at the time. The obvious racism shown in these articles, although written some forty years ago, reflects attitudes that have largely gone unchallenged even today.

Bibliographers also frequently find themselves confronted with titles that can only provoke the curious to determine what the author had in mind when selecting a title. Some examples of these are:

Land of poco tiempo
The old equalizer
Spirit fathers and paternal lovers
Going home again: The new American scholarship boy

Then, of course, there are articles which by their title imply strong cultural significance which can only really be understood by a person knowledgeable of the cultural implications of the title. For example, we have the following:

El tecato
The "low riders: Portrait of an urban youth subculture
Zoot suiters and Mexicans: Symbols in crowd behavior
Susto revisited: Illness as a strategic role
Fifteen cases of embrujada combining medication and suggestion in treatment
The curandero's apprentice: A theraputic integration of folk and medical healing

Regardless of what ultimately motivated our efforts, we have sought to design a bibliography that would suit the needs of researchers, practitioners, and students interested in Hispanic mental health. We have tried not to be too limiting in our search or too broad. Within a range that seemed comfortable, we gathered citations that seemed to us to be of potential interest to users of the bibliography.

REFERENCES

Abad, V, Ramos, J., & Boyce, E. A model for delivery of mental health services to Spanish-speaking minorities. American Journal of Orthopsychiatry, 1974, 44(4), 584-595.

Abad, V., Ramos, J., & Boyce, E. Clinical issues in the psychiatric treatment of Puerto Ricans. In E.R. Padilla & A.M. Padilla (eds.), Transcultural Psychiatry: An Hispanic Perspective (Monograph No. 4). Los Angeles: University of California, Spanish Speaking Mental Health Research Center, 1977.

Acosta, F. X. Client ethnicity and preferences as critical variables in psychotherapy: The Mexican American. Unpublished manuscript, Department Psychiatry, School of Medicine, University of Southern California, 1975.

Aiello, J. R., & Jones, S. E. Field study of the proxemic behavior of young school children in three subcultural groups. Journal of Personality and Social Psychology, 1971, 19(3), 351-356.

Allinsmith, W., & Goethals, G. W. Cultural factors in mental health: An anthropological perspective. Review of Educational Research, 1956, 26(5), 429-450.

Anderson, J. G., & Evans, F. B. Family socialization and educational achievement in two cultures: The Mexican American and Anglo American (Working paper 58). Lafayette, Ind.: Institute for the Study of Social Change, Purdue University, 1973. (ERIC Document Reproduction Service No. ED 077 813.)

Ardila, R., & Finley, G. Psychology in Latin America: A bibliography. Revista Interamericana de Psicologia, 1975, 9(3-4), whole number.

Carlos, M. L., & Sellers, L. Family, kinship structure and modernization in Latin America. Latin American Research Review, 1972, 7(2), 95-124.

Favazza, A. R., & Oman, M. Anthropological and Cross-Cultural Themes in Mental Health: An Annotated Bibliography, 1925-1974. Columbia, Mo.: University of Missouri Press, 1977.

Hernandez, N. G. Variables affecting achievement of middle school Mexican American students. Review of Educational Research, 1973, 43(1), 1-39.

Keefe, S. E., Padilla, A. M., & Carlos, M. L. The Mexican American extended family as an emotional support system. Human Organization, 1979, 38(2), 144-152.

Padilla, A. M., & Aranda, P. Latino Mental Health: Bibliography and Abstracts (DHEW Publication No. (HSM) 73-9144). Washington, D.C.: U.S. Government Printing Office, 1974.

Padilla, A. M., Olmedo, E. L., Lopez, S., & Perez, R. Hispanic Mental Health Bibliography II (Monograph No. 6). Los Angeles: University of California, Spanish Speaking Mental Health Research Center, 1978.

Sanchez, G. I. Group differences in Spanish-speaking children: A critical review. Journal of Applied Psychology, 1932a, 16(5), 549-558

Sanchez, G. I. Scores of Spanish-speaking children on repeated tests. Journal of Genetic Psychology, 1932b, 40(1), 223-231.

Sanchez, G. I. Bilingualism and mental measures. Journal of Applied Psychology, 1934a, 18(6), 765-772.

Sanchez, G. I. The implications of a basal vocabulary to the measurement of the abilities of bilingual children. Journal of Social Psychology, 1934b, 5(3), 395-402.

Weaver, J. L. Health care as a political issue: A Chicano perspective. Paper presented at the Annual Meeting of the Western Political Science Association, Albuquerque, New Mexico, 1971.

DICTIONARY OF DESCRIPTOR TERMS

ABILITY TESTING Studies dealing with variables described as affecting validity or reliability of tests designed to measure one or more aspects of intellectual functioning, especially as applied to Hispanic populations. The term applies to the testing of specific abilities or aptitudes, as opposed to the assessment of global intelligence.

ACCULTURATION (1) Process of change or adaptation from one culture to another. (2) Studies specifically measuring, manipulating, or making reference to the process of acculturation.

ACHIEVEMENT MOTIVATION (1) Motivation or desire of individual or group for occupational or personal achievement. (2) Studies measuring or making inferences about achievement motivation or some subtype thereof. (3) Term may be used in combination with subtypes specifically identifying the type of achievement desired (e.g., occupational aspirations).

ACHIEVEMENT TESTING Any of a series of standardized tests given to determine a student's level of academic performance relative to some national norm (e.g., Metropolitan Achievement Test, Stanford Achievement Test, etc.).

ADMINISTRATORS (1) Those individuals who serve as directors or managers. (2) To be used in reference to studies detailing the administration of mental health Centers, education facilities, or social service centers.

ADOLESCENTS Any study including subjects between ages 13 and 18.

ADULT EDUCATION Any educational program primarily directed at a population over 18 years of age.

ADULTS Studies involving subjects over the age of 18.

AGGRESSION Forceful or hostile behavior.

ALCOHOLISM Studies commenting on the causes or effects of excessive alcohol consumption.

ALABAMA (see STATE).

ALASKA (see STATE).

ALTRUISM Any conduct that helps others in the absence of anticipated external rewards for the helping deed.

ANOMIE Lack of purpose, identity, or ethical values in an individual or in a society; rootlessness.

ANXIETY Studies dealing with the measurement, etiology, process or treatment of anxiety. Subject population may be, but need not necessarily be, defined as clinically ill.

ARIZONA (see STATE).

ARKANSAS (see STATE).

ARMY GENERAL CLASSIFICATION TEST

ART Papers commenting on or criticizing any form of artistic expression.

ASSERTIVENESS (1) Articles measuring assertive behavior, as distinct from AGGRESSION. (2) Articles dealing with assertiveness training, in which interpersonal skills are taught which increase self-assertive behavior (related BEHAVIOR THERAPY).

ATTITUDES (1) Articles specifically mentioning, measuring, or, manipulating notions toward some object or idea. (2) The term should always be followed by an index term specifically identifying the object of attitude.

ATTRIBUTION OF RESPONSIBILITY Articles specifically measuring, manipulating, or making inferences to attribution of responsibility (i.e., self vs. other; internal vs. external, etc.).

ATTRIBUTION THEORY (1) Heider's theory that we give both meaning and predictability to the events of our lives. (2) Articles dealing with development or specific applications of attribution theory.

AUTHORITARIANISM A set of attitudes and personality characteristics typically including ethnocentrism, deference to authority, and a requirement for rigid obedience from subordinate individuals. Often reported as a cultural factor in Latino family roles. (See also FAMILY ROLES, CULTURAL FACTORS, ROLE EXPECTATIONS.)

BEHAVIOR MODIFICATION Studies reporting the modification of behavior through alteration of some aspect of the subject's natural environment.

BEHAVIOR THERAPY Studies reporting the process or outcome of a specific application of a psychotherapeutic technique generally considered to be derived directly from learning principles (e.g., systematic desensitization and implosive therapy).

BENDER VISUAL-MOTOR GESTALT TEST

BIBLIOGRAPHY To be used to describe the type of reference with a collection of citations pertaining to a specific subject area.

BILINGUAL Studies which, while not making inference to the more general topic of bilingualism, use subjects who are fluent in two or more languages.

BILINGUAL-BICULTURAL EDUCATION Education which is not only bilingual, but is also bicultural (knowledgeable and respectful of both cultures).

BILINGUAL-BICULTURAL PERSONNEL Personnel employed in any human services setting who are both bilingual (fluent in two languages) and bicultural (knowledgeable and respectful of both cultures).

BILINGUALISM Studies specifically making inference to the process of acquisition and use of a language as seen in individuals speaking more than one language. (See also BILINGUAL, LANGUAGE ACQUISITION, LANGUAGE LEARNING.)

BIRTH CONTROL Studies dealing with any aspect of contraception--e.g., attitudes, methods, etc.

BOOK Term referring to a bound volume, as distinct from articles,s, chapters, or papers contained within volumes or works which are unbound.

CALIFORNIA (see STATE).

CALIFORNIA ACHIEVEMENT TESTS

CALIFORNIA PSYCHOLOGICAL INVENTORY (CPI)

CALIFORNIA TEST OF MENTAL MATURITY

CAPITALISM (1) The economic system in which the means of production and distribution are privately owned and operated for the profit of a few by methods of exploitation of the labor force. (2) Those articles mentioning this form of economic technique.

CARIBBEAN Articles making specific mention of or using subject populations from any of the Caribbean islands, but excluding Puerto Rico and Cuba.

CASE STUDY An uncontrolled, naturalistic observation of an individual or small group; commonly used in exploratory and psychoanalytic studies.

CATTELL CULTURE-FREE INTELLIGENCE TEST

CENSUS Studies reporting on the reliability or validity of U.S. Census data. Term should not be used for discussion of survey research methodology in general (see SURVEY, RESEARCH METHODOLOGY), or for discussion of results of such surveys (see SURVEY, DEMOGRAPHIC).

CENTRAL AMERICA Articles making specific mention of, or using subject populations from, any of the countries of Central America.

CHICANO MOVEMENT A social/political movement which includes as a goal the increase of ethnic pride or identity among Mexican Americans. Other socially relevant goals may be included as well.

CHILD ABUSE (1) Physical and/or mental cruelty shown to a child. (2) physical or mental neglect shown to a child.

CHILDREARING PRACTICES General term for values, attitudes, behaviors, etc., used by parents in raising of children. (See also FAMILY RELATIONS, FAMILY STRUCTURE, SOCIALIZATION.)

CHILDREN (1) Those persons within the age range of 2 to 12 years. (2) Any articles making reference to or including subjects from ages 2 to 12.

CLASSROOM BEHAVIOR Term used to describe studies

measuring and/or observing specific behaviors of students within a classroom setting.

COGNITIVE DEVELOPMENT The development of those processes by which individuals think, know, and gain an awareness of objects and events.

COGNITIVE DISSONANCE (1) Principle that incongruous cognitions motivate the individual to reduce the perceived inconsistency so as to achieve greater consonance. (2) Any study which uses cognitive disonance to explain its findings.

COGNITIVE STYLE The individual's characteristic style of perceiving the environment (e.g., habitual tendency to scan the entire picture vs. focusing on fine details). Term is often associated with the concept of field dependence.

COLLEGE STUDENTS Those articles which make reference to or include as subjects adults enrolled in institutions of higher education.

COLORADO (see STATE).

COMMUNITY Term used to describe studies which focus on a specific geographical region--e.g., barrio, neighborhood, catchment area, etc.

COMMUNITY INVOLVEMENT (1) Involvement by community figures in educational or therapeutic programs aimed at the solution of societal problems. (2) Study of any phase of a program stressing or including community involvement (i.e., recruitment, training, use, evaluation, etc.).

COMPETITION (1) Behavior or attitudes stressing individual rather than joint efforts. Orientation toward individual success and achievement rather than group or humanitarian values. (2) Studies stressing competition as a value or behavior in children or adults. (See also COOPERATION.)

COMPOUND-COORDINATE DISTINCTION Term used to describe bilingual acquisition, whether the second language was learned conjointly with the first (Compound) or whether the second language was learned separately in different environs (Coordinate).

CONFLICT RESOLUTION (1) Conflict is a state that ensues when an individual or group is faced with two or more incompatible responses. Conflict resolution is therefore a characteristic style used by an individual or group to resolve such conflicts. (2) A major focus of the study must be the exploration of conflict resolution or one of its synonyms.

CONFORMITY Term used in social/psychological research as the adherence of attitudes, values and/or behaviors to social norms.

CONNECTICUT (see STATE).

COOPERATION (1) Behavior or attitudes stressing joint rather than individual efforts. Orientation toward humanitarian values or group success rather than individual success or achievement. (2) Studies stressing cooperation as a value or behavior in children or adults. (See also COMPETITION.)

COPING MECHANISMS (1) Typical responses developed by an individual to reduce threat or anxiety. (2) Studies describing development, uses, or consequences of behaviors which are specifically defined as a coping mechanism.

CORRECTIONS Studies dealing with any aspect of the judicial correctional system (e.g., probation, parole, jail, prison). Studies dealing with the science of penology. (See also CRIMINOLOGY, DELINQUENCY.)

CRIMINOLOGY (1) Studies of crime, criminals, and penology. Social, psychiatric, and psychological aspects are usually considered relevant. (2) Term would include studies of psychological or social aspects of individuals defined as criminals. (See also CORRECTIONS, DELINQUENCY.)

CROSS CULTURAL Studies making comparisons between two or more separate ethnic groups or cultures.

CROSS GENERATIONAL Studies making comparisons between two or more generations (i.e., 1st, 2nd, 3rd, etc.) of individuals who share the same ethnic heritage.

CUBAN Studies using or commenting on a population identified as being of Cuban descent.

CULTURAL CHANGE Studies observing the process of change as applied to the entire culture--i.e., shifts in U.S. or Mexican culture. Not to be confused with acculturation, which is a process occurring with an individual.

CULTURAL FACTORS Specific uses of the superordinate term culture. The term is typically used in relation to some specific area (e.g., intelligence testing, mental health, etc.)

CULTURAL PLURALISM Studies and practices affirming the right of minority groups to maintain their own communal identity and subcultural values. Practices and studies which interpret society as consisting of several cultures, rather than the monocultural/melting-pot theory. Term includes articles on biculturalism, a specific aspect of this superordinate term.

CULTURE (1) That complex whole referring to the laws, customs, and beliefs acquired as a function of membership in society. (2) Term is used to index review articles and essays discussing culture as an abstract concept rather than as a concept affecting some specific function--such articles are indexed under the term CULTURAL FACTORS.

CULTURE-FAIR TESTS Intelligence, personality, and/or achievement tests which are reportedly reliable and valid across ethnic groups.

CURANDERISMO The practice of folk medicine among individuals of Mexican descent.

CURRICULUM Studies describing the course content taught at any level or type of education. Term is generally used in conjunction with descriptors detailing the particular level or type of education involved.

DEATH (1) Cessation of life. (2) Studies commenting on differing cultural conceptions of death (e.g., its causes, customs surrounding it, etc.).

DELAWARE (see STATE).

DELINQUENCY (1) Studies of crime, criminality, and penology in which the subject population is under age 18. (2) Term would include studies of social, psychological, and psychiatric characteristics of these individuals. (See also CRIMINOLOGY, CORRECTIONS, GANGS.)

DEMOGRAPHIC Studies which, using survey research techniques, make inference to the incidence or prevalence of various conditions (e.g., fertility rate, mortality rate, etc.) in various populations; rates should be based on or refer to some standardized population group (e.g., an SMSA, state, etc.).

DEPRESSION Studies dealing with the etiology, process, measurement, or treatment of depression. The disorder may be, but need not necessarily be, found in clinical populations.

DEVIANCE (1) Behavior which differs from average, standard, or accepted behaviors. The study must specifically focus on the development or use of any of the various sociological theories of deviance. (2) Studies of secondary deviance (deviance caused by societal reaction to primary deviance) would be included in this term.

DISCRIMINATION Studies or reports describing a partiality or prejudice in treatment or policies, especially policies directed against the welfare of some minority group.

DISEASE (1) A state of physical illness or bodily dysfunction. (2) Studies commenting on either cultural conceptions of disease and/or on differing social roles associated with well and sick roles in different cultures.

DREAMS Studies describing dreams or using dreams in psychotherapy (particularly as applied to Latinos).

DRUG ABUSE (1) Studies involving nonmedical use of drugs, often with deleterious consequences for the individual involved. Physiological addiction is not involved, though psychological dependence may be present. (2) Studies may deal either with the practice of drug abuse or with individuals engaging in said practice.

DRUG ADDICTION (1) Studies involving individuals physically addicted to psychoactive substances. (2) Studies may deal either with the practice of drug addiction or with individuals so addicted.

DYADIC INTERACTION (1) Studies dealing with face-to-face interaction between two individuals. (2) Note that stress is placed on formal analysis of the quantitative aspects of interaction (e.g., interpersonal distance, rate of speech) as well as the qualitative aspects of interaction (e.g., affect).

EARLY CHILDHOOD EDUCATION Educational projects of any type directed at a population 1 to 6 years of age.

EAST Geographic area in which a study was conducted, including the following states: Connecticut, Delaware, Maine, Maryland, Massachusetts, New Hampshire, New Jersey, New York, Pennsylvania, Rhode Island, Vermont, Washington D.C.

ECONOMIC FACTORS Factors dealing with the production, distribution, and consumption of wealth, and the satisfaction or dissatisfaction of the material needs of the people.

EDUCATION (1) A system in society established to train and instruct individuals in certain required skills. (2) Studies making reference to the general construct of the educational system.

EDUCATIONAL ASSESSMENT Studies dealing with variables affecting any of the various educational assessment techniques (e.g., teacher's grades, standardized achievement test), especially as applied to Latino populations.

EDUCATIONAL COUNSELING Counseling and guidance within an educational setting. It often focuses on career or educational goals, though it may focus, when necessary, on personal concerns.

EDUCATIONAL MATERIALS Materials used by teachers in an instructional setting (e.g., textbooks, films, etc.)

EMPIRICAL Any study involving actual collection of data.

EMPLOYMENT (1) Studies commenting on rates or types of employment found in various population subgroups. (2) Studies commenting on psychological and social effects of unemployment.

ENVIRONMENTAL FACTORS Factors of the physical conditions, circumstances, and influences surrounding and affecting the development of an organism or a group of organisms (i.e., the interaction between the physical environment and the individual or group).

EQUAL OPPORTUNITY Studies or reports dealing with formal efforts to increase access to societal resources for minority groups.

ESCALA DE INTELIGENCIA WECHSLER Spanish version of the Wechsler Intelligence Scale for Children (WISC) and the Wechsler Adult Intelligence Scale (WAIS).

ESPIRITISMO Spiritism; the traditional healing practice among Puerto Ricans.

ESSAY (1) Articles which, rather than reporting the collection of original data, attempt to integrate, analyze, or comment upon the existing literature. (2) An opinionated article.

ETHNIC IDENTITY (1) To be used in reference to studies investigating the self- identification process of individuals, with specific focus on ethinic and/or racial attributes of the process. (2) Person's identification as member of an ethnic group.

EXAMINER EFFECTS Effects on intelligence, personality, or other test performance of variables attributable to the personality, behavior, or presence of the examiner.

EXTENDED FAMILY (1) Family members more distantly related than the nuclear family. (2) Studies mentioning or making inferences about the extended family. (See also FAMILY ROLES, FAMILY STRUCTURE.)

FAMILY PLANNING (1) Studies reporting the process or outcome of programs which provide instruction about the regulation of family size. (2) Studies reporting individuals' or groups' attitudes or utilization of family planning services.

FAMILY ROLES Term describing role expectations within family settings. Characteristic behavior expected of person occupying a particular position in the family.

FAMILY STRUCTURE Formal organizational aspects of a person's family life (e.g., extent of contact with extended vs. nuclear family; age at which individuals move from home; size and composition of family).

FAMILY THERAPY Articles referring to the treatment of more than one member of the family simultaneously in the same session.

FARM LABORERS Rural working class engaged in agricultural labor. (See also MIGRANTS, RURAL, UNDOCUMENTED WORKERS.)

FATALISM The attitude that man has little control over his fate. This variable is believed to be closely associated with one's cultural group and can be considered a cultural factor.

FATHER-CHILD INTERACTION Studies dealing with or making inferences to the interaction between father and child.

FEMALE (1) Studies making reference to some attribute of female gender, not related to sex roles. (2) Studies which have an exclusively female subject population.

FERTILITY Studies dealing with any aspect of reproduction rates (e.g., rates across different groups; beliefs; etc.).

FICTIVE KINSHIP Anthropological term used to describe those relationships between non-bloodline relations (e.g., godparents in the baptism ceremony).

FIELD DEPENDENCE-INDEPENDENCE An individual's characteristic mode of perceiving the environment. Dependence is where the field (context, environment) dominates the perception of its parts; Independence is where the parts are seen as discreet from the organized field. (related FATALISM, COGNITIVE STYLE, ATTRIBUTION OF RESPONSIBILITY, LOCUS OF CONTROL.)

FINANCING Articles that have to do with supplying money, credit, or capital.

FLORIDA (see STATE).

FOLK MEDICINE (1) Healing practices relying on superstitious, cultural, or religious beliefs. (See also CURANDERISMO, ESPIRITISMO.)

GANGS Studies specifically mentioning the social, psychological, or psychiatric aspects of juvenile gangs and their members. (See also DELINQUENCY, CRIMINOLOGY.)

GENDER IDENTITY Those studies which describe the process and/or measure an individual's identification with either sex.

GEORGIA (see STATE).

GERONTOLOGY The study of old age, embracing the sciences of geriatrics, psychology, sociology, anthropology as they apply to the study of individuals over the age of 60.

GOODENOUGH DRAW-A-MAN TEST

GRAMMAR (1) A superordinate term dealing with word forms (morphology), word order in sentences (syntax), language sounds (phonology), and word meaning (semantics). The system of words and word order of a language. (2) Articles mentioning either the concept of grammar or any of its subordinate terms (SYNTAX, PHONOLOGY, SEMANTICS) should be indexed under this term.

GROUP DYNAMICS (1) Studies involving the effects of membership in some group (e.g., family, peer group, or play group) on the attitudes, beliefs, or behavior of group members. (2) Stress here is placed on group's effect on the individual and the individual's effect on the group.

HAWAII (see STATE).

HEALTH Articles in which a major topic is the assessment, improvement, or comment on the state of the physical health of the subjects. Articles dealing with cultural conceptions of health, illness, and the societal roles associated with each state.

HEALTH DELIVERY SYSTEMS Studies dealing with organizational variables (e.g., staffing patterns, service location, hours of operation) affecting effectiveness of delivery of physical or mental health care.

HEALTH EDUCATION (1) Programs designed to increase the general public's knowledge of factors affecting either physical or mental health. (2) Studies dealing with any aspect of health education--i.e., planning, development, implementation, or evaluation.

HIGHER EDUCATION Any study which has college, university (i.e., postsecondary) education as a major topic.

HISTORY Articles which provide background information on a subject or issue.

HOMOSEXUALITY Those articles which make reference to an individual's or group's sexual desire for those of the same sex.

HOUSING (1) The physical structure in which people live. (2) To be used in reference to the condition of housing, urban renewal, relocation, etc.

IDAHO (see STATE).

ILLINOIS (see STATE).

ILLINOIS TEST OF PSYCHOLINGUISTIC ABILITY (ITPA)

IMAGERY Research utilizing mental images, for example, the use of imagery in therapy.

IMMIGRATION Movement across national boundaries with or without approval of governments concerned.

IMPAIRMENT Studies dealing with developmental, emotional, and/or physical disabilities.

INDIANA (see STATE).

INDIGENOUS POPULATIONS Articles mentioning any of the aboriginal peoples of North America, South America, or the West Indies, or their cultures.

INFANCY The first two years of human life.

INHALANT ABUSE Studies commenting on the causes or effects of deliberate inhalation of volatile substances (e.g., gasoline or paint fumes).

INSTITUTIONALIZATION Studies detailing the unintended and often detrimental effects of placement of an individual into a residential institution (e.g., reinforcement of passive behavior). Can also refer to such effects as they occur in nonresidential institutions.

INSTRUCTIONAL TECHNIQUES Studies dealing with actual instructor or teacher procedures used in the instructional situation.

INTEGRATION To remove legal or social barriers imposing segregation or discrimination.

INTELLIGENCE (1) The global capacity to profit from experience. It is a complex mental ability that includes such primary abilities as verbal comprehension, space visualization, reasoning ability, and numerical ability. (2) To be used to describe studies which discuss the construct of intelligence and not intelligence testing.

INTELLIGENCE TESTING Studies dealing with variables described as affecting the validity or reliability of intelligence tests, especially as applied to Latino populations.

INTERMARRIAGE Studies dealing with any aspect of interethnic group marriages (i.e., marriages outside of one's own ethnic group).

INTERPERSONAL ATTRACTION The term used to describe liking between individuals. Commonly used in social psychological research measuring similarity, attractiveness, etc.

INTERPERSONAL RELATIONS (1) Study of face-to-face verbal and nonverbal interactions between more than two individuals. (2) Note that stress is placed on qualitative (e.g., affect) and quantitative (e.g., interpersonal distance, rate of speech) aspects of the interaction.

INTERPERSONAL SPACING Studies showing any of the effects of the degree of physical crowding on behavior.

JOB PERFORMANCE The actual performance and/or execution of one's duties while at work, or the measurement thereof.

JUDICIAL PROCESS A process which is allowed, enforced, or set by order of a judge or court of law.

KANSAS (see STATE).

KENTUCKY (see STATE).

LABOR FORCE (1) Wage-earning workers as a group, distinguished from capital or management. (2) Those articles dealing specifically with the labor force.

LANGUAGE ACQUISITION Studies observing or making inference to the normal process of acquisition of language. Term implies absence of formal INSTRUCTION. Language as taught by parents, siblings, peers or others.

LANGUAGE ASSESSMENT Studies with a major focus on the development, validation, or use of a measure of any of the various language abilities.

LANGUAGE COMPREHENSION (1) A global term encompassing the various processes involved in understanding of language. (2) Term will be used in conjunction with other descriptors, such as SYNTAX, SEMANTICS, or PHONOLOGY.

LANGUAGE LEARNING Studies observing or making inference to the process of acquiring a language (generally, though not necessarily a second language) as a result of formalized (i.e., classroom) instruction.

LEADERSHIP Studies measuring, manipulating, or making inferences to the leadership qualities of a group or an individual.

LEARNING Studies measuring or manipulating the individual's actual degree of success at retaining new information. Stress is placed on actual success at a task rather than on the degree of potential success. (See also INTELLIGENCE, INTELLIGENCE TESTING.)

LEARNING DISABILITIES (1) A subcategory of SPECIAL EDUCATION that focuses upon specific perceptual dysfuntions (e.g., mirror vision, auditory problems, etc.). (2) Must not be confused with MENTAL RETARDATION. A learning disabled student can, and does, have an IQ above 80.

LEGISLATION The making of a law or laws and the process thereof; this includes the proposal, enactment, and implementation of laws.

LINGUISTIC COMPETENCE (1) Studies measuring or making an inference to a generalized construct of language performance. Term implies the combination of the various linguistic constructs (grammar, syntax, semantics, phonology, etc.) into one generalized measure. (2) Term should be used only in the presence of a clear inference to a global construct of language competence.

LINGUISTICS (1) Studies discussing, in a general sense, the structure of development of a particular language. (2) This superordinate term would be used in conjunction with other descriptors, such as syntax, semantics, etc., which more accurately describe the content of the study. (3) Studies dealing with or commenting on the science of linguistics.

LOCUS OF CONTROL Used for studies which measure internal vs. external control of reinforcement, whether reinforcement is contingent on own efforts and behavior or the result of powerful others, fate or luck (related FATALISM, COGNITIVE STYLE, ATTRIBUTION OF RESPONSIBILITY).

LOUISIANA (see STATE).

MACHISMO A set of values and personality traits attributed to Hispanic men, including a strong sense of manliness, honor, and self-respect. Stereotypically, machismo also connotes sexual prowess, overindulgence in alcohol, and physical aggressiveness.

MAINE (see STATE).

MALE (1) Studies making reference to some attribute of male gender not related to sex roles (e.g., number of males in certain occupation, etc.). (2) Studies which have an exclusively male subject population.

MARITAL STABILITY Studies dealing with levels or patterns of marital stability in various populations (e.g., divorce levels, relationship of ethnicity or age to the length of marriage, etc.).

MARRIAGE Studies commenting on the social institution of marriage--its rates in various groups; its effects on participants, attitudes and customs concerning marriage.

MARXIAN THEORY The theory that the structures and systems of modes of production are a determinate combination of economic, political, and ideological levels. Moreover, economic level takes primacy.

MARYLAND (see STATE).

MASS MEDIA Studies dealing with any aspect of the mass media and its relationship to Latinos (e.g., stereotypes portrayed in the mass media, or educational programs carried through mass media).

MASSACHUSETTS (see STATE).

MATHEMATICS (1) Studies involving as a relevant variable the teaching, learning, or use of any mathematical construct. (2) Studies involving an attempt to teach mathematical concepts to children.

MEDICAL STUDENTS Those articles which refer to individuals enrolled in medical schools.

MEMORY Articles measuring or making a specific inference to the individual's memory function

MENTAL HEALTH (1) Articles having as a major topic the assessment or improvement of persons' mental or emotional well-being. (2) Articles commenting on cultural conceptions of mental health or illness.

MENTAL HEALTH PROFESSION Articles specifically dealing with one or more of the mental health professions (i.e., psychology, psychiatry, social work, or nursing).

MENTAL RETARDATION Any study involving subjects defined as mentally subnormal. Mental subnormality in Anglo populations is typically defined in terms of an IQ of less than 70 points.

METHADONE MAINTENANCE (1) A specific treatment for opiate addiction involving periodic administration of small quantities of methadone. (2) Any study including methadone maintenance as a relevant variable.

METROPOLITAN ACHIEVEMENT TEST

METROPOLITAN READINESS TEST

METROPOLITAN READING READINESS TEST

MEXICAN Studies using or commenting on a population identified as being Mexican.

MEXICAN AMERICAN Studies using or commenting on a population identified as being of Mexican descent and living in the United States.

MEXICO To be used in studies that discuss particular aspects of this country (e.g., economy, unemployment, history, etc.). Only to be used in reference to the entire country and not to individuals from this country.

MICHIGAN (see STATE).

MIDWEST Geographic area in which a study was conducted, including the following states: Illinois, Indiana, Iowa, Kansas, Michigan, Minnesota, Missouri, Nebraska, North Dakota, Ohio, Oklahoma, South Dakota, Wisconsin.

MIGRANTS Articles commenting on or having as research subjects that portion of the farm labor population that follows the seasonal cycle of planting and harvesting across the United States.

MIGRATION Movement within national boundaries (e.g., between states).

MILITARY Articles making specific mention of, or using subject populations from, any branch of the armed forces.

MINNESOTA (see STATE).

MINNESOTA MULTIPHASIC PERSONALITY INVENTORY (MMPI)

MISSISSIPPI (see STATE).

MISSOURI (see STATE).

MODELING (1) A method of learning by relying on the imitation of responses emitted by another. (2) Studies specifically mentioning or making inference to modeling as a method of learning.

MONTANA (see STATE).

MOTHER-CHILD INTERACTION Studies dealing with or making inference to the interaction between a mother and her child.

MUSIC Term used for studies which describe the music of a particular group.

NEBRASKA (see STATE).

NEUROSIS Studies of any of the functional (i.e., nonorganic) mental disorders. Study must specifically identify its population as neurotic (or some variation thereof), and must attempt some comment on the process, etiology, or treatment of the neurosis.

NEVADA (see STATE).

NEW HAMPSHIRE (see STATE).

NEW JERSEY (see STATE).

NEW MEXICO (see STATE).

NEW YORK (see STATE).

NORTH CAROLINA (see STATE).

NORTH DAKOTA (see STATE).

NURSING Articles dealing with nurses, nursing schools, psychiatric nursing, or other facets of the nursing profession.

NUTRITION Studies dealing with dietary or eating habits of Latinos, or any consequences thereof.

OCCUPATIONAL ASPIRATIONS Desires, whether judged as realistic or not, of a person regarding his ultimate occupational attainment. The status which one expects or hopes to achieve within the occupational setting.

OHIO (see STATE).

OKLAHOMA (see STATE).

OREGON (see STATE).

PARAPROFESSIONALS (1) An individual without professional training performing certain specified functions in the areas of counseling, psychotherapy, or education under the direction of a qualified professional. (2) Studies commenting on the selection, training, or use of paraprofessionals.

PARENTAL INVOLVEMENT (1) Involvement by parental figure (mother, father, guardian, godparent) in educational or therapeutic activities aimed at the welfare of a child. (2) Studies of any phase of programs employing parental involvement (i.e., recruitment of parents, training of parents, evaluation program, etc.). (3) Studies using parents as behavior change agents in attempts to modify the behavior of children (i.e., parent training programs).

PEABODY PICTURE-VOCABULARY TEST

PEER GROUP (1) The group with which an individual associates (one's peers). (2) Studies including some aspect of the peer group as an independent or dependent variable.

PENNSYLVANIA (see STATE).

PERCEPTION (1) A field of psychology studying cognitive processes used in depicting physical characteristics of objects. (2) Studies specifically mentioning any of the processes of perception of stimuli (e.g., cognitive style) as seen in Latinos.

PERFORMANCE EXPECTATIONS (1) Expectations regarding the quantity or quality of another's performance. (2) Note that stress is placed on another's performance.

PERSONALITY (1) A field of psychology concentrating on individual differences in behavior; the characteristic behavior of an individual. (2) Studies making specific inference to the concept or study of personality.

PERSONALITY ASSESSMENT Studies dealing with variables described as affecting reliability or validity of personality assessment devices (e.g., MMPI, RORSCHACH TEST), especially as applied to the Latino population.

PERSONNEL Articles dealing with personnel availiability in terms of numbers or distribution, to be followed by the term to which it applies, such as PHYSICIAN, MENTAL HEALTH PROFESSION, etc.

PHONOLOGY Studies measuring or making inference to phonetics (speech sounds) in a language or dialect. (See also GRAMMAR, BILINGUALISM, LANGUAGE LEARNING.)

PHYSICAL DEVELOPMENT Process of regular, age-related, sequential development of physical skills and strengths in children. Studies commenting on the relative level of these age-related changes within or across different populations (e.g., level of physical coordination in different groups).

PHYSICIANS (1) Studies measuring or manipulating the attitudes or judgment of physicians toward their service populations (e.g., diagnosis of similar complaints across different ethnic groups; physicians' conception of their social role). (2) Studies measuring or manipulating attitudes of a service population toward their physicians (e.g., conceptions of the physician's role). (3) Articles referring to the number of physicians, distribution, availability are to be indexed under this term in conjunction with the term PERSONNEL.

POLICE-COMMUNITY RELATIONS Studies dealing with any aspect of the relationship between a police force and the population it serves. Includes articles dealing with police patrol or riot control tactics as these affect the community's relations to the police.

POLICY Principle, plan, or course of action to be followed; normative or accepted procedural guidelines, or proposed new guidelines.

POLITICAL POWER Those studies describing the nature and/or acquisition of political influence. This is commonly used in reference to minority groups' need for further political power to correct social injustices.

POLITICS Those articles dealing with the science of government, political affairs and/or political methods or tactics.

POVERTY (1) The state of economic and material deprivation. (2) Articles making specific reference to poverty or any of its synonyms (e.g., low SES, poor, etc.).

PREJUDICE (1) A cluster of learned beliefs, attitudes, and values (usually negative) that bias an individual toward the members of a particular group. (2) Can be used in conjunction with discrimination only when the attitudes or prejudice are discussed along with the act of discrimination.

PRIMARY PREVENTION Studies or programs which focus primarily on either the identification and/or treatment of individuals before the development of psychopathology or the identification and alleviation of societal conditions ultimately causing such psychopathology. In either case, the primary goal is the prevention of psychopathology before its occurrence.

PROCEEDINGS Description of the type of article. One of a collection of articles that were presented at a professional conference.

PROFESSIONAL TRAINING Instruction designed to improve one's understanding and application of any profession (e.g., education, mental health). Usually this term is used in reference to those professions which require graduate training.

PROGRAM EVALUATION (1) Studies reporting results, intended or accidental, of any intervention of any type. This term may be used in conjunction with the term PSYCHOTHERAPY OUTCOME to report results of psychotherapy. (2) Studies reporting or commenting on methodology for making program evaluations. In this case, the term may be used in conjunction with the term RESEARCH METHODOLOGY.

PROJECTIVE TESTING (1) A type of personality testing involving presentation of highly ambiguous materials to the subject. (2) Studies involving the use, validation, or development of projective tests.

PSYCHIATRIC STATUS SCHEDULE

PSYCHOPATHOLOGY Studies or articles dealing in a general sense with the behaviors or characteristics of the various mental disorders.

PSYCHOPHARMACOLOGY Studies of the physiological or behavioral effects of psychoactive drugs.

PSYCHOSIS Studies dealing with any of the severe mental disorders in which sense of or contact with reality is lost and the personality becomes quite disordered. Study must specifically define its subjects as psychotic and must attempt some statement about the process of psychotic disorder in the subject population.

PSYCHOSOCIAL ADJUSTMENT (1) A generalized construct indicating the individual's personal and social adjustment within his environment. (2) Studies making a major inference about psychosocial adjustment, either as a generalized construct or as measured by some specific referent of an individual or group.

PSYCHOTHERAPISTS Studies which measure, manipulate, or make some inference to variables subsumed in the personality or behavior of the qualified person offering psychotherapeutic services.

PSYCHOTHERAPY Treatment of mental disorders by counseling, psychoanalysis, etc. Treatment can be administered in inpatient or outpatient setting, group or individual context, and can use any accepted theoretical orientation (e.g., behavior modification, client-centered therapy, etc.).

PSYCHOTHERAPY OUTCOME Studies dealing with the results, intended or unintended, of any psychotherapeutic intervention. Term will be used in combination with other descriptor terms (e.g., BEHAVIOR MODIFICATION) to specifically describe the type of intervention.

PUERTO RICAN-I Studies using or commenting on a population identified as being on the island of Puerto Rico.

PUERTO RICAN-M Studies using or commenting on a population identified as being of Puerto Rican descent and living on the United States mainland.

RAVEN PROGRESSIVE MATRICES

READING (1) Study of techniques for teaching or increasing reading capability. (2) Study commenting on reading ability of some population.

REHABILITATION The restoration to a normal or optimum state of health and/or constructive activity by medical treatment and physical or psychological therapy.

RELIGION (1) Belief in a spiritual being, power, or divine creator. (2) Studies including as a major variable or making inferences on the basis of a person's religion.

REPRESENTATION To be used as a general term including over- and underrepresentation, with specific reference to numbers of minority-group persons in mental health professions.

RESEARCH METHODOLOGY (1) The design and selection of experimental materials, pretesting, study administration, data analysis, and interpretation of study results. (2) Studies, a major focus of which is the analysis of the above topics as they affect research on Latino populations.

RESOURCE UTILIZATION Studies which focus on the rate of usage of various facilities or services (e.g., psychotherapy, hospitalization, etc.).

REVIEW (1) Articles which, while not involving collection of any data themselves, attempt to systematically integrate and summarize the literature of a given topic area. (2) Secondary research.

RHODE ISLAND (see STATE).

ROLE EXPECTATIONS (1) Expectations related to the behavior shown by an individual occupying a certain social position or role. (2) Note that stress is placed on qualitative aspects of the role performance.

RORSCHACH TEST

ROTTER INTERNAL-EXTERNAL SCALE A commonly used scale for the measurement of degree of internal or external locus of control; it is often referred to as the 'I-E Scale'. (See also LOCUS OF CONTROL.)

RURAL Studies which include the population's rural residence as a relevant variable.

SCHIZOPHRENIA Those studies which refer to the study of the process, etiology, or treatment of schizophrenia.

SCHOLASTIC ACHIEVEMENT Studies measuring or making inference to an individual or group's level of skill, practice, success, or other accomplishments in an educational institution.

SCHOLASTIC APTITUDE TEST The examination used to determine incoming college students' ability to succeed.

SCHOLASTIC ASPIRATIONS The status which one expects or wishes to achieve within the school setting.

SELF CONCEPT Pertaining to a person's view of themself in relation to the world, his peers, cultural group, etc. The individual's awareness of his/her own body, including all of the individual's thoughts, feelings, attitudes, etc. A differentiated portion of the phenomenological field. The individual's definition of his/her self.

SEMANTICS (1) Studies measuring, or making inference to, the relationship between symbols (i.e., words) and the meanings given them by their users. (2) Studies dealing with word meanings and changes in word meanings. (3) Studies coded under this term should also be coded under the term GRAMMAR.

SES (1) The relative rank of an individual's and/or a group's educational, economic, and social attainment. (2) Studies specifically focusing on any of the various causes or effects of socioeconomic status.

SEX COMPARISON Studies including sex as an independent variable.

SEX ROLES Behavior expected of an individual by reason of his or her sex. (See also FAMILY ROLES.)

SEXUAL BEHAVIOR Studies mentioning frequency or type of various sexual practices (e.g., premarital intercourse, homosexuality) in various population groups.

SOCIAL MOBILITY Movement by an individual or group up or down in socioeconomic status.

SOCIAL SCIENCES (1) Those articles whose area of study stems from a sociological and/or anthropological perspective. (2) Articles discussing the characteristics, problems, etc., of any of the social sciences.

SOCIAL SERVICES To be used for those articles which discuss welfare-community advocacy programs. This is not to be used for mental health or health-related articles unless there is specific mention of welfare-community advocacy programs.

SOCIAL STRUCTURE The pattern of interrelated statuses and roles found in a society or other group at a particular time and constituting a relatively stable set of social relations. The organized pattern of interrelated rights and obligations of persons and groups in a system of interaction as analyzed in terms of statuses, roles, social norms, and social institutions.

SOCIALIZATION General term describing the child's experience in society, including influences from parents, peers, teachers, police, etc. (See also CHILDREARING PRACTICES, FAMILY STRUCTURE.)

SOUTH Geographic area in which a study was conducted, including the following states: Alabama, Arkansas, Florida, Georgia, Kentucky, Louisiana, Mississippi, North Carolina, South Carolina, Tennessee, Virginia, West Virginia

SOUTH AMERICA Articles making specific mention of or using subject populations from any of the countries of South America.

SOUTH CAROLINA (see STATE).

SOUTH DAKOTA (see STATE).

SOUTHWEST Geographic area in which a study was conducted, including the following states: Arizona, California, Colorado, New Mexico, Texas.

SPANISH SURNAMED Studies which, while using some fairly vague term to identify their population as being of Latino origin, do not identify the specific ethnic grouping of the subjects.

SPECIAL EDUCATION A specific branch of education that instructs students that have lower IQs and are learning disabled and/or physically handicapped. (Also to include Remedial Education.)

STANFORD ACHIEVEMENT TEST

STANFORD-BINET INTELLIGENCE TEST

STATE The index term specifically identifies any one of the 50 states or Washington D.C. Reference is to the state in which a study was conducted or about which an article focuses.

STEREOTYPES Fixed, often inaccurate, ideas about the appearance, behavior, etc., of a certain group. The assignment of identical characteristics to all members of a given group.

STRESS Studies including physical and/or mental tension or strain as a major variable.

SUICIDE Those articles which focus on the act of self-inflicted murder.

SURVEY Studies utilizing survey research methods to obtain data. Term can be applied to literature commenting on planning, pretesting, and administering survey instruments. Term is a subset of the more general term RESEARCH METHODOLOGY.

SYMPTOMATOLOGY Studies which measure or make inference to the degree or nature of symptoms expressed across or within various cultural groups.

SYNTAX (1) Studies measuring or making inference to the arrangement of words as elements in a sentence. (2) The organization and interrelationship of words, phrases, clauses, and sentences. (3) Studies indexed under this term should also be indexed under the term GRAMMAR.

TEACHERS Articles discussing teachers or any other group of professional personnel employed in an educative role in the school setting.

TENNESSEE (see STATE).

TEST RELIABILITY (1) Complex property of a testing instrument or process that assures similar results on repetition of the process--considered to be dependent on the degree to which the measure is free of random influence. (2) Term should be used for any article making or implying any statement about the reliability of any measuring or testing instrument.

TEST VALIDITY (1) A property of a testing instrument or procedure ensuring that the obtained scores accurately measure that which they are supposed to measure. (2) Term should be used for any study making or implying any statement about the validity of any testing instrument.

TEXAS (see STATE).

THEMATIC APPERCEPTION TEST (TAT)

THEORETICAL (1) An article which includes a large number of interrelated propositions and provides a conceptual scheme within which human behavior can be explained. (2) To be used for articles that deal only with theory.

THERAPEUTIC COMMUNITY Treatment approaches which, by manipulating all aspects of a person's life, seek to modify his behavior. Stress is placed on the totality of control over the environment (e.g., hospital or institutional environment).

TIME ORIENTATION Man's perception of time and its relationship to life; a specific variable that is thought to be closely associated with one's cultural group.

UNDOCUMENTED WORKERS Immigrants from one of the Latin American countries who reside in the United States, either temporarily or permanently, and engage in productive labor but who do not possess legal proof of their immigration or resident status.

URBAN (1) Articles which make specific reference to residence within a city. (2) Articles in which the urban residence of the population, though not specifically mentioned, is important to the article.

UTAH (see STATE).

VALUES (1) An individual's or group's beliefs concerning the relative worth, utility, or importance of concepts, objects, etc. (2) Studies making specific mention or measurement of individuals' or groups' values.

VERMONT (see STATE).

VETERANS (1) Articles making specific mention of organizations or institutions serving former members of the armed forces. (2) Studies using as subject populations former members of the armed forces.

VIRGINIA (SEE STATE).

VOCATIONAL COUNSELING The guidance and assistance provided to others in developing and enhancing job skills and, at times, in obtaining employment.

WASHINGTON (see STATE).

WASHINGTON D.C. (see STATE).

WECHSLER ADULT INTELLIGENCE SCALE (WAIS)

WECHSLER INTELLIGENCE SCALE FOR CHILDREN (WISC)

WECHSLER MENTAL ABILITY SCALE

WECHSLER-BELLEVUE INTELLIGENCE SCALE

WEST Geographic area in which a study was conducted, including the following states: Alaska, Hawaii, Idaho, Montana, Nevada, Oregon, Utah, Washington, Wyoming.

WEST VIRGINIA (see STATE).

WISCONSIN (see STATE).

WYOMING (see STATE).

INDEX

1662, 1726, 1753, 1837, 1873, 1874, 1878, 1884, 1896, 1926, 1975

DEATH 18, 19, 143, 501, 503, 504, 896, 897, 918, 1191, 1411, 1475, 1520, 1532, 1533, 1561, 1563, 1912

DELINQUENCY 112, 113, 167, 207, 476, 531, 544, 549, 578, 582, 602, 718, 814, 835, 857, 961, 1093, 1144, 1208, 1235, 1303, 1347, 1394, 1536, 1543, 1569, 1572, 1584, 1671, 1773, 1783, 1794, 1800, 1818, 1820, 1831, 1832, 1913

DEMOGRAPHIC 6, 24, 47, 75, 76, 112, 113, 121, 133, 134, 147, 159, 170, 174, 189, 201, 220, 229, 257, 307, 325, 344, 364, 384, 385, 386, 436, 443, 469, 488, 503, 504, 505, 511, 515, 521, 528, 535, 537, 538, 544, 561, 601, 620, 684, 690, 699, 700, 706, 727, 730, 731, 733, 734, 740, 744, 747, 759, 761, 775, 777, 790, 835, 837, 839, 843, 844, 861, 862, 894, 895, 896, 910, 914, 917, 945, 966, 969, 980, 986, 1019, 1023, 1028, 1029, 1031, 1065, 1080, 1081, 1082, 1085, 1092, 1122, 1123, 1131, 1143, 1165, 1197, 1200, 1202, 1212, 1222, 1226, 1236, 1248, 1249, 1251, 1256, 1261, 1274, 1281, 1283, 1295, 1315, 1318, 1328, 1334, 1342, 1356, 1369, 1384, 1385, 1396, 1459, 1471, 1472, 1513, 1516, 1517, 1518, 1522, 1524, 1533, 1538, 1566, 1579, 1609, 1610, 1627, 1638, 1653, 1655, 1659, 1676, 1683, 1684, 1697, 1703, 1713, 1714, 1747, 1776, 1778, 1801, 1832, 1849, 1850, 1851, 1852, 1853, 1854, 1855, 1856, 1857, 1858, 1859, 1860, 1861, 1862, 1863, 1864, 1877, 1879, 1880, 1881, 1882, 1890, 1897, 1902, 1906, 1908, 1909, 1911, 1912, 1937, 1946, 1966

DEPRESSION 1, 147, 177, 312, 382, 456, 497, 503, 557, 582, 691, 732, 797, 820, 836, 843, 937, 959, 961, 982, 1122, 1123, 1226, 1414, 1421, 1588, 1679, 1770, 1834, 1835, 1921

DEVIANCE 1, 113, 159, 287, 288, 289, 290, 443, 472, 578, 691, 693, 721, 729, 748, 835, 857, 934, 963, 1025, 1029, 1049, 1061, 1145, 1245, 1377, 1385, 1478, 1587, 1649, 1671, 1811

DISCRIMINATION 4, 6, 14, 25, 42, 68, 69, 77, 88, 89, 93, 109, 110, 166, 167, 168, 176, 190, 200, 202, 213, 215, 219, 221, 231, 241, 242, 248, 254, 262, 264, 266, 286, 296, 297, 299, 300, 301, 304, 309, 319, 341, 348, 358, 359, 383, 384, 399, 414, 449, 487, 488, 503, 534, 535, 538, 560, 561, 583, 585, 586, 601, 603, 611, 640, 651, 652, 655, 679, 683, 684, 687, 690, 695, 701, 704, 706, 708, 709, 712, 726, 744, 746, 751, 752, 757, 764, 788, 806, 827, 828, 837, 857, 873, 877, 909, 911, 912, 926, 984, 1007, 1011, 1016, 1019, 1066, 1070, 1076, 1115, 1140, 1142, 1164, 1169, 1170, 1188, 1219, 1236, 1250, 1258, 1263, 1269, 1270, 1273, 1276, 1277, 1278, 1280, 1281, 1283, 1290, 1293, 1298, 1313, 1321, 1323, 1332, 1348, 1359, 1363, 1375, 1377, 1396, 1398, 1406, 1413, 1416, 1419, 1437, 1445, 1462, 1534, 1546, 1605, 1610, 1613, 1615, 1617, 1623, 1625, 1653, 1659, 1663, 1676, 1684, 1690, 1707, 1731, 1746, 1775, 1776, 1778, 1837, 1848, 1864, 1866, 1867, 1869, 1870, 1871, 1872, 1883, 1885, 1895, 1898, 1901, 1906, 1941, 1953, 1954, 1955, 1965, 1971, 1972, 1983

DISEASE 23, 27, 404, 410, 503, 504, 516, 576, 588, 597,

654, 685, 839, 959, 1161, 1191, 1308, 1309, 1373, 1506, 1517, 1522, 1585, 1626, 1628, 1674, 1687, 1732, 1801, 1810, 1891, 1951

DREAMS 197, 198, 478, 897, 1104, 1105, 1374, 1561, 1562, 1563

DRUG ABUSE 107, 112, 114, 138, 147, 160, 199, 218, 218, 229, 310, 324, 401, 403, 425, 482, 498, 511, 561, 581, 582, 594, 606, 669, 674, 700, 723, 724, 837, 879, 961, 973, 978, 979, 993, 1009, 1031, 1111, 1149, 1152, 1157, 1223, 1226, 1228, 1283, 1284, 1292, 1305, 1306, 1314, 1315, 1328, 1347, 1394, 1404, 1421, 1440, 1466, 1511, 1514, 1516, 1582, 1598, 1630, 1639, 1649, 1671, 1722, 1786, 1787, 1790, 1823, 1909, 1949, 1950, 1985

DRUG ADDICTION 88, 112, 114, 115, 116, 199, 210, 229, 230, 310, 325, 401, 425, 432, 482, 575, 606, 643, 648, 669, 837, 977, 979, 986, 987, 993, 1009, 1032, 1226, 1228, 1282, 1292, 1315, 1328, 1394, 1511, 1514, 1516, 1598, 1630, 1639, 1671, 1680, 1722, 1823, 1950, 1985, 1989, 1990

DYADIC INTERACTION 21, 108, 148, 151, 335, 755, 765, 767, 874, 998, 1055, 1301, 1412, 1478, 1757, 1942

EARLY CHILDHOOD EDUCATION 14, 33, 220, 278, 345, 371, 416, 417, 437, 459, 460, 536, 540, 607, 644, 662, 696, 713, 742, 750, 780, 794, 804, 845, 863, 864, 942, 972, 1020, 1049, 1184, 1185, 1325, 1375, 1388, 1455, 1538, 1662, 1747, 1754, 1757, 1772, 1816, 1916, 1925, 1993, 1997

EAST 1, 2, 13, 21, 23, 51, 53, 54, 67, 87, 105, 107, 109, 110, 111, 147, 158, 162, 163, 164, 187, 203, 204, 210, 224, 227, 240, 242, 265, 272, 319, 341, 347, 355, 356, 369, 370, 408, 425, 433, 436, 437, 438, 446, 464, 467, 468, 469, 470, 471, 472, 473, 503, 548, 554, 555, 557, 558, 559, 560, 561, 563, 571, 574, 578, 581, 582, 583, 594, 602, 614, 620, 621, 622, 623, 624, 625, 642, 644, 645, 669, 672, 674, 687, 688, 691, 703, 713, 714, 718, 725, 729, 730, 731, 732, 738, 739, 744, 758, 759, 810, 838, 840, 842, 858, 872, 874, 879, 898, 912, 928, 929, 945, 946, 985, 986, 987, 991, 993, 994, 998, 1009, 1011, 1017, 1020, 1031, 1043, 1045, 1048, 1083, 1092, 1122, 1123, 1137, 1142, 1146, 1147, 1148, 1157, 1212, 1223, 1235, 1236, 1237, 1261, 1288, 1299, 1301, 1309, 1328, 1338, 1339, 1369, 1399, 1408, 1413, 1421, 1430, 1454, 1463, 1477, 1478, 1511, 1515, 1530, 1535, 1556, 1568, 1591, 1595, 1596, 1597, 1598, 1599, 1600, 1601, 1602, 1613, 1619, 1628, 1654, 1672, 1682, 1716, 1718, 1727, 1741, 1805, 1811, 1812, 1814, 1816, 1825, 1834, 1856, 1858, 1902, 1911, 1925, 1942, 1943, 1947, 1964, 1969, 1984, 1989, 1990

ECONOMIC FACTORS 23, 31, 47, 66, 78, 98, 121, 134, 146, 147, 165, 169, 170, 185, 200, 201, 209, 214, 215, 229, 232, 235, 241, 250, 254, 265, 309, 325, 332, 370, 384, 405, 428, 449, 488, 490, 491, 496, 510, 514, 534, 537, 560, 561, 569, 573, 584, 601, 613, 616, 618, 622, 644, 653, 659, 682, 684, 686, 690, 694, 706, 722, 744, 747, 751, 761, 776, 777, 817, 835, 873, 884, 885, 912, 913, 928, 957, 975, 1007, 1029, 1041, 1042, 1043, 1080, 1101, 1115, 1121, 1140, 1143, 1144, 1164, 1192, 1197, 1200, 1232, 1236, 1238, 1243, 1266, 1270, 1271,

247, 254, 269, 535, 623, 649, 650, 698, 699, 739, 747, 807, 821, 898, 901, 913, 929, 970, 971, 987, 1005, 1037, 1045, 1061, 1069, 1144, 1177, 1200, 1236, 1252, 1253, 1254, 1258, 1263, 1304, 1315, 1334, 1368, 1408, 1427, 1433, 1437, 1443, 1456, 1529, 1612, 1622, 1659, 1696, 1698, 1699, 1784, 1821, 1847, 1919, 1977

OHIO 511, 835, 1442

OKLAHOMA 626, 1221, 1897, 1898

OREGON 1177, 1895

PARAPROFESSIONALS 1, 2, 4, 5, 9, 29, 44, 45, 171, 173, 256, 265, 310, 352, 467, 475, 482, 533, 549, 571, 581, 639, 643, 647, 655, 686, 689, 738, 740, 766, 796, 858, 863, 903, 908, 968, 1013, 1031, 1055, 1083, 1224, 1276, 1292, 1294, 1323, 1327, 1384, 1386, 1405, 1426, 1493, 1595, 1596, 1597, 1599, 1639, 1651, 1691, 1692, 1777, 1786, 1790, 1799, 1816, 1830, 1900, 1940

PARENTAL INVOLVEMENT 11, 20, 32, 55, 83, 127, 207, 215, 247, 253, 270, 276, 278, 344, 437, 607, 728, 742, 750, 780, 782, 789, 826, 845, 863, 864, 903, 939, 1131, 1142, 1180, 1184, 1185, 1213, 1262, 1286, 1325, 1459, 1483, 1571, 1577, 1729, 1772, 1866, 1888, 1895, 1923

PEABODY PICTURE-VOCABULARY TEST 155, 374, 649, 650, 785, 804, 852, 972, 1120, 1148, 1217, 1233, 1325, 1455, 1538, 1710, 1753, 1816, 1817

PEER GROUP 114, 279, 421, 422, 476, 532, 545, 582, 672, 709, 857, 880, 985, 1077, 1189, 1271, 1287, 1363, 1399, 1423, 1428, 1429, 1440, 1466, 1535, 1586, 1587, 1709, 1722, 1773, 1794, 1808, 2000

PENNSYLVANIA 838, 840, 945, 1142, 1235, 1591, 1628, 1969

PERCEPTION 57, 85, 86, 224, 354, 415, 589, 758, 875, 941, 942, 958, 971, 974, 1063, 1209, 1335, 1644, 1781, 1947, 1967

PERFORMANCE EXPECTATIONS 3, 194, 246, 269, 297, 527, 539, 540, 547, 640, 806, 832, 898, 916, 1159, 1192, 1216, 1346, 1406, 1624, 1636, 1705, 1722, 1780, 1844, 1845, 1907, 1931

PERSONALITY 73, 125, 187, 206, 285, 287, 311, 320, 357, 450, 451, 452, 454, 455, 457, 461, 462, 466, 478, 528, 540, 578, 672, 674, 736, 737, 803, 816, 817, 818, 821, 822, 833, 850, 851, 856, 880, 884, 885, 887, 889, 899, 900, 931, 944, 951, 963, 970, 976, 986, 1001, 1009, 1027, 1042, 1060, 1062, 1067, 1086, 1090, 1091, 1094, 1102, 1120, 1124, 1131, 1147, 1166, 1167, 1168, 1171, 1190, 1208, 1215, 1217, 1233, 1239, 1288, 1297, 1304, 1307, 1342, 1344, 1347, 1451, 1457, 1458, 1469, 1476, 1490, 1507, 1510, 1562, 1565, 1594, 1603, 1645, 1647, 1728, 1784, 1831, 1832, 1844, 1942, 1954, 1963, 1969, 1989

PERSONALITY ASSESSMENT 39, 44, 85, 104, 150, 188, 252, 433, 446, 552, 663, 670, 691, 721, 785, 815, 818, 865, 899, 900, 925, 931, 1001, 1012, 1059, 1060, 1114, 1147, 1167, 1168, 1171, 1172, 1190, 1205, 1226, 1245, 1279, 1289, 1307, 1344, 1347, 1357, 1360, 1364, 1378, 1396, 1397, 1414, 1430, 1457, 1458, 1476, 1521, 1550, 1572, 1717, 1723, 1846, 1847

PERSONNEL 230, 254, 269, 341, 475, 503, 643, 849, 904, 1096, 1108, 1340, 1401, 1514, 1522, 1598, 1647, 1723, 1793, 1778, 1801, 1866, 1915

PHONOLOGY 57, 86, 99, 157, 224, 344, 373, 423, 608, 609, 725, 875, 1011, 1053, 1174, 1176, 1193, 1311, 1350, 1353, 1458, 1662, 1805, 1958, 1968

PHYSICAL DEVELOPMENT 85, 424, 654, 749, 776, 864, 981, 1130, 1208, 1294, 1419, 1662, 1951, 1973

PHYSICIANS 4, 146, 179, 322, 475, 500, 503, 521, 523, 537, 587, 620, 765, 778, 905, 906, 928, 947, 1089, 1102, 1103, 1154, 1191, 1196, 1210, 1258, 1259, 1269, 1385, 1425, 1464, 1465, 1511, 1522, 1599, 1628, 1640, 1660, 1801

POLICE-COMMUNITY RELATIONS 249, 264, 341, 444, 481, 482, 488, 835, 1277, 1281, 1283, 1284, 1327, 1515, 1602, 1716, 1723, 1773, 1946

POLICY 14, 120, 173, 179, 200, 202, 217, 249, 255, 297, 301, 302, 313, 314, 317, 324, 327, 341, 346, 359, 431, 445, 474, 480, 482, 511, 539, 569, 582, 588, 594, 596, 601, 611, 612, 618, 652, 653, 655, 681, 683, 684, 685, 688, 694, 695, 733, 751, 764, 766, 773, 791, 798, 802, 825, 837, 839, 849, 904, 910, 967, 1014, 1021, 1024, 1031, 1064, 1066, 1075, 1077, 1102, 1109, 1111, 1113, 1115, 1140, 1141, 1149, 1155, 1156, 1157, 1160, 1201, 1218, 1219, 1222, 1225, 1236, 1260, 1266, 1267, 1268, 1269, 1280, 1281, 1284, 1311, 1313, 1329, 1331, 1381, 1383, 1386, 1388, 1426, 1439, 1475, 1483, 1499, 1501, 1506, 1512, 1530, 1581, 1592, 1595, 1597, 1598, 1600, 1601, 1602, 1605, 1609, 1618, 1619, 1626, 1627, 1644, 1684, 1734, 1774, 1786, 1790, 1792, 1796, 1866, 1873, 1883, 1888, 1901, 1909, 1975, 1996

POLITICAL POWER 34, 78, 144, 165, 176, 266, 281, 334, 506, 511, 526, 534, 561, 567, 573, 580, 585, 613, 666, 687, 690, 706, 726, 777, 802, 825, 921, 1007, 1093, 1115, 1121, 1125, 1126, 1140, 1150, 1155, 1157, 1201, 1229, 1232, 1270, 1276, 1293, 1300, 1312, 1322, 1323, 1359, 1377, 1381, 1445, 1475, 1481, 1482, 1483, 1527, 1542, 1554, 1556, 1623, 1639, 1653, 1756, 1807, 1862, 1885, 1911, 1930, 1945, 1983, 1984, 1994

POLITICS 34, 69, 120, 176, 196, 249, 281, 307, 330, 334, 341, 342, 436, 506, 537, 563, 610, 613, 690, 706, 726, 777, 802, 826, 921, 1007, 1093, 1101, 1115, 1121, 1125, 1126, 1198, 1201, 1229, 1230, 1232, 1269, 1271, 1276, 1293, 1300, 1312, 1323, 1445, 1554, 1556, 1618, 1639, 1641, 1653, 1661, 1689, 1726, 1748, 1756, 1764, 1807, 1862, 1871, 1930, 1983, 1984

POVERTY 1, 6, 26, 42, 60, 71, 74, 86, 88, 112, 121, 135, 146, 147, 168, 169, 176, 186, 190, 193, 199, 200, 202, 214, 215, 220, 221, 232, 235, 242, 249, 270, 294, 297, 302, 309, 310, 311, 319, 353, 367, 384, 400, 413, 436, 442, 459, 475, 492, 503, 512, 513, 514, 515, 521, 522, 526, 538, 561, 563, 565, 623, 644, 654, 667, 681, 684, 693, 701, 706, 727, 737, 738, 744, 750, 753, 762, 764, 774, 776, 781, 800, 807, 813, 814, 820, 842, 843, 844, 873, 874, 898, 901, 906, 913, 915, 946, 951, 959, 968, 969, 985, 987, 990, 995, 1008, 1011, 1020, 1022, 1023, 1025, 1027, 1029, 1030, 1039, 1040, 1042, 1043, 1044, 1045, 1064, 1066, 1071, 1079, 1085, 1093, 1112, 1115,

384, 395, 407, 409, 443, 451, 452, 454, 456, 470, 470, 472, 473, 480, 495, 528, 531, 534, 561, 568, 608, 615, 640, 643, 662, 666, 681, 685, 705, 734, 735, 751, 767, 769, 788, 792, 799, 803, 817, 822, 837, 868, 873, 883, 884, 910, 920, 926, 935, 941, 955, 957, 973, 980, 986, 992, 997, 1007, 1010, 1023, 1057, 1068, 1072, 1089, 1092, 1094, 1131, 1140, 1141, 1150, 1158, 1161, 1176, 1182, 1207, 1211, 1214, 1216, 1218, 1222, 1231, 1234, 1238, 1243, 1252, 1264, 1268, 1280, 1282, 1283, 1284, 1290, 1294, 1298, 1299, 1312, 1329, 1354, 1356, 1357, 1359, 1368, 1370, 1375, 1376, 1378, 1382, 1388, 1396, 1397, 1398, 1405, 1418, 1435, 1452, 1456, 1475, 1477, 1481, 1484, 1490, 1491, 1492, 1501, 1502, 1513, 1518, 1522, 1546, 1564, 1567, 1570, 1582, 1594, 1604, 1607, 1608, 1609, 1610, 1616, 1629, 1634, 1638, 1643, 1650, 1655, 1662, 1684, 1685, 1692, 1734, 1742, 1743, 1764, 1791, 1792, 1802, 1827, 1829, 1879, 1892, 1893, 1899, 1906, 1911, 1936, 1945, 1962, 1987, 1995

ROLE EXPECTATIONS 6, 7, 8, 10, 22, 228, 248, 332, 421, 454, 463, 531, 582, 598, 759, 767, 823, 857, 858, 903, 905, 906, 936, 939, 947, 971, 1044, 1089, 1103, 1149, 1151, 1175, 1195, 1200, 1267, 1279, 1304, 1307, 1335, 1368, 1374, 1429, 1435, 1452, 1559, 1657, 1743, 1829, 2000, 2001

RORSCHACH TEST 211, 251, 415, 648, 865, 899, 900, 1397, 1989

ROTTER INTERNAL-EXTERNAL SCALE 204, 292, 357, 466, 634, 635, 638, 674, 1027, 1347, 1546, 1678, 1770

RURAL 96, 169, 170, 185, 190, 200, 214, 215, 254, 273, 276, 280, 282, 283, 321, 327, 417, 459, 525, 526, 529, 563, 568, 588, 617, 622, 641, 658, 659, 690, 697, 701, 706, 722, 724, 727, 763, 768, 769, 839, 842, 843, 844, 855, 855, 856, 857, 859, 875, 880, 882, 887, 888, 890, 907, 928, 956, 957, 966, 968, 969, 970, 971, 990, 1006, 1008, 1040, 1042, 1044, 1046, 1062, 1064, 1087, 1089, 1091, 1098, 1101, 1107, 1152, 1182, 1187, 1192, 1193, 1229, 1230, 1232, 1257, 1290, 1295, 1304, 1305, 1306, 1318, 1353, 1415, 1420, 1421, 1445, 1467, 1468, 1506, 1510, 1513, 1525, 1526, 1548, 1560, 1585, 1626, 1661, 1674, 1682, 1724, 1808, 1821, 1822, 1849, 1850, 1851, 1853, 1858, 1860, 1878, 1883, 1963, 1977, 2002

SCHIZOPHRENIA 1, 51, 210, 240, 251, 425, 497, 515, 518, 519, 541, 543, 648, 691, 703, 813, 937, 945, 992, 1026, 1065, 1117, 1119, 1122, 1123, 1202, 1204, 1226, 1414, 1476, 1477, 1524, 1555, 1557, 1558, 1559, 1655, 1668, 1914

SCHOLASTIC ACHIEVEMENT 11, 13, 20, 30, 42, 48, 55, 58, 59, 60, 60, 61, 62, 63, 76, 95, 117, 142, 150, 168, 169, 186, 187, 194, 221, 222, 234, 242, 246, 253, 254, 259, 261, 262, 270, 276, 278, 292, 296, 297, 298, 300, 301, 302, 321, 343, 369, 371, 419, 422, 460, 485, 508, 512, 530, 532, 538, 539, 540, 552, 553, 565, 591, 599, 615, 619, 626, 628, 630, 637, 640, 649, 650, 651, 660, 675, 677, 678, 706, 715, 718, 723, 737, 741, 745, 779, 781, 783, 784, 792, 794, 808, 812, 822, 828, 829, 840, 846, 850, 851, 854, 855, 856, 877, 881, 886, 893, 898, 911, 930, 933, 938, 939, 952, 974, 976, 988, 1006, 1022, 1024, 1027, 1043, 1045, 1047, 1070, 1076, 1077, 1079, 1093, 1095, 1129, 1134, 1169, 1170, 1172, 1180,

1181, 1200, 1205, 1210, 1216, 1244, 1255, 1276, 1343, 1349, 1396, 1398, 1399, 1416, 1420, 1434, 1437, 1447, 1462, 1476, 1482, 1491, 1500, 1504, 1505, 1516, 1545, 1546, 1552, 1605, 1624, 1637, 1646, 1675, 1698, 1699, 1706, 1717, 1718, 1733, 1735, 1736, 1745, 1746, 1791, 1795, 1797, 1798, 1800, 1816, 1818, 1838, 1845, 1849, 1851, 1859, 1860, 1863, 1872, 1873, 1874, 1878, 1880, 1911, 1917, 1918, 1919, 1920, 1926, 1933, 1952, 1958, 1970, 1974, 1987

SCHOLASTIC APTITUDE TEST 595, 678, 679, 1079

SCHOLASTIC ASPIRATIONS 58, 59, 67, 202, 241, 253, 354, 512, 539, 637, 649, 650, 752, 783, 788, 789, 792, 807, 821, 846, 881, 898, 939, 970, 971, 976, 1022, 1024, 1037, 1045, 1047, 1069, 1177, 1205, 1252, 1254, 1255, 1263, 1343, 1437, 1446, 1447, 1612, 1622, 1624, 1696, 1699, 1784, 1803, 1850, 1918, 1919, 1977

SELF CONCEPT 3, 13, 20, 48, 58, 60, 61, 62, 77, 85, 88, 125, 153, 191, 192, 208, 219, 297, 299, 302, 357, 374, 383, 399, 425, 427, 489, 501, 512, 532, 538, 553, 578, 582, 610, 641, 642, 649, 650, 664, 668, 672, 674, 707, 721, 737, 770, 785, 789, 792, 808, 823, 836, 952, 970, 972, 974, 977, 984, 1005, 1006, 1012, 1033, 1035, 1036, 1059, 1060, 1086, 1112, 1114, 1140, 1150, 1169, 1170, 1172, 1175, 1184, 1185, 1217, 1230, 1233, 1245, 1288, 1291, 1302, 1321, 1347, 1380, 1398, 1421, 1423, 1440, 1441, 1444, 1473, 1491, 1507, 1510, 1534, 1546, 1550, 1551, 1577, 1624, 1690, 1728, 1730, 1804, 1808, 1818, 1819, 1820, 1826, 1883, 1886, 1887, 1944, 1960, 1986, 1990, 1995, 1996, 1998

SEMANTICS 154, 157, 158, 224, 373, 379, 466, 608, 633, 787, 933, 1003, 1039, 1072, 1073, 1159, 1162, 1174, 1664, 1815, 1964

SES 1, 4, 6, 8, 10, 11, 13, 21, 22, 23, 26, 27, 34, 42, 44, 45, 46, 47, 50, 52, 53, 59, 60, 61, 63, 66, 67, 68, 69, 71, 77, 83, 85, 86, 89, 96, 104, 109, 110, 112, 115, 121, 123, 131, 132, 133, 134, 135, 136, 137, 138, 139, 140, 142, 143, 146, 147, 164, 168, 169, 176, 178, 179, 186, 187, 190, 192, 193, 199, 202, 209, 212, 214, 215, 220, 224, 225, 229, 230, 232, 235, 236, 241, 242, 246, 250, 253, 254, 258, 259, 264, 265, 270, 271, 279, 282, 283, 284, 287, 290, 291, 292, 298, 300, 310, 311, 319, 325, 326, 332, 336, 340, 342, 355, 356, 358, 364, 368, 384, 399, 401, 405, 407, 409, 412, 414, 422, 427, 430, 444, 445, 446, 452, 454, 456, 458, 459, 469, 470, 472, 473, 474, 475, 485, 489, 494, 496, 503, 506, 508, 515, 517, 518, 519, 521, 524, 526, 528, 529, 530, 532, 535, 538, 553, 557, 559, 565, 570, 574, 578, 582, 585, 586, 595, 601, 613, 616, 618, 620, 622, 623, 626, 634, 635, 637, 643, 645, 652, 654, 658, 667, 672, 674, 675, 680, 682, 684, 686, 690, 691, 694, 694, 696, 697, 699, 700, 701, 706, 713, 715, 716, 722, 723, 728, 729, 730, 731, 734, 735, 737, 743, 744, 747, 748, 752, 753, 755, 761, 762, 768, 769, 770, 772, 774, 775, 776, 777, 781, 783, 790, 792, 796, 797, 798, 799, 800, 801, 807, 810, 812, 813, 815, 816, 817, 818, 820, 821, 829, 835, 839, 842, 843, 844, 846, 850, 851, 853, 855, 856, 858, 861, 862, 871, 874, 875, 884, 885, 888, 896, 903, 911, 912, 913, 914, 916, 917, 919, 920, 928, 929, 930, 939, 940, 943, 945, 946, 951, 954, 956, 959, 968, 971, 974, 975, 976, 980,

985, 987, 990, 991, 994, 998, 999, 1000, 1005, 1008, 1011, 1012, 1013, 1015, 1018, 1020, 1022, 1027, 1029, 1030, 1034, 1039, 1042, 1044, 1045, 1053, 1056, 1058, 1062, 1067, 1069, 1070, 1071, 1077, 1079, 1085, 1093, 1095, 1101, 1102, 1112, 1114, 1115, 1120, 1121, 1122, 1123, 1129, 1131, 1139, 1144, 1146, 1171, 1174, 1176, 1177, 1178, 1179, 1180, 1181, 1184, 1185, 1190, 1193, 1195, 1196, 1199, 1200, 1202, 1203, 1204, 1205, 1208, 1209, 1211, 1217, 1218, 1219, 1220, 1230, 1233, 1236, 1240, 1241, 1245, 1248, 1252, 1253, 1254, 1255, 1256, 1271, 1274, 1288, 1291, 1295, 1296, 1304, 1311, 1315, 1324, 1333, 1334, 1336, 1339, 1342, 1343, 1353, 1358, 1360, 1363, 1369, 1380, 1385, 1394, 1399, 1408, 1409, 1410, 1416, 1418, 1419, 1427, 1433, 1434, 1437, 1439, 1442, 1455, 1458, 1459, 1461, 1462, 1465, 1466, 1469, 1471, 1476, 1477, 1482, 1500, 1507, 1511, 1513, 1516, 1518, 1519, 1520, 1524, 1528, 1534, 1535, 1537, 1538, 1546, 1555, 1557, 1558, 1565, 1568, 1571, 1574, 1598, 1611, 1612, 1613, 1618, 1621, 1622, 1624, 1628, 1629, 1630, 1638, 1639, 1641, 1644, 1646, 1647, 1650, 1653, 1654, 1655, 1656, 1658, 1659, 1662, 1671, 1672, 1673, 1675, 1676, 1678, 1679, 1682, 1683, 1686, 1690, 1695, 1697, 1698, 1699, 1700, 1713, 1718, 1719, 1722, 1724, 1729, 1744, 1745, 1747, 1748, 1757, 1758, 1762, 1764, 1767, 1769, 1778, 1783, 1787, 1789, 1797, 1798, 1800, 1801, 1806, 1807, 1808, 1811, 1812, 1818, 1821, 1831, 1839, 1842, 1845, 1849, 1850, 1851, 1852, 1853, 1854, 1855, 1856, 1857, 1858, 1859, 1860, 1863, 1881, 1886, 1887, 1889, 1890, 1894, 1896, 1899, 1901, 1909, 1911, 1913, 1914, 1919, 1928, 1929, 1930, 1931, 1935, 1950, 1952, 1959, 1960, 1964, 1965, 1966, 1969, 1987

SEX COMPARISON 10, 13, 21, 33, 48, 49, 53, 67, 76, 84, 103, 114, 115, 129, 136, 143, 146, 152, 155, 192, 197, 198, 204, 212, 218, 228, 237, 257, 259, 261, 279, 295, 325, 329, 340, 355, 357, 358, 400, 413, 420, 443, 446, 452, 456, 461, 462, 484, 504, 509, 514, 517, 523, 542, 553, 558, 559, 572, 585, 591, 599, 611, 612, 620, 624, 627, 642, 643, 660, 674, 699, 700, 706, 707, 716, 722, 723, 724, 728, 730, 739, 743, 749, 754, 755, 770, 775, 811, 816, 819, 822, 835, 840, 843, 844, 851, 852, 856, 857, 874, 880, 882, 885, 886, 887, 888, 889, 894, 895, 901, 934, 943, 953, 954, 958, 959, 968, 970, 971, 974, 978, 979, 989, 999, 1000, 1001, 1005, 1011, 1012, 1028, 1033, 1034, 1035, 1039, 1048, 1053, 1055, 1058, 1060, 1061, 1062, 1067, 1080, 1081, 1091, 1098, 1122, 1123, 1128, 1146, 1150, 1159, 1162, 1167, 1168, 1171, 1189, 1197, 1202, 1206, 1215, 1219, 1221, 1226, 1233, 1245, 1254, 1255, 1257, 1261, 1306, 1324, 1328, 1334, 1339, 1342, 1353, 1362, 1363, 1369, 1420, 1421, 1440, 1456, 1460, 1466, 1469, 1475, 1476, 1489, 1503, 1505, 1518, 1519, 1521, 1525, 1526, 1535, 1561, 1563, 1628, 1645, 1646, 1662, 1670, 1671, 1672, 1675, 1681, 1685, 1715, 1719, 1727, 1735, 1742, 1745, 1746, 1760, 1764, 1767, 1783, 1804, 1831, 1832, 1834, 1839, 1849, 1850, 1851, 1858, 1859, 1860, 1862, 1917, 1918, 1924, 1928, 1929, 1950, 1952, 1959, 1971, 1999, 2002

SEX ROLES 2, 6, 14, 21, 27, 31, 46, 47, 73, 93, 106, 108, 125, 140, 152, 165, 169, 190, 198, 204, 220, 221, 222, 257, 261, 265, 279, 287, 288, 289, 290, 292, 309, 319, 320, 332, 334, 365, 381, 393, 395, 396, 397, 405, 421, 435, 443, 452, 453, 488, 517, 524, 542, 545, 565, 570,

577, 587, 591, 597, 612, 616, 623, 641, 642, 643, 659, 668, 680, 691, 693, 706, 709, 719, 720, 721, 763, 768, 769, 805, 811, 830, 832, 836, 873, 917, 925, 956, 990, 1012, 1044, 1067, 1086, 1090, 1094, 1102, 1149, 1158, 1159, 1189, 1195, 1202, 1212, 1227, 1231, 1236, 1248, 1249, 1250, 1263, 1264, 1265, 1267, 1297, 1333, 1335, 1358, 1368, 1374, 1396, 1420, 1435, 1460, 1463, 1510, 1537, 1553, 1555, 1568, 1587, 1613, 1643, 1685, 1742, 1743, 1755, 1756, 1766, 1775, 1784, 1809, 1826, 1844, 1881, 1882, 1891, 1960, 1994

SEXUAL BEHAVIOR 213, 221, 287, 288, 289, 290, 319, 405, 410, 442, 445, 507, 582, 597, 691, 768, 771, 832, 925, 963, 987, 1071, 1144, 1195, 1248, 1249, 1255, 1524, 1568, 1649

SOCIAL MOBILITY 6, 104, 171, 202, 209, 247, 255, 283, 292, 332, 442, 443, 473, 500, 534, 535, 616, 622, 623, 645, 728, 744, 764, 846, 913, 929, 970, 971, 976, 980, 1005, 1011, 1029, 1069, 1101, 1139, 1140, 1144, 1177, 1200, 1229, 1231, 1253, 1263, 1274, 1290, 1427, 1433, 1434, 1435, 1438, 1468, 1553, 1577, 1611, 1622, 1646, 1650, 1696, 1697, 1699, 1719, 1720, 1784, 1821, 1880, 1885, 1919, 1945, 1952

SOCIAL SCIENCES 34, 79, 80, 144, 254, 281, 330, 451, 616, 684, 777, 803, 841, 857, 1110, 1275, 1285, 1356, 1401, 1402, 1403, 1454, 1485, 1564, 1604, 1607, 1663, 1823, 1892, 1893, 1899, 1937, 1969

SOCIAL SERVICES 23, 87, 93, 94, 121, 147, 169, 196, 229, 232, 239, 245, 254, 265, 278, 319, 353, 358, 400, 403, 427, 428, 436, 445, 465, 482, 511, 533, 549, 561, 581, 603, 644, 653, 656, 684, 686, 687, 727, 748, 764, 767, 839, 849, 910, 955, 1014, 1113, 1141, 1149, 1152, 1198, 1223, 1236, 1266, 1271, 1276, 1295, 1323, 1329, 1334, 1381, 1399, 1407, 1442, 1445, 1511, 1515, 1542, 1603, 1618, 1639, 1656, 1716, 1724, 1729, 1732, 1748, 1786, 1843, 1902, 1915, 1976

SOCIAL STRUCTURE 176, 282, 346, 447, 537, 570, 616, 624, 690, 746, 965, 1010, 1011, 1031, 1044, 1101, 1217, 1273, 1353, 1565, 1587, 1612, 1682, 1686, 1763, 1764, 1779, 1894, 1900

SOCIALIZATION 3, 40, 48, 58, 204, 219, 265, 301, 313, 314, 315, 357, 393, 449, 483, 507, 512, 532, 540, 572, 577, 616, 718, 823, 829, 838, 857, 963, 1011, 1024, 1045, 1067, 1102, 1184, 1185, 1200, 1209, 1217, 1257, 1304, 1343, 1363, 1399, 1411, 1435, 1460, 1484, 1497, 1498, 1503, 1504, 1551, 1577, 1612, 1662, 1681, 1704, 1707, 1730, 1759, 1806, 1923, 1943, 1962, 1963, 1999

SOUTH 139, 223, 307, 325, 360, 432, 466, 498, 575, 589, 598, 614, 648, 785, 806, 808, 978, 979, 989, 994, 998, 1014, 1015, 1056, 1064, 1092, 1286, 1307, 1369, 1414, 1467, 1468, 1537, 1649, 1650, 1651, 1656, 1720, 1787, 1788, 1789, 1790, 1858, 1901

SOUTH AMERICA 79, 80, 139, 203, 283, 334, 345, 389, 404, 576, 910, 1023, 1124, 1143, 1182, 1238, 1290, 1427, 1454, 1464, 1465, 1539, 1619, 1713, 1855, 1861

SOUTHWEST 7, 8, 9, 10, 11, 12, 13, 14, 15, 16, 17, 19, 20, 22, 28, 29, 30, 31, 33, 34, 35, 36, 37, 38, 41, 46, 47, 48, 49, 52, 57, 58, 59, 60, 61, 62, 63, 65, 69, 74, 75, 82,

83, 84, 85, 86, 88, 90, 93, 95, 96, 101, 106, 108, 112, 113, 119, 122, 123, 130, 131, 132, 133, 134, 135, 137, 138, 142, 143, 144, 146, 149, 150, 157, 165, 167, 169, 170, 174, 178, 180, 181, 182, 183, 185, 188, 189, 194, 197, 198, 200, 205, 206, 207, 212, 214, 215, 216, 220, 225, 226, 229, 230, 231, 232, 233, 235, 236, 237, 238, 239, 242, 243, 244, 245, 246, 247, 253, 255, 256, 257, 261, 263, 264, 266, 267, 271, 275, 276, 278, 279, 284, 292, 294, 295, 296, 297, 298, 299, 302, 303, 304, 312, 316, 317, 318, 321, 325, 326, 327, 329, 330, 335, 338, 339, 340, 342, 343, 344, 356, 359, 363, 364, 365, 372, 373, 377, 381, 382, 383, 385, 386, 390, 397, 400, 401, 410, 411, 413, 414, 416, 417, 418, 420, 422, 423, 427, 429, 430, 431, 434, 435, 439, 440, 441, 443, 444, 445, 450, 452, 454, 461, 475, 478, 479, 481, 482, 483, 484, 485, 487, 488, 489, 490, 491, 492, 493, 495, 496, 497, 499, 504, 507, 509, 512, 513, 515, 517, 518, 519, 521, 522, 523, 524, 526, 527, 528, 529, 530, 531, 538, 539, 540, 547, 549, 552, 553, 556, 564, 565, 566, 568, 572, 573, 577, 580, 585, 590, 591, 596, 599, 600, 604, 608, 609, 613, 618, 619, 626, 627, 628, 630, 632, 633, 635, 636, 637, 638, 643, 647, 649, 650, 656, 658, 659, 660, 663, 667, 671, 673, 675, 676, 677, 678, 679, 680, 686, 690, 693, 694, 696, 697, 700, 705, 706, 707, 708, 715, 721, 722, 723, 724, 726, 728, 740, 741, 743, 747, 748, 749, 750, 751, 752, 753, 754, 755, 756, 757, 760, 762, 763, 764, 765, 766, 770, 771, 772, 773, 774, 775, 776, 779, 780, 782, 783, 784, 786, 787, 789, 794, 797, 798, 802, 804, 808, 809, 811, 812, 814, 815, 816, 817, 818, 819, 820, 821, 822, 825, 827, 834, 835, 836, 842, 843, 844, 845, 851, 852, 853, 854, 855, 856, 857, 859, 860, 861, 863, 864, 865, 866, 867, 868, 869, 870, 871, 875, 877, 878, 880, 882, 886, 887, 888, 889, 890, 891, 892, 893, 894, 895, 896, 897, 899, 900, 902, 905, 906, 907, 908, 909, 911, 915, 916, 917, 919, 920, 921, 922, 923, 924, 932, 933, 935, 940, 943, 947, 948, 949, 950, 952, 953, 954, 956, 957, 958, 960, 961, 966, 967, 968, 970, 971, 972, 974, 976, 977, 981, 983, 984, 994, 998, 999, 1000, 1001, 1002, 1003, 1005, 1006, 1007, 1008, 1012, 1013, 1018, 1019, 1022, 1024, 1029, 1037, 1047, 1049, 1050, 1051, 1052, 1054, 1055, 1057, 1058, 1062, 1065, 1067, 1069, 1070, 1071, 1073, 1075, 1077, 1078, 1079, 1080, 1081, 1082, 1084, 1085, 1087, 1088, 1092, 1093, 1095, 1096, 1097, 1098, 1099, 1100, 1101, 1102, 1103, 1107, 1108, 1112, 1120, 1121, 1128, 1129, 1130, 1131, 1133, 1134, 1139, 1141, 1149, 1152, 1154, 1159, 1162, 1174, 1179, 1184, 1185, 1186, 1188, 1191, 1192, 1193, 1194, 1196, 1199, 1200, 1202, 1204, 1205, 1206, 1208, 1209, 1211, 1214, 1217, 1218, 1219, 1220, 1221, 1224, 1227, 1228, 1230, 1231, 1232, 1233, 1235, 1238, 1241, 1244, 1245, 1246, 1248, 1249, 1251, 1252, 1253, 1254, 1255, 1256, 1263, 1270, 1271, 1274, 1276, 1277, 1281, 1282, 1283, 1284, 1287, 1289, 1291, 1292, 1293, 1296, 1302, 1303, 1308, 1310, 1311, 1312, 1318, 1323, 1324, 1325, 1327, 1330, 1331, 1332, 1333, 1334, 1335, 1336, 1337, 1341, 1350, 1352, 1353, 1358, 1361, 1362, 1363, 1364, 1365, 1369, 1371, 1384, 1385, 1387, 1391, 1395, 1404, 1407, 1409, 1410, 1415, 1416, 1419, 1420, 1423, 1424, 1425, 1427, 1428, 1429, 1433, 1434, 1438, 1439, 1440, 1441, 1443, 1446, 1448, 1449, 1451, 1453, 1455, 1456, 1457, 1458, 1462, 1466, 1467, 1469, 1470, 1472, 1474, 1475, 1476, 1482, 1483, 1489, 1490, 1494, 1500, 1505, 1509, 1512, 1514, 1516, 1517, 1518, 1519, 1520, 1521, 1525, 1526, 1532, 1533, 1538, 1543, 1544, 1552, 1565, 1567, 1573, 1574, 1575, 1576, 1577, 1585, 1587, 1590, 1620, 1626, 1627, 1628, 1630, 1631, 1633, 1635, 1637, 1645, 1657, 1659, 1661, 1669, 1670, 1673, 1674, 1675, 1678, 1679, 1680, 1681, 1686, 1687, 1688, 1701, 1709, 1711, 1715, 1719, 1723, 1736, 1737, 1745, 1746, 1747, 1749, 1750, 1751, 1753, 1757, 1762, 1763, 1764, 1766, 1768, 1770, 1773, 1774, 1777, 1779, 1783, 1791, 1795, 1797, 1798, 1800, 1801, 1804, 1806, 1807, 1808, 1809, 1810, 1817, 1818, 1819, 1820, 1822, 1828, 1829, 1831, 1833, 1836, 1838, 1839, 1842, 1845, 1846, 1847, 1848, 1850, 1852, 1853, 1854, 1858, 1860, 1863, 1864, 1867, 1868, 1869, 1870, 1871, 1872, 1873, 1874, 1876, 1882, 1885, 1889, 1894, 1900, 1903, 1904, 1905, 1906, 1915, 1918, 1919, 1920, 1922, 1923, 1924, 1926, 1930, 1931, 1932, 1934, 1938, 1949, 1951, 1954, 1955, 1957, 1958, 1959, 1960, 1965, 1966, 1971, 1972, 1973, 1976, 1984, 2001

SPANISH SURNAMED 17, 23, 24, 25, 27, 32, 39, 41, 44, 45, 50, 52, 56, 62, 63, 72, 82, 89, 91, 99, 102, 103, 118, 120, 121, 133, 136, 165, 173, 179, 203, 210, 215, 216, 218, 220, 225, 227, 235, 240, 242, 260, 261, 262, 263, 274, 312, 314, 327, 336, 341, 347, 348, 353, 358, 373, 374, 375, 378, 387, 388, 402, 418, 427, 441, 456, 480, 486, 490, 491, 492, 504, 507, 511, 513, 532, 536, 556, 564, 571, 576, 583, 592, 593, 599, 600, 614, 639, 657, 659, 661, 662, 666, 667, 668, 672, 676, 680, 681, 703, 705, 714, 715, 725, 733, 735, 736, 747, 748, 752, 754, 755, 757, 760, 761, 764, 770, 776, 777, 787, 790, 794, 795, 798, 812, 828, 835, 840, 847, 857, 858, 859, 862, 866, 867, 869, 899, 900, 926, 927, 938, 940, 943, 947, 948, 951, 959, 969, 974, 978, 979, 991, 1018, 1021, 1029, 1036, 1038, 1039, 1057, 1065, 1086, 1092, 1105, 1108, 1131, 1136, 1137, 1145, 1153, 1181, 1197, 1201, 1212, 1223, 1226, 1229, 1232, 1235, 1251, 1260, 1266, 1268, 1275, 1289, 1291, 1300, 1302, 1305, 1306, 1309, 1312, 1313, 1314, 1316, 1317, 1319, 1337, 1349, 1354, 1355, 1356, 1359, 1362, 1364, 1383, 1386, 1389, 1390, 1396, 1400, 1407, 1412, 1414, 1429, 1446, 1451, 1465, 1485, 1513, 1514, 1520, 1529, 1530, 1538, 1539, 1544, 1566, 1567, 1594, 1595, 1597, 1600, 1604, 1606, 1607, 1609, 1610, 1617, 1619, 1626, 1634, 1635, 1636, 1637, 1640, 1641, 1642, 1660, 1661, 1664, 1672, 1688, 1703, 1719, 1734, 1738, 1739, 1741, 1752, 1755, 1783, 1784, 1789, 1792, 1796, 1804, 1813, 1817, 1822, 1840, 1843, 1846, 1849, 1850, 1851, 1852, 1853, 1854, 1855, 1856, 1857, 1859, 1860, 1861, 1862, 1863, 1866, 1875, 1877, 1884, 1885, 1886, 1887, 1890, 1901, 1905, 1910, 1917, 1921, 1923, 1924, 1937, 1938, 1952, 1967

SPECIAL EDUCATION 11, 14, 118, 150, 193, 210, 219, 303, 318, 327, 354, 359, 361, 464, 595, 627, 652, 903, 988, 1018, 1049, 1127, 1214, 1217, 1218, 1220, 1222, 1365, 1706, 1939

STANFORD ACHIEVEMENT TEST 11, 262, 337, 781, 808, 851, 855, 856, 1134, 1547, 1637

STANFORD-BINET INTELLIGENCE TEST 52, 219, 284, 362, 407, 409, 416, 417, 477, 612, 800, 801, 848, 853, 864, 933, 1207, 1218, 1219, 1390, 1455, 1547, 1629, 1636, 1702, 1705, 1736

BIBLIOGRAPHY

1   AUTH   **ABAD, V., RAMOS, J., & BOYCE, E.**
    TITL   CLINICAL ISSUES IN THE PSYCHIATRIC TREAT-
           MENT OF PUERTO RICANS.
    SRCE   *IN E. R. PADILLA & A. M. PADILLA (EDS.), TRAN-*
           SCULTURAL PSYCHIATRY: AN HISPANIC PER-
           SPECTIVE (MONOGRAPH NO. 4). LOS ANGE-
           LES: UNIVERSITY OF CALIFORNIA, SPANISH
           SPEAKING MENTAL HEALTH RESEARCH CEN-
           TER, 1977, PP. 25-34.
    INDX   PSYCHOPATHOLOGY,   SYMPTOMATOLOGY,
           POVERTY, SES, RELIGION, CULTURAL FAC-
           TORS, SCHIZOPHRENIA, CHILDREARING PRAC-
           TICES, LINGUISTIC COMPETENCE, CHILD
           ABUSE, DEVIANCE, DEPRESSION, ANXIETY, AL-
           COHOLISM, BILINGUAL-BICULTURAL PERSON-
           NEL, PARAPROFESSIONALS, ESSAY, ACCUL-
           TURATION, ESPIRITISMO, PUERTO RICAN-M,
           CONNECTICUT, EAST
    ABST   CLINICAL ISSUES AND PROBLEMS FACED BY
           THE CONNECTICUT MENTAL HEALTH CENTER'S
           CLINICA HISPANA ARE IDENTIFIED, BASED ON
           FOUR YEARS OF CLINICAL EXPERIENCE WHILE
           SERVICING THE PUERTO RICAN POPULATION
           OF NEW HAVEN (APPROXIMATELY 15,000). THE
           MOST COMMONLY OBSERVED CLINICAL PROB-
           LEMS ARE: (1) SOMATIC COMPLAINTS (E.G.,
           DOLOR DE CEREBRO); (2) PSEUDO-HALLUCI-
           NATIONS; (3) SCHIZOPHRENIA; (4) IMPAIRED
           IMPULSE CONTROL; (5) SUICIDE; (6) ALCOHOL-
           ISM; AND (7) ATAQUE. INTERVENTIONS FOUND
           EFFECTIVE FOR EACH PROBLEM ARE DIS-
           CUSSED IN RELATION TO CULTURAL TRAITS,
           CHILD-REARING   PRACTICES,   SOCIOECO-
           NOMIC CONDITIONS, MIGRATION, LANGUAGE
           BARRIERS AND MISDIAGNOSIS. CLINICAL IS-
           SUES RAISED ARE: (1) MULTIPLICITY OF CLIENT
           PROBLEMS; (2) ADVOCACY ROLE OF CLINI-
           CIANS; (3) TRAINING AND USE OF PARA-
           PROFESSIONALS (ADVANTAGES AND DISAD-
           VANTAGES   OF   TWO   MODELS   UTILIZING
           PARAPROFESSIONAL STAFF ARE DISCUSSED);
           AND (4) IMPORTANCE OF ESPIRITISMO IN
           THERAPY. BY SHARING CLINICAL IM-
           PRESSIONS OF PUERTO RICAN PSYCHIATRIC
           PATIENTS, MENTAL HEALTH CENTERS SERVING
           THIS CULTURALLY DIVERSE POPULATION WILL
           DEVELOP MORE RELEVANT SERVICES AND
           CLINICAL TRAINING PROGRAMS. 16 REFER-
           ENCES.
    ACCN   000001

2   AUTH   **ABAD, V., RAMOS, J., & BOYCE, E.**
    TITL   A MODEL FOR DELIVERY OF MENTAL HEALTH
           SERVICES TO SPANISH-SPEAKING MINORITIES.
    SRCE   *AMERICAN JOURNAL OF ORTHOPSYCHIATRY,*
           1974, 44(4), 584-595.
    INDX   HEALTH DELIVERY SYSTEMS, PUERTO RICAN-
           M, MEXICAN AMERICAN, BILINGUAL-BICUL-
           TURAL PERSONNEL, MENTAL HEALTH, SEX
           ROLES, CULTURAL FACTORS, FICTIVE KINSHIP,
           PARAPROFESSIONALS, ESPIRITISMO, CON-
           NECTICUT, EAST
    ABST   A MENTAL HEALTH PROGRAM FOR SPANISH-
           SPEAKING MINORITIES IS DESCRIBED WHICH
           TAKES INTO ACCOUNT UNIQUE HISPANIC CUL-
           TURAL AND LINGUISTIC CHARACTERISTICS.
           THE SPANISH CLINIC AT THE CONNECTICUT
           MENTAL HEALTH CENTER IN NEW HAVEN PRO-
           VIDES SERVICES TO THE HISPANIC POPULA-
           TION, MOSTLY PUERTO RICAN, WITHIN A
           FRAMEWORK RELEVANT TO THEIR NEEDS, EX-
           PECTATIONS, AND CULTURAL PATTERNS. ITS
           USE OF BILINGUAL STAFF, A WALK-IN CLINIC,
           EDUCATIONAL AND PREVENTIVE PROGRAMS,
           COLLABORATION WITH FAITH HEALERS, AS
           WELL AS LOCAL POLITICAL AND RELIGIOUS
           LEADERS ARE DISCUSSED. 20 REFERENCES.
           (JOURNAL ABSTRACT MODIFIED)
    ACCN   000002

3   AUTH   **ABOUD, F. E.**
    TITL   SELF-EVALUATION: INFORMATION SEEKING
           STRATEGIES FOR INTERETHNIC SOCIAL COM-
           PARISONS.
    SRCE   *JOURNAL OF CROSS-CULTURAL PSYCHOLOGY,*
           1976, 7(3), 289-300.
    INDX   SELF CONCEPT, SOCIALIZATION, CROSS CUL-
           TURAL, EMPIRICAL, ATTITUDES, CHILDREN,
           CULTURAL FACTORS, ETHNIC IDENTITY, MEXI-
           CAN AMERICAN, PERFORMANCE EXPECTA-
           TIONS, WASHINGTON, WEST
    ABST   ETHNIC MINORITY AND MAJORITY STUDENTS
           WERE GIVEN THE OPPORTUNITY TO RECEIVE
           SCORE INFORMATION ABOUT THEIR OWN AND
           THE OTHER ETHNIC GROUP AFTER THEY
           THEMSELVES HAD TAKEN A TEST. YOUNG MA-
           JORITY WHITE CHILDREN GENERALLY CHOSE
           TO LOOK AT OTHER WHITES' SCORES. A LARGE
           PORTION OF YOUNG CHICANOS ALSO SOUGHT
           WHITE SCORE INFORMATION, OR SOUGHT CHI-
           CANOS WHO HAD PERFORMED BETTER AND
           WHITES WHO HAD PERFORMED WORSE THAN
           THEY. THIS GROUP ENHANCEMENT STRATEGY
           WAS ALSO PREVALENT AMONG COLLEGE
           BLACKS. ETHNIC INFORMATION SEEKING IS
           DISCUSSED IN TERMS OF THREE STRATEGIES—
           SEEKING IN-GROUP INFORMATION, SEEKING
           OUT-GROUP INFORMATION, AND SEEKING
           GROUP-ENHANCEMENT INFORMATION—AND
           THE DIFFERENTIAL USE OF THESE STRATEGIES
           BY MINORITY AND MAJORITY STUDENTS. 15
           REFERENCES. (JOURNAL ABSTRACT)
    ACCN   000003

4   AUTH   **ACOSTA, F. X.**
    TITL   BARRIERS BETWEEN MENTAL HEALTH SER-
           VICES AND MEXICAN AMERICANS: AN EXAMI-
           NATION OF A PARADOX.

SRCE   *AMERICAN JOURNAL OF COMMUNITY PSY-CHOLOGY, 1979, 7(5), 503-519.*

INDX   HEALTH DELIVERY SYSTEMS, ESSAY, ACCUL-TURATION, DISCRIMINATION, BILINGUAL-BI-CULTURAL PERSONNEL, RESOURCE UTILIZA-TION, STEREOTYPES, CURANDERISMO, FOLK MEDICINE, MENTAL HEALTH, STRESS, SES, PSY-CHOTHERAPY OUTCOME, CULTURAL FAC-TORS, PARAPROFESSIONALS, PSYCHOTHER-APY, PHYSICIANS, BILINGUALISM, MEXICAN AMERICAN, PSYCHOTHERAPISTS

ABST   ALTHOUGH MEXICAN AMERICANS LIVE UNDER HIGH LEVELS OF PSYCHOLOGICAL AND ENVI-RONMENTAL STRESS THAT WOULD ORDINAR-ILY LEAD TO MENTAL HEALTH PROBLEMS, THEY CONSISTENTLY UNDERUTILIZE MENTAL HEALTH SERVICES. POSSIBLE BARRIERS TO UTILIZA-TION ARE THEREFORE EXAMINED—SUCH AS THE RELATIONSHIP BETWEEN SOCIAL CLASS AND TREATMENT OFFERED; STEREOTYPES CONCERNING MEXICAN AMERICAN FOLK PSY-CHIATRY; LIMITATIONS IMPOSED BY LAN-GUAGE DIFFERENCES; AND THE EFFECTS OF STEREOTYPES BETWEEN ANGLOS AND MEXI-CAN AMERICANS. THIS EXAMINATION REVEALS THAT RECENT EMPIRICAL FINDINGS DEMON-STRATE (1) THAT MEXICAN AMERICANS ARE NOT PREJUDICED AGAINST SEEING ANGLO THERAPISTS, AND (2) THAT CURANDEROS (FOLK HEALERS) ARE NOT WIDELY UTILIZED. IT IS CONCLUDED THAT ERRONEOUS ASSUMP-TIONS ABOUT MEXICAN AMERICAN STEREO-TYPES, PREFERENCES, AND RESOURCES HAVE PERMITTED THE DOMINANT CULTURE TO MINI-MIZE THE SIGNIFICANCE OF MEXICAN AMERI-CAN UNDERUTILIZATION. RECOMMENDATIONS FOR FUTURE RESEARCH AND IMPROVEMENT IN THE DELIVERY OF MENTAL HEALTH SER-VICES ARE PRESENTED. IN PARTICULAR, IT IS NOTED THAT THE FEW FACILITIES THAT HAVE INCREASED BILINGUAL-BICULTURAL STAFFING HAVE EXPERIENCED INCREASED MEXICAN AMERICAN UTILIZATION AND THUS PROVIDE THE MOST ENCOURAGING MODELS. 49 REF-ERENCES.

ACCN   002000

5   AUTH   **ACOSTA, F. X.**

TITL   CLIENT ETHNICITY AND PREFERENCES AS CRITICAL VARIABLES IN PSYCHOTHERAPY: THE MEXICAN-AMERICAN.

SRCE   *UNPUBLISHED MANUSCRIPT, DEPARTMENT OF PSYCHIATRY, UNIVERSITY OF SOUTHERN CALI-FORNIA SCHOOL OF MEDICINE, 1975.*

INDX   MEXICAN AMERICAN, PSYCHOTHERAPY, BILIN-GUAL-BICULTURAL PERSONNEL, PARAPRO-FESSIONALS, PSYCHOTHERAPISTS, CULTURAL FACTORS, REVIEW, MENTAL HEALTH, RE-SOURCE UTILIZATION

ABST   REASONS FOR THE SPARSE UTILIZATION OF MENTAL HEALTH SERVICES BY MEXICAN AMERICANS ARE EXPLORED. NO DEFINITIVE UNDERSTANDING OF WHY THE MEXICAN IS SO MINIMALLY INVOLVED IN PSYCHOLOGICAL SERVICES IS EVIDENT IN THE LITERATURE, AL-THOUGH THE CONDITIONS OF POVERTY AND DISCRIMINATION DO PLACE THE MEXICAN AMERICAN PEOPLE IN A PARTICULARLY VUL-

NERABLE POSITION TO EXPERIENCE PSYCHO-LOGICAL DISTRESS. RESEARCH AND THEORY ON THE IMPORTANCE OF THE CLIENT'S PER-CEPTIONS OF PSYCHOTHERAPISTS ARE CRITI-CALLY REVIEWED, AND THE RECENT CONTRI-BUTIONS FROM CLINICAL AND SOCIAL PSYCHOLOGICAL RESEARCH ON MEXICAN AMERICAN CLIENTS' PERCEPTIONS AND PREF-ERENCES FOR PSYCHOTHERAPISTS ARE CON-SIDERED. SUCH CLIENT FACTORS AS CLIENT ETHNICITY AND PREFERENCE MAY BE IMPOR-TANT TO THE SUCCESSFUL INITIATION AND PROCESS OF PSYCHOTHERAPY. 58 REFER-ENCES. (AUTHOR ABSTRACT MODIFIED)

ACCN   000004

6   AUTH   **ACOSTA, F. X.**

TITL   ETHNIC VARIABLES IN PSYCHOTHERAPY: THE MEXICAN AMERICAN.

SRCE   *IN J. L. MARTINEZ (ED.), CHICANO PSY-CHOLOGY. NEW YORK: ACADEMIC PRESS, 1977, PP. 215-232.*

INDX   RESOURCE UTILIZATION, MENTAL HEALTH, PSYCHOTHERAPY, DEMOGRAPHIC, CULTURAL FACTORS, ACCULTURATION, SES, POVERTY, SOCIAL MOBILITY, DISCRIMINATION, LINGUIS-TIC COMPETENCE, FAMILY STRUCTURE, FAMILY ROLES, SEX ROLES, ETHNIC IDENTITY, ATTI-TUDES, ROLE EXPECTATIONS, FOLK MEDICINE, CURANDERISMO, HEALTH DELIVERY SYSTEMS, BILINGUAL-BICULTURAL PERSONNEL, REVIEW, ESSAY

ABST   RECENT EMPIRICAL FINDINGS AND CLINICAL REPORTS INDICATE THAT MEXICAN AMERI-CANS HAVE A GREAT NEED FOR PSYCHOTH-ERAPEUTIC INTERVENTION AND THAT THEY EX-PRESS POSITIVE ATTITUDES TOWARD PSYCHOTHERAPISTS AND MENTAL HEALTH SERVICES. YET THEY REMAIN CONSISTENTLY UNDERREPRESENTED IN MENTAL HEALTH SER-VICES. MUCH REMAINS UNKNOWN IN THIS AREA, ESPECIALLY REGARDING THE INTERAC-TIVE EFFECTS ON THE SUCCESS OF PSY-CHOTHERAPY WITH MEXICAN AMERICANS BY SUCH VARIABLES AS GENERATION, AGE, SEX, LANGUAGE USAGE, TREATMENT ATTITUDES AND EXPECTATIONS, TREATMENT AP-PROACHES, AND THERAPIST ATTITUDES AND CHARACTERISTICS. THE DEGREE TO WHICH STEREOTYPES AND PREJUDICE MAY EXIST AMONG PSYCHOTHERAPISTS NEEDS FURTHER EXAMINATION. IMPROVED SERVICES AND TREATMENT OUTCOMES WILL COME FROM THE FOLLOWING: (1) CONTINUED CLINICAL RESEARCH; (2) DEVELOPMENT OF GREATER AWARENESS AND UNDERSTANDING OF THE CULTURAL AND ETHNIC CHARACTERISTICS OF THE MEXICAN AMERICAN; (3) COMMUNICA-TION OF MORE ACCURATE INFORMATION TO THERAPISTS, TRAINEES AND SUPERVISORS; (4) MORE SUPERVISED EXPERIENCE IN WORKING WITH MEXICAN AMERICAN PATIENTS; AND (5) INCREASED BILINGUAL/BICULTURAL STAFFING OF CLINICS AND PSYCHOLOGY DEPART-MENTS. 51 REFERENCES.

ACCN   000005

7   AUTH   **ACOSTA, F. X.**

TITL MEXICAN AMERICAN AND ANGLO AMERICAN REACTIONS TO ETHNICALLY SIMILAR AND DISSIMILAR PSYCHOTHERAPISTS.

SRCE *IN R. ALVAREZ (ED.), DELIVERY OF SERVICES FOR LATINO COMMUNITY MENTAL HEALTH (MONOGRAPH NO. 2). LOS ANGELES: UNIVERSITY OF CALIFORNIA, SPANISH SPEAKING MENTAL HEALTH RESEARCH CENTER, APRIL 1975, PP. 51-80.*

INDX PSYCHOTHERAPY, PSYCHOTHERAPISTS, ROLE EXPECTATIONS, EMPIRICAL, PSYCHOTHERAPY OUTCOME, MEXICAN AMERICAN, COLLEGE STUDENTS, CALIFORNIA, SOUTHWEST, CROSS CULTURAL

ABST ONE HUNDRED EIGHTY-SEVEN MEXICAN AMERICAN AND ANGLO COLLEGE STUDENTS WERE PRESENTED DIFFERENTIAL INTRODUCTIONS TO A TAPED THERAPIST WITH CONTRASTING SPEECH ACCENT. THE TWO MATCHED THERAPY TAPES PRESENTED A THERAPIST WORKING WITH A DEPRESSED, AND AT TIMES ANGRY YOUNG MAN. IN ONE TAPE THE THERAPIST SPOKE FLUENT ENGLISH WITH A STANDARD AMERICAN ACCENT, IN THE OTHER HE SPOKE FLUENT ENGLISH WITH A SLIGHT SPANISH ACCENT. THE THERAPIST WAS IDENTIFIED AS BEING ONE OF FOUR CATEGORIES: ANGLO AMERICAN PROFESSIONAL, ANGLO AMERICAN NONPROFESSIONAL, MEXICAN AMERICAN PROFESSIONAL, MEXICAN AMERICAN NONPROFESSIONAL. AFTER HEARING A TAPE, SUBJECTS WERE ASKED TO INDICATE ON A SELF-DISCLOSURE SCALE THEIR DEGREE OF WILLINGNESS TO TALK TO THE THERAPIST THEY HAD JUST HEARD AND INDICATE ON A RATING SCALE THEIR ATTITUDES TOWARD THE THERAPIST. ADDITIONAL DATA INCLUDED RATING ATTITUDES TOWARD PSYCHOTHERAPY AND TEST SCORES ON SELF-ESTEEM. THROUGH AN ANALYSIS OF VARIANCE, SIGNIFICANT DIFFERENCES IN THE DEGREE OF SELF-DISCLOSURE TO THERAPISTS OF DIFFERENT ETHNICITY AND PROFESSIONAL LEVEL WERE FOUND BETWEEN ANGLOS AND MEXICAN AMERICANS. THE FINDING THAT MEXICAN AMERICANS SHOWED LESS SELF-DISCLOSURE THAN ANGLO AMERICANS TO BOTH CHICANO AND ANGLO THERAPISTS WAS IN SUPPORT OF THE STUDY'S GENERAL HYPOTHESIS. SEVERAL RECOMMENDATIONS FOR FUTURE RESEARCH WITH THE MEXICAN AMERICAN IN THE AREA OF CLIENT-THERAPIST INTERACTIONS ARE MADE. 41 REFERENCES.

ACCN 000006

8 AUTH **ACOSTA, F. X.**

TITL PRETHERAPY EXPECTATIONS AND DEFINITIONS OF MENTAL ILLNESS AMONG MINORITY AND LOW-INCOME PATIENTS.

SRCE *HISPANIC JOURNAL OF BEHAVIORAL SCIENCES, 1979, 1(4), 403-410.*

INDX MENTAL HEALTH, MEXICAN AMERICAN, CROSS CULTURAL, EMPIRICAL, ATTITUDES, ADULTS, CALIFORNIA, SOUTHWEST, URBAN, PSYCHOTHERAPY, PSYCHOTHERAPISTS, ROLE EXPECTATIONS, RESOURCE UTILIZATION, SES, CULTURAL FACTORS

ABST TO FATHOM LOW-INCOME MEXICAN AMERI-

CANS' (MA) AND ANGLO AMERICANS' (AA) UNDERUTILIZATION OF MENTAL HEALTH SERVICES, 92 OUTPATIENTS (44 MA, 48 AA) AT AN EAST LOS ANGELES NEIGHBORHOOD MENTAL HEALTH CLINIC WERE INTERVIEWED. CONDUCTED PRIOR TO SUBJECTS' FIRST THERAPY SESSION, THE INTERVIEWS FOCUSED ON THE SUBJECTS' (1) EXPECTATIONS OF THERAPIST BEHAVIOR, (2) EXPECTED TIME IN THERAPY, AND (3) DEFINITIONS OF MENTAL ILLNESS. RESULTS SHOWED THAT NEARLY 50% OF BOTH MA AND AA SUBJECTS EXPECTED THE THERAPIST TO ENGAGE THEM IN ACTIVE DIALOGUE TO SOLVE THEIR PROBLEMS; ONLY SECONDARILY DID THEY EXPECT A PASSIVE, LISTENING THERAPIST. SECOND, BOTH MA'S AND AA'S ANTICIPATED HAVING ABOUT 20 THERAPY SESSIONS—MORE THAN FOUR TIMES THE AVERAGE NUMBER OF THERAPY SESSIONS FOR CLIENTS IN THE UNITED STATES. THIRD, MA'S AND AA'S WERE QUITE SIMILAR IN THEIR DEFINITIONS OF "EMOTIONAL PROBLEMS." HOWEVER, THERE WAS A SLIGHT INTER-ETHNIC DIFFERENCE IN THE DEFINITION OF "EMOTIONALLY DISTURBED," AND A MARKED DIFFERENCE IN THE DEFINITION OF "MENTAL ILLNESS." IT IS CONCLUDED THAT LOW-INCOME MA'S AND AA'S HOLD MANY SIMILAR AND SOPHISTICATED PERCEPTIONS OF PSYCHOTHERAPY; YET THERE ARE SOME IMPORTANT DIFFERENCES IN THEIR DEFINITIONS OF MENTAL DISORDERS—DIFFERENCES WHICH REQUIRE THERAPISTS TO BE MORE PRUDENT AND CULTURALLY SENSITIVE IN THEIR USE OF THE "MENTAL ILLNESS" LABEL. 17 REFERENCES.

ACCN 001757

9 AUTH **ACOSTA, F. X., & SHEEHAN, J. G.**

TITL PREFERENCE TOWARD MEXICAN AMERICAN AND ANGLO AMERICAN PSYCHOTHERAPISTS.

SRCE *JOURNAL OF CONSULTING AND CLINICAL PSYCHOLOGY, 1976, 44(2), 272-279.*

INDX MEXICAN AMERICAN, PSYCHOTHERAPY, PSYCHOTHERAPISTS, PARAPROFESSIONALS, ADULTS, EMPIRICAL, CROSS CULTURAL, MENTAL HEALTH, BILINGUAL-BICULTURAL PERSONNEL, CALIFORNIA, SOUTHWEST

ABST THERAPIST PREFERENCES AND ATTITUDES TOWARD PSYCHOTHERAPY WERE EXAMINED AMONG 94 MEXICAN AMERICAN AND 93 ANGLO COMMUNITY COLLEGE STUDENTS. EACH LISTENED TO ONE OF TWO MATCHED THERAPY AUDIOTAPES. USING THE SAME DIALOGUE, IN ONE TAPE THE THERAPIST SPOKE FLUENT ENGLISH WITH A SLIGHT SPANISH ACCENT, AND IN THE OTHER TAPE HE SPOKE FLUENT ENGLISH WITH A STANDARD AMERICAN ACCENT. THE THERAPIST WAS IDENTIFIED AS BEING IN ONE OF FOUR CATEGORIES: ANGLO PROFESSIONAL, ANGLO NONPROFESSIONAL, MEXICAN AMERICAN PROFESSIONAL, OR MEXICAN AMERICAN NONPROFESSIONAL. BOTH ETHNIC GROUPS ATTRIBUTED MORE SKILL, UNDERSTANDING, TRUSTWORTHINESS, AND ATTRACTIVENESS TO THE ANGLO PROFESSIONAL AND TO THE MEXICAN AMERICAN NONPROFESSIONAL. THE MEXICAN AMERICAN PROFESSIONAL WAS SEEN BY BOTH GROUPS LESS FA-

VORABLY THAN WAS THE MEXICAN AMERICAN NONPROFESSIONAL. MEXICAN AMERICANS SHOWED A MORE FAVORABLE ATTITUDE TOWARD THE USEFULNESS OF THERAPY THAN DID ANGLOS. IMPLICATIONS OF THE FINDINGS FOR THE FIELD OF PSYCHOTHERAPY AND FOR THE DELIVERY OF PSYCHOLOGICAL SERVICES TO MEXICAN AMERICANS AND OTHER MINORITIES ARE DISCUSSED. 14 REFERENCES. (JOURNAL ABSTRACT MODIFIED)

ACCN   000007

10   AUTH   **ACOSTA, F. X., & SHEEHAN, J. G.**
      TITL   PSYCHOTHERAPIST ETHNICITY AND EXPERTISE AS DETERMINANTS OF SELF-DISCLOSURE.
      SRCE   *IN M. R. MIRANDA (ED.), PSYCHOTHERAPY WITH THE SPANISH SPEAKING: ISSUES IN RESEARCH AND SERVICE DELIVERY (MONOGRAPH NO. 3). LOS ANGELES: UNIVERSITY OF CALIFORNIA, SPANISH SPEAKING MENTAL HEALTH RESEARCH CENTER, 1976, PP. 51-59.*
      INDX   PSYCHOTHERAPY, PSYCHOTHERAPISTS, ROLE EXPECTATIONS, EMPIRICAL, PSYCHOTHERAPY OUTCOME, MEXICAN AMERICAN, COLLEGE STUDENTS, CROSS CULTURAL, SEX COMPARISON, SES, CALIFORNIA, SOUTHWEST
      ABST   A COMPARISON OF SELF-DISCLOSURE TENDENCIES OF 94 MEXICAN AMERICAN AND 93 ANGLO JUNIOR COLLEGE STUDENTS WAS MADE USING A QUESTIONNAIRE DESIGNED TO MEASURE SELF-DISCLOSURE. THE QUESTIONNAIRE WAS ADMINISTERED FOLLOWING THE PLAYING OF TWO TAPES WHICH PRESENTED A THERAPIST WORKING WITH A CLIENT. IN ONE TAPE, THE THERAPIST SPOKE FLUENT ENGLISH WITH A SLIGHT SPANISH ACCENT; IN THE OTHER TAPE, HE SPOKE FLUENT ENGLISH WITH A STANDARD AMERICAN ACCENT. RESULTS INDICATE THAT MEXICAN AMERICANS DIFFER SIGNIFICANTLY FROM ANGLO AMERICANS IN THEIR OVERALL SELF-DISCLOSURE TENDENCY. WHILE BOTH ETHNIC GROUPS SHOWED SOME POSITIVE WILLINGNESS TO DISCLOSE TO A THERAPIST, MEXICAN AMERICANS SHOWED SIGNIFICANTLY LESS WILLINGNESS THAN DID ANGLO AMERICANS OF SIGNIFICANCE IS THAT WHILE MEXICAN AMERICANS ARE SELF-DISCLOSING, UTILIZATION OF MENTAL HEALTH SERVICES BY MEXICAN AMERICANS IS LIMITED. 8 REFERENCES.

      ACCN   000008

11   AUTH   **ACOSTA, R. T.**
      TITL   FACTORS CONTRIBUTING TO THE SUCCESSFUL REMEDIATION OF READING DISABILITIES IN MEXICAN-AMERICAN THIRD GRADERS (DOCTORAL DISSERTATION, UNIVERSITY OF CALIFORNIA, LOS ANGELES, 1971).
      SRCE   *DISSERTATION ABSTRACTS INTERNATIONAL, 1972, 32(7), 3658A. (UNIVERSITY MICROFILMS NO.72-02,767.)*
      INDX   MEXICAN AMERICAN, ACCULTURATION, SCHOLASTIC ACHIEVEMENT, SPECIAL EDUCATION, CHILDREN, EMPIRICAL, READING, SES, TEACHERS, STANFORD ACHIEVEMENT TEST, PARENTAL INVOLVEMENT, CALIFORNIA, SOUTHWEST
      ABST   TO IDENTIFY FACTORS THAT APPEAR TO BE

CONTRIBUTING TO SUCCESSFUL REMEDIATION OF READING DISABILITIES IN MEXICAN AMERICAN CHILDREN IN MILLER-UNRUH READING PROGRAMS, TWO GROUPS OF 30 THIRD-GRADE STUDENTS FROM THE TWO CALIFORNIA SCHOOL DISTRICTS MAKING THE HIGHEST AND LOWEST MEAN AND MEDIAN GAINS ON THE STANFORD ACHIEVEMENT READING TEST (SART) WERE EXAMINED. THE FOLLOWING HYPOTHESES WERE TESTED: (1) THE SUCCESS OF MEXICAN AMERICAN CHILDREN ON THE SART IS POSITIVELY CORRELATED WITH THEIR PARENTS' DEGREE OF ACCULTURATION, INCOME LEVEL, EDUCATIONAL ATTAINMENT, AND EDUCATIONAL AND OCCUPATIONAL ASPIRATIONS FOR THEIR CHILD; AND (2) THE TEACHERS OF SUCCESSFULLY REMEDIATED MEXICAN AMERICAN CHILDREN PROVIDE RICHER METHODS AND MATERIALS FOR READING INSTRUCTION AND HAVE A HIGHER DEGREE OF PREPARATION AND EXPERIENCE IN TEACHING MEXICAN AMERICAN CHILDREN THAN TEACHERS OF STUDENTS WHO MADE LOWER SART GAIN SCORES. RESULTS INDICATE THAT (1) PARENTS INCOME AND ASPIRATIONS FOR CHILD ARE SIGNIFICANTLY CORRELATED WITH THEIR CHILDREN'S SART GAIN SCORES, AND (2) THAT ALL FIVE HOME ENVIRONMENTAL VARIABLES ARE HIGHLY INTERCORRELATED. DIFFERENCES BETWEEN READING METHODS USED IN THE TWO SCHOOLS, ONE WITH HIGH GAINS AND THE OTHER WITH LOW GAINS, WERE NOT SIGNIFICANT. HOWEVER, IN THE SCHOOL WITH HIGH GAINS, THE TEACHERS USED THE DIAGNOSTIC AND PRESCRIPTIVE APPROACH TO TEACHING READING MORE FREQUENTLY AND WERE FOUND TO HAVE A HIGHER DEGREE OF PREPARATION AND MORE YEARS OF EXPERIENCE TEACHING CHILDREN OF MEXICAN DESCENT. CONCLUSIONS REGARDING THE INAPPROPRIATENESS OF THE SART FOR MEXICAN AMERICAN CHILDREN AND THE IMPLICATIONS FOR TEACHERS ARE DISCUSSED. 100 REFERENCES. (AUTHOR SUMMARY MODIFIED)

ACCN   000009

12   AUTH   **ADAMS, R. L., KOBOS, J. C., & PRESTON J.**
      TITL   EFFECT OF RACIAL ETHNIC GROUPING, AGE AND IQ RANGE ON THE VALIDITY OF THE SATZ-MOGEL SHORT FORM OF THE WECHSLER ADULT INTELLIGENCE SCALE.
      SRCE   *JOURNAL OF CONSULTING AND CLINICAL PSYCHOLOGY, 1977, 45(3), 498-499.*
      INDX   WAIS, TEST VALIDITY, INTELLIGENCE TESTING, MEXICAN AMERICAN, EMPIRICAL, TEXAS, CROSS CULTURAL, ADULTS, SOUTHWEST
      ABST   TO CROSS-VALIDATE THE EFFECTIVENESS OF THE SATZ-MOGEL SHORT FORM OF THE WECHSLER ADULT INTELLIGENCE SCALE (WAIS), 342 BLACK, MEXICAN AMERICAN, AND WHITE TEXAS HOSPITAL PATIENTS WERE TESTED ON THE ENTIRE WAIS. DATA ANALYSIS CONTROLLED FOR THE INFLUENCE OF AGE, RACIAL/ETHNIC GROUP, AND IQ RANGE, AND THE RECORDS WERE RECORDED USING THE SATZ-MOGEL PROCEDURE. RESULTS SUGGEST THAT THE SHORT FORM IS EQUALLY VALID FOR ES-

TIMATING COMPLETE WAIS IQ'S FOR ALL ETH-
NIC AND AGE GROUPS, BUT NOT ALL IQ
RANGES. IN THE 110-129 PERFORMANCE IQ
RANGE THE CORRECTED PART-WHOLE COR-
RELATION WAS ONLY .37, COMPARED TO A
CORRELATION OF .61 FOR THE 90-109 RANGE
AND .67 FOR THE 70-89 RANGE. THIS PROBLEM
CAN BE ELIMINATED, HOWEVER, BY ADMINIS-
TERING THE REMAINING COMPLETE WAIS ITEMS
IN THOSE CASES. 5 REFERENCES. (AUTHOR
ABSTRACT MODIFIED)

ACCN   002002

13   AUTH   **ADKINS, D. D., PAYNE, F. D., & BALLIF, B. L.**
     TITL   MOTIVATION FACTOR SCORES AND RESPONSE
SET SCORES FOR TEN ETHNIC-CULTURAL
GROUPS OF PRESCHOOL CHILDREN.
     SRCE   *AMERICAN EDUCATIONAL RESEARCH JOUR-
NAL, 1972, 9(4), 557-572.*
     INDX   CROSS CULTURAL, CHILDREN, MEXICAN
AMERICAN, PUERTO RICAN-M, ACHIEVEMENT
TESTING, ACHIEVEMENT MOTIVATION, EMPIRI-
CAL, SELF CONCEPT, SES, RESEARCH METH-
ODOLOGY, SEX COMPARISON, EAST, WEST,
SOUTHWEST, SCHOLASTIC ACHIEVEMENT
     ABST   A TOTAL OF 1,588 HEADSTART CHILDREN IN
SEVEN STATES ACROSS THE COUNTRY WERE
ADMINISTERED AN OBJECTIVE-PROJECTIVE
TEST DEVISED BY THE AUTHORS TO MEASURE
ACHIEVEMENT MOTIVATION IN PRESCHOOL-
ERS. THE CHILDREN COMPRISED 2 SES AND 10
ETHNIC-CULTURAL GROUPS—(1) MIDDLE-
CLASS: MORMON, JEWISH, CATHOLIC; AND (2)
LOWER-CLASS: PUERTO RICAN, NEGRO-UR-
BAN, WHITE-RURAL, HAWAIIAN, ORIENTAL (WEST
COAST), MEXICAN AMERICAN, AND AMERICAN
INDIAN. THE TEST CENTERS AROUND THE AC-
TIVITIES OF IMAGINARY FIGURES, "GUMP-
GOOKIES," DEPICTED VERBALLY AND THROUGH
ILLUSTRATIONS AS BEHAVING IN WAYS IN-
TENDED TO SHOW MOTIVATIONAL DIFFER-
ENCES IN INSTRUMENTAL ACTIVITIES, SCHOOL
ACTIVITIES, AND SELF-EVALUATION. WHEN
CORRELATED WITH ETHNIC-CULTURAL AND
SEX DIFFERENCES, ONLY THE ETHNIC-CUL-
TURAL GROUP VARIABLE WAS SIGNIFICANT IN
ALL THREE ACHIEVEMENT MOTIVATION RE-
SPONSES. THE THREE MIDDLE-CLASS SAMPLES
HAD HIGHER MEAN SCORES THAN THE OTHER
GROUPS. AMONG THE LOWER-CLASS SAMPLES,
THE NEGRO-URBAN, WHITE-RURAL, AND
PUERTO RICAN CHILDREN EMERGED WITH
SUBSTANTIALLY HIGHER ACHIEVEMENT MOTI-
VATION SCORES THAN THE MEXICAN AMERI-
CAN, ORIENTAL, AMERICAN INDIAN, AND HA-
WAIIAN SAMPLES. FURTHERMORE, A
SIGNIFICANT BUT WEAK TENDENCY FOR GIRLS
TO EXHIBIT HIGHER SCORES THAN BOYS ON
SCHOOL ENJOYMENT EMERGED. A CONCLUD-
ING COMMENT IS THAT TEST RELIABILITY DATA
MAKE IT CLEAR THAT PERSONS WHO ARE DE-
VELOPING COGNITIVE OR AFFECTIVE TESTS
FOR CHILDREN CANNOT IGNORE THE EFFECT
OF RESPONSE SETS ON FACTOR SCORES. 17
REFERENCES.
     ACCN   000010

14   AUTH   **ADKINS, P., & YOUNG, R. G.**
     TITL   CULTURAL PERCEPTIONS IN THE TREATMENT
OF HANDICAPPED SCHOOL CHILDREN OF
MEXICAN-AMERICAN PARENTAGE.
     SRCE   *JOURNAL OF RESEARCH AND DEVELOPMENT
IN EDUCATION, 1976, 9(4), 83-90.*
     INDX   SEX ROLES, DISCRIMINATION, HEALTH, ATTI-
TUDES, MENTAL HEALTH, FAMILY THERAPY,
CHILDREARING PRACTICES, CHILDREN, CUL-
TURE, EARLY CHILDHOOD EDUCATION, ESSAY,
FAMILY ROLES, FAMILY STRUCTURE, MENTAL
RETARDATION, MEXICAN AMERICAN, MOTHER-
CHILD INTERACTION, SPECIAL EDUCATION,
TEXAS, SOUTHWEST, RELIGION, IMPAIRMENT,
RESOURCE UTILIZATION, POLICY, PROGRAM
EVALUATION, HEALTH DELIVERY SYSTEMS,
CULTURAL FACTORS
     ABST   THE EARLY LEARNING CENTER FOR THE
HANDICAPPED IN EL PASO, TEXAS, HAS EN-
COUNTERED SPEECH, LANGUAGE, RELI-
GIOUS, FAMILIAL, AND CULTURAL DIFFER-
ENCES AMONG THE MEXICAN AMERICAN
POPULATION WHICH REQUIRE SPECIAL CON-
SIDERATION FOR EFFECTIVE PARENT TRAINING
AND PARTICIPATION. CASE HISTORIES WERE
REVIEWED, REVEALING THE RELATIONSHIP OF
ATTITUDES TOWARD FAMILY AND HEALTH
WHICH AFFECT THE DELIVERY OF SERVICES
TO HANDICAPPED MEXICAN AMERICAN CHIL-
DREN. AMONG THE CHARACTERISTICS NOTED
TO INTERFERE WITH MEDICAL CARE AND EDU-
CATION ARE: (1) A STRONG SENSE OF FAMILY
PRIDE (I.E., THE HANDICAPPED CHILD MAY BE
SHELTERED AND HIDDEN FROM PUBLIC SCRU-
TINY); (2) RELIGIOUS BELIEFS (I.E., CARE MAY
BE DENIED IF NOT SANCTIONED BY THE PRIEST);
(3) THE MACHISMO MODEL (I.E., DISRUPTIVE
HYPERACTIVE BEHAVIOR EXHIBITED BY A MALE
CHILD MAY BE INTERPRETED BY THE MEXICAN
AMERICAN FATHER AS NORMAL); (4) FAMILY
VALUES ENCOURAGING CHILDHOOD PASSIV-
ITY (I.E., THE PATHOLOGICALLY WITHDRAWN
CHILD MAY BE UNRECOGNIZED); AND (5) SU-
PERSTITION AND LACK OF KNOWLEDGE ABOUT
MEDICAL TECHNOLOGY (I.E., NEEDED DIAG-
NOSTIC PROCEDURES MAY BE MISUNDER-
STOOD AND REJECTED). MEXICAN AMERICAN
PARENTS, OFTEN DISCRIMINATED AGAINST BY
STEREOTYPING, HUMILIATION, OR MISUNDER-
STANDING, ARE SENSITIVE AND HIGHLY EMO-
TIONAL WITH REGARD TO THEIR HANDI-
CAPPED CHILD. STAFF MUST BE VERY
SUPPORTIVE AND REINFORCING TO COMBAT
POTENTIAL NEGATIVISM FROM THE EXTENDED
FAMILY AND FRIENDS. IT IS CONCLUDED THAT
USING SPANISH-SPEAKING PARENTS AS OR-
IENTERS FOR NEW FAMILIES, A HOME-CEN-
TERED APPROACH, PARENT DISCUSSION
GROUPS, AND STAFF TRAINED IN THE AREAS
OF SOCIOLOGY, PSYCHOLOGY, AND ANTHRO-
POLOGY WILL FURTHER THE EFFECTIVE SER-
VICING OF THE MEXICAN AMERICAN POPULA-
TION. 9 REFERENCES.
     ACCN   002003

15   AUTH   **ADORNO, W.**
     TITL   THE ATTITUDES OF SELECTED MEXICAN AND
MEXICAN-AMERICAN PARENTS IN REGARDS TO
BILINGUAL/BICULTURAL EDUCATION (DOC-

48

TORAL DISSERTATION, UNITED STATES INTER-
NATIONAL UNIVERSITY, 1973).

SRCE   *DISSERTATION ABSTRACTS INTERNATIONAL,
1973, 34(4), 1574A. (UNIVERSITY MICROFILMS
NO.73-22,653.)*

INDX   ADULTS, MEXICAN AMERICAN, ATTITUDES, BI-
LINGUAL-BICULTURAL EDUCATION, CALIFOR-
NIA, SOUTHWEST

ABST   THE EFFECTIVENESS OF BILINGUAL/BICUL-
TURAL PROGRAMS IN MEETING THE NEEDS OF
NON-ENGLISH-SPEAKING STUDENTS DE-
PENDS UPON EDUCATORS' BEING INFORMED
ABOUT THE ATTTIUDES OF STUDENTS' PAR-
ENTS REGARDING THEIR PROGRAMS. THE
FINDINGS RESULTING FROM INTERVIEWING 75
MEXICAN AMERICAN PARENTS WHOSE CHIL-
DREN ARE ENROLLED IN THREE DIFFERENT
CALIFORNIA METROPOLITAN PRE-SCHOOLS OR
ELEMENTARY SCHOOLS THAT HAVE A BILIN-
GUAL/BICULTURAL PROGRAM INDICATED THAT:
(1) PARENTS FELT THAT KNOWLEDGE OF TWO
LANGUAGES IS VALUED IN OUR SOCIETY AND
ALSO WOULD GIVE THEIR CHILDREN GREATER
UPWARD MOBILITY; (2) PARENTS WANTED THEIR
CHILDREN TO LEARN ABOUT THE CULTURE OF
MEXICO; (3) IT DID NOT APPEAR THAT THE PAR-
ENTS WERE AWARE OF THE PROBLEM OF
NEGATIVE SELF-IMAGE ; AND (4) SOME SOCIO-
CULTURAL AND DEMOGRAPHIC VARIABLES DO
INFLUENCE PARENTS' ATTITUDES CONCERN-
ING BILINGUAL/BICULTURAL EDUCATION. 54
REFERENCES.

ACCN   000011

16   AUTH   **AGUILAR, I.**
TITL   INITIAL CONTACTS WITH MEXICAN-AMERICAN
FAMILIES.
SRCE   *SOCIAL WORK, 1972, 17(3), 66-70.*
INDX   MEXICAN AMERICAN, CULTURAL FACTORS, EX-
TENDED FAMILY, PREJUDICE, MENTAL HEALTH,
PSYCHOTHERAPY, CASE STUDY, CALIFORNIA,
SOUTHWEST
ABST   SOCIAL WORKERS IN THEIR INITIAL CONTACT
WITH MEXICAN AMERICANS MUST CONSIDER
THE CULTURAL VALUES, BEHAVIOR PATTERNS,
AND THE BARRIERS TO ASSIMILATION EXPERI-
ENCED BY THIS GROUP. IN ORDER FOR SOCIAL
WORKERS TO INITIATE AND MAINTAIN COOP-
ERATION WITH MEXICAN AMERICAN CLIENTS,
DIFFERENT CULTURAL AND SOCIAL EXPECTA-
TIONS SHOULD BE ACCOUNTED FOR. A CASE
EXAMPLE OF A MEXICAN AMERICAN FAMILY IL-
LUSTRATES HOW ADAPTATION BY THE SOCIAL
WORKER IN THE INITIAL CONTACTS ENCOUR-
AGES EFFECTIVE COUNSELING AND AN
AGENCY-CLIENT PARTNERSHIP. PREPARING
SOCIAL WORKERS TO SERVE SUCH FAMILIES
DURING THEIR TRAINING IS RECOMMENDED.
(JOURNAL ABSTRACT MODIFIED)
ACCN   000012

17   AUTH   **AGUILAR, I.**
TITL   PSYCHONOVELA: FACT OR FICTION.
SRCE   *PRESENTED AT THE FIRST SYMPOSIUM ON CHI-
CANO PSYCHOLOGY, UNIVERSITY OF CALIFOR-
NIA, IRVINE, MAY 16, 1976.*
INDX   PSYCHOTHERAPY, CULTURAL FACTORS, CASE

STUDY, SPANISH SURNAMED, MEXICAN AMERI-
CAN, ADULTS, CALIFORNIA, SOUTHWEST
ABST   THE USE OF PSYCHODRAMA, MODIFIED TO IN-
CLUDE CULTURAL CUES AND EXPERIENCES
FAMILIAR TO SPANISH-SPEAKING PERSONS, IS
PROPOSED. APPLICATION OF THIS TECHNIQUE
AT THE CLINICA DE SALUD MENTAL XIPE-TO-
TEC AT METROPOLITAN STATE HOSPITAL IN
NORWALK, CALIFORNIA, IS VIVIDLY DESCRIBED
IN A CASE EXAMPLE OF A PSYCHOTIC MIDDLE-
AGED MEXICAN WOMAN. LABELED 'PSYCHON-
OVELA' BECAUSE IT IS PATERNED AFTER
SPANISH LANGUAGE TELEVISION SOAP OP-
ERAS CALLED TELENOVELA, THE TECHNIQUE
DESCRIBED IN THIS CASE STUDY INCLUDED:
(1) SETTING THE MOOD FOR THE DRAMA; (2)
DESCRIBING THE INCIDENT TO BE ACTED OUT
BY THE PATIENTS; (3) CHOOSING PATIENTS TO
ACT AND CORRECTING PATIENTS' PERCEP-
TIONS AND MISINTERPRETATIONS; AND (4) RE-
VIEWING GROUP AND INDIVIDUAL REACTIONS
TO THE PSYCHONOVELA SESSIONS.
ACCN   000013

18   AUTH   **AGUILAR, I., & WOOD, V. N.**
TITL   ASPECTS OF DEATH, GRIEF AND MOURNING IN
THE TREATMENT OF SPANISH-SPEAKING MEN-
TAL PATIENTS.
SRCE   *JOURNAL OF THE NATIONAL ASSOCIATION OF
SOCIAL WORKERS, 1976, 21, 49-54.*
INDX   MENTAL HEALTH, CULTURAL FACTORS, MEXI-
CAN AMERICAN, ESSAY, DEATH, CULTURE
ABST   THE MEXICAN'S PERVASIVE RESPECT FOR
DEATH, THE SIGNIFICANCE OF BURIAL, AND
THE SYMBOLISM SURROUNDING THESE EVENTS
HAVE BEEN USED TO DEVELOP A RITUAL-
DRAMA (AT THE XIPE-TOTEC CLINICA DE SALUD
MENTAL, METROPOLITAN STATE HOSPITAL,
NORWALK, CALIFORNIA) TO FACILITATE CA-
THARSIS IN SPANISH-SPEAKING MENTAL PA-
TIENTS. THE EFFECTIVENESS OF AMBIENCE
AND GROUP COOPERATION IN THE MOURNING
RITUAL IS EMPHASIZED. (AUTHOR ABSTRACT
MODIFIED)
ACCN   000014

19   AUTH   **AGUILAR, I., & WOOD, V. N.**
TITL   THERAPY THROUGH A DEATH RITUAL.
SRCE   *SOCIAL WORK, 1976, 21(1), 49-54.*
INDX   CULTURAL FACTORS, DEATH, ESSAY, FOLK
MEDICINE, INSTITUTIONALIZATION, MENTAL
HEALTH, MEXICAN AMERICAN, PSYCHOSOCIAL
ADJUSTMENT, PSYCHOTHERAPY OUTCOME,
CALIFORNIA, SOUTHWEST, THERAPEUTIC
COMMUNITY
ABST   A PROGRAM FOR SPANISH-SPEAKING PA-
TIENTS IN A CALIFORNIA STATE MENTAL HOS-
PITAL IS DESCRIBED, WHICH PLACES SPANISH-
SPEAKING PATIENTS IN A FAMILIAR CULTURAL
SETTING. THE AIM IS TO RELAX PATIENTS AND
REMOVE ADDITIONAL STRESS CAUSED
THROUGH CONFLICT WITH ANGLO AMERICAN
CULTURE. WHEN THERE IS REASON TO SUS-
PECT THAT PATIENTS HAVE UNRESOLVED FEEL-
INGS ABOUT THE DEATH OF SOMEONE CLOSE
WHICH MAY HAVE PRECIPITATED THEIR CON-
DITION, PARTICIPATION IN A RITUAL FUNERAL
DRAMA FREQUENTLY HAS A CURATIVE EFFECT.

THE RITUAL DRAMA, EMBODYING MEXICAN CUSTOMS RELATED TO DEATH AND MOURNING, STRIVES TO PRODUCE EMOTIONAL CATHARSIS FOR THE INDIVIDUAL AS WELL AS A COLLECTIVE RESPONSE AND THE DEVELOPMENT OF GROUP COHESIVENESS. 11 REFERENCES. (NCMHI ABSTRACT)

ACCN   002325

20 AUTH   **AGUIRRE, R. W.**
    TITL   THE EFFECTS OF A PARENTAL INVOLVEMENT PROGRAM ON SELF CONCEPTS AND SCHOOL ATTITUDES OF MEXICAN-AMERICAN FIRST GRADE CHILDREN (DOCTORAL DISSERTATION, UNIVERSITY OF HOUSTON, 1972).
    SRCE   *DISSERTATION ABSTRACTS INTERNATIONAL, 1973, 34(3), 1056A. (UNIVERSITY MICROFILMS NO.73-06,366.)*
    INDX   PARENTAL INVOLVEMENT, ATTITUDES, EDUCATION, SELF CONCEPT, CHILDREN, EMPIRICAL, SCHOLASTIC ACHIEVEMENT, MEXICAN AMERICAN, TEXAS, SOUTHWEST
    ABST   THE PURPOSE OF THIS STUDY WAS TO DETERMINE THE EFFECTS OF A STRUCTURED PARENTAL INVOLVEMENT PROGRAM ON THE SELF CONCEPT AND SCHOOL ATTITUDE OF FIRST-GRADE MEXICAN AMERICAN CHILDREN. AN EXPERIMENTAL AND A CONTROL GROUP OF CHILDREN WERE ADMINISTERED TWO TEST INSTRUMENTS (SCHOOL SENTIMENT INDEX AND SELF APPRAISAL INDEX) BEFORE AND AFTER THE EXPERIMENTAL GROUP PARENTS ATTENDED TRAINING SESSIONS. THE TESTS WERE GIVEN ORALLY IN ENGLISH AND SPANISH. FINDINGS SHOWED NO EFFECTS OF PARENTAL INVOLVEMENT ON CHILDREN'S ATTITUDES AND SELF CONCEPT. OBSERVATIONS OF ATTENDING PARENTS, HOWEVER, INDICATED THAT PARENTAL ATTITUDES ARE MORE LIKELY TO CHANGE THAN THOSE OF CHILDREN, AND THAT THIS MAY BE A MORE CRITICAL FACTOR THAN PARENTS BEING PHYSICALLY INVOLVED IN THE SCHOOL. 41 REFERENCES. (AUTHOR ABSTRACT MODIFIED)
    ACCN   000015

21 AUTH   **AIELLO, J. R., & JONES, S. E.**
    TITL   FIELD STUDY OF THE PROXEMIC BEHAVIOR OF YOUNG SCHOOL CHILDREN IN THREE SUBCULTURAL GROUPS.
    SRCE   *JOURNAL OF PERSONALITY AND SOCIAL PSYCHOLOGY, 1971, 19(3), 351-356.*
    INDX   PUERTO RICAN-M, CHILDREN, INTERPERSONAL SPACING, SEX COMPARISON, SEX ROLES, EMPIRICAL, DYADIC INTERACTION, CROSS CULTURAL, SES, INTERPERSONAL RELATIONS, NEW YORK, EAST
    ABST   THE PROXEMIC RELATIONSHIPS OF INTERACTING PAIRS OF FIRST- AND SECOND-GRADE CHILDREN FROM THREE SUBCULTURAL GROUPS WERE OBSERVED IN SCHOOL PLAYGROUNDS. INTERACTION DISTANCE AND DIRECTIONS OF SHOULDER ORIENTATION (AXIS) WERE RECORDED. MIDDLE-CLASS WHITE CHILDREN STOOD FARTHER APART THAN LOWER-CLASS BLACK AND PUERTO RICAN CHILDREN. SEX DIFFERENCES AMONG WHITE CHILDREN IN DISTANCE SCORES AND CUL-

TURE AND SEX DIFFERENCES IN AXIS SCORES WERE ALSO FOUND. THE RESULTS SUGGEST THAT PROXEMIC PATTERNS ARE ACQUIRED EARLY IN LIFE AND SUPPORT THE CONTENTION THAT DIFFERENCES BETWEEN THE DOMINANT CULTURE AND OTHER GROUPS IN THE USE OF SPACE ARE BASIC, WITH THE QUALIFICATION THAT SEX ROLES ALSO INFLUENCE PROXEMIC BEHAVIOR. 8 REFERENCES.

ACCN   000016

22 AUTH   **AIKEN, T. W., STUMPHAUZER, J. S., & VELOZ, E. V.**
    TITL   BEHAVIORAL ANALYSIS OF NON-DELINQUENT BROTHERS IN A HIGH JUVENILE CRIME COMMUNITY.
    SRCE   *BEHAVIORAL DISORDERS, 1977, 2, 212-222.*
    INDX   EMPIRICAL, CASE STUDY, COMMUNITY, GANGS, ROLE EXPECTATIONS, SES, MALE, ADOLESCENTS, CALIFORNIA, SOUTHWEST, MEXICAN AMERICAN, RESEARCH METHODOLOGY, ATTITUDES, MODELING, ENVIRONMENTAL FACTORS
    ABST   TO EXAMINE THE BEHAVIOR OF YOUTHS WHO STAY OUT OF TROUBLE IN A HIGH GANG DENSITY AREA, TWO BROTHERS WERE INTERVIEWED. CAESAR, 23, AND RICHARD, 14, BOTH INTERACT SUCCESSFULLY WITH LOCAL GANG MEMBERS, YET THEY OPENLY DISAVOW ANY PARTICIPATION IN DELINQUENT BEHAVIOR. A BEHAVIOR ANALYSIS OF THE BROTHERS WAS CONDUCTED IN THEIR BARRIO, CONSISTING OF (1) A STRUCTURED BUT OPEN-ENDED INTERVIEW AND OBSERVATION TECHNIQUE PLUS (2) A REINFORCEMENT SURVEY CENTERING ON THE PEOPLE, PLACES, ACTIVITIES, AND SOCIAL SITUATIONS THAT THESE INDIVIDUALS FIND MOST AND LEAST REWARDING. THESE ANALYSES REVEALED AN EXTENSIVE SERIES OF TROUBLE-AVOIDING AND POSITIVELY REINFORCING BEHAVIORS IN THE TWO SUBJECTS. IN PARTICULAR, EMPHASIS WAS PLACED BY BOTH BROTHERS ON AN EX-OFFENDER, MALE ADULT WHO WAS A BARRIO COUNSELOR AND A POWERFUL ROLE MODEL. SECONDLY, THE BROTHERS HAD POSITIVE ATTITUDES ABOUT THE COMMUNITY, SCHOOLS, AND TEACHERS, AND BOTH EXPRESSED A DESIRE TO REMAIN IN THE COMMUNITY SO THEY CAN CONTRIBUTE POSITIVELY TO IT. THESE NON-DELINQUENT ATTITUDES AND BEHAVIORS WERE OBSERVED TO BE MAINTAINED BY SUCCESSFUL EXPERIENCES AND A GOOD DEAL OF SOCIAL AND SELF-REINFORCEMENT. RESULTS SUGGEST THAT NON-DELINQUENT, ADAPTIVE BEHAVIOR IS BEING TAUGHT AND LEARNED IN THIS HIGH JUVENILE CRIME AREA, AND THAT NATURAL MEDIATORS SUCH AS THESE TWO BROTHERS COULD GO ON TO TEACH THIS BEHAVIOR TO OTHER YOUNG PEOPLE IN A COMMUNITY-BASED DELINQUENCY PREVENTION PROGRAM. 20 REFERENCES.
    ACCN   002004

23 AUTH   **AILINGER, R. L.**
    TITL   A STUDY OF ILLNESS REFERRAL IN A SPANISH-SPEAKING COMMUNITY.

SRCE   *NURSING RESEARCH, 1977, 26(1), 53-56.*

INDX   ATTITUDES, ACCULTURATION, ADULTS, CULTURAL FACTORS, DISEASE, ECONOMIC FACTORS, EMPIRICAL, ESPIRITISMO, EXTENDED FAMILY, FICTIVE KINSHIP, HEALTH, HEALTH DELIVERY SYSTEMS, FEMALE, MEXICAN AMERICAN, NURSING, RESOURCE UTILIZATION, SES, SOCIAL SERVICES, SPANISH SURNAMED, URBAN, EAST

ABST   LATIN AMERICAN IMMIGRANT FAMILIES LIVING IN A COOPERATIVE IN A SUBURB OF AN EASTERN METROPOLIS WERE STUDIED OVER A 14-MONTH PERIOD. BY MEANS OF PARTICIPANT OBSERVATION, A FAMILY HEALTH CALENDAR, AND INTERVIEWS, THREE PHASES OF ILLNESS REFERRAL WERE ASCERTAINED: (1) THERE WAS EXTENDED USE OF SELF-TREATMENT; (2) REFERRALS WERE MADE TO THE SOCIAL NETWORK, PARTICULARLY TO PEOPLE FROM THE SAME COUNTRY OF ORIGIN; AND (3) REFERRALS TO THE PROFESSIONAL NETWORK WERE MADE TO PROFESSIONALS WITH THE SAME CULTURAL HERITAGE. A CLOSE LOOK AT THE FAMILY HEALTH CALENDAR REVEALED THAT MOST ILLNESSES REPORTED BY FAMILIES DID NOT GO BEYOND SELF-TREATMENT. IN CONCLUSION, SUCH CULTURAL INFLUENCES AS LANGUAGE, SOCIAL NETWORKS, AND PRIORITIES OF DAILY LIVING ARE DISCUSSED IN TERMS OF THE SPECIFIC ALTERNATIVES SELECTED BY FAMILIES WHEN ACTUAL ILLNESS INCIDENTS OCCUR. 13 REFERENCES. (AUTHOR ABSTRACT MODIFIED)

ACCN   002399

24   AUTH   **ALBA, R. D.**

TITL   ETHNIC NETWORKS AND TOLERANT ATTITUDES.

SRCE   *PUBLIC OPINION QUARTERLY, 1978, 42(1), 1-16.*

INDX   ATTITUDES, AUTHORITARIANISM, ETHNIC IDENTITY, IMMIGRATION, CHILDREARING PRACTICES, REVIEW, DEMOGRAPHIC, CROSS CULTURAL, ACCULTURATION, INTERMARRIAGE, SPANISH SURNAMED, PUERTO RICAN-M, CULTURAL CHANGE, RESEARCH METHODOLOGY, ADULTS, CULTURAL FACTORS, EMPIRICAL, RELIGION, ACCULTURATION

ABST   THE EMPIRICAL ASSOCIATION BETWEEN ATTITUDES OF AUTHORITARIANISM AND THE ETHNIC HOMOGENEITY OF AN INDIVIDUAL'S NETWORK OF PRIMARY RELATIONS WAS EXAMINED UTILIZING DATA FROM GREELEY AND ROSSI'S 1966 CATHOLIC AMERICANS STUDY. THE SAMPLE CONSISTED OF 2,071 CATHOLIC AMERICANS OF 10 ETHNIC BACKGROUNDS. PUERTO RICANS AND OTHER SPANISH SURNAME PERSONS WERE INCLUDED IN A GROUP LABELED HISPANIC. IT IS ARGUED THAT THE ATTITUDINAL DIFFERENCES BETWEEN THOSE IN HOMOGENEOUS AND HETEROGENEOUS FAMILY NETWORKS REFLECT A PROCESS OF ACCULTURATION PARALLELING SOCIAL ASSIMILATION. ACCORDING TO FINDINGS PRESENTED IN FOUR TABLES, DESCENDANTS OF EARLIER GROUPS OF IMMIGRANTS FROM NORTHERN AND WESTERN EUROPE ARE GENERALLY MORE TOLERANT AND LESS AUTHORITARIAN THAN MEMBERS OF MORE RECENTLY

IMMIGRATED ETHNIC GROUPS. SIMILARLY, THE DIFFERENCE BETWEEN ETHNIC GROUPS EXPRESSING INTOLERANT ATTITUDES AND THOSE WITH MORE TOLERANT VIEWPOINTS DECREASED AS SOCIAL ASSIMILATION INCREASED. FINALLY, A DECLINE IN ETHNIC DIFFERENTIATION AND AN INCREASE IN DIFFERENTIATION BASED ON OTHER CHARACTERISTICS (SUCH AS EDUCATION, AGE, AND SEX) ACCOMPANIED SOCIAL ASSIMILATION. SINCE EXTENSIVE OR INCREASING ASSIMILATION WAS FOUND AMONG ALL GROUPS, IT IS SUSPECTED THAT EXTENSIVE CULTURAL CHANGES ARE OCCURRING AS WELL. PREVIOUS RESEARCH ON ETHNIC PERSISTENCE HAS UTILIZED SOCIOCULTURALLY HETEROGENEOUS ETHNIC CATEGORIES, THUS OBSCURING CULTURAL CHANGE. THIS STUDY RAISES BOTH IMPORTANT ISSUES IN THE ASSESSMENT OF ETHNICITY AS WELL AS SERIOUS DOUBTS REGARDING CLAIMS OF PERSISTING ETHNIC DIVERSITY IN THE UNITED STATES. 19 REFERENCES.

ACCN   002005

25   AUTH   **ALBA, R. D.**

TITL   SOCIAL ASSIMILIATION AMONG AMERICAN CATHOLIC NATIONAL-ORIGIN GROUPS.

SRCE   *AMERICAN SOCIOLOGICAL REVIEW, 1976, 41(6), 1030-1046.*

INDX   ACCULTURATION, INTERPERSONAL ATTRACTION, INTERPERSONAL RELATIONS, SPANISH SURNAMED, INTERMARRIAGE, DISCRIMINATION, INTEGRATION, CULTURAL PLURALISM, ETHNIC IDENTITY, ESSAY, REVIEW, RELIGION

ABST   THE CURRENT RESURGENCE OF INTEREST IN WHITE ETHNICITY LARGELY HAS TAKEN THE FORM OF ASSERTING THE CONTINUED VITALITY OF ETHNIC COMMUNITIES. CURRENT SCHOLARS, FOLLOWING GORDON'S (1964) WELL KNOWN DISTINCTION BETWEEN ACCULTURATION AND SOCIAL ASSIMILATION, ACKNOWLEDGE THE GREAT EXTENT OF ACCULTURATION BUT MAINTAIN THAT SOCIAL ASSIMILATION HAS NOT TAKEN PLACE. THEY CLAIM THAT PRIMARY RELATIONSHIPS ARE GENERALLY BETWEEN INDIVIDUALS OF LIKE ETHNICITY. THIS PAPER, USING DATA ABOUT CATHOLIC NATIONAL-ORIGIN GROUPS IN THE EARLY 1960'S, FINDS LITTLE SUPPORT FOR THESE PRESENT ASSERTIONS OF ETHNIC VITALITY. RATES OF MIXED ANCESTRY AND INTERETHNIC MARRIAGE ARE DISCUSSED ALONG WITH VARIATION TRENDS IN THE RATE BY GENERATION AND AGE AND THE RELATIONSHIP OF ANCESTRY AND MARRIAGE TO SOCIAL ASSIMILATION. 37 REFERENCES. (JOURNAL ABSTRACT MODIFIED)

ACCN   000017

26   AUTH   **ALCOCER, A. M.**

TITL   ALCOHOLISM AMONG CHICANOS.

SRCE   *IN A. M. PADILLA & E. R. PADILLA (EDS.), IMPROVING MENTAL HEALTH AND HUMAN SERVICES FOR HISPANIC COMMUNITIES: SELECTED PRESENTATIONS FROM REGIONAL CONFERENCES. WASHINGTON, D.C.: NATIONAL COALITION OF HISPANIC MENTAL*

HEALTH AND HUMAN SERVICE ORGANIZA-
TIONS (COSSMHO), 1977, PP. 35-42.

INDX   ALCOHOLISM, MEXICAN AMERICAN, ACCUL-
TURATION, POVERTY, SES, MALE, REHABILITA-
TION, ESSAY

ABST   A CURSORY OVERVIEW OF THE LITERATURE
ON ALCOHOLISM AMONG CHICANOS IS PRE-
SENTED. THE PREVALENCE OF ALCOHOLISM
AMONG THE CHICANO POPULATION IS ESTAB-
LISHED BY INDIRECT MEASURES, SUCH AS
PERCENTAGES OF LIVER DISORDERS, NUM-
BERS OF INTOXICATION AND DRUNK DRIVING
ARRESTS, AND BY MEANS OF PRACTITIONER
EXPERIENCE IN THE FIELD. THE RATE OF CHI-
CANO ALCOHOLISM IS ESTIMATED TO BE
HIGHER THAN COMPARABLE ANGLO POPULA-
TIONS. SOME CONTRIBUTING FACTORS ARE
REVIEWED WITH SPECIAL FOCUS ON CUL-
TURAL SHOCK, POVERTY, AND THE AVAIL-
ABILITY OF ALCOHOL WITHIN THE COMMU-
NITY. IT IS CONCLUDED THAT SERVICES FOR
THE CHICANO ALCOHOLIC ARE INEFFECTIVE
AND INADEQUATE. ASPECTS OF PREVENTION,
TREATMENT, REHABILITATION AND RESEARCH
ARE DISCUSSED. 6 REFERENCES. (AUTHOR
SUMMARY MODIFIED)

ACCN   000018

27 AUTH   **ALCOCER, A. M.**
TITL   A REVIEW OF LITERATURE ON SPANISH SPEAK-
ING ALCOHOL RELATED PROBLEMS.

SRCE   *ALHAMBRA, CALIF.: TECHNICAL SYSTEMS IN-
STITUTE, UNDATED.*

INDX   MEXICAN AMERICAN, ALCOHOLISM, SPANISH
SURNAMED, REVIEW, ADULTS, MALE, FEMALE,
ADOLESCENTS, CULTURAL FACTORS, DIS-
EASE, REHABILITATION, SES, ATTITUDES, AC-
CULTURATION, SEX ROLES, PRIMARY PREVEN-
TION, RESOURCE UTILIZATION

ABST   THE REVIEW COVERS THREE MAIN AREAS OF
ALCOHOL RELATED PROBLEMS AMONG THE
SPANISH SPEAKING: (1) PREVALENCE; (2) CON-
TRIBUTING FACTORS; AND (3) PREVENTION,
TREATMENT AND REHABILITATION. THE LIT-
ERATURE GENERALLY SUPPORTS THE EXIS-
TENCE OF ALCOHOL RELATED PROBLEMS
AMONG THE SPANISH SPEAKING AND CITES
ACCULTURATION PROBLEMS, SES, AND MI-
NORITY STATUS AS DETERMINANTS OF ALCO-
HOL ABUSE. IN THE AREA OF TREATMENT AND
REHABILITATION OF ALCOHOL RELATED PROB-
LEMS, UNDERUTILIZATION OF HEALTH SER-
VICES, AND A LACK OF CULTURALLY RELEVANT
SERVICES ARE DOCUMENTED. 124 REFER-
ENCES.

ACCN   000019

28 AUTH   **ALEGRIA, D., GUERRA, E., MARTINEZ, C., JR.,
& MEYER, G. G.**
TITL   EL HOSPITAL INVISIBLE: A STUDY OF CURAN-
DERISMO.

SRCE   *ARCHIVES OF GENERAL PSYCHIATRY, 1977, 34,
1354-1357.*

INDX   CURANDERISMO, TEXAS, SOUTHWEST, FOLK
MEDICINE, HEALTH DELIVERY SYSTEMS,
HEALTH, MENTAL HEALTH, RELIGION, EMPIRI-
CAL, ADULTS, MEXICAN AMERICAN, CULTURAL
FACTORS

ABST   THIS REPORT PRESENTS THE RESULTS OF IN-
TERVIEWS WITH 16 MEXICAN AMERICAN FOLK
HEALERS (CURANDEROS AND CURANDERAS)
IN SAN ANTONIO, TEXAS. CURANDERISMO WAS
FOUND TO BE ALIVE AND WELL IN SAN ANTO-
NIO, THOUGH ITS PRACTITIONERS TEND TO BE
OLDER AND ITS FUTURE UNCLEAR. SEVERAL
SALIENT CHARACTERISTICS OF THE PRACTI-
TIONERS WERE CLARIFIED SUCH AS THE PRO-
CESS OF BECOMING A HEALER, REFERRAL
PRACTICES, TYPES OF DISORDERS TREATED,
AND TREATMENT OF THE TRADITIONAL FOLK
ILLNESSES. A BASICALLY CONSERVATIVE PO-
SITION IS TAKEN ON WHETHER CURANDEROS
CAN EVER BE INCORPORATED INTO THE HEALTH
CARE DELIVERY SYSTEM. HOWEVER, THIS
STUDY CONFIRMS THAT THE PRACTITIONERS
AND THEIR CLIENTS SIMULTANEOUSLY UTILIZE
THE FOLK MEDICAL SYSTEM AND THE SCIEN-
TIFIC MEDICAL SYSTEM. 14 REFERENCES.
(JOURNAL ABSTRACT)

ACCN   002006

29 AUTH   **ALEXANDER, D. J., & NAVA, A.**
TITL   A PUBLIC POLICY ANALYSIS OF BILINGUAL
EDUCATION IN CALIFORNIA.

SRCE   *SAN FRANCISCO: R AND E RESEARCH ASSOCI-
ATES, 1976.*

INDX   BILINGUAL-BICULTURAL EDUCATION, BILIN-
GUAL-BICULTURAL PERSONNEL, BILINGUAL-
ISM, MEXICAN AMERICAN, LANGUAGE LEARN-
ING, PARAPROFESSIONALS, LEGISLATION,
JUDICIAL PROCESS, CALIFORNIA, SOUTHWEST

ABST   AN OVERVIEW OF BILINGUAL EDUCATIONAL
PROGRAMS AND THE CHANGES IN CALIFOR-
NIA STATE LAWS AND EDUCATIONAL PHILOSO-
PHIES AFFECTING THE ESTABLISHMENT OF
SUCH PROGRAMS IS PRESENTED. THE IMPACT

s6480F   BILINGUAL EDUCATION ON THE EDUCA-
TIONAL PROCESS, SOCIETY AND GOVERN-
MENT IS DISCUSSED. DESIGNED TO MEET THE
NEEDS OF LOCAL SCHOOL DISTRICT ADMINIS-
TRATORS AND SCHOOL BOARD MEMBERS AS
THEY FORMULATE BILINGUAL EDUCATION
POLICIES AND PROGRAMS FOR THEIR DIS-
TRICTS, THIS REPORT PRESENTS: (1) AN HIS-
TORICAL ANALYSIS AND OVERALL VIEW OF
THE CURRENT BILINGUAL NEEDS IN CALIFOR-
NIA; (2) A COMPARISON OF TEACHING METH-
ODS AND MODELS; (3) LEGAL AND LEGISLA-
TIVE RESPONSIBILITIES; (4) AN ANALYSIS OF
AVAILABLE STATE AND FEDERAL PROGRAMS;
AND (5) A SET OF RECOMMENDATIONS FOR
SCHOOL DISTRICT POLICYMAKERS. 30 REFER-
ENCES.

ACCN   000020

30 AUTH   **ALLEN, B. V.**
TITL   PAYING STUDENTS TO LEARN.

SRCE   *PERSONNEL AND GUIDANCE JOURNAL, 1975,
53(10), 774-778.*

INDX   EDUCATIONAL COUNSELING, ACHIEVEMENT
MOTIVATION, SCHOLASTIC ACHIEVEMENT,
COLLEGE STUDENTS, MEXICAN AMERICAN,
ADOLESCENTS, CROSS CULTURAL, EMPIRI-
CAL, CALIFORNIA, SOUTHWEST

ABST   TEN HIGH SCHOOL AND COMMUNITY COL-
LEGE STUDENTS (4 MEXICAN AMERICAN AND

6 BLACK) WERE FOLLOWED OVER A 9 YEAR PE-
RIOD. DURING THE FIRST YEAR, STUDENTS RE-
CEIVED MONETARY AND OTHER REWARDS IN A
SPECIAL BEHAVIOR MODIFICATION PROGRAM
DESIGNED TO ENCOURAGE THEM TO DE-
VELOP STUDY HABITS, COMPLETE HOME-
WORK ASSIGNMENTS AND RAISE THEIR GRADE
AVERAGES. THE ROLE OF THE COUNSELOR
AND CHANGING OF THE BEHAVIORAL INCEN-
TIVES IN RESPONSE TO SUBJECT'S NEEDS ARE
DESCRIBED. AT THE END OF THE FIRST YEAR
ALL THE STUDENTS HAD ALTERED THEIR
GRADES FROM BELOW TO ABOVE A C AVER-
AGE. AT THE END OF 8 MORE YEARS, IT WAS
FOUND THAT ALL THE HIGH SCHOOL SUB-
JECTS HAD GRADUATED, AND 5 WENT ON TO
COLLEGE. SUBJECTS WHO BEGAN THE PRO-
GRAM AS HIGH SCHOOL STUDENTS COM-
PLETED MORE YEARS OF COLLEGE THAN
THOSE WHO STARTED AFTER HIGH SCHOOL.
THE INFLUENCE OF THE PROGRAM ON THE
STUDENTS, THEIR PARENTS AND SIBLINGS IS
ALSO DISCUSSED. THE IMPORTANCE OF EARLY
INTERVENTION IS ESPECIALLY EMPHASIZED. 3
REFERENCES.

ACCN   000022

31   AUTH   **ALLEN, R. A.**
     TITL   MEXICAN PEON WOMEN IN TEXAS.
     SRCE   *SOCIOLOGY AND SOCIAL RESEARCH, 1931,*
           16(2), 131-142.
     INDX   MEXICAN AMERICAN, FARM LABORERS, SEX
           ROLES, FAMILY ROLES, EMPIRICAL, FEMALE,
           IMMIGRATION, ECONOMIC FACTORS, SURVEY,
           TEXAS, SOUTHWEST
     ABST   FINDINGS IN A LATE 1920'S SURVEY OF THE IN-
           DUSTRIAL AND ECONOMIC POSITION OF 294
           MEXICAN IMMIGRANT FARM WOMEN IN 5 CEN-
           TRAL TEXAS COUNTIES ARE REVIEWED. THE
           INFLUENCE OF FEMININE SUBSERVIENCE, TEN-
           ANT FARMING AND POVERTY ON THE DAILY
           LIVES AND PROBABLE FUTURE OF THESE
           WOMEN ARE DISCUSSED.
     ACCN   000023

32   AUTH   **ALLINSMITH, W., & GOETHALS, G. W.**
     TITL   CULTURAL FACTORS IN MENTAL HEALTH: AN
           ANTHROPOLOGICAL PERSPECTIVE.
     SRCE   *REVIEW OF EDUCATIONAL RESEARCH, 1956,*
           26(5), 429-450.
     INDX   CULTURAL FACTORS, MENTAL HEALTH, CUL-
           TURE, REVIEW, EDUCATION, PARENTAL IN-
           VOLVEMENT, ACCULTURATION, SPANISH SUR-
           NAMED, CHILDREARING PRACTICES, PSY-
           CHOSOCIAL ADJUSTMENT
     ABST   A REVIEW OF ANTHROPOLOGICAL LITERA-
           TURE IS UNDERTAKEN TO FOCUS ON PROB-
           LEMS OF MENTAL HEALTH IN RELATION TO
           EDUCATION. FOUR SECTIONS OF THE ARTICLE
           ADDRESS: (1) THE PRINCIPLES OF MENTAL
           HEALTH AS RELATED TO THE INDIVIDUAL AND
           HIS CULTURE; (2) KEY MENTAL HEALTH PROB-
           LEMS, AS EXEMPLIFIED BY ANTHROPOLOGI-
           CAL FINDINGS; (3) IMPLICATIONS FOR AMERI-
           CAN EDUCATION; AND (4) A TECHNIQUE FOR
           ASSESSING THEORY AND DERIVING NEW IN-
           SIGHTS INTO HUMAN BEHAVIOR. IT IS SUG-
           GESTED THAT THE RESULTS OF CROSS-CUL-

TURAL METHODS OF RESEARCH WILL BE OF
CRUCIAL IMPORTANCE TO EDUCATORS, AND
WILL CLARIFY THE CONDITIONS THAT PRO-
MOTE HEALTHY PERSONALITY DEVELOPMENT
AND GENUINE PSYCHOLOGICAL WELL-BEING.
67 REFERENCES.

ACCN   000024

33   AUTH   **ALSTON, H. L., & DOUGHTIE, E. B.**
     TITL   CORRESPONDENCE OF CONSTRUCTS MEA-
           SURED BY THE KINDERGARTEN SCREENING
           INVENTORY BY SEX AND ETHNIC GROUP.
     SRCE   *PSYCHOLOGY IN THE SCHOOLS, 1975, 12(4),*
           428-429.
     INDX   CHILDREN, EARLY CHILDHOOD EDUCATION,
           SEX COMPARISON, ETHNIC IDENTITY, CROSS
           CULTURAL, MEXICAN AMERICAN, COGNITIVE
           DEVELOPMENT, EMPIRICAL, ACHIEVEMENT
           TESTING, TEXAS, SOUTHWEST
     ABST   THIS STUDY INVESTIGATED WHETHER THE
           CONSTRUCTS MEASURED BY THE KINDER-
           GARTEN SCREENING INVENTORY (KSI) WERE
           THE SAME FOR MALES AND FEMALES AND FOR
           ANGLO AMERICAN, NEGRO AMERICAN, AND
           MEXICAN AMERICAN GROUPS. SUBJECTS WERE
           1,527 KINDERGARTEN CHILDREN FROM THE
           INDEPENDENT SCHOOL DISTRICT OF HOUS-
           TON, TEXAS. THE FACTOR-RELATING PROCE-
           DURE PROPOSED BY H. F. KAISER, ET AL. (1969)
           TO DETERMINE THE EXTENT TO WHICH THE
           SAME CONSTRUCTS WERE MEASURED WITH
           DIFFERENT GROUPS WAS USED. THE CORRE-
           SPONDENCE BETWEEN THE CONSTRUCTS
           MEASURED BY THE KSI FOR MALES AND FE-
           MALES AND FOR THE ANGLO AMERICAN AND
           NEGRO AMERICAN AND MEXICAN AMERICAN
           GROUPS WAS VERY SIMILAR. FINDINGS INDI-
           CATE THAT SUBSTANTIALLY THE SAME CON-
           STRUCTS ARE BEING MEASURED BY THE KSI
           FOR BOTH SEXES AND ALL ETHNIC GROUPS. 5
           REFERENCES. (PASAR ABSTRACT MODIFIED)
     ACCN   000025

34   AUTH   **ALTHEIDE, D. L., & GILMORE, R. P.**
     TITL   THE CREDIBILITY OF PROTEST.
     SRCE   *AMERICAN SOCIOLOGICAL REVIEW, 1972, 37(1),*
           99-108.
     INDX   SES, SOCIAL SCIENCES, SURVEY, ETHNIC IDEN-
           TITY, COLLEGE STUDENTS, ADULTS, MEXICAN
           AMERICAN, COMMUNITY INVOLVEMENT, POLI-
           TICS, POLITICAL POWER, EMPIRICAL, COLO-
           RADO, SOUTHWEST
     ABST   AFTER A STUDENT PROTEST OVER THE SALE
           OF A PARTICULAR BRAND OF BEER AT A COL-
           LEGE CAMPUS (COLORADO STATE COLLEGE
           IN PUEBLO), THE AUTHORS EXAMINED THE
           PUBLIC PERCEPTION OF THE PROTEST USING
           3 HYPOTHESES DERIVED FROM TURNER (1969).
           A TOTAL OF 486 PERSONS (284 STUDENTS, 27
           FACULTY, 16 COLLEGE ADMINISTRATORS AND
           159 CITY RESIDENTS) COMPLETED QUESTION-
           NAIRES ABOUT THEIR PERCEPTIONS OF THE
           PROTEST (I. E., TYPE AND NUMBER OF PER-
           SONS INVOLVED, REPRESENTATION OF MEXI-
           CAN AMERICANS, APPROVAL OR DISAP-
           PROVAL). THE HYPOTHESES TESTED WERE (1)
           THE MORE PARTICIPANTS ARE SEEN CONSTI-
           TUTING A MAJOR PART OF THE GROUP WHOSE

GRIEVANCES ARE KNOWN, THE MORE CREDIBLE THEY ARE AS PROTESTERS; (2) MORE ADVANTAGED GROUPS WILL MORE READILY ACCEPT THE CLAIMS OF INJUSTICE THAN WILL THE LESS ADVANTAGED GROUPS; (3) THE MORE PEOPLE VIEW SOCIETY AS UNSTABLE AND WITH AN INDIVIDUALISTIC ORIENTATION, THE LESS LIKELY THEY WILL BE TO CONSIDER COLLECTIVE ACTION AS LEGITIMATE. WITH ONE EXCEPTION, ALL THE HYPOTHESES WERE IN THE PREDICTED DIRECTION. THE EXCEPTION WAS THAT MIDDLE-CLASS PEOPLE WERE NOT MORE LIKELY THAN OTHER CLASSES TO DEFINE THE EVENT AS A PROTEST. THE MOST IMPORTANT PREDICTOR VARIABLE WAS ETHNICITY: MEXICAN AMERICANS WERE MOST LIKELY TO VIEW THE INCIDENT FAVORABLY. OTHER VARIABLES THAT AFFECTED THE PUBLIC PERCEPTION OF THE EVENT ARE DISCUSSED. 21 REFERENCES. (JOURNAL ABSTRACT MODIFIED)

ACCN   000026

35   AUTH   **ALTUS, G. T.**
TITL   WISC PATTERNS OF A SELECTIVE SAMPLE OF BILINGUAL SCHOOL CHILDREN.
SRCE   *JOURNAL OF GENETIC PSYCHOLOGY, 1953, 83(1), 241-248.*
INDX   WISC, INTELLIGENCE TESTING, MEXICAN AMERICAN, CHILDREN, EMPIRICAL, BILINGUAL, INTELLIGENCE, CROSS CULTURAL, CALIFORNIA, SOUTHWEST
ABST   A COMPARISON OF THE INTELLIGENCE TEST PATTERNING OF A MEXICAN DESCENT BILINGUAL GROUP TO THAT OF A UNILINGUAL ENGLISH-SPEAKING SAMPLE IS EQUATED ON THE BASIS OF AGE, SEX, AND PERFORMANCE IQ. THE WECHSLER INTELLIGENCE SCALE FOR CHILDREN IS UTILIZED IN THIS STUDY. SUBJECTS WERE REFERRALS FOR PRELIMINARY SCREENING FOR MENTALLY RETARDED SPECIAL CLASSES OR PARTICIPANTS IN A RESEARCH READING SURVEY. THE CONCLUSION IS THAT THE PERFORMANCE IQ DIFFERENCE IS STATISTICALLY INSIGNIFICANT WHILE THE VERBAL IQ DISSIMILARITY OF 17 POINTS IS HIGHLY SIGNIFICANT IN FAVOR OF THE UNILINGUALS. VERBAL SUBTESTS INDICATE STATISTICALLY SIGNIFICANT DISCREPANCIES BETWEEN THE GROUPS. A UNIQUE SUBTEST PATTERNING IS EVIDENT WHICH IS DISCORDANT TO THE CONVENTIONAL ADULT WECHSLER PATTERN FOR THE MENTALLY RETARDED. THE BILINGUAL GROUP SCORED IN THE PSYCHOMETRICALLY RETARDED RANGE IN VERBAL SKILLS (ENGLISH); HOWEVER, MUCH OF THIS RETARDATION IS ATTRIBUTED TO A LINGUISTIC HANDICAP AND DOES NOT ACCURATELY REFLECT THE CHILD'S POTENTIAL CAPACITY. THESE RESULTS MIGHT BE BENEFICIAL IN THE DIAGNOSIS OF BORDERLINE CASES OF PSYCHOMETRIC MENTAL RETARDATION WITHIN THE BILINGUALS AND MIGHT PRESENT EVIDENCE AS TO THE HANDICAPPING INFLUENCES OF BILINGUALISM. FURTHER LONGITUDINAL RESEARCH IS NEEDED TO DETERMINE THE MAGNITUDE OF SUCH DIFFERENCES AND THE BILINGUAL STUDENT'S ABILITY TO CHANGE AS

A RESULT OF CONTINUAL SCHOOLING. 8 REFERENCES.

ACCN   000027

36   AUTH   **ALTUS, W. D.**
TITL   THE AMERICAN MEXICAN: THE SURVIVAL OF A CULTURE.
SRCE   *JOURNAL OF SOCIAL PSYCHOLOGY, 1949, 29(2), 211-220.*
INDX   CULTURE, MEXICAN AMERICAN, EMPIRICAL, INTELLIGENCE, BILINGUALISM, ACCULTURATION, ADULTS, SOUTHWEST, WEST, MILITARY
ABST   IN 1943, ALL NEWLY-INDUCTED SOLDIERS WHO WERE FOUND TO BE FUNCTIONALLY ILLITERATE BY ARMY STANDARDS WERE SENT TO A SPECIAL TRAINING CENTER WHERE THEY EITHER ATTAINED A SET LITERARY STANDARD WITHIN 12 WEEKS OR WERE DISCHARGED. IN THE NINTH SERVICE COMMAND SPECIAL TRAINING CENTER, WHICH SERVICED THE EIGHT WESTERNMOST STATES, MANY MEXICAN TRAINEES WERE PRESENT. THE LINGUISTIC ASPECTS OF MEXICAN CULTURE STRIKINGLY PERSISTED AMONG THESE TRAINEES. ALL SPOKE SPANISH, NO MATTER HOW MANY GENERATIONS THEIR ANCESTORS MAY HAVE LIVED IN THE UNITED STATES. EXPLANATIONS FOR THE PERSISTENCE OF THE MEXICAN CULTURE INCLUDE: THE GEOGRAPHIC PROXIMITY OF THE HOMELAND; AN INDIGENOUS DIET; RELIGION; THE PRESENCE OF MEXICAN MOVIES AND NEWSPAPERS; THE PURSUIT OF UNSKILLED OOCUPATIONS IN COMPANY WITH OTHER MEXICANS; AND FINALLY, THE OCCASIONAL ANTAGONISM OF THE MAJORITY POPULATION WHICH CAUSES THE MEXICAN TO CLOSE RANKS ABOUT HIS CULTURE. 2 REFERENCES.

ACCN   000028

37   AUTH   **ALTUS, W. D.**
TITL   A NOTE ON GROUP DIFFERENCES IN INTELLIGENCE AND THE TYPE OF TEST USED.
SRCE   *JOURNAL OF CONSULTING PSYCHOLOGY, 1948, 12(3), 194-195.*
INDX   CROSS CULTURAL, WECHSLER MENTAL ABILITY SCALE, MEXICAN AMERICAN, EMPIRICAL, INTELLIGENCE TESTING, ARMY GENERAL CLASSIFICATION TEST, ADULTS, INDIGENOUS POPULATIONS, WEST, SOUTHWEST
ABST   A COMPARISON OF RACIAL GROUP DIFFERENCES IN INTELLIGENCE AND THE EFFECT OF A PARTICULAR TYPE OF TEST IS PRESENTED. EACH ANGLO, NEGRO, MEXICAN AND INDIAN GROUP WAS ADMINISTERED THE FOLLOWING TESTS: THE WECHSLER MENTAL ABILITY SCALE B, FORM B SUBTESTS (INFORMATION ARITHMETIC COMPREHENSION AND SIMILARITIES), THE ARMY GENERAL CLASSIFICATION TEST (AGCT), AND THE MECHANICAL APTITUDE TEST (MAT). SUBJECTS WERE ALL CLASSIFIED AS ILLITERATE UPON ENTERING THE ARMY AND ALL MET COMMON CRITERION FOR GRADUATION ON THE BASIS OF TWO READING AND MATH OBJECTIVE TESTS. VERBAL SUBTEST RESULTS SHOW THAT THE MEAN SCORES FOR ANGLO AND NEGRO GROUPS ARE SUPERIOR TO THAT OF THE MEXICAN AND INDIAN GROUPS. THE AGCT REVEALS THE MEAN SCORE OF THE AN-

GLO TO BE SUPERIOR TO THAT OF THE MEXI-CAN, AND THE NEGRO MEAN SCORE IS INFE-RIOR TO THE MEXICAN, BUT SUPERIOR TO THE INDIAN. RESULTS OF THE MAT DISCLOSE SU-PERIOR MAINTENANCE OF ANGLO MEAN SCORE IN COMPARISON TO THE OTHER GROUPS. THE MEXICAN MAT GROUP MEAN SCORE IS BETTER THAN THE NEGRO AND IN-DIAN GROUP SCORES. IT IS CONCLUDED THAT GROUP INFERIORITY OR SUPERIORITY IS, IN PART, A FUNCTION OF THE TEST EMPLOYED. AN ASSUMPTION IS MADE THAT CERTAIN GROUP DIFFERENCES IN IQ REPORTED IN PRE-VIOUS RESEARCH FOR NATIONAL, LINGUISTIC, OR RACIAL GROUPS MIGHT BE COMPLETELY CONTRADICTED IF THE TYPE OF MEASURE IS CHANGED. NO REFERENCES.

ACCN   000029

38 AUTH   **ALTUS, W. D.**
    TITL   RACIAL AND BILINGUAL GROUP DIFFERENCES IN PREDICTABILITY AND IN MEAN APTITUDE TEST SCORES IN AN ARMY SPECIAL TRAINING CENTER.
    SRCE   *PSYCHOLOGICAL BULLETIN, 1945, 42(5), 310-320.*
    INDX   INTELLIGENCE TESTING, WECHSLER MENTAL ABILITY SCALE, CROSS CULTURAL, MEXICAN AMERICAN, BILINGUALISM, ARMY GENERAL CLASSIFICATION TEST, EMPIRICAL, ADULTS, WEST, SOUTHWEST
    ABST   AN EXAMINATION OF THE AMERICAN MEXICAN AND THE SURVIVAL OF HIS CULTURE IS PRE-SENTED. THE LINGUISTIC ASPECTS OF MEXI-CAN CULTURE PERSIST AMONG THOSE AMERI-CAN CITIZENS OF MEXICAN ANCESTRY FOUND IN AN AMERICAN SPECIAL TRAINING CENTER. ALL TRAINEES OF MEXICAN ANCESTRY SPOKE SPANISH NO MATTER HOW MANY GENERA-TIONS THEIR ANCESTORS MAY HAVE LIVED IN THE UNITED STATES. WHILE MANY ATTENDED ENGLISH-SPEAKING SCHOOLS AND COULD NOT READ OR WRITE IN ENGLISH, THEY COULD READ AND WRITE IN SPANISH, A LANGUAGE THEY HAD NOT FORMALLY STUDIED IN SCHOOL. THE NATIVE-BORN AND REARED NON-ENGLISH MEXICAN HAS BEEN SHOWN TO BE MORE MA-LADJUSTED AND LESS INTELLIGENT THAN THE NON-ENGLISH FOREIGN-BORN AND EDU-CATED SPANISH-SPEAKING SUBJECT. THE PROPINQUITY OF MEXICO, RELIGION, DIETS, MEXICAN MOVIES, AND SPANISH NEWSPAPERS ALL AID IN THE PERSISTENCE OF HIS ORIGINAL LANGUAGE. DISCUSSION OF HISTORICAL IN-STITUTIONS OF THE MEXICAN AND TWO CASE STUDIES ARE PRESENTED TO FURTHER EX-PLAIN THE PERSISTENCE OF THE CULTURE AND LANGUAGE. IT IS SUGGESTED THAT SPAN-ISH PERSISTS WITH GREATER HARDINESS AMONG AMERICAN MEXICANS THAN DOES ANY OTHER NON-ENGLISH TONGUE AMONG COMPARABLE GROUPS OF AMERICAN CITI-ZENS. 2 REFERENCES.

ACCN   000030

39 AUTH   **ALTUS, W. D., & CLARK, J. H.**
    TITL   THE EFFECT OF ADJUSTMENT PATTERNS ON THE INTERCORRELATION OF INTELLIGENCE SUBTEST VARIABLES.
    SRCE   *JOURNAL OF SOCIAL PSYCHOLOGY, 1949, 30(1), 39-48.*
    INDX   PERSONALITY ASSESSMENT, INTELLIGENCE TESTING, PSYCHOSOCIAL ADJUSTMENT, CROSS CULTURAL, SPANISH SURNAMED, ADULTS, EM-PIRICAL, MMPI, WAIS, MILITARY
    ABST   AN INVESTIGATION OF THE EFFECT OF AD-JUSTMENT PATTERNS UPON THE INTERCOR-RELATION OF INTELLIGENCE SUBTEST VARI-ABLES IS PRESENTED. THREE GROUPS OF ARMY ILLITERATES, TWO ANGLO SAMPLES AND ONE SPANISH-SPEAKING SAMPLE WERE AD-MINISTERED AN ADJUSTMENT TEST CONSIST-ING OF THE MINNESOTA MULTIPHASIC PER-SONALITY INVENTORY AND BELL'S ADJUSTMENT INVENTORY. IN ADDITION, THE WECHSLER ADULT INTELLIGENCE SCALE WAS GIVEN. THE DATA SHOW THAT SUBJECTS CLASSED AS MALADJUSTED HAVE A HIGHER ORDER OF INTERCORRELATION AMONG THEIR ABILITIES (WHEN ABILITIES ARE DEFINED BY A SCORE ON INDIVIDUAL SUBTESTS OF THE WAIS) THAN DO THE WELL-ADJUSTED TRAIN-EES. CONFIRMATION OF THIS FINDING WAS OBTAINED ON A "BRIGHT NORMAL" GROUP OF VETERANS UNDERGOING COUNSELING. A NUMBER OF HYPOTHESES WHICH MIGHT EX-PLAIN THE FINDINGS ARE EXAMINED. ONE HY-POTHESIS OFFERED TO EXPLAIN THE CONSIS-TENT INTERCORRELATION TRENDS OF THE MALADJUSTED IS THAT HE IS STILL EMOTION-ALLY AND INTELLECTUALLY A CHILD WITH UN-DIFFERENTIATED ABILITIES. 6 REFERENCES.

ACCN   000031

40 AUTH   **ALVAREZ, M. G.**
    TITL   THE USE OF QUESTIONS IN DISCOURSE.
    SRCE   *UNPUBLISHED MANUSCRIPT, DEPARTMENT OF PSYCHOLOGY, UNIVERSITY OF CALIFORNIA, LOS ANGELES, 1977.*
    INDX   MEXICAN AMERICAN, SOCIALIZATION, LIN-GUISTICS, EMPIRICAL, MOTHER-CHILD INTER-ACTION, CHILDREN, ADULTS
    ABST   AN EXAMINATION OF QUESTIONS AS KEY ELE-MENTS OF SOCIAL INTERACTION BETWEEN CHILD AND MOTHER, AND CHILD AND ADULT WAS MADE. THIS EXPLORATORY STUDY ALSO ATTEMPTED TO ASCERTAIN THE "CLASSIFIA-BILITY" OF QUESTIONS AND THEIR ROLE IN DISCOURSE. THE CONVERSATIONS OF TWO PRE-SCHOOL CHILDREN WITH THEIR MOTH-ERS WERE INDEPENDENTLY CODED BY EXPER-IMENTERS. THIS WAS THE INITIAL STAGE OF A PLANNED LONGITUDINAL STUDY. THE TAPED CONVERSATIONS WERE THEN USED TO INVES-TIGATE THE FOLLOWING: (1) THE TYPES OF QUESTIONS USED; (2) WHO THEY WERE DI-RECTED TO; AND (3) HOW THEY WERE AN-SWERED. QUESTION TYPES WERE THOSE DE-VELOPED BY HOLZMAN AND CORSARO. HOLZMAN'S CLASSIFICATIONS WERE CLARIFI-CATION, CONFIRMATION, INFORMATION, LEAD-ING QUESTIONS AND NON-QUESTION. COR-SARO'S CLASSIFICATIONS WERE PERMISSION, QUESTION WITH ANSWER AND TAG QUESTION. IT WAS FOUND THAT CHILDREN PRIMARILY

USED INFORMATION REQUESTS WHILE INTER-ACTING. THE ADULTS USED CLARIFICATION REQUESTS MORE OFTEN THAN THE CHILDREN. ADULTS RESPONDED TO ALMOST ALL OF THE CHILDREN'S QUESTIONS, WHEREAS THE CHILDREN'S RESPONSES SOMETIMES DEPENDED UPON WHO ASKED THE QUESTION AND WHAT TYPE OF INTERROGATIVE WAS USED. THE STUDY INDICATES THAT CLASSIFICATION OF QUESTIONS ACCORDING TO THEIR FORM AND FUNCTION IS A USEFUL TOOL IN DISCOURSE ANALYSIS AND THAT QUESTIONS PLAY A PRIMARY ROLE IN INTERACTION. 5 REFERENCES.

ACCN   000032

41   AUTH   **ALVAREZ, R.**
      TITL   A MENTAL HEALTH RESEARCH PROGRAM FOR THE SPANISH SPEAKING.
      SRCE   *IN A. M. PADILLA & E. R. PADILLA (EDS.), IMPROVING MENTAL HEALTH AND HUMAN SERVICES FOR HISPANIC COMMUNITIES: SELECTED PRESENTATIONS FROM REGIONAL CONFERENCES. WASHINGTON, D.C.: NATIONAL COALITION OF HISPANIC MENTAL HEALTH AND HUMAN SERVICE ORGANIZATIONS (COSSMHO), 1977, PP. 57-59.*
      INDX   ESSAY, SPANISH SURNAMED, RESEARCH METHODOLOGY, PROFESSIONAL TRAINING, MENTAL HEALTH, CALIFORNIA, SOUTHWEST
      ABST   THE SPANISH SPEAKING MENTAL HEALTH RESEARCH AND DEVELOPMENT PROGRAM (NOW CALLED THE SPANISH SPEAKING MENTAL HEALTH RESEARCH CENTER) AT THE UNIVERSITY OF CALIFONIA, LOS ANGELES WAS ESTABLISHED TO MEET THE MENTAL HEALTH NEEDS OF THE SPANISH SPEAKING COMMUNITY IN THREE SPECIFIC WAYS. THESE ARE: (1) RESEARCH EVALUATION OF MENTAL HEALTH NEEDS FROM A PERSPECTIVE CULTURALLY INDIGENOUS TO THE SPANISH SPEAKING COMMUNITY; (2) DEVELOPMENT OF RESEARCH SCHOLARS IN THE MENTAL HEALTH AREA WHO ARE THEMSELVES MEMBERS OF THE CULTURAL COMMUNITY AND CAN THEREFORE GENERATE CULTURALLY INDIGENOUS PERSPECTIVES IN THEIR SCIENTIFIC WORK; AND (3) PROVISION OF TECHNICAL ASSISTANCE OF A RESEARCH NATURE TO COMMUNITY ORGANIZATIONS IN THE MENTAL HEALTH FIELD. THE PROGRAM'S PHILOSOPHY EMPHASIZES THE DISCOVERY AND ANALYSIS OF POSITIVE AND CONSTRUCTIVE ASPECTS OF ECONOMIC, SOCIAL AND CULTURAL STRUCTURES WITHIN THE COMMUNITY. FOR THIS PURPOSE A TYPOLOGY WAS DEVELOPED TO CLASSIFY AND EVALUATE RESEARCH ON THE SPANISH SPEAKING IN THESE THREE AREAS: (1) REVIEW OF EXISTING KNOWLEDGE PERTINENT TO CHICANO SELF DETERMINATION AND ITS IMPLICATIONS FOR MENTAL HEALTH; (2) DEVELOPMENT OF NEW INDIGENOUS PERSPECTIVES TO GENERATE POLICY-RELEVANT KNOWLEDGE; AND (3) VERIFICATION OF PAST RESEARCH, CORRECTION OF ERRORS AND DEVELOPMENT OF NEW RESEARCH FROM THESE PROBLEMS. THE TECHNICAL ASSISTANCE, AS DIFFERENTIATED FROM SERVICE, PROGRAM HAS PROVIDED COMMUNITY ORGANIZATIONS WITH AN EVALUATION MECHANISM FOR THEIR PROGRAMS, AS WELL AS DISSEMINATED RELEVANT MATERIALS ON MENTAL HEALTH AS IT PERTAINS TO THE SPANISH SPEAKING POPULATION. (AUTHOR SUMMARY MODIFIED)

ACCN   000034

42   AUTH   **ALVAREZ, R.**
      TITL   THE PSYCHO-HISTORICAL AND SOCIOECONOMIC DEVELOPMENT OF THE CHICANO COMMUNITY IN THE UNITED STATES.
      SRCE   *IN N. R. YETMAN & C. H. STEELE (EDS.), MAJORITY AND MINORITY: THE DYNAMICS OF RACIAL AND ETHNIC RELATIONS. BOSTON: ALLYN & BACON, 1975, PP. 192-206.*
      INDX   HISTORY, MEXICAN AMERICAN, ACCULTURATION, PREJUDICE, DISCRIMINATION, STEREOTYPES, POVERTY, SES, MIGRATION, IMMIGRATION, EMPLOYMENT, FARM LABORERS, SCHOLASTIC ACHIEVEMENT, ESSAY, CULTURAL CHANGE, CROSS GENERATIONAL
      ABST   FOUR HISTORICAL PERIODS IN MEXICAN AMERICAN HISTORY ARE IDENTIFIED WITH THE PURPOSE OF DESCRIBING THE SOCIALIZATION EXPERIENCES PREDOMINANT IN EACH GENERATION. FACTS AND INTERPRETATIONS NOT TRADITIONALLY TAKEN INTO ACCOUNT IN MEXICAN AMERICAN HISTORY ARE PRESENTED IN ORDER TO GENERATE HYPOTHESES REGARDING THE PSYCHO-HISTORICAL AND SOCIOECONOMIC DEVELOPMENT OF THE PRESENT CHICANO GENERATION OF THE 1960'S. THE EFFECTS OF AMERICAN IMPERIALISM ON THE CREATION GENERATION (1800'S), MIGRANT GENERATION (EARLY-1900'S), AND MEXICAN AMERICAN GENERATION (POST-WW II) ARE RELATED TO THE ASPIRATIONS AND CONCERNS OF THE FOURTH GENERATION—THE CHICANO GENERATION OF THE 1960'S. EMPHASIS IS PLACED ON THE NEW CONSCIOUSNESS OF MEXICAN AMERICANS SINCE THE LATE 1960'S, SIMILARITIES BETWEEN THE CHICANO AND THE CREATION GENERATIONS, AND THE SOCIAL AND ECONOMIC PROBLEMS YET TO BE RESOLVED BY THIS FOURTH GENERATION OF MEXICAN AMERICANS.

ACCN   000035

43   AUTH   **ALVAREZ, R.**
      TITL   THE UNIQUE PSYCHO-HISTORICAL EXPERIENCE OF THE MEXICAN-AMERICAN PEOPLE.
      SRCE   *SOCIAL SCIENCE QUARTERLY, 1971, 52, 15-29.*
      INDX   MEXICAN AMERICAN, HISTORY, ESSAY, ACCULTURATION, CULTURE
      ABST   IN THIS BOOK REVIEW, FOUR STRENGTHS OF GREBLER, MOORE, AND GUZMAN'S (1970) "THE MEXICAN AMERICAN PEOPLE" ARE DISCUSSED. (1) THE EXTENSIVE GEOGRAPHICAL AREA AND RANGE OF DEMOGRAPHIC VARIABLES SYSTEMATICALLY COMPARED FOR FIVE SOUTHWESTERN STATES AND ONE MIDWESTERN CITY IS VIEWED AS A UNIQUE, INITIAL STEP TOWARD A COMPREHENSIVE UNDERSTANDING OF THE MEXICAN AMERICAN (MA) POPULATION OF THIS COUNTRY. (2) THE BOOK IS SEEN AS A GENUINE ATTEMPT TO INCLUDE MANY DISCIPLINARY POINTS OF VIEW TO INTERPRET THE DEMOGRAPHIC VARIABLES, THUS

AVOIDING THE PITFALL OF LIMITED PERSPEC-
TIVES AND INADEQUATE DATA INTERPRETA-
TION. (3) NON-DEMOGRAPHIC DATA ON SEX,
FAMILY ROLES AND OTHER SOCIOLOGICAL
AND PSYCHOSOCIAL VARIABLES ARE ALSO IN-
CLUDED, WHICH WILL DO MUCH TO DISPEL
OLD STEREOTYPES AND RAISE FURTHER
QUESTIONS FOR RESEARCH. (4) FINALLY, THE
BOOK MAY BECOME THE BEDROCK TOOL OF
FUTURE RESEARCH ON MEXICAN AMERICANS
BECAUSE OF ITS COMPREHENSIVE DATA
ANALYSES, COMPETENTLY COMPILED BIBLI-
OGRAPHY, AND PRESENTATION OF OTHER
HELPFUL RESEARCH MATERIALS SUCH AS
MAPS, TABLES AND APPENDICES. AN ASPECT
OF MA DEVELOPMENT WHICH THE BOOK NE-
GLECTED IS THE PSYCHO-HISTORICAL EXPERI-
ENCE OF THE MA PEOPLE PRE-1900. PRE-1900
HISTORICAL, POLITICAL, RELIGIOUS, ECO-
NOMIC AND LANGUAGE FACTORS WHICH
GREATLY INFLUENCED POST-1900 EXPERI-
ENCES ARE DISCUSSED AT LENGTH.

ACCN 000036

44 AUTH **ALVAREZ, R. (ED.)**
    TITL DELIVERY OF SERVICES FOR LATINO COMMU-
          NITY MENTAL HEALTH (MONOGRAPH NO. 2).
    SRCE *LOS ANGELES: UNIVERSITY OF CALIFORNIA,*
          SPANISH SPEAKING MENTAL HEALTH RE-
          SEARCH AND DEVELOPMENT PROGRAM, 1975.
    INDX HEALTH DELIVERY SYSTEMS, MENTAL HEALTH,
          FOLK MEDICINE, CULTURAL FACTORS, SPAN-
          ISH SURNAMED, PUERTO RICAN-M, MEXICAN
          AMERICAN, PARAPROFESSIONALS, REVIEW,
          PERSONALITY ASSESSMENT, PROJECTIVE
          TESTING, BILINGUAL-BICULTURAL PERSON-
          NEL, PSYCHOTHERAPY, SES, MENTAL HEALTH
          PROFESSION, EMPIRICAL, BOOK
    ABST THREE AREAS VITAL TO THE DELIVERY OF SER-
          VICES TO LATINO COMMUNITIES ARE EXAM-
          INED. (1) EXISTING HEALTH CARE SYSTEMS
          ARE OVERVIEWED, WITH SUGGESTIONS FOR
          INNOVATIONS AT THE ORGANIZATIONAL LEVEL.
          (2) PERSONALITY ASSESSMENT AND RESULT
          INTERPRETATIONS ARE CRITICALLY REVIEWED,
          AND SUGGESTIONS FOR DIFFERENT WAYS OF
          INTERPRETING RESULTS WHEN DEALING WITH
          LATINOS ARE OFFERED. SOME DIRECTIONS
          FOR THE DEVELOPMENT OF MORE RELEVANT
          TESTS ARE ALSO SUGGESTED. (3) THE THIRD
          AREA IS CONCERNED WITH THE DEVELOP-
          MENT OF PROFESSIONAL PERSONNEL. AN EM-
          PIRICAL EXPERIMENT IS RECOMMENDED ON
          THE ETHNIC CHARACTERISTICS OF THERA-
          PISTS AND THE IMPACT THAT ETHNIC CUES
          MIGHT HAVE ON PATIENTS. SUGGESTIONS FOR
          DEVELOPING A CULTURALLY SENSITIVE THER-
          APEUTIC RELATIONSHIP BETWEEN PATIENT AND
          THERAPIST ARE MADE. (AUTHOR SUMMARY
          MODIFIED)
    ACCN 000033

45 AUTH **ALVAREZ, R., DE HOYOS, L., DIEPPA, I., MEJIA,**
          K., MEJIA, R., PADILLA, A. M., TORRES, C.,
          TRINIDAD, I., & VALDEZ, R.
    TITL LATINO COMMUNITY MENTAL HEALTH (MONO-
          GRAPH NO. 1).

    SRCE *LOS ANGELES: UNIVERSITY OF CALIFORNIA,*
          SPANISH SPEAKING MENTAL HEALTH RE-
          SEARCH AND DEVELOPMENT PROGRAM, 1974.
    INDX COMMUNITY, HEALTH DELIVERY SYSTEMS,
          MENTAL HEALTH, MENTAL HEALTH PROFES-
          SION, REVIEW, CULTURAL FACTORS, SES, PAR-
          APROFESSIONALS, BILINGUAL-BICULTURAL
          PERSONNEL, SPANISH SURNAMED, BOOK
    ABST THE RESULTS OF A STUDY BY THE LATINO
          TASK FORCE ON COMMUNITY MENTAL HEALTH
          TRAINING ARE PRESENTED. THE IDENTIFI-
          CATION OF THE MENTAL HEALTH PROBLEMS
          OF THE LATINO .COMMUNITY AND THEIR
          CAUSES, PRIMARILY CULTURAL CONFLICT AND
          OPPRESSION, ARE FOCUSED ON IN ORDER TO
          FORMULATE VIABLE RECOMMENDATIONS FOR
          COMMUNITY MENTAL HEALTH PROGRAMS, RE-
          SEARCH AND TRAINING. AN EVALUATION OF
          THE RELEVANCY AND EFFECTIVENESS OF EX-
          ISTING SERVICES LEADS TO THESE RECOM-
          MENDATIONS AMONG SEVERAL OTHERS: (1)
          HOUSING OF LATINO ADVOCATE OFFICES IN
          ALL MAJOR PUBLIC SERVICE INSTITUTIONS SO
          THAT EFFICIENCY AND COORDINATION CAN BE
          MAXIMIZED; (2) UTILIZING TECHNIQUES FOR
          IDENTIFYING SOCIAL AND CULTURAL CON-
          FLICTS WHICH PRODUCE LATINO CLIENTS; (3)
          PROMOTING SERVICES THAT ARE COMPATIBLE
          WITH AND SUPPORTIVE OF LATINO SOCIAL
          AND CULTURAL STRUCTURES SUCH AS EX-
          TENDED FAMILY, RELIGION AND FOLK MEDI-
          CINE PRACTICES; (4) STAFFING OF PROGRAMS
          WITH INDIGENOUS RESOURCE PERSONS AND
          SUPPORTING COMMUNITY PARTICIPATION IN
          HIRING STAFF SENSITIVE TO LATINO VALUES
          AND ACTIVE IN THE LATINO COMMUNITY.
          TRAINING RECOMMENDATIONS INCLUDE: (1)
          CURRICULUM CHANGES THAT INCLUDE STUDY
          OF LATINO VALUES AND CULTURAL PERSPEC-
          TIVES, AND (2) IN-SERVICE PROGRAMS THAT
          RE-ORIENT AND SENSITIZE PROFESSIONALS
          TO LATINO BEHAVIOR PATTERNS AND PREFER-
          ENCES. RESEARCH RECOMMENDATIONS IN-
          CLUDE: (1) INVOLVING LATINO FACULTY, STU-
          DENTS AND COMMUNITY IN PLANNING AND
          IMPLEMENTING MENTAL HEALTH RESEARCH IN
          THE BARRIOS, AND (2) TAKING STEPS TO CON-
          DUCT RESEARCH ON THE APPLICABILITY AND
          REFINEMENT OF THE CULTURE-CONFLICT
          THEORY. THE STUDY IS WRITTEN TO APPEAL
          TO BOTH COMMUNITY WORKERS AND MENTAL
          HEALTH PROFESSIONALS. 22 REFERENCES.
    ACCN 000037

46 AUTH **ALVIREZ, D.**
    TITL THE EFFECTS OF FORMAL CHURCH AFFILIA-
          TION AND RELIGIOSITY ON THE FERTILITY PAT-
          TERNS OF MEXICAN AMERICAN CATHOLICS.
    SRCE *DEMOGRAPHY, 1973, 10(1), 19-36.*
    INDX FERTILITY, RELIGION, MEXICAN AMERICAN,
          BIRTH CONTROL, SES, ACCULTURATION, CROSS
          CULTURAL, SEX ROLES, ADULTS, EMPIRICAL,
          TEXAS, SOUTHWEST
    ABST THE EFFECTS OF RELIGION ON THE FERTILITY
          PATTERNS OF MEXICAN AMERICANS ARE EX-
          AMINED WITH TWO DIFFERENT PATH MODELS,
          THE INSTITUTIONAL MODEL USING FORMAL
          AFFILIATION WITH THE ROMAN CATHOLIC

CHURCH AS A MEASURE OF RELIGION, AND THE RELIGIOSITY MODEL USING AN INFORMAL MEASURE OF RELIGIOSITY. EACH MODEL, TESTED SEPARATELY FOR HUSBANDS AND WIVES, EXAMINES THE EFFECTS OF RELIGION ON CONTRACEPTIVE METHODS USED AND ON DESIRED FAMILY SIZE. ALTHOUGH THE MAJORITY OF MEXICAN AMERICANS ARE CATHOLICS AND TEND TO HAVE LARGE FAMILIES, RELIGION DOES NOT SEEM TO HAVE THE SAME EFFECT ON THEIR FERTILITY PATTERNS AS ON THAT OF OTHER CATHOLICS IN THE UNITED STATES. AMONG THE MEN, NEITHER FORMAL AFFILIATION NOR RELIGIOSITY AFFECT THE FERTILITY PATTERNS IN ANY WAY, WHILE AMONG THE WOMEN THE EFFECT IS SLIGHT. CONSIDERING THE CATHOLIC CHURCH'S POSITION ON CONTRACEPTIVE USAGE, IT IS ESPECIALLY NOTEWORTHY THAT RELIGION DOES NOT AFFECT THE USE OR NON-USE OF THE MORE EFFECTIVE MEANS OF CONTRACEPTION, A FACTOR CONTRIBUTING TO THE GENERALLY WEAK ASSOCIATION BETWEEN THE MEASURES OF RELIGION AND WANTED FAMILY SIZE. A PARTIAL EXPLANATION OF THE STUDY RESULT IS ATTEMPTED AS NEITHER OF THE TWO MODELS PROVED TO BE POWERFUL PREDICTORS OF FERTILITY DIFFERENTIALS AMONG MEXICAN AMERICANS. 18 REFERENCES. (JOURNAL ABSTRACT MODIFIED)

ACCN 000038

47 AUTH **ALVIREZ, D., & BEAN, F. D.**
TITL THE MEXICAN AMERICAN FAMILY.
SRCE *IN C. H. MINDEL & R. N. HABERSTEIN (EDS.), ETHNIC FAMILIES IN AMERICA: PATTERNS AND VARIATIONS. NEW YORK: ELSEVIER SCIENTIFIC PUBLISHING CO., 1976, PP. 271-291.*
INDX ACCULTURATION, CULTURAL CHANGE, CULTURAL FACTORS, DEMOGRAPHIC, ECONOMIC FACTORS, ESSAY, EMPLOYMENT, FAMILY ROLES, FAMILY STRUCTURE, FERTILITY, HISTORY, MEXICAN AMERICAN, SES, SEX ROLES, SOUTHWEST, STEREOTYPES, ENVIRONMENTAL FACTORS, TIME ORIENTATION
ABST AN HISTORICAL OVERVIEW, A DESCRIPTION OF ETHNIC FACTORS, AND A DEMOGRAPHIC CHARACTERIZATION OF MEXICAN AMERICANS ARE COMBINED IN AN EFFORT TO PORTRAY THE CHANGING MEXICAN AMERICAN FAMILY. THREE MEXICAN AMERICAN PERSONALITY TRAITS SAID TO STRONGLY REFLECT FAMILY PATTERNS ARE THE EMPHASIS ON PERSONS RATHER THAN GOALS, A DE-EMPHASIS OF MATERIALISM AND COMPETITION, AND A PRESENT TIME ORIENTATION. IN ADDITION, THE MEXICAN AMERICAN FAMILY STRUCTURE IS, TO A GREAT EXTENT, INFLUENCED BY FAMILISM (THE DEEP IMPORTANCE OF FAMILY TO ALL OF ITS MEMBERS), MALE DOMINANCE, AND THE SUBORDINATION OF YOUNGER PERSONS TO OLDER PERSONS. FINALLY, DEMOGRAPHIC CHARACTERISTICS OF THE MODERN MEXICAN AMERICAN FAMILY THAT DIFFER FROM THOSE OF ANGLOS INCLUDE: (1) HIGHER FERTILITY; (2) LOWER SES, AS MEASURED BY OCCUPATION, INCOME, AND EDUCATION; (3) LOWER FEMALE PARTICIPATION IN THE WORK FORCE;

(4) MALE UNDERREPRESENTATION IN WHITE COLLAR JOBS; AND (5) LOWER MEDIAN FAMILY INCOME. IN GENERALIZING ABOUT ETHNIC DIFFERENCES, IT IS DIFFICULT TO SORT OUT THE EFFECTS OF ETHNICITY VERSUS SES BECAUSE MEXICAN AMERICAN FAMILIES OF HIGH AND LOW SES DIFFER IN PLACE OF RESIDENCE, ACCULTURATION, RETENTION OF SPANISH LANGUAGE, AND SEX ROLES. MOREOVER, CONSIDERABLE DIVERSITY AND HETEROGENEITY OCCUR AMONG MEXICAN AMERICAN FAMILIES BECAUSE MEXICAN AMERICANS DO NOT CONFORM TO STEREOTYPES ASSIGNED TO THEM AND BECAUSE THE MEXICAN AMERICAN FAMILY HAS EXPERIENCED CHANGES RELATED TO GENERATION, CLASS DIFFERENCES, AND INCREASING URBANIZATION. AS MEXICAN AMERICAN FAMILIES HAVE BEEN EXPOSED TO AND PARTICIPATED IN URBAN, MIDDLE CLASS LIFE STYLES AND CULTURE, THE INTERNAL STRUCTURE OF THE FAMILY HAS CHANGED AND CAN BE EXPECTED TO CHANGE IN THE FUTURE. 26 REFERENCES.
ACCN 002007

48 AUTH **AMARO, H.**
TITL MULTIDIMENSIONAL SELF-CONCEPT OF ANGLO AND CHICANO CHILDREN.
SRCE *UNPUBLISHED MANUSCRIPT, DEPARTMENT OF PSYCHOLOGY, UNIVERSITY OF CALIFORNIA, LOS ANGELES, 1977.*
INDX SELF CONCEPT, CHILDREN, MEXICAN AMERICAN, CROSS CULTURAL, SEX COMPARISON, EMPIRICAL, ETHNIC IDENTITY, ACHIEVEMENT MOTIVATION, SOCIALIZATION, EDUCATION, SCHOLASTIC ACHIEVEMENT, CALIFORNIA, SOUTHWEST
ABST THE EFFECTS OF ETHNICITY, AGE AND SEX OF SUBJECT ON ETHNIC PREFERENCE WERE THE FOCUS OF THIS STUDY OF 432 SANTA BARBARA SCHOOL AGE CHILDREN. SIX DIMENSIONS OF SELF CONCEPT WERE INCLUDED IN THE FACTORIAL ANALYSIS: (1) SELF PERCEPTION; (2) SOCIAL SKILLS; (3) ACADEMIC SKILLS; (4) FUTURE ACHIEVEMENT; (5) TEACHER ATTITUDE/SCHOOL BEHAVIOR; AND (6) PHYSICAL/ATHLETIC SKILLS. PICTURES OF BLACK, ANGLO AND CHICANO CHILDREN WERE SHOWN TO THE SUBJECTS AS THEY WERE PRESENTED WITH THE SELF-CONCEPT QUESTIONS. SUBJECTS ANSWERED BY CHOOSING THE BLACK, ANGLO OR CHICANO PICTURE. ANALYSIS OF VARIANCE WITH REPEATED MEASURES ON CHOICE OF PICTURE YIELDED DIFFERENTIAL RESULTS FOR THE SIX DIMENSIONS. A DEVELOPMENTAL TREND OF INCREASING ANGLO CHOICES FOR SCHOOL AND ACHIEVEMENT-RELATED DIMENSIONS WAS EVIDENT TOGETHER WITH A SIMILAR TREND OF INCREASING ETHNIC CHOICES FOR ATHLETIC AND SOCIAL DIMENSIONS. 41 REFERENCES. (AUTHOR ABSTRACT MODIFIED)
ACCN 000039

49 AUTH **AMATORE, B., & LOYA, F.**
TITL AN ANALYSIS OF MINORITY AND WHITE SUICIDE RATES IN DENVER: 1960-1970.
SRCE *PAPER PRESENTED AT THE ANNUAL MEETING*

OF THE ROCKY MOUNTAIN PSYCHOLOGICAL ASSOCIATION, LAS VEGAS, 1973. (AVAILABLE FROM DR. FRED LOYA, DEPARTMENT OF PSYCHIATRY, NPI, UNIVERSITY OF CALIFORNIA, LOS ANGELES, CA 90024.)

INDX   SUICIDE, MEXICAN AMERICAN, CROSS CULTURAL, SEX COMPARISON, ADOLESCENTS, ADULTS, EMPIRICAL, COLORADO, SOUTHWEST

ABST   THE DATA PRESENTED FOR DENVER INDICATE THAT BLACK AND CHICANO SUICIDE RATES HAVE INCREASED FIVE TIMES AS RAPIDLY AS THOSE OF THE WHITE POPULATION. THE MAJORITY OF BLACK AND CHICANO SUICIDES OCCURRED BEFORE 40 YEARS OF AGE. THIS CONTRASTS WITH THE ANGLO AGE DISTRIBUTION PATTERN WHICH SHOWS THE MAJORITY OF SUICIDES OCCURRING AFTER 40. THE ASSESSMENT OF SUICIDE LETHALITY FOR MINORITY POPULATIONS MUST BE RE-DEFINED WITH REGARD TO THE MORE YOUTHFUL INCIDENCE OF SUICIDE AMONG MINORITY PERSONS. THE IMPLICATIONS OF THESE FINDINGS REGARDING THE URGENT NEED FOR CRISIS TREATMENT, FOLLOW-UP, AND OUTREACH CARE ARE DISCUSSED.

ACCN   000040

50   AUTH   **AMERICAN NURSES ASSOCIATION.**

TITL   MEMBERSHIP INCREASES CITED FOR ETHNIC NURSES OF COLOR.

SRCE   *THE AMERICAN NURSE, SEPTEMBER 1976, P. 10.*

INDX   NURSING, SES, SPANISH SURNAMED, REPRESENTATION, FEMALE

ABST   THIS BRIEF ARTICLE CITES RECENT INCREASES OF "ETHNIC NURSES OF COLOR." ON JULY 31, 1976, THE AMERICAN NURSES' ASSOCIATION (ANA) MEMBERSHIP TOTALED 197,310. THE ONE TABLE PROVIDED SHOWS THE PERCENTAGE DISTRIBUTION OF ANA MEMBERS BY RACE/ETHNICITY. THE LARGEST NONWHITE CATEGORIES IN ORDER ARE BLACK, FILIPINO, JAPANESE, AND SPANISH SURNAME. TOGETHER, ALL NONWHITE CATEGORIES ACCOUNT FOR 6.9% OF MEMBERSHIP, OR MORE THAN 13,500 MEMBERS. SINCE DECEMBER, 1973, EVERY CATEGORY OF NONWHITE MEMBERS EXCEPT AMERICAN INDIAN HAS GROWN FASTER THAN WHITE MEMBERSHIP. DURING THIS PERIOD, THE ASSOCIATION HAS EXPERIENCED A NET GROWTH OF 10,818 MEMBERS, OF WHICH 23.1% CONSISTED OF NONWHITE MEMBERS (1.9% SPANISH SURNAMED). THESE FIGURES DEMONSTRATE THAT, WHILE A LARGE MAJORITY OF ANA MEMBERS ARE WHITE, THE AMERICAN NURSES' ASSOCIATION IS EXPERIENCING SUCCESS IN RECRUITING NURSES ON THE VARIOUS NONWHITE ETHNIC CATEGORIES. OF NOTE, HOWEVER, IS THE FACT THAT SPANISH SURNAME MEMBER FIGURES ARE LOWER THAN ANY OTHER RACIAL/ETHNIC GROUP.

ACCN   002008

51   AUTH   **AMIN, A. E.**

TITL   CULTURE AND THE POST-HOSPITAL COMMUNITY ADJUSTMENT OF LONG-TERM HOSPITALIZED PUERTO RICAN SCHIZOPHRENIC PATIENTS IN NEW YORK CITY (DOCTORAL DISSERTATION, COLUMBIA UNIVERSITY, 1974).

SRCE   *DISSERTATION ABSTRACTS INTERNATIONAL, 1974, 35, 5964B. (UNIVERSITY MICROFILMS NO. 74-26,579).*

INDX   SCHIZOPHRENIA, MALE, PUERTO RICAN-M, EMPIRICAL, COMMUNITY, VALUES, INSTITUTIONALIZATION, PSYCHOSOCIAL ADJUSTMENT, ACCULTURATION, INTERPERSONAL RELATIONS, NEW YORK, EAST

ABST   THIS STUDY INVESTIGATES THE RELATIONSHIP BETWEEN CULTURAL VALUES AND THE POST-HOSPITAL COMMUNITY ADJUSTMENT OF MALE SCHIZOPHRENIC PUERTO RICAN EX-PATIENTS. THE HYPOTHESIS TESTED IS: EX-PATIENTS WHO HAVE RETAINED THEIR NATIVE CULTURAL VALUES ARE MORE LIKELY TO SHOW BETTER COMMUNITY READJUSTMENT PATTERNS THAN THOSE WHO DO NOT RETAIN THESE VALUES. THIS HYPOTHESIS WAS CONFIRMED. INFLUENCE OF THE INDIVIDUAL'S LIVING ARRANGEMENTS AND LENGTH OF LIVING IN THE U.S. ON HIS POST-HOSPITAL ADJUSTMENT ARE DISCUSSED. 169 REFERENCES. (AUTHOR ABSTRACT MODIFIED)

ACCN   000041

52   AUTH   **AMMONS, R. B., & AGUERO, A.**

TITL   THE FULL RANGE PICTURE VOCABULARY TEST: VII. RESULTS FOR A SPANISH AMERICAN SCHOOL AGED POPULATION

SRCE   *JOURNAL OF SOCIAL PSYCHOLOGY, 1950, 32(1), 3-10*

INDX   STANFORD-BINET INTELLIGENCE TEST, INTELLIGENCE TESTING, CHILDREN, EMPIRICAL, ADOLESCENTS, SPANISH SURNAMED, SES, BILINGUAL, COLORADO, SOUTHWEST

ABST   TO OBTAIN NORMS FOR SPANISH-AMERICAN (SA) CHILDREN ON THE FULL RANGE PICTURE VOCABULARY TEST (FRPVT), 80 SA CHILDREN FROM GRADES 1 TO 10 WERE TESTED ON BOTH THE FRPVT AND THE 1937 STANFORD-BINET. THE SAMPLE POPULATION WAS REPRESENTATIVE OF THE DENVER, COLORADO SA POPULATION WITH RESPECT TO OCCUPATIONS OF THE PARENTS. RELIABILITY COEFFICIENTS DISCLOSED THAT SCORES ON FORM A AND FORM B OF THE PICTURE VOCABULARY CORRELATED .86, .85, AND .82, RESPECTIVELY, WITH THE BINET VOCABULARY TEST RAW SCORES. THERE IS AN INDICATION OF REGULAR AGE PROGRESSION IN SCORES WHILE NO SEX DIFFERENCES IN PERFORMANCE WERE NOTED. THE PICTURE VOCABULARY TEST SCORES REVEAL LITTLE BILINGUAL HANDICAP AT THE EARLIER AGE LEVELS. IT IS FOUND THAT THE TEST HAS CONSIDERABLE INTEREST VALUE AND CAN BE ADMINISTERED IN A SHORT TIME. IT IS SUGGESTED THAT THE FRPVT CAN BE PROFITABLY USED IN THE INDIVIDUAL TESTING OF SPANISH-AMERICAN CHILDREN AND THAT THE SEPARATE NORMS FOR SA'S SHOULD BE USED WHEREVER INDICATED. 20 REFERENCES.

ACCN   000042

53   AUTH   **ANASTASI, A., & CORDOVA, F. D.**

TITL   SOME EFFECTS OF BILINGUALISM ON INTELLI-

GENCE TEST PERFORMANCE OF PUERTO RICAN SCHOOL CHILDREN IN NEW YORK CITY.

SRCE   *JOURNAL OF EDUCATIONAL PSYCHOLOGY, 1953, 44(1), 1-19.*

INDX   BILINGUALISM, INTELLIGENCE TESTING, PUERTO RICAN-M, CHILDREN, EMPIRICAL, CATTELL CULTURE-FREE INTELLIGENCE TEST, SEX COMPARISON, SES, ACCULTURATION, NEW YORK, EAST

ABST   ADMINISTRATION OF THE CATTELL "CULTURE FREE" TEST TO SPANISH-SPEAKING CHILDREN PROVIDES THE SETTING FOR EXAMINING THE EFFECTS OF BILINGUALISM UPON INTELLIGENCE TEST PERFORMANCE. TWO FORMS (2A AND 2B) OF THE TEST WERE GIVEN TO 176 PUERTO RICAN CHILDREN IN SPANISH AND IN ENGLISH USING A 2 BY 2 LATIN SQUARE DESIGN. AN ANALYSIS OF VARIANCE REVEALED SIGNIFICANT F-RATIOS FOR SUBJECTS, SESSIONS, AND ORDER-SEX INTERACTION. THE MOST OUTSTANDING FINDING IS THE MARKED IMPROVEMENT FROM FIRST TO SECOND TESTING SESSION, REGARDLESS OF LANGUAGE. ALTHOUGH THERE IS NO OVERALL SEX DIFFERENCE IN SCORE, THE GIRLS PERFORMED BETTER WHEN THE TESTING ORDER WAS SPANISH-ENGLISH, THE BOYS WHEN IT WAS ENGLISH-SPANISH. THIS ORDER-SEX INTERACTION IS ATTRIBUTED MAINLY TO THE RAPPORT BETWEEN THE CHILDREN AND EXAMINER. THE OVERALL PERFORMANCE OF THE GROUP IS CONSIDERABLY BELOW THE TEST NORMS REPORTED BY CATTELL. SOME REASONS ADVANCED FOR SUCH A DISCREPANCY ARE: THE VERY LOW SOCIOECONOMIC LEVEL OF THE PUERTO RICAN CHILDREN, THEIR BILINGUALISM WHICH MAKES THEM DEFICIENT IN BOTH LANGUAGES, THEIR EXTREME LACK OF TEST SOPHISTICATION, AND THEIR POOR EMOTIONAL ADJUSTMENT TO THE SCHOOL SITUATION. IT IS SUGGESTED THAT THE FIRST STEP FOR THE EFFECTIVE EDUCATION OF MIGRANT PUERTO RICAN CHILDREN IS TO FIND A SOLUTION FOR THE LANGUAGE PROBLEM WHICH GIVES RISE TO THE CHILDREN'S MALADJUSTMENT. 32 REFERENCES.

ACCN   000043

54   AUTH   **ANASTASI, A., & DEJESUS, C.**

TITL   LANGUAGE DEVELOPMENT AND NONVERBAL IQ OF PUERTO RICAN PRESCHOOL CHILDREN IN NEW YORK CITY.

SRCE   *JOURNAL OF ABNORMAL AND SOCIAL PSYCHOLOGY, 1953, 48(3), 357-366.*

INDX   CHILDREN, EMPIRICAL, PUERTO RICAN-M, GOODENOUGH DRAW-A-MAN TEST, LANGUAGE ACQUISITION, BILINGUALISM, INTELLIGENCE TESTING, NEW YORK, EAST

ABST   LANGUAGE DEVELOPMENT AND NONVERBAL IQ WERE MEASURED IN 50 5-YEAR-OLD PUERTO RICAN CHILDREN IN NEW YORK CITY. EACH CHILD'S LANGUAGE WAS RECORDED IN BOTH SPANISH AND ENGLISH, BUT ALL TESTING WAS CONDUCTED BY A PUERTO RICAN EXAMINER WHO SPOKE IN SPANISH EXCLUSIVELY. IT WAS FOUND THAT CHILDREN USED SPANISH ALMOST ENTIRELY; ONLY ABOUT 2 PERCENT OF THEIR WORDS AND LESS THAN 1 PERCENT OF

THEIR SENTENCES WERE SPOKEN IN ENGLISH. THE PERFORMANCE OF THE PUERTO RICAN CHILDREN WAS COMPARED TO THAT OF 50 WHITE AND 50 NEGRO 5-YEAR-OLD CHILDREN TESTED WITH THE SAME PROCEDURES IN AN EARLIER STUDY BY ANASTASI AND D'ANGELO. ALTHOUGH THE EDUCATIONAL AND OCCUPATIONAL LEVELS OF THE PUERTO RICAN PARENTS WERE LOWER THAN THOSE OF WHITE AND NEGRO PARENTS, THE PUERTO RICAN CHILDREN DID NOT DIFFER SIGNIFICANTLY FROM THE WHITE OR NEGRO GROUPS IN THE GOODENOUGH DRAW-A-MAN TEST. THE PUERTO RICAN CHILDREN SUPERSEDED THE WHITE AND NEGRO GROUPS IN MEAN SENTENCE LENGTH AND IN MATURITY OF SENTENCE STRUCTURE. IT IS SUGGESTED THAT THE GREATER EXTENT OF ADULT CONTACT IN THE HOME ENVIRONMENT OF PUERTO RICAN CHILDREN IS A POSSIBLE EXPLANATION FOR THEIR SUPERIORITY IN EARLY LINGUISTIC DEVELOPMENT. 18 REFERENCES.

ACCN   000044

55   AUTH   **ANCHOR, K. N., & ANCHOR, F. N.**

TITL   SCHOOL FAILURE AND PARENTAL SCHOOL INVOLVEMENT IN AN ETHNICALLY MIXED SCHOOL.

SRCE   *JOURNAL OF COMMUNITY PSYCHOLOGY, 1974, 2(3), 265-267.*

INDX   MEXICAN AMERICAN, PARENTAL INVOLVEMENT, SCHOLASTIC ACHIEVEMENT, CROSS CULTURAL

ABST   RESULTS OF A SURVEY WHICH INVESTIGATED THE RELATIONSIP BETWEEN SCHOOL FAILURE AND PARENTAL INVOLVEMENT INDICATE THAT PARENTS OF CHILDREN WITH LOW SUCCESS WERE FEWER IN ATTENDANCE AT SCHEDULED PARENT-TEACHER CONFERENCES THAN PARENTS OF CHILDREN WITH HIGH SUCCESS. THIS FINDING WAS MORE PRONOUNCED FOR MEXICAN AMERICAN PARENTS. RESULTS ARE DISCUSSED IN TERMS OF THE FUTURE APPLICATION OF LEARNING THEORY AS A POSSIBLE ALTERNATIVE TO THE PRESENT EDUCATIONAL STRUCTURE AND ITS PREDOMINANT SUCCESS-FAILURE APPROACH TO STUDENT PERFORMANCE. 7 REFERENCES.

ACCN   000045

56   AUTH   **ANDERS, A., PARLADE, R., CHATEL, J., & PEELE, R.**

TITL   WHY WE DID NOT ESTABLISH A SEPARATE COMPLETE PROGRAM FOR SPANISH SPEAKING PATIENTS.

SRCE   *IN E. R. PADILLA & A. M. PADILLA (EDS.), TRANSCULTURAL PSYCHIATRY: AN HISPANIC PERSPECTIVE (MONOGRAPH NO. 4). LOS ANGELES: UNIVERSITY OF CALIFORNIA, SPANISH SPEAKING MENTAL HEALTH RESEARCH CENTER, 1977, PP. 63-66.*

INDX   ACCULTURATION, BILINGUAL, SPANISH SURNAMED, ADMINISTRATORS, ESSAY, CASE STUDY, PSYCHOTHERAPY

ABST   THE PROCESS BEHIND A DECISION NOT TO ESTABLISH A SEPARATE HOSPITAL UNIT FOR SPANISH-SPEAKING PATIENTS IS DISCUSSED. BASICALLY, TWO POSITIONS AND THEIR SUPPORTIVE ARGUMENTS ARE PRESENTED: (1) A

TOTALLY SEPARATE UNIT WILL PROVIDE ALL SERVICES IN A MANNER CULTURALLY SENSITIVE AND RESPONSIVE TO LATINOS; AND (2) A BILINGUAL/BICULTURAL COORDINATOR AND OTHER BILINGUAL/BICULTURAL STAFF WILL PROVIDE SUFFICIENT SERVICES TO LATINO PATIENTS. AN INTERESTING ASPECT OF THIS PROCESS IS THAT THE SPANISH-SPEAKING CLINICIANS WERE STRONGLY AGAINST THE SEPARATE UNIT FOR THESE REASONS: (1) PLACING ALL SPANISH-SPEAKING PATIENTS ON ONE WARD WOULD BE DISCRIMINATORY; AND (2) THE PATIENTS ARE AMERICAN AND NOT INTERESTED IN SEGREGATION. TWO ASPECTS OF THE DECISION WERE EMPHASIZED: (1) THAT THE SPANISH-SPEAKING PROFESSIONALS WERE LIKELY TO BE THE ONES WHO ADJUSTED WELL TO AMERICAN SOCIETY; AND (2) THAT THE PATIENTS AND THEIR COMMUNITY SHOULD BE CONSULTED REGARDING THEIR DESIRE FOR SEPARATE FACILITIES. 2 REFERENCES.

ACCN   000046

57   AUTH   **ANDERSON, A. H., & NOVINA, J.**
     TITL   A STUDY OF THE RELATIONSHIP OF THE TESTS OF CENTRAL AUDITORY ABILITIES AND THE ILLINOIS TEST OF PSYCHOLINGUISTIC ABILITIES.
     SRCE   *JOURNAL OF LEARNING DISABILITIES, 1973, 6(3), 46-48.*
     INDX   ITPA, CALIFORNIA, SOUTHWEST, CHILDREN, MEXICAN AMERICAN, CROSS CULTURAL, TEST RELIABILITY, TEST VALIDITY, ABILITY TESTING, LANGUAGE ACQUISITION, LANGUAGE ASSESSMENT, LINGUISTIC COMPETENCE, PHONOLOGY, PERCEPTION, EMPIRICAL
     ABST   TO EXAMINE THE RELATIONSHIP OF THE FLOWERS-COSTELLO TESTS OF CENTRAL AUDITORY ABILITIES (TCAA) AND THE ILLINOIS TEST OF PSYCHOLINGUISTIC ABILITIES (ITPA), 17 MEXICAN AMERICAN AND 3 BLACK KINDERGARTEN CHILDREN IN SOUTHERN CALIFORNIA WERE ADMINISTERED BOTH TESTS. PEARSON PRODUCT-MOMENT CORRELATION COEFFICIENTS REVEALED SIGNIFICANT RELATIONSHIPS BETWEEN THE TCAA AND THE ITPA AUDITORY SUBTESTS. FURTHER, THE TWO SUBTESTS OF THE TCAA INDICATED DIFFERENT SENSITIVITY TO ABILITIES USED ON THE ITPA, SUGGESTING THAT SEPARATE SUBTEST NORMS AND TOTAL RAW SCORE NORMS BOTH WOULD ENHANCE THE FUTURE DIAGNOSTIC UTILITY OF THE TCAA. 2 REFERENCES. (JOURNAL ABSTRACT MODIFIED)
     ACCN   000047

58   AUTH   **ANDERSON, J. G., & EVANS, F. B.**
     TITL   FAMILY SOCIALIZATION AND EDUCATIONAL ACHIEVEMENT IN TWO CULTURES: MEXICAN AMERICAN AND ANGLO AMERICAN.
     SRCE   *SOCIOMETRY, 1976, 39(3), 209-222.*
     INDX   MEXICAN AMERICAN, ADOLESCENTS, SOCIALIZATION, CHILDREARING PRACTICES, ACHIEVEMENT MOTIVATION, SELF CONCEPT, SCHOLASTIC ACHIEVEMENT, FATALISM, SCHOLASTIC ASPIRATIONS, INSTRUCTIONAL TECHNIQUES, CROSS CULTURAL, EMPIRICAL, NEW MEXICO, SOUTHWEST
     ABST   THIS STUDY EXAMINED VARIATIONS IN FAMILY

SOCIALIZATION PRACTICES AMONG ANGLO AMERICANS AND MEXICAN AMERICANS AND THE EFFECT OF THESE PRACTICES ON ACHIEVEMENT VALUES, SELF-CONCEPT AND EDUCATIONAL ACHIEVEMENT. DATA WERE COLLECTED FROM 102 JUNIOR HIGH SCHOOL STUDENTS AND THEIR FAMILIES. THE MEXICAN AMERICANS APPARENTLY EXPERIENCED MUCH LESS INDEPENDENCE TRAINING AND WERE GRANTED LITTLE AUTONOMY IN DECISION MAKING; THEY WERE FOUND TO HAVE LITTLE CONFIDENCE IN THEIR ABILITY TO SUCCEED IN SCHOOL AND TO BE SOMEWHAT FATALISTIC ABOUT THEIR FUTURE DESPITE THE HIGH LEVEL OF ACHIEVEMENT TRAINING THEY WERE EXPOSED TO IN THE HOME. RESULTS ALSO SUGGEST THAT DIRECT ATTEMPTS TO ENCOURAGE GREATER ACADEMIC EFFORT ON THE PART OF THE STUDENTS MAY ACTUALLY INHIBIT ACADEMIC PERFORMANCE. IN CONTRAST, PARENTAL INDEPENDENCE TRAINING RESULTS IN SIGNIFICANT GAINS IN ACHIEVEMENT AMONG BOTH GROUPS OF STUDENTS BY INCREASING THE STUDENT'S CONFIDENCE IN COPING WITH HIS PHYSICAL AND SOCIAL ENVIRONMENT. SUCH TRAINING MAY BE CRITICAL AMONG MEXICAN AMERICAN STUDENTS IF THEY ARE TO PERFORM WELL IN CLASSROOMS WHICH REQUIRE THAT THEY WORK LARGELY ON THEIR OWN INITIATIVE. 55 REFERENCES. (JOURNAL ABSTRACT)

ACCN   000048

59   AUTH   **ANDERSON, J. G., & JOHNSON, W. H.**
     TITL   SOCIAL AND CULTURAL CHARACTERISTICS OF MEXICAN-AMERICAN FAMILIES LIVING IN SOUTH EL PASO, TEXAS.
     SRCE   *PAPER PREPARED FOR THE JOINT MEETING OF THE AMERICAN ASSOCIATION FOR THE ADVANCEMENT OF SCIENCES WITH THE NATIONAL COUNCIL OF TEACHERS OF MATHEMATICS, DALLAS, DECEMBER 27, 1968. (ERIC DOCUMENT REPRODUCTION SERVICE NO. ED 026 175)*
     INDX   CULTURE, FAMILY STRUCTURE, MEXICAN AMERICAN, ATTITUDES, EDUCATION, SCHOLASTIC ACHIEVEMENT, SCHOLASTIC ASPIRATIONS, TEACHERS, ACHIEVEMENT MOTIVATION, CULTURAL FACTORS, MATHEMATICS, SES, TEXAS, SOUTHWEST, URBAN
     ABST   A STUDY OF URBAN SPANISH-SPEAKING CHILDREN AND THEIR FAMILIES IN SOUTH EL PASO, TEXAS SOUGHT TO IDENTIFY CULTURAL AND SOCIAL CHARACTERISTICS OF THE CHILDREN WITH RESPECT TO LANGUAGE PATTERNS, BASIC ATTITUDES TOWARDS SCHOOL AND MATHEMATICS, SELF-CONCEPT OF ABILITY, ATTITUDES TOWARDS PEERS, AND ACHIEVEMENT MOTIVATION. GENERAL CHARACTERISTICS OF THE STUDENT'S FAMILY WITH RESPECT TO SOCIOECONOMIC STATUS, LANGUAGE PATTERNS, ATTITUDES TOWARD SCHOOL AND MATHEMATICS, AND THE AMOUNT OF SUPPORT GIVEN TO THE CHILD TO ASSIST HIM IN HIS SCHOOL WORK WERE ALSO INVESTIGATED. ALTHOUGH THE STUDENTS CAME FROM LARGE, IMPOVERISHED FAMILIES WHERE PARENTS' EDUCATIONAL LEVELS WERE RELA-

TIVELY LOW, HIGHER EDUCATIONAL ASPIRATION FOR THE CHILDREN WAS EVIDENT. ALTHOUGH LACK OF SUPPORT OF THE CHILDREN IN SCHOOL WAS APPARENT, PARENTS FELT THAT EVERYTHING THE CHILDREN STUDY WILL BE VALUABLE TO THEM OUTSIDE SCHOOL. IT IS CONCLUDED THAT MOTIVATIONAL FACTORS ARE FAR MORE IMPORTANT IN PREDICTING SUCCESS IN MATHEMATICS THAN ARE THE EDUCATIONAL LEVEL OR LANGUAGE OF THE PARENTS. (RIE ABSTRACT MODIFIED)

ACCN   000050

60   AUTH   **ANDERSON, J. G., & JOHNSON, W. H.**
     TITL   SOCIOCULTURAL DETERMINANTS OF ACHIEVEMENT AMONG MEXICAN-AMERICAN STUDENTS.
     SRCE   *LAS CRUCES, NEW MEXICO: NEW MEXICO STATE UNIVERSITY, 1968. (ERIC DOCUMENT REPRODUCTION SERVICE NO. ED 017 394)*
     INDX   EDUCATION, SCHOLASTIC ACHIEVEMENT, BILINGUALISM, LANGUAGE LEARNING, CULTURE, CULTURAL FACTORS, POVERTY, SES, MEXICAN AMERICAN, SELF CONCEPT, ACHIEVEMENT MOTIVATION, SCHOLASTIC ACHIEVEMENT, EMPIRICAL, SOUTHWEST
     ABST   THE PRELIMINARY FINDINGS OF THE SOUTHWEST EDUCATIONAL DEVELOPMENT LABORATORY'S MATHEMATICS PROJECT ARE PRESENTED IN THIS MONOGRAPH. IN THE FIRST PHASE OF THE PROJECT, AN ATTEMPT WAS MADE TO IDENTIFY THOSE CHARACTERISTICS OF MEXICAN AMERICAN FAMILIES THAT MAY AFFECT THE EDUCATIONAL ACHIEVEMENT OF THEIR CHILDREN. DATA WERE COLLECTED AND ANALYZED FOR 263 HIGH SCHOOL STUDENTS (GRADES 7-12) IN A SOUTHWESTERN COMMUNITY. THE STUDENT QUESTIONNAIRE REVEALED 9 INDEPENDENT FACTORS CHARACTERIZING THE EMPHASIS THAT PARENTS PLACE ON EDUCATION, THE LANGUAGE USED IN THE HOME, AND THE CHILD'S SELF-IMAGE AND ACADEMIC MOTIVATION. THE RESULTS SUGGEST THAT MEXICAN AMERICAN CHILDREN MAY NOT HAVE AS MUCH CONFIDENCE IN THEIR ABILITY TO SUCCEED IN SCHOOL AS THEIR CLASSMATES. FOR EXAMPLE, ACHIEVEMENT IN BOTH ENGLISH AND MATHEMATICS APPEARS TO BE HIGHLY AFFECTED BY THE CHILD'S CONFIDENCE IN HIS ABILITY TO SUCCEED IN SCHOOL AND BY THE EMPHASIS THE PARENTS PLACE ON EDUCATION, WHILE HIS MASTERY OF ENGLISH APPEARS TO BE INFLUENCED BY THE LANGUAGE SPOKEN IN THE HOME AND BY THE FATHER'S EDUCATIONAL BACKGROUND. IN CONTRAST, ACHIEVEMENT IN MATHEMATICS APPEARS TO BE RELATED TO THE STUDENT'S DESIRE TO ACHIEVE IN SCHOOL. THE RESULTS OF THIS STUDY SUGGEST THAT IT MAY BE POSSIBLE TO IMPROVE THE ACADEMIC PERFORMANCE OF MANY MEXICAN AMERICAN CHILDREN BY PROPER DESIGN OF EDUCATIONAL PROGRAMS. 44 REFERENCES. (RIE ABSTRACT MODIFIED)

ACCN   000051

61   AUTH   **ANDERSON, J. G., & JOHNSON, W. H.**
     TITL   STABILITY AND CHANGE AMONG THREE GEN-

ERATIONS OF MEXICAN AMERICANS: FACTORS AFFECTING ACHIEVEMENT.
     SRCE   *AMERICAN EDUCATIONAL RESEARCH JOURNAL, 1971, 8(2), 285-309.*
     INDX   MEXICAN AMERICAN, SCHOLASTIC ACHIEVEMENT, ACHIEVEMENT MOTIVATION, SELF CONCEPT, SES, CULTURAL FACTORS, EDUCATION, ADOLESCENTS, SURVEY, EMPIRICAL, BILINGUAL, ACCULTURATION, CROSS CULTURAL, CROSS GENERATIONAL, SOUTHWEST, NEW MEXICO
     ABST   AN EXAMINATION OF SOCIOCULTURAL CHANGE AND THE INFLUENCE OF THE HOME ENVIRONMENT ON THE ACHIEVEMENT OF MEXICAN AMERICAN (MA) CHILDREN IN THE EDUCATIONAL SYSTEM IS PRESENTED. A STRATIFIED SAMPLE OF 163 JUNIOR AND SENIOR HIGH SCHOOL STUDENTS WERE ADMINISTERED A QUESTIONNAIRE TO ASSESS THE ACHIEVEMENT CHARACTERISTICS OF EACH CHILD IN THE FAMILY. THE NINE FACTORS IN THE QUESTIONNAIRE ARE AS FOLLOWS: (1) LANGUAGE USAGE IN THE FAMILY; (2) STUDENT'S DESIRE TO ACHIEVE IN SCHOOL; (3) PARTICIPATION IN EXTRACURRICULAR ACTIVITIES; (4) PARENTAL STRESS ON ACADEMIC ACHIEVEMENT; (5) PARENTAL STRESS ON COMPLETING HIGH SCHOOL; (6) PARENTAL STRESS ON ATTENDING COLLEGE; (7) PARENTAL ASSISTANCE WITH SCHOOL WORK; (8) SELF-CONCEPT OF ABILITY; AND (9) STUDENT'S EDUCATIONAL ASPIRATIONS. IT IS DISCLOSED THAT THERE IS LITTLE DIFFERENCE BETWEEN MA FAMILIES AND OTHER FAMILIES WITH RESPECT TO THE AMOUNT OF EMPHASIS ON EDUCATION THAT THE CHILD EXPERIENCES IN THE HOME. THIS CONTRADICTS THE NOTION THAT MA FAMILIES PLACE LITTLE EMPHASIS ON EDUCATION AND ACHIEVEMENT. THE MOST SIGNIFICANT FINDING IS THAT MA CHILDREN MAY HAVE LESS CONFIDENCE IN THEIR ABILITY TO SUCCESSFULLY FULFILL THE EXPECTATIONS OF THEIR PARENTS AND THE SCHOOL THAN THEIR PEERS. IT IS SUGGESTED THAT DESIGNING EDUCATIONAL PROGRAMS THAT DIRECTLY ATTEMPT TO IMPROVE THE DEGREE OF CONFIDENCE THAT MA CHILDREN HAVE IN THEIR ABILITY TO SUCCEED IN SCHOOL MAY IMPROVE THEIR ACADEMIC PERFORMANCE. 21 REFERENCES.

ACCN   000052

62   AUTH   **ANDERSON, J. G., & SAFAR, D.**
     TITL   THE INFLUENCE OF DIFFERENTIAL COMMUNITY PERCEPTION ON THE PROVISION OF EQUAL EDUCATIONAL OPPORTUNITIES.
     SRCE   *SOCIOLOGY OF EDUCATION, 1967, 40(3), 219-230.*
     INDX   EQUAL OPPORTUNITY, EDUCATION, CROSS CULTURAL, SPANISH SURNAMED, ATTITUDES, SCHOLASTIC ACHIEVEMENT, ACHIEVEMENT MOTIVATION, SELF CONCEPT, EMPIRICAL, ADULTS, SOUTHWEST, INDIGENOUS POPULATIONS
     ABST   EXTENSIVE INTERVIEWS WITH COMMUNITY MEMBERS AND SCHOOL PERSONNEL IN TWO MULTICULTURAL SOUTHWESTERN COMMUNITIES DEMONSTRATE THE IMPORTANCE OF PERCEPTIONS AND ATTITUDES IN THE PROVISION

OF EQUAL EDUCATIONAL OPPORTUNITY FOR SPANISH AMERICAN AND INDIAN CHILDREN. THE FINDINGS REVEAL A UBIQUITOUS FEELING THAT SPANISH AMERICAN AND INDIAN CHILDREN ARE LESS CAPABLE OF ACHIEVING DESIRABLE GOALS THAN ARE THEIR ANGLO PEERS. THIS LACK OF ACHIEVEMENT OF THE MINORITY GROUPS APPEARS, IN A LARGE PART, TO BE PERCEIVED AS A LACK OF INNATE ABILITY AND SUPPORT RATHER THAN AS THE FAULT OF INADEQUATE SCHOOL PROGRAMS. MOREOVER, THIS FEELING OF INFERIORITY APPEARS TO BE INTERNALIZED BY THE MINORITY GROUPS THEMSELVES, THUS CREATING AN INSIDIOUS NEGATIVE CLIMATE FOR THEIR CHILDREN. 21 REFERENCES.

ACCN   000053

63   AUTH   **ANDERSON, M.**

TITL   A COMPARATIVE STUDY OF THE ENGLISH SPEAKING AND SPANISH SPEAKING BEGINNERS IN THE PUBLIC SCHOOLS.

SRCE   *SAN FRANCISCO: R AND E RESEARCH ASSOCIATES, 1976. (REPRINTED FROM AN UNPUBLISHED MASTER'S THESIS, UNIVERSITY OF TEXAS, 1951.)*

INDX   SCHOLASTIC ACHIEVEMENT, SES, SPANISH SURNAMED, ACHIEVEMENT TESTING, INTELLIGENCE, EDUCATION, CROSS CULTURAL, EMPIRICAL, ENVIRONMENTAL FACTORS, CHILDREN, TEXAS, SOUTHWEST, MEXICAN AMERICAN

ABST   THE ABILITY, SOCIOECONOMIC STATUS, AND ACHIEVEMENT OF THE BEGINNING PUPILS OF THE ELEMENTARY PUBLIC SCHOOLS OF MCALLEN, HIDALGO COUNTY, TEXAS, IN 1950 WERE STUDIED. THE OBJECTIVE WAS TO UNDERSTAND THE PROBLEMS IN THOSE SCHOOLS WHERE BOTH ENGLISH-SPEAKING AND SPANISH-SPEAKING PUPILS ARE ENROLLED IN LARGE NUMBERS. TEST DATA OF TWO KINDS WERE OBTAINED: (1) MEASURES OF APTITUDE AT THE BEGINNING OF THE YEAR; AND (2) MEASURES OF ACHIEVEMENT AT THE END OF THE YEAR. SOCIOECONOMIC STATUS WAS DETERMINED BY HOME VISITS AND RATED BY THE INDEX OF STATUS CHARACTERISTICS AND THE INDEX OF CLASS-TYPED VALUE ATTITUDES. THE MAJOR CONCLUSIONS ARE: (1) ENGLISH-SPEAKING STUDENTS HOLD A DECIDED ADVANTAGE OVER SPANISH-SPEAKING STUDENTS IN SOCIOECONOMIC STATUS, IN GENERAL MENTAL ABILITY AS MEASURED BY THE TEST USED, AND IN ACHIEVEMENT AS MEASURED BY TEST SCORES AND SCHOOL MARKS; (2) THE SIGNIFICANT CORRELATION OF EVERY FACTOR EXCEPT ONE WITH THE SOCIAL STATUS OF THE SPANISH-SPEAKING PUPILS SUGGESTS THAT IN ALL PROBABILITY A REMOVAL OF THE ENVIRONMENTAL HANDICAPS WOULD BE FOLLOWED BY AN INCREASE IN SCORES ON BOTH GENERAL MENTAL ABILITY AND ACHIEVEMENT; (3) VERY LOW CORRELATIONS BETWEEN SCHOOL MARKS AND THE OTHER FACTORS INDICATE THAT TEACHERS OF THE SPANISH-SPEAKING PUPILS FIND IT MORE DIFFICULT THAN TEACHERS OF THE ENGLISH-SPEAKING STUDENTS TO ASSIGN PROPER SCHOOL RATINGS; AND (4)

THE TESTS OF GENERAL MENTAL ABILITY ARE BETTER PREDICTORS OF READING SUCCESS WITH ENGLISH-SPEAKING STUDENTS THAN WITH SPANISH-SPEAKING STUDENTS. 27 REFERENCES. (AUTHOR SUMMARY MODIFIED)

ACCN   000054

64   AUTH   **ANDERSSON, T., & BOYER, M.**

TITL   BILINGUAL SCHOOLING IN THE UNITED STATES (2ND. ED.).

SRCE   *AUSTIN, TEXAS: NATIONAL EDUCATIONAL LABORATORY PUBLICATIONS, 1978.*

INDX   BILINGUALISM, BILINGUAL-BICULTURAL EDUCATION, BILINGUAL-BICULTURAL PERSONNEL, LEGISLATION, CURRICULUM, INSTRUCTIONAL TECHNIQUES, IMMIGRATION, REVIEW, PROFESSIONAL TRAINING, TEACHERS, MEXICAN AMERICAN, PUERTO RICAN-M, CUBAN, BIBLIOGRAPHY, BOOK

ABST   BILINGUAL EDUCATION (B.E.) AS A PROMISING MOVEMENT TOWARDS EQUALIZING ACCESS TO EDUCATION FOR BOTH NON-ENGLISH-SPEAKING AND ENGLISH-SPEAKING CHILDREN IS PRESENTED. AN HISTORICAL OVERVIEW OF B.E. AND THE DYNAMICS OF IMPLEMENTING B.E. PROGRAMS ARE DISCUSSED IN RELATION TO THE FOLLOWING: (1) WHAT IS BILINGUALISM?; (2) BILINGUAL SCHOOLING IN THE UNITED STATES; (3) A RATIONALE FOR BILINGUAL SCHOOLING; (4) PLANNING A BILINGUAL PROGRAM; (5) THE PROGRAM; AND (6) PRESCHOOL BILINGUAL EDUCATION. AN ANALYSIS OF THE OVERALL IMPLICATIONS OF B.E. ON EDUCATION AND SOCIETY SUGGESTS THAT THE FOLLOWING SHORT TERM BENEFITS SHOULD OCCUR WITHIN THE NEXT FIVE YEARS: (1) NON-ENGLISH-SPEAKING CHILDREN WILL ACQUIRE CONFIDENT SELF IMAGES, READING AND SKILLS IN TWO LANGUAGES, FLUENT ENGLISH-SPEAKING SKILLS, CULTURAL AWARENESS, AND CROSS-CULTURAL UNDERSTANDING; (2) INCREASED COMMUNITY SUPPORT THROUGH THE SUCCESS OF B.E. PROGRAMS; AND (3) EXPANDED LEGISLATION TO ASSURE B.E. RESOURCES IN EDUCATION. THE TWO MOST POWERFUL FACTORS AFFECTING THE CURRENT DEVELOPMENT OF B.E. ARE WIDESPREAD ETHNOCENTRISM AND SHORT-SIGHTED ECONOMIC VIEWS. FOR B.E. TO BECOME A SUCCESSFUL METHOD OF EDUCATION, CULTURAL PLURALISM AND HOME EDUCATION MUST OCCUR. INCLUDED ARE 13 APPENDICES OF NATIONAL AND INTERNATIONAL B.E. CONCERNS AND AN INDEPTH BIBLIOGRAPHY OF 870 SOURCES WITH A BIBLIOGRAPHY INDEX.

ACCN   000055

65   AUTH   **ANDRULIS, D. P.**

TITL   ETHNICITY AS A VARIABLE IN THE UTILIZATION AND REFERRAL PATTERNS OF A COMPREHENSIVE MENTAL HEALTH CENTER.

SRCE   *JOURNAL OF COMMUNITY PSYCHOLOGY, 1977, 5, 231-237.*

INDX   ADOLESCENTS, CROSS CULTURAL, CULTURAL FACTORS, EMPIRICAL, MENTAL HEALTH, MEXICAN AMERICAN, NEUROSIS, PSYCHOSIS, PSYCHOTHERAPISTS, PSYCHOTHERAPY OUT-

COME, RESOURCE UTILIZATION, TEXAS, SOUTHWEST, HEALTH DELIVERY SYSTEMS, ADULTS, PSYCHOTHERAPY, SYMPTOMA-TOLOGY

ABST   A 50% SAMPLE OF THE 1972 POPULATION OF TERMINATED CASES AT A SAN ANTONIO, TEXAS, COMPREHENSIVE MENTAL HEALTH CENTER WAS EXAMINED FOR UTILIZATION AND REFERRAL PATTERNS OF BLACK (N = 87), MEXICAN AMERI-CAN (N = 567), AND ANGLO (N = 496) CLIENTS. IT WAS EXPECTED THAT THE MEXICAN AMERI-CANS WOULD BE REFERRED BY FAMILY OR FRIENDS LESS OFTEN, AND THAT MEXICAN AMERICAN AND BLACK CLIENTS WOULD BE CLASSIFIED AS PSYCHOTIC WHILE ANGLOS AS NEUROTIC. ADDITIONALLY, DUE TO THE DIFFI-CULTIES IN PROVIDING RELEVANT SERVICES TO THE MINORITY GROUPS, IT WAS PREDICTED THAT MEXICAN AMERICAN AND BLACK CLIENTS WOULD TERMINATE TREATMENT EARLIER AND, AS A RESULT, RECEIVE FEWER REFERRALS TO OTHER FACILITIES OR CARETAKERS IN THE COMMUNITY. IN ACCORD WITH THE EXPECTA-TIONS, MEXICAN AMERICANS TENDED TO BE REFERRED TO THE CENTER LESS OFTEN BY FAMILY OR FRIENDS. SECOND, AT THE CENTER, YOUNG MEXICAN AMERICAN CLIENTS TENDED TO BE DIAGNOSED AS HAVING TRANSIENT SITUATIONAL DISORDERS, WITH A SUBSTAN-TIAL NUMBER ALSO CLASSIFIED AS HAVING PERSONALITY DISORDERS. IT WAS ALSO FOUND THAT BETWEEN THEIR DIAGNOSIS AND DIS-CHARGE, CERTAIN FACTORS CAUSED THE MEXICAN AMERICANS TO DROP OUT PREMA-TURELY, WHILE ANGLOS CONTINUED IN TREAT-MENT LONG ENOUGH TO RECEIVE CLOSED-CASE EVALUATIONS. THIS DISILLUSIONMENT THAT MEXICAN AMERICANS HAD WITH THE MENTAL HEALTH SYSTEM AND THEIR PREMA-TURE TERMINATION OF SERVICES MAY RESULT FROM: (1) CULTURAL DIFFERENCES BETWEEN STAFF AND THE YOUNG MEXICAN AMERICAN CLIENT; (2) DIFFERENT PERCEPTIONS OF MEN-TAL ILLNESS; OR (3) THE MEXICAN AMERICAN RELIANCE ON THE EXTENDED FAMILY FOR SUPPORT AND GUIDANCE. IN VIEW OF THIS, THE DIFFICULTIES IN PROVIDING EFFECTIVE AND CONTINUOUS CARE, ESPECIALLY TO YOUNG CLIENTS, ARE DISCUSSED. 13 REFER-ENCES. (JOURNAL ABSTRACT MODIFIED)

ACCN   002009

66 AUTH **ANGLE, J.**

TITL   MAINLAND CONTROL OF MANUFACTURING AND REWARD FOR BILINGUALISM IN PUERTO RICO.

SRCE *AMERICAN SOCIOLOGICAL REVIEW, 1976, 41(2), 289-307.*

INDX PUERTO RICAN-I, ECONOMIC FACTORS, BILIN-GUALISM, SES, ADULTS, REVIEW, PREJUDICE, LABOR FORCE

ABST   THE LITERATURE ON LANGUAGE GROUP/RE-LATIONS IN THE ECONOMY OF QUEBEC PROV-INCE SUGGESTS THAT MORE FRENCH CANA-DIANS ARE BILINGUAL THAN ENGLISH CANADIANS BECAUSE MANY BUSINESSES USE ENGLISH AND ARE OWNED OR OPERATED BY ENGLISH CANADIANS. BILINGUAL FRENCH CA-NADIANS ARE REWARDED, ON THE AVERAGE,

BY PLACEMENT INTO BETTER OCCUPATIONS. THE HYPOTHESIS IS MADE THAT A SIMILAR RE-WARD EXISTS FOR BILINGUALISM IN ENGLISH IN THE SPANISH MOTHER TONGUE LABOR FORCE IN PUERTO RICO. THE 1970 CENSUS OF POPULATION IN PUERTO RICO PROVIDED DATA FOR A TEST OF THIS HYPOTHESIS IN WHICH THE REWARD IS DEMONSTRATED. IT IS ALSO HYPOTHESIZED THAT IT IS MAINLAND AMERI-CAN OWNERSHIP OF BUSINESSES WHICH AC-COUNTS FOR THIS REWARD. THESE HYPOTHE-SES WERE TESTED ON THE LABOR FORCE IN MANUFACTURING AND WERE NOT CON-FIRMED. 27 REFERENCES. (JOURNAL AB-STRACT MODIFIED)

ACCN   000056

67 AUTH **ANTONOVSKY, A.**

TITL   ASPIRATIONS, CLASS AND RACIAL-ETHNIC MEMBERSHIP.

SRCE *JOURNAL OF NEGRO EDUCATION, 1967, 36(4), 385-393.*

INDX ADOLESCENTS, EMPIRICAL, PUERTO RICAN-M, CROSS CULTURAL, SES, ACHIEVEMENT MOTI-VATION, FAMILY STRUCTURE, URBAN, SCHO-LASTIC ASPIRATIONS, SEX COMPARISON, EAST

ABST   A COMPARISON OF THE LEVEL OF ASPIRATION AMONG MIDDLE- AND LOWER-CLASS ANGLO AMERICAN, NEGRO, AND PUERTO RICAN TENTH-GRADE MALE AND FEMALE HIGH SCHOOL STUDENTS IS PRESENTED. THE 378 SUBJECTS WERE ADMINISTERED A QUESTION-NAIRE RELATED TO THEIR FUTURE SOCIOECO-NOMIC-EDUCATIONAL ASPIRATIONS. FIND-INGS INDICATE THAT MIDDLE-CLASS ANGLO AMERICANS CLEARLY HAVE A HIGHER LEVEL OF ASPIRATION THAN THE OTHER FIVE GROUPS. THE LOWER-CLASS PUERTO RICANS TEND TO HAVE A RELATIVELY LOW ASPIRATIONAL LEVEL AND THEY ALSO REPORT FEWEST SUCCESS MODELS. THERE IS A SUBSTANTIAL SIMILARITY IN PATTERNS OF RESPONSE OF THE TWO NE-GRO, THE LOWER-CLASS ANGLO AMERICAN, AND THE MIDDLE-CLASS PUERTO RICAN GROUPS. A COMPARISON OF NEGRO AND AN-GLO AMERICAN BOYS, HOLDING CLASS CON-STANT, DOES NOT CHANGE THE RESULTS. THE ANGLO AMERICAN MIDDLE-CLASS BOYS CON-SISTENTLY HAVE HIGHER ASPIRATIONS THAN THE OTHER GROUPS. 11 REFERENCES.

ACCN   000058

68 AUTH **ANTUNES, G., GORDON, C., GAITZ, C. M., & SCOTT, J.**

TITL   ETHNICITY, SOCIOECONOMIC STATUS, AND THE ETIOLOGY OF PSYCHOLOGICAL DISTRESS.

SRCE *SOCIOLOGY AND SOCIAL RESEARCH, 1974, 58(4), 361-368.*

INDX SES, CROSS CULTURAL, MEXICAN AMERICAN, ADULTS, EMPIRICAL, SYMPTOMATOLOGY, STRESS, DISCRIMINATION, SURVEY

ABST   TO IDENTIFY THE MECHANISMS RESPONSIBLE FOR THE INVERSE ASSOCIATION BETWEEN SO-CIAL CLASS AND PSYCHOLOGICAL DISTRESS, A RESEARCH DESIGN CREATED BY DOHREN-WEND AND DOHRENWEND WAS USED TO COMPARE THE DISTRESS LEVEL OF ANGLOS, BLACKS AND MEXICAN AMERICANS FOR TWO

LEVELS OF SOCIOECONOMIC STATUS. THE MECHANISMS DISCUSSED ARE: (1) THE SOCIAL SELECTION HYPOTHESIS; AND (2) THE SOCIAL STRESS HYPOTHESIS. DATA CONTRADICT THE SOCIAL STRESS INTERPRETATION, AND SUPPORT THE SOCIAL SELECTION PROCESS, IN WHICH PSYCHOLOGICALLY IMPAIRED PERSONS TEND TO DECLINE IN SOCIOECONOMIC STATUS WHILE THE LOWER STATUS IMPAIRED FAIL TO RISE. THIS IS IN CONTRAST TO THE SOCIAL STRESS THEORY WHICH PREDICTS PSYCHOLOGICAL PROBLEMS AS A COMMON CONSEQUENCE OF HIGH LEVELS OF ENVIRONMENTAL STRESS. 25 REFERENCES. (JOURNAL ABSTRACT MODIFIED)

ACCN 000059

69 AUTH **ANTUNES, G., & GAITZ, C. M.**
TITL ETHNICITY AND PARTICIPATION: A STUDY OF MEXICAN-AMERICANS, BLACKS, AND WHITES.
SRCE *AMERICAN JOURNAL OF SOCIOLOGY, 1975, 80(5), 1192-1211.*
INDX CROSS CULTURAL, EMPIRICAL, MEXICAN AMERICAN, SES, ADULTS, DISCRIMINATION, COMMUNITY INVOLVEMENT, POLITICS, ETHNIC IDENTITY, TEXAS, SOUTHWEST
ABST THIS STUDY HYPOTHESIZES THAT, BECAUSE OF A PROCESS OF "COMPENSATION" OR "ETHNIC IDENTIFICATION," MEMBERS OF DISADVANTAGED ETHNIC GROUPS HAVE HIGHER LEVELS OF SOCIAL AND POLITICAL PARTICIPATION THAN PERSONS OF THE SAME SOCIAL CLASS WHO ARE MEMBERS OF THE DOMINANT SOCIAL GROUP. REPLICATING THE STUDIES OF ORUM (1966) AND OLSEN (1970), ANALYSIS OF THE DATA TAKEN FROM THIS COMMUNITY SURVEY ONLY PARTIALLY SUPPORTS THE HYPOTHESIS WITH REGARD TO 11 PARTICIPATION VARIABLES. WHEN SOCIAL CLASS IS CONTROLLED, BLACK LEVELS OF PARTICIPATION GENERALLY EXCEED OR EQUAL THOSE OF WHITES; HOWEVER, LEVELS OF PARTICIPATION AMONG MEXICAN AMERICANS TEND TO BE LOWER THAN THOSE OF WHITES. SEVERAL EXPLANATIONS WHICH MIGHT ACCOUNT FOR THESE DISCREPANT FINDINGS ARE DISCUSSED. 27 REFERENCES. (JOURNAL ABSTRACT)

ACCN 000060

70 AUTH **APODACA, B.**
TITL TEACHER-CHILD INTERACTION AND COGNITIVE DEVELOPMENT.
SRCE *PAPER PRESENTED AT THE 1ST SYMPOSIUM ON CHICANO PSYCHOLOGY, UNIVERSITY OF CALIFORNIA, IRVINE, MAY 16, 1976.*
INDX REVIEW, TEACHERS, PROFESSIONAL TRAINING, MODELING, CLASSROOM BEHAVIOR, INSTRUCTIONAL TECHNIQUES, COMMUNITY INVOLVEMENT, EDUCATION, LEARNING, COGNITIVE DEVELOPMENT, ENVIRONMENTAL FACTORS
ABST TEACHER EDUCATION PROGRAMS THROUGHOUT THE NATION HAVE ATTEMPTED A WIDE VARIETY OF CURRICULAR REFORMS PERTAINING TO CHILDREN'S LEARNING IN THE CLASSROOM. THIS PAPER PROVIDES A THEORETICAL INTERPRETATION (PLUS ADVICE FOR THE APPROPRIATE USE) OF AN OBSERVATIONAL

TRAINING MODEL FOR STUDENT TEACHERS. THE MODEL IS DESIGNED TO ENHANCE THE TEACHING/LEARNING SITUATION THROUGH A SYSTEM OF IN-CLASS SUPERVISION WHICH INVOLVES TEACHERS' AND STUDENT TEACHERS' STUDY OF THEIR OWN BEHAVIOR. BASED ON SOCIAL LEARNING THEORY, THE MODEL INCLUDES FIVE COMPONENTS: (1) THE PROFESSIONAL RESPONSE; (2) THE TEACHER AS A TECHNICAL SUPERVISOR; (3) THE TEACHER AS A MEDIATOR OF THE ENVIRONMENT; (4) INDIVIDUALIZATION; AND (5) COMMUNITY INVOLVEMENT. THE ROLES OF THE SUPERVISOR, COOPERATING TEACHERS, AND STUDENT TEACHERS ARE ALSO DISCUSSED. 46 REFERENCES. (AUTHOR ABSTRACT MODIFIED)

ACCN 000061

71 AUTH **ARAGON, J. A.**
TITL THE CHALLENGE OF CULTURAL PLURALISM: CULTURALLY DIFFERENT EDUCATORS TEACHING CULTURALLY DIFFERENT CHILDREN.
SRCE *IN A. CASTANEDA, M. RAMIREZ III, C. E. CORTES & M. BARRERA (EDS.), MEXICAN AMERICANS AND EDUCATIONAL CHANGE. NEW YORK: ARNO PRESS, 1974, PP. 258-267.*
INDX EDUCATION, PROFESSIONAL TRAINING, TEACHERS, BILINGUAL-BICULTURAL EDUCATION, BILINGUAL-BICULTURAL PERSONNEL, MEXICAN AMERICAN, CULTURAL PLURALISM, POVERTY, SES, CULTURAL FACTORS, ACCULTURATION, ESSAY
ABST ARGUMENTS FOR THE DEVELOPMENT AND FUNDING OF GRADUATE PROGRAMS TO PRODUCE CREDENTIALED DOCTORATE LEVEL CHICANO PROFESSORS TO TAKE POSITIONS IN BICULTURAL EDUCATION AT ALL LEVELS OF GOVERNMENT AND ACADEMIA ARE PRESENTED. RATHER THAN RETRAINING TRADITIONALLY ORIENTED UNIVERSITY FACULTY, IT IS PROPOSED THAT MEXICAN AMERICAN PROFESSORS PROVIDE THE TRAINING TO TEACHERS WHO WILL BE WORKING WITH MEXICAN AMERICAN STUDENTS. DIFFERENCES BETWEEN THE CULTURE OF POVERTY AND ETHNICITY ARE DISCUSSED. THE AUTHOR ALSO OFFERS A DEFINITION OF CULTURE, INCLUDING LANGUAGE, DIET, COSTUMES, SOCIAL PATTERNS, AND ETHICS, WHICH COULD BE USED IN TEACHERS' PRESERVICE AND INSERVICE CLASSES.

ACCN 000062

72 AUTH **ARAGON, J. A., & ULIBARRI, S. R.**
TITL LEARN, AMIGO, LEARN.
SRCE *PERSONNEL AND GUIDANCE JOURNAL, 1971, 50(2), 87-89.*
INDX ESSAY, EDUCATIONAL COUNSELING, CULTURAL FACTORS, PROFESSIONAL TRAINING, CULTURAL PLURALISM, SPANISH SURNAMED, EDUCATION, CULTURE
ABST THE PROBLEMS THAT CONFRONT GUIDANCE PERSONNEL IN THEIR RELATIONSHIP WITH CULTURALLY DIFFERENT CLIENTS ARE DISCUSSED IN TERMS OF THE FOLLOWING CULTURAL CHARACTERISTICS: (1) LANGUAGE; (2) DIET; (3) MANNER OF DRESS; (4) SOCIAL PATTERNS, ESPECIALLY THE EXTENDED FAMILY

SYSTEM AMONG HISPANICS; AND (5) ETHICS. WHEN COUNSELORS FAIL TO RECOGNIZE THESE CHARACTERISTICS OF CULTURAL GROUPS, CULTURALLY DIFFERENT STUDENTS MAY BECOME EMOTIONALLY CRIPPLED. IT IS THEREFORE CONCLUDED THAT COUNSELORS' INSERVICE PREPARATION SHOULD INCLUDE EXPERIENCES THAT WILL FAMILIARIZE THEM WITH THE TRAITS OF VARIOUS CULTURAL GROUPS. COUNSELORS MUST FIND WAYS TO REINFORCE A POSITIVE SELF-IMAGE IN THEIR CLIENTS AND ALSO PROMOTE MUTUAL RESPECT AMONG CULTURALLY DIVERSE PEOPLE.

ACCN   000063

73 AUTH **ARAMONI, A.**
    TITL MACHISMO.
    SRCE *PSYCHOLOGY TODAY, JANUARY 1972, PP. 69-72.*
    INDX SEX ROLES, ESSAY, CULTURE, MEXICAN, FAMILY ROLES, MALE, PERSONALITY, COPING MECHANISMS, MACHISMO
    ABST AN INVESTIGATION OF MACHISMO AS A BEHAVIORAL PATTERN AMONG MALES IN MEXICO IS PRESENTED. MACHISMO IS A PARADOXICAL BEHAVIOR IN WHICH THE MALE SEEKS HYPERMANLINESS TO PROVE HIMSELF A "MAN." ALTHOUGH NOT A UNIVERSAL TRAIT OF MEXICANS, MACHISMO IS FOUND IN CERTAIN SOCIOECONOMIC CLASSES. IN GENERAL, MACHISMO IS AN ATTITUDE TOWARD EXISTENCE WHICH REFLECTS THE WAY A SPECIAL TYPE OF MAN RESPONDS TO CONDITIONS OF LIFE. OVER-COMPENSATING FOR HIS ACUTE INNER FEELINGS OF INADEQUACY AND GUILT, THE MACHISTA STRUTS THROUGH LIFE, GIVING AND SEEKING CHALLENGES. THERE IS A POSITIVE STRIVING IN THIS STRUGGLE THAT EPITOMIZES THE FUNDAMENTAL PROBLEM OF ANY PERSON WHO IS TRYING TO EMERGE FROM A PROFOUND SYMBIOSIS. THAT IS, THE MACHISTA IS IMPELLED TO DOMINATE OTHERS IN ORDER TO DENY HIS OWN WEAKNESS, EXTREME DEPENDENCY, AND REGRESSIVE UNDERTOW. PASSAGES FROM RURAL MEXICAN SONGS ARE CITED TO INDICATE THE CHARACTERISTICS OF MACHISMO. IT IS CONCLUDED THAT MACHISMO IS A QUEST FOR INDIVIDUATION, DIGNITY, AND RELATEDNESS. THERE ARE MANY DIFFERENT WAYS IN WHICH A PERSON CAN RESPOND TO AN ENTRENCHED SENSE OF FEAR AND INADEQUACY. THE RESPONSE OF THE MACHISTA IS TO TRANSCEND THE UNIVERSALLY UNBEARABLE FEAR OF ALONENESS AND WEAKNESS THROUGH ACTING BIGGER, STRONGER, AND MORE GLORIOUS.

ACCN   000064

74 AUTH **ARANDA, R. G.**
    TITL THE MEXICAN-AMERICAN SYNDROME.
    SRCE *AMERICAN JOURNAL OF PUBLIC HEALTH, 1971, 61(1), 104-109.*
    INDX MEXICAN AMERICAN, POVERTY, CHICANO MOVEMENT, COMMUNITY INVOLVEMENT, HEALTH DELIVERY SYSTEMS, ESSAY, STEREOTYPES, HEALTH EDUCATION, COMMUNITY, CALIFORNIA, SOUTHWEST
    ABST ANGLO PREJUDICE AND HEALTH PROBLEMS WITHIN THE BARRIO HAVE LED TO THE

STEREOTYPED MEXICAN AMERICAN (MA) SYNDROME IN WHICH THE MA IS DESCRIBED AS DUMB, DIRTY, AND LAZY. THE CHICANO MOVEMENT HAS DONE MUCH TO COMBAT THIS STEREOTYPE BY IMPROVING THE HEALTH OF THE COMMUNITY. ACTION HAS BEEN TAKEN AT THE GRASS-ROOTS LEVEL IN THE AREAS OF NARCOTICS REHABILITATION AND PREVENTION, FREE CLINICS, HOME ECONOMICS CLASSES, BIRTH CONTROL INFORMATION, FACILITIES FOR THE RETARDED, AND THE ESTABLISHMENT OF THE EAST LOS ANGELES HEALTH TASK FORCE. IT IS CONCLUDED THAT THE MA SYNDROME IS BEING REPLACED BY THE MORE POSITIVE CHICANO IDENTITY EMPHASIZING PRIDE, ACTION, SELF-BETTERMENT, AND SELF-DETERMINATION. 11 REFERENCES.

ACCN   000065

75 AUTH **ARANDA, R. G., & ACOSTA, P. B.**
    TITL MIGRATION, CULTURE AND HEALTH OF MEXICAN AMERICANS IN AN ACCULTURATION GRADIENT.
    SRCE *WASHINGTON, D.C.: OFFICE OF ECONOMIC OPPORTUNITY, 1971. (ERIC DOCUMENT REPRODUCTION SERVICES NO. ED 055 722)*
    INDX ACCULTURATION, ADULTS, DEMOGRAPHIC, EMPIRICAL, FEMALE, MEXICAN, MEXICAN AMERICAN, SOUTHWEST, HEALTH, FERTILITY, IMMIGRATION, MALE, EMPLOYMENT
    ABST TWO GROUPS OF MEXICAN AMERICAN FAMILIES CALIFORNIA (26 IN EAST LOS ANGELES, 101 IN SAN YSIDRO) WITH CHILDREN IN HEAD START RESPONDED TO A QUESTIONNAIRE GATHERING DATA ON BIRTHPLACE, FAMILY INCOME, DIETARY HABITS, AND PREGNANCY HISTORY OF THE MOTHERS. THIS REPORT FOCUSES ON FAMILY HISTORY AND PREGNANCY. (1) FAMILY HISTORY. IN EAST LOS ANGELES, 31% OF THE MOTHERS AND 35% OF THE FATHERS WERE MEXICAN-BORN. MEAN FAMILY SIZE IN BOTH SETTINGS WAS 5.8. (2) PREGNANCY. MEXICAN-BORN WOMEN WERE IN POORER HEALTH DURING PREGNANCY THAN U.S.-BORN WOMEN AND SOUGHT MORE MEDICAL CARE. FURTHERMORE, MEXICAN-BORN WOMEN HAD MORE COMPLICATIONS DURING PREGNANCY THAN DID U.S.-BORN WOMEN. HOWEVER, A HIGHER PERCENTAGE OF MEXICAN-BORN WOMEN IN LOS ANGELES HAD MEDICAL PROBLEMS THAN MEXICAN-BORN IN SAN YSIDRO. CONTRARY TO THESE FINDINGS, PREMATURITY RATES IN BOTH SETTINGS WERE FOUND TO BE WELL BELOW THE NATIONAL AVERAGE. 16 REFERENCES.

ACCN   000066

76 AUTH **ARCE, C. H.**
    TITL CHICANOS IN HIGHER EDUCATION.
    SRCE *INTEGRATED EDUCATION, 1976, 14(3), 14-18.*
    INDX REVIEW, EDUCATION, HIGHER EDUCATION, MEXICAN AMERICAN, DEMOGRAPHIC, REPRESENTATION, SEX COMPARISON, HISTORY, COLLEGE STUDENTS, SCHOLASTIC ACHIEVEMENT
    ABST THIS OVERVIEW PRESENTS A STATISTICAL SKETCH OF CHICANOS WITH REGARD TO THEIR PRESENT AND FUTURE EDUCATIONAL NEEDS AND TRENDS. DEMOGRAPHIC DATA ARE BASED

ON THE 1974 CURRENT POPULATION SURVEYS OF THE U.S. CENSUS BUREAU. THE ROLE OF CHICANO FACULTY IN THE OVERALL SYSTEM OF AMERICAN HIGHER EDUCATION IS DISCUSSED, ALONG WITH A BRIEF HISTORY OF CHICANO PARTICIPATION IN HIGHER EDUCATION. 5 REFERENCES.

ACCN   000067

77 AUTH **ARCE, C. H.**
    TITL   NATIONAL CHICANO IDENTITY AND MENTAL HEALTH PROJECT.
    SRCE   *UNPUBLISHED MANUSCRIPT, 1976. (AVAILABLE FROM AUTHOR, SURVEY RESEARCH CENTER, INSTITUTE FOR SOCIAL RESEARCH, UNIVERSITY OF MICHIGAN, ANN ARBOR, MICHIGAN 48106.)*
    INDX   ETHNIC IDENTITY, ACCULTURATION, SURVEY, RESEARCH METHODOLOGY, CROSS CULTURAL, MEXICAN AMERICAN, MENTAL HEALTH, PSYCHOPATHOLOGY, SELF CONCEPT, RESOURCE UTILIZATION, ATTITUDES, THEORETICAL, REPRESENTATION, DISCRIMINATION, SES, CENSUS, EMPIRICAL
    ABST   THE MAJOR OBJECTIVES OF THIS RESEARCH PROPOSAL ARE TO CONDUCT A NATIONAL STUDY OF THE MENTAL HEALTH IMPLICATIONS OF ETHNIC IDENTITY AND CONSCIOUSNESS ON PERSONS OF MEXICAN ORIGIN, AND TO DEVELOP A NATIONAL RESOURCE OF SURVEY DATA FOR MINORITY SCHOLARS. TOPICS COVERED INCLUDE: (1) A CRITICAL REVIEW OF SOCIAL SCIENCE RESEARCH ON CHICANOS AND THE NEED FOR NEW RESEARCH; (2) A THEORETICAL FRAMEWORK FOR THE PROPOSED RESEARCH AND REVIEW OF LITERATURE, COVERING GROUP IDENTIFICATION, ASSIMILATION, MODELS OF ETHNIC CONSCIOUSNESS, SOCIOCULTURAL INFLUENCES ON MENTAL HEALTH STATUS, UTILIZATION OF MENTAL HEALTH RESOURCES, AND ATTITUDES TOWARDS TRADITIONAL AND ALTERNATIVE AGENCIES; AND (3) METHODS OF PROCEDURE, SAMPLING METHODS, AND DATA ANALYSIS. THIS PROPOSED STUDY WILL PROVIDE NEEDED DATA ON THE MENTAL HEALTH STATUS, SELF-DEFINITION OF PROBLEMS, AND UTILIZATION OF MENTAL HEALTH SERVICES BY CHICANOS TO FORMAL AGENCIES AND INSTITUTIONS, COMMUNITY ORGANIZATIONS, AND OTHERS. IT WILL ALSO FACILITATE THE TRAINING OF CHICANO SCHOLARS AND THE DEVELOPMENT OF AN INNOVATIVE METHODOLOGY. 174 REFERENCES.
    ACCN   000068

78 AUTH **ARCINIEGA, T. A.**
    TITL   WHY THE RECENT RODRIGUEZ, SERRANO, AND SIMILAR COURT ACTIONS AREN'T ENOUGH: A CRITIQUE OF PUBLIC EDUCATION.
    SRCE   *JOURNAL OF INSTRUCTIONAL PSYCHOLOGY, 1975, 2(4), 2-13.*
    INDX   EDUCATION, POLITICAL POWER, CHILDREN, BILINGUAL-BICULTURAL EDUCATION, ADOLESCENTS, ESSAY, MEXICAN AMERICAN, JUDICIAL PROCESS, LEGISLATION, ECONOMIC FACTORS, CULTURAL PLURALISM
    ABST   THE RECENT EMPHASIS ON EQUAL OPPORTUNITY HAS EXPANDED THE ROLE OF PUBLIC EDUCATION TO INCLUDE IMPROVING SOCIAL CONDITIONS OF DISADVANTAGED MINORITIES IN OUR SOCIETY. HOWEVER, ANY CHANGES WITHIN THE EDUCATIONAL STRUCTURE HAVE BEEN AT THE SUPERFICIAL LEVEL. THIS APPROACH CAN BE TERMED THE TRADITIONAL TRACTIVE RESPONSE, AND ASSUMES A CULTURAL DEFICIT RATIONALE SINCE IT ATTEMPTS TO CHANGE STUDENTS TO MEET THE REQUIREMENTS OF THE MAJORITY CULTURE. WHAT IS NEEDED IS A SYSTEM-CHANGE RESPONSE BASED UPON CULTURAL PLURALISM. THIS APPROACH WOULD ENCOURAGE SCHOOLS TO USE THE MINORITY LANGUAGE, INCLUDE CHICANO CULTURE IN THE CURRICULUM, INVOLVE THE MINORITY COMMUNITY IN MAKING EDUCATIONAL POLICIES, ESTABLISH MINORITY REPRESENTATION THROUGHOUT THE SCHOOL ORGANIZATIONAL STRUCTURE, AND ADEQUATELY ADDRESS THE ISSUE OF CULTURAL BIAS EXISTING IN COUNSELING AND TESTING PROGRAMS. 10 REFERENCES.
    ACCN   000069

79 AUTH **ARDILA, R.**
    TITL   PSYCHOLOGY IN LATIN AMERICA.
    SRCE   *AMERICAN PSYCHOLOGIST, 1968, 23, 567-574.*
    INDX   ESSAY, HISTORY, SOUTH AMERICA, MEXICO, SOCIAL SCIENCES, MENTAL HEALTH PROFESSION, PROFESSIONAL TRAINING
    ABST   THIS ESSAY PROVIDES AN OVERVIEW OF THE GROWING SCIENCE AND PROFESSION OF PSYCHOLOGY IN LATIN AMERICA AND ALSO OFFERS A COMPARISON TO BEEBE-CENTER AND MCFARLAND'S DESCRIPTION OF THE DISCIPLINE IN 1941. FIRST, A BRIEF HISTORY IS PRESENTED, BEGINNING IN 1898 WITH THE ESTABLISHMENT OF THE FIRST PSYCHOLOGICAL LABORATORY. NEXT, IT IS REPORTED THAT THE NUMBER OF PSYCHOLOGISTS HAS INCREASED FROM 100 IN 1941 TO 1,800 IN 1968, AND THE PRINCIPAL SUBDISCIPLINES ARE CLINICAL PSYCHOLOGY, CROSS-CULTURAL STUDIES, AND PSYCHOMETRICS. AT PRESENT THERE ARE 15 PROFESSIONAL PSYCHOLOGICAL SOCIETIES, AS WELL AS 39 LATIN AMERICAN JOURNALS (MOSTLY DEVOTED TO GENERAL AND APPLIED PSYCHOLOGY). FINALLY, FIVE TABLES PROVIDE DATA ON THE STATUS OF PSYCHOLOGICAL RESEARCH, DEGREES OFFERED, LEGAL RECOGNITION, ETC., IN EACH LATIN AMERICAN COUNTRY. IT IS CONCLUDED THAT MANY ASPECTS OF PROFESSIONAL TRAINING, ORGANIZATIONS, AND PUBLICATIONS NEED IMPROVEMENT SO THAT LATIN AMERICAN PSYCHOLOGY CAN TAKE ITS PLACE IN THE MODERN WORLD. 6 REFERENCES.
    ACCN   002011

80 AUTH **ARDILA, R., & FINLEY, G.**
    TITL   PSYCHOLOGY IN LATIN AMERICA: A BIBLIOGRAPHY.
    SRCE   *INTERAMERICAN JOURNAL OF PSYCHOLOGY, 1975, 9(3-4), 1-171.*
    INDX   BIBLIOGRAPHY, SOUTH AMERICA, CENTRAL AMERICA, MEXICO, MENTAL HEALTH, SOCIAL SCIENCES, MENTAL HEALTH PROFESSION
    ABST   TO PROVIDE A MEDIUM WHEREBY THE INTER-

AMERICAN COMMUNITY OF PSYCHOLOGISTS MAY BECOME FAMILIAR WITH EACH OTHER'S WORK, RESEARCH DONE BY LATIN AMERICAN PSYCHOLOGISTS AND FOREIGN PSYCHOLOGISTS WORKING WITH LATIN AMERICAN POPULATIONS IS LISTED. ALL NATIONS SOUTH OF THE RIO GRANDE AND THE CARIBBEAN ARE INCLUDED. OVER 2000 PUBLISHED ARTICLES FROM 1960 TO 1975 (WITH A FEW BEFORE 1960) COVER THE AREAS OF GENERAL PSYCHOLOGY, METHODOLOGY AND PSYCHOMETRICS, PHYSIOLOGICAL AND COMPARATIVE PSYCHOLOGY, PERCEPTION, LEARNING, MOTIVATION, THINKING AND LANGUAGE, PERSONALITY, DEVELOPMENTAL PSYCHOLOGY, SOCIAL PSYCHOLOGY, CLINICAL PSYCHOLOGY, EDUCATIONAL PSYCHOLOGY, INDUSTRIAL PSYCHOLOGY, BEHAVIOR MODIFICATION, AND PSYCHOANALYSIS. ALL TITLES ARE PRESENTED IN THE ORIGINAL LANGUAGE (ENGLISH, SPANISH, OR PORTUGESE). (NCMHI ABSTRACT MODIFIED)

ACCN   002012

81 AUTH   **ARELLANO, E. (ED.)**
    TITL   EL CUADERNO: DE VEZ EN CUANDO.
    SRCE   *DIXON, N.M.: LA ACADEMIA DE LA NUEVA RAZA, 1976.*
    INDX   HISTORY, MENTAL HEALTH, CULTURAL FACTORS, MEXICAN AMERICAN, ESSAY, ART, BOOK
    ABST   LA ACADEMIA DE LA NUEVA RAZA, FOUNDED TO DEVELOP A BODY OF KNOWLEDGE MEANINGFUL TO LA RAZA, IS AN EDUCATION-ACTION AND RESEARCH INSTITUTE THAT HAS ASSUMED A STRONG ROLE IN EDUCATION FOR COMMUNITY LIVING. EL CUADERNO IS A JOURNAL THAT CARRIES THE "EMERGING PHILOSOPHY" FROM THE BARRIO. THE JOURNAL CONTAINS A BODY OF KNOWLEDGE FROM THE CHICANO EXPERIENCE, USING THE PARAMETERS OF PERSONAL HISTORY, ORAL HISTORY, FOLKLORE AND THE ARTS IN AN EFFORT TO REFLECT THE ACTIONS OF PRIOR AND CURRENT INDIVIDUAL AND SOCIETAL EXPERIENCES. THROUGH A THOUGHT AND ACTION DIALECTICAL PROCESS, INDIVIDUALS PARTICIPATING IN THE DIALOGUE NOT ONLY CONTRIBUTE TO THEIR EXPERIENCE, BUT ALSO ANALYZE THE SOCIETAL FORCES THAT MAY BE IMPAIRING OR ENHANCING THEIR ULTIMATE FULFILLMENT AS PERSONS. (AUTHOR SUMMARY MODIFIED)
    ACCN   000070

82 AUTH   **ARIAS, R. R.**
    TITL   THE INFLUENCE OF CHICANO CULTURE ON HEALTH CARE (SPECIAL REPORT NO. 4).
    SRCE   *IN COMMUNITY HEALTH BULLETIN. LOS ANGELES: EAST LOS ANGELES HEALTH SYSTEM INC., UNDATED.*
    INDX   HEALTH, FOLK MEDICINE, CURANDERISMO, RELIGION, CULTURAL FACTORS, HEALTH DELIVERY SYSTEMS, REVIEW, SPANISH SURNAMED, CALIFORNIA, SOUTHWEST
    ABST   THIS BULLETIN SUMMARIZES THE PURPOSE AND MOST PREVALENT FINDINGS DOCUMENTED IN AN EXHAUSTIVE LITERATURE REVIEW BY THE EAST LOS ANGELES HEALTH SYS-

TEM. CATHOLICISM AND CURANDERISMO ARE THE TWO ISSUES DISCUSSED IN RELATION TO CULTURALLY DETERMINED ATTITUDES IN A SPANISH SURNAMED POPULATION WHICH AFFECT THEIR UTILIZATION OF EMERGENCY MEDICAL SERVICES AND HEALTH SERVICES IN GENERAL.

ACCN   000071

83 AUTH   **ARMOR, D., CONRY-OSEGUERA, P., COX, M., KING, N., MCDONNELL, L., PASCAL, A., PAULY, E., & ZELLMAN, G.**
    TITL   ANALYSIS OF THE SCHOOL PREFERED READING PROGRAM IN SELECTED LOS ANGELES MINORITY SCHOOLS.
    SRCE   *SANTA MONICA, CALIF.: THE RAND CORPORATION, AUGUST 1976.*
    INDX   CROSS CULTURAL, MEXICAN AMERICAN, READING, EMPIRICAL, CHILDREN, SES, HEALTH, PARENTAL INVOLVEMENT, EDUCATION, COMMUNITY, CALIFORNIA, SOUTHWEST, PROGRAM EVALUATION, CHILDREN
    ABST   OVERALL FINDINGS OF THIS REPORT SUPPORT THE CONTINUATION OF THE LOS ANGELES SCHOOL DISTRICT'S USE OF THE SCHOOL PREFERRED READING PROGRAM IN PREDOMINANTLY MINORITY SCHOOLS. ALTHOUGH FACTORS SUCH AS SOCIOECONOMIC STATUS, HEALTH, ETHNICITY, ATTENDANCE AND EARLIER READING SCORES WERE FOUND TO ACCOUNT FOR THE LARGEST PART OF THE VARIATION IN 6TH GRADE READING SCORES, OTHER VARIABLES REFLECTING PARTICULAR SCHOOL, TEACHER AND CLASSROOM EXPERIENCES ALSO HAD A SIGNIFICANT INFLUENCE FOR BOTH BLACK AND MEXICAN AMERICAN CHILDREN. THE INABILITY TO IDENTIFY SPECIFIC FACTORS ASSOCIATED WITH THE READING GAINS OF MA STUDENTS, WHICH WERE ALMOST IDENTICAL TO THE GAINS REGISTERED BY BLACK STUDENTS, WAS PROBABLY DUE TO FAILURE TO INCLUDE OR MEASURE SOME KEY VARIABLES.
    ACCN   000072

84 AUTH   **ARMSTRONG, R. A.**
    TITL   TEST BIAS FROM THE NON-ANGLO VIEWPOINT: A CRITICAL EVALUATION OF INTELLIGENCE TEST ITEMS BY MEMBERS OF THREE CULTURAL MINORITIES (DOCTORAL DISSERTATION, UNIVERSITY OF ARIZONA, 1972).
    SRCE   *DISSERTATION ABSTRACTS INTERNATIONAL, 1972, 33(4), 1502A. (UNIVERSITY MICROFILMS NO.72-25,504.)*
    INDX   CROSS CULTURAL, INTELLIGENCE TESTING, EMPIRICAL, TEST VALIDITY, ARIZONA, SOUTHWEST, COLLEGE STUDENTS, SEX COMPARISON, CULTURE-FAIR TESTS, ADULTS
    ABST   SIXTY-THREE MEMBERS OF THREE CULTURAL MINORITIES (BLACK, NATIVE AMERICAN, AND MEXICAN AMERICAN) WERE ASKED TO RESPOND TO A NUMBER OF SET ITEM TYPES SIMILAR TO ITEM TYPES FOUND ON VARIOUS STANDARDIZED INTELLIGENCE TESTS. ALL RESPONDENTS WERE ALSO ASKED TO EVALUATE EACH TYPE OF TEST ITEM ON FAIRNESS OR APPROPRIATENESS FOR THEIR PARTICULAR MINORITY. A SMALL NUMBER OF MIDDLE CLASS

ANGLOS WERE ALSO ASKED TO EVALUATE THE SAME SET OF ITEM TYPES FOR BIAS AGAINST NON-ANGLOS, TO COMPARE WITH THE NON-ANGLO GROUP. THE RESULTS SHOW THAT PERSONS OF ONE CULTURE FIND IT EXTREMELY DIFFICULT TO JUDGE BIAS AGAINST ANOTHER CULTURE, THUS SUPPORTING THE UNDERLYING PREMISE OF THE STUDY. THE INVESTIGATION ALSO SUPPORTED A NUMBER OF INTELLIGENCE TEST CRITICISMS FOUND IN LITERATURE ON CROSS CULTURAL TESTING: (1) THE ITEMS REQUIRED A HIGH DEGREE OF VERBAL FACILITY; (2) CONTAINED MATERIAL INAPPROPRIATE TO THE GROUP'S BACKGROUND; AND (3) TAPPED SKILLS NOT GENERALLY TAUGHT BY A PARTICULAR CULTURE. WHEN COMPARING THE ANGLO AND NON-ANGLO RATINGS, LITTLE AGREEMENT WAS FOUND BETWEEN THE TWO GROUPS. FROM THE TEST ITEMS IDENTIFIED IN THIS EXPLORATORY STUDY, THE FIRST PROTOTYPE OF A CROSS CULTURAL TEST WAS DEVELOPED. A NUMBER OF SUGGESTIONS FOR FUTURE RESEARCH ARE PRESENTED. 61 REFERENCES.

ACCN   000073

85   AUTH   **ARNHEIM, D. D., & SINCLAIR, W. A.**
     TITL   THE EFFECT OF A MOTOR DEVELOPMENT PROGRAM ON SELECTED FACTORS IN MOTOR ABILITY, PERSONALITY, SELF-AWARENESS, AND VISION.
     SRCE   *AMERICAN CORRECTIVE THERAPY JOURNAL, 1974, 28(6), 167-171.*
     INDX   GOODENOUGH DRAW-A-MAN TEST, CHILDREN, URBAN, CALIFORNIA, SOUTHWEST, MEXICAN AMERICAN, CROSS CULTURAL, PHYSICAL DEVELOPMENT, READING, PERSONALITY ASSESSMENT, SELF CONCEPT, SES, EMPIRICAL, PERCEPTION, ABILITY TESTING
     ABST   TO DETERMINE THE BENEFITS OF A MOTOR DEVELOPMENT PROGRAM, A YEAR-LONG PRE- AND POST-TEST STUDY WAS CONDUCTED ON 73 CHILDREN IN TWO LOS ANGELES ELEMENTARY SCHOOLS. LINCOLN ELEMENTARY, HAVING A MOTOR DEVELOPMENT PROGRAM, WAS LARGELY COMPRISED OF LOW SES, CULTURALLY DISADVANTAGED STUDENTS; THE SCHOOL HAD A MULTIETHNIC MIX OF MEXICAN AMERICAN, ANGLO, BLACK, AND ORIENTAL CHILDREN. COLLINS ELEMENTARY DID NOT HAVE A MOTOR DEVELOPMENT PROGRAM, AND HAD PRIMARILY MIDDLE-CLASS ANGLO STUDENTS. THE FOLLOWING AREAS WERE TESTED: (1) PERSONALITY (CALIFORNIA TEST OF PERSONALITY); (2) SENSORY MOTOR AND MOVEMENT SKILLS; (3) SELF-IMAGE (GOODENOUGH DRAW-A-MAN TEST); AND (4) READING ABILITY. RESULTS DEMONSTRATED THAT THE LINCOLN STUDENTS IMPROVED SIGNIFICANTLY IN ALL FOUR AREAS IN COMPARISON TO THE COLLINS STUDENTS. SPECIFICALLY, THEY IMPROVED IN (1) PERSONAL AND SOCIAL ADJUSTMENT, (2) DEXTERITY, AGILITY, BALANCE, AND OTHER MOTOR SKILLS, (3) AWARENESS OF THEIR BODIES, AND (4) THEIR EYE MOVEMENTS AND ABILITY TO COMPREHEND WHEN READING. IT IS CONCLUDED THAT A MOTOR DEVELOPMENT PROGRAM CAN MAKE MANY POSITIVE CHANGES IN SCHOOL CHILDREN. 14 REFERENCES.

ACCN   000074

86   AUTH   **ARNOLD, R. D., & WIST, A. H.**
     TITL   AUDITORY DISCRIMINATION ABILITIES OF DISADVANTAGED ANGLO AND MEXICAN-AMERICAN CHILDREN.
     SRCE   *ELEMENTARY SCHOOL JOURNAL, 1970, 70(6), 295-299.*
     INDX   LEARNING DISABILITIES, MEXICAN AMERICAN, EMPIRICAL, CHILDREN, POVERTY, PHONOLOGY, BILINGUALISM, PERCEPTION, TEXAS, SOUTHWEST, CROSS CULTURAL, SES
     ABST   TWO DISADVANTAGED ETHNIC GROUPS, 90 ANGLO AMERICANS (AA) AND 93 MEXICAN AMERICANS (MA), DIVIDED INTO THREE AGE GROUPS (6-9 YEARS OF AGE) WERE ADMINISTERED A TEST OF 40 WORD-PART PHONEMIC DISCRIMINATIONS. THE TEST WAS DEVISED IN PART FROM THE WEPMAN AUDITORY DISCRIMINATION TEST AND CONSISTED OF THREE SCALES. THE MA SCALE CONTAINED 20 ITEMS WHICH WERE PHONEMES JUDGED TO BE DIFFICULT FOR THE MA AND AA CHILDREN. THE AA SCALE CONTAINED 10 ITEMS FROM THE WEPMAN TEST, WHILE AN ADDITIONAL 10 WERE CONTROL ITEMS. EACH WORD PAIR REQUIRED ORAL DISCRIMINATION IN THE INITIAL, MEDIAL, OR FINAL POSITION. FOR EACH ITEM OF EACH OF THE THREE SCALES, ITEM DIFFICULTIES AND ITEM INTERCORRELATIONS WERE COMPUTED. ON THE MA SCALE (20 ITEMS), THE MEAN ERROR SCORES FOR AA'S WERE CONSISTENTLY LOWER THAN THE SCORES OF MA'S. THE RESULTS FAVORED THE AA SUBJECTS OF ALL AGE GROUPS. THE AA SCALE (10 ITEMS) RESULTS WERE ALSO FAVORABLE FOR THE AA SUBJECTS. THE FINDINGS APPEAR TO SUPPORT PREVIOUS STUDIES WHICH SHOW A HIGHER INCIDENCE OF PROBLEMS IN AUDITORY DISCRIMINATION AMONG CHILDREN OF LOW SOCIOECONOMIC LEVELS. THERE IS AN INDICATION THAT MEMBERSHIP IN A MINORITY ETHNIC GROUP ALSO INCREASES THE CHANCES THAT CHILDREN WILL HAVE PROBLEMS IN AUDITORY DISCRIMINATION. ONE EDUCATIONAL IMPLICATION IS THAT DISADVANTAGED MA CHILDREN NEED CONSIDERABLY MORE PRACTICE WITH ENGLISH, THEIR SECOND LANGUAGE. 12 REFERENCES.

ACCN   000075

87   AUTH   **ARON, B., MORALES, P. A., & AMELAR, R.**
     TITL   COMMUNITY RESPONSE TO FREE VASECTOMY.
     SRCE   *NEW YORK JOURNAL OF MEDICINE, 1973, 73(18), 2270-2275.*
     INDX   SOCIAL SERVICES, COMMUNITY, CULTURAL FACTORS, EMPIRICAL, BIRTH CONTROL, PUERTO RICAN-M, NEW YORK, EAST, HEALTH EDUCATION
     ABST   ELECTIVE VASECTOMY CONSTITUTED ONLY 37% OF STERILIZATION OPERATIONS IN 1967. TUBAL LIGATION, DESPITE ITS COMPLEXITIES, WAS MORE POPULAR. BELLEVUE HOSPITAL VASECTOMY SERVICE PROVIDED FREE OR INEXPENSIVE VASECTOMIES TO THE MEDICALLY

INDIGENT OF LOWER MANHATTAN, AND THE INITIAL RESPONSE OF THE COMMUNITY IS REPORTED. IN THE SERIES OF 116 PATIENTS, RELATIVELY FEW WERE POOR, BLACK, OR PUERTO RICAN. INADEQUATE INFORMATION OR CULTURAL FACTORS MAY ACCOUNT FOR THE RELUCTANCE, AND INTENSIFIED EDUCATION AND RESEARCH MAY RESULT IN GREATER ACCEPTANCE. 7 REFERENCES. (PASAR ABSTRACT)

ACCN   000076

88   AUTH   **ARON, W. S., ALGER, N., & GONZALEZ, R. T.**
     TITL   CHICANOIZING THE THERAPEUTIC COMMUNITY.
     SRCE   *JOURNAL OF PSYCHEDELIC DRUGS, 1974, 6(3), 321-327.*
     INDX   REHABILITATION, THERAPEUTIC COMMUNITY, MEXICAN AMERICAN, DRUG ADDICTION, POVERTY, DISCRIMINATION, SELF CONCEPT, ESSAY, CULTURAL FACTORS, INSTRUCTIONAL TECHNIQUES, CALIFORNIA, SOUTHWEST, URBAN
     ABST   THE PROBLEM OF DRUG ADDICTION, ITS ANTECEDENT CONDITIONS IN A CHICANO POPULATION (LA COLONIA IN OXNARD, CA.), AND THERAPEUTIC INTERVENTIONS SUGGESTED BY THESE CONDITIONS ARE EXAMINED ALONG WITH HOW THEY MIGHT BE INCORPORATED INTO A THERAPEUTIC COMMUNITY PROGRAM SPECIALLY DESIGNED TO MEET THE NEEDS OF CHICANO DRUG ADDICTS. POVERTY, LACK OF EDUCATION, AND DISCRIMINATION ARE THE IDENTIFIED CAUSES OF DRUG ABUSE. CONDITIONS RESULTING FROM THESE CAUSES— NEGATIVE SELF-IMAGE AND HIGH UNEMPLOYMENT— MUST BE DEALT WITH IF A PROGRAM IS TO BE SUCCESSFUL. SUGGESTIONS FOR CONCEPTS (E.G., "EL GRUPO," ROLLA" AND "LA REALIDAD) RELEVANT TO A REHABILITATION PROGRAM SERVING CHICANO ADDICTS ARE EXPLAINED. ALSO DISCUSSED IS THE RATIONALE FOR A SEPARATE THERAPEUTIC PROGRAM (MODELED AFTER SYNANON) FOR ETHNIC MINORITIES. 26 REFERENCES.
     ACCN   000077

89   AUTH   **ARROYO, L. E.**
     TITL   INDUSTRIAL AND OCCUPATIONAL DISTRIBUTION OF CHICANA WORKERS.
     SRCE   *IN R. SANCHEZ & R. M. CRUZ (EDS.), ESSAYS ON LA MUJER, (ANTHOLOGY NO. 1). LOS ANGELES: UNIVERSITY OF CALIFORNIA, CHICANO STUDIES CENTER, 1977, PP. 150-187.*
     INDX   REPRESENTATION, SES, LABOR FORCE, EQUAL OPPORTUNITY, CAPITALISM, REVIEW, FEMALE, MEXICAN AMERICAN, SPANISH SURNAMED, TEXAS, CALIFORNIA, DISCRIMINATION, EMPLOYMENT, LEADERSHIP, EMPIRICAL, ADULTS
     ABST   TO DOCUMENT THE OPPRESSION OF CHICANAS IN U.S. SOCIETY, THIS REPORT PROFILES THE OCCUPATIONAL STATUS AND DISTRIBUTION OF 139,138 CHICANA WORKERS IN CALIFORNIA AND TEXAS. INFORMATION WAS DERIVED FROM THE U.S. GOVERNMENT EQUAL EMPLOYMENT OPPORTUNITY REPORT OF 1969, BASED ON REPORTS OF EMPLOYERS AND CORPORATIONS EMPLOYING 100 OR MORE PERSONS. THE DATA ARE LIMITED DUE TO

CATEGORIZATIONS OF SPANISH SURNAME AND MINORITIES, DIFFERENT METHODOLOGIES IN GATHERING DATA, AND SUSPECTED UNDERCOUNTING. NINE TABLES DESCRIBE THE OCCUPATIONAL DISTRIBUTION OF THE CHICANA POPULATION FOR THE U.S.—INCLUDING (1) PROPORTION OF EMPLOYMENT BY INDUSTRIAL SECTOR, (2) EMPLOYMENT BY CATEGORY AND DISTRIBUTION OF CHICANAS AS PERCENT OF TOTAL CHICANA EMPLOYMENT FOR NATION, SOUTHWEST, CALIFORNIA, AND TEXAS, (3) INDUSTRIES IN WHICH THE CHICANA BLUE-COLLAR WORKER, WHITE-COLLAR WORKER, OR SERVICE WORKER ACCOUNTED FOR OVER 50% OF THE CHICANAS EMPLOYED, AND (4) INDUSTRIES IN WHICH CHICANAS ACCOUNT FOR A SUBSTANTIAL PERCENTAGE OF THE TOTAL FEMALES EMPLOYED. THE STATISTICS INDICATE THAT CHICANAS ARE CONSISTENTLY EMPLOYED IN THE LOWEST PAID CATEGORIES OF THE LABOR FORCE. A BRIEF REVIEW OF LITERATURE ON THE FARAH GARMENT WORKERS STRIKE OF 1972-1974 GIVES INSIGHTS INTO THE TYPES OF PRESSURES AND DISCRIMINATION FACED BY THE 4,000 STRIKING WORKERS AND REVEALS THE CHICANAS AS LEADERS, ORGANIZERS, AND ACTIVE PARTICIPANTS. AN APPENDIX PROVIDES A COMPLETE BREAKDOWN OF SPANISH SURNAMED FEMALE EMPLOYMENT BY INDUSTRY AND OCCUPATION FOR CALIFORNIA AND TEXAS. 15 REFERENCES.

ACCN   002013

90   AUTH   **ASHER, J. J., & GARCIA, R.**
     TITL   THE OPTIMAL AGE TO LEARN A FOREIGN LANGUAGE.
     SRCE   *MODERN LANGUAGE JOURNAL, 1969, 53(5), 334-341.*
     INDX   LANGUAGE ACQUISITION, CUBAN, CHILDREN, ADOLESCENTS, EMPIRICAL, BILINGUALISM, CALIFORNIA, SOUTHWEST
     ABST   USING 71 7-19 YEAR-OLD CUBAN IMMIGRANTS, AN ATTEMPT WAS MADE TO DETERMINE WHICH FACTORS WERE RELATED TO THE ACHIEVEMENT OF A NATIVE PRONUNCIATION OF ENGLISH. THE FACTORS WERE AGE OF THE CHILDREN WHEN THEY ENTERED THE UNITED STATES, LENGTH OF TIME IN THE UNITED STATES, SEX, AND ANY INTERACTION BETWEEN THE VARIABLES. THE RESULTS SHOWED THAT ALTHOUGH NO CUBAN CHILD ACHIEVED A NATIVE PRONUNCIATION OF ENGLISH, A NEAR-NATIVE PRONUNCIATION WAS MOST APT TO OCCUR IF THE BOY OR GIRL WAS 6 OR YOUNGER WHEN COMING TO THE UNITED STATES, AND LIVED IN THIS COUNTRY BETWEEN 5 AND 8 YEARS. A BIOLOGICAL EXPLANATION IS PROPOSED TO ACCOUNT FOR THE FINDINGS.
     ACCN   000078

91   AUTH   **ASSOCIATION OF AMERICAN MEDICAL COLLEGES.**
     TITL   MEDICAL SCHOOL ADMISSION REQUIREMENTS 1977-1978.
     SRCE   *WASHINGTON, D.C.: ASSOCIATION OF AMERICAN MEDICAL COLLEGES, 1977.*

INDX PROFESSIONAL TRAINING, REPRESENTATION, SPANISH SURNAMED, MEDICAL STUDENTS

ABST INFORMATION VALUABLE TO MINORITY GROUP STUDENTS CONSIDERING ENTERING MEDICAL SCHOOL IS PRESENTED FOR QUICK, EASY REFERENCE IN CHAPTERS 7 AND 11. INCLUDED ARE: (1) AAMC STATEMENT ON MEDICAL EDUCATION OF MINORITY GROUP STUDENTS; (2) TABLES SHOWING MINORITY ENROLLMENT BY SCHOOL AND YEAR; (3) NAMES OF RESOURCE PERSONS AT EVERY U.S. MEDICAL SCHOOL; AND (4) FINANCIAL AID INFORMATION. 9 REFERENCES.

ACCN 000079

92 AUTH **ATENCIO, T. C.**
TITL MENTAL HEALTH AND THE SPANISH SPEAKING.
SRCE *IN S. G. RILEY (ED.), MENTAL HEALTH PLANNING CONFERENCE FOR THE SPANISH SPEAKING. ROCKVILLE, MD.: NATIONAL INSTITUTE OF MENTAL HEALTH, 1972, PP. 19-32.*
INDX MEXICAN AMERICAN, ESSAY, MENTAL HEALTH, CULTURE, HEALTH, CULTURAL FACTORS
ABST AN ANALYSIS OF MENTAL HEALTH IN THE SPANISH-SPEAKING (SS) COMMUNITY IS PRESENTED IN THREE PARTS. THE FIRST DESCRIBES THE RELATIONSHIP BETWEEN MENTAL HEALTH AND LA ACADEMIA DE LA NUEVA RAZA (LALNR). LA ACADEMIA IS ENGAGED IN A PROCESS OF COLLECTING A BODY OF KNOWLEDGE AND TRANSFORMING IT INTO AN EDUCATIONAL PROCESS. IT IS NOTED THAT KNOWLEDGE ON NORMATIVE BEHAVIOR OF THE SS MUST BE STUDIED. SECOND, THE PROBLEMS WITH INSTITUTIONS AND GOVERNMENT AGENCIES IN RELATION TO THE SS ARE DISCUSSED. SPECIFICALLY, THE SS HAVE TO FORM COUNTER-INSTITUTIONS AND NOT EMULATE THE AMERICAN INSTITUTIONS—AND THIS INCLUDES COUNTER-INSTITUTIONAL METHODS TO DO RESEARCH AND TRAINING BY MAKING USE OF THE "TOTAL BARRIO EXPERIENCE." A CONSOLIDATION OF THIS KNOWLEDGE INTO A CONSTITUENCY PLANNING PROGRAM FOR MENTAL HEALTH WILL PROVIDE IMPORTANT INFORMATION ON HOW THE SS VIEW THE WORLD AND CATEGORIZE THEIR ILLNESSES. LASTLY, SEVERAL CASE ILLUSTRATIONS THAT DESCRIBE VARYING DEGREES OF ILLNESS IN TERMS OF SS DIAGNOSTIC TERMINOLOGY ARE REPORTED. IT IS IMPORTANT TO RECOGNIZE THE WAY PEOPLE DESCRIBE THEIR BEHAVIOR BECAUSE THEIR ASSESSMENT OFFERS SOLUTIONS TO THEIR PROBLEMS.
ACCN 000080

93 AUTH **ATENCIO, T. C.**
TITL NO ESTAN TODOS LOS QUE SON, NO SON TODOS LOS QUE ESTAN.
SRCE *IN E. ARELLANO (ED.), EL CUADERNO: DE VEZ EN CUANDO. DIXON, N.M.: LA ACADEMIA DE LA NUEVA RAZA, 1976, PP. 51-61.*
INDX MENTAL HEALTH, ESSAY, MEXICAN AMERICAN, SOCIAL SERVICES, CULTURE, SEX ROLES, DISCRIMINATION, FATALISM, HISTORY, FOLK MEDICINE, NEW MEXICO, SOUTHWEST
ABST RACIAL DISCRIMINATION, IMPERIALISM AND

DOMESTIC COLONIALISM AFFECT THE MENTAL HEALTH OF THE PEOPLE OF LA RAZA. ANTHROPOLOGICAL AND SOCIOLOGICAL STUDIES FREQUENTLY REACH CONCLUSIONS THAT HAVE LITTLE TO DO WITH THE STYLE OF LIFE AND CULTURE OF THE MEXICAN AMERICANS. A BETTER APPROACH WOULD BE TO ANALYZE THE LIFESTYLE OF THE PEOPLE OF LA RAZA IN TERMS OF THEIR LIFE EXPERIENCES, CULTURE, LORE, AND ORAL HISTORY FROM THE VILLAGES OF NORTHERN NEW MEXICO, AND THE SOCIAL, POLITICAL AND ECONOMIC CONDITIONS THAT AFFECT THEIR LIVES. THIS INFORMATION CAN THEN BE USED TO DEVELOP NEW METHODS OF PREVENTION AND TREATMENT OF MENTAL AND SOCIAL PROBLEMS.
ACCN 000082

94 AUTH **ATENCIO, T. C.**
TITL THE SURVIVAL OF LA RAZA DESPITE SOCIAL SERVICES.
SRCE *SOCIAL CASEWORK, 1971, 52(5), 262-268.*
INDX SOCIAL SERVICES, MEXICAN AMERICAN, ESSAY, COMMUNITY INVOLVEMENT, CULTURE
ABST AN APPEAL IS MADE TO SOCIAL WORKERS TO REPLACE THEIR AURA OF PROFESSIONALISM WITH A SPIRIT OF BROTHERHOOD IN ORDER TO CREATE A NEW HUMANITY. THE PHILOSOPHICAL FOUNDATIONS ON WHICH SOCIAL WORK AND ITS TRAINING ARE BASED ARE EXAMINED, ALONG WITH THE CONCEPTS OF INDIVIDUALIZATION, AUTONOMY, SELF-DETERMINATION, AND SOCIAL CONTROL IN THE CONTEXT OF SOCIAL WORK. IT IS SUGGESTED THAT THE SOCIAL WORKER MUST EMERGE AS A MODEL OF A NEW MAN WHO IS AWARE, RESPONSIBLE, AND CAPABLE OF WORKING WITHIN THE INSTITUTIONALIZED FRAMEWORK TO CREATE A NEW HUMANITY. ONE ALTERNATIVE IS TO IMPLEMENT AN EDUCATIONAL PLAN MEANINGFUL TO LA RAZA. LA ACADEMIA DE LA RAZA IS AN EDUCATION-ACTION-RESEARCH INSTITUTE THAT SERVES TO EDUCATE AND TO RESOLVE CONFLICT IN THE COMMUNITY. LEARNING MATERIAL DERIVED FROM AN INDIVIDUAL'S LIFE EXPERIENCE, CULTURE, AND ORAL HISTORY ARE EMPLOYED TO MAKE A PERSON COGNIZANT OF THE SOCIAL, POLITICAL, AND ECONOMIC CONDITIONS THAT AFFECT HIS LIFE. FROM THIS KNOWLEDGE, AN INDIVIDUAL DEVELOPS A SKILL FOR COPING WITH LIVING CONDITIONS. 7 REFERENCES.
ACCN 000083

95 AUTH **ATENCIO, T. C., & ARELLANO, E.**
TITL MINING AND PROCESSING EL ORO DEL BARRIO.
SRCE *AGENDA, SPRING 1975, PP. 16-21.*
INDX EDUCATION, MEXICAN AMERICAN, COLLEGE STUDENTS, CULTURE, SCHOLASTIC ACHIEVEMENT, HISTORY, CULTURAL FACTORS, MASS MEDIA, ART, CULTURAL CHANGE, ESSAY, NEW MEXICO, SOUTHWEST
ABST THIS PHILOSOPHICAL DISCUSSION ARGUES FOR THE CREATION OF AN ALTERNATIVE TO EXISTING EDUCATIONAL INSTITUTIONS. UNIVERSITIES HAVE UNDERGONE CONSIDERABLE CHANGE SINCE THEIR BEGINNING IN THIS

COUNTRY. AS THE INDUSTRIAL EPOCH MOVED TOWARD THE TECHNICAL, THE PURPOSES AND METHODS OF UNIVERSITIES CHANGED. THE QUESTION POSED BY THE AUTHORS FOR INDO-HISPANOS TO CONSIDER IS THIS: TO WHAT END, WHAT EPOCH, AND FOR WHOM ARE FUTURE INSTITUTIONS TO CHANGE? THE AUTHORS PROPOSE THAT THEIR LA ACADEMIA DE LA NUEVA RAZA LOCATED IN DIXON, NEW MEXICO, IS A CREATIVE ALTERNATIVE TO PRESENT EDUCATIONAL INSTITUTIONS. THE ACADEMIA'S ADVOCACY ROLE IN COMMUNITY ISSUES ILLUSTRATES HOW THEIR APPROACH HAS BEEN HELPFUL IN EXPOSING INJUSTICES AND PRODUCING CHANGE. THE PROCESS FOR UNCOVERING THE POTENTIAL "ORO" (GOLD) IN EACH INDIVIDUAL INCLUDES: (1) PERSONAL HISTORY; (2) ORAL HISTORY; (3) FOLKLORE; AND (4) THE ARTS.

ACCN   000084

96 AUTH **AVELLAR, J., & KAGAN, S.**
    TITL DEVELOPMENT OF COMPETITIVE BEHAVIORS IN ANGLO AMERICAN AND MEXICAN AMERICAN CHIDLREN.
    SRCE *PSYCHOLOGICAL REPORTS, 1976, 39, 191-198.*
    INDX COMPETITION, CHILDREN, MEXICAN AMERICAN, CROSS CULTURAL, EMPIRICAL, SES, CALIFORNIA, SOUTHWEST, CULTURAL FACTORS, RURAL
    ABST TO CLARIFY THE NATURE OF THE DIFFERENCES IN SOCIAL MOTIVES OF ANGLO AND MEXICAN AMERICAN CHILDREN OF THE SAME ECONOMIC LEVEL, 112 CHILDREN WERE ASSESSED USING 6 TWO-PERSON CHOICE CARDS. FIFTY-SIX ANGLO AND 56 MEXICAN AMERICAN CHILDREN (14 PAIRS OF BOYS AND 14 PAIRS OF GIRLS, AGES 5 TO 6 AND 7 TO 9) PARTICIPATED IN THE EXPERIMENT. THE SUBJECTS CAME FROM SEMIRURAL COMMUNITIES 35 MILES EAST OF LOS ANGELES. IN THE ABSENCE OF THE POSSIBILITY OF ABSOLUTE GAINS, SIGNIFICANT CULTURAL AND AGE DIFFERENCES WERE OBSERVED: ANGLOS AND OLDER CHILDREN MORE OFTEN CHOSE TO GIVE THEIR PEERS FEWER REWARDS THAN DID MEXICAN AMERICAN AND YOUNGER CHILDREN. THE CULTURAL DIFFERENCES INCREASED WITH AGE. THE OBSERVED CULTURAL DIFFERENCES COULD NOT BE ATTRIBUTED TO ECONOMIC LEVEL AND, CONTRARY TO THE CONCLUSIONS OF PREVIOUS RESEARCH, WERE PROBABLY RELATED TO A CONCERN FOR RELATIVE GAINS AND NOT RIVALRY. 8 REFERENCES. (JOURNAL ABSTRACT MODIFIED)
    ACCN 001733

97 AUTH **AVILES ROIG, C. A.**
    TITL ASPECTOS SOCIOCULTURALES DEL PROBLEMA DE ALCOHOLISMO EN PUERTO RICO. (SOCIOCULTURAL ASPECTS OF THE PROBLEM OF ALCOHOLISM IN PUERTO RICO.)
    SRCE *IN E. TONGUE, R. T. LAMBO & B. BLAIR (EDS.), PROCEEDINGS OF THE INTERNATIONAL CONFERENCE ON ALCOHOLISM AND DRUG ABUSE, SAN JUAN, PUERTO RICO, 1973. LAUSANNE, SWITZERLAND: INTERNATIONAL COUNCIL ON*

ALCOHOL AND ADDICTION, 1975, PP. 78-85. (SPANISH)
    INDX ESSAY, PUERTO RICAN-I, ALCOHOLISM, CULTURAL FACTORS, FAMILY STRUCTURE, FAMILY THERAPY, REHABILITATION, MACHISMO
    ABST THIS SUBJECTIVE DISCUSSION OF THE TREATMENT OF ALCOHOLICS IN PUERTO RICO FOCUSES ON THOSE SOCIOCULTURAL COMPONENTS THAT PROMOTE DRINKING AND THOSE WHICH HELP CURE THE PROBLEM. THE FACTORS WHICH PROMOTE ALCOHOLISM INCLUDE (1) THE "CULT OF MACHISMO," (2) THE RECENT SO-CALLED "SOCIAL FRIDAYS" DURING WHICH MEN STAY AWAY FROM HOME ALL WEEKEND AND DRINK TO THE POINT OF INTOXICATION, AND (3) ADVERTISEMENTS WHICH EQUATE LIQUOR WITH SUCCESS, SEXUAL GRATIFICATION, AND THE PUERTO RICAN IDENTITY. THESE FACTORS COMBINED ARE SEEN AS CAUSING THE HIGH NUMBER OF ALCOHOLICS IN THE ISLAND—ESTIMATED AT 100,000 IN 1972. REGARDING THOSE FACTORS WHICH ASSIST IN THE CURE OF ALCOHOLISM, FAMILY SUPPORT IS CONSIDERED THE MOST IMPORTANT. USUALLY IT IS A DEVOTED FAMILY MEMBER WHO BRINGS THE ALCOHOLIC IN FOR TREATMENT, AND THIS PERSON OFTEN REMAINS TO ASSIST IN THE DETOXIFICATION PROGRAM AND TO HELP THE ALCOHOLIC ESTABLISH A POSITIVE ATTITUDE. SUCH FAMILY SUPPORT FACILITATES THE USE OF AMBULATORY SERVICES AND THEREBY REDUCES THE NEED FOR HOSPITALIZATION. (AUTHOR ABSTRACT MODIFIED)
    ACCN 002014

98 AUTH **AVRITCH, R.**
    TITL THE FAMILY IN PUERTO RICO AS A SOCIO-ECONOMIC UNIT.
    SRCE *JOURNAL OF EDUCATION, 1967, 150(2), 15-22.*
    INDX FAMILY STRUCTURE, CULTURE, ECONOMIC FACTORS, PUERTO RICAN-I, EDUCATION, CASE STUDY
    ABST NATIVE PUERTO RICAN INFORMANTS WITH VARYING BACKGROUNDS WERE ASKED THEIR VIEWS ON THE ROLE OF THE PUERTO RICAN FAMILY AS A SOCIOECONOMIC UNIT BY A VISITING ANGLO TEACHER. USING ANTHROPOLOGICAL FIELDWORK METHODS, THE INVESTIGATOR QUESTIONED OVER FORTY PERSONS ON THE CULTURAL CONFLICTS AFFECTING FAMILIES AND THE RESULTING CHANGE IN FAMILY VALUES AND GOALS. FINALLY, THE CONCLUSIONS AND IMPLICATIONS OF THIS STUDY ON REDUCING ETHNOCENTRISM IN THE TEACHER WHO WORKS WITH PUERTO RICAN IMMIGRANTS ARE DISCUSSED. 4 REFERENCES.
    ACCN 000086

99 AUTH **AXELROD, J.**
    TITL SOME PRONUNCIATION AND LINGUISTIC PROBLEMS OF SPANISH-SPEAKING CHILDREN IN AMERICAN CLASSROOMS.
    SRCE *ELEMENTARY ENGLISH, 1974, 51(2), 203-206.*
    INDX LINGUISTIC COMPETENCE, SPANISH SURNAMED, CHILDREN, PHONOLOGY, BILINGUALISM, ESSAY

ABST ERRORS IN PRONOUNCING WRITTEN ENGLISH WORDS MAY BE TRACED TO ONE OF TWO VERY DIFFERENT SOURCES. (1) A SPANISH-SPEAKING CHILD HAS A LINGUISTIC PROBLEM IF, IN TRYING TO PRONOUNCE A WRITTEN ENGLISH WORD, HE APPLIES SPANISH LANGUAGE PHONICS LAWS WHICH DO NOT APPLY TO ENGLISH. (2) A SPANISH-SPEAKING CHILD HAS A PRONUNCIATION PROBLEM IF HE TRIES TO APPLY ENGLISH PHONICS LAWS TO ENGLISH WORDS AND STILL MISPRONOUNCES THEM. THE HIGH PERCENTAGE OF PRONUNCIATION PROBLEMS IN LEARNING TO SPEAK ENGLISH HAS TWO PROMINENT CAUSES: (1) THE PLACEMENT OF THE SPEECH ORGANS IS DIFFERENT IN SPANISH AND ENGLISH; AND (2) CHILDREN HAVE HAD NO PRACTICE IN PRONOUNCING SOUNDS NOT USED IN THEIR OWN LANGUAGE. TEACHERS AND SPEECH THERAPISTS, PREFERABLY BILINGUAL, MUST CAREFULLY DIAGNOSE THE PROBLEM AND USE THE APPROPRIATE REMEDIAL INSTRUCTIONS IN TREATING THESE CHILDREN. 10 REFERENCES.

ACCN 000087

100 AUTH **AYALA, P.**
TITL FOLK PRACTICES, FOLK MEDICINE AND CURANDERISMO ON THE WEST SIDE OF CHICAGO.
SRCE *PAPER PRESENTED AT THE ANNUAL MEETING OF THE SOCIETY FOR APPLIED ANTHROPOLOGY, MIAMI, APRIL 1972.*
INDX FOLK MEDICINE, CURANDERISMO, PSYCHOTHERAPISTS, MENTAL HEALTH, ESPIRITISMO, ESSAY, CASE STUDY, ILLINOIS, MIDWEST, MEXICAN AMERICAN
ABST VARIOUS FORMS OF FOLK MEDICINE AS PRACTICED BY MEXICAN AMERICANS IN CHICAGO BARRIOS ARE DESCRIBED. CURANDEROS ARE DIFFERENTIATED FROM ESPIRITISTAS BOTH IN THE AILMENTS THEY TREAT AND CURES THEY USE. EMOTIONAL ILLNESSES TREATED BY BOTH FOLK HEALERS ARE EL OJO MALO, SUSTO, AND EMBRUJADO. DUE TO THE RELUCTANCE OF THE BARRIO RESIDENTS TO DISCLOSE THEIR FOLK MEDICINE PREFERENCES TO STRANGERS, IT IS IMPOSSIBLE TO SURVEY THE USE PATTERNS, BUT AN EXPERIENCED GUESS ESTIMATES BETWEEN 60-80% OF THE POPULATION RELY ON FOLK RESOURCES FOR AT LEAST SOME ILLNESSES. FOLK MEDICINE IS, THEREFORE, A FORCE TO BE RECKONED WITH BY CLINICIANS WORKING WITH MEXICAN AMERICANS IN CHICAGO AS WELL AS OTHER MEXICAN-ORIGIN COMMUNITIES.

ACCN 000088

101 AUTH **BACA, G. M.**
TITL FORTY FAMILIES: A COMPARATIVE STUDY OF MEXICAN-AMERICAN AND ANGLO PARENTS OF AN INSTITUTIONALIZED RETARDED CHILD (DOCTORAL DISSERTATION, UNIVERSITY OF DENVER, 1975).
SRCE *DISSERTATION ABSTRACTS INTERNATIONAL, 1975, 36(5), 3128A. (UNIVERSITY MICROFILMS NO.75-25,310.)*
INDX MEXICAN AMERICAN, CROSS CULTURAL, EMPIRICAL, ADULTS, MENTAL RETARDATION, IMPAIRMENT, INSTITUTIONALIZATION, CULTURE,

CULTURAL FACTORS, NEW MEXICO, SOUTHWEST
ABST THIS CROSS-CULTURAL, EXPLORATORY STUDY COMPARED 20 MEXICAN AMERICAN AND 20 ANGLO FAMILIES IN NEW MEXICO WHO HAD INSTITUTIONALIZED A RETARDED CHILD. LENGTHY PERSONAL INTERVIEWS WITH THESE FAMILIES PROVIDED THE DATA. THE RESEARCH OBJECTIVE WAS TO COMPARE THE EXPERIENCES, BELIEFS, ATTITUDES AND PERCEPTIONS OF THE TWO GROUPS CONCERNING THEIR RETARDED CHILD. FIVE AREAS WERE INVESTIGATED: (1) BELIEFS ABOUT THE ETIOLOGY OF MENTAL RETARDATION; (2) ATTITUDES TOWARD INSTITUTIONALIZATION; (3) THEIR PREINSTITUTIONAL ACTIVITIES ON BEHALF OF THE CHILD; (4) CONCERNS WITHIN THE NUCLEAR FAMILY; AND (5) HOPES AND FEARS FOR THE CHILD'S FUTURE. CONTENT ANALYSIS WAS THE PRIMARY ANALYSIS METHOD. ONE OF THE MOST IMPORTANT FINDINGS WAS THAT MEXICAN AMERICAN AND ANGLO PARENTS UNDERGO SIMILAR EXPERIENCES IN TRYING TO COMPREHEND THEIR CHILD'S DISABILITY AND TO COPE WITH THE PROBLEM. 86 REFERENCES. (AUTHOR ABSTRACT MODIFIED)

ACCN 000089

102 AUTH **BACA, J. E.**
TITL SOME HEALTH BELIEFS OF THE SPANISH SPEAKING.
SRCE *AMERICAN JOURNAL OF NURSING, 1969, 69(10), 2172-2176.*
INDX FOLK MEDICINE, ESSAY, FATALISM, HEALTH, CULTURAL FACTORS, SPANISH SURNAMED, CURANDERISMO
ABST TRADITIONAL BELIEFS AND PRACTICES CONCERNING HEALTH AND ILLNESSES ARE STILL AN IMPORTANT FACTOR IN WORKING WITH SPANISH AMERICANS WHO RETAIN THEIR CULTURAL HERITAGE. THREE GENERAL CLASSIFICATIONS OF DISEASE RECOGNIZED BY SPANISH AMERICANS ARE: (1) NATURAL DISEASES; (2) MAGICAL DISEASES; AND (3) PSYCHOLOGICAL DISEASES. BRIEF DESCRIPTIONS OF MAL AIRE, MAL OJO, SUSTO, EMPACHO, AND CAIDA DE LA MOLLERA AND THEIR FOLK TREATMENTS ARE GIVEN. THE FUNCTIONS OF THE CURANDERO (FOLK HEALER), SOBADOR (MASSEUR), AND ALBOLARIO (SPECIALIST IN WITCHCRAFT ILLNESSES) ARE DESCRIBED. 10 REFERENCES.

ACCN 000090

103 AUTH **BACHRACH, L. L.**
TITL UTILIZATION OF STATE AND COUNTY MENTAL HOSPITALS BY SPANISH AMERICANS IN 1972 (STATISTICAL NOTE 116).
SRCE *ROCKVILLE, MD.: NATIONAL INSTITUTE OF MENTAL HEALTH, DIVISION OF BIOMETRY, JUNE 1975.*
INDX SPANISH SURNAMED, EMPIRICAL, RESOURCE UTILIZATION, MENTAL HEALTH, INSTITUTIONALIZATION, SEX COMPARISON, MALE, FEMALE, SURVEY, CROSS CULTURAL
ABST SPANISH AMERICAN ADMISSIONS TO MENTAL HOSPITALS NATIONWIDE ARE EXAMINED WITH THE PURPOSE OF SHOWING IF AND HOW THEY

DIFFER FROM ADMISSIONS OF OTHER ETHNIC GROUPS IN TERMS OF THE FOLLOWING VARIABLES: (1) AGE, (2) SEX, (3) MARITAL STATUS, (4) SOCIOECONOMIC LEVEL, (5) DIAGNOSIS, (6) LEGAL STATUS UPON ADMISSION, AND (7) LOCALE OF PREVIOUS PSYCHIATRIC CARE. THE DATA, REPRESENTING A SMALL SAMPLE OF STATE AND COUNTY MENTAL HOSPITAL ADMISSIONS FOR 1972, FAIL TO SHOW HIGHER UTILIZATION BY SPANISH AMERICANS—EXCEPT FOR THE AGE 65+ POPULATION. SEVERAL POSSIBLE EXPLANATIONS ARE DISCUSSED. 30 REFERENCES.

ACCN 000091

104 AUTH **BACK, K. W.**
TITL THE CHANGE-PRONE PERSON IN PUERTO RICO.
SRCE *PUBLIC OPINION QUARTERLY, 1958, 22(3), 330-340.*
INDX PUERTO RICAN-I, EMPIRICAL, SES, SOCIAL MOBILITY, HOUSING, URBAN, PERSONALITY ASSESSMENT, ADULTS
ABST THE RELATIONSHIP BETWEEN CHANGEABILITY AND RESIDENTIAL MOBILITY IN A SAMPLE OF 405 SUBJECTS FROM SLUM AREAS IN THE DIFFERENT STAGES OF THE HOUSING RELOCATION PROCESS IS INVESTIGATED. THE INTERVIEW CONSISTED OF THE FOLLOWING FIVE PERSONALITY MEASURES RELATING TO ACCEPTANCE OF CHANGE: THE ROLE-PLAYING TEST INVESTIGATING "CREATIVITY" IN HUMAN RELATION SITUATIONS; A SENTENCE COMPLETION TEST GIVING SCORES FOR "OPTIMISM" AND "AMBITION; INTERVIEW INDICES MEASURING ATTITUDES TOWARD "MODERNISM; AND RECORDS OF BEHAVIORAL "VARIABILITY." THE CHARACTERISTICS OF CHANGE-PRONE RESPONDENTS INDICATE THAT "CHANGERS" ARE MORE LIKELY TO BE YOUNG, EDUCATED MEN. MOST RECEPTIVE TOWARD CHANGE ARE HEADS OF FAMILIES WHO EITHER HAVE HIGH-STATUS JOBS OR A JOB ADAPTED TO THE INDUSTRIALIZATION OF THE COUNTRY. OPPOSITION TO CHANGE OCCURS IN FAMILIES OF LABORERS AND SERVICE WORKERS. CHANGEABILITY POINTS TO PERSONS WITH AN OPPORTUNITY FOR SOCIAL MOBILITY WHO ARE YOUNG ENOUGH TO LOOK TO THE FUTURE AND WHO FIT INTO THE GOVERNMENT PROGRAMS FOR EDUCATION AND ECONOMIC CHANGE. THE RELATION BETWEEN CHANGEABILITY AND RESIDENTIAL MOBILITY SHOWS LITTLE CORRELATION WITH ACCEPTANCE TO CHANGE. THE PROPORTION OF PERSONS WHO HAVE MOVED OUT OF THE SLUMS INTO HOUSING PROJECTS IS NOT POSITIVELY RELATED TO THE CHANGEABILITY SCORES. WHILE THE PERSONALITY MEASURES SHOW NO RELATIONSHIP TO MOBILITY, MODERNISM AND VARIABILITY HAVE SIGNIFICANT POSITIVE RELATIONSHIPS WITH THE INDEX OF RESIDENTIAL MOBILITY. 4 REFERENCES.
ACCN 000092

105 AUTH **BACKNER, B. L.**
TITL COUNSELING BLACK STUDENTS: ANY PLACE FOR WHITEY?

SRCE *JOURNAL OF HIGHER EDUCATION, 1970, 41(7), 630-637.*
INDX PUERTO RICAN-M, HIGHER EDUCATION, COLLEGE STUDENTS, EMPIRICAL, EDUCATIONAL COUNSELING, NEW YORK, EAST, CROSS CULTURAL
ABST BLACK AND PUERTO RICAN STUDENTS FROM A SPECIAL EDUCATIONAL PROGRAM PROVIDED DATA ON ATTITUDES AND OPINIONS REGARDING ETHNIC SIMILARITY OF THEIR COUNSELORS. THREE SAMPLINGS WERE OBTAINED IN SEPARATE PROJECTS, EACH WITH ITS OWN PURPOSE, EACH UTILIZING A DIFFERENT METHOD OF SAMPLING, AND ALL THREE VARYING WIDELY IN RELIABILITY AND VALIDITY. RESULTS FROM THE FIRST STUDY INDICATE THAT SEX AND AGE ARE MORE IMPORTANT FACTORS THAN RACIAL BACKGROUND WHEN SELECTING A COUNSELOR. THE SECOND STUDY SHOWED STUDENTS TO HAVE A PREFERENCE FOR A COUNSELOR OF SIMILAR ETHNIC BACKGROUND, ALTHOUGH SOME OF THEM INDICATED DISSATISFACTION WITH COUNSELOR EFFECTIVENESS. THE THIRD STUDY REVEALED THAT THE ONLY STUDENTS DESIRING A COUNSELOR FROM THEIR OWN ETHNIC BACKGROUND WERE STUDENTS WHO WERE ALREADY WORKING WITH A COUNSELOR WHOSE ETHNIC BACKGROUND WAS SIMILAR TO THEIRS. THE THREE SAMPLINGS PROVIDE EVIDENCE THAT BLACK AND PUERTO RICAN STUDENTS FEEL THAT SIMILARITY OF ETHNIC BACKGROUND BETWEEN COUNSELOR AND STUDENT "DOESN'T MATTER." THE FINDINGS SUGGEST THAT EVEN WHEN A STUDENT SAYS THAT HE DOES FEEL THAT HIS COUNSELOR'S BACKGROUND IS IMPORTANT, THIS OFTEN HAS MORE TO DO WITH THE STUDENT'S FEELING ABOUT THE COUNSELOR AS A PERSON. 2 REFERENCES.
ACCN 000093

106 AUTH **BADAINES, J.**
TITL IDENTIFICATION, IMITATION AND SEX ROLE PREFERENCE IN FATHER-PRESENT AND FATHER-ABSENT BLACK AND CHICANO BOYS.
SRCE *THE JOURNAL OF PSYCHOLOGY, 1976, 92(FIRST HALF), 15-24.*
INDX EMPIRICAL, CHILDREN, MALE, SEX ROLES, MEXICAN AMERICAN, FATHER-CHILD INTERACTION, CROSS CULTURAL, TEXAS, SOUTHWEST, MODELING
ABST THIS TWO PART STUDY WAS CONCERNED WITH IDENTIFICATION AND IMITATION IN 52 BLACK AND CHICANO 7 YEAR-OLD BOYS. PART 1 INVESTIGATED THE EFFECT OF RACE OF MODEL AND SUBJECT ON IMITATION BEHAVIOR. PART 2 INVESTIGATED THE EFFECT OF PATERNAL PRESENCE ON CHOICE OF A MALE OR FEMALE MODEL AND MASCULINE SEX-ROLE PREFERENCE. AFTER VIEWING FILMED MODELS, BLACK BOYS EXPRESSED A SIGNIFICANT PREFERENCE FOR THE BLACK MODE, BUT FOR CHICANO BOYS NO SIGNIFICANT PREFERENCES AMONG BLACK, WHITE OR CHICANO MODELS WERE OBTAINED. FATHER-PRESENT SUBJECTS HAD A SIGNIFICANTLY HIGHER MALE SEX-ROLE PREFERENCE SCORE AS COMPARED TO

FATHER-ABSENT. BOTH FATHER-ABSENT AND FATHER-PRESENT SUBJECTS IMITATED THE MALE MODEL SIGNIFICANTLY MORE THAN THE FEMALE, BUT THESE SCORES DID NOT CORRELATE SIGNIFICANTLY WITH THE SEX-ROLE PREFERENCE SCORE. BY AGE SEVEN, MASCULINE PREFERENCE APPEARED WELL ESTABLISHED, BUT IT WAS MORE MARKED FOR THE FATHER-PRESENT BOYS. 23 REFERENCES. (JOURNAL ABSTRACT MODIFIED)

ACCN   000094

107 AUTH **BAILEY, W. C., & KOVAL, M.**
     TITL   DIFFERENTIAL PATTERNS OF DRUG ABUSE AMONG WHITE ACTIVISTS AND NONWHITE MILITANT COLLEGE STUDENTS.
     SRCE   *INTERNATIONAL JOURNAL OF THE ADDICTIONS, 1972, 7(2), 191-199.*
     INDX   DRUG ABUSE, COLLEGE STUDENTS, SURVEY, CROSS CULTURAL, CULTURAL FACTORS, EMPIRICAL, PUERTO RICAN-M, NEW YORK, EAST
     ABST   A PILOT STUDY WAS CONDUCTED TO TEST THE HYPOTHESIS THAT WHITE STUDENT ACTIVISTS WOULD SHOW A GREATER INVOLVEMENT WITH DRUGS THAN NONWHITE STUDENT MILITANTS. QUESTIONNAIRE RESPONSES WERE OBTAINED FROM COLLEGE STUDENTS CLASSIFIED AS BLACK MILITANTS OR NONMILITANTS (76), WHITE ACTIVISTS OR NONACTIVISTS (57), AND PUERTO RICAN MILITANTS OR NONMILITANTS (19). CHI-SQUARE ANALYSIS FOR THE TOTAL SAMPLE REVEALS THAT THE MAJORITY OF SUBJECTS WERE DRUG USERS, WITH A SLIGHTLY HIGHER PROPORTION AMONG WHITES. BETWEEN-GROUP ANALYSIS SHOWS THAT WHITE ACTIVISTS WERE THE MOST INVOLVED AND BLACK NONMILITANTS THE LEAST INVOLVED WITH DRUGS. COMPARISON BETWEEN NONWHITE MILITANTS AND WHITE ACTIVISTS SUPPORTS THE HYPOTHESIS; WHITE ACTIVISTS REPORTED SIGNIFICANTLY MORE USE OF OPIATES AND LSD-TYPE DRUGS. MARIJUANA WAS THE MOST FREQUENTLY USED DRUG AMONG NONWHITE MILITANTS (46%). CULTURAL VALUES CONTRIBUTING TO SUBGROUP DIFFERENCES IN DRUG USE ARE DISCUSSED. 3 REFERENCES. (PASAR ABSTRACT MODIFIED)

ACCN   000095

108 AUTH **BAKER, G.**
     TITL   DECISION PROFILES OF MEXICAN-DESCENT.
     SRCE   *PAPER PRESENTED AT THE ANNUAL CONFERENCE OF THE NATIONAL COUNCIL ON FAMILY RELATIONS, ST. LOUIS, 1974. (ERIC DOCUMENT REPRODUCTION SERVICE NO. ED 103 730)*
     INDX   MEXICAN AMERICAN, CROSS CULTURAL, EMPIRICAL, FAMILY ROLES, SEX ROLES, ARIZONA, SOUTHWEST, DYADIC INTERACTION
     ABST   AN EXPLORATORY STUDY OF DECISION MAKING IN FAMILIES OF MEXICAN HERITAGE WAS CARRIED OUT IN PHOENIX, ARIZONA. A NORMATIVE MODEL OF DECISION RATIONALITY AND MEASUREMENT (FAMILY PROBLEM INSTRUMENT-FPI) WAS ADAPTED FROM PREVIOUS RESEARCH. TAPE RECORDED DATA WERE PROVIDED BY 27 FAMILIES. HUSBANDS AND WIVES RESPONDED SEPARATELY TO FAMILY DECISION SITUATIONS WHICH WERE CONSTRUCTED AND REVISED IN SEVERAL STAGES. RESULTS INDICATED THAT DECISION RATIONALITY LEVELS VARIED BY PROBLEM AREA, BY DECISION DIMENSION, AND BY FAMILY ROLE. IN GENERAL, FAMILIES REACHED A MIDDLE LEVEL OF DECISION RATIONALITY, AS MEASURED WITHIN THE LIMITATIONS IMPOSED BY A NORMATIVE MODEL OF DECISION MAKING. BASED ON THE FINDINGS, FAMILY PROFILES OR CASE STUDIES WERE CONSTRUCTED. THESE MAY BE USEFUL TO THOSE INTERESTED IN UNDERSTANDING THE DYNAMICS OF DECISION MAKING IN FAMILIES OF MEXICAN DESCENT. 21 REFERENCES. (RIE ABSTRACT MODIFIED)

ACCN   000096

109 AUTH **BAKER, S. H., & LEVENSON, B.**
     TITL   EARNING PROSPECTS OF BLACK AND WHITE WORKING-CLASS WOMEN.
     SRCE   *SOCIOLOGY OF WORK AND OCCUPATIONS, 1976, 3(2), 123-149.*
     INDX   EMPLOYMENT, DISCRIMINATION, EDUCATION, LABOR FORCE, SES, NEW YORK, EAST, URBAN, VOCATIONAL COUNSELING, EMPIRICAL, FEMALE, PUERTO RICAN-M, ADULTS, ADOLESCENTS, REPRESENTATION, CROSS CULTURAL, EQUAL OPPORTUNITY
     ABST   EARNINGS OF 1,100 BLACK, PUERTO RICAN, AND WHITE FEMALE GRADUATES OF A NEW YORK CITY VOCATIONAL HIGH SCHOOL WERE ANALYZED FOR A PERIOD OF FIVE YEARS AFTER GRADUATION. ANALYSIS OF WORK HISTORIES (BASED ON RECORDS OBTAINED FROM BOTH THE SOCIAL SECURITY ADMINISTRATION AND THE HIGH SCHOOL OF FASHION INDUSTRIES) REVEALED THAT BLACK AND PUERTO RICAN GRADUATES WHO COMPLETED THE SAME CURRICULUM AS WHITES EARN CONSIDERABLY LESS UPON ENTRY INTO THE LABOR MARKET. THE INITIAL UNEMPLOYMENT RATE WAS FIVE TIMES AS HIGH FOR NON-WHITES, AND EARNINGS IMPROVED LITTLE DURING THE FIVE YEARS AFTER GRADUATION. FACTORS FOUND TO CONTRIBUTE TO EARNING DIFFERENCES WERE RACE, INDUSTRIAL LOCATION OF JOB PLACEMENT, AND ACCESS TO EMPLOYMENT WITH GREATER EARNINGS POTENTIAL. COMPONENT ANALYSIS SUGGESTS THAT PRE-EMPLOYMENT INTERVENTION OFFERS LITTLE POTENTIAL FOR BRINGING BLACK AND PUERTO RICAN WORKERS UP TO PARITY. OF THE DIFFERENCES AMONG BLACK AND WHITE HIGH-EARNING GRADUATES, 72% RESULTED FROM DIFFERENCES IN INCOME MOBILITY RATES BETWEEN THE FIRST AND SECOND QUARTER AFTER GRADUATION, WHILE 22% WAS DUE TO FIRST JOB PAY-SCALE DIFFERENCES, AND ONLY 5% RESULTED FROM DIFFERENCES IN CURRICULUM PLACEMENT. IT IS DOUBTFUL, THEREFORE, THAT EQUALIZED TRAINING AND EDUCATION OF WHITES AND MINORITY GROUPS WILL LEAD TO COMPARABLE EARNINGS AND JOB OPPORTUNITIES. 33 REFERENCES.

ACCN   002015

110 AUTH **BAKER, S. H., & LEVENSON, B.**
TITL JOB OPPORTUNITIES OF BLACK AND WHITE WORKING-CLASS WOMEN.
SRCE *SOCIAL PROBLEMS, 1975, 22(4), 510-533.*
INDX PUERTO RICAN-M, EMPLOYMENT, FEMALE, EMPIRICAL, ADULTS, DISCRIMINATION, LABOR FORCE, EQUAL OPPORTUNITY, SES, CROSS CULTURAL, URBAN, NEW YORK, EAST, VOCATIONAL COUNSELING, REPRESENTATION, STEREOTYPES
ABST ENTRY EMPLOYMENT OF BLACK, PUERTO RICAN, AND WHITE GRADUATES OF THE SAME VOCATIONAL SCHOOL AND CURRICULA ARE EXAMINED IN ORDER TO ASSESS HOW OPEN THE EMPLOYMENT STRUCTURE IS FOR YOUNG WORKING-CLASS WOMEN. THE DATA DEMONSTRATE THAT FROM THE START MINORITY WOMEN DO NOT SHARE THE OCCUPATIONAL SUCCESS OF THEIR WHITE COUNTERPARTS. FACTORS AFFECTING THEIR CAREER SUCCESS ARE ANALYZED. FIRST, THE SCHOOL AND STATE EMPLOYMENT SERVICE REFERRAL AND PLACEMENT ACTIVITIES RESTRICT RATHER THAN EXPAND THE LABOR MARKET OPPORTUNITIES AVAILABLE TO THEM; THE REASONS ARE EXAMINED. SECOND, INDUSTRIAL PATTERNS OF RECRUITMENT ARE FOUND TO BE RACIALLY DISCRIMINATORY. FINALLY, THE RELATIONSHIP BETWEEN MARKET PLACE RECRUITMENT AND SCHOOL REFERRAL IS EXPLORED. THE FINDINGS CONCERNING EQUALITY OF OPPORTUNITY AMONG THESE WORKING-CLASS WOMEN ARE NOT OPTIMISTIC. 24 REFERENCES. (AUTHOR ABSTRACT)
ACCN 002016

111 AUTH **BALIAN, P., CARDONA, L., GARCIA, M., & ORTIZ, R.**
TITL INTRODUCTION OF THE PUERTO RICAN FAMILY IN NEW YORK CITY SCHOOLS OF SOCIAL WORK.
SRCE *SOCIAL WORK EDUCATION REPORTER, 1971, 19(1), 41-42.*
INDX MENTAL HEALTH PROFESSION, PUERTO RICAN-M, HIGHER EDUCATION, ESSAY, NEW YORK, EAST, PROFESSIONAL TRAINING
ABST THE PROBLEMS AND ISSUES RELATED TO PUERTO RICAN FACULTY OF NEW YORK SCHOOLS OF SOCIAL WORK ARE PRESENTED BRIEFLY. IT IS ARGUED THAT SCHOOLS WILL NOT ATTRACT PUERTO RICAN STUDENTS IF PUERTO RICAN FACULTY ARE NOT AVAILABLE. GRADUATES FROM SUCH SCHOOLS ARE BADLY NEEDED TO WORK WITHIN PUERTO RICAN COMMUNITIES TO PLAN AND IMPLEMENT RELEVANT PROGRAMS. A LIST OF DEMANDS INCLUDES (1) MORE ACTIVE RECRUITMENT OF PUERTO RICAN FACULTY, (2) POLICY CHANGES REGARDING TENURE PROMOTION, AND (3) AN INTERNSHIP PROGRAM FOR POTENTIAL PUERTO RICAN FACULTY CANDIDATES.
ACCN 000097

112 AUTH **BALK, D.**
TITL THE CATCHMENT AREA AND ITS TARGET POPULATIONS: A NEEDS ASSESSMENT SYNTHESIS.
SRCE *PHOENIX, ARIZ.: PHOENIX SOUTH COMMUNITY MENTAL HEALTH CENTER, 1976.*
INDX HEALTH DELIVERY SYSTEMS, MENTAL HEALTH, COMMUNITY, CHILDREN, ADULTS, DEMOGRAPHIC, DELINQUENCY, SES, POVERTY, GERONTOLOGY, PSYCHOPATHOLOGY, DRUG ADDICTION, DRUG ABUSE, ALCOHOLISM, EMPIRICAL, MEXICAN AMERICAN, CROSS CULTURAL, ARIZONA, SOUTHWEST
ABST ASSESSMENT OF NEEDS HAS BECOME RECOGNIZED AS A SIGNIFICANT ELEMENT IN THE PLANNING, DELIVERY AND EVALUATION OF COMMUNITY MENTAL HEALTH SERVICES. THIS SYNTHESIS DESCRIBES THE STUDIES CONDUCTED BY THE RESEARCH DEPARTMENT OF THE PHOENIX SOUTH COMMUNITY MENTAL HEALTH CENTER FROM 1973 THROUGH 1975. METHODS USED FOR GATHERING DATA (I.E., KEY INFORMANT, COMMUNITY FORUM, RATES UNDER TREATMENT, SOCIAL INDICATORS AND FIELD SURVEY) AS WELL AS DESCRIPTIVE SUMMARIES OF THE TARGET, HIGH-RISK POPULATIONS (I.E., CHILDREN AND YOUTH, ELDERLY, CHRONICALLY ILL AND SOCIALLY DISABLED, DRUG AND ALCOHOL ABUSERS) AND THEIR ASSESSED NEEDS ARE DISCUSSED IN DEPTH. MAPS AND GRAPHIC PLATES ILLUSTRATE HOW THE NEEDS ASSESSMENT DATA ARE APPLIED TO PREVENTION AND TREATMENT PLANNING AND EVALUATION. 37 REFERENCES.
ACCN 000098

113 AUTH **BALK, D., & BATES, J.**
TITL CHILD LIFE IN SOUTH PHOENIX: CENSUS TRACT 1167.
SRCE *PHOENIX, ARIZ.: PHOENIX SOUTH COMMUNITY MENTAL HEALTH CENTER, 1976.*
INDX CHILDREN, MENTAL HEALTH, DEVIANCE, EMPIRICAL, DEMOGRAPHIC, COMMUNITY, CROSS CULTURAL, MEXICAN AMERICAN, DELINQUENCY, HEALTH DELIVERY SYSTEMS, ARIZONA, SOUTHWEST
ABST THIS STUDY OF CHILD LIFE PRESENTS NEEDS ASSESSMENT DATA FROM ONE CENSUS TRACT OF THE PHOENIX SOUTH CATCHMENT AREA IN 1976. THE DATA COLLECTION EMPHASIZED IDENTIFYING WHICH BEHAVIORS ARE CONSIDERED PROBLEMS BY FAMILY MEMBERS AND NEIGHBORHOOD ADULTS AND WHICH BEHAVIORS ARE PERCEIVED AS STRENGTHS IN 5 TO 12 YEAR-OLD CHILDREN. THE ASSESSMENT RESULTS ARE DISCUSSED IN RELATION TO FURTHER RESEARCH, PROGRAM PLANNING, AND INFORMATION DISSEMINATION.
ACCN 000099

114 AUTH **BALL, J. C.**
TITL MARIJUANA SMOKING AND THE ONSET OF HEROIN USE.
SRCE *IN J. O. COLE & J. R. WITTENBORN (EDS.), DRUG ABUSE: SOCIAL AND PSYCHOPHARMACOLOGICAL ASPECTS. SPRINGFIELD, ILL.: CHARLES C. THOMAS, 1969, PP. 117-128.*
INDX DRUG ABUSE, DRUG ADDICTION, PUERTO RICAN-I, ADULTS, SEX COMPARISON, PEER GROUP, EMPIRICAL
ABST A STUDY WAS MADE OF THE ONSET OF HEROIN USE BY PUERTO RICAN ADDICTS. THE FOLLOWING QUESTIONS WERE CONSIDERED: WHO PROVIDED THE ILLEGAL DRUG? HOW WERE THE TECHNIQUES OF ADMINISTRATION

LEARNED? FROM WHOM? WHERE DID THE EVENT OCCUR? WERE THERE PERCURSORS? HOW IS OPIATE ADDICTION SPREAD AMONG JUVENILES? HEROIN USE BEGAN IN AN UNSUPERVISED STREET SETTING, WHILE THE SUBJECTS WERE STILL TEENAGERS. THE INITIATES HAD USUALLY SMOKED MARIJUANA BEFORE USING OPIATES. THERE WAS NO EVIDENCE THAT THE ONSET OF DRUG USE WAS A CONSEQUENCE OF PROSELYTIZING, COERCION, OR SEDUCTION. ONSET WAS A GROUP PROCESS. THE INCIPIENT ADDICT WILLINGLY SOUGHT TO JOIN THE ADDICT GROUP AND LEARN THE TECHNIQUES AND NORMS OF THE DRUG SUBCULTURE. HE WAS NOT MISLED BY MERCENARY FRAUD. THE INTERPERSONAL AND SITUATIONAL FACTORS ASSOCIATED WITH THE ONSET OF MARIJUANA SMOKING AND OPIATE USE AMONG THE PUERTO RICAN ADDICTS OF THIS STUDY HAVE NOT CHANGED DURING THE PAST 40 YEARS. ALTHOUGH THE INCIDENCE AND PREVALENCE OF DRUG ABUSE IN PUERTO RICO MAY HAVE CHANGED DURING THIS PERIOD, THE EVIDENCE SUGGESTS THAT THE PEER-GROUP BEHAVIOR LEADING TO THE ONSET OF DRUG ADDICTION HAS REMAINED UNCHANGED. 20 REFERENCES.

ACCN   000100

115 AUTH   **BALL, J. C., & PABON, D. O.**
     TITL   LOCATING AND INTERVIEWING NARCOTIC ADDICTS IN PUERTO RICO.
     SRCE   *SOCIOLOGY AND SOCIAL RESEARCH, 1965, 49(4), 401-411.*
     INDX   RESEARCH METHODOLOGY, PUERTO RICAN-I, DRUG ADDICTION, ADULTS, EMPIRICAL, SES, SEX COMPARISON
     ABST   THE INTERVIEW PROCEDURE EMPLOYED AND THE FIELD EXPERIENCES WHICH TOOK PLACE DURING THE 2-YEAR FOLLOWUP STUDY OF 243 FORMER NARCOTIC ADDICTS IN PUERTO RICO ARE DISCUSSED. POST-HOSPITAL INFORMATION WAS SECURED FOR 97% OF THE SUBJECTS; 109 OF THE FORMER ADDICTS WERE LOCATED AND INTERVIEWED IN PUERTO RICO. IT WAS FOUND THAT THE FORMER FEMALE ADDICTS, MOST OF WHOM WERE ENGAGED IN PROSTITUTION, WERE MORE DIFFICULT TO LOCATE THAN THE FORMER MALE ADDICTS. SUBJECTS FROM MIDDLE- OR UPPER-CLASS FAMILIES, FROM RURAL AREAS, AND THOSE NOT ACTIVELY ENGAGED IN "LIFE ON THE STREET" WERE MORE READILY INTERVIEWED THAN OTHERS. PRELIMINARY ANALYSIS OF THE RESEARCH FINDINGS REVEALS THAT MORE THAN HALF OF THE SUBJECTS WERE EITHER INCARCERATED OR USING OPIATES AT THE TIME OF THE INTERVIEW. OF THOSE "ON THE STREET," ONE-THIRD WERE USING OPIATES. THE SUBJECT'S OCCUPATION WAS ASSOCIATED WITH HIS ADDICTION STATUS. THUS, THOSE MALES ENGAGED IN ILLEGAL OCCUPATIONS WERE MOST LIKELY TO BE DRUG USERS, TO HAVE ARREST RECORDS, AND TO BE IMPRISONED OR HOSPITALIZED. 11 REFERENCES.
     ACCN   000101

116 AUTH   **BALL, J. C., & SNARR, R. W.**
     TITL   A TEST OF THE MATURATION HYPOTHESIS WITH RESPECT TO OPIATE ADDICTION.
     SRCE   *BULLETIN ON NARCOTICS, 1969, 21(4), 9-13.*
     INDX   DRUG ADDICTION, PUERTO RICAN-I, ADULTS, EMPIRICAL, CRIMINOLOGY, REHABILITATION
     ABST   THE RESULTS OF FOLLOWUP STUDIES ON 242 PUERTO RICAN OPIUM ADDICTS INDICATE THAT 67% WERE STILL USING HEROIN OR WERE INCARCERATED. WITH CONTINUED USE OF THE DRUG, THE EXTENT OF CRIMINALITY AND SOCIAL IMPAIRMENT INCREASED. A SIZABLE MINORITY, 20% TO 40%, OF THE ADDICTS BECAME ABSTINENT AND REASONABLY PRODUCTIVE CITIZENS. THUS, TWO MAJOR PATTERNS WERE FOUND AMONG HEROIN ADDICTS: NONPRODUCTIVE CRIMINALITY, OR MATURATION TO A POINT OF ABSTINENCE. 12 REFERENCES.
     ACCN   000102

117 AUTH   **BALLENTINE, L., & LEVINE, D. U.**
     TITL   RESEARCH NOTE: HOME ENVIRONMENT AND READING PERFORMANCE AMONG AFRO, ANGLO AND MEXICAN KINDERGARTEN STUDENTS IN AN INNER CITY SCHOOL.
     SRCE   *UNPUBLISHED MANUSCRIPT, MISSOURI UNIVERSITY, KANSAS CITY, CENTER FOR THE STUDY OF METROPOLITAN PROBLEMS IN EDUCATION, AUGUST 1971. (ERIC DOCUMENT REPRODUCTION SERVICE NO. ED 058 943)*
     INDX   READING, SCHOLASTIC ACHIEVEMENT, CROSS CULTURAL, MEXICAN AMERICAN, EMPIRICAL, URBAN, FAMILY ROLES, KANSAS, MIDWEST
     ABST   THIS EXPLORATORY STUDY EXAMINED THE RELATIONSHIP BETWEEN READING PERFORMANCE SCORES AND THREE MEASURES OF HOME ENVIRONMENT AMONG KINDERGARTEN STUDENTS OF DIFFERENT RACIAL AND ETHNIC BACKGROUND. IT ALSO DETERMINED WHETHER THERE WAS EVIDENCE THAT PARTICIPATION IN A FOLLOW THROUGH PROGRAM HAD BEEN EFFECTIVE IN OVERCOMING EDUCATIONAL DISADVANTAGES ASSOCIATED WITH NONSUPPORTIVE HOME ENVIRONMENTS. SUBJECTS IN THE STUDY WERE KINDERGARTEN STUDENTS WHO HAD FINISHED THEIR FIRST YEAR IN A FOLLOW THROUGH PROGRAM; 11 WERE MEXICAN AMERICAN, 10 WERE ANGLO AMERICAN, AND 9 WERE AFRO-AMERICAN. FOUR OF THE MEXICAN AMERICAN, SEVEN OF THE AFRO-AMERICAN, AND FOUR OF THE ANGLO AMERICAN STUDENTS HAD BEEN IN A PRE-KINDERGARTEN HEAD START PROGRAM THE YEAR BEFORE. HOME ENVIRONMENT MEASURES USED WERE: (1) A MODIFIED 40-ITEM VERSION OF THE DAVE AND WOLF INTERVIEW SCHEDULE FOR ASSESSING HOME INFLUENCES ON ACHIEVEMENT AND INTELLIGENCE; (2) INTERVIEWER'S RATING OF THE ORDERLINESS OF THE LIVING ROOM IN EACH SUBJECT'S HOME; AND (3) THE FREQUENCY WITH WHICH THE SUBJECT'S MOTHER ATTENDED CHURCH. RESULTS SHOW THAT THE STRONGEST CORRELATIONS BETWEEN HOME-ENVIRONMENT MEASURES AND READING LEVEL WERE AMONG THE ANGLO AMERICAN AND AFRO-AMERICAN STUDENTS. MOST IMPORTANT OF THE FINDINGS WAS THAT MEASURES OF HOME ENVI-

RONMENT CORRELATED WITH READING LEVEL AMONG THE SAMPLE OF ECONOMICALLY DISADVANTAGED STUDENTS FINISHING KINDERGARTEN. 2 REFERENCES. (RIE ABSTRACT)

ACCN 000103

118 AUTH **BALLESTEROS, D.**
TITL TOWARD AN ADVANTAGED SOCIETY: BILINGUAL EDUCATION IN THE 70'S.
SRCE *THE NATIONAL ELEMENTARY PRINCIPAL, 1970, 50(2), 25-28.*
INDX BILINGUAL-BICULTURAL EDUCATION, SPANISH SURNAMED, CHILDREN, ESSAY, EQUAL OPPORTUNITY, SPECIAL EDUCATION
ABST SCHOOLS MUST CHANGE THEIR PROGRAMS TO MEET THE NEEDS OF STUDENTS INSTEAD OF TRYING TO CHANGE THE STUDENTS TO MEET THE NEEDS OF SCHOOLS. THIS POINT IS PARTICULARLY CLEAR IN RELATION TO SPANISH-SPEAKING CHILDREN WHO ARE PLACED IN CLASSES FOR THE MENTALLY RETARDED IN DISPROPORTIONATE NUMBERS OR SUFFER DISCOURAGEMENT AND LOW MORALE AS A RESULT OF THE TREATMENT THEY RECEIVE IN SCHOOL. BILINGUAL EDUCATION SHOULD BE SEEN AS A POSITIVE FORCE IN SCHOOL PROGRAMS BECAUSE IT (1) REDUCES RETARDATION THROUGH STUDENTS' ABILITY TO IMMEDIATELY LEARN IN THE MOTHER TONGUE, (2) REINFORCES SCHOOL-HOME RELATIONS THROUGH A COMMON COMMUNICATION BOND, (3) PROJECTS THE CHILD INTO AN ATMOSPHERE OF PERSONAL EDUCATION, SELF-WORTH AND ACHIEVEMENT, AND (4) PRESERVES AND ENRICHES THE CULTURAL AND HUMAN RESOURCES OF A PEOPLE. THE ENACTMENT OF THE BILINGUAL EDUCATION ACT, TITLE VII OF THE ELEMENTARY AND SECONDARY EDUCATION ACT, GIVES IMPETUS TO THE EDUCATION OF THE SPANISH-SPEAKING STUDENT. THE FIRST PRIORITY OF THIS ACT IS TO STRENGTHEN THE EDUCATION OF BILINGUAL CHILDREN, PARTICULARLY FROM LOW INCOME FAMILIES; SECOND, TO PROMOTE BILINGUALISM AMONG ALL STUDENTS. BILINGUAL EDUCATION MUST BE VIEWED AS AN ASSET, NOT A LIABILITY OR REMEDIAL PROGRAM, IF THE PROGRAM IS TO BE SUCCESSFUL.
ACCN 000104

119 AUTH **BARBERIO, R.**
TITL THE RELATIONSHIP BETWEEN ACHIEVEMENT MOTIVATION AND ETHNICITY IN ANGLO AMERICAN AND MEXICAN AMERICAN JUNIOR HIGH SCHOOL STUDENTS.
SRCE *PSYCHOLOGICAL RECORD, 1967, 17(2), 263-266.*
INDX ACHIEVEMENT MOTIVATION, ADOLESCENTS, CROSS CULTURAL, EMPIRICAL, INTELLIGENCE, MEXICAN AMERICAN, TEXAS, SOUTHWEST
ABST IN AN EFFORT TO DETERMINE NEED ACHIEVEMENT (N-ACH), 342 ANGLO AMERICAN AND MEXICAN AMERICAN STUDENTS 12-14 YEARS OF AGE WERE PROVIDED A SET OF THREE 4X5-INCH STIMULUS PICTURES AND A TEST BOOKLET TO WRITE A STORY FOR EACH OF THE PICTURES. EACH PICTURE HAD FIVE RELATED QUESTIONS THAT THE SUBJECTS WERE TO EX-

POUND UPON. AFTER ALL 342 OF THE TESTS HAD BEEN ADMINISTERED AND SCORED, THEN THE TEST BOOKLETS OF 69 MEXICAN AMERICAN SUBJECTS WERE RANDOMLY SELECTED AND MATCHED WITH A LIKE GROUP OF ANGLO AMERICAN SUBJECTS HAVING THE SAME INTELLIGENCE. IT WAS CONCLUDED THAT THERE IS NO STATISTICALLY SIGNIFICANT DIFFERENCE IN THE MEAN NEED TO ACHIEVE BETWEEN ANGLO AND MEXICAN AMERICAN EIGHTH-GRADE STUDENTS HAVING THE SAME INTELLIGENCE. THIS SUGGESTS THAT DIFFERENCES IN N-ACH NORMALLY ATTRIBUTED TO ETHNIC GROUP MEMBERSHIP ARE DUE RATHER TO DIFFERENCES IN INTELLIGENCE. 3 REFERENCES.

ACCN 000105

120 AUTH **BARCELO, C. J., JR.**
TITL FEDERAL ADVISORY BODIES. . . WHO ASKS HISPANICS FOR ADVICE?
SRCE *AGENDA, JANUARY/FEBRUARY 1977, PP. 17-20.*
INDX POLITICS, REPRESENTATION, SPANISH SURNAMED, ADMINISTRATORS, POLICY
ABST ADVISORY COMMITTEES ARE A COMMON AND WIDESPREAD BUREAUCRATIC PHENOMENON WHOSE EXISTENCE AND ACTIVITIES ARE LITTLE KNOWN AND POORLY PUBLICIZED. SINCE 1972 WHEN CONGRESS PASSED THE FEDERAL ADVISORY ACT REQUIRING GREATER ACCOUNTABILITY AND PUBLIC ACCESSIBILITY FROM THESE COMMITTEES, REPORTS REVEAL THE SIGNIFICANT LACK OF HISPANIC REPRESENTATION ON THESE COMMITTEES. THIS BRIEF ARTICLE SUMMARIZES THE FINDINGS OF THE 1976 SENATE COMMITTEE ON GOVERNMENT OPERATIONS WHICH DOCUMENTS A PATTERN OF SEVERE UNDERREPRESENTATION OF WOMEN AND MINORITIES, ESPECIALLY HISPANICS.
ACCN 000106

121 AUTH **BARCELO, C. J., JR., & BREITER, T.**
TITL HISPANICS ON WELFARE—THE FACTS AND FIGURES.
SRCE *AGENDA, MARCH/APRIL 1977, PP. 4-10.*
INDX POVERTY, SPANISH SURNAMED, MEXICAN AMERICAN, PUERTO RICAN-M, SOCIAL SERVICES, ECONOMIC FACTORS, EMPIRICAL, DEMOGRAPHIC, EMPLOYMENT, NUTRITION, HOUSING, SES
ABST AN OVERVIEW OF HISPANIC PARTICIPATION RATES IN SPECIFIC WELFARE PROGRAMS IS PRESENTED. ALTHOUGH DATA ON PARTICIPATION RATES BY ETHNIC GROUP ARE NOT COMPLETE, THREE NATIONWIDE PROGRAMS ARE EXAMINED: (1) AID TO FAMILIES WITH DEPENDENT CHILDREN (AFDC); (2) FOOD STAMP PROGRAM; AND (3) PUBLIC HOUSING ASSISTANCE. THE PAUCITY OF AVAILABLE DATA DOES NOT ALLOW CONCLUSIONS TO BE MADE ABOUT THE HISTORICAL AND CULTURAL DISLIKE BY MOST HISPANICS FOR DEPENDENCE ON ASSISTANCE AGENCIES. REFORMS IN WELFARE PROGRAMS CANNOT BE SENSITIVE AND RESPONSIVE TO THE HISPANIC SEGMENT OF THE POPULATION WITHOUT MORE ACCURATE DATA AND CONSIDERATION OF VARIABLES SUCH AS

CULTURAL IDENTIFICATION AND ATTITUDES TOWARD ASSISTANCE PROGRAMS.

ACCN 000107

122 AUTH **BARKER, G. C.**

TITL SOCIAL FUNCTIONS OF LANGUAGE IN A MEXICAN-AMERICAN COMMUNITY.

SRCE *ACTA AMERICANA, 1947, 5(3), 185-202.*

INDX LINGUISTICS, BILINGUALISM, ACCULTURATION, INTERPERSONAL RELATIONS, CASE STUDY, MEXICAN AMERICAN, ARIZONA, BILINGUAL, SOUTHWEST

ABST AN INQUIRY INTO THE LANGUAGE FUNCTION OF A BILINGUAL MINORITY GROUP IN THE PROCESS OF CULTURAL CHANGE IS PRESENTED. INFORMAL OBSERVATIONS, QUESTIONNAIRES, AND INTERVIEWS OVER A PERIOD OF 6 MONTHS EXAMINED THE LANGUAGE USAGE OF THE INDIVIDUALS FROM AN IN-GROUP AND OUT-GROUP RELATIONS PERSPECTIVE. DATA INDICATE A DIVISION OF THE SOCIAL FUNCTIONS OF LANGUAGE WITHIN THE SPECIFIC AREAS OF INTIMATE OR FAMILY RELATIONS, INFORMAL RELATIONS, FORMAL RELATIONS, AND ANGLO-MEXICAN RELATIONS. CONGRUITY OF THE INDIVIDUAL'S LINGUISTIC BEHAVIOR IS PATTERNED WITH HIS SOCIAL RELATIONS, AND FOUR VARYING DEGREES OF BILINGUAL TYPES ARE DESCRIBED. IN ADDITION, CONGRUITY OF THE GROUP'S LINGUISTIC BEHAVIOR IS PATTERNED WITH ITS SOCIAL RELATIONS. THE GROUP TENDS TO PRESERVE SPANISH AS THE LANGUAGE FOR FAMILY RELATIONS WHILE RESERVING ENGLISH FOR IMPERSONAL RELATIONS. A CORRELATION OF LINGUISTIC BEHAVIOR PATTERNS WITH BASIC ACCULTURATION CONDITIONS REVEALS DIVERGENT TYPES OF CULTURAL ORIENTATIONS. THUS, LINGUISTIC BEHAVIOR IS CONCERNED NOT SO MUCH WITH WHAT AN INDIVIDUAL STATES ARE HIS ATTITUDES AND VALUES AS WITH HOW HE USES AND REACTS TO THE LINGUISTIC SYMBOL SYSTEMS AT HIS COMMAND IN THE DAILY COURSE OF HIS SOCIAL CONTACTS.

ACCN 000108

123 AUTH **BARNES, R. F.**

TITL CONFLICTS OF CULTURAL TRANSCRIPTION: A REVIEW OF DILEMMAS FACED BY THE MEXICAN AMERICAN WORKER AND HIS FAMILY.

SRCE *UNPUBLISHED MANUSCRIPT, UNIVERSITY OF CALIFORNIA AT DAVIS, DEPARTMENT OF APPLIED BEHAVIORAL SCIENCES, MAY 1969. (ERIC DOCUMENT REPRODUCTION SERVICE NO. ED 030 522)*

INDX REVIEW, ACCULTURATION, MEXICAN AMERICAN, FAMILY STRUCTURE, SES, FARM LABORERS, MIGRATION, CALIFORNIA, SOUTHWEST

ABST MEXICAN TRADITIONS AND CUSTOMS AND CHANGES ENCOUNTERED IN THE UNITED STATES ARE REVIEWED INDICATING THE EFFECT OF MIGRATION ON THE FAMILY UNIT. DISCUSSION INCLUDES FAMILY LIFE IN MEXICO, THE STATUS OF MEXICAN WOMEN, FAMILY LIFE IN A DIFFERENT CULTURE, THE CALIFORNIA FARM LABOR SITUATION, AND LEGISLATION AFFECTING THE FARM WORKER. EMPLOYMENT

OPPORTUNITIES, HEALTH AND WELFARE SERVICES, FRINGE BENEFITS, AND HOUSING ARE TOPICS CONSIDERED IN PRESENTING CURRENT AND FUTURE NEEDS OF CALIFORNIA'S FARM WORKERS. EDUCATIONAL PROBLEMS AND EDUCATIONAL NEEDS OF THE MEXICAN AMERICAN ARE POINTED OUT IN CONCLUDING SECTIONS. 19 REFERENCES. (RIE ABSTRACT MODIFIED)

ACCN 000109

124 AUTH **BARRERA, M.**

TITL MEXICAN-AMERICAN MENTAL HEALTH SERVICE UTILIZATION: A CRITICAL EXAMINATION OF SOME PROPOSED VARIABLES.

SRCE *COMMUNITY MENTAL HEALTH JOURNAL, 1978, 14(1), 35-45.*

INDX MEXICAN AMERICAN, BILINGUAL-BICULTURAL PERSONNEL, MENTAL HEALTH, RESOURCE UTILIZATION, REVIEW, CULTURAL FACTORS, PSYCHOTHERAPY, ESSAY

ABST A NUMBER OF REPORTS INDICATE THAT MEXICAN AMERICANS HAVE A LOWER PREVALENCE OF MENTAL HEALTH SERVICE USAGE THAN OTHER ETHNIC GROUPS. ALTHOUGH A NUMBER OF FACTORS HAVE BEEN PROPOSED TO ACCOUNT FOR THEIR UNDERUTILIZATION, NONE OF THE FACTORS HAVE BEEN ADEQUATELY SUPPORTED BY EXISTING RESEARCH. VARIABLES ASSOCIATED WITH THE RESPONSIVENESS AND QUALITY OF MENTAL HEALTH SERVICES, PARTICULARLY THE AVAILABILITY OF BILINGUAL-BICULTURAL STAFF, ARE ADVOCATED AS THE MOST RELEVANT AREAS FOR FUTURE RESEARCH. 43 REFERENCES. (AUTHOR ABSTRACT)

ACCN 000110

125 AUTH **BATT, C. E.**

TITL MEXICAN CHARACTER: AN ADLERIAN INTERPRETATION.

SRCE *JOURNAL OF INDIVIDUAL PSYCHOLOGY, 1969, 25(2), 183-201.*

INDX PERSONALITY, MEXICAN, ESSAY, SELF CONCEPT, HISTORY, REVIEW, SEX ROLES, ALCOHOLISM, CHILDREN, FAMILY ROLES, THEORETICAL

ABST THE FIRST PART OF THIS LITERATURE REVIEW DESCRIBING MEXICAN NATIONAL CHARACTER EXAMINES THE VIEWS OF SAMUEL RAMOS AND OCTAVIO PAZ. THE EMPIRICAL DATA FROM OSCAR LEWIS AND THE AUTHOR COMPOSE THE SECOND PART OF THE REVIEW. RAMOS PERCEIVES MEXICAN CHARACTER IN TERMS OF THE ADLERIAN INFERIORITY COMPLEX AND THE BASIC STRIVING FOR SECURITY AND SUPERIORITY. HE SEES THE FEELING OF INFERIORITY AS UNDENIABLY INFLUENCED BY EXTERNAL CIRCUMSTANCES, BUT ULTIMATELY DEPENDENT ON THE DEGREE OF CONFIDENCE THAT THE INDIVIDUAL HAS IN HIMSELF. THIS SELF-CONFIDENCE CAN BE GREATLY UNDERMINED WHEN A PERSON'S GOAL OVERREACHES HIS ABILITY. THEN, HE CAN ACHIEVE ONLY AN ILLUSION OF SUPERIORITY BY DOMINATING OR POWER STRIVING. PAZ VIEWS THE MEXICAN AS LIVING IN A SOCIETY WHICH GIVES HIM NO SENSE OF COMMUNITY AND

THEREFORE DOES NOT ENABLE HIM TO FEEL OR EXPRESS THE EQUIVALENT OF ADLER'S SOCIAL INTEREST. THE EMPIRICAL DATA OF LEWIS AND OTHERS HAVE ADDED TO THE "CULT OF MANLINESS," AN ADLERIAN DYNAMIC, WITH THE DISCUSSIONS OF MASCULINE PROTEST AND MAN'S FEAR FOR HIS STATUS, AND AS A COUNTERPART, THE FEMALE MARTYR COMPLEX AND THE OCCASIONAL DEFIANT FEMALE. THE DATA HAVE SHOWN THAT THESE CHARACTERISTICS DEVELOP NOT SO MUCH FROM THE MEXICAN HISTORICOCULTURAL SITUATION AS FROM THE CHILDHOOD EXPERIENCES WITHIN THE STRUCTURE OF THE LATIN FAMILY. THESE OBSERVATIONS STILL APPLY TO THE CURRENT SCENE IN MEXICO. 32 REFERENCES.

ACCN 000112

126 AUTH **BAUERMEISTER, J. J., FERNANDEZ DE CINTRON, C. F., & RIVERA-MEDINA, E.**

TITL COMMUNITY PSYCHOLOGY IN PUERTO RICO: MEETING THE CHALLENGE OF A RAPIDLY CHANGING SOCIETY.

SRCE *IN I. ISCOE, B. L. BLOOM, & C. D. SPEILBERGER (EDS.), COMMUNITY PSYCHOLOGY IN TRANSITION. NEW YORK: HEMISPHERE PUBLISHING CORP., 1977, PP. 301-307.*

INDX COLLEGE STUDENTS, COMMUNITY INVOLVEMENT, CURRICULUM, EDUCATION, ESSAY, HIGHER EDUCATION, MENTAL HEALTH PROFESSION, PROFESSIONAL TRAINING, PUERTO RICAN-I

ABST THE DEPARTMENT OF PSYCHOLOGY OF THE UNIVERSITY OF PUERTO RICO REVISED THE TRAINING OBJECTIVES OF ITS MASTERS DEGREE PROGRAM IN 1974-75 IN RESPONSE TO THE MENTAL HEALTH NEEDS OF A SOCIETY IMMERSED IN THE PROBLEMS OF RAPID GROWTH AND CHANGE. A COMMUNITY PSYCHOLOGY TRAINING MODEL WAS CREATED WITH THE FOLLOWING OBJECTIVES: (1) TO TRAIN STUDENTS TO IDENTIFY, UNDERSTAND, AND INVESTIGATE THE PSYCHO-SOCIAL PROCESSES AND NEEDS OF COMMUNITIES, AND TO GAIN KNOWLEDGE ABOUT ATTITUDES, LEADERSHIP, VALUES, SOCIALIZATION PROCESSES, PROPAGANDA, SOCIAL CHANGE, AND PLANNING; (2) TO PREPARE STUDENTS TO IDENTIFY AND DEVELOP AVAILABLE COMMUNITY RESOURCES TO MEET THE NEEDS OF THE POPULATION; (3) TO DEVELOP SKILLS IN PRIMARY PREVENTION WITH GROUPS, RECOGNIZING THE SOCIAL FORCES THAT EXIST IN THE COMMUNITY; AND (4) TO DEVELOP SKILLS IN CONSULTATION AND IN THE EVALUATION OF MENTAL HEALTH AND SOCIAL PROGRAMS: COURSEWORK FOR THE FOUR SEMESTER PROGRAM IS DESCRIBED—INCLUDING SOCIAL AND COMMUNITY PSYCHOLOGY WITH SPECIFIC REFERENCE TO PUERTO RICO; SUPERVISED PRACTICUM EXPERIENCES IN COMMUNITY INTERVENTIONS; AND A THESIS PROJECT. A KEY COMPONENT OF THE PROGRAM IS THE OPPORTUNITY FOR FIELD TRAINING AT A NEWLY ESTABLISHED COMMUNITY CENTER PROVIDING PSYCHO-SOCIAL SERVICES AND USING INNOVATIVE MODELS OF PROFESSIONAL INTERVENTION.

ACCN 002018

127 AUTH **BAUERMEISTER, J. J., & JEMAIL, J. A.**

TITL MODIFICATION OF "ELECTIVE MUTISM" IN THE CLASSROOM SETTING: A CASE STUDY.

SRCE *BEHAVIOR THERAPY, 1975, 6, 246-250.*

INDX BEHAVIOR MODIFICATION, PUERTO RICAN-I, CHILDREN, CASE STUDY, TEACHERS, INSTRUCTIONAL TECHNIQUES, CLASSROOM BEHAVIOR, PARENTAL INVOLVEMENT

ABST OPERANT CONDITIONING TECHNIQUES WERE APPLIED TO A CASE OF "ELECTIVE MUTISM—A PARTICULAR VERBAL BEHAVIOR PROBLEM IN WHICH FULLY DEVELOPED SPEECH IS EMITTED IN THE PRESENCE OF SOME PERSONS BUT SUPPRESSED IN THE PRESENCE OF OTHERS. THE CHILD WAS AN 8 YEAR-OLD, THIRD GRADE PUERTO RICAN BOY WHO REFUSED TO PARTICIPATE IN CLASSROOM ACTIVITIES WHICH REQUIRED VERBAL COMMUNICATION. OUTSIDE THE CLASSROOM SETTING, HOWEVER, HE WAS OBSERVED TO COMMUNICATE FREELY AND WITHOUT DIFFICULTY. THE TREATMENT WAS ADMINISTERED IN PUERTO RICO BY CLASSROOM TEACHERS IN THE CLASSROOM SETTING THROUGHOUT APPROXIMATELY 20 SCHOOL DAYS. THE CHILD'S VERBAL EXPRESSION IN THE CLASSROOM WAS CONSIDERABLY INCREASED BY MAKING SOCIAL AND TANGIBLE REINFORCERS CONTINGENT UPON HAND RAISING, ANSWERING QUESTIONS, AND READING ALOUD; COMPLETION OF CLASSROOM ASSIGNMENTS WAS SIMILARLY IMPROVED. PARENTAL COOPERATION WAS ELICITED IN THE PROGRAM. AT THE TIME THE STUDY WAS COMPLETED HIS GRADES HAD IMPROVED TO SUCH A DEGREE THAT HIS TEACHERS RECOMMENDED HIS PROMOTION TO THE FOURTH GRADE. FOLLOW-UP OBSERVATION A YEAR LATER INDICATED THAT TREATMENT GAINS HAD BEEN MAINTAINED. 14 REFERENCES. (JOURNAL ABSTRACT MODIFIED)

ACCN 002019

128 AUTH **BAUERMEISTER, J. J., & JEMAIL, J. A.**

TITL TEACHERS AS EXPERIMENTERS AND BEHAVIORAL ENGINEERS: AN EXTENSION AND CROSS-CULTURAL REPLICATION.

SRCE *INTERAMERICAN JOURNAL OF PSYCHOLOGY, 1976, 10, 41-55.*

INDX BEHAVIOR MODIFICATION, CHILDREN, TEACHERS, CLASSROOM BEHAVIOR, INSTRUCTIONAL TECHNIQUES, EMPIRICAL, CASE STUDY, PUERTO RICAN-I

ABST THREE EXPERIMENTS IN THE SYSTEMATIC APPLICATION OF BEHAVIOR PRINCIPLES IN THE CLASSROOM SETTING WERE CONDUCTED BY ELEMENTARY SCHOOL TEACHERS IN PUERTO RICO. THE FIRST TWO EXPERIMENTS DEMONSTRATED THE MODIFICATION OF NON-COMPLETION OF WRITTEN ASSIGNMENTS AND OUT-OF-SEAT BEHAVIORS AMONG FIRST-GRADERS, WITH COMPLETION OF ASSIGNMENTS AND IN-SEAT BEHAVIOR REINFORCED BY CONTINGENT RECOGNITION AND PRAISE. THE MEAN PERCENT OF WORK COMPLETED ROSE FROM 9% TO 92.6% DURING THE 42 DAYS OF THE FIRST EXPERIMENT. IN THE SECOND CASE, OUT-OF-SEAT BEHAVIOR DECLINED FROM A MEAN FREQUENCY OF 15.66 TO 3.55 PER 50-MINUTE PE-

RIOD AFTER 25 DAYS OF MODIFICATION. IN EX-PERIMENT THREE, A MULTIPLE BASELINE DESIGN WAS EMPLOYED TO ILLUSTRATE THE MODIFICATION OF NON-COMPLETION OF WRITTEN ASSIGNMENTS AND THE QUALITY (NEATNESS) OF WRITTEN WORK. THE REIN-FORCEMENT CONTINGENCIES (I.E., APPROVAL, STARS, AND PARTICIPATION IN A PUPPET SHOW) RESULTED IN AN INCREASE OF FROM 2.85% TO 84% ASSIGNED WORK COMPLETED, AND IN A LATER PHASE, MARKED IMPROVEMENT IN THE PRESENTATION OF THE WORK. THESE FIND-INGS SUPPORT THE RELIABILITY AND APPLI-CABILITY OF BEHAVIOR ANALYSIS PRINCIPLES, AND DEMONSTRATE THAT TEACHERS, PAR-ENTS, AND OTHER MEMBERS OF COMMUNI-TIES IN WHICH THE SHORTAGE OF BEHAV-IORAL SCIENCE PROFESSIONALS IS A CRITICAL PROBLEM CAN BE TRAINED AS BEHAVIORAL ENGINEERS. 35 REFERENCES. (JOURNAL AB-STRACT MODIFIED)

ACCN   002020

129 AUTH   **BAXTER, J. C.**
     TITL   INTERPERSONAL SPACING IN NATURAL SET-TINGS.
     SRCE   *SOCIOMETRY, 1970, 33(4), 444-456.*
     INDX   INTERPERSONAL SPACING, CROSS CULTURAL, SEX COMPARISON, MEXICAN AMERICAN, IN-TERPERSONAL RELATIONS
     ABST   DIFFERENT SPATIAL ARRANGEMENTS WERE EXAMINED AMONG THREE SUBCULTURAL GROUPINGS, THREE SEX COMBINATIONS, AND THREE AGE LEVELS IN TWO OBSERVATIONAL SETTINGS. SUBJECTS (819 PAIRS) WERE CLASSIFIED ACCORDING TO: (1) ANGLO, BLACK, OR MEXICAN AMERICAN (MA) ETHNIC GROUP; (2) ADULT, ADOLESCENT, OR CHILD AGE LEVEL; (3) MALE-MALE, FEMALE-FEMALE, MALE-FE-MALE SEX COMBINATION; AND (4) INDOOR OR OUTDOOR OBSERVATION SETTING. RATINGS OF INTERPERSONAL DISTANCE WERE MADE FROM AN UNOBTRUSIVE LOCATION IN EACH SETTING. DATA INDICATE THE TENDENCY FOR MA SUBJECTS OF ALL AGES AND SEX GROUP-INGS TO INTERACT MORE PROXIMALLY THAN THE OTHER TWO GROUPS. MA'S NOT ONLY STAND CLOSER TOGETHER, BUT THEY TOUCH EACH OTHER MORE OFTEN. THE TENDENCY FOR BLACKS TO STAND AT GREATER DIS-TANCES IS CONSISTENT WITH EARLIER STUD-IES. AGE-GROUP COMPARISONS REVEAL THAT THE ETHNIC GROUP DIFFERENCES IN SPACING ARE PRESENT EVEN IN THE YOUNGEST SUB-JECT GROUPS. WHILE THE SIZE OF THESE DIF-FERENCES INCREASES WITH AGE, THEIR PRES-ENCE IN THE CHILDREN'S GROUP SUGGESTS THAT SCHEMATA OF APPROPRIATE SPATIAL AR-RANGEMENTS ARE LEARNED EARLY IN CHILD-HOOD AND PERSIST INTO ADULTHOOD. IMPLI-CATIONS OF THE FINDINGS IN THE AREAS OF INTERPERSONAL AND ENVIRONMENTAL DE-SIGN ARE DISCUSSED. 22 REFERENCES.

ACCN   000113

130 AUTH   **BAY AREA BILINGUAL EDUCATION LEAGUE AND THE MULTILINGUAL ASSESSMENT PRO-GRAM**
     TITL   BILINGUAL TESTING AND ASSESSMENT.
     SRCE   *PROCEEDINGS OF BABEL WORKSHOP AND PRELIMINARY FINDINGS MULTILINGUAL AS-SESSMENT PROGRAM. BERKELEY: BABEL, JUNE 1972.*
     INDX   BILINGUAL-BICULTURAL EDUCATION, INTELLI-GENCE TESTING, TEST RELIABILITY, TEST VA-LIDITY, ACHIEVEMENT TESTING, PROCEED-INGS, CULTURE-FAIR TESTS, EDUCATIONAL ASSESSMENT, CALIFORNIA, SOUTHWEST, ABILITY TESTING
     ABST   THE PROCEEDINGS FROM THE FIRST ANNUAL BILINGUAL-BICULTURAL TESTING AND AS-SESSMENT WORKSHOP ARE REPORTED. EIGHT INSTRUMENTS (WECHSLER INTELLIGENCE SCALE FOR CHILDREN, COMPREHENSIVE TEST OF BASIC SKILLS, COOPERATIVE PRIMARY, LORGE-THORNDIKE, INTER-AMERICAN SERIES-GENERAL ABILITY, CULTURE-FAIR INTELLI-GENCE TEST, MICHIGAN ORAL PRODUCTION TEST, AND THE PEABODY PICTURE-VOCABU-LARY TEST) ARE EXAMINED IN TERMS OF THEIR APPLICABILITY TO BILINGUAL-BICULTURAL STUDENTS. A CRITICAL REVIEW OF THE NEW INTER-AMERICAN SERIES TEST OF GENERAL ABILITY AND TESTS OF READING SHOWS THAT THE TEST AUTHORS AND PUBLISHERS ARE GROSSLY NEGLIGENT IN THE LACK OF RELIA-BILITY AND VALIDITY OF THIS LARGE SCALE TEST. A BRIEF DESCRIPTION OF A CRITERION-REFERENCED SYSTEM FOR THE ASSESSMENT OF A BILINGUAL CURRICULUM PROVIDES A STIMULUS FOR FURTHER INVESTIGATION AND EXPERIMENTATION WITH THIS METHODOLOGY. A PRESENTATION OF "SOME CAUTIONARY NOTES ON ATTEMPTING TO ADAPT I.Q. TEST FOR USE WITH MINORITY CHILDREN AND A NEO-PIAGETIAN APPROACH TO INTELLECTUAL ASSESSMENT: PARTIAL REPORT OF PRELIMI-NARY FINDINGS" CLEARLY DISCLOSES THE COMPLEXITIES INVOLVED IN TESTING AND AS-SESSMENT OF BILINGUAL-BICULTURAL CHIL-DREN. RESOLUTIONS AND FINDINGS ARE PRO-VIDED. 23 REFERENCES.

ACCN   000114

131 AUTH   **BAYARD, M. P.**
     TITL   ETHNIC IDENTITY AND STRESS: THE SIGNIFI-CANCE OF SOCIOCULTURAL CONTEXT.
     SRCE   *IN J. M. CASAS & S. E. KEEFE (EDS.), FAMILY AND MENTAL HEALTH IN THE MEXICAN AMERI-CAN COMMUNITY (MONOGRAPH NO. 7). LOS ANGELES: UNIVERSITY OF CALIFORNIA, SPAN-ISH SPEAKING MENTAL HEALTH RESEARCH CENTER, 1978, PP. 109-123.*
     INDX   ACCULTURATION, STRESS, MEXICAN AMERI-CAN, CASE STUDY, MENTAL HEALTH, SES, PRO-CEEDINGS, CALIFORNIA, SOUTHWEST, EMPIRI-CAL
     ABST   CASE HISTORIES OF FOUR MEXICAN AMERI-CANS ARE PRESENTED WITHIN THE HYPOTHE-TICAL FRAMEWORK THAT THE POTENTIAL FOR CULTURAL STRESS IN A POPULATION OF MEXI-CAN AMERICANS VARIES ACROSS LEVELS OF ACCULTURATION. THE DATA GATHERED OVER SEVERAL MONTHS FROM NUMEROUS MEET-INGS WITH EACH SUBJECT ILLUSTRATE SEV-ERAL POINTS: (1) MEXICAN AMERICANS ARE A

HETEROGENEOUS GROUP AND ACCULTURA-
TION IS ONE FACTOR WHICH CONTRIBUTES TO
VARIATIONS IN STRESS; (2) THE KINDS OF
STRESS A MEMBER OF THIS GROUP MAY BE
SUSCEPTIBLE TO VARIES ACCORDING TO
WHERE IN THE ACCULTURATION PROCESS THE
PERSON MAY BE; (3) THERE ARE OTHER
SOURCES OF STRESS WHICH COMBINE WITH
CULTURAL STRESS ELEMENTS TO CREATE A
COMPLEX INTERACTION; AND (4) THIS INTER-
ACTION MUST BE TAKEN INTO ACCOUNT BY
THE CLINICIAN IN ORDER TO PROVIDE MEAN-
INGFUL TREATMENT AND CORRECT THE SERI-
OUS UNDERUTILIZATION OF MENTAL HEALTH
SERVICES BY THIS GROUP. 10 REFERENCES.
(AUTHOR SUMMARY MODIFIED)

ACCN   000115

132 AUTH   **BEAN, F. D.**
    TITL   COMPONENTS OF INCOME AND EXPECTED
            FAMILY SIZE AMONG MEXICAN AMERICANS.
    SRCE   *SOCIAL SCIENCE QUARTERLY, 1973, 54(1), 103-*
            116.
    INDX   SES, ADULTS, EMPIRICAL, MEXICAN AMERI-
            CAN, FAMILY STRUCTURE, FERTILITY, MAR-
            RIAGE, TEXAS, SOUTHWEST
    ABST   TWO CONTRADICTORY HYPOTHESES MAY BE
            FOUND IN THE LITERATURE CONCERNING THE
            INCOME-FERTILITY RELATIONSHIP. USING DATA
            FROM THE 1969 AUSTIN FAMILY SURVEY, THIS
            STUDY ANALYZES THE INFLUENCE OF TWO
            COMPONENTS OF INCOME—SOCIAL STATUS
            INCOME AND RELATIVE INCOME—ON THE FER-
            TILITY OF 348 MEXICAN AMERICAN COUPLES.
            THE TWO COMPONENTS OF INCOME RELATE
            TO FERTILITY IN DIFFERENT WAYS; AGE AT
            MARRIAGE RELATES IN OPPOSITE DIREC-
            TIONS. THE STUDY REINFORCES THE NOTION
            THAT SOCIAL PROCESSES OF A REFERENCE
            GROUP MAY UNDERLIE FERTILITY BEHAVIOR, A
            POSSIBILITY WHICH NEEDS MORE CONSID-
            ERATION IN A SOCIOECONOMIC THEORY OF
            FAMILY FORMATION. 37 REFERENCES.
    ACCN   000116

133 AUTH   **BEAN, F. D. & BRADSHAW, B. S.**
    TITL   INTERMARRIAGE BETWEEN PERSONS OF
            SPANISH AND NON-SPANISH SURNAME:
            CHANGES FROM MID-NINETEENTH TO MID-
            TWENTIETH CENTURY.
    SRCE   *SOCIAL SCIENCE QUARTERLY, 1970, 51(2), 389-*
            395.
    INDX   SPANISH SURNAMED, CROSS CULTURAL, FAMILY
            STRUCTURE, EMPIRICAL, ADULTS, MARRIAGE,
            INTERMARRIAGE, TEXAS, SOUTHWEST, DEMO-
            GRAPHIC, SES, CULTURAL FACTORS, MEXICAN
            AMERICAN
    ABST   UTILIZING DATA FROM SELECTED MID-19TH
            AND MID-20TH CENTURY TIME PERIODS,
            CHANGES IN THE INCIDENCE OF INTERMAR-
            RIAGE BETWEEN SPANISH SURNAMED (SS)
            AND NON-SPANISH SURNAMED (NSS) PER-
            SONS IN BEXAR COUNTY, TEXAS, ARE STUD-
            IED. IT IS HYPOTHESIZED THAT THE EXTENT OF
            INTERMARRIAGE BETWEEN THE TWO POPULA-
            TIONS MAY BE SEEN AS A FUNCTION OF CUL-
            TURAL NORMS AND DEMOGRAPHIC FACTORS.

TO DETERMINE IF THE INCIDENCE OF INTER-
MARRIAGE BETWEEN SS AND NSS HAS
CHANGED INDEPENDENTLY OF DEMOGRAPHIC
EFFECTS, THE EXPECTED INCIDENCE OF IN-
TERMARRIAGE WAS CALCULATED AS A
PROBABILITY BASED ON SELECTED VARIABLES
AND COMPARED WITH THE ACTUAL INCI-
DENCE OF INTERMARRIAGE. THE DATA ARE
PRESENTED IN TABULAR FORM FOR OVER 10,-
000 MARRIAGES THAT WERE RECORDED IN
1850, 1860, 1950, AND 1960. IT WAS FOUND
THAT EXOGAMOUS MARRIAGES OCCURRED AT
A HIGHER THAN EXPECTED RATE AS PRE-
DICTED FROM DEMOGRAPHIC FACTORS ALONE
IN THE 1950-1960 DATA. THIS SUPPORTS THE
HYPOTHESIS THAT NORMATIVE FACTORS WHICH
INHIBITED INTERMARRIAGE IN THE 1850-1860'S
HAVE SINCE WEAKENED. IT IS SUGGESTED
THAT HISTORICAL CIRCUMSTANCES, SUCH AS
SOCIAL STRATIFICATION IN THE SS POPULA-
TION AS WELL AS THE SPLIT BETWEEN NATIVE
ANGLOS AND ANGLO IMMIGRANTS IN THE NSS
POPULATION, DEPRESSED THE RATE OF INTER-
MARRIAGE IN THE EARLIER TIME PERIOD. 14
REFERENCES. (AUTHOR SUMMARY MODIFIED)

ACCN   000160

134 AUTH   **BEAN, F. D., & WOOD, C. H.**
    TITL   ETHNIC VARIATIONS IN THE RELATIONSHIP BE-
            TWEEN INCOME AND FERTILITY.
    SRCE   *DEMOGRAPHY, 1974, 11(4), 629-640.*
    INDX   SES, FERTILITY, MEXICAN AMERICAN, CROSS
            CULTURAL, DEMOGRAPHIC, EMPIRICAL,
            ADULTS, TEXAS, CALIFORNIA, NEW MEXICO,
            ARIZONA, COLORADO, SOUTHWEST, ECO-
            NOMIC FACTORS
    ABST   THE EFFECTS OF HUSBAND'S POTENTIAL AND
            RELATIVE INCOMES ON COMPLETED FERTILITY,
            AS WELL AS THEIR EFFECTS ON CERTAIN PAR-
            ITY PROGRESSION PROBABILITIES, WERE EX-
            AMINED WITHIN SAMPLES OF ANGLOS, BLACKS,
            AND MEXICAN AMERICANS FROM THE FIVE
            SOUTHWESTERN STATES. THE RESULTS RE-
            VEAL DIFFERENT PATTERNS OF RELATIONSHIP
            BY ETHNICITY BETWEEN INCOME AND FERTIL-
            ITY MEASURES. THE EFFECTS ON COMPLETED
            FERTILITY OF THE INCOME MEASURES WERE
            POSITIVE FOR ANGLOS, NEGATIVE FOR BLACKS,
            WHILE FOR MEXICAN AMERICANS THE EFFECT
            OF POTENTIAL INCOME WAS NEGATIVE AND
            THAT OF RELATIVE INCOME WAS POSITIVE. IN-
            COME EFFECTS ON THE PARITY PROGRESSION
            PROBABILITIES FOLLOW A SIMILAR PATTERN.
            41 REFERENCES. (JOURNAL ABSTRACT MODI-
            FIED)
    ACCN   000117

135 AUTH   **BEASLEY, R. M., & ANTUNES, G.**
    TITL   THE ETIOLOGY OF CRIME: AN ECOLOGICAL
            ANALYSIS.
    SRCE   *CRIMINOLOGY, 1974, 1(4), 439-461.*
    INDX   URBAN, CRIMINOLOGY, GROUP DYNAMICS,
            POVERTY, SES, EMPLOYMENT, MEXICAN
            AMERICAN, CROSS CULTURAL, COMMUNITY,
            ENVIRONMENTAL FACTORS, EMPIRICAL, TEXAS,
            SOUTHWEST
    ABST   CONCLUDING FROM PREVIOUS RESEARCH THAT
            THE IMPORTANT CORRELATES OF SERIOUS

CRIME CAN BE REDUCED TO THREE TYPES— MEASURES OF SOCIOECONOMIC STATUS, MEASURES OF CROWDING, AND MEASURES OF ETHNIC OR SUBCULTURE SEGREGATION— DATA FOR EACH OF THESE INDEPENDENT VARIABLES WERE COLLECTED FROM 1970 CENSUS RECORDS FOR THE CITY OF HOUSTON AND COMPARED TO THE HOUSTON POLICE RECORDS FOR CRIMES REPORTED DURING THE SAME YEAR. BECAUSE PREVIOUS RESEARCH DID NOT PRODUCE PREDICTIVE CONCLUSIONS USING TECHNIQUES SUCH AS FACTOR ANALYSIS, THE DATA HERE WERE ANALYZED WITH A VARIETY OF REGRESSION TECHNIQUES, INCLUDING BIVARIATE, MULTIPLE, AND POLYNOMIAL REGRESSION. RESULTS INDICATE THAT THE FEW VARIABLES SELECTED ON THE THEORETICAL GROUNDS CHOSEN (I.E., MEDIAN INCOME, POPULATION DENSITY AND PERCENTAGE OF MINORITY POPULATION) CAN STATISTICALLY ACCOUNT FOR ALMOST ALL OF THE VARIANCE IN THE RATES OF MAJOR CRIMES EXAMINED. THE APPLICATION AND LEVEL OF PREDICTABILITY ACHIEVED FOR EACH TYPE OF REGRESSION ANALYSIS USED ARE DISCUSSED. 20 REFERENCES.

ACCN   000118

136 AUTH   **BECKWITH, L., & THOMPSON, S. K.**
     TITL   RECOGNITION OF VERBAL LABELS OF PICTURED OBJECTS AND EVENTS BY 17- TO 30-MONTH-OLD INFANTS.
     SRCE   *JOURNAL OF SPEECH AND HEARING RESEARCH, 1976, 19(4), 690-699.*
     INDX   COGNITIVE DEVELOPMENT, SPANISH SURNAMED, LANGUAGE ASSESSMENT, LINGUISTIC COMPETENCE, LANGUAGE COMPREHENSION, EMPIRICAL, SES, SEX COMPARISON, INFANCY, CROSS CULTURAL, RESEARCH METHODOLOGY, TEST VALIDITY, TEST RELIABILITY
     ABST   A TECHNIQUE FOR EFFICIENTLY PRESENTING A LARGE NUMBER OF VOCABULARY ITEMS WAS DEVELOPED FOR THE TESTING OF VOCABULARY COMPREHENSION IN CHILDREN YOUNGER THAN TWO YEARS. THE TECHNIQUE, INCORPORATING SLIDES OF REAL OBJECTS, HAD THE ADVANTAGES OF MAINTAINING THE CHILD'S ATTENTION, MOTIVATING TASK CONTINUATION, AND OVERCOMING THE EXTRANEOUS CONTEXTUAL CUES OF TEST MATERIALS. THE SUBJECTS WERE 106 CHILDREN, AGED 17 TO 30 MONTHS, FROM A WIDE RANGE OF SOCIAL STATUS GROUPS AND FROM BOTH ENGLISH AND SPANISH LANGUAGE FAMILIES. RESULTS INDICATED SIGNIFICANT STABILITY OVER TIME AS WELL AS A SIGNIFICANT RELATIONSHIP TO MATERNAL REPORT. ANALYSIS OF ERRORS SUGGESTED THAT COMPREHENSION DEVELOPS SIMILARLY TO PRODUCTION, IN THAT SIMPLE NOUNS WERE THE EASIEST ITEMS, VERBS WERE MORE DIFFICULT, AND MODIFIERS AND LOCATIVES WERE THE MOST DIFFICULT. THERE WERE NO SIGNIFICANT MAIN EFFECTS OF SEX OR SOCIAL STATUS. HOWEVER, SPECIFIC ENVIRONMENTAL VARIABLES, SUCH AS PARENTAL ATTITUDES AND PLAYMATE PATTERNS, WERE SIGNIFICANTLY CORRELATED WITH TEST PERFORMANCE. MORE FLEXIBLE

FAMILY CONTROL SYSTEMS AND MORE INTERACTION WITH PEERS WERE BOTH ASSOCIATED WITH BETTER VOCABULARY COMPREHENSION IN FIRST BORN CHILDREN. 13 REFERENCES. (JOURNAL ABSTRACT)

ACCN   002021

137 AUTH   **BEIGEL, A., HUNTER, E. J., TAMERIN, J. S., CHAPIN, E. H., & LOWERY, M. J.**
     TITL   PLANNING FOR THE DEVELOPMENT OF COMPREHENSIVE COMMUNITY ALCOHOLISM SERVICES: I. THE PREVALENCE SURVEY.
     SRCE   *AMERICAN JOURNAL OF PSYCHIATRY, 1974, 131(10), 1112-1116.*
     INDX   ALCOHOLISM, COMMUNITY, RESEARCH METHODOLOGY, SURVEY, EMPIRICAL, MEXICAN AMERICAN, SES, ARIZONA, SOUTHWEST, HEALTH
     ABST   A SHORT TERM, LOW COST METHOD FOR ASSESSING THE EXTENT OF A COMMUNITY'S ALCOHOLISM PROBLEM IS PRESENTED ALONG WITH EXAMPLES OF HOW THESE DATA CAN BE USED IN PLANNING A RATIONAL PROGRAM. THE PIMA COUNTY ALCOHOLISM TASK FORCE IN TUCSON, ARIZONA, DESIGNED THEIR SURVEY TO IDENTIFY THE "VISIBLE" PROBLEM DRINKER AND ALSO TO OBTAIN INFORMATION ABOUT HIS/HER LOCATION, SOCIOECONOMIC STATUS, AGE, AND ETHNIC GROUP WITHIN THE TIME AND FINANCIAL LIMITATIONS OF AN NIMH INITIATION AND DEVELOPMENT GRANT. 10 REFERENCES. (JOURNAL ABSTRACT MODIFIED)

ACCN   000119

138 AUTH   **BEIGEL, A., MCCABE, T. R., TAMERIN, J. S., LOWERY, M. J., CHAPIN, E. H., & HUNTER, E. J.**
     TITL   PLANNING FOR THE DEVELOPMENT OF COMPREHENSIVE COMMUNITY ALCOHOLISM SERVICES: II. ASSESSING COMMUNITY AWARENESS AND ATTITUDES.
     SRCE   *AMERICAN JOURNAL OF PSYCHIATRY, 1974, 131(10), 1116-1121.*
     INDX   ALCOHOLISM, COMMUNITY, ATTITUDES, MEXICAN AMERICAN, CROSS CULTURAL, SURVEY, EMPIRICAL, SES, HEALTH, DRUG ABUSE, ARIZONA, SOUTHWEST
     ABST   IN DEVELOPING AN EFFECTIVE COMMUNITY EDUCATION AND TREATMENT PROGRAM FOR ALCOHOLISM, THE FOLLOWING DIMENSIONS NEED TO BE ASSESSED: (1) ATTITUDES TOWARD ALCOHOL USE AND ABUSE; (2) DRINKING HABITS; (3) AWARENESS OF AVAILABLE SERVICES AND FACILITIES FOR THE ALCOHOLIC; (4) EXTENT OF PERSONAL DRINKING PROBLEMS; AND (5) COMPARATIVE PERCEPTIONS OF ALCOHOL ABUSE IN DIFFERENT ETHNIC GROUPS. THE METHODOLOGY USED TO GATHER THESE DATA IS EXPLAINED AS IT WAS APPLIED BY THE ALCOHOL TASK FORCE OF PIMA COUNTY, ARIZONA. THE RESULTS OF THIS SURVEY REVEALED ETHNIC DIFFERENCES IN ATTITUDES AND DEGREE OF AWARENESS OF COMMUNITY SERVICES. THE IMPORTANCE OF INDIVIDUALIZED COMMUNITY EDUCATION AND TREATMENT PROGRAMS IS EMPHASIZED. 11 REFERENCES. (JOURNAL ABSTRACT MODIFIED)

ACCN   000120

139 AUTH **BELCHER, J. C.**
    TITL A CROSS-CULTURAL HOUSEHOLD LEVEL-OF-
          LIVING SCALE.
    SRCE *RURAL SOCIOLOGY, 1972, 37(2), 208-220.*
    INDX RESEARCH METHODOLOGY, SES, PUERTO RI-
          CAN-I, CROSS CULTURAL, EMPIRICAL, HOUS-
          ING, TEST RELIABILITY, TEST VALIDITY, GEOR-
          GIA, SOUTH, SOUTH AMERICA
    ABST LEVEL-OF-LIVING AND RELATED SOCIOECO-
          NOMIC INDICES PREVIOUSLY USED IN SOCIAL
          SCIENCE RESEARCH HAVE BEEN CULTURE
          BOUND AND INADEQUATE FOR LONGITUDINAL
          STUDIES; THEY HAVE BEEN BASED ON POS-
          SESSION OF ITEMS RATHER THAN ON THEIR
          FUNCTIONAL USE. TO DEVELOP IN THIS STUDY
          A CROSS-CULTURALLY VALID MEASURE, A LIST
          OF FUNCTIONS WERE GIVEN WEIGHTS; FUNC-
          TIONAL ALTERNATIVES TO THE ITEM LISTED
          ARE PREMITTED. THE RESULTING 14-ITEM
          SCALE WAS TESTED BY USE OF DATA FROM
          RURAL GEORGIA, PUERTO RICO, AND THE DO-
          MINICAN REPUBLIC. EVIDENCE IS PRESENTED
          THAT THE INSTRUMENT IS A VALID AND RELI-
          ABLE MEASURE OF LEVEL-OF-LIVING. 18 REF-
          ERENCES. (JOURNAL ABSTRACT MODIFIED)
    ACCN 000121

140 AUTH **BELCHER, J. C., & CRADER, K. W.**
    TITL SOCIAL CLASS, STYLE OF LIFE AND FERTILITY
          IN PUERTO RICO.
    SRCE *SOCIAL FORCES, 1974, 52(4), 488-495.*
    INDX SES, FERTILITY, PUERTO RICAN-I, ADULTS, SEX
          ROLES, EMPIRICAL
    ABST STYLES OF LIFE ARE VIEWED AS BEHAVIORAL
          CONSTELLATIONS SELECTED AMONG AVAIL-
          ABLE CULTURAL ALTERNATIVES AND MANI-
          FESTED IN THE MANNER IN WHICH GOODS ARE
          CONSUMED. COMPONENTS INDICATING LIFE
          STYLE WERE SELECTED BY PRINCIPAL COM-
          PONENTS SOLUTION AND VARIMAX ROTATION.
          THESE COMPONENTS WERE: (1) MIDDLE CLASS
          SYNDROME; (2) MALE DOMINANCE; (3) AGRI-
          CULTURAL SELF-SUFFICIENCY; AND (4) EVE-
          NING LEISURE. CROSS TABULATIONS WERE
          MADE ON COMPLETED FERTILITY BY EMPLOY-
          ING BOTH HOLLINGSHEAD'S SOCIAL CLASSES
          AND THE STYLE OF LIFE TYPOLOGY. THE STYLE
          OF LIFE APPROACH SYSTEMATICALLY DIFFER-
          ENTIATES FERTILITY PATTERNS WITHIN WHAT
          THE HOLLINGSHEAD PROCEDURE WOULD IN-
          DICATE TO BE A HOMOGENEOUS GROUP. 22
          REFERENCES. (JOURNAL ABSTRACT MODI-
          FIED)
    ACCN 000122

141 AUTH **BELSASSO, G.**
    TITL THE HISTORY OF PSYCHIATRY IN MEXICO.
    SRCE *HOSPITAL AND COMMUNITY PSYCHIATRY, 1969,
          20(11), 342-344.*
    INDX MENTAL   HEALTH   PROFESSION,   HISTORY,
          MEXICO, ESSAY
    ABST THE DEVELOPMENT OF PSYCHIATRY IN MEXICO
          IS INTIMATELY CONNECTED WITH THE HISTORI-
          CAL DEVELOPMENT OF THE COUNTRY. INFLU-
          ENCES FROM SPAIN, AFRICA, FRANCE, AND
          THE U.S. OVER THE PAST FOUR CENTURIES

HAVE AFFECTED THE BASIC INDIAN HERITAGE.
EACH OF THESE ERAS AND THEIR MAJOR PSY-
CHIATRIC PRACTICES ARE BRIEFLY DIS-
CUSSED. FACILITIES AND PROGRAMS DEVEL-
OPED SINCE 1947 ARE MOST THOROUGHLY
DESCRIBED.
    ACCN 000123

142 AUTH **BENDER, P. S., & RUIZ, R. A.**
    TITL RACE AND CLASS AS DIFFERENTIAL DETERMI-
          NANTS OF UNDERACHIEVEMENT AND UNDER-
          ASPIRATION AMONG MEXICAN AMERICANS.
    SRCE *JOURNAL OF EDUCATIONAL RESEARCH, 1974,
          68(2), 51-56.*
    INDX SCHOLASTIC ACHIEVEMENT, OCCUPATIONAL
          ASPIRATIONS, CROSS CULTURAL, COGNITIVE
          STYLE, SES, TIME ORIENTATION, ADOLES-
          CENTS, MEXICAN AMERICAN, LOCUS OF CON-
          TROL, TEXAS, SOUTHWEST
    ABST THIS STUDY COMPARES MEXICAN AMERICAN
          AND ANGLO ELEVENTH-GRADE HIGH SCHOOL
          STUDENTS FROM THE LOWER AND MIDDLE SO-
          CIOECONOMIC CLASSES WITH RESPECT TO (1)
          LOCUS OF CONTROL, ADEQUATE ACHIEVE-
          MENT REALITY ORIENTATION, AND TEMPORAL
          ORIENTATION AS POTENTIAL CORRELATES OF
          (2) CURRENT SCHOLASTIC PERFORMANCE AND
          FUTURE   EDUCATIONAL   AND   VOCATIONAL
          GOALS. IN GENERAL, THIS STUDY INDICATED
          THAT MEMBERSHIP IN SOCIAL CLASS RATHER
          THAN RACIAL GROUP WAS THE CRITICAL FAC-
          TOR IN DETERMINING CURRENT ACADEMIC
          ACHIEVEMENT, EDUCATIONAL ASPIRATIONS,
          AND BELIEF IN ONE'S ABILITY TO CONTROL HIS
          ENVIRONMENT. INFERENCES EMERGE THAT
          GENERALIZATIONS FROM ONE ETHNIC MI-
          NORITY GROUP AND/OR SOCIOECONOMIC
          CLASS TO ANOTHER GROUP OR CLASS MAY
          NOT NECESSARILY BE VALID. IN ADDITION,
          PROGRAMS DESIGNED TO INVOLVE LOW-
          ACHIEVING AND LOW-ASPIRING STUDENTS
          SHOULD TAKE RELEVANT VARIABLES, SUCH AS
          SOCIAL CLASS, INTO ACCOUNT IN THEIR DE-
          VELOPMENT. 14 REFERENCES. (JOURNAL AB-
          STRACT)
    ACCN 000124

143 AUTH **BENGSTON, V. L., CUELLAR, J. B., & RAGAN,
          P. K.**
    TITL STRATUM CONTRASTS AND SIMILARITIES IN
          ATTITUDES TOWARD DEATH.
    SRCE *JOURNAL OF GERONTOLOGY, 1977, 32(1), 76-
          78.*
    INDX GERONTOLOGY, DEATH, ATTITUDES, SES, CROSS
          CULTURAL,   SEX   COMPARISON,   MEXICAN
          AMERICAN, EMPIRICAL, ADULTS, CALIFORNIA,
          SOUTHWEST, URBAN
    ABST BOTH SURVEY AND ETHNOGRAPHIC DATA WERE
          USED TO EXPLORE ATTITUDES TOWARD DEATH
          AMONG 1,269 INDIVIDUALS OF VARYING SO-
          CIAL CATEGORIES DEFINED BY AGE, SOCIAL
          CLASS, SEX, AND RACE (WHITE, BLACK, MEXI-
          CAN AMERICAN). THE SURVEY CONSISTED OF
          STRUCTURED INTERVIEWS FOCUSING ON
          THREE ASPECTS OF ORIENTATION TO DEATH
          AND DYING: (1) EXPRESSED FEAR OF DEATH;
          (2) REPORTED FREQUENCY OF THOUGHTS
          ABOUT DEATH; AND (3) PERCEIVED PROXIMITY

OF DEATH. THE FOUR SOCIAL STRATUM VARIABLES TAKEN TOGETHER EXPLAINED RELATIVELY LITTLE VARIATION IN ATTITUDES TOWARD DEATH, SUGGESTING GREATER SIMILARITY ACROSS SOCIAL CATEGORIES THAN HAD BEEN ANTICIPATED. HOWEVER, ANALYSIS BY AGE RESULTED IN SUBSTANTIAL DIFFERENCES, WITH MIDDLE-AGED RESPONDENTS (45-54 YEARS) EXPRESSING GREATEST FEARS OF DEATH AND THE ELDERLY (65-74) EXPRESSING THE LEAST. THE PATTERN OF DECREASED FEAR BY AGE WAS PRONOUNCED AMONG THE TWO MINORITY GROUPS—MIDDLE-AGED MEXICAN AMERICANS AND BLACKS EXPRESSED THE GREATEST FEAR OF DEATH, AND ELDERLY MEXICAN AMERICANS THE LEAST. CONTRASTS BETWEEN RACIAL GROUPS WERE ALSO EVIDENT IN PERCEIVED PROXIMITY OF DEATH, WITH THE BLACK SUBSAMPLE HAVING THE GREATEST EXPECTATIONS OF LONGEVITY AND THE MEXICAN AMERICAN THE LEAST. FOUR THEMES ARE SUMMARIZED AS THE RESULTS: (1) THE MIDDLE-AGED CRISIS EVIDENCED BY MANY INDIVIDUALS IN CONFRONTING DEATH, AND THE APPARENT RESOLUTION EXHIBITED BY ELDERLY RESPONDENTS; (2) THE EFFECTS OF BIOGRAPHICAL AND HISTORICAL EVENTS IN SHAPING INDIVIDUAL ORIENTATIONS TOWARD DEATH; (3) CULTURAL HETEROGENEITY WITHIN, AS WELL AS AMONG, GROUPS IN DEATH-RELATED ATTITUDES; AND (4) AGE AS A LEVELER OF PRIOR SOCIAL DISTINCTIONS, AS AGING INDIVIDUALS FROM VARIOUS SOCIAL CATEGORIES DEAL WITH THE INEVITABILITY OF IMPENDING DEATH. 35 REFERENCES. (JOURNAL ABSTRACT MODIFIED)

ACCN   002022

144 AUTH   **BENGSTON, V. L., GRIGSBY, E., CORRY, E. M., & HRUBY, M.**
     TITL   RELATING ACADEMIC RESEARCH TO COMMUNITY CONCERNS: A CASE STUDY IN COLLABORATIVE EFFORT.
     SRCE   *JOURNAL OF SOCIAL ISSUES, 1977, 33(4), 75-92.*
     INDX   COMMUNITY INVOLVEMENT, CASE STUDY, RESEARCH METHODOLOGY, MEXICAN AMERICAN, CALIFORNIA, SOUTHWEST, COMMUNITY, GERONTOLOGY, SOCIAL SCIENCES, CONFLICT RESOLUTION, POLITICAL POWER
     ABST   TO OFFER ADVICE ABOUT THE PITFALLS AND ADVANTAGES OF COMMUNITY INVOLVEMENT IN STUDIES OF MINORITY COMMUNITIES, THIS PAPER DESCRIBES THE EXPERIENCES OF ONE SUCH PROJECT. THE STUDY WAS A FIVE-YEAR INVESTIGATION IN LOS ANGELES OF ANGLO, BLACK, AND MEXICAN AMERICAN ELDERLY (AGES 45-74). INITIALLY THERE WAS NO COMMUNITY INPUT, BUT WHEN COMMUNITY ADVOCATES LEARNED OF THE STUDY THEY QUICKLY PROTESTED, DEMANDING THE HIRING OF MINORITY STAFF AS WELL AS A DECISION-MAKING ROLE IN ALL PROJECT ACTIVITIES. CONFLICTS RAPIDLY DEVELOPED (STEMMING LARGELY FROM ACCUSATIONS OF ACADEMIC "ELITISM"), BUT EVENTUALLY A PROCESS FOR CONFLICT RESOLUTION EVOLVED. THERE WERE MEETINGS BETWEEN THE RESEARCH STAFF,

FUNDING AGENCY STAFF, AND COMMUNITY REPRESENTATIVES; THEN A COMMUNITY RESEARCH PLANNING COMMITTEE WAS FORMED WHICH HAD ADVISORY AND SOME DECISION-MAKING POWERS. THESE EXPERIENCES TAUGHT THE RESEARCH STAFF SEVERAL IMPORTANT LESSONS ABOUT COMMUNITY RESEARCH: (1) IN THE REVIEW PROCESS, INVOLVE PERSONS FROM THE LAY COMMUNITY AND FROM FEDERAL AGENCIES; (2) TO AVOID CONFLICTS WITH THE COMMUNITY, STRATEGIES FOR CONFLICT RESOLUTION MUST BE PLANNED AS CAREFULLY AS THE RESEARCH DESIGN AND METHODOLOGY; AND (3) COMMUNITY OR ACTION RESEARCHERS MUST ADOPT A FLEXIBLE STANCE. IT IS CONCLUDED THAT ALTHOUGH COLLABORATION BETWEEN ACADEMICIANS AND COMMUNITY ADVOCATES HAS BEEN RARE IN THE PAST, IT WILL BECOME INCREASINGLY FREQUENT AND ESSENTIAL—REFLECTING THE CHANGING NATURE OF ACCOUNTABILITY IN SOCIAL SCIENCE RESEARCH. 25 REFERENCES.

     ACCN   001808

145 AUTH   **BERGLAND, B. W., & LUNDQUIST, G. W.**
     TITL   THE VOCATIONAL EXPLORATION GROUP AND MINORITY YOUTH: AN EXPERIMENTAL OUTCOME STUDY.
     SRCE   *JOURNAL OF VOCATIONAL BEHAVIOR, 1975, 7(3), 289-296.*
     INDX   EMPLOYMENT, VOCATIONAL COUNSELING, ADOLESCENTS, MEXICAN AMERICAN, ACHIEVEMENT MOTIVATION, ATTITUDES, PSYCHOTHERAPY OUTCOME, OCCUPATIONAL ASPIRATIONS, EMPIRICAL
     ABST   THIS STUDY WAS DESIGNED TO INVESTIGATE EXPERIMENTALLY THE EFFECTIVENESS OF THE VOCATIONAL EXPLORATION GROUP IN ASSISTING STUDENTS TO BECOME MORE AWARE OF THE WORLD OF WORK AND ITS RELEVANCE FOR THEM. SIXTY MALE, MEXICAN AMERICAN, JUNIOR HIGH STUDENTS WERE RANDOMLY ASSIGNED TO ONE OF THREE GROUPS: (1) VOCATIONAL EXPLORATION GROUP (VEG); (2) VEG WITHOUT INTERACTION; OR (3) CONTROL. UPON COMPLETION OF TREATMENTS SUBJECTS WERE POST-TESTED WITH AN INSTRUMENT DESIGNED TO ASSESS KNOWLEDGE OF FACTORS SUCH AS DIFFERING FUNCTIONS OF JOBS, INTERESTS AND SKILLS NEEDED IN DIFFERENT JOBS, AND SATISFACTIONS AVAILABLE FROM WORK. ANALYSES REVEALED NO STATISTICALLY SIGNIFICANT DIFFERENCES AMONG GROUPS. 5 REFERENCES. (JOURNAL ABSTRACT)
     ACCN   000125

146 AUTH   **BERKANOVIC, E., & REEDER, L. G.**
     TITL   ETHNIC, ECONOMIC, AND SOCIAL PSYCHOLOGICAL FACTORS IN THE SOURCE OF MEDICAL CARE.
     SRCE   *SOCIAL PROBLEMS, 1973, 21(2), 246-259.*
     INDX   ATTITUDES, CROSS CULTURAL, CULTURAL FACTORS, ECONOMIC FACTORS, EMPIRICAL, HEALTH, HEALTH DELIVERY SYSTEMS, SURVEY, URBAN, MEXICAN AMERICAN, PHYSICIANS, POVERTY, RESOURCE UTILIZATION, SES, SEX

COMPARISON, CALIFORNIA, SOUTHWEST, ADULTS

ABST TO ASSESS THE IMPACT OF CULTURAL AND ACCESS FACTORS ON HEALTH BEHAVIOR, A MULTISTAGE AREA PROBABILITY SAMPLE OF APPROXIMATELY 1,600 L.A. COUNTY RESIDENTS WERE SURVEYED REGARDING MEDICAL SERVICE UTILIZATION. THE DEPENDENT VARIABLE WAS THE SOURCE OF MEDICAL CARE DURING A ONE-YEAR PERIOD, AND THE INDEPENDENT VARIABLES WERE INCOME AND ETHNICITY. A REVIEW OF THE LITERATURE REVEALED THREE ALTERNATIVE MODELS OF THE DETERMINANTS OF HEALTH BEHAVIOR: (1) UNEQUAL ACCESS; (2) CULTURE OF POVERTY; AND (3) CULTURAL AND SOCIAL PSYCHOLOGICAL DIFFERENCES RELATED TO ETHNICITY AND SOCIOECONOMIC STATUS. DATA ON SOURCE OF MEDICAL CARE BY BOTH INCOME AND ETHNICITY (BLACK, N = 3; WHITE, N = 84; MEXICAN, N = 7) REVEALED A COMPLEX PATTERN IN WHICH INCOME AND ETHNICITY DID NOT COMBINE LINEARLY, BUT IN WHICH SPECIFIC COMBINATIONS OF THESE VARIABLES LED TO LARGE DIFFERENCES IN THE PERCENTAGE DISTRIBUTION OF SOURCE OF CARE. THIS INTERACTION CANNOT BE EXPLAINED EITHER BY THE HYPOTHESIS OF UNEQUAL ACCESS TO CARE OR BY THE CULTURE OF POVERTY HYPOTHESIS. INSTEAD, IT APPEARS THAT ETHNICITY AND SES CREATE DIFFERENTIAL LIFE EXPERIENCES, WHICH, AMONG OTHER THINGS, LEAD TO DIFFERENCES IN VALUE PREFERENCES. WITH RESPECT TO PROGRAM PLANNING, THE DATA IMPLY THE NEED FOR PLURALISM IN THE ORGANIZATION OF HEALTH SERVICES AND A NEED FOR TRAINING HEALTH PROFESSIONALS TO SERVE SPECIFIC TARGET GROUPS IN THE POPULATION. 35 REFERENCES.

ACCN 002023

147 AUTH **BERLE, B. M.**
TITL 80 PUERTO RICAN FAMILIES IN NEW YORK CITY: HEALTH AND DISEASE STUDIED IN CONTEXT.
SRCE *NEW YORK: COLUMBIA UNIVERSITY PRESS, 1958.*
INDX PUERTO RICAN-M, MIGRATION, HEALTH, ACCULTURATION, ALCOHOLISM, ANOMIE, ANXIETY, BILINGUAL, CASE STUDY, CHILDREARING PRACTICES, COMMUNITY, CONFLICT RESOLUTION, CULTURE, ESPIRITISMO, DEMOGRAPHIC, DRUG ABUSE, ECONOMIC FACTORS, EMPIRICAL, EMPLOYMENT, ENVIRONMENTAL FACTORS, ETHNIC IDENTITY, FICTIVE KINSHIP, BIRTH CONTROL, FAMILY STRUCTURE, FAMILY ROLES, HEALTH DELIVERY SYSTEMS, MENTAL HEALTH, DEPRESSION, POVERTY, SES, SOCIAL SERVICES, URBAN, NEW YORK, EAST, BOOK
ABST A STUDY OF THE RELATIONSHIP BETWEEN HEALTH, DISEASE, AND THE ENVIRONMENT AMONG PUERTO RICANS WAS CONDUCTED BY CLINICIANS IN A MANHATTAN SLUM NEIGHBORHOOD. DATA COLLECTED FROM A SAMPLE OF 80 PUERTO RICAN FAMILIES PERTAINED TO MIGRATION, FAMILY STRUCTURE, LANGUAGE, LEVEL OF EDUCATION, RELIGION, PHYSICAL

APPEARANCE, HOUSING, AND LEVEL AND TYPE OF INCOME. ATTENTION WAS FOCUSED ON THE RELATIONSHIP BETWEEN SOCIAL AND ENVIRONMENTAL FACTORS, SUSCEPTIBILITY TO ILLNESS, AND THE MANAGEMENT OF ILLNESS WITHIN THE SAMPLE. FINDINGS REVEALED PUERTO RICANS DEMONSTRATE A HIGH SUSCEPTIBILITY TO ILLNESS, WITH HIGH INCIDENCES OF TUBERCULOSIS AND HIGH ADMISSION RATES TO MENTAL HOSPITALS. THIS IS ATTRIBUTED TO THE IMPACT OF CHANGE IN THE SOCIAL STRUCTURE OF THIS POPULATION. AMONG THIS SAMPLE, TRADITIONAL WAYS HAVE BEEN DISRUPTED BY MIGRATION TO THE U.S. AND THE ACCULTURATION PROCESS. IN ADDITION, BY MIGRATING TO THE U.S., PUERTO RICANS HOPE TO ACHIEVE UPWARD MOBILITY, AND ILLNESS IS OFTEN PERCEIVED AS A FAILURE TO PROGRESS ECONOMICALLY. THE EMOTIONAL AND PSYCHOLOGICAL IMPACT ON ILLNESS AMONG THIS SAMPLE MUST BE CONSIDERED FOR MORE EFFECTIVE HEALTH SERVICES. 40 REFERENCES.

ACCN 000126

148 AUTH **BERNAL Y DEL RIO, V.**
TITL IMITATION, IDENTIFICATION AND IDENTITY.
SRCE *PAPER PRESENTED AT THE HERMAN GOLDMAN INTERNATIONAL LECTURE SERIES, NEW YORK MEDICAL COLLEGE, MAY 14, 1971.*
INDX ESSAY, PUERTO RICAN-M, PUERTO RICAN-I, PSYCHOTHERAPY, CULTURAL FACTORS, MENTAL HEALTH, TIME ORIENTATION, DYADIC INTERACTION
ABST A COMPARISON OF SELECTED BEHAVIORS BY NATIVE PUERTO RICANS AND MAINLAND AMERICANS AS OBSERVED IN TWO SETTINGS IS PRESENTED. HAND SHAKING, LATENESS, AND EXPRESSION OF HOSTILITY WERE SELECTED BECAUSE THEY ARE EASILY RECORDED AND OBSERVED BOTH IN A SOCIAL SETTING AND IN THE PSYCHOTHERAPY TREATMENT SETTING. THE FOUR GROUPS COMPARED WERE (1) SOPHISTICATED PUERTO RICANS, (2) LOWER INCOME PUERTO RICANS, (3) TRANSIENT CONTINENTALS, AND (4) REPLANTED CONTINENTALS. THE INFLUENCE OF CULTURE AND SETTING ON BEHAVIORAL IMITATION AND IDENTIFICATION ARE DESCRIBED THROUGH CLINICAL AND SOCIAL EXPERIENCES. 7 REFERENCES.

ACCN 000127

149 AUTH **BERNAL, E. M.**
TITL COMPARATIVE CONCEPT LEARNING AMONG ANGLO, BLACK AND MEXICAN-AMERICAN CHILDREN UNDER STANDARD AND FACILITATION CONDITIONS OF TASK ADMINISTRATION.
SRCE *PRESENTED AT THE MEETING OF THE AMERICAN PSYCHOLOGICAL ASSOCIATION, WASHINGTON, D.C., 1971.*
INDX CROSS CULTURAL, MEXICAN AMERICAN, CHILDREN, EMPIRICAL, INTELLIGENCE, LEARNING, COGNITIVE DEVELOPMENT, PROCEEDINGS, TEXAS, SOUTHWEST, ABILITY TESTING, CULTURE-FAIR TESTS
ABST THE EFFECTS OF A STANDARD TASK ADMINISTRATION VERSUS A COMPLEX FACILITATION

STRATEGY ON THE CONCEPT LEARNING (CL) OF MONOLINGUAL, ENGLISH-SPEAKING MEXI-CANS (MAI), BILINGUAL MEXICAN AMERICANS (MAII), ANGLO AMERICANS (AA), AND BLACK AMERICANS (BA) WERE COMPARED. THE THREE HYPOTHESES GENERATED WERE: (1) FACILITA-TION STRATEGIES WILL HAVE LITTLE EFFECT FOR AA'S IN THEIR PERFORMANCE UNDER STANDARD CL TEST CONDITIONS; (2) ETHNIC MINORITIES WILL SCORE HIGHER ON CL TASKS WITH FACILITATION STRATEGIES THAN WITH THE STANDARD CL ADMINISTRATION; (3) UN-DER EQUAL FACILITATIVE CONDITIONS, THE AA GROUP WILL NOT PERFORM SIGNIFICANTLY BETTER ON CL TASKS THAN DO THE BA, MAI, OR MAII STUDENTS. ONE HUNDRED NINETY-TWO SUBJECTS (EIGHTH GRADERS FROM 3 PUBLIC SCHOOLS AND 6 PRIVATE SCHOOLS IN SAN ANTONIO, TEXAS) WERE ADMINISTERED THE MODIFIED VERSION OF THE LETTER SETS TEST AND THE NUMBER SERIES TEST. THE RE-SULTS SHOW THAT THE HYPOTHESES WERE SUPPORTED. THE AA GROUP WAS NOT AF-FECTED BY THE INTERVENTION TECHNIQUE, WHEREAS THE ETHNIC GROUPS HAD A SIG-NIFICANT DIFFERENCE IN THE PREDICTED DI-RECTION. MOREOVER, WITH THE FACILITATION TECHNIQUE THE ETHNIC MINORITY GROUPS PERFORMED AS WELL AS THE AA'S. IT IS CON-CLUDED THAT, CONTRARY TO THE HEREDITAR-IAN POSITION, ETHNICALLY APPROPRIATE EN-VIRONMENTAL INTERVENTION CAN EFFECTIVELY ELIMINATE THE SIGNIFICANT CL-PERFORM-ANCE DIFFERENCES ACROSS ETHNIC POPU-LATIONS. 73 REFERENCES.

ACCN   000128

150 AUTH   **BERNAL, E. M.**
     TITL   GIFTED MEXICAN CHILDREN: AN ETHNO-SCI-ENTIFIC PERSPECTIVE.
     SRCE   *CALIFORNIA JOURNAL OF EDUCATIONAL RE-SEARCH, 1974, 25(5), 261-273.*
     INDX   SPECIAL EDUCATION, CHILDREN, INTELLI-GENCE TESTING, WISC, PERSONALITY ASSESS-MENT, ETHNIC IDENTITY, COGNITIVE DEVELOP-MENT, SCHOLASTIC ACHIEVEMENT, URBAN, MEXICAN AMERICAN, EMPIRICAL, TEXAS, SOUTHWEST
     ABST   THE IDENTIFICATION OF GIFTED, BILINGUAL MEXICAN AMERICAN CHILDREN IN THE EARLY ELEMENTARY GRADES THROUGH TRADI-TIONAL TECHNIQUES (PRINCIPALLY IQ TEST) HAS BEEN DIFFICULT AND LARGELY IMPRACTI-CAL. THIS RESEARCH WAS UNDERTAKEN TO DETERMINE IF BEHAVIORAL DESCRIPTORS AB-STRACTED FROM INTERVIEWS WITH MEXICAN AMERICAN BARRIO RESIDENTS COULD BE USED TO DIFFERENTIATE GIFTED CHICANO CHIL-DREN FROM THEIR AVERAGE PEERS. A PUR-POSIVE SAMPLE OF 54 GIFTED AND AVERAGE CHILDREN, FIVE TO NINE YEARS OF AGE, WAS SELECTED FROM TWO TEXAS CITIES AND TESTED WITH THREE DIFFERENT INSTRU-MENTS—THE WISC, THE TORRANCE VERBAL AND FIGURAL TESTS OF CREATIVITY, AND THE CARTOON CONSERVATION SCALES. THEIR RATINGS ON 43 BEHAVIORS WERE SUBJECTED TO MULTIPLE DISCRIMINANT ANALYSIS, AND

THE RESULTS INDICATED THAT NINE ITEMS HAD HIGH DISCRIMINANT POWER. CHICANO VIEWS ON GIFTEDNESS ARE SUMMARIZED, AND IMPLICATIONS FOR CROSS CULTURAL RE-SEARCH AND EDUCATION ARE DISCUSSED. 27 REFERENCES. (JOURNAL ABSTRACT)

ACCN   000129

151 AUTH   **BERNAL, M. E., NORTH, J. A., ROSEN, P. M. DELFINI, L. F., & SCHULTZ, L. A.**
     TITL   OBSERVER ETHNICITY EFFECTS ON CHICANO MOTHERS AND SONS.
     SRCE   *HISPANIC JOURNAL OF BEHAVIORAL SCI-ENCES, 1979, 1(2), 151-164.*
     INDX   MEXICAN AMERICAN, CHILDREN, EMPIRICAL, EXAMINER EFFECTS, MOTHER-CHILD INTER-ACTION, RESEARCH METHODOLOGY, DYADIC INTERACTION, BEHAVIOR THERAPY, AGGRES-SION
     ABST   TEN CHICANO BOYS, AGES 5 TO 7, WHO WERE DEFINED IN SCHOOL AS HAVING SOCIALLY AG-GRESSIVE BEHAVIOR PROBLEMS WERE OB-SERVED BY FOUR FEMALES (2 ANGLOS, 2 CHI-CANAS) IN THEIR HOMES IN INTERACTIONS WITH THEIR MOTHERS. THIS REPORT FOCUSES ON ONE FACET OF THE LARGER STUDY— NAMELY, THE POSSIBLE BIASING INFLUENCE OF OBSERVER ETHNICITY. ASSIGNED AT RAN-DOM TO THE HOMES, THE OBSERVERS USED A TIME-SAMPLING TECHNIQUE TO OBSERVE AND CODE THE FOLLOWING BEHAVIORS: (1) THE COMPLIANT, DESIRABLE, ANNOYING, AND DE-VIANT BEHAVIOR OF THE BOYS; AND (2) THE COMMANDS AND TYPES OF ATTENTION GIVEN BY THE MOTHERS. RESULTS REVEALED THAT THE BOYS WERE SLIGHTLY LESS COMPLIANT AND MORE NONVERBALLY ABUSIVE IN THE PRESENSE OF THE ANGLO THAN CHICANA OB-SERVERS, BUT THE DIFFERENCE WAS NOT STA-TISTICALLY SIGNIFICANT. IN POST-EXPERIMENT INTERVIEWS, THE MOTHERS REPORTED NO AP-PRECIABLE REACTIVITY TO THE OBSERVER'S ETHNICITY. IT IS THEREFORE CONCLUDED THAT IN CONTRAST TO PSYCHOTHERAPY OR TEST-ING SITUATIONS, OBSERVER ETHNICITY MAY BE OF NEGLIGIBLE IMPORTANCE IN NATURAL-ISTIC OBSERVATION STUDIES. STILL, IT IS CAU-TIONED THAT UNTIL FUTURE RESEARCH TAKES INTO ACCOUNT THE HETEROGENEITY WITHIN THE CHICANO POPULATION AS WELL AS THE MANY COMPLEX FACTORS INVOLVED IN NA-TURALISTIC SETTINGS, THE PRESENT FIND-INGS CANNOT BE GENERALIZED TO CHICA-NOS AS A GROUP. IT IS ALSO NOTED THAT THE PRESENT STUDY OFFERS A GOOD MODEL FOR FUTURE EVALUATIONS OF EXPERIMENTER-ETHNICITY EFFECTS. 9 REFERENCES.

ACCN   001758

152 AUTH   **BERNAT, G. S.**
     TITL   CHICANO RACIAL ATTITUDES MEASURE (CRAM): STANDARDIZATION AND RESULTS OF AN INI-TIAL STUDY.
     SRCE   *UNPUBLISHED MASTER'S THESIS, UNIVERSITY OF ARIZONA, DEPARTMENT OF PSYCHOLOGY, 1976.*
     INDX   ACCULTURATION, MEXICAN AMERICAN, CHIL-DREN, CROSS CULTURAL, ETHNIC IDENTITY,

EMPIRICAL, SEX COMPARISON, TEST RELIABIL-
ITY, PREJUDICE, SEX ROLES, ATTITUDES

ABST THE CHICANO RACIAL ATTITUDE MEASURE
(CRAM), DESIGNED TO MEASURE RACIAL ATTI-
TUDES TOWARD CHICANOS BY CHICANO AND
ANGLO CHILDREN WAS TESTED AND STAN-
DARDIZED. ADAPTED FROM THE PRESCHOOL
RACIAL ATTITUDE MEASURE (PRAM II) DE-
SIGNED TO MEASURE RACIAL ATTITUDES TO-
WARDS BLACKS, IT USES PICTURES TO ELICIT
RACIAL AND SEX ROLE ATTITUDES. RESULTS
DEMONSTRATE AN OVERWHELMINGLY PRO-
ANGLO, ANTI-CHICANO BIAS AMONG BOTH
THE ANGLO AND CHICANO CHILDREN TESTED.
SEVERAL ANALYSES OF VARIANCE DEMON-
STRATE THAT RACIAL ATTITUDE TOWARDS CHI-
CANOS WAS NOT AFFECTED BY ETHNICITY,
SEX, OR AGE OF SUBJECT. TESTS WERE ALSO
CONDUCTED TO ESTABLISH STANDARDS FOR
THE CRAM WITH THE HOPE THAT OTHER RE-
SEARCHERS WILL BE ABLE TO USE THE IN-
STRUMENT. 19 REFERENCES. (AUTHOR AB-
STRACT MODIFIED)

ACCN 000130

153 AUTH **BERNAT, G., & BALCH, P.**
TITL THE CHICANO RACIAL ATTITUDE MEASURE
(CRAM): RESULTS OF AN INITIAL INVESTIGA-
TION.
SRCE *AMERICAN JOURNAL OF COMMUNITY PSY-
CHOLOGY, 1979, 7(2), 137-146.*
INDX ATTITUDES, MEXICAN AMERICAN, ETHNIC
IDENTITY, CHILDREN, EMPIRICAL, SELF CON-
CEPT, CROSS CULTURAL, PREJUDICE
ABST THE CHICANO RACIAL ATTITUDE MEASURE
(CRAM) IS DESIGNED TO MEASURE THE ATTI-
TUDES OF CHICANO AND ANGLO CHILDREN
TOWARDS CHICANOS. IT IS ADAPTED FROM
THE PRESCHOOL RACIAL ATTITUDE MEASURE
(PRAM II) WHICH MEASURES RACIAL ATTI-
TUDES TOWARDS BLACKS. AS AN INITIAL AS-
SESSMENT OF THE CRAM, IT WAS ADMINIS-
TERED TO 120 CHILDREN, AGES 5 TO 7; 60
WERE CHICANO, 60 ANGLO, AND BOTH
GROUPS WERE EVENLY DIVIDED BY SEX.
TWENTY-FOUR RACIAL ATTITUDE PICTURES
WERE USED, EACH PICTURE SHOWING ONE
CHICANO AND ONE ANGLO FIGURE. ACCOM-
PANYING EACH PICTURE WAS A BRIEF STORY
CONTAINING EITHER A POSITIVE OR A NEGA-
TIVE EVALUATIVE ADJECTIVE (PEA OR NEA, RE-
SPECTIVELY). AS A CONTROL FOR COGNITIVE
DEVELOPMENT, 12 SEX-ROLE PICTURES WERE
ALSO INCLUDED. THE CHILDREN WERE TESTED
INDIVIDUALLY. THE RESULTS DEMONSTRATED
AN OVERWHELMING PRO-ANGLO, ANTI-CHI-
CANO BIAS AMONG BOTH THE ANGLO AND
CHICANO CHILDREN. RACIAL ATTITUDE TO-
WARDS CHICANOS WAS NOT AFFECTED BY
RACE, SEX, OR AGE OF SUBJECT. THE IMPLI-
CATIONS OF THESE FINDINGS FOR COMMU-
NITY-BASED RESEARCH AND INTERVENTION
ARE DISCUSSED. 11 REFERENCES. (JOURNAL
ABSTRACT MODIFIED)

ACCN 001825

154 AUTH **BERNEY, D., COOPER, R. L., & FISHMAN, J. A.**

TITL SEMANTIC INDEPENDENCE AND THE DEGREE
OF BILINGUALISM IN TWO PUERTO RICAN
COMMUNITIES.
SRCE *REVISTA INTRAMERICANA DE PSICOLOGIA, 1968,
2(4), 289-294.*
INDX BILINGUALISM, PUERTO RICAN-M, PUERTO RI-
CAN-I, BILINGUAL, SEMANTICS, LANGUAGE
ASSESSMENT, EMPIRICAL
ABST AN INVESTIGATION OF A MEASURE OF SEMAN-
TIC INDEPENDENCE WHICH CAN BE DERIVED
FROM VERBAL FLUENCY MEASURES OF DE-
GREE OF BILINGUALISM IS DESCRIBED. THE
SPANISH AND ENGLISH WORD-NAMING AND
WORD-ASSOCIATION RESPONSES OF TWO
GROUPS OF PUERTO RICAN RESPONDENTS,
ONE LIVING ON THE ISLAND AND THE OTHER
ON THE MAINLAND, WERE ANALYZED. THE
ANALYSIS WAS IN TERMS OF THE PROPORTION
OF TRANSLATION-EQUIVALENT PAIRS TO THE
NUMBER OF WORDS PRODUCED IN THE
WEAKER LANGUAGE FOR EACH OF FIVE SO-
CIETAL DOMAINS. THE RESPONDENTS LIVING
ON THE ISLAND GAVE SIGNIFICANTLY HIGHER
TRANSLATION-EQUIVALENT RATIOS THAN DID
THOSE LIVING ON THE MAINLAND. THE DO-
MAINS OF THE FAMILY AND NEIGHBORHOOD
EXHIBITED THE SMALLEST TRANSLATION-
EQUIVALENT RATIOS AND THE DOMAINS OF
EDUCATION AND RELIGION THE LARGEST. SE-
MANTIC INDEPENDENCE AND RELATIVE BILIN-
GUAL PROFICIENCY WERE FOUND TO BE
LARGELY INDEPENDENT DIMENSIONS, WITH
THE FORMER REFLECTING THE COORDINATE-
NESS OF THE BILINGUAL'S LANGUAGE SYS-
TEM. 6 REFERENCES.
ACCN 000131

155 AUTH **BETANCOURT, R.**
TITL SEX DIFFERENCES IN LANGUAGE PROFI-
CIENCY OF MEXICAN-AMERICAN THIRD AND
FOURTH GRADERS.
SRCE *JOURNAL OF EDUCATION, 1976, 158(2), 55-65.*
INDX MEXICAN AMERICAN, CHILDREN, LINGUISTIC
COMPETENCE, PEABODY PICTURE-VOCABU-
LARY TEST, BILINGUALISM, SEX COMPARISON,
CULTURAL FACTORS, EMPIRICAL
ABST MEXICAN AMERICAN THIRD AND FOURTH
GRADERS (N = 62) WERE ADMINISTERED A
LANGUAGE PROFICIENCY TEST (MORENO TEST
OF ORAL PROFICIENCY) AND VOCABULARY
TEST (PEABODY PICTURE VOCABULARY) IN
ENGLISH AND SPANISH ON TWO OCCASIONS.
MALES SCORED SIGNIFICANTLY HIGHER ON
SPANISH PROFICIENCY CONTRARY TO GEN-
ERAL RESEARCH FINDINGS. THE SAMPLE WAS
FURTHER DIVIDED INTO HIGH AND LOW SPAN-
ISH ABILITY GROUPS AND ANALYZED WITH
PARALLEL RESULTS. HOWEVER, FEMALE
SCORES ON SPANISH PROFICIENCY WERE EVEN
LOWER FOR THE HIGH GROUP THAN THE LOW.
A CULTURAL INHIBITION HYPOTHESIS WAS
PROPOSED BASED, IN PART, ON MACOBY'S IN-
TEGRATIVE HYPOTHESIS TO ACCOUNT FOR
THESE RESULTS. 25 REFERENCES. (JOURNAL
ABSTRACT)
ACCN 000132

156 AUTH **BIKSON, T. K.**

TITL DO THEY TALK THE SAME LANGUAGE? LEXICAL INTERFACE AND ETHNICITY.

SRCE *SANTA MONICA, CA.: THE RAND CORPORATION, 1977.*

INDX LANGUAGE ASSESSMENT, MEXICAN AMERICAN, EMPIRICAL, CROSS CULTURAL, CHILDREN, LINGUISTIC COMPETENCE

ABST SPONTANEOUS SPEECH PERFORMANCE OF ETHNICALLY DIVERSE SUBJECTS IS INVESTIGATED BY MEASURING WITHIN- AND BETWEEN-GROUP LEXICAL INTERFACE AND BY ASSESSING DIRECTION OF VOCABULARY OVERLAP. INTERVIEW DATA WERE COLLECTED FROM 144 ELEMENTARY SCHOOL CHILDREN, COMPRISING EQUAL WHITE, CHICANO AND BLACK SUBSAMPLES EVENLY DIVIDED AMONG LOWER AND UPPER GRADES. ANALYSES FOCUS ON WHETHER TEXTS EXHIBIT A SINGLE LEXICON BETTER ACCESSED BY WHITE S'S OR RATHER GENERATE PLURAL LEXICA ACCESSED WITH COMPARABLE ADEQUACY BY EACH ETHNIC GROUP. SIMILAR WITHIN-GROUP LEXICAL STYLES EMERGED. HOWEVER, INTERFACE EXPLORATION—I.E., THE PROPORTION OF COMMON WORDS TO TOTAL ENTRIES IN A SUBJECT'S LEXICON PLUS ENTRIES IN A RELEVANT GROUP LEXICON—FOUND MINORITY LEXICA TO BE DIFFERENT FROM AND BROADER THAN THE WHITE LEXICON THEY PARTIALLY SUBSUME. SINCE THE LANGUAGE OF BLACK AND CHICANO S'S IN SPONTANEOUS SPEECH REVEALS A BROADER WORKING VOCABULARY THAN THAT OF WHITE AGE-MATES, IT IS CONCLUDED THAT ASSESSMENTS BASED ON MAJORITY USAGE MAINTAIN RACE AND CLASS DIFFERENTIATION OF OUTCOMES BY FAILING TO REPRESENT THE RANGE OF MINORITY LEXICAL STYLE. 8 REFERENCES. (AUTHOR ABSTRACT MODIFIED)

ACCN 002025

157 AUTH **BIKSON, T. K.**

TITL MINORITY SPEECH AS OBJECTIVELY MEASURED AND SUBJECTIVELY EVALUATED.

SRCE *PERSONALITY AND SOCIAL PSYCHOLOGY BULLETIN, 1974, 1(1), 336-338.*

INDX LINGUISTICS, CHILDREN, MEXICAN AMERICAN, CROSS CULTURAL, SEMANTICS, PHONOLOGY, COGNITIVE DEVELOPMENT, TEACHERS, EMPIRICAL, CALIFORNIA, SOUTHWEST

ABST SPONTANEOUS SPEECH PERFORMANCE OF ETHNICALLY DIVERSE SUBJECTS WAS INVESTIGATED BY WAY OF OBJECTIVE LINGUISTIC MEASURES AND TEACHER EVALUATIONS. INTERVIEW DATA WERE COLLECTED FROM 144 ELEMENTARY SCHOOL CHILDREN, COMPRISING EQUAL WHITE, CHICANO, AND BLACK SUBSAMPLES EVENLY DIVIDED AMONG LOWER AND HIGHER GRADES. SPEECH EVALUATORS WERE 60 WHITE TEACHERS. ANALYSIS FOCUSED ON WHETHER MINORITY CHILDREN ARE, OR ARE PERCEIVED AS, LINGUISTICALLY DEFICIENT COMPARED WITH WHITE AGE MATES. OBJECTIVE MEASURES INDICATE MINORITY SPEECH PERFORMANCE EQUALS OR EXCELS WHITE PERFORMANCE, BUT TEACHERS HEAR IT AS SIGNIFICANTLY INFERIOR. EVIDENCE SUGGESTS THAT SYSTEMATIC UNDER-

REPRESENTATION OF MINORITY LANGUAGE PROFICIENCY STEMS FROM DISCRIMINATION DIFFICULTIES AND ETHNIC STEREOTYPING. 5 REFERENCES. (AUTHOR ABSTRACT)

ACCN 000133

158 AUTH **BLANK, M., & FRANK, S. M.**

TITL STORY RECALL IN KINDERGARTEN CHILDREN: EFFECT OF METHOD OF PRESENTATION ON PSYCHOLINGUISTIC PERFORMANCE.

SRCE *CHILD DEVELOPMENT, 1971, 42(1), 299-312.*

INDX SYNTAX, SEMANTICS, PUERTO RICAN-M, CHILDREN, CROSS CULTURAL, EMPIRICAL, INTELLIGENCE, LINGUISTIC COMPETENCE, MEMORY, NEW YORK, EAST

ABST A STORY-RETELLING TASK WAS USED TO TEST SYNTACTIC AND SEMANTIC ASPECTS OF LANGUAGE PERFORMANCE IN 34 KINDERGARTNERS. TWO GROUPS OF SUBJECTS WERE MATCHED FOR AGE, IQ, AND ETHNIC BACKGROUND (NEGRO, PUERTO RICAN, AND WHITE SUBJECTS IN EACH GROUP). SYNTACTIC RECALL WAS REDUCED IN AMOUNT AND VARIED IN PATTERN FROM THE COMMONLY USED SINGLE-SENTENCE IMITATION TASK. SEVERAL FACTORS APPEARED TO BE RESPONSIBLE, INCLUDING SUCH VARIABLES AS SEMANTIC CONTENT AND "STRESS" (THE NEED TO RETAIN LARGE AMOUNTS OF INFORMATION). LINGUISTIC PERFORMANCE, INCLUDING BOTH SEMANTIC AND SYNTACTIC RECALL, WAS ENHANCED BY VARYING THE METHOD OF PRESENTATION SO THAT THE SUBJECT WAS REQUIRED TO PLAY A MORE ACTIVE ROLE IN THE SITUATION. IN ADDITION TO THE METHOD OF PRESENTATION, INTELLIGENCE WAS FOUND TO INFLUENCE PERFORMANCE IN THAT SUBJECTS WITH HIGHER MENTAL AGES SHOWED SIGNIFICANTLY BETTER RECALL. 16 REFERENCES.

ACCN 000134

159 AUTH **BLOOM, B. L.**

TITL A CENSUS TRACT ANALYSIS OF SOCIALLY DEVIANT BEHAVIORS.

SRCE *MULTIVARIATE BEHAVIORAL RESEARCH, 1966, 1(3), 307-320.*

INDX RESEARCH METHODOLOGY, CENSUS, DEMOGRAPHIC, DEVIANCE, PSYCHOPATHOLOGY, COMMUNITY, CROSS CULTURAL, HOUSING, ENVIRONMENTAL FACTORS, RESOURCE UTILIZATION, FEMALE, WEST, URBAN

ABST THE ECOLOGICAL CORRELATES OF VARIOUS FORMS OF SOCIAL DISEQUILIBRIUM IN 15 CENSUS TRACT CHARACTERISTICS WERE INVESTIGATED. NINE MEASURES OF SOCIAL DISEQUILIBRIUM, FAMILIAL DISRUPTION, MARITAL DISRUPTION, ECONOMIC DISRUPTION (ENVIRONMENTAL DISRUPTION, EDUCATIONAL DISRUPTION, JUVENILE DELINQUENCY, PSYCHIATRIC DISRUPTION-PUBLIC, PSYCHIATRIC DISRUPTION-PRIVATE, AND SUICIDE RATE) WERE FOUND TO BE HIGHLY INTERCORRELATED OVER THE TRACTS. OF THE NINE MEASURES OF SOCIAL DISEQUILIBRIUM, PUBLIC PSYCHIATRIC HOSPITAL ADMISSION RATES WERE SIGNIFICANTLY RELATED TO MOST OF THE CENSUS TRACT CHARACTERISTICS. WHERE SIGNIFICANT RELATIONSHIPS EXIST, THESE TYPES OF

SOCIAL DISEQUILIBRIUM ARE WITHOUT EXCEPTION HIGH IN THOSE CENSUS TRACTS CHARACTERIZED BY HIGH PROPORTIONS OF SPANISH SURNAMES, FOREIGN BORNS, AND FEMALES. IN ADDITION, THESE CENSUS TRACTS CAN ALSO BE DESCRIBED AS HAVING LOW COMMUNITY PARTICIPATION, LOW POPULATION LEVEL PER HOUSEHOLD, LOW EDUCATIONAL LEVEL, LOW ECONOMIC LEVEL, FEW SOUND HOUSING UNITS, AND A HIGH INCIDENCE OF TUBERCULOSIS. THE FINDINGS CONFIRM PREVIOUS STUDIES REGARDING THE DEMOGRAPHIC STRUCTURE OF URBAN COMMUNITIES AND THE PATTERNS OF SOCIALLY DEVIANT BEHAVIOR. ATTENTION IS GIVEN TO THE METHODOLOGICAL PROBLEMS AND POSSIBILITIES IN THE USE OF CORRELATIONAL DATA TO SUGGEST CAUSE-EFFECT RELATIONSHIPS. 21 REFERENCES.

ACCN   000135

160 AUTH **BLOOM, D., & PADILLA, A. M.**
    TITL A PEER-INTERVIEWER MODEL IN CONDUCTING SURVEYS AMONG MEXICAN AMERICAN YOUTH.
    SRCE *JOURNAL OF COMMUNITY PSYCHOLOGY, 1979, 7, 129-136. (ALSO PUBLISHED AS OCCASIONAL PAPER NO. 8. LOS ANGELES: UNIVERSITY OF CALIFORNIA, SPANISH SPEAKING MENTAL HEALTH RESEARCH CENTER, 1979.)*
    INDX RESEARCH METHODOLOGY, SURVEY, ADOLESCENTS, REVIEW, DRUG ABUSE
    ABST RECENT STUDIES INDICATE AN INCREASE IN SUBSTANCE ABUSE AMONG MEXICAN AMERICAN YOUTH. DUE TO THE SENSITIVITY OF INVESTIGATING SUBSTANCE ABUSE AMONG YOUNG PEOPLE AND THE DIFFICULTY IN GAINING ACCESS TO MINORITY COMMUNITIES, AN ALTERNATIVE METHOD OF OBTAINING SURVEY DATA IS PROPOSED: THE PEER-INTERVIEWER APPROACH. THE REPORT INCLUDES A REVIEW OF DRUG SURVEYS AND AN ANALYSIS OF THE SPECIAL PROBLEMS OF CONDUCTING RESEARCH IN MINORITY AREAS. THEN THE PROCEDURES INVOLVED IN IMPLEMENTING THE PROPOSED PEER-INTERVIEWER MODEL ARE ELABORATED, WITH SPECIAL EMPHASIS ON (1) THE MODEL'S THEORETICAL RATIONALE, (2) THE MANNER FOR SELECTING AND TRAINING INTERVIEWERS, (3) SPECIAL CONSIDERATIONS IN DEVELOPING A SURVEY INSTRUMENT, AND (4) THE PROBLEMS AND ADVANTAGES IN USING THIS MODEL. IT IS CONCLUDED THAT THE PEER-INTERVIEWER MODEL IS NOT ONLY FEASIBLE, BUT ALSO ADVANTAGEOUS FOR RESEARCH FOCUSING ON MINORITY ADOLESCENTS. MOREOVER, THE MODEL SHOULD PROVE EFFECTIVE FOR STUDIES OF TOPICS OTHER THAN SUBSTANCE ABUSE—SUCH AS GANG ACTIVITY, SEXUAL PRACTICES, AND OTHER ADOLESCENT SUBCULTURAL BEHAVIOR. 22 REFERENCES. (AUTHOR ABSTRACT MODIFIED)
    ACCN 001796

161 AUTH **BLOOMBAUM, M., YAMAMOTO, J., & JAMES, Q.**
    TITL CULTURAL STEREOTYPING AMONG PSYCHOTHERAPISTS.

    SRCE *JOURNAL OF CONSULTING AND CLINICAL PSYCHOLOGY, 1968, 32(1), 99.*
    INDX PSYCHOTHERAPISTS, EMPIRICAL, PREJUDICE, CULTURAL FACTORS, STEREOTYPES, PSYCHOTHERAPY, CROSS CULTURAL, MEXICAN AMERICAN, ATTITUDES
    ABST STEREOTYPICAL ATTITUDES AMONG PSYCHOTHERAPISTS ABOUT SEX, RACE, RELIGION OR SOCIOECONOMIC STATUS AND THEIR POSSIBLE EFFECTS ON PATIENTS ARE DISCUSSED. THE AUTHORS CAUTION THAT THE PSYCHOTHERAPIST MUST BE AWARE THAT CERTAIN BEHAVIORS DISPLAYED DURING THE PSYCHOTHERAPEUTIC PROCESS MIGHT SUGGEST THAT HE HOLDS PREJUDICIAL ATTITUDES—ATTITUDES THAT CAN BE NEGATIVELY PERCEIVED BY PATIENTS. ONE-HALF HOUR STRUCTURED INTERVIEWS WERE OBTAINED WITH 16 PRACTICING PSYCHOTHERAPISTS IN WHICH THEIR ATTITUDES TOWARD MEXICAN AMERICANS, NEGROES, JAPANESE AMERICANS, CHINESE AMERICANS, AND JEWS WERE INVESTIGATED. OF ALL RESPONSES, 22.6 PERCENT WERE CULTURALLY STEREOTYPIC IN TERMS OF IMPUTATIONS OF SUPERSTITIOUSNESS, CHANGEABILITY IN IMPULSE, GRASP OF ABSTRACT IDEAS, AND DISTINCTION BETWEEN ILLUSION AND FACT. MEXICAN AMERICANS ARE MOST FREQUENTLY THE OBJECTS OF SUCH STEREOTYPES, WITH NEGROES, JEWS, CHINESE AMERICANS, AND JAPANESE AMERICANS FOLLOWING IN THAT ORDER. OF ALL RESPONSES, 79.2 PERCENT INDICATED THE PRESENCE OF MORE SUBTLE STEREOTYPIC ATTITUDES. THE RACIAL DISTANCE SCALE FROM BOGARDUS' SOCIAL DISTANCE SCALE WAS ALSO ADMINISTERED. PSYCHOTHERAPISTS DIFFERENTIATED AMONG FIVE ETHNIC GROUPS WITH RESPECT TO THE DEGREES OF SOCIAL DISTANCE THEY MAINTAINED. THEY LEAST OFTEN PREFERRED TO INTERMARRY WITH NEGROES, NEXT WITH CHINESE AMERICANS, AND THEN MEXICAN AMERICANS, THEN JAPANESE AMERICANS, AND MOST OFTEN WITH JEWS. IT IS CONCLUDED THAT THE PSYCHOTHERAPISTS MAY BE SAID TO REFLECT THE GENERAL CULTURE OF WHICH THEY ARE A PART; AND THEY ARE, THEREFORE, NOT TO BE CONSIDERED IMMUNE TO CULTURAL CONDITIONING. 1 REFERENCE.
    ACCN 000136

162 AUTH **BLUESTONE, H., BISI, R., & KATZ, A. J.**
    TITL THE ESTABLISHMENT OF A MENTAL HEALTH SERVICE IN A PREDOMINANTLY SPANISH-SPEAKING NEIGHBORHOOD OF NEW YORK CITY.
    SRCE *BEHAVIORAL NEUROPSYCHIATRY, 1969, 1(5), 12-16.*
    INDX PUERTO RICAN-M, HEALTH DELIVERY SYSTEMS, MENTAL HEALTH, PSYCHOTHERAPY, ESSAY, NEW YORK, EAST, PROGRAM EVALUATION
    ABST COMMUNITY MENTAL HEALTH PROGRAMS ARE CURRENTLY MAKING CONTACT WITH LARGE NUMBERS OF PUERTO RICAN PATIENTS WHO EITHER SPEAK NO ENGLISH OR WHOSE COMMAND OF ENGLISH IS LIMITED. SINCE SPANISH-SPEAKING PSYCHOTHERAPISTS ARE IN SHORT SUPPLY, SOME CLINICS HAVE FOUND

DIFFICULTY IN TREATING THESE PATIENTS. OB-
SERVATION OF MANY PUERTO RICAN PATIENTS
WHO EVIDENCE LONG TERM AVOIDANCE OF
ENGLISH SUGGESTS A CONNECTION BE-
TWEEN SUCH AVOIDANCE AND EMOTIONAL
PROBLEMS RELATED TO PHOBIC AVOIDANCE
OF THE ENVIRONMENT. THE DEMONSTRATION
PROGRAM DESCRIBED IN THIS REPORT WAS
DEVELOPED TO EXPLORE THE USE OF A
TRANSLATOR AS A FUNCTIONAL SOLUTION TO
THE LANGUAGE BARRIER. THE PSYCHIATRIST
HAD NO COMMAND OF SPANISH AND HE WAS
ASSISTED BY A BILINGUAL AIDE. A NONPARTI-
CIPANT, SPANISH-COMPREHENDING PSYCHIA-
TRIST OBSERVER MADE AN INDEPENDENT DI-
AGNOSIS. HIGH CORRELATION BETWEEN THE
TWO DIAGNOSES OFFERS SUPPORT FOR THE
USE OF THE INTERPRETER-TRANSLATOR IN DI-
AGNOSIS WITH NON-ENGLISH-SPEAKING PA-
TIENTS. THE CONCLUSIONS SEEM TO INDI-
CATE A VALID ROLE FOR THE TRANSLATOR IN
BOTH DIAGNOSIS AND GROUP PSYCHOTHER-
APY. THE PRACTICAL DIFFICULTIES, SUCH AS
HOW MUCH THE INTERPRETER SHOULD INTER-
ACT WITH PATIENTS AND WHERE HE SHOULD
SIT IN RELATION TO THE PSYCHOTHERAPIST,
ARE ALSO DISCUSSED. (JOUNAL ABSTRACT
MODIFIED)

ACCN 000137

163 AUTH **BLUESTONE, H., & PURDY, B.**
TITL PSYCHIATRIC SERVICES TO PUERTO RICAN PA-
TIENTS IN THE BRONX.
SRCE *IN E. R. PADILLA & A. M. PADILLA (EDS.), TRAN-*
SCULTURAL PSYCHIATRY: AN HISPANIC PER-
SPECTIVE (MONOGRAPH NO. 4). LOS ANGE-
LES: UNIVERSITY OF CALIFORNIA, SPANISH
SPEAKING MENTAL HEALTH RESEARCH CEN-
TER, 1977, PP. 45-49.
INDX LINGUISTIC COMPETENCE, BILINGUAL-BICUL-
TURAL PERSONNEL, SYMPTOMATOLOGY, FOLK
MEDICINE, PROFESSIONAL TRAINING, PSY-
CHOTHERAPY, CULTURAL FACTORS, PSYCHO-
PATHOLOGY, ACCULTURATION, PUERTO RI-
CAN-I, NEW YORK, EAST
ABST PSYCHIATRIC SERVICES TO PUERTO RICAN
PEOPLE MUST ALLOW FOR ADAPTATION TO
LANGUAGE AND CULTURAL FACTORS. HOW
THESE FACTORS HAVE BEEN CONSIDERED IN
THE DEVELOPMENT OF SERVICES BY THE
BRONX-LEBANON HOSPITAL CENTER IN NEW
YORK IS DESCRIBED. THE INFLUENCE OF LAN-
GUAGE AND CULTURE ON CLINICAL SYMP-
TOMS AND DIAGNOSIS ARE DISCUSSED BRIEFLY
ALONG WITH IMPLICATIONS FOR PATIENT CARE
AND STAFF TRAINING. 2 REFERENCES.
ACCN 000138

164 AUTH **BOARD OF EDUCATION, CITY OF NEW YORK.**
TITL THE PUERTO RICAN STUDY: 1953-1957.
SRCE *NEW YORK: AUTHOR, 1958.*
INDX RESEARCH METHODOLOGY, PUERTO RICAN-
M, BILINGUALISM, LANGUAGE LEARNING,
CURRICULUM, INSTRUCTIONAL TECHNIQUES,
ADOLESCENTS, CHILDREN, ACCULTURATION,
SES, PSYCHOSOCIAL ADJUSTMENT, STRESS,
EMPIRICAL, URBAN, NEW YORK, EAST
ABST THE RESULTS OF A FOUR YEAR INQUIRY ON

THE IMPACT THAT INCREASED NUMBERS OF
PUERTO RICANS HAVE HAD ON THE NEW YORK
CITY PUBLIC SCHOOLS ARE PRESENTED. THE
STUDY ADDRESSED ITSELF TO TWO ISSUES: (1)
MORE EFFECTIVE METHODS AND MATERIALS
NEEDED FOR TEACHING ENGLISH TO SPANISH-
SPEAKING PUERTO RICAN CHILDREN; AND (2)
MORE RAPID AND SUCCESSFUL ADJUSTMENT
OF PUERTO RICAN PARENTS AND CHILDREN
TO NEW COMMUNITIES. FOUR PHASES CHAR-
ACTERIZED THE STUDY. FIRST, DURING THE EX-
PLORATORY STAGE AN INTENSIVE STUDY OF
SEVEN REPRESENTATIVE SCHOOLS, WHICH IN-
CLUDED AN ETHNIC-EDUCATIONAL SURVEY
AND A TESTING PROGRAM, WAS CONDUCTED.
SECOND, THE EXPERIMENTAL PHASE IN-
CLUDED AN EMPHASIS ON THE ADOPTION
AND CONSTRUCTION OF TESTS AND TECH-
NIQUES FOR ASSESSMENT OF THE ABILITIES
OF PUERTO RICAN CHILDREN. THE THIRD AND
FOURTH PHASES WERE USED TO DEVELOP,
PRODUCE, AND IMPROVE CURRICULUM MATE-
RIALS RELEVANT TO THE PUERTO RICAN CHILD.
THE BOOK IS DIVIDED INTO THREE PARTS
WHICH PARALLEL THE PHASES OF THE PROJ-
ECT. PART I PRESENTS THE DEVELOPMENT OF
METHODS AND MATERIALS FOR TEACHING EN-
GLISH TO NON-ENGLISH-SPEAKING CHIL-
DREN. PART II REVIEWS STUDIES CONDUCTED
ON PUERTO RICAN PUPILS IN NEW YORK CITY
SCHOOLS AND THE SCHOOL'S ROLE IN THEIR
EDUCATIONAL-SOCIAL-CULTURAL ADJUST-
MENT. PART III SNYTHESIZES THE CONCLU-
SIONS OF THE STUDY AND THEIR RELATION TO
POLICY PLANNING AND LONG RANGE PRO-
GRAMS. RESULTS, ACHIEVEMENTS, AND RE-
SEARCH MATERIALS ARE EXTENSIVELY DE-
TAILED THROUGHOUT THE CHAPTERS WHICH
DOCUMENT THE STUDY'S 4-YEAR PROGRESS.
ACCN 000139

165 AUTH **BODINE, J. J.**
TITL A TRI-ETHNIC TRAP: THE SPANISH AMERICAN
IN TAOS.
SRCE *IN J. HELM (ED.), SPANISH-SPEAKING PEOPLE*
IN THE UNITED STATES. PROCEEDINGS OF THE
1968 ANNUAL SPRING MEETING OF THE
AMERICAN ETHNOLOGICAL SOCIETY. SEATTLE:
UNIVERSITY OF WASHINGTON PRESS, 1968, PP.
145-153.
INDX CROSS CULTURAL, SPANISH SURNAMED, AC-
CULTURATION, HISTORY, ECONOMIC FACTORS,
RELIGION, ESSAY, SEX ROLES, INDIGENOUS
POPULATIONS, POLITICAL POWER, PROCEED-
INGS, NEW MEXICO, SOUTHWEST
ABST CULTURAL AND HISTORICAL FACTORS THAT
DEFINE THE RELATIONSHIPS AMONG THE
THREE ETHNIC GROUPS—INDIAN, SPANISH
AMERICAN AND ANGLO—OF TAOS,NEW
MEXICO, ARE EXAMINED. UNLIKE SIMILAR TRI-
ETHNIC COMMUNITIES IN THE U.S. WHERE THE
INDIAN GROUPS HAVE USUALLY BEEN LOOKED
DOWN UPON AS THE LOWEST GROUP BY THE
OTHER TWO, IN TAOS THE SPANISH AMERI-
CANS ARE VIEWED AS THE LOWEST GROUP.
ANGLOS, WHO DOMINATE MOST OF THE
TOWN'S BUSINESS, SEE THE INDIAN CULTURE
AS A MYSTERIOUS, BEAUTIFUL, NATURAL PRO-

CESS TO BE STUDIED AND PRESERVED, WHILE THE SPANISH AMERICANS AND THEIR CULTURAL UNIQUENESS ARE EITHER IGNORED OR DEGRADED. IN SPITE OF THESE PREJUDICES, THE SPANISH AMERICANS HAVE MAINTAINED POLITICAL CONTROL IN TAOS, AND VIA THIS AUTHORITY HAVE THWARTED SEVERAL INDIAN ATTEMPTS TO GAIN MORE LAND OR GOVERNMENT MONIES. THE STUDY OF THIS COMMUNITY EMPHASIZES THE NEED TO UNDERSTAND ETHNOCENTRISM AS A FACTOR IN MULTICULTURAL CONTACT AND CONFLICT. 18 REFERENCES.

ACCN 000140

166 AUTH **BOGARDUS, E. S.**
TITL CULTURAL PLURALISM AND ACCULTURATION.
SRCE *SOCIOLOGY AND SOCIAL RESEARCH, 1949, 34, 125-159.*
INDX CULTURAL PLURALISM, ACCULTURATION, DISCRIMINATION, MEXICAN AMERICAN, ESSAY, THEORETICAL
ABST CULTURAL PLURALISM IS THE FUNCTIONING OF TWO OR MORE CULTURE SYSTEMS AT THE SAME TIME WITHIN THE SAME NATIONAL UNIT OF HUMAN SOCIETY. TO UNDERSTAND ITS SIGNIFICANCE IT MAY BE CONSIDERED WITHIN ITS NATURAL FRAMEWORK, THAT IS, AS AN ASPECT OF ACCULTURATION. A BRIEF EXAMINATION OF ACCULTURATION AND ITS VARIOUS TYPES IS DESCRIBED. ACCULTURATION IS A PROCESS OF DEVELOPING ONE CULTURE SYSTEM OUT OF TWO OR MORE CULTURE SYSTEMS WHOSE HUMAN REPRESENTATIVES ARE IN CONTACT WITH EACH OTHER. IT IS EXPRESSED IN THREE OR MORE OVERLAPPING TYPES OF ACCULTURATION: (1) BLIND, (2) IMPOSED, AND (3) DEMOCRATIC. 8 REFERENCES. (JOURNAL ABSTRACT MODIFIED)

ACCN 000141

167 AUTH **BOGARDUS, E. S.**
TITL GANGS OF MEXICAN-AMERICAN YOUTH.
SRCE *SOCIOLOGY AND SOCIAL RESEARCH, 1943-1944, 28, 55-66.*
INDX GANGS, MEXICAN AMERICAN, ADOLESCENTS, DELINQUENCY, DISCRIMINATION, ESSAY, CALIFORNIA, SOUTHWEST
ABST THE SOCIAL BEHAVIOR OF MEXICAN AMERICAN (MA) GANG MEMBERS IN LOS ANGELES DURING THE 1940'S IS EXAMINED. THE GANGSTERISM OF SOME MA YOUTHS SHOULD BE VIEWED AS A PART OF A TOTAL SPECTRUM OF GANGS WHOSE MEMBERSHIP INCLUDES INDIVIDUALS OF DIFFERENT RACIAL AND CULTURAL BACKGROUNDS FROM ALL PARTS OF THE WORLD. THE UNDERLYING FACTOR OF GANG BEHAVIOR FOR THIS PARTICULAR ETHNIC SUBGROUP IS THE CONFLICT OF CULTURES IN WHICH MA'S ARE MADE TO FEEL OSTRACIZED AND INFERIOR. IN ADDITION, THE EDUCATIONAL SYSTEM CREATES PROBLEMS FOR MA YOUTHS. AFTER DROPPING OUT OF SCHOOL AND ENCOUNTERING EMPLOYMENT DISCRIMINATION, MA YOUTH DRIFT INTO A VICIOUS CYCLE OF DELINQUENCY AND CRIME. IT IS RECOMMENDED THAT MORE SOCIAL WORK IS NEEDED IN THE MA HOME AND THAT JOB

TRAINING PROGRAMS FOR DELINQUENT YOUTH ARE VITAL. ATTITUDES OF SOCIAL TOLERANCE AND UNDERSTANDING ON THE PART OF POLICE OFFICERS, NEWS MEDIA, AND THE GENERAL PUBLIC ARE ALSO NECESSARY. MA DELINQUENTS AND GANGSTERS SHOULD NOT BE TREATED AS "MEXICANS" BUT AS ANTISOCIAL YOUTH WHO ARE SUBJECT TO PREVAILING NEGATIVE CULTURAL PATTERNS IN THEIR IMPOVERISHED NEIGHBORHOODS. 1 REFERENCE.

ACCN 000142

168 AUTH **BOGARDUS, E. S.**
TITL THE MEXICAN IMMIGRANT AND SEGREGATION.
SRCE *AMERICAN JOURNAL OF SOCIOLOGY, 1930, 36, 74-80.*
INDX DISCRIMINATION, PREJUDICE, MEXICAN AMERICAN, SES, POVERTY, MIGRATION, SCHOLASTIC ACHIEVEMENT, BILINGUALISM, ESSAY
ABST THE NUMBER OF MEXICAN IMMIGRANTS WHO HAVE TAKEN OUT CITIZENSHIP PAPERS IS IS VERY SMALL, AND THIS IS REGARDED AS A RESULT OF SEGREGATION. THE MEXICAN, WHEN QUESTIONED ABOUT THIS, ANSWERS THAT AMERICANS IN MEXICO DO NOT BECOME MEXICAN CITIZENS; OR HE IS EXPECTING TO RETURN TO MEXICO, BUT HE RARELY DOES. THE MEXICAN BRINGS WITH HIM A HIGH DEGREE OF LOYALTY TO HIS NATIVE COUNTRY. OFTEN THE EDUCATED AND PROSPEROUS MEXICAN IS PREVENTED BY PROPERTY OWNERS FROM OWNING PROPERTY IN THE BETTER NEIGHBORHOODS. THE MEXICAN CAN SECURE JUSTICE FROM THE MEXICAN CONSUL MORE EASILY THAN IN THE COURTS OF THE UNITED STATES. FINALLY, THE MEXICAN SAYS THAT EVEN IF HE BECAME A CITIZEN, AMERICANS WOULD STILL CALL HIM A "DIRTY GREASER." (JOURNAL ABSTRACT)

ACCN 000143

169 AUTH **BOGARDUS, E. S.**
TITL THE MEXICAN IMMIGRANT.
SRCE *JOURNAL OF APPLIED SOCIOLOGY, 1927, 11, 470-488.*
INDX MEXICAN AMERICAN, IMMIGRATION, RURAL, URBAN, INTERPERSONAL RELATIONS, SEX ROLES, EMPLOYMENT, FARM LABORERS, CULTURAL FACTORS, NUTRITION, SCHOLASTIC ACHIEVEMENT, MIGRATION, LABOR FORCE, ACCULTURATION, AGGRESSION, SOCIAL SERVICES, ESSAY, SES, POVERTY, HISTORY, CALIFORNIA, SOUTHWEST, ECONOMIC FACTORS
ABST THE ECOLOGICAL, CULTURAL, AND SOCIAL PATTERNS OF MEXICAN IMMIGRANTS IN SOUTHERN CALIFORNIA DURING THE 1920'S ARE EXAMINED. COMMUNITY ORGANIZATION AND BASIC OCCUPATIONS ARE DESCRIBED AS SIMPLE AND EASILY MANIPULATED BY AMERICAN EXPLOITATION. HEALTH, EATING AND SPENDING PATTERNS ARE IMPROVED AS CULTURAL ATTITUDES CHANGE. THE INCENTIVE FOR MEXICANS TO MIGRATE IS PRIMARILY ECONOMIC OPPORTUNITY. THE IMPACT OF THIS ON LABOR ADJUSTMENTS, SOCIAL DISORGANIZATION, AND LACK OF OPPORTUNITY TO LEARN WORK SKILLS IS BLAMED FOR MOST

OF THE IMMIGRANT PROBLEMS. THE ROLE OF CHARITY AND PUBLIC RELIEF AGENCIES IS PERCEIVED AS BOTH RELIEVING AND CAUSING FINANCIAL DEPENDENCE BY POOR IMMIGRANTS. BEHAVIOR PROBLEMS SUCH AS DELINQUENCY, THIEVING AND PERSONAL VIOLENCE ARE CAUSED BY DIFFERENCES IN MEXICAN AND AMERICAN STANDARDS AND CUSTOMS AS WELL AS THE SOCIALLY DISORGANIZING PROCESS OF IMMIGRATION. ACCOMODATION AND ASSIMILATION ARE MEASURED IN TERMS OF LEARNING ENGLISH, OWNING PROPERTY, AND INCREASING RESPONSIBILITY.

ACCN   000144

170 AUTH **BOGARDUS, E. S.**
    TITL THE MEXICAN IN THE UNITED STATES.
    SRCE *SAN FRANCISCO: R AND E RESEARCH ASSOCIATES, 1970. (REPRINTED FROM UNIVERSITY OF SOUTHERN CALIFORNIA, SCHOOL OF RESEARCH STUDIES NUMBER FIVE, 1934.)*
    INDX ACCULTURATION, ADULT EDUCATION, HISTORY, CRIMINOLOGY, CULTURAL FACTORS, DEMOGRAPHIC, ECONOMIC FACTORS, EDUCATION, PREJUDICE, RELIGION, RURAL, URBAN, MEXICAN AMERICAN, MIGRATION, HEALTH, CALIFORNIA, SOUTHWEST
    ABST BASED ON LIFE HISTORIES, INTERVIEW DATA AND PSYCHO-SOCIAL ANALYSIS, THIS STUDY EXAMINES THE MEXICAN IMMIGRANT AND THE SOCIAL SITUATIONS HE HAS KNOWN IN MEXICO AND IN THE UNITED STATES. CULTURAL CONFLICT IS EXPLAINED AS LACK OF UNDERSTANDING BY AMERICANS OF MEXICANS AND VICE VERSA. DISTINCTIONS ARE MADE BETWEEN GENERATIONS AND NEWLY ARRIVED IMMIGRANTS AND HOW THIS INFLUENCES THE CONFLICT AND ADJUSTMENT PROCESS. SEPARATE CHAPTERS DEAL WITH SUCH TOPICS AS COMMUNITY AND CAMP LIFE, HEALTH, LABOR, AMUSEMENTS, RELIGION, CHILD WELFARE, CITIZENSHIP, REPATRIATION AND LEGISLATION. 183 REFERENCES.
    ACCN 000145

171 AUTH **BOK, M.**
    TITL MARGINALITY IN MINORITY GROUP NONPROFESSIONAL STATUS.
    SRCE *PROCEEDINGS OF THE 81ST ANNUAL CONVENTION OF THE AMERICAN PSYCHOLOGICAL ASSOCIATION, 1973, 8, 961-962.*
    INDX OCCUPATIONAL ASPIRATIONS, CURRICULUM, SOCIAL MOBILITY, PROFESSIONAL TRAINING, PARAPROFESSIONALS, EMPLOYMENT, PUERTO RICAN-M, EMPIRICAL
    ABST THE AWARENESS THAT INDIGENOUS PEOPLE CAN CONTRIBUTE TO THE SOLUTION OF SOCIAL PROBLEMS HAS LED TO THE INCREASED USE OF NONPROFESSIONALS BY SERVICE ORGANIZATIONS. BUT AS THEIR NUMBER HAS GROWN AND THEIR ACTIVITIES MULTIPLIED, THE PROBLEMS INVOLVED HAVE BECOME MORE APPARENT. ONE OF THE MOST SALIENT CHARACTERISTICS OF INDIGENOUS NONPROFESSIONALS IS THEIR MARGINALITY. THIS STUDY IDENTIFIES AND DISCUSSES SELECTED CHARACTERISTICS OF MINORITY GROUP NON-

PROFESSIONALS (MAINLY BLACKS AND PUERTO RICANS) TRAINED IN A UNIVERSITY-BASED, NONCREDIT, HUMAN SERVICES PROGRAM. AGE, PRIOR WORK EXPERIENCE, CURRENT EMPLOYMENT STATUS, AND EDUCATION ARE EMPHASIZED AS EXAMPLES OF INDIGENOUS NONPROFESSIONAL CHARACTERISTICS WHICH REFLECT THEIR MARGINALITY AND CONTINUED DISCRIMINATION. 3 REFERENCES.

ACCN   000146

172 AUTH **BONNHEIM, M. L.**
    TITL FAMILY INTERACTION AND ACCULTURATION AMONG MEXICAN AMERICAN INHALANT USERS.
    SRCE *UNPUBLISHED DOCTORAL DISSERTATION, UNIVERSITY OF TEXAS HEALTH SCIENCE CENTER AT DALLAS, 1977.*
    INDX ACCULTURATION, INHALANT ABUSE, FAMILY STRUCTURE, FAMILY ROLES, INTERPERSONAL RELATIONS, ADOLESCENTS, ETHNIC IDENTITY, FATHER-CHILD INTERACTION, MOTHER-CHILD INTERACTION, STRESS, COPING MECHANISMS, EMPIRICAL, MEXICAN AMERICAN, REVIEW
    ABST TO ELUCIDATE THE RELATIONSHIP BETWEEN FAMILY STRUCTURE AND DRUG INHALANT ABUSE AMONG MEXICAN AMERICANS, BOTH FAMILY INTERACTION AND LEVEL OF ACCULTURATION WERE INVESTIGATED AMONG 20 MEXICAN AMERICAN FAMILIES. TEN FAMILIES HAD A MALE ADOLESCENT WHO WAS AN INHALANT ABUSER AND 10 FAMILIES HAD A MALE ADOLESCENT WHO HAD NEVER USED INHALANTS BUT MATCHED ON THE USE OF OTHER DRUGS. AN ACCULTURATION QUESTIONNAIRE WAS ADMINISTERED TO EACH FAMILY, AND EACH FAMILY ALSO PARTICIPATED IN A VIDEOTAPED INTERVIEW DESIGNED TO REVEAL THE NATURE OF FAMILY INTERACTION. FURTHERMORE, ALL FAMILIES WERE RATED BY TWO BILINGUAL MENTAL HEALTH PROFESSIONALS ON 113 ITEMS OF THE FAMILY INTERACTION Q-SORT, AND THE RATINGS WERE THEN CORRELATED WITH AN "OPTIMALLY HEALTHY MEXICAN AMERICAN FAMILY" STEREOTYPE. DATA ANALYSIS REVEALED THAT 23 ITEMS DIFFERENTIATED THE INHALANT USER FROM NON-USER FAMILIES. USER FAMILIES WERE MORE INCONSISTENT, NEGATIVISTIC, UNFOCUSED, CONFUSED, INTERNALLY CONFLICTED, ANXIOUS, AND DEFENSIVE. THE NON-USER FAMILIES SEEMED TO HAVE A GREATER SENSE OF FAMILY UNITY, HEALTHIER PARENTAL COALITIONS, AND CLEAR COMMUNICATIONS; THEY WERE ALSO MORE TRUSTING, SKILLED, COOPERATIVE, AND PRODUCTIVE. SECONDLY, IT WAS FOUND THAT DIFFERENCES IN ACCULTURATION LEVELS BETWEEN FAMILY MEMBERS DID NOT DIFFERENTIATE USER FROM NON-USER FAMILIES. STILL, IT IS CONCLUDED THAT THE QUALITY OF FAMILY COPING SKILLS, COMBINED WITH THE ACCULTURATION PROCESS, MAY BE LINKED TO INHALANT ABUSE AMONG MEXICAN AMERICAN ADOLESCENTS. THIS DISSERTATION INCLUDES AN EXTENSIVE LITERATURE REVIEW ON INHALANT ABUSE, ACCULTURATION, AND FAMILY ASSESSMENT, AS WELL AS 11 TABLES AND 10 APPENDICES COVERING

RESEARCH INSTRUMENTS AND RESULTS. 121 REFERENCES.

ACCN 000147

173 AUTH **BOOTH, R. F., & BERRY, N. H.**
TITL MINORITY GROUP DIFFERENCES IN THE BACKGROUND, PERSONALITY, AND PERFORMANCE OF NAVY PARAMEDICAL PERSONNEL.
SRCE *JOURNAL OF COMMUNITY PSYCHOLOGY, 1978, 6, 60-68.*
INDX ABILITY TESTING, CROSS CULTURAL, EDUCATIONAL ASSESSMENT, EMPIRICAL, EQUAL OPPORTUNITY, JOB PERFORMANCE, PARAPROFESSIONALS, PROFESSIONAL TRAINING, SPANISH SURNAMED, POLICY, MILITARY
ABST A COMPARISON OF 1,091 BLACK PERSONS, 192 HISPANIC PERSONS, 186 ASIAN PERSONS, AND A RANDOM SAMPLE OF 1,785 WHITE PERSONS WHO ENTERED NAVY HOSPITAL CORPSMAN AND DENTAL TECHNICIAN TRAINING REVEALED SIGNIFICANT BETWEEN-GROUP DIFFERENCES ON A NUMBER OF APTITUDE, BACKGROUND, AND PERSONALITY MEASURES. WHEN PARTICIPANTS IN THIS RESEARCH WERE DIVIDED INTO THOSE INDIVIDUALS WHO HAD BEEN FULLY QUALIFIED FOR PARAMEDICAL TRAINING (HIGH APTITUDE), THOSE WHO HAD BEEN ONLY MARGINALLY QUALIFIED FOR TRAINING (MEDIUM APTITUDE), AND THOSE WHO HAD BEEN ACCEPTED FOR TRAINING DESPITE THE FACT THAT THEY HAD NOT BEEN QUALIFIED (LOW APTITUDE), BETWEEN-GROUP COMPARISONS REVEALED THAT MINORITY GROUP MEMBERS AT THE LOW AND MEDIUM APTITUDE LEVELS TENDED TO PERFORM BETTER, BOTH IN TRAINING AND ON THE JOB, THAN DID THE WHITES AT COMPARABLE APTITUDE LEVELS. THE PERFORMANCE OF INDIVIDUALS WITH HIGH APTITUDE TEST SCORES WAS NOT RELATED TO MINORITY GROUP STATUS. THESE FINDINGS SUGGEST THAT CONSIDERATION SHOULD BE GIVEN TO MINORITY GROUP MEMBERSHIP IN SCREENING CANDIDATES FOR THESE PARAMEDICAL JOBS AND THAT AFFIRMATIVE ACTION PROGRAMS, AT LEAST WHEN THEY ARE EVALUATED IN TERMS OF TRAINING PERFORMANCE AND JOB TURNOVER, CAN PRODUCE SIGNIFICANT BENEFITS FOR THE INDIVIDUALS CONCERNED AND FOR THE ORGANIZATION. 14 REFERENCES. (JOURNAL ABSTRACT)

ACCN 002026

174 AUTH **BORAH, W., & COOK, S. F.**
TITL MARRIAGE AND LEGITIMACY IN MEXICAN CULTURE: MEXICO AND CALIFORNIA.
SRCE *CALIFORNIA LAW REVIEW, 1966, 54(2), 946-1008.*
INDX MARRIAGE, MEXICAN, MEXICAN AMERICAN, CULTURAL FACTORS, EMPIRICAL, DEMOGRAPHIC, CHILDREN, MARITAL STABILITY, HISTORY, INTERMARRIAGE, RELIGION, CALIFORNIA, SOUTHWEST, MEXICO, FEMALE
ABST AN HISTORICAL AND STATISTICAL INQUIRY IS MADE INTO THE MARRIAGE AND LEGITIMACY PATTERNS IN MEXICAN CULTURE BOTH NORTH AND SOUTH OF THE U.S.-MEXICO BORDER FROM THE TIME OF THE SPANISH EXPLORERS THROUGH CONTEMPORARY U.S. WELFARE SERVICES. COMPOSED OF TWO PARTS, THE FIRST DESCRIBES THE CULTURAL AND POLITICAL EVENTS WHICH INFLUENCED MARRIAGE AND LEGITIMACY BEHAVIORS IN MEXICO THROUGH THESE PERIODS: (1) THE INDIGENOUS PATTERNS BEFORE SPANISH COLONIZATION (PRE-1600); (2) THE COLONIAL PERIOD OF SPANISH AND EUROPEAN INFLUENCE (1600-1850); (3) THE NEW LEGISLATION AFTER MEXICO GAINED INDEPENDENCE FROM SPAIN (1850-1910) WHICH INCLUDED SEPARATION OF CHURCH AND STATE; AND (4) CONDITIONS SINCE THE REVOLUTION OF 1910. PART TWO ANALYZES THE SAME BEHAVIORS AS THEY ARE FOUND AMONG MEXICAN AMERICANS IN SANTA CLARA COUNTY, CALIFORNIA. EMPIRICAL DATA FROM SEVERAL SOURCES IN BOTH MEXICO AND CALIFORNIA ARE SUMMARIZED IN TABLES. SOME OF THE MAJOR CONCLUSIONS REGARDING ANGLO AND MEXICAN AMERICAN PATTERNS IN SANTA CLARA ARE: (1) MEXICAN AMERICANS BORN IN MEXICO DO NOT SIGNIFICANTLY DIFFER FROM THOSE BORN IN THE U.S. IN USING WELFARE OR IN BEING LEGALLY MARRIED; (2) MEXICAN AMERICAN WOMEN ARE FAR MORE FREQUENTLY PARTNERS IN COMMON LAW MARRIAGE THAN ANGLO WOMEN; (3) IN BOTH ETHNIC GROUPS, THE OLDER WOMEN HAVE FEWER COMMON LAW MARRIAGES RECORDED THAN THE YOUNGER WOMEN; (4) THERE IS A STRONG PREFERENCE BY MEXICAN AMERICAN COUPLES TO MARRY EITHER IN JUDICIAL OR PROTESTANT CEREMONIES RATHER THAN IN THE CATHOLIC CHURCH. OVERALL, IT IS CONCLUDED THAT THE STUDY SUPPORTS THE HYPOTHESIS THAT MEXICAN AMERICAN BEHAVIOR IN MARRIAGE AND FAMILY UNION IS CONDITIONED BY CULTURAL CARRY-OVER FROM MEXICAN CUSTOMS AND LAWS IN MARRIAGE AND LEGITIMACY. 97 REFERENCES. (AUTHOR SUMMARY MODIFIED)

ACCN 000148

175 AUTH **BORRELLO, M. A., & MATHIAS, E.**
TITL BOTANICAS: PUERTO RICAN FOLK PHARMACIES.
SRCE *NATURAL HISTORY, AUGUST/SEPTEMBER 1977, PP. 66-72.*
INDX CULTURAL FACTORS, CULTURE, ESPIRITISMO, FOLK MEDICINE, PUERTO RICAN-M, RELIGION, NEW YORK, URBAN, ESSAY, MENTAL HEALTH
ABST BOTANICAS (HERBAL-RELIGIOUS SUPPLY SHOPS) ARE EVIDENCE OF THE BIFURCATED RELIGIOUS SYSTEM OF PUERTO RICANS RESIDING IN SPANISH HARLEM, NEW YORK. MOST PUERTO RICANS ARE ROMAN CATHOLIC BUT MANY ARE INVOLVED WITH SPIRITISM, WHICH IS A MIXTURE OF CATHOLICISM, YORUBA RELIGION (AFRICAN), AND TEACHINGS OF THE FRENCH SPIRITIST-PHILOSOPHER, HIPPOLYTE RIVEL. SPIRITIST TEACHING CONSISTS OF WAYS TO CONTACT SPIRITS TO ENLIST AID AND PROVIDE REASON FOR THE UNEXPLAINED. THERE ARE ALSO SPECIAL SAINTS WHICH ARE VENERATED WITH AMULETS, OILS, LOTIONS, CANDLES, BEADED NECKLACES, AND INCENSE

PURCHASED AT A BOTANICA. SPIRITIST MEET-INGS ARE ATTENDED AT A CENTRO (RELIGIOUS CENTER) AND PRESIDED OVER BY A MEDIUM WHO HAS THE ABILITY TO COMMUNICATE WITH THE SPIRIT WORLD. THE MEDIUM CAN SEE PAST, PRESENT, AND FUTURE EVENTS IN VISIONS AND THEREBY PRESCRIBE PRAYERS AND CEREMONICAL RITES TO SOLVE PROB-LEMS. THE BOTANICA CONTRIBUTES TO THIS SYSTEM BY FUNCTIONING AS A FOLK PHAR-MACY, THROUGH WHICH THE MEDIUM MINIS-TERS TO THE PHYSICAL AND SPIRITUAL HEALTH OF THE COMMUNITY. IN NEW YORK, THE POPU-LARITY OF THE BOTANICAS DEMONSTRATES THAT A MINORITY SUBCULTURE HAS MAN-AGED TO MAINTAIN A SUBSTANTIAL LEVEL OF ETHNIC AND SPIRITUAL UNITY.

ACCN   002027

176 AUTH   **BORRERO, M., CUADRADO, L., & RODRIGUEZ, P.**

TITL   THE PUERTO RICAN ROLE IN INTEREST-GROUP POLITICS.

SRCE   *SOCIAL CASEWORK, 1974, 55(2), 94-99.*

INDX   CAPITALISM, POLITICS, PUERTO RICAN-M, ES-SAY, POVERTY, COMMUNITY INVOLVEMENT, DISCRIMINATION, MENTAL HEALTH PROFES-SION, SOCIAL STRUCTURE, COOPERATION, COMPETITION, SES, GROUP DYNAMICS, CUL-TURAL PLURALISM, POLITICAL POWER

ABST   IF PUERTO RICAN PROFESSIONALS IN THE U.S. ALLOW THEMSELVES TO FOCUS SOLELY ON THE PROBLEMS OF PUERTO RICANS, RATHER THAN BROADENING THEIR CONCERNS BE-YOND THEIR OWN INTEREST GROUP, THEY WILL FIND THEMSELVES PERPETUATING A CAP-ITALISTIC SYSTEM THAT HAS KEPT MINORITIES POOR, DIVIDED, AND OPPRESSED. POTENTIAL POLITICAL AND ECONOMIC POWER LIES IN THE COALITION OF THE VARIOUS GROUPS— E.G., HISPANICS, BLACK, THE ELDERLY, POOR WHITES—WHO MAKE UP THE 24%-30% OF THE POPULATION WHO LIVE BELOW THE POVERTY LINE. ALTHOUGH THIS PROPOSAL IS BASED ON THE ASSUMPTION THAT THESE GROUPS WOULD BE WILLING TO IDENTIFY AND WORK WITH ONE ANOTHER, AND COULD COOPERATE EFFECTIVELY ONCE ORGANIZED, THE AU-THORS CONTEND THAT IT IS ACTUALLY SO-CIALIZED PATTERNS OF BEHAVIOR WHICH HAVE PERPETUATED A SYSTEM OF INEQUALITIES AND KEPT GROUPS FROM UNITING IN A COM-MON CAUSE. ONCE THE GOAL OF A UNITED FRONT HAS BEEN IDENTIFIED, THE NEXT STEP IS TO WORK ON THE PROCESS. THE PERSPEC-TIVE WHICH PUERTO RICANS HAVE AS NEW-COMERS TO NORTH AMERICA (I.E., LESS COM-PETITIVE AND MORE COOPERATIVE IN ORIENTATION AND POSSESSING A DIVERSE HUMANISTIC CULTURAL HERITAGE) WILL PRO-VIDE THE BASIC VALUES NEEDED TO UNIFY OP-PRESSED GROUPS. THE CONTINUATION OF PUERTO RICAN INTEREST-GROUP MENTALITY, ON THE OTHER HAND, LEADS ONLY TO A TO-KEN PARTICIPATION IN AND REINFORCEMENT OF A DESTRUCTIVE SYSTEM. IT IS THE PUERTO RICAN PROFESSIONAL, ESPECIALLY THOSE IN

THE HUMAN SERVICE FIELDS, WHO MUST TAKE THE FIRST STEP. 14 REFERENCES.

ACCN   002028

177 AUTH   **BOULETTE, T. R.**

TITL   ASSERTIVE TRAINING WITH LOW INCOME MEX-ICAN AMERICAN WOMEN.

SRCE   *IN M. R. MIRANDA (ED.), PSYCHOTHERAPY WITH THE SPANISH SPEAKING: ISSUES IN RESEARCH AND SERVICE DELIVERY (MONOGRAPH NO. 3). LOS ANGELES: UNIVERSITY OF CALIFORNIA, SPANISH SPEAKING MENTAL HEALTH RE-SEARCH CENTER, 1976, PP. 67-71.*

INDX   PSYCHOPATHOLOGY, ANXIETY, DEPRESSION, MARRIAGE, FAMILY ROLES, BEHAVIOR THER-APY, MODELING, PSYCHOTHERAPY, PSYCHO-THERAPISTS, BILINGUAL-BICULTURAL PER-SONNEL, MEXICAN AMERICAN, ADULTS, FEMALE, MENTAL HEALTH, HEALTH, REVIEW, ESSAY, ASSERTIVENESS

ABST   ASSERTIVE TRAINING HAS BEEN FOUND TO BE WELL ACCEPTED AND WELL UTILIZED BY LOW INCOME MEXICAN AMERICAN WOMEN WHO DEMONSTRATE PSYCHOPHYSIOLOGICAL SYMPTOMS, DEPRESSION AND GENERALIZED ANXIETY. SPECIFIC TECHNIQUES USED IN AS-SERTIVE TRAINING AND THE MODIFICATIONS FOUND USEFUL WITH MEXICAN AMERICAN WOMEN ARE ILLUSTRATED. GUIDELINES AND SUGGESTIONS FOR THE USE OF THIS TECH-NIQUE ARE PRESENTED.

ACCN   000150

178 AUTH   **BOULETTE, T. R.**

TITL   DETERMINING NEEDS AND APPROPIATE COUNSELING APPROACHES FOR MEXICAN-AMERICAN WOMEN: A COMPARISON OF THER-APEUTIC LISTENING AND BEHAVIORAL RE-HEARSAL.

SRCE   *SAN FRANCISCO: R AND E RESEARCH ASSOCI-ATES, 1976. (REPRINTED FROM AN UNPUB-LISHED DOCTORAL DISSERTATION, UNIVER-SITY OF CALIFORNIA AT SANTA BARBARA, 1975.)*

INDX   REVIEW, EMPIRICAL, MENTAL HEALTH, CUL-TURAL FACTORS, BEHAVIOR THERAPY, FE-MALE, MEXICAN AMERICAN, SES, PSYCHOTH-ERAPY, COMMUNITY, ADULTS, HEALTH DELIVERY SYSTEMS, RESOURCE UTILIZATION, PSY-CHOTHERAPY OUTCOME, CALIFORNIA, SOUTHWEST

ABST   TWO INDIVIDUAL COUNSELING STRATEGIES, THERAPEUTIC LISTENING AND BEHAVIOR RE-HEARSAL, WITH LOW INCOME MEXICAN AMERICAN WOMEN WERE TESTED EXPERIMEN-TALLY AND COMPARED TO DETERMINE WHICH WOULD BE MORE EFFECTIVE IN PROMOTING CLIENT ATTAINMENT OF SPECIFIC GOALS. RANDOMIZATION PROCEDURES WERE USED TO ASSIGN 36 VOLUNTARY PATIENTS TO ONE OF TWO TREATMENT CONDITIONS FOR EIGHT WEEKLY COUNSELING SESSIONS AND TO ONE OF THREE COUNSELORS. THE SUBJECTS WERE FOUND TO BE DISADVANTAGED, SPEAK EN-GLISH INFREQUENTLY, REPORT HIGH RATES OF SEVERE MARITAL DISHARMONY, AND DEMON-STRATE SYMPTOMS CONSISTENT WITH THE CLINICAL DIAGNOSIS OF DEPRESSION. NEI-THER TREATMENT MODEL WAS CONSISTENTLY

EFFECTIVE IN PROMOTING FAVORABLE TREATMENT OUTCOMES. IT MAY WELL BE THAT THESE WOMEN CANNOT PROFIT FROM EXPOSURE TO MORE ABSTRACT COUNSELING PROCEDURES UNTIL THEIR IMMEDIATE ECONOMIC AND SOCIAL CRISES ARE RESOLVED. 69 REFERENCES.

ACCN   000151

179   AUTH   **BOULETTE, T. R.**
TITL   PARENTING: SPECIAL NEEDS OF LOW-INCOME SPANISH-SURNAMED FAMILIES.
SRCE   *PEDIATRIC ANNALS, 1977, 6(9), 95-107.*
INDX   CULTURAL FACTORS, MIGRANTS, CHILDREN, CHILDREARING PRACTICES, COPING MECHANISMS, SES, ESSAY, FAMILY ROLES, FATHER-CHILD INTERACTION, HEALTH, HEALTH DELIVERY SYSTEMS, MOTHER-CHILD INTERACTION, SPANISH SURNAMED, STEREOTYPES, PHYSICIANS, CULTURAL PLURALISM, POLICY

ABST   THIS REVIEW OF THE FACTORS WHICH THE PEDIATRICIAN WILL WANT TO CONSIDER IN WORKING WITH HISPANIC CHILDREN ASSERTS THAT INTERVENTION STRATEGIES WITH THE LOW-INCOME SPANISH-SPEAKING OR SPANISH SURNAMED POPULATION MUST BE BASED ON THE REALITY THAT WE CURRENTLY KNOW VERY LITTLE ABOUT THEIR CORE CULTURE, FAMILY, AND CHILDREARING VALUES AND PRACTICES. INAPPROPRIATE GENERALIZATIONS DERIVED FROM POORLY DESIGNED STUDIES, ANECDOTAL REPORTS OF ISOLATED ENCLAVES, AND AUTHORS' ROMANTIC OR DEPRECATORY STEREOTYPICAL VIEWS ARE THE ESSENCE OF OUR CURRENT KNOWLEDGE. IN ADDITION, THERE HAS BEEN LOW AWARENESS OF THE ACTUAL INFLUENCES OF POVERTY, PREJUDICE, SOCIAL CLASS, NATIVITY, BICULTURATION, AND FAMILY DIFFERENCES WHICH CAN IMPINGE ON ACTUAL PHYSICAL AND MENTAL HEALTH. THE HEALTH PROFESSIONAL MUST BE SENSITIVE TO THESE CONSIDERATIONS AND SHOULD AVOID DESTRUCTIVE "HELPER" BEHAVIORS, SUCH AS MYTH-BUILDING, CULTURE BLAMING, AND INSENSITIVITY TO THE CONSEQUENCES OF SOCIAL CONDITIONS THAT VICTIMIZE THE SPANISH SURNAMED AND PROMOTE DESTRUCTIVE PARENTING. SUCH FACTORS CITED AND DISCUSSED ARE: (1) MATERNAL DEPRIVATION; (2) FATHER ABSENCE AND STRESSFUL FATHERING; (3) EXCESSIVE ATTACHMENT BETWEEN MOTHER AND CHILD; (4) EARLY BURDENING OF THE OLDER CHILD WITH REARING OF SIBLINGS; (5) USE OF CHILDREN AS INTERPRETERS; (6) EXCESSIVE WORK REQUIREMENTS; (7) DEGRADING PUNISHMENTS; (8) PUNISHMENTS THAT DISCOURAGE THE EXPRESSION OF EMOTION; AND (9) LIMITED EDUCATION AND LIMITED ABILITY TO SPEAK ENGLISH. CONSEQUENTLY, IN WORKING WITH THESE POPULATIONS THE HEALTH COUNSELOR SHOULD BECOME AWARE OF COURTESY-INTERACTION STYLES OF CLIENTS AND INDIVIDUAL CULTURAL DIFFERENCES AND STRENGTHS; AND HE MUST ALSO AVOID CULTURAL GENERALIZATIONS IF HE HOPES TO WORK EFFECTIVELY WITH THESE FAMILIES. 24 REFERENCES.

ACCN   002030

180   AUTH   **BOULETTE, T. R.**
TITL   PREVENTIVE MENTAL HEALTH STRATEGIES FOR THE LOW INCOME SPANISH-SPEAKING.
SRCE   *IN A. M. PADILLA & E. R. PADILLA (EDS.), IMPROVING MENTAL HEALTH AND HUMAN SERVICES FOR HISPANIC COMMUNITIES: SELECTED PRESENTATIONS FROM REGIONAL CONFERENCES. WASHINGTON, D.C.: NATIONAL COALITION OF HISPANIC MENTAL HEALTH AND HUMAN SERVICE ORGANIZATIONS (COSSMHO), 1977, PP. 51-56.*
INDX   PRIMARY PREVENTION, MEXICAN AMERICAN, PSYCHOPATHOLOGY, MASS MEDIA, ESSAY, CALIFORNIA, SOUTHWEST
ABST   SOCIAL AND ECONOMIC OPPRESSION AND THE RESULTANT POVERTY CONDITIONS HAVE SERIOUS DELETERIOUS PSYCHOLOGICAL CONSEQUENCES FOR THE SPANISH-SPEAKING. SUCH SOCIALLY OPPRESSIVE INFLUENCES HAVE A MORE DAMAGING EFFECT ON FAMILIES WHO ARE MOST VULNERABLE. MENTAL HEALTH PROGRAMS DESIGNED TO STRENGTHEN FAMILY UNIT, AND THEREBY DECREASE ITS VULNERABILITY, HAVE BEEN DESIGNED AND USED SUCCESSFULLY IN SANTA BARBARA COUNTY, CALIFORNIA. BY USING PRIMARY PREVENTION STRATEGIES BASED ON COPLAN'S THEORIES OF PREVENTIVE PSYCHIATRY AND MODIFIED TO FIT THE LIFESTYLE OF THE SPANISH-SPEAKING FAMILY, THESE PROGRAMS HAVE BEEN EFFECTIVE IN STRENGTHENING THE POSITIVE MENTAL HEALTH OF THE FAMILIES SERVED. THREE SERVICE MODALITIES ARE DESCRIBED: (1) A BILINGUAL BOOK (UNA FAMILIA SANA) AND TELEVISION SERIES THAT DESCRIBES, EXPLAINS AND ENCOURAGES USE OF AVAILABLE RESOURCES; (2) EDUCATIONAL COFFEE KLATCHES (MERIENDAS EDUCATIVAS) WHICH ENCOURAGE USE OF MENTAL HEALTH SERVICES AND PROVIDE BASIC MENTAL HEALTH EDUCATION TO LOW INCOME SPANISH-SPEAKING MOTHERS; AND (3) A FAMILY CARE CENTER (EL CENTRO FAMILIAR) WHICH PROVIDES A COMPREHENSIVE TRAINING, SERVICES AND ENRICHMENT PROGRAM FOR FAMILIES.

ACCN   000152

181   AUTH   **BOULETTE, T. R.**
TITL   PROBLEMAS FAMILIARES: EDUCATIONAL MENTAL HEALTH TELEVISION PROGRAMMING IN SPANISH.
SRCE   *PAPER PRESENTED AT THE ANNUAL CONVENTION OF THE CALIFORNIA STATE PSYCHOLOGICAL ASSOCIATION, FRESNO, CALIFORNIA, JANUARY 1974.*
INDX   MASS MEDIA, MENTAL HEALTH, HEALTH EDUCATION, MEXICAN AMERICAN, ESSAY, PRIMARY PREVENTION, CALIFORNIA, SOUTHWEST
ABST   THE WIDENING GAP BETWEEN HIGH NEED AND LOW UTILIZATION OF PUBLIC OUT- PATIENT PSYCHIATRIC SERVICES BY THE MEXICAN AMERICAN POPULATION IS WELL DOCUMENTED. COMBINED WITH THE EFFORTS OF MAKING EXISTING SERVICES MORE RELEVANT (I.E., RECRUITING BILINGUAL PROFESSIONALS) IS THE NEED FOR EDUCATING MEXICAN AMERICAN CONSUMERS TO THE EXISTENCE

AND APPROPRIATE USES OF MENTAL HEALTH SERVICES. THE USE OF MULTIPLE ETHNIC AND CLASS SPECIFIC EDUCATIONAL, PREVENTIVE AND TREATMENT PROGRAMS WITH THE MEXICAN AMERICAN POPULATION OF SANTA BARBARA COUNTY IS DISCUSSED. AMONG THESE PROGRAMS ARE: (1) "MERIENDAS EDUCATIVAS" (EDUCATIONAL COFFEE KLATCHES); (2) "FIESTAS EDUCATIVAS" (EDUCATIONAL PARTIES); AND (3) "CLASES DE SALUD MENTAL" (INFORMAL GROUP COUNSELING IN CHURCHES AND OTHER CENTERS). A MOST IMPORTANT AND APPARENTLY SUCCESSFUL PART OF THIS EDUCATIONAL ENDEAVOR IS THE USE OF OVER 30 SHORT, CULTURALLY RELEVANT TELEVISION PROGRAMS WHICH PRESENT SUCH MENTAL HEALTH THEMES AS "UN MATRIMONIO SANO" (A HEALTHY MARRIAGE) AND "LOS NINOS APRENDEN LO QUE VEN" (CHILDREN LEARN WHAT THEY SEE). ALTHOUGH EDUCATIONAL TELEVISION PROGRAMMING IN SPANISH CANNOT BE CONSIDERED THE ONLY SOLUTION TO INCREASING THE UTILIZATION OF SERVICES BY MEXICAN AMERICANS, ITS EDUCATIONAL AS WELL AS PRIMARY AND SECONDARY PREVENTION FUNCTIONS MERIT FURTHER EXPLORATION.

ACCN 000153

182 AUTH **BOULETTE, T. R.**
TITL PROBLEMAS FAMILIARES: TELEVISION PROGRAMS IN SPANISH FOR MENTAL HEALTH EDUCATION.
SRCE *HOSPITAL AND COMMUNITY PSYCHIATRY, 1974, 25(5), 282.*
INDX MASS MEDIA, HEALTH EDUCATION, MENTAL HEALTH, PRIMARY PREVENTION, MEXICAN AMERICAN, ESSAY, CALIFORNIA, SOUTHWEST
ABST THE NEED FOR INFORMING SPANISH-SPEAKING CONSUMERS ABOUT THE EXISTENCE AND APPROPRIATE USES OF MENTAL HEALTH SERVICES CAN BE MET BY PRODUCING SHORT, EDUCATIONAL TELEVISION PROGRAMS DEALING WITH INFORMATION ABOUT MENTAL HEALTH. THESE PRODUCTIONS IN CONJUNCTION WITH AN AGGRESSIVE ADVERTISING PROGRAM HAVE RECEIVED FREQUENT AND POSITIVE VIEWER RESPONSE IN THE SANTA BARBARA COUNTY, CALIFORNIA, AREA. THE VALUE OF TELEVISION AS AN EDUCATIONAL DEVICE, AS WELL AS A TOOL IN PRIMARY AND SECONDARY PREVENTION OF MENTAL HEALTH PROBLEMS, MERITS FURTHER EXPLORATION.
ACCN 000154

183 AUTH **BOULETTE, T. R.**
TITL SOME EFFECTS OF OPERANT CONDITIONING WITH A MEXICAN-AMERICAN MALE.
SRCE *IN R. E. HOSFORD & C. S. MOSS (EDS.), THE CRUMBLING WALLS: TREATMENT AND COUNSELING OF PRISONERS (VOL. 14). URBANA, ILL.: UNIVERSITY OF ILLINOIS PRESS, 1975, PP. 121-135.*
INDX BEHAVIOR MODIFICATION, LEARNING, INSTITUTIONALIZATION, MEXICAN AMERICAN, MALE, ATTITUDES, AGGRESSION, CRIMINOLOGY, TEXAS, SOUTHWEST, CORRECTIONS, BEHAVIOR THERAPY, EMPIRICAL, CASE STUDY

ABST THIS CASE STUDY DESCRIBES SOME EFFECTS OF OPERANT CONDITIONING METHODS ON A 23 YEAR-OLD, UNMARRIED, TEXAS-BORN, FIRST GENERATION CHICANO INCARCERATED IN A FEDERAL CORRECTIONAL FACILITY. ALTHOUGH LIMITATIONS OF THE CASE STUDY METHOD IN SOCIAL RESEARCH PREVENT UNDUE CERTAINTY AND GENERALIZATION OF ANY FINDINGS, IT IS HOPED THAT THIS CASE WILL SERVE IN SOME WAY TO STIMULATE SCHOLARLY ENDEAVORS AND PERTINENT RESEARCH IN THE NEGLECTED AREA OF THE MENTAL HEALTH CARE OF LOW INCOME AND/OR INCARCERATED MEXICAN AMERICANS. 23 REFERENCES. (AUTHOR ABSTRACT)
ACCN 000155

184 AUTH **BOULETTE, T. R.**
TITL UNA FAMILIA SANA—A HEALTHY FAMILY.
SRCE *SANTA BARBARA, CALIF.: DEPARTMENT OF MENTAL HEALTH OF SANTA BARBARA COUNTY, MARCH 1975.*
INDX MASS MEDIA, HEALTH EDUCATION, MENTAL HEALTH, MARITAL STABILITY, PRIMARY PREVENTION, FAMILY ROLES, CHILDREARING PRACTICES, ESSAY, MARRIAGE
ABST PREPARED BY A NURSE-EDUCATOR AND A PSYCHIATRIC TECHNICIAN, THIS BOOKLET IS WRITTEN ESPECIALLY FOR LOW INCOME, SPANISH-SPEAKING PARENTS TO PROMOTE FAMILY MENTAL HEALTH. IN SIMPLE LANGUAGE AND FRANK STATEMENTS, BASIC MENTAL HEALTH CONCEPTS ARE PRESENTED, IN BOTH SPANISH AND ENGLISH, ON SIX TOPICS: MARRIAGE, BIRTH, MOTHER, FATHER, CHILD-REARING, AND SCHOOL EXPERIENCE. THE IMPORTANCE OF PREVENTING MARITAL, EMOTIONAL AND DEVELOPMENTAL ILLNESS AS WELL AS SEEKING COUNSELING AS SOON AS POSSIBLE IS RECOGNIZED AND EMPHASIZED. INDICATORS OF EMOTIONAL PROBLEMS BOTH IN CHILDREN AND PARENTS ARE LISTED ALONG WITH EXPLANATIONS OF HOW TREATMENT WILL FACILITATE UNDERSTANDING AND RESOLVING THESE PROBLEMS. OVERALL, THIS EDUCATIONAL FORMAT DECREASES THE MYSTERIOUS OR FRIGHTENING ASPECTS OF THE CAUSE AND TREATMENT OF EMOTIONAL PROBLEMS AND ENCOURAGES POSITIVE EFFORT TO IMPROVE FAMILY LIFE BY MEETING THE PHYSICAL, EMOTIONAL AND SPIRITUAL NEEDS OF FAMILY MEMBERS.
ACCN 000156

185 AUTH **BOWDEN, S.**
TITL NUTRITIONAL BELIEFS AND FOOD PRACTICES OF MEXICAN-AMERICAN MOTHERS.
SRCE *UNPUBLISHED MASTER'S THESIS, FRESNO STATE COLLEGE, 1968. (ERIC DOCUMENT REPRODUCTION SERVICE NO. ED 050 837)*
INDX MEXICAN AMERICAN, NUTRITION, EMPIRICAL, FAMILY ROLES, ECONOMIC FACTORS, RURAL, FARM LABORERS, HEALTH EDUCATION, FEMALE, CALIFORNIA, SOUTHWEST
ABST IN THE LOCALE OF HANFORD, CALIFORNIA, THIS 1968 NUTRITIONAL STUDY WAS MADE TO EXPLORE AND EVALUATE THE NUTRITIONAL BELIEFS AND FOOD PRACTICES OF MEXICAN

AMERICAN MOTHERS AMONG LOW-INCOME AGRICULTURAL WORKING FAMILIES. SOME 35 MOTHERS WHOSE CHILDREN ATTENDED THE HANFORD CHILD DAY-CARE CENTER WERE INTERVIEWED AT HOME TO DETERMINE FAMILY CHARACTERISTICS AND FOOD- BUYING AND MENU PLANNING PRACTICES. OPEN-ENDED QUESTIONS PROVIDED INFORMATION ABOUT DIETARY ESSENTIALS AND THE MOTHER'S FAMILIARITY WITH THE 4 BASIC DAILY FOODS. RESULTS OF THE STUDY ARE PRESENTED IN TERMS OF GROCERY BUYING AND MENU PLANNING, HOME FOOD PRODUCTION AND PRESERVATION, INFLUENCE OF CHILD DAY-CARE CENTER TRAINING, MOTHER'S 24-HOUR RECALL OF HER DIET, A DIETARY QUESTIONNAIRE, AND DAILY DIETARY ESSENTIALS (FOLK BELIEFS, ETC.). IN SUMMARY, IT IS NOTED THAT: (1) ADVANCED PLANNING OF MEALS WAS NOT THE RULE, WITH THE MAJORITY OF MOTHERS DECIDING ON MENUS JUST BEFORE STARTING MEAL PREPARATION; (2) APPROXIMATELY ONE-HALF OF THE FAMILIES PRODUCED SOME TYPE OF FOOD AT HOME, AND ONE-THIRD PRESERVED SOME FOOD BY CANNING; AND (3) MENU EVALUATION REVEALED DEFICIENCIES IN MILK, FRUITS, AND VEGETABLES. 44 REFERENCES. (RIE ABSTRACT)

ACCN   000157

186 AUTH **BOWERS, T. (PRODUCER)**
     TITL MENTAL HEALTH MATTERS.
     SRCE *ROCKVILLE, MD.: ALCOHOL, DRUG ABUSE AND MENTAL HEALTH ADMINISTRATION, 1977.*
     INDX SES, POVERTY, PSYCHOPATHOLOGY, EDUCATION, SCHOLASTIC ACHIEVEMENT, PSYCHOTHERAPY, CULTURAL FACTORS, FAMILY STRUCTURE, FAMILY ROLES, ACCULTURATION, BILINGUAL-BICULTURAL PERSONNEL, BILINGUAL-BICULTURAL EDUCATION, ESSAY, MEXICAN AMERICAN, BILINGUALISM
     ABST THIS TRANSCRIPT OF A 15-MINUTE RADIO PROGRAM FEATURING DR. AMADO PADILLA AS GUEST SPEAKER HIGHLIGHTS SOME CAUSES OF MENTAL HEALTH PROBLEMS AMONG SPANISH-SPEAKING PEOPLE IN THE U.S. THE SPECIAL PROBLEMS OF LATINOS WHICH HAVE A BEARING ON THEIR MENTAL STABILITY ARE IDENTIFIED AS SOCIOECONOMIC LEVEL, UNEMPLOYMENT AND EDUCATIONAL LEVEL. THE TIGHTER, MORE INTEGRATED FAMILIAL NETWORK OF LATINO FAMILIES IS IDENTIFIED AS BOTH A POSITIVE SUPPORT FOR PERSONS UNDERGOING A CRISIS AS WELL AS A DETERRENT TO THEIR SEEKING OUTSIDE PROFESSIONAL HELP. LANGUAGE IS DESCRIBED AS A SOCIAL BARRIER FOR LATINOS, ESPECIALLY FOR CHILDREN ENTERING SCHOOL AND FOR PERSONS SEEKING TREATMENT FROM MENTAL HEALTH CENTERS THAT DO NOT HAVE BILINGUAL STAFF.
     ACCN 000158

187 AUTH **BOXHILL, C. J., KALARICKAL, T. V., & CURICO, M. L.**
     TITL CERTAIN EXPRESSED MORAL BELIEFS OF THREE GROUPS OF EARLY ADOLESCENT BOYS.

     SRCE *NATIONAL CATHOLIC GUIDANCE JOURNAL, 1969, 14(1), 21-24.*
     INDX ADOLESCENTS, SES, PUERTO RICAN-M, CROSS CULTURAL, SCHOLASTIC ACHIEVEMENT, PERSONALITY, EMPIRICAL, NEW YORK, EAST, MALE
     ABST THE HYPOTHESIS THAT THERE IS NO DIFFERENCE IN EXPRESSED MORAL BELIEFS OF NEGRO, PUERTO RICAN, AND WHITE EARLY ADOLESCENT BOYS LIVING IN A LOW SOCIOECONOMIC AREA WAS TESTED. THE SUBJECTS—111 NEGRO, 116 PUERTO RICAN, AND 78 WHITE EIGHTH-GRADE BOYS—WERE ADMINISTERED THE STUDENT BELIEF INVENTORY. RESULTS INDICATE THAT THE WHITE GROUP SCORED HIGHER THAN THE NEGRO AND PUERTO RICAN GROUPS ON THE TRAITS OF HONESTY AND RESPONSIBILITY. NO SIGNIFICANT DIFFERENCE WAS FOUND BETWEEN ANY GROUPS IN THE TRAITS OF FRIENDLINESS, LOYALTY, AND MORAL COURAGE. 12 REFERENCES.
     ACCN 000159

188 AUTH **BRADFORD, A., FARRAR, D., & BRADFORD, G.**
     TITL EVALUATION REACTIONS OF COLLEGE STUDENTS TO DIALECT DIFFERENCES IN THE ENGLISH OF MEXICAN-AMERICANS.
     SRCE *LANGUAGE AND SPEECH, 1974, 17(3), 255-270.*
     INDX ATTITUDES, COLLEGE STUDENTS, EMPIRICAL, MEXICAN AMERICAN, PERSONALITY ASSESSMENT, CALIFORNIA, SOUTHWEST, STEREOTYPES, PREJUDICE, LINGUISTIC COMPETENCE
     ABST IN LOS ANGELES, AN ASSESSMENT WAS MADE OF THE ATTITUDES OF 48 ANGLO COLLEGE STUDENTS TOWARDS MEXICAN AMERICANS SPEAKING STANDARD ENGLISH VERSUS THOSE SPEAKING A CHICANO DIALECT OF ENGLISH. STUDENTS RATED 4 PAIRS OF MATCHED GUISE VOICES ON 15 SEMANTIC DIFFERENTIAL SCALES. DIALECT DIFFERENCES CONSISTENTLY AFFECTED THEIR RATINGS. SPEECH APPROACHING CHICANO ENGLISH WAS NEGATIVELY STEREOTYPED BY THE ANGLO STUDENTS ON SCALES RELATED TO SUCCESS, ABILITY, AND SOCIAL AWARENESS. RATERS ALSO ATTENDED TO NON-DIALECT VOICE DIFFERENCES, ESPECIALLY FOR MORE STANDARD ENGLISH VOICES. IN RATING STANDARD ENGLISH, STUDENTS USED A DIFFERENT, MORE COMPLEX PROCEDURE FOR JUDGING PERSONALITY. STUDY FINDINGS INDICATE THAT SPEAKERS OF A NON-STANDARD DIALECT ARE NEGATIVELY STEREOTYPED. THE IMPLICATIONS OF THESE RESULTS FOR EDUCATIONAL POLICIES FOR MEXICAN AMERICAN STUDENTS ARE BRIEFLY DISCUSSED. 10 REFERENCES. (AUTHOR ABSTRACT MODIFIED)
     ACCN 002351

189 AUTH **BRADSHAW, B. S., & BEAN, F. D.**
     TITL TRENDS IN THE FERTILITY OF MEXICAN AMERICANS.
     SRCE *SOCIAL SCIENCE QUARTERLY, 1973, 53(4), 688-696.*
     INDX FERTILITY, MEXICAN AMERICAN, DEMOGRAPHIC, EMPIRICAL, CROSS CULTURAL, SOUTHWEST
     ABST THE TRENDS IN MEXICAN AMERICAN FERTIL-

ITY IN COMPARISON TO ANGLO AMERICAN FERTILITY FROM 1950 TO 1970 IN THE SOUTHWESTERN STATES ARE EXAMINED. THE PROBLEM OF NON-COMPARABILITY BETWEEN DEFINED POPULATIONS FROM DECADE TO DECADE IS RESOLVED BY USING DATA FOR BOTH THE "MEXICAN ORIGIN" POPULATION AND THE SPANISH LANGUAGE OR SURNAME POPULATION. IN GENERAL, MEXICAN AMERICANS AND ANGLO AMERICANS IN THE SOUTHWEST HAVE FOLLOWED SIMILAR TRENDS IN FERTILITY SINCE 1950. THE AVERAGE FERTILITY OF WOMEN IN BOTH GROUPS WAS HIGHER IN 1960 THAN IN 1950. CONSIDERING THE EXTENSIVELY DOCUMENTED HIGH FERTILITY OF THE MEXICAN AMERICAN POPULATION, THESE TRENDS PROVIDE LITTLE EVIDENCE TO SUPPORT THE THESIS THAT THE FERTILITY LEVELS OF THE TWO POPULATIONS HAVE SUBSTANTIALLY CONVERGED FROM 1950 TO 1970. IN FACT, THE 1969 MEXICAN ORIGIN AND 1970 SPANISH LANGUAGE OR SURNAME AGE-ADUSTED FERTILITY MEASURES ARE VERY NEARLY THE SAME AS THOSE FOR THE 1950 SPANISH SURNAME POPULATION. 19 REFERENCES. (AUTHOR SUMMARY MODIFIED)

ACCN   000161

190 AUTH **BRAM, J.**
　　　TITL THE LOWER STATUS PUERTO RICAN FAMILY.
　　　SRCE *IN J. C. STONE & D. P. DENEVI (EDS.), TEACHING MULTICULTURAL POPULATIONS: FIVE HERITAGES. NEW YORK: VAN NOSTRAND, 1971, PP. 130-140.*
　　　INDX PUERTO RICAN-M, FAMILY ROLES, FAMILY STRUCTURE, POVERTY, SES, SEX ROLES, CULTURE, MIGRATION, CULTURAL FACTORS, HEALTH, RURAL, URBAN, FARM LABORERS, DISCRIMINATION, MARRIAGE, ACCULTURATION, PUERTO RICAN-I, ESSAY
　　　ABST SOME OF THE LOCAL HISTORICAL PECULIARITIES OF THE LOWER STATUS PUERTO RICAN ARE DISCUSSED WITH THE INTENT OF BETTER UNDERSTANDING THIS SEGMENT OF THE SPANISH SPEAKING WESTERN WORLD. MARITAL ARRANGEMENTS, THE ROLE OF CHILDREN IN FAMILY RELATIONSHIPS, STATUS DIFFERENCES BETWEEN MAINLAND AND ISLAND GROUPS, ECONOMIC ADVANCES MADE BY THE ISLAND SOCIETY AND THE EFFECT OF PREJUDICE AGAINST PUERTO RICANS ARE DISCUSSED. IN ORDER TO UNDERSTAND ANY ONE PUERTO RICAN FAMILY GROUP, IT IS NECESSARY TO "LOCATE" IT ON THE OVERALL MAP OF SOCIAL CHANGE WHICH THIS ETHNIC GROUP IS EXPERIENCING. 13 REFERENCES. (AUTHOR SUMMARY MODIFIED)
　　　ACCN 000162

191 AUTH **BRANCH, C. H., & MARTINEZ, F. H.**
　　　TITL TRAINING "ANGLOS" TO WORK WITH "CHICANO" HEROIN ADDICTS IN A METHADONE PROGRAM.
　　　SRCE *EXCHANGE, 1975, 3(1), 29-32.*
　　　INDX REVIEW, STEREOTYPES, HEALTH DELIVERY SYSTEMS, MEXICAN AMERICAN, MENTAL HEALTH, CULTURAL FACTORS, PSYCHOTHER-

APY, ETHNIC IDENTITY, SELF CONCEPT, METHADONE MAINTENANCE, ESSAY
　　　ABST THERE IS AN URGENT NEED FOR A SYSTEMATIC RESEARCH PROGRAM TO DEVELOP PARADIGMS BY WHICH THE CHICANO PATIENT CAN BE EVALUATED FOR AND PLACED IN TREATMENT MODALITIES WHICH ACCOUNT FOR CULTURAL AND ETHNIC VARIABLES AS WELL AS PSYCHODYNAMIC VARIABLES. A RE-EXAMINATION OF THE SELF-CONCEPT MODEL AS IT PERTAINS TO CHICANO HETEROGENEITY IS A LOGICAL WAY TO BEGIN TO ESTABLISH THE CHICANO PATIENT'S CLINICAL IDENTITY. PENALOSA'S (1970) OPERATIONAL DEFINITION OF THE MEXICAN AMERICAN IS BASED ON THE EXTENT TO WHICH THE PERSON PERCEIVES HIMSELF AS ETHNICALLY DIFFERENT. USING HIS DEFINITION "AMERICANS OF MEXICAN DESCENT" WOULD BE AMENABLE TO AN ANGLO THERAPIST, WHILE MOST "MEXICAN AMERICANS" AND ALL "CHICANOS" WOULD REQUIRE A BILINGUAL AND BICULTURAL THERAPIST IF SERVICES WERE TO BE TRULY RELEVANT. OTHER PROBLEMS WHICH NEED EXAMINATION AND CORRECTION, IF ANGLOS ARE GOING TO BE EVEN MINIMALLY EFFECTIVE WITH CHICANO PATIENTS, ARE: (1) THE TENDENCY TO CONTAMINATE CULTURAL FACTORS WITH CHARACTERISTICS ATTRIBUTABLE TO POVERTY AND WITH DYNAMICS ASSOCIATED WITH MENTAL ILLNESS; (2) THE INCORPORATION OF MISINTERPRETED OR OVEREMPHASIZED "KNOWLEDGE" OF MEXICAN AMERICAN CULTURE, SUCH AS MACHISMO OR CURANDERISMO, INTO THE THERAPY SITUATION; AND (3) THE UNDERESTIMATION OF LANGUAGE DIFFERENCES IN WORKING WITH CHICANO PATIENTS. IT IS THUS EVIDENT THAT NO "COOKBOOK" APPROACH TO INTERCULTURAL DELIVERY OF HEALTH SERVICES CAN REALLY BE USEFUL. 8 REFERENCES.
　　　ACCN 000163

192 AUTH **BRAND, E. S., & RUIZ, R. A.**
　　　TITL ETHNIC ESTEEM AMONG ANGLO, BLACK AND CHICANO SECOND GRADE AND FIFTH GRADE CHILDREN.
　　　SRCE *UNPUBLISHED MANUSCRIPT, UNDATED. (AVAILABLE FROM DR. R. A. RUIZ, DEPARTMENT OF PSYCHOLOGY, UNIVERSITY OF MISSOURI, KANSAS CITY, MO., 64110).*
　　　INDX ETHNIC IDENTITY, SELF CONCEPT, CROSS CULTURAL, MEXICAN AMERICAN, CHILDREN, EXAMINER EFFECTS, RESEARCH METHODOLOGY, SEX COMPARISON, SES, EMPIRICAL, MIDWEST
　　　ABST PATTERNS OF ETHNIC IDENTIFICATION AND PREFERENCE AMONG ANGLO, BLACK AND CHICANO SECOND AND FIFTH GRADE CHILDREN WERE EXAMINED. THE STUDENTS' TASK WAS TO RELATE TWELVE STATEMENTS BASED UPON THE SELF-ESTEEM ANTECEDENTS OF COMPETENCE, SIGNIFICANCE, VIRTUE, AND POWER TO ETHNIC CUES PRESENTED IN A PHOTOGRAPHIC AND SOCIOMETRIC MODALITY. THE FOLLOWING VARIABLES WERE CONTROLLED: SEX AND ETHNICITY OF EXAMINERS; RELATIVE ATTRACTIVENESS OF PHOTOGRAPHS EMPLOYED IN THE PHOTOGRAPHIC

MODALITY; AND SEX, AGE, AND SOCIOECO-NOMIC LEVEL OF SUBJECTS. WHEN RESULTS FROM SIXTY TESTS OF SIGNIFICANCE WERE CONSIDERED COMPOSITELY, BLACKS INDICA-TIED HIGHER OWN-GROUP PREFERENCE THAN ANGLOS. PATTERNS OF ETHNIC PREFERENCE WERE INFLUENCED BY AGE AND SEX OF THE CHILDREN AND ETHNICITY OF EXAMINER. 34 REFERENCES. (AUTHOR ABSTRACT MODIFIED)

ACCN   000164

193 AUTH **BRANSFORD, L.**
     TITL   MENTAL RETARDATION AND THE MEXICAN-AMERICAN.
     SRCE   *SAN FERNANDO, CALIF.: MONTAL EDUCA-TIONAL ASSOCIATES, 1972.*
     INDX   MENTAL RETARDATION, MEXICAN AMERICAN, INTELLIGENCE, SES, SPECIAL EDUCATION, POVERTY, CHILDREN, REVIEW, INTELLIGENCE TESTING, BILINGUAL, BILINGUAL-BICULTURAL EDUCATION
     ABST   A DISCUSSION OF SIGNIFICANT ISSUES CON-CERNING THE CLASSIFICATION OF MEXICAN AMERICAN (MA) CHILDREN AS MENTALLY RE-TARDED IS PRESENTED. ONE OF THE MOST SE-RIOUS INEQUITIES IN OUR EDUCATIONAL SYS-TEM IS THE MISDIAGNOSIS OF MA CHILDREN AND THEIR DIFFERENTIAL TREATMENT. THERE IS NO GENETIC REASON WHY THE RATE OF IN-CIDENCE OF MENTAL RETARDATION AMONG THE MA POPULATION SHOULD BE GREATER THAN AMONG THE POPULATION AS A WHOLE. WHAT IS KNOWN, HOWEVER, IS THAT: (1) MOST MENTALLY RETARDED CHILDREN IN PUBLIC SCHOOLS ARE MILDLY RETARDED; (2) LOWER SOCIOECONOMIC COMMUNITIES CONTRIB-UTE A GREATER SHARE OF MENTALLY RE-TARDED CHILDREN; (3) CERTAIN ETHNIC GROUPS TEND TO HAVE A LARGE PROPOR-TION OF THEIR POPULATION IN LOWER SOCIO-ECONOMIC COMMUNITIES; AND (4) THE MEM-BERS OF SOME OF THESE ETHNIC GROUPS ARE BILINGUAL. A CRITICAL ANALYSIS OF THESE FOUR FACTS AS THEY RELATE TO THE MIS-PLACEMENT OF MA CHILDREN CONCLUDES THAT INTERVENTION AND REMEDIAL PRO-GRAMS WHICH EMPHASIZE BILINGUAL-BICUL-TURAL TRAINING AND PARENTAL INVOLVE-MENT ARE ABSOLUTELY NECESSARY FOR LONG-RANGE GAINS. 15 REFERENCES.

ACCN   000166

194 AUTH **BRAWNER, M. R.**
     TITL   MIGRATION AND EDUCATIONAL ACHIEVEMENT OF MEXICAN AMERICANS.
     SRCE   *SOCIAL SCIENCE QUARTERLY, 1973, 53(4), 727-737.*
     INDX   MIGRATION, SCHOLASTIC ACHIEVEMENT, MEX-ICAN AMERICAN, ACHIEVEMENT MOTIVATION, CHILDREN, EMPIRICAL, WISCONSIN, MIDWEST, TEXAS, SOUTHWEST, ATTITUDES, ADULTS, MENTAL RETARDATION, PERFORMANCE EX-PECTATIONS, EDUCATION, ENVIRONMENTAL FACTORS, MIGRANTS
     ABST   A LONGITUDINAL STUDY OF MEXICAN AMERI-CAN SCHOOL CHILDREN AND THEIR PARENTS IN RACINE, WISCONSIN, IS REPORTED. QUES-TIONNAIRES WERE ADMINISTERED IN 1959-60

TO 209 MEXICAN AMERICAN MALE AND FE-MALE HEADS OF HOUSEHOLDS OR THEIR FE-MALE SPOUSES. THE FOLLOWING YEAR, THOSE FROM THE PREVIOUS SAMPLE WHO HAD CHIL-DREN UP TO THE AGE OF 21 WERE REINTER-VIEWED ALONG WITH OTHER SUBJECTS FROM REPRESENTATIVE SCHOOL DISTRICTS. 175 BOYS AND 196 GIRLS FROM THE FAMILIES OF PAR-ENTS INTERVIEWED IN 1959-60 WERE STUDIED IN 1969. A MATCHED CONTROL GROUP FROM COTUALLS, TEXAS, ONE OF THE TOWNS FROM WHICH MANY OF THE SUBJECTS HAD ORIGI-NALLY MIGRATED, WAS USED. THE FINAL SAMPLE WITH THOSE IN TEXAS REVEALED THAT THE MIGRANTS' CHILDREN HAD A CLEAR ADVANTAGE IN TERMS OF POSTGRADUATE EDUCATION, GRADES COMPLETED AND LOWER DROPOUT RATE. SEVERE RETARDATION (3 OR MORE YEARS) WAS FOUND MUCH MORE OFTEN IN TEXAS THAN IN THE WISCONSIN SAMPLE. DATA FROM THE ORIGINAL RACINE STUDY SUGGESTS THAT THE ATTITUDES AND PERCEP-TIONS OF THE MEXICAN AMERICAN PARENTS INTERVIEWED DID NOT INDICATE THAT THEY WERE LIKELY TO PRODUCE HIGH ACHIEVING CHILDREN. THE HIGHER ACHIEVEMENT OF THE RACINE STUDENTS (VS. THE TEXAS STUDENTS) IS ATTRIBUTED TO THE HIGHER LEVEL OF EX-PECTATIONS OF TEACHERS AND ADMINISTRA-TORS IN RACINE. THE RACINE SCHOOL SYS-TEM HAS SUBSTANTIALLY BETTER RESOURCES AT ITS COMMAND WHICH MAKE POSSIBLE A WIDER RANGE OF ACADEMIC AND VOCA-TIONAL COURSES, TEAM SPORTS, AND SOCIAL SERVICES. THE RACINE STUDENTS WOULD, THEREFORE, NOT ONLY HAVE MORE OPPOR-TUNITIES BUT WOULD BE UNDER GREATER PRESSURE TO TAKE ADVANTAGE OF THIS. FINDINGS ARE BRIEFLY DISCUSSED. 16 REFER-ENCES. (SOCIOLOGY ABSTRACT)

ACCN   000167

195 AUTH **BRAZELTON, T. B.**
     TITL   IMPLICATIONS OF INFANT DEVELOPMENT AMONG THE MAYAN INDIANS OF MEXICO.
     SRCE   *HUMAN DEVELOPMENT, 1972, 15(2), 90-111.*
     INDX   CHILDREN, CHILDREARING PRACTICES, IN-DIGENOUS POPULATIONS, MEXICO, CROSS CULTURAL, HEALTH, COGNITIVE DEVELOP-MENT, CULTURAL FACTORS, EMPIRICAL, MOTHER-CHILD INTERACTION, INFANCY
     ABST   TWELVE NEONATAL OBSERVATIONS, 93 TESTS OF LATER INFANT DEVELOPMENT USING BAY-LEY AND KNOBLICK-PASAMANICK SCALES, AND 12 FOUR-HOUR OBSERVATIONS OF CHILD-REARING PRACTICES WERE RECORDED AMONG THE ZINACANTECA INDIANS OF SOUTHEAST-ERN MEXICO. THESE MAYAN DESCENDENTS BEAR QUIET, ALERT INFANTS FITTED TO THE CHILD-REARING PRACTICES TO WHICH THEY ARE EXPOSED IN THEIR MOTHER'S BELLY CINCH, THE REBOZO. DESPITE A VERY DIFFER-ENT KIND OF CHILD-REARING STIMULATION, THESE INFANTS SHOW PARALLEL PROGRESS COMPARED TO AMERICAN INFANTS IN MOTOR, MENTAL AND SOCIAL PARAMETERS. THE IN-TRAUTERINE CONDITIONS OF (1) SUBCLINICAL NUTRITION, (2) FREQUENT INFECTION, AND (3)

MILD HYPOXIA OF HIGH ALTITUDE ARE SUGGESTED AS POWERFUL INFLUENCES ON THE NEONATE'S BEHAVIOR. 27 REFERENCES. (JOURNAL ABSTRACT MODIFIED)

ACCN 000168

196 AUTH **BREITER, T.**
TITL HISPANICS AND THE ROMAN CATHOLIC CHURCH.
SRCE *AGENDA, JANUARY/FEBRUARY 1977, PP. 4-9.*
INDX RELIGION, PREJUDICE, REPRESENTATION, SOCIAL SERVICES, ACCULTURATION, POLITICS, HISTORY, MEXICAN AMERICAN, PUERTO RICAN-M, ESSAY, PROFESSIONAL TRAINING
ABST OF ALL INSTITUTIONS WHICH AFFECT THE LIVES OF HISPANICS, THE ROMAN CATHOLIC CHURCH IS PROBABLY THE ONE WHICH LEAVES THE MOST DEEPLY INGRAINED AND PERVASIVE IMPRESSIONS. THE EMOTIONAL AND PSYCHOLOGICAL IMPACT OF THE CHURCH DATES BACK TO THE CONQUISTADORS. THE CHURCH SENT PRIESTS TO HELP THE SOLDIERS DOMINATE THE NATIVES, AND THAT SENSE OF DOMINATION CONTINUES TODAY. THE CHURCH HAS FAILED TO RECOGNIZE AND SUPPORT THE TEMPORAL NEEDS OF ITS LARGEST MINORITY—HISPANICS. HISPANIC PRIESTS AND NUNS ARE GREATLY UNDERREPRESENTED IN THE CHURCH HIERARCHY. THE FEW HISPANIC BISHOPS WHO HAVE RECENTLY BEEN APPOINTED CANNOT PROVIDE THE SPANISH-SPEAKING PARISHIONERS WITH THE GUIDANCE AND PROGRAMS THEY ARE BEGINNING TO DEMAND. FORMAL ACTIVITY TO BROADEN THE CHURCH'S ASSISTANCE TO HISPANIC CATHOLICS HAS INCREASED SINCE THE 1960'S, WHEN THE FIRST OFFICIAL SUPPORT GIVEN TO A POLITICAL AND SOCIAL ISSUE OF IMPORTANCE TO HISPANICS—THE CHAVEZ GRAPE BOYCOTT—RECEIVED CHURCH BACKING. SINCE THEN, AN HISPANIC CAUCUS AT THE NATIONAL CATHOLIC CONFERENCE LEVEL HAS MADE THE CHURCH INCREASINGLY AWARE OF ITS HISPANIC MEMBERS.
ACCN 000169

197 AUTH **BRENNEIS, C. B., & ROLL, S.**
TITL DREAM PATTERNS IN ANGLO AND CHICANO YOUNG ADULTS.
SRCE *PSYCHIATRY, 1976, 39, 280-289.*
INDX ADULTS, COLLEGE STUDENTS, CROSS CULTURAL, CULTURAL FACTORS, DREAMS, EMPIRICAL, MEXICAN AMERICAN, SEX COMPARISON, FEMALE, MALE, NEW MEXICO, SOUTHWEST
ABST THE LAST IN A SERIES OF EXPLORATORY CROSS-CULTURAL INVESTIGATIONS OF DREAMS, THIS STUDY EXAMINES DIFFERENCES IN THE ORGANIZATION AND CONTENT OF DREAMS OF ANGLO AND CHICANO MEN AND WOMEN. SUBJECTS WERE 42 CHICANO MALES, 65 CHICANO FEMALES, 61 ANGLO MALES, AND 74 ANGLO FEMALES, ALL VOLUNTEERS FROM THE UNIVERSITY OF NEW MEXICO. A TOTAL OF 1,123 DREAMS WERE COLLECTED AND ANALYZED IN TERMS OF ERICKSON'S FRAMEWORK FOR EXAMINING THE MANIFEST CONTENT OF DREAMS. AMONG ANGLOS, THE MAJOR SEX DIFFERENCES WERE THAT FE-

MALES MORE OFTEN CONSTRUCTED ENCLOSED, "SAFE" SETTINGS WITH FAMILIAR CHARACTERS, WHILE THE MALES REPORTED MORE OPEN AND UNFAMILIAR SETTINGS. ANGLOS OF BOTH SEXES REPORTED GREATER LOCOMOTION AND MORE DREAMS IN WHICH THEY WERE THE CENTRAL FIGURES THAN THE CHICANOS. WITH CHICANOS, THE FEMALES REPORTED SIMILAR SAFE, ENCLOSED SETTINGS AS DID ANGLO FEMALES, WITH NURTURANT THEMES; CHICANO MALES REPORTED MORE PHYSICAL EXERTION AND AGGRESSIVE AND SEXUAL THEMES. BOTH MALE AND FEMALE CHICANOS REPORTED GREATER EMPHASIS ON DEATH, A LESSER SENSE OF PHYSICAL DESTINATION, AND MORE FAMILIAR CHARACTERS THAN DID THE ANGLOS. DISCUSSION OF THESE CROSS-CULTURAL DIFFERENCES EMPHASIZES THE CONGRUENCE OF CHICANO THEMES WITH DOMINANT HISPANIC VALUES AND COSMOLOGY. THE AUTHORS CAUTION, HOWEVER, THAT THEIR WORK IS NOT READILY GENERALIZABLE SINCE IT PERTAINS TO ONLY ONE OF THE LIFE-STAGES (YOUNG ADULTHOOD). 10 REFERENCES.

ACCN 002479

198 AUTH **BRENNEIS, C. B., & ROLL, S.**
TITL EGO MODALITIES IN THE MANIFEST DREAMS OF MALE AND FEMALE CHICANOS.
SRCE *PSYCHIATRY, 1975, 38(2), 172-185.*
INDX SEX COMPARISON, DREAMS, MEXICAN AMERICAN, COLLEGE STUDENTS, EMPIRICAL, CULTURAL FACTORS, SEX ROLES, SOUTHWEST
ABST STRIKING DIFFERENCES BETWEEN MALE AND FEMALE DREAMS WERE FOUND IN THE AREAS OF SETTING, CHARACTERS, INTERACTION, SELF, INSTINCTUAL MODALITIES, AND REALISM. THE MANIFEST CONTENT OF YOUNG ADULT MALE AND FEMALE CHICANOS WERE EXAMINED THROUGH AN INVENTORY OF DREAM CONTENT AND PATTERN. GENERALLY SPEAKING, THE MEN'S INTERNAL PSYCHIC WORLD, AS VIEWED THROUGH THEIR DREAMS, TENDED TO BE ORGANIZED AROUND A HIGHLY VISIBLE AND DEMARCATED SELF SEEN AS ROBUSTLY ACTIVE, RANDOMLY IN MOTION, AND OFTEN CONTENTIOUSLY INVOLVED WITH UNRELATED OTHERS. THE CONFINES OF THIS INTERNAL WORLD ARE BROAD, OCCUPIED BY BOUNDARIES AND BARRIERS, AND OFTEN SUBJECT TO UNPREDICTABLE EVENTS. IN CONTRAST, THE WOMEN'S INTERNAL WORLD CONTAINED A LESS SHARPLY DEFINED, LESS ACTIVE, LESS CONTENTIOUS SELF, WITH A GREATER RANGE OF INTERACTIONS AND MORE FAMILIAR CHARACTERS. NARROWER CONFINES WERE MATCHED BY LESS EMPHASIS ON BOUNDARIES, GREATER PREDICTABILITY, AND MORE GOAL DIRECTED LOCOMOTION. 27 REFERENCES. (AUTHOR ABSTRACT MODIFIED)
ACCN 000170

199 AUTH **BRENNER, J. H., COLES, R., & MEAGHER, D.**
TITL DRUGS AND YOUTH: MEDICAL, PSYCHIATRIC AND LEGAL FACTS.
SRCE *NEW YORK: LIVERIGHT PUBLISHING CORPORATION, 1970.*

INDX DRUG ADDICTION, POVERTY, CROSS CUL-
TURAL, ESSAY, PUERTO RICAN-M, SES, DRUG
ABUSE, URBAN, COLLEGE STUDENTS

ABST THE RACIAL AND SOCIOECONOMIC ASPECTS
OF MARIJUANA USE ARE DISCUSSED. BLACKS
AND PUERTO RICANS HAVE ALWAYS FUR-
NISHED THE LARGE MAJORITY OF TRADI-
TIONAL ADDICTS. NEARLY THREE OUT OF EVERY
FOUR ADDICTS ARE BLACK, AND OVER HALF
OF ALL THE NATION'S ADDICTS LIVE IN NEW
YORK CITY. BUT MARIJUANA USE THAT FOR-
MERLY MARKED GHETTO YOUTHS NOW EXISTS
AMONG COLLEGE STUDENTS AND SUBURBAN
YOUTHS. NARCOTICS ARE USED BY THE
GHETTO POOR TO ESCAPE THEIR KNOWL-
EDGE OF THE INACCESSIBILITY TO A MIDDLE-
CLASS STANDARD OF LIFE AND VALUES—THE
SAME VALUES AND STANDARDS FROM WHICH
THE RICH YOUTH ARE ESCAPING WITH PSY-
CHEDELIC DRUGS. MANY GHETTO YOUTHS
FIND MARIJUANA NOT AN EXCITING PATH TO
"SELF-DISCOVERY," BUT AN INEVITABLE AS-
PECT OF A FIERCE AND BRUTISH LIFE. ON THE
OTHER SIDE OF THE GHETTO WALL, SELF-CON-
SCIOUS AFFLUENT STUDENTS TELL PSYCHIA-
TRISTS THAT THE WORLD IS EVIL, HYPOCRITI-
CAL, AND MUST AT ALL COSTS BE FLED. THE
THEME ON CAMPUS, AS IN THE GHETTO, IS ES-
CAPE. THE AMERICAN SOCIAL AND ECONOMIC
SYSTEM, WHICH MAKES THE GHETTO POS-
SIBLE, APPARENTLY FINDS VINDICTIVE LEGIS-
LATION AGAINST ADDICTS EASIER THAN ANY
REAL EFFORT TO CHANGE LIFE IN THE GHETTO.

ACCN 000171

200 AUTH **BRIGGS, V. M., JR.**
TITL CHICANOS AND RURAL POVERTY.
SRCE *BALTIMORE: JOHNS HOPKINS UNIVERSITY
PRESS, 1973.*
INDX FARM LABORERS, MEXICAN AMERICAN, UN-
DOCUMENTED WORKERS, POVERTY, RURAL,
DISCRIMINATION, IMMIGRATION, MIGRATION,
ECONOMIC FACTORS, POLICY, ESSAY, SOUTH-
WEST, BOOK
ABST PUBLIC POLICY HAS CONTINUOUSLY BEEN RE-
SPONSIVE TO THE INTERESTS OF CORPORATE
FARM OWNERS WHILE BEING UNRESPONSIVE
TO MINIMAL WAGE AND WELFARE NEEDS OF
SOUTHWEST FARMWORKERS, WHO ARE PRI-
MARILY CHICANOS. THE ECONOMIC PLIGHT OF
RURAL CHICANOS IS A CLASSIC EXAMPLE OF
ADMINISTERED SOCIAL OPPRESSION WHICH IS
AGGRAVATED BY THE USE OF "GREEN-CAR-
DERS," "WHITE-CARDERS" AND BORDER COM-
MUTERS. THE AUTHOR SUGGESTS ALTERNA-
TIVE AGRICULTURAL AND EMPLOYMENT
POLICIES TO ALLEVIATE THE PRESENT POV-
ERTY AND TO AVOID THE EXODUS OF RURAL
CHICANOS TO URBAN BARRIOS. IF BETTER
ECONOMIC OPPORTUNITIES FOR CHICANOS
ARE NOT OPENED UP IN THE AGRICULTURAL
AND NONFARM RURAL SECTORS, OTHER SUP-
PORTIVE PROGRAMS MUST BE DEVISED.
ACCN 000174

201 AUTH **BRIGGS, V. M., JR.**
TITL ILLEGAL IMMIGRATION AND THE AMERICAN
LABOR FORCE: THE USE OF SOFT DATA FOR
ANALYSIS.
SRCE *AMERICAN BEHAVIORAL SCIENTIST, 1976, 19(3),
351-363.*
INDX IMMIGRATION, UNDOCUMENTED WORKERS,
MEXICAN, ECONOMIC FACTORS, RESEARCH
METHODOLOGY, LABOR FORCE, DEMO-
GRAPHIC, ESSAY
ABST THE LACK OF ACCURATE KNOWLEDGE RE-
GARDING THE CONTEMPORARY IMPACT OF IL-
LEGAL IMMIGRATION, PRIMARILY BY MEXI-
CANS, ON THE LABOR FORCE OF THE UNITED
STATES IS EXAMINED. IT IS ARGUED THAT SO-
CIAL SCIENTISTS MUST PURSUE THIS "KNOWL-
EDGE CRISIS" IF SOCIETY IS TO BE INFORMED
AS TO THE VALIDITY OF AN EMERGING SOCIAL
ISSUE. THE DEFICIENCIES IN THE DATA COL-
LECTED BY THE IMMIGRATION AND NATURALI-
ZATION SERVICE ARE POINTED OUT, AND SUG-
GESTIONS MADE FOR USING OTHER DATA
SOURCES SUCH AS UNEMPLOYMENT AND
SCHOOL DROPOUT RATES, LEVEL OF FOOD
STAMP USE, AND UNION ACTIVITY. MORE IN-
TUITIVE, INVESTIGATIVE, AND DESCRIPTIVE
ANALYTICAL METHODS ARE SUGGESTED IN
THE STUDY OF THIS COMPLEX HUMAN DI-
LEMMA. 14 REFERENCES.
ACCN 000172

202 AUTH **BRIGGS, V. M., JR.**
TITL IMPLICATIONS OF NONINSTITUTIONAL CON-
SIDERATIONS UPON THE EFFECTIVENESS OF
MANPOWER PROGRAMS FOR CHICANOS.
SRCE *AUSTIN: UNIVERSITY OF TEXAS, CENTER FOR
THE STUDY OF HUMAN RESOURCES, 1973.*
INDX LABOR FORCE, POVERTY, SES, LINGUISTIC
COMPETENCE, CULTURAL FACTORS, ADULT
EDUCATION, EDUCATION, OCCUPATIONAL AS-
PIRATIONS, SCHOLASTIC ASPIRATIONS, ESSAY,
REVIEW, SOCIAL MOBILITY, VOCATIONAL
COUNSELING, CROSS CULTURAL, DISCRIMI-
NATION, EQUAL OPPORTUNITY, PROGRAM
EVALUATION, POLICY
ABST THE NEED TO TAILOR MANPOWER PROGRAMS
TO THE SPECIAL CULTURAL ATTRIBUTES OF
THOSE SERVED IS DISCUSSED. ALTHOUGH
DATA THAT COMPARE THE RESULTS OF VOCA-
TIONAL EDUCATION AND TRAINING OF THE
SPANISH-SPEAKING AS A DISTINCT GROUP
ARE QUITE LIMITED, THOSE STUDIES THAT ARE
AVAILABLE ARE UNANIMOUS IN THEIR CON-
CLUSIONS: RETURNS ON INVESTMENT IN THE
DEVELOPMENT OF THE EMPLOYMENT POTEN-
TIAL OF CHICANOS ARE HIGHER THAN THOSE
FOR BLACKS AND, IN SOME INSTANCES, EVEN
FOR ANGLOS. THE THESIS THAT RACIAL
SUBGROUPS REQUIRE SPECIAL ATTENTION
IMPLIES THAT THERE IS A DIFFERENTIAL IN THE
ECONOMIC EXPERIENCE BETWEEN THE VARI-
OUS SUBGROUPS. THESE DIFFERENCES ARE
DUE TO BARRIERS PRESENTED BY THE OPER-
ATION OF SOCIETY'S INSTITUTIONS AND TO
CULTURAL AND SOCIAL CHARACTERISTICS OF
THE GROUPS WHICH RESTRICT ASSIMILATION.
THUS IT IS POSITED THAT THERE IS A DEFINITE
NEED FOR FRAGMENTED POLICY, RATHER THAN
ONE HOMOGENEOUS PROGRAM, IF ASSUR-
ANCES OF EQUAL ECONOMIC OPPORTUNITY

ARE TO BE PROVIDED TO ALL RACIAL GROUPS. THE PAST SUCCESS OF PROGRAMS SUCH AS JOB CORPS AND OPERATION SER (A MAN-POWER AGENCY FUNDED BY U.S. DEPT. OF LA-BOR TO PROMOTE EMPLOYMENT OF LATINOS) IS DISCUSSED. 17 REFERENCES.

ACCN   000173

203 AUTH **BRISK, M. E.**
     TITL THE ACQUISITION OF SPANISH GENDER BY FIRST-GRADE SPANISH-SPEAKING CHILDREN.
     SRCE *IN G. D. KELLER, R. V. TESCHNER & S. VIERA (EDS.), BILINGUALISM IN THE BICENTENNIAL AND BEYOND. NEW YORK: BILINGUAL PRESS, 1976, PP. 143-160.*
     INDX SOUTH AMERICA, CROSS CULTURAL, BILIN-GUAL, PUERTO RICAN-M, GRAMMAR, LAN-GUAGE ACQUISITION, CHILDREN, SYNTAX, SPANISH SURNAMED, EMPIRICAL, MASSACHU-SETTS, EAST
     ABST TWENTY-ONE SPANISH-SPEAKING FIRST GRADERS (16 IN BOSTON, 5 IN ARGENTINA) WERE TESTED FOR THE FOLLOWING RELA-TIONSHIPS: (1) THE NUMBER OF ERRORS AND CONSISTENCY OF NOUN ENDING WITH GEN-DER; (2) SPECIFIC KINDS OF ERRORS IN AC-QUIRING GENDER; AND (3) EFFECT OF SEX ON ACQUISITION OF GENDER. ALL OF THE CHIL-DREN WERE GIVEN A LIST OF 10 SPANISH-ORI-GIN NOUNS WHILE THE BOSTON SAMPLE WAS ADMINISTERED AN ADDITIONAL 13 NOUN LIST IN SPANISH CONTAINING WORDS FROM EN-GLISH WITH AND WITHOUT SPANISH MOR-PHOLOGY. THE RESULTS INDICATE THAT THESE FIRST-GRADE CHILDREN HAVE NOT YET FULLY ACQUIRED GRAMMATICAL GENDER AND HAVE MORE DIFFICULTY WITH NEUTRAL AND NON-CORRESPONDING NOUN ENDINGS. THE IN-FLUENCE OF ENGLISH DOES NOT MAKE A DIF-FERENCE, ALTHOUGH THERE ARE INCREASED ERRORS FOR THE BORROWED WORDS. IN GENERAL, IDENTIFICATION OF "EL" AND "LA" AS AN IMPORTANT GRAMMATICAL CATEGORY IS DIFFICULT FOR THIS AGE GROUP, EVEN THOUGH THEY USE IT CONSISTENTLY WITHIN THE CONTEXT OF A SENTENCE. 1 REFERENCE.

ACCN   000175

204 AUTH **BRITAIN, S. D., & ABAD, M.**
     TITL FIELD-INDEPENDENCE: A FUNCTION OF SEX AND SOCIALIZATION IN A CUBAN AND AN AMERICAN GROUP.
     SRCE *PERSONALITY AND SOCIAL PSYCHOLOGY BUL-LETIN, 1974, 1(1), 319-320.*
     INDX COGNITIVE STYLE, ETHNIC IDENTITY, CROSS CULTURAL, CULTURAL FACTORS, SEX ROLES, SEX COMPARISON, CUBAN, SOCIALIZATION, EMPIRICAL, LOCUS OF CONTROL, ROTTER IN-TERNAL-EXTERNAL SCALE, FIELD DEPEN-DENCE-INDEPENDENCE, URBAN, NEW JERSEY, EAST, ADOLESCENTS
     ABST THE RELATIONSHIP BETWEEN FIELD-DEPEN-DENCE AND CULTURAL BIASES TOWARD CON-TROL AND DISCIPLINE PRACTICES WAS EX-PLORED USING 72 CUBAN- AND U.S.- BORN ADOLESCENTS FROM AN INNER CITY HIGH SCHOOL IN NEW JERSEY. IT WAS HYPOTHE-SIZED THAT THE STRICT CONTROL PRACTICES

DESCRIBED FOR THE CUBAN CULTURE WOULD FOSTER GREATER FIELD-DEPENDENCE IN THEIR ADOLESCENTS THAN WOULD THE PRACTICES OF THE U.S. GROUP. A BATTERY OF TESTS WAS ADMINISTERED INCLUDING THE HIDDEN FIG-URES TEST, DRAW-A-PERSON TEST, AND THE ROTTER INTERNAL-EXTERNAL CONTROL SCALE. FINDINGS SUPPORT THE HYPOTHESIS THAT THE CUBAN SOCIALIZATION PROCESS DOES NOT FACILITATE AUTONOMY OR FIELD-INDE-PENDENCE; U.S. MALES WERE MOST FIELD-IN-DEPENDENT, FOLLOWED BY U.S. FEMALES, CUBAN MALES AND FEMALES. FURTHERMORE, MALES OF BOTH CULTURES WERE AWARE OF DIFFERENTIAL SOCIALIZATION OF THE SEXES. SEX DIFFERENCES IN FIELD-DEPENDENCE WERE NOT LARGER IN THE CUBAN SAMPLE, AND ANALYSIS OF VARIANCE REVEALED NO DIFFER-ENCES IN LOCUS OF CONTROL. 13 REFER-ENCES. (AUTHOR ABSTRACT MODIFIED)

ACCN   000176

205 AUTH **BRODY, G. H., & BRODY, J. A.**
     TITL VICARIOUS LANGUAGE INSTRUCTION WITH BI-LINGUAL CHILDREN THROUGH SELF-MODEL-ING.
     SRCE *CONTEMPORARY EDUCATIONAL PSYCHOLOGY, 1976, 1, 138-145.*
     INDX BILINGUALISM, LANGUAGE ACQUISITION, MODELING, MEXICAN AMERICAN, CHILDREN, EMPIRICAL, BILINGUAL, ARIZONA, SOUTH-WEST
     ABST THE PRESENT EXPERIMENT WAS CONDUCTED TO DETERMINE THE EFFECTIVENESS OF A SELF-MODELING PROCEDURE AND A SELF-MODEL-ING PROCEDURE COMBINED WITH SOCIAL RE-INFORCEMENT ON THE LANGUAGE ACQUISI-TION OF BILINGUAL CHILDREN. IN THE SELF-MODELING CONDITION THE CHILDREN WERE PROMPTED TO MIMIC PORTIONS OF SEN-TENCES ON AUDIOTAPE. THESE FRAGMENTS WERE EDITED INTO COMPLETE SENTENCES AND SERVED AS MODELS DURING INSTRUC-TION. CHILDREN IN THE SELF- MODELING GROUP DISPLAYED SIGNIFICANTLY MORE AD-JECTIVE USAGE AND ADOPTED MORE OF THE MODELED CONTENT THAN CHILDREN WHOSE SELF-MODELED RESPONSES WERE SOCIALLY REINFORCED OR WHO WERE ASSIGNED TO THE TWO CONTROL CONDITIONS. ENHANCED EXPOSURE TO VERBALIZED MODELS LEADS TO INCREASED GENERALIZATION AND IN-CREASED LANGUAGE ACQUISITION IN BILIN-GUAL HISPANIC CHILDREN. 19 REFERENCES. (JOURNAL ABSTRACT MODIFIED)

ACCN   000177

206 AUTH **BRONSON, L., & MEADOW, A.**
     TITL THE NEED ACHIEVEMENT ORIENTATION OF CATHOLIC AND PROTESTANT MEXICAN-AMERI-CANS.
     SRCE *REVISTA INTERAMERICANA DE PSICOLOGIA, 1968, 2(3), 159-168.*
     INDX ACHIEVEMENT MOTIVATION, RELIGION, MEXI-CAN AMERICAN, EMPIRICAL, TIME ORIENTA-TION, PERSONALITY, ADULTS, SOUTHWEST, AT-TITUDES, VALUES
     ABST THE NEED ACHIEVEMENT ORIENTATIONS OF 54

PROTESTANT AND 54 CATHOLIC MEXICAN AMERICAN SUBJECTS OF SIMILAR LEVELS OF ACCULTURATION AND SOCIOECONOMIC BACKGROUND ARE REPORTED. IT WAS HYPOTHESIZED THAT VALUES RELATED TO THE PROTESTANT ETHIC WOULD BE REFLECTED BY PROTESTANT SUBJECTS. DATA INDICATE THAT THE ROSEN SCALE, EVALUATING BASIC ACHIEVEMENT MOTIVATION, REFLECTS AN EQUAL DRIVE IN BOTH GROUPS. THE MCCLELLAND FOUR-NEED ACHIEVEMENT CARDS, REFLECTING VALUES AND ATTITUDES, SHOW THE PROTESTANTS TO HAVE ACHIEVEMENT GOALS MORE RELATED TO AN ACTIVISTIC-INDIVIDUALISTIC-FUTURE ORIENTATION. IT IS SUGGESTED THAT CERTAIN ELEMENTS OF THE PROTESTANT RELIGION (SUCH AS STEWARDSHIP, INDIVIDUAL RESPONSIBILITY, ASCETICISM, AND SELF-DISCIPLINE) ARE RESPONSIBLE FOR THE ATTITUDE DIFFERENCES EXPRESSED BY PROTESTANT SUBJECTS. 7 REFERENCES.

ACCN   000178

207 AUTH   BROOKS, B. D.
     TITL   CONTINGENCY MANAGEMENT WITH A MEXICAN AMERICAN FAMILY FOR TRUANCY REDUCTION: A CASE REPORT.
     SRCE   JOURNAL OF INSTRUCTIONAL PSYCHOLOGY, 1975, 2(2), 2-5.
     INDX   PARENTAL INVOLVEMENT, FAMILY ROLES, ADOLESCENTS, EDUCATION, ACHIEVEMENT MOTIVATION, BEHAVIOR THERAPY, DELINQUENCY, CASE STUDY, PSYCHOTHERAPY, PSYCHOTHERAPY OUTCOME, MEXICAN AMERICAN, CALIFORNIA, SOUTHWEST, BEHAVIOR MODIFICATION
     ABST   THIS CASE REPORT DEMONSTRATES THE USE OF A CONTINGENCY CONTRACT WITH A MEXICAN AMERICAN FAMILY IN AN EFFORT TO INCREASE A FAMILY MEMBER'S SCHOOL ATTENDANCE. RESULTS SUPPORT THE PREMISE THAT MEXICAN AMERICAN PARENTS, SOMETIMES THOUGHT OF AS PLACING EDUCATION AS A LOW PRIORITY, WILL RESPOND FAVORABLY TO THE SCHOOL ESTABLISHMENT WHEN THEY ARE AWARE OF THE EXPECTATIONS PLACED ON THEM BY THE SCHOOL. SCHOOL ATTENDING BEHAVIOR SIGNIFICANTLY INCREASED AS A RESULT OF THE USE OF A SYSTEMATIC CONTINGENCY MANAGEMENT PROGRAM. 2 REFERNCES. (JOURNAL ABSTRACT)
     ACCN   000179

208 AUTH   BROOKS, B. D., & MERINO, S.
     TITL   STRATEGIES FOR TEACHING WITHIN A BICULTURAL SETTING.
     SRCE   READING IMPROVEMENT, 1976, 13(2), 86-91.
     INDX   BILINGUAL-BICULTURAL EDUCATION, CULTURAL PLURALISM, CULTURAL FACTORS, MEXICAN AMERICAN, COMPETITION, COOPERATION, SELF CONCEPT, ESSAY, ATTITUDES, TEACHERS
     ABST   THE MULTI-CULTURAL NATURE OF THE AMERICAN SOCIAL STRUCTURE REQUIRE THAT EDUCATORS BECOME AWARE OF CULTURAL DIFFERENCES. THE STATEMENT, I TREAT ALL MY STUDENTS ALIKE CAN NO LONGER BE AC-

CEPTED AS A VIABLE ATTITUDE AMONG TEACHERS. CULTURAL PLURALISM DICTATES THAT TEACHERS BECOME AWARE OF CULTURAL VARIATIONS AND DEVELOP STRATEGIES FOR DEALING WITH THESE DIFFERENCES. THIS ARTICLE POINTS OUT SOME OF THESE VARIATIONS, GIVES EXAMPLES OF HOW THESE DIFFERENCES ARE MANIFEST IN STUDENT BEHAVIOR, AND PRESENTS SOME METHODS FOR DEALING WITH BICULTURAL SITUATIONS AMONG MEXICAN AMERICAN STUDENTS. 6 REFERENCES. (JOURNAL ABSTRACT)

ACCN   000180

209 AUTH   BROOM, L., & SHEVKY, E.
     TITL   MEXICANS IN THE UNITED STATES: A PROBLEM IN DIFFERENTIATION.
     SRCE   SOCIOLOGY AND SOCIAL RESEARCH, 1951, 36(3), 150-158.
     INDX   MEXICAN AMERICAN, ACCULTURATION, SOCIAL MOBILITY, MIGRATION, ECONOMIC FACTORS, SES, URBAN, MEXICAN, RELIGION, ESSAY, INTEGRATION
     ABST   AN ATTEMPT TO SPECIFY AN ANALYTIC APPROACH TO THE STUDY OF MEXICANS IN THE UNITED STATES IS PRESENTED. THE FOUR MAIN HEADINGS UNDER WHICH THE DISCUSSION IS OUTLINED ARE: (1) ECONOMIC FUNCTION AND MOBILITY; (2) ACCULTURATION AND URBANIZATION; (3) STATUS AND ASSIMILATION; AND (4) MODES OF ISOLATION AND INTEGRATION. THE FIRST TASK CENTERS ON THE PROBLEM OF DIFFERENTIATING THE POPULATION WITH REGARD TO ITS SOURCE AND MIGRATION HISTORY. GEOGRAPHIC ORIGINS OF THE POPULATION, PRIOR OCCUPATIONAL STATUS CHARACTERISTICS, AND ACCULTURATION ARE EXAMINED. ANOTHER SECTION OF THE STUDY INVOLVES THE DIFFERENTIATION OF THE POPULATION WITH RESPECT TO ITS PRESENT SOCIOECONOMIC STATUS, URBANIZATION, AND ACCULTURATION TO AMERICAN NORMS. FINALLY, MODES OF CULTURAL AND INSTITUTIONAL ISOLATION OR FUNCTIONAL INTEGRATION ARE POSTULATED AS FOLLOWS: (1) THE CONTINUED ISOLATION OF ATOMISTIC ENCLAVES; (2) THE EMERGENCE OF AN INTEGRATED ETHNIC COMMUNITY; AND (3) REDUCTION IN THE ISOLATION OF THE MEXICAN AMERICAN POPULATION, THEIR INCORPORATION IN THE LARGER SOCIETY, AND THE PROGRESSIVE LIQUIDATION OF THE ETHNIC ENCLAVES. 14 REFERENCES.
     ACCN   000181

210 AUTH   BROWN, E., & RODRIGUEZ, R.
     TITL   BLACK AND HISPANIC CAUCUS: FINAL REPORT.
     SRCE   UNPUBLISHED MANUSCRIPT PREPARED FOR THE NEW YORK STATE DEPARTMENT OF MENTAL HYGIENE TASK FORCE FOR THE DEVELOPMENT OF COMMUNITY RESIDENTIAL AND REHABILITATIVE PROGRAMS, FEBRUARY 1975.
     INDX   MENTAL RETARDATION, DRUG ADDICTION, MENTAL HEALTH, SPANISH SURNAMED, ESSAY, EDUCATION, JUDICIAL PROCESS, CHILDREN, ADULTS, PUERTO RICAN-M, SCHIZOPHRENIA, MIGRATION, GERONTOLOGY, ALCOHOLISM, PRIMARY PREVENTION, COMMUNITY, PREJU-

DICE, NEW YORK, EAST, PROGRAM EVALUATION, HEALTH DELIVERY SYSTEMS, SPECIAL EDUCATION

ABST WHEN THE BLACK AND HISPANIC MEMBERS OF THE NEW YORK STATE DEPARTMENT OF MENTAL HYGIENE TASK FORCE FOR THE DEVELOPMENT OF COMMUNITY AND REHABILITATIVE PROGRAMS REALIZED THAT THEIR CONCERNS WERE BEING IGNORED BY THE OTHER TASK FORCE MEMBERS, THEY FORMED A BLACK AND HISPANIC CAUCUS. THIS CAUCUS PRODUCED A SPECIAL REPORT ADDRESSING THE ISSUES OF RACISM AND POLITICAL DETERMINISM WITHIN THE MENTAL HEALTH DELIVERY SYSTEM OF NEW YORK STATE. THE REPORT STATES THAT EXISTING TREATMENT METHODS AND PROFESSIONAL ATTITUDES MUST CHANGE IF THE SYSTEM IS TO BE AT ALL RELEVANT TO BLACKS AND HISPANICS. SEVERAL AREAS OF PARTICULAR CONCERN ARE IDENTIFIED AND DISCUSSED: (1) THE SOCIAL GENESIS OF MENTAL DISABILITY; (2) THE EFFECT OF EUROPEAN PSYCHIATRY AND THE POLITICS OF THE WHITE SYSTEM OF DOMINANCE ON DELIVERY OF SERVICES TO BLACK AND HISPANIC CLIENTS; (3) BLACK AND HISPANIC PSEUDO-RETARDATES—THE SOCIAL AND POLITICAL CAUSES AND RAMIFICATIONS OF LABELING CHILDREN MENTALLY RETARDED; AND (4) THE CLINICAL AGGRESSION AGAINST BLACK AND HISPANIC PATIENTS AND PRISONERS WHICH IS CALLED DRUG THERAPY, BEHAVIOR MODIFICATION, RESEARCH, NORMALIZATION AND OTHER METHODS THAT ARE DEFINED OR CONTROLLED BY WHITES. DEMANDS FOR CHANGES INCLUDE: (1) FUNDING AND CONTROL OF COMMUNITY-BASED ORGANIZATIONS THAT ARE COMPATIBLE WITH THE COMMUNITY SERVED; (2) THE DEVELOPMENT OF A PERMANENT INSTITUTE TO STUDY RACISM AND MENTAL HYGIENE IN THE STATE; AND (3) A HIGHER PRIORITY FOR DEALING WITH THE PROBLEMS OF YOUTH, ALCOHOLISM AND SENIOR CITIZENS IN BLACK AND HISPANIC COMMUNITIES. 31 REFERENCES.

ACCN 000182

211 AUTH **BROWN, F.**
TITL INTELLIGENCE TEST PATTERNS OF PUERTO RICAN PSYCHIATRIC PATIENTS.
SRCE *JOURNAL OF SOCIAL PSYCHOLOGY, 1960, 52(2), 225-230.*
INDX INTELLIGENCE, WECHSLER-BELLEVUE INTELLIGENCE SCALE, RORSCHACH TEST, PUERTO RICAN-M, EMPIRICAL, ADULTS, INTELLIGENCE TESTING, PSYCHOPATHOLOGY
ABST A SAMPLE OF 59 PUERTO RICAN PSYCHIATRIC PATIENTS WAS EVALUATED FOR INTELLECTUAL LEVEL AND FUNCTIONING BY CONVERTING WECHSLER-BELLEVUE (W-B) SUBTEST SCORES TO IQ EQUIVALENTS AND BY CERTAIN RORSCHACH DETERMINANTS. VERBAL, PERFORMANCE, AND FULL-SCALE IQ'S WERE TAKEN DIRECTLY FROM THE W-2 TEST PROTOCOLS. THE NUMBER OF CASES FOR EACH SUBTEST RANGED FROM 45 TO 49. FINDINGS INDICATE THAT THE GROUP AS A WHOLE IS CLASSIFIED

AS DULL NORMAL INTELLIGENCE (15TH PERCENTILE) WHEN COMPARED WITH STANDARDIZATION NORMS. ALSO, AS A GROUP THEY ARE MUCH MORE VARIABLE THAN MEMBERS OF THE GENERAL POPULATION. SUBTEST ANALYSIS REVEALS A SIGNIFICANTLY LOW THRESHOLD FOR ANXIETY AS REFLECTED IN A BORDERLINE RATING FOR THE FACTOR DESIGNATED AS FREEDOM FROM DISTRACTION. VERBAL COMPREHENSION IS AT THE LOW AVERAGE RANGE AND IS AIDED BY AVERAGE SENSITIVITY TO SOCIAL SEQUENCES AS A RESOURCE IN DEALING WITH SOCIAL SITUATIONS. PERCEPTUAL ORGANIZATION IS AT THE DULL NORMAL LEVEL AND MAY ALSO REFLECT ANXIETY. THE ESTIMATED IQ MEAN OF 103, BASED ON RORSCHACH DETERMINANTS, SUGGESTS A POTENTIAL FOR AVERAGE INTELLECTUAL FUNCTIONING. AVERAGE INTELLECTUAL FUNCTIONING WAS OBTAINED DESPITE A CONSTRICTIVE CONFINEMENT AS REFLECTED IN LOW PRODUCTION OF HUMAN RESPONSES ON THE RORSCHACH. 9 REFERENCES.

ACCN 000183

212 AUTH **BROWN, R. L.**
TITL SOCIAL DISTANCE PERCEPTION AS A FUNCTION OF MEXICAN-AMERICAN AND OTHER ETHNIC IDENTITY.
SRCE *SOCIOLOGY AND SOCIAL RESEARCH, 1973, 57(3), 273-287.*
INDX ETHNIC IDENTITY, CROSS CULTURAL, MEXICAN AMERICAN, COLLEGE STUDENTS, EMPIRICAL, RELIGION, SES, TEXAS, SOUTHWEST, ATTITUDES, SEX COMPARISON
ABST SLIGHTLY MODIFIED BOGARDUS SOCIAL DISTANCE SCALES WERE ADMINISTERED TO 423 ANGLO, ASIAN AMERICAN, BLACK, MEXICAN AMERICAN, AND NATIVE AMERICAN STUDENTS IN SOCIOLOGY CLASSES OF A SOUTH TEXAS UNIVERSITY. EMPHASIS WAS ON COMPARISONS BETWEEN OTHER WHITES AND MEXICAN AMERCANS. HYPOTHESES THAT RACIAL DISTANCE INDICES WOULD REFLECT THE STUDENT'S OWN ETHNIC GROUP, RELATED ETHNIC GROUPS AND REGIONAL SUBCULTURAL FEATURES WERE BORNE OUT. ADDITIONALLY, MAJOR DIFFERENCES WERE FOUND TO BE DUE TO ETHNICITY RATHER THAN SOCIAL CLASS. 22 REFERENCES. (AUTHOR ABSTRACT MODIFIED)

ACCN 000184

213 AUTH **BROWNING, H. L.**
TITL THE REPRODUCTIVE BEHAVIOR OF MINORITY GROUPS IN THE USA.
SRCE *IN W. MONTAGNA & W. A. SADLER (EDS.), REPRODUCTIVE BEHAVIOR. NEW YORK: PLENUM, 1974, PP. 299-317.*
INDX SEXUAL BEHAVIOR, DISCRIMINATION, FERTILITY, MEXICAN AMERICAN, CROSS CULTURAL, CULTURAL FACTORS, BIRTH CONTROL, REVIEW, FAMILY PLANNING, VALUES
ABST IN AN ATTEMPT TO UNDERSTAND THE ETHNIC COMPONENT OF MINORITY FERTILITY AS DISTINGUISHABLE FROM THE SOCIOECONOMIC COMPONENTS, THE AUTHOR REVIEWS FERTILITY LITERATURE AND SPECIFIC CENSUS DATA

ON U.S. BLACKS AND MEXICAN AMERICANS. EMPHASIS IS GIVEN TO THE INDEPENDENT EFFECT OF CULTURAL FACTORS (NORMS, VALUES, BELIEFS, AND LIFESTYLES) AS OPPOSED TO STRUCTURAL FACTORS (EDUCATION, OCCUPATION, AND INCOME) ON THE DIFFERENTIAL FERTILITY OF MEXICAN AMERICANS. IT IS POSITED THAT ETHNICITY DOES HAVE AN INDEPENDENT EFFECT ON FERTILITY. THE ISOLATION OF THIS EFFECT DOES NOT TAKE INTO ACCOUNT THE GREAT DIFFERENCES IN FERTILITY RATES AMONG MEXICAN AMERICAN SUBCULTURES. IN SUMMARY, NEITHER HYPOTHESIS—ETHNIC HOMOGENEITY NOR MODERNIZATION—IS FOUND TO EXPLAIN MINORITY FERTILITY SATISFACTORILY. IMPLICATIONS FOR THOSE WORKING ON FERTILITY PROBLEMS (I.E., FAMILY PLANNING PROGRAMS) ARE DISCUSSED. 19 REFERENCES.

ACCN   000185

214 AUTH **BRUHN, C. M., & PANGBORN, R. M.**
     TITL   FOOD HABITS OF MIGRANT FARM WORKERS IN CALIFORNIA.
     SRCE   *JOURNAL OF THE AMERICAN DIETETIC ASSOCIATION, 1971, 59(4), 347-355.*
     INDX   ADULTS, CROSS CULTURAL, CULTURAL FACTORS, ECONOMIC FACTORS, EMPIRICAL, FARM LABORERS, FEMALE, MEXICAN AMERICAN, NUTRITION, POVERTY, SES, CALIFORNIA, SOUTHWEST, RURAL, MALE, MIGRANTS
     ABST   SIXTY-FIVE MIGRANT AGRICULTURE FAMILIES OF MEXICAN DESCENT AND 26 FAMILIES OF ANGLO HERITAGE WERE INTERVIEWED IN THEIR LABOR CAMP IN NORTHERN CALIFORNIA, CONCERNING THEIR FOOD PURCHASING PATTERNS, FOOD PREFERENCES, COOKING PRACTICES, THE EMOTIONAL SIGNIFICANCE OF FOODS, AND THEIR DESIRE FOR CHANGING THEIR FOOD HABITS. THE MEXICAN FAMILIES SHOPPED ONCE A WEEK, WHILE MOST ANGLO FAMILIES SHOPPED EVERY DAY, SPENDING $40.00 AND $50.00 PER WEEK, RESPECTIVELY. BOTH GROUPS DEMONSTRATED SIMILAR FOOD HABITS DUE TO LOW INCOME, BUT ALSO REVEALED DIFFERENCES DUE TO ETHNIC FACTORS. THE SIMILARITIES OF POVERTY WERE REFLECTED IN BOTH GROUPS' HIGH CONSUMPTION OF BEANS, WHITE BREAD OR TORTILLAS, IN THEIR EMPATHY FOR OTHERS WHO WERE POOR, AND IN THEIR RELUCTANCE TO WITHHOLD FOOD FROM CHILDREN. ETHNIC DIFFERENCES WERE REFLECTED IN FOODS PREFERRED, THE FREQUENCY OF CONSUMPTION, AND THEIR FOOD-RELATED FOLKLORE ABOUT MENSTRUATION, PREGNANCY, AND VIRILITY. THE STRONG FAMILY TIES AND LIMITED ENGLISH OF THE MEXICAN FAMILIES MINIMIZED THEIR EXPOSURE TO THE EATING HABITS OF OTHERS. ANGLO FAMILIES, ON THE OTHER HAND, COULD READILY OBTAIN THE INGREDIENTS FOR THE FOODS OF THEIR CHOICE AND HAD A WIDER EXPOSURE TO THE FOOD HABITS OF THE PEOPLE AMONG WHOM THEY CIRCULATED. 16 REFERENCES.

ACCN   002480

215 AUTH **BRUHN, J. G.**

TITL   HEALTH MANPOWER NEEDS AMONG MEXICAN-AMERICANS IN TEXAS.
SRCE   *TEXAS REPORT ON BIOLOGY AND MEDICINE, 1974, 32(3 & 4), 633-647.*
INDX   ATTITUDES, CHILDREN, CULTURAL FACTORS, ECONOMIC FACTORS, EQUAL OPPORTUNITY, HEALTH, HEALTH EDUCATION, HIGHER EDUCATION, MEXICAN AMERICAN, NURSING, PARENTAL INVOLVEMENT, POVERTY, SES, SPANISH SURNAMED, TEXAS, SOUTHWEST, URBAN, RURAL, DISCRIMINATION, HEALTH DELIVERY SYSTEMS
ABST   BOTH A SHORTAGE AND AN INAPPROPRIATE DISTRIBUTION OF CERTAIN HEALTH PERSONNEL IN TEXAS ARE REVEALED BY A COMPARISON BETWEEN THE NUMBER OF ACTIVE "PATIENT-CARE PHYSICIANS," DENTISTS, PHARMACISTS, REGISTERED NURSES, AND OCCUPATIONAL AND PHYSICAL THERAPISTS PER 1,000 POPULATION IN THE STATE AND NATIONAL RATIO. THE SITUATION IS MOST ACUTE IN THE 28 TEXAS COUNTIES WITH PREDOMINANTLY MEXICAN AMERICAN POPULATIONS, WHERE, EXCEPT FOR THE 6 PREDOMINANTLY URBAN COUNTIES, HEALTH MANPOWER SHORTAGES ARE SEVERE. TWENTY-FOUR OF THESE COUNTIES HAVE FEWER "PATIENT-CARE PHYSICIANS" THAN THE STATE RATIO AND 4 HAVE NO PHYSICIANS AT ALL. NINE OF THE COUNTIES HAVE NO DENTISTS AND 6 HAVE FEWER THAN THE STATE RATIO. SIMILAR STATISTICS EXIST FOR PHARMACISTS, REGISTERED NURSES, AND OCCUPATIONAL AND PHYSICAL THERAPISTS. THESE COUNTIES ARE ALSO PREDOMINANTLY RURAL, EXCEED THE STATE PERCENTAGES OF INCOMES BELOW THE POVERTY LEVEL, AND HAVE YOUNG POPULATIONS WITH LOWER MEDIAN YEARS OF SCHOOL THAN THE MEDIAN FOR THE STATE. EDUCATION OF MEXICAN AMERICANS IS VIEWED AS A FIRST STEP IN AMELIORATING THE PROBLEM. IN THAT REGARD, THE AREA HEALTH EDUCATION CENTER (AHEC) IS PRESENTED AS A POSITIVE ACTION PROGRAM WHOSE GOALS ARE: (1) TO ENHANCE THE SKILLS AND RESOURCES OF LOCAL AND EDUCATIONAL AND HEALTH CARE PERSONNEL; (2) TO ASSIST IN DEVELOPING HEALTH CAREER CURRICULA AND CLINICAL TRAINING SITES; (3) TO INCREASE STUDENTS' KNOWLEDGE OF HEALTH CAREERS AND TO ENHANCE PREPARATION AND RECRUITMENT INTO THOSE CAREERS; AND (4) THROUGH THE ABOVE EFFORTS, TO PROVIDE A REGIONAL IMPETUS TOWARD IMPROVING HEALTH SERVICES AND THE QUALITY OF HEALTH CARE. 8 REFERENCES.

ACCN   002031

216 AUTH **BRUHN, J. G., FUENTES, R. G., TREVINO, F. M., & WILLIAMS, L. B., JR.**
     TITL   FOLLOW-UP OF MINORITY PREMEDICAL STUDENTS ATTENDING SUMMER ENRICHMENT PROGRAMS IN A MEDICAL SETTING.
     SRCE   *TEXAS MEDICINE, 1976, 72(8), 87-90.*
     INDX   COLLEGE STUDENTS, EDUCATION, EDUCATIONAL COUNSELING, EMPIRICAL, HEALTH, MEDICAL STUDENTS, PROFESSIONAL TRAIN-

ING, PROGRAM EVALUATION, SPANISH SUR-
NAMED, TEXAS, SOUTHWEST, REPRESENTA-
TION

ABST   CAREER OUTCOMES OF 112 PREMEDICAL MI-
NORITY STUDENTS (60 BLACKS, 51 MEXICAN
AMERICANS, 1 AMERICAN INDIAN), WHO PAR-
TICIPATED IN A 9-WEEK SUMMER ENRICHMENT
PROGRAM AT THE UNIVERSITY OF TEXAS MED-
ICAL BRANCH IN GALVESTON, WERE SUR-
VEYED AFTER THE PROGRAM'S 6TH YEAR.
QUESTIONNAIRES HAD BEEN MAILED TO THE
STUDENTS ONE YEAR AFTER THEY ATTENDED
THE FIRST SUMMER PROGRAM TO OBTAIN
THEIR ASSESSMENT OF THE PROCEEDINGS
AND THEIR CURRENT CAREER PLANS. THERE-
AFTER, DATA WERE UPDATED AT YEARLY IN-
TERVALS. FURTHER INFORMATION WAS
GLEANED FROM STUDENT CORRESPONDENCE
WITH THE AUTHORS AT VARIOUS POINTS, ASK-
ING FOR ADVICE IN THEIR CAREERS, OR AT-
TESTING TO THE PERSONAL SIGNIFICANCE OF
THEIR SUMMER EXPERIENCE. BY STATISTICAL
ANALYSIS, 81 OF ALL STUDENTS WHO AT-
TENDED THE SUMMER PROGRAMS WERE
STUDYING OR WORKING IN SOME AREA OF
THE HEALTH PROFESSIONS, AND AN ADDI-
TIONAL 5 WERE PURSUING GRADUATE DE-
GREES IN NONHEALTH AREAS. RESULTS INDI-
CATE THAT: (1) SUMMER ENRICHMENT,
REINFORCEMENT, AND WORK-STUDY PRO-
GRAMS HAVE HELPED INCREASE THE NUMBER
OF BLACK AND MEXICAN AMERICAN STU-
DENTS APPLYING FOR ADMISSION TO HEALTH
PROFESSIONAL SCHOOLS; AND (2) THE TOTAL
IMPACT OF THE SUMMER EXPERIENCE ON
MEDICAL STUDENTS AND FACULTY IS DIFFI-
CULT TO EVALUATE. 8 REFERENCES. (NCMHI
ABSTRACT MODIFIED)

ACCN   002033

217 AUTH   **BRUHN, J. G., & FUENTES, R. G., JR.**
TITL   CULTURAL FACTORS AFFECTING UTILIZATION
OF SERVICES BY MEXICAN AMERICANS.
SRCE   *PSYCHIATRIC ANNALS, 1977, 7(12), 20-29.*
INDX   MEXICAN AMERICAN, FOLK MEDICINE, HEALTH
DELIVERY SYSTEMS, POLICY, CULTURAL PLU-
RALISM, ESSAY, ACCULTURATION, CURANDER-
ISMO, PREJUDICE, RESOURCE UTILIZATION,
CULTURAL FACTORS
ABST   THOUGH FACTORS ASSOCIATED WITH ACCUL-
TURATION TEND TO INCREASE MEXICAN
AMERICANS' USE OF MODERN HEALTH CARE
SYSTEMS, AN ALTERNATE SYSTEM—ROOTED
IN FOLK MEDICINE AND FAMILIAL HOME CARE—
CONTINUES TO FLOURISH. BUT INSTEAD OF
RECOGNIZING THE CULTURAL BASIS AND
VALUE OF SUCH A SYSTEM, MANY ANGLO
HEALTH PROFESSIONALS URGE MEXICAN
AMERICAN PATIENTS TO ABANDON THEIR TRA-
DITIONAL BELIEFS AND PRACTICES ABOUT ILL-
NESS. TO COUNTERACT THIS SITUATION, THE
PRESENT ESSAY SUGGESTS THAT IT SHOULD
BE POSSIBLE FOR THE TWO HEALTH CARE SYS-
TEMS TO WORK TOGETHER SO THAT MEXICAN
AMERICANS CAN BENEFIT FROM BOTH AT THE
SAME TIME. FIRST, THE TWO HEALTH SYSTEMS
SHOULD BE VIEWED AS COMPLEMENTARY,
NOT ANTAGONISTIC, SINCE THE MEXICAN

AMERICAN SYSTEM IS DESIGNED TO HELP
PSYCHOLOGICAL AND SPIRITUAL NEEDS WHILE
THE ANGLO HEALTH CARE SYSTEM IS AIMED
PRIMARILY AT PHYSICAL AILMENTS. SECOND,
THE LARGER ANGLO SYSTEM SHOULD BE
FLEXIBLE ENOUGH TO ACCOMMODATE PA-
TIENTS WHO USE TWO SUCH DISPARATE BUT
MUTUALLY BENEFICIAL APPROACHES TO
HEALING. IN CONCLUSION, IT IS RECOM-
MENDED THAT ANGLO HEALTH CARE PROFES-
SIONALS SHOULD STRIVE TO BECOME MORE
INFORMED ABOUT THE POSSIBLE COMPLE-
MENTARITY OF THESE TWO HEALTH CARE SYS-
TEMS. 20 REFERENCES.

ACCN   002032

218 AUTH   **BRUNSWICK, A. F.**
TITL   HEALTH NEEDS OF ADOLESCENTS: HOW THE
ADOLESCENT SEES THEM.
SRCE   *AMERICAN JOURNAL OF PUBLIC HEALTH, 1969,
59(9), 1730-1745.*
INDX   ADOLESCENTS, ATTITUDES, CROSS CUL-
TURAL, DRUG ABUSE, EMPIRICAL, FATALISM,
HEALTH, PUERTO RICAN-M, NUTRITION, UR-
BAN, SEX COMPARISON, NEW YORK, MALE, FE-
MALE, SURVEY, DRUG ABUSE, ALCOHOLISM,
SPANISH SURNAMED
ABST   A PROBABILITY SAMPLE OF 122 ADOLES-
CENTS, 12 TO 17 YEARS-OLD AND LIVING IN
THE WASHINGTON HEIGHTS SECTION OF NEW
YORK CITY, WERE INTERVIEWED IN JUNE, 1967,
TO ASCERTAIN SELF-IDENTIFIED HEALTH
PROBLEMS. THE SAMPLE WAS ETHNICALLY
HETEROGENEOUS WITH REPRESENTATION
FROM NEGROES, WHITES, PUERTO RICANS,
AND OTHER LATIN AMERICANS. TRAINED IN-
TERVIEWERS, MATCHED TO RESPONDENTS BY
ETHNICITY AND SEX, USED A STRUCTURED
QUESTIONNAIRE TO INTERVIEW TEENS IN THEIR
HOMES. FINDINGS INDICATE THAT ADOLES-
CENTS ARE CONCERNED ABOUT THEIR HEALTH
AND ARE ABLE TO PROVIDE DETAILED INFOR-
MATION ABOUT THEIR OWN FEELINGS AND
PERCEPTIONS REGARDING HEALTH MATTERS.
ONE IN SIX ADOLESCENTS CONSIDERED HIS
GENERAL HEALTH TO BE LESS THAN GOOD.
NEGRO GIRLS AND SPANISH BOYS WERE MOST
OFTEN CRITICAL OF THEIR GENERAL STATE OF
HEALTH. PERSONAL HEALTH PRACTICES WHICH
ADOLESCENTS WERE CONCERNED ABOUT IN-
CLUDED: (1) LACK OF EXERCISE; (2) POOR EAT-
ING HABITS; (3) SMOKING; AND (4) INADE-
QUATE SLEEP. MAJOR HEALTH AND MEDICAL
PROBLEMS REPORTED FOR ADOLESCENTS IN
GENERAL WERE CIGARETTE SMOKING (44),
DRUGS (34), DRINKING (32), AND AIR POLLU-
TION (18). IN CONCLUSION, OF SIGNIFICANCE
TO THOSE INTERESTED IN IMPROVING HEALTH
SERVICES AND HEALTH PRACTICES IS THAT
FOUR-FIFTHS OF THE SPANISH AND NEGRO
YOUNGSTERS SAID THAT BEING HEALTHY MAT-
TERED A LOT TO THEM; MOREOVER, SPANISH
BOYS INDICATED CONSIDERABLE FATALISM
ABOUT THE AVOIDABILITY OF ILLNESS. 13 REF-
ERENCES.

ACCN   002034

219 AUTH   **BRUSSELL, C. B.**

TITL COGNITIVE AND INTELLECTUAL FUNCTIONING OF SPANISH-SPEAKING CHILDREN.

SRCE *IN J. C. STONE & D. P. DENEVI (EDS.), TEACHING MULTICULTURAL POPULATIONS: FIVE HERITAGES. NEW YORK: VAN NOSTRAND, 1971, PP. 267-271.*

INDX INTELLIGENCE, INTELLIGENCE TESTING, MEXICAN AMERICAN, CHILDREN, CROSS CULTURAL, STANFORD-BINET INTELLIGENCE TEST, ADOLESCENTS, BILINGUALISM, WISC, SOCIALIZATION, SPECIAL EDUCATION, DISCRIMINATION, STEREOTYPES, SELF CONCEPT, REVIEW

ABST LITERATURE CONCERNING THE PERFORMANCE OF SPANISH-SPEAKING CHILDREN AS MEASURED BY STANDARD INTELLIGENCE TESTS IS REVIEWED. IT IS SUGGESTED THAT, ALTHOUGH SUCH IQ TESTS ARE NOT APPROPRIATE OR VALID FOR MEASURING THE COGNITIVE AND INTELLECTUAL LEVEL OF SPANISH-SPEAKING CHILDREN, THEY MAY STILL HAVE SOME PREDICTIVE VALUE UNDER SPECIFIC CONDITIONS IN CERTAIN AREAS. RATHER THAN TOTALLY DISCARDING THESE TESTS, IT IS PROPOSED THAT TEACHERS BE ENCOURAGED TO VIEW THEIR RESULTS AS FLEXIBLE INDICATORS OF EXPECTED OPERATIONAL LEVEL AT A GIVEN TIME AND NOT ESTABLISHED MENTAL ABILITY. 32 REFERENCES. (AUTHOR SUMMARY MODIFIED)

ACCN 000186

220 AUTH **BRUSSELL, C. B.**

TITL DISADVANTAGED MEXICAN AMERICAN CHILDREN AND EARLY EDUCATIONAL EXPERIENCE.

SRCE *AUSTIN, TEXAS: SOUTHWEST EDUCATIONAL DEVELOPMENT CORPORATION, 1968. (ERIC DOCUMENT REPRODUCTION SERVICE NO. ED030517)*

INDX SPANISH SURNAMED, MEXICAN AMERICAN, HISTORY, CULTURE, SES, DEMOGRAPHIC, FAMILY STRUCTURE, CENSUS, IMMIGRATION, MIGRATION, EMPLOYMENT, POVERTY, ACCULTURATION, FATALISM, AUTHORITARIANISM, TIME ORIENTATION, SEX ROLES, FOLK MEDICINE, HEALTH, BILINGUALISM, INTELLIGENCE TESTING, INTELLIGENCE, COGNITIVE DEVELOPMENT, COGNITIVE STYLE, CULTURE-FAIR TESTS, TEXAS, SOUTHWEST, BIBLIOGRAPHY, EARLY CHILDHOOD EDUCATION, EDUCATION, TEACHERS, REVIEW

ABST A SYNTHESIS OF LITERATURE ON THE MEXICAN AMERICANS OF TEXAS AND THE SOUTHWEST PROVIDES AN OVERVIEW OF THE GENERAL RESEARCH FINDINGS. THE VOLUME IS INTENDED AS A RESOURCE FOR TEACHERS AND OTHERS WHO WORK WITH MEXICAN AMERICAN CHILDREN. PART 1 IS A CONCISE HISTORY OF THE POPULATION. PART II PRESENTS A SYNTHESIS OF CURRENT LITERATURE ON THE SOCIAL CHARACTERISTICS OF THE MEXICAN AMERICAN. PART III IDENTIFIES PROBLEMS IN THE EDUCATION OF SPANISH-SPEAKING CHILDREN. PART IV PRESENTS A RATIONALE FOR EARLY CHILDHOOD EDUCATION PROGRAMS AS A PARTIAL SOLUTION TO THE PROBLEMS OF EDUCATING A DISADVANTAGED POPULATION. PART V GIVES BRIEF DESCRIPTIONS OF A NUMBER OF CURRENT PROJECTS

DEALING WITH THE EDUCATIONALLY DISADVANTAGED SECTOR OF THE MEXICAN AMERICAN POPULATION. PART VI IS A SUMMARY OF THE MAJOR IDEAS PRESENTED IN EACH SECTION. THE APPENDICES CONTAIN AN EXTENSIVE BIBLIOGRAPHY FOR EACH OF THE FIRST 5 SECTIONS. (DK) 153 REFERENCES. (RIE ABSTRACT)

ACCN 000188

221 AUTH **BRUSSELL, C. B.**

TITL SOCIAL CHARACTERISTICS AND PROBLEMS OF THE SPANISH-SPEAKING ATOMISTIC SOCIETY.

SRCE *IN J. C. STONE & D. P. DENEVI (EDS.), TEACHING MULTICULTURAL POPULATIONS: FIVE HERITAGES. NEW YORK: VAN NOSTRAND, 1971, PP. 169-196.*

INDX MEXICAN AMERICAN, CULTURE, FAMILY ROLES, FAMILY STRUCTURE, INTERPERSONAL RELATIONS, SEX ROLES, SEXUAL BEHAVIOR, MARRIAGE, FICTIVE KINSHIP, ACCULTURATION, ACHIEVEMENT MOTIVATION, EDUCATION, SCHOLASTIC ACHIEVEMENT, POVERTY, BILINGUALISM, STEREOTYPES, DISCRIMINATION, FATALISM, TIME ORIENTATION, HEALTH, FOLK MEDICINE, CURANDERISMO, BILINGUAL-BICULTURAL EDUCATION, REVIEW

ABST A BROAD OVERVIEW OF MEXICAN AMERICAN CULTURE-IS PRESENTED WITH PARTICULAR ATTENTION TO: FAMILY AND COMMUNITY STRUCTURE; VIEWS OF ANGLOS; PERCEPTION OF TIME, ACHIEVEMENT, AND ILLNESS; LANGUAGE SKILLS AND HOW THEY AFFECT EDUCATION; AND ACCULTURATION. EACH OF THESE FACTORS IS DISCUSSED IN TERMS OF ITS INFLUENCE ON THE NUCLEAR FAMILY. THE SOCIAL SYSTEM OF SPANISH-SPEAKING PEOPLES IS DESCRIBED AS AN "ATOMISTIC SOCIETY" WHICH (1) CONSIDERS THE NUCLEAR FAMILY AS THE BASIC UNIT OUT OF WHICH INDIVIDUALS PURSUE ECONOMIC AND SOCIAL ENDS, (2) SEES THE RELATIONSHIPS BEYOND THE FAMILY AS BEING BETWEEN ONE INDIVIDUAL AND ANOTHER, RATHER THAN BETWEEN AN INDIVIDUAL AND GROUPS OF OTHERS, AND (3) SEES THE RELATIONSHIP BETWEEN INDIVIDUALS AND OTHERS AS CHARACTERIZED BY A HIGH DEGREE OF PERSONALISM. 34 REFERENCES.

ACCN 000187

222 AUTH **BRYANT, B., & MEADOW, A.**

TITL SCHOOL-RELATED PROBLEMS OF MEXICAN-AMERICAN ADOLESCENTS.

SRCE *JOURNAL OF SCHOOL PSYCHOLOGY, 1976, 14(2), 139-150.*

INDX MEXICAN AMERICAN, ADOLESCENTS, SCHOLASTIC ACHIEVEMENT, CULTURAL FACTORS, EDUCATION, AUTHORITARIANISM, FAMILY ROLES, SEX ROLES, COOPERATION, COMPETITION, EXTENDED FAMILY, REVIEW

ABST SELECTED ASPECTS OF THE SCHOOL PROBLEMS OF MEXICAN AMERICAN ADOLESCENTS ARE EXPLAINED BY AN ANALYSIS OF MAJOR CULTURAL THEMES. THE DATA PRESENTED SUGGEST THAT FOR SOME MEXICAN AMERI-

CAN ADOLESCENTS SCHOOL HAS AT LEAST THESE FOUR MEANINGS: (1) A PLACE WHERE TEACHERS ARE FREQUENTLY PERCEIVED AND TREATED AS AUTHORITY FIGURES SIMILAR TO THEIR FATHERS, AND THERFORE, ARE TARGETS OF REBELLION; (2) A PLACE LACKING STRICT EXTERNAL PROHIBITION OF ENCOUNTERS WITH THE OPPOSITE SEX; (3) A PUBLIC ARENA OF ACTIVITY WHERE ONE CAN BRING HONOR OR SHAME TO ONE'S FAMILY; AND (4) AN INSTITUTION WHICH EXPECTS PARTICIPATING INDIVIDUALS TO VALUE INDIVIDUAL COMPETITION AND SUCCESS. PROBLEMS OF MEXICAN AMERICAN FEMALE ADOLESCENTS REGARDING DIRECT EXPRESSION OF ANGER ARE ALSO DISCUSSED. 24 REFERENCES. (JOURNAL ABSTRACT MODIFIED)

ACCN   000189

---

223 AUTH **BRYANT, C. A.**
TITL   THE PUERTO RICAN MENTAL HEALTH UNIT.
SRCE   *PSYCHIATRIC ANNALS, 1975, 5(8), 66-75.*
INDX   PUERTO RICAN-M, MENTAL HEALTH, HEALTH DELIVERY SYSTEMS, ESSAY, ESPIRITISMO, COMMUNITY INVOLVEMENT, CULTURAL FACTORS, FLORIDA, SOUTH, PROGRAM EVALUATION
ABST   THE OBJECTIVES OF THE PUERTO RICAN MENTAL HEALTH UNIT IN DADE COUNTY, FLORIDA, ARE TO IMPROVE THE COPING CAPABILITY OF PERSONS UNDERGOING MENTAL HEALTH CRISES AND TO RAISE THE MENTAL HEALTH LEVEL OF THE PUERTO RICAN COMMUNITY. STRATEGIES THAT HAVE EMERGED FOR ACHIEVING THESE GOALS ARE: (1) TO BUILD SUPPORT NETWORKS IN THE COMMUNITY FOR PREVENTION AND AFTERCARE OF MENTAL HEALTH CASUALTIES; (2) TO FACILITATE INDIGENOUS SOCIAL ACTION AND COMMUNITY DEVELOPMENT; (3) TO ACT AS MEDIATORS BETWEEN PSYCHIATRIC PERSONNEL AND PATIENTS; (4) TO PARTICIPATE IN TRAINING PROGRAMS FOR MENTAL HEALTH PERSONNEL, PROVIDING THEM WITH INFORMATION NEEDED TO DELIVER CULTURALLY APPROPRIATE CARE TO PUERTO RICANS; AND (5) TO PROVIDE AGENCIES SERVING THE COMMUNITY WITH INFORMATION THAT WILL ENABLE THEM TO SERVE PUERTO RICAN FAMILIES MORE EFFECTIVELY. THE AUTHOR, A MEDICAL ANTHROPOLOGIST, EMPHASIZES THAT THIS PROGRAM IS BUILT ON TWO ASSUMPTIONS. FIRST, IN ORDER FOR THE MENTAL HEALTH UNIT TO HAVE A LASTING EFFECT ON COMMUNITY MENTAL HEALTH IT MUST BUILD ON THE CULTURAL VALUES, SOCIAL SYSTEMS AND SOCIAL ACTION PRESENT IN THE PUERTO RICAN COMMUNITY; AND SECOND, THE PROGRAM SHOULD SERVE ONLY AS A TEMPORARY SYSTEM TO BE SUPERSEDED BY A COMPREHENSIVE NETWORK OF COMMUNITY SUPPORT SYSTEMS THAT IS WELL INTEGRATED WITH THE MENTAL HEALTH CARE DELIVERY SYSTEM THROUGHOUT THE COUNTY. 11 REFERENCES. (AUTHOR SUMMARY MODIFIED)

ACCN   000190

---

224 AUTH **BRYEN, D. N.**

TITL   SPEECH-SOUND DISCRIMINATION ABILITY ON LINGUISTICALLY UNBIASED TESTS.
SRCE   *EXCEPTIONAL CHILDREN, 1976, 42(4), 195-201.*
INDX   CULTURE-FAIR TESTS, PHONOLOGY, LINGUISTICS, SEMANTICS, PERCEPTION, BILINGUAL-BICULTURAL EDUCATION, CHILDREN, SES, CROSS CULTURAL, EMPIRICAL, PUERTO RICAN-M, RESEARCH METHODOLOGY, EDUCATIONAL ASSESSMENT, TEST VALIDITY, EAST, BILINGUAL
ABST   TRADITIONAL TESTING PRACTICES ARE CONSIDERED BY SOME EDUCATORS TO BE DISCRIMINATORY AGAINST MINORITY GROUPS. IN RESPONSE TO THIS PROBLEM, ONE PARTICULAR LANGUAGE ABILITY, SPEECH-SOUND DISCRIMINATION, WAS ASSESSED USING A BILINGUAL PERSPECTIVE RATHER THAN ONE STRESSING THE RIGHTNESS OF STANDARD ENGLISH. THREE PARALLEL FORMS OF SPEECH-SOUND DISCRIMINATION (STANDARD ENGLISH, BLACK ENGLISH, AND SPANISH) WERE EACH ADMINISTERED TO A SAMPLE OF LOWER SOCIOECONOMIC WHITE, BLACK AND PUERTO RICAN CHILDREN. RESULTS INDICATE THAT EACH GROUP DID BEST ON THE DISCRIMINATION FORM THAT MOST CLOSELY APPROXIMATED THE PHONOLOGICAL STRUCTURE OF ITS OWN LANGUAGE. THERE WERE NO SIGNIFICANT DIFFERENCES IN ABILITY AMONG THE THREE GROUPS WHEN PERFORMANCES ACROSS ALL LANGUAGE FORMS WERE TESTED. EDUCATIONAL IMPLICATIONS FOR ASSESSMENT ARE DISCUSSED. 23 REFERENCES. (JOURNAL ABSTRACT MODIFIED)

ACCN   000191

---

225 AUTH **BUCKHOUT, R.**
TITL   TOWARD A TWO-CHILD NORM: CHANGING FAMILY PLANNING ATTITUDES.
SRCE   *AMERICAN PSYCHOLOGIST, 1972, 27(1), 16-25.*
INDX   BIRTH CONTROL, ATTITUDES, CROSS CULTURAL, EMPIRICAL, SPANISH SURNAMED, COLLEGE STUDENTS, RELIGION, SES, CALIFORNIA, SOUTHWEST, SURVEY, FAMILY PLANNING
ABST   FAMILY PLANNING ATTITUDES AMONG YOUNG UNMARRIED UNDERGRADUATE STUDENTS OF VARIOUS ETHNIC BACKGROUNDS ARE EXAMINED. THE SAMPLE (80.9% WHITE, 9.1% BLACK, 5.3% SPANISH SURNAME (SS), 3.0% ORIENTAL, AND 1.5% NATIVE AMERICAN) WAS STRATIFIED BY RACE ACCORDING TO CALIFORNIA'S POPULATION DISTRIBUTION. SUBJECTS CONSISTED OF AN EQUAL NUMBER OF MALES AND FEMALES WITH A MEAN AGE OF 22 YEARS. IN ADDITION, EXPANDED SUB-SAMPLE GROUPS OF SS AND BLACKS WERE SURVEYED TO FACILITATE COMPARISONS AGAINST THE MAIN SAMPLE. A QUESTIONNAIRE WITH A 10-POINT PREFERENCE SCALE DESIGNED TO COLLECT STANDARD DEMOGRAPHIC DATA, BIOGRAPHICAL INFORMATION, FAMILY PLANNING IDEAS, AND ATTITUDES TOWARD STERILIZATION, ABORTION, AND BIRTH CONTROL WAS ADMINISTERED TO THE SUBJECTS BY 16 INTERVIEWERS. THE FINDINGS REVEAL: (1) THE IDEAL NUMBER OF CHILDREN DESIRED BY ANGLOS IS 2.45, WHILE BLACKS AND THE SS DESIRE LARGER FAMILIES, 4.1 AND 4.0 CHILDREN RE-

SPECTIVELY; (2) LITTLE ENTHUSIASM FOR POPULATION ALTERNATIVES SUCH AS ABORTIONS, STERILIZATION, AND THE PILL IS INDICATED BY BLACKS AND SS CATHOLICS; AND (3) THE SS GROUP DIFFERED FROM THE MAIN SAMPLE ON THE ITEMS "IDEAL NUMBER OF CHILDREN" AND "VOLUNTARY STERILIZATION OF SPOUSE." IT IS CONCLUDED THAT THE FINDINGS SIGNAL A SHIFT TOWARD A TWO-CHILD NORM FOR ONLY THE YOUNG ANGLO SUBJECTS. THE IMPLICATION OF THESE FINDINGS IS THAT MINORITY-GROUP MEMBERS SHOULD SET THEIR OWN TIMETABLE FOR DEALING WITH OVERPOPULATION. ALSO, MANDATORY STERILIZATION SHOULD BE RULED OUT AND THE NOTION THAT EVERY CHILD BE WANTED SHOULD BE EMPHASIZED. 24 REFERENCES.

ACCN   000192

226 AUTH   **BUCKHOUT, R.**
     TITL   THE WAR ON PEOPLE: A SCENARIO FOR POPULATION CONTROL.
     SRCE   *ENVIRONMENT AND BEHAVIOR, 1971, 3(3), 322-344.*
     INDX   BIRTH CONTROL, ATTITUDES, CROSS CULTURAL, EMPIRICAL, MEXICAN AMERICAN, COLLEGE STUDENTS, CALIFORNIA, SOUTHWEST
     ABST   A 1970 SURVEY OF ATTITUDES TOWARD POPULATION CONTROL WAS GUIDED BY THE QUESTION WHETHER THE PRESENT GENERATION, LIKE PREVIOUS GENERATIONS, WANTS TOO MANY CHILDREN AND WHETHER THEY WOULD TAKE STEPS TO REDUCE FAMILY SIZE TO REPLACEMENT LEVELS. FOR A STRATIFIED SAMPLE OF 267 UNMARRIED UNDERGRADUATES, COMPARABLE DEMOGRAPHICALLY WITH THE GENERAL POPULATION OF CALIFORNIA, THE IDEAL NUMBER OF CHILDREN DESIRED WAS 2.6 (RECENTLY 2.45), WHICH IS LOWER THAN THE USUAL 3.0. SUBJECTS GENERALLY ACCEPTED A 2-CHILD FAMILY NORM. MOST SUBJECTS FAVORED ARTIFICIAL BIRTH CONTROL BUT NOT VOLUNTARY STERILIZATION OR ABORTION, AND FAVORED ADOPTION ONLY IF CLEARLY INFERTILE THEMSELVES. MOST REGARDED POPULATION GROWTH AS VERY SERIOUS, WOULD SUPPORT VOLUNTARY LIMITATIONS OF FAMILY SIZE, FAVORED INCENTIVES FOR ADOPTIONS, BUT WERE STRONGLY OPPOSED TO MANDATORY STERILIZATION. ADDDITIONAL DATA CONTRASTS BLACK AND CHICANO SAMPLES WITH THE REPRESENTATIVE SAMPLE. THE FORMER, BY COMPARISON, TEND TO FAVOR LARGER FAMILIES AND TO REGARD POPULATION GROWTH AS LESS SERIOUS. IT IS SUGGESTED THAT CHILDREN IMPLY SOCIAL POWER TO CHICANOS, AND MASCULINITY TO UNMARRIED BLACKS. 22 REFERENCES. (SOCIOLOGY ABSTRACT)
     ACCN   000193

227 AUTH   **BUDOFF, M., CORMAN, L., & GIMON, A.**
     TITL   AN EDUCATIONAL TEST OF LEARNING POTENTIAL ASSESSMENT WITH SPANISH-SPEAKING YOUTH.
     SRCE   *INTERAMERICAN JOURNAL OF PSYCHOLOGY, 1976, 10, 13-24.*

INDX   SPANISH SURNAMED, BILINGUAL, INTELLIGENCE, CHILDREN, WISC, RAVEN PROGRESSIVE MATRICES, TEST VALIDITY, INTELLIGENCE TESTING, RESEARCH METHODOLOGY, EMPIRICAL, EAST
ABST   THE LEARNING POTENTIAL (LP) PROCEDURE REPRESENTS AN ALTERNATIVE METHOD OF MEASURING THE GENERAL ABILITY OF SPANISH-SPEAKING STUDENTS WHO TEND TO SCORE LOW ON TRADITIONAL IQ TESTS. POSTTEACHING SCORES ON AN ELECTRICITY CURRICULUM UNIT TEST WERE USED AS CRITERIA TO COMPARE THE RELATIVE PREDICTIVE POWER OF LP AND IQ MEASURES FOR SPANISH-SPEAKING STUDENTS. SUBJECTS WERE ADMINISTERED THE RAVEN LP PROCEDURE, THE SEMANTIC TEST OF INTELLIGENCE, THE WISC PERFORMANCE SCALE IN SPANISH, AND THE WISC VOCABULARY SUBTEST IN SPANISH AND ENGLISH. BEFORE AND AFTER PARTICIPATION IN AN ELECTRICITY UNIT, SUBJECTS TOOK THE ELECTRICITY UNIT EVALUATION INSTRUMENT. POSTTRAINING RAVEN LP SCORES SIGNIFICANTLY PREDICTED PERFORMANCE ON THE MINIMALLY VERBAL SYMBOLIC LEVEL OF THE ELECTRICITY INSTRUMENT. IQ SCORES WERE NOT POSITIVELY RELATED TO POSTTEACHING ELECTRICITY SCORES. THE LP PROCEDURE RESULTED IN INCREASED LEVELS OF PERFORMANCE ON A REASONING TASK. 15 REFERENCES. (JOURNAL ABSTRACT)
ACCN   000194

228 AUTH   **BUEHLER, M. H., WIEGERT, A. J., & THOMAS, D. L.**
     TITL   CORRELATES OF CONJUGAL POWER: A FIVE CULTURE ANALYSIS OF ADOLESCENT PERCEPTIONS.
     SRCE   *JOURNAL OF COMPARATIVE FAMILY STUDIES, 1974, 5(1), 5-16.*
     INDX   MARRIAGE, ADOLESCENTS, FAMILY STRUCTURE, CROSS CULTURAL, MARITAL STABILITY, ATTRIBUTION THEORY, INTERPERSONAL RELATIONS, ROLE EXPECTATIONS, CULTURAL FACTORS, RELIGION, SEX COMPARISON, AGGRESSION, EMPIRICAL, PUERTO RICAN-I, THEORETICAL, MEXICAN
     ABST   TWO THEORETICAL FRAMEWORKS DOMINATE THE EXPLANATION OF THE RELATIVE POWER OF HUSBAND AND WIFE: IDEOLOGICAL THEORY WHICH EMPHASIZES NORMS; AND RESOURCE THEORY WHICH EMPHASIZES PERSONAL ATTRIBUTES AND POSSESSIONS. BOTH ORIENTATIONS HAVE RECEIVED SOME SUPPORT IN EMPIRICAL RESEARCH, BUT THE SUPPORT HAS BEEN MIXED. THIS STUDY, USING THE SCALED RESPONSES OF ADOLESCENTS FROM CATHOLIC HIGH SCHOOLS IN 5 COUNTRIES (U.S., GERMANY, PUERTO RICO, SPAIN AND MEXICO) ABOUT THEIR PARENTS' DECISION-MAKING POWERS, CORROBORATES SELECTED PAST FINDINGS, BUT FAILS TO ANSWER CRUCIAL ISSUES CONCERNING THE RELATIVE EXPLANATORY POTENTIAL OF RESOURCE VERSUS IDEOLOGY THEORY. THE STUDY FINDS THAT ADOLESCENT MALES IN FIVE CULTURAL CONTEXTS PERCEIVE FATHER AS HAVING MORE POWER THAN MOTHER, AND ATTRIBUTE MORE

POWER TO FATHER THAN DO FEMALE RESPONDENTS. INTERCULTURAL COMPARISON ON AN INDUSTRIALIZATION CONTINUUM SHOWS A TENDENCY FOR INDUSTRIALIZATION TO REDUCE HUSBAND'S POWER. INTRACULTURAL CORRELATIONS PARTIALLY REPLICATE THE FINDINGS THAT HUSBAND'S OCCUPATION IS POSITIVELY RELATED TO HIS POWER, AND THAT WIFE'S EMPLOYMENT OUTSIDE THE HOME IS NEGATIVELY RELATED TO HUSBAND'S POWER. IN GENERAL, THE RELIGIOSITY OF EITHER PARENT IS POSITIVELY ASSOCIATED WITH HUSBAND'S POWER. HUSBAND'S AND WIFE'S EDUCATION GIVE MIXED RESULTS. 36 REFERENCES. (AUTHOR SUMMARY MODIFIED)

ACCN   000195

229   AUTH   **BULLINGTON, B.**
TITL   HEROIN USE IN THE BARRIO.
SRCE   *LEXINGTON, MASS.: LEXINGTON BOOKS, 1977.*
INDX   ATTITUDES, CULTURAL FACTORS, DEMOGRAPHIC, DRUG ABUSE, DRUG ADDICTION, ECONOMIC FACTORS, ENVIRONMENTAL FACTORS, ESSAY, LEGISLATION, MENTAL HEALTH, METHADONE MAINTENANCE, MEXICAN AMERICAN, SES, SOCIAL SERVICES, CALIFORNIA, SOUTHWEST, URBAN, CORRECTIONS, REVIEW, BOOK
ABST   THE CULTURAL SETTING IN WHICH DRUG USE TAKES PLACE IS EXAMINED, WITH A FOCUS ON THE DRUG USE BEHAVIOR OF CHICANOS RESIDING IN ONE EAST L.A. COMMUNITY. RESEARCH WAS CONDUCTED BETWEEN 1967-1972 IN THE NARCOTICS PREVENTION PROJECT, A COMMUNITY-BASED DRUG PREVENTION AND USE INTERVENTION PROGRAM LOCATED IN BOYLE HEIGHTS, EAST LOS ANGELES. SIX TOPICS FORM THE SUBSTANCE OF THE BOOK: (1) A REVIEW OF THE HISTORY OF DRUG USE DOCUMENTS AND THE TRANSFORMATION OF ATTITUDES, POLICIES, AND PROCEDURES FOR DEALING WITH THE NARCOTICS PROBLEM; (2) THE INFLUENCE OF CHICANO CULTURE AND BARRIO LIFE ON DRUG USING BEHAVIOR; (3) AN OVERVIEW OF PUNITIVE/TREATMENT PROCEDURES THAT HAVE BEEN ATTEMPTED FROM 1914 TO THE PRESENT; (4) A DESCRIPTION OF DATA COLLECTION ON DRUG USE IN THE BARRIO (I.E., PERSONAL INTERVIEWS CONDUCTED BY EX-ADDICTS) AND A REVIEW OF RESULTING DEMOGRAPHIC CHARACTERISTICS OF DRUG USERS; (5) A DESCRIPTION OF THE CHICANO ADDICT PERSONALITY TYPE AND DRUG USE PATTERNS; AND (6) AN ACCOUNT OF SOCIAL ORGANIZATIONS DESIGNED TO AMELIORATE THE DRUG PROBLEM (COURTS, POLICE, PROBATION AND PAROLE, AND CORRECTIONS) AND THEIR INFLUENCE ON DRUG USE PATTERNS. IT IS CONCLUDED THAT THE VERY AGENCIES THAT HAVE BEEN ASSIGNED TO MITIGATE THE SEVERITY OF THE PROBLEM ARE IN FACT AGGRAVATING IT, THEREBY ENCOURAGING MANY OF THE MYTHS AND STEREOTYPES REGARDING DRUG USERS, THEIR LIFESTYLES, AND THEIR REHABILITATION POTENTIAL. 170 REFERENCES.

ACCN   002035

230   AUTH   **BULLINGTON, B., MUNNS, J. G., & GEIS, G.**
TITL   PURCHASE OF CONFORMITY: EX-NARCOTIC ADDICTS AMONG THE BOURGEOISIE.
SRCE   *SOCIAL PROBLEMS, 1969, 16(4), 456-463.*
INDX   REHABILITATION, DRUG ADDICTION, ADULTS, MEXICAN AMERICAN, SES, CALIFORNIA, SOUTHWEST, CASE STUDY, EMPIRICAL, CROSS CULTURAL, PERSONNEL, ATTITUDES, EMPLOYMENT
ABST   THE HYPOTHESIS THAT A DECENT SALARY AND SOCIAL SERVICE STATUS WOULD BE SUFFICIENT TO LEAD EX-ADDICT CASEWORKERS INTO ACCEPTANCE OF MIDDLE-CLASS VALUES AND LIFESTYLES WAS INVESTIGATED. DATA WERE OBTAINED FROM 31 EX-ADDICTS THROUGH INTERVIEWS AND FIELD OBSERVATION. IT IS CONCLUDED THAT THE LURES OF SALARY AND PRESTIGE STATUS ALONE ARE NOT SUFFICIENT TO INSURE MIDDLE-CLASS ATTITUDES AND BEHAVIOR. SEVERAL UNIQUE CROSS-PRESSURES PREVENT TOTAL ABSORPTION OF THE SUBJECTS INTO THE BOURGEOISIE; AMONG THESE ARE ADMINISTRATIVE PRESSURES TO MAINTAIN A STREET STYLE AND EMPATHY WITH CLIENTS AND DAILY ASSOCIATION WITH PRACTICING ADDICTS. 11 REFERENCES. (JOURNAL ABSTRACT MODIFIED)

ACCN   000196

231   AUTH   **BULLOCK, P.**
TITL   EMPLOYMENT PROBLEMS OF THE MEXICAN AMERICAN.
SRCE   *INDUSTRIAL RELATIONS, 1964, 3(2), 37-50.*
INDX   MEXICAN AMERICAN, LABOR FORCE, ESSAY, DISCRIMINATION, ADULTS, SOUTHWEST, EMPLOYMENT, CROSS CULTURAL, CULTURAL FACTORS
ABST   SOME OF THE CAUSES AND POSSIBLE SOLUTIONS OF MEXICAN AMERICAN EMPLOYMENT PROBLEMS ARE REVIEWED. THE LIMITED AMOUNT OF INFORMATION AVAILABLE ABOUT THE PROBLEMS AND THE LACK OF RECOGNITION OF THE PROBLEMS BY THE LARGER SOCIETY ARE DISCUSSED. CULTURAL FORCES AFFECTING UNDEREMPLOYMENT, EDUCATION AND TRAINING DEFICIENCIES, AND DISCRIMINATION IN EMPLOYMENT ARE PRESENTED ALONG WITH A BRIEF PROFILE OF THE MEXICAN AMERICAN WORKER IN THE FIVE SOUTHWESTERN STATES. A SIGNIFICANT ASPECT OF THE REVIEW IS ITS DISCUSSION OF THE SIMILARITIES AND DIFFERENCES BETWEEN THE MOVEMENTS IN THE BLACK AND MEXICAN AMERICAN COMMUNITIES FOR MORE AND BETTER JOBS. 12 REFERENCES.

ACCN   000197

232   AUTH   **BULLOUGH, B.**
TITL   POVERTY, ETHNIC IDENTITY AND PREVENTIVE HEALTH CARE.
SRCE   *JOURNAL OF HEALTH AND SOCIAL BEHAVIOR, 1972, 13(4), 347-359.*
INDX   SES, ECONOMIC FACTORS, ETHNIC IDENTITY, MENTAL HEALTH, HEALTH, PSYCHOSOCIAL ADJUSTMENT, MEXICAN AMERICAN, CROSS CULTURAL, CULTURAL FACTORS, RESOURCE UTILIZATION, SOCIAL SERVICES, COMMUNITY

INVOLVEMENT, POVERTY, CALIFORNIA, SOUTH-WEST, URBAN, FEMALE, ANOMIE, FAMILY PLAN-NING

ABST LOW-INCOME MOTHERS FROM THREE LOS AN-GELES POVERTY AREAS, REPRESENTING THREE ETHNIC GROUPS (BLACK, MEXICAN AMERICAN AND ANGLO), WERE QUESTIONED ABOUT THE PREVENTIVE HEALTH CARE THEY OBTAINED FOR THEMSELVES AND THEIR CHILDREN. THE STUDY INVESTIGATED THE ROLE OF THREE TYPES OF ALIENATION (POWERLESSNESS, HOPELESSNESS AND SOCIAL ISOLATION) AS BARRIERS TO THE UTILIZATION OF PREVEN-TIVE HEALTH SERVICES. IT WAS FOUND THAT THE MORE WELL KNOWN BARRIERS TO THE UTILIZATION OF PREVENTIVE SERVICES SUCH AS LOW SOCIOECONOMIC STATUS AND LOW EDUCATION LEVEL ARE REINFORCED BY THESE TYPES OF ALIENATION. FAMILY PLANNING BE-HAVIOR WAS FOUND TO BE THE TYPE OF PRE-VENTIVE CARE MOST INFLUENCED BY ALIENA-TION. 43 REFERENCES. (JOURNAL ABSTRACT MODIFIED)

ACCN 000198

233 AUTH **BUNKER, G. L., & JOHNSON, M. A.**
TITL ETHNICITY AND RESISTANCE TO COMPENSA-TORY EDUCATION: A COMPARISON OF MOR-MON AND NON-MORMON ETHNIC ATTITUDES.
SRCE *REVIEW OF RELIGIOUS RESEARCH, 1975, 16(2), 74-82.*
INDX RELIGION, ATTITUDES, PREJUDICE, UTAH, CALIFORNIA, SOUTHWEST, WEST, EMPIRICAL, MEXICAN AMERICAN, ADOLESCENTS, COL-LEGE STUDENTS
ABST AN ATTEMPT WAS MADE TO ASSESS WHETHER RELIGIOUS TEACHINGS WITHIN THE CHURCH OF JESUS CHRIST OF LATTER-DAY SAINTS (MORMON CHURCH) ARE GENERATING SECU-LAR RACIAL TOLERANCE OR INTOLERANCE TOWARD NEGROES, AMERICAN INDIANS, AND/ OR MEXICAN AMERICANS. SECULAR RACIAL ATTITUDES WERE ASSESSED BY AN INSTRU-MENT MEASURING ATTITUDES TOWARD COM-PENSATORY EDUCATION FOR VARIOUS ETHNIC GROUPS AS A MEASURE OF GROUP TOLER-ANCE. THE SUBJECT POPULATIONS INCLUDED ONE HIGH SCHOOL AND ONE COLLEGE IN UTAH AND TWO HIGH SCHOOLS AND TWO COLLEGES IN CALIFORNIA (TOTAL N = 616).THE MAJOR DIFFERENCES BETWEEN SCHOOLS WERE THEIR GEOGRAPHICAL LOCATIONS AND THE RELIGIOUS PREFERENCES OF THE STU-DENTS. THE TWO UTAH SCHOOLS WERE FROM 94% TO 96% MORMON WHILE THE CALIFORNIA SCHOOLS WERE LESS THAN 1% MORMON. THE DATA INDICATED THAT THE MORMONS, COM-PARED TO OTHERS IN THE "GENERAL CUL-TURE," ARE NOT SIGNIFICANTLY DIFFERENT IN THEIR SECULAR RACIAL ATTITUDES. 10 REF-ERENCES. (AUTHOR ABSTRACT MODIFIED)
ACCN 002036

234 AUTH **BURBACH, H. J., & THOMPSON, M. A.**
TITL NOTE ON ALIENATION, RACE, AND COLLEGE ATTRITION.
SRCE *PSYCHOLOGICAL REPORTS, 1973, 33(1), 273-274.*

INDX COLLEGE STUDENTS, PSYCHOSOCIAL AD-JUSTMENT, PUERTO RICAN-M, CROSS CUL-TURAL, MENTAL HEALTH, EMPIRICAL, SCHO-LASTIC ACHIEVEMENT, ANOMIE
ABST WHEN COLLEGE PERSISTERS (23 PUERTO RI-CANS, 61 BLACKS, 377 WHITES) AND NONPER-SISTERS (20 PUERTO RICANS, 36 BLACKS, AND 91 WHITES) WERE COMPARED BY RACE ON AL-IENATION AND THREE OF ITS COMPONENTS, POWERLESSNESS, NORMLESSNESS, AND SO-CIAL ISOLATION, NO SIGNIFICANT DIFFER-ENCES WERE FOUND. 6 REFERENCES. (JOUR-NAL ABSTRACT)
ACCN 000199

235 AUTH **BURGOYNE, R. W., WOLKON, G. H., STAPLES, F., KLINE, F., & POWERS, M.**
TITL WHICH PATIENTS RESPOND TO A MENTAL HEALTH CONSUMER SURVEY.
SRCE *AMERICAN JOURNAL OF COMMUNITY PSY-CHOLOGY, 1977, 5(3), 355-361.*
INDX ADULTS, CROSS CULTURAL, CULTURAL FAC-TORS, ECONOMIC FACTORS, EMPIRICAL, MEN-TAL HEALTH, MEXICAN AMERICAN, POVERTY, CALIFORNIA, SES, SOUTHWEST, SPANISH SUR-NAMED, URBAN, PSYCHOTHERAPY
ABST CHARACTERISTICS OF PATIENTS AT THE LOS ANGELES COUNTY UNIVERSITY OF SOUTHERN CALIFORNIA MEDICAL CENTER, ADULT PSY-CHIATRIC OUTPATIENT CLINIC WHO RE-SPONDED TO A LOS ANGELES COUNTY VOL-UNTARY "CLIENT SATISFACTION SURVEY" QUESTIONNAIRE WERE COMPARED WITH THOSE WHO DID NOT. AS THEY ARRIVED AT THE CLINIC ON A GIVEN DAY, 128 CONSECU-TIVE PATIENTS WERE HANDED THE QUESTION-NAIRE AND OBSERVED BY THE REGISTRATION CLERKS AS EITHER RETURNING THE QUES-TIONNAIRE TO A MARKED COLLECTION BOX IN THE WAITING ROOM OR FAILING TO DO SO. COMPARISONS BETWEEN THOSE WHO DID AND THOSE WHO DID NOT WERE MADE ON THE VARIABLES OF ETHNICITY, EDUCATION, TYPE OF MEDICATION, SEX, AGE, INCOME, MARITAL STATUS, PRIOR PSYCHIATRIC HOSPI-TALIZATION, RELIGION, ENGLISH- OR SPANISH-SPEAKING, TYPE OF TREATMENT, FREQUENCY OF TREATMENT, LENGTH OF TREATMENT, AT-TENDANCE, AND PSYCHIATRIC DIAGNOSIS. THREE SIGNIFICANT DIFFERENCES EMERGED: IF AN INDIVIUAL WAS (1) A MEMBER OF A MI-NORITY GROUP (BLACK OR SPANISH SUR-NAMED), (2) HAD LESS THAN A HIGH SCHOOL EDUCATION, AND (3) WAS TAKING ANTIPSY-CHOTIC MEDICATION, HIS CHANCE OF RE-TURNING A QUESTIONNAIRE TO A WAITING ROOM COLLECTION BOX WAS 79%, COM-PARED TO THE 30% CHANCE OF RETURNING IT IF HE HAD NONE OF THESE CHARACTERISTICS. YOUNGER PATIENTS AND "ANGLOS" MORE OFTEN USED THE U.S. MAIL THAN THE COL-LECTION BOX. THE STUDY SUGGESTS THAT DEPENDENCE PRODUCED BY RELATIVE SO-CIOCULTURAL INADEQUACY IS ONE OF THOSE STIMULI THAT PLACE PATIENTS IN A PER-CEIVED STATE OF DIMINISHED FREEDOM. THIS DIMINISHED FREEDOM MIGHT ACCOUNT FOR THE GROUP'S IMMEDIATE CONFORMITY IM-

PLIED IN THEIR INCREASED RATE OF RETURN-
ING QUESTIONNAIRES TO THE COLLECTION
BOX AT THE AGENCY. 6 REFERENCES.

ACCN 002037

236 AUTH **BURGOYNE, R. W., WOLKON, G., & STAPLES, F.**

TITL DO LATINOS AND BLACKS PARTICIPATE IN OUTPATIENT SERVICES CONSUMER SURVEYS?

SRCE *IN E. R. PADILLA & A. M. PADILLA (EDS.), TRAN-SCULTURAL PSYCHIATRY: AN HISPANIC PER-SPECTIVE (MONOGRAPH NO. 4). LOS ANGE-LES: UNIVERSITY OF CALIFORNIA, SPANISH SPEAKING MENTAL HEALTH RESEARCH CEN-TER, 1977, PP. 79-83.*

INDX RESEARCH METHODOLOGY, SURVEY, SES, MEXICAN AMERICAN, PROGRAM EVALUATION, EMPIRICAL, CALIFORNIA, MENTAL HEALTH, SOUTHWEST

ABST IN MARCH 1975 THE DEPARTMENT OF EVALUA-TION AND RESEARCH OF THE LOS ANGELES COUNTY MENTAL HEALTH DEPARTMENT CON-DUCTED A CLIENT SATISFACTION SURVEY AT ALL COUNTY FUNDED FACILITIES. TO DETER-MINE THE TYPE OF PATIENTS WHO VOLUNTAR-ILY RETURNED THE FORM, THIS STUDY EXAM-INED THE PORTION OF THE COUNTY-WIDE SURVEY THAT WAS DONE AT ONE CLINIC. AVAILABLE CHARACTERISTICS OF THE PA-TIENTS WHO RETURNED THE QUESTIONNAIRE WERE COMPARED WITH THOSE WHO DID NOT. THE FINDING THAT ETHNIC MINORITIES, THE LESS EDUCATED, AND THOSE ON ANTIPSY-CHOTIC MEDICATION RESPONDED MORE OFTEN REFUTES A COMMON VIEW THAT CON-SUMER SURVEYS EXCLUDE THE VIEWS OF ETH-NIC MINORITY PATIENTS. 6 REFERENCES.

ACCN 000200

237 AUTH **BURIEL, R.**

TITL COGNITIVE STYLES AMONG THREE GENERA-TIONS OF MEXICAN CHILDREN.

SRCE *JOURNAL OF CROSS-CULTURAL PSYCHOLOGY, 1975, 6(4), 417-429.*

INDX COGNITIVE STYLE, MEXICAN AMERICAN, AC-CULTURATION, CHILDREN, CROSS CULTURAL, EMPIRICAL, CALIFORNIA, SOUTHWEST, CROSS GENERATIONAL, FIELD DEPENDENCE-INDE-PENDENCE, SEX COMPARISON

ABST A COMPARISON OF FIRST, SECOND, AND THIRD GENERATION MEXICAN AMERICAN CHILDREN REGARDING FIELD DEPENDENCE-INDEPEN-DENCE IS PRESENTED. IT WAS HYPOTHESIZED THAT THE COGNITIVE STYLES OF MEXICAN AMERICAN CHILDREN WOULD BECOME IN-CREASINGLY MORE FIELD INDEPENDENT FROM THE FIRST TO THIRD GENERATION. ALSO, A DE-CLINE IN SEX DIFFERENCES WAS EXPECTED TO FOLLOW A SIMILAR PATTERN. A COMPARISON GROUP OF ANGLO AMERICAN CHILDREN WAS INCLUDED IN THE STUDY. RESULTS DID NOT SUPPORT THE HYPOTHESIS: ANGLO CHILDREN WERE THE MOST FIELD INDEPENDENT AND SHOWED THE SMALLEST SEX DIFFERENCE WHILE SECOND, FIRST, AND THIRD GENERA-TION MEXICAN AMERICAN CHILDREN FOL-LOWED RESPECTIVELY. THE UNEXPECTED RE-SULTS ARE DISCUSSED AS THE POSSIBLE

OUTCOME OF SELECTIVE MIGRATION AND COMMUNITY ACCULTURATION PROCESSES. 20 REFERENCES. (JOURNAL ABSTRACT MODI-FIED)

ACCN 000201

238 AUTH **BURIEL, R.**

TITL RELATIONSHIP OF THREE FIELD-DEPENDENCE MEASURES TO THE READING AND MATH ACHIEVEMENT OF ANGLO AMERICAN AND MEXICAN AMERICAN CHILDREN.

SRCE *JOURNAL OF EDUCATIONAL PSYCHOLOGY, 1978, 70(2), 167-174.*

INDX ACHIEVEMENT TESTING, CHILDREN, COGNI-TIVE DEVELOPMENT, CROSS CULTURAL, TEST VALIDITY, EMPIRICAL, FIELD DEPENDENCE-IN-DEPENDENCE, LEARNING, MEXICAN AMERI-CAN, CALIFORNIA, WISC, READING, MATHE-MATICS, INTELLIGENCE TESTING, SOUTHWEST, TEST RELIABILITY

ABST A COMPREHENSIVE TEST OF THE RELATION-SHIP BETWEEN FIELD DEPENDENCE AND ACHIEVEMENT COMPARED 40 MEXICAN AMERICAN 40 ANGLO AMERICAN CHILDREN FROM FIRST THROUGH FOURTH GRADE ON THREE COMMONLY USED MEASURES OF FIELD DEPENDENCE: (1) THE PORTABLE ROD-AND-FRAME TEST; (2) THE CHILDREN'S EMBEDDED FIGURES TEST, AND (3) THE WECHSLER INTEL-LIGENCE SCALE FOR CHILDREN BLOCK-DE-SIGN SUBTEST. DATA WERE ANALYZED IN THREE STEPS TO DETERMINE THE RELIABILITY OF THE THREE FIELD-DEPENDENCE TESTS IN MEASUR-ING CULTURAL DIFFERENCES IN FIELD DEPEN-DENCE, THE INTERCORRELATION AMONG THE THREE TESTS FOR MEMBERS OF BOTH CUL-TURAL GROUPS, AND THE RELATIONSHIP OF EACH OF THE THREE TESTS TO THE READING AND MATH ACHIEVEMENT OF MEXICAN AMERI-CAN AND ANGLO CHILDREN. RESULTS GEN-ERALLY FAILED TO SUPPORT THE ASSUMP-TIONS THAT (1) MEXICAN AMERICAN CHILDREN ARE MORE FIELD DEPENDENT THAN ANGLO AMERICAN CHILDREN, (2) INTERCORRELA-TIONS BETWEEN THE THREE FIELD-DEPEN-DENCE TESTS SHOULD BE SIGNIFICANT AND COMPARABLE FOR MEMBERS OF BOTH CUL-TURAL GROUPS, AND (3) FIELD DEPENDENCE IS OF SUBSTANTIAL IMPORTANCE TO THE SCHOOL ACHIEVEMENT OF ANGLO AMERICAN AND MEXICAN AMERICAN CHILDREN. IT IS CONCLUDED THAT THE ADMINISTRATION OF ONLY A SINGLE INSTRUMENT TO MEASURE FIELD DEPENDENCE MAY RESULT IN AN INAC-CURATE ASSESSMENT OF CHILDREN'S ACA-DEMIC POTENTIAL, ESPECIALLY THOSE FROM DIFFERENT CULTURAL BACKGROUNDS. 31 REFERENCES.

ACCN 002038

239 AUTH **BURIEL, R., LOYA, P., GONDA, T., & KLESSEN, K.**

TITL CHILD ABUSE AND NEGLECT REFERRAL PAT-TERNS OF ANGLO AND MEXICAN AMERICANS.

SRCE *HISPANIC JOURNAL OF BEHAVIORAL SCI-ENCES, 1979, 1(3), 215-227.*

INDX MEXICAN AMERICAN, CROSS CULTURAL, CHILD ABUSE, CALIFORNIA, SOUTHWEST, EMPIRICAL,

RESOURCE UTILIZATION, SOCIAL SERVICES, TEACHERS, STEREOTYPES, VALUES

ABST TO ASCERTAIN DIFFERENCES IN THE WAYS ANGLOS AND MEXICAN AMERICANS (MA) GET REFERRED TO CHILD PROTECTION AGENCIES FOR CASES OF CHILD ABUSE AND NEGLECT (C.A.N.), 225 CASES EACH FOR BOTH ETHNIC GROUPS WERE RANDOMLY SELECTED FROM THE 1974 THROUGH 1977 RECORDS OF TWO SUCH COUNTY AGENCIES IN SOUTHERN CALIFORNIA. THE DATA SHOWED THAT MA'S WERE REFERRED FOR C.A.N. SIGNIFICANTLY MORE OFTEN BY NONPROFESSIONAL COMMUNITY SOURCES. A MORE PRECISE BREAKDOWN REVEALED: (1) MA'S WERE TWICE AS LIKELY AS ANGLOS TO BE REFERRED BY SCHOOL PERSONNEL; (2) THERE WAS NO APPRECIABLE ETHNIC GROUP DIFFERENCE IN THE RATE OF REFERRAL BY FAMILY MEMBERS; AND (3) MA'S WERE SIGNIFICANTLY LESS LIKELY TO BE REFERRED BY NEIGHBORS, FRIENDS, OR ANONYMOUS COMMUNITY SOURCES. NO FIRM CONCLUSIONS ARE PROVIDED, AND INSTEAD THE DISCUSSION SECTION OFFERS THREE ALTERNATIVE INTERPRETATIONS OF THE FINDINGS. (1) THE TEACHERS' PROPENSITY FOR MAKING REFERRALS EITHER BETRAYS A BIASED ATTITUDE THAT MA PARENTS ARE CHILD ABUSERS, OR ELSE THAT TEACHERS ARE MORE AWARE OF C.A.N. CASES DUE TO THEIR PROLONGED CONTACT WITH THE CHILDREN. (2) THE ABSENCE OF A DIFFERENCE IN THE RATE OF REFERRALS BY FAMILY MEMBERS MAY REFLECT MA'S INCREASING ACCULTURATION TO THE AMERICAN CUSTOM OF SEEKING OUTSIDE HELP. (3) ON THE OTHER HAND, THE RARITY OF REFERRALS BY FRIENDS AND NEIGHBORS MAY BE DUE TO THE PERSISTENCE OF A MEXICAN AMERICAN CULTURAL VALUE—NAMELY, THE VALUE OF NONINTERFERENCE IN FAMILY MATTERS BY OUTSIDERS. IT IS CONCLUDED THAT MORE RESEARCH IS NECESSARY TO INVESTIGATE THESE SEVERAL QUESTIONS. 16 REFERENCES.

ACCN 001759

240 AUTH **BURKE, J. L., LAFAVE, H. G., & KURTZ, G. E.**
TITL MINORITY GROUP MEMBERSHIP AS A FACTOR IN CHRONICITY.
SRCE *PSYCHIATRY, 1965, 28, 235-238.*
INDX SCHIZOPHRENIA, PSYCHOTHERAPY, BILINGUAL, BILINGUAL-BICULTURAL PERSONNEL, PSYCHOTHERAPY OUTCOME, ACCULTURATION, SPANISH SURNAMED, PSYCHOPATHOLOGY, MENTAL HEALTH, MASSACHUSETTS, EAST
ABST THE STUDY IS A REPORT ON A SPECIALIZED REHABILITATION PROGRAM FOR CHRONIC SCHIZOPHRENICS IN WHICH THOSE WHO BELONG TO A MINORITY GROUP OR WHO SPEAK ANOTHER LANGUAGE BETTER THAN THEY SPEAK ENGLISH WERE TREATED WITHIN A TOTAL REHABILITATION PROGRAM. INCLUDED IN THIS STUDY WERE 85 MINORITY GROUP MEMBERS. THE RESULTS OF THIS STUDY INDICATE THAT ONE OF THE FACTORS THAT MAY BE INVOLVED IN CHRONICITY IS THAT OF BELONGING TO A MINORITY GROUP OR SPEAKING A LANGUAGE OTHER THAN THAT SPOKEN BY

STAFF, WHICH PREVENTS ADEQUATE COMMUNICATION AND UNDERSTANDING, AND, IN MANY INSTANCES, MAKES IT EASIER FOR STAFF TO IGNORE THE PATIENTS CONCERNED. 8 REFERENCES. (JOURNAL ABSTRACT)

ACCN 000202

241 AUTH **BURKE, Y. B.**
TITL MINORITY ADMISSIONS TO MEDICAL SCHOOLS: PROBLEMS AND OPPORTUNITIES.
SRCE *JOURNAL OF MEDICAL EDUCATION, 1977, 52(9), 731-738.*
INDX CULTURAL FACTORS, DISCRIMINATION, ECONOMIC FACTORS, EDUCATION, EQUAL OPPORTUNITY, ESSAY, HEALTH EDUCATION, HIGHER EDUCATION, LEGISLATION, MEDICAL STUDENTS, MEXICAN AMERICAN, OCCUPATIONAL ASPIRATIONS, PROFESSIONAL TRAINING, SCHOLASTIC ASPIRATIONS, SES, REPRESENTATION
ABST THE CONGRESS AND THE ASSOCIATION OF AMERICAN MEDICAL COLLEGES (AAMC) HAVE THE COMMON OBJECTIVE OF ENSURING THAT ALL AMERICANS WILL ENJOY A HIGH LEVEL OF MEDICAL CARE. IN FURTHERANCE OF THAT OBJECTIVE, AN AAMC TASK FORCE IN 1970 RECOMMENDED THAT REPRESENTATION OF MINORITY GROUPS IN M.D. PROGRAMS BE INCREASED FROM 2.8% TO 12% BY 1975-76. WHILE THAT GOAL WAS NOT REALIZED, SUBSTANTIAL PROGRESS HAS BEEN MADE. FORMIDABLE BARRIERS (INCLUDING HIGHER GRADUATE EDUCATION TUITION, LIMITED SCHOLARSHIPS FUNDS, AND INADEQUATE ACADEMIC PREPARATION) REMAIN FOR MANY MINORITY STUDENTS WHO WANT TO ENTER THE HEALTH PROFESSIONS. PERHAPS THE GREATEST BARRIER CONSISTS OF THE SUBTLE DISCRIMINATORY PRESSURES THAT MANIFEST THEMSELVES IN ALL INSTITUTIONS OF THE COUNTRY. THE PHRASE "REVERSE DISCRIMINATION" POSES A NEW POLITICAL OBSTACLE TO THE ELIMINATION OF SUCH PRESSURES. A SERIES OF COURT DECISIONS HAS BEGUN TO ERODE THE SPECIAL ADMISSIONS PROGRAMS THAT ARE ATTEMPTING TO OPEN UP PROFESSIONAL SCHOOLS TO MEMBERS OF MINORITY GROUPS. 6 REFERENCES. (JOURNAL ABSTRACT MODIFIED)

ACCN 002039

242 AUTH **BURMA, J. H.**
TITL SPANISH-SPEAKING GROUPS IN THE UNITED STATES.
SRCE *LONDON: DUKE UNIVERSITY PRESS, 1954.*
INDX MIGRATION, IMMIGRATION, SPANISH SURNAMED, MEXICAN AMERICAN, CUBAN, PUERTO RICAN-M, HISTORY, LABOR FORCE, FARM LABORERS, SCHOLASTIC ACHIEVEMENT, BILINGUALISM, DISCRIMINATION, PREJUDICE, RELIGION, ACCULTURATION, EDUCATION, POVERTY, SES, ESSAY, REVIEW, NEW YORK, NEW MEXICO, EAST, SOUTHWEST, BOOK
ABST THE SPANISH SPEAKING GROUPS UNDER STUDY IN THIS BOOK ARE THE HISPANOS OF NEW MEXICO, MEXICAN AMERICANS FROM THE SOUTHWEST, FILIPINO AMERICANS FROM THE WEST COAST, AND PUERTO RICANS FROM NEW

YORK. ALL GROUPS ARE SYMPATHETICALLY PORTRAYED THROUGH THEIR HISTORY, MIGRATION, CULTURAL CHARACTERISTICS, EMPLOYMENT AND ECONOMIC STATUS, ASSIMILATION PATTERNS, RELIGION, ORGANIZATIONS, AND POLITICAL LOYALTIES. MEXICAN AMERICANS COMPRISE THE LARGEST OF THE GROUPS STUDIED AND PRESENT CERTAIN FEATURES UNIQUE IN THE HISTORY OF HUMAN MIGRATION. VARIOUS ASPECTS OF ATTITUDES OF THE RECEIVING SOCIETY (E.G., PREJUDICES, DISCRIMINATION, AND SOCIAL STRATIFICATION) ARE DISCUSSED. SOCIAL PROBLEMS OF EACH GROUP ARE SEEN AS STEMMING FROM ECONOMIC DEPRIVATION, MINIMAL ACCESS TO POLITICS, POOR EDUCATION, ANTIMINORITY VIEWS, AND SOCIAL STEREOTYPES. THE FINAL CHAPTER DEALS WITH "LOS HERMANOS PENITENTES—A FLAGELLANT BROTHERHOOD SOCIETY WHICH IS DISCUSSED IN TERMS OF ITS SIGNIFICANCE TO MEXICAN CULTURAL HERITAGE. 159 REFERENCES.

ACCN 000203

243 AUTH **BURRUEL, G.**
TITL LA FRONTERA, A MENTAL HEALTH CLINIC IN THE CHICANO COMMUNITY.
SRCE *IN THE REPORT OF THE SOUTHWEST STATES CHICANO CONSUMER CONFERENCE ON HEALTH. ROCKVILLE, MD.: U.S. DEPARTMENT OF HEALTH, EDUCATION AND WELFARE, 1972, PP. 27-33.*
INDX MENTAL HEALTH, HEALTH DELIVERY SYSTEMS, MEXICAN AMERICAN, COMMUNITY, PROGRAM EVALUATION, FINANCING, ARIZONA, SOUTHWEST, ESSAY
ABST LA FRONTERA, A MENTAL HEALTH OUTPATIENT CLINIC, IS PART OF A RECENTLY FORMED NETWORK OF MENTAL HEALTH SERVICES IN THE TUCSON, ARIZONA, AREA ESPECIALLY DESIGNED TO SERVE THE LARGE CHICANO POPULATION OF THAT AREA. CONTRARY TO THE LITERATURE ON MEXICAN AMERICANS' USE OF MENTAL HEALTH FACILITIES, LA FRONTERA IS SUCCESSFUL IN ATTRACTION AND TREATING SPANISH- SPEAKING CLIENTS. THE PAPER TRACES THE DEVELOPMENT OF THIS PROGRAM, ITS CURRENT FUNCTIONING, AND FEATURES IN THE HOPE THAT IT MAY BE HELPFUL TO OTHERS IN PLANNING AND DEVELOPING PROGRAMS TO SERVE CHICANOS. PROPOSAL DEVELOPMENT, FUNDING ARRANGEMENTS, PRESENT STATUS OF THE PROGRAM, AND FUTURE PLANS ARE DISCUSSED.
ACCN 000206

244 AUTH **BURRUEL, G., & CHAVEZ, N.**
TITL INDIVIDUAL INVOLVEMENT IN THE CHICANO MOVEMENT.
SRCE *IN M. M. MANGOLD (ED.), LA CAUSA CHICANA: THE MOVEMENT FOR JUSTICE. NEW YORK: FAMILY SERVICE ASSOCIATION OF AMERICA, 1971, PP. 30-41.*
INDX MEXICAN AMERICAN, CHICANO MOVEMENT, ETHNIC IDENTITY, ADULTS, SURVEY, ATTITUDES, SOUTHWEST
ABST THE MAJOR TASK OF THIS STUDY WAS TO DE-

TERMINE WHY AND HOW INDIVIDUALS BECOME INVOLVED IN THE CHICANO MOVEMENT. NEW INSIGHTS INTO THIS PROCESS WERE GAINED FROM DATA COLLECTED VIA LENGTHY, UNSTRUCTURED INTERVIEWS WITH 18 CHICANOS WHO WERE KNOWN TO HAVE VARIOUS RELATIONSHIPS WITH THE MOVEMENT. RANGING IN AGE FROM 22 TO 70 AND LIVING IN THE SOUTHWEST, THE SUBJECTS WERE ASKED ABOUT THEIR PRESENT SITUATION, PAST BACKGROUND, AND FEELINGS AND ATTITUDES TOWARD THE MOVEMENT. THE TYPOLOGY WHICH EVOLVED FROM THE INTERVIEW DATA INCLUDED THESE FOUR DIMENSIONS OF INVOLVEMENT: (1) NEGATIVELY AFFECTIVELY INVOLVED; (2) POSITIVELY AFFECTIVELY INVOLVED; (3) INDIRECTLY BEHAVIORALLY INVOLVED; AND (4) DIRECTLY BEHAVIORALLY INVOLVED. THOUGH NOT AN EXHAUSTIVE TYPOLOGY, IT ALLOWS ANALYSIS OF INDIVIDUAL INVOLVEMENT IN RELATION TO SOCIAL-PERSONAL SITUATION, ADJUSTMENT TO LIVING IN AN ANGLO SOCIETY, PERCEPTION OF THE MEXICAN AMERICAN SITUATION, AND PERCEPTION OF THE MOVEMENT. THE FOLLOWING CONDITIONS APPEAR TO BE NECESSARY BEFORE AN INDIVIDUAL BECOMES INVOLVED: (1) SOME DEGREE OF EXPLICIT AWARENESS OF THE PROBLEMS FACING MEXICAN AMERICANS; (2) TRANSITION FROM IDENTIFICATION AS AN INDIVIDUAL TO THAT OF A MEMBER OF THE BROADER ETHNIC GROUP EXPERIENCING PROBLEMS; AND (3) DECISION OF THE INDIVIDUAL TO DO SOMETHING ABOUT THE PROBLEMS FACING MEXICAN AMERICANS. 12 REFERENCES. (AUTHOR SUMMARY MODIFIED)

ACCN 000207

245 AUTH **BURRUEL, G., & CHAVEZ, N.**
TITL MENTAL HEALTH OUTPATIENT CENTERS: RELEVANT OR IRRELEVANT TO MEXICAN AMERICANS.
SRCE *IN A. B. TULIPAN, C. L. ATTNEAVE & E. KINGSTONE (EDS.), BEYOND CLINIC WALLS. UNIVERSITY, ALA.: UNIVERSITY OF ALABAMA PRESS, 1974, PP. 108-129.*
INDX MENTAL HEALTH, HEALTH DELIVERY SYSTEMS, SOCIAL SERVICES, MEXICAN AMERICAN, CULTURAL FACTORS, COMMUNITY, MENTAL HEALTH PROFESSION, ARIZONA, SOUTHWEST, ESSAY
ABST ISSUES CONCERNING THE IRRELEVANCY OF MENTAL HEALTH CLINICS TO MEXICAN AMERICANS ARE IDENTIFIED AND DISCUSSED. REASONS FOR THE INEFFECTIVENESS AND UNDERUTILIZATION OF AVAILABLE SERVICES BY MEXICAN AMERICANS ARE: (1) CONTINUED USE OF TRADITIONAL PSYCHIATRIC SERVICES; (2) DIFFERENCES IN SYMPTOM CATEGORIZATION; (3) LACK OF BILINGUAL/BICULTURAL CAREGIVERS; (4) DIFFERENCES IN VIEWING TREATMENT; (5) THE LOW VISIBILITY OF MENTAL HEALTH DISORDERS AMONG MEXICAN AMERICANS; AND (6) LOCATION OF SERVICES. A DESCRIPTION OF THE DEVELOPMENT AND SUCCESS OF LA FRONTERA, A MENTAL HEALTH OUTPATIENT CLINIC IN TUCSON, DEMONSTRATES HOW EVERY ONE OF THE OBSTACLES

TO BETTER SERVICE LISTED ABOVE HAS BEEN OVERCOME. IT IS CONCLUDED THROUGH THE ACCOMPLISHMENTS OF THIS CLINIC THAT MENTAL HEALTH CENTERS CAN BE RELEVANT TO MEXICAN AMERICANS. 22 REFERENCES.

ACCN 000208

246 AUTH **BURRUEL, J. M.**
TITL A STUDY OF MEXICAN-AMERICAN TENTH-GRADE STUDENTS SHOWING THE RELATIONSHIP BETWEEN PARENTAL ATTITUDES AND SOCIOECONOMIC LEVEL (DOCTORAL DISSERTATION, ARIZONA STATE UNIVERSITY, 1970).
SRCE *DISSERTATION ABSTRACTS INTERNATIONAL, 1970, 32(1), 114A. (UNIVERSITY MICROFILMS NO. 71-13,241.)*
INDX SCHOLASTIC ACHIEVEMENT, SES, MEXICAN AMERICAN, ADOLESCENTS, ADULTS, ATTITUDES, EMPIRICAL, EDUCATION, PERFORMANCE EXPECTATIONS, TEACHERS, ADMINISTRATORS, ARIZONA, SOUTHWEST
ABST TO DETERMINE THE EFFECT OF PARENTAL ATTITUDES AND SOCIO-ECONOMIC LEVEL (SES) ON THE LENGTH OF TIME THEIR CHILDREN REMAIN IN SCHOOL, A SAMPLE OF ONE HUNDRED HOUSEHOLDS WAS SELECTED REPRESENTING PARENTS OF TENTH-GRADE STUDENTS WHO HAD EITHER DROPPED OUT OR WERE STILL IN THE PHOENIX SCHOOL SYSTEM. A THREE-WAY ANALYSIS OF VARIANCE WAS PERFORMED ON SCHOOL STATUS, SES, AND PARENTS, AND DISCRIMINANT ANALYSIS WAS PERFORMED USING ATTITUDE SCORES TO PREDICT SCHOOL STATUS. THE DATA REVEALED THE FOLLOWING: (1) ATTITUDE OF PARENTS WAS INFLUENCED BY BOTH SCHOOL STATUS OF CHILD AND SES; (2) ALL PARENTS HAD POSITIVE ATTITUDES TOWARD ALL LEVELS OF EDUCATION, SCHOOL TEACHERS AND ADMINISTRATORS, AND SCHOOL PRACTICES EXCEPT FOR DROPPING OUT PRACTICES; (3) PARENTS WITH HIGHER SES WITH CHILDREN STILL IN SCHOOL HAD MORE POSITIVE ATTITUDE TOWARDS HOMEWORK THAN PARENTS WHOSE CHILDREN HAVE DROPPED OUT OF SCHOOL; AND (4) PARENTS, OVERALL, PERCEIVE AND EXPECT THEIR CHILDREN TO ACT DOMINEERING AND AFFECTIONATE INSTEAD OF PASSIVE OR HOSTILE. THESE FINDINGS INDICATE THE NEED FOR FURTHER STUDIES TO EXAMINE WAYS SCHOOLS CAN IMPROVE THE EDUCATIONAL ENVIRONMENT FOR MEXICAN AMERICAN STUDENTS. 65 REFERENCES.
ACCN 000205

247 AUTH **BURSTEIN, A. G., & KOBOS, J.**
TITL PSYCHOLOGICAL TESTING AS A DEVICE TO FOSTER SOCIAL MOBILITY.
SRCE *AMERICAN PSYCHOLOGIST, 1971, 26(11), 1041-1042.*
INDX SOCIAL MOBILITY, PARENTAL INVOLVEMENT, ADOLESCENTS, CATTELL CULTURE-FREE INTELLIGENCE TEST, OCCUPATIONAL ASPIRATIONS, INTELLIGENCE TESTING, MEXICAN AMERICAN, TEXAS, SOUTHWEST
ABST THE INITIATION BY A UNIVERSITY GROUP OF A HEALTH CAREER OPPORTUNITIES PROGRAM IN COLLABORATION WITH A LOCAL HIGH SCHOOL IS DISCUSSED. THE ESSENCE OF THE PROGRAM WAS LINKING MEDICAL AND NURSING STUDENTS WITH A POPULATION OF HIGH SCHOOL STUDENTS, MAINLY CHICANO, AND TESTING SERVICES WERE OFFERED AND THE RESULTS MADE AVAILABLE TO THE STUDENTS AND THEIR PARENTS. THE PROGRAM IS CONCLUDED TO BE SUCCESSFUL IN TERMS OF STUDENT-PARENT-TEACHER-PSYCHOLOGY TRAINEE INVOLVEMENT, AND IT IS NOTED THAT PSYCHOLOGICAL TESTING WAS USED POSITIVELY TO MAXIMIZE THE SUBJECTS' EFFECTIVE FREEDOM TO CHOOSE AMONG REALISTIC GOALS.
ACCN 000204

248 AUTH **BUSH, J. A.**
TITL THE MINORITY ADMINISTRATOR: IMPLICATIONS FOR SOCIAL WORK EDUCATION.
SRCE *JOURNAL OF EDUCATION FOR SOCIAL WORK, 1977, 13(1), 15-22.*
INDX ADMINISTRATORS, ADULTS, ATTITUDES, CROSS CULTURAL, DISCRIMINATION, EMPIRICAL, EMPLOYMENT, EQUAL OPPORTUNITY, JOB PERFORMANCE, HIGHER EDUCATION, ROLE EXPECTATIONS, MEXICAN AMERICAN, SURVEY, PROFESSIONAL TRAINING
ABST SINCE THERE IS EVIDENCE OF DISCRIMINATION IN ETHNIC MINORITIES' (PARTICULARLY BLACKS AND CHICANOS) EXPERIENCES IN ADMINISTRATIVE SOCIAL WORK POSITIONS, 30 TOP LEVEL MINORITY SOCIAL SERVICE ADMINISTRATORS WERE INTERVIEWED FROM ACROSS THE NATION, WITH A CONCENTRATION IN SOUTHERN CALIFORNIA. THE SAMPLE INCLUDED MEN (N = 26) AND WOMEN (N = 4), AND 15 BLACK AND 15 CHICANO ADMINISTRATORS. ALSO, THE SAMPLE WAS LOOSELY STRATIFIED TO REPRESENT PUBLIC AND PRIVATE ORGANIZATIONS, PUBLIC AND NON-PROFIT ORGANIZATIONS, SERVICE AND BUSINESS ORGANIZATIONS, AND ANGLO-RUN AND MINORITY-RUN ORGANIZATIONS. ADMINISTRATORS WERE ASKED 28 QUESTIONS ABOUT THEMSELVES, THEIR AGENCIES, AND THEIR PERSONAL EXPERIENCES AS MINORITY ADMINISTRATORS. IN DISCUSSING PERSONAL EXPERIENCES, THEY WERE ASKED TO DESCRIBE A SERIES OF ISSUES: COMPETENCE, APPOINTMENT, COMPARATIVE QUALIFICATIONS, PREPARATION FOR ASSIGNED DUTIES, AND STAFF AND PEER RELATIONSHIPS. THE FINDINGS SHOW THAT THE ADMINISTRATORS PERCEIVE THEMSELVES AS BEING REQUIRED TO HAVE GREATER JOB ENTRANCE CAPABILITIES, RECEIVING LESS ORGANIZATIONAL SUPPORT, HAVING LESS INTRINSIC AUTHORITY, AND HAVING LIMITED OPPORTUNITIES FOR UPWARD MOVEMENT IN COMPARISON WITH THEIR ANGLO PEERS, AS WELL AS HAVING LIMITED CHANNELS FOR COMMUNICATION. RECOMMENDATIONS FOR SOCIAL WORK EDUCATION ARE GIVEN. 8 REFERENCES. (NCMHI ABSTRACT MODIFIED)
ACCN 002041

249 AUTH **BUSTAMANTE, J. A.**

TITL   THE IMMIGRANT WORKER: A SOCIAL PROBLEM OR A HUMAN RESOURCE.

SRCE   *EL MIRLO CANTA DE NOTICATLAN, 1977, 4(7-8), 1-4. (PUBLICATION OF CHICANO STUDIES CENTER, UNIVERSITY OF CALIFORNIA, LOS ANGELES.)*

INDX   UNDOCUMENTED WORKERS, IMMIGRATION, MEXICO, POLICY, ESSAY, POVERTY, POLITICS, POLICE-COMMUNITY RELATIONS

ABST   THE PHENOMENON OF UNDOCUMENTED IMMIGRATION FROM MEXICO STEMS FROM TWO INTERRELATED FACTORS: (1) A DEMAND FOR CHEAP LABOR IN THE UNITED STATES; AND (2) UNEMPLOYMENT, ECONOMIC DEPENDENCY, AND POVERTY IN MEXICO. THIS MEANS THAT WHATEVER MEASURE IS TAKEN BY ONE COUNTRY WITHOUT TAKING INTO ACCOUNT INTERVENING FACTORS ON THE OTHER SIDE OF THE BORDER WILL NOT ONLY MAINTAIN THE PROBLEM BUT MAY WORSEN IT. ANY APPROACH TO THE PROBLEM, THEN, MUST BE BINATIONAL. RESTRICTIVE MEASURES—SUCH AS REINFORCING POLICE TYPE PROGRAMS AND/OR LAUNCHING MASSIVE DEPORTATIONS—HAVE FAILED IN THE PAST PRECISELY BECAUSE THEY ARE UNILATERAL IN APPROACH. MEXICO SHOULD NOT PASSIVELY ACCEPT U.S. INTERNAL MEASURES OF DEPORTATIONS OF MEXICAN NATIONALS WHICH, IN TURN, RESULT IN FURTHER INCREASES IN MEXICO'S ALREADY HIGH UNEMPLOYMENT. INSTEAD, IN THE EVENT OF NEW CHANGES IN U.S. IMMIGRATION POLICIES TOWARD MEXICO (LIKE P.L. 94-571, SIGNED ON OCTOBER 20, 1976), THE MEXICAN GOVERNMENT SHOULD EXPLORE VARIOUS COUNTER-MEASURES—E.G., INSTITUTING A DEFENSE OF HUMAN RIGHTS OF THE MEXICAN IMMIGRANT IN THE CONTEXT OF U.S.-LATIN AMERICAN RELATIONS, SIMILAR TO WHAT HAS BEEN EFFECTED IN THE PANAMA CANAL; OR SEEKING EXPRESSIONS OF SOLIDARITY FROM U.S. MINORITY GROUPS, PARTICULARLY THOSE OF MEXICAN DESCENT. IN TERMS OF EFFICIENCY, THESE STRATEGIES MIGHT NOT BE MORE EFFECTIVE THAN INTERNATIONAL NEGOTIATIONS BETWEEN THE TWO GOVERNMENTS; BUT THEY MIGHT BE THE ONLY KIND OF ALTERNATIVES LEFT FOR A COUNTRY THAT FACES LIMITATIONS IN OFFERING UNDOCUMENTED NATIVES CONDITIONS OF HUMAN DIGNITY AND SELF-DETERMINATION THAT WOULD KEEP THEM IN THE LAND OF THEIR ANCESTORS. 9 REFERENCES.

ACCN   002042

250 AUTH   **BUSTAMANTE, J. A.**

TITL   STRUCTURAL AND IDEOLOGICAL CONDITIONS OF THE MEXICAN UNDOCUMENTED IMMIGRATION TO THE UNITED STATES.

SRCE   *AMERICAN BEHAVIORAL SCIENTIST, 1976, 19(3), 364-376.*

INDX   SES, UNDOCUMENTED WORKERS, MARXIAN THEORY, IMMIGRATION, HISTORY, ESSAY, MEXICAN, CROSS CULTURAL, LABOR FORCE, ECONOMIC FACTORS, CAPITALISM, GANGS, MEXICAN AMERICAN

ABST   A MYTH THAT ATTRIBUTES HIGH UNEMPLOYMENT TO IMMIGRANTS COMING INTO THE UNITED STATES HAS EXISTED FROM THE TIME OF THE 1830'S IRISH IMMIGRATION. PERMEATED BY AN ETHNIC BIAS AGAINST FOREIGN "DEVIANT" GROUPS, THIS MYTH HAS GROWN OUT OF THE DIALECTICAL RELATIONSHIP BETWEEN SOCIETY'S ECONOMIC BASE AND ITS FUNCTIONS; AND IT HAS SERVED TO FRAGMENT WORKERS AND DAMPEN THEIR PROTESTS BY IMPUTING TO OUTSIDERS THE CAUSE OF ECONOMIC INEQUALITIES. AT THE SAME TIME IT HAS ENABLED GOVERNMENT AGENCIES TO PROTECT THE ECONOMIC INTERESTS OF DOMINANT GROUPS AND PROVIDED A BASIS FOR DEMONSTRATING CONCERN FOR WORKERS' INTERESTS BY DEPORTING ILLEGAL IMMIGRANTS OR BY RESTRICTING IMMIGRATION. THE INFLUENCE OF THIS MYTH ON PUBLIC POLICY AND INDUSTRIAL EXPANSION IS DISCUSSED. 14 REFERENCES. (AUTHOR SUMMARY MODIFIED)

ACCN   000210

251 AUTH   **BUSTAMENTE, J. A.**

TITL   CULTURAL FACTORS IN HYSTERIAS WITH SCHIZOPHRENIC CLINICAL PICTURE.

SRCE   *INTERNATIONAL JOURNAL OF SOCIAL PSYCHIATRY, 1968, 14(2), 113-118.*

INDX   CULTURAL FACTORS, SCHIZOPHRENIA, CUBAN, RELIGION, RORSCHACH TEST, ESSAY, PSYCHOPATHOLOGY, EMPIRICAL, CARIBBEAN

ABST   AN ANTHROPOLOGIC-CLINICAL STUDY OF 127 PATIENTS WITH DISSOCIATIVE SCHIZOPHRENIC REACTION IN A HAVANA, CUBA, PSYCHIATRIC CLINIC IS PRESENTED. THE SAMPLE INCLUDED PATIENTS OF BOTH SEXES AND ANGLO, BLACK, AND MULATTO RACES WHO SHOWED A MYSTICAL OR PERSECUTORY DELUSION WITH VISUAL HALLUCINATIONS. EMPLOYING RORSCHACH AND MIRA LOPEZ' MIOKINETIC PSYCHODIAGNOSTIC TESTS, THESE PATIENTS ARE DESCRIBED AS HAVING A DISSOCIATIVE REACTION (HYSTERIA) IN WHICH CHANGES IN THE PATIENT'S CONSCIOUS PATTERN APPEAR TO BE A PSYCHOTIC DISTURBANCE DURING WHICH LOGICAL THINKING AND MAGICAL THOUGHTS OCCUR SIMULTANEOUSLY. WHEN THIS DISSOCIATIVE REACTION OCCURS IT IS IMPOSSIBLE TO KEEP BOTH THOUGHT PROCESSES APART, AND THE TOTAL MAGIC INFLUENCE OF RELIGIOUS BELIEF APPEARS AS A DELUSION. THIS PROCESS IS RELATED TO THE PARTICULAR MIXTURE OF SPANISH CATHOLICISM AND AFRICAN YORUBA RELIGION COMMON TO THE CUBAN NATIVES ATTENDING THE CLINIC. THIS TYPE OF PSYCHIATRIC PROBLEM AND THE CULTURAL FACTORS WHICH CAN CHANGE THE CLASSICAL NOSOLOGICAL PICTURE ARE A PRACTICAL EXAMPLE OF WHAT TRANSCULTURAL PSYCHIATRIC RESEARCH HAS TO OFFER. 18 REFERENCES.

ACCN   000211

252 AUTH   **BUTCHER, J. N., & GARCIA, R. E.**

TITL   CROSS-NATIONAL APPLICATION OF PSYCHOLOGICAL TESTS.

SRCE   *PERSONNEL AND GUIDANCE JOURNAL, 1978, 56(8), 472-475.*

INDX   CROSS CULTURAL, CULTURAL FACTORS, CUL-

TURE-FAIR TESTS, ESSAY, EXAMINER EFFECTS, INTELLIGENCE TESTING, MMPI, PERSONALITY ASSESSMENT, TEST RELIABILITY, TEST VALIDITY, RESEARCH METHODOLOGY

ABST A REVIEW OF PRACTICAL ISSUES INVOLVED IN THE ADAPTATION AND APPLICATION OF ENGLISH LANGUAGE PERSONALITY INVENTORIES CROSS-NATIONALLY IS MADE WITH SPECIFIC REFERENCE TO THE MINNESOTA MULTIPHASIC PERSONALITY INVENTORY (MMPI). METHODOLOGICAL PROBLEMS ENCOUNTERED IN THE CROSS-CULTURAL STUDY OF PERSONALITY INCLUDE: (1) DIFFERENCES IN PERSONALITY CHARACTERISTICS; (2) NONEQUIVALENCE OF PSYCHOLOGICAL CONSTRUCTS; (3) LANGUAGE DIFFERENCES; (4) BEHAVIOR DIFFERENCES RELATED TO CULTURAL CONTEXTS; (5) APPROPRIATENESS OF TEST INSTRUMENTS; (6) DIFFICULTIES IN RANDOM SELECTION OR STRATIFIED SAMPLING PROCEDURES; AND (7) PROBLEMS OF DETERMINING APPROPRIATE EVALUATION CRITERIA. IN TRANSLATING PERSONALITY INVENTORIES, ONE ENCOUNTERS LINGUISTIC PROBLEMS (E.G., IDIOMATIC SPEECH, AND DIFFERENCES IN GRAMMAR AND SYNTAX) AND PROBLEMS IN DETERMINING THE CULTURAL AND PSYCHOLOGICAL EQUIVALENCY OF TEST ITEMS. TO MINIMIZE THESE DIFFICULTIES, TRANSLATORS MUST BE VERY FAMILIAR WITH BOTH THE ORIGINAL AND THE TARGET LANGUAGE. ALTHOUGH CROSS-CULTURAL TEST GENERALIZATION AND VALIDITY ARE DIFFICULT TO ESTABLISH, ADAPTATION OF PSYCHOLOGICAL INSTRUMENTS ENABLES PROFESSIONAL PSYCHOLOGISTS IN COUNTRIES WHERE FINANCIAL RESOURCES ARE LIMITED TO HAVE A PSYCHOTECHNOLOGY THAT THEY WOULD OTHERWISE NOT HAVE. IN ADDITION, IT ALLOWS THE DEVELOPMENT OF TECHNIQUES FOR CROSS-CULTURALLY COMPARING PERSONALITY DEVELOPMENT IN TERMS OF DIFFERING ENVIRONMENTAL VARIABLES. 8 REFERENCES.

ACCN 002043

253 AUTH **BUYS, C. J., FIELD, T. K., & SCHMIDT, M. M.**
TITL A COMPARISON OF LOW SOCIO-ECONOMIC MEXICAN AMERICAN STUDENTS' AND PARENTS' ATTITUDES TOWARD COLLEGE EDUCATION.
SRCE *PERSONALITY AND SOCIAL PSYCHOLOGY BULLETIN, 1976, 2(3), 294-298.*
INDX MEXICAN AMERICAN, SES, COLLEGE STUDENTS, SCHOLASTIC ACHIEVEMENT, EDUCATION, EDUCATIONAL COUNSELING, PARENTAL INVOLVEMENT, ATTITUDES, ACHIEVEMENT MOTIVATION, EMPIRICAL, HIGHER EDUCATION, NEW MEXICO, SOUTHWEST, SCHOLASTIC ASPIRATIONS
ABST ATTITUDES TOWARD EDUCATION AMONG A GROUP OF LOW SOCIOECONOMIC (SES) MEXICAN AMERICAN STUDENTS (N⅞0) AND THEIR PARENTS WERE ASSESSED AND COMPARED. QUESTIONNAIRES AND INTERVIEWS FROM A SAMPLE SURVEY SHOWED THAT LOW-SES MEXICAN AMERICAN STUDENTS HELD FAVORABLE ATTITUDES TOWARD COLLEGE EDUCATION. STUDENTS, HOWEVER, WHEN COM-

PARED WITH THEIR PARENTS HELD SIGNIFICANTLY LESS FAVORABLE ATTITUDES TOWARD COLLEGE EDUCATION. THE FACT THAT OVER ONE-HALF OF THE STUDENTS IN THIS SAMPLE DID NOT PLAN TO ATTEND COLLEGE REFLECTED THIS ATTITUDE. THE DISCREPANCY BETWEEN THE STUDENTS' AND THE PARENTS' ATTITUDES WAS ATTRIBUTED TO GENERATIONAL DIFFERENCES. THE DISCREPANCY BETWEEN THE STUDENTS' FAVORABLE ATTITUDES TOWARD COLLEGE AND THEIR HESITANCY TO ENROLL IN COLLEGE WAS ATTRIBUTED TO A GROWING DISCONTENTMENT WITH COLLEGE EDUCATION. THE IMPORTANCE OF A STUDENT'S PERCEIVING HIS HOME ENVIRONMENT AS CONDUCIVE TO EDUCATION IS ALSO DISCUSSED. 9 REFERENCES. (AUTHOR ABSTRACT MODIFIED)

ACCN 000212

254 AUTH **BYRNE, D., MALDONADO, L., & RIVERA, O.**
TITL CHICANOS IN UTAH.
SRCE *SALT LAKE CITY: THE UTAH STATE BOARD OF EDUCATION, 1976.*
INDX ACCULTURATION, CULTURAL FACTORS, EDUCATION, REPRESENTATION, MEXICAN AMERICAN, EMPIRICAL, EQUAL OPPORTUNITY, ECONOMIC FACTORS, SES, SOCIAL SERVICES, INTELLIGENCE TESTING, SCHOLASTIC ACHIEVEMENT, DISCRIMINATION, THEORETICAL, SOCIAL SCIENCES, RURAL, URBAN, OCCUPATIONAL ASPIRATIONS, ATTITUDES, LABOR FORCE, COMMUNITY, PROGRAM EVALUATION, PERSONNEL, ADULTS, CHILDREN, ACHIEVEMENT TESTING, CULTURAL PLURALISM, EMPLOYMENT, UTAH, WEST
ABST USING THE MODEL OF INTERNAL COLONIALISM—IDENTIFIED BY (A) THE MINORITY GROUP'S MODE OF ENTRY INTO THE SOCIETY, (B) THE FORCED ALTERATION OF THE COLONIZED PEOPLES' INSTITUTIONS BY THE DOMINANT GROUP, (C) THE EXTERNAL ADMINISTRATION CARRIED OUT BY THE DOMINANT SOCIETY, AND (D) ENDEMIC RACIST PATTERNS OF BEHAVIOR WITHIN SOCIETAL INSTITUTIONS—THIS STUDY EXAMINES THE SOCIAL CONDITIONS OF CHICANOS IN AN AREA WHERE THEY CONSTITUTE A NUMERICALLY MINOR PORTION OF THE POPULATION. RESEARCH FOCUSED ON (1) OCCUPATIONAL HISTORY, ASPIRATIONS AND EDUCATIONAL LEVELS OF 1,783 CHICANO CLIENTS OF THE STATE EMPLOYMENT AGENCY, (2) DEMOGRAPHIC CHARACTERISTICS, VALUES, AND ATTITUDES OF 270 SOCIAL SERVICE AGENCY PERSONNEL, (3) THE PERSPECTIVES OF 2,691 AGENCY CLIENTS ON SOCIAL SERVICE AGENCIES, (4) FAMILY BIOGRAPHIC INFORMATION, RESULTS OF IQ AND STANDARDIZED ACHIEVEMENT TESTS, AND GRADE POINT AVERAGE OF 1,479 CHICANO STUDENTS, AND (5) THE EDUCATORS' VIEW OF CHICANO STUDENTS. THE SAMPLE SELECTED REPRESENTED A GEOGRAPHIC AND ECONOMIC CROSS-SECTION OF THE ENTIRE STATE. FINDINGS IN THIS STUDY PARALLELED THOSE IN AREAS WHERE THE SPANISH-SPEAKING CONSTITUTE A LARGE PROPORTION OF THE POPULATION. ALTHOUGH THE SOCIAL SITUATION OF THE CHI-

CANO HAS HISTORICALLY BEEN ANALYZED IN TERMS OF AN ASSIMILATIONIST PERSPECTIVE, IT IS CONCLUDED THAT A MORE ACCURATE EXPLANATION CAN BE MADE FROM THE PERSPECTIVE OF INTERNAL COLONIALISM. 27 REFERENCES.

ACCN   000213

255   AUTH   **CABRERA, Y. A.**
      TITL   SCHIZOPHRENIA IN THE SOUTHWEST: MEXICAN AMERICANS IN ANGLO-LAND.
      SRCE   *IN M. P. DOUGLASS (ED.), CLAREMONT READING CONFERENCE: THIRTY-FIRST YEARBOOK. CLAREMONT, CALIF.: CLAREMONT GRADUATE SCHOOL AND UNIVERSITY CENTER, 1967, PP. 101-106.*
      INDX   CULTURE, HISTORY, ETHNIC IDENTITY, SOCIAL MOBILITY, ACCULTURATION, ESSAY, CROSS CULTURAL, EDUCATION, POLICY, MEXICAN AMERICAN, CULTURAL PLURALISM, SOUTHWEST
      ABST   THE HYPOTHESIS THAT MEXICAN AMERICANS (MA) AND ANGLO AMERICANS (AA) LIVE IN WORLDS OF UNREALITY WITH REFERENCE TO EACH OTHER IS EXAMINED. THE LIFE OF THE MA IS COMPLICATED BY THE THREE WORLDS THEY LIVE IN: ONE WORLD HAS ITS HISTORICAL FOUNDATIONS IN EUROPE, THE OTHER IS INDO-MEXICAN WITH ITS FOLK-CULTURE CHARACTERISTICS, AND THE LAST IS ANGLO AMERICAN. THE BASIC PROBLEM IN ATTEMPTING TO UNDERSTAND THIS CIRCUMSTANCE IS THAT NONE OF THESE WORLDS IS A FULL REALITY FOR MA'S. THESE WORLDS ARE MIXTURES OF FACT AND FANTASY IN THE LIFE OF THE MA. IT IS SHOWN THAT MA'S REFLECT DEGREES OF ORIENTATIONS FROM A MEXICAN TO AA CULTURE. MA'S WHO ARE SOCIALLY MOBILE ARE NOT EXACT COUNTERPARTS OF AA MIDDLE CLASS, AND THOSE WHO ARE MIDDLE CLASS SEEM TO LOSE THEIR ETHNIC-GROUP IDENTITY. AA'S TEND TO VIEW SOCIALLY DISADVANTAGED MA'S IN TERMS OF FOLK-CULTURE TRAITS AND APPEAR TO BE GENERALLY UNAWARE OF THE CONCERNS OF MA'S. IT IS CONCLUDED THAT AA'S AND MA'S IN THE SOUTHWEST DO NOT UNDERSTAND EACH OTHER VERY WELL. A MAJOR IMPLICATION OF THIS CIRCUMSTANCE IS THAT INSTRUCTIONAL OBJECTIVES IN OUR SCHOOLS WILL CONTINUE TO FALTER UNLESS EDUCATORS RECOGNIZE THE IMPORTANCE OF UNDERSTANDING CULTURE AND LANGUAGE DIFFERENCES AS WELL AS ETHNIC AND RACIAL DIVERSITY IN SCHOOL CHILDREN. 6 REFERENCES.
      ACCN   000214

256   AUTH   **CAGEL, W. P.**
      TITL   THE USE OF COMMUNITY WORKERS IN A SPANISH SPEAKING COMMUNITY.
      SRCE   *IN E. R. PADILLA & A. M. PADILLA (EDS.), TRANSCULTURAL PSYCHIATRY: AN HISPANIC PERSPECTIVE (MONOGRAPH NO. 4). LOS ANGELES: UNIVERSITY OF CALIFORNIA, SPANISH SPEAKING MENTAL HEALTH RESEARCH CENTER, 1977, PP. 67-71.*
      INDX   PARAPROFESSIONALS, BILINGUAL-BICULTURAL PERSONNEL, COMMUNITY, COMMUNITY

INVOLVEMENT, PRIMARY PREVENTION, ESSAY, CALIFORNIA, SOUTHWEST, MENTAL HEALTH, PROGRAM EVALUATION

      ABST   THE UTILIZATION OF COMMUNITY WORKERS BY OLIVE VIEW COMMUNITY MENTAL HEALTH CENTER IN SAN FERNANDO, LOS ANGELES COUNTY, IS DESCRIBED. THE SUCCESS OF THE CENTER IN TREATING SPANISH-SPEAKING PATIENTS SINCE THE WORKERS JOINED THE STAFF IN 1971 IS DOCUMENTED. THE UNIQUE WAYS IN WHICH COMMUNITY WORKERS CAN BE USED INCLUDE COMMUNITY RELATIONS, OUTREACH, CONTINUITY OF CARE, HOME VISITS, LIAISON WITH OTHER COMMUNITY AGENCIES, AND THERAPY.
      ACCN   000215

257   AUTH   **CAHALAN, D.**
      TITL   ETHNORELIGIOUS GROUP DIFFERENCES: 1974 CALIFORNIA DRINKING SURVEY.
      SRCE   *UNPUBLISHED MANUSCRIPT, SCHOOL OF PUBLIC HEALTH, UNIVERSITY OF CALIFORNIA, BERKELEY, 1975.*
      INDX   ALCOHOLISM, DEMOGRAPHIC, SEX ROLES, SEX COMPARISON, MARITAL STABILITY, HEALTH, EMPLOYMENT, JUDICIAL PROCESS, AGGRESSION, ATTITUDES, SURVEY, EMPIRICAL, MEXICAN AMERICAN, PRIMARY PREVENTION, CALIFORNIA, SOUTHWEST
      ABST   PREPARED AS A SUPPLEMENTARY REPORT TO THE 1974 "FINDINGS OF A STATEWIDE CALIFORNIA SURVEY ON ATTITUDES RELATED TO CONTROL OF DRINKING PROBLEMS," THIS REPORT PROVIDES ADDITIONAL DETAIL ON SOME KEY ITEMS ON DRINKING ATTITUDES AND BEHAVIOR AS ANALYZED BY A COMBINATION OF ETHNIC AND RELIGIOUS CLASSIFICATIONS. THE CATEGORIES JEWISH, PROTESTANT, CATHOLIC, ASIATIC, BLACK, ANGLO, AND CHICANO ARE DISCUSSED IN RELATION TO: (1) QUANTITY/FREQUENCY OF DRINKING; (2) DRINKING PROBLEMS DURING LAST THREE YEARS; (3) SERIOUSNESS OF PROBLEM; (4) SEVERITY OF ALCOHOL PROBLEMS WITH RESPECT TO OTHER SOCIAL PROBLEMS; (5) ATTITUDE TOWARD PUBLIC EDUCATION AND PUBLIC MEDIA CAMPAIGNS; AND (6) RELATIVE POPULARITY OF VARIOUS PREVENTION MEASURES. SUBSTANTIAL DIFFERENCES AMONG THE GROUPS WERE FOUND IN HEAVY DRINKING AND INCIDENCE OF PROBLEMS RELATED TO DRINKING. IN GENERAL, IRISH CATHOLICS, CHICANOS, AND BLACKS (ESPECIALLY BLACK FEMALES) EXHIBITED FAIRLY HIGH RATES OF HEAVY DRINKING, INTOXICATION, AND DRINKING PROBLEMS, WHILE JEWS AND ASIATICS HAD RELATIVELY LOW RATES. ON THE OTHER HAND, ETHNORELIGIOUS GROUPS WERE NOT FOUND TO DIFFER IN THEIR PERCEPTION OF ALCOHOLISM AS A SERIOUS PROBLEM, NOR IN THEIR SUPPORT OF MEASURES TO PREVENT OR MINIMIZE DRINKING PROBLEMS, EXCEPT FOR A SLIGHT MAJORITY OF BLACKS WHO FELT "ALCOHOL TAXES ARE HIGH ENOUGH." A MAJORITY OF WHITE PROTESTANTS, JEWS, AND ASIATICS SAID THEY WOULD FAVOR INCREASING ALCOHOL TAXES FOR PROVIDING MORE TREATMENT

AND PREVENTION. (AUTHOR SUMMARY MODI-FIED)

ACCN   000216

258 AUTH **CAHILL, I. D.**
     TITL   CHILD-REARING PRACTICES IN LOWER SOCIO-ECONOMIC ETHNIC GROUPS (DOCTORAL DISSERTATION, COLUMBIA UNIVERSITY, 1967).
     SRCE   *DISSERTATION ABSTRACTS INTERNATIONAL, 1967, 27(9), 3139A. (UNIVERSITY MICROFILMS NO. 67-02,788.)*
     INDX   SES, CHILDREARING PRACTICES, MEXICAN AMERICAN, CROSS CULTURAL, EMPIRICAL, FEMALE, MOTHER-CHILD INTERACTION
     ABST   SIXTY MOTHERS OF THE LOWER SOCIOECONOMIC GROUP WERE INTERVIEWED ABOUT THE CHILD-REARING PRACTICES THEY HAD USED ON A FIVE YEAR-OLD CHILD FROM BIRTH TO THE TIME OF INTERVIEW. THE SCHEDULE USED WAS ONE DESIGNED BY SEARS, MACCOBY AND LEVINE. INTERVIEWS WERE COLLECTED ON THE MATERNITY WARD OF A HOSPITAL SEVERAL DAYS AFTER THE BIRTH OF A BABY FROM MOTHERS REPRESENTING PUERTO RICAN, BLACK AND WHITE GROUPS EQUALLY. THE MOTHERS' RESPONSES, AS WELL AS INFORMATION OBTAINED FROM OBSERVATIONS, WERE BROKEN DOWN INTO 82 DEPENDENT VARIABLES WHICH CONSISTED OF 5 OR MORE CATEGORIES FOR SCALING. TWO HYPOTHESES WERE TESTED. (1) THERE ARE DIFFERENCES IN THE CHILD-REARING PRACTICES OF PUERTO RICAN, BLACK AND WHITE FAMILIES OF THE LOWER SOCIOECONOMIC GROUP. THIS HYPOTHESIS WAS REJECTED. (2) THERE ARE DIFFERENCES BETWEEN THE CHILD-REARING PRACTICES OF THE FAMILIES IN THIS STUDY AND THOSE OF THE WORKING-CLASS AND MIDDLE-CLASS MOTHERS AS REPORTED BY SEARS, MACCOBY AND LEVINE IN PATTERNS OF CHILD-REARING. THIS HYPOTHESIS WAS ACCEPTED, AND IT WAS CONCLUDED THAT SOCIOECONOMIC STATUS IS MORE IMPORTANT THAN ETHNICITY IN REGARD TO CHILD-REARING PRACTICES. THE RELATIONSHIP OF TOILET TRAINING, WEANING, DISCIPLINE, AGGRESSION, PERMISSIVENESS AND OTHER VARIABLES ARE DISCUSSED AT LENGTH. 126 REFERENCES. (AUTHOR SUMMARY MODIFIED)
     ACCN   000217

259 AUTH **CAIN, M. A.**
     TITL   A STUDY OF THE RELATIONSHIPS BETWEEN SELECTED FACTORS AND THE SCHOOL ACHIEVEMENT OF MEXICAN AMERICAN MIGRANT CHILDREN (DOCTORAL DISSERTATION, MICHIGAN STATE UNIVERSITY, 1970).
     SRCE   *DISSERTATION ABSTRACTS INTERNATIONAL, 1971, 31(8), 3947A. (UNIVERSITY MICROFILMS NO. 71-02,043.)*
     INDX   SCHOLASTIC ACHIEVEMENT, FARM LABORERS, CHILDREN, SES, MEXICAN AMERICAN, FAMILY ROLES, MOTHER-CHILD INTERACTION, FATHER-CHILD INTERACTION, SEX COMPARISON, EMPIRICAL, CHILDREARING PRACTICES, MIGRANTS, MICHIGAN, MIDWEST, READING, MATHEMATICS
     ABST   THE POSSIBLE RELATIONSHIPS OF AGE, SEX,

PARENT-CHILD RELATIONS, AND MODES OF PROBLEM RESPONSE TO THE SCHOOL ACHIEVEMENT OF MEXICAN AMERICAN MIGRANT CHILDREN WERE INVESTIGATED. SUBJECTS WERE 58 MEXICAN AMERICAN MIGRANT BOYS AND GIRLS, RANGING IN AGE FROM 7 THROUGH 13, WHO ATTENDED A SUMMER SCHOOL PROGRAM IN MICHIGAN. IT WAS FOUND THAT ARITHMETIC ACHIEVEMENT EQUALED OR EXCELLED READING ACHIEVEMENT AT EACH AGE LEVEL. ALL ACHIEVEMENT DECREASED BEYOND THE 9-YEAR-OLD LEVEL. NO DIFFERENCES WERE NOTED BETWEEN ACHIEVEMENT OF BOYS AND GIRLS. PARENT-CHILD RELATIONS WERE PERCEIVED AS SIGNIFICANTLY LOVING AND PROTECTING. THE CHILD-REARING DIMENSIONS OF REJECTION AND NEGLECT WERE SIGNIFICANTLY LESS PREVALENT THAN OTHER DIMENSIONS. CHILDREN SAW THEMSELVES AS MORE REWARDED THAN PUNISHED. MOTHERS WERE SEEN AS MORE PROTECTING, MORE DEMANDING, MORE REWARDING, AND MORE PUNISHING THAN FATHERS. RELATIVELY LOWER ARITHMETIC AND READING SCORES WERE SIGNIFICANTLY RELATED TO MOTHER'S REJECTION, NEGLECT, AND CASUALNESS. FATHER'S LOVE WAS POSITIVELY RELATED TO ARITHMETIC ACHIEVEMENT, WHILE THEIR CASUALNESS WAS NEGATIVELY CORRELATED WITH READING AND PERFORMANCE. IT WAS FOUND THAT 41 PERCENT OF CHILDREN'S STORY COMPLETIONS WERE GOAL ORIENTED, GRATIFICATION DEFERRING, MIDDLE CLASS SOLUTIONS; 34 PERCENT USED WITHDRAWAL FROM PROBLEMS AND 25 PERCENT INCLUDED APPEALS TO AUTHORITY, USE OF FANTASY, OR ANTISOCIAL AGGRESSION. THE SOLUTIONS HAD NO RELATIONSHIPS TO SCHOOL ACHIEVEMENT.

ACCN   000218

260 AUTH **CALDWELL, F. F., & MOWRY, M. D.**
     TITL   THE ESSAY VERSUS THE OBJECTIVE EXAMINATION AS MEASURES OF ACHIEVEMENT OF BILINGUAL CHILDREN.
     SRCE   *JOURNAL OF EDUCATIONAL PSYCHOLOGY, 1933, 24(9), 696-702.*
     INDX   ACHIEVEMENT TESTING, SPANISH SURNAMED, CHILDREN, BILINGUAL, LEARNING, EMPIRICAL, CROSS CULTURAL, TEST VALIDITY, LINGUISTIC COMPETENCE, ABILITY TESTING
     ABST   A COMPARISON OF THE ESSAY AND OBJECTIVE EXAMINATIONS AS MEASURES OF ACHIEVEMENT AMONG ANGLO AMERICAN (AA) AND SPANISH AMERICAN (SA) CHILDREN IS PRESENTED. PUPILS WERE TESTED IN THE AREAS OF ENGLISH AND HISTORY. A TOTAL OF 643 SUBJECTS WERE EXAMINED AND THE RESULTS FROM 4,646 TESTS WERE USED AS A BASIS FOR THE CONCLUSIONS. THE DATA INDICATE THAT LANGUAGE DIFFICULTY OPERATES TO PENALIZE SA PUPILS WHEN EITHER THE OBJECTIVE OR THE ESSAY TYPE OF EXAMINATION IS USED AS A MEASUREMENT OF ACHIEVEMENT. THERE IS CONSIDERABLY MORE HANDICAP EXPERIENCED WITH THE ESSAY THAN WITH THE OBJECTIVE TEST. THIS IS BECAUSE ESSAY TESTS DEMAND A "RECALL" OF VO-

CABULARY, WHEREAS THE OBJECTIVE EXAMINATION REQUIRES LARGELY A "RECOGNITION" OF UNFAMILIAR WORDS. THERE IS A GREATER HANDICAP EXPERIENCED BY SA CHILDREN WHEN TESTS ARE GIVEN IN HISTORY RATHER THAN IN ENGLISH. IT IS POSSIBLE THAT THE APPLICATION OF ENGLISH IN A SITUATION OTHER THAN IN THE FIELD OF ENGLISH MIGHT TEND TO INCREASE THE LANGUAGE DIFFICULTY. THE SA CHILD SCORES RELATIVELY HIGHER ON THE OBJECTIVE TEST THAN ON THE ESSAY. IT IS SUGGESTED THAT TEACHERS SHOULD EMPLOY THE OBJECTIVE TYPE OF TEST IN ORDER TO INSURE THE LANGUAGE HANDICAPPED SA A MORE RELIABLE MEASURE OF ACHIEVEMENT.

ACCN   000219

261 AUTH   **CALDWELL, F. F., & MOWRY, M. D.**
     TITL   SEX DIFFERENCES IN SCHOOL ACHIEVEMENT AMONG SPANISH-AMERICAN AND ANGLO-AMERICAN CHILDREN.
     SRCE   *JOURNAL OF EDUCATIONAL SOCIOLOGY, 1935, 8(3), 168-173.*
     INDX   SEX COMPARISON, SCHOLASTIC ACHIEVEMENT, CROSS CULTURAL, SPANISH SURNAMED, CHILDREN, BILINGUAL, EMPIRICAL, SEX ROLES, ACHIEVEMENT TESTING, NEW MEXICO, SOUTHWEST
     ABST   AN ATTEMPT WAS MADE TO DETERMINE: (1) WHETHER TEACHERS' GRADES ASSIGNED TO BILINGUAL CHILDREN ARE AS FAIR CRITERIA OF SCHOOL ACHIEVEMENT AS GRADES ASSIGNED TO THE ENGLISH-SPEAKING GROUP; AND (2) WHETHER THERE IS A TENDENCY FOR TEACHERS TO GRADE THIS BILINGUAL GROUP CONSISTENTLY HIGHER OR LOWER THAN KNOWLEDGE OF SUBJECT MATTER WOULD JUSTIFY. A TOTAL OF 167 ANGLO AMERICANS AND 216 SPANISH AMERICANS WERE TESTED IN ENGLISH WHILE 153 ANGLO AMERICANS AND 146 SPANISH AMERICANS WERE TESTED IN HISTORY BY MEANS OF OBJECTIVE AND ESSAY TESTING PROCEDURES. THE OBJECTIVE TEST AND THE NEW STANFORD ACHIEVEMENT TEST (NSAT) SCORES CORRELATED HIGHLY IN BOTH LANGUAGE GROUPS, WHILE CORRELATION COEFFICIENTS OF THE ESSAY TEST AND THE NSAT WERE MARKEDLY LOWER IN THE SPANISH AMERICAN GROUP. THE STUDY INDICATES THAT THE OBJECTIVE TEST IS A MORE RELIABLE MEASURE OF GENERAL SCHOOL ACHIEVEMENT FOR SPANISH AMERICAN CHILDREN WHILE THE ESSAY TEST IS A MORE RELIABLE MEASURE OF ANGLO CHILDREN. IT WAS FOUND THAT TEACHERS' GRADES FOR THE BILINGUAL GROUP ARE NOT AS RELIABLE CRITERIA OF ACHIEVEMENT AS THOSE GRADES ASSIGNED TO ANGLO CHILDREN. IN EFFECT, SPANISH AMERICAN CHILDREN ARE BEING GRADED CONSISTENTLY LOWER THAN THEIR ACTUAL KNOWLEDGE OF SUBJECT MATTER JUSTIFIES. IT IS RECOMMENDED THAT FURTHER STUDY OF THESE MIXED CLASSES SHOULD DETERMINE THE NATURE OF BIASES, PREJUDICES, AND EMOTIONAL OR SENTIMENTAL INFLUENCES THAT ARE IN OPERATION. THE DEGREE TO WHICH THESE FACTORS OPERATE TO INFLUENCE CLASSROOM METHODS AND PROCEDURES MIGHT ALSO BE STUDIED.

ACCN   000220

262 AUTH   **CALDWELL, F. F., & MOWRY, M. D.**
     TITL   TEACHERS' GRADES AS CRITERIA OF ACHIEVEMENT OF BILINGUAL CHILDREN.
     SRCE   *JOURNAL OF APPLIED PSYCHOLOGY, 1934, 18(3), 288-292.*
     INDX   EDUCATIONAL ASSESSMENT, SCHOLASTIC ACHIEVEMENT, CHILDREN, BILINGUAL, SPANISH SURNAMED, STANFORD ACHIEVEMENT TEST, TEACHERS, DISCRIMINATION, EMPIRICAL
     ABST   SEX DIFFERENCES IN SCHOOL ACHIEVEMENT AMONG 340 SPANISH AMERICAN (SA) AND 283 ANGLO AMERICAN (AA) CHILDREN ARE EXAMINED. SUBJECTS WERE ADMINISTERED 3,000 SHORT OBJECTIVE AND ESSAY TESTS. ALL OF THE TESTS WERE CHECKED TWICE. THE FOLLOWING ITEMS WERE TO BE STUDIED: THE DIFFERENCES IN MEAN SCORES EARNED BY MALES AND FEMALES FROM EACH GROUP AND THE RELATIVE AMOUNT OF LANGUAGE HANDICAP EXPERIENCED BY SA FEMALES AS COMPARED TO SA MALES. AN EXAMINATION OF THE DATA REVEALS THAT AA FEMALES EXCEED AA MALES ENROLLED IN SCHOOL BY 16.3 PERCENT. IT IS NOTED THAT AA PARENTS MAY BE MORE INCLINED TO ENCOURAGE THEIR BOYS TO QUIT SCHOOL AND TO GO TO WORK WHEREAS SA PARENTS ENCOURAGE THEIR GIRLS TO STAY HOME AND CONTRIBUTE TO THE FAMILY SUPPORT AT AN EARLIER AGE THAN IS REQUIRED OF BOYS. THE CRITICAL RATIOS INDICATE THAT THERE ARE NO SEX DIFFERENCES IN RESPONDING TO THE TWO TYPES OF TESTS SUFFICIENTLY LARGE TO BE CONSIDERED STATISTICALLY SIGNIFICANT, ALTHOUGH SA MALES EARN SLIGHTLY HIGHER SCORES ON THE ESSAY TEST THAN SA FEMALES. THIS IS PROBABLY DUE TO MORE SOCIAL CONTACT WITH AA'S IN SPORT ACTIVITIES AND SOCIAL FUNCTIONS.

ACCN   000221

263 AUTH   **CALHOUN, J. P.**
     TITL   DEVELOPMENTAL AND SOCIOCULTURAL ASPECTS OF IMAGERY IN THE PICTURE-WORD PAIRED-ASSOCIATE LEARNING OF CHILDREN.
     SRCE   *DEVELOPMENTAL PSYCHOLOGY, 1974, 10(3), 357-366.*
     INDX   CHILDREN, SPANISH SURNAMED, CROSS CULTURAL, LEARNING, MEMORY, IMAGERY, EMPIRICAL, NEW MEXICO, SOUTHWEST
     ABST   THE STUDY INVESTIGATES THE EFFECTS OF PICTURES AS COMPARED TO CONCRETE NOUNS IN BOTH STIMULUS AND RESPONSE POSITIONS THROUGH PAIRED-ASSOCIATE LEARNING. TWO HUNDRED FIFTY-SIX SUBJECTS, 128 MIDDLE-CLASS ANGLO AND 128 LOW-SES SPANISH AMERICAN CHILDREN, LEARNED PAIRED-ASSOCIATE LISTS IN WHICH PICTURES AND ORALLY PRESENTED WORDS WERE LEARNED AS COMBINATIONS OF PICTURE-PICTURE, PICTURE-WORD, WORD-PICTURE, AND WORD-WORD. HALF OF THE SUBJECTS WERE PLACED IN A RECALL TEST DURING

LEARNING TRIALS, AND HALF IN A RECOGNITION CONDITION. ONE WEEK AFTER ORIGINAL LEARNING, THE SUBJECTS WERE RETESTED. MAJOR FINDINGS INDICATED THAT: (1) PICTURES IN THE STIMULUS POSITION GREATLY FACILITATED LEARNING, WHEREAS PICTURES IN THE RESPONSE TERM PRODUCED NEGATIVE EFFECTS BUT ONLY IN THE RECALL CONDITION; (2) PICTURES PRODUCED BETTER LONG-TERM RETENTION IN BOTH STIMULUS AND RESPONSE POSITIONS THAN DID WORDS; AND (3) NO SIGNIFICANT DIFFERENCES BETWEEN SOCIOCULTURAL GROUPS IN OVERALL PAIRED-ASSOCIATE PERFORMANCE APPEARED, BUT LONG-TERM RETENTION WAS SIGNIFICANTLY BETTER FOR ANGLO SUBJECTS. 32 REFERENCES. (JOURNAL ABSTRACT MODIFIED)

ACCN   000222

264 AUTH   **CALIFORNIA STATE ADVISORY COMMITTEE TO THE UNITED STATES COMMISSION ON CIVIL RIGHTS.**

TITL   POLICE-COMMUNITY RELATIONS IN EAST LOS ANGELES, CALIFORNIA.

SRCE   *CALIFORNIA STATE ADVISORY COMMITTEE TO THE UNITED STATES COMMISSION ON CIVIL RIGHTS, OCTOBER 1970. (AVAILABLE FROM MEXICAN-AMERICAN LEGAL DEFENSE FUND, 145 NINTH STREET, SAN FRANCISCO, CA 94103.)*

INDX   POLICE-COMMUNITY RELATIONS, SES, ESSAY, MEXICAN AMERICAN, DISCRIMINATION, CALIFORNIA, SOUTHWEST, URBAN

ABST   RELATIONS BETWEEN THE MEXICAN AMERICAN COMMUNITY OF LOS ANGELES AND LOCAL LAW ENFORCEMENT AGENCIES ARE DISCUSSED. LAW ENFORCEMENT AGENCIES HISTORICALLY HAVE BEEN COMPOSED OF INDIVIDUALS WHOSE CULTURAL ORIENTATION IS BASICALLY ANGLO AND WHO HAVE VERY LITTLE UNDERSTANDING OF THE CULTURE, LIFESTYLE, AND LANGUAGE OF THE COMMUNITY WHICH THEY ARE ASSIGNED TO SERVE. INVESTIGATION OF EVENTS SURROUNDING THE DEATH OF THE CHICANO COMMUNITY'S LEADING SPOKESMAN DURING THE RIOTOUS NATIONAL CHICANO MORATORIUM MARCH IN AUGUST, 1970 REVEALED A DANGEROUS BREAKDOWN IN COMMUNICATION BETWEEN THE COMMUNITY AND THE POLICE. EXISTING POLICE COMMUNITY RELATIONS PROGRAMS ARE COMPLETELY INEFFECTIVE, AND A FEELING THAT THE POLICE ARE DOING THEIR JOB WELL IS GENERALLY LACKING. THE TWO MAIN ATTITUDES TOWARD POLICE ARE ANGER AND FEAR. RECOMMENDATIONS INCLUDE: (1) THOROUGH INVESTIGATION AND PUBLIC AIRING OF THE SITUATION AS A MINIMUM STARTING POINT; (2) ESTABLISHMENT OF AN OFFICE WITH POLICE REPRESENTATION BUT OPERATING INDEPENDENTLY OF AND WITH AUTHORITY OVER LAW ENFORCEMENT PERSONNEL TO ACCEPT AND ACT UPON CITIZENS' COMPLAINTS AGAINST POLICE OFFICERS; (3) U.S. DEPARTMENT OF JUSTICE-COMMUNITY RELATIONS SERVICE OBSERVATION, MONITORING, AND EVALUATION OF POLICE-COMMUNITY RELATIONS IN THE CHICANO COMMUNITY FOR A YEAR; AND (4) ESTABLISHMENT OF A COMMITTEE OF MEXICAN AMERICANS AND LOCAL POLICE TO CONDUCT APPROPRIATE INVESTIGATIONS AND RECOMMEND CHANGES IN CURRENT LAW ENFORCEMENT PROCEDURES AND POLICE-COMMUNITY RELATIONS PROGRAMS.

ACCN   000223

265 AUTH   **CALLAN, J. P.**

TITL   MEETING MENTAL HEALTH NEEDS OF PUERTO RICAN FAMILIES.

SRCE   *HOSPITAL AND COMMUNITY PSYCHIATRY, 1973, 24(5), 330-333.*

INDX   ACCULTURATION, COMMUNITY INVOLVEMENT, COPING MECHANISMS, CULTURAL FACTORS, ECONOMIC FACTORS, ENVIRONMENTAL FACTORS, ESSAY, FAMILY ROLES, FAMILY STRUCTURE, HEALTH DELIVERY SYSTEMS, MENTAL HEALTH, IMMIGRATION, PARAPROFESSIONALS, PSYCHOPATHOLOGY, PSYCHOSIS, PSYCHOSOCIAL ADJUSTMENT, PUERTO RICAN-M, PUERTO RICAN-I, SES, SEX ROLES, SOCIALIZATION, SOCIAL SERVICES, CONNECTICUT, EAST, THERAPEUTIC COMMUNITY, STRESS, PSYCHOTHERAPY, RESOURCE UTILIZATION, URBAN, BILINGUAL-BICULTURAL PERSONNEL

ABST   AN INCREASING NUMBER OF PUERTO RICANS BEGAN APPEARING AT HARTFORD, CONNECTICUT, AREA HOSPITALS AND AT A LOCAL SOCIAL WORK AGENCY WITH SYMPTOMS OF EMOTIONAL DISTRESS. IN MANY CASES THE SYMPTOMS WERE CAUSED BY THE STRESSES OF LIVING ON THE MAINLAND AND THE EROSION OF FAMILIAR CUSTOMS AND MORES. IN JUNE, 1972, THE SOCIAL WORK AGENCY AND THE PSYCHIATRIC CLINIC OF A LOCAL HOSPITAL ESTABLISHED A SPECIAL PROGRAM TO PROVIDE PSYCHIATRIC SERVICES FOR THEM. EIGHT SPANISH-SPEAKING SOCIAL WORKERS AND CASE WORKERS PARTICIPATING IN THE PROGRAM ACCEPTED REFERRALS FROM SCHOOLS, HOSPITALS, AND RELIGIOUS AND SOCIAL ORGANIZATIONS. CASE WORKERS CONSULTED WITH A PSYCHIATRIC DIRECTOR WEEKLY TO DISCUSS CASE MANAGEMENT. A PRAGMATIC THERAPEUTIC APPROACH WAS USED, FOCUSING ON INDIVIDUAL AND FAMILIAL STRENGTHS RATHER THAN PSYCHOPATHOLOGY AND EMPHASIZING ENVIRONMENTAL MANIPULATION. PATIENTS WERE SEEN BY A PSYCHIATRIST IF INDICATED. HOSPITALIZATION WAS FOUND TO BE REQUIRED IN ABOUT 10 OF THE CASES. COMMON PROBLEMS REVOLVED AROUND DOMESTIC DISHARMONY, ADOLESCENT ACTING OUT, LACK OF MONEY, AGGRESSIVE BEHAVIOR, AND OTHER PROBLEMS ASSOCIATED WITH HIGH DENSITY LIVING. THE AUTHOR DESCRIBES THE CHARACTERISTICS AND CULTURE OF PUERTO RICAN FAMILIES, THE PROBLEMS THEY ENCOUNTER ON THE MAINLAND, AND SOME OF THE DIFFICULTIES ENCOUNTERED IN WORKING WITH THEM. (AUTHOR ABSTRACT MODIFIED)

ACCN   002328

266 AUTH   **CAMARILLO, A. M.**

TITL   RESEARCH NOTE ON CHICANO COMMUNITY LEADERS: THE G. I. GENERATION.

SRCE *AZTLAN: CHICANO JOURNAL OF THE SOCIAL SCIENCES AND THE ARTS, 1971, 2(2), 145-150.*

INDX MEXICAN AMERICAN, COMMUNITY INVOLVEMENT, COMMUNITY, RELIGION, MALE, DISCRIMINATION, POLITICAL POWER, LEADERSHIP, CASE STUDY, CALIFORNIA, SOUTHWEST

ABST THE NEW POLITICAL ACTIVITY AND AWARENESS WITHIN THE CHICANO COMMUNITY HAS BEEN ATTRIBUTED TO THE CHICANO LEADERS BEING VETERANS OF WORLD WAR II OR THE KOREAN WAR. AFTER INTERVIEWING NINE MEN HAVING LEADERSHIP POSITIONS IN ORGANIZATIONS OR COMMUNITY AFFAIRS (SEVEN OF WHOM WERE WAR VETERANS), IT IS CONCLUDED THAT THE MOTIVATING FACTOR FOR THEIR ACTIVISM STEMS FROM CHILDHOOD OR ADOLESCENT EXPERIENCES OF SOCIAL INEQUALITY. THE MAJORITY OF THESE MEN HAD: (1) SEEN THE CATHOLIC CHURCH AS A SOURCE OF OPPRESSION AGAINST CHICANOS; (2) BEEN INVOLVED IN COMMUNITY ORGANIZATIONAL ACTIVITIES PRIOR TO THESE WARS; AND (3) COME FROM FAMILIES WHO WERE ACTIVE IN SOCIAL AND POLITICAL ISSUES. PARTICIPATION IN THE WAR MERELY PROVIDED AN ADDITIONAL CATALYST FOR THEIR ACTIVISM AND THEREFORE IS NOT THE UNDERLYING FACTOR FOR THEIR POLITICAL AND SOCIAL INVOLVEMENT.

ACCN 000224

267 AUTH **CAMARILLO, M. R., & DEL BUONO, A.**

TITL UTILIZING BARRIO EXPERTISE IN SOCIAL WORK EDUCATION.

SRCE *IN M. M. MANGOLD (ED.), LA CAUSA CHICANA: THE MOVEMENT FOR JUSTICE. NEW YORK: FAMILY SERVICE ASSOCIATION OF AMERICA, 1971, PP. 115-125.*

INDX MENTAL HEALTH PROFESSION, PROFESSIONAL TRAINING, HIGHER EDUCATION, PREJUDICE, MEXICAN AMERICAN, REPRESENTATION, COMMUNITY, ESSAY, CALIFORNIA, SOUTHWEST

ABST UTILIZING BARRIO EXPERIENCES AND DEVELOPING BARRIO PERSPECTIVES COULD VASTLY IMPROVE SOCIAL WORK EDUCATION. A BRIEF ANALYSIS OF SOCIAL WORK EDUCATION AS A PART OF THE TOTAL HIGHER EDUCATION SYSTEM IS PRESENTED TO ELUCIDATE ITS EFFECTS ON CHICANOS. THE NECESSITY FOR SOCIAL WORK EDUCATION TO REFLECT THE NEEDS OF CHICANOS HAS BEEN RECOGNIZED BY SAN JOSE STATE COLLEGE; THEIR PHILOSOPHY AND CERTIFICATION PROGRAM FOR BARRIO PROFESSORS IS DISCUSSED. IN CONCLUSION, IT IS POSITED THAT INCLUSION OF BARRIO EXPERIENCES IN THE SOCIAL WORK STUDENT'S TRAINING WILL RESULT IN A MORE SENSITIVE, RESPONSIVE, AND EFFECTIVE SOCIAL WORKER ABLE TO DELIVER CRITICALLY NEEDED SERVICES. 14 REFERENCES. (AUTHOR SUMMARY MODIFIED)

ACCN 000225

268 AUTH **CAMPBELL, J. T.**

TITL TESTS ARE VALID FOR MINORITY GROUPS TOO.

SRCE *PUBLIC PERSONNEL MANAGEMENT, 1973, 2(1), 70-73.*

INDX EMPLOYMENT, JOB PERFORMANCE, TEST VALIDITY, MEXICAN AMERICAN, CROSS CULTURAL, ACHIEVEMENT TESTING, EMPIRICAL

ABST POPULAR OPINION TO THE CONTRARY, THIS STUDY FOUND THAT APTITUDE TESTS WHICH PREDICT JOB PERFORMANCE FOR ONE ETHNIC GROUP USUALLY WILL PREDICT ABOUT AS WELL FOR OTHER ETHNIC GROUPS. CONVERSELY, THOSE TESTS WHICH DO NOT PREDICT JOB PERFORMANCE FOR ONE GROUP WILL PROBABLY NOT PREDICT FOR OTHER ETHNIC GROUPS. THREE OCCUPATIONS WERE TESTED—MEDICAL TECHNICIAN, CARTOGRAPHIC TECHNICIAN AND INVENTORY MANAGEMENT SPECIALIST. THE STUDY INCLUDED JOB ANALYSIS, INSTRUMENT DEVELOPMENT AND DATA ANALYSIS. 1 REFERENCE. (AUTHOR SUMMARY MODIFIED)

ACCN 000226

269 AUTH **CAMPBELL, J. T., CROOKS, L. A., MAHONEY, M. H., & ROCK, D. A.**

TITL AN INVESTIGATION OF SOURCES OF BIAS IN THE PREDICTION OF JOB PERFORMANCE: A SIX YEAR STUDY. (FINAL PROJECT REPORT PR-73-37)

SRCE *PRINCETON, N.J.: EDUCATIONAL TESTING SERVICE, 1973.*

INDX ABILITY TESTING, ACHIEVEMENT TESTING, ADULTS, CROSS CULTURAL, CULTURE-FAIR TESTS, EMPLOYMENT, EMPIRICAL, EQUAL OPPORTUNITY, EXAMINER EFFECTS, JOB PERFORMANCE, LABOR FORCE, MEXICAN AMERICAN, OCCUPATIONAL ASPIRATIONS, PERFORMANCE EXPECTATIONS, PERSONNEL, PREJUDICE

ABST IN RESPONSE TO CONCERNS ABOUT FAIRNESS OF TESTING PRACTICES USED FOR GOVERNMENT AND INDUSTRY PROMOTION, THE U.S. CIVIL SERVICE COMMISSION AND EDUCATIONAL TESTING SERVICE CONDUCTED A SIX YEAR STUDY (1966-1972) TO EXAMINE THE RELATIONSHIP BETWEEN BACKGROUND AND ABILITY MEASURES AND JOB PERFORMANCE FOR THREE ETHNIC GROUPS (MEXICAN AMERICANS, BLACK, AND CAUCASIANS). THREE OCCUPATIONS WITH ETHNIC REPRESENTATION WERE SELECTED FOR STUDY—MEDICAL TECHNICIANS, CARTOGRAPHIC TECHNICIANS, AND INVENTORY MANAGERS. RESEARCHERS ANALYZED JOBS TO DETERMINE FACTORS NECESSARY FOR SUCCESSFUL JOB PERFORMANCE, THEN THEY ADMINISTERED APTITUDE/ABILITY TEST BATTERIES AND BACKGROUND DATA/JOB ACTIVITY QUESTIONNAIRES. FINALLY, CRITERION MEASURES FOR JOB PERFORMANCE WERE DEVELOPED WHICH INCLUDED SUPERVISORS' OVERALL RATINGS, JOB KNOWLEDGE TESTING, AND WORK SAMPLE INSPECTION. APTITUDE TESTS WERE FOUND TO HAVE EQUAL VALIDITY FOR THE THREE ETHNIC GROUPS, AND REGRESSION EQUATIONS DEVELOPED ON MAJORITY GROUP DATA PREDICTED ALMOST EQUALLY WELL FOR MINORITY GROUPS. THE USE OF SUPERVISORS' RATINGS AS A CRITERION OF JOB PERFORMANCE IS QUESTIONED SINCE INTERACTION EFFECTS WERE FOUND BETWEEN ETHNIC GROUP MEMBER-

SHIP OF RATER AND RATEES. STUDY FINDINGS HAVE IMPLICATIONS FOR EMPLOYERS, BEHAVIORAL SCIENTISTS, AND OTHERS CONCERNED WITH SOCIAL AND PUBLIC POLICY ISSUES. 42 REFERENCES.

ACCN   002045

270 AUTH   **CAMPBELL, W.**
    TITL   PARENTS' PERCEPTIONS OF THEIR POWERLESSNESS IN LOWER CLASS WHITE, MIDDLE CLASS WHITE AND LOWER CLASS MEXICAN AMERICAN HOMES AND THE RESULTING INFLUENCE ON STUDENT ACHIEVEMENT (DOCTORAL DISSERTATION, UNIVERSITY OF TOLEDO, 1972).
    SRCE   *DISSERTATION ABSTRACTS INTERNATIONAL, 1972, 33(1), 70A. (UNIVERSITY MICROFILMS NO. 72-20,178.)*
    INDX   SCHOLASTIC ACHIEVEMENT, SES, POVERTY, MEXICAN AMERICAN, CROSS CULTURAL, EMPIRICAL, ANOMIE, PARENTAL INVOLVEMENT, ADULTS, MIDWEST
    ABST   THE PURPOSE OF THIS STUDY WAS TO DISCOVER FEELINGS OF MASTERY OR POWERLESSNESS OF PARTICULAR GROUPS OF PARENTS IN RELATION TO SOCIETY AT LARGE AND THE LOCAL SCHOOL SYSTEM. THREE RANDOMLY CHOSEN GROUPS OF PARENTS (LOWER AND MIDDLE CLASS ANGLOS, LOWER CLASS MEXICAN AMERICANS), WITH CHILDREN IN GRADES SIX TO NINE, WERE GIVEN TWO POWERLESSNESS SCALES AND A BACKGROUND DATA QUESTIONNAIRE. PARENTAL POWERLESSNESS SCORES WERE COMPARED AMONG THE THREE GROUPS, THEN STUDENT GRADE POINT AVERAGES AND ACHIEVEMENT TEST SCORES WERE CORRELATED WITH PARENTAL POWERLESSNESS SCORES. DATA ANALYSIS INDICATED NO SIGNIFICANT DIFFERENCES BETWEEN THE THREE PARENT GROUPS IN RELATION TO THE LOCAL SCHOOL SYSTEM; BUT THERE WERE SIGNIFICANT DIFFERENCES IN POWERLESSNESS SCORES RELATED TO MASS SOCIETY ISSUES. THE ONLY SIGNIFICANT CORRELATIONS BETWEEN PARENTAL POWERLESSNESS AND STUDENT ACHIEVEMENT WERE IN THE LOWER CLASS WHITE SAMPLE. CONCLUSIONS RELATING TO PARENTAL SES LEVEL AND ETHNICITY AND STUDENT SCHOOL ACHIEVEMENT ARE DISCUSSED. 30 REFERENCES. (AUTHOR SUMMARY MODIFIED)
    ACCN   000227

271 AUTH   **CAMPION, J. E., BRUGNOLI, G. A., & GREENER, J. M.**
    TITL   JOB SATISFACTION OF MEXICAN-AMERICAN BLUE-COLLAR EMPLOYEES.
    SRCE   *JSAS CATALOG OF SELECTED DOCUMENTS IN PSYCHOLOGY, 1976, 6, 10. (MS. NO. 1182)*
    INDX   EMPLOYMENT, JOB PERFORMANCE, ATTITUDES, MEXICAN AMERICAN, MALE, SES, CROSS CULTURAL, EMPIRICAL, URBAN, ADULTS, SOUTHWEST
    ABST   THE JOB ATTITUDES OF MEXICAN AMERICAN EMPLOYEES WERE DETERMINED IN A SAMPLE OF 58 MEXICAN AMERICAN AND 48 WHITE, BLUE-COLLAR MALE EMPLOYEES OF A FOOD PROCESSING COMPANY LOCATED IN A LARGE SOUTHWESTERN CITY. A MODIFIED VERSION OF PORTER'S NEED SATISFACTION QUESTIONNAIRE WAS USED TO MEASURE NEEDS, ESTEEM NEEDS, AUTONOMY NEEDS, AND SELF-ACTUALIZATION NEEDS. IT WAS FOUND THAT NEED SATISFACTION AND IMPORTANCE WERE VERY SIMILAR FOR THESE TWO GROUPS. ONLY 2 OF 26 COMPARISONS WERE STATISTICALLY SIGNIFICANT. THE MEXICAN AMERICAN EMPLOYEES WERE MORE SATISFIED WITH JOB PRESTIGE OUTSIDE THE COMPANY, AND COMPARED TO THE NONMINORITY GROUP, THEY PERCEIVED OPPORTUNITY FOR FRIENDSHIP AS MORE IMPORTANT. THE HIERARCHIES OF NEED SATISFACTION AND IMPORTANCE WERE ALSO QUITE SIMILAR FOR THE TWO GROUPS. OVERALL, IT IS PROPOSED THAT MEXICAN AMERICAN EMPLOYEES PERCEIVE AND EVALUATE THEIR JOBS IN A MANNER VERY SIMILAR TO THAT OF NONMINORITY EMPLOYEES IN COMPARABLE JOBS. THESE FINDINGS ARE DISCUSSED IN RELATION TO EARLIER WORK THAT HAD FOUND DIFFERENCES IN NEED SATISFACTION AND IMPORTANCE BETWEEN EMPLOYEES IN MEXICO AND THE U.S. (NCMHI ABSTRACT)
    ACCN   000228

272 AUTH   **CAMPOS, A. P.**
    TITL   PROPOSED STRATEGY FOR THE 1970'S.
    SRCE   *SOCIAL CASEWORK, 1974, 55, 111-116.*
    INDX   MENTAL HEALTH PROFESSION, NEW YORK, EAST, THEORETICAL, ESSAY, IMMIGRATION, FINANCING, PROGRAM EVALUATION, PUERTO RICAN-M
    ABST   THIS EVALUATION OF THE PUERTO RICAN COMMUNITY DEVELOPMENT PROJECT INDICATES THE NEED FOR MORE EFFECTIVE PLANNING DIRECTED TOWARD INSTITUTIONAL CHANGE. IN RESPONSE TO THE ECONOMIC OPPORTUNITY ACT OF 1964, A GROUP OF PUERTO RICAN LEADERS IN NEW YORK CITY PROPOSED A NUMBER OF SELF-HELP PROGRAMS TO EXPAND JOB OPPORTUNITIES, PROVIDE VOCATIONAL TRAINING, IMPROVE BILINGUAL ELEMENTARY AND PRE-SCHOOL EDUCATION, AND ENHANCE YOUTH DEVELOPMENT. THE PROJECT IS CRITICIZED ON THE FOLLOWING GROUNDS: (1) ITS DEVELOPERS VIEWED POVERTY PRIMARILY AS THE MISFORTUNE OF INDIVIDUALS RATHER THAN AS SOCIAL INJUSTICE IN THE FORM OF SYSTEMATIC DEPRIVATION; (2) PROGRAMS WERE BASED ON A PHILOSOPHY OF REHABILITAIVE SERVICES RATHER THAN INSTITUTIONAL CHANGE; (3) THE PROPOSED NEW BUREAUCRACY WAS ADMINISTRATIVELY CUMBERSOME AND MADE DECISION-MAKING DIFFICULT; AND (4) IN PLANNING TO UTILIZE THE ETHNIC COMMUNITY, THE PLANNERS FAILED TO REALIZE BASIC DIFFERENCES BETWEEN PUERTO RICANS AND THE IMMIGRANTS WHO PROCEEDED THEM. A NEW STRATEGY IS SUGGESTED FOR THE 1970'S—A CHANGE OF EMPHASIS FROM A CULTURAL STRATEGY TO ONE OF POLITICAL POWER. ONLY THROUGH POLITICAL POWER WILL PUERTO RICANS BE ASSURED FULL PARTICIPATION IN DECISIONS THAT AFFECT THE

124

WELFARE STATE AND THE BENEFITS IT PRO-
VIDES. 11 REFERENCES.
ACCN   000229

273 AUTH **CANCIAN, F. M.**
     TITL   INTERACTION IN ZINACANTECO INDIANS.
     SRCE   *AMERICAN SOCIOLOGICAL REVIEW, 1964, 29(4),
            540-550.*
     INDX   MEXICO, INDIGENOUS POPULATIONS, RURAL,
            INTERPERSONAL RELATIONS
     ABST   TEN INDIAN FAMILIES IN ZINACANTAN, MEXICO,
            WERE OBSERVED AND THE QUALITY AND
            QUANTITY OF INTERACTION WITHIN EACH
            FAMILY RECORDED. THESE DATA WERE USED
            TO TEST SIX HYPOTHESES BASED ON SMALL
            GROUP RESEARCH AND ON THE THEORY OF
            SELF-OTHER PATTERNS. THE HYPOTHESES
            PREDICT THAT WITHIN FAMILY DYADS (1) AF-
            FECTION ELICITS AFFECTION, (2) DOMINANCE
            ELICITS SUBMISSION, AND (3) HIGH INTERAC-
            TION RATE IS RELATED TO AFFECTION; MORE-
            OVER, WITHIN EACH FAMILY ALL INDIVIDUALS
            WILL EXHIBIT (4) THE SAME DEGREE OF AFFEC-
            TION, (5) THE SAME DEGREE OF DOMINANCE-
            SUBMISSION, AND (6) THE SAME INTERACTION
            RATE. HYPOTHESES 1, 2, 4, AND 5 ARE SUP-
            PORTED. 30 REFERENCES. (JOURNAL AB-
            STRACT)
     ACCN   000230

274 AUTH **CANDELARIA, C.**
     TITL   THE FUTURE OF BILINGUAL MULTICULTURAL
            EDUCATION.
     SRCE   *AGENDA, MARCH/APRIL 1977, PP. 30-33.*
     INDX   BILINGUAL-BICULTURAL EDUCATION, EDUCA-
            TION, SPANISH SURNAMED, PROGRAM
            EVALUATION, LEGISLATION, ESSAY
     ABST   HOPE IN THE FUTURE FOR LATINOS RESTS ON
            THE STRENGTH OF PUBLIC EDUCATION'S BI-
            LINGUAL MULTICULTURAL PROGRAMS. THREE
            SIGNIFICANT ASPECTS OF BILINGUAL EDUCA-
            TION ARE DISCUSSED. FIRST, ALTHOUGH MA-
            JOR FEDERAL LAWS AUTHORIZING BILINGUAL
            EDUCATION DATE BACK ONLY TO 1974 AND
            1968, FORMAL BILINGUAL PROGRAMS IN
            AMERICAN PUBLIC SCHOOLS HAVE HAD A
            LONGER HISTORY IN SOME STATES, AND THE
            BILINGUAL MULTICULTURAL PROGRAMS OF
            FOREIGN COUNTRIES ARE GAINING RECOGNI-
            TION. SECOND, THE CONTINUING GROWTH
            AND DEVELOPMENT OF PROGRAMS PROVE
            THAT NEGATIVISM AMONG EDUCATORS AND
            THE PUBLIC CAN BE BROKEN DOWN. THIRD,
            BECAUSE THE HISTORY OF BILINGUAL PRO-
            GRAMS HAS BEEN SO DIFFICULT, IT IS IMPERA-
            TIVE THAT SELF-EVALUATION AND PRIORITY-
            SETTING BE CONTINUED AND EVEN INTENSI-
            FIED IN ORDER TO PROVIDE EFFECTIVE AND
            RELEVANT PROGRAMS FOR PARTICULAR AREAS
            OF THE COUNTRY.
     ACCN   000231

275 AUTH **CANEDO, O. O.**
     TITL   PERFORMANCE OF MEXICAN AMERICAN STU-
            DENTS ON A MEASURE OF VERBAL INTELLI-
            GENCE (DOCTORAL DISSERTATION, UNITED
            STATES INTERNATIONAL UNIVERSITY, 1972).
     SRCE   *DISSERTATION ABSTRACTS INTERNATIONAL,*

*1972, 33(3), 1016A. (UNIVERSITY MICROFILMS
NO. 72-23,489.)*
INDX   INTELLIGENCE TESTING, INTELLIGENCE, CHIL-
        DREN, MEXICAN AMERICAN, WISC, CULTURAL
        FACTORS, TEST VALIDITY, CALIFORNIA, SOUTH-
        WEST
ABST   TO ASSESS THE APPROPRIATENESS OF ITEMS
        CONTAINED IN THE VERBAL SECTION OF THE
        WECHSLER INTELLIGENCE SCALE FOR CHIL-
        DREN (WISC) WHEN USED TO TEST MEXICAN
        AMERICAN STUDENTS, AN ANALYSIS OF MISSED
        ITEMS ON THE VERBAL SECTION OF THE WISC
        TAKEN BY MEXICAN AMERICAN AND ANGLO
        STUDENTS, AGES 11 AND 12, WAS CON-
        DUCTED. RESULTS LED TO A MODIFICATION OF
        THE VERBAL SECTION OF THE WISC BY IDEN-
        TIFYING AND REPLACING 37 ITEMS INDICATING
        LANGUAGE BIAS. THREE MODIFIED VERBAL
        FORMS OF THE WISC VOCABULARY TEST WERE
        DEVELOPED AND THEN ANALYZED AS TO THEIR
        VALIDITY AS INSTRUMENTS FOR ASSESSING
        INTELLIGENCE OF MEXICAN AMERICAN STU-
        DENTS RESIDING IN CALIFORNIA. FINDIGS IN-
        DICATE THAT MEXICAN AMERICANS WILL NOT
        PERFORM SIGNIFICANTLY BETTER ON THE SAME
        TEST MATERIAL THAT HAS MERELY BEEN
        TRANSLATED FROM ENGLISH INTO SPANISH.
        HOWEVER, A TEST THAT ACCOUNTS FOR THEIR
        CULTURAL AND LINGUISTIC BACKGROUND WILL
        PRODUCE POSITIVE RESULTS IN FAVOR OF
        THIS GROUP. IMPLICATIONS FOR THE USE OF
        SUCH TESTS IN SCHOOLS AND THE NEED FOR
        FURTHER TEST DEVELOPMENT AND RE-
        SEARCH ARE DISCUSSED. 69 REFERENCES.
        (AUTHOR SUMMARY MODIFIED)
ACCN   000233

276 AUTH **CANTU, I. S.**
     TITL   THE EFFECTS OF FAMILY CHARACTERISTICS,
            PARENTAL INFLUENCE, LANGUAGE SPOKEN,
            SCHOOL EXPERIENCE AND SELF MOTIVATION
            ON THE LEVEL OF EDUCATIONAL ACHIEVE-
            MENT AMONG MEXICAN AMERICANS (DOC-
            TORAL DISSERTATION, UNIVERSITY OF MICHI-
            GAN, ANN ARBOR, 1975).
     SRCE   *DISSERTATION ABSTRACTS INTERNATIONAL,
            1975, 36(6), 3261A. (UNIVERSITY MICROFILMS
            NO. 75-29,186.)*
     INDX   SCHOLASTIC ACHIEVEMENT, BILINGUAL, FAMILY
            ROLES, MEXICAN AMERICAN, EMPIRICAL,
            ACHIEVEMENT MOTIVATION, PARENTAL IN-
            VOLVEMENT, EDUCATION, RURAL, TEXAS,
            SOUTHWEST, CHILDREN
     ABST   THE EFFECTS OF FAMILY CHARACTERISTICS,
            PARENTAL INFLUENCE, LANGUAGE SPOKEN,
            SCHOOL EXPERIENCES, AND SELF-MOTIVA-
            TION ON THE EDUCATIONAL ATTAINMENT OF
            MEXICAN AMERICANS WAS INVESTIGATED
            THROUGH A QUESTIONNAIRE CONSISTING OF
            43 QUESTIONS ADMINISTERED TO 73 RAN-
            DOMLY SELECTED MEXICAN AMERICANS FROM
            THE LOWER RIO GRANDE VALLEY OF TEXAS.
            THE FINDINGS INDICATE THAT A MAJOR FAC-
            TOR IN THE EDUCATION OF MEXICAN AMERI-
            CAN CHILDREN IS THE SOCIOECONOMIC CON-
            DITIONS OF THE FAMILY. PARENTAL INFLUENCE
            AND THE SCHOOL THE CHILD ATTENDS HAVE
            INORDINATE INFLUENCES IN MOTIVATING AND

ASSURING THAT THE MEXICAN AMERICAN STUDENT WILL SUCCEED IN HIS EDUCATIONAL ENDEAVORS. SCHOOLS ALSO PLAY AN IMPORTANT ROLE IN ASSURING THAT MEXICAN AMERICAN STUDENTS ARE GIVEN AN EQUAL OPPORTUNITY TO SUCCEED. 51 REFERENCES. (AUTHOR SUMMARY MODIFIED)

ACCN 000234

277 AUTH **CARDENAS, D. N.**
TITL COMPOUND AND COORDINATE BILINGUAL-ISM/BICULTURALISM IN THE SOUTHWEST.
SRCE *IN R. W. EWTON & J. ORNSTEIN (EDS.), STUDIES IN LANGUAGE AND LINGUISTICS. EL PASO: TEXAS WESTERN PRESS, 1972, PP. 165-180.*
INDX COMPOUND-COORDINATE DISTINCTION, BILINGUALISM, COGNITIVE DEVELOPMENT, LANGUAGE ACQUISITION, LINGUISTICS, CULTURE, CULTURAL PLURALISM, RESEARCH METHODOLOGY, ESSAY
ABST COMPOUND AND COORDINATE BILINGUALISM ARE DEFINED AND OPERATIONALIZED VIA EXAMPLES IN AN ATTEMPT TO EXPLAIN SOME OF THE DYNAMICS OF MULTILINGUAL INDIVIDUALS' BEHAVIOR. BILINGUALISM AND BICULTURALISM AS DISTINCT AND RELATED CONCEPTS ARE USED TO SCHEMATIZE THE ACCULTURATION PROCESS AND ITS VARIATIONS. BILINGUALISM AND ITS RELATIONSHIP TO BICULTURALISM IS DISCUSSED ALONG WITH SUGGESTIONS FOR MAKING THE INEVITABLE ASSIMILATION PROCESS MORE TOLERABLE AND COMPREHENSIBLE TO THOSE EXPERIENCING IT. 10 REFERENCES.

ACCN 000235

278 AUTH **CARDENAS, E., MIYADE, F., ALVARADO, C., & SCHIFF, S.**
TITL PROGRESS REPORT OF PROGRAM ACTIVITIES: 1976-1977.
SRCE *UNPUBLISHED MANUSCRIPT, SANTA BARBARA FAMILY CARE CENTER, SANTA BARBARA, CALIF., 1977.*
INDX MEXICAN AMERICAN, ESSAY, BILINGUAL-BICULTURAL EDUCATION, SCHOLASTIC ACHIEVEMENT, EARLY CHILDHOOD EDUCATION, PARENTAL INVOLVEMENT, CHILDREARING PRACTICES, PRIMARY PREVENTION, MENTAL HEALTH, CALIFORNIA, SOUTHWEST, SOCIAL SERVICES
ABST THE CENTRO FAMILIAR DE SANTA BARBARA, A PRIVATE NONPROFIT ORGANIZATION PROVIDING SOCIAL AND EDUCATIONAL PROGRAMS TO LOW-INCOME MEXICAN AMERICAN MOTHERS AND CHILDREN, IS DESCRIBED. INCLUDED ARE BRIEF SUMMARIES OF THE HISTORY, PHILOSOPHY, AND OBJECTIVES OF THE PROGRAM, THE AVAILABLE FACILITIES, AND THE CHARACTERISTICS OF THE POPULATION SERVED. LENGTHY REPORTS ON THE SPECIFIC PROGRAMS FOR MOTHERS, CHILDREN AND PARENTING CLASSES ARE ALSO PRESENTED.

ACCN 000236

279 AUTH **CARILLO-BERON, C.**
TITL CHANGING ADOLESCENT SEX-ROLE IDEOLOGY THROUGH SHORT TERM BICULTURAL GROUP PROCESS.
SRCE *SAN FRANCISCO: R AND E RESEARCH ASSOCIATES, 1977.*
INDX SEX ROLES, SEX COMPARISON, ADOLESCENTS, RESEARCH METHODOLOGY, STEREOTYPES, CULTURAL FACTORS, CROSS CULTURAL, CALIFORNIA, SOUTHWEST, SES, GROUP DYNAMICS, URBAN, PEER GROUP, MEXICAN AMERICAN, EMPIRICAL, ATTITUDES, MALE, FEMALE
ABST TO ASSESS A GROUP-CENTERED METHOD OF INTERVENTION AS AN AID TO CHICANO YOUTHS' ACCEPTANCE OF MORE EGALITARIAN SEX ROLES, 96 HIGH SCHOOL STUDENTS (EQUAL NUMBERS OF CHICANOS AND ANGLOS, MALES AND FEMALES) FROM A LOWER SOCIOECONOMIC AREA NEAR SAN FRANCISCO WERE STUDIED. HALF WERE ASSIGNED TO FOUR SESSIONS OF SMALL GROUP DISCUSSION WHICH FOCUSED ON SEX ROLE BEHAVIOR EXPECTATIONS, AND THE REMAINDER SERVED AS A CONTROL GROUP. IT WAS EXPECTED THAT THE CHICANOS WOULD IDENTIFY WITH MORE TRADITIONAL VALUES THAN THE ANGLOS AND CONSEQUENTLY EXHIBIT GREATER POST-INTERVENTION VALUE CHANGE. FEMALES WERE EXPECTED TO EXHIBIT GREATER CHANGE IN THE DIRECTION OF EGALITARIAN VALUES THAN THE MALES. THE ASSESSMENT INSTRUMENTS WERE (1) THE ATTITUDE-INTEREST ANALYSIS TEST TO ASSESS SEX ROLE ATTITUDES, (2) AN SES SCALE, (3) THE VALUE-ORIENTATION SCHEDULE TO DETERMINE TRADITIONALISM, AND (4) THE LORR GROUP PROCESS MEASURE TO ASSESS BEHAVIORAL CHANGE. DATA WERE ANALYZED IN A 2X2X2X2 ANOVA FRAMEWORK WITH TREATMENT, SEX, ETHNICITY, AND TIME AS THE INDEPENDENT VARIABLES. THE VALUE-ORIENTATION SCHEDULE REVEALED NO DIFFERENCES BETWEEN THE TWO ETHNIC GROUPS, BUT SIGNIFICANT DIFFERENCES WERE FOUND IN THE PREDICTED DIRECTION ON THE ATTITUDE-INTEREST ANALYSIS TEST FOR POST-TEST BY TREATMENT, SEX, AND ETHNICITY. ALTHOUGH THE LORR SCORING METHOD DID NOT YIELD SUFFICIENT OBJECTIVE SUPPORT OF BEHAVIORAL CHANGE DUE TO THE GROUP PROCESS, 33 OF THE UNIVARIATE TESTS DID SHOW A SIGNIFICANT DIFFERENCE, AND COMMENTS OF THE PARTICIPANTS POINTED TO THE EFFICACY OF THE INTERVENTION. DATA ARE PRESENTED IN 40 TABLES AND 11 FIGURES. 57 REFERENCES.

ACCN 002046

280 AUTH **CARLOS, M. L.**
TITL FICTIVE KINSHIP AND MODERNIZATION IN MEXICO: A COMPARATIVE ANALYSIS.
SRCE *ANTHROPOLOGICAL QUARTERLY, 1973, 46(2), 75-91.*
INDX FICTIVE KINSHIP, MEXICO, CULTURE, REVIEW, RELIGION, INDIGENOUS POPULATIONS, FAMILY STRUCTURE, RURAL, URBAN, EXTENDED FAMILY
ABST THIS PAPER ANALYZES THE IMPACT OF MODERNIZATION ON COMPADRAZGO (I.E., FICTIVE KINSHIP) IN MEXICO. THE PURPOSE IS TO DESCRIBE AND EXPLAIN HOW MODERNIZATION SYSTEMATICALLY ALTERS THE STRUCTURAL

DIMENSIONS, FUNCTIONS AND DYNAMICS OF THE INSTITUTION. IN ADDITION, A FULL ACCOUNT IS GIVEN OF THE MAJOR PATTERNS AND TRENDS IN COMPADRAZGO IN RURAL AND URBAN SETTINGS. FINALLY, THE EARLY WORK OF ROBERT REDFIELD ON MEXICAN COMPADRAZGO IS REVIEWED, MODIFIED, AND UPDATED. 51 REFERENCES. (JOURNAL ABSTRACT)

ACCN 000237

281 AUTH **CARLOS, M. L.**
     TITL A MODEL OF BROKER, CONSTITUENCY AND NETWORK POLITICS IN MEXICAN COMMUNITIES AND REGIONS.
     SRCE *PAPER PRESENTED AT THE ANNUAL MEETINGS OF THE AMERICAN ANTHROPOLOGICAL ASSOCIATION, WASHINGTON, D.C., NOVEMBER 1976.*
     INDX MEXICO, POLITICS, POLITICAL POWER, SOCIAL SCIENCES, ESSAY
     ABST A MODEL WHICH DEMONSTRATES THE INTERACTION BETWEEN POWER CENTERS AND LEVELS OF NATIONAL AND SUB-NATIONAL ACTIVITIES OF MEXICAN POLITICAL LIFE IS PRESENTED. REGIONAL AND COMMUNITY ASPECTS OF THE SYSTEM ARE EXAMINED AS WELL AS THE POLITICAL BROKERAGE AND NETWORK POLITICS WHICH LINK THESE LEVELS AND CENTERS. THE AUTHOR HOPES TO BROADEN THE VIEW THAT LOCAL, STATE AND NATIONAL REPRESENTATION IN THE MEXICAN POLITICAL SYSTEM IS LIMITED TO SOCIAL ELITES, THE NATIONAL PARTY AND THE RULING REGIME. IT IS ARGUED THAT GRASS-ROOTS INTERESTS ARE REPRESENTED VIA POLITICAL BROKERS AND NETWORK POLITICS, AND THAT THESE MUST BE STUDIED AND THEIR CONSTITUENCY DOCUMENTED IN ORDER TO IDENTIFY THE KINDS OF INTERESTS AND GRASS-ROOTS PRESSURE TO WHICH THE MEXICAN GOVERNMENT IS MOST RESPONSIVE. 7 REFERENCES. (AUTHOR SUMMARY MODIFIED)

ACCN 000238

282 AUTH **CARLOS, M. L.**
     TITL TRADITIONAL AND MODERN FORMS OF COMPADRAZGO AMONG MEXICANS AND MEXICAN-AMERICANS: A SURVEY OF CONTINUITIES AND CHANGES.
     SRCE *ATTIDEL XL CONGRESSO INTERNAZIONALE DEGLI AMERICANISTI, ROMA-GENOVA, SEPTEMBER 3-10, 1972.*
     INDX MEXICAN, MEXICAN AMERICAN, REVIEW, FICTIVE KINSHIP, ACCULTURATION, SES, URBAN, RURAL, INDIGENOUS POPULATIONS, MEXICO, SOCIAL STRUCTURE, CULTURAL CHANGE
     ABST TRENDS IN MEXICAN AND MEXICAN AMERICAN PATTERNS OF COMPADRAZGO ARE IDENTIFIED, WITH DICUSSION FOCUSING ON SUCH VARIABLES AS COMMUNITY TYPE, CLASS, ETHNICITY, URBANIZATION AND SOCIAL STRATIFICATION AS THEY AFFECT THE FORM OF COMPADRAZGO USED. A COMPARATIVE ANALYSIS OF THE CONTINUITIES AND CHANGES IN COMPADRAZGO AS IT IS PRACTICED IN MEXICO AND THE UNITED STATES IS PRESENTED. THE GENERAL CHARACTERISTICS OF MODERN AND

TRADITIONAL FORMS OF COMPADRAZGO AMONG THESE TWO POPULATIONS ARE IDENTIFIED, AND IT IS POSITED THAT THE FICTIVE KINSHIP SYSTEM OF COMPADRAZGO DOES AND WILL CONTINUE TO ADAPT STRUCTURALLY AND FUNCTIONALLY TO THE EFFECTS OF MODERNIZATION IN TRADITIONAL MEXICAN COMMUNITIES BOTH IN MEXICO AND THE U.S. THE LITERATURE IS EXTENSIVELY REVIEWED AND COMPARED REGARDING COMPADRAZGO IN INDIAN VILLAGES, HETEROGENEOUS COMMUNITIES, AND CITIES IN MEXICO AND THE U.S. 65 REFERENCES. (AUTHOR SUMMARY MODIFIED)

ACCN 000239

283 AUTH **CARLOS, M. L., & SELLERS, L.**
     TITL FAMILY, KINSHIP STRUCTURE, AND MODERNIZATION IN LATIN AMERICA.
     SRCE *LATIN AMERICAN RESEARCH REVIEW, 1972, 7(2), 95-124.*
     INDX FICTIVE KINSHIP, ACCULTURATION, EXTENDED FAMILY, SES, CENTRAL AMERICA, SOUTH AMERICA, CULTURE, REVIEW, RURAL, URBAN, SOCIAL MOBILITY, ESSAY, MEXICO, CULTURAL CHANGE
     ABST AN ANALYSIS OF FAMILY AND KINSHIP PATTERNS IN LATIN AMERICA AMONG DISTINCT SOCIOECONOMIC GROUPS IN URBAN AND RURAL SETTINGS IS PRESENTED. THE LITERATURE ON WHICH THE ANALYSIS RESTS IS ALSO CRITICALLY EXAMINED. MUCH OF THE FOCUS IS ON THOSE ASPECTS OF THE MATERIAL WHICH DEAL WITH EXTENDED FAMILY (PARENTESCO) RELATIONS AND WITH FICTIVE KINSHIP (COMPADRAZGO) TIES; LESS ATTENTION IS GIVEN TO STUDIES AND COMPONENTS OF THE NUCLEAR FAMILY. THE CENTRAL THEME DEVELOPED IN THE ESSAY IS THAT FAMILIAL TIES AND THE INSTITUTION OF FICTIVE KINSHIP ARE NOT BREAKING DOWN UNDER THE IMPACT OF MODERNIZATION, DESPITE THEORIES AND INTERPRETATIONS OF URBANIZATION AND INDUSTRIALIZATION WHICH MAINTAIN THAT THE OPPOSITE IS TRUE. 115 REFERENCES. (AUTHOR SUMMARY)

ACCN 000240

284 AUTH **CARLSON, H. B., & HENDERSON, N.**
     TITL THE INTELLIGENCE OF AMERICAN CHILDREN OF MEXICAN PARENTAGE.
     SRCE *JOURNAL OF ABNORMAL AND SOCIAL PSYCHOLOGY, 1950, 45, 544-551.*
     INDX INTELLIGENCE, INTELLIGENCE TESTING, CALIFORNIA TEST OF MENTAL MATURITY, STANFORD-BINET INTELLIGENCE TEST, MEXICAN AMERICAN, EMPIRICAL, CHILDREN, CROSS CULTURAL, SES, CALIFORNIA, SOUTHWEST
     ABST TO ASCERTAIN ALLEGED GROUP DIFFERENCES IN INTELLIGENCE BETWEEN ANGLO- AND MEXICAN-DESCENT ELEMENTARY SCHOOL CHILDREN, 115 MEXICANS AND 105 ANGLO AMERICANS WERE ADMINISTERED THE FOLLOWING INTELLIGENCE TESTS: DETROIT BEGINNING FIRST GRADE, DETROIT PRIMARY, PINTNER-CUNNINGHAM, KUHLMAN-ANDERSON, CALIFORNIA TEST OF MENTAL MATURITY (ELEMENTARY SHORT FORM) AND THE STAN-

FORD-BINET (1937 REVISION). THE MEXICAN CHILDREN WERE FOUND TO HAVE CONSISTENTLY LOWER MEAN IQ SCORES THAN THE ANGLO GROUP. THE DIFFERENCE BETWEEN THE TWO GROUPS INCREASED IN MAGNITUDE FROM THE FIRST TO THE LAST TESTING PERIODS OVER A SPAN OF 5 1/2 YEARS, PRIMARILY BECAUSE OF A DROP IN MEAN IQ OF THE MEXICAN CHILDREN. WHILE THESE DISSIMILARITIES MIGHT BE DUE TO HEREDITARY FACTORS, IT WAS SUGGESTED THAT UNCONTROLLED ENVIRONMENTAL FACTORS REMAINED. THEREFORE, NO FINAL STATEMENT OF THE RELATIVE NATIVE SUPERIORITY OF ONE NATIONAL GROUP COULD BE MADE. IT IS CONCLUDED THAT WHEN SCORES WERE OBTAINED FROM VARIOUS TESTS AND THEN TREATED AS A SINGLE VARIABLE, THE POSSIBILITY OF PREDICTION OF LATER TEST SCORES WAS LESS FOR THE MEXICAN GROUP. THIS FINDING QUESTIONS THE APPROPRIATENESS OF THE COMMON PRACTICE IN SCHOOLS OF RECORDING FOR PREDICTIVE PURPOSES AN INDEX OF INTELLECTUAL BRIGHTNESS FOR A CHILD WHO IS NOT A MEMBER OF THE CULTURAL GROUP UPON WHICH THE TEST IS STANDARDIZED, AND ESPECIALLY SO WHEN THE INDEX IS TO BE USED AT SOME TIME SUBSEQUENT TO THE TESTING PERIOD. 26 REFERENCES.

ACCN   000241

285 AUTH   **CARR, L. G., & HAUSER, W. J.**
     TITL   ANOMIE AND RELIGIOSITY: AN EMPIRICAL RE-EXAMINATION.
     SRCE   *JOURNAL FOR THE SCIENTIFIC STUDY OF RELIGION, 1976, 15(1), 69-74.*
     INDX   ANOMIE, CONFORMITY, PERSONALITY, RELIGION, CROSS CULTURAL, CULTURAL FACTORS, PUERTO RICAN-M, MEXICAN AMERICAN, EMPIRICAL, MIDWEST
     ABST   THE HYPOTHESIS THAT RELIGIOSITY REDUCES ANOMIE IN MODERN SOCIETY IS RE-EXAMINED. ANOMIE WAS NOT FOUND TO BE INVERSELY RELATED TO RELIGIOSITY, NOR WAS AN INVERSE RELATIONSHIP BETWEEN ANOMIE AND CLASS REDUCED BY RELIGIOSITY. CONTROLS FOR ACQUIESCENT AND SOCIAL DESIRABILITY MEASUREMENT ERROR DID NOT ALTER THIS FINDING NOR DID THE SUBSTITUTION OF AN ALTERNATIVE MEASURE (POWERLESSNESS) FOR ANOMIE. IN SUM, CURRENT EMPIRICAL RESEARCH DOES NOT SUPPORT THOSE WHO HAVE INTERPRETED DURKHEIM TO SAY THAT RELIGION REDUCES ANOMIE IN MODERN SOCIETY. 24 REFERENCES. (JOURNAL ABSTRACT MODIFIED)
     ACCN   000242

286 AUTH   **CARRANZA, M. A., & RYAN, E. B.**
     TITL   EVALUATIVE REACTIONS OF BILINGUAL ANGLO AND MEXICAN AMERICAN ADOLESCENTS TOWARD SPEAKERS OF ENGLISH AND SPANISH.
     SRCE   *LINGUISTICS: AN INTERNATIONAL REVIEW, 1975, 166, 84-104.*
     INDX   DISCRIMINATION, BILINGUALISM, BILINGUAL, ADOLESCENTS, MEXICAN AMERICAN, ATTITUDES, CROSS CULTURAL, EMPIRICAL, BILINGUAL-BICULTURAL EDUCATION
     ABST   THE MATCHED GUISE TECHNIQUE WAS USED WITH MEXICAN AMERICAN AND ANGLO HIGH SCHOOL STUDENTS WHO HAD TAKEN SPANISH CLASSES TO DETERMINE THEIR EVALUATIVE REACTIONS TOWARD SPEAKERS OF ENGLISH AND SPANISH. IT WAS ASSUMED THAT THE STUDENTS' REACTIONS WOULD BE INFLUENCED BY (1) CONTEXT OF SPEECH (HOME OR SCHOOL) AND (2) TYPE OF RATING SCALE (STATUS AND SOLIDARITY). THE MAJOR HYPOTHESES TESTED WERE THAT MEXICAN AMERICANS WOULD RATE SPANISH HIGHER IN THE HOME CONTEXT AND ENGLISH HIGHER IN THE SCHOOL, WITH ANGLOS RATING ENGLISH HIGHER IN BOTH CONTEXTS. RESULTS FOUND SPANISH WAS RATED HIGHER IN THE HOME CONTEXT WITH ENGLISH RATED HIGHER IN THE SCHOOL CONTEXT BY BOTH MEXICAN AMERICAN AND ANGLO STUDENTS. THIS IS AS EXPECTED FOR THE MEXICAN AMERICANS BUT CONTRARY TO PREDICTIONS FOR ANGLOS. POSSIBLE INTERPRETATIONS FOR THIS FINDING ARE THAT THE FAVORABLE REACTIONS TOWARD SPANISH SPEAKERS BY ANGLO STUDENTS IS RELATED TO THEIR ATTENDING SPANISH CLASSES IN SCHOOL AND THAT EXPOSURE TO A FOREIGN LANGUAGE HAS INCREASED THEIR REGARD FOR A NON-ENGLISH LANGUAGE. THE IMPLICATIONS OF THESE FINDINGS FOR BILINGUAL EDUCATION ARE DISCUSSED. 42 REFERENCES.
     ACCN   000243

287 AUTH   **CARRIER, J. M.**
     TITL   CULTURAL FACTORS AFFECTING MALE MEXICAN HOMOSEXUAL BEHAVIOR.
     SRCE   *ARCHIVES OF SEXUAL BEHAVIOR, 1976, 5, 103-124.*
     INDX   URBAN, MALE, SEX ROLES, SEXUAL BEHAVIOR, GENDER IDENTITY, SES, DEVIANCE, PERSONALITY, EMPIRICAL, SURVEY, MEXICAN, HOMOSEXUALITY, CULTURAL FACTORS
     ABST   SOME ASPECTS OF THE MESTIZOIZED URBAN CULTURE IN MEXICO ARE LINKED TO MALE HOMOSEXUALITY IN SUPPORT OF THE THEORY THAT CULTURAL FACTORS PLAY AN IMPORTANT ROLE IN THE KIND OF LIFE STYLES AND SEX PRACTICES OF HOMOSEXUAL MALES. THE FOLLOWING FACTORS ARE CONSIDERED RELEVANT: THE SHARP DICHOTOMIZATION OF GENDER ROLES, DUAL CATEGORIZATION OF FEMALES AS GOOD OR BAD, SEPARATE SOCIAL NETWORKS MAINTAINED BY MALES BEFORE AND AFTER MARRIAGE, PROPORTION OF UNMARRIED MALES, AND DISTRIBUTION OF INCOME. ONE RESULT OF THE SHARP DICHOTOMIZATION OF SEX ROLES IS THE WIDELY HELD BELIEF THAT EFFEMINATE MALES GENERALLY PREFER TO PLAY THE FEMALE ROLE RATHER THAN THE MALE. EFFEMINACY AND HOMOSEXUALITY ARE ALSO LINKED BY THE BELIEF THAT AS A RESULT OF THIS ROLE PREFERENCE EFFEMINATE MALES ARE SEXUALLY INTERESTED ONLY IN MASCULINE MALES WITH WHOM THEY PLAY THE PASSIVE SEX ROLE. THE PARTICIPATION OF MASCULINE MALES IN HOMOSEXUAL

ENCOUNTERS IS RELATED IN PART TO A RELA-
TIVELY HIGH LEVEL OF SEXUAL AWARENESS IN
COMBINATION WITH THE LACK OF STIGMATI-
ZATION OF THE INSERTOR ROLE AND IN PART
TO THE RESTRAINTS PLACED ON ALTERNATIVE
SEXUAL OUTLETS BY AVAILABLE INCOME AND/
OR MARITAL STATUS. 19 REFERENCES. (JOUR-
NAL ABSTRACT MODIFIED)

ACCN   000244

288 AUTH   **CARRIER, J. M.**
    TITL   FAMILY ATTITUDES AND MEXICAN MALE HO-
            MOSEXUALITY.
    SRCE   *URBAN LIFE, 1976, 5, 359-375.*
    INDX   SEX ROLES, SEXUAL BEHAVIOR, FAMILY ROLES,
            DEVIANCE, INTERPERSONAL RELATIONS, MASS
            MEDIA, MEXICAN, CULTURE, EMPIRICAL, GEN-
            DER IDENTITY, MALE, URBAN, HOMOSEXUAL-
            ITY, ATTITUDES, CULTURAL FACTORS
    ABST   SOME OF THE WAYS IN WHICH FAMILY PER-
            SPECTIVES ON HOMOSEXUALITY AFFECT THE
            BEHAVIOR OF SINGLE MEXICAN MALES WERE
            EXPLORED VIA INTERVIEW DATA WITH INDE-
            PENDENT INFORMANTS, FRIENDSHIP CIRCLES
            AND FAMILIES. MEXICAN ATTITUDES TOWARD
            HOMOSEXUALITY ARE CONSIDERED HIGHLY
            NEGATIVE AND YET MEXICAN SOCIETY GEN-
            ERALLY ACCEPTS THE INEVITABILITY OF HO-
            MOSEXUAL CONTACTS BETWEEN MEN AND
            DOESN'T DIFFERENTIATE BETWEEN HOMOSEX-
            UALITY AND OTHER SEXUAL OUTLETS AS LONG
            AS THEY ARE CARRIED OUT WITH DISCRETION.
            FAMILY DEMANDS AND INFLUENCES ARE DE-
            SCRIBED AS CAUSING RESPONDENTS TO BE
            CONCERNED OVER HOW MUCH THEIR PAR-
            ENTS AND SIBLINGS KNOW AND TO FEAR
            BEING SEEN WITH KNOWN HOMOSEXUALS.
            HOMOSEXUALLY INVOLVED MASCULINE MALES
            FACE DIFFERENT FAMILY RESPONSES THAN DO
            EFFEMINATE ONES. GENERALLY MASCULINE
            MALES WHO PLAY THE "ACTIVE" INSERTOR
            ROLE ARE NOT IDENTIFIED AS HOMOSEXUALS
            UNLESS THEY USE THIS SEXUAL OUTLET EX-
            CLUSIVELY. THE LACK OF A WIDESPREAD HO-
            MOSEXUAL SUBCULTURE IS ALSO PARTLY DUE
            TO FAMILY INFLUENCES. OVERALL, THE MEXI-
            CAN FAMILY PLAYS A LARGER ROLE IN HOMO-
            SEXUAL BEHAVIOR THAN DOES THE ANGLO
            AMERICAN FAMILY. 11 REFERENCES.
    ACCN   000245

289 AUTH   **CARRIER, J. M.**
    TITL   PARTICIPANTS IN URBAN MEXICAN MALE HO-
            MOSEXUAL ENCOUNTERS.
    SRCE   *ARCHIVES OF SEXUAL BEHAVIOR, 1971, 1(4),*
            279-291.
    INDX   ADULTS, CULTURAL FACTORS, EMPIRICAL,
            GENDER IDENTITY, HOMOSEXUALITY, MALE,
            MEXICAN, SEXUAL BEHAVIOR, URBAN, DEVI-
            ANCE, SEX ROLES, CROSS CULTURAL
    ABST   PRELIMINARY DATA ARE PRESENTED ON 53
            URBAN MEXICAN MALES INTERVIEWED DUR-
            ING 1970-1971 IN A STUDY OF HOMOSEXUAL
            ENCOUNTERS IN A LARGE MEXICAN CITY. THESE
            DATA ARE COMPARED WITH DATA FROM RE-
            CENT STUDIES IN THE UNITED STATES AND EN-
            GLAND OF MALE HOMOSEXUAL BEHAVIOR. AL-
            THOUGH PRELIMINARY AND LIMITED, THE

MEXICAN DATA INDICATE THAT CULTURAL FAC-
TORS ARE IMPORTANT DETERMINANTS OF LIFE
STYLES AND SEX PRACTICES OF HOMOSEX-
UAL MALES. FORTY-EIGHT OF THE 53 (90) PRE-
FERRED AND USUALLY PRACTICED ANAL IN-
TERCOURSE, FOUR PREFERRED ORAL
CONTACTS, AND ONE PREFERRED MUTUAL
MASTURBATION. INTERVIEWEES WERE ALSO
GROUPED ACCORDING TO MAJOR TYPE OF
SEX ACTIVITY DURING THE FIRST SUSTAINED
YEAR OF HOMOSEXUAL ACTIVITY AFTER PU-
BERTY. ONE INTRAGROUP COMPARISON INDI-
CATES SIGNIFICANT DIFFERENCES BETWEEN
THE ACTIVE AND ANAL PASSIVE INTERVIEW-
EES. FOR EXAMPLE, AS CHILDREN ANAL PAS-
SIVE SUBJECTS HAD SIGNIFICANTLY MORE HO-
MOSEXUAL CONTACTS WITH ADULTS; THEY
ALSO CONSIDERED THEMSELVES MORE EF-
FEMINATE AND AS CHILDREN WERE MORE IN-
VOLVED WITH FEMALE SEX-TYPED ACTIVITIES.
COMPARISON OF DATA FROM THE ENGLISH
AND UNITED STATES STUDIES WITH THE PRES-
ENT DATA SUGGESTS THAT PREFERENCE FOR
A PARTICULAR SEXUAL TECHNIQUE IS NOT AS
DEVELOPED IN THE FORMER TWO COUNTRIES;
WHEN THERE IS A PREFERENCE, IT IS NOT
USUALLY FOR ANAL INTERCOURSE. 8 REFER-
ENCES. (AUTHOR ABSTRACT)

ACCN   002047

290 AUTH   **CARRIER, J. M.**
    TITL   "SEX ROLE PREFERENCE" AS AN EXPLANA-
            TORY VARIABLE IN HOMOSEXUAL BEHAVIOR.
    SRCE   *ARCHIVES OF SEXUAL BEHAVIOR, 1977, 6, 53-*
            65.
    INDX   SEX ROLES, SEXUAL BEHAVIOR, MALE, EMPIR-
            ICAL, MEXICAN, MEXICAN AMERICAN, CROSS
            CULTURAL, SES, DEVIANCE, INTERPERSONAL
            RELATIONS, GENDER IDENTITY, URBAN, HO-
            MOSEXUALITY, CULTURAL FACTORS
    ABST   SEX ROLE PREFERENCES BY MALES INVOLVED
            IN HOMOSEXUAL ENCOUNTERS MUST BE
            CONSIDERED A POTENTIALLY IMPORTANT AS-
            PECT OF THEIR BEHAVIOR CONSIDERING THE
            CROSS CULTURAL DATA PRESENTED IN THIS
            PAPER. WHETHER OR NOT SEX ACTS ARE AC-
            COMPANIED BY OR GENERATE FEELINGS OF A
            ROLE BEING PLAYED DEPENDS ON BOTH THE
            EXPECTATIONS OF THE CULTURE AND THE
            PERSONALITY DYNAMICS OF THE INVOLVED
            INDIVIDUALS. ALTHOUGH THE RELATIVE EF-
            FECTS OF CULTURAL EXPECTATIONS AND PER-
            SONALITY ON DEVELOPMENT OF SEX-ROLE
            PREFERENCES CANNOT BE ASSESSED WITH
            AVAILABLE DATA, IT SEEMS CLEAR THAT IN SO-
            CIETIES LIKE MEXICO, BRAZIL AND TURKEY,
            CULTURAL EXPECTATIONS GREATLY AFFECT
            HOMOSEXUAL BEHAVIORS. ESPECIALLY INFLU-
            ENTIAL IN SEVERAL COUNTRIES IS THE SHARPLY
            DICHOTOMIZED GENDER ROLES AND THE
            CULTURAL FORMULATION LINKING EFFEMI-
            NACY AND HOMOSEXUALITY THAT APPEAR TO
            PROVIDE THE NECESSARY CONDITIONS FOR
            SEX-ROLE PREFERENCE DEVELOPMENT. 23
            REFERENCES. (AUTHOR SUMMARY MODIFIED)
    ACCN   000246

291 AUTH   **CARRILLO, C.**

TITL CHICANOS AND PSYCHOTHERAPY: ISSUES AND TRENDS.

SRCE *PAPER PRESENTED AT THE SPANISH-SPEAKING MENTAL HEALTH RESEARCH CENTER COLLOQUIUM SERIES, UNIVERSITY OF CALIFORNIA, LOS ANGELES, 1977.*

INDX PSYCHOTHERAPY, REVIEW, MEXICAN AMERICAN, SES, PSYCHOTHERAPY OUTCOME, RESEARCH METHODOLOGY, MENTAL HEALTH, HEALTH DELIVERY SYSTEMS, RESOURCE UTILIZATION

ABST THE INCREASING LITERATURE ON MENTAL HEALTH ISSUES PERTAINING TO CHICANOS HAS (1) EMPHASIZED BARRIERS TO AVAILABLE SERVICES, (2) RAISED LEGISLATIVE AND PROFESSIONAL AWARENESS OF CHICANO NEEDS, AND (3) DEVELOPED THE NEED FOR A CRITICAL EXAMINATION OF OTHER ISSUES INVOLVED IN THE DELIVERY OF PSYCHOTHERAPEUTIC SERVICES TO CHICANOS. THE VALIDITY AND EFFECTIVENESS OF PSYCHOTHERAPY WITH CHICANOS BY CHICANO THERAPISTS IS AN ESPECIALLY RICH AREA FOR STUDY. THIS PAPER REVIEWS PSYCHOTHERAPY AND ITS PROBLEMS IN ORDER TO CONSTRUCT A CONTEXT WITHIN WHICH TO VIEW THE SEMINAL WORK OF CHICANO PRACTITIONERS. ADDITIONALLY, THE GROWING NEED TO AVAIL THE CHICANO COMMUNITY OF PSYCHOTHERAPEUTIC SERVICES IS DISCUSSED. TRENDS IN CHICANO PSYCHOTHERAPY AS DESCRIBED IN THE LITERATURE ARE SURVEYED AND ISSUES PERTINENT TO THE DELIVERY AND EVALUATION OF PSYCHOTHERAPY TO CHICANOS IS REVIEWED. IN CONCLUSION, AN INTEGRATION OF SOCIO-ECO-POLITICAL CONCEPTS TOWARDS THE EVOLUTION OF A CHICANO PSYCHOTHERAPY IS PRESENTED. (AUTHOR SUMMARY MODIFIED)

ACCN 000247

292 AUTH **CARRILLO-BERON, C.**

TITL A COMPARISON OF ANGLO AND CHICANO WOMEN.

SRCE *SAN FRANCISCO: R AND E RESEARCH ASSOCIATES, 1974.*

INDX FEMALE, SEX ROLES, FAMILY STRUCTURE, AUTHORITARIANISM, FATALISM, ACCULTURATION, FAMILY ROLES, ATTRIBUTION OF RESPONSIBILITY, ROTTER INTERNAL-EXTERNAL SCALE, SOCIAL MOBILITY, SES, SCHOLASTIC ACHIEVEMENT, EMPIRICAL, LOCUS OF CONTROL, AUTHORITARIANISM, CALIFORNIA, SOUTHWEST

ABST TO COMPARE THE DIFFERENCES IN CHICANO AND ANGLO WOMEN REGARDING INTERNAL AND EXTERNAL LOCUS OF CONTROL, AND TO RELATE THESE DIFFERENCES TO CHICANOS' TRADITIONAL FAMILY IDEOLOGY, 25 CHICANO AND 25 ANGLO WOMEN WERE ADMINISTERED TESTS MEASURING AUTHORITARIANISM, INTERNAL-EXTERNAL CONTROL AND SOCIO-ECONOMIC LEVEL. IT WAS HYPOTHESIZED THAT: (1) CHICANOS WOULD SCORE SIGNIFICANTLY HIGHER ON THE AUTHORITARIAN SCALES THAN ANGLOS; (2) CHICANOS WOULD SCORE SIGNIFICANTLY MORE EXTERNALLY THAN ANGLO SUBJECTS; AND (3) THERE WOULD BE A SIGNIFICANT RELATIONSHIP BETWEEN THE AU-

THORITARIAN AND INTERNAL-EXTERNAL SCORES. THE FIRST HYPOTHESIS WAS CONFIRMED; THERE WAS NO SIGNIFICANT DIFFERENCE ON THE TWO GROUPS' I-E SCORES DUE TO HIGH EXTERNAL SCORES FOR BOTH THE ANGLO AND CHICANO SUBJECTS. THIS STUDY AND ITS AUTHORITARIAN TRADITIONAL FAMILY IDEOLOGY SCALE, IF FURTHER DEVELOPED, MAY HAVE PRACTICAL USES AS A METHOD OF EVALUATING TRADITIONALISM AND ACCULTURATION OF CHICANO FAMILY STRUCTURE. 55 REFERENCES. (AUTHOR SUMMARY MODIFIED)

ACCN 000248

293 AUTH **CARRINGER, D. C.**

TITL CREATIVE THINKING ABILITIES OF MEXICAN YOUTH: THE RELATIONSHIP OF BILINGUALISM.

SRCE *JOURNAL OF CROSS CULTURAL PSYCHOLOGY, 1974, 5(4), 492-503.*

INDX BILINGUALISM, MEXICAN, COMPOUND-COORDINATE DISTINCTION, ADOLESCENTS, EMPIRICAL, BILINGUAL, COGNITIVE STYLE

ABST TO EXAMINE THE RELATIONSHIP OF BILINGUALISM TO THE CREATIVE THINKING ABILITIES OF MEXICAN YOUTH, SUBTESTS FROM THE TORRANCE TESTS OF CREATIVE THINKING WERE ADMINISTERED TO SPANISH-ENGLISH COORDINATE BILINGUAL AND SPANISH MONOLINGUAL SUBJECTS FROM TWO PRIVATE HIGH SCHOOLS IN TORREON, COAHUILA, MEXICO. IT WAS HYPOTHESIZED THAT THE SPANISH-ENGLISH COORDINATE BILINGUALS WOULD SCORE SIGNIFICANTLY HIGHER ON THE DEPENDENT MEASURES OF FIGURAL FLUENCY, FIGURAL FLEXIBILITY, FIGURAL ORIGINALITY, VERBAL FLUENCY, VERBAL FLEXIBILITY, AND VERBAL ORIGINALITY THAN THE SPANISH MONOLINGUALS. A MULTIVARIATE ANALYSIS INDICATED THAT THE MAIN EFFECT OF LANGUAGE GROUP WAS SIGNIGICANT IN FAVOR OF THE BILINGUALS. NEITHER THE MAIN EFFECT OF SEX NOR THE INTERACTION EFFECT WAS SIGNIFICANT. UNIVARIATE ANALYSIS INDICATED THAT THE DEPENDENT MEASURES OF VERBAL FLEXIBILITY AND ORIGINALITY, AND FIGURAL ORIGINALITY WERE SIGNIFICANT AT THE .05 LEVEL IN FAVOR OF THE BILINGUALS, AND THE DEPENDENT MEASURE OF FIGURAL FLUENCY WAS SIGNIFICANT AT THE .01 LEVEL IN FAVOR OF THE BILINGUALS. 23 REFERENCES. (JOURNAL ABSTRACT)

ACCN 000249

294 AUTH **CARROW, E.**

TITL COMPREHENSION OF ENGLISH AND SPANISH BY PRESCHOOL MEXICAN AMERICAN CHILDREN.

SRCE *THE MODERN LANGUAGE JOURNAL, 1971, 55(5), 299-306.*

INDX MEXICAN AMERICAN, CHILDREN, EMPIRICAL, BILINGUAL, LANGUAGE COMPREHENSION, EDUCATION, POVERTY, TEXAS, SOUTHWEST, BILINGUALISM

ABST THE AUDITORY COMPREHENSION OF ENGLISH AND SPANISH BY PRESCHOOL MEXICAN AMERICAN CHILDREN WAS STUDIED IN 99 CHILDREN FROM HOUSTON DAY-CARE CEN-

TERS SERVING BELOW POVERTY LEVEL FAMILIES. SUBJECTS WERE ADMINISTERED THE AUDITORY TEST FOR LANGUAGE COMPREHENSION IN BOTH SPANISH AND ENGLISH. RESULTS WERE COMPARED WITH THOSE OF A CONTROL GROUP COMPOSED OF ENGLISH-SPEAKING CHILDREN OF ALL SOCIOECONOMIC LEVELS SELECTED FROM NURSERIES AND DAY-CARE CENTERS IN SAN ANTONIO. GENERAL FINDINGS DISCUSSED INCLUDE: (1) MEXICAN AMERICAN CHILDREN ARE, LINGUISTICALLY SPEAKING, A VERY HETEROGENEOUS GROUP WITH A WIDE VARIATION OF COMPREHENSION OF THE TWO LANGUAGES; (2) THE GREATER PROPORTION UNDERSTAND ENGLISH BETTER THAN SPANISH; (3) BOTH LANGUAGES IMPROVE AS THE CHILDREN BECOME OLDER; AND (4) THE SEQUENCE OF LANGUAGE DEVELOPMENT IS SIMILAR IN BOTH GROUPS AND WITHIN THE MEXICAN AMERICAN GROUP IN BOTH SPANISH AND ENGLISH. ALTHOUGH ANALYSIS OF PERFORMANCE ON SPECIFIC ITEMS MAY LEAD ONE TO CONCLUDE THAT MEXICAN AMERICAN CHILDREN AS A GROUP DID NOT COMPREHEND ENGLISH AS WELL AS THE CONTROL GROUP, THIS CONCLUSION IS NOT WARRANTED AS THE BILINGUAL GROUP HAD SOME CHILDREN WHO SPOKE PRACTICALLY NO ENGLISH AND THE ENTIRE GROUP REPRESENTED A LOWER SES LEVEL THAN THE CONTROL GROUP. THE IMPLICATIONS OF THESE FINDINGS FOR PLANNING LANGUAGE DEVELOPMENT PROGRAMS AND FURTHER RESEARCH ARE DISCUSSED. 11 REFERENCES.

ACCN   000250

295 AUTH   **CARROW, M. A.**
     TITL   LINGUISTIC FUNCTIONING OF BILINGUAL AND MONOLINGUAL CHILDREN.
     SRCE   *JOURNAL OF SPEECH AND HEARING DISORDERS, 1957, 22(3), 371-380.*
     INDX   BILINGUALISM, LANGUAGE ASSESSMENT, CALIFORNIA ACHIEVEMENT TESTS, SOUTHWEST, CHILDREN, BILINGUAL, SEX COMPARISON, LINGUISTIC COMPETENCE, READING, TEXAS, MEXICAN AMERICAN
     ABST   A COMPARISON OF ENGLISH LANGUAGE ABILITY AND ACHIEVEMENT WAS MADE BETWEEN A MONOLINGUAL AND A BILINGUAL GROUP OF CHILDREN. SUBJECTS WERE THIRD-GRADE YOUTHS OF SIMILAR SOCIOECONOMIC STATUS, AGE, AND INTELLIGENCE. THE FOLLOWING LANGUAGE INDICES WERE EMPLOYED: THE CALIFORNIA TEST OF ACHIEVEMENT, THE DURRELL SULLIVAN READING CAPACITY TEST, THE GILLMORE ORAL READING TEST, AND THE FAIRBANKS TEST OF ARTICULATION FOR NONREADERS. RESULTS INDICATE THAT THERE WAS A SIGNIFICANT DIFFERENCE BETWEEN THE LANGUAGE GROUPS—IN FAVOR OF THE MONOLINGUAL GROUP—IN THE TESTS OF ORAL READING ACCURACY, ORAL READING COMPREHENSION, HEARING VOCABULARY, ARITHMETIC REASONING, AND SPEAKING VOCABULARY. NO SIGNIFICANT DIFFERENCES WERE FOUND BETWEEN GROUPS ON SILENT READING

VOCABULARY, ORAL READING RATE, SPELLING, VERBAL OUTPUT, LENGTH OF CLAUSE, AND DEGREE OF SUBORDINATION. THE BILINGUAL GROUP MADE MORE AND DIFFERENT TYPES OF ARTICULATORY AND GRAMMATICAL ERRORS THAN THE MONOLINGUAL GROUP. THE MALES DID NOT DIFFER SIGNIFICANTLY FROM THE FEMALES IN ANY OF THE MEASURES OF LANGUAGE FUNCTIONING EXCEPT THAT OF ORAL READING RATE. EDUCATIONAL AND RESEARCH IMPLICATIONS ARE PROVIDED FOR FURTHER STUDY OF BILINGUALISM. 16 REFERENCES.

ACCN   000251

296 AUTH   **CARTER, T. P.**
     TITL   MEXICAN AMERICANS IN SCHOOL: A HISTORY OF EDUCATIONAL NEGLECT.
     SRCE   *IN J. C. STONE & D. P. DENEVI (EDS.), TEACHING MULTICULTURAL POPULATIONS: FIVE HERITAGES. NEW YORK: VAN NOSTRAND, 1971, PP. 197-246.*
     INDX   EDUCATION, SCHOLASTIC ACHIEVEMENT, MEXICAN AMERICAN, BILINGUALISM, BILINGUAL-BICULTURAL EDUCATION, BILINGUAL-BICULTURAL PERSONNEL, DISCRIMINATION, PREJUDICE, EQUAL OPPORTUNITY, LEGISLATION, INSTRUCTIONAL TECHNIQUES, CURRICULUM, TEACHERS, REVIEW, SOUTHWEST
     ABST   THE PRESENT SCHOOL IS INAPPROPRIATE FOR MANY MEXICAN AMERICANS. THIS FACT IS RECOGNIZED BY A SIGNIFICANT NUMBER OF EDUCATORS, AND SOME ADVOCATE RADICAL INSTITUTIONAL CHANGES. FACTORS PARTICULARLY DISADVANTAGEOUS ARE DE FACTO SEGREGATION, ISOLATION, DEPENDENCE ON ENGLISH-SPEAKING AND INADEQUATE TEACHERS. LESS OBVIOUS FACTORS INCLUDE RIGIDITY OF SCHOOL PRACTICES AND POLICIES, CURRICULAR IRRELEVANCY, CULTURE CONFLICT AND NEGATIVE PERCEPTIONS OF EDUCATORS. THE AGGREGATE OF THESE FACTORS PRODUCES A GENERALLY NEGATIVE SCHOOL ENVIRONMENT, A FACTOR RECOGNIZED AS CRUCIAL TO SCHOOL SURVIVAL AND SUCCESS. SELECTED STATISTICAL AND DESCRIPTIVE DATA ARE INCLUDED AS DOCUMENTATION THAT SCHOOLS INADVERTENTLY DISCOURAGE MEXICAN AMERICAN CHILDREN FROM DOING WELL. (AUTHOR SUMMARY MODIFIED)

ACCN   000252

297 AUTH   **CARTER, T. P.**
     TITL   MEXICAN AMERICANS IN SCHOOL: A HISTORY OF EDUCATIONAL NEGLECT.
     SRCE   *PRINCETON, N.J.: COLLEGE ENTRANCE EXAMINATION BOARD, 1970.*
     INDX   CALIFORNIA, TEXAS, SOUTHWEST, EDUCATION, DISCRIMINATION, PREJUDICE, TEACHERS, ADMINISTRATORS, EMPIRICAL, CHILDREN, SCHOLASTIC ACHIEVEMENT, CULTURE, CULTURAL FACTORS, BILINGUALISM, ATTITUDES, PERFORMANCE EXPECTATIONS, INTELLIGENCE TESTING, POVERTY, SELF CONCEPT, HISTORY, PROGRAM EVALUATION, POLICY, BOOK
     ABST   TO ACCOUNT FOR THE GENERAL FAILURE OF

MEXICAN AMERICAN (MA) CHILDREN IN SCHOOL, SEMISTRUCTURED INTERVIEWS WERE CONDUCTED WITH OVER 250 SCHOOL PERSONNEL (I.E., TEACHERS, ADMINISTRATORS, SCHOOL BOARD MEMBERS) IN RURAL AND URBAN SCHOOLS IN THE FIVE SOUTHWESTERN STATES. THE DATA ARE PRESENTED IN THE FORM OF DISCUSSIONS OF FIVE TOPICS: (1) THE NATURE OF MA'S POOR ACHIEVEMENT AND PARTICIPATION IN SCHOOL; (2) MA CULTURAL VALUES AND THE PROBLEMS ASSOCIATED WITH POVERTY AND BILINGUALISM; (3) FLAWS IN THE SCHOOL SYSTEM; (4) MA PERCEPTIONS OF THE SCHOOL SYSTEM; AND (5) BICULTURAL TEACHER TRAINING, REMEDIAL PROGRAMS, AND OTHER CORRECTIVE MEASURES TO AID THE MA PUPIL. THE RESULTS SUGGEST, FIRST OF ALL, THAT THE DISCRIMINATORY NATURE OF LOCAL SOCIAL SYSTEMS GIVES THE MA LITTLE INCENTIVE TO ACHIEVE. SECOND, THE QUALITY OF EDUCATION IS OFTEN SEPARATIST AND SUBSTANDARD, AND THEREFORE IT DISCOURAGES AND DEMORALIZES THE MA CHILD. THIRD, ALTHOUGH SOME CHANGES ARE OCCURRING, ROTE TEACHING, BIASED INSTRUCTORS, WIDESPREAD DISCOURAGEMENT OF SPANISH, AND RIGID INSISTENCE UPON CONFORMITY TO ANGLO MIDDLE-CLASS VALUES ARE STILL THE RULE RATHER THAN THE EXCEPTION. MOREOVER, MOST OF THE EXISTING SPECIAL PROGRAMS FOR MA CHILDREN ARE DESIGNED TO CHANGE THE CHILD INSTEAD OF THE SCHOOL SYSTEM. THE AUTHOR CONCLUDES THAT DRASTIC CHANGES ARE REQUIRED IN SCHOOLS, AND HE ADVOCATES THE USE OF COMMUNITY GROUP PRESSURE TO PROMOTE SUCH CHANGES. 180 REFERENCES.

ACCN   001746

298 AUTH   **CARTER, T. P.**
     TITL   MEXICAN AMERICANS: HOW THE SCHOOLS HAVE FAILED THEM.
     SRCE   *COLLEGE BOARD REVIEW, 1970, 75(SPRING), 5-11.*
     INDX   SCHOLASTIC ACHIEVEMENT, MEXICAN AMERICAN, EDUCATION, CHILDREN, ESSAY, CROSS CULTURAL, SES, HIGHER EDUCATION, COLLEGE STUDENTS, REVIEW, IMMIGRATION, SOUTHWEST
     ABST   THE "FAILURE" OF THE MEXICAN AMERICAN MINORITY IS DUE IN LARGE PART TO THE AMERICAN SCHOOL SYSTEM. AMERICAN SOCIETY, OVERALL, HAS SERVED TO PROMOTE CONDITIONS, POLICIES AND PRACTICES THAT DISCOURAGE SCHOOL ACHIEVEMENT AND ENCOURAGE EARLY SCHOOL TERMINATION BY MINORITIES. IT IS ARGUED THAT THE RURAL AGRICULTURAL ECONOMY OF THE SOUTHWEST HAS NURTURED THE "ETHNIC CASTE SYSTEM" AND KEPT MEXICAN AMERICANS IN UNSKILLED AND LOWER ECONOMIC STATUS POSITIONS. THIS, IN TURN, IS REFLECTED IN POOR SCHOOL PERFORMANCE AND LIMITED OPPORTUNITIES FOR THE CHILDREN. THE EFFECT OF IMMIGRATION AND THE ECONOMIC HISTORY OF THE SOUTHWEST ON THE PRESENT SCHOOL SITUATION ARE DISCUSSED.

SOME STATISTICAL DATA REGARDING YEARS OF SCHOOL, DROP OUT RATES AND HIGHER EDUCATION ENROLLMENTS ARE PRESENTED. ALTHOUGH THE UNDERLYING PHILOSOPHY OF EDUCATORS HAS BEEN TO ASSIMILATE MEXICAN AMERICAN CHILDREN, THE ALTERATION OF THE CULTURAL AND FAMILY PATTERNS OF THESE CHILDREN CAN NO LONGER BE TOLERATED. 2 REFERENCES.

ACCN   000253

299 AUTH   **CARTER, T. P.**
     TITL   THE NEGATIVE SELF-CONCEPT OF MEXICAN-AMERICAN STUDENTS.
     SRCE   *SCHOOL AND SOCIETY, 1968, 96(2300), 217-219.*
     INDX   SELF CONCEPT, CROSS CULTURAL, EMPIRICAL, MEXICAN AMERICAN, DISCRIMINATION, ADOLESCENTS, EDUCATION, CALIFORNIA, SOUTHWEST
     ABST   MOST EDUCATORS WHO DEAL WITH MEXICAN AMERICAN CHILDREN ARE CONVINCED THAT THIS GROUP CONTAINS A LARGER THAN NORMAL PERCENTAGE OF INDIVIDUALS WHO VIEW THEMSELVES NEGATIVELY. A NEGATIVE SELF-IMAGE IS SEEN AS A PRIMARY REASON FOR THE GROUP'S LACK OF EDUCATIONAL SUCCESS. THREE SETS OF SOCIOPSYCHOLOGICAL INSTRUMENTS WERE ADMINISTERED TO 190 MEXICAN AMERICAN AND 98 ANGLO HIGH SCHOOL NINTH GRADERS. PROFILES DRAWN OF THE GROUP RESULTS WERE ALMOST IDENTICAL. IN SOME CASES, A SLIGHTLY LARGER PERCENTAGE OF THE MEXICAN AMERICANS RATED THEMSELVES ON THE POSITIVE EXTREME. THE INTERVIEWED STUDENTS SUPPORTED THE NOTION THAT AS A GROUP THEY DID NOT SUFFER FROM A NEGATIVE VIEW OF THEMSELVES. IT WAS SUGGESTED THAT THE SUPPOSED NEGATIVE-IMAGE OF THE MEXICAN AMERICAN IS IN REALITY AN ANGLO STEREOTYPE PROJECTED ON THIS ETHNIC GROUP. THE IMPLICATIONS OF A NEGATIVE SELF-IMAGE ARE DISCUSSED. MEXICAN AMERICANS ARE A HETEROGENEOUS GROUP OF PEOPLE, AND EDUCATORS MUST REEXAMINE THE SCHOOL AND THE STUDENTS THEY SERVE TO TEST SUCH CURRENTLY HELD BELIEFS AS THE GROUP NEGATIVE SELF-IMAGE. THE ACCEPTANCE OF THESE NOTIONS SERVES TO PROTECT EDUCATORS FROM AN INDEPTH EXAMINATION OF OTHER PROBLEMS RELATED TO SUCCESS AND FAILURE OF MEXICAN AMERICAN STUDENTS IN THE "ANGLO" SCHOOL. 1 REFERENCE.

ACCN   000254

300 AUTH   **CARTER, T. P.**
     TITL   THE PERSISTENCE OF A PERSPECTIVE.
     SRCE   *IN A. CASTANEDA, M. RAMIREZ III, C. E. CORTES & M. BARRERA (EDS.), MEXICAN AMERICANS AND EDUCATIONAL CHANGE. NEW YORK: ARNO PRESS, 1974, PP. 268-284.*
     INDX   SES, MEXICAN AMERICAN, EDUCATION, SCHOLASTIC ACHIEVEMENT, ACCULTURATION, CULTURAL PLURALISM, CULTURAL FACTORS, BILINGUAL-BICULTURAL EDUCATION, CURRICULUM, INSTRUCTIONAL TECHNIQUES,

BILINGUALISM, DISCRIMINATION, ENVIRON-
MENTAL FACTORS

ABST   ONE PERSPECTIVE CONTINUES TO PERMEATE
EDUCATIONAL THINKING CONCERNING THE
SCHOOLING OF MEXICAN AMERICAN CHIL-
DREN. THE "CULTURAL DEPRIVATION" THEORY
AND ITS DEPENDENT "COMPENSATORY EDU-
CATION" PROGRAMS REMAIN THE ONLY COM-
PREHENSIVE MODELS AVAILABLE OR PER-
PETUATED BY PRESENT SCHOOL SYSTEMS.
THIS PAPER PRESENTS A FOUR-DIMENSIONAL
TYPOLOGY OF VIEWS OF MINORITY GROUP
LIFE STYLES AND COROLLARY EDUCATIONAL
APPROACHES DERIVED FROM THE SOCIAL SCI-
ENCES. CAUSES AND CONSEQUENCES OF MI-
NORITY GROUP LIFE STYLES ARE CLASSIFIED
AS EXTERNAL OR INTERNAL AND POSITIVE OR
NEGATIVE. ALTERNATIVES TO THE PREVALENT
"CULTURAL   DEPRIVATION—COMPENSATORY
EDUCATION" MODEL FOR EACH CLASSIFICA-
TION ARE TENTATIVELY SUGGESTED. AL-
THOUGH THE FOUR WAY SCHEME PRESENTS
MANY LIMITATIONS, IT IS HOPED THIS FRAME-
WORK WILL STIMULATE ANALYSIS AND NEW
SCHOOL PROGRAMS AND APPROACHES. 6
REFERENCES. (AUTHOR SUMMARY MODIFIED)

ACCN   000255

301 AUTH   **CARTER, T. P.**
     TITL   WHERE TO FROM HERE?
     SRCE   IN J. C. STONE & D. P. DENEVI (EDS.), TEACHING
            MULTICULTURAL POPULATIONS: FIVE HERI-
            TAGES. NEW YORK: VAN NOSTRAND, 1971, PP.
            272-284.

     INDX   EDUCATION, SCHOLASTIC ACHIEVEMENT,
            CULTURE, CULTURAL FACTORS, MEXICAN
            AMERICAN, STEREOTYPES, PREJUDICE, DIS-
            CRIMINATION, CULTURAL CHANGE, ENVIRON-
            MENTAL FACTORS, SOCIALIZATION, BILIN-
            GUAL-BICULTURAL PERSONNEL, TEACHERS,
            REVIEW, POLICY, EQUAL OPPORTUNITY

     ABST   AMERICAN SOCIETY AND ITS SCHOOLS CON-
            TINUE TO PRODUCE AN ADULT MEXICAN
            AMERICAN POPULATION THAT IS PREPARED
            FOR PARTICIPATION IN LITTLE MORE THAN THE
            AGRICULTURAL ECONOMY OF THE TRADI-
            TIONAL SOUTHWEST. THIS ECONOMY, HOW-
            EVER, HAS CHANGED DRASTICALLY SINCE
            WORLD WAR II. POLITICAL AND OTHER LEAD-
            ERS NOW REALIZE THAT MAINTAINING AN EVER
            INCREASING MEXICAN AMERICAN POPULA-
            TION WITH LOW STATUS AND POOR EDUCA-
            TION IS A SERIOUS THREAT TO NATIONAL ECO-
            NOMIC STABILITY. IT IS POSITED THAT CHANGES
            ARE NECESSARY IN THREE AREAS, ALL OF
            WHICH ARE INEXORABLY INTERRELATED AND
            DEPENDENT ON SOCIETAL AND LOCAL MORES.
            THE AREAS REQUIRING CHANGE ARE: (1) SO-
            CIETY'S MORES AND UNDERSTANDING OF
            CULTURAL DIFFERENCES; (2) THE SCHOOL'S
            POSITION ON THE KIND AND QUALITY OF EDU-
            CATION AVAILABLE TO MEXICAN AMERICANS
            AND ITS ROLE IN PLANNING FOR EQUAL OP-
            PORTUNITIES; AND (3) THE EFFECT OF PRES-
            ENT AND PROPOSED SCHOOL PROGRAMS ON
            MEXICAN AMERICAN CHILDREN. RECOMMEN-
            DATIONS FOR NECESSARY CHANGES IN EACH
            AREA ARE DISCUSSED. 6 REFERENCES.

ACCN   000256

302 AUTH   **CARTER, T. P., & SEGURA, R. D.**
     TITL   MEXICAN AMERICANS IN SCHOOL: A DECADE
            OF CHANGE.
     SRCE   PRINCETON, N.J.: COLLEGE ENTRANCE EXAMI-
            NATION BOARD, 1979.

     INDX   MEXICAN AMERICAN, EDUCATION, CHILDREN,
            REVIEW, CULTURAL FACTORS, CULTURAL PLU-
            RALISM, POLICY, TEACHERS, ADMINISTRA-
            TORS, SCHOLASTIC ACHIEVEMENT, BOOK,
            PREJUDICE, ATTITUDES, ENVIRONMENTAL
            FACTORS, BILINGUAL-BICULTURAL EDUCA-
            TION, CULTURE, VALUES, POVERTY, SELF CON-
            CEPT, BILINGUALISM, TEXAS, CALIFORNIA,
            SOUTHWEST

     ABST   EXPRESSLY INTENDED AS AN UPDATE OF
            CARTER'S "MEXICAN AMERICANS IN SCHOOL"
            PUBLISHED IN 1970, THIS VOLUME OFFERS A
            COMPREHENSIVE   ASSESSMENT   OF   THE
            SCHOOL SYSTEM'S CHANGES OVER THE PAST
            TEN YEARS WITH REGARD TO MEXICAN AMERI-
            CAN (MA) CHILDREN IN THE SOUTHWEST. THE
            REPORT IS BASED UPON AN EXTENSIVE RE-
            VIEW OF THE LITERATURE, INTERVIEWS WITH
            MANY EDUCATORS AND LAY PERSONS IN CALI-
            FORNIA' AND TEXAS, PLUS THE AUTHORS' OB-
            SERVATIONS IN CLASSROOMS AND SPECIAL
            SCHOOL PROGRAMS. EIGHT PRINICIPAL TOP-
            ICS ARE ADDRESSED IN THE TEXT: (1) THE MA'S
            HISTORY OF EDUCATIONAL NEGLECT; (2) MA'S
            ACADEMIC ACHIEVEMENT, INCLUDING THEIR
            PERFORMANCE ON STANDARDIZED TESTS AND
            THEIR REPRESENTATION IN HIGHER EDUCA-
            TION; (3) SOCIOCULTURAL AND COGNITIVE
            FACTORS INFLUENCING MA CHILDREN'S
            LEARNING ABILITY; (4) DE FACTO SEGREGA-
            TION AND OTHER ANTI-HISPANIC PRACTICES
            IN SCHOOLS; (5) ENVIRONMENTAL FACTORS
            INHIBITING MA CHILDREN'S MOTIVATION; (6)
            SCHOOL PROGRAMS DESIGNED TO CHANGE
            THE MA CHILD (E.G., ESL, REMEDIAL READ-
            ING); (7) EFFORTS TO CHANGE THE EDUCA-
            TIONAL SYSTEM (E.G., BILINGUAL-BICULTURAL
            AND MIGRANT EDUCATIONAL PROGRAMS); AND
            (8) SPECULATION ABOUT THE MA CHILD'S
            EDUCATIONAL FUTURE. IT IS CONCLUDED THAT
            DESPITE SOME IMPROVEMENTS, LITTLE PROG-
            RESS HAS BEEN MADE IN SCHOOLS SINCE
            1970. IT IS ARGUED, THEREFORE, THAT MA'S
            HOPE FOR THE FUTURE LIES IN THEIR OWN
            SELF-DETERMINATION TO EFFECT POLITICAL
            AND PROGRAMMATIC CHANGES IN THE EDU-
            CATIONAL SYSTEM. SIX APPENDICES COM-
            PLETE THE VOLUME, INCLUDING REVIEWS OF
            SEVERAL IMPORTANT EDUCATIONAL STUDIES,
            PLUS THE "PLAN ESPIRITUAL ATZLAN" WHICH
            IDENTIFIES KEY CHICANO POLITICAL GOALS.
            381 REFERENCES.

ACCN   001840

303 AUTH   **CARVAJAL, T. L., & LANE, J. M.**
     TITL   THE EDUCATIONALLY NEGLECTED.
     SRCE   REGIONAL TRAINING PROGRAM TO SERVE THE
            BILINGUAL BICULTURAL EXCEPTIONAL CHILD.
            SAN FERNANDO, CALIF.: MONTAL EDUCA-
            TIONAL ASSOCIATES, 1972.

     INDX   SPECIAL EDUCATION, ESSAY, EDUCATION,

PROFESSIONAL TRAINING, TEACHERS, MEXI-
CAN AMERICAN, TEST VALIDITY, INTELLIGENCE
TESTING, CURRICULUM, EQUAL OPPORTU-
NITY, SOUTHWEST, EDUCATIONAL ASSESS-
MENT

ABST THE CASE OF THE EDUCATIONALLY NE-
GLECTED MEXICAN AMERICAN (MA) POPULA-
TION IN THE SOUTHWEST IS PRESENTED. IN-
ADEQUATE EDUCATION IS SEEN AS A
CONTRIBUTING FACTOR THAT HAS DE-
PRESSED THE MA POPULATION TO THE LOWER
ECHELONS OF SOCIETY. EFFORTS THAT WILL
STRESS EVALUATION OF THE "EDUCATIONAL
SYSTEM" RATHER THAN THE CHILD ARE NEC-
ESSARY. EVALUATION OF SPECIAL EDUCA-
TIONAL CLASSES AND CURRICULUM FOR THE
MENTALLY RETARDED IS ESSENTIAL. YOUNG-
STERS WHO HAVE BEEN CATEGORIZED AS
"DISADVANTAGED" EITHER SOCIALLY, EDUCA-
TIONALLY, OR CULTURALLY ARE EDUCATION-
ALLY NEGLECTED. THE TERM CONNOTES NEG-
LIGENCE, COMPLACENCY, INSENSITIVITY, AND
SOMETIMES APATHY. THE "PROBLEM" TEACHER
IS ONE WHO REALLY MUST BE EVALUATED.
THESE ARE HIS CHARACTERISTICS: 1) APA-
THETIC, 2) INSENSITIVE, 3) SENSATIONALISTIC,
4) COMPLACENT, AND 5) PERPLEXED. DISCUS-
SION OF THE TEACHING PROFESSION AND ITS
PHILOSOPHY OF CONCERN FOR PEOPLE IS
PRESENTED. THE TEACHER PREPARATION
TRAINING IN COLLEGES AND UNIVERSITIES
AND THE LOCAL SCHOOL DISTRICTS' ADMIN-
ISTRATIVE ATTEMPTS TO HELP THEIR TEACH-
ERS ARE TWO AREAS THAT MUST BE IM-
PROVED. AN EXAMINATION OF IMPROPER
DIAGNOSTIC TECHNIQUES AND THE SERIOUS
CONSEQUENCE OF MISPLACED CHILDREN RE-
VEALS THAT THE INTELLECTUAL MEASURE-
MENT OF MINORITY CHILDREN HAS BEEN
ABUSED. THE WECHSLER INTELLIGENCE SCALE
FOR CHILDREN AND THE WECHSLER ADULT IN-
TELLIGENCE SCALE CAN BE USED TO ASSESS
THE PLACEMENT OF MA CHILDREN IN CLASSES
FOR THE RETARDED. THERE SHOULD BE A
CAREFUL EXAMINATION, HOWEVER, OF TEST
PROFILES THAT INDICATE A 15-POINT, OR MORE,
SPREAD BETWEEN LOW VERBAL AND HIGH
PERFORMANCE TEST SCORES. 6 REFERENCES.

ACCN 000257

304 AUTH **CARVER, C. S., GLASS, D. C., SNYDER, M. L.,
& KATZ, I.**

TITL FAVORABLE EVALUATIONS OF STIGMATIZED
OTHERS.

SRCE *PERSONALITY AND SOCIAL PSYCHOLOGY BUL-
LETIN, 1977, 3(2), 232-235.*

INDX ATTITUDES, MEXICAN AMERICAN, COLLEGE
STUDENTS, SOUTHWEST, PREJUDICE, MALE,
EMPIRICAL, DISCRIMINATION

ABST TO DETERMINE IF ATTITUDINAL AMBIVALENCE
TOWARD MINORITY GROUP INDIVIDUALS CON-
TRIBUTES TO AN AMPLIFICATION EFFECT IN
WHICH THE RESPONSE TOWARD THE OBJECT
OF AMBIVALENCE IS EXAGGERATED, WHITE
SOUTHWEST MALE COLLEGE STUDENTS WERE
ASKED TO RATE A STIMULUS PERSON ON THE
BASIS OF TRANSCRIPTS OF BOGUS INTER-
VIEWS. IN THE FIRST THREE EXPERIMENTS,

BLACKS WERE RATED MORE POSITIVELY THAN
WHITES BY THREE GROUPS OF STUDENTS
(N = 106, N = 73, AND N = 107), EVEN THOUGH
BOTH BLACKS AND WHITES WERE UNFAVORA-
BLY PORTRAYED. IN THE FOURTH EXPERIMENT
(N = 109), NO DIFFERENCES WERE FOUND BE-
TWEEN THE RATINGS OF WHITES AND CHICA-
NOS. THE LACK OF CONSISTENCY BETWEEN
THESE FINDINGS AND PREVIOUS RESEARCH
BY DIENSTBIER (1970) MAY BE ATTRIBUTED TO
THE SUBJECTS' DESIRE NOT TO APPEAR
PREJUDICED, OR TO THEIR WILLINGNESS TO
CREDIT BLACK INTERVIEWEES FOR THEIR
STRUGGLE AGAINST AN OPPRESSIVE ENVI-
RONMENT. THE ABSENCE OF THIS EFFECT FOR
CHICANOS MAY REFLECT LESS SALIENCE OF
DISCRIMINATION. IT IS POSSIBLE THAT THE
MERE LABELING OF A STIMULUS PERSON AS A
MEMBER OF A STIGMATIZED GROUP FAILS TO
AROUSE FULLY THE AMBIVALENT ATTITUDES
ON WHICH AMPLIFICATION IS PRESUMED TO
DEPEND. 10 REFERENCES. (NCMHI ABSTRACT
MODIFIED)

ACCN 002048

305 AUTH **CARVER, R. P.**

TITL THE COLEMAN REPORT: USING INAPPRO-
PRIATELY DESIGNED ACHIEVEMENT TESTS.

SRCE *AMERICAN EDUCATIONAL RESEARCH JOUR-
NAL, 1975, 12(1), 77-86.*

INDX ACHIEVEMENT TESTING, EQUAL OPPORTU-
NITY, EDUCATION, INTEGRATION, EMPIRICAL,
METROPOLITAN READINESS TEST, CHILDREN

ABST THE DATA IN THE COLEMAN REPORT HAVE
BEEN INTERPRETED BY SOME AS INDICATING
THAT DIFFERENCES BETWEEN SCHOOLS HAVE
LITTLE IMPACT ON ACHIEVEMENT. THIS INTER-
PRETATION IS DERIVED FROM THE FACT THAT
ONLY ABOUT 10 OF THE VARIANCE IN THE
TEST SCORES WAS ASSOCIATED WITH DIFFER-
ENCES BETWEEN SCHOOLS, WHILE ABOUT 90
WAS ASSOCIATED WITH DIFFERENCES BE-
TWEEN INDIVIDUALS WITHIN SCHOOLS. IF THE
VARIANCE ASSOCIATED WITH SCHOOL DIFFER-
ENCES IS APPROPRIATELY COMPARED TO THE
VARIANCE ASSOCIATED WITH ATTENDING
SCHOOL ONE YEAR, THEN SCHOOL DIFFER-
ENCES ARE QUITE LARGE. IT IS NOT APPRO-
PRIATE TO DRAW CONCLUSIONS ABOUT
ACHIEVEMENT WHEN THE CONCLUSIONS ARE
BASED ON RESULTS OF TESTS THAT WERE DE-
SIGNED TO MAXIMIZE INDIVIDUAL DIFFER-
ENCES. THE COLEMAN RESULTS MAKE A GREAT
DEAL MORE SENSE WHEN THE TEST SCORES
ARE INTERPRETED AS REFLECTING APTITUDE
INSTEAD OF ACHIEVEMENT. 7 REFERENCES.
(JOURNAL ABSTRACT)

ACCN 000258

306 AUTH **CARVER, R. P.**

TITL TWO DIMENSIONS OF TESTS: PSYCHOMETRIC
AND EDUMETRIC.

SRCE *AMERICAN PSYCHOLOGIST, 1974, 29(7), 512-
518.*

INDX EDUCATIONAL ASSESSMENT, RESEARCH
METHODOLOGY, TEST RELIABILITY, TEST VA-

LIDITY, EDUCATION, ESSAY, INTELLIGENCE TESTING, ACHIEVEMENT TESTING

ABST THE DIFFERENCES BETWEEN PSYCHOMETRIC AND EDUMETRIC TESTS ARE SUMMARIZED REGARDING: (1) PURPOSE, (2) ITEM SELECTION, (3) VALIDITY, AND (5) SCORE INTERPRETATION. IT IS POSITED THAT TESTS MEASURING DIFFERENCES BETWEEN INDIVIDUALS (PSYCHOMETRIC) AND WITHIN INDIVIDUALS (EDUMETRIC) ARE QUITE DIFFERENT IN THEIR DEVELOPMENT AND STANDARDIZATION BECAUSE THEY MEASURE DIFFERENT DIMENSIONS—THE FIRST MEASURES APTITUDE AND THE OTHER ACHIEVEMENT. A TEST THAT IS BEST AT MEASURING ONE DIMENSION SHOULD NOT BE USED TO MEASURE THE OTHER AS IT WILL NOT BE SENSITIVE TO THAT DIMENSION AND WILL GIVE AN INACCURATE MEASURE OF A PERSON'S ABILITIES OR GAINS. THIS ISSUE IS ESPECIALLY IMPORTANT IN SCHOOL EDUCATIONAL TESTING WHERE TEST RESULTS ARE USED TO PLAN CHANGES AND EVALUATE TEACHING PROGRAMS. IT IS HOPED THAT THE CONFUSION BETWEEN THESE TWO TEST DIMENSIONS WILL BE RESOLVED AND THAT FUTURE TESTS WILL BE DEVELOPED WITH AN AWARENESS OF BOTH DIMENSIONS. 15 REFERENCES.

ACCN 000259

307 AUTH **CASAL, L. & HERNANDEZ, A. R.**
TITL CUBANS IN THE U.S.: A SURVEY OF THE LITERATURE.
SRCE *UNIVERSITY OF PITTSBURGH, CENTER FOR LATIN AMERICAN STUDIES, 1975, 5(2), 25-51.*
INDX ACCULTURATION, CUBAN, BIBLIOGRAPHY, CULTURAL FACTORS, DEMOGRAPHIC, EMPLOYMENT, CULTURAL CHANGE, MENTAL HEALTH, FAMILY STRUCTURE, POLITICS, IMMIGRATION, REVIEW, SOUTH
ABST A REVIEW OF THE LITERATURE REGARDING CUBAN AMERICANS (NUMBERING APPROXIMATELY 750,000 IN 1970) FOCUSES ON THE FOLLOWING AREAS: (1) CAUSES OF IMMIGRATION; (2) DEMOGRAPHIC COMPOSITION; (3) EXILES AS SOURCES OF INFORMATION ABOUT THE SOCIETY OF ORIGIN; (4) ASSIMILATION AND ACCULTURATION OF CUBAN EXILES; (5) POLITICAL BEHAVIOR AND ATTITUDES OF THE EXILES; (6) CHANGES IN BOTH THE FAMILY AND SEX ROLES; (7) MENTAL HEALTH; (8) OCCUPATIONAL ADJUSTMENT, SKILL TRANSFERABILITY, AND SOCIAL MOBILITY; (9) YOUTH PROBLEMS; (10) CUBANS ON WELFARE AND OTHER "AT RISK" GROUPS; (11) THE RELATIONSHIP OF CUBANS TO OTHER ETHNIC/RACIAL GROUPS; AND (12) THE IMPACT OF THE CUBAN IMMIGRATION ON THE HOST SOCIETY AND REFUGEE PROGRAMS. A CRITICAL REVIEW OF THE RESEARCH DESIGN AND FINDINGS OF THE ARTICLES IN EACH OF THESE AREAS IS PRESENTED. IT IS CONCLUDED THAT FUTURE RESEARCH ON CUBAN COMMUNITIES SHOULD FOCUS ON THEIR POWER STRUCTURE, LEADERSHIP PATTERNS, AND LINKAGES WITH NONCUBAN POWER STRUCTURES. MOREOVER, AN APPEAL IS MADE FOR MORE SYSTEMATIC EFFORTS AT MAKING RESEARCH ON CUBANS

RELEVANT TO GENERAL THEORETICAL ISSUES IN THE SOCIAL SCIENCES. AN ANNOTATED BIBLIOGRAPHY OF 22 ARTICLES IS APPENDED. 39 REFERENCES.

ACCN 002049

308 AUTH **CASAS, J. M.**
TITL APPLICABILITY OF A BEHAVIORAL MODEL IN SERVING THE MENTAL HEALTH NEEDS OF THE MEXICAN AMERICAN.
SRCE *IN M. R. MIRANDA (ED.), PSYCHOTHERAPY WITH THE SPANISH SPEAKING: ISSUES IN RESEARCH AND SERVICE DELIVERY (MONOGRAPH NO. 3). LOS ANGELES: UNIVERSITY OF CALIFORNIA, SPANISH SPEAKING MENTAL HEALTH RESEARCH CENTER, 1976, PP. 61-65.*
INDX CASE STUDY, ANXIETY, MEXICAN AMERICAN, ADULTS, SYMPTOMATOLOGY, CULTURAL FACTORS, PSYCHOTHERAPY, BEHAVIOR THERAPY
ABST PREVALENT THERAPEUTIC PRACTICES AND THEIR FAILURE TO MEET THE PSYCHOLOGICAL AND CULTURAL NEEDS OF THE MEXICAN AMERICAN ARE DISCUSSED. CONTENDING THAT THERAPEUTIC SHORTCOMINGS ARE THE RESULT OF A BASIC ETHNOCENTRIC BELIEF SYSTEM THAT PERMEATES THIS SOCIETY AND ITS VARIOUS FIELDS OF SOCIAL SCIENCE, THE AUTHOR OFFERS AN ALTERNATIVE MODEL FOR PROVIDING EFFECTIVE THERAPY FOR THE MEXICAN AMERICAN. THE FRAMEWORK FOR THIS MODEL IS BASED ON A RESPECTFUL UNDERSTANDING AND ACCEPTANCE OF PSYCHOCULTURAL DIFFERENCES IN HUMAN-RELATIONAL, INCENTIVE-MOTIVATIONAL, AND LEARNING STYLES. BESIDES ENCOMPASSING VARIED GOALS, THIS MODEL ALLOWS USE OF A VARIETY OF THERAPEUTIC TECHNIQUES. DEPENDING ON THE CLIENT'S NEEDS AND GOALS, THE THERAPIST IS FREE TO DIRECT ATTENTION SOLELY OR IN COMBINATION WITH THE BEHAVIORAL, THE EMOTIONAL, OR THE COGNITIVE REALMS. STRENGTHS AND WEAKNESSES OF THE MODEL ARE IDENTIFIED AND DISCUSSED. 6 REFERENCES.

ACCN 000260

309 AUTH **CASAVANTES, E.**
TITL PRIDE AND PREJUDICE: A MEXICAN AMERICAN DILEMMA.
SRCE *CIVIL RIGHTS DIGEST, 1970, 3(1), 22-27.*
INDX ESSAY, MEXICAN AMERICAN, CULTURE, STEREOTYPES, POVERTY, SEX ROLES, DISCRIMINATION, PREJUDICE, ECONOMIC FACTORS, EDUCATION
ABST THE ATTRIBUTES OF PEOPLE LIVING IN THE CULTURE OF POVERTY AND, SPECIFICALLY, THE QUALITIES OF THE MEXICAN AMERICAN (MA) PEOPLE ARE EXAMINED. SOCIAL SCIENTISTS WHO STUDY MA'S FOCUS ON THEIR POVERTY AND IGNORE THE IMPACT OF ENVIRONMENTAL FACTORS ON THE TOTALITY OF THEIR LIVES. THIS SCIENTIFIC OVERSIGHT HAS RESULTED IN THE PERPETUATION OF VERY DAMAGING STEREOTYPES. EIGHT QUALITIES WHICH HAVE BEEN INVALIDLY ATTRIBUTED TO MA'S AS PART OF THEIR ETHNICITY ARE LISTED. WHILE THESE ATTRIBUTES HAVE BEEN USED TO CHARACTERIZE THE MA, THEY ARE REALLY DE-

SCRIPTIVE OF PEOPLE, REGARDLESS OF ETH-NICITY, LIVING IN POVERTY. IN THIS CONTEXT, THESE ATTRIBUTES ARE VALID. THE DANGER, HOWEVER, IS IN ASSIGNING THESE ATTRI-BUTES AS THE UNIQUE POSSESSION OF ONE ETHNIC GROUP. THREE DIFFERENT SETS OF AT-TRIBUTES OF THE MA INCLUDE: (1) A SET OF FALSE ATTRIBUTES USUALLY ASCRIBED TO HIM BECAUSE HE IS POOR; (2) NATIONAL ORI-GIN, CULTURE, CUSTOMS, AND RELIGION; AND (3) DEMOGRAPHIC DATA ON EDUCATIONAL AT-TAINMENT AND INCOME WHICH CHARACTER-IZE THE MA WITHIN THE CULTURE OF POVERTY CONCEPT. IT IS CONCLUDED THAT POVERTY, MORE THAN ETHNICITY, SEEMS TO ACCOUNT FOR MANY FAILURES OF MA CHILDREN IN THE CLASSROOMS AND FOR A FATHER'S FAILURE IN VOCATIONAL ENDEAVORS. A RECOMMEN-DATION IS MADE TO IMPROVE THE SELF-IMAGE OF THE MA SO THAT NEITHER HE NOR THOSE HE ENCOUNTERS ACT OUT A NEGATIVE SELF-FULFILLING PROPHECY. NO REFERENCES.

ACCN   000261

310 AUTH   **CASAVANTES, E. J.**
     TITL   EL TECATO: SOCIAL AND CULTURAL FACTORS AFFECTING DRUG USE AMONG CHICANOS (2ND ED.).
     SRCE   *WASHINGTON, D.C.: NATIONAL COALITION OF HISPANIC MENTAL HEALTH AND HUMAN SER-VICES ORGANIZATIONS (COSSMHO), 1976.*
     INDX   CULTURAL FACTORS, DRUG ADDICTION, MEXI-CAN AMERICAN, POVERTY, RELIGION, SES, CASE STUDY, EMPIRICAL, PARAPROFESSIONALS, RE-HABILITATION, DRUG ABUSE, BIBLIOGRAPHY
     ABST   FORMAL INTERVIEWS OF 26 PERSONS LAST-ING FROM ONE TO TWO HOURS WERE MADE IN AN ATTEMPT TO ASSOCIATE CULTURAL FAC-TORS WITH DRUG USE. HALF OF THOSE INTER-VIEWED WERE CURRENT DRUG REHABILITA-TION PROGRAM COUNSELORS WHO HAD THEMSELVES BEEN DRUG ADDICTS AT ONE TIME. OTHERS INTERVIEWED (IN ORDER TO SERVE AS AN INFORMAL "CONTROL GROUP) WERE NON-ADDICTS, PHYSICIANS, PH.D'S, COLLEGE GRADUATES AND PROGRAM DIREC-TORS. RESPONDENTS WERE NOT A RANDOM SAMPLE. INTERVIEWS WERE TAPE RECORDED AND TRANSCRIBED VERBATIM. RESPONDENTS WERE ASKED TO EXPRESS THEIR OPINIONS ON TOPICS SUCH AS MACHISMO AND DRUG USE, THE DIRECT EFFECT OF POVERTY ON DRUGS, AND STRESS FACTORS AND PREDISPOSITION TO DRUG USE. THE INVESTIGATION ALSO IN-CLUDED CONTRIBUTIONS IN THE AREAS OF PERCEIVED RELATIONSHIPS BETWEEN: EDU-CATION, POVERTY, AND DRUG USE IN THE CHI-CANO COMMUNITY; PERCEPTIONS OF RELI-GION AND RELIGIOUS INSTITUTIONS AND DRUG USE; PERCEPTIONS OF THE COUNSELORS CONCERNING THE CHICANO FAMILY AND ITS INFLUENCE ON DRUG ABUSE; PERCEIVED UNIQUENESS OF THE CHICANO ADDICT; PER-SONALITY AND PSYCHOPATHOLOGY FACTORS AND DRUG ADDICTION; AND SOME RECOM-MENDATIONS FOR TREATMENT. THE AUTHOR REFUTES ANY IMPLICATION THAT MEXICAN/CHICANO CULTURE "CAUSES" DRUG USE OR

DRUG ABUSE. A SELECTED ANNOTATED BIBLI-OGRAPHY ON DRUG ABUSE AMONG THE SPANISH-SPEAKING IS ALSO INCLUDED. 91 REFERENCES.

ACCN   000262

311 AUTH   **CASAVANTES, E. J.**
     TITL   A NEW LOOK AT THE ATTRIBUTES OF THE MEX-ICAN AMERICAN.
     SRCE   *ALBUQUERQUE, N.M.: SOUTHWESTERN COOP-ERATIVE EDUCATIONAL LABORATORY, INC., 1969.*
     INDX   CULTURE, MEXICAN AMERICAN, SES, POVERTY, ESSAY, ETHNIC IDENTITY, STEREOTYPES, ATTI-TUDES, ACCULTURATION, PERSONALITY, ETH-NIC IDENTITY, REVIEW, THEORETICAL, VALUES
     ABST   THE WORKS OF W. MADSEN, C. HELLER, O. LEWIS, AND OTHER SOCIAL SCIENTISTS WHO HAVE WRITTEN ON THE CHARACTERISTICS OF MEXICAN AMERICANS ARE EXAMINED. IT IS FELT THAT THESE AUTHORS HAVE DRAWN CONCLUSIONS THAT ARE INADEQUATE BE-CAUSE OF PARTIAL OR BIASED SAMPLING TECHNIQUES. THE MAIN CONTENTION IS THAT ALTHOUGH THESE STUDIES MAY PROVIDE AN ACCURATE DESCRIPTION OF A FEW CHICANOS IN A PARTICULAR AREA OF THE COUNTRY, THEY ALMOST INVARIABLY FAIL TO TAKE INTO ACCOUNT TWO IMPORTANT CO-EXISTING SO-CIOCULTURAL VARIABLES: (1) THE EFFECT OF SOCIOECONOMIC CLASS ON THE BEHAVIOR OF THE MEXICAN AMERICAN; AND (2) THE EF-FECT OF ETHNICITY ON THE BEHAVIOR OF THE MEXICAN AMERICAN. MANY OF THE CHARAC-TERISTICS USED TO DESCRIBE THE MEXICAN AMERICAN ARE BASICALLY DESCRIPTIONS OF INDIVIDUALS FROM THE LOWEST SOCIOECO-NOMIC CLASS COMMONLY REFERRED TO AS THE CULTURE OF POVERTY. A NEW CONCEP-TUAL MODEL FOR STUDYING THE ATTRIBUTES OF MEXICAN AMERICANS IS PROPOSED. BASED ON A SCHEMA CALLED EL CHICANO BELIEF SYSTEMS, THE MODEL INTEGRATES RE-GIONAL, SOCOECONOMIC, AND OTHER VAL-UES (I.E., CHURCH, CHILD-REARING, MAR-RIAGE, EDUCATION, HEALTH, ETC.) INTO AN OVERALL METHOD BY WHICH TO STUDY AND UNDERSTAND INDIVIDUAL DIFFERENCES BE-TWEEN CHICANOS. IMPLICATIONS OF THIS MODEL FOR RESEARCH AND EDUCATION RE-GARDING MEXICANS ARE DISCUSSED. 23 REF-ERENCES.
     ACCN   000263

312 AUTH   **CASPER, E. G., & PHILIPPUS, M. J.**
     TITL   FIFTEEN CASES OF EMBRUJADA: COMBINING MEDICATION AND SUGGESTION IN TREAT-MENT.
     SRCE   *HOSPITAL AND COMMUNITY PSYCHIATRY, 1975, 26(5), 271; 274.*
     INDX   FOLK MEDICINE, CURANDERISMO, SPANISH SURNAMED, CASE STUDY, COLORADO, SOUTHWEST, HEALTH DELIVERY SYSTEMS, ANXIETY, DEPRESSION, MENTAL HEALTH, PRO-GRAM EVALUATION, PSYCHOTHERAPY, PSY-CHOTHERAPY OUTCOME
     ABST   THE TREATMENT APPROACH FOUND EFFEC-TIVE WITH 15 MEXICAN AND MEXICAN AMERI-

CAN PATIENTS WITH EMBRUJADA (HEXED) IS DISCUSSED. WHEN THE STAFF AT A DENVER MENTAL HEALTH CLINIC WERE FACED WITH THE SYMPTOMS ACCOMPANYING EMBRUJADA IN 13 FEMALE AND 2 MALE PATIENTS, THEY FORMULATED A TREATMENT PLAN FOLLOWING THE RITUALS USED BY CURANDEROS, THE HEALERS OF MEXICAN FOLK MEDICINE. THE SELECTION OF A MEDICATION APPROPRIATE TO THE MIXED SYMPTOMS OF ANXIETY AND DEPRESSION IN THESE PATIENTS AND THE USE OF SUGGESTION IN EXPLAINING THE MEDICATION'S SOURCE AND EFFECT ARE DESCRIBED AS IMITATING THE CURANDERO'S ACTIVITIES. THE APPARENT IMPROVEMENT OF 13 OF THE 15 CASES USING THIS TREATMENT SEEMS TO INDICATE THAT THE SUGGESTION ASPECT OF THIS TREATMENT APPROACH WORKED IN A MANNER SIMILAR TO THAT OF THE CURANDERO'S. IT IS HOPED THAT FURTHER USE OF SIMILAR METHODS AND REPORTS OF THEIR RESULTS BY OTHER CLINICS WILL ASCERTAIN THE VALUE OF THIS TREATMENT METHOD WITH PATIENTS COMPLAINING OF EMBRUJADA. 5 REFERENCES.

ACCN 000264

313 AUTH **CASTANEDA, A.**

TITL MELTING POTTERS VS. CULTURAL PLURALISTS: IMPLICATIONS FOR EDUCATION.

SRCE *IN A. CASTANEDA, M. RAMIREZ III, C. E. CORTES & M. BARRERA (EDS.), MEXICAN AMERICANS AND EDUCATIONAL CHANGE. NEW YORK: ARNO PRESS, 1974, PP. 22-39.*

INDX CULTURAL PLURALISM, CULTURE, ACCULTURATION, MEXICAN AMERICAN, EDUCATION, ETHNIC IDENTITY, LEGISLATION, JUDICIAL PROCESS, SOCIALIZATION, CHILDREARING PRACTICES, BILINGUALISM, CURRICULUM, INSTRUCTIONAL TECHNIQUES, POLICY

ABST DEMOCRATIC CULTURAL PLURALISM, MEANING THE CULTURALLY DEMOCRATIC RIGHT OF A CHILD TO EXPLORE THE MAINSTREAM CULTURAL ENVIRONMENT WITH THOSE CULTURAL FORMS AND LOYALTIES HE HAS LEARNED AT HOME AND IN HIS OWN COMMUNITY, ALSO CALLED BICULTURALISM, IS ADVOCATED AS A POINT OF FOCUS FOR EDUCATORS AND OTHERS CONCERNED WITH EDUCATIONAL CHANGE. ASSUMPTIONS UNDERLYING THE GOAL OF EDUCATIONAL BICULTURALISM ARE EXPLORED AS A BASIS FOR THE BICULTURAL MODEL PROPOSED. THESE ASSUMPTIONS ARE DISCUSSED IN TERMS OF: (1) VARIATIONS IN CULTURAL VALUES; (2) SOCIALIZATION PRACTICES OF HOME AND COMMUNITY; (3) LEARNING STYLES OF CHILDREN; AND (4) AREAS OF CHANGE FOR CREATING A CULTURALLY DEMOCRATIC EDUCATIONAL ENVIRONMENT. SPECIFIC AREAS FOR CHANGE IN THE SCHOOL ENVIRONMENT DEALING WITH CULTURALLY DIVERSE STUDENTS ARE IDENTIFIED AS: (1) COMMUNICATION (LANGUAGE, DOMINANT, SECONDARY); (2) MODES OF HUMAN RELATIONS; (3) INCENTIVE-MOTIVATION PREFERENCES; AND (4) TEACHING AND CURRICULUM METHODS REFLECTING MODES OF THINKING, PERCEIVING, REMEMBERING AND PROBLEM

SOLVING IN DIFFERENT CULTURES. THE MELTING POT THEORIES, RANGING FROM ANGLO CONFORMITY TO THE MANDATORY CULTURAL PLURALIST FORMS, ARE ALL SEEN AS PROMOTING ANGLO SUPERIORITY. CULTURAL DEMOCRACY IS THE RESPONSIBILITY OF ALL SCHOOLS TEACHING CHILDREN WHO ARE CULTURALLY DIFFERENT FROM THE MAINSTREAM. 8 REFERENCES.

ACCN 000265

314 AUTH **CASTANEDA, A., HEROLD, P. L., & RAMIREZ, M., III.**

TITL NEW APPROACHES TO BILINGUAL, BICULTURAL EDUCATION: A NEW PHILOSOPHY OF EDUCATION (NO. 1).

SRCE *AUSTIN: THE DISSEMINATION CENTER FOR BILINGUAL BICULTURAL EDUCATION, 1974.*

INDX BILINGUAL-BICULTURAL EDUCATION, CULTURAL PLURALISM, CHILDREN, SPANISH SURNAMED, ACCULTURATION, POLICY, EDUCATION, SOCIALIZATION, ESSAY

ABST THIS MANUAL IS THE FIRST IN A SERIES OF SEVEN TEACHER-TRAINING UNITS DEVELOPED ESPECIALLY FOR THE USE OF BILINGUAL-BICULTURAL PROJECTS. FUNDED UNDER AN E.S.E.A. (ELEMENTARY AND SECONDARY EDUCATION ACT) TITLE VII GRANT, THE MATERIALS PROPOSE A NEW PHILOSOPHY OF EDUCATION CALLED "CULTURAL DEMOCRACY" WHICH RECOGNIZES THE INDIVIDUALITY OF BOTH TEACHERS AND STUDENTS AND WHICH PROVIDES INFORMATION ABOUT THE EDUCATION OF CULTURALLY DIVERSE CHILDREN. THIS FIRST PART OF THE SERIES COVERS FIVE ISSUES RELATED TO PUBLIC EDUCATION AND THE MEXICAN AMERICAN CHILD: (1) EDUCATIONAL PHILOSOPHY APPROPRIATE TO CULTURAL DEMOCRACY; (2) ACCULTURATION PRESSURES AND THE MELTING POT THEORY; (3) FACETS OF CULTURAL EXCLUSION POLICY; (4) SOCIALIZATION PRESSURES IN AMERICAN EDUCATION; AND (5) THE COMPENSATORY EDUCATION MOVEMENT. 8 REFERENCES. (AUTHOR SUMMARY MODIFIED)

ACCN 000266

315 AUTH **CASTANEDA, A., RAMIREZ, M., III, & HEROLD, P. L.**

TITL CULTURALLY DEMOCRATIC LEARNING ENVIRONMENTS: A COGNITIVE STYLES APPROACH.

SRCE *MULTI-LINGUAL ASSESSMENT PROJECT. RIVERSIDE, CALIF.: SYSTEMS AND EVALUATIONS IN EDUCATION, 1972.*

INDX EDUCATION, CULTURAL PLURALISM, ESSAY, TEACHERS, INSTRUCTIONAL TECHNIQUES, MEXICAN AMERICAN, CHILDREARING PRACTICES, COGNITIVE STYLE, SOCIALIZATION, CHILDREN, FIELD DEPENDENCE-INDEPENDENCE

ABST THIS MANUAL FOR TEACHERS OF CULTURALLY DIFFERENT CHILDREN HAS TWO OBJECTIVES. THE FIRST IS IMPROVING TEACHER EFFECTIVENESS AND EQUIPPING TEACHERS WITH A TEACHING STRATEGY THAT WILL MAKE LEARNING ENJOYABLE AND SUCCESSFUL FOR CHILDREN WHO PRESENTLY FAIL. THE SECOND PURPOSE IS TO PRESERVE IN TODAY'S EDU-

CATIONAL SYSTEM THE CONCEPT OF CULTURAL DEMOCRACY— THAT IS, THE RIGHT OF ANY AMERICAN CHILD TO REMAIN IDENTIFIED WITH HIS OWN ETHNIC GROUP WHILE ADOPTING MAINSTREAM AMERICAN VALUES AND LIFESTYLES. CULTURALLY DEMOCRATIC LEARNING ENVIRONMENTS CAN BE PRESERVED BY SCHOOLS AND TEACHERS THROUGH THE IMPLEMENTATION OF COGNITIVE STYLES OF LEARNING THAT ARE CULTURALLY APPROPRIATE TO EACH CHILD. SINCE CHILDREN DEVELOP PREFERRED MODES OF LEARNING IN EARLY YEARS AT HOME, CULTURALLY DEMOCRATIC LEARNING ENVIRONMENTS (SCHOOLS) MUST INTEGRATE THE CHILD'S HOME LEARNING MODE. AS A GENERAL RULE, CHILDREN ARE MORE LIKELY TO BE FIELD-DEPENDENT THAN FIELD-INDEPENDENT IF THEY ARE MEMBERS OF ETHNIC GROUPS THAT EMPHASIZE FAMILY LOYALTY AND CLOSE PERSONAL TIES AMONG THE FAMILY MEMBERS. IT IS HYPOTHESIZED THAT THE PRIMARY REASON EDUCATIONAL INSTITUTIONS HAVE FAILED THE MAJORITY OF MEXICAN AMERICANS AND OTHER ETHNIC MINORITY GROUPS IS THE INSENSITIVITY OF SCHOOL PERSONNEL TO THE COGNITIVE STYLES OF THESE PEOPLE. IT IS CRITICALLY IMPORTANT THAT EDUCATIONAL INSTITUTIONS BE SUFFICIENTLY FLEXIBLE TO OPERATE IN BOTH FIELD-DEPENDENT AND FIELD-INDEPENDENT COGNITIVE STYLES AND TO RESPECT THE PERSON REGARDLESS OF HIS STYLE. 6 REFERENCES.

ACCN   000267

316 AUTH **CASTRO, F. G.**
TITL DISCONTINUATION IN PSYCHOTHERAPY AS RELATED TO DEGREE OF ACCULTURATION AMONG MEXICAN AMERICAN PATIENTS IN AN ADULT OUTPATIENT PSYCHIATRIC CLINIC.
SRCE *UNPUBLISHED MASTER'S THESIS, DEPARTMENT OF SOCIAL WELFARE, UNIVERSITY OF CALIFORNIA AT LOS ANGELES, JUNE 1976.*
INDX PSYCHOTHERAPY, MEXICAN AMERICAN, ACCULTURATION, PSYCHOTHERAPY OUTCOME, RESOURCE UTILIZATION, MENTAL HEALTH, CULTURAL FACTORS, ADULTS, EMPIRICAL, CALIFORNIA, SOUTHWEST, FATALISM
ABST THE RESULTS OF SEVERAL STUDIES HAVE INDICATED THAT ETHNIC MINORITY AND/OR LOW SOCIOECONOMIC STATUS PATIENTS DROP OUT OF PSYCHOTHERAPY SOONER THAN HAVE MIDDLE-CLASS ANGLO AMERICAN PATIENTS. OTHER STUDIES OF UNDERUTILIZATION OF MENTAL HEALTH SERVICES BY MEXICAN AMERICANS AND OTHER SPANISH-SPEAKING PEOPLES IMPLY THAT THERE MAY BE A COMMON FACTOR RESPONSIBLE FOR THIS TREND. IT WAS HYPOTHESIZED THAT MEXICAN AMERICAN PATIENTS LOW IN DEGREE OF ACCULTURATION WOULD DROP OUT OF PSYCHOTHERAPY SOONER THAN WOULD MEXICAN AMERICAN PATIENTS HIGH IN DEGREE OF ACCULTURATION. IN GENERAL, THIS HYPOTHESIS WAS NOT CONFIRMED. SEVERAL SIGNIFICANT DIFFERENCES WERE FOUND BETWEEN CONTINUOUS AND DISCONTINUOUS PATIENTS HOWEVER. DISSATISFIED PATIENTS WERE MORE

FATALISTIC, AND THIS ATTITUDE SEEMED TO INFLUENCE EARLY TERMINATION. A WIDER CONCEPTION OF PSYCHOTHERAPY IN WORKING WITH MEXICAN AMERICAN PATIENTS IS STRESSED, AND THIS INCLUDES PLACING THE RESPONSIBILITY FOR PSYCHOTHERAPEUTIC OUTCOME ON THE THERAPIST, NOT THE PATIENT. 60 REFERENCES. (AUTHOR ABSTRACT MODIFIED)
ACCN   000268

317 AUTH **CASTRO, F. G.**
TITL LEVEL OF ACCULTURATION AND RELATED CONSIDERATIONS IN PSYCHOTHERAPY WITH SPANISH SPEAKING/SURNAMED CLIENTS (OCCASIONAL PAPER NO. 3).
SRCE *LOS ANGELES: UNIVERSITY OF CALIFORNIA, SPANISH SPEAKING MENTAL HEALTH RESEARCH CENTER, 1977.*
INDX PSYCHOTHERAPY, MEXICAN AMERICAN, ACCULTURATION, PSYCHOTHERAPY OUTCOME, RESOURCE UTILIZATION, MENTAL HEALTH, CULTURAL FACTORS, ADULTS, EMPIRICAL, CALIFORNIA, SOUTHWEST, POLICY
ABST THIS MONOGRAPH (1) PRESENTS A FIELD STUDY OF THE EFFECTS OF THE LEVEL OF ACCULTURATION ON THE SPANISH-SPEAKING/SURNAMED (SS/S) PATIENT'S DESIRE TO CONTINUE OR DISCONTINUE IN PSYCHOTHERAPY AND (2) DISCUSSES THE TYPES OF PSYCHOTHERAPY THOUGHT TO BE MOST APPROPRIATE AND BENEFICIAL TO THE NEEDS OF THESE CLIENTS. AFTER INTERVIEWING 32 VOLUNTARY SUBJECTS WHO WERE PATIENTS AT THE EAST LOS ANGELES ADULT PSYCHIATRIC CLINIC, IT WAS FOUND THAT (1) DISSATISFIED CLIENTS EXHIBITED A SIGNIFICANTLY LESSER SENSE OF PERSONAL CONTROL THAN DID SATISFIED CLIENTS, (2) DISSATISFIED CLIENTS EXHIBITED A TREND TOWARDS A SHORTER FUTURE TIME PERSPECTIVE THAN DID SATISFIED CLIENTS, AND (3) DISCONTINUOUS CLIENTS EXHIBITED A TREND TOWARDS A MORE PASSIVE CONCEPTION OF PSYCHOTHERAPY AS OPPOSED TO A MORE ACTIVE CONCEPTION BY CONTINUOUS CLIENTS. IMPAIRED COMMUNICATION AND DIMINISHED FAVORABLE EXPECTANCIES ARE THE TWO FACTORS IDENTIFIED AS LEADING TO DISSATISFACTION WITH THERAPY AND PREMATURE TERMINATION BY SS/S CLIENTS. FOR THESE CLIENTS, A TWO PHASE PROCESS OF PSYCHOTHERAPY INVOLVING THE ESTABLISHMENT OF A TRUSTING PATIENT-THERAPIST RELATIONSHIP AND THE USE OF AN ACTION PROBLEM SOLVING TECHNIQUE IS SEEN TO BE MOST BENEFICIAL. A CREATIVE BLEND OF CRISIS INTERVENTION TECHNIQUES COUPLED WITH ASSERTIVE TRAINING TECHNIQUES IS PROPOSED AS THE MOST EFFECTIVE COMBINATION FOR PROVIDING QUALITY PSYCHOTHERAPEUTIC AID FOR SS/S CLIENTS. 60 REFERENCES. (AUTHOR SUMMARY MODIFIED)
ACCN   000269

318 AUTH **CATE, C. C.**
TITL TEST BEHAVIOR OF ESL STUDENTS.
SRCE *CALIFORNIA JOURNAL OF EDUCATIONAL RESEARCH, 1967, 18(4), 184-187.*

INDX WAIS, WISC, CHILDREN, EMPIRICAL, CATTELL CULTURE-FREE INTELLIGENCE TEST, RAVEN PROGRESSIVE MATRICES, INTELLIGENCE TESTING, SPECIAL EDUCATION, CALIFORNIA, SOUTHWEST

ABST THE RELATIONSHIP AMONG SEVERAL GROUP ABILITY TESTS AND A PERFORMANCE PORTION OF AN INDIVIDUAL TEST IS REPORTED. ONE HUNDRED TWENTY-ONE NATIVE SPANISH-SPEAKING STUDENTS (ETHNICITY NOT SPECIFIED) ENROLLED IN ENGLISH AS A SECOND LANGUAGE (ESL) CLASSES WERE ADMINISTERED THE PERFORMANCE SCALE OF EITHER THE WISC OR WAIS AS APPROPRIATE TO THEIR AGE. IN ADDITION, THE TESTS OF GENERAL ABILITY (TOGA), RAVEN PROGRESSIVE MATRICES (RPM), CATTELL CULTURE FREE INTELLIGENCE TEST (CCF), AND THE TEST RAPIDO BARRANQUILLA (BARSIT) WERE ALSO GIVEN. RESULTS SHOW THAT THE CORRELATIONS BETWEEN TOGA, RPM, CCF, BARSIT, AND THE WISC PERFORMANCE SCALE WERE .64, .69, .57, AND .77 RESPECTIVELY. THE RESULTS FURTHER INDICATE THAT GROUP TESTS CAN BE USED FOR THE PURPOSE OF ESTABLISHING A BASELINE IN ABILITY AND FOR POSSIBLE IDENTIFICATION OF STUDENTS TO BE SCREENED FOR SPECIAL EDUCATION CLASSES. NO REFERENCES.

ACCN 000270

319 AUTH **CAYO SEXTON, P.**
TITL FROM SPANISH HARLEM.
SRCE *IN J. C. STONE & D. P. DENEVI (EDS.), TEACHING MULTICULTURAL POPULATIONS: FIVE HERITAGES. NEW YORK: VAN NOSTRAND, 1971, PP. 118-129.*
INDX URBAN, PUERTO RICAN-M, SES, POVERTY, CULTURAL CHANGE, IMMIGRATION, LEADERSHIP, AGGRESSION, SEX ROLES, SEXUAL BEHAVIOR, RELIGION, DISCRIMINATION, MASS MEDIA, SOCIAL SERVICES, ESSAY, NEW YORK, EAST, CENSUS
ABST EAST HARLEM, TWO SQUARE MILES OF MANHATTAN ISLAND, NEW YORK, IS HOME FOR THOUSANDS OF PUERTO RICANS, NEGROES AND ITALIANS. THE PROBLEMS OF SLUMS (E.G., DISEASE, UNEMPLOYMENT, AND CROWDING) ARE DISCUSSED WITH EMPHASIS ON THE PUERTO RICAN POPULATION. RACE AND ETHNICITY ARE RECOGNIZED AS THE CAUSE OF MOST OF THE OPEN AND HIDDEN CONFLICT IN THIS AREA, BUT COMMONALITIES BETWEEN NEIGHBORHOODS ARE ALSO POINTED OUT. IMMIGRATION AND HOMELAND INFLUENCES ON PUERTO RICANS IN THIS AREA ARE IDENTIFIED AND DESCRIBED. SOME CENSUS AND SOCIOECONOMIC DATA ARE PROVIDED. 4 REFERENCES.

ACCN 000271

320 AUTH **CAZARES, M. L.**
TITL FAMILY LIFE IN A MEXICAN PRISON.
SRCE *PAPER PRESENTED AT THE SPANISH SPEAKING MENTAL HEALTH RESEARCH CENTER COLLOQUIM SERIES, UNIVERSITY OF CALIFORNIA, LOS ANGELES, 1977.*
INDX MEXICO, CORRECTIONS, HISTORY, ESSAY, FICTIVE KINSHIP, PERSONALITY, SEX ROLES, FAMILY STRUCTURE, FAMILY ROLES, MEXICAN

ABST ISLAS MARIAS, A MEXICAN PENAL COLONY, ALLOWS ITS PRISONERS TO HAVE THEIR FAMILIES LIVE WITH THEM ON THE PENITENTIARY GROUNDS UNTIL THEIR PRISON SENTENCES ARE COMPLETED. IN FACT, FAMILY LIFE THERE APPROXIMATES NORMAL FAMILIAL CONDITIONS AS THEY EXIST THROUGHOUT THE MEXICAN REPUBLIC. THE PRISON'S HISTORY AND THE RECENT ATTEMPTS OF THE MEXICAN GOVERNMENT TO RESOLVE THE PROBLEM OF FAMILY DISINTEGRATION RELATED TO IMPRISONMENT ARE DESCRIBED. FAMILY LIFE STYLES, MALE-FEMALE RELATIONSHIPS, COMPRADRAZGO AND OTHER CUSTOMS AS FOLLOWED BY THE PRISONERS' FAMILIES ARE DESCRIBED. THE PENAL COLONY DEMONSTRATES THE MEXICAN GOVERNMENT'S ATTEMPTS TO IMPROVE PRISON CONDITIONS WHILE MAINTAINING CONCERN FOR FAMILY UNITY. 21 REFERENCES.

ACCN 000272

321 AUTH **CEJA, M. V.**
TITL METHODS OF ORIENTATION OF SPANISH SPEAKING CHILDREN TO AN AMERICAN SCHOOL.
SRCE *SAN FRANCISCO: R AND E RESEARCH ASSOCIATES, 1973. (REPRINTED FROM AN UNPUBLISHED MANUSCRIPT, UNIVERSITY OF SOUTHERN CALIFORNIA, 1957.)*
INDX EDUCATION, SCHOLASTIC ACHIEVEMENT, LANGUAGE LEARNING, HISTORY, MEXICAN AMERICAN, CHILDREN, BILINGUALISM, CURRICULUM, BILINGUAL-BICULTURAL EDUCATION, ESSAY, CALIFORNIA, SOUTHWEST, RURAL, INTEGRATION
ABST THE RATIONALE AND PLAN FOR A PROGRAM TO INTEGRATE SPANISH-SPEAKING CHILDREN IN THE SCHOOLS OF WESTMORELAND SCHOOL DISTRICT, IMPERIAL COUNTY, CALIFORNIA ARE PRESENTED. THE BELIEF THAT STEPS MUST BE TAKEN TO ADJUST THE MEXICAN AMERICAN MINORITY TO THE AMERICAN PATTERN OF LIVING AND THAT THIS CHALLENGE MUST BE MET IN THE SCHOOLS IS FORWARDED. THIS STUDY INCLUDES: (1) A DISCUSSION OF THE BASIC NEEDS OF CHILDREN AND THEIR RELATION TO THE UNIQUE NEEDS OF THE SPANISH-SPEAKING CHILD; (2) AN HISTORICAL REVIEW OF METHODS USED BY SOME SCHOOL DISTRICTS IN ORIENTING THE SPANISH-SPEAKING CHILD (ETHNIC GROUPING, ALSO KNOWN AS SEGREGATION; SPECIAL TRAINING OR AMERICANIZATION CLASSES; AND DIRECT INTEGRATION); (3) A DESCRIPTION OF THE COMMUNITY OF WESTMORELAND AND ITS SCHOOL DISTRICT'S USE OF GROUPING AND SPECIAL TRAINING TO ORIENT SPANISH-SPEAKING CHILDREN; (4) AN EVALUATION OF THESE METHODS AND THE CAUSES THAT FORCED THEIR DISCONTINUANCE; AND (5) THE RECOMMENDED PROGRAM FOR FUTURE USE BY THE WESTMORELAND SCHOOL—DIRECT INTEGRATION. 29 REFERENCES.

ACCN 000273

322 AUTH **CENTRO DE DOCUMENTACION SOBRE EL AL-COHOLISMO Y ABUSO DE ALCOHOL.**

TITL EL PROGRAMA DE ACCION CONTRA EL ALCO-HOLISMO Y EL ABUSO DEL ALCOHOL EN MEXICO. (THE ACTION PROGRAM AGAINST AL-COHOLISM AND DRUG ABUSE IN MEXICO.)

SRCE *MEXICO, D.F.: CENTRO DE DOCUMENTACION SOBRE EL ALCOHOLISMO Y EL ABUSO DEL AL-COHOL, DIRECCION GENERAL DEL SALUD MENTAL DE LA S.S.A. Y UNIDAD XOCHIMILCO DE LA UNIVERSIDAD METROPOLITANA, BOLE-TIN NO. 1, OCTUBRE 1976. (SPANISH)*

INDX ALCOHOLISM, REHABILITATION, HEALTH, JU-DICIAL PROCESS, LEGISLATION, PRIMARY PRE-VENTION, MENTAL HEALTH, PHYSICIANS, ES-SAY, MEXICO, MEXICAN

ABST "EL CONSEJO DE SALUBRIDAD GENERAL" (BOARD OF GENERAL WELFARE) WILL IMPLE-MENT NATIONAL PROGRAMS THROUGHOUT MEXICO TO FIGHT ALCOHOLISM, BASED ON A CAMPAIGN OF SCIENTIFIC ORIENTATION ON THE EFFECTS OF ALCOHOLISM ON HEALTH AND SOCIAL RELATIONS. ALCOHOLISM DOES NOT RECOGNIZE SOCIOECONOMIC LEVELS, SEX, OR GEOGRAPHIC DISTRIBUTION, BUT IT AFFECTS THE POOR MORE THAN THE WEALTHY. THIS PROGRAM IS BASED ON THE REALIZA-TION THAT ALCOHOLISM IS A SOCIAL AND PUBLIC HEALTH PROBLEM OF SERIOUS MEDI-CAL, SOCIAL, ECONOMIC, AND ETHICAL CON-SEQUENCES. ALCOHOLISM CAN BE PRE-VENTED AND PEOPLE THAT SUFFER THIS SICKNESS CAN BE REHABILITATED. THE NUM-BER OF MEXICANS THAT SUFFER FROM ALCO-HOLISM PLACES THIS PROBLEM AMONG THE PRINCIPAL SICKNESSES IN URGENT NEED OF ATTENTION.

ACCN 000274

323 AUTH **CERAME, A.**

TITL PROGRAMA GENERAL PARA EL DISENO Y CON-STRUCCION DE CENTROS DE SALUD MENTAL. (GENERAL PROGRAM FOR THE DESIGN AND CONSTRUCTION OF MENTAL HEALTH CEN-TERS.)

SRCE *IN J. A. ROSSELLO (ED.), MANUAL DE PSIQUIA-TRIA SOCIAL. SPAIN: INDUSTRIAS GRAFICAS "DIARIO-DIA, 1968, PP. 465-492. (SPANISH)*

INDX ESSAY, PUERTO RICAN-I, MENTAL HEALTH, RE-HABILITATION, RESOURCE UTILIZATION, HEALTH DELIVERY SYSTEMS

ABST BASED UPON THE MODEL OF RIO PIEDRAS, THE MOST COMPLETE MENTAL HEALTH CEN-TER IN PUERTO RICO, A PROGRAM IS OFFERED FOR THE PLANNING AND CONSTRUCTION OF OTHER CENTERS THROUGHOUT THE ISLAND. THE FIVE MAJOR ASPECTS OF SUCH MENTAL HEALTH CENTERS ARE DISCUSSED: (1) AN IN-PATIENT CENTER; (2) AMBULATORY TREAT-MENT; (3) DAY-CARE; (4) 24-HOUR EMERGENCY SERVICE; AND (5) AN EDUCATIONAL COMMU-NITY OUTREACH PROGRAM. IN ALL CASES, THESE FACILITIES SHOULD BE INTEGRATED AS MUCH AS POSSIBLE WITH THE OUTSIDE WORLD. SECOND, PROLONGED, ISOLATED INSTITU-TIONALIZATION SHOULD BE AVOIDED. THIRD, INPATIENTS SHOULD BE ENCOURAGED TO CARRY ON AS MANY ACTIVITIES AS POSSIBLE.

FINALLY, CONSIDERATIONS ARE ALSO PRE-SENTED CONCERNING DIAGNOSTIC FACILI-TIES, VOCATIONAL-REHABILITATION CENTERS, AND ADMINISTRATIVE AREAS. 18 REFERENCES.

ACCN 002272

324 AUTH **CERAME, A., DE RODRIGUEZ, F. C., & DE ABRUNA, M. C.**

TITL LA ADICCION A DROGAS Y ESTADISTICAS RE-LACIONADAS. (DRUG ADDICTION AND RE-LATED STATISTICS.)

SRCE *IN J. A. ROSSELLO (ED.), MANUAL DE PSIQUIA-TRIA SOCIAL. SPAIN: INDUSTRIAS GRAFICAS "DIARIO-DIA, 1968, PP. 373-434. (SPANISH)*

INDX PUERTO RICAN-I, ESSAY, DRUG ABUSE, PRO-GRAM EVALUATION, POLICY, HEALTH DELIVERY SYSTEMS, REHABILITATION

ABST THE TREATMENT AND PREVENTION OF DRUG ADDICTION IN PUERTO RICO ARE DISCUSSED AT LENGTH, SUPPLEMENTED BY GRAPHS AND STATISTICS ON DRUG ABUSE RATES AND THE TREATMENT PROVIDED BY VARIOUS HOSPI-TALS AND CENTERS ON THE ISLAND. THE SER-VICES PROVIDED BY THESE CLINICS, DAY CEN-TERS, AND INTENSIVE-TREATMENT CENTERS ARE SOCIALLY ORIENTED, AIMED AT HELPING THE ADDICT MAINTAIN HIS SOCIAL AND ECO-NOMIC TIES AND RESPONSIBILITIES. IT IS SUG-GESTED THAT THESE SERVICES CAN BE IM-PROVED BY CONDUCTING GENERAL EVALUATIONS OF EXISTING PROGRAMS, IN-CREASING THE NUMBER OF STAFF MEMBERS AND FACILITIES, PROVIDING SEPARATE FACILI-TIES FOR FEMALE ADDICTS, AND INCREASING DRUG EDUCATION EFFORTS AMONG ADOLES-CENTS AND THE COMMUNITY AT LARGE.

ACCN 002273

325 AUTH **CHAMBERS, C. D., CUSKEY, W. R., & MOFFETT, A. D.**

TITL DEMOGRAPHIC FACTORS IN OPIATE ADDIC-TION AMONG MEXICAN AMERICANS.

SRCE *PUBLIC HEALTH REPORTS, 1970, 85(6), 523-531.*

INDX DEMOGRAPHIC, DRUG ADDICTION, MEXICAN AMERICAN, EMPIRICAL, RELIGION, SEX COM-PARISON, MARITAL STABILITY, SES, ADULTS, ECONOMIC FACTORS, TEXAS, SOUTHWEST, KENTUCKY, SOUTH

ABST TO ISOLATE ANY CHANGES WHICH MAY HAVE OCCURRED IN MEXICAN AMERICAN (MA) DRUG ADDICTS IN RECENT YEARS, THE HISTORIES OF THE 106 MA ADDICTS ADMITTED TO THE FEDERAL HOSPITALS AT LEXINGTON, KEN-TUCKY, AND FORT WORTH, TEXAS, IN THE FIRST 6 MONTHS OF 1961 WERE COMPARED STATISTICALLY, BY SEX, WITH THE HISTORIES OF THE 169 MA'S ADMITTED DURING THE SAME PERIOD OF 1967. THE STUDY SHOWED THAT THE INCIDENCE OF MA ADDICTS AMONG ALL ADDICTS ADMITTED TO THE TWO HOSPITALS DOUBLED BETWEEN 1961 AND 1967, EVEN THOUGH THE TOTAL NUMBER OF HOSPITAL ADMISSIONS DECREASED BY ALMOST 20 PER-CENT. THE INCREASE, HOWEVER, WAS ONLY AMONG THE MALE ADDICTS. FEMALE REPRE-SENTATION IN 1967, WAS LESS THAN HALF THAT OF 1961. THE MAJORITY OF MA'S IN 1967 RESIDED IN TEXAS; IN 1961 CALIFORNIA WAS

THE LARGEST CONTRIBUTOR OF MA ADDICTS. AN OVERWHELMING MAJORITY OF THE MA ADDICTS, REGARDLESS OF SEX, WERE SCHOOL DROPOUTS. A LARGE MAJORITY OF THE MA OPIATE ADDICTS IN 1967 HAD HISTORIES OF SMOKING MARIJUANA, HISTORIES WHICH USUALLY HAD PRECEDED THEIR USE OF OPIATES. OPIATE USE MOST OFTEN BEGAN DURING THE ADOLESCENT YEARS. THE MA ADDICTS WERE MOST FREQUENTLY FOUND TO BE YOUNG ADULTS; MEAN AGE DECREASED BETWEEN 1961 AND 1967. ALMOST ALL WERE ADDICTED TO HEROIN, WHICH THEY PURCHASED FROM ILLEGAL SOURCES; ALMOST ALL USED IT INTRAVENOUSLY. EVEN THOUGH THE MA ADDICTS SUPPLEMENTED THEIR INCOMES FROM ILLEGAL SOURCES, THE MAJORITY MAINTAINED SOME LEGAL OCCUPATIONAL ROLE WHILE ADDICTED. ALL HAD BEEN ARRESTED; THE FIRST ARREST MOST FREQUENTLY HAD PRECEDED THE USE OF OPIATES. BY 1967, RECIDIVISM WAS INCREASING, AND READMISSIONS WERE MORE LIKELY TO BE VOLUNTARY RATHER THAN ENFORCED. 16 REFERENCES.

ACCN 000275

---

326 AUTH **CHANDLER, C. R.**
TITL VALUE ORIENTATIONS AMONG MEXICAN AMERICANS IN A SOUTHWESTERN CITY.
SRCE *SOCIOLOGY AND SOCIAL RESEARCH, 1974, 58(3), 262-271.*
INDX MEXICAN AMERICAN, URBAN, CULTURE, SES, ADULTS, ACCULTURATION, FATALISM, SOUTHWEST, SURVEY, EMPIRICAL
ABST VALUE ORIENTATION QUESTIONS RELATED TO ACTIVITY, INTEGRATION WITH KIN, TRUST, AND OCCUPATIONAL PRIMACY WERE ASKED OF A RANDOM SAMPLE OF 300 MEXICAN AMERICAN MEN AND WOMEN IN AN URBAN SETTING. AS HYPOTHESIZED, "MODERN" ORIENTATIONS WERE EXPRESSED BY YOUNGER RESPONDENTS WITH MORE FORMAL SCHOOLING AND HIGHER STATUS OCCUPATIONS. OTHERS, AND IN FACT THE MAJORITY, GAVE "TRADITIONAL" RESPONSES. THE RESULTS ARE DISCUSSED IN RELATION TO OTHER STUDIES AND IN LIGHT OF "MODERNISM" THEORY. 14 REFERENCES. (JOURNAL ABSTRACT)
ACCN 000276

---

327 AUTH **CHANDLER, J. T., & PLAKOS, J.**
TITL SPANISH SPEAKING PUPILS CLASSIFIED AS EDUCABLE MENTALLY RETARDED.
SRCE *SACRAMENTO: CALIFORNIA STATE DEPARTMENT OF EDUCATION, DIVISION OF INSTRUCTION, 1969.*
INDX MENTAL RETARDATION, CHILDREN, EDUCATION, WISC, ESCALA DE INTELIGENCIA WECHSLER, RURAL, URBAN, INTELLIGENCE, EMPIRICAL, MEXICAN AMERICAN, CALIFORNIA, SOUTHWEST, SPANISH SURNAMED, INTELLIGENCE TESTING, SPECIAL EDUCATION, POLICY
ABST A TOTAL OF 47 PUPILS ENROLLED IN GRADES THREE TO EIGHT WERE ADMINISTERED THE ESCALA DE INTELIGENCIA WECHSLER PARA NINOS WHICH IS THE SPANISH VERSION OF THE WECHSLER INTELLIGENCE SCALE FOR CHILDREN (WISC). THE RESULTS OF THE STUDY SHOWED THAT THE MEAN GAIN BETWEEN THE PRIOR ENGLISH TEST SCORES AND THE SUBSEQUENT SPANISH TEST SCORES WAS 13.15 IQ POINTS. THE AVERAGE IQ ON THE ENGLISH VERSION OF THE WISC WAS 68.61 AND 81.76 ON THE SPANISH VERSION. THESE FINDINGS INDICATE THAT WHEN THESE PUPILS ARE ABLE TO PERFORM IN THEIR PRIMARY LANGUAGE, THEIR IQ TEST PERFORMANCE IS, IN MANY CASES, ABOVE THE CUTOFF LEVEL (IQ OF 75) FOR PLACEMENT IN A CLASS FOR THE EDUCABLE MENTALLY RETARDED (EMR). IT IS RECOMMENDED THAT SCHOOL DISTRICT PERSONNEL SHOULD REVIEW THE CASES OF SPANISH SURNAMED PUPILS ENROLLED IN EMR CLASSES, AND THOSE STUDENTS WHOSE PRIMARY LANGUAGE IS SPANISH SHOULD BE RETESTED WITH THE SPANISH VERSION OF THE WISC. A "TRANSITION" PROGRAM SHOULD BE PROVIDED FOR PUPILS WHO NEED SPECIAL INSTRUCTION IN THE USE OF THE ENGLISH LANGUAGE. LONG RANGE PLANS SHOULD BE MADE TO IMPROVE THE PRESENT METHODS AND INSTRUMENTS USED FOR ASSESSING PUPILS PRIOR TO REFERRAL TO EMR CLASSES, PARTICULARLY THOSE PUPILS WITH DIFFERENT CULTURAL AND LINGUISTIC BACKGROUNDS.
ACCN 000277

---

328 AUTH **CHAPA, R.**
TITL OBSERVATIONS ON THE CHICANO MENTAL HEALTH MOVEMENT.
SRCE *IN A. M. PADILLA & E. R. PADILLA (EDS.), IMPROVING MENTAL HEALTH AND HUMAN SERVICES FOR HISPANIC COMMUNITIES: SELECTED PRESENTATIONS FROM REGIONAL CONFERENCES. WASHINGTON, D.C.: NATIONAL COALITION OF HISPANIC MENTAL HEALTH AND HUMAN SERVICE ORGANIZATIONS (COSSMHO), 1977, PP. 15-17.*
INDX CHICANO MOVEMENT, MENTAL HEALTH, ESSAY, HISTORY, COMMUNITY INVOLVEMENT, MEXICAN AMERICAN, HEALTH DELIVERY SYSTEMS, PROCEEDINGS
ABST A BRIEF SUMMARY OF THE FOUR CONFERENCES DEALING WITH THE CHICANO MENTAL HEALTH MOVEMENT SINCE 1969 IS PROVIDED. THE HIGH POINTS OF EACH CONFERENCE AND THE OVERALL TREND OF THE MOVEMENT ARE DISCUSSED. EXPECTATIONS FOR THE FIFTH CONFERENCE (1975) ARE ESTABLISHED AS (1) THE EXAMINATION AND CHANGE OF ATTITUDES WHICH LIMIT INVOLVEMENT, AND (2) THE DEFINITION OR REDEFINITION OF ROLES, NEEDS, COMMITMENTS, PRIORITIES, AND STRATEGIES WITHIN THE HUMAN SERVICES DELIVERY APPARATUS.
ACCN 000278

---

329 AUTH **CHERLIN, A., & REEDER, L. G.**
TITL THE DIMENSIONS OF PSYCHOLOGICAL WELL-BEING: A CRITICAL REVIEW.
SRCE *SOCIOLOGICAL METHODS AND RESEARCH, 1975, 4(2), 189-214.*
INDX MENTAL HEALTH, RESEARCH METHODOLOGY, TEST VALIDITY, TEST RELIABILITY, REVIEW, SUR-

VEY, CALIFORNIA, CROSS CULTURAL, MEXICAN AMERICAN, SEX COMPARISON, THEORETICAL, SOUTHWEST, ADULTS, STRESS, PSYCHOSOCIAL ADJUSTMENT, URBAN

ABST DATA FROM TWO INDEPENDENT LOS ANGELES METROPOLITAN AREA SURVEYS (LAMAS) WHICH PARTIALLY REPLICATE BRADBURN'S STUDIES IN PSYCHOLOGICAL WELL-BEING ARE PRESENTED. TEN ITEMS IN THE REVISED AFFECT BALANCE SCALE WERE INCLUDED IN LAMAS V'S 1,078 INTERVIEWS AND LAMAS VI'S 1,008 INTERVIEWS OF LOS ANGELES AREA HOUSEHOLDS. ALPHA RELIABILITIES WERE VERY SIMILAR FOR BOTH SEXES AND FOR ANGLOS AND BLACKS. MEXICAN AMERICANS SHOWED A SOMEWHAT LOWER RELIABILITY IN LAMAS V AND A SOMEWHAT HIGHER RELIABILITY IN LAMAS VI. BRADBURN'S THEORETICAL, SOCIAL PSYCHOLOGICAL MODEL IS CRITICALLY EXAMINED AND THE FINDINGS PLACED IN THE MORE GENERAL CONTEXT OF MEASURES OF DIMENSIONS OF EMOTION AND RELATED VARIABLES. SEVERAL PROBLEMS IN INTERPRETATION ARE DISCUSSED: (1) THE RELATIVELY SIMPLE NOTIONS OF POSITIVE AND NEGATIVE AFFECT MAY MASK A COMPLEXITY OF EMOTIONS WHICH INVALIDATE A STRAIGHT-FORWARD INTERPRETATION OF THE BRADBURN ITEMS; (2) THE SITUATIONALLY SPECIFIC FOCUS OF MANY OF THE ITEMS AND THE EMPHASIS ON THE OCCURRENCE OF CERTAIN FEELINGS MAY CONTRIBUTE TO THE INDEPENDENCE OF THE TWO AFFECT DIMENSIONS; AND (3) THE ADDED UTILITY OF THE AFFECT BALANCE SCALE AND THE BALANCE MODEL HAVE YET TO BE SATISFACTORILY DEMONSTRATED. RECOGNIZING THE CONSIDERABLE VALUE OF SUBJECTIVE MEASURES IN THE ASSESSMENT OF THE PUBLIC STATE OF WELL-BEING, THE DEVELOPMENT OF MULTIPLE INDICATORS OF PSYCHOLOGICAL WELL-BEING ARE SUGGESTED. 56 REFERENCES.

ACCN 002051

330 AUTH **CHICANO COORDINATING COUNCIL ON HIGHER EDUCATION.**

TITL EL PLAN DE SANTA BARBARA: A CHICANO PLAN FOR HIGHER EDUCATION.

SRCE *SANTA BARBARA, CALIF.: LA CAUSA PUBLICATIONS, 1970.*

INDX HIGHER EDUCATION, CHICANO MOVEMENT, EDUCATION, CURRICULUM, MEXICAN AMERICAN, SOCIAL SCIENCES, COMMUNITY, REPRESENTATION, HISTORY, POLITICS, BIBLIOGRAPHY, CALIFORNIA, SOUTHWEST

ABST A PLAN OF ACTION FOR CHICANOS IN HIGHER EDUCATION RECOGNIZING CHICANO ACCESS TO THE UNIVERSITY AS A CRITICAL DIMENSION OF THE CHICANO MOVEMENT AND INTEGRAL TO THE DEVELOPMENT OF THE CHICANO COMMUNITY (CC) IS PRESENTED. THE INSTITUTIONALIZATION OF CHICANO PROGRAMS WITHIN THE UNIVERSITY IS THE FIRST STEP IN ACHIEVING THE FOLLOWING OBJECTIVES: (1) COLLEGES/UNIVERSITIES MUST BE A MAJOR INSTRUMENT IN LIBERATING THE CC; (2) COLLEGES/UNIVERSITIES ARE RESPONSIBLE FOR THE EDUCATION OF, RESEARCH ON, AND PRO-

VISION OF PUBLIC SERVICES TO THE CC; AND (3) INTERESTS OF THE CC WILL ONLY BE SERVED BY PROGRAMS INSTITUTED BY AND FOR CHICANOS. OUTLINES AND DISCUSSIONS FOR THE ORGANIZATION OF CHICANO PROGRAMS INCLUDE: (1) CHICANO STUDIES AS AN ACCREDITED ACADEMIC DISCIPLINE; (2) RECRUITMENT AND ADMISSION OF CHICANO STUDENTS, FACULTY, ADMINISTRATORS, AND UNIVERSITY STAFF; (3) SUPPORT PROGRAMS SUCH AS COLLEGE ORIENTATION, ACADEMIC COUNSELING, TUTORIAL ASSISTANCE, AND FINANCIAL AID; (4) POLITICAL ACTION PROGRAMS TO INFLUENCE THE DECISION-MAKING PROCESS AT THE UNIVERSITY; AND (5) MECHA AS A NETWORK OF STUDENT ACTIVISM TO POLITICIZE AND SOCIALIZE STUDENTS TO THE ULTIMATE GOALS OF THE MOVEMENT. A SELECTED BIBLIOGRAPHY OF 102 REFERENCES IS ALSO INCLUDED.

ACCN 000279

331 AUTH **CHRISTENSEN, E. W.**

TITL COUNSELING PUERTO RICANS: SOME CULTURAL CONSIDERATIONS.

SRCE *THE PERSONNEL AND GUIDANCE JOURNAL, 1975, 53(5), 349-356.*

INDX PUERTO RICAN-M, EDUCATIONAL COUNSELING, CULTURAL FACTORS, EXTENDED FAMILY, FATALISM, STEREOTYPES, ESSAY

ABST SOME FACTS ABOUT PUERTO RICO, NATIVE-BORN AND MAINLAND-RAISED PUERTO RICANS, AND CULTURAL CHARACTERISTICS SUCH AS FATALISMO, RESPETO, DIGNIDAD, MACHISMO AND HUMANISMO ARE PRESENTED. PRACTICAL SUGGESTIONS FOR THE COUNSELOR TO CONSIDER ARE LISTED: (1) EXAMINE YOUR OWN PREJUDICES; (2) CALL STUDENTS BY THEIR RIGHT NAMES (MANY USE BOTH THEIR FATHER'S AND MOTHER'S FAMILY NAME); (3) FIND WAYS TO WORK WITH THE FAMILY; (4) UNDERSTAND THE CONCEPT OF HIJO DE CRIANZA, WHICH REFERS TO PARENTS RAISING OTHER THAN THEIR OWN CHILDREN AND IS PART OF THE EXTENDED FAMILY CONCEPT; AND (5) BE PATIENT AND WORK AT DEMONSTRATING CREDIBILITY, HONESTY AND RELIABILITY IN THE CLIENT-COUNSELOR RELATIONSHIP. A GLOSSARY OF SPANISH TERMS USED IN THE ARTICLE IS PROVIDED. 12 REFERENCES.

ACCN 000280

332 AUTH **CHRISTENSEN, E. W.**

TITL THE PUERTO RICAN WOMAN: THE CHALLENGE OF A CHANGING SOCIETY.

SRCE *CHARACTER POTENTIAL, 1975, 7(2), 89-96.*

INDX FEMALE, PUERTO RICAN-I, CULTURAL CHANGE, CHILDREARING PRACTICES, SOCIAL MOBILITY, SEX ROLES, ESSAY, ROLE EXPECTATIONS, ECONOMIC FACTORS, SES, EMPIRICAL, CONFLICT RESOLUTION

ABST PUERTO RICAN WOMEN ON THE ISLAND ARE DESCRIBED BASED ON PERSONAL OBSERVATION, 10 YEARS OF CLINICAL EXPERIENCE, AND A LARGE RESEARCH SAMPLE. COMPARED TO OTHER LATIN AMERICAN COUNTRIES, PUERTO RICAN CHILD-REARING PRACTICES FACILITATE THE FEMALE'S MOVEMENT INTO

WORK AND EDUCATION; PUERTO RICAN WOMEN HAVE THUS MADE UNIQUE PROGRESS AND HOLD IMPORTANT POSITIONS IN THE ISLAND'S SOCIETY. THEY HAVE NOT WITHDRAWN FROM THE TRADITIONAL ROLES AND CONSEQUENTLY OFTEN EXPERIENCE CONFLICT BETWEEN THE VALUES OF THE SOCIETY AND THEIR OWN PERSONAL VALUES AND ASPIRATIONS. THE STRENGTHS OF THE PUERTO RICAN WOMAN BRING CONFLICTS AND DILEMMAS IN DECISIONS INVOLVED IN ACCEPTING AND SEEKING NEW ROLES WITHOUT RELINQUISHING OLD ROLES. CONFLICTS ARE PERPETUATED BECAUSE PUERTO RICAN MALES ARE INADEQUATELY AND UNREALISTICALLY PREPARED FOR THE WOMEN'S SUCCESS. THE PATTERNS OF CONFLICT CAN BE OVERCOME IF THE CHILD-REARING ATTITUDES, EXPECTATIONS, AND BEHAVIORS BECOME CONSISTENT WITH THE NEW SITUATION ON THE ISLAND. 7 REFERENCES. (AUTHORS SUMMARY MODIFIED.)

ACCN   000281

333 AUTH   **CHRISTENSEN, E. W.**
    TITL   WHEN COUNSELING PUERTO RICANS . . .
    SRCE   *THE PERSONNEL AND GUIDANCE JOURNAL, 1977, 55(7), 412-415.*
    INDX   PUERTO RICAN-M, PSYCHOTHERAPY, EDUCATIONAL COUNSELING, CULTURE, FAMILY STRUCTURE, MOTHER-CHILD INTERACTION, FAMILY THERAPY, ESSAY
    ABST   COUNSELORS WORKING WITH PUERTO RICAN CLIENTS SHOULD WORK WITHIN THE FRAMEWORK OF THE PUERTO RICAN CULTURE. THE STRENGTHS OF THIS CULTURE ARE MANY, BUT WITH REGARD TO COUNSELING TWO ARE ESPECIALLY RELEVANT: (1) THE FAMILY SYSTEM; AND (2) THE UNIQUE AND INFLUENTIAL ROLE OF THE MOTHER. THE COUNSELOR CAN BECOME MORE INVOLVED WITH THE FAMILY SYSTEM BY (1) TALKING AND ASKING ABOUT THE COUNSELEE'S FAMILY, (2) UTILIZING FAMILY MEMBERS AS CONSULTANTS ABOUT HIS COUNSELEE, AND (3) BECOMING INVOLVED IN COMMUNITY ACTIVITIES ATTENDED BY COUNSELEES AND THEIR FAMILIES. THE IMPORTANCE OF THE MOTHER IN THE PUERTO RICAN CULTURE GIVES HER A UNIQUE STATUS AS A POTENTIAL ALLY FOR ANY COUNSELOR WORKING WITH PUERTO RICAN CLIENTS. SHE IS THE PRIME SOURCE OF HELP FOR PERSONAL PROBLEMS OR PLANNING OF A STUDENT'S FUTURE. THE COUNSELOR CAN BECOME INVOLVED WITH MOTHERS AS A DEVELOPMENTAL CONSULTANT PROVIDING ADVICE AND INSIGHT INTO CHILD-REARING FUNCTIONS, AND AS AN EDUCATOR HELPING THE MOTHER TO UNDERSTAND THE MAINLAND CULTURE. CAUTION IS GIVEN REGARDING WORKING WITHIN ESTABLISHED FAMILY ROLES AND RECOGNIZING DIFFERENCES BETWEEN MAINLAND AND NATIVE PUERTO RICANS. 15 REFERENCES.

ACCN   000282

334 AUTH   **CHRISTIAN, C. C., JR.**
    TITL   CARACTERIZACION DE LOS TEMAS CULTUR-

ALES EN HISPANOAMERICA. (CHARACTERIZATION OF CULTURAL THEMES IN HISPANOAMERICA).
    SRCE   *REVISTA DE CIENCIAS SOCIALES, 1970, 14, 379-398.*
    INDX   ART, CULTURE, SEX ROLES, POLITICS, POLITICAL POWER, SOUTH AMERICA, MEXICO, ESSAY, CENTRAL AMERICA, MALE
    ABST   EVERY CULTURAL SYSTEM CAN BE CHARACTERIZED BY CERTAIN PREVAILING THEMES. THESE THEMES GUIDE MEMBERS OF PARTICULAR CULTURAL GROUPS AND ORIENT THEM TO THE SALIENT FEATURES OF THEIR CULTURE. THE MOST IMPORTANT THEMES IN THE HISPANIC CULTURE ARE DISCUSSED IN AN ATTEMPT TO DISCOVER AND EXPLAIN THE TOTALITY OF THE CULTURE THROUGH ITS MOST CHARACTERISTIC ASPECTS. THE NUCLEUS OF THE REFERENCE POINTS IN THE HISPANIC CULTURE CAN BE LOCALIZED IN A THREE-DIMENSIONAL SPACE: TOWARDS THE INDIVIDUAL, TOWARDS THE CONCRETE, AND TOWARDS THE EMOTIONAL. MAN AS AN INDIVIDUAL IS RARELY CONCEIVED AS A MEMBER OF A COLLECTIVE, "A SOCIAL UNIT," BUT RATHER AS A BIOLOGICAL INDIVIDUAL WITH NEEDS AND IMPULSES SIMILAR TO THOSE OF ANIMALS. THIS IS THE CONCRETE MAN, THE MAN OF FLESH AND BONES WITH HIS SEXUAL IMPULSES AND HIS DESIRES TO RULE OVER OTHERS. THE CONCRETE MAN IS ALSO CONCEIVED AS AN EMOTIONAL BEING. THE HISTORICAL PROCESSES THAT HAVE CULMINATED IN THE DEVELOPMENT OF HIS UNIQUE AND PERSONAL IDENTITY ARE THE MOST IMPORTANT ASPECT OF HIS PERSONALITY.

ACCN   000283

335 AUTH   **CHRISTIAN, N. E. JR., & GREENE, J. E.**
    TITL   ETHNICITY AS AN IMPUT VARIABLE TO EQUITY THEORY.
    SRCE   *JOURNAL OF PSYCHOLOGY, 1976, 94(2), 237-243.*
    INDX   EMPIRICAL, NEW MEXICO, SOUTHWEST, COLLEGE STUDENTS, MALE, DYADIC INTERACTION, COOPERATION, THEORETICAL, MEXICAN AMERICAN, PREJUDICE, CROSS CULTURAL
    ABST   THE EQUITY MODEL (USED TO ACCOUNT FOR SHARING OF REWARDS AMONG MEMBERS OF A DYAD WORKING IN PARTNERSHIP) IS A PLAUSIBLE MEANS OF VIEWING AND STUDYING ETHNIC RELATIONS. THE PRIMARY HYPOTHESIS WAS THAT WITHIN A HOMOGENEOUS DYAD (COMPOSED OF MEMBERS OF THE SAME ETHNIC GROUP) GREATER EQUITY OCCURS THAN IN A HETEROGENEOUS DYAD (COMPOSED OF MEMBERS OF DIFFERENT ETHNIC GROUPS). A SUBHYPOTHESIS WAS THAT GREATER EQUITY OCCURS IN A DYAD COMPOSED OF MEMBERS OF TWO DIFFERENT MINORITY GROUPS THAN IN A DYAD COMPOSED OF A MINORITY GROUP MEMBER AND A WHITE INDIVIDUAL. THE SUBJECTS OF THE STUDY WERE 18 ANGLO, 18 BLACK, AND 18 CHICANO MALE COLLEGE STUDENTS AGED 17 TO 34. THE TASK INVOLVED A SUBJECT AND A STOOGE WORKING IN PARTNERSHIP TO IDENTIFY CORRECTLY 18 AMERICAN SLANG WORDS FOR A REWARD. THE RE-

SULTS OF AN ANALYSIS OF VARIANCE INDICATED PARTIAL SUPPORT FOR THE PRIMARY HYPOTHESIS, IN THAT HOMOGENEOUS CHICANO DYADS WERE THE MOST EQUITABLE. THESE FINDINGS SHOW THAT EQUITY THEORY CAN BE EMPLOYED AS A USEFUL FRAMEWORK FOR STUDYING INTER-GROUP RELATIONS. 17 REFERENCES. (JOURNAL ABSTRACT MODIFIED)

ACCN   002052

---

336   AUTH   **CHRISTIANSEN, T., & LIVERMORE, G.**

TITL   A COMPARISON OF ANGLO AMERICAN AND SPANISH AMERICAN CHILDREN ON THE WISC.

SRCE   *JOURNAL OF SOCIAL PSYCHOLOGY, 1970, 81(1), 9-14.*

INDX   INTELLIGENCE TESTING, CROSS CULTURAL, SPANISH SURNAMED, WISC, EMPIRICAL, SES, ADOLESCENTS, INTELLIGENCE, ENVIRONMENTAL FACTORS

ABST   THE INFLUENCE OF ENVIRONMENTAL VARIABLES IN THE DEVELOPMENT OF INTELLIGENCE SUGGESTS A RELATIONSHIP BETWEEN SOCIAL CLASS AND INTELLIGENCE. THE PERFORMANCE OF LOWER- AND MIDDLE-CLASS ANGLO AMERICANS WITH LOWER- AND MIDDLE-CLASS SPANISH AMERICANS ON THE WISC IS COMPARED. NINETY-TWO ANGLO-AMERICAN AND SPANISH-AMERICAN CHILDREN, 13-14 YEARS OF AGE, NONE OF WHOM WERE ENROLLED IN SPECIAL EDUCATION CLASSES, WERE CLASSIFIED ON THE BASIS OF SOCIAL CLASS AND ETHNIC ORIGIN INTO FOUR GROUPS. COMPARISONS WERE MADE OF THE FOLLOWING: (1) THE FULL SCALE IQ SCORES; (2) THE VERBAL SCALE IQ SCORES; (3) THE PERFORMANCE SCALE IQ SCORES; AND (4) THE INTELLECTIVE FACTORS OF VERBAL COMPREHENSION, FREEDOM FROM DISTRACTIBILITY, PRECEPTUAL ORGANIZATION AND RELEVANCE. DATA REVEALED THAT MIDDLE-CLASS CHILDREN IN BOTH ETHNIC GROUPS SCORED SIGNIFICANTLY HIGHER THAN THE LOWER-CLASS CHILDREN ON EACH OF THE WISC MEASURES EXAMINED. ON THOSE MEASURES WHERE ETHNIC ORIGIN WAS A FACTOR, ANGLO AMERICANS SCORED SIGNIFICANTLY HIGHER THAN SPANISH AMERICANS. SOCIAL CLASS WAS A MORE IMPORTANT FACTOR IN DIFFERENTIATING AMONG SUBJECTS ON THE WISC MEASURES THAN ETHNIC ORIGIN. IT IS CONCLUDED THAT GENERAL INTELLIGENCE AND THE DEVELOPMENT OF VERBAL ABILITIES, INCLUDING THE ABILITY TO UTILIZE ACQUIRED VERBAL SKILLS IN NEW SITUATIONS, ARE RELATED TO ETHNIC ORIGIN AND SOCIAL CLASS. NONVERBAL ABILITIES, PERCEPTUAL ORGANIZATION ABILITY, AND THE ABILITY TO CONCENTRATE ON A TASK WERE FOUND TO RELATE ONLY TO MEMBERSHIP IN A PARTICULAR SOCIAL CLASS. 11 REFERENCES.

ACCN   000284

---

337   AUTH   **CICIRELLI, V. G., GRANGER, R., SCHEMMEL, O., COOPER, W., & HOLTHOUSE, N.**

TITL   PERFORMANCE OF DISADVANTAGED PRIMARY-GRADE CHILDREN ON THE REVISED ILLINOIS TEST OF PSYCHOLINGUISTIC ABILITIES.

SRCE   *PSYCHOLOGY IN THE SCHOOLS, 1971, 8(3), 240-246.*

INDX   ITPA, CHILDREN, CROSS CULTURAL, MEXICAN AMERICAN, STANFORD ACHIEVEMENT TEST, METROPOLITAN READINESS TEST, LINGUISTIC COMPETENCE, LANGUAGE ASSESSMENT, MEMORY, EMPIRICAL

ABST   THE PERFORMANCE OF DISADVANTAGED PRIMARY SCHOOL CHILDREN IN GRADES ONE, TWO, AND THREE SUBDIVIDED INTO WHITE, BLACK, AND MEXICAN AMERICAN GROUPS IS REPORTED BASED ON THE USE OF THE REVISED ILLINOIS TEST OF PSYCHOLINGUISTIC ABILITIES (ITPA). WHEN COMPARED TO EXISTING NORMS FOR MIDDLE-CLASS WHITES, THE GROUP AS A WHOLE TENDS TO BE BELOW AVERAGE AT EACH GRADE LEVEL ON THE ITPA; THE MEANS ARE SMALLER, AND THE STANDARD DEVIATIONS ARE LARGER. THE ITPA TEST PROFILES REVEAL STRONG POINTS IN THE ABILITIES THAT USE THE VISUAL CHANNEL IN MANUAL EXPRESSION AND IN AUDITORY SEQUENTIAL MEMORY. THESE CHILDREN ARE WEAKEST IN ABILITIES THAT INVOLVE THE AUDITORY CHANNEL AND THE TWO ABILITIES ASSOCIATED WITH LANGUAGE. FOR THE RACIAL ETHNIC SUBGROUPS, THE PATTERN IS SIMILAR EXCEPT THAT THE RANGE OF DEVIATION FOR THE WHITES IS SMALLER; THE MEXICAN AMERICANS EXCEL IN VISUAL SEQUENTIAL MEMORY; AND IN CONTRAST, THE BLACKS EXCEL IN AUDITORY SEQUENTIAL MEMORY. THE INTERCORRELATIONS AMONG THE SUBTESTS OF THE ITPA ARE SIMILAR TO THOSE REPORTED IN THE TEST MANUAL. INTERCORRELATIONS OF THE ITPA SUBTESTS WITH THE METROPOLITAN READINESS TEST AND STANFORD ACHIEVEMENT TEST SCORES INDICATE THAT THE STRONGEST ABILITIES OF THE CHILDREN ARE LEAST CORRELATED WITH READINESS AND ACHIEVEMENT, WHILE THEIR WEAKEST ABILITIES ARE MOST CORRELATED. THE ABILITIES THAT ARE HIGHLY RELATED TO SCHOOL ACHIEVEMENT ARE THOSE IN WHICH THEY SHOW THE GREATEST DEFICIENCY. TWO IMPORTANT QUESTIONS ARISE CONCERNING WHY THERE IS SUCH A CONTRAST IN THE PROFILES OF THE WHITES, BLACKS, AND MEXICAN AMERICANS WITH REGARD TO THE MEMORY ABILITIES. WHETHER THE DIFFERENCE IS CULTURAL OR INNATE IS DISCUSSED. 13 REFERENCES.

ACCN   000285

---

338   AUTH   **CLARK, M., KAUFMAN, S., & PIERCE, R.**

TITL   EXPLORATIONS OF ACCULTURATION: TOWARD A MODEL OF ETHNIC IDENTITY.

SRCE   *HUMAN ORGANIZATION, 1976, 35(3), 231-238.*

INDX   ACCULTURATION, ETHNIC IDENTITY, EMPIRICAL, CULTURAL PLURALISM, CULTURE, MEXICAN AMERICAN, CROSS CULTURAL, RESEARCH METHODOLOGY, CROSS GENERATIONAL, CALIFORNIA, SOUTHWEST

ABST   THIS PAPER EXAMINES INTERVIEW DATA FROM A THREE GENERATION SAMPLE DRAWN FROM TWO ETHNIC MINORITY GROUPS (JAPANESE AMERICANS AND MEXICAN AMERICANS) IN THE SAN FRANCISCO BAY AREA. FIRST, THE

HISTORY OF THE CONCEPT ACCULTURATION, COMBINING BOTH "CLASSIC" LITERATURE AND THE NEWER "ETHNIC IDENTITY" LITERATURE, IS REVIEWED. SECOND, SIX ETHNIC IDENTITY PROFILE TYPES ARE PRESENTED, WITH CASE SUMMARIES ILLUSTRATING THE CHARACTERISTICS SHARED BY MEMBERS OF EACH PROFILE TYPE. A COMPARISON OF (1) THE COMPOSITION OF THE VARIABLES INCLUDED IN EACH TYPE, AND (2) THE TWO PROFILE TYPES OF EACH GENERATION, REVEAL THE INFLUENCE OF INDIVIDUAL CHOICE IN THE EXPRESSION OF ETHNIC IDENTITY. 41 REFERENCES. (JOURNAL ABSTRACT MODIFIED)

ACCN   000286

339 AUTH   **CLARK, M., & MENDELSON, M.,**
    TITL   MEXICAN-AMERICAN AGED IN SAN FRANCISCO: A CASE DESCRIPTION.
    SRCE   *GERONTOLOGIST, 1969, 9(2), 90-95.*
    INDX   MEXICAN AMERICAN, GERONTOLOGY, ADULTS, CASE STUDY, IMMIGRATION, CULTURAL FACTORS, FAMILY STRUCTURE, FAMILY ROLES, ACCULTURATION, EXTENDED FAMILY, CALIFORNIA, SOUTHWEST, FEMALE
    ABST   A CASE DESCRIPTION OF THE MEXICAN AMERICAN AGED IN SAN FRANCISCO IS PRESENTED. MOST ELDERLY PERSONS OF MEXICAN DESCENT WHO NOW LIVE IN SAN FRANCISCO CAME FROM VILLAGES IN MEXICO. BECAUSE OF THE PATTERN OF IMMIGRATION, THE OLDER PERSONS OF MEXICAN DESCENT HAVE BEEN EXPOSED TO THE COMBINED PROCESSES OF ACCULTURATION AND URBANIZATION. THE COMPOSITION AND LIFE STYLE OF ONE RELATIVELY UNACCULTURATED FAMILY IS DESCRIBED, WITH A FOCUS ON THE 71 YEAR-OLD GRANDMOTHER. THIS ELDERLY WOMAN'S TWO SONS AND DAUGHTER WORK, WHILE SHE ASSUMES RESPONSIBILITY FOR ALL THE HOUSEKEEPING AND COOKING, AS WELL AS CARE OF THE GRANDCHILDREN. THE EVIDENCE OF HER CONTINUED IMPORTANCE IN THE FAMILY PLEASES HER, AND SHE SEEMS TO BE IN HER ELEMENT WITH A HOUSE FULL OF FAMILY AND FRIENDS. SHE ALSO CARRIES ON AN ACTIVE TRADE BETWEEN THIS COUNTRY AND GUADALAJARA. SECOND ONLY TO HER DELIGHT IN HER TRADING TRIPS TO MEXICO IS HER PENCHANT FOR GAMBLING. THIS FAMILY IS RELATIVELY UNACCULTURATED, AS THEY MANIFEST TRADITIONAL MEXICAN PATTERNS TO A SOMEWHAT GREATER EXTENT THAN MANY MORE ANGLICIZED FAMILES. IT IS CONCLUDED THAT THE MAJOR TASK IN MENTAL HEALTH TODAY IS TO SEEK A WAY OF HELPING PEOPLE TO ESTABLISH AND MAINTAIN SENSE OF SELF, MEANING, AND WORTH, WITHOUT RECOURSE TO ARBITRARY HIERARCHICAL ARRANGEMENTS IN WHICH ONE ASSURES HIS OWN COMPETENCE AND VALUE BY THE DEVALUATION OF OTHERS. 8 REFERENCES.

ACCN   000287

340 AUTH   **CLELAND, C. C., ISCOE, I., & PATTON, W. F.**
    TITL   CLIMATOLOGICAL INFLUENCES IN MENTAL DEFICIENCY AS RELATED TO THREE ETHNIC GROUPS.

SRCE   *REVISTA INTERAMERICANA DE PSICOLOGIA, 1967, 1(1), 13-25.*
INDX   ENVIRONMENTAL FACTORS, MENTAL RETARDATION, CROSS CULTURAL, MEXICAN AMERICAN, EMPIRICAL, SES, SEX COMPARISON, TEXAS, SOUTHWEST
ABST   AN INVESTIGATION OF THE RELATIONSHIP BETWEEN SEASON OF CONCEPTION AND SUBSEQUENT BIRTH OF MENTAL DEFECTIVES IN TEXAS IS PRESENTED. UTILIZATION OF THE TEXAS INSTITUTIONALIZED POPULATION AFFORDS A DIFFERENTIAL ASSESSMENT OF THE EFFECTS OF TEMPERATURE SINCE THIS STATE IS WARMER IN CONTRAST TO THE STATES WHERE SIMILAR STUDIES WERE CONDUCTED. SUBJECTS NUMBERING 11,000 WERE GROUPED ACCORDING TO ETHNICITY (ANGLO, NEGRO, MEXICAN AMERICAN), LEVEL OF RETARDATION, SEX, AND PATERNAL EDUCATIONAL LEVEL. ANALYSIS INDICATES THAT MORE RETARDATES SEEM TO HAVE BEEN CONCEIVED IN THE HOTTER MONTHS OF THE YEAR FROM THE MA SAMPLE. THOSE SUBJECTS WITH IQ'S LESS THAN 20 ALSO SEEM TO HAVE BEEN CONCEIVED IN GREATER NUMBERS DURING HOTTER MONTHS. NO SUCH TREND WAS FOUND FOR THE TOTAL 11,000 RETARDATES. SEASONAL VARIATIONS IN SEASON OF CONCEPTION AMONG RETARDATES ALSO REFLECT WIDE DIFFERENCES WITH RESPECT TO PATERNAL EDUCATIONAL LEVEL. THESE FINDINGS PROVIDE MODEST SUPPORT FOR PREVIOUS STUDIES RELATING SEASON OF BIRTH TO INCIDENCE OF RETARDATION. 11 REFERENCES.
ACCN   000288

341 AUTH   **COALITION OF CONCERNED BLACK AMERICANS.**
    TITL   A PRELIMINARY REPORT OF THE EXPERIENCES OF THE MINORITY JUDICIARY IN THE CITY OF NEW YORK.
    SRCE   *HOWARD LAW JOURNAL, 1975, 18(3), 495-542.*
    INDX   JUDICIAL PROCESS, REPRESENTATION, CORRECTIONS, URBAN, SURVEY, POLITICS, EMPIRICAL, PERSONNEL, NEW YORK, EAST, ADULTS, DISCRIMINATION, ATTITUDES, SPANISH SURNAMED, PUERTO RICAN-M, POLICE-COMMUNITY RELATIONS, POLICY
    ABST   THIS REPORT EXAMINES THE INEQUITIES IN THE REPRESENTATION AND STATUS OF BLACK AND HISPANIC CITIZENS WITHIN THE JUDICIAL SYSTEM AS PERCEIVED BY MINORITY JUDGES. PARTICULAR ATTENTION IS DIRECTED TOWARD ADMINISTRATIVE POLICIES WHICH CURTAIL THE EFFECTIVENESS OF THESE JUDGES AND DIMINISH THEIR IMPACT WITHIN THE LEGAL SYSTEM. PRELIMINARY RESULTS ARE PRESENTED BASED ON A SURVEY AND IN-DEPTH INTERVIEWS WITH 24 OUT OF 39 PARTICIPATING JUDGES (37 BLACK AND 2 HISPANIC) AND COVER SELECTION AND ASSIGNMENT OF JUDGES, PRESSURES ON THE JUDICIARY, RACISM, COURTROOM FACILITIES AND PERSONNEL, PLEA BARGAINING, THE BAIL SYSTEM, AND TRENDS PERCEIVED IN THE ADMINISTRATION OF JUSTICE. ALTHOUGH BOTH THE APPOINTIVE AND ELECTIVE SYSTEMS OF JUDICIAL SELECTION HAVE INCREASED THE

NUMBER OF MINORITY JUDGES, BLACKS AND HISPANICS ACCOUNT FOR LESS THAN 10 OF THE JUDGES IN NEW YORK CITY. HOWEVER, 70-85 OF THE DEFENDANTS SEEN IN COURTS ARE NON-WHITE. THE RESPONDENTS COMMENTED ON THE PERVASIVE RACISM WITHIN THE AMERICAN LEGAL SYSTEM. PLEA BARGAINING AND THE BAIL SYSTEM WERE CONSIDERED TO BE PARTICULARLY UNFAIR TO MINORITIES. THE PRESENT SYSTEM OF JUDICIAL ASSIGNMENT, ALTHOUGH ALLOWING FOR SOME FAVORIT-ISM, WAS NOT FELT TO INTERFERE WITH JUDI-CIAL INDEPENDENCE. MANY OF THE RESPON-DENTS EXPRESSED THE OPINION THAT SOME JUDGES WERE DISCIPLINED FOR BEING TOO LENIENT OR EXPRESSING PARTISAN OPINIONS. OVERALL, THEIR VIEW OF TRENDS IN THE AD-MINISTRATION OF MINORITY JUSTICE WAS NOT OPTIMISTIC. SUGGESTIONS ARE MADE FOR EF-FECTIVE UTILIZATION OF THE STUDY'S FIND-INGS THROUGH CONTACT WITH BAR ASSOCIA-TIONS, THE LEGISLATURE, CIVIL RIGHTS ORGANIZATIONS AND THE NEWS MEDIA. A COPY OF THE RESEARCH INSTRUMENT IS IN-CLUDED. 24 REFERENCES.

ACCN   002053

342 AUTH   **COBAS, J. A.**
     TITL   STATUS CONSCIOUSNESS AND LEFTISM: A STUDY OF MEXICAN-AMERICAN ADOLES-CENTS.
     SRCE   *SOCIAL FORCES, 1977, 55(4), 1028-1042.*
     INDX   MEXICAN AMERICAN, ADOLESCENTS, ETHNIC IDENTITY, POLITICS, SES, ATTRIBUTION OF RE-SPONSIBILITY, PREJUDICE, EMPIRICAL, TEXAS, SOUTHWEST
     ABST   USING DATA COLLECTED AMONG MEXICAN AMERICAN ADOLESCENTS IN A TEXAS HIGH SCHOOL, THIS PAPER TESTS A MODEL WHICH PREDICTS THE RELATIONSHIP BETWEEN STA-TUS CONSCIOUSNESS AND POLITICAL LEF-TISM. THE RELATIONSHIP IS SUMMARIZED AS FOLLOWS: SYSTEM BLAME HAS A POSITIVE EF-FECT ON POLITICAL LEFTISM; ETHNIC CON-SCIOUSNESS HAS A POSITIVE EFFECT ON SYS-TEM BLAME. FOR THE SAMPLE AS A WHOLE, RESULTS SUPPORT THE MODEL, ALTHOUGH THE EFFECT OF SYSTEM BLAME ON LEFTISM IS WEAK. FURTHER ANALYSIS REVEALS AN INTER-ACTIVE RELATIONSHIP SUCH THAT SYSTEM BLAME HAS A SIGNIFICANT EFFECT ON LEF-TISM AMONG RESPONDENTS WHOSE FATHER'S OCCUPATION IS NOT LOW, BUT NO EFFECT AMONG RESPONDENTS WHOSE FATHER'S OC-CUPATION IS LOW. THE INTERACTION IS APPAR-ENTLY DUE TO A GREATER RELEVANCE OF SYS-TEM BLAME ITEMS TO HIGHER OCCUPATION LEVEL RESPONDENTS. THIS SUGGESTS THE PRESENCE OF OTHER DETERMINANTS OF LEF-TISM AND THAT POLITICAL ATTITUDES OF SIG-NIFICANT OTHERS ARE AMONG THESE DETER-MINANTS. 50 REFERENCES. (JOURNAL ABSTRACT MODIFIED)

ACCN   000289

343 AUTH   **COERS, W. C.**
     TITL   COMPARATIVE ACHIEVEMENT OF WHITE AND MEXICAN JUNIOR HIGH SCHOOL PUPILS.
     SRCE   *PEABODY JOURNAL OF EDUCATION, 1935, 12(4), 157-162.*
     INDX   SCHOLASTIC ACHIEVEMENT, ACHIEVEMENT TESTING, INTELLIGENCE, EMPIRICAL, MEXI-CAN AMERICAN, CROSS CULTURAL, ADOLES-CENTS, TEXAS, SOUTHWEST
     ABST   AN ATTEMPT IS MADE TO DETERMINE THE RELATIVE ACHIEVEMENT OF THE WHITE AND MEXICAN CHILDREN AS DETERMINED BY STAN-DARD TESTS. SUBJECTS WERE DISTRIBUTED AS FOLLOWS: 66 WHITES AND 66 MEXICANS IN THE SIXTH-GRADE; 18 WHITES AND 18 MEXI-CANS IN SEVENTH GRADE; 13 WHITES AND 13 MEXICANS IN THE EIGHTH GRADE. SCORES WERE OBTAINED ON THE KUHLMANN-ANDER-SON TEST, A GROUP INTELLIGENCE TEST, AND THE PUBLIC SCHOOL ACHIEVEMENT TEST, BATTERY A, A MEASURE OF SCHOLASTIC ACHIEVEMENT FOR THE SUBJECTS. ON THE BASIS OF THE ANALYSIS OF ALL DATA OB-TAINED, THE FOLLOWING CONCLUSIONS ARE REACHED: (1) THE MEXICAN GROUP IN ALL THREE GRADES ACHIEVE MORE IN PROPOR-TION TO THEIR MENTAL ABILITY THAN THE WHITE GROUP ON ALL PARTS OF THE ACHIEVE-MENT TEST EXCEPT LANGUAGE USAGE; (2) THE RELATIVE ACHIEVEMENT OF THE MEXICAN GROUPS IS GREATEST ON THE ARITHMETIC COMPUTATION TEST, FOLLOWED CLOSELY BY THE RELATIVE ACHIEVEMENT OF THE SPELL-ING TEST; (3) THE MEXICAN GROUPS IN ALL THREE GRADES SHOW HIGHER AND CONSIS-TENT CORRELATION COEFFICIENTS THAN THE WHITE GROUP BETWEEN ABILITY TO SCORE ON THE INTELLIGENCE TEST AND ABILITY TO SCORE ON THE ACHIEVEMENT TEST; (4) THE SIXTH-GRADE MEXICAN GROUP SHOWS MOST CONSISTENT AND DEFINITE RELATIONSHIPS ON ALL PARTS OF THE ACHIEVEMENT TEST; AND (5) THE INFERIOR PUPILS (ACCORDING TO THEIR TESTED MENTAL ABILITY) OF BOTH WHITE AND MEXICAN GROUPS IN EACH GRADE ARE WORKING MORE UP TO THEIR CAPACITY THAN ARE THE SUPERIOR PUPILS, BUT THERE IS NO APPRECIABLE DIFFERENCE IN EFFICIENCY OF ACHIEVEMENT BETWEEN THE WHITE AND MEX-ICAN GROUPS AT VARIOUS INTELLIGENCE LEV-ELS. NO REFERENCES.

ACCN   000291

344 AUTH   **COHEN, A. D.**
     TITL   MEXICAN-AMERICAN EVALUATIONAL JUDG-MENTS ABOUT LANGUAGE VARIETIES.
     SRCE   *INTERNATIONAL JOURNAL OF THE SOCIOLOGY OF LANGUAGE, 1974, 3, 33-51.*
     INDX   MEXICAN AMERICAN, LINGUISTICS, IMMIGRA-TION, ATTITUDES, DEMOGRAPHIC, PHONOL-OGY, LANGUAGE COMPREHENSION, PAREN-TAL INVOLVEMENT, SURVEY, CALIFORNIA, SOUTHWEST
     ABST   A SAMPLE OF PREDOMINANTLY IMMIGRANT MEXICAN-AMERICAN PARENTS (N 81 FAMILIES) WERE INTERVIEWED TO DETERMINE ATTITUDES TOWARD THE BEST VARIETIES OF SPANISH AND ENGLISH. LANGUAGE PROFI-CIENCY AND USE, LANGUAGE PREFERENCE ATTITUDES, AND DEMOGRAPHIC VARIABLES WERE ALSO ASSESSED. THE MAJORITY OF RE-

SPONDENTS FELT THE BEST SPANISH/ENGLISH WAS SPOKEN IN MEXICO AND THE U.S., RESPECTIVELY, WHILE SMALLER GROUPS CHOSE SPAIN FOR THE BEST SPANISH AND ENGLAND FOR THE BEST ENGLISH. THE LATTER RESPONSES WERE MORE PREVALENT AMONG MALES, PARENTS WITH A HIGHER SOCIOECONOMIC LEVEL, PARENTS MORE PROFICIENT IN SPANISH AND ENGLISH, AND PARENTS MORE CONCERNED WITH THEIR CHILDREN LEARNING ENGLISH FOR INSTRUMENTAL PURPOSES. THE APPROPRIATENESS OF THIS DIRECT APPROACH TO ASSESS LANGUAGE ATTITUDES IS DISCUSSED. 10 REFERENCES. (PASAR ABSTRACT)

ACCN   000292

345 AUTH   **COHEN, A., & LAOSA, L. M.**
    TITL   SECOND LANGUAGE INSTRUCTION: SOME RESEARCH CONSIDERATIONS.
    SRCE   *CURRICULUM STUDIES, 1976, 8(2), 149-165.*
    INDX   LANGUAGE LEARNING, MEXICAN AMERICAN, RESEARCH METHODOLOGY, REVIEW, SOUTH AMERICA, TEACHERS, BILINGUAL-BICULTURAL EDUCATION, BILINGUALISM, CROSS CULTURAL, EARLY CHILDHOOD EDUCATION, EDUCATION, INSTRUCTIONAL TECHNIQUES, PROGRAM EVALUATION

    ABST   A REVIEW OF THE LITERATURE ON METHODS IN A VARIETY OF COUNTRIES FOR TEACHING A SECOND LANGUAGE (SOUTH AFRICA, SOUTH AMERICA, THE PHILIPPINES, IRELAND, WALES, CANADA, AND THE U.S.) INDICATES THE SUCCESS OF DIFFERENT APPROACHES TO THE TEACHING OF PRELITERACY AND LITERACY SKILLS AND SUBJECT MATTER ACQUISITION. HOWEVER, THE LITERATURE ON THE EFFECTS OF BILINGUAL EDUCATION IS CONTRADICTORY, AND THE CONFUSION IS POSTULATED TO BE DUE TO DIFFERENCES IN (1) THE EDUCATIONAL TREATMENTS INVESTIGATED, (2) THE CHARACTERISTICS OF THE STUDENTS IN THE SAMPLES INVESTIGATED, (3) THE CONTEXTS IN WHICH THE PROGRAMS TOOK PLACE, (4) THE RESEARCH DESIGNS AND METHODS EMPHASIZED, AND (5) THE INTERACTIONS AMONG FACTORS 1-4. TO ILLUSTRATE THESE STUDY DIFFERENCES AND THE NEED FOR CAREFUL RESEARCH DESIGN AND METHODOLOGY, TWO EMPIRICAL STUDIES ARE EXAMINED: THE REDWOOD CITY BILINGUAL EDUCATION PROGRAM, DESIGNED FOR SPANISH-SPEAKING MEXICAN AMERICAN CHILDREN; AND THE CULVER CITY SPANISH IMMERSION PROGRAM, DESIGNED FOR ENGLISH-SPEAKING ANGLO AMERICAN CHILDREN. THE RESULTS EMPHASIZE THE NEED TO CONTROL FOR A NUMBER OF VARIABLES BEFORE COMPARING DIFFERENT PROGRAM OUTCOMES. FURTHERMORE, THE ROLE OF THE RESEARCHER OR EVALUATOR SHOULD BE TO IDENTIFY, DEFINE, AND ADEQUATELY MEASURE THE TREATMENT, STUDENT, AND CONTEXT VARIABLES AND TO EXPLORE THE EFFECTS OF DIFFERENT CONFIGURATIONAL COMBINATIONS OF THESE VARIABLES UPON STUDENTS' OUTCOMES. 57 REFERENCES.

    ACCN   002054

346 AUTH   **COHEN, L. M.**
    TITL   GIFTS TO STRANGERS: PUBLIC POLICY AND THE DELIVERY OF HEALTH SERVICES TO ILLEGAL ALIENS.
    SRCE   *ANTHROPOLOGICAL QUARTERLY, 1973, 46(3), 183-195.*
    INDX   IMMIGRATION, UNDOCUMENTED WORKERS, HEALTH, HEALTH DELIVERY SYSTEMS, LEGISLATION, JUDICIAL PROCESS, POLICY, SOCIAL STRUCTURE
    ABST   AN INCREASING COMMITMENT TO UNIVERSAL HEALTH COVERAGE IN THE UNITED STATES CALLS FOR EXAMINATION OF THE POLICY PROBLEMS INVOLVED IN DECISIONS TO EXTEND OR TO WITHHOLD HEALTH SERVICES TO "OUTSIDER" GROUPS SUCH AS ILLEGAL ALIENS. CONGRESSIONAL HEARINGS AND OTHER DOCUMENTS OFFER SOURCE MATERIAL TO IDENTIFY AREAS OF CONSENSUS AND CONFLICT INVOLVED IN THE EXCHANGE PATTERNS BETWEEN SPECIAL INTERST GROUPS AND THESE ALIENS. FAILURES TO ACHIEVE CONSENSUS IN POLICIES TOWARDS THESE ALIENS ARE ASSOCIATED WITH CONTRASTING VALUES AND NORMS REGARDING THE "LEGAL" AND THE "MORAL," THE "WORTHY" AND THE "UNWORTHY" IN OUR SOCIETY. THE WORK OF M. MAUSS ON RECIPROCITY AND GIFT GIVING CONTRIBUTES TO AN UNDERSTANDING OF THE RELATIONSHIP BETWEEN ECONOMIC "VALUE" AND ALTRUISTIC BEHAVIOR TOWARDS ALIENS. G. SIMMEL'S ANALYSIS OF THE FUNCTION OF SECRECY IN SOCIAL LIFE UNDERSCORES THE NEED TO UNDERTAKE STUDIES OF HIDDEN GROUPS WHOSE RELATIONS WITH SOCIETY OFFER A BROAD VISION OF SOCIAL REALITY. 18 REFERENCES. (JOURNAL ABSTRACT)
    ACCN   000293

347 AUTH   **COHEN, L. M., & FERNANDEZ, C. L.**
    TITL   ETHNIC IDENTITY AND PSYCHOCULTURAL ADAPTATION OF SPANISH-SPEAKING FAMILIES.
    SRCE   *CHILD WELFARE, 1974, 53(7), 413-421.*
    INDX   ESSAY, IMMIGRATION, ETHNIC IDENTITY, SPANISH SURNAMED, CENTRAL AMERICA, CULTURAL CHANGE, FAMILY STRUCTURE, PSYCHOSOCIAL ADJUSTMENT, COPING MECHANISMS, URBAN, WASHINGTON D. C., EAST, ACCULTURATION, CHILDREN, ADULTS, CROSS GENERATIONAL
    ABST   IN ADJUSTING TO AMERICAN URBAN LIFE, SPANISH-SPEAKING IMMIGRANT FAMILIES UNDERGO SOCIAL AND PSYCHOCULTURAL CHANGES THAT AFFECT THEIR ETHNIC IDENTITY. ONE HUNDRED SUCH FAMILIES LIVING IN WASHINGTON, D.C. WERE INTERVIEWED CONCERNING THEIR OCCUPATIONAL CAREERS AND HELP-SEEKING PATTERNS. IN OVER 75 PERCENT OF THE FAMILIES STUDIED, FINDINGS REVEALED THAT SELECTION AND ACCOMODATION ARE KEY FACTORS IN UTILIZING COMMUNITY HEALTH SERVICES. EGO-ADAPTIVE MECHANISMS ASSOCIATED WITH CULTURAL CHANGES TEND TO OCCUR AT A MODERATE RATE AND VARY DEPENDING ON THE PERSON'S AGE. ACTING AS AGENTS OF CULTURAL LINK-

AGES FOR THEIR PARENTS, CHILDREN REINFORCE THEIR OWN IDENTIFICATION, BUT THEY NEED TO HAVE ACCESSIBLE MODELS ALLOWING THEM TO LEARN EXPECTATIONS, MEANINGS, AND ACTIVITIES CONSIDERED NORMAL IN AMERICAN SOCIETY. HOWEVER, IN RAPIDLY ADAPTING TO URBAN LIFE, CHILDREN TEND TO REJECT THEIR CULTURAL HERITAGE. FURTHER STUDIES OF ADJUSTMENT PATTERNS ARE NECESSARY TO ASCERTAIN THE DIFFERENT WAYS IMMIGRANTS ADAPT OR REJECT THEIR CULTURAL IDENTITY. 8 REFERENCES.

ACCN   000294

348 AUTH **COHEN, R. E.**
    TITL BORDERLINE CONDITIONS: A TRANSCULTURAL PERSPECTIVE.
    SRCE *UNPUBLISHED MANUSCRIPT, HARVARD MEDICAL SCHOOL, UNDATED.*
    INDX PSYCHOPATHOLOGY, CULTURAL FACTORS, PSYCHOTHERAPY, MENTAL HEALTH, SYMPTOMATOLOGY, STEREOTYPES, DISCRIMINATION, SPANISH SURNAMED, REVIEW, ADULTS, VALUES
    ABST FACTORS AFFECTING THE INTERACTION BETWEEN THERAPIST AND PATIENTS WITH BORDERLINE CONDITIONS ARE DISCUSSED WITHIN THE TRANSCULTURAL FRAMEWORK OF PSYCHIATRIC DIAGNOSIS AND TREATMENT OF BORDERLINE STATES. IT IS RECOGNIZED THAT THERAPISTS GENERALLY CLASSIFY AND TREAT SYMPTOMS BASED ON THE VALUES AND EXPERIENCES OF THEIR OWN CULTURE AND PSYCHIATRIC TRAINING. IT IS POSITED THAT WHEN THERAPISTS AND PATIENTS COME FROM DIFFERENT CULTURAL BACKGROUNDS POTENTIAL PROBLEMS AND AREAS OF DISSONACE OCCUR. IN ORDER TO BETTER UNDERSTAND THE INFLUENCE OF TRANSCULTURAL FACTORS ON THE SUCCESS OF THERAPEUTIC INTERVENTION IN BORDERLINE CASES THE AUTHOR FOCUSES ON THE FOLLOWING AREAS: (1) ATTEMPTING TO IDENTIFY THE SOCIO-CULTURAL FACTORS THAT INFLUENCE AND MODIFY THE DOCTOR-PATIENT RELATIONSHIP IN THE TREATMENT OF BORDERLINE STATES; (2) INDICATING THE NEED TO RECONCEPTUALIZE THE THEORY OF DYNAMIC PSYCHOTHERAPY IN THE LIGHT OF DIVERSE CULTURAL AND SOCIAL FACTORS; AND (3) EMPHASIZING THE NEED TO DEVELOP INTERVENTIVE SKILLS INCORPORATING SOCIOLOGICAL AND ANTHROPOLOGICAL FINDINGS. 37 REFERENCES. (AUTHOR SUMMARY MODIFIED)
    ACCN 000295

349 AUTH **COHEN, R. E.**
    TITL PREVENTIVE MENTAL HEALTH PROGRAMS FOR ETHNIC MINORITY POPULATIONS: A CASE IN POINT.
    SRCE *PAPER PRESENTED AT THE 39TH CONGRESO INTERNACIONAL DE AMERICANISTAS, LIMA, PERU, AUGUST 2-9, 1970.*
    INDX PRIMARY PREVENTION, MENTAL HEALTH, CULTURAL FACTORS, PUERTO RICAN-M, ESSAY, TIME ORIENTATION, FAMILY ROLES, HEALTH EDUCATION, LEGISLATION, HEALTH DELIVERY SYSTEMS, PROFESSIONAL TRAINING, COPING MECHANISMS, PSYCHOSOCIAL ADJUSTMENT, VALUES
    ABST EXPERIENCES WITH LOW-INCOME PUERTO RICAN FAMILIES WHICH CHALLENGE MENTAL HEALTH PROFESSIONALS TO THINK IN TERMS OF COMPREHENSIVE PREVENTIVE MENTAL HEALTH PROGRAMS ARE OFFERED. IT WAS LEARNED THAT: (1) AN INDIVIDUAL CAN ENCOUNTER SERIOUS PERSONAL PROBLEMS WHEN HE TRIES TO ADAPT TO THE SOCIAL MORES OF AN ALIEN CULTURE; (2) PROBLEM SOLVING AND PERSONAL DEVELOPMENT CAN BE FACILITATED OR IMPEDED BY ONE'S HERITAGE; (3) INTERACTIONS WITH REPRESENTATIVES OF SOCIAL SYSTEMS CAN STRONGLY AFFECT THE INDIVIDUAL'S SELF-ESTEEM; (4) COPING MECHANISMS FOR THE MASTERY OF ADAPTATIONAL CRISIS NEED TO BE DEVELOPED BY THE CULTURAL-ALIEN INDIVIDUAL; (5) THE ALIEN INDIVIDUAL NEEDS TO INCREASE HIS ABILITY TO DEVELOP VALUES AND STYLES OF BEHAVIOR WHICH ARE ADAPTIVELY ADEQUATE FOR HIS NEW SOCIAL CONDITIONS; (6) PROFESSIONALS AND SOCIAL INSTITUTIONS WHO UNDERSTAND THE IMPORTANCE OF DIFFERENCES IN VALUE ORIENTATION MUST SUPPORT AND STRENGTHEN INDIVIDUAL COMPETENCY AND AUTONOMY OF CULTURAL ALIENS; AND (7) A LOVING RELATIONSHIP WITHIN A SECURE, FAMILIAR ENVIRONMENT FOR HEALTHY PERSONALITY DEVELOPMENT NEEDS TO BE ESTABLISHED FOR CULTURAL ALIENS. ENCOURAGING SUGGESTIONS FOR MEETING SOME OF THESE OBJECTIVES ARE: (1) FOR COMMUNITIES TO PROVIDE ASSISTANCE DURING THE TRANSITIONAL PERIODS—I.E., FREEDOM FROM WANT AND ALIENATION; (2) TO ACQUIRE ADEQUATE ROLE MODELS THROUGH RELATIONS OF TRUST AND IDENTIFICATION WITH OTHERS; AND (3) TO ESTABLISH MENTAL HEALTH PROGRAMS WITH ACTIVITIES SUCH AS EDUCATION, INTERVENTION, PARTICIPATION, EXERCISE INPUTS, DEVELOPMENT OF MENTAL HEALTH MANPOWER, RESEARCH AND DATA GATHERING, AND WORKING WITH THE COMMUNITY. 29 REFERENCES.
    ACCN 000297

350 AUTH **COHEN, R. E.**
    TITL PRINCIPLES OF PREVENTIVE MENTAL HEALTH PROGRAMS FOR ETHNIC MINORITY POPULATIONS: THE ACCULTURATION OF PUERTO RICANS TO THE UNITED STATES.
    SRCE *AMERICAN JOURNAL OF PSYCHIATRY, 1972, 128(12), 1529-1533.*
    INDX PRIMARY PREVENTION, MENTAL HEALTH, HEALTH DELIVERY SYSTEMS, PUERTO RICAN-M, ACCULTURATION, CULTURAL FACTORS, IMMIGRATION, URBAN, ESSAY, VALUES
    ABST THIS PAPER PRESENTS CONCEPTS AND METHODS BY WHICH MENTAL HEALTH PROFESSIONALS CAN PLAN EFFECTIVE INTERVENTIONS WHICH TAKE INTO ACCOUNT THE HISTORICAL, PSYCHOLOGICAL, SOCIOLOGICAL AND CULTURAL VALUES OF THE IMMIGRANTS. THESE CONCEPTS AND METHODS ARE DRAWN FROM KLUCKHOHN'S THEORY ON THE VARIATION OF VALUE ORIENTATIONS. BY DEVELOPING A

MODEL FOR COMPARISON OF PUERTO RICAN AND AMERICAN MIDDLE-CLASS URBAN VALUE SYSTEMS, THE SOURCES OF CONFLICT CAN BE IDENTIFIED, UNDERSTOOD, AND WITH APPROPRIATE INTERVENTIONS, PREVENTED. METHODS FOR THE DESIGN AND IMPLEMENTATION OF MENTAL HEALTH PROGRAMS BUILT ON THIS MODEL ARE DISCUSSED. AN ONGOING PREVENTIVE PROGRAM IS ENVISIONED AS INCLUDING THE FOLLOWING ACTIVITIES: (1) EDUCATION FOR BOTH CAREGIVERS AND RECIPIENTS OF SERVICES IN MENTAL HEALTH PRINCIPLES; (2) MENTAL HEALTH MANPOWER TRAINING FOR BILINGUAL NATIVE PUERTO RICANS WHO WOULD ACT AS PARAPROFESSIONALS; (3) PARTICIPATION AND COLLABORATION ON THE PART OF MENTAL HEALTH PROFESSIONALS WITH OTHER SERVICE AGENCIES AT ALL GOVERNMENT LEVELS IN AMELIORATING STRESSFUL CONDITIONS FOR PUERTO RICAN FAMILIES WITH EDUCATION, HOUSING, EMPLOYMENT AND OTHER NEEDS; (4) CONSULTATION WITH OTHER CARE GIVING PROFESSIONALS TO DEVELOP EFFECTIVE POLICIES CONSISTENT WITH THE NEEDS OF MINORITIES SERVED; (5) ACTION AS LINKING AGENTS BETWEEN SPANISH SPEAKING AND NON-SPANISH SPEAKING GROUPS TO BREAK DOWN LANGUAGE AND CULTURE DIFFERENCES; (6) PARTICIPATION IN THE ORGANIZATION OF NEW MODELS OF HEALTH CARE DELIVERY THAT MAY BE ADAPTED TO THE NEEDS AND BEHAVIOR PATTERNS OF ETHNIC MINORITY GROUPS; AND (7) RESEARCH AND DATA GATHERING TO DETERMINE THE MOST APPROPRIATE MEANS FOR PROVIDING SERVICES TO PUERTO RICAN AND OTHER IMMIGRANTS. 26 REFERENCES.

ACCN   000298

351 AUTH   **COHEN, R. E.**
    TITL   PROBLEMAS ENTRE PADRES Y HIJOS. (PROBLEMS BETWEEN PARENTS AND CHILDREN.)
    SRCE   *EL NOTICIERO, SEPTEMBER 1970, 10. (SPANISH)*
    INDX   FATHER-CHILD INTERACTION, MOTHER-CHILD INTERACTION, PUERTO RICAN-M, ESSAY, MENTAL HEALTH, CHILDREARING PRACTICES, FAMILY ROLES
    ABST   PARENTS AND CHILDREN OF THE HISPANIC COMMUNITY MAY SUFFER EMOTIONAL CONFLICTS, AS THEY NOT ONLY HAVE TO ADAPT THEMSELVES TO A CONTINUALLY CHANGING SOCIETY, BUT TO A SOCIETY BASICALLY DIFFERENT FROM THEIR OWN. PARENTS REACT TO THEIR OWN DISORIENTATION BY EXERCISING A RIGID FORM OF AUTHORITY TOWARDS THEIR CHILDREN AS A WAY TO COMPENSATE FOR THE FEELING THAT TRADITIONAL VALUES ARE DISAPPEARING FROM THEIR HOMES. CHILDREARING PRACTICES GROW MORE AND MORE INCONSISTENT AND THEIR CHILDREN GROW UP NOT KNOWING WHICH VALUES TO INCORPORATE. SOCIAL RULES APPEAR TO BE CONFUSING AND FULL OF CONTRADICTIONS AND THERE IS A PROGRESSIVE DEVIATION FROM THE FAMILIAR BASE. IN ORDER TO PREVENT THESE PROBLEMS, PARENTS MUST BE AWARE OF THE CULTURAL DIFFERENCES AND

OPEN TO NEW METHODS TO RAISE THEIR CHILDREN, RESOLVE PROBLEMS AND IMPLEMENT NEW FEMININE AND MASCULINE ROLES THAT CAN BE BETTER IDENTIFIED WITH THE NEW SOCIAL SITUATION.

ACCN   000300

352 AUTH   **COHEN, R. E.**
    TITL   A PROCESS MODEL TO ORGANIZE CHILD ABUSE/NEGLECT SERVICES: A PROBLEM SOLVING APPROACH.
    SRCE   *UNPUBLISHED MANUSCRIPT, HARVARD MEDICAL SCHOOL, JANUARY 1976.*
    INDX   CHILD ABUSE, HEALTH DELIVERY SYSTEMS, COMMUNITY, PRIMARY PREVENTION, ESSAY, PARAPROFESSIONALS, COMMUNITY INVOLVEMENT
    ABST   THE IMPLEMENTATION OF THE CHILD ABUSE PREVENTION AND TREATMENT ACT REQUIRES AN INTERDEPENDENT AND INTERORGANIZATIONAL MODEL THAT UTILIZES AVAILABLE PSYCHOLOGICAL AND SOCIAL SUPPORT SYSTEMS. CONCEPTUAL GUIDELINES IN ADMINISTERING CHILD ABUSE/NEGLECT PROGRAMS NEED TO INTEGRATE A SYSTEMATIC NETWORK OF HUMAN RESOURCES, DECISION MAKING, AND COMMUNICATION. SINCE COMMUNITIES VARY IN LEVEL OF NEEDS AND RESOURCES, THE MODEL SUGGESTS THAT A GROUP OR INDIVIDUAL COORDINATE THE VARIOUS SERVICES. A COORDINATING SYSTEM THAT IS BOTH HORIZONTAL AND VERTICAL WILL FACILITATE TRANSFER OF RESOURCES, RESPONSIBILITY, AND INTERVENTION WITH FAMILIES AND THUS PROVIDE AN EFFECTIVE COMMUNITY CHILD ABUSE/NEGLECT PROGRAM.

ACCN   000301

353 AUTH   **COHEN, R. E., ADAMS, G., & GOMEZ, A.**
    TITL   THE LACK OF FIT BETWEEN CATEGORICAL FEDERAL FUNDING PATTERNS AND THE COMPREHENSIVE PLANNING NEEDS OF A SPANISH SPEAKING MINORITY POPULATION.
    SRCE   *UNPUBLISHED MANUSCRIPT, HARVARD MEDICAL SCHOOL, DEPARTMENT OF PSYCHIATRY, BOSTON, UNDATED.*
    INDX   SPANISH SURNAMED, HEALTH, HEALTH DELIVERY SYSTEMS, SOCIAL SERVICES, PROFESSIONAL TRAINING, EDUCATION, BILINGUAL-BICULTURAL EDUCATION, PUERTO RICAN-M, REHABILITATION, CUBAN, HOUSING, EMPLOYMENT, SURVEY, POVERTY, FINANCING
    ABST   FINDINGS FROM A STUDY CONDUCTED IN THE SOUTH END OF BOSTON WHERE A LARGE PERCENTAGE OF THE RESIDENTS ARE SPANISH-SPEAKING (SS) INDICATE THAT FEDERAL AND PRIVATE FUNDING FOR SS PROGRAMS IS INADEQUATE TO MEET THIS GROUP'S NEEDS. FEDERAL FUNDING FOR EDUCATION, HEALTH, WELFARE, EMPLOYMENT AND HOUSING FOR ANY GROUP OF RESIDENTS, BUT ESPECIALLY FOR MINORITIES, IS STRUCTURED TO MEET THE CATEGORICAL NEEDS OF EACH OF THESE COMPONENTS BUT WITH LITTLE OR NO COORDINATION BETWEEN THEM. THIS RESULTS IN LACK OF SPECIFIC PROGRAMS FOR THE SS AT THE FEDERAL LEVEL AND LACK OF FEDERAL

FUNDING FOR PRIVATE OR SELF-HELP GROUPS AT THE LOCAL LEVEL. AFTER INTERVIEWING ADMINISTRATORS AND STAFF AT SEVERAL AGENCIES OPERATING UNDER DHEW, REGIONAL OFFICE, NEW ENGLAND STATES, AND GATHERING CLIENT, STAFF AND SERVICES DATA FROM 25 GREATER BOSTON NEIGHBORHOOD HEALTH CENTERS, TWO MAJOR CONCLUSIONS WERE DETERMINED: (1) THERE ARE NO SPECIFIC PROGRAMS FOR SS PEOPLE CURRENTLY FUNDED BY THE FEDERAL GOVERNMENT THROUGH THE REGIONAL OFFICE, ALTHOUGH FEDERAL FUNDS DO GO TO HEALTH CENTERS PROVIDING SERVICES TO SS, TO UNIVERSITIES AND MEDICAL SCHOOLS PROVIDING MINORITY TRAINING PROGRAMS, AND TO OTHER ORGANIZATIONS OR INSTITUTIONS FOR CONSTRUCTION, STAFFING AND TRAINING; AND (2) MOST LOCAL SELF-HELP OR PRIVATE AGENCIES HAVE NEITHER THE PERSONNEL NOR EXPERTISE TO CUT THROUGH THE RED TAPE OF PUTTING TOGETHER A COMPREHENSIVE PROGRAM OR TO DEVELOP GRANTS FOR FUNDING SPECIAL PROGRAMS. RECOMMENDATIONS FOR CORRECTING THESE DISCREPANCIES ARE DISCUSSED.

ACCN   000302

354 AUTH   **COHEN, S. A., & COOPER, T.**
     TITL   SEVEN FALLACIES: READING RETARDATION AND THE URBAN DISADVANTAGED BEGINNING READER.
     SRCE   *READING TEACHER, 1972, 26(1), 38-45.*
     INDX   READING, SPECIAL EDUCATION, TEACHERS, SCHOLASTIC ASPIRATIONS, LEARNING DISABILITIES, PUERTO RICAN-M, CROSS CULTURAL, CULTURAL FACTORS, PERCEPTION, LINGUISTICS, URBAN, REVIEW, CURRICULUM
     ABST   A REVIEW OF THE RESEARCH INDICATES THAT MANY EXCUSES FOR NOT REACHING BLACK AND PUERTO RICAN URBAN POOR ARE FALLACIOUS. SEVEN FALLACIES ARE DISCUSSED: (1) URBAN BLACK CHILDREN TEND TO BE LESS VERBAL THAN MIDDLE-CLASS CHILDREN; (2) LITTLE VERBAL INTERACTION TAKES PLACE BETWEEN THE DISADVANTAGED CHILD AND HIS PARENTS OR OTHER ADULTS; (3) BLACK ENGLISH IS A SUBSTANDARD FORM OF STANDARD ENGLISH; (4) THE MISMATCH BETWEEN BLACK ENGLISH SYNTAX AND STANDARD ENGLISH SYNTAX REQUIRES THE BLACK CHILD TO TRANSLATE WRITTEN STANDARD ENGLISH INTO SPOKEN BLACK ENGLISH; (5) THE DISADVANTAGED CHILD'S DEFICIENT CONCEPTUAL AND USABLE VOCABULARY INTERFERES WITH HIS LEARNING TO READ; (6) IMPROVEMENT OF ORAL LANGUAGE PATTERNS OF DISADVANTAGED CHILDREN WILL HELP THEM READ BETTER; AND (7) POOR ARTICULATION CONTRIBUTES TO AUDITORY DISCRIMINATION DEFICIENCIES, AND THIS REFLECTS IN THE DIFFICULTY OF LEARNING PHONIC SKILLS. 33 REFERENCES. (PASAR ABSTRACT MODIFIED)

ACCN   000303

355 AUTH   **COHEN, S. M., & KAPSIS, R. E.**
     TITL   PARTICIPATION OF BLACKS, PUERTO RICANS, AND WHITES IN VOLUNTARY ASSOCIATIONS: A TEST OF CURRENT THEORIES.
     SRCE   *SOCIAL FORCES, 1978, 56(4), 1053-1071.*
     INDX   ADULTS, ATTITUDES, COMMUNITY INVOLVEMENT, CROSS CULTURAL, CULTURAL FACTORS, EDUCATION, EMPIRICAL, INTERPERSONAL RELATIONS, PUERTO RICAN-M, SES, SEX COMPARISON, NEW YORK, EAST, SURVEY, URBAN, THEORETICAL
     ABST   TO INTERPRET THE RELATIVELY HIGH RATES OF VOLUNTARY ORGANIZATION AMONG BLACKS, THEORISTS HAVE DEVELOPED DEPRIVATION AND NORMATIVE CAUSAL THEORIES. ACCORDING TO THE DEPRIVATION THEORY, A MINORITY GROUP SUBJECTED TO OBJECTIVE CONDITIONS OF DEPRIVATION SHOULD EXHIBIT COMPARABLE LEVELS OF ORGANIZATIONAL INVOLVEMENT BECAUSE OF COMPENSATORY AND ETHNIC COMMUNITY PROCESSES. THE NORMATIVE THEORY STATES THAT DEPRIVED MINORITY GROUP STATUS WILL LEAD TO SOCIAL AND POLITICAL ACTIVISM THROUGH ETHNIC SOLIDARITY ONLY IF THE NORMS OF THE COMMUNITY STRESS SUCH ACTIVISM. THE ORGANIZATIONAL BEHAVIOR OF PUERTO RICANS, BLACK, AND WHITES WAS EXAMINED IN ORDER TO TEST SEVERAL KEY POSTULATES FROM BOTH THE DEPRIVATION AND NORMATIVE THEORIES. DATA WERE COLLECTED BY THE NEW YORK NEIGHBORHOOD STUDY OF THE BUREAU OF APPLIED SOCIAL RESEARCH, COLUMBIA UNIVERSITY, IN 1972. TRAINED INTERVIEWERS EMPLOYED A BLOCK QUOTA SAMPLE DESIGN TO INTERVIEW 1,683 RESIDENTS OF SEVEN NEW YORK NEIGHBORHOODS. RESPONDENTS WERE ASKED TO IDENTIFY THEIR ANCESTRY, AGE, SEX, EDUCATIONAL ATTAINMENT, AND ORGANIZATIONAL AFFILIATIONS. THREE MEASURES OF ETHNIC IDENTIFICATION WERE EMPLOYED IN THE ANALYSIS: ETHNIC ENDOGAMY, INTRA-ETHNIC FRIENDSHIP, AND ETHNIC IN-GROUP SOLIDARITY. REGRESSION COEFFICIENTS WERE CALCULATED FOR MALES AND FEMALES. IN NO GROUP DID ETHNIC IDENTIFICATION APPEAR TO MOBILIZE INDIVIDUALS INTO VOLUNTARY ORGANIZATIONS. AS RESULTS ARE INCOMPATIBLE WITH BOTH THE DEPRIVATION AND NORMATIVE THEORY, FURTHER INQUIRIES INTO THE MECHANISMS WHICH PREDISPOSE A MINORITY POPULATION TO BE MORE INVOLVED IN VOLUNTARY ORGANIZATIONS ARE NEEDED. 24 REFERENCES.

ACCN   002055

356 AUTH   **COLE, D. L., & COLE, S.**
     TITL   COUNTERNORMATIVE BEHAVIOR AND LOCUS OF CONTROL.
     SRCE   *JOURNAL OF SOCIAL PSYCHOLOGY, 1977, 101(1), 21-28.*
     INDX   COLLEGE STUDENTS, CROSS CULTURAL, CULTURAL FACTORS, LOCUS OF CONTROL, SES, FEMALE, MALE, CALIFORNIA, SOUTHWEST, EAST, MEXICAN, MEXICO, EMPIRICAL
     ABST   TWO STUDIES TESTED THE HYPOTHESIS THAT PERSONS TAKING ACTION AIMED AT SELF-IMPROVEMENT, IN CULTURAL CONTEXTS WHERE SUCH ACTIONS ARE COUNTERNORMATIVE,

SHOULD SHOW DIFFERENCES IN LOCUS OF CONTROL WHEN CONTRASTED WITH PERSONS FOR WHOM SUCH ACTIONS ARE NOT COUNTERNORMATIVE. THE FIRST STUDY CONTRASTED LOCUS OF CONTROL SCORES BETWEEN 109 MALE AND FEMALE MEXICAN BUSINESS ADMINISTRATION MAJORS IN A UNIVERSITY IN MEXICO AND 61 AMERICAN MALE AND FEMALE BUSINESS ADMINISTRATION STUDENTS IN A CATHOLIC UNIVERSITY IN CALIFORNIA. THE SECOND CONTRASTED LOCUS OF CONTROL SCORES BETWEEN 67 MALE AND FEMALE AMERICAN LIBERAL ARTS STUDENTS FROM AN ECONOMICALLY DEPRESSED MOUNTAIN REGION OF APPALACHIA WITH 226 SUCH STUDENTS FROM AN ECONOMICALLY ADVANTAGED AREA IN CALIFORNIA. THE INSTRUMENT USED WAS THE LEVENSON IPC SCALES, WHICH PROVIDES THREE SCORES: ONE FOR INTERNAL LOCUS OF CONTROL (I), A SECOND FOR CONTROL BY POWERFUL OTHERS (P), AND A THIRD FOR CONTROL BY FATE OR CHANCE (C). FOR USE WITH THE MEXICAN SUBJECTS, THE TEST INSTRUMENT WAS TRANSLATED INTO SPANISH AND TRANSLATED BACK INTO ENGLISH TO CHECK ON THE ACCURACY OF THE ORIGINAL TRANSLATION. IN BOTH THE MEXICAN AND THE ECONOMICALLY DISADVANTAGED LIBERAL ARTS GROUPS, PURSUIT OF SUCH GOALS WAS MARKEDLY MORE COUNTERNORMATIVE FOR WOMEN. IN EACH STUDY, WOMEN IN THE COUNTERNORMATIVE GROUP SHOWED STRONGER REJECTION OF CONTROL BY POWERFUL OTHERS OR BY FATE OR CHANCE THAN DID SUBJECTS IN CONTEXTS WHEREIN SUCH ACTIONS WERE NOT SO COUNTERNORMATIVE. 18 REFERENCES. (JOURNAL ABSTRACT MODIFIED)

ACCN   002056

357 AUTH   **COLE, D., & COLES, S.**
     TITL   LOCUS OF CONTROL AND CULTURAL CONFORMITY: ON GOING AGAINST THE NORM.
     SRCE   *PERSONALITY AND SOCIAL PSYCHOLOGY BULLETIN, 1974, 1(1), 351-353.*
     INDX   CONFORMITY, COPING MECHANISMS, CULTURAL FACTORS, CROSS CULTURAL, MEXICAN AMERICAN, SELF CONCEPT, PERSONALITY, SOCIALIZATION, EMPIRICAL, ATTRIBUTION THEORY, SEX COMPARISON, COLLEGE STUDENTS, LOCUS OF CONTROL, ROTTER INTERNAL-EXTERNAL SCALE
     ABST   THE ROTTER INTERNAL-EXTERNAL SCALE (I-E) AND THE LEVENSON INTERNAL, POWERFUL OTHERS, AND CHANCE SCALES (IPC) WERE ADMINISTERED TO 235 MEXICAN, 111 CATHOLIC AMERICAN, AND 339 LIBERAL ART MAJOR AMERICAN STUDENTS; IN ADDITION, THE I-E SCALE ALONE WAS ADMINISTERED TO 44 GERMAN STUDENTS. EXCEPT FOR THE U.S. LIBERAL ARTS STUDENTS, THE MAJORITY OF THE SUBJECTS WERE CATHOLIC BUSINESS MAJORS. A COMPARISON OF LOCUS OF CONTROL SCORES ACROSS THESE FOUR SAMPLES DEMONSTRATED SUPPORT FOR THE STUDY'S HYPOTHESIS THAT A SENSE OF INTERNAL CONTROL AND A REJECTION OF EXTERNAL CONTROL ARE GREATER WHEN THE INDI-

VIDUAL ASSUMES COUNTER NORMATIVE BEHAVIOR (IN THIS CASE, AMBITION BEING A DEPARTURE FROM MEXICAN CULTURAL NORMS). THE MOST SIGNIFICANT FINDING WAS THAT MEXICAN FEMALE STUDENTS SHOWED A GREATER DEGREE OF INTERNALITY, INDICATING THE EXTENT TO WHICH THEY ARE OPPOSING THE OVERT CULTURAL NORM IN A MALE-ORIENTED SOCIETY. OVERALL, COUNTER NORMATIVE BEHAVIOR WHICH IS AT A CONSCIOUS LEVEL IS SEEN AS PROVIDING A SENSE OF INTERNAL CONTROL, DEPENDING ON THE EXTENT TO WHICH STATUS AS A COLLEGE STUDENT REPRESENTS A DEPARTURE FROM THE NORMS OF THE SOCIETY. (PASAR ABSTRACT MODIFIED)

ACCN   000304

358 AUTH   **COLE, J., & PILISUK, M.**
     TITL   DIFFERENCES IN THE PROVISION OF MENTAL HEALTH SERVICES BY RACE.
     SRCE   *AMERICAN JOURNAL OF ORTHOPSYCHIATRY, 1976, 46(3), 510-525.*
     INDX   ADULTS, CROSS CULTURAL, DISCRIMINATION, EMPIRICAL, HEALTH DELIVERY SYSTEMS, MALE, MENTAL HEALTH, MEXICAN AMERICAN, PREJUDICE, PSYCHOTHERAPY, SES, SOCIAL SERVICES, SPANISH SURNAMED, STEREOTYPES, FEMALE, SEX COMPARISON
     ABST   DIFFERENCES IN THE PROVISION OF MENTAL HEALTH SERVICES OFFERED TO WHITE AND THIRD WORLD CLIENTS IN A CRISIS CLINIC WERE STUDIED AND COMPARED. HANDWRITTEN RECORDS OF MENTAL HEALTH WORKERS FOR 94 CLIENTS (50 BLACKS, 9 CHICANOS, 32 WHITES, 2 ASIANS, AND 1 ARAB) WERE EXAMINED FOR: (1) DIAGNOSIS; (2) CASE DISPOSITION; (3) MEDICATION; (4) DESCRIPTIVE LABELS; (5) NUMBER OF VISITS AND TERMINATION OF TREATMENT; (6) WORKER'S OPINION OF THE PATIENT; AND (7) CASE MANAGEMENT AND SUPPLEMENTAL SERVICES. CLEAR AND CONSISTENT DIFFERENCES WERE FOUND. WHITE MEN IN THIS SAMPLE WERE MORE LIKELY TO RECEIVE PSYCHOTHERAPY, TO BE TREATED WITHOUT MEDICATION, TO RECEIVE LONG-TERM THERAPY, TO TERMINATE TREATMENT THEMSELVES, AND TO BE DESCRIBED AS BRIGHT OR VERBAL. THIRD WORLD MEN WERE MORE LIKELY TO BE DESCRIBED AS HOSTILE OR PARANOID. SUPPORTIVE SERVICES (E.G., OUTREACH AND FOLLOWUP) WHILE UNCOMMON, WERE GIVEN AS FREQUENTLY TO THIRD WORLD CLIENTS AS TO WHITES. THE PATTERNS FOR WOMEN DID NOT SUPPORT THE HYPOTHESIS OF RACIAL DIFFERENCES. SUGGESTED REASONS FOR THIS DISCREPANCY INCLUDE INADEQUATE UNDERSTANDING OF THE PROBLEMS OF RACE ON THE PART OF THE STAFF AND THE FACT THAT DISTURBED MINORITY MALES ARE PERCEIVED AS DANGEROUS AND NOT SUITED TO TRADITIONAL THERAPIES. 18 REFERENCES. (NCMHI ABSTRACT MODIFIED)

ACCN   002057

359 AUTH   **COMITE ESTATAL DE CALIFORNIA DE LA**

COMISION DE DERECHOS CIVILES DE LOS ESTADOS UNIDOS.

TITL LAS ESCUELAS DE GUADALUPE: UN LEGADO DE OPRESION EDUCACIONAL. (THE SCHOOLS OF GUADALUPE: A LEGACY OF EDUCATIONAL OPPRESSION.)

SRCE *WASHINGTON, D.C.: U.S. COMMISSION ON CIVIL RIGHTS, FEBRUARY 1974. (SPANISH)*

INDX EDUCATION, DISCRIMINATION, PREJUDICE, MEXICAN AMERICAN, CASE STUDY, EMPIRICAL, TEACHERS, CHILDREN, SPECIAL EDUCATION, COMMUNITY INVOLVEMENT, POLICY, CALIFORNIA, SOUTHWEST

ABST THE SCHOOL DISTRICT AND COMMUNITY OF "GUADALUPE" (A PSEUDONYM) WERE ACCUSED BY THE CALIFORNIA COMMITTEE OF THE UNITED STATES CIVIL RIGHTS COMMISSION OF GROSS VIOLATIONS OF THE EDUCATIONAL AND CIVIL RIGHTS OF THE MEXICAN AMERICAN COMMUNITY. THE CALIFORNIA STATE COMMITTEE STARTED ITS INVESTIGATIONS DURING THE SPRING OF 1972 AS A RESULT OF ALLEGATIONS BROUGHT TO THE COMMITTEE BY MEXICAN AMERICAN RESIDENTS. THE MOST IMPORTANT ALLEGATIONS WERE: (1) INFERIOR QUALITY OF THE EDUCATION; (2) FAILURE IN HIRING MEXICAN AMERICAN BILINGUAL AND BICULTURAL PROFESSIONAL STAFF; (3) EXCESSIVE CORPORAL PUNISHMENT; (4) FAILURE TO INCLUDE MEXICAN AMERICAN PARENTS IN THE ACTIVITIES OF THE SCHOOL; AND (5) PERSECUTION OF THE INDIVIDUALS THAT COMPLAINED OF THE DISTRICT'S EDUCATIONAL PRACTICES. THE COMMISSION'S MAJOR RECOMMENDATIONS TO THE SCHOOL DISTRICT WERE: (1) THE UNITED STATES OFFICE OF EDUCATION SHOULD INITIATE A REVIEW OF THE DISTRICT'S EDUCATIONAL PRACTICES AS THEY RELATE TO MEXICAN AMERICAN STUDENTS; (2) MORE BILINGUAL, BICULTURAL MEXICAN AMERICANS SHOULD BE HIRED; (3) SCHOOL BOARDS SHOULD PROMULGATE THE POLICY FORBIDDING THE USE OF CORPORAL PUNISHMENT; AND (4) THE UNITED STATES DEPARTMENT OF JUSTICE SHOULD INVESTIGATE A PATTERN OF CIVIL RIGHTS VIOLATIONS TO TAKE NECESSARY ACTION TO INSURE THAT THESE RIGHTS ARE RESTORED. THIS REPORT WAS PREPARED BY THE STATE COMMITTEE TO BE SUBMITTED TO THE UNITED STATES CIVIL RIGHTS COMMISSION.

ACCN 000305

360 AUTH **CONCHA, P., GARCIA, L., & PEREZ, A.**

TITL COOPERATION VERSUS COMPETITION: A COMPARISON OF ANGLO-AMERICAN AND CUBAN-AMERICAN YOUNGSTERS IN MIAMI.

SRCE *THE JOURNAL OF SOCIAL PSYCHOLOGY, 1975, 95(SECOND HALF-APRIL), 273-274.*

INDX CUBAN, COOPERATION, COMPETITION, ADOLESCENTS, CHILDREN, EMPIRICAL, ACCULTURATION, FLORIDA, SOUTH

ABST STUDIES ON COOPERATION AND COMPETITION OF SUBCULTURES, WHILE FOCUSING ON EDUCATIONAL AND SOCIAL INFLUENCES, HAVE NEGLECTED TO ASK IF THE DIFFERENCES MAY BE DUE TO AGE. A RANDOM SAMPLE OF 96 STUDENTS REPRESENTING THREE AGE LEVELS WERE SELECTED FROM SIX MIAMI SCHOOLS. TWO MADSEN COOPERATION BOARDS WERE USED TO TEST GROUP DIFFERENCES BETWEEN COOPERATION AND COMPETITION. ANALYSIS OF VARIANCE FOR REPEATED MEASURES SHOWED A SIGNIFICANT EFFECT FOR ETHNICITY. AS AGE INCREASED SO DID THE COOPERATIVE BEHAVIOR FOR BOTH NATIONALITIES. THUS, AS CUBAN CHILDREN BECOME MORE ACCULTURATED IN AMERICAN SOCIETY THEY TEND TO DEMONSTRATE GREATER COOPERATION. 2 REFERENCES.

ACCN 000306

361 AUTH **CONRY-OSEGUERA, P.**

TITL BEYOND THE IQ TESTS: PROBLEMS IN ALTERNATIVE TESTING PROCEDURES WITH CHICANO CHILDREN.

SRCE *THRESHOLDS, 1976, 2(2), 22-32.*

INDX INTELLIGENCE TESTING, SPECIAL EDUCATION, CULTURAL FACTORS, CASE STUDY, REVIEW, BILINGUAL-BICULTURAL PERSONNEL, MEXICAN AMERICAN, CHILDREN, BILINGUALISM

ABST EDUCATORS AND PSYCHOLOGISTS IN DEVELOPING ALTERNATIVES TO PREVIOUSLY USED STANDARDIZED TESTS TO ASSESS INTELLECTUAL ABILITIES OF MINORITY CHILDREN FAIL TO RECOGNIZE THAT THESE NEW TESTS ARE NOT "CULTURE FREE." ALTERNATIVE METHODS STILL HAVE THE FOLLOWING BIAS: (1) NONVERBAL TESTS REFLECT PERCEPTUAL SKILLS AND EXPERIENCES THAT ARE ACQUIRED IN A SPECIFIC CULTURAL ENVIRONMENT; (2) TRANSLATING STANDARDIZED TESTS INTO SPANISH ASSUMES SPANISH-SPEAKING CHILDREN TO BE A HOMOGENEOUS GROUP WITH THE SAME SPEECH PATTERNS AND VOCABULARY; (3) BILINGUAL CHILDREN COMMUNICATING IN A MIXTURE OF BOTH SPANISH AND ENGLISH CANNOT BE ASSESSED ADEQUATELY WITH A TEST THAT IS ALL ENGLISH OR ALL SPANISH; AND (4) ANY TEST MEASURING COGNITIVE ABILITY IS IN ITSELF BIASED SINCE COGNITION IS CULTURALLY RELATIVE. UNTIL INSTRUMENTS ARE DEVELOPED THAT ARE SENSITIVE TO CULTURALLY DIFFERENT CHILDREN, EXTREME CAUTION MUST BE USED IN PLACING CHILDREN IN A PROGRAM FOR THE MENTALLY RETARDED. 24 REFERENCES.

ACCN 000307

362 AUTH **COOK, J. M., & ARTHUR, G.**

TITL INTELLIGENCE RATINGS FOR 97 MEXICAN CHILDREN IN ST. PAUL, MINN.

SRCE *JOURNAL OF THE INTERNATIONAL COUNCIL FOR EXCEPTIONAL CHILDREN, 1951, 18(1), 14-15.*

INDX INTELLIGENCE TESTING, MEXICAN AMERICAN, CHILDREN, EMPIRICAL, STANFORD-BINET INTELLIGENCE TEST, MINNESOTA, MIDWEST

ABST AN INVESTIGATION TO DETERMINE THE DIFFERENT RATINGS BETWEEN A VERBAL SCALE AND A NONVERBAL SCALE FOR MEXICAN SCHOOL CHILDREN IS PRESENTED. NINETY-SEVEN SUBJECTS RANGING FROM GRADES ONE TO NINE WERE EXAMINED WITH BOTH THE STANFORD-BINET (SB) AND THE POINT SCALE PERFORMANCE TEST (PSPT). THE PSPT INDI-

CATED A MEAN IQ OF 101.06 (SD 17.35), AND THE SB REVEALED A MEAN IQ OF 83.77 (SD 14.14). THE DIFFERENCE BETWEEN THE VERBAL AND NONVERBAL RATINGS WAS SIGNIFICANT. IT IS CONCLUDED THAT EDUCATIONAL AND VOCATIONAL GUIDANCE FOR MEXICAN SCHOOL CHILDREN SHOULD BE BASED UPON RESULTS FROM NONVERBAL INTELLIGENCE SCALES AS WELL AS ON THE MORE COMMONLY USED VERBAL SCALES. IN MANY CASES, THE PSPT REVEALS A HIGH DEGREE OF POTENTIAL ABILITY THAT IS NOT INDICATED BY EITHER THE SB OR GROUP TESTS. 2 REFERENCES.

ACCN   000308

363 AUTH   **COOKSEY, R. C.**
    TITL   PARENTAL ROLE PERCEPTION BY THE YOUNG MEXICAN AMERICAN CHILD (DOCTORAL DISSERTATION, UNIVERSITY OF TEXAS, AUSTIN, 1974).
    SRCE   *DISSERTATION ABSTRACTS INTERNATIONAL, 1974, 35(5), 2754A. (UNIVERSITY MICROFILMS NO.74-24,842.)*
    INDX   FAMILY ROLES, MEXICAN AMERICAN, CHILDREN, ATTITUDES, EMPIRICAL, RESEARCH METHODOLOGY, TEXAS, SOUTHWEST
    ABST   IN ORDER FOR TEACHERS TO PREPARE READING MATERIALS THAT WILL SUPPORT THE PERSONALITY DEVELOPMENT AND ACCULTURATION OF YOUNG MEXICAN AMERICAN CHILDREN, INFORMATION ABOUT CHILDREN'S PERCEPTION OF PARENTAL ROLES, RESPONSIBILITIES, ATTRIBUTES, AND PRIVILEGES IS NEEDED. THIS STUDY TESTS THE EFFECTIVENESS OF ONE INSTRUMENT, A CHILDREN'S INTERVIEW SCHEDULE COMPOSED OF 55 PARTIALLY OPEN-ENDED QUESTIONS, IN OBTAINING INFORMATION FROM 60 FIVE YEAR-OLD MEXICAN AMERICAN CHILDREN ABOUT PARENTAL ROLES IN THEIR SOCIETY. IT IS CONCLUDED: (1) THAT THE INSTRUMENT DOES ELICIT RESPONSES FROM CHILDREN AT THE RATE OF 89 OR GREATER IN 7 OUT OF THE 9 RESPONSE AREAS; (2) THAT THE RESPONSES ARE INTERPRETABLE IN TERMS OF PARENTAL TASKS AND QUALITIES; AND (3) THAT PARENTAL ROLES AS PERCEIVED BY THE CHILDREN CAN BE DESCRIBED FROM THE DATA OBTAINED. THE FINDINGS INDICATE THAT OF THE SEVERAL INDEPENDENT VARIABLES, ONLY SEX AND MIGRANT STATUS SHOWED SIGNIFICANT GROUP DIFFERENCES IN THE CHILDREN'S PERCEPTION OF THEIR PARENTS. 157 REFERENCES.

ACCN   000309

364 AUTH   **COONEY, R. S.**
    TITL   CHANGING LABOR FORCE PARTICIPATION OF MEXICAN AMERICAN WIVES: A COMPARISON WITH ANGLOS AND BLACKS.
    SRCE   *SOCIAL SCIENCE QUARTERLY, 1975, 56(2), 252-261.*
    INDX   LABOR FORCE, FEMALE, CROSS CULTURAL, MEXICAN AMERICAN, MARRIAGE, SES, CENSUS, DEMOGRAPHIC, CULTURAL FACTORS, EMPIRICAL, ADULTS, SOUTHWEST
    ABST   THIS STUDY EXAMINES WHETHER THE DIFFERENCES BETWEEN THE LABOR FORCE PARTICI-

PATION RATES OF MEXICAN AMERICAN MARRIED WOMEN, AGED 15-54, IN THE SOUTHWEST IN 1960 AND 1970 AND COMPARABLE ANGLO AND BLACK FEMALES CAN BE ACCOUNTED FOR BY DIFFERENCES IN SOCIOECONOMIC FACTORS. AFTER CONTROLLING FOR SES, THE DIFFERENCE BETWEEN MEXICAN AMERICAN AND ANGLO PARTICIPATION RATES WAS REDUCED BY 79 PERCENT IN 1960 AND 95 PERCENT IN 1970. FOR THE MEXICAN AMERICAN-BLACK COMPARISONS, 35 AND 65 PERCENT OF THESE DIFFERENCES IN 1960 AND 1970, RESPECTIVELY, CAN BE ACCOUNTED FOR BY SOCIOECONOMIC FACTORS. THESE RESULTS NOT ONLY SUBSTANTIATE THE IMPORTANCE OF SOCIOECONOMIC FACTORS FOR EXPLAINING INTERETHNIC, ESPECIALLY MEXICAN AMERICAN AND ANGLO, VARIATIONS IN FEMALE LABOR FORCE PARTICIPATION, BUT ALSO ARE CONSISTENT WITH THE HYPOTHESIS THAT THE IMPORTANCE OF FAMILISM FOR THE MEXICAN AMERICAN POPULATION HAS DECLINED. 17 REFERENCES. (AUTHOR ABSTRACT MODIFIED)

ACCN   000310

365 AUTH   **COONEY, R. S.**
    TITL   THE MEXICAN AMERICAN FEMALE IN THE LABOR FORCE.
    SRCE   *UNPUBLISHED MANUSCRIPT, FORDHAM UNIVERSITY, 1975.*
    INDX   MEXICAN AMERICAN, FEMALE, ADULTS, EMPIRICAL, LABOR FORCE, CROSS CULTURAL, CULTURE, EMPLOYMENT, CENSUS, SEX ROLES, SOUTHWEST, REPRESENTATION
    ABST   THIS STUDY INVESTIGATES THE SIMILARITIES AND DIFFERENCES IN LABOR MARKET PARTICIPATION AMONG ANGLOS, BLACKS, AND MEXICAN AMERICANS IN THE SOUTHWEST. U.S. CENSUS DATA FOR THE YEARS 1960 AND 1970 WERE USED, AND FEMALES AGE 18 TO 65, MARRIED WITH A SPOUSE PRESENT, WERE SELECTED. AGE AND CHILDREN PRESENT RATHER THAN SOCIOECONOMIC STATUS WAS USED AS AN INDEPENDENT FACTOR IN ASSESSING ETHNIC DIFFERENCES IN THE PARTICIPATION RATES. THE RESULTS REVEAL THAT THE PRESENCE OF PRESCHOOL CHILDREN IS MORE OF A DETERRENT FOR ANGLOS WORKING THAN FOR MEXICAN AMERICANS AND BLACKS. OVERALL, THE FINDINGS INDICATE THE FOLLOWING TRENDS: (1) ALL THREE GROUPS INCREASED IN CLERICAL-SALES EMPLOYMENT; (2) MEXICAN AMERICANS HAD THE GREATEST OVERALL INCREASE IN LABOR PARTICIPATION; AND (3) COMPARED TO THE OTHER GROUPS, BLACKS INCREASED PROPORTIONATELY IN THEIR REPRESENTATION IN WHITE-COLLAR OCCUPATIONS. 10 REFERENCES.

ACCN   000311

366 AUTH   **COPPOLILLO, H. P.**
    TITL   THE ABUSED AND NEGLECTED CHILD: A SUMMARY OF A PANEL DISCUSSION.
    SRCE   *IN E. R. PADILLA & A. M. PADILLA (EDS.), TRANSCULTURAL PSYCHIATRY: AN HISPANIC PERSPECTIVE (MONOGRAPH NO. 4). LOS ANGELES: UNIVERSITY OF CALIFORNIA, SPANISH*

SPEAKING MENTAL HEALTH RESEARCH CENTER, 1977, PP. 105-108.

INDX CHILD ABUSE, CORRECTIONS, CHILDREN, PSYCHOTHERAPY, LEGISLATION, ESSAY, PRIMARY PREVENTION

ABST THE FOLLOWING ISSUES SURROUNDING CHILD ABUSE AND NEGLECT ARE DISCUSSED BRIEFLY: (1) FACTORS INFLUENCING DETECTION; (2) REPORTING AND TREATMENT; AND (3) MEASURES FOR PREVENTING AND TREATING CHILD ABUSE AS A CULTURAL AND SOCIAL ILLNESS. FOUR MAJOR STEPS IN PROGRAM PLANNING AND DEVELOPMENT ARE PROPOSED, INCLUDING ADEQUATE LEGISLATION, CHILD AND FAMILY SUPPORT SYSTEMS, RECRUITMENT AND COMPENSATION OF WELL TRAINED PERSONNEL, AND THE DEVELOPMENT OF MODELS FROM EXISTING. EFFECTIVE PROGRAMS. ALL SEGMENTS OF SOCIETY MUST MAKE A CONCERTED EFFORT TO PREVENT CHILD ABUSE AND NEGLECT SINCE CHILDREN REPRESENT A FUTURE RESOURCE FOR ALL SOCIETY.

ACCN 000312

367 AUTH **CORDASCO, F.**

TITL EDUCATIONAL ENLIGHTENMENT OUT OF TEXAS: TOWARD BILINGUALISM.

SRCE *IN J. C. STONE & D. P. DENEVI (EDS.), TEACHING MULTICULTURAL POPULATIONS: FIVE HERITAGES. NEW YORK: VAN NOSTRAND, 1971, PP. 19-23.*

INDX BILINGUALISM, BILINGUAL-BICULTURAL EDUCATION, BILINGUAL-BICULTURAL PERSONNEL, POVERTY, MEXICAN AMERICAN, PUERTO RICAN-M, EDUCATION, LEGISLATION, ESSAY

ABST IN THIS INTRODUCTION TO STONE AND DENEVI'S BOOK, THE HISTORY OF THE LAW PASSED BY THE 90TH CONGRESS WHICH PROVIDES FUNDING FOR BILINGUAL EDUCATION (TITLE VII OF THE ELEMENTARY AND SECONDARY EDUCATION ACT) IS DESCRIBED. TWO POINTS ARE EMPHASIZED: (1) THAT THE LAW IN ITS ORIGINAL FORM WAS INITIATED BY A TEXAS SENATOR WHO PROPOSED THE ESTABLISHMENT OF BILINGUAL PROGRAMS TO CHILDREN WHOSE PARENTS WERE BORN IN MEXICO OR PUERTO RICO OR WHO HAD SPANISH SURNAMES; AND (2) THAT THE LAW PROVIDES AID TO PROGRAMS BENEFITING LOW INCOME NON-ENGLISH-SPEAKING CHILDREN. THIS LAW HAS BEEN A POWERFUL CHANGE AGENT IN BRINGING ABOUT THE RECOGNITION OF THE SCHOOL AS A PLACE WHICH SERVES THE CHILDREN OF AN OPEN SOCIETY AND AS SUCH MUST BUILD ON THE CULTURAL STRENGTHS, ANCESTRAL PRIDE AND NATIVE LANGUAGE THOSE CHILDREN BRING TO THE CLASSROOM. 1 REFERENCE.

ACCN 000313

368 AUTH **CORDASCO, F.**

TITL THE EQUALITY OF EDUCATIONAL OPPORTUNITY: A BIBLIOGRAPHY OF SELECTED REFERENCES.

SRCE *TOTOWA, N.J.: LITTLEFIELD, ADAMS AND CO., 1973.*

INDX EDUCATION, EQUAL OPPORTUNITY, PUERTO RICAN-M, ACCULTURATION, BILINGUAL-BICULTURAL EDUCATION, URBAN, SES, LEGISLATION, CROSS CULTURAL, BIBLIOGRAPHY, MIGRANTS, INDIGENOUS POPULATIONS

ABST FROM THE VAST LITERATURE SPAWNED IN THE 1960'S AND EARLY 1970'S DEALING WITH AMERICAN SCHOOLS AND THE CHILDREN OF THE POOR, THIS BIBLIOGRAPHY COLLECTS THOSE TITLES MOST RELEVANT TO THESE ISSUES: (1) MINORITY CHILDREN (BLACKS, PUERTO RICANS, MEXICAN AMERICANS, INDIANS, THE APPALACHIAN POOR, ETHNICS, AND MIGRANTS); (2) DESEGREGATION OF URBAN SCHOOLS; (3) MULTIFARIOUS EDUCATIONAL EXPERIMENTS AND FAILING INNOVATIVE DESIGN; (4) INCREASED COMMUNITY INVOLVEMENT; AND (5) ALIENATION AND DISAFFECTION. THE BIBLIOGRAPHY'S ENTRIES ARE ARRANGED UNDER FIVE MAIN CATEGORIES: (1) ROLE OF THE SCHOOL; (2) DROPOUTS AND DELINQUENCY; (3) CHARACTERISTICS OF THE DISADVANTAGED STUDENT; (4) TEACHERS AND TEACHER EDUCATION; AND (5) PROGRAMS AND MATERIALS. THE AUTHOR HAS ANNOTATED SOME OF THE TITLES AND PROVIDED A PREFACE AND BIBLIOGRAPHICAL ESSAY WHICH SKETCHES THE SOCIOECONOMIC AND POLITICAL CONTEXTS WITHIN WHICH EDUCATIONAL HISTORY HAS TAKEN PLACE. A PROFILE OF THE PUERTO RICAN COMMUNITY'S DIFFICULTIES IN SEEKING EDUCATIONAL OPPORTUNITY AS WELL AS A SUMMARY OF THE 1969 REPORT OF THE URBAN EDUCATION TASK FORCE ARE ALSO INCLUDED. THESE MATERIALS ARE INTENDED AS A GUIDE TO THE LITERATURE ON THE EQUALITY OF EDUCATIONAL OPPORTUNITY AS IT HAS DEVELOPED OVER THE LAST DECADE. (AUTHOR SUMMARY MODIFIED)

ACCN 000314

369 AUTH **CORDASCO, F.**

TITL THE PUERTO RICAN CHILD IN THE AMERICAN SCHOOL.

SRCE *JOURNAL OF NEGRO EDUCATION, 1967, 36(2), 181-186. (REPRINTED IN J. C. STONE & D. P. DENEVI (EDS.), TEACHING MULTICULTURAL POPULATIONS: FIVE HERITAGES. NEW YORK: VAN NOSTRAND, 1971, PP. 141-147.)*

INDX PUERTO RICAN-M, MIGRATION, EDUCATION, EMPIRICAL, SCHOLASTIC ACHIEVEMENT, CHILDREN, COMMUNITY INVOLVEMENT, ACCULTURATION, ETHNIC IDENTITY, NEW YORK, EAST

ABST THE PUERTO RICAN MIGRATION PRESENTS UNIQUE PROBLEMS FOR THE AMERICAN SCHOOLS. WITH THE INCREASING MIGRATION AND THE RECURRENT PATTERN OF GHETTOIZATION OF NEW ARRIVALS, THE MIGRANT CHILD, NON-ENGLISH-SPEAKING AND NURTURED BY A DIFFERENT CULTURE, POSES A NEW CHALLENGE. THE PUERTO RICAN CHILD IS ASKED TO ADAPT TO A "CULTURAL AMBIANCE" WHICH IS UNFAMILIAR AND HE REMAINS FURTHER BURDENED BY ALL THE NEGATIVE PRESSURES OF A GHETTO MILIEU. IN 1960 MORE THAN 52.9 OF PUERTO RICANS IN NEW YORK CITY 25 YEARS AND OLDER HAD LESS THAN AN EIGHTH-GRADE EDUCATION. THERE IS EVIDENCE THAT PUERTO RICANS

MORE THAN ANY OTHER GROUP ARE STILL SEVERELY HANDICAPPED IN ACHIEVING AN EDUCATION IN NEW YORK CITY PUBLIC SCHOOLS. AS A REMEDIAL MEASURE, AN EDUCATIONAL PROGRAM TO MEET THE NEEDS OF PUERTO RICAN CHILDREN HAS PROVIDED IMPROVEMENT OF EDUCATIONAL OPPORTUNITIES AND IN TEACHING STRATEGIES. THE PROBLEM WHICH IS MOST IMPORTANT TO PUERTO RICAN CHILDREN IS THE PROCESS OF ACCULTURATION AND ITS SUBSEQUENT EFFECT ON THEIR IDENTITY, LANGUAGE, AND CULTURE. 31 REFERENCES.

ACCN   000316

370   AUTH   **CORDASCO, F.**
      TITL   SPANISH SPEAKING CHILDREN IN AMERICAN SCHOOLS.
      SRCE   *INTERNATIONAL MIGRATION REVIEW, 1975, 9(3), 379-382.*
      INDX   BILINGUAL-BICULTURAL EDUCATION, CHILDREN, ECONOMIC FACTORS, EDUCATION, ESSAY, PUERTO RICAN-M, EAST, NEW YORK, PROGRAM EVALUATION
      ABST   A BRIEF DESCRIPTION IS PRESENTED OF A FEDERALLY DECREED (1974) PROGRAM FOR THE NON-ENGLISH-SPEAKING CHILDREN IN NEW YORK CITY—A PROGRAM WHICH ACKNOWLEDGES THE UNMET NEEDS OF SPANISH-SPEAKING CHILDREN NOT ONLY IN NEW YORK CITY BUT IN ALL AMERICAN SCHOOLS. THE PROGRAM'S MANDATE TO "ESTABLISH A MAJOR NEW PROGRAM TO IMPROVE THE EDUCATION OF ALL SPANISH-SPEAKING PUPILS" ECHOES THE U.S. SENATE SELECT COMMITTEE'S 1972 REPORT WHICH CONCLUDED THAT "SOME OF OUR MOST DRAMATIC, WHOLESALE FAILURES OF THE PUBLIC SCHOOL SYSTEMS OCCUR AMONG MEMBERS OF LANGUAGE MINORITIES." THE NEW YORK PROGRAM, ADMINISTERED BY THE BOARD'S OFFICE OF BILINGUAL EDUCATION, AND PIONEERED BY P.S.#25, DISTRICT 7—THE FIRST COMPLETELY BILINGUAL SCHOOL IN THE HISTORY OF NEW YORK CITY, AND A MODEL FOR THE PROPOSED CITYWIDE PROGRAM—IS SUPPORTED ENTHUSIASTICALLY BY THE PUERTO RICAN COMMUNITY. HISTORICALLY, HOWEVER, IT IS ONLY THE LATEST IN A NUMBER OF SUCH PROPOSALS EXTENDING BACK TO 1947—EACH OF WHICH WAS HAILED AS THE WAY TO AMELIORATE THE PROBLEMS OF PUERTO RICAN PUPILS ENROLLED IN NEW YORK CITY SCHOOLS. BECAUSE OF THEIR FAILURE TO IMPROVE CONDITIONS FOR PUERTO RICAN STUDENTS, THE FEDERAL COURT CONSENT DECREE CAN ONLY BE MONITORED, BOTH IN AND OUTSIDE NEW YORK CITY, WITH CAUTIOUS OPTIMISM. 5 REFERENCES.

ACCN   002329

371   AUTH   **CORDASCO, F. M., & COVELLO, L.**
      TITL   STUDIES OF PUERTO RICAN CHILDREN IN AMERICAN SCHOOLS: A PRELIMINARY BIBLIOGRAPHY.
      SRCE   *JOURNAL OF HUMAN RELATIONS, 1968, 16, 264-285. (ERIC DOCUMENT REPRODUCTION SERVICE NO. ED021910)*

      INDX   EDUCATION, SCHOLASTIC ACHIEVEMENT, INSTRUCTIONAL TECHNIQUES, CURRICULUM, CROSS CULTURAL, ACHIEVEMENT TESTING, BILINGUALISM, BILINGUAL-BICULTURAL EDUCATION, BILINGUAL-BICULTURAL PERSONNEL, ADMINISTRATORS, BILINGUALISM, PUERTO RICAN-M, BIBLIOGRAPHY, EARLY CHILDHOOD EDUCATION, CHILDREN
      ABST   THIS PRELIMINARY BIBLIOGRAPHY IS A HANDY LIST OF STUDIES ON PUERTO RICAN CHILDREN AND THEIR EXPERIENCES IN AMERICAN MAINLAND SCHOOLS. ALSO INCLUDED ARE (1) A BIBLIOGRAPHIC NOTE ON THOSE TITLES WHICH CONSTITUTE A WORKING LIST FROM THE OVERALL STUDY OF THE MIGRATION AND EXPERIENCE OF PUERTO RICANS ON THE AMERICAN MAINLAND, AND (2) A SHORT LIST OF SUGGESTED SOURCES FOR THE STUDY OF THE "DISADVANTAGED CHILD." SINCE THE BIBLIOGRAPHY IS ESSENTIALLY LIMITED TO THE PUERTO RICAN EXPERIENCE IN MAINLAND SCHOOLS, NEITHER ANNOTATION NOR SUBJECT CAPTIONING APPEARED TO BE PRACTICAL OR NECESSARY. OTHER SOURCES OF INFORMATION CONCERNING PUERTO RICANS ARE CITED.

ACCN   000317

372   AUTH   **CORDOVA, R. R.**
      TITL   ASSESSING ATTITUDES AND PERFORMANCES OF STUDENT TEACHERS IN MEXICAN-AMERICAN SCHOOLS (DOCTORAL DISSERTATION, UNIVERSITY OF CALIFORNIA, LOS ANGELES, 1970).
      SRCE   *DISSERTATION ABSTRACTS INTERNATIONAL, 1971, 32(1), 279A. (UNIVERSITY MICROFILMS NO. 71-16,303.)*
      INDX   MEXICAN AMERICAN, CHILDREN, EMPIRICAL, TEACHERS, ATTITUDES, CALIFORNIA, SOUTHWEST
      ABST   THE PURPOSE OF THIS STUDY WAS TO MEASURE THE ATTITUDES OF STUDENT TEACHERS TOWARD CULTURALLY DIFFERENT CHILDREN IN THE ELEMENTARY SCHOOLS. HYPOTHESIZED WAS THAT: (1) TEACHERS' ATTITUDE TOWARD CHILDREN IN GENERAL AND THEIR ATTITUDES TOWARD CULTURALLY DIFFERENT CHILDREN ARE RELATED; AND (2) TEACHER ETHNIC BACKGROUND AND ATTITUDES ARE RELATED. THESE ATTITUDES WERE MEASURED BY TWO INSTRUMENTS: THE MINNESOTA TEACHER ATTITUDE INVENTORY (MTAI), AND THE CULTURAL ATTITUDE INVENTORY (CAI). THE RELATIONSHIP BETWEEN PERFORMANCE AND ATTITUDES WAS ASSESSED THROUGH THE USE OF OBSERVED MICRO-LESSONS. RESULTS REVEAL THAT SCORES ON THE MTAI AND THE CAI WERE SIGNIFICANTLY RELATED, AS WERE ETHNIC BACKGROUND AND CAI SCORES. ANGLO STUDENT TEACHERS CONSISTENTLY SCORED HIGHER THAN MEXICAN AMERICAN AND SPANISH SURNAME TEACHERS. THE STRONGEST RELATIONSHIP FOUND WAS THAT BETWEEN GROUP AND MICROTEACHING, AND GROUP AND THE SCORES ON THE MTAI. TEACHERS WHO VOLUNTEERED TO TEACH IN A CULTURALLY DIFFERENT SCHOOL SCORED HIGHER ON THE MTAI AND THE MI-

CRO-TEACHING THAN THOSE WHO HAD BEEN ASSIGNED TO TEACH THERE. RESULTS SUGGEST THAT TEACHERS WHO VOLUNTEER TO TEACH IN A MEXICAN AMERICAN SCHOOL GENERALLY TEND TO BE WARMER, TO HAVE BETTER STUDENT-TEACHER RAPPORT, AND TO BE MORE SUCCESSFUL IN TEACHING MEXICAN AMERICAN CHILDREN. 39 REFERENCES.

ACCN   000318

373 AUTH   **CORNEJO, R. J.**
    TITL   THE ACQUISITION OF LEXICON IN THE SPEECH OF BILINGUAL CHILDREN.
    SRCE   *IN P. R. TURNER (ED.), BILINGUALISM IN THE SOUTHWEST. TUCSON, ARIZ.: THE UNIVERSITY OF ARIZONA PRESS, 1973, PP. 67-93.*
    INDX   BILINGUALISM, CHILDREN, PHONOLOGY, SYNTAX, GRAMMAR, EMPIRICAL, LINGUISTICS, BILINGUAL-BICULTURAL EDUCATION, SEMANTICS, SPANISH SURNAMED, TEXAS, SOUTHWEST
    ABST   THE SPEECH OF SPANISH-ENGLISH BILINGUAL 5 YEAR-OLD CHILDREN IN TEXAS WAS STUDIED TO DETERMINE THE LEXICON OF THESE CHILDREN BEFORE THEY ENTER FIRST GRADE. AFTER RECORDING THE SPEECH OF 100 CHILDREN IN INTERVIEW, DIALOGUE, AND CONVERSATION SETTINGS, 24 CHILDREN WERE SELECTED FOR ANALYSIS OF THEIR SYNTAX, PHONOLOGY, LEXICON, AND SEMANTICS. ANALYSIS SHOWS THE FOLLOWING LANGUAGE CHARACTERISTICS: (1) ENGLISH IS THE DOMINANT LANGUAGE; (2) SPANISH IS USED AT HOME, BUT SPANISH STRUCTURE AND PHONOLOGY ARE INFLUENCED BY ENGLISH; (3) PARENTS AND CHILDREN SHOW A SYSTEMATIC PATTERN IN THEIR LANGUAGE DOMAIN; (4) THERE IS SIGNIFICANT INTERFERENCE FROM ENGLISH TO SPANISH; (5) INTERFERENCE FROM SPANISH TO ENGLISH IS HIGHLY SIGNIFICANT AT THE PHONOLOGICAL LEVEL, MINOR AT THE LEXICAL AND GRAMMATICAL LEVELS; (6) THERE IS A BELOW AGE LEVEL PATTERN IN THE FLUENCY AND ARTICULATION OF COMMON SPANISH WORDS; AND (7) THE HOMES IN RURAL AREAS SEEM TO BE MORE "LITERATE" AND FAMILIAR WITH TRADITIONAL CHILDREN'S LITERATURE THAN THOSE IN URBAN AREAS. RECOMMENDATIONS FOR CURRICULUM DEVELOPMENT, TEACHER TRAINING, USE OF MATERIALS AND NEEDED RESEARCH IN BILINGUAL EDUCATION ARE MADE. 10 REFERENCES.
    ACCN   000319

374 AUTH   **CORNETT, J. D., AINSWORTH, L., & ASKINS, B.**
    TITL   EFFECT OF AN INTERVENTION PROGRAM ON "HIGH RISK" SPANISH AMERICAN CHILDREN.
    SRCE   *JOURNAL OF EDUCATIONAL RESEARCH, 1974, 67(8), 342-343.*
    INDX   LINGUISTIC COMPETENCE, SELF CONCEPT, SPANISH SURNAMED, CHILDREN, BILINGUAL, PEABODY PICTURE-VOCABULARY TEST, BILINGUAL-BICULTURAL EDUCATION, EMPIRICAL, IMPAIRMENT
    ABST   MENTAL ABILITY, LANGUAGE DEVELOPMENT (ENGLISH AND SPANISH), AND SELF-IMAGE CHANGES WERE STUDIED AS EFFECTS OF AN EARLY INTERVENTION PROGRAM FOR PRE-

SCHOOL CHILDREN. THE SUBJECTS WERE FIFTY BILINGUAL CHILDREN (AGES 3 TO 5) FROM DISADVANTAGED BACKGROUNDS. SUBJECTS EXHIBITED A NUMBER OF ADDITIONAL HANDICAPPING FACTORS. DIFFERENCES BETWEEN GROUPS (N = 30 FOR EXPERIMENTAL AND N = 20 FOR CONTROL) WERE ANALYZED BY MEANS OF A COVARIANCE TECHNIQUE WHICH USED PRETEST SCORES AS COVARIATES. RESULTS INDICATED THAT INTERVENTION SUBJECTS MADE SIGNIFICANTLY GREATER GAINS IN MENTAL ABILITY AND IN ENGLISH AND SPANISH LANGUAGE ABILITY. IN ADDITION, INTERVENTION SUBJECTS DEMONSTRATED A POSITIVE GROWTH IN SELF-IMAGE. 5 REFERENCES. (JOURNAL ABSTRACT MODIFIED)

ACCN   000320

375 AUTH   **CORTES, C. E.**
    TITL   NEW APPROACHES TO BILINGUAL, BICULTURAL EDUCATION: CONCEPTS AND STRATEGIES FOR TEACHING THE MEXICAN AMERICAN EXPERIENCE (NO. 7).
    SRCE   *AUSTIN, TEXAS: THE DISSEMINATION CENTER FOR BILINGUAL BICULTURAL EDUCATION, 1974.*
    INDX   BILINGUAL-BICULTURAL EDUCATION, SPANISH SURNAMED, CHILDREN, CULTURAL PLURALISM, INSTRUCTIONAL TECHNIQUES, CURRICULUM
    ABST   SEVENTH AND LAST IN A SERIES OF TEACHER-TRAINING MANUALS FOR IMPLEMENTATION OF CULTURAL DEMOCRACY IN AMERICAN SCHOOLS, THIS COMPONENT FOCUSES ON THE TEACHING OF THE MEXICAN AMERICAN EXPERIENCE. SIX TRADITIONAL FRAMES OF REFERENCE ARE IDENTIFIED AS HINDERING THE STUDY OF THE CHICANO EXPERIENCE: (1) THE IDEA THAT U.S. HISTORY IS A UNIDIRECTIONAL EAST-TO-WEST PHENOMENON; (2) THE LABELING OF THE CHICANO EXPERIENCE AS "JUST LIKE" THAT OF OTHER IMMIGRANT GROUPS; (3) THE VIEW OF THE CHICANO EXPERIENCE AS HOMOGENOUS; (4) THE ASSUMPTION THAT MEXICAN AMERICANS ARE A SOCIAL PROBLEM; (5) THE CONCEPT OF THE "AWAKENING MEXICAN AMERICAN" ARISING FROM A CENTURY LONG SIESTA; AND (6) THE ATTEMPT TO EXPLAIN THE CHICANO EXPERIENCE BY PRESENTING A FEW CHICANO HEROES OR SUCCESS STORIES. ALTERNATIVES FOR EACH OF THESE ERRONEOUS FRAMES OF REFERENCE ARE DISCUSSED UNDER SIX RESPECTIVE EXPLORATORY CONCEPTS: (1) GREATER AMERICA CONCEPT; (2) COMPARATIVE ETHNIC EXPERIENCES; (3) CHICANO DIVERSITY; (4) SOCIETY AS A PROBLEM; (5) HISTORY OF ACTIVITY; AND (6) THE CHICANO PEOPLE. THE TEACHING STRATEGIES RECOMMENDED FOR IMPLEMENTING THESE CONCEPTS INCLUDE THE SELECTIVE USE OF MEXICAN AMERICAN SUPPLEMENTARY MATERIALS, THE CONSTANT USE OF LOCAL COMMUNITY RESOURCES, AND THE PARTICIPATION IN THE CHICANO EXPERIENCE. THE EXPLORATORY CONCEPTS PROVIDE A MEANS FOR ORGANIZING KNOWLEDGE IN WAYS WHICH SHED NEW LIGHT ON THE CHICANO AND HELP ERADICATE COMMON MISCONCEPTIONS. THE TEACHING

STRATEGIES SHOULD BE USEFUL IN OPERATIONALIZING THE STUDY OF THE MEXICAN AMERICAN IN A MANNER WHICH CAN BOTH STIMULATE STUDENTS AND DEVELOP IN THEM A GREATER UNDERSTANDING OF THE CHICANO EXPERIENCE. PROMOTING CULTURAL DEMOCRACY IS THE MORAL AND INTELLECTURAL OBLIGATION OF ALL TEACHERS. (AUTHOR SUMMARY MODIFIED)

ACCN   000321

376 AUTH **CORTES, C. E.**
     TITL REVISING THE "ALL AMERICAN SOUL COURSE: A BICULTURAL AVENUE TO EDUCATIONAL REFORM.
     SRCE *IN A. CASTANEDA, M. RAMIREZ III., C. E. CORTES & M. BARRERA (EDS.), MEXICAN AMERICANS AND EDUCATIONAL CHANGE. NEW YORK: ARNO PRESS, 1974, PP. 314-339.*
     INDX MEXICAN AMERICAN, BILINGUAL-BICULTURAL EDUCATION, CULTURAL PLURALISM, HISTORY, EDUCATION, PREJUDICE, STEREOTYPES, EDUCATIONAL MATERIALS, ESSAY
     ABST CRITICISM IS DIRECTED AGAINST THE U.S. EDUCATIONAL SYSTEM'S CONTINUING FAILURE TO ERADICATE, OR EVEN QUESTION, THE PREJUDICE TO WHICH MEXICAN AMERICANS ARE SUBJECTED IN SCHOOLS. PARTICULAR ATTENTION IS GIVEN TO THE ANTI-HISPANIC THEMES IN THE MEDIA AND LITERATURE, INCLUDING ADVERTISING, TELEVISION, MOVIES, AS WELL AS TEXTBOOKS. THE STEADY BOMBARDMENT OF THESE THEMES HAS LED TO DAMAGING STEREOTYPES OF MEXICAN AMERICANS, AND THEREBY CONTRIBUTED TO MEXICAN AMERICANS' EDUCATIONAL DIFFICULTIES. TO PROMOTE A POSITIVE FORCE FOR REDUCING SUCH PREJUDICE AND FOR CREATING BETTER INTER-ETHNIC UNDERSTANDING, SEVERAL BICULTURAL REFORMS ARE PROPOSED: (1) CRITICAL BICULTURAL ANALYSIS OF TEXTBOOKS; (2) SELECTION OF BICULTURAL MATERIALS FOR COURSE BALANCE; AND (3) DEVELOPMENT OF BICULTURAL MATERIALS THROUGH THE USE OF COMMUNITY RESOURCES. SUGGESTIONS FOR OPERATIONALIZING THESE REFORMS ARE OFFERED. 22 REFERENCES.

ACCN   000322

377 AUTH **CORTESE, M.**
     TITL BEHAVIOR MODIFICATION PRINCIPLES APPLIED TO THE TREATMENT OF HYSTERIAL SPASMODIC TORTICOLLIS.
     SRCE *UNPUBLISHED MANUSCRIPT, UNIVERSITY OF CALIFORNIA AT LOS ANGELES, SPRING 1976.*
     INDX BEHAVIOR MODIFICATION, MEXICAN, CASE STUDY, EMPIRICAL, MENTAL HEALTH, ADULTS, CULTURAL FACTORS, FEMALE, CALIFORNIA, SOUTHWEST
     ABST BEHAVIOR MODIFICATION PRINCIPLES IN CONJUNCTION WITH CHEMOTHERAPY AND GROUP THERAPY WERE USED IN TREATING A CASE OF HYSTERICAL SPASMODIC TORTICOLLIS IN A 47 YEAR-OLD MEXICAN FEMALE PATIENT IN AN OUTPATIENT MENTAL HEALTH SETTING. A TREATMENT PROGRAM WAS DESIGNED USING A BEHAVIORAL PERSPECTIVE WHICH IN-

CLUDED EXERCISES IN THE PATIENT'S HOME, FAMILY INVOLVEMENT IN THE EXERCISES, AND REINFORCEMENT FOR THE PATIENT. DATA COLLECTED REVEALED GRADUAL IMPROVEMENT. IT WAS INFERRED, THOUGH SEVERE METHODOLOGICAL LIMITATIONS WERE RECOGNIZED, THAT THE ADDITION OF THE BEHAVIORALLY-BASED TREATMENT WAS EFFECTIVE IN TREATING WHAT IS GENERALLY CONSIDERED A REFRACTORY SYMPTOM. 11 REFERENCES. (AUTHOR ABSTRACT MODIFIED)

ACCN   000323

378 AUTH **CORTESE, M.**
     TITL INTERVENTION RESEARCH WITH HISPANIC AMERICANS: A REVIEW.
     SRCE *HISPANIC JOURNAL OF BEHAVIORAL SCIENCES, 1979, 1(1), 4-20.*
     INDX SPANISH SURNAMED, ETHNIC IDENTITY, RESEARCH METHODOLOGY, REVIEW, PSYCHOTHERAPY, BEHAVIOR MODIFICATION, PROGRAM EVALUATION, CULTURAL FACTORS, CROSS CULTURAL, PSYCHOTHERAPISTS
     ABST THIS EVALUATION OF 15 PUBLISHED STUDIES OF PSYCHOTHERAPY AND BEHAVIOR MODIFICATION RESEARCH ON HISPANICS EXAMINES THE CONTENTION THAT INTERVENTION THERAPIES SHOULD BE MODIFIED TO ACCOMODATE CRITICAL SOCIAL, CULTURAL, OR ETHNIC VARIABLES. THREE EVALUATION CRITERIA ARE USED: (1) THE MANNER OF CLASSIFYING THE SUBJECTS BY ETHNICITY; (2) THE STAGE OF INTERVENTION; AND (3) THE EXPERIMENTAL DESIGN. SOME OF THE STUDIES SUGGEST THAT METHODOLOGIES WHICH DEEMPHASIZE SELF-DISCLOSURE OR CLIENT INTERACTION ARE MORE EFFECTIVE WITH HISPANICS; OTHERS CHALLENGE THE NOTION THAT MATCHING THE CLIENT AND COUNSELOR BY ETHNICITY IS ALWAYS PREFERRED BY THE HISPANIC CLIENT. HOWEVER, IT IS ARGUED IN THIS REVIEW THAT NO FIRM CONCLUSIONS CAN BE DERIVED BECAUSE OF THE PAUCITY OF RESEARCH AND THE FAILURE OF RESEARCHERS TO PROPERLY DEFINE THE VARIABLE OF ETHNICITY. MORE RESEARCH IS URGED, AND SIX RECOMMENDATIONS FOR THE ACCURATE DETERMINATION OF CLIENT ETHNICITY ARE OFFERED. 44 REFERENCES.

ACCN   001760

379 AUTH **CORTESE, M., & SMYTH, P.**
     TITL A NOTE ON THE TRANSLATION TO SPANISH OF A MEASURE OF ACCULTURATION.
     SRCE *HISPANIC JOURNAL OF BEHAVIORAL SCIENCES, 1979, 1(1), 65-68.*
     INDX EMPIRICAL, ACCULTURATION, RESEARCH METHODOLOGY, BILINGUAL, ETHNIC IDENTITY, TEST VALIDITY, TEST RELIABILITY, MEXICAN AMERICAN, SEMANTICS
     ABST BACK TRANSLATION, DECENTERING, AND STATISTICAL TECHNIQUES WERE USED TO PRODUCE A SPANISH-LANGUAGE VERSION OF A SEMANTIC DIFFERENTIAL PAPER-AND-PENCIL TEST THAT MEASURES LEVEL OF ACCULTURATION ON A MEXICAN-TO-AMERICAN CONTINUUM. DEVELOPED BY OLMEDO (1978), THE TEST MEASURES THE AFFECTIVE MEANING OF

FOUR CONCEPTS (I.E., MOTHER, FATHER, MALE, FEMALE) ON 15 PAIRS OF BIPOLAR ADJECTIVES. THE INSTRUMENT ALSO USES A SOCIOCULTURAL APPROACH BY COLLECTING DEMOGRAPHIC AND PERSONAL DATA RELEVANT TO LEVEL OF ACCULTURATION. THE TEST WAS ADMINISTERED TWICE, ONCE IN ENGLISH AND ONCE IN SPANISH, TO 21 BILINGUAL COLLEGE STUDENTS SO THAT THE LINGUISTIC EQUIVALENCE OF THE TWO VERSIONS COULD BE ASCERTAINED. THE TEST-RETEST AND ENGLISH-SPANISH TEST CORRELATIONS WERE WELL WITHIN ACCEPTABLE LIMITS, THEREBY AFFIRMING THE EQUIVALENCE OF THE ENGLISH AND SPANISH VERSIONS. THIS SUCCESSFUL TRANSLATION SHOULD BE PARTICULARLY USEFUL TO RESEARCHERS WHO WISH TO INCLUDE LEVEL OF ACCULTURATION IN THEIR EXPERIMENTAL DESIGNS AND WHO WISH TO INCLUDE SUBJECTS WHO ARE MONOLINGUAL IN SPANISH OR ENGLISH. 3 REFERENCES. (JOURNAL ABSTRACT MODIFIED)

ACCN   001761

380   AUTH   **COSTA, A. L.**
TITL   THE EFFECTS OF DEPRIVATION ON CHILDREN'S LANGUAGE AND THOUGHT PROCESSES WITH SOME IMPLICATIONS FOR CURRICULA.
SRCE   *UNPUBLISHED MANUSCRIPT, SACRAMENTO COUNTY SCHOOLS, UNDATED.*
INDX   CHILDREN, MEXICAN AMERICAN, ESSAY, CURRICULUM, COGNITIVE DEVELOPMENT, LANGUAGE LEARNING, ENVIRONMENTAL FACTORS, THEORETICAL
ABST   ENVIRONMENTAL FACTORS INFLUENCING CHILDREN'S LANGUAGE AND COGNITIVE LEARNING (SUCH AS PARENTAL PRESENCE OR ABSENCE, CROWDING, TEMPORAL AND STIMULUS DEPRIVATION) ARE EXPLORED BY MEANS OF PIAGETIAN LEARNING AND DEVELOPMENT THEORY. GUIDELINES FOR CURRICULUM DEVELOPMENT, ENRICHMENT EXPERIENCES AND REMEDIAL LEARNING. EDUCATIONAL GOALS FOR DEPRIVED LEARNERS ALSO DERIVED FROM PIAGETIAN THEORY ARE: (1) TO DEVELOP A MORE CONCEPTUAL, EXTENDED, MEANINGFUL LANGUAGE; (2) TO DEVELOP THINKING PROCESSES FOR PROBLEM SOLVING, GENERALIZING, CLASSIFYING AND CATEGORIZING; (3) TO SPEAK CLEARLY IN ACCEPTABLE COLLOQUIAL LANGUAGE; (4) TO ENJOY LEARNING; (5) TO LISTEN AND ATTEND PRODUCTIVELY; AND (6) TO VIEW THE ADULT AS A SOURCE OF INFORMATION. QUESTIONS REGARDING USE OF THE PROPOSED MODEL IN PRESENT SCHOOL SYSTEMS ARE DISCUSSED. 22 REFERENCES.

ACCN   000324

381   AUTH   **COSTELLO, R. M.**
TITL   "CHICANA LIBERATION" AND THE MEXICAN AMERICAN MARRIAGE.
SRCE   *PSYCHIATRIC ANNALS, 1977, 7(12), 64-73.*
INDX   TEXAS, SOUTHWEST, SEX ROLES, FAMILY STRUCTURE, MENTAL HEALTH, CHICANO MOVEMENT, ESSAY, CULTURAL CHANGE, FEMALE, CURANDERISMO, MARRIAGE, CASE STUDY, FAMILY THERAPY, CHILDREN, CUL-

TURAL FACTORS, MEXICAN AMERICAN, BILINGUAL-BICULTURAL PERSONNEL, MENTAL HEALTH PROFESSION, THERAPEUTIC COMMUNITY, ATTITUDES, FAMILY ROLES, MARITAL STABILITY
ABST   IF MENTAL HEALTH PROFESSIONALS ARE TO INTERVENE IN SITUATIONS OF MARITAL DISCORD, AN UNDERSTANDING OF THE SOCIOCULTURAL CONTEXT IS ESSENTIAL. IN THE PAST, MEXICAN AMERICAN WOMEN EXPERIENCING MARITAL DISSATISFACTION EITHER ENDURED THEIR SITUATION OR ATTEMPTED TO INFLUENCE THEIR HUSBANDS' BEHAVIOR THROUGH CURANDERISMO. TODAY, THE CHICANA LIBERATION MOVEMENT, THE WELFARE SYSTEM, INCREASED EMPLOYMENT OPPORTUNITIES, AND CONTACT WITH NON-HISPANIC MENTAL HEALTH PROFESSIONALS HAVE ENCOURAGED MORE WOMEN TO SEEK DIVORCE AND FREEDOM. THESE WOMEN, HOWEVER, FACE OPPOSITION FROM THE CHICANO FAMILY NETWORK AND THE TRADITIONAL VALUES ESPOUSED BY THE COMMUNITY AND MEXICAN AMERICAN HEALTH CLINIC STAFF. THREE CASE STUDIES DESCRIBE THE TENSION PRODUCED BY CONFLICTING CULTURAL VALUES, AS WELL AS HOW CLIENTS' BEHAVIOR CAN BE A SENSITIVE BAROMETER OF THE INTENSITY OF DEMANDS MADE BY THE SYSTEM. IT IS SUGGESTED THAT COMMUNITY MENTAL HEALTH PROFESSIONALS RECOGNIZE THEIR ROLE IN THE DEVELOPMENT OF A MORE HUMANE SOCIETY. IN PARTICULAR, THEY SHOULD INVOLVE CHILDREN IN THEIR PARENTS' THERAPY IN ORDER TO PREVENT FUTURE MENTAL HEALTH PROBLEMS AND THEREBY MAINTAIN POSITIVE CULTURAL CHANGE.

ACCN   002059

382   AUTH   **COSTELLO, R. M., VARGAS, L. A., BAILLARGEON, J. G., & HERNANDEZ, M. C.**
TITL   MEXICAN AMERICAN BEHAVIORAL ADJUSTMENTS IN AN ANGLO HOSPITAL.
SRCE   *PSYCHIATRIC ANNALS, 1977, 7(12), 82-85.*
INDX   ALCOHOLISM, COPING MECHANISMS, CROSS CULTURAL, CULTURAL FACTORS, DEPRESSION, EMPIRICAL, ENVIRONMENTAL FACTORS, HEALTH, MENTAL HEALTH, MEXICAN AMERICAN, PROGRAM EVALUATION, MALE, SOUTHWEST, TEXAS, EMPIRICAL, THERAPEUTIC COMMUNITY, MILITARY
ABST   IN A SAN ANTONIO VETERAN'S ADMINISTRATION HOSPITAL ALCOHOL TREATMENT UNIT WITH A MIXED PATIENT POPULATION (ANGLOS, 60 ; MEXICAN AMERICANS, 40), THE EFFECTS OF ETHNICITY ON SOCIAL ADJUSTMENT WERE EXAMINED. THE INSTRUMENT WAS A STANDARD BEHAVIOR RATING SCALE DEVELOPED TO ORGANIZE THE PERCEPTIONS OF 7 STAFF MEMBERS CONCERNING PATIENT BEHAVIOR. BEHAVIOR PROFILES WERE FACTOR ANALYZED ACCORDING TO THE DIMENSIONS OF COMMUNICATION AND MOOD. INITIAL PROFILES ON THE TWO GROUPS REVEALED THAT THE MEXICAN AMERICANS WERE MORE POORLY EDUCATED, HAD MORE UNEMPLOYMENT, A LOWER MILITARY RANK, A LOWER AVERAGE AGE WHEN FIRST HOSPITALIZED, AND WERE

ALSO MORE FREQUENTLY LIVING WITH AN-OTHER PERSON BEFORE ADMISSION. DESPITE THIS PREPONDERANCE OF NEGATIVE VARI-ABLES, THE MEXICAN AMERICAN PATIENTS WERE RATED EQUAL TO THE ANGLOS ON THE COMMUNICATION DIMENSION AND RATED SU-PERIOR TO THE ANGLOS ON THE MOOD SCALE. TO DISCOVER POSSIBLE CAUSES FOR THIS FINDING, THE BIOGRAPHICAL DATA WERE REANALYZED AND PRODUCED ONE KEY VARI-ABLE: LIVING STATUS BEFORE ADMISSION. THIS SINGLE FACTOR (BY ITSELF AND IN INTER-ACTION WITH ETHNICITY) IS BELIEVED TO BE CRITICAL IN EXPLAINING BOTH DIMENSIONS OF WARD BEHAVIOR. THE GROUP OF PATIENTS WHO WERE FOUND TO BE THE MOST CONVER-SATIONAL AND IN THE MOST EUPHORIC MOOD WERE THOSE LIVING WITH OTHERS BEFORE HOSPITALIZATION. THE GROUP FOUND TO BE LEAST CONVERSATIONAL AND MOST GLOOMY WERE ANGLOS LIVING ALONE. 1 REFERENCE.

ACCN   002060

383 AUTH **COTA-ROBLES DE SUAREZ, C.**
     TITL SKIN COLOR AS A FACTOR OF RACIAL IDENTI-FICATION AND PREFERENCE OF YOUNG CHI-CANO CHILDREN.
     SRCE *AZTLAN, 1971, 2(1), 107-150.*
     INDX ETHNIC IDENTITY, MEXICAN AMERICAN, SELF CONCEPT, PREJUDICE, CHILDREN, DISCRIMI-NATION, CULTURAL FACTORS, EDUCATION, EMPIRICAL, CALIFORNIA, SOUTHWEST
     ABST AN INVESTIGATION ON THE RESPONSES TO RACIAL AWARENESS AND ATTITUDES OF THE CHICANO CHILD, AGES 4 TO 5, IS PRESENTED. THE SUBJECTS WERE 28 LOW-INCOME CHIL-DREN IN TWO HEADSTART CLASSES. ALL SUB-JECTS WERE GIVEN THE CHOICE TEST, WHICH CONSISTS OF TWO PICTURES, ONE DEPICTING AN ANGLO AND ANOTHER A CHICANO. THE CHILDREN WERE TO GIVE THEIR PREFERENCE FOR A FRIEND AND A PLAYMATE. IN ADDITION, THE COLORING TEST, WHICH CONSISTS OF AN UNCOLORED COPY OF A BOY (IF THE SUBJECT WAS A GIRL THE DRAWING GIVEN WOULD ALSO BE A GIRL), WAS ALSO GIVEN. THE TASK WAS TO COLOR THE FACE USING THE SAME COLOR AS THEIR SKIN COLOR AND, ON A SEC-OND DRAWING, TO COLOR THE FACE WITH WHAT THEY LIKE BOYS AND GIRLS TO BE. RE-SULTS SHOW THAT 75 PERCENT OF THE CHIL-DREN IN CLASS A AND 50 PERCENT IN CLASS B IDENTIFIED THEIR SKIN COLOR, YET 70 PER-CENT IN BOTH CLASSES DID NOT SHOW A PREFERENCE FOR THE COLOR BROWN. AL-THOUGH THE CHILDREN ACCURATELY IDENTI-FIED THE COLORS OF THE CRAYONS USED, THEY OVERWHELMINGLY CHOSE BIZARRE COLORS AS SKIN COLOR PREFERENCES. THEIR REFUSAL TO CHOOSE AN APPROPRIATE COLOR FOR THEMSELVES OR AS SKIN PREFERENCES IS INDICATIVE OF EMOTIONAL ANXIETY AND CONFLICT. WHEN THE CHILD REJECTS THE DARK COLOR, HE KNOWS THAT HE MUST BE IDENTIFIED WITH THAT WHICH HE REJECTS AND THEREFORE IS IN CONFLICT. THE WHITE RACISM AND ETHNOCENTRISM IN OUR SOCI-ETY HAS MANY IMPLICATIONS FOR THE EDU-

CATOR. THE EDUCATOR MUST DEVELOP A PROGRAM THAT WILL PRESENT CHICANO LAN-GUAGE AND CULTURE TO THE CHICANO CHILD IN A POSITIVE MANNER. THIS CAN ONLY BE AC-COMPLISHED BY OFFERING THE CHICANO CHILD A PHYSICAL ENVIRONMENT AND EMO-TIONAL CLIMATE THAT IS CONDUCIVE TO MEANINGFUL LEARNING EXPERIENCES. 86 REFERENCES.

ACCN   000325

384 AUTH **COUNCIL ON INTERRACIAL BOOKS FOR CHILDREN.**
     TITL FACT SHEETS ON INSTITUTIONAL RACISM.
     SRCE *NEW YORK: COUNCIL ON INTERRACIAL BOOKS FOR CHILDREN, 1978. (AVAILABLE FROM FOUNDATION FOR CHANGE, 1841 BROADWAY (60TH ST), NEW YORK, N.Y., 10023.)*
     INDX DISCRIMINATION, PREJUDICE, ECONOMIC FACTORS, SES, POVERTY, HEALTH DELIVERY SYSTEMS, MASS MEDIA, HOUSING, URBAN, EMPLOYMENT, LABOR FORCE, DEMOGRAPHIC, REPRESENTATION, EQUAL OPPORTUNITY, RE-VIEW, EDUCATION, CULTURAL PLURALISM
     ABST THIS 22-PAGE BOOKLET PRESENTS STATISTI-CAL EVIDENCE OF INSTITUTIONAL RACISM IN THE UNITED STATES AND IDENTIFIES THE ECO-NOMIC BENEFITS DERIVED BY THE WHITE POPULATION FROM THE SUBORDINATION, EX-CLUSION, AND EXPLOITATION OF NON-WHITE GROUPS. INFORMATION, INCLUDING ELEVEN TABLES, IS DRAWN FROM CURRENT MAGA-ZINES, JOURNALS, NEWSPAPERS, AND GOV-ERNMENT REPORTS. WHITES OVERWHELM-INGLY CONTROL AMERICAN ECONOMY THROUGH THE OWNERSHIP OF CORPORA-TIONS, BUSINESSES, LAND, BANKS, AND THE INSURANCE INDUSTRY AS WELL AS THROUGH THE CONTROL OF LABOR UNIONS AND THE STOCK EXCHANGE. IN CONTRAST, THE BLACKS, NATIVE AMERICANS, PERSONS OF SPANISH ORIGIN, AND OTHER MINORITIES IN THE U.S. LIVE IN POVERTY. THESE GROUPS ARE EX-PLOITED THROUGH LOWER WAGES, HIGHER PRICES, HIGHER RENTS, LESS DESIRABLE CREDIT TERMS, SUBSTANDARD HOUSING, AND HAZARDOUS WORKING CONDITIONS. AL-THOUGH MINORITIES REPRESENT ABOUT 20 OF THE U.S. POPULATION, THEY ACCOUNT FOR 11 OF THE EMPLOYED AND 24 OF THE UNEMPLOYED LABOR FORCE. THE U.S. COM-MISSION ON CIVIL RIGHTS FOUND THAT MI-NORITIES ARE SYSTEMATICALLY EXCLUDED FROM SUBURBAN AREAS AND ISOLATED WITHIN DECAYING INNER CITIES. IN MOST LARGE CIT-IES, WHITE STUDENTS ARE OUTNUMBERED BY RACIAL-ETHNIC MINORITIES; NEVERTHELESS, THE PREPONDERANT MAJORITY OF HIGH LEVEL ADMINISTRATORS AND TEACHERS IN THESE CITIES ARE WHITE. SIMILAR FINDINGS OBTAIN IN THE AREAS OF HEALTH, GOVERNMENT, AND THE MEDIA. ALTHOUGH NO EXPLICIT RECOM-MENDATIONS ARE MADE, IT IS STATED THAT THE CLEAR IDENTIFICATION OF ALL ASPECTS OF WHITE CONTROL AND MINORITY OPPRES-SION IS A NECESSARY STEP IN WEAKENING THE POWER OF RACISM.

ACCN   000491

385 AUTH **COUNTY OF LOS ANGELES, DEPARTMENT OF HEALTH SERVICES, MENTAL HEALTH SERVICES.**

TITL PATIENT AND SERVICE STATISTICS (REPORT NO. 10).

SRCE *LOS ANGELES: COUNTY OF LOS ANGELES, DEPARTMENT OF HEALTH SERVICES, JANUARY 1973.*

INDX MENTAL HEALTH, PROGRAM EVALUATION, HEALTH DELIVERY SYSTEMS, REHABILITATION, CALIFORNIA, SOUTHWEST, DEMOGRAPHIC, SURVEY, EMPIRICAL

ABST PATIENT AND SERVICE STATISTICS REPORTS HAVE BEEN THE MENTAL HEALTH SERVICES MAJOR TOOL FOR MAINTAINING AN OVERVIEW OF THE DIVERSE SERVICES DELIVERED AND THE CHARACTERISTICS OF THE PATIENTS TO WHOM THE SERVICES ARE DELIVERED. THIS REPORT COMPILES DATA FROM 113 COUNTY REPORTING UNITS OVER THE FISCAL YEAR 1971-72, WHICH RECEIVED STATE AND COUNTY FUNDING FOR SHORT-DOYLE SERVICES. AS THIS REPORT WAS WRITTEN BEFORE AND DURING THE ORGANIZATION OF THE NEW DEPARTMENT OF HEALTH SERVICES SOME OF THE REFERENCES AND STATEMENTS ARE NOT COMPLETELY UPDATED. POPULATION AND MENTAL HEALTH REGION CHARACTERISTICS ANALYZED INCLUDE THE FOLLOWING: SEX, AGE, RACE, EDUCATION, MARITAL STATUS, DIAGNOSIS, BIRTH AND DEATH RATES, SUICIDE AND ALCOHOLISM RATES, AND ADULT AND JUVENILE DRUG RATES. INPATIENT AND OUTPATIENT RATES BY DISTRICT AND COST ARE ANALYZED ALONG WITH SEVERAL OTHER VARIABLES. PROJECTED PROBLEM AREAS AND REQUIRED SERVICES ARE ALSO PRESENTED FOR THE ENTIRE COUNTY AND BY SEPARATE DISTRICTS.

ACCN 000326

386 AUTH **COUNTY OF LOS ANGELES, DEPARTMENT OF HEALTH SERVICES, MENTAL HEALTH SERVICES.**

TITL 1973-1974 PATIENT AND SERVICES STATISTICS (REPORT NO. 11).

SRCE *LOS ANGELES: COUNTY OF LOS ANGELES, DEPARTMENT OF HEALTH SERVICES, SEPTEMBER 1975.*

INDX HEALTH DELIVERY SYSTEMS, MENTAL HEALTH, REHABILITATION, PROGRAM EVALUATION, DEMOGRAPHIC, CALIFORNIA, SOUTHWEST

ABST INFORMATION ON CLIENT CHARACTERISTICS AND TYPES OF MANDATED MENTAL HEALTH (SHORT-DOYLE ACT) SERVICES PROVIDED TO CLIENTS ADMITTED AND DISCHARGED DURING FISCAL YEAR 1973-74 IN LOS ANGELES COUNTY ARE REPORTED. DATA ARE BASED ON INFORMATION CONTAINED IN STANDARD ADMISSION AND DISCHARGE DOCUMENTS SUBMITTED BY 140 COUNTY REPORTING UNITS. THE VARIABLES INCLUDED FOR ANALYSIS ARE AGE, FAMILY MONTHLY INCOME, SEX, NUMBER OF PERSONS DEPENDENT ON INCOME, ETHNIC ORIGIN, MARITAL STATUS, SOURCE OF REFERRAL, PROBLEM AREA, LEGAL STATUS AT

ENTRY AND EXIT, NUMBER AND TYPE OF SERVICE, FINAL PRIMARY DIAGNOSIS, AND REFERRAL OUT RECOMMENDATION. THESE PATIENT AND SERVICE STATISTICS ARE INTENDED TO AID IN PROGRAM EVALUATION AND PLANNING OF SERVICES.

ACCN 000327

387 AUTH **COX, B. G., RAMIREZ, M., III, HEROLD, P. L., & CASTANEDA, A.**

TITL NEW APPROACHES TO BILINGUAL, BICULTURAL EDUCATION: SELF-ASSESSMENT UNITS (NO. 8).

SRCE *AUSTIN, TEXAS: THE DISSEMINATION CENTER FOR BILINGUAL BICULTURAL EDUCATION, 1974.*

INDX CULTURAL PLURALISM, BILINGUAL-BICULTURAL EDUCATION, SPANISH SURNAMED, CHILDREN, EDUCATIONAL MATERIALS, CURRICULUM, EDUCATION, FIELD DEPENDENCE-INDEPENDENCE

ABST AS PART OF A SEVEN COMPONENT SERIES OF TEACHER-TRAINING MATERIALS DEVELOPED UNDER AN ELEMENTARY AND SECONDARY EDUCATION ACT (E.S.E.A.) TITLE VII GRANT FOR BILINGUAL-BICULTURAL PROJECTS, THIS COMPONENT CONTAINS 21 SELF-ASSESSMENT UNITS COVERING A WIDE RANGE OF TOPICS INCLUDING: (1) A NEW PHILOSOPHY OF EDUCATION; (2) MEXICAN AMERICAN VALUES AND CULTURALLY DEMOCRATIC EDUCATIONAL ENVIRONMENTS; (3) INTRODUCTION TO COGNITIVE STYLES; (4) FIELD SENSITIVITY AND FIELD DEPENDENCE IN CHILDREN; (5) FIELD SENSITIVE AND FIELD INDEPENDENT TEACHING STRATEGIES; (6) DEVELOPING COGNITIVE FLEXIBILITY; AND (7) CONCEPTS AND STRATEGIES FOR TEACHING THE MEXICAN AMERICAN EXPERIENCE.

ACCN 000328

388 AUTH **CRANSTON, A., KENNEDY, E., & MONTOYA, R.**

TITL BILINGUAL HEALTH EDUCATION AND SERVICES AMENDMENTS TO THE PUBLIC HEALTH SERVICE ACT. SENATE BILL S. 3280.

SRCE *CONGRESSIONAL RECORD, PROCEEDINGS AND DEBATES OF THE 93RD CONGRESS, SECOND SESSION, MAY 29, 1974, 120(75), 1-6.*

INDX BILINGUAL-BICULTURAL PERSONNEL, HEALTH, PROFESSIONAL TRAINING, HIGHER EDUCATION, MENTAL HEALTH PROFESSION, RESOURCE UTILIZATION, SPANISH SURNAMED, HEALTH EDUCATION, REPRESENTATION, LEGISLATION, ESSAY, COMMUNITY INVOLVEMENT

ABST SENATE BILL S.3543 WAS DESIGNED TO AMEND PUBLIC HEALTH SERVICE ACT S.3280, WHICH WOULD INCLUDE THE TRAINING OF BILINGUAL PERSONS IN THE MENTAL HEALTH PROFESSIONS AND THE ESTABLISHMENT OF BILINGUAL-BICULTURAL COMMUNITY HEALTH, MENTAL HEALTH AND MIGRANT HEALTH CENTERS. THE PROPOSED CHANGES WERE SUBMITTED BY SENATORS CRANSTON, KENNEDY, AND MONTOYA TO MORE ADEQUATELY MEET THE NEEDS OF MINORITY COMMUNITIES. EXAMPLES OF TYPICAL HEALTH PROBLEMS ENCOUNTERED BY THE NON-ENGLISH-SPEAKING PERSON WITH RESPECT TO THE PRESENT SERVICES AVAILABLE AND THE LACK OF BILIN-

GUAL-BICULTURAL TRAINED MENTAL HEALTH PERSONNEL ARE REPORTED. IT IS CONCLUDED THAT THE NEEDS OF THOSE WITH LIMITED ENGLISH-SPEAKING ABILITY CAN ONLY BE MET BY TRAINING BILINGUAL PERSONS IN HEALTH AREAS AND BY ESTABLISHING CULTURALLY SENSITIVE HEALTH CENTERS.

ACCN   000329

389   AUTH   **CRAPANZANO, V., & GARRISON, V. (EDS.)**
TITL   CASE STUDIES IN SPIRIT POSSESSION.
SRCE   *NEW YORK: JOHN WILEY AND SONS, 1977.*
INDX   ESPIRITISMO, PUERTO RICAN-I, FOLK MEDICINE, MENTAL HEALTH, CROSS CULTURAL, CASE STUDY, CURANDERISMO, SOUTH AMERICA, INDIGENOUS POPULATIONS, CULTURE, BOOK
ABST   THIS VOLUME CONTAINS TEN DETAILED INDIVIDUAL CASE HISTORIES OF SPIRIT POSSESSION. WRITTEN BY ANTHROPOLOGISTS, THESE ORIGINAL STUDIES RANGE IN APPROACH FROM THE PSYCHOANALYTIC TO THE SOCIAL ANTHROPOLOGICAL, FROM THE PHENOMENOLOGICAL TO THE SOCIAL STRATEGIC. MATERIAL FROM MOROCCO, SENEGAL, EGYPT, ETHIOPIA, SRI LANKA, MALAYSIA, BRAZIL, PUERTO RICO, AND THE UNITED STATES IS PRESENTED. THESE CASE HISTORIES REINFORCE THE VIEW THAT POSSESSION STATES AND OTHER NON-WESTERN HEALING TECHNIQUES ARE VERY WORTHWHILE APPROACHES TO TREATING TROUBLED PEOPLE. INSIGHTS AND KNOWLEDGE DRAWN FROM THESE STUDIES ARE AN IMPORTANT SOURCE OF UNDERSTANDING THE DIMENSIONS OF THIS PHENOMENON THROUGHOUT THE CULTURES OF THE WORLD. (AUTHOR SUMMARY MODIFIED)

ACCN   000330

390   AUTH   **CRAWFORD, A. N.**
TITL   THE CLOZE PROCEDURE AS A MEASURE OF THE READING COMPREHENSION OF ELEMENTARY LEVEL MEXICAN-AMERICAN AND ANGLO-AMERICAN CHILDREN (DOCTORAL DISSERTATION, UNIVERSITY OF CALIFORNIA, LOS ANGELES, 1971).
SRCE   *DISSERTATION ABSTRACTS INTERNATIONAL, 1971, 31(7), 3162A. (UNIVERSITY MICROFILMS NO. 71-00610.)*
INDX   READING, RESEARCH METHODOLOGY, CROSS CULTURAL, MEXICAN AMERICAN, CHILDREN, EMPIRICAL, TEST VALIDITY, TEST RELIABILITY, BILINGUALISM, CALIFORNIA, SOUTHWEST
ABST   A STUDY INVESTIGATING THE VALIDITY, RELIABILITY, AND APPROPRIATENESS OF CLOZE TESTS AS A MEASURE OF THE READING COMPREHENSION OF THIRD- AND SIXTH-GRADE MEXICAN AMERICAN AND ANGLO AMERICAN CHILDREN IS REPORTED. CORRELATIONS BETWEEN SCORES ON CLOZE TESTS AND ON STANDARDIZED READING TESTS AND ORAL READING TESTS WERE SIGNIFICANT FOR MEXICAN AMERICAN STUDENTS, WHETHER THEIR HOME LANGUAGE WAS ENGLISH OR SPANISH, AND FOR ANGLO AMERICAN CHILDREN. CORRELATIONS WERE SIGNIFICANT FOR GROUPS CLASSIFIED AS MORE ABLE OR LESS ABLE EXCEPT WHERE LOW VARIABILITY WAS PRO-

DUCED BY RESTRICTION OF THE RANGE OF SCORES. THE RELIABILITY COEFFICIENTS OF ALL GROUPS, EXCEPT THE SIXTH-GRADE MEXICAN AMERICANS, WITH ENGLISH AS HOME LANGUAGE WERE ABOVE 0.70. 57 REFERENCES.

ACCN   000331

391   AUTH   **CRESON, D. L., MCKINLEY, C., & EVANS, R.**
TITL   FOLK MEDICINE IN THE MEXICAN-AMERICAN SUBCULTURE.
SRCE   *DISEASES OF THE NERVOUS SYSTEM, 1969, 30(4), 264-266.*
INDX   FOLK MEDICINE, CURANDERISMO, ADULTS, EMPIRICAL, MEXICAN AMERICAN, ACCULTURATION
ABST   TWENTY-FIVE PATIENTS WITH SPANISH SURNAMES WERE INTERVIEWED IN A SEMISTRUCTURED SESSION THAT FOCUSED ON PERSONAL HISTORY, FAMILIARITY AND UTILIZATION OF FOLK HEALERS AND REMEDIES, AND COLLECTION OF ANECDOTAL INFORMATION. IT WAS APPARENT THAT FOR THIS GROUP, WHICH WAS PREDOMINANTLY OF LOW SOCIOECONOMIC CLASS, THE CONCEPT OF FOLK ILLNESS WAS DEEPLY ENTRENCHED AND RESISTANT TO THE INFLUENCE OF ANGLO AMERICAN CULTURE AND ITS SCIENTIFIC MEDICINE. IT IS SUGGESTED THAT FAILURE OF A PHYSICIAN TO RECOGNIZE THE CULTURAL IMPLICATIONS OF FOLK MEDICINE CAN RESULT IN FAULTY DIAGNOSIS AND INAPPROPRIATE AND COSTLY TREATMENT PROCEDURES. IT IS CONCLUDED THAT NO CLEAR UNDERSTANDING OF PSYCHOLOGICAL PATHOLOGY CAN BE FORTHCOMING WHEN SYMPTOMS ARE EVALUATED IN ALIEN TERMS. THE INCIDENCE AND SIGNIFICANCE OF FOLK MEDICINE IS, AS YET, POORLY UNDERSTOOD AND THE UNDERLYING CULTURAL FACTORS ARE INADEQUATELY STUDIED. CLARIFYING CULTURAL FACTORS AND THE CONFLICTS IMPLICIT IN ACCULTURATION WILL MAKE IT POSSIBLE TO PROVIDE A BETTER STANDARD OF CARING FOR THE PHYSICALLY AND MENTALLY ILL IN THE LATIN AMERICAN SUBCULTURE. 5 REFERENCES.

ACCN   000332

392   AUTH   **CRESPIN, B. J.**
TITL   FACILITATION OF BILINGUAL BICULTURAL EDUCATION.
SRCE   *READING IMPROVEMENT, 1976, 13(2), 96-97.*
INDX   BILINGUAL-BICULTURAL EDUCATION, MEXICAN AMERICAN, ESSAY, EDUCATION, CHILDREN, BILINGUAL-BICULTURAL PERSONNEL, FINANCING, TEACHERS
ABST   BILINGUAL EDUCATION IN WHICH THE CHILD'S DOMINANT LANGUAGE AND CULTURE ARE RESPECTED, IS THE ONLY INNOVATIVE PROGRAM THAT CAN CHANGE THE PRESENT SYSTEM. THE PROBLEM LIES IN NOT HAVING ENOUGH OF THESE PROGRAMS FOR THE STUDENTS THAT REALLY NEED THEM. SEVERAL STATES ARE WORKING TOWARD BILINGUAL TEACHER CERTIFICATION, BUT TOO MANY EDUCATORS STILL SEE BILINGUAL EDUCATION AS A RADICAL FORM OF EDUCATION. BILINGUAL PROGRAMS ARE NEITHER NEW NOR RADICAL, YET

THE MONEY FOR BILINGUAL EDUCATION HAS NOT YET REACHED THE CHILDREN FOR WHOM IT WAS MANDATED AND APPROPRIATED. THERE IS A GROWING TREND, HOWEVER, TO TRAIN MORE BILINGUAL TEACHERS AND ADMINISTRATORS AND TO PROVIDE SPANISH AND MEXICAN HISTORY TO ALL TEACHERS WORKING WITH MEXICAN AMERICAN STUDENTS.

ACCN   000333

393 AUTH   **CROMWELL, R. E., CORRALES, R., & TORSIELLO, P. M.**

TITL   NORMATIVE PATTERNS OF MARITAL DECISION MAKING POWER AND INFLUENCE IN MEXICO AND THE UNITED STATES: A PARTIAL TEST OF RESOURCE AND IDEOLOGY THEORY.

SRCE   *JOURNAL OF COMPARATIVE FAMILY STUDIES, 1973, 4(AUTUMN), 175-196.*

INDX   MARRIAGE, MARITAL STABILITY, MEXICAN, FAMILY STRUCTURE, EMPIRICAL, CROSS CULTURAL, CULTURAL FACTORS, THEORETICAL, SEX ROLES, SOCIALIZATION, MINNESOTA, MIDWEST, MEXICO

ABST   SELF-REPORT RESPONSES FROM HUSBANDWIFE PAIRS IN MEXICO AND THE UNITED STATES WERE ANALYZED TO (1) DETERMINE NORMATIVE PATTERNS OF DECISION-MAKING POWER AND INFLUENCE FOR HUSBANDS AND WIVES WITHIN EACH CULTURE, AND (2) TEST THE EXPLANATORY POWER OF RESOURCE THEORY AND IDEOLOGICAL THEORY AS EACH RELATES TO NORMATIVE EXPECTATIONS ABOUT WHO SHOULD MAKE DECISIONS. FINDINGS WERE AS ANTICIPATED, AS THE IMPACT OF RESOURCES (JOB, EDUCATION, INCOME) AND IDEOLOGY (SOCIAL CLASS, AGE AND DEGREE OF INDUSTRIALIZATION) IS TOWARD EGALITARIANISM IN BOTH MEXICO AND THE UNITED STATES. INCREASED ROLE AMBIGUITY IS PREDICTED AS MARITAL NORMS CHANGE IN RESPONSE TO THE CHANGING ROLES OF MEN AND WOMEN IN FAMILY GROUPS. METHODOLOGICAL AND CONCEPTUAL WEAKNESSES ARE DISCUSSED. 35 REFERENCES.

ACCN   000334

394 AUTH   **CROMWELL, R. E., VAUGHAN, C. E., & MINDEL, C. H.**

TITL   ETHNIC MINORITY FAMILY RESEARCH IN AN URBAN SETTING: A PROCESS OF EXCHANGE.

SRCE   *THE AMERICAN SOCIOLOGIST, 1975, 10(3), 141-150.*

INDX   COMMUNITY, URBAN, SURVEY, COMMUNITY INVOLVEMENT, RESEARCH METHODOLOGY, MEXICAN AMERICAN, CROSS CULTURAL, CULTURAL FACTORS

ABST   SOCIAL SCIENTISTS HAVE BEEN INCREASING THEIR INTEREST IN CONDUCTING RESEARCH IN ETHNIC MINORITY URBAN COMMUNITIES BUT ACCOMPLISHING SURVEYS IN THESE COMMUNITIES HAS BECOME MORE DIFFICULT. MEMBERS OF MINORITY COMMUNITIES ARE BEGINNING TO QUESTION WHY AND FOR WHAT PURPOSE THEY ARE BEING SURVEYED. EMPLOYING PROCEDURES ALLOWING FOR COMMUNITY INPUT CAN REDUCE THE EXTENT OF RESISTANCE ENCOUNTERED BY RESEARCHERS. THAT THIS APPROACH IS NOT ALWAYS

SUCCESSFUL IS ATTESTED BY A CASE EXAMPLE IN WHICH THE EXCHANGE PROCESS WAS INCORPORATED IN THE RESEARCH DESIGN TO EXAMINE THE RELATIONSHIP BETWEEN FAMILY STRUCTURE, VALUES, AND "SUCCESSFUL URBAN LIVING; AND THE METHOD FOR OBTAINING DATA HAD TO BE ALTERED DUE TO ORGANIZED COMMUNITY RESISTENCE. RESEARCHERS, IN UTILIZING THE EXCHANGE PROCESS, MUST OBTAIN SUPPORT AND INVOLVEMENT FROM THE COMMUNITY DURING THE ACTUAL PLANNING PHASE OF THE PROJECT, OTHERWISE THEY WILL PROBABLY ENCOUNTER OBSTACLES PREVENTING THE SUCCESSFUL COMPLETION OF THEIR RESEARCH. 14 REFERENCES.

ACCN   000335

395 AUTH   **CROMWELL, R. E., & RUIZ, R. A.**

TITL   THE MYTH OF MACHO DOMINANCE IN DECISION MAKING WITHIN MEXICAN AND CHICANO FAMILIES.

SRCE   *HISPANIC JOURNAL OF BEHAVIORAL SCIENCES, 1979, 1(4), 355-373.*

INDX   MEXICAN, MEXICAN AMERICAN, REVIEW, SEX ROLES, FAMILY ROLES, MALE, FEMALE, ADULTS, STEREOTYPES, CROSS CULTURAL, CULTURAL FACTORS, MACHISMO

ABST   THE PATRIARCHAL HISPANIC FAMILY STRUCTURE CHARACTERIZED BY MACHO DOMINANCE IN MARITAL DECISION MAKING IS A MYTH WHICH STILL PREVAILS IN THE SOCIAL SCIENCE LITERATURE. THIS MYTH, WHICH IS PERPETUATED AND DISSEMINATED THROUGH IMPRESSIONISTIC ESSAYS, IS VERY COMPATIBLE WITH THE "SOCIAL DEFICIT" MODEL OF HISPANIC FAMILY LIFE AND CULTURE. TO CHALLENGE THIS MYTH, AN INTENSIVE ANALYSIS WAS CONDUCTED OF FOUR STUDIES OF HUSBAND-WIFE DECISION-MAKING IN MEXICAN AND CHICANO FAMILIES. THIS REVIEW OF THESE EMPIRICAL DATA FAIL TO SUPPORT THE NOTION OF MALE DOMINANCE. BASICALLY, THE RESULTS SUGGEST THAT WHILE WIVES MAKE THE FEWEST UNILATERAL DECISIONS AND HUSBANDS MAKE MORE, JOINT DECISIONS ARE BY FAR THE MOST COMMON IN MEXICAN AND CHICANO FAMILIES. IT IS CONCLUDED THAT THE MACHO MYTH IS REFUTED BY THE DATA, AND WHAT IS THEREFORE REQUIRED ARE MORE SOPHISTICATED RESEARCH DESIGNS CONCERNING SEX ROLE BEHAVIOR OF HISPANIC MEN AND WOMEN—WITH SPECIAL EMPHASIS ON HOW SEX ROLES INFLUENCE FAMILY LIFE AND MARRIAGE. 34 REFERENCES. (JOURNAL ABSTRACT MODIFIED)

ACCN   001762

396 AUTH   **CROMWELL, R. E., & WIETING, S. G.**

TITL   MULTIDIMENSIONALITY OF CONJUGAL DECISION MAKING INDICES.

SRCE   *JOURNAL OF COMPARATIVE FAMILY STUDIES, 1975, 6(2), 139-152.*

INDX   MARRIAGE, INTERPERSONAL RELATIONS, FAMILY STRUCTURE, CROSS CULTURAL, EMPIRICAL, FAMILY ROLES, SEX ROLES, RESEARCH METHODOLOGY

ABST   THE GENERAL HYPOTHESIS THAT ADDITIVE IN-

DICES OF CONJUGAL DECISION-MAKING OF THE BLOOD AND WOLFE (1960) TYPE YIELD A UNIDIMENSIONAL MEASURE IS TESTED. ON A THEORETICAL LEVEL IT IS BELIEVED SCALE ITEMS ARE MULTIDIMENSIONAL BY NATURE. TO PROVIDE AN EMPIRICAL TEST OF THE RELATIVE DIMENSIONALITY OF CONJUGAL DECISION-MAKING, INTER-ITEM CORRELATION MATRICES WERE COMPUTED AND FACTOR ANALYZED FOR FIVE SEPARATE SAMPLES USING BLOOD AND WOLFE TYPE ADDITIVE INDICES. THE RESULTS DO NOT SUPPORT A UNIDIMENSIONAL CONCLUSION BUT INDICATE A MULTIDIMENSIONAL PATTERN. ALSO, SOME DISTINCT MALE AND FEMALE PATTERNS IN THE DATA SETS ARE INDICATED. IMPLICATIONS FOR THEORY AND RESEARCH ON FAMILY POWER ARE DISCUSSED. 61 REFERENCES. (AUTHOR SUMMARY MODIFIED)

ACCN   000336

397 AUTH   **CROMWELL, V. T.**

TITL   A STUDY OF ETHNIC MINORITY COUPLES: AN EXAMINATION OF DECISION MAKING STRUCTURES, PATRIARCHY, AND TRADITIONAL SEX ROLE STEREOTYPES WITH IMPLICATIONS FOR COUNSELING.

SRCE   *UNPUBLISHED DOCTORAL DISSERTATION, UNIVERSITY OF MISSOURI, KANSAS CITY, 1976.*

INDX   MARRIAGE, SEX ROLES, MEXICAN AMERICAN, CROSS CULTURAL, EMPIRICAL, INTERPERSONAL RELATIONS, STEREOTYPES, PSYCHOTHERAPY, CULTURAL FACTORS, KANSAS, SOUTHWEST

ABST   THE STRUCTURE OF DECISION-MAKING, PATRIARCHY, AND TRADITIONAL SEX ROLE STEREOTYPES OF ANGLO, BLACK, AND CHICANO COUPLES WAS INVESTIGATED, WITH ETHNICITY, SEX, WIFE'S EMPLOYMENT STATUS, EDUCATIONAL LEVEL OF BOTH HUSBAND AND WIFE AND FAMILY SIZE AS INDEPENDENT VARIABLES. 137 MARRIED COUPLES FROM KANSAS CITY WERE QUESTIONED ABOUT THEIR DECISION-MAKING STRUCTURE AND BELIEFS ABOUT SEX ROLES. A MAJOR FOCUS OF THE STUDY WAS TO DRAW IMPLICATIONS FROM THE FINDINGS FOR COUNSELING. NO SUPPORT FOR THE PRIMARY HYPOTHESIS—THAT THE DEGREE OF PATRIARCHY IN ANGLO, BLACK, AND CHICANO COUPLES WILL BE GREATEST AMONG CHICANOS, INTERMEDIARY AMONG ANGLOS, AND LEAST AMONG BLACKS—WAS FOUND. INSTEAD, IT WAS FOUND THAT EGALITARIANISM IS PREVALENT ACROSS AND WITHIN ALL ETHNIC GROUPS. THE MOST SIGNIFICANT DIFFERENCES ARE BETWEEN HUSBANDS AND WIVES WITHIN GROUPS, DEMONSTRATING THAT ALL MARRIAGES ARE DIFFERENT, REGARDLESS OF ETHNIC MEMBERSHIP. THE RESULTS REVEALED: (1) HUSBANDS PERCEIVE MORE SYNCRATIC DECISION THAN DO WIVES; (2) HUSBANDS OF EACH ETHNIC GROUP ATTRIBUTED MORE DECISION-MAKING POWER TO THEMSELVES THAN TO THEIR WIVES OR, CONVERSELY, THAN THEIR WIVES ATTRIBUTED TO THEM; (3) HUSBANDS REPORTED MORE TRADITIONAL SEX ROLE STEREOTYPING THAN THEIR WIVES; (4) WIVES SEEMED TO BE IN

CONFLICT BETWEEN TRADITIONAL AND NONTRADITIONAL VIEWS; (5) WIVES ACROSS EACH ETHNIC GROUP MANIFESTED SIGNIFICANT DIFFERENCES BETWEEN EDUCATION LEVEL AND MEAN SCORES ON SEX ROLE STEREOTYPES; AND (6) WIVES WITH A HIGHER EDUCATIONAL LEVEL WERE MORE NONTRADITIONAL IN SEX ROLE ATTITUDES THAN WIVES WITH A LOWER LEVEL OF EDUCATION. THE FINDINGS ALSO SUGGEST THAT ANGLO AND CHICANO COUPLES TEND TO AGREE REGARDING THE POWER STRUCTURE WITHIN THEIR MARRIAGE MORE THAN BLACK COUPLES. 98 REFERENCES. (AUTHOR ABSTRACT MODIFIED)

ACCN   000337

398 AUTH   **CROOKS, L. A.**

TITL   AN INVESTIGATION OF SOURCES OF BIAS IN THE PREDICTION OF JOB PERFORMANCE: A SIX YEAR STUDY.

SRCE   *PROCEEDINGS OF INVITATIONAL CONFERENCE. PRINCETON, N.J.: EDUCATIONAL TESTING SERVICE, 1972.*

INDX   JOB PERFORMANCE, MEXICAN AMERICAN, CROSS CULTURAL, ACHIEVEMENT TESTING, PROCEEDINGS, CULTURE-FAIR TESTS, EMPIRICAL, ABILITY TESTING

ABST   AN ATTEMPT TO INVESTIGATE APTITUDE AND ABILITY FACTORS CONSIDERED CRITICAL TO JOB PERFORMANCE IN BOTH INDUSTRY AND GOVERNMENT AMONG THREE ETHNIC GROUPS IS PRESENTED. 465 BLACKS, ANGLOS AND MEXICAN AMERICANS WERE ADMINISTERED A SERIES OF TESTS. SCORES WERE OBTAINED ON THE FRENCH, ET AL.,KIT OF REFERENCE TESTS FOR COGNITIVE FACTORS, A CIVIL SERVICE TEST AND A DETAILED QUESTIONNAIRE DESIGNED TO OBTAIN INFORMATION ON THE SUBJECTS' PERSONAL HISTORY. WORK PERFORMANCE WAS MEASURED BY MEANS OF A DETAILED TASK CHECKLIST DEVELOPED FROM INTERVIEWS AND OBSERVATIONS OF JOB PERFORMANCE. THE CHECKLIST DETERMINED THE INTENSITY, IMPORTANCE, AND RELATIVE COMPLEXITY OF THE TASKS PERFORMED BY THE SUBJECTS TESTED. MEDICAL TECHNICIAN, CARTOGRAPHIC TECHNICIAN, AND INVENTORY MANAGEMENT SPECIALIST WERE THE RESPECTIVE JOB CLASSIFICATIONS ALL SUBJECTS HELD DURING TIME OF TESTING. ON THE BASIS OF THE ANALYSIS OF ALL DATA OBTAINED, THE FOLLOWING CONCLUSIONS ARE REACHED: (1) APTITUDE TESTS WHICH HAVE VALIDITY IN RELATION TO JOB PERFORMANCE FOR ONE ETHNIC GROUP GENERALLY SHOW VALIDITY FOR OTHER ETHNIC GROUPS; (2) TESTS WHICH ARE VALID AGAINST A RATING CRITERION ALSO SHOW VALIDITY AGAINST MORE OBJECTIVE CRITERION MEASURES; (3) MULTIPLE REGRESSION WEIGHTS DETERMINED ON A SINGLE ETHNIC GROUP HOLD UP ON CROSS-VALIDATION ACROSS DIFFERENT ETHNIC GROUPS; AND (4) ETHNIC GROUP RATER-RATEE COMBINATIONS INTERACT TO AFFECT THE RATINGS ASSIGNED, BUT THE EFFECT APPEARS TO BE COMPLEX AND PROBABLY DIFFERS FROM ONE ETHNIC GROUP TO ANOTHER. CONTAINED IN THE STUDY ARE A NUM-

BER OF WRITTEN IMPLICATIONS FOR EMPLOY-ERS IN GOVERNMENT, EMPLOYERS IN INDUS-TRY, FOR BLACKS AND SPANISH AMERICANS AND GOVERNMENTAL REGULATIVE AGENCIES. A TECHNICAL CRITIQUE DEMONSTRATING THE NEED FOR FUTURE RESEARCH IS ALSO IN-CLUDED. 13 REFERENCES.

ACCN   000338

399 AUTH   **CROSS, W. C., & MALDONADO, B.**
    TITL   THE COUNSELOR, THE MEXICAN-AMERICAN, AND THE STEREOTYPE.
    SRCE   *ELEMENTARY SCHOOL GUIDANCE AND COUN-SELING, 1971, 6(1), 27-31.*
    INDX   MEXICAN AMERICAN, STEREOTYPES, DIS-CRIMINATION, ESSAY, SES, SELF CONCEPT, CHILDREN, EDUCATION, CULTURAL FACTORS, EDUCATIONAL COUNSELING, ADULTS
    ABST   THE SCHOOL COUNSELOR SHOULD BE AWARE THAT THE DISPARITY BETWEEN THE DEMANDS OF THE ANGLO SOCIETY AND THE BASIC POSI-TIVE VALUES TO WHICH THE TRADITIONAL MEXICAN AMERICAN ADHERES TENDS TO CRE-ATE SCHIZOID CONDITIONS IN WHICH HE MUST FUNCTION. HE IS SERIOUSLY HANDICAPPED UNTIL HE LEARNS TO UNDERSTAND AND TO ACCEPT THE CULTURAL DIFFERENCES OF A PEOPLE WHO HAVE BEEN ACCUSED BY MANY OF HAVING NO CULTURE. AN OVERVIEW OF SOME OF THESE CULTURAL DIFFERENCES IS OFFERED. THE ANGLO AMERICAN SEES THE MEXICAN AMERICAN AS IMMORAL, VIOLENT, GIVEN TO FIGHTING, UNINTELLIGENT, IMPROV-IDENT, IRRESPONSIBLE, AND LAZY. USUALLY BILINGUAL, THE MEXICAN AMERICAN GENER-ALLY HAS A SPANISH SURNAME, IS ROMAN CATHOLIC, IS LIKELY TO MARRY WITHIN HIS OWN GROUP AND LIVE IN A SOCIALLY SEGRE-GATED COMMUNITY, AND HAS LESS THAN 5 YEARS OF SCHOOLING. HE HAS A LARGE NUM-BER OF CHILDREN AND A HOUSEHOLD WHICH INCLUDES VARIOUS NUCLEAR FAMILIES OF DIFFERING GENERATIONS. HIS LIFE EXPECT-ANCY IS SHORTER THAN THAT OF THE ANGLO. MODEST BUT PROUD, HE IS ORIENTED TO-WARD THE PRESENT RATHER THAN THE FU-TURE AND DEMONSTRATES A MARKED INCLI-NATION TOWARD DEPENDENCY UPON HIS KINSMEN AND COMPADRES. HE TOLERATES THE STATUS QUO RATHER THAN ATTEMPTING TO MANIPULATE OR CHANGE THE ENVIRON-MENT. ALTHOUGH HE DOES NOT ALWAYS ECO-NOMICALLY MEET THE CHALLENGES OF LIFE, HE DOES CARE MORE ABOUT HIS FAMILY MEM-BERS THAN ANYONE ELSE. 15 REFERENCES.

ACCN   000341

400 AUTH   **CROUCH, B. M.**
    TITL   AGE AND INSTITUTIONAL SUPPORT: PERCEP-TIONS OF OLDER MEXICAN AMERICANS.
    SRCE   *JOURNAL OF GERONTOLOGY, 1972, 27(4), 524-529.*
    INDX   GERONTOLOGY, MEXICAN AMERICAN, ADULTS, HEALTH DELIVERY SYSTEMS, SOCIAL SER-VICES, RESOURCE UTILIZATION, RELIGION, POVERTY, ATTITUDES, FAMILY ROLES, HEALTH, SEX COMPARISON, SURVEY, EMPIRICAL, TEXAS, SOUTHWEST

ABST   OLDER MEXICAN AMERICANS WERE SUR-VEYED TO DETERMINE THEIR ATTITUDES TO-WARD AGING AND TOWARD SUPPORT FOR THE AGED FROM FAMILY, CHURCH AND GOVERN-MENT. AGING WAS VIEWED NEGATIVELY AND WAS PERCEIVED TO BEGIN AT AGE SIXTY OR BELOW. THE CHURCH AND GOVERNMENT, RATHER THAN THE FAMILY, WERE SEEN AS EX-PECTED SOURCES OF SUPPORT FOR THE AGED. ANALYSIS BY AGE AND SEX GROUPS DID NOT REVEAL ANY DIFFERENCES ON THESE ATTI-TUDES. OLDER MEXICAN AMERICANS DID NOT APPEAR TO BE SUBSTANTIALLY DIFFERENT FROM OTHER OLDER AMERICANS, THOUGH THE PROVISION OF EXTRA FAMILIAL SOURCES OF SUPPORT FOR THE MEXICAN AMERICAN EL-DERLY SHOULD TAKE INTO ACCOUNT BOTH THEIR LOW SOCIOECONOMIC STATUS AND THEIR LANGUAGE BARRIER. 10 REFERENCES.

ACCN   000342

401 AUTH   **CROWTHER, B.**
    TITL   PATTERNS OF DRUG USE AMONG MEXICAN AMERICANS.
    SRCE   *THE INTERNATIONAL JOURNAL OF THE ADDIC-TIONS, 1972, 7(4), 637-647.*
    INDX   MEXICAN AMERICAN, DRUG ABUSE, DRUG ADDICTION, SES, EMPIRICAL, ADULTS, CRIMI-NOLOGY, CROSS CULTURAL, SOUTHWEST, TEXAS
    ABST   PATTERNS OF DRUG USE WERE COMPARED FOR MEXICAN AMERICAN AND ANGLO NAR-COTIC ADDICTS. THE MEXICAN AMERICANS SHOWED MUCH LESS EXPERIMENTATION IN THEIR DRUG USE, WITH THE MOST TYPICAL PATTERN BEING FIRST MARIJUANA AND THEN HEROIN USE. THE DIFFERENCES ARE MAIN-TAINED WHEN MEDICAL USE, SOCIAL CLASS, AND PRIOR DELINQUENCY HISTORIES ARE CONTROLLED. A SPECULATIVE HYPOTHESIS FOR THIS FINDING CONCERNS CULTURAL DIF-FERENCES IN THE PERCEPTION OF THE VALUE OF THE DRUGS. 6 REFERENCES. (JOURNAL AB-STRACT)

ACCN   000343

402 AUTH   **CUCA, J.**
    TITL   APA SURVEY RESULTS: GRADUATE ENROLL-MENTS LEVELING OFF.
    SRCE   *APA MONITOR, NOVEMBER 1974, PP. 16; 19.*
    INDX   MENTAL HEALTH PROFESSION, PROFESSIONAL TRAINING, REPRESENTATION, SPANISH SUR-NAMED, SURVEY, EMPIRICAL, CROSS CUL-TURAL, EQUAL OPPORTUNITY, FEMALE
    ABST   THE FOURTH ANNUAL APA SURVEY EXAMIN-ING THE TREND OF GRADUATE ENROLLMENT IN PSYCHOLOGY INDICATES THAT THERE WAS A 25% DROP IN ENROLLMENT IN 1970-71, A 12% DROP IN 1971-72, AND A TAPERING OFF TO 3% IN 1972-73. BUT DESPITE THE DE-CREASE, WOMEN—BUT NOT MINORITIES—HAVE HAD INCREASED REPRESENTATION IN PSY-CHOLOGY GRADUATE PROGRAMS. WITH RE-GARD TO THE VARIOUS FIELDS IN PSY-CHOLOGY, THE CLINICAL AREA HAS ATTRACTED THE HIGHEST PROPORTION OF STUDENTS, ES-PECIALLY IN MASTER'S PROGRAMS. STATIS-TICS ALSO REVEAL THAT ALTHOUGH THERE IS

ONLY A 6% UNEMPLOYMENT RATE FOR THOSE WITH M.A. DEGREES, THE UNEMPLOYMENT LEVEL IS AROUND 20% FOR THOSE WITH DOCTORATES.

ACCN   000344

403 AUTH   **CURREN, D. J., RIVERA, J. J., & SANCHEZ, R. B.**

TITL   PROCEEDINGS OF PUERTO RICAN CONFERENCES ON HUMAN SERVICES.

SRCE   *WASHINGTON, D.C.: NATIONAL COALITION OF HISPANIC MENTAL HEALTH AND HUMAN SERVICES ORGANIZATIONS (COSSMHO), 1975.*

INDX   PUERTO RICAN-M, PUERTO RICAN-I, HEALTH DELIVERY SYSTEMS, MENTAL HEALTH, CULTURAL FACTORS, GERONTOLOGY, ALCOHOLISM, DRUG ABUSE, HEALTH, ATTITUDES, RESEARCH METHODOLOGY, INTELLIGENCE TESTING, JUDICIAL PROCESS, SOCIAL SERVICES, FOLK MEDICINE, ESPIRITISMO, PROCEEDINGS

ABST   IN NOVEMBER, 1974 TWO CONFERENCES WERE SPONSORED BY THE NATIONAL COALITION OF SPANISH-SPEAKING MENTAL HEALTH ORGANIZATIONS RELATED TO THE HEALTH AND MENTAL HEALTH NEEDS OF MAINLAND AND NATIVE PUERTO RICANS. THIS VOLUME PRESENTS THE PROCEEDINGS OF BOTH CONFERENCES, THE FIRST HELD IN CAGUAS, PUERTO RICO, AND THE SECOND IN NEW YORK CITY. THE PURPOSE OF THESE CONFERENCES WAS TO PROVIDE A COMPREHENSIVE PERSPECTIVE ON THE NEEDS AND RESOURCES OF THE PUERTO RICAN PEOPLE. THE MAJOR THEMES AND ISSUES OF THE CONFERENCES INCLUDED: (1) THE DOCUMENTATION OF NEED AND THE SETTING OF PRIORITIES THAT CONSIDER THE CULTURE AND LANGUAGE PATTERNS OF PUERTO RICANS; AND (2) THE DEVELOPMENT AND USE OF NEW, INNOVATIVE SERVICES FREE FROM THE REPRESSIVE AND POLITICAL "BENIGN NEGLECT" CHARACTERISTICS OF PAST MINORITY-ANGLO PROFESSIONAL RELATIONSHIPS. DIVIDED INTO TWO PARTS, THE BOOK FIRST GIVES A COMPLETE OVERVIEW OF THE BROAD SPECTRUM OF PROBLEMS COMMON TO BOTH ISLAND AND MAINLAND PUERTO RICAN HUMAN SERVICES. SECONDLY, IT PROVIDES A PENETRATING ANALYSIS OF THE CAUSE, PREVALENCE AND IMPACT OF THESE CONCERNS ON THE PUERTO RICAN COMMUNITY AND ITS RESOURCES. BY THE NATURE OF ITS SUBJECT MATTER AND SCOPE OF PRESENTATION THIS BOOK PROVIDES VALUABLE INFORMATION TO HUMAN SERVICE WORKERS DESIRING CURRENT LITERATURE PERTAINING TO WHAT THE PUERTO RICANS PERCEIVE AS THEIR ACTUAL NEEDS. IT ALSO PROVIDES THE GUIDELINES FOR COLLECTING AND UTILIZING DATA VITAL TO DEVELOPING RELEVANT SERVICES FOR PUERTO RICANS. THIRTY CONTRIBUTORS ARE PRESENTED AND EIGHT SPECIAL WORKSHOPS ARE SUMMARIZED.

ACCN   000345

404 AUTH   **CURRIER, R. L.**

TITL   THE HOT-COLD SYNDROME AND SYMBOLIC BALANCE IN MEXICAN AND SPANISH-AMERICAN FOLK MEDICINE.

SRCE   *ETHNOLOGY, 1966, 5(3), 251-263.*

INDX   FOLK MEDICINE, MEXICAN AMERICAN, CENTRAL AMERICA, SOUTH AMERICA, MEXICO, ESSAY, DISEASE

ABST   AN EXAMINATION OF THE HOT-COLD SYNDROME AND SYMBOLIC BALANCE IN MEXICAN AND SPANISH-AMERICAN FOLK MEDICINE IS PRESENTED. ON A CONSCIOUS LEVEL, THE HOT-COLD SYNDROME IS A BASIC PRINCIPLE OF HUMAN PHYSIOLOGY AND IT FUNCTIONS AS A LOGICAL SYSTEM FOR CONFRONTING THE PROBLEMS OF DISORDER AND DISEASE. ON A SUBCONSCIOUS LEVEL THE HOT-COLD SYNDROME IS A MODEL OF SOCIAL RELATIONS. IN THIS LATTER SENSE, THE HOT-COLD SYNDROME IS CALLED A PROJECTIVE SYSTEM. THE NATURE OF PEASANT SOCIETY IS A CONTINUOUS ATTEMPT TO ACHIEVE A BALANCE BETWEEN TWO OPPOSING FORCES: THE TENDENCY TOWARD INTIMACY AND THAT TOWARD WITHDRAWAL. IT IS CONTENDED THAT THE INDIVIDUAL'S PREOCCUPATION WITH SUSTAINING SUCH A BALANCE BETWEEN HOT AND COLD IS A WAY OF REENACTING, IN SYMBOLIC TERMS, A FUNDAMENTAL ACTIVITY IN SOCIAL RELATIONS. A DESCRIPTION IS GIVEN OF THE HOT-COLD SYNDROME AS A MEDICAL BELIEF THAT DEFINES CALIDAD (I.E., QUALITY) IN THE CLASSIFICATION OF FOODS, AND A LIST OF THE MANY TYPES OF ILLNESSES CAUSED BY COLD OR HOT QUALITIES ENTERING THE BODY. FOLK BELIEFS AND THEIR RELATION TO THE HOT-COLD SYNDROME ARE ALSO DISCUSSED. THE HOT-COLD SYNDROME AS A PROJECTIVE SYSTEM IS DESCRIBED IN RELATION TO CHILD DEVELOPMENT IN MEXICAN PEASANT SOCIETY. 25 REFERENCES.

ACCN   000346

405 AUTH   **CURTIS, F. L. S.**

TITL   OBSERVATIONS OF UNWED PREGNANT ADOLESCENTS.

SRCE   *AMERICAN JOURNAL OF NURSING, 1974, 74(1), 100-102.*

INDX   ADOLESCENTS, FAMILY STRUCTURE, SURVEY, PUERTO RICAN-M, CULTURAL FACTORS, ECONOMIC FACTORS, SEXUAL BEHAVIOR, SEX ROLES, INTERPERSONAL RELATIONS, SES, FEMALE

ABST   A QUESTIONNAIRE WAS ADMINISTERED TO 30 PREGNANT AND 20 NONPREGNANT ADOLESCENTS TO FIND OUT ABOUT THEIR INTERPERSONAL RELATIONSHIPS AND INTERESTS. RESULTS SHOWED NONPREGNANT GIRLS PARTICIPATED IN MORE GAMES AND SPORTS THAN DID THE PREGNANT GROUP. THE TENDENCY OF THE PREGNANT GIRLS WAS TOWARD SOLITARY OR NO ACTIVITIES. IN THE NONPREGNANT GROUP, ALL THE GIRLS HAD DEVELOPED A HOBBY, WHILE IN THE PREGNANT GROUP ONLY 9 GIRLS OUT OF 30 HAD DEVELOPED A HOBBY. IT IS RECOMMENDED THAT YOUNG PEOPLE BE ENCOURAGED BY FAMILIES AND COMMUNITY LEADERS TO BE INVOLVED IN USEFUL ACTIVITIES. 4 REFERENCES.

ACCN   000347

406 AUTH **DALTON, S.**
     TITL LANGUAGE DOMINANCE AND BILINGUAL RE-
           CALL.
     SRCE *THE JOURNAL OF PSYCHOLOGY, 1973, 84(JULY),*
           257-265.
     INDX BILINGUALISM, COLLEGE STUDENTS, MEMORY,
           COMPOUND-COORDINATE DISTINCTION, EM-
           PIRICAL, LINGUISTIC COMPETENCE, BILIN-
           GUAL
     ABST BOTH UNILINGUAL AND BILINGUAL WORD LISTS
           WERE RECALLED BY 98 BILINGUAL SUBJECTS.
           ALL WERE TESTED IN SMALL GROUPS, RAN-
           DOMLY ASSIGNED TO ONE OF THE FOUR EX-
           PERIMENTAL GROUPS, AND PRESENTED WITH
           FOUR 16-WORD LISTS REFLECTING THREE
           LANGUAGE CONDITIONS: SPANISH, ENGLISH,
           OR MIXED. FINDINGS SHOWED THAT A DIRECT
           RELATIONSHIP BETWEEN DOMINANCE AND
           RECALL WHICH OCCURS UNDER BILINGUAL
           CONDITIONS DISAPPEARED UNDER THE BILIN-
           GUAL CONDITIONS OF THE EXPERIMENT. BI-
           LINGUAL LISTS WERE RECALLED AS WELL AS
           UNILINGUAL LISTS, AND LED TO SUPERIOR RE-
           CALL OF SPANISH FOR NEARLY ALL SUBJECTS.
           8 REFERENCES. (JOURNAL ABSTRACT MODI-
           FIED)
     ACCN 000348

407 AUTH **DARCY, N. T.**
     TITL BILINGUALISM AND THE MEASUREMENT OF IN-
           TELLIGENCE: REVIEW OF A DECADE OF RE-
           SEARCH.
     SRCE *JOURNAL OF GENETIC PSYCHOLOGY, 1963,*
           103, 259-282.
     INDX BILINGUALISM, INTELLIGENCE TESTING, IN-
           TELLIGENCE, REVIEW, PUERTO RICAN-M, MEX-
           ICAN AMERICAN, WISC, CATTELL CULTURE-FREE
           INTELLIGENCE TEST, GOODENOUGH DRAW-A-
           MAN TEST, STANFORD-BINET INTELLIGENCE
           TEST, CROSS CULTURAL, SES
     ABST A DECADE OF RESEARCH CONCERNED WITH
           THE EFFECTS OF BILINGUALISM ON THE MEA-
           SUREMENT OF INTELLIGENCE IS REVIEWED.
           SOME OF THE PROBLEMS IN THIS FIELD ARE
           CONSIDERED TO BE: (1) DIVERGENT DEFINI-
           TIONS FOR BILINGUALISM; (2) DETERMINING
           DEGREES OF BILINGUALISM; (3) TYPES OF IN-
           TELLIGENCE TESTS USED; (4) ISOLATION FROM
           OTHER ENVIRONMENTAL FACTORS; (5) TESTS
           WITH TIME LIMITS; (6) OPTIMAL AGE TO LEARN
           ANOTHER LANGUAGE; AND (7) RELATION OF
           LANGUAGE TO CONCEPTUAL THINKING. THE
           RESULTS CONFIRM THAT BILINGUALISM IS NOT
           UNIFORM AS TO KIND, AND THAT ITS INFLU-
           ENCE ON INDIVIDUALS OF DIFFERENT RACES
           AND IN DIFFERENT ENVIRONMENTS CANNOT
           BE PREDICTED WITHOUT MORE RESEARCH.
           THE INCONSISTENCY OF STUDIES DEALING
           WITH BILINGUALISM AND ITS RELATION TO THE
           MEASUREMENT OF INTELLIGENCE CAN FRE-
           QUENTLY BE RESOLVED BY REFERRING TO
           SEVERAL IMPORTANT FACTORS. THESE IN-
           CLUDE THE AGE OF BEGINNING THE SECOND
           LANGUAGE, THE SOCIOECONOMIC AND CUL-
           TURAL BACKGROUNDS OF THE SUBJECTS,
           THE INSTRUMENTS USED FOR MEASURING

THE DEGREES OF BILINGUALISM, AS WELL AS
VERBAL AND NONVERBAL INTELLIGENCE, AND
THE METHODS EMPLOYED IN TEACHING THE
SECOND LANGUAGE. IT IS SUGGESTED THAT
CAREFULLY CONTROLLED RESEARCH, SOME
OF WHICH SHOULD BE OF A LONGITUDINAL
NATURE, IS NEEDED. 43 REFERENCES.
     ACCN 000349

408 AUTH **DARCY, N. T.**
     TITL THE PERFORMANCE OF BILINGUAL PUERTO
           RICAN CHILDREN ON VERBAL AND ON NON-
           LANGUAGE TESTS OF INTELLIGENCE.
     SRCE *JOURNAL OF EDUCATIONAL RESEARCH, 1952,*
           45(7), 499-506.
     INDX INTELLIGENCE TESTING, BILINGUALISM, CHIL-
           DREN, PUERTO RICAN-M, BILINGUAL, INTELLI-
           GENCE, EMPIRICAL, NEW YORK, EAST
     ABST THE PERFORMANCE OF BILINGUAL PUERTO
           RICAN CHILDREN ON A VERBAL AND NONVER-
           BAL TEST OF INTELLIGENCE IS INVESTIGATED.
           THE FOLLOWING QUESTIONS WERE POSITED
           BY THE INVESTIGATOR: (1) IS THERE A SIGNIFI-
           CANT DIFFERENCE BETWEEN THE MEAN IQ
           ACHIEVED ON THE PINTNER GENERAL ABILITY
           TEST (PGAT), VERBAL SERIES, AND THE MEAN
           IQ ACHIEVED ON THE PGAT, NON-LANGUAGE
           SERIES, WHEN ADMINISTERED TO A BILINGUAL
           PUERTO RICAN POPULATION IN GRADES FIVE
           AND SIX?; (2) IS THERE A SIGNIFICANT DIFFER-
           ENCE IN THE MEAN MENTAL AGES OF THESE
           SUBJECTS AS MEASURED BY THE TWO TESTS?;
           AND (3) CAN THE TWO TESTS BE USED INTER-
           CHANGEABLY FOR THIS POPULATION? THE
           SUBJECTS CONSISTED OF 235 CHILDREN, 117
           BOYS AND 118 GIRLS. RESULTS SHOW THAT
           THE OBTAINED MEAN IQ DIFFERENCE BE-
           TWEEN THE LANGUAGE AND NONLANGUAGE
           TESTS IS SIGNIFICANT IN FAVOR OF THE PINT-
           NER NON-LANGUAGE TEST. SIMILARLY, THE
           DIFFERENCE BETWEEN THE MEAN MENTAL
           AGES FOR THE TWO TESTS IS SIGNIFICANT IN
           FAVOR OF THE PINTNER NON-LANGUAGE TEST.
           THE COEFFICIENTS OF CORRELATION BE-
           TWEEN THE IQ'S ACHIEVED ON THE TWO TESTS
           ARE TOO LOW TO WARRANT THE SUBSTITU-
           TION OF ONE TEST FOR THE OTHER. IT IS CON-
           CLUDED, HOWEVER, THAT THE TWO TESTS ARE
           MEASURING THE SAME FUNCTIONS TO A FAIRLY
           LARGE EXTENT, SINCE THE COEFFICIENT OF
           CORRELATION BETWEEN THE IQ'S IS MORE
           THAN 19 TIMES ITS PROBABLE ERROR AND
           THE COEFFICIENT OF CORRELATION BETWEEN
           THE MENTAL AGES IS MORE THAN 10 TIMES ITS
           PROBABLE ERROR. THE IMPLICATION IS THAT
           THE ADMINISTRATION OF INTELLIGENCE TESTS
           OF BOTH VERBAL AND NONLANGUAGE TYPES
           WOULD YIELD A MORE VALID PICTURE OF THE
           INTELLIGENCE OF A BILINGUAL POPULATION
           THAN EITHER ONE ALONE. 1 REFERENCE.
     ACCN 000350

409 AUTH **DARCY, N. T.**
     TITL A REVIEW OF THE LITERATURE ON THE EFFECT
           OF BILINGUALISM UPON THE MEASUREMENT
           OF INTELLIGENCE.
     SRCE *JOURNAL OF GENETIC PSYCHOLOGY, 1953,*
           82(1), 21-57.

INDX   BILINGUALISM, INTELLIGENCE TESTING, RE-
VIEW, INTELLIGENCE, CROSS CULTURAL, STAN-
FORD-BINET INTELLIGENCE TEST, MEXICAN,
SES

ABST   A REVIEW OF A REPRESENTATIVE NUMBER OF
STUDIES THAT DEALT WITH THE EFFECTS OF
BILINGUALISM UPON THE MEASUREMENT OF
INTELLIGENCE IS PRESENTED. THE STUDIES
ARE CLASSIFIED UNDER THE FOLLOWING
HEADINGS: (1) WHERE BILINGUALISM HAS A
FAVORABLE EFFECT UPON THE MEASURE-
MENT OF INTELLIGENCE; (2) WHERE BILIN-
GUALISM HAS AN UNFAVORABLE EFFECT UPON
THE MEASUREMENT OF INTELLIGENCE; AND
(3) WHERE BILINGUALISM HAS NO EFFECT
UPON THE MEASUREMENT OF INTELLIGENCE.
THE FINDINGS CLEARLY INDICATE THAT STUD-
IES WHICH CONCLUDE THAT BILINGUALISM
HAS A FAVORABLE EFFECT ON THE MEASURE-
MENT OF INTELLIGENCE ARE IN THE MINORITY.
SINCE LITTLE ATTEMPT HAS BEEN MADE TO
CONTROL VARIABLES SUCH AS SOCIOECO-
NOMIC STATUS AND DEGREE OF BILINGUAL-
ISM, THE RESULTS OF THESE STUDIES MAY BE
QUESTIONED. MOST OF THE LITERATURE SUG-
GESTS THAT BILINGUALS SUFFER FROM A
LANGUAGE HANDICAP WHEN MEASURED BY
VERBAL TESTS OF INTELLIGENCE. HOWEVER,
THERE IS NO INDICATION OF THE INFERIORITY
OF BILINGUAL SUBJECTS WHEN THEIR PER-
FORMANCE ON NONLANGUAGE TESTS OF IN-
TELLIGENCE IS MEASURED AGAINST THAT OF
MONOLINGUAL SUBJECTS. A FEW STUDIES RE-
PORT THAT BILINGUALISM DOES NOT SERVE
AS ANY HANDICAP WHEN VERBAL TESTS ARE
USED TO MEASURE INTELLIGENCE. 110 REF-
ERENCES.

ACCN   000351

410   AUTH   **DARROW, W. W.**
TITL   VENEREAL INFECTIONS IN THREE ETHNIC
GROUPS IN SACRAMENTO.
SRCE   *AMERICAN JOURNAL OF PUBLIC HEALTH, 1976,*
66(5), 446-450.
INDX   DISEASE, CROSS CULTURAL, SEXUAL BEHAV-
IOR, MEXICAN AMERICAN, SYMPTOMATOLOGY,
EMPIRICAL, CALIFORNIA, SOUTHWEST
ABST   BLACKS TREATED IN SACRAMENTO COUNTY
CLINICS WERE MOST LIKELY TO HAVE GONOR-
RHEA, CHICANOS WERE SLIGHTLY MORE LIKELY
TO HAVE NONSPECIFIC URETHRITIS AND OTHER
SEXUALLY TRANSMITTED DISEASES, AND
WHITES WERE MOST LIKELY TO BE UNIN-
FECTED. WHITES TENDED TO NAME GREATER
NUMBERS OF DIFFERENT SEXUAL PARTNERS,
BUT DIFFERENCES AMONG THE THREE GROUPS
WERE NOT STATISTICALLY SIGNIFICANT. BLACK
MEN MORE FREQUENTLY REPORTED TO CLIN-
ICS WITH GENITOURINARY SYMPTOMS AND
DELAYED SIGNIFICANTLY LONGER BEFORE
SEEKING TREATMENT. FUTURE RESEARCH
SHOULD ASSESS THE RELATIVE CONTRIBU-
TIONS OF SEXUAL AND HEALTH BEHAVIORS TO
THE DISTRIBUTIONS OF DIFFERENT SEXUALLY
TRANSMITTED DISEASES IN DIFFERENT
GROUPS. 24 REFERENCES. (JOURNAL AB-
STRACT)
ACCN   000352

411   AUTH   **DAVENPORT, E. L.**
TITL   THE INTELLIGENCE QUOTIENTS OF MEXICAN
AND NONMEXICAN SIBLINGS.
SRCE   *SCHOOL AND SOCIETY, 1932, 36(923), 304-306.*
INDX   MEXICAN AMERICAN, INTELLIGENCE TESTING,
EMPIRICAL, GOODENOUGH DRAW-A-MAN TEST,
EDUCATION, CHILDREN, CROSS CULTURAL,
TEXAS, SOUTHWEST
ABST   THE INTERPRETATION OF TEST SCORES ON
THE BASIS OF THE STABILITY OF THE INTELLI-
GENCE QUOTIENTS (IQ'S) OF ELEMENTARY
SCHOOL MEXICAN AND NON-MEXICAN CHIL-
DREN IS REPORTED. TWO HUNDRED TEN MEX-
ICAN AND 62 PAIRS OF NON-MEXICAN SIB-
LINGS IN THE FIRST THREE GRADES OF
ELEMENTARY SCHOOL FROM SAN ANTONIO,
TEXAS, WERE TESTED WITH THE GOODEN-
OUGH DRAW-A-MAN TEST. WITH THIS TEST THE
FACTOR OF LANGUAGE DIFFICULTY FOR THE
MEXICAN GROUP IS ELIMINATED. THE FIND-
INGS SHOW THAT THE CORRELATION OF THE
IQ'S OF OLDER AND YOUNGER MEXICAN CHIL-
DREN IS .25, WHILE THAT OF THE NON-MEXI-
CAN SIBLINGS IS .51. THE DIFFERENCE BE-
TWEEN THE MEAN IQ'S OF THE OLDER AND
YOUNGER SIBLINGS IN THE TWO LANGUAGE
GROUPS SUGGESTS THE HYPOTHESIS THAT
THE OLDER MEXICAN SIBLINGS GAINED IN IQ
SINCE SCHOOL ENTRANCE. THIS HYPOTHESIS
IS SUPPORTED BY THE FACT THAT ALTHOUGH
THE MEXICAN SIBLINGS, BOTH OF WHOM WERE
JUST BEGINNING SCHOOL, WERE ALMOST
EQUAL IN IQ, THERE IS A SIGNIFICANT DIFFER-
ENCE WHEN THE OLDER MEXICAN SIBLING
HAS ATTENDED SCHOOL AND THE YOUNGER
HAS NOT. IT IS CONCLUDED THAT PROGNOSIS
ON THE BASIS OF THE GOODENOUGH IQ TEST
AT SCHOOL ENTRANCE IS LIKELY TO UNDER-
ESTIMATE THE FUTURE ABILITIES OF THE MEX-
ICAN CHILD.
ACCN   000353

412   AUTH   **DAVIDSON, A. R., JACCARD, J. J., TRIANDIS,**
H. C., MORALES, M. L., & DIAZ-GUERRERO, R.
TITL   CROSS-CULTURAL MODEL TESTING: TOWARD
A SOLUTION OF THE ETIC-EMIC DILEMMA.
SRCE   *INTERNATIONAL JOURNAL OF PSYCHOLOGY,*
1976, 11(1), 1-13.
INDX   CROSS CULTURAL, RESEARCH METHOD-
OLOGY, MEXICAN, FEMALE, EMPIRICAL, FER-
TILITY, ATTITUDES, SES, ADULTS, BIRTH CON-
TROL
ABST   A MODEL FOR THE PREDICTION OF FERTILITY
BEHAVIOR FROM ATTITUDINAL COMPONENTS,
DEVELOPED BY TRIANDIS, WAS TESTED WITH
SAMPLES OF U.S. AND MEXICAN WOMEN. THREE
BEHAVIORS WERE STUDIED: (1) THE INTEN-
TION TO HAVE A TWO CHILD FAMILY; (2) THE
INTENTION TO USE BIRTH CONTROL PILLS;
AN (3) THE INTENTION TO HAVE A CHILD IN
THE NEXT TWO YEARS. THE ELEMENTS OF THE
TESTED MODEL ARE ETIC, BUT THE OPERA-
TIONALIZATION OF THE VARIABLES WAS DONE
EMICALLY. RESULTS SUPPORT THE MODEL IN
BOTH CULTURES. WHILE THE PREDICTIVE
UTILITY OF THE MODEL IS EQUIVALENT IN TWO
CULTURES, THERE ARE SOCIAL CLASS DIFFER-
ENCES ON WHICH COMPONENT OF THE MODEL

IS MOST EMPHASIZED. THE U.S. UPPER-MIDDLE CLASS SAMPLE AND THE MEXICAN UPPER-MIDDLE CLASS SAMPLE EMPHASIZED THE PERSON'S ATTITUDE TOWARD AN ACT, WHILE THE MEXICAN LOWER SES SAMPLE EMPHASIZED THE PERSON'S NORMATIVE BELIEFS (MORAL OBLIGATIONS). 25 REFERENCES. (JOURNAL ABSTRACT MODIFIED)

ACCN 000354

413 AUTH **DAVIDSON, C., & GAITZ, C. M.**
TITL ARE THE POOR DIFFERENT? A COMPARISON OF WORK BEHAVIOR AND ATTITUDES AMONG THE URBAN POOR AND NON-POOR.
SRCE *SOCIAL PROBLEMS, 1974, 22(2), 229-245.*
INDX TEXAS, SOUTHWEST, CROSS CULTURAL, POVERTY, URBAN, MEXICAN AMERICAN, LABOR FORCE, JOB PERFORMANCE, EMPLOYMENT, EMPIRICAL, ATTITUDES, SEX COMPARISON, MALE, FEMALE,
ABST TO DETERMINE WHETHER POVERTY IS THE RESULT OF A WORK ORIENTATION PECULIAR TO THE POOR, A SECONDARY ANALYSIS OF DATA OBTAINED FROM A STRATIFIED SAMPLE OF THE HOUSTON POPULATION WAS CONDUCTED. ETHNICITY (BLACK, MEXICAN AMERICAN, ANGLO) AND SEX WERE CONTROLLED, AND AGE WAS STANDARDIZED. THE FINDINGS CAST DOUBT ON THE CULTURE OF POVERTY HYPOTHESIS INSOFAR AS IT PERTAINS TO WORK HABITS AND ATTITUDES. THE ASSUMPTION THAT THE POOR WORK LESS THAN THE NONPOOR WAS FOUND TO BE UNWARRANTED IN THE CASES OF MEXICAN AMERICAN MALES AND OF WOMEN OF WHATEVER ETHNICITY. THE EMPLOYMENT RATE AMONG MEXICAN AMERICAN IMPOVERISHED MALES WAS HIGHER THAN AMONG THE ANGLO NONPOOR. NO SIGNIFICANT DIFFERENCES IN ATTITUDES TOWARD WORK WERE FOUND TO EXIST BETWEEN THE POOR AND NONPOOR WITHIN ANY ETHNIC GROUP. CONTRARY TO A POPULAR VIEW, THE MINORITY POOR WERE FOUND TO BE AS WORK-ORIENTED AS THE ANGLO NONPOOR. 32 REFERENCES. (AUTHOR ABSTRACT)

ACCN 002061

414 AUTH **DAVIDSON, C., & GAITZ, C. M.**
TITL ETHNIC ATTITUDES AS A BASIS FOR MINORITY COOPERATION IN A SOUTHWESTERN METROPOLIS.
SRCE *SOCIAL SCIENCE QUARTERLY, 1973, 53(4), 738-748.*
INDX CROSS CULTURAL, EMPIRICAL, ADULTS, SES, DISCRIMINATION, MEXICAN AMERICAN, ATTITUDES, INTEGRATION, EQUAL OPPORTUNITY, CROSS GENERATIONAL, INTERMARRIAGE, TEXAS, SOUTHWEST
ABST WHILE SURVEYS INDICATE THAT ETHNIC INTERGROUP COOPERATION IN TEXAS IS INCREASING, MINORITY YOUTHS TEND TO REFLECT A SEPARATIST ATTITUDE AGAINST WHITES. A STUDY OF AGE-RELATED ATTITUDES CONCERNING APPROVED SOCIAL INTERACTION AND ETHNIC ATTITUDES TOWARDS EQUALITY REVEALED THAT MEXICAN AMERICANS IN HOUSTON WERE (1) MORE TOLERANT OF BLACKS THAN WERE WHITES, (2) MORE APT

TO TO SEE BLOCKAGE TO MINORITY OPPORTUNITIES THAN WHITES, AND (3) MORE SUPPORTIVE OF MEANS TO ACHIEVE MINORITY EQUALITY THAN WHITES. AGE WAS NOT FOUND TO BE A FACTOR OF ATTITUDAL DIFFERENCES WITHIN ETHNIC GROUPS. YOUNGER GROUPS WERE AT TIMES MORE CONSERVATIVE, BUT THEY WERE MORE APT TO ACCEPT INTERRACIAL MARRIAGE AMONG WHITES THAN WERE THE OLDER GROUPS. IT APPEARS THAT BLACKS MORE SO THAN MEXICAN AMERICANS PERCEIVED THEIR OWN GROUP AS UNEQUAL, CONSIDERED QUOTAS AND DEMONSTRATIONS AS MEANS TO OBTAIN EQUALITY, AND WERE UNHAPPY WITH THE GOVERNMENT'S PROGRESS IN CIVIL RIGHTS. 16 REFERENCES.

ACCN 000355

415 AUTH **DAVIS, E. E., & EKWALL, E. E.**
TITL MODE OF PERCEPTION AND FRUSTRATION IN READING.
SRCE *JOURNAL OF CLINICAL PSYCHOLOGY, 1976, 32(4), 798-800.*
INDX READING, PERCEPTION, CHILDREN, MEXICAN AMERICAN, STRESS, ANXIETY, INSTRUCTIONAL TECHNIQUES, WISC, BENDER VISUAL-MOTOR GESTALT TEST, RORSCHACH TEST, EMPIRICAL, CROSS CULTURAL
ABST DUE TO THE CLOSE RELATIONSHIP BETWEEN PERCEPTION AND READING, IT WAS HYPOTHESIZED THAT OBSERVED MODES OF PERCEPTION (AS MEASURED BY THE WISC, THE BENDER VISUAL MOTOR-GESTALT TEST, THE RORSCHACH INK BLOT TEST, AND THE HOUSE-TREE-PERSON TECHNIQUE) COULD BE EMPLOYED EFFECTIVELY TO PREDICT THE FRUSTRATION READING LEVEL FOR ELEMENTARY SCHOOL CHILDREN. INVESTIGATIONS WERE MADE OF READING FRUSTRATION LEVELS (I.E., THE DEGREE OF FAILURE SUFFICIENT TO CAUSE PHYSIOLOGICAL INDICATIONS OF EMOTIONAL STRESS ON POLYGRAPH RECORDINGS) IN 62 ELEMENTARY SCHOOL CHILDREN. APPROXIMATELY EQUAL NUMBERS OF ANGLOS, BLACKS, AND MEXICAN AMERICANS PARTICIPATED. IT WAS FOUND THAT MOST CHILDREN WITH A LESS RESTRICTED, MORE EXPANSIVE MODE OF PERCEPTION BEGIN TO SHOW SIGNS OF FRUSTRATION UPON REACHING 6-9 ORAL READING ERRORS. FOR PUPILS WHO ARE JUDGED TO BE MORE RESTRICTED IN THEIR MODE OF PERCEPTION, THE DEGREE OF FAILURE NEEDED TO CAUSE INDICATIONS OF FRUSTRATION IS TWICE AS GREAT. THE IMPLICATION IS THAT, FOR MOST CHILDREN, READING PASSAGES FOR INSTRUCTIONAL PURPOSES MUST BE NO MORE DIFFICULT THAN TO ALLOW FOR ABOUT 5 ORAL READING ERRORS. 12 REFERENCES.

ACCN 002062

416 AUTH **DAVIS, E. E., & ROWLAND, T.**
TITL A REPLACEMENT FOR THE VENERABLE STANFORD-BINET.
SRCE *JOURNAL OF CLINICAL PSYCHOLOGY, 1974, 30(4), 517-521.*
INDX INTELLIGENCE TESTING, ETHNIC IDENTITY, MEXICAN AMERICAN, TEST VALIDITY, STANFORD-BINET INTELLIGENCE TEST, EARLY

CHILDHOOD EDUCATION, CROSS CULTURAL, TEXAS, SOUTHWEST

ABST CURRENT INTEREST IN EARLY CHILDHOOD EDUCATION HAS SPURRED EFFORTS TO PRODUCE TESTS OF THE GENERAL MENTAL ABILITY OF YOUNG CHILDREN THAT WILL BE AS PRODUCTIVE AS THE STANFORD-BINET AND YET AT THE SAME TIME AVOID SOME OF ITS WEAKNESSES WHICH HAVE BECOME EVIDENT OVER THE YEARS. RESULTS OF TESTING 33 CHILDREN WITH BOTH THE MCCARTHY SCALES OF CHILDREN'S ABILITIES AND THE STANFORD-BINET INTELLIGENCE SCALES PROVIDE THE BASIS FOR A DISCUSSION OF THE TWO TESTS. MANY WORKERS PROBABLY WILL PREFER THE STRUCTURE OF THE MSCA, AND EVIDENCE IS PRESENTED FOR THE TENTATIVE JUDGMENT THAT THE NEW TEST YIELDS SCORES THAT PARALLEL BINET IQ'S. 11 REFERENCES. (AUTHOR SUMMARY)

ACCN 000356

417 AUTH **DAVIS, E. E., & WALKER, C.**
TITL VALIDITY OF THE MCCARTHY SCALES FOR SOUTHWESTERN RURAL CHILDREN.
SRCE *PERCEPTION AND MOTOR SKILLS, 1976, 42, 563-567.*
INDX ABILITY TESTING, CHILDREN, CULTURAL FACTORS, CULTURE-FAIR TESTS, EARLY CHILDHOOD EDUCATION, EMPIRICAL, INTELLIGENCE TESTING, ITPA, MEXICAN AMERICAN, STANFORD-BINET INTELLIGENCE TEST, TEXAS, SOUTHWEST, TEST VALIDITY, RURAL
ABST A STUDY ASSESSING THE VALIDITY OF THE MCCARTHY SCALES OF CHILDREN'S ABILITIES FOR AMERICAN SOUTHWESTERN RURAL CHILDREN IS PRESENTED. MCCARTHY SCORES WERE COMPARED WITH SCORES ON THE STANFORD-BINET INTELLIGENCE SCALE, THE ILLINOIS TEST OF PSYCHOLINGUISTIC ABILITIES, AND THE TEST FOR AUDITORY COMPREHENSION OF LANGUAGE FOR 49 KINDERGARTEN CHILDREN ABOUT 5.5 YEARS OF AGE. THE MAJORITY OF THE CHILDREN HAD BEEN STRONGLY INFLUENCED BY THE SPANISH LANGUAGE AND MEXICAN CULTURE. ALTHOUGH THE MEANS FOR THE TESTS WERE MOSTLY LOW, INTERCORRELATIONS WITH OTHER TESTS AND WITH PREVIOUS RESULTS WERE SATISFACTORY. IT IS CONCLUDED THAT THESE INTERCORRELATIONS ARE EVIDENCE OF THE CONCURRENT VALIDITY OF THE MCCARTHY SCALES. 19 REFERENCES. (NCHHI ABSTRACT)
ACCN 002063

418 AUTH **DAVIS, O. L., JR., & PERSONKE, C. R., JR.**
TITL EFFECTS OF ADMINISTERING THE METROPOLITAN READINESS TEST IN ENGLISH AND SPANISH TO SPANISH SPEAKING SCHOOL ENTRANTS.
SRCE *JOURNAL OF EDUCATIONAL MEASUREMENT, 1968, 5(3), 231-234.*
INDX METROPOLITAN READINESS TEST, TEST VALIDITY, CHILDREN, EMPIRICAL, SPANISH SURNAMED, INTELLIGENCE TESTING, TEXAS, SOUTHWEST
ABST THE METROPOLITAN READINESS TEST WAS ADMINISTERED BOTH IN ENGLISH AND SPAN-

ISH TO 88 CHILDREN WITH SPANISH SURNAMES. MOST OF THE MEAN DIFFERENCES WERE NOT STATISTICALLY SIGNIFICANT. IT IS CONCLUDED THAT LANGUAGE ITSELF IS NOT THE CRITICAL COMPONENT OF CULTURE-FAIRNESS IN THE TESTING OF THESE CHILDREN. IT IS SUGGESTED THAT PREVIOUS LEARNING, SPECIFICALLY THE INADEQUACY OF EXPERIENTIAL BACKGROUND, PROBABLY IS A MORE IMPORTANT DETERMINANT OF LOW PERFORMANCE THAN THE LANGUAGE IN WHICH THE TEST IS ADMINISTERED. 5 REFERENCES.

ACCN 000357

419 AUTH **DAY, R. C., & CHADWICK, B. A.**
TITL PROGRAMMED REINFORCEMENT IN THE CLASSROOM: THE EFFECTS OF TANGIBLE AND SOCIAL REWARDS ON THE EDUCATIONAL ACHIEVEMENT OF MEXICAN AMERICAN AND BLACK CHILDREN. (GRANT NO. MH-14497).
SRCE *FINAL REPORT PRESENTED TO THE NATIONAL INSTITUTE OF MENTAL HEALTH, 1970.*
INDX BEHAVIOR MODIFICATION, CLASSROOM BEHAVIOR, MIGRANTS, WASHINGTON, WEST, CROSS CULTURAL, MEXICAN AMERICAN, CHILDREN, EMPIRICAL, INSTRUCTIONAL TECHNIQUES, SCHOLASTIC ACHIEVEMENT
ABST FINDINGS FROM PRELIMINARY AND FOLLOWUP STUDIES ON THE EFFECTIVENESS OF SYSTEMATICALLY SCHEDULED REINFORCEMENT, COMBINING MATERIAL AND SOCIAL REINFORCERS TO IMPROVE THE ACADEMIC PERFORMANCE OF POORLY MOTIVATED, UNDERACHIEVING MEXICAN AMERICAN AND BLACK CHILDREN WITH CLASSROOM BEHAVIORAL PROBLEMS, ARE PRESENTED. THE MEXICAN AMERICAN CHILDREN WERE FROM MIGRANT FARM LABOR FAMILIES OR FROM FAMILIES THAT HAD RECENTLY DROPPED OUT OF THE MIGRANT STREAM TO SETTLE IN PASCO OR KENNEWICK, WASHINGTON, ON A RELATIVELY PERMANENT BASIS. THE BLACK CHILDREN WERE FROM FAMILIES THAT MIGRATED TO THE PASCO AREA DURING AND FOLLOWING WORLD WAR II TO WORK IN DEFENSE-RELATED INDUSTRIES. THE OBJECTIVES OF THE STUDY WERE AS FOLLOWS: (1) TO TEST THE EFFECTS OF PROGRAMMED REINFORCEMENT IN THE CLASSROOM PERFORMANCE OF 25 UNDERACHIEVING, DISRUPTIVE CHILDREN FROM ECONOMICALLY DEPRIVED, MINORITY-GROUP BACKGROUNDS; (2) TO TEST THE EFFECT AND STRENGTH OF TEACHER MEDIATED SOCIAL REINFORCERS ON THE CHILDREN'S ACADEMIC AND SOCIAL RESPONSES; (3) TO EXPLORE THE PARENTAL ATTITUDES ABOUT THEIR CHILDREN'S ACADEMIC AND SOCIAL PERFORMANCE; AND (4) TO ASSESS THE CHANGE IN STUDENT ATTITUDES TOWARD SELF, SCHOOL, THE TEACHER, AND VARIOUS ACADEMIC ACTIVITIES AS A CONSEQUENCE OF PARTICIPATION IN THE PROGRAMMED REINFORCEMENT SYSTEM. 53 REFERENCES.
ACCN 000358

420 AUTH **DE AVILA, E. A., & HAVASSY, B. E.**
TITL PIAGETIAN ALTERNATIVE TO IQ: MEXICAN-AMERICAN STUDY.

SRCE *IN N. HOBBS (ED.), ISSUES IN THE CLASSIFICA-TION OF EXCEPTIONAL CHILDREN. SAN FRAN-CISCO: JOSSEY-BASS PUBLISHERS, 1975, PP. 246-265.*

INDX INTELLIGENCE, MEXICAN AMERICAN, INTELLI-GENCE TESTING, TEST VALIDITY, COGNITIVE DEVELOPMENT, COGNITIVE STYLE, RESEARCH METHODOLOGY, CROSS CULTURAL, SEX COM-PARISON, CHILDREN, EMPIRICAL, NEW MEXICO, COLORADO, TEXAS, CALIFORNIA, SOUTHWEST

ABST USING PIAGETIAN MEASURES OF COGNITIVE DEVELOPMENT TO ASSESS THE LEVEL OF IN-TELLECTUAL FUNCTIONING OF DIFFERENT AGE GROUPS WITHIN A MEXICAN AMERICAN POPU-LATION, IT WAS FOUND THAT MEXICAN AMERI-CAN CHILDREN PERFORMED AT COGNITIVE LEVELS APPROPRIATE FOR THEIR CHRONO-LOGICAL AGE. MOREOVER, NO DIFFERENCES IN LEVEL OF COGNITIVE DEVELOPMENTAL PERFORMANCE WERE FOUND BETWEEN AN-GLO AND MEXICAN AMERICAN CHILDREN. DATA ALSO SHOW THE SAME DEVELOPMENTAL CURVES FOR BOTH ETHNIC GROUPS. FROM THESE FINDINGS IT IS CONCLUDED: (1) THAT MEXICAN AMERICAN CHILDREN DEVELOP COGNITIVELY THE SAME AS, AND AT BASICALLY THE SAME RATE AS, ANGLO CHILDREN; (2) THAT THE FAILURE OF MEXICAN AMERICAN CHILDREN TO PERFORM WELL ON STANDARD-IZED TESTS MUST BE ATTRIBUTED TO REA-SONS OTHER THAN THEIR ALLEGED COGNI-TIVE INABILITY; AND (3) THAT THE REASONS FOR POOR PERFORMANCE BY MINORITY CHIL-DREN ON STANDARDIZED TESTS LIES IN THE TEST BIASES AND THE CURRICULUM USED IN MOST SCHOOLS. 31 REFERENCES. (AUTHOR SUMMARY MODIFIED)

ACCN 000360

421 AUTH **DE HOYOS, A., & DE HOYOS, G.**

TITL THE AMIGO SYSTEM AND ALIENATION OF THE WIFE IN THE CONJUGAL MEXICAN FAMILY.

SRCE *IN B. FARBER (ED.), KINSHIP AND FAMILY OR-GANIZATION. NEW YORK: JOHN WILEY AND SONS, 1966, PP. 102-115.*

INDX ANOMIE, MEXICAN, FAMILY STRUCTURE, FAMILY ROLES, EMPIRICAL, CULTURAL FACTORS, ROLE EXPECTATIONS, MARRIAGE, PEER GROUP, SEX ROLES, MALE, FEMALE

ABST THE AMIGO SYSTEM, INFORMAL GROUPS OF MALE PEERS WHICH SIGNIFICANTLY INFLU-ENCE THE SOCIALIZATION OF MEXICAN MALES, WAS INVESTIGATED IN RELATION TO THE AL-IENATION OF THE WIFE IN THE MEXICAN CON-JUGAL SYSTEM. IT WAS HYPOTHESIZED THAT IN THOSE FAMILIES WHERE THE HUSBAND KEEPS CLOSE INVOLVEMENT WITH HIS AMIGO SYSTEM, ALIENATION OF THE WIFE IS PRESENT. THE PRINCIPAL ASSUMPTION WAS THAT CON-FLICT BETWEEN THE AMIGO SYSTEM AND THE CONJUGAL SYSTEM IS BASED ON THESE FOUR FACTORS: (1) COMPETITION FOR SCARCE RE-SOURCES—E.G., TIME, MONEY AND LOYALTY; (2) CONFLICTING VALUE ORIENTATIONS OF THE HUSBAND AND WIFE; (3) RELATIVE LOW STATUS OF MARRIAGE IN THE CULTURE; AND (4) DIFFERENTIAL STATUS OF MALE AND FE-MALE IN THE CULTURE. SCALE RESPONSES

MEASURING HUSBAND'S PARTICIPATION IN THE AMIGO SYSTEM AND ALIENATION IN THE WIFE FROM 101 MARRIED WOMEN LIVING IN CIUDAD JUAREZ WERE ANALYZED BY CORRELATION ANALYSIS AND ANALYSIS OF VARIANCE. RE-SULTS SHOW A STATISTICALLY SIGNIFICANT POSITIVE ASSOCIATION BETWEEN THE HUS-BAND'S PARTICIPATION IN THE AMIGO SYSTEM AND THE ALIENATION OF THE WIFE. OTHER FINDINGS ARE DISCUSSED IN TERMS OF THE SPOUSE'S SOCIAL CLASS, EDUCATION, AGE, NUMBER OF CHILDREN, AND YEARS MARRIED. ALSO DISCUSSED ARE THE SOCIAL PRO-CESSES OF ADAPTATION, GOAL ACHIEVEMENT, INTEGRATION AND PATTERN MAINTENANCE AS THEY AFFECT THE AMIGO SYSTEM AND MEXI-CAN FAMILY LIFE. 19 REFERENCES.

ACCN 000367

422 AUTH **DE LA VEGA, M.**

TITL SOME FACTORS AFFECTING LEADERSHIP OF MEXICAN AMERICANS IN A HIGH SCHOOL.

SRCE *SAN FRANCISCO: R AND E RESEARCH ASSOCI-ATES, 1974. (REPRINTED FROM AN UNPUB-LISHED MASTER'S THESIS, UNIVERSITY OF SOUTHERN CALIFORNIA, 1951.)*

INDX MEXICAN AMERICAN, ADOLESCENTS, LEAD-ERSHIP, FAMILY ROLES, AUTHORITARIANISM, SES, RELIGION, ACHIEVEMENT MOTIVATION, EDUCATION, ATTITUDES, PEER GROUP, EMPIR-ICAL, SCHOLASTIC ACHIEVEMENT, TEACHERS, CALIFORNIA, SOUTHWEST, ENVIRONMENTAL FACTORS

ABST CONDITIONS THAT AID OR PREVENT THE DE-VELOPMENT OF LEADERSHIP IN MEXICAN AMERICAN STUDENTS WERE STUDIED THROUGH INTERVIEWS WITH 22 MEXICAN AMERICAN AND NON-MEXICAN AMERICAN STUDENTS FROM A WHITTIER, CALIFORNIA, HIGH SCHOOL IN 1951. INTERVIEW QUESTIONS COVERED LANGUAGE HANDICAP, NEED FOR BELONGING, ATTITUDE TOWARD TEACHERS AND MEXICAN AMERICAN STUDENT LEADERS AND RELATIONSHIP TO PARENTS. EDITED TRANSCRIPTS OF THE STUDENT INTERVIEWS ARE INCLUDED. FIVE MAJOR CONCLUSIONS ARE DISCUSSED: (1) THE EMOTIONAL NEED FOR BELONGING AND FOR ACHIEVEMENT ARE FRUSTRATED IN THESE MEXICAN AMERICAN HIGH SCHOOL STUDENTS; (2) THERE ARE IN-DICATIONS THAT IMPROVEMENT OF COMMU-NICATION BETWEEN TEACHER AND STUDENT MAY BRING ABOUT A BETTER MOTIVATION OF MEXICAN AMERICAN STUDENTS AT THE SEC-ONDARY LEVEL; (3) THE GREATEST HANDICAP IS NOT OF LANGUAGE BUT RATHER CULTURE AND SOCIAL CLASS (EXTREME DISSIMILARITY OF ENVIRONMENTS FAMILIAR TO MEXICAN AMERICAN STUDENTS AND MAJORITY CUL-TURE TEACHERS); (4) THAT THIS PARTICULAR SCHOOL SITUATION IS BASICALLY NO DIFFER-ENT FROM THAT EXISTING ELSEWHERE IN THE COUNTRY WITH RESPECT TO CURRICULUM ORGANIZATION (COLLEGE PREPARATORY, GENERAL AND COMMERCIAL); AND (5) EN-ROLLMENT IN EACH TYPE OF COURSE IS RE-LATED VERY SIGNIFICANTLY TO STUDENT SO-CIAL CLASS STATUS. IN LIGHT OF THESE

OBSERVATIONS, IT SEEMS THAT THE PROBLEMS OF MEXICAN AMERICAN ADJUSTMENT IN THE SECONDARY SCHOOLS AND THE LACK OF LEADERSHIP DO NOT NECESSARILY ARISE FROM A PURELY ETHNIC SOURCE, BUT MAY HAVE ROOTS IN THE SOCIAL CLASS STRUCTURE OF AMERICAN LIFE. 20 REFERENCES. (AUTHOR SUMMARY MODIFIED)

ACCN   000361

423 AUTH **DE LA ZERDA FLORES, N., & HOPPER, R.**
     TITL   MEXICAN AMERICAN'S EVALUATIONS OF SPOKEN SPANISH AND ENGLISH.
     SRCE   *SPEECH MONOGRAPHS, 1974, 42(2), 91-98.*
     INDX   LINGUISTICS, BILINGUALISM, PHONOLOGY, MEXICAN AMERICAN, ATTITUDES, ACCULTURATION, ADOLESCENTS, ADULTS, COGNITIVE DEVELOPMENT, BILINGUAL, TEXAS, SOUTHWEST
     ABST   RELATIONSHIPS BETWEEN THE DEGREE OF ACCULTURATION OF MEXICAN AMERICANS AND THEIR ATTITUDES TOWARD THE LANGUAGES (STANDARD ENGLISH, STANDARD SPANISH, ACCENTED ENGLISH, AND TEXAN MEXICAN) COMMONLY USED WITHIN THE MEXICAN AMERICAN AND ANGLO AMERICAN CULTURES ARE EXAMINED. IT IS HYPOTHESIZED THAT MEXICAN AMERICANS WOULD REACT IN VARIED WAYS TO EACH LANGUAGE GUISE ACCORDING TO (1) THE EXTENT TO WHICH THEY IDENTIFY WITH THE SPEECH COMMUNITY REPRESENTED BY EACH DIALECT, AND (2) PERSONAL STEREOTYPES HELD ABOUT EACH OF THE SPEECH COMMUNITIES. SIXTY-TWO MEXICAN AMERICAN ADULTS RESPONDED TO TAPED SAMPLES OF THE FOUR LANGUAGE GUISES. THEIR LANGUAGE EVALUATION SCORES WERE CORRELATED TO ACCULTURATION AND ATTITUDE VARIABLES MEASURED BY (1) ETHNIC SELF-REFERENT, (2) AMOUNT OF SPANISH USED, (3) INCOME AND OCCUPATION, (4) TIES WITH MEXICO, (5) LEVEL OF EDUCATION, (6) AGE, AND (7) POLICY OF SCHOOL TOWARD SPANISH (FOR STUDENT PARTICIPANTS). FINDINGS SUPPORT THE HYPOTHESIS THAT LISTENERS REACT DIFFERENTLY TO DIFFERENT SPEECH SAMPLES. THE MOST SIGNIFICANT DIFFERENCE WAS DETERMINED BY THE VARIABLES OF AGE AND PREFERRED SELF-REFERENT. THE MOST IMPORTANT FINDING WAS THAT SPANISH AS THE LANGUAGE OF LA RAZA IS STILL VIEWED POSITIVELY BY MOST MEXICAN AMERICANS. 11 REFERENCES.
     ACCN   000362

424 AUTH **DE LAZARIN, A. N.**
     TITL   THE CHICANO: PERSPECTIVES FOR EDUCATION.
     SRCE   *ENCUENTRO FEMENIL, 1973, 1(1), 34-61.*
     INDX   ATTITUDES, CULTURAL FACTORS, EDUCATION, EDUCATIONAL COUNSELING, ESSAY, MEXICAN AMERICAN, PHYSICAL DEVELOPMENT, ADOLESCENTS, PREJUDICE, RELIGION, STEREOTYPES, CASE STUDY
     ABST   INTENDED PRIMARILY FOR COUNSELOR PRACTITIONERS WISHING TO ENHANCE THEIR SKILLS IN WORKING WITH MEXICAN AMERICAN YOUTHS, THIS BOOK HAS THE FOLLOWING OBJECTIVES: (1) TO EXAMINE AND MINIMIZE STEREOTYPES THAT HAVE PERPETUATED FOR MANY YEARS AND TO EMPHASIZE THE UNIQUENESS, DIGNITY, AND WORTH OF EACH INDIVIDUAL MEXICAN AMERICAN; (2) TO DESCRIBE VARIOUS LEGITIMATE CHARACTERISTICS, CONCERNS, AND PROBLEMS OF MEXICAN AMERICAN ADOLESCENTS; (3) TO DESCRIBE AND EXAMINE THE THEORETICAL AND PRACTICAL ASPECTS OF THE PROCESS OF COUNSELING AS A MEANS OF HELPING MEXICAN AMERICAN YOUTHS RESOLVE THESE CONCERNS AND PROBLEMS; (4) TO DESCRIBE AND EXAMINE THE VARIOUS FUNCTIONS AND ROLES THAT COUNSELORS OF MEXICAN AMERICAN ADOLESCENTS CAN ASSUME IN ATTEMPTING TO HELP THESE YOUTHS; AND (5) TO PROVIDE COUNSELORS WITH EXAMPLES OF ACTUAL COUNSELING CASES INVOLVING MEXICAN AMERICAN YOUTHS. THE FIVE CHAPTERS COVER: (1) THE SOCIAL PSYCHOLOGY OF THE MEXICAN AMERICAN; (2) THE DEVELOPMENTAL, BIOLOGICAL, PSYCHOLOGICAL, AND SOCIOLOGICAL CHARACTERISTICS OF ADOLESCENTS WITH EMPHASIS GIVEN TO PROBLEMS UNIQUE TO MEXICAN AMERICAN YOUTHS; (3) THE INGREDIENTS OF EFFECTIVE COUNSELING; (4) PROCEDURAL ASPECTS OF COUNSELING INCLUDING THE VARIOUS ROLES THAT COUNSELORS SHOULD ASSUME; (5) A PRESENTATION OF FOUR COUNSELING CASES INVOLVING MEXICAN AMERICANS; AND (6) A DESCRIPTION OF THE FUTURE OF COUNSELING FOR MEXICAN AMERICAN YOUTHS. 42 REFERENCES.
     ACCN   000363

425 AUTH **DE LEON, G.**
     TITL   PHOENIX HOUSE THERAPEUTIC COMMUNITY: THE INFLUENCE OF TIME IN PROGRAM ON CHANGE IN RESIDENT DRUG ADDICTS.
     SRCE   *PROCEEDINGS OF THE 81ST ANNUAL CONVENTION OF THE AMERICAN PSYCHOLOGICAL ASSOCIATION, 1973, 8, 397-398.*
     INDX   THERAPEUTIC COMMUNITY, DRUG ABUSE, DRUG ADDICTION, MENTAL HEALTH, ADULTS, SCHIZOPHRENIA, SELF CONCEPT, ATTITUDES, PSYCHOTHERAPY OUTCOME, PROGRAM EVALUATION, PUERTO RICAN-M, NEW YORK, EAST, URBAN, REHABILITATION
     ABST   THREE DIFFERENT STUDIES INVOLVING ANGLO, BLACK AND PUERTO RICAN PATIENTS AT THE NEW YORK CITY TREATMENT COMMUNITY, PHOENIX HOUSE, ARE REVIEWED. THOUGH EACH USES DIFFERENT INDICATORS FOR MEASURING CHANGE IN DRUG ADDICTS (I.E., CRIMINAL ACTIVITY, PSYCHOPATHOLOGICAL SIGNS AND EMOTIONALITY), EACH STUDY SHOWED THAT THE ADDICTS WHO ATTENDED THE PROGRAM IMPROVED. THE EXTENT OF OVERALL THERAPEUTIC EFFECT INCREASED WITH LENGTH OF RESIDENCE. THESE FINDINGS ARE PARTICULARLY STRIKING IN THAT THEY WERE OBTAINED WITH DIFFERENT SAMPLES ACROSS SEVERAL YEARS OF RESEARCH AND WITH DIFFERENCES IN MEASURES AND METHODS. A MOST IMPORTANT IM-

PLICATION DRAWN FROM THE ABOVE FINDING IS THAT ASSESSMENT OF THE EFFICACY OF A THERAPEUTIC COMMUNITY PROGRAM MUST INCLUDE STUDIES NOT ONLY OF ITS GRADU-ATES OR CURES, BUT ALSO THE MANY INDI-VIDUALS WHO DROP OUT OF THE PROGRAM AGAINST CLINICAL ADVICE. FOLLOW-UPS OF THESE PATIENTS CAN PROVIDE DATA ON THE DIFFERENCES BETWEEN DRUG ABUSERS AND GRADATIONS IN TREATMENT CRITERIA. 3 REF-ERENCES.

ACCN   000364

426 AUTH **DE LEON, O., SEVILLA, E., & SALAS, G.**
     TITL   ASPECTOS TRANSCULTURALES DE LA QUEJA SOMATICA: FACTORES SOCIALES Y DE PER-SONALIDAD. (TRANSCULTURAL ASPECTS OF THE SOMATIC COMPLAINT: PERSONALITY AND SOCIAL FACTORS.)
     SRCE   *REVISTA DE NEURO-PSIQUIATRIA (LIMA), 1976, 39(1), 10-23. (SPANISH)*
     INDX   MEXICAN AMERICAN, CROSS CULTURAL, EM-PIRICAL, ADULTS, FEMALE, ILLINOIS, MIDWEST, CULTURAL FACTORS, HEALTH, MENTAL HEALTH, IMMIGRATION, PSYCHOPATHOLOGY, SYMP-TOMATOLOGY
     ABST   TO ASCERTAIN SOCIOCULTURAL DIFFER-ENCES IN THE EXPRESSION OF PSYCHOSO-MATIC SYMPTOMATIC BEHAVIOR, A COMPARI-SON WAS MADE BETWEEN TWO CULTURALLY DISTINCT SETS OF FEMALE PSYCHIATRIC OUT-PATIENTS WHO LIVED IN THE SAME LOWER-CLASS NEIGHBORHOOD IN CHICAGO. 28 SUB-JECTS WERE RECENT IMMIGRANTS FROM MEXICO (AVERAGE AGE OF 40.8 YEARS) AND 34 WERE CENTRAL EUROPEAN IMMIGRANTS WHO HAD SPENT MANY YEARS IN THE U.S. (AV-ERAGE AGE OF 52.7YEARS). SUBJECTS WERE ASSESSED BY MEANS OF THE CORNELL MEDI-CAL INDEX (CMI), THE EYSENCK PERSONALITY INVENTORY (EPI), AND THE WHITELEY INDEX OF HYPOCHONDRIASIS (WIH). NO SIGNIFICANT DIFFERENCE DUE TO ETHNICITY WAS FOUND, AS BOTH GROUPS EXHIBITED SIMILAR PRO-FILES ON THE CMI, EPI, AND WIH. ALTHOUGH IT IS NORMALLY ASSUMED THAT PSYCHOSO-MATIC COMPLAINTS INCREASE WITH AGE, AGE WAS FOUND TO BE OF NO IMPORTANCE AMONG THESE SUBJECTS AS THE YOUNGER AND OLDER GROUPS HAD SIMILAR TEST RESULTS. ALSO, INCOME AND EDUCATION WERE NOT FOUND TO BE ASSOCIATED WITH PSYCHOSO-MATIC COMPLAINTS. ONE DIFFERENCE, HOW-EVER, WAS THAT THE MEXICAN AMERICAN SUBJECTS HAD A HIGHER PROPORTION OF COMPLAINTS. THIS CAN BE EXPLAINED BY THE RECENCY OF THEIR IMMIGRATION AND THEIR SLIGHT COMMAND OF ENGLISH. IN CONCLU-SION, THESE PSYCHOSOMATIC COMPLAINTS ARE CONSIDERED TO BE EGO ADAPTIVE DE-VICES IN RESPONSE TO THE PROCESS OF EN-CULTURATION AND THE INTERNALIZATION OF NORMATIVE ELEMENTS OF THE HOST CUL-TURE. 37 REFERENCES. (AUTHOR ABSTRACT MODIFIED)

ACCN   002064

427 AUTH **DE RIOS, M. D., & FELDMAN, D. J.**

TITL   SOUTHERN CALIFORNIAN MEXICAN AMERI-CAN DRINKING PATTERNS: SOME PRELIMINARY OBSERVATIONS.
SRCE   *JOURNAL OF PSYCHEDELIC DRUGS, 1977, 9(2), 151-158.*
INDX   ALCOHOLISM, ACCULTURATION, ADULTS, ATTI-TUDES, COPING MECHANISMS, CROSS GEN-ERATIONAL, CULTURAL FACTORS, EMPIRICAL, HEALTH, MALE, MENTAL HEALTH, MEXICAN, MEXICAN AMERICAN, RESOURCE UTILIZATION, SELF CONCEPT, SES, SOCIAL SERVICES, SPAN-ISH SURNAMED, URBAN, SOUTHWEST, CALI-FORNIA, STRESS
ABST   A STUDY OF MEXICAN AMERICAN ALCOHOL USE IN SOUTHERN CALIFORNIA WAS MADE TO DETERMINE WHY THE TREATMENT RECORD FOR THIS POPULATION IS SO POOR. CON-DUCTED DURING A 14-MONTH PERIOD, RE-SEARCH WAS CARRIED OUT VIA DAY-TO-DAY INTERVIEWING AND PARTICIPANT OBSERVA-TION IN A VARIETY OF NEIGHBORHOOD SET-TINGS—INCLUDING SPANISH-SPEAKING AL-COHOLICS ANONYMOUS MEETINGS, PERIODIC THERAPY GROUPS WITH MEXICAN AMERICAN ALCOHOLICS, AND LOCAL BARS WHERE IN-FORMAL INTERVIEWS WERE CONDUCTED BOTH WITH PATRONS AND WITH MEXICAN AMERICAN BARTENDERS, WAITERS, AND WAITRESSES RE-GARDING CLIENT DRINKING PATTERNS. IN AD-DITION, INTERVIEWS WERE CONDUCTED WITH SPANISH-SPEAKING COUNSELORS IN LOCAL MENTAL HEALTH CENTERS AND WITH MEXICAN AMERICAN MENTAL HEALTH WORKERS EM-PLOYED BY THE COUNTY, REGARDING THEIR OBSERVATIONS ON SOCIAL AND CULTURAL FACTORS INFLUENCING MEXICAN AMERICAN ALCOHOLISM. FROM THESE DATA PLUS PER-SONAL BIOGRAPHIES OF SELF-DISCLOSED MEXICAN AMERICAN ALCOHOLICS, THE REA-SONS FOR THE POOR TREATMENT RECORD WERE FOUND TO BE MOSTLY CULTURAL ONES. AMONG THEM WERE: (1) VARIATIONS IN FORM AND STRUCTURE OF LIFESTYLE IN THE MEXI-CAN AMERICAN COMMUNITY; (2) A TRADITION OF LEARNING ACCULTURATION AND COPING MECHANISMS THROUGH INTERACTIONS AT LOCAL BARS; (3) A DISTRUST AND SUSPICION ON THE PART OF MINORITY GROUP PEOPLE TOWARD ESTABLISHMENT AGENCIES; AND (4) MENTAL STRESSES RELATED TO MINORITY GROUP STATUS USED AS JUSTIFICATION FOR ALCOHOL USE. IT IS CONCLUDED THAT THE MOST EFFECTIVE TREATMENT WOULD BE ONE THAT OFFERS THE INDIVIDUAL A MORE SATIS-FYING PAYOFF FOR NOT DRINKING THAN THE ONE PRESENTLY RECEIVED FROM DRINKING. 31 REFERENCES.
ACCN   002065

428 AUTH **DE RODRIGUEZ, L. V.**
TITL   SOCIAL WORK PRACTICE IN PUERTO RICO.
SRCE   *SOCIAL WORK, 1973, 18(2), 32-40.*
INDX   MENTAL HEALTH, SOCIAL SERVICES, PUERTO RICAN-I, ENVIRONMENTAL FACTORS, CUL-TURAL FACTORS, ESSAY, ECONOMIC FACTORS
ABST   THE CONCEPT OF SELF-DETERMINATION POSES SERIOUS QUESTIONS FOR THE SOCIAL WORKER IN PUERTO RICO. IN ATTEMPTING TO HELP

CLIENTS MAKE DECISIONS, THE SOCIAL WORKER ENCOUNTERS ATTITUDES, LIFE STYLES, AND ECONOMIC AND SOCIAL CONDITIONS QUITE DIFFERENT FROM THOSE ON THE MAINLAND. THESE DIFFERENCES ARE IDENTIFIED AND DISCUSSED IN TERMS OF 3 MAIN FACTORS: (1) HISTORICAL DEVELOPMENT OF THE ISLAND; (2) GEOGRAPHIC LIMITATIONS; AND (3) DEVELOPMENT OF SOCIAL WORK UNDER GOVERNMENT AUSPICES. IT IS CONCLUDED THAT PUERTO RICAN SOCIAL WORKERS HAVE TO DEVELOP SERVICES THAT ARE ADAPTED TO THE LIFE STYLE OF THE ISLAND IF THEY ARE TO FULFILL THEIR CLIENTS' EXPECTATIONS.

ACCN   000365

429 AUTH   **DEAN, R. S.**
     TITL   INTERNAL CONSISTENCY OF THE PIAT WITH MEXICAN-AMERICAN CHILDREN.
     SRCE   *PSYCHOLOGY IN THE SCHOOLS, 1977, 14(2), 167-171.*
     INDX   ACHIEVEMENT TESTING, CHILDREN, CROSS CULTURAL, CULTURE-FAIR TESTS, EMPIRICAL, MEXICAN AMERICAN, ARIZONA, SOUTHWEST, TEST RELIABILITY, TEST VALIDITY
     ABST   AN INVESTIGATION TO DETERMINE THE RELIABILITY AND THE STANDARD ERROR OF MEASUREMENT OF THE PEABODY INDIVIDUAL ACHIEVEMENT TEST (PIAT) WHEN ADMINISTERED TO SEPARATE SAMPLES OF 30 ANGLO AND 30 MEXICAN AMERICAN CHILDREN (6 TO 16 YEARS-OLD) IS REPORTED. SPLIT-HALF RELIABILITIES FOR BOTH GROUPS WERE SIMILAR TO STABILITY RELIABILITIES FOUND IN STANDARDIZATION. INDICES OF INTERNAL CONSISTENCY AND STANDARD ERRORS OF MEASUREMENT WERE GENERALLY EQUIVALENT FOR THE TWO GROUPS. IT IS CONCLUDED THAT THE PIAT IS AS RELIABLE WITH MEXICAN AMERICAN CHILDREN AS WITH THEIR ANGLO COUNTERPARTS. 3 REFERENCES. (NCHHI ABSTRACT)
     ACCN   002067

430 AUTH   **DEAN, R. S.**
     TITL   V. RELIABILITY OF THE WISC-R WITH MEXICAN-AMERICAN CHILDREN.
     SRCE   *JOURNAL OF SCHOOL PSYCHOLOGY, 1977, 15(3), 267-268.*
     INDX   ABILITY TESTING, CHILDREN, EDUCATION, EDUCATIONAL ASSESSMENT, LANGUAGE ASSESSMENT, LEARNING, EMPIRICAL, SES, MEXICAN AMERICAN, TEST RELIABILITY, TEST VALIDITY, WISC, INTELLIGENCE TESTING, ARIZONA, SOUTHWEST
     ABST   BECAUSE THERE IS EVIDENCE THAT STANDARDIZED TESTS ADMINISTERED TO MEMBERS OF MINORITY POPULATIONS MAY BE SUBJECT TO VARIOUS DISTORTIONS, THIS STUDY EXAMINED THE RELIABILITY OF THE WISC-R SUBTESTS AND IQ SCALES WHEN ADMINISTERED TO MEXICAN AMERICAN CHILDREN. FURTHER, IN AN EFFORT TO EXTRAPOLATE THESE FINDINGS TO THE INDIVIDUAL CHILD, THE STUDY ASCERTAINED THE STANDARD ERRORS OF MEASUREMENT FOR EACH SUBTEST AND IQ SCALE. THE SUBJECTS WERE 53 (28 MALE AND 25 FEMALE) ECONOMICALLY DISADVANTAGED MEXICAN AMERICAN CHILDREN ATTENDING SCHOOL IN THE PHOENIX, ARIZONA, AREA. ALL SUBJECTS HAD BEEN REFERRED FOR PSYCHOLOGICAL EVALUATION RESULTING FROM LEARNING DIFFICULTIES IN THE REGULAR CLASSROOM. THE SUBJECTS (MEAN AGE = 11.14) WERE INDIVIDUALLY ADMINISTERED THE 10 REGULAR SUBTESTS OF THE WISC-R OVER A 12-MONTH PERIOD BY ANGLO EXAMINERS; AND THEIR WISC-R FULL SCALE IQ SCORES RANGED FROM 86 TO 108. RESULTS WERE THAT THE RELIABILITIES OBTAINED WERE NOT SIGNIFICANTLY DIFFERENT THAN THOSE REPORTED IN THE WISC-R (1974) MANUAL FOR 11.5 YEAR-OLD CHILDREN. MOREOVER, ALTHOUGH THE STANDARD ERRORS OF MEASUREMENT EXCEEDED THOSE FOUND IN THE STANDARDIZED 1974 SAMPLE, THEY WERE LESS THAN FIVE POINTS ON ALL THREE IQ SCALES. THESE RESULTS, THOUGH PRELIMINARY IN SCOPE, CLEARLY DEMONSTRATE THE WISC-R TO BE A RELIABLE INSTRUMENT IN EVALUATING MEXICAN AMERICAN CHILDREN. 4 REFERENCES.
     ACCN   002068

431 AUTH   **DEANDA, R., & LOCKETT, V.**
     TITL   INTRODUCING BLACK AND CHICANO CONTENT INTO A SOCIAL WORK CURRICULUM: A RECOMMENDATION.
     SRCE   *SOCIAL WORK EDUCATION REPORTER, 1972, 20(3), 28-31.*
     INDX   PROFESSIONAL TRAINING, MENTAL HEALTH PROFESSION, CURRICULUM, MEXICAN AMERICAN, CROSS CULTURAL, ESSAY, REPRESENTATION, HIGHER EDUCATION, TEXAS, SOUTHWEST, POLICY
     ABST   TO IMPROVE THE PROFESSIONAL CALIBER OF GRADUATE STUDENTS AND TO IMPROVE DELIVERY OF SOCIAL SERVICES TO THE BLACK AND CHICANO COMMUNITIES THE FOLLOWING RECOMMENDATIONS WERE SUBMITTED TO THE FACULTY AND ADMINISTRATION OF THE GRADUATE SCHOOL OF SOCIAL WORK OF THE UNIVERSITY OF HOUSTON BY THE BLACK/BROWN COALITION (BBC) REPRESENTING GRADUATE MINORITY STUDENTS IN SOCIAL WORK. CONSIDERING HOUSTON'S LARGE MINORITY COMMUNITY, THE UNIVERSITY'S CURRICULUM IN THE FIELD OF SOCIAL WORK SHOULD EMPHASIZE THE CULTURAL, PSYCHOSOCIAL AND HISTORICAL ASPECTS OF THESE GROUPS IN A SEQUENCE OF COURSES ON HUMAN BEHAVIOR, SOCIAL ENVIRONMENT AND SOCIAL WORK PRACTICE, POLICY AND RESEARCH. THE SUCCESSFUL IMPLEMENTATION OF THIS CURRICULUM ALSO DEPENDS UPON THE FOLLOWING: (1) SENSITIZING THE FACULTY AND ADMINISTRATION TO MINORITY NEEDS; (2) REPRESENTATION OF MINORITY COMMUNITY MEMBERS ON CURRICULUM COMMITTEES AND CREATION OF AN ETHNIC MINORITIES SEQUENCE COMMITTEE; (3) HIRING OF BLACK AND CHICANO FACULTY; (4) OFFERING COURSES WHICH WOULD SENTISIZE ALL STUDENTS TO THE STRENGTHS, PROBLEMS, AND NEEDS OF MINORITIES; AND (5) PROVISION OF SUFFICIENT FUNDING BY THE

UNIVERSITY TO ENSURE THE CONTINUING IMPROVEMENT OF THE ETHNIC CONTENT OF THE CURRICULUM.

ACCN   000359

432 AUTH   **DEFLEUR, L. B., BALL J. C., & SNARR, R. W.**
     TITL   THE LONG-TERM SOCIAL CORRELATES OF OPIATE ADDICTION.
     SRCE   *SOCIAL PROBLEMS, 1969, 17(2), 225-234.*
     INDX   DRUG ADDICTION, PUERTO RICAN-I, REHABILITATION, CRIMINOLOGY, EMPIRICAL, ADULTS, MALE, KENTUCKY, SOUTH
     ABST   A FOLLOW-UP STUDY WAS UNDERTAKEN OF FORMER HEROIN ADDICTS FROM PUERTO RICO WHO HAD BEEN FEDERAL PRISONERS AT THE U.S. PUBLIC HEALTH HOSPITAL IN LEXINGTON BETWEEN 1935 AND 1962. EXTENSIVE DATA WERE OBTAINED FOR EACH SUBJECT BY MEANS OF A FIELD INTERVIEW, A URINALYSIS TO CHECK ON ADDICTION STATUS, AND A CURRENT FBI RECORD. WITH THESE DATA THE LONG-TERM SOCIAL CORRELATES OF HEROIN ADDICTION WERE EXAMINED. FIRST, DRUG USE, ARRESTS, AND OCCUPATIONAL CAREERS OF THE SUBJECTS OVER TIME WERE TRACED. SECOND, BY BRINGING TOGETHER A NUMBER OF PRE-ADDICTION AND POST-ADDICTION CHARACTERISTICS, THE LIFE PATTERNS OF THE SUBJECTS WERE ANALYZED. 10 REFERENCES. (JOURNAL ABSTRACT)

ACCN   000366

433 AUTH   **DEL CASTILLO, J. C.**
     TITL   THE INFLUENCE OF LANGUAGE UPON SYMPTOMATOLOGY IN FOREIGN BORN PATIENTS.
     SRCE   *THE AMERICAN JOURNAL OF PSYCHIATRY, 1970, 127(2), 242-244.*
     INDX   PSYCHOPATHOLOGY, SYMPTOMATOLOGY, BILINGUAL-BICULTURAL PERSONNEL, PERSONALITY ASSESSMENT, PSYCHOSIS, PSYCHOTHERAPY, PSYCHOTHERAPISTS, ESSAY, PUERTO RICAN-M, ADULTS, AGGRESSION, NEW JERSEY, EAST, BILINGUAL, BILINGUALISM
     ABST   BASED UPON EXPERIENCES WITH BILINGUAL PATIENTS WHO SHOWED PSYCHOTIC SYMPTOMS IN INTERVIEWS HELD IN THEIR NATIVE LANGUAGE BUT NOT IN THOSE CONDUCTED IN FOREIGN LANGUAGES, THE AUTHOR SUGGESTS THAT A THEORETICAL EXPLANATION CAN BE FOUND WHICH WILL BE HELPFUL IN TREATING THE PATIENTS AS WELL AS UNDERSTANDING THE PHENOMENON. IT IS POSTULATED THAT THE EFFORT OF COMMUNICATING IN ANOTHER LANGUAGE PRODUCES UNCONSCIOUS VIGILANCE OVER THE EMOTIONS. (JOURNAL ABSTRACT MODIFIED)

ACCN   000368

434 AUTH   **DEL CASTILLO, R. G.**
     TITL   A PRELIMINARY COMPARISON OF CHICANO, IMMIGRANT AND NATIVE BORN FAMILY STRUCTURES, 1850-1880.
     SRCE   *AZTLAN: INTERNATIONAL JOURNAL OF CHICANO STUDIES RESEARCH, 1975, 6(1), 87-96.*
     INDX   MEXICAN AMERICAN, FAMILY STRUCTURE, IMMIGRATION, ACCULTURATION, EMPIRICAL, CROSS CULTURAL, CALIFORNIA, SOUTHWEST, MICHIGAN, MIDWEST
     ABST   IN AN ATTEMPT TO STUDY THE HISTORICAL EXPERIENCE OF NATIONAL ETHNIC GROUPS IN THE UNITED STATES, THIS ESSAY COMPARES DATA ON FAMILY ORGANIZATION AND STRUCTURE FOR CHICANOS IN LOS ANGELES DURING THE PERIOD 1850-1880 WITH SIMILAR DATA ON THE EUROPEAN IMMIGRANT AND NATIVE-BORN IN DETROIT DURING THE SAME YEARS. THE COMPARABILITY OF LOS ANGELES AND DETROIT AS WELL AS THE SELECTION OF FAMILY STRUCTURE VARIABLES IS DISCUSSED. THE STUDY TENTATIVELY EXPLORES COMPARATIVE RELATIONSHIPS SUGGESTED BY THE DATA AND OFFERS A NUMBER OF HYPOTHETICAL STATEMENTS THAT CAN SERVE AS A STARTING POINT FOR FURTHER INVESTIGATIONS OF THE RELATIVE PROGRESS OR LACK OF PROGRESS EXPERIENCED BY CHICANO COMMUNITIES AS COMPARED TO OTHER ETHNIC GROUPS. 10 REFERENCES. (AUTHOR SUMMARY MODIFIED)

ACCN   000369

435 AUTH   **DELGADO, A. V.**
     TITL   A STUDY OF THE CONCEPT OF MACHISMO.
     SRCE   *PAPER PRESENTED AT THE ROCKY MOUNTAIN SOCIAL SCIENCE ASSOCIATION CONFERENCE, EL PASO, TEXAS, APRIL 25-27, 1974.*
     INDX   SEX ROLES, RESOURCE UTILIZATION, CULTURAL FACTORS, MEXICAN AMERICAN, MALE, EMPIRICAL, COLORADO, SOUTHWEST, MACHISMO
     ABST   THE PURPOSE OF THIS RESEARCH IS TWOFOLD: (1) TO CONSTRUCT A MEASUREMENT SCALE THAT WILL MEASURE THE CONCEPT OF MACHO, AND (2) TO TEST THE THEORETICAL HYPOTHESIS THAT MACHO IS A CONTRIBUTING DETERRENT ELEMENT IN THE UTILIZATION OF HEALTH CARE DELIVERY. TO DATE, THE PREDICTIVE UTILIZATION RATE OF HEALTH SERVICES AVAILABLE TO THE LOW-INCOME CHICANO POPULATION HAS BEEN ONE OF SPECULATION. THE DATA PRESENTED IN THIS ANALYSIS STRONGLY SUGGEST A HIGH CORRELATION BETWEEN THOSE WHO SCORED HIGH ON THE MACHO SCALE AND THOSE WHO ARE NON-USERS OF HEALTH SERVICES. CONVERSELY, THESE DATA REFLECT A HIGH CORRELATION BETWEEN THOSE WHO SCORED LOW ON THE MACHO SCALE, AND THOSE WHO ARE USERS OF HEALTH SERVICES. THIS INTERPRETATION SUGGESTS THAT THE MACHO SCALE HAS A HIGH DEGREE OF PREDICTABILITY IN RELATION TO THE UTILIZATION OF HEALTH CARE SERVICES BY LOW-INCOME CHICANOS. THESE FINDINGS SUBSEQUENTLY MAY HAVE SOCIOLOGICAL APPLICABILITY TO THE FIELD OF MEDICINE. 30 REFERENCES. (AUTHOR ABSTRACT)

ACCN   000370

436 AUTH   **DELGADO, M.**
     TITL   SOCIAL WORK AND THE PUERTO RICAN COMMUNITY.
     SRCE   *SOCIAL CASEWORK, 1974, 55(2), 117-123.*
     INDX   SOCIAL SERVICES, PUERTO RICAN-M, POVERTY, MENTAL HEALTH, HEALTH DELIVERY SYSTEMS, DEMOGRAPHIC, ENVIRONMENTAL FAC-

TORS, PROFESSIONAL TRAINING, EMPIRICAL, POLITICS, ESSAY, URBAN, CULTURAL FACTORS, NEW YORK, EAST, ESSAY

ABST THE PROFESSIONAL EDUCATION AND PRACTICE OF PUERTO RICAN SOCIAL WORKERS ARE DESCRIBED AS FAILING TO MEET THE NEEDS OF PUERTO RICANS IN NEW YORK CITY AND OTHER COMMUNITIES. SUPPORTED BY DEMOGRAPHIC DATA AND PERSONAL EXPERIENCES, THE AUTHOR DISCUSSES HOW SOCIAL WORK EDUCATION DOES NOT ADEQUATELY TRAIN SOCIAL WORKERS TO DEAL WITH SYSTEMIC PROBLEMS (E.G., HEALTH, HOUSING AND EMPLOYMENT) WHICH THE POOR ARE POWERLESS TO OBTAIN ON THEIR OWN. IT IS CONCLUDED THAT PUERTO RICAN STUDENTS COULD PROBABLY PROVIDE MORE EFFECTIVE ADVOCACY IN OTHER PROFESSIONS SUCH AS LAW, EDUCATION AND ADMINISTRATION, SINCE THE SOCIAL WORK PROFESSION HAS TURNED AWAY FROM THE POOR AND THEIR PROBLEMS. 17 REFERENCES.

ACCN 000371

437 AUTH **DELGADO, M., & MONTALVO, S.**

TITL PREVENTIVE MENTAL HEALTH SERVICES FOR PRESCHOOL CHILDREN.

SRCE *CHILDREN TODAY, 1979, JANUARY-FEBRUARY, 6-8; 34.*

INDX CHILDREN, COMMUNITY INVOLVEMENT, EARLY CHILDHOOD EDUCATION, MENTAL HEALTH, PARENTAL INVOLVEMENT, PUERTO RICAN-M, MASSACHUSETTS, PRIMARY PREVENTION, EAST, ESSAY, EDUCATIONAL COUNSELING, MOTHER-CHILD INTERACTION, TEACHERS

ABST THE DEVELOPMENT OF A COMMUNITY MENTAL HEALTH PROGRAM FOCUSING ON THE NEEDS OF PUERTO RICAN PRESCHOOL CHILDREN IN WORCHESTER, MASSACHUSETTS, IS DESCRIBED. THE PROGRAM, WHICH PROVIDES CONSULTATION/INTERVENTION SERVICES TO THE CHILDREN'S PARENTS, DAY-CARE TEACHERS, AND FAMILY DAY-CARE PROVIDERS, IS CONDUCTED THROUGH THE HISPANIC PROGRAM OF THE WORCHESTER YOUTH GUIDANCE CENTER. CONSULTANTS MAKE HOME VISITS TO ASSIST MOTHERS WITH PROBLEMS RELATED TO CHILD DEVELOPMENT, DAY-CARE PLACEMENT, AND STRATEGIES FOR TEACHING THEIR PRESCHOOL CHILDREN. CONSULTATIVE VISITS ARE ALSO MADE TO DAY-CARE FACILITIES TO ASSIST TEACHERS WHO WORK WITH PUERTO RICAN PARENTS AND CHILDREN. THE UTILIZATION OF DAY-CARE FACILITIES BY PUERTO RICANS HAS INCREASED SINCE THE INITIATION OF THE PROGRAM. (JOURNAL ABSTRACT MODIFIED)

ACCN 001803

438 AUTH **DELGADO, M., & SCOTT, J. F.**

TITL STRATEGIC INTERVENTION: A MENTAL HEALTH PROGRAM FOR THE HISPANIC COMMUNITY.

SRCE *JOURNAL OF COMMUNITY PSYCHOLOGY, 1979, 7, 187-197.*

INDX HEALTH DELIVERY SYSTEMS, MENTAL HEALTH, PUERTO RICAN-M, ESSAY, COMMUNITY INVOLVEMENT, HEALTH EDUCATION, RESOURCE UTILIZATION, MASSACHUSETTS, EAST, COMMUNITY, PRIMARY PREVENTION

ABST A MULTIFACTED MENTAL HEALTH PROGRAM DIRECTED TO THE HISPANIC (MOSTLY PUERTO RICAN) COMMUNITY OF WORCHESTER, MASSACHUSETTS, IS DESCRIBED. THE MODEL ON WHICH THE PROGRAM IS BASED RESTS HEAVILY ON KNOWLEDGE OF HISPANIC LIFESTYLES AS WELL AS ON EXTENSIVE EXPLORATORY CONTACTS WITH KEY HISPANIC COMMUNITY LEADERS WHO PROVIDED INFORMATION ABOUT COMMUNITY NEEDS. THE CENTER'S HISPANIC PROGRAM CONSISTS OF FIVE COMPONENTS: (1) COMMUNITY EDUCATION; (2) CLINICAL CONSULTATION; (3) PROGRAM CONSULTATION; (4) RESEARCH; AND (5) CLINICAL INTERVENTION AND CASE MANAGEMENT. THESE COMPONENTS OF THE PROGRAM ARE DESCRIBED IN DETAIL AND THE RATIONALE FOR STRATEGIC INTERVENTION IS PRESENTED. IN ADDITION, THE PROGRAM IS ORIENTED AROUND FIVE GOALS TO SERVICE DELIVERY: (1) FLEXIBILITY IN PROGRAM DESIGN TO ACCOMMODATE CHANGING COMMUNITY NEEDS; (2) PRIMARY PREVENTION PROGRAMS AS AN INTEGRAL PART OF SERVICE DELIVERY; (3) MULTIFACTED PROGRAMMING; (4) COMMUNITY-BASED SERVICES ACCESSIBLE TO ALL GEOGRAPHICAL AREAS AND SEGMENTS OF THE POPULATION; AND (5) COUNSELING IN GENERIC SETTINGS TO AVOID THE STIGMA ASSOCIATED WITH MENTAL HEALTH SERVICES. 57 REFERENCES. (JOURNAL ABSTRACT MODIFIED)

ACCN 001799

439 AUTH **DEMOS, G. D.**

TITL ATTITUDES OF MEXICAN AMERICAN AND ANGLO AMERICAN GROUPS TOWARDS EDUCATION.

SRCE *JOURNAL OF SOCIAL PSYCHOLOGY, 1962, 57(2), 249-256.*

INDX ATTITUDES, EDUCATION, CROSS CULTURAL, MEXICAN AMERICAN, ADOLESCENTS, EMPIRICAL, CALIFORNIA, SOUTHWEST

ABST THE PURPOSE OF THIS STUDY WAS TO ASCERTAIN WHETHER OR NOT SIGNIFICANT ATTITUDINAL DIFFERENCES EXIST TOWARD EDUCATION BETWEEN MEXICAN AMERICAN AND ANGLO AMERICAN PUPILS (GRADES 7-12) WHEN MATCHED ON SOCIOECONOMIC LEVEL, INTELLIGENCE, AGE, GRADE, AND SEX, AND IF THESE DIFFERENCES ARE A FUNCTION OF ETHNIC GROUP MEMBERSHIP. RESPONSES TO 29 ISSUES RELATED TO EDUCATION BY A STRATIFIED SAMPLE OF 105 MEXICAN AMERICANS WERE COMPARED TO (1) 105 RANDOMLY SELECTED ANGLO AMERICANS AND (2) 105 ANGLO AMERICANS THAT WERE MATCHED WITH THE MEXICAN AMERICAN SAMPLE. DIFFERENCES IN ATTITUDE WERE FOUND AMONG THE MEXICAN AMERICAN AND ANGLO AMERICAN GROUPS. THERE WERE MORE DIFFERENCES BETWEEN THE RANDOMLY SELECTED ANGLO AMERICANS AND MEXICAN AMERICANS THAN BETWEEN THE MATCHED ANGLO AMERICANS AND MEXICAN AMERICANS. IN EVERY CASE WHERE A DIFFERENCE WAS FOUND BETWEEN

THE RANDOM SAMPLES, THE ANGLO AMERICAN GROUP HAD THE MORE DESIRABLE ATTITUDE TOWARD EDUCATION. MATCHING OF THE MEXICAN AMERICAN AND ANGLO AMERICAN GROUPS WITH REGARD TO AGE, GRADE, SEX, SOCIAL CLASS, AND INTELLIGENCE DOES REDUCE THE NUMBER OF DIFFERENCES OF ATTITUDE BETWEEN THE TWO GROUPS. HOWEVER THERE STILL EXIST SIGNIFICANT DIFFERENCES THAT MAY BE ACCOUNTED FOR AS DIFFERENCES DUE TO MEXICAN AMERICAN ETHNIC GROUP MEMBERSHIP.

ACCN   000372

440 AUTH   **DEMPSEY, A. D.**
    TITL   TIME CONSERVATION ACROSS CULTURES.
    SRCE   *INTERNATIONAL JOURNAL OF PSYCHOLOGY, 1971, 6(2), 115-120.*
    INDX   COGNITIVE DEVELOPMENT, CROSS CULTURAL, MEXICAN AMERICAN, EMPIRICAL, CHILDREN, INDIGENOUS POPULATIONS, ARIZONA, SOUTHWEST
    ABST   DIFFERENCES ARE EXAMINED AMONG FIVE INDIAN TRIBES, MEXICAN AMERICANS (MA) AND MIDDLE-CLASS ANGLOS IN THEIR ABILITY TO CONSERVE CERTAIN ASPECTS OF TIME. SUBJECTS WERE 7, 9, AND 11 YEARS-OLD. FIFTEEN CHILDREN FROM EACH AGE GROUP WERE SELECTED FOR A TOTAL SAMPLE OF 315. EACH CHILD WAS SEEN INDIVIDUALLY BY THE EXAMINER AND WAS GIVEN FOUR TESTS FOR THE CONSERVATION OF TIME—TWO FOR EVENTS. THE TASKS WERE BASED ON LOVELL AND SLATER'S (1960) REPLICATION OF PIAGET'S CONSERVATION OF TIME EXPERIMENTS. THE RESULTS INDICATE THAT NO GROUP TESTED WAS ABLE TO CONSERVE SIMULTANEITY ON ANY OF THE TESTS USED. ON THE SIMPLE ORDER OF EVENT TASKS, ONLY ANGLO CHILDREN WERE ABLE TO CONSERVE TIME AT AGE 7. BY AGE 9 ALL EXCEPT NAVAJO AND APACHE CHILDREN CONSERVE TIME, AND BY AGE 11 ALL EXCEPT APACHE CHILDREN CONSERVE TIME. ON THE HARDER ORDER OF EVENTS TEST, NONE OF THE GROUPS ACHIEVED CONSERVATION BY AGE 9 AND ONLY ANGLO, MA, AND PIMA INDIANS ACHIEVED CONSERVATION OF TIME BY AGE 11. THE EFFECT OF CULTURE ON THE CONSERVATION OF TIME APPEARS TO BE AMPLY DEMONSTRATED BY THIS STUDY. 22 REFERENCES.
    ACCN   000373

441 AUTH   **DENNER, B., FREED, H. M., & SCHENSUL, S. L.**
    TITL   LATINO UTILIZATION OF COMMUNITY MENTAL HEALTH OUTPOSTS.
    SRCE   *UNPUBLISHED MANUSCRIPT, SONOMA COUNTY MENTAL HEALTH SERVICES, SANTA ROSA, CALIF., UNDATED.*
    INDX   EMPIRICAL, MEXICAN AMERICAN, CHILDREN, ADULTS, MENTAL HEALTH, RESOURCE UTILIZATION, COMMUNITY, CROSS CULTURAL, CULTURAL FACTORS, HEALTH DELIVERY SYSTEMS, SPANISH SURNAMED, CALIFORNIA, SOUTHWEST
    ABST   THE NOTION THAT ADDING LATINO STAFF TO INNER-CITY, MULTI-PURPOSE HUMAN SERVICE AGENCIES SERVING SPANISH-SPEAKING/SUR-NAMED (SSS) CLIENTS WOULD INCREASE THE NUMBER OF CLIENT OPENINGS WAS EVALUATED BY STUDYING STAFF COMPOSITION AND REPORTED CASE OPENINGS IN TWO OUTPOSTS ASSOCIATED WITH AN INNER-CITY COMMUNITY MENTAL HEALTH CENTER SERVING A PREDOMINANTLY MEXICAN AMERICAN POPULATION DURING 1969 TO 1973. DATA ANALYSIS DID NOT SUPPORT THE HYPOTHESIS. THE OUTPOST WITH MORE LATINO STAFF SERVING A GREATER NUMBER OF SSS CLIENTS DEMONSTRATED A NEGATIVE LINEAR REGRESSION BETWEEN INCREASE IN LATINO STAFF AND DECREASE IN SSS CLIENTS. THE CONCLUSION WAS THAT CONVENTIONAL WAYS OF RECORDING CLIENT CONTACTS IS INAPPROPRIATE IN AN AGENCY COMMITTED TO COMMUNITY DEVELOPMENT. 5 REFERENCES. (AUTHOR ABSTRACT)
    ACCN   000374

442 AUTH   **DERBYSHIRE, R. L.**
    TITL   ADAPTATION OF ADOLESCENT MEXICAN AMERICANS TO UNITED STATES SOCIETY.
    SRCE   *IN E. B. BRODY (ED.), BEHAVIOR IN NEW ENVIRONMENTS: ADAPTATION OF MIGRANT POPULATIONS. BEVERLY HILLS: SAGE PUBLICATIONS, 1970, PP. 275-290.*
    INDX   ADOLESCENTS, MEXICAN AMERICAN, PSYCHOSOCIAL ADJUSTMENT, IMMIGRATION, ACCULTURATION, POVERTY, FAMILY ROLES, SEXUAL BEHAVIOR, EDUCATION, MENTAL HEALTH, ATTITUDES, EMPIRICAL, ETHNIC IDENTITY, SOCIAL MOBILITY
    ABST   A COMPARISON OF ATTITUDES AND BEHAVIORS OF LOWER-CLASS MEXICAN AMERICAN ADOLESCENTS WHO WERE BORN AND REARED, OR WHOSE PARENTS WERE BORN AND REARED, IN THE UNITED STATES IS MADE WITH THOSE ADOLESCENTS WHO IMMIGRATED, OR WHOSE PARENTS IMMIGRATED, FROM MEXICO TO THE U.S. THE SAMPLE WAS COMPOSED OF 89 ADOLESCENTS—41 IN THE MIGRANT CATEGORY AND 48 IN THE NONMIGRANT CATEGORY. A 34-PAGE QUESTIONNAIRE WHICH COVERED PERSONAL AND FAMILY HISTORY, FEELING AND ATTITUDES TOWARD PERSONS, AND VALUES SIGNIFICANT IN THE LIFE OF AN ADOLESCENT WAS ADMINISTERED TO THE SUBJECTS. FINDINGS SHOW THAT SIGNIFICANT DIFFERENCES BETWEEN CATEGORIES DO NOT APPEAR ON ATTITUDES CONCERNING FAMILY, FATHER, MOTHER, AND MEXICAN CULTURAL PATTERNS. HOWEVER, LARGE DIFFERENCES EXIST IN ATTITUDES CONCERNING PREMARITAL SEX. THE NONMIGRANT ADOLESCENTS DO NOT HAVE A DUAL STANDARD FOR PREMARITAL SEXUAL RELATIONS WHILE THE MIGRANT CATEGORY MAINTAINS A DUAL STANDARD. NONMIGRANTS VIEW FORMAL EDUCATION AS A MEANS FOR UPWARD MOBILITY WHILE THE MIGRANT ADOLESCENTS LESS FREQUENTLY SEE EDUCATION IN THIS MANNER. SIGNIFICANTLY FEWER MIGRANTS SEE WORK IN TERMS OF FUTURE ORIENTATION AS OPPOSED TO ESTABLISHED ADOLESCENTS. WORK IS VIEWED BY MIGRANTS AS PRESENT-ORIENTED PHENOMENA. MOST OF THE YOUNGSTERS FROM BOTH

CATEGORIES VIEW MENTAL ILLNESS AS A "MIS-FORTUNE, AN ILLNESS WHICH "CAN BE CURED, AND SOMETHING FOR WHICH "ONE SHOULD NOT BE PUNISHED. FINDINGS ON A NUMBER OF OTHER ATTITUDES AND BEHAVIORS BE-TWEEN BOTH GROUPS ARE DISCUSSED. 23 REFERENCES.

ACCN 000375

443 AUTH **DERBYSHIRE, R. L.**
TITL ADOLESCENT IDENTITY CRISIS IN URBAN MEX-ICAN AMERICANS IN EAST LOS ANGELES.
SRCE *IN E. B. BRODY (ED.), MINORITY GROUP ADO-LESCENTS IN THE UNITED STATES. BALTIMORE: THE WILLIAMS AND WILKINS COMPANY, 1968, PP. 73-110.*
INDX MEXICAN AMERICAN, ADOLESCENTS, SEX ROLES, CHILDREARING PRACTICES, DEMO-GRAPHIC, CULTURE, SOCIAL MOBILITY, RE-VIEW, ACCULTURATION, SEX COMPARISON, EMPIRICAL, DEVIANCE, PSYCHOSOCIAL ADJUSTMENT, ETHNIC IDENTITY, URBAN, CALI-FORNIA, SOUTHWEST
ABST FUNCTIONAL RELATIONS BETWEEN SIMULTA-NEOUS MEMBERSHIP IN SOCIALLY AND CUL-TURALLY EXCLUDED MINORITIES AND THEIR EFFECT UPON ADOLESCENT IDENTITY CRISIS IN MEXICAN AMERICAN ADOLESCENTS ARE EXAMINED VIA DATA GATHERED FROM 89 EAST LOS ANGELES TEENAGERS. THE COMBINED EFFECT OF ADOLESCENT IDENTITY CRISIS AND CULTURAL IDENTITY CRISIS SUGGESTS THAT MEXICAN AMERICAN ADOLESCENTS ARE PAR-TICULARLY VULNERABLE TO DEVIANT BEHAV-IOR. ACCORDING TO THIS INVESTIGATION, FORCED ACCULTURATION OF MINORITIES BY THE DOMINANT GROUP MAY IMPEDE INTEGRA-TION OF DOMINANT VALUE ORIENTATIONS AND BEHAVIORS. PRIDE IN ONE'S CULTURAL HERI-TAGE APPEARS FUNCTIONAL AS AN INTEGRA-TIVE TECHNIQUE FOR REDUCING ADOLES-CENT IDENTITY AND ROLE CONFLICT. 40 REFERENCES. (AUTHOR SUMMARY MODIFIED)
ACCN 000376

444 AUTH **DERBYSHIRE, R. L.**
TITL CHILDREN'S PERCEPTIONS OF THE POLICE: A COMPARATIVE STUDY OF ATTITUDES AND AT-TITUDE CHANGE.
SRCE *JOURNAL OF CRIMINAL LAW, CRIMINOLOGY AND POLICE SCIENCE, 1968, 59(2), 183-190. (ALSO IN N. N. WAGNER & M. J. HAUG (EDS.), CHICANOS: SOCIAL AND PSYCHOLOGICAL PERSPECTIVES: SAINT LOUIS: C. V. MOSBY, 1971, PP. 175-183.)*
INDX POLICE-COMMUNITY RELATIONS, CHILDREN, ATTITUDES, CROSS CULTURAL, MEXICAN AMERICAN, SES, AUTHORITARIANISM, URBAN, EMPIRICAL, CALIFORNIA, SOUTHWEST
ABST IN AN EFFORT TO DETERMINE THE EFFECTIVE-NESS OF ATTITUDE CHANGE OF CHILDREN TO-WARD POLICE, LOW-SES NEGRO CHILDREN WERE CHOSEN TO PARTICIPATE IN A "POLICE-MAN BILL" PROGRAM. IN ADDITION, TWO OTHER DIVERGENT ETHNIC GROUPS (MEXICAN AMERICAN AND WHITE) FROM AVERAGE- AND HIGH-SOCIAL-CLASS CATEGORIES, RESPEC-TIVELY, WERE ADMINISTERED THE PRETEST

ONLY. THE HYPOTHESES EXPLORED WERE: (1) CHILDREN FROM LOW SOCIOECONOMIC AREAS WILL DESCRIBE A POLICEMAN WITH GREATER ANTIPATHY THAN WILL YOUNGSTERS FROM A SIGNIFICANTLY HIGHER SOCIOECONOMIC AREA; AND (2) LOWER-CLASS CHILDREN WHO PARTICIPATE IN THE "POLICEMAN BILL PRO-GRAM WILL CHANGE THEIR PERCEPTIONS OF THE POLICE. NINETY CHILDREN, 30 FROM EACH ETHNIC GROUP, WERE ASKED TO DRAW PIC-TURES OF A POLICEMAN AT WORK. AFTER PRE-SENTATION OF THE "POLICEMAN BILL" PRO-GRAM, THE NEGRO CHILDREN WERE ASKED TO DRAW ANOTHER PICTURE OF THE POLICE-MAN PERFORMING HIS TASKS. THROUGH TWO INDEPENDENT MEASURES (I.E., INDEPENDENT RATERS AND PICTURE CONTENT) THE NEGRO CHILDREN DISPLAYED SIGNIFICANTLY LESS ANTIPATHY TOWARD THE POLICE ON THE PRE-TEST. CHILDREN FROM THE THREE DIFFERENT ETHNIC AND SOCIAL CLASS CATEGORIES DIS-PLAYED SIGNIFICANTLY DIFFERENT ATTITUDES TOWARD THE POLICE. MEXICAN AMERICAN CHILDREN SHOWED GREATER ANTIPATHY SCORES AND WHITE CHILDREN SHOWED THE LEAST. THE GREATER SCORES OF ANTIPATHY BY THE MEXICAN AMERICANS ARE INTER-PRETED NOT AS A FEELING OF ANTIPATHY FOR POLICE BUT AS A NEGATIVE REACTION TO AN IMPERSONAL, UNIVERSALISTIC INSTITUTION AND ITS REPRESENTATIVES. IT IS CONCLUDED THAT THE "POLICEMAN BILL" PROGRAM BE CONTINUED AND INTENSIFIED THROUGHOUT THE LOS ANGELES SCHOOLS. 10 REFER-ENCES.

ACCN 000377

445 AUTH **DERBYSHIRE, R. L.**
TITL MENTAL HEALTH NEEDS AND RESOURCE UTI-LIZATION AMONG MEXICAN AMERICANS IN EAST LOS ANGELES (REPORT NO. IR11, MH-01539).
SRCE *LOS ANGELES: WELFARE PLANNING COUNCIL, 1967.*
INDX ACCULTURATION, ADOLESCENTS, ADULTS, BI-LINGUAL, COPING MECHANISMS, CROSS CUL-TURAL, CULTURAL FACTORS, POLICY, EMPIRI-CAL, ETHNIC IDENTITY, FAMILY ROLES, SURVEY, COMMUNITY, HEALTH EDUCATION, MENTAL HEALTH, MEXICAN AMERICAN, SES, SEXUAL BEHAVIOR, SOCIAL SERVICES, PSYCHOTHER-APY, SOUTHWEST, URBAN, CALIFORNIA
ABST ATTITUDES TOWARD AND UTILIZATION OF MENTAL HEALTH RESOURCES AMONG SUB-SETS OF MEXICAN AMERICANS OF EAST LOS ANGELES ARE EXPLORED. THE STUDY'S OVER-ALL DATA-GATHERING TECHNIQUE WAS THE QUESTIONNAIRE INTERVIEW, CONDUCTED IN A LOS ANGELES HOSPITAL AND IN EAST LOS AN-GELES NEIGHBORHOODS BY A SMALL STAFF HOUSED IN A COMMUNITY CENTER. INCLUDED IN THE STUDY WERE: (1) A SAMPLE SURVEY OF MEXICAN AMERICAN MENTAL PATIENTS AND THEIR FAMILIES AT METROPOLITAN STATE HOSPITAL; (2) AN INQUIRY INTO ADOLESCENT ATTITUDES TOWARD MENTAL ILLNESS, AU-THORITY, FAMILY, AND MEXICAN CULTURE; (3) A

COMPARATIVE STUDY OF MEXICAN AMERICAN, NEGRO, AND CAUCASIAN CHILDREN'S ATTITUDES TOWARD THE POLICE; (4) A DEMONSTRATION OF GROUP WORK WITH A SMALL NUMBER OF MEXICAN AMERICAN WOMEN EXPERIENCING PROBLEMS WITH THEIR ADOLESCENT CHILDREN; (5) A SURVEY OF POWER AND INFLUENCE AMONG MEXICAN AMERICANS; AND (6) ANALYSIS OF SOCIAL AGENCY FUNCTIONS, WITH PARTICULAR EMPHASIS ON THE AGENCIES' VIEWS OF PROBLEMS IN EACH SUBSTUDY. A SUMMARY OF THESE FINDINGS AND RECOMMENDATIONS POINT TO THE CONCLUSION THAT THE GAP BETWEEN THIS POPULATION AND THEIR UNDERUTILIZATION OF MENTAL HEALTH SERVICES IS MAINLY AGENCY-BASED. MAKING SERVICES MORE RELEVANT TO THE PEOPLE'S RATHER THAN THE AGENCY'S NEEDS COULD MAKE THE MENTALLY ILL BOTH MORE VISIBLE AND MORE AMENABLE TO SERVICE. SAMPLES OF THE STUDY'S QUESTIONNAIRES ARE APPENDED. 12 REFERENCES.

ACCN 002069

---

446 AUTH **DEREN, S.**
TITL AN EMPIRICAL EVALUATION OF THE VALIDITY OF THE DRAW-A-FAMILY TEST.
SRCE *JOURNAL OF CLINICAL PSYCHOLOGY, 1975, 31(3), 542-546.*
INDX TEST VALIDITY, CROSS CULTURAL, ETHNIC IDENTITY, SES, SEX COMPARISON, PERSONALITY ASSESSMENT, PROJECTIVE TESTING, EMPIRICAL, PUERTO RICAN-M, NEW YORK, EAST
ABST TO DETERMINE THE VALIDITY OF THE DRAW-A-FAMILY TEST (DAF), DRAWINGS WERE OBTAINED FROM 239 MEMBERS OF 91 FAMILIES (30 BLACK, 30 PUERTO RICAN, 30 WHITE, AND 10 OTHER) AND SCORED FOR SIZE, DETAIL, AND NUMBER OF FIGURES. SOME SUPPORT OF THE VALIDITY OF INTERPRETATIONS OF THE DAF WAS FOUND; ETHNICITY WAS RELATED TO SIGNIFICANT DIFFERENCES ON THE SIZE VARIABLE, FOR SPECIFIED SUBGROUPS FAMILY DRAWINGS WERE LESS FREQUENTLY REPRESENTATIVE OF ACTUAL FAMILY SIZE, AND THE SIZE AND DETAIL VARIABLES WERE HIGHLY CORRELATED. FURTHER RESEARCH USING DISTINCT CRITERIA GROUPS TO ASSESS THE EFFECTS OF SEX AND SOCIOECONOMIC LEVEL IS NEEDED. 22 REFERENCES. (PASAR ABSTRACT)
ACCN 000378

---

447 AUTH **DI PAOLO, M. D.**
TITL NATIVISM IN PUERTO RICO: THE INDEPENDENCE MOVEMENT.
SRCE *JOURNAL OF EDUCATION, 1967, 150(2), 35-38.*
INDX PUERTO RICAN-I, ACCULTURATION, CULTURAL CHANGE, SOCIAL STRUCTURE, ESSAY
ABST THE CONCEPT OF NATIVISM IS DEFINED AS A LARGE SCALE REACTION THAT OPPOSES ANY PROCESS THREATENING TO ASSIMILATE THE INDIGENOUS CULTURE. FROM AN ANTHROPOLOGICAL PERSPECTIVE THE IMPLICATIONS OF NATIVISM WITH RESPECT TO PUERTO RICO'S INDEPENDENCE MOVEMENT MUST BE UNDERSTOOD IN TERMS OF THE FORCES ACTING ON THE PUERTO RICANS. REACTIONS AGAINST UNITED STATES INTERVENTION AND THE INCREASED ACCULTURATION THAT CONTINUES TO ALTER THE PUERTO RICAN WAY OF LIFE WERE DISCUSSED AMONG 20 STUDENTS, TEACHERS, ADMINISTRATORS, LOCAL LEADERS, AND PRIVATE CITIZENS. THE NATIVISTIC ATTITUDE PERMEATES THE POLITICAL, SOCIAL, AND CULTURAL ASPECTS OF PUERTO RICAN SOCIETY. IN ADDITION, IT HAS CREATED CULTURAL CONFLICT AMONG VARIOUS MEMBERS WITHIN THE SOCIETY. THE NATIVISM REACTION MUST BE CONSIDERED AS A COMPOSITE OF THE VARIOUS ISSUES OF ASSIMILATION, ACCULTURATION, EXPLICIT AND IMPLICIT CULTURAL LEVELS, FORCE, AND INNOVATION. IT IS SUGGESTED THAT WITH INCREASED CULTURE CONFLICT WITH THE UNITED STATES, INTRA-CULTURE CONFLICT WILL ALSO INCREASE.
ACCN 001218

---

448 AUTH **DIAZ, A. V.**
TITL TEST RAPIDO BARRANQUILLA Y REVISED BETA EXAMINATION EN SUJETOS PUERTORRIQUENOS. (BARRANQUILLA RAPID SURVEY TEST AND REVISED BETA EXAMINATION ON PUERTO RICAN SUBJECTS.)
SRCE *REVISTA INTERAMERICANA DE PSICOLOGIA, 1977, 11(1), 14-17. (SPANISH)*
INDX PUERTO RICAN-I, EMPIRICAL, INTELLIGENCE TESTING, TEST VALIDITY, ADULTS
ABST TO DETERMINE WHICH OF TWO INTELLIGENCE TESTS WOULD BE MORE VALID AND APPROPRIATE FOR THE PUERTO RICAN POPULATION—THE BARRANQUILLA RAPID TEST (BARSIT) OR THE REVISED BETA EXAMINATION—19 MALE AND 12 FEMALE PUERTO RICANS AT A VOCATIONAL REHABILITATION CENTER WERE ADMINISTERED BOTH TESTS. BARSIT RAW SCORES WERE CONVERTED INTO WECHSLER-TYPE IQ SCORES AND THEN COMPARED TO THE BETA IQ SCORES. RESULTS SHOWED A BARSIT MEAN IQ OF 93.71 WHILE THE BETA MEAN IQ SCORE FOR THE SAMPLE WAS 84. THIS DIFFERENCE WAS STATISTICALLY SIGNIFICANT. SECONDLY, THE BARSIT IQ SCORES WERE FOUND TO CORRELATE SIGNIFICANTLY WITH THE SUBJECTS' EDUCATIONAL LEVELS WHEREAS THE BETA SCORES DID NOT. IN THIS VEIN, BECAUSE THE UNIVERSITY STUDENTS IN THE SAMPLE OBTAINED A MEAN BETA SCORE OF ONLY 87, COMPARED TO A MEAN BARSIT SCORE OF 112.53, IT WAS CONCLUDED THAT THE BARSIT IS PROBABLY A MORE ACCURATE INDICATOR OF THEIR INTELLIGENCE. IT IS RECOMMENDED THAT MORE SUBJECTS BE TESTED IN ORDER TO SUBSTANTIATE THE ACCURACY OF THESE RESULTS FOR THE PUERTO RICAN POPULATION IN GENERAL. 8 REFERENCES. (AUTHOR ABSTRACT MODIFIED)
ACCN 002070

---

449 AUTH **DIAZ, M. N.**
TITL THE INFANT IN MEXICAN-AMERICAN CULTURE.
SRCE *BIRTH DEFECTS, 1974, 10(2), 153-166.*
INDX MEXICAN AMERICAN, FAMILY ROLES, INFANCY, CHILDREN, ESSAY, STEREOTYPES, SOCIALIZATION, CULTURAL FACTORS, DISCRIMINATION,

ENVIRONMENTAL FACTORS, ECONOMIC FACTORS

ABST LIFE IN THE UNITED STATES FOR A MEXICAN AMERICAN INFANT OFTEN DOES NOT HOLD A PLEASANT FUTURE. THE CONCEPT OF TRADITIONAL CULTURE HAS FREQUENTLY BEEN USED TO PERPETUATE THE STEREOTYPE OF MEXICAN AMERICANS, FROM BIRTH THROUGH ADULTHOOD, AS AN AHISTORIC PEOPLE WHO ARE CONSTANTLY UNDERGOING AND REACTING TO ACCULTURATION, BUT WHO DO NOT GENERATE THEIR OWN HISTORY. THIS VIEW OF CULTURE AS THE DETERMINANT OF ALL ACTS IS QUESTIONED. RATHER CULTURE IS THAT ENTITY WHICH IS AFFECTED NOT ONLY BY FAMILY AND COMMUNITY, BUT ALSO BY POLICY MAKERS WHO LIMIT OR ENLARGE THE DAILY CHOICES AND OPPORTUNITIES, THE ECONOMIC, SOCIAL AND POLITICAL SITUATIONS IN WHICH THE INDIVIDUAL MUST FUNCTION. WITH THIS FRAMEWORK, THE LIFE SITUATIONS A MEXICAN AMERICAN WILL FACE ARE DESCRIBED: POPULATION GROWTH, INCREASED URBANIZATION, AGRICULTURAL EMPLOYMENT, MIGRATORY LABOR PATTERNS, PARENTAL INCOME, HEALTH BEHAVIORS, MATERNAL NUTRITION, FAMILY STRUCTURE, HOUSING, EDUCATIONAL DISCRIMINATION, AND LANGUAGE PROBLEMS. THE DEFENSIVE STRATEGIES WHICH WILL MAKE IT POSSIBLE FOR THE YOUNG MEXICAN AMERICAN TO FUNCTION IN THIS UNEQUAL AND UNFAIR LIFE SITUATION ARE LEARNED AT A VERY YOUNG AGE. IT IS POSITED THAT REPEATED EXPERIENCES OF DEFEAT AND LACK OF OPPORTUNITY WITHIN THE OVERALL AMERICAN SOCIAL STRUCTURE, NOT THE TRADITIONAL CONCEPT OF CULTURE, LIMIT THE LIFE CAREERS OF YOUNG MEXICAN AMERICANS. 11 REFERENCES.

ACCN 000379

450 AUTH **DIAZ-GUERRERO, R.**
TITL THE ACTIVE AND THE PASSIVE SYNDROMES.
SRCE *REVISTA INTERAMERICANA DE PSICOLOGIA, 1967, 1(4), 263-272.*
INDX CROSS CULTURAL, PERSONALITY, CULTURAL FACTORS, TEST RELIABILITY, TEST VALIDITY, COLLEGE STUDENTS, EMPIRICAL, MEXICAN, MEXICO, TEXAS, SOUTHWEST
ABST ACTIVE AND PASSIVE SYNDROMES ARE PRESENTED AS EXPLANATORY CONSTRUCTS FOR THE STUDY OF THE EFFECTS OF CULTURE ON PERSONALITY AND ETHNICITY. THESE CONSTRUCTS ARE MEDIATED BY SOCIOCULTURAL PREMISES THAT ARE CULTURALLY SIGNIFICANT STATEMENTS HELD BY A MAJORITY OF THE MEMBERS OF A SOCIETY. TO ILLUSTRATE THESE CONSTRUCTS, THE UNITED STATES WAS IDENTIFIED AS AN "ACTIVE" CULTURE AND MEXICO AS A "PASSIVE" ONE. A SERIES OF 112 STATEMENTS, DICHOTOMIZED ON THE ACTIVE-PASSIVE DIMENSION, WERE PRESENTED TO GRADUATE STUDENTS IN THE TWO COUNTRIES. THE RESULTS SHOWED 101 OF THE STATEMENTS TO HAVE HIGH INTERJUDGE RELIABILITY AND A DIFFERENTIAL FACE VALIDITY.

ACCN 000380

451 AUTH **DIAZ-GUERRERO, R.**
TITL A MEXICAN PSYCHOLOGY.
SRCE *AMERICAN PSYCHOLOGIST, 1977, 32(11), 934-944.*
INDX CULTURAL FACTORS, CULTURE, CROSS CULTURAL, ESSAY, MEXICO, SOCIAL SCIENCES, PERSONALITY, COGNITIVE STYLE, ADOLESCENTS, REVIEW, THEORETICAL, ATTITUDES
ABST AMERICAN PSYCHOLOGY'S CLAIM TO UNIVERSALITY IS CHALLENGED BY DATA SUGGESTING A SOCIOCULTURAL PSYCHOLOGY OF PERSONALITY. SPECIFIC FACTORIAL SCALES OF MEXICAN SOCIOCULTURAL PREMISES HAVE BEEN FOUND TO BE MEANINGFULLY ASSOCIATED WITH A NUMBER OF RELIABLE MEASURES OF PSYCHOLOGICAL DIMENSIONS. A COMPOSITE PORTRAIT OF MEXICAN YOUTH ON THE BASIS OF INTRA- AND CROSS-CULTURAL STUDIES IS PRESENTED, AND FROM THE EVIDENCE IT IS PROPOSED THAT CULTURE CAN ACCOUNT FOR SIGNIFICANT VARIANCE OF BONA FIDE PSYCHOLOGICAL AND BEHAVIORAL DIMENSIONS. THUS, THERE IS A BASIS TO SPEAK ABOUT SOCIOCULTURAL PSYCHOLOGIES (E.G., A MEXICAN PSYCHOLOGY), PARTICULARLY WITH REFERENCE TO CULTURALLY BOUND PERCEPTUAL AND COPING STYLES AS THEY RELATE TO PERSONALITY AND COGNITION. 39 REFERENCES. (JOURNAL ABSTRACT MODIFIED)

ACCN 002071

452 AUTH **DIAZ-GUERRERO, R.**
TITL MEXICANS AND AMERICANS: TWO WORLDS, ONE BORDER...AND ONE OBSERVER.
SRCE *IN S. R. ROSS, (ED.), VIEWS ACROSS THE BORDER: THE UNITED STATES AND MEXICO. ALBUQUERQUE: UNIVERSITY OF NEW MEXICO PRESS, 1978, PP. 283-307.*
INDX ESSAY, REVIEW, HISTORY, CULTURAL FACTORS, ATTITUDES, GROUP DYNAMICS, SES, AUTHORITARIANISM, SOUTHWEST, TEXAS, MEXICO, MEXICAN, CROSS CULTURAL, ACCULTURATION, CULTURAL CHANGE, CHILDREARING PRACTICES, SEX COMPARISON, PERSONALITY, EDUCATION, COGNITIVE STYLE, COOPERATION, COMPETITION, FATALISM, FAMILY ROLES, SEX ROLES, ADULTS, ADOLESCENTS, VALUES
ABST FACTUAL EVIDENCE POINTS TO DIFFERENCES BETWEEN THE AMERICAN AND MEXICAN SOCIOCULTURES AND TO DIFFUSION OF CULTURAL VALUES ACROSS THE BORDER. THE HISTORICAL BACKGROUNDS OF THE TWO COUNTRIES DIFFER IN ATTITUDES AND BEHAVIOR TOWARD RELIGIOUS AND STATE AUTHORITY, AND THIS IS REFLECTED IN THEIR WORLD VIEWS. SIGNIFICANT DIFFERENCES IN A NUMBER OF PSYCHOLOGICAL VARIABLES HAVE ALSO BEEN MEASURED. IN ONE STUDY, BOYS IN MEXICO CITY CONSISTENTLY SUBSCRIBED TO AFFILIATIVE OBEDIENCE AS A SOCIOCULTURAL PREMISE, WHILE THREE COMPARABLE ENGLISH-SPEAKING GROUPS IN CHICAGO, AUSTIN, AND LONDON, ENGLAND, PREFERRED ACTIVE SELF-ASSERTION. FOR SOME VARIABLES, HOWEVER, THE MEXICAN UPPER AND LOWER CLASSES, AND MALES AND FEMALES, DIFFERED MORE THAN DID MEXICANS AND AMERICANS. TWO OTHER PER-

SONALITY DIFFERENCES CLOSELY RELATED TO CONTRASTING ASPECTS OF THE TWO CULTURES ARE DISCUSSED: AMERICANS TEND TO BE MORE COMPLEX AND DIFFERENTIATED IN THEIR COGNITIVE STRUCTURES; MEXICANS TEND TO BE MORE FAMILY-CENTERED, MORE COOPERATIVE, AND MORE PESSIMISTIC. SOME DIFFUSION OF VALUES AND ATTITUDES ACROSS THE BORDER HAS BEEN DEMONSTRATED, AND ALTHOUGH SOCIAL INTERACTION BETWEEN THE TWO NATIONALITIES IN BORDER REGIONS HAS NOT BEEN SYSTEMATICALLY EXPLORED, THE AUTHOR FEELS THAT SELECTIVE ASSIMILATION OF EACH OTHER'S CULTURE IS MUTUALLY BENEFICIAL. RESEARCH ON INTERPERSONAL AND GROUP INTERACTION WOULD ASSIST IN UNDERSTANDING PATTERNS OF ACCULTURATION AND INTERACTION ACROSS CULTURES. 30 REFERENCES.

ACCN 002072

453 AUTH **DIAZ-GUERRERO, R.**
TITL NEUROSIS AND THE MEXICAN FAMILY STRUCTURE.
SRCE *AMERICAN JOURNAL OF PSYCHIATRY, 1955, 112(6), 411-417.*
INDX MEXICAN, NEUROSIS, EMPIRICAL, FAMILY ROLES, FAMILY STRUCTURE, VALUES, SEX ROLES, PSYCHOPATHOLOGY, STRESS, MALE, FEMALE, MACHISMO
ABST AN ANALYSIS IS MADE OF THE CULTURAL ASSUMPTIONS WHICH, IT IS BELIEVED, UNDERLIE SEX ROLES IN THE MEXICAN FAMILY AND WHICH ALSO LEAD TO NEUROSIS AMONG MEXICAN MEN AND WOMEN. THE DATA ARE BASED ON THE AUTHOR'S EXPERIENCE AS A PSYCHOTHERAPIST PLUS A SURVEY QUESTIONNAIRE COMPLETED BY 294 MEN AND WOMEN IN MEXICO CITY. THE KEY FACTOR IN THIS ANALYSIS IS THE MEXICAN "EXISTENTIAL" VALUE ORIENTATION WHICH IMPLIES A NATURAL SUPERIORITY OF THE MALE. THE PRODUCT OF THIS ORIENTATION IS A MASCULINE-FEMININE SOCIOCULTURAL DICHOTOMY THAT, IN THE MALE, CAUSES A BATTLE BETWEEN THE SUPEREGO AND THE ID—THAT IS, AN AMIBVALENCE BETWEEN THE "MALE SET AND "FEMALE SET OF CULTURAL VALUES. IN THE FEMALE, THE MAIN AREA OF STRESS IS HER VARIABLE SUCCESS IN LIVING UP TO THE STIFF REQUIREMENTS THAT THE CULTURAL PREMISES DEMAND. IT IS CONCLUDED THAT MANY OF THE NEUROSIS-PROVOKING CONFLICTS IN THE MEXICAN ARE "INNER CONFLICTS CAUSED MORE BY CLASHES OF VALUES THAN BY CLASHES OF THE INDIVIDUAL WITH REALITY. 7 REFERENCES. (AUTHOR SUMMARY MODIFIED)
ACCN 000381

454 AUTH **DIAZ-GUERRERO, R.**
TITL PSYCHOLOGY OF THE MEXICAN: CULTURE AND PERSONALITY.
SRCE *AUSTIN: UNIVERSITY OF TEXAS PRESS, 1975.*
INDX MEXICO, MEXICAN, REVIEW, SURVEY, CROSS CULTURAL, COLLEGE STUDENTS, ADULTS, FAMILY ROLES, ACHIEVEMENT MOTIVATION, ROLE EXPECTATIONS, SES, MEXICAN AMERICAN, ACCULTURATION, PERSONALITY, ATTI-

TUDES, CULTURAL FACTORS, CULTURE, BOOK, MENTAL HEALTH, INTERPERSONAL RELATIONS, STRESS, NEUROSIS, TEXAS, SOUTHWEST, MOTHER-CHILD INTERACTION
ABST THE DIFFERENTIAL EFFECT ON PERSONALITY OF AMERICAN AND MEXICAN SOCIOCULTURAL SYSTEMS IS THE THEME OF THIS VOLUME OF DIAZ-GUERRERO'S COLLECTED WORKS—PRIMARILY SURVEY AND/OR QUESTIONNAIRE STUDIES IN MEXICO AND THE UNITED STATES. IN THE INTRODUCTORY REMARKS THE FUNDAMENTAL PROPOSITION IS THAT AMERICANS ARE MOTIVATED BY POWER AND ACHIEVEMENT, WHILE MEXICANS BY AFFILIATION AND LOVE. THE ENSUING 10 CHAPTERS THEN PROBE VARIOUS FACETS OF THIS DICHOTOMY: (1) CULTURAL ASSUMPTIONS UNDERLYING ROLE PLAYING IN THE MEXICAN FAMILY; (2) MEXICAN ASSUMPTIONS ABOUT INTERPERSONAL RELATIONS; (3) 10 MOTIVATING NEEDS OF THE MEXICAN WORKER (RANGING IN INTENSITY FROM HUNGER TO THE NEED TO BELONG); (4) THE MENTAL HEALTH OF MEXICO CITY'S RESIDENTS; (5) THE MEANING OF "RESPECT" AMONG MEXICANS AND AMERICANS; (6) AN EVALUATION OF VARIOUS "ROLES" IN MEXICO AND THE U.S.; (7) THE PROBLEM OF STRESS ENCOUNTERED IN THESE TWO COUNTRIES; (8) THE PASSIVE-ACTIVE DICHOTOMY IN THESE TWO COUNTRIES; (9) THE PRELIMINARY RESULTS OF SOCIOLOGICAL RESEARCH IN MEXICO; AND (10) THE DIMENSIONS OF SOCIO-ECONOMIC DEVELOPMENT IN THE U.S. AND MEXICO. BEYOND THESE ISSUES, THE AUTHOR'S SPECIAL CONCERN IS THE ACCULTURATING MEXICAN AMERICAN, IN WHOM BROAD CHANGES IN ATTITUDES AND CUSTOMS ARE NECESSARILY TAKING PLACE. FOR THIS PERSON, THE AUTHOR RECOMMENDS THE DEVELOPMENT OF A SECOND "MESTIZAGE" ("CROSSBREEDING") WHICH EMBODIES THE BEST OF THE TWO PARENT CULTURES, THEREBY RETAINING FUNDAMENTAL GOALS WHILE ALLOWING FOR THE MASTERY OF SKILLS AND TECHNOLOGIES IMPORTANT FOR THE ADVANCEMENT OF ALL PEOPLES. 107 REFERENCES.
ACCN 001755

455 AUTH **DIAZ-GUERRERO, R.**
TITL SOCIO-CULTURAL PREMISES, ATTITUDES AND CROSS CULTURAL RESEARCH.
SRCE *INTERNATIONAL JOURNAL OF PSYCHOLOGY, 1967, 2(2), 79-87.*
INDX MEXICAN, CROSS CULTURAL, CULTURE, STRESS, COPING MECHANISMS, ESSAY, PERSONALITY
ABST THE ACTIVE-PASSIVE ENDURER OF STRESS DICHOTOMY IS EMPLOYED TO EXAMINE THE DIFFERENT SOCIOCULTURAL PREMISES FOUND IN AMERICAN AND MEXICAN POPULATIONS. AMERICANS ARE CLASSIFIED AS ACTIVE ENDURERS OF STRESS AND MEXICANS AS PASSIVE ENDURERS OF STRESS. THE TWO SOCIOCULTURAL PREMISES ARE THAT THE MEXICANS WANT TO AVOID STRESS AND AMERICANS WANT TO FACE STRESS. IN CROSS-CULTURAL RESEARCH, THE NEED TO ASCERTAIN SOCIOCULTURAL PREMISES OF WORLDWIDE VALUE

SO AS TO CLASSIFY CULTURES ACCORDING TO THEM IS EMPHASIZED BECAUSE CROSS-CULTURAL RESEARCH IN THE ACTIVE-PASSIVE STRESS DICHOTOMY HAS IMPORTANT IMPLICATIONS FOR ECONOMIC DEVELOPMENT AND SOCIAL CHANGE. SPECIFICALLY, IT IS PREDICTED THAT "UNDERDEVELOPED NATIONS WILL HAVE PASSIVE-ENDURER-OF-STRESS CULTURES. 11 REFERENCES.

ACCN   000382

456 AUTH   **DIAZ-GUERRERO, R.**
     TITL   TEST ANXIETY AND GENERAL ANXIETY IN MEXICAN AND AMERICAN SCHOOL CHILDREN.
     SRCE   IN C. D. SPIELBERGER & R. DIAZ-GUERRERO (EDS.), CROSS CULTURAL ANXIETY. WASHINGTON, D.C.: HEMISPHERE PUBLISHING, 1976, PP. 135-142.
     INDX   ATTITUDES, ANXIETY, CHILDREN, CONFORMITY, CROSS CULTURAL, CULTURAL FACTORS, DEPRESSION, EMPIRICAL, MENTAL HEALTH, MEXICAN, NEUROSIS, SES, SEX COMPARISON, FEMALE, SPANISH SURNAMED, TEST VALIDITY, REVIEW, PROJECTIVE TESTING
     ABST   THIS CHAPTER PROVIDES AN OVERVIEW OF RECENTLY DEVELOPED METHODS FOR TESTING ANXIETY IN BOTH ENGLISH AND SPANISH, AND REPORTS ON RESULTS OBTAINED FROM THE ADMINISTRATION OF THE TEST ANXIETY SCALE FOR CHILDREN (TASC) TO MEXICAN AMERICAN AND AMERICAN SCHOOL CHILDREN. IT ALSO DISCUSSES RESULTS OBTAINED FROM "AX," A VARIABLE OF THE HOLTZMAN INKBLOT TEST (HIT) THAT MEASURES ANXIETY IN FANTASY. THE SAMPLE CONSISTED OF A TOTAL OF 392 CHILDREN, HALF OF THEM MEXICAN AND HALF AMERICAN, WHO WERE IN 1ST, 4TH, OR 7TH GRADE AND WHO WERE PAIRED BY SEX, SES, AND SCHOOL GRADE AT THE TIME OF TESTING. AGES OF THE PAIRS WERE 6.7, 9.7, AND 12.7 YEARS. RESULTS OF THE TASC ANXIETY SCALE PROVED HIGHLY SIGNIFICANT FOR CULTURE, SES, AND SEX. MEXICAN SUBJECTS SCORED HIGHER ON ALL TASC SCALES THAN DID THE AMERICAN SUBJECTS. ACROSS CULTURES, SUBJECTS FROM THE LOWER SOCIOECONOMIC CLASS SCORED HIGHER ON THE ANXIETY SCALE THAN THOSE FROM THE UPPER SOCIOECONOMIC LEVEL. ALSO, REGARDLESS OF CULTURE, GIRLS SCORED HIGHER ON THE TASC BUT SHOWED A STRONGER TENDENCY FOR THE SCORES TO DIMINISH WITH AGE. THE MEAN HIT AX SCORE FOR AMERICANS WAS 9.1 COMPARED TO ONLY 5.6 FOR THE MEXICAN CHILDREN, INDICATING THAT WHILE MEXICAN CHILDREN SHOWED GREATER TEST ANXIETY, AMERICAN CHILDREN REVEALED HIGHER SCORES ON UNDERLYING SYMBOLIC ANXIETY. FINALLY, SPIELBERGER'S STATE-TRAIT ANXIETY INVENTORY FOR CHILDREN (STAIC), THE USE OF INKBLOTS AS POSSIBLE TOOLS FOR CROSS-CULTURAL ANXIETY STUDIES, AND THE CONSONANCE BETWEEN CULTURAL TRAITS AND TEST RESULTS ARE EXPLORED. 16 REFERENCES.

ACCN   002472

457 AUTH   **DIAZ-GUERRERO, R.**

     TITL   UNA ESCALA FACTORIAL DE PREMISAS HISTORICO-SOCIOCULTURALES DE LA FAMILIA MEXICANA. (A FACTORIAL SCALE OF HISTORICAL AND SOCIOCULTURAL PREMISES OF THE MEXICAN FAMILY.)
     SRCE   REVISTA LATINOAMERICANA DE PSICOLOGIA, 1972, 6(3-4), 235-244. (SPANISH)
     INDX   ADOLESCENTS, CULTURE, EMPIRICAL, RESEARCH METHODOLOGY, PERSONALITY, FAMILY ROLES, ATTITUDES, MEXICAN, MEXICO
     ABST   A FACTORIAL SCALE OF HISTORICAL AND SOCIOCULTURAL PREMISES IS DEVELOPED IN ORDER TO MEASURE CULTURAL VALUES IN MEXICAN SOCIETY. A GROUP OF 190 SUBJECTS DIVIDED ACCORDING TO THREE AGE GROUPS, TWO SOCIAL CLASSES AND SEX WAS STUDIED IN MEXICO CITY. THE AGE GROUPS WERE 12, 15 AND 18 YEARS OF AGE, AND THE SUBJECTS WERE SECONDARY SCHOOL STUDENTS. ALL OF THE SUBJECTS RESPONDED TO A QUESTIONNAIRE CONTAINING 22 STATEMENTS OF HISTORIC-SOCIOCULTURAL PREMISES CONCERNING THE MEXICAN FAMILY. A PRINCIPAL AXIS FACTOR ANALYSIS OF THE RESPONSES RESULTED IN ONLY ONE FACTOR ACCOUNTING FOR 61% OF THE VARIANCE. THIS FACTOR WAS CALLED "TRADITIONALISM IN THE MEXICAN FAMILY. THIS STUDY CONTENDS THAT THIS TYPE OF QUESTIONNAIRE USED TO MEASURE CULTURAL VARIABLES IS OF GREATER VALUE IN THE EXPLANATION OF HUMAN BEHAVIOR THAN ARE THE AFFIRMATIONS AND DEDUCTIONS OF MANY OTHER THEORIES NOW IN VOGUE. THE SCALE SHOULD BE USEFUL IN MEASURING THE DEGREE OF TRADITIONALISM AMONG GROUPS WITH SIMILAR DEMOGRAPHIC CHARACTERISTICS. 7 REFERENCES. (AUTHOR ABSTRACT MODIFIED)

ACCN   000383

458 AUTH   **DIAZ-GUERRERO, R., LICHTSZAJN, J., & LAGUNES, I. R.**
     TITL   ALIENACION DE LA MADRE, PSICOPATOLOGIA Y LA PRACTICA CLINICA EN MEXICO. (ALIENATION FROM THE MOTHER, PSYCHOPATHOLOGY, AND CLINICAL PRACTICE IN MEXICO.)
     SRCE   HISPANIC JOURNAL OF BEHAVIORAL SCIENCES, 1979, 1(2), 117-133. (SPANISH)
     INDX   MEXICAN, MEXICO, ADOLESCENTS, EMPIRICAL, ATTITUDES, VALUES, SES, CULTURAL FACTORS, MOTHER-CHILD INTERACTION, PSYCHOPATHOLOGY, INTERPERSONAL RELATIONS
     ABST   BEGINNING WITH THE RECOGNITION OF THE IMPORTANCE AND INFLUENCE OF CULTURE IN THE PERSONALITY AND BEHAVIOR OF THE INDIVIDUAL, THIS STUDY RELATES THE ROLE OF THE MATERNAL FIGURE TO THE AFFECTIVE BEHAVIOR OF THE MEXICAN. TWO HUNDRED ADOLESCENTS OF BOTH SEXES AND OF DIFFERENT SOCIOECONOMIC LEVELS IN MEXICO CITY SERVED AS SUBJECTS. THEY WERE ADMINISTERED A SERIES OF QUESTIONNAIRES WHICH IDENTIFIED VARIOUS ASPECTS OF TRADITIONAL MEXICAN CULTURE. SUBJECTS WERE ASKED TO JUDGE THE CONCEPT OF "INSULT TO THE MOTHER IN RELATION TO OTHER, SIMILARLY CHARGED AFFECTIVE CONCEPTS, SUCH AS "DEATH, "SUICIDE, AND "DRUNKENNESS.

RESULTS SHOW THAT "INSULT TO THE MOTHER IS VIEWED VERY NEGATIVELY. THE CLINICAL INTERESTS OF THE RESEARCHERS FOCUSES ON THOSE INDIVIDUALS WHO VIEWED THE CONCEPT OF "INSULT TO THE MOTHER LESS NEGATIVELY, AND ON THOSE WHO VIEWED IT AS EXTREMELY NEGATIVE. 26 REFERENCES. (JOURNAL ABSTRACT)

ACCN   001763

459 AUTH   **DIAZ-GUERRERO, R., REYES-LAGUNES, I., WITZKE, D. B., & HOLTZMAN, W. H.**
    TITL   PLAZA SESAMO IN MEXICO: AN EVALUATION.
    SRCE   *JOURNAL OF COMMUNICATION, 1976, 26(2), 145-154.*
    INDX   ABILITY TESTING, CHILDREN, CLASSROOM BEHAVIOR, COGNITIVE DEVELOPMENT, CURRICULUM, EARLY CHILDHOOD EDUCATION, EDUCATION, EDUCATIONAL MATERIALS, EMPIRICAL, ENVIRONMENTAL FACTORS, INSTRUCTIONAL TECHNIQUES, LEARNING, LINGUISTIC COMPETENCE, MASS MEDIA, MEXICAN, MEXICO, POVERTY, RURAL, SES, URBAN
    ABST   THE IMPACT OF PLAZA SESAMO (A PRODUCTION OF SESAME STREET ADAPTED TO LATIN CULTURE) UPON COGNITIVE AND PERCEPTUAL DEVELOPMENT WAS ASSESSED UNDER FIELD CONDITIONS TO SEE IF POSITIVE FINDINGS FROM EARLIER EXPERIMENTALLY CONTROLLED STUDIES COULD BE CONFIRMED. 1,-113 FOUR AND FIVE YEAR-OLDS FROM THREE SOCIOECONOMIC GROUPS PARTICIPATED IN THE STUDY. CHILDREN OF THE LOWER CLASS AND MIDDLE CLASS WERE SELECTED FROM 12 DAY-CARE CENTERS WITHIN THE HEALTH DEPT. OF MEXICO CITY. CHILDREN FROM RURAL, ECONOMICALLY DEPRIVED FAMILIES WERE SELECTED FROM THREE SMALL VILLAGES OF CENTRAL MEXICO. HOME VISITS AND INTERVIEWS WERE CONDUCTED WITH ALL PARENTS IN BOTH URBAN AND RURAL SAMPLES. THE EXPERIMENT LASTED 12 MONTHS, WITH ONE-HALF OF THE CHILDREN VIEWING PLAZA SESAMO WHILE THE OTHER HALF (THE CONTROL GROUP) WATCHED CARTOONS. SIXTEEN TESTS OF 7 COGNITIVE SKILLS WERE EMPLOYED TO EVALUATE THE CHILDREN AT THREE POINTS IN THE EXPERIMENT. NEGATIVE RESULTS CONCERNING THE VALUE OF EXPOSURE TO PLAZA SESAMO WERE OBTAINED FOR ALL CHILDREN EXCEPT THE URBAN, LOWER-CLASS FOUR YEAR-OLDS. OVERALL, THE 12-MONTH GAIN IN THE LEARNING SCORE FOR THE PLAZA SESAMO VIEWERS WAS ONLY SLIGHTLY GREATER THAN THE GAINS ACHIEVED BY THE CHILDREN WHO ONLY WATCHED CARTOONS. THESE FINDINGS CONTRADICT EARLIER CONTROLLED EXPERIMENTAL RESULTS WHICH SHOWED THAT VIEWING PLAZA SESAMO WAS ASSOCIATED WITH IMPROVED COGNITIVE DEVELOPMENT. 4 REFERENCES.

ACCN   002073

460 AUTH   **DIAZ-GUERRERO, R., & HOLTZMAN, W. H.**
    TITL   LEARNING BY TELEVISED PLAZA SESAMO IN MEXICO.
    SRCE   *JOURNAL OF EDUCATIONAL PSYCHOLOGY, 1974, 66(5), 632-643.*

INDX   ACHIEVEMENT TESTING, CHILDREN, COGNITIVE DEVELOPMENT, EARLY CHILDHOOD EDUCATION, EDUCATIONAL MATERIALS, EMPIRICAL, MEXICAN, SCHOLASTIC ACHIEVEMENT, MASS MEDIA, LEARNING
ABST   A CONTROLLED EXPERIMENTAL STUDY WAS MADE OF THE EFFECTS OF "PLAZA SESAMO", A SPANISH VERSION OF "SESAME STREET," DURING ITS FIRST TELECAST SEASON IN MEXICO CITY. A TOTAL OF 221 CHILDREN FROM THREE DIFFERENT LOWER-CLASS DAY-CARE CENTERS, EQUALLY DIVIDED BY AGES 3, 4, AND 5, AND BY SEX, WERE RANDOMLY ASSIGNED TO EXPERIMENTAL AND CONTROL GROUPS. COMPLETE DATA WERE LATER OBTAINED ON 173 OF THESE CHILDREN. A BATTERY OF NINE TESTS WAS INDIVIDUALLY ADMINISTERED PRE-, DURING, AND POSTTELECAST. MEASURES OF ATTENTION TO THE PROGRAM AND OF ATTENDANCE WERE ALSO TAKEN. HIGHLY SIGNIFICANT DIFFERENCES WERE FOUND FOR SPECIFIC ACHIEVEMENT TESTS DEALING WITH GENERAL KNOWLEDGE, NUMBERS, LETTERS, AND WORDS AS TAUGHT BY "PLAZA SESAMO." SIGNIFICANT DIFFERENCES WERE ALSO FOUND FOR FIVE COGNITIVE TESTS ONLY INDIRECTLY RELATED TO "PLAZA SESAMO AS WELL AS FOR ORAL COMPREHENSION, A TEST COMPLETELY INDEPENDENT OF THE PROGRAM CONTENT. THE LARGEST DIFFERENCES OCCURRED IN 4 YEAR-OLDS, THE SMALLEST IN 3 YEAR-OLDS. THE RATE OF LEARNING WAS CONSISTENTLY FASTER FOR THE EXPERIMENTAL GROUPS THAN THE CONTROLS ACROSS THE THREE TESTING PERIODS. AMOUNT OF ATTENTION CORRELATED AS HIGH AS .49 WITH GAINS AS MEASURED BY SEVERAL TESTS. LOW BUT SIGNIFICANT CORRELATIONS WERE FOUND BETWEEN ATTENDANCE AND AMOUNT OF GAIN. 5 REFERENCES. (AUTHOR ABSTRACT)
ACCN   002074

461 AUTH   **DIAZ-GUERRERO, R., & PECK, R. F.**
    TITL   RESPETO Y POSICION SOCIAL EN DOS CULTURAS. (RESPECT AND SOCIAL STATUS IN TWO CULTURES.)
    SRCE   *ANUARIO DE PSICOLOGIA, 1962, 1, 37-62. (SPANISH)*
    INDX   MEXICAN, CULTURE, CROSS CULTURAL, FAMILY ROLES, COLLEGE STUDENTS, EMPIRICAL, PERSONALITY, ATTITUDES, EXTENDED FAMILY, MEXICO, TEXAS, SOUTHWEST, SEX COMPARISON
    ABST   THE RELATIONSHIP BETWEEN RESPECT AND SOCIAL STATUS IS INVESTIGATED IN TWO CULTURES TO DETERMINE IF A PERSON'S STATUS WITHIN HIS SOCIETY INCREASES WITH THE AMOUNT OF RESPECT SHOWN. UNIVERSITY STUDENTS IN MEXICO AND IN THE UNITED STATES WERE ADMINISTERED A 60-ITEM QUESTIONNAIRE TO DETERMINE THE FREQUENCY WITH WHICH MALES AND FEMALES OF BOTH CULTURES CONSIDER CERTAIN INDIVIDUAL TRAITS AND ROLES AS DESERVING OF RESPECT. THE MEXICAN SAMPLE CONSISTED OF 216 MALE AND 82 FEMALE STUDENTS, AT THE PREPARATORY LEVEL, FROM THE NATIONAL AUTONOMOUS UNIVERSITY OF MEXICO (UNAM). THE UNITED STATES SAMPLE, TAKEN FROM

THE FIRST AND SECOND YEAR CLASSES AT THE UNIVERSITY OF TEXAS, CONSISTED OF 176 MALES AND 164 FEMALES. FOR ANALYSIS, THE RESULTS WERE FIRST CATEGORIZED INTO THE FOLLOWING QUALITATIVE MEASURES: AGE AND SEX, IMMEDIATE FAMILY, EXTENDED FAMILY, FRIENDS, NEIGHBORS, OCCUPATIONS, ECONOMIC STATUS, AND MISCELLANEOUS DATA. THE QUANTITATIVE MEASURES WERE ANALYZED ACCORDING TO FREQUENCY OF POSITIVE RESPONSE, IN THE FOLLOWING MANNER: (1) ITEMS RESPONDED TO POSITIVELY BY MORE THAN 50 PERCENT OF THE SUBJECTS WERE LABELED HIGH RESPECT (HR), (2) POSITIVE RESPONSES BY 50 PERCENT OF THE SUBJECTS WERE CLASSIFIED MEDIUM RESPECT (MR), AND (3) LESS THAN 50 PERCENT POSITIVE RESPONSE TO ANY ITEM WAS CONSIDERED AS LITTLE RESPECT (LR). NUMEROUS CROSS-CULTURAL COMPARISONS ARE PRESENTED PERTAINING TO THE SIMILARITIES AND DIFFERENCES IN THE CONCEPT OF RESPECT. HYPOTHETICAL CONSIDERATIONS FROM THESE RESULTS SUGGEST THAT THE RACIAL DISCRIMINATION PROBLEMS FOUND IN THE UNITED STATES CAN BE LINKED TO THE SOCIOCULTURAL PREMISE THAT "RESPECT IS GIVEN ONLY TO THOSE WHO TAKE ADVANTAGE OF THE OPPORTUNITY TO BECOME ECONOMICALLY STRONG. 16 REFERENCES.

ACCN   000384

462   AUTH   **DIAZ-GUERRERO, R., & TAPIA, L. L.**
     TITL   DIFERENCIAS SEXUALES EN EL DESARROLLO DE LA PERSONALIDAD DEL ESCOLAR MEXICANO. (SEX DIFFERENCES IN THE PERSONALITY DEVELOPMENT OF THE MEXICAN SCHOLAR.)
     SRCE   *REVISTA LATINOAMERICANA DE PSICOLOGIA, 1972, 4(3), 345-351. (SPANISH)*
     INDX   CHILDREN, EMPIRICAL, PROJECTIVE TESTING, CULTURE, PERSONALITY, SEX COMPARISON, MEXICAN, MEXICO
     ABST   DIFFERENCES ATTRIBUTED TO SEX IN THE DEVELOPMENT OF THE PERSONALITY WERE INVESTIGATED. IN A FACTORIAL STUDY OF 442 MEXICAN SCHOOL CHILDREN—THREE AGE LEVELS AND BOTH SEXES—IT WAS FOUND THAT BOYS DIFFERED FROM GIRLS IN 7 OF THE 21 VARIABLES OF THE HOLTZMAN INKBLOT TECHNIQUE (HIT). IN 5 OF THESE VARIABLES THE DIFFERENCE WAS EXACTLY THE SAME AS THAT PREVIOUSLY FOUND BY THE AUTHOR BETWEEN U.S. AND MEXICAN SUBJECTS. THE FINDINGS ARE EXPLAINED IN TERMS OF THE ACTIVE-PASSIVE DIMENSION: MEXICAN MEN ARE MORE ACTIVE THAN MEXICAN WOMEN, IN THE SAME WAY IN WHICH NORTH AMERICANS ARE MORE ACTIVE THAN MEXICANS. 13 REFERENCES. (JOURNAL ABSTRACT MODIFIED)
     ACCN   000385

463   AUTH   **DIAZ-ROYO, A. T.**
     TITL   DIGNIDAD AND RESPETO: TWO CORE THEMES IN THE TRADITIONAL PUERTO RICAN FAMILY CULTURE.
     SRCE   *PAPER PRESENTED AT THE FOURTEENTH SEMINAR OF THE COMMITTEE ON FAMILY RESEARCH OF THE INTERNATIONAL SOCIOLOGI-*

CAL ASSOCIATION, CURACAO, NETHERLAND ANTILLES, SEPTEMBER 3, 1975.
     INDX   PUERTO RICAN-I, ROLE EXPECTATIONS, FAMILY ROLES, ESSAY, CULTURE, INTERPERSONAL RELATIONS, ACCULTURATION
     ABST   DIGNIDAD AND RESPETO ARE CULTURAL VALUES OF GREAT IMPORTANCE IN THE PUERTO RICAN FAMILY BUT GENERALLY IGNORED IN SOCIAL RESEARCH. DIGNIDAD IS SYMBOLIC OF MORAL AND TRADITIONAL VALUES REFLECTED IN THE PERSONAL CRITERIA FOR SELF-EVALUATION AND IN THE PUBLIC PRESENTATION OF ONESELF. RESPETO DICTATES THE BEHAVIOR IN PUBLIC PLACES IN WHICH THE RECIPROCITY OF ACTORS IN A SITUATION ASSUMES A NORMATIVE HIERARCHICAL PATTERN. THESE TWO THEMES ARE INTERRELATED IN THAT RESPETO LEGITIMIZES THE CULTURAL BELIEF SYSTEM WHILE DIGNIDAD SYMBOLICALLY REPRESENTS THE ETHICAL CODE AMONG PUERTO RICANS. IMPLICIT WITHIN THESE TWO CULTURAL CONCEPTS IS A DUALITY OF THE PRIVATE AND PUBLIC SELF AND IN WHICH MORALITY IS CONSIDERED AN OBJECTIVE CRITERIA BY WHICH A PERSON'S BEHAVIOR IS EVALUATED. 36 REFERENCES.
     ACCN   000386

464   AUTH   **DICKER, A.**
     TITL   PROJECT "DO YOUR OWN THING AN EXPERIMENT IN INFORMAL EDUCATION FOR THE RETARDED.
     SRCE   *JOURNAL FOR SPECIAL EDUCATORS OF THE MENTALLY RETARDED, 1971, 7(3), 150-155.*
     INDX   PUERTO RICAN-M, SPECIAL EDUCATION, CROSS CULTURAL, ESSAY, INSTRUCTIONAL TECHNIQUES, CHILDREN, NEW YORK, EAST, MENTAL RETARDATION
     ABST   THE TRADITIONAL, FORMALLY STRUCTURED CLASSROOM ENVIRONMENT HAS BEEN ABANDONED IN AN EXPERIMENTAL PROGRAM FOR 14 CHILDREN WITH RETARDED MENTAL DEVELOPMENT. THE 10 BOYS AND 4 GIRLS IN THIS CLASS, ALL BLACK OR PUERTO RICAN FROM A LOW-SOCIOECONOMIC AREA OF NEW YORK CITY, RANGE IN AGE FROM 10 TO 13, AND IN MENTAL AGE FROM 6 TO 9. INFORMALITY IS THE KEYNOTE IN THIS CLASSROOM AND THE PUPILS ARE PROVIDED WITH FAMILIAR, COMMONPLACE ARTICLES AND MATERIALS WITH WHICH TO "DO THEIR OWN THING IN ADDITION TO CONVENTIONAL MODERN TEACHING AIDS. ALTHOUGH THE TECHNIQUE USED HERE HAS SHOWN THAT A CLASSROOM ENVIRONMENT FOR THE MENTALLY RETARDED CAN BE AT THE SAME TIME HUMANE AND EDUCATIONAL, IT IS STRESSED THAT FINDING THE PROPER BALANCE BETWEEN THE FORMAL AND INFORMAL APPROACH IS NECESSARY FOR BOTH THE TEACHER AND THE PUPIL.
     ACCN   000387

465   AUTH   **DIEPPA, I.**
     TITL   CHICANOS: ISSUES IN SOCIAL WORK EDUCATION REGARDING STUDENTS, FACULTY, AND CURRICULUM ENRICHMENT.
     SRCE   *SOCIAL WORK EDUCATION REPORTER, 1972, 20(1), 56-59.*

INDX   MEXICAN AMERICAN, PROFESSIONAL TRAINING, MENTAL HEALTH PROFESSION, CURRICULUM, ESSAY, COMMUNITY INVOLVEMENT, SOCIAL SERVICES, CULTURAL PLURALISM

ABST   SERVING THE NEEDS OF THE CHICANO POPULATION DEPENDS UPON A RELEVANT SOCIAL WORK CURRICULUM WHICH ACTIVELY RECRUITS CHICANO STUDENTS (PROVIDING THEM WITH SUFFICIENT FINANCIAL ASSISTANCE), HIRES CHICANO FACULTY, AND INCLUDES CHICANOS ON THE COUNCIL OF SOCIAL WORK EDUCATION (CSWE). THE ACADEMIC CURRICULUM SHOULD: (1) CONTAIN COURSES DEALING WITH CHICANO LIFE AND EXPERIENCE IN AMERICAN SOCIETY; (2) INTEGRATE CHICANO CONTENT INTO THE REQUIRED COURSES; (3) ESTABLISH A WORKING RELATIONSHIP WITH THE CHICANO STUDIES PROGRAM ALREADY ON CAMPUS; AND (4) ENCOURAGE FIELD WORK IN THE BARRIOS INDEPENDENT OF EXISTING SOCIAL WELFARE DELIVERY SERVICES. TOKENISM WILL NOT RESOLVE EXISTING INADEQUACIES OF THE SOCIAL WORK CURRICULUM. ONLY BY INTEGRATING THE CHICANO AND CHICANO CONTENT INTO THE OVERALL SOCIAL WORK CURRICULUM WILL SOCIAL WORKERS DEVELOP THE SKILLS NECESSARY TO MEET THE NEEDS OF THE CHICANO COMMUNITY.

ACCN   000388

466 AUTH   **DIXON, J. C., GARCIA-ESTEVE, J., & SIGVARTSEN, M. L.**

TITL   PERSONALITY AND LANGUAGE STRUCTURE IN TWO LANGUAGES.

SRCE   *REVISTA INTERAMERICANA DE PSICOLOGIA, 1968, 2(1), 13-23.*

INDX   BILINGUALISM, PERSONALITY, PUERTO RICAN-I, GRAMMAR, SEMANTICS, CROSS CULTURAL, ROTTER INTERNAL-EXTERNAL SCALE, ATTRIBUTION OF RESPONSIBILITY, COLLEGE STUDENTS, FATALISM, FLORIDA, SOUTH

ABST   THE RELATIONSHIP BETWEEN PERSONALITY AND DIFFERENTIAL USE OF VARIOUS GRAMMATICAL STRUCTURES WAS STUDIED IN A GROUP OF 162 FLORIDA AND 201 PUERTO RICAN COLLEGE STUDENTS OF BOTH SEXES. THE PERSONALITY MEASURES INCLUDED THE INTERNAL-EXTERNAL SCALE AND AN ADAPTATION OF THE ATTRIBUTION OF RESPONSIBILITY SCALE. THE LANGUAGE MEASURES WERE DERIVED FROM AN ADAPTATION OF THE SEMANTIC DIFFERENTIAL TECHNIQUE TO ASSESS THE ACTIVE-POTENT DIMENSION OF MEANING OF FIRST-PERSON SUBJECT AND OBJECT PRONOUNS. IN ADDITION, 40 SELECTED VERBS WERE PROVIDED WITH INSTRUCTIONS TO USE THESE IN MAKING 40 ORAL SENTENCES. THE MOST SIGNIFICANT FINDING WAS THE FAILURE, IN 264 COMPARISONS, TO FIND A SINGLE SIGNIFICANT RELATIONSHIP BETWEEN PERSONALITY MEASURES AND MEASURES OF GRAMMATICAL AND SEMANTIC STRUCTURE. ANOTHER SIGNIFICANT FINDING WAS THAT THE ATTITUDE OF PASSIVE ACCEPTANCE OF "EL DESTINO (DESTINY) IS CLEARLY NOT AN IMMUTABLE PART OF "SPANISH CHARACTER, NOR IS THE SPANISH

LANGUAGE NECESSARILY A DETERMINANT OF SUCH AN ATTITUDE. 16 REFERENCES.

ACCN   000389

467 AUTH   **DOHEN, D.**

TITL   A NEW JUVENILE COURT ROLE IN AN ETHNICALLY CONTROLLED COMMUNITY AGENCY.

SRCE   *SOCIAL WORK, 1971, 16(2), 25-29.*

INDX   JUDICIAL PROCESS, PUERTO RICAN-M, ESSAY, PARAPROFESSIONALS, COMMUNITY INVOLVEMENT, NEW YORK, EAST, ADOLESCENTS

ABST   THE MULTIFACETED COURTWORKER ROLE DEVELOPED BY THE NEW YORK CITY JUVENILE COURT SERVICES PROGRAMS—A PROJECT SPONSORED BY A PRIVATE, CITYWIDE ANTI-POVERTY AGENCY RUN BY AND FOR PUERTO RICANS—IS DESCRIBED. THE NEW ROLE FOR THE NONPROFESSIONAL YOUTHS AT COURT COMPRISED FOUR MAJOR ACTIVITIES: (1) CASE FINDING; (2) CROSS-CULTURAL INTERPRETATION; (3) REPRESENTING THE PUERTO RICAN SOCIAL ENVIRONMENT; AND (4) ACTING AS A BRIDGEMAN BETWEEN THE PUERTO RICAN COMMUNITY AND NEW YORK CITY AGENCIES. 4 REFERENCES. (AUTHOR ABSTRACT MODIFIED)

ACCN   000390

468 AUTH   **DOHRENWEND, B. P.**

TITL   EPIDEMIOLOGICAL DATA FOR MENTAL HEALTH CENTER PLANNING—A SYMPOSIUM. II. PSYCHIATRIC DISORDER IN GENERAL POPULATIONS: PROBLEM OF THE UNTREATED "CASE.

SRCE   *AMERICAN JOURNAL OF PUBLIC HEALTH AND THE NATION'S HEALTH, 1970, 60(6), 1052-1064.*

INDX   PSYCHOPATHOLOGY, SURVEY, EMPIRICAL, CROSS CULTURAL, PUERTO RICAN-M, COMMUNITY, URBAN, MENTAL HEALTH, ADULTS, PSYCHIATRIC STATUS SCHEDULE, IMPAIRMENT, NEW YORK, EAST, SYMPTOMATOLOGY

ABST   AN INVESTIGATION OF WHETHER THE TYPICAL UNTREATED "CASES IN THE GENERAL POPULATION SUFFER FROM PSYCHIATRIC CONDITIONS COMPARABLE TO THOSE OF TYPICAL CASES IN PSYCHIATRIC TREATMENT WAS CONDUCTED. REPRESENTED IN THE SAMPLE WERE WHITE PROTESTANTS, JEWS, IRISH, NEGROES, PUERTO RICANS, COMMUNITY LEADERS, HEADS OF FAMILIES, OUTPATIENTS, AND INPATIENTS. THE RESPONDENTS WERE SPLIT INTO TWO GROUPS; HALF WERE GIVEN THE STRUCTURED INTERVIEW SCHEDULE (SIS) AND THE OTHER HALF THE PSYCHIATRIC STATUS SCHEDULE (PSS). BOTH QUESTIONNAIRES WERE DESIGNED TO ELICIT EVIDENCE OF PSYCHIATRIC SYMPTOMATOLOGY AND ATTENDANT IMPAIRMENT OF FUNCTIONING IN WORK, MARITAL AND SEXUAL RELATIONS, CHILDREARING, HOUSEKEEPING, FRIENDSHIP, AND LEISURE ACTIVITIES. TOWARD THE END OF THE INTERVIEW A PSYCHIATRIC INTERVIEWER RATED THEM ON "CASENESS AND "IMPAIRMENT. ADDITIONAL RATINGS ON THESE SCALES WERE MADE OF THE WRITTEN RECORDS OF THE INTERVIEWS WITH SUBSAMPLES OF RESPONDENTS. REGARDING BOTH "CASENESS AND "IMPAIRMENT, THERE WAS A SHARP CONTRAST BETWEEN THE PATIENT AND NONPATIENT

GROUPS. THE CONTRASTS WERE MORE PRO-NOUNCED WHEN THE SIS WAS USED THAN WHEN THE PSS WAS USED. 28 REFERENCES.

ACCN   000391

469 AUTH   **DOHRENWEND, B. P.**
     TITL   SOCIAL STATUS AND PSYCHOLOGICAL DISOR-DER: AN ISSUE OF SUBSTANCE AND AN ISSUE OF METHOD.
     SRCE   *AMERICAN SOCIOLOGICAL REVIEW, 1966, 31(1), 14-34. (REPRINTED IN L. C. KOLB, V. W. BER-NARD & B. P. DOHRENWEND (EDS.), URBAN CHALLENGES TO PSYCHIATRY. BOSTON: LITTLE, BROWN & COMPANY, 1969, PP. 375-410.)*
     INDX   SES, PSYCHOPATHOLOGY, CROSS CULTURAL, ADULTS, DEMOGRAPHIC, STRESS, NEW YORK, EAST, PUERTO RICAN-M, ESSAY
     ABST   THE MOST CONSISTENT DEMOGRAPHIC FIND-ING REPORTED IN SOCIAL PSYCHIATRIC FIELD STUDIES IS AN INVERSE RELATION BETWEEN SOCIAL CLASS AND PSYCHOLOGICAL DISOR-DER. THIS RELATIONSHIP IS INTERPRETED ON THE ONE HAND AS EVIDENCE OF SOCIAL CAU-SATION, WITH LOW STATUS PRODUCING DIS-ORDER, AND ON THE OTHER HAND AS EVI-DENCE OF SOCIAL SELECTION, WITH THE PREEXISTING DISORDER DETERMINING SO-CIAL STATUS. WHETHER NEGROES AND PUERTO RICANS IN NEW YORK CITY HAVE HIGHER OR LOWER RATES OF DISORDER THAN THEIR CLASS COUNTERPARTS IN MORE ADVAN-TAGED ETHNIC GROUPS IS DISCUSSED. THE FACTS ARE NOT AVAILABLE FROM EXISTING RESEARCH. THE RESULTS OF FIELD STUDIES CONTAIN CLUES TO GROUP DIFFERENCES IN MODES EXPRESSING DISTRESS, INCLUDING SOME THAT INVOLVE PROBLEMS OF RE-SPONSE BIAS, BUT THE EVIDENCE IS FAR FROM CLEAR ABOUT THE RELATION OF THE SYMPTOMS REPORTED TO THE UNDERLYING PSYCHIATRIC CONDITION OF INDIVIDUALS. TWO MAJOR QUESTIONS CONFRONT FURTHER WORK IN THIS FIELD. FIRST, WHAT ARE THE CULTURAL AND SITUATIONAL FACTORS THAT LEAD TO DIFFERENT MODES OF EXPRESSING PSYCHOLOGICAL SYMPTOMS? SECOND, UN-DER WHAT CONDITIONS DOES SYMPTOMATIC EXPRESSION OF PSYCHOLOGICAL DISTRESS BECOME EVIDENCE OF UNDERLYING PERSON-ALITY DEFECT? MEASUREMENT OF PSYCHO-LOGICAL DISORDER IN DIFFERENT GROUPS WITH SOME HOPE OF RESOLVING THE CRU-CIAL ETIOLOGICAL ISSUE OF CAUSATION VS. SOCIAL SELECTION IS DEPENDENT ON THE ANSWERS TO THESE TWO QUESTIONS. 44 REF-ERENCES.
     ACCN   000392

470 AUTH   **DOHRENWEND, B. P.**
     TITL   SOCIAL STATUS, STRESS AND PSYCHOLOGI-CAL SYMPTOMS.
     SRCE   *MILBANK MEMORIAL FUND QUARTERLY, 1969, 47(1), 137-150.*
     INDX   PSYCHOPATHOLOGY, SES, PUERTO RICAN-M, CROSS CULTURAL, EMPIRICAL, REVIEW, STRESS, SYMPTOMATOLOGY, ADULTS, REVIEW, NEW YORK, EAST, CULTURAL FACTORS, SURVEY, UR-BAN

ABST   THIS STUDY EXAMINED THE INCIDENCE OF PSYCHIATRIC DISORDER AMONG NEGRO AND PUERTO RICAN GROUPS RELATIVE TO THEIR SOCIAL CLASS COUNTERPARTS IN MORE AD-VANTAGED ETHNIC GROUPS IN THE WASHING-TON HEIGHTS AREA OF NEW YORK CITY. SUB-JECTS CONSISTED OF A SAMPLE FROM THE GENERAL POPULATION OF APPROXIMATELY 1,000 21 TO 59 YEAR-OLD ADULTS, OF WHOM 150 WERE SEEN FOR FOLLOWUP. IN ADDITION, ABOUT 100 PSYCHIATRIC OUTPATIENTS SERVED AS SUBJECTS. RESULTS GENERALLY CONFIRM EARLIER REPORTS OF AN INVERSE RELATION-SHIP BETWEEN SOCIAL CLASS AND PSYCHO-LOGICAL DISORDER. HOWEVER, PUERTO RI-CAN SUBJECTS SHOWED LARGER PROPORTIONS OF SYMPTOMS THAN THEIR COUNTERPARTS IN OTHER GROUPS. NEGRO SUBJECTS DID NOT SHOW HIGHER RATES THAN JEWISH OR IRISH ETHNIC GROUPS. FIND-INGS SUGGEST THAT THERE ARE STRONG ETHNIC AND CLASS DIFFERENCES IN MODES OF EXPRESSING DISTRESS. 17 REFERENCES.

ACCN   000394

471 AUTH   **DOHRENWEND, B. P., CHIN-SHONG, E. T., ERGI, G., MENDELSOHN, F. S., & STOKES, J.**
     TITL   MEASURES OF PSYCHIATRIC DISORDER IN CONTRASTING CLASS AND ETHNIC GROUPS: A PRELIMINARY REPORT OF ONGOING RE-SEARCH.
     SRCE   *IN E. H. HARE & J. K. WING (EDS.), PSYCHIATRIC EPIDEMIOLOGY. LONDON: OXFORD UNIVER-SITY PRESS, 1970, PP. 159-202.*
     INDX   CROSS CULTURAL, RESEARCH METHOD-OLOGY, PSYCHIATRIC STATUS SCHEDULE, PUERTO RICAN-M, ADULTS, EMPIRICAL, NEW YORK, EAST, SYMPTOMATOLOGY, PSYCHO-PATHOLOGY, SURVEY, CULTURAL FACTORS
     ABST   THE RELATIVE IMPORTANCE OF SOCIAL CAU-SATION VS. SOCIAL SELECTION FACTORS IN SOCIAL-CLASS DIFFERENCES IN RATES OF PSYCHOPATHOLOGY IS INVESTIGATED. A SAMPLE OF 580 SUBJECTS, AGES 21 TO 64, CAME FROM FIVE ETHNIC GROUPS: WHITE AN-GLO-SAXON PROTESTANT, JEWISH, IRISH, BLACK, AND PUERTO RICAN. INFORMATION WAS OBTAINED FROM THE STRUCTURED IN-TERVIEW SCHEDULE (SIS) AND THE PSYCHIAT-RIC STATUS SCHEDULE (PSS). THE SUBJECTS WERE RANDOMLY ALTERNATED BETWEEN THE TWO INSTRUMENTS WHICH PROBED PSYCHI-ATRIC SYMPTOMATOLOGY AND IMPAIRMENT OF FUNCTIONING. MAJOR FINDINGS WERE: (1) BOTH JUDGMENTAL AND PRELIMINARY OB-JECTIVE MEASURES OF DISORDER DISCRIMI-NATE SHARPLY BETWEEN COMMUNITY LEAD-ERS, PSYCHIATRIC PATIENTS, AND COMMUNITY RESPONDENTS; (2) TYPICAL "CASES IN THE COMMUNITY ARE NOT THE SAME TYPICAL CASES IN THE PSYCHIATRIC CLINIC OR HOSPI-TAL; (3) THE TWO TYPES OF INTERVIEWS PRES-ENT DIFFERENT PICTURES TO PSYCHIATRISTS OF THE PSYCHIATRIC CONDITIONS OF THE COMMUNITY RESPONDENTS; (4) COMMUNITY RESPONDENTS APPEAR MORE SERIOUSLY ILL TO PSYCHIATRISTS ON THE BASIS OF A WRIT-TEN RECORD FROM WHICH CLUES TO SOCIAL

AND PATIENT STATUS HAVE BEEN REMOVED THAN THEY APPEAR IN A FACE-TO-FACE INTERVIEW; (5) COMMUNITY RESPONDENTS ADMIT MORE SYMPTOMS TO PSYCHIATRISTS THAN THEY ADMIT TO LAY INTERVIEWERS. THE CLASS AND ETHNIC DIFFERENCES FOUND IN THE TWO INSTRUMENTS SUGGEST THAT SUCH SUBCULTURAL DIFFERENCES MAY BE RELATED NOT ONLY TO THE TYPES OF SYMPTOMS PROBED BUT ALSO TO THE TYPES OF QUESTIONING PROCEDURES USED TO ASK ABOUT THE SYMPTOMS. 19 REFERENCES.

ACCN   000395

472 AUTH   **DOHRENWEND, B. P., & CHIN-SHONG, E. T.**
    TITL   SOCIAL STATUS AND ATTITUDES TOWARD PSYCHOLOGICAL DISORDER: THE PROBLEM OF TOLERANCE OF DEVIANCE.
    SRCE   *AMERICAN SOCIOLOGICAL REVIEW, 1967, 32(3), 417-433.*
    INDX   SES, ATTITUDES, PSYCHOPATHOLOGY, DEVIANCE, REVIEW, PUERTO RICAN-M, NEW YORK, EAST, MENTAL HEALTH
    ABST   THE HYPOTHESES THAT THERE IS A GROWING ACCEPTANCE OF A MENTAL HEALTH ORIENTATION TOWARD PROBLEMS OF DEVIANT BEHAVIOR AMONG HIGH-STATUS GROUPS AND A GREATER TOLERANCE OF DEVIANCE IN LOW-STATUS GROUPS WERE TESTED. RESULTS INDICATE THAT, WHILE THERE MAY BE AN INCREASING TENDENCY TO USE THE LABEL "MENTALLY ILL FOR DESCRIBING DIFFERENT TYPES OF DEVIANT BEHAVIOR, SHARP DIFFERENCES IN JUDGMENTS OF THE SERIOUSNESS OF THE PROBLEMS REMAIN. THE PSYCHIATRISTS' EVALUATION FOCUSED ON THE INDIVIDUAL'S UNDERLYING PSYCHOPATHOLOGY WHILE THE COMMUNITY RESPONDENTS JUDGED SERIOUSNESS IN TERMS OF WHETHER OR NOT IT THREATENED OTHERS, RATHER THAN ON THE NATURE OF THE INTRAPSYCHIC PATHOLOGY. ATTITUDES TOWARD MENTAL ILLNESS APPEAR TO BE RELATED TO A COMPLEX INTERACTION OF ETHNICITY AND EDUCATION. THE APPEARANCE OF GREATER TOLERANCE OF DEVIANT BEHAVIOR IN LOW-STATUS GROUPS IS AN ARTIFACT OF VIEWING THEIR ATTITUDES WITHIN A HIGH-STATUS FRAME OF REFERENCE—THAT IS, THEIR DEFINITION OF SERIOUS MENTAL ILLNESS IS NARROWER THAN THAT OF HIGHER STATUS GROUPS. WHEN BOTH LOWER AND UPPER STATUS GROUPS DEFINE A PATTERN OF BEHAVIOR AS SERIOUSLY DEVIANT, LOWER STATUS GROUPS ARE LESS TOLERANT. MOREOVER, THE RELATIVELY TOLERANT POLICY OF UPPER STATUS GROUPS APPEARS TO BE A CONSEQUENCE OF THEIR GENERALLY MORE LIBERAL ORIENTATION RATHER THAN OF COMPREHENSION OF THE NATURE OF PSYCHOPATHOLOGY IN PSYCHIATRIC TERMS. 25 REFERENCES.

ACCN   000396

473 AUTH   **DOHRENWEND, B. P., & DOHRENWEND, B. S.**
    TITL   SOCIAL STATUS AND PSYCHOLOGICAL DISORDER: A CASUAL INQUIRY.
    SRCE   *NEW YORK: JOHN WILEY & SONS, 1969.*
    INDX   PSYCHOPATHOLOGY, SES, PUERTO RICAN-M,

CROSS CULTURAL, EMPIRICAL, REVIEW, STRESS, SYMPTOMATOLOGY, ADULTS, NEW YORK, EAST, SOCIAL MOBILITY, URBAN, SURVEY, BOOK
    ABST   A REVIEW OF THE LITERATURE CONSISTENTLY INDICATES AN INVERSE RELATION BETWEEN SOCIAL CLASS AND REPORTED RATE OF PSYCHOLOGICAL DISORDER. TWO HYPOTHESES ARE OFFERED FOR THIS FINDING: (1) SOCIAL CAUSATION, THE ENVIRONMENTAL PRESSURES ASSOCIATED WITH LOW SOCIAL STATUS CAUSE PSYCHOPATHOLOGY; AND (2) SOCIAL SELECTION, PREEXISTING PSYCHOLOGICAL DISORDER LEADS TO LOW SOCIAL STATUS. SINCE NEITHER SOCIAL ENVIRONMENTAL NOR GENETICALLY ORIENTED INVESTIGATORS HAVE PRESENTED CONCLUSIVE EVIDENCE FOR THE CAUSAL FACTOR IN PSYCHOPATHOLOGY, THE AUTHORS PRESENT A RESEARCH STRATEGY BASED ON PROCESSES OF ETHNIC-GROUP ASSIMILATION IN OPEN-CLASS SOCIETIES. THE STRATEGY IS BASED ON THREE ASSUMPTIONS: (1) THERE IS AN ALMOST UNIVERSALLY SHARED NORM IN OPEN-CLASS SOCIETIES THAT UPWARD SOCIAL MOBILITY IS DESIRABLE; (2) SERIOUS PSYCHOLOGICAL DISORDER INVOLVES DISABILITY THAT DECREASES THE PROBABILITY OF UPWARD SOCIAL MOBILITY AND INCREASES THE PROBABILITY OF DOWNWARD SOCIAL MOBILITY; AND (3) THERE IS GREATER DOWNWARD SOCIAL PRESSURE ON MEMBERS OF DISADVANTAGED ETHNIC GROUPS THAN ON THEIR SOCIAL CLASS COUNTERPARTS IN MORE ADVANTAGED ETHNIC GROUPS. INTERVIEWS CONCERNING GENERAL PSYCHOLOGICAL DISORDER WITH NEGRO, PUERTO RICAN, JEWISH, AND IRISH SUBJECTS IN THE WASHINGTON HEIGHTS SECTION OF NEW YORK CITY SUPPORTED THE SOCIAL ENVIRONMENTAL HYPOTHESIS. THIS WAS DUE MAINLY TO THE STRONG AND CONSISTENTLY HIGHER RATES OF SYMPTOMS ON ALL MEASURES REPORTED BY PUERTO RICANS RELATIVE TO THEIR CLASS COUNTERPARTS IN THE MORE ADVANTAGED ETHNIC GROUPS. A PROBLEM OF RESPONSE SET, HOWEVER, SUGGESTS THAT THE CONSISTENTLY HIGH RATES OF SYMPTOMS AMONG PUERTO RICANS MAY INVALIDATE THE INTERPRETATION OF HIGHER RATES OF PSYCHOLOGICAL DISORDER AMONG THIS GROUP. OTHER QUESTIONS CONCERNING THE VALIDITY OF THE MEASUREMENT INSTRUMENTS THEMSELVES CALL INTO QUESTION THE FINDINGS. THUS, ALTHOUGH THE LOW SOCIAL STATUS OF DISADVANTAGED ETHNIC GROUPS DOES RESULT IN GREATER STRESS, THE RELATIONSHIP OF PSYCHOPATHOLOGY NECESSITATES ADDITIONAL RESEARCH. 325 REFERENCES.

ACCN   000397

474 AUTH   **DOMINGUEZ-YBARRA, A., & GARRISON, J.**
    TITL   TOWARDS ADEQUATE PSYCHIATRIC CLASSIFICATION AND TREATMENT OF MEXICAN AMERICAN PATIENTS.
    SRCE   *PSYCHIATRIC ANNALS, 1977, 7(12), 86-96.*
    INDX   ACCULTURATION, ADULTS, BILINGUAL, COPING MECHANISMS, CULTURAL FACTORS, FAMILY

ROLES, FAMILY STRUCTURE, FOLK MEDICINE, HEALTH, MENTAL HEALTH, MEXICAN AMERI-CAN, PSYCHOTHERAPY, PSYCHOTHERAPISTS, RELIGION, CURANDERISMO, SES, ESSAY, POLICY

ABST CHRONIC UNDERREPRESENTATION OF MEXI-CAN AMERICANS AMONG PATIENTS RECEIVING ALL FORMS OF PSYCHIATRIC TREATMENT IN THE U.S. CAN BE TRACED TO: (1) BAD EXPERI-ENCES IN THE PAST WITH MENTAL HEALTH IN-STITUTIONS; (2) EMBARRASSMENT IN DIS-CUSSING MATTERS RELATED TO MENTAL HEALTH; AND (3) MORE IMMEDIATE SUPPORT WITHIN THE EXTENDED FAMILY NETWORK. THE CLINICIAN CHARGED WITH TREATING PER-SONS FROM THIS POPULATION IS ADVISED TO ASSESS THE CULTURAL LEVEL OF A MEXICAN AMERICAN PATIENT BY ASCERTAINING PLACE OF RESIDENCE, LENGTH OF STAY IN THE NEIGHBORHOOD, FLUENCY IN ENGLISH AND SPANISH, CONVICTIONS ABOUT RELIGION, AND TRADITIONAL FOLK ILLNESS BELIEFS. IN TREATMENT, THE CLINICIAN SHOULD CON-SIDER UTILIZING THE FAMILY SUPPORT NET-WORK; AND WHEN BELIEF IN CURANDERSIMO HAS BEEN ESTABLISHED, THE CLINICIAN MIGHT FIND COLLABORATION WITH A CURANDERO PROFITABLE. FOR EXAMPLE, THE POVERTY-LEVEL, ACCULTURATING MEXICAN AMERICAN MAY SUFFER FROM "VERGUENZA (A GUILT-LADEN STATE OF ALIENATION). CULTURALLY APPROPRIATE THERAPY CAN REDUCE "VER-GUENZA TO A MANAGEABLE STATE BY PRO-VIDING THE CLIENT BOTH WITH A LINK TO HIS MEXICAN TRADITIONS AND A METHOD OF UN-DERSTANDING AND COPING WITH HIS PROB-LEMS. 20 REFERENCES.

ACCN 002075

475 AUTH **DONDERO, A. S.**

TITL LOS ANGELES COUNTY MENTAL HEALTH SER-VICES TO THE CHICANO POPULATION: A SUR-VEY (DOCTORAL DISSERTATION, CALIFORNIA SCHOOL OF PROFESSIONAL PSYCHOLOGY, LOS ANGELES, 1973).

SRCE *DISSERTATION ABSTRACTS INTERNATIONAL, 1973, 34, 5164B. (UNIVERSITY MICROFILMS NO. 74-7926).*

INDX HEALTH DELIVERY SYSTEMS, PSYCHOTHER-APY, MENTAL HEALTH PROFESSION, PSYCHO-THERAPISTS, PHYSICIANS, PARAPROFESSION-ALS, SES, POVERTY, REPRESENTATION, SURVEY, MEXICAN AMERICAN, ADULTS, EMPIRICAL, BI-LINGUAL-BICULTURAL PERSONNEL, PERSON-NEL, CALIFORNIA, SOUTHWEST, PROGRAM EVALUATION

ABST THE EXTENT TO WHICH THE SPANISH SUR-NAMED MINORITY IS CURRENTLY UNDER-SERVED BY THE LOS ANGELES COUNTY MEN-TAL HEALTH DELIVERY SYSTEM WITH RESPECT TO MENTAL HEALTH PATIENT POPULATION AND MENTAL HEALTH PROFESSIONAL STAFF COM-POSITION WAS INVESTIGATED. THE RESULTS OF THIS SURVEY DEMONSTRATED THAT PRES-ENT MENTAL HEALTH SERVICES IN LOS ANGE-LES COUNTY ARE NOT MEETING THE NEEDS OF THIS LARGE SEGMENT OF THE POPULA-TION AND ARE ESPECIALLY INADEQUATE FOR THOSE WHO SPEAK ONLY SPANISH. THE SPAN-

ISH SURNAME GROUP ACCOUNTED FOR 18% OF THE TOTAL COUNTY POPULATION WHILE ONLY 7% OF THE PROFESSIONAL DIRECT SER-VICES STAFF HAD SPANISH SURNAMES. IN NONE OF THE REGIONS DID THE PATIENT POPULATION PROPORTIONATELY APPROXI-MATE THE GENERAL REGIONAL POPULATION. FOR THE MOST PART, THE MENTAL HEALTH CENTERS WERE UNDERSTAFFED, OPERATED ON A VERY LIMITED BUDGET, AND HAD TRANS-PORTATION PROBLEMS IN ALL THE REGIONS MAKING THE CENTERS INACCESSIBLE TO LARGE NUMBERS OF CHICANOS. INDICATED WAS AN IMPERATIVE NEED FOR MENTAL HEALTH EDUCATION AND BETTER COORDINATION OF MENTAL HEALTH SERVICES. THERE IS ALSO A NEED FOR RESEARCH SO THAT REALISTIC PROGRAMS CAN BE DESIGNED. FINALLY, THERE IS A CRUCIAL NEED TO EDUCATE THE EXIST-ING STAFF TO THE CULTURE, NEEDS, AND LIFE-STYLE OF THIS POPULATION. 54 REFERENCES. (AUTHOR ABSTRACT MODIFIED)

ACCN 000398

476 AUTH **DOOB, C. B.**

TITL FAMILY BACKGROUND AND PEER GROUP DE-VELOPMENT IN A PUERTO RICAN DISTRICT.

SRCE *THE SOCIOLOGICAL QUARTERLY, 1970, 11, 523-532.*

INDX DELINQUENCY, PUERTO RICAN-M, URBAN, PEER GROUP, INTERPERSONAL RELATIONS, FAMILY STRUCTURE, FAMILY ROLES, MOTHER-CHILD INTERACTION, FATHER-CHILD INTERACTION, GANGS, GROUP DYNAMICS, CASE STUDY, THEORETICAL, EMPIRICAL

ABST A NINE-MONTH PARTICIPANT-OBSERVATION STUDY IN EAST HARLEM, NEW YORK, EXAM-INED THE LIFE STYLES OF 10 PUERTO RICAN BOYS RANGING IN AGE FROM 10 TO 18. FORTY-EIGHT OTHERS WERE OBSERVED LESS INTEN-SIVELY. TWO HYPOTHESES EMERGED FROM THE OBSERVATION THAT A BOYS' PEER GROUP CHOICE IS A PRODUCT OF THE FAMILY OF ORI-GIN: (1) THE COHESION OF THE PEER GROUP IN WHICH THE BOYS SEEK MEMBERSHIP WILL BE SIMILAR TO THAT IN THE FAMILY OF ORIGIN; AND (2) THE RANGE OF THE BOYS' PEER GROUP CONTACTS CORRESPONDS TO THOSE MAINTAINED BY THE PARENTS. IT IS PROPOSED THAT THESE HYPOTHESES BE TESTED SUBSE-QUENTLY WITH A SURVEY DESIGN. THROUGH THIS STUDY OF PEER AFFILIATIONS, THE AU-THOR HAS BEGUN TO EXAMINE THE EXTENT TO WHICH A DIFFERENTIATION OF INTEREST AND ORIENTATION IS TAKING PLACE WITHIN ETHNIC GROUPS AND THE SOCIAL ANTECED-ENTS TO THIS PROCESS. 19 REFERENCES.

ACCN 000399

477 AUTH **DOUGLAS, J. W. B., INGLEBY, J. D., ROSS, J. M., & TILLOTT, J. M.**

TITL BEHAVIORAL STYLES OF 4 1/2 YEAR-OLD BOYS WHEN RESPONDING TO TEST DEMANDS.

SRCE *EDUCATIONAL RESEARCH, 1972, 14(3), 208-212.*

INDX COGNITIVE STYLE, CHILDREN, STANFORD-BI-NET INTELLIGENCE TEST, EXAMINER EFFECTS, IMMIGRATION, CROSS CULTURAL, INTELLI-

GENCE TESTING, PUERTO RICAN-M, MALE, EMPIRICAL

ABST A METHOD FOR MEASURING THE RESPONSE STYLE OF PRESCHOOL CHILDREN PERFORMING COGNITIVE TASKS (THE STANFORD-BINET INTELLIGENCE TEST, FORM L) WAS INVESTIGATED. IT WAS NOT POSSIBLE TO RECORD BEHAVIOR IN ADEQUATE DETAIL USING THE METHOD OF A HANDWRITTEN PROTOCOL, SO A MODIFIED PROCEDURE WAS ADOPTED WHICH CLASSIFIED RESPONSES DIRECTLY BY THEIR TYPE AND RECORDED THEM IN CODE. USING THIS METHOD, RELIABILITY WAS FOUND TO BE HIGH. MOREOVER, OVER A 4-6 WEEK PERIOD THERE WAS SUBSTANTIAL CONSISTENCY IN THE STYLE OF BEHAVIOR SHOWN BY THESE CHILDREN WHEN DEALING WITH TEST DEMANDS. SINCE THERE WERE ETHNIC DIFFERENCES IN THE 32 CHILDREN, IT WAS ALSO OF INTEREST TO DISCOVER WHETHER CHILDREN OF IMMIGRANT AND U.S.-BORN PARENTS WOULD SHOW DIFFERENCES IN BEHAVIOR COMPARABLE TO THE DIFFERENCES BETWEEN PUERTO RICAN AND MIDDLE-CLASS AMERICAN CHILDREN. SOME BEHAVIORAL DIFFERENCES WERE FOUND, BUT THESE APPEARED TO BE WHOLLY A FUNCTION OF DIFFERING TEST PERFORMANCE. 1 REFERENCE. (PASAR ABSTRACT MODIFIED)

ACCN 000400

478 AUTH **DOUGLAS, R. R.**
TITL HYPNOTIC RESISTANCE IN THE VICTORIAN CONSCIENCE.
SRCE *JOURNAL OF THE AMERICAN INSTITUTE OF HYPNOSIS, 1974, 15(3), 112-115.*
INDX PSYCHOTHERAPY, ATTITUDES, PERSONALITY, PSYCHOTHERAPY OUTCOME, MEXICAN AMERICAN, CROSS CULTURAL, PSYCHOPATHOLOGY, HISTORY, DREAMS, CASE STUDY, ARIZONA, SOUTHWEST
ABST FREUD AND OTHER PRACTITIONERS IN THE VICTORIAN PERIOD CRITICIZED HYPNOSIS AS A LIMITED TECHNIQUE WITH MANY WEAKNESSES. THIS WAS BASED ON HYPNOSIS AS IT THEN WAS PRACTICED, AND AS SUCH REFLECTED THE RIGID, REPRESSIVE QUALITIES OF THE VICTORIAN ERA. AN ATTEMPT HAS BEEN MADE TO CHECK THIS THEORY BY COMPARING TEN MEXICANS (VICTORIAN), EIGHT MEXICAN AMERICANS (SEMI-VICTORIAN), AND TEN ANGLOS (NON-VICTORIAN) PATIENTS IN TUCSON AND NOGALES, ARIZONA WITH REGARD TO THEIR RESPONSES TO HYPNOSIS. MEXICAN CLIENTS SAW THE HYPNOTIST AS AN AUTHORITY AND SEEMED TO UNDERGO A SPLIT BETWEEN THE TRANCE EXPERIENCE AND CONSCIOUS AWARENESS. THEIR RESPONSES WERE SIMILAR TO ONES NOTED BY VICTORIAN HYPNOTISTS. MEXICAN AMERICANS SHOWED INCREASING ABILITY TO COMBINE TRANCE AND CONSCIOUS AWARENESS AND FELT THEY WERE PARTICIPATING IN THE HYPNOTIC PROCESS. REACTIONS IN THIS GROUP VARIED ACCORDING TO AGE AND DEGREE OF AMERICANIZATION. ANGLOS, ON THE OTHER HAND, APPROACHED HYPNOSIS WITH BOTH ACCEPTANCE OF CAUSE AND EFFECT IN EMOTIONAL PROBLEMS AND WERE APT TO BE MORE ANALYTIC AND CRITICAL OF THE TECHNIQUE. ANGLOS RESPONDED THE BEST OF ALL THE GROUPS TO THE HYPNOTIC TREATMENT. THESE CASE STUDIES INDICATE THAT FOR THOSE HAVING A MORE "MODERN CONSCIENCE, HYPNOSIS WOULD BE EFFECTIVE IN AN ONGOING PSYCHOTHERAPY PROGRAM. 5 REFERENCES. (AUTHOR SUMMARY MODIFIED)

ACCN 000401

479 AUTH **DRAKE, R. H.**
TITL A COMPARATIVE STUDY OF THE MENTALITY AND ACHIEVEMENT OF MEXICAN AND WHITE CHILDREN.
SRCE *SAN FRANCISCO: R AND E RESEARCH ASSOCIATES, 1972. (REPRINTED FROM AN UNPUBLISHED MASTER'S THESIS, UNIVERSITY OF SOUTHERN CALIFORNIA, 1927.)*
INDX INTELLIGENCE, INTELLIGENCE TESTING, EDUCATION, EMPIRICAL, MEXICAN AMERICAN, CROSS CULTURAL, BILINGUALISM, TEST RELIABILITY, ARIZONA, SOUTHWEST, ADOLESCENTS
ABST TO DETERMINE WHAT DIFFERENCES IN INTELLIGENCE, IF ANY, THERE ARE BETWEEN MEXICAN AMERICAN AND WHITE CHILDREN, 317 7TH AND 8TH GRADERS IN A TUCSON, ARIZONA, SCHOOL WERE GIVEN THE FOLLOWING TESTS: (1) PINTER NON-LANGUAGE; (2) NATIONAL INTELLIGENCE TESTS, SCALE A, FORMS 1 AND 2; AND (3) STANFORD ACHIEVEMENT TEST, FORMS A AND B. DATA ARE PRESENTED IN TABULAR AND GRAPH FORM. THE TEST RESULTS INDICATE THAT THE WHITES WERE SUPERIOR IN INTELLIGENCE TO THE MEXICAN AMERICANS, AND THAT THE ACHIEVEMENT OF THE WHITES IN ACADEMIC SUBJECTS WAS GREATER THAN THAT OF THE MEXICAN AMERICANS. ASSESSMENT OF THE TEST INSTRUMENTS REVEALED THAT THE PINTER WAS NOT RELIABLE FOR EITHER WHITE OR MEXICAN AMERICAN SUBJECTS, WHILE THE NATIONAL INTELLIGENCE AND STANFORD TESTS PROVED TO BE RELIABLE FOR BOTH GROUPS. 30 REFERENCES. (AUTHOR SUMMARY MODIFIED)

ACCN 000402

480 AUTH **DUBOIS, B. L.**
TITL CULTURAL AND SOCIAL FACTORS IN THE ASSESSMENT OF LANGUAGE CAPABILITIES.
SRCE *ELEMENTARY ENGLISH, 1974, 51(2), 257-261.*
INDX LANGUAGE ASSESSMENT, CULTURAL FACTORS, BILINGUALISM, ESSAY, REVIEW, LINGUISTIC COMPETENCE, SPANISH SURNAMED, CROSS CULTURAL, POLICY
ABST IN PLANNING LANGUAGE COURSES FOR ANY GROUP OF STUDENTS, THE TEACHER SHOULD FIRST ASSESS THE STUDENTS' LANGUAGE COMPETENCE. WHEN TEACHING STUDENTS WHO USE MORE THAN ONE LANGUAGE, ASSESSMENT OF THEIR LANGUAGE SKILLS CANNOT BE DONE WITHOUT ASSESSMENT OF LANGUAGE DOMINANCE. THE ACCURACY OF THIS ASSESSMENT MAY BE SERIOUSLY IMPAIRED BY (1) INAPPROPRIATE CONDITIONS OF OBSERVATION, AND (2) THE ASSESSORS' LACK OF KNOWLEDGE REGARDING LANGUAGE DOMI-

NANCE IN BILINGUALS. THESE TWO SITUATIONS ARE DISCUSSED USING EXAMPLES DRAWN FROM THE LITERATURE. 11 REFERENCES. (AUTHOR SUMMARY MODIFIED)

ACCN 000403

481 AUTH **DUNLAP, R. L., BEIGEL, A., & ARMON, V.**
TITL YOUNG CHILDREN AND THE WATTS REVOLT.
SRCE *COMMUNITY MENTAL HEALTH JOURNAL, 1968, 4(3), 201-210.*
INDX STRESS, CHILDREN, EMPIRICAL, URBAN, MEXICAN AMERICAN, CROSS CULTURAL, ATTITUDES, POLICE-COMMUNITY RELATIONS, CALIFORNIA, SOUTHWEST
ABST IMMEDIATELY FOLLOWING THE WATTS RACE RIOT IN LOS ANGELES, AUGUST 1965, SEMISTRUCTURED INTERVIEWS WERE OBTAINED WITH 107 BLACK, 23 MEXICAN AMERICAN, AND 52 WHITE PRESCHOOL CHILDREN. RESPONSE DATA WERE USED TO ASSESS THE CHILDREN'S AWARENESS OF RIOT EVENTS, THEIR FEARS OR OTHER AFFECTIVE REACTIONS, AND THEIR ATTITUDES TOWARD THE RIOT PARTICIPANTS. OVER 70 PERCENT IN EACH GROUP WERE AWARE OF THE RIOTING, AND APPROXIMATELY 50 PERCENT GAVE EVIDENCE OF RIOT-RELATED FEAR. ATTITUDES OF BLACK AND WHITE CHILDREN TOWARD THE RIOTERS VARIED IN POSITIVE-NEGATIVE DIRECTION AND INTENSITY, WHILE THE SMALL MEXICAN AMERICAN GROUP WAS MORE UNIFORMLY HOSTILE-FEARFUL. 13 REFERENCES.

ACCN 000404

482 AUTH **DURAN, R., (ED.)**
TITL SALUBRIDAD CHICANA: SU PRESERVACION Y MANTENIMIENTO. THE CHICANO PLAN FOR MENTAL HEALTH.
SRCE *BOULDER, COLO.: WESTERN INTERSTATE COMMISSION OF HIGHER EDUCATION, 1975.*
INDX MENTAL HEALTH, FAMILY STRUCTURE, CULTURE, ALCOHOLISM, DRUG ADDICTION, POLICE-COMMUNITY RELATIONS, URBAN, COMMUNITY, HOUSING, EDUCATION, CHILDREN, SOCIAL SERVICES, ACCULTURATION, UNDOCUMENTED WORKERS, PROFESSIONAL TRAINING, DRUG ABUSE, REHABILITATION, PARAPROFESSIONALS, RESOURCE UTILIZATION, HEALTH DELIVERY SYSTEMS, BILINGUAL-BICULTURAL PERSONNEL, BILINGUAL-BICULTURAL EDUCATION, LEGISLATION, CULTURAL PLURALISM, POLICY, COMMUNITY INVOLVEMENT, SOUTHWEST, BOOK
ABST THE RECOMMENDATIONS BY THE TASK FORCE COVER A WIDE SPECTRUM OF ISSUES CONSIDERED RELEVANT IN DEVELOPING EFFECTIVE AND ADEQUATE MENTAL HEALTH SERVICES FOR THE SPANISH-SPEAKING COMMUNITIES IN THE SOUTHWEST. IN ASSESSING THE NEEDS OF THE CHICANO POPULATION THE FOLLOWING AREAS WERE ADDRESSED: (1) LA FAMILIA; (2) THE URBAN BARRIO; (3) MENTAL HEALTH NEEDS OF MIGRANT WORKERS; (4) DRUG USE; (5) ALCOHOLISM; (6) EDUCATION; (7) LEGAL PROCUREMENT OF MENTAL HEALTH SERVICES; AND (8) CRITERIA TO EVALUATE SERVICES. SOME OF THE RECOMMENDATIONS RELATE TO THE IMPORTANCE OF BILINGUAL-

BICULTURAL EDUCATION, IMPROVING EQUAL OPPORTUNITIES, HAVING COMMUNITY-BASED MONITORING SYSTEMS, AND THE NEED FOR SCIENTISTS TO DEVELOP "CULTURE FREE TESTS AND PROVIDE AN OVERALL CHICANO THEORY OF MENTAL HEALTH.

ACCN 000405

483 AUTH **DURRETT, M. E., O'BRYANT, S., & PENNEBAKER, J. W.**
TITL CHILD-REARING REPORTS OF WHITE, BLACK, AND MEXICAN-AMERICAN FAMILIES.
SRCE *DEVELOPMENTAL PSYCHOLOGY, 1975, 11(6), 871.*
INDX CHILDREARING PRACTICES, SOCIALIZATION, FATHER-CHILD INTERACTION, MOTHER-CHILD INTERACTION, EMPIRICAL, ATTITUDES, ADULTS, AUTHORITARIANISM, ACHIEVEMENT MOTIVATION, CROSS CULTURAL, MEXICAN AMERICAN, TEXAS, SOUTHWEST
ABST ALTHOUGH ETHNIC DIFFERENCES HAVE BEEN NOTED IN THE SOCIALIZATION PROCESS, LITTLE INFORMATION HAS BEEN OBTAINED REGARDING CHILD REARING PRACTICES AMONG WHITES, BLACKS AND MEXICAN AMERICANS. INTERVIEWS CONDUCTED USING BLOCK'S CHILD REARING PRACTICES REPORT (CRPR) REVEALED THAT FOR 90 LOW INCOME FAMILES, EACH HAVING A 5 YEAR-OLD CHILD IN HEADSTART, FAMILIES USED THE SAME TECHNIQUES BUT FOR DIFFERENT REASONS. WHITE AND BLACK PARENTS WERE MORE AUTHORITIVE THAN MEXICAN AMERICAN PARENTS. HOWEVER, MEXICAN AMERICAN PARENTS WERE MORE CONSISTENT IN REWARD AND PUNISHMENT PRACTICES, STRESSED GREATER CONTROL OVER EMOTIONS, AND WERE MORE PROTECTIVE THAN THE WHITE AND BLACK PARENTS. 1 REFERENCE.

ACCN 000406

484 AUTH **DURRETT, M. E., & DAVY, A. J.**
TITL RACIAL AWARENESS IN YOUNG MEXICAN-AMERICAN, NEGRO AND ANGLO CHILDREN.
SRCE *YOUNG CHILDREN, 1970, 26(1), 16-24.*
INDX ETHNIC IDENTITY, MEXICAN AMERICAN, CROSS CULTURAL, SEX COMPARISON, EMPIRICAL, CHILDREN, CALIFORNIA, SOUTHWEST
ABST THE DOLL TECHNIQUE WAS PRESENTED TO 30 ANGLO, 30 MEXICAN AMERICAN AND 25 NEGRO CHILDREN ATTENDING INTERRACIAL PREKINDERGARTEN PROGRAMS. IT WAS FOUND THAT THE ANGLO SUBJECTS EXPRESSED THE GREATEST OWN-RACE PREFERENCE BOTH IN IDENTIFICATION AND PLAYMATE CHOICE. THE NEGRO SUBJECTS SHOWED THE LEAST OWN-GROUP PREFERENCE, PARTICULARLY IN THE CHOICE OF PLAYMATE. THE MEXICAN AMERICAN SUBJECTS WERE HIGHLY AWARE OF THE RACIAL DIFFERENCES BETWEEN NEGROES AND ANGLOS AND APPEARED TO HAVE APPLIED POSITIVE VALUE TERMS TO THE ANGLO GROUP. SOME POSITIVE CHANGES THAT APPEAR TO HAVE EVOLVED DURING THE PAST 10 YEARS INCLUDE: (1) LESS OWN-RACE REJECTION BY THE NEGRO SUBJECTS AS SHOWN BY THE INCREASED PROPORTION OF SUBJECTS MAKING OWN-RACE CHOICES IN IDENTIFICATION; AND

(2) LESS EVIDENCE OF DEROGATORY RE-
MARKS AND HOSTILE ATTITUDES EXPRESSED
BY EITHER THE ANGLO OR NEGRO CHILDREN.
ALTHOUGH POSITIVE CHANGES HAVE BEEN
NOTED, MANY NEGRO CHILDREN, PARTICU-
LARLY BOYS, NEED HELP IN DEVELOPING MORE
POSITIVE OWN-RACE ACCEPTANCE. 12 REFER-
ENCES. (AUTHOR SUMMARY MODIFIED)

ACCN   000407

485 AUTH **DURRETT, M. E., & KIM, C. C.**
     TITL   A COMPARATIVE STUDY OF BEHAVIORAL MA-
            TURITY IN MEXICAN-AMERICAN AND ANGLO
            PRESCHOOL CHILDREN.
     SRCE   *JOURNAL OF GENETIC PSYCHOLOGY, 1973,*
            123(1), 55-62.
     INDX   CHILDREN, CROSS CULTURAL, MEXICAN
            AMERICAN, SCHOLASTIC ACHIEVEMENT, IN-
            TERPERSONAL RELATIONS, SES, PSYCHOSO-
            CIAL ADJUSTMENT, CALIFORNIA, SOUTHWEST
     ABST   THE PURPOSES OF THIS STUDY WERE TO
            COMPARE (1) THE DEGREE OF BEHAVIORAL
            MATURITY OF MEXICAN AMERICAN PRE-
            SCHOOL CHILDREN AND ANGLO CHILDREN
            AND (2) THE FACTOR STRUCTURE OF BEHAV-
            IORAL MATURITY AT THIS AGE LEVEL IN THESE
            TWO GROUPS OF CHILDREN. ONE HUNDRED
            THIRTY-THREE MEXICAN AMERICAN CHILDREN
            WHO WERE ENROLLED IN PRE-KINDERGARTEN
            PROGRAMS IN THE PUBLIC SCHOOLS AND 139
            ANGLO PRESCHOOL CHILDREN SERVED AS
            SUBJECTS. THE TEACHERS RATED THE CHIL-
            DREN ENROLLED IN THEIR CLASSES ON AN 18-
            ITEM BEHAVIORAL MATURITY SCALE. THE MEX-
            ICAN AMERICAN GROUP, AS A WHOLE, WAS
            LESS MATURE THAN THE ANGLO GROUP, EVEN
            THOUGH THEY SHOWED A HIGHER DEGREE OF
            MATURITY ON CERTAIN SPECIFIC ITEMS. AT
            THIS AGE LEVEL, AN EMOTIONAL FACTOR, AN
            INTERPERSONAL FACTOR, AND TWO ACA-
            DEMIC MATURITY FACTORS EMERGED IN MEX-
            ICAN AMERICAN CHILDREN, EVEN THOUGH
            THE ACADEMIC MATURITY FACTOR LACKED A
            CLEAR DEFINITION. FOR ANGLO CHILDREN,
            TWO EMOTIONAL FACTORS, TWO INTERPER-
            SONAL FACTORS, AND AN ACADEMIC FACTOR
            EMERGED. THE ACADEMIC MATURITY FACTOR
            WAS NOT AS CLEARLY DEFINED IN THE ANGLO
            GROUP AS WAS THE CASE FOR THE MEXICAN
            AMERICAN GROUP AT THIS AGE LEVEL. AS A
            WHOLE, THE FACTOR STRUCTURE OF BEHAV-
            IORAL MATURITY IN THE ANGLO CHILDREN
            WAS MORE COMPLEX AND LESS CLEAR COM-
            PARED WITH THE BEHAVIORAL MATURITY
            STRUCTURE OF THE MEXICAN AMERICAN
            CHILDREN. 6 REFERENCES. (AUTHOR SUM-
            MARY)

ACCN   000408

486 AUTH **DUVAL, M. K.**
     TITL   LATINOS AND HEALTH CARE: THE QUEST FOR
            EQUITY.
     SRCE   *PAPER PRESENTED AT THE NATIONAL HEALTH*
            MANPOWER EDUCATION CONFERENCE FOR
            SPANISH SURNAMED, CHICAGO, OCTOBER 21,
            1972.
     INDX   SPANISH SURNAMED, HEALTH, PROFESSIONAL

TRAINING, REPRESENTATION, LEGISLATION,
ESSAY
     ABST   THIS OPENING ADDRESS TO THE NATIONAL
            HEALTH MANPOWER EDUCATION CONFER-
            ENCE FOR THE SPANISH SURNAMED (SS) PRO-
            VIDES (1) A BRIEF OVERVIEW OF THE CONTRI-
            BUTIONS OF LATINO FOLK MEDICINE TO
            MODERN AMERICAN MEDICINE, (2) STATISTI-
            CAL DOCUMENTATION OF THE SEVERE SHORT-
            AGE OF SPANISH SURNAMED HEALTH PROFES-
            SIONALS AND THE UNDERREPRESENTATION
            OF SS STUDENTS IN MEDICAL, DENTAL AND
            NURSING SCHOOLS THROUGHOUT THE
            COUNTRY, AND (3) A SUMMARY OF RECENT
            NATIONAL LEGISLATION FOR INCREASING
            SPANISH SURNAMED AMERICANS IN HEALTH
            MANPOWER PROFESSIONAL TRAINING AND
            HEALTH SERVICES. IT IS CONTENDED THAT THE
            ESTABLISHMENT OF THE OFFICE OF THE SPE-
            CIAL ASSISTANT ON HEALTH NEEDS OF SPAN-
            ISH SURNAMED AMERICANS (1970) HAS IN-
            CREASED THE RECOGNITION AT THE
            DEPARTMENT OF HEALTH, EDUCATION AND
            WELFARE OF THE UNIQUE PROBLEMS OF THE
            SS IN THE HEALTH FIELD. THIS INCREASED
            AWARENESS WILL, IDEALLY, BE FOLLOWED BY
            AN EVALUATION OF PRESENT NEEDS AND IM-
            PLEMENTATION OF A COMPREHENSIVE HEALTH
            SERVICES AND HEALTH MANPOWER DEVEL-
            OPMENT PROGRAM.

ACCN   000409

487 AUTH **DWORKIN, A. G.**
     TITL   NATIONAL ORIGIN AND GHETTO EXPERIENCE
            AS VARIABLES IN MEXICAN AMERICAN STER-
            EOTYPY.
     SRCE   *IN N. N. WAGNER & M. J. HAUG (EDS.), CHICA-*
            NOS: SOCIAL AND PSYCHOLOGICAL PERSPEC-
            TIVES. ST. LOUIS: C. V. MOSBY COMPANY, 1971,
            PP. 136-139.
     INDX   ACCULTURATION, MEXICAN AMERICAN,
            STEREOTYPES, ADULTS, DISCRIMINATION, MI-
            GRATION, EMPIRICAL, CALIFORNIA, COLO-
            RADO, SOUTHWEST, IMMIGRATION
     ABST   THIS INVESTIGATION EXAMINED WHETHER THE
            FOREIGN-BORN MEXICAN AMERICAN (FBMA)
            LIVING IN THE BARRIO RETAINS FAVORABLE
            STEREOTYPES OF ANGLOS OR ACQUIRES UN-
            FAVORABLE IMAGES HELD BY NATIVE-BORN
            MEXICAN AMERICAN (NBMA) COUNTERPARTS.
            A SAMPLE OF 131 MA'S LIVING IN THE LOS AN-
            GELES AND DENVER STANDARD METROPOLI-
            TAN STATISTICAL AREAS WAS DIVIDED INTO
            THREE GROUPS—78 NBMA'S, 32 FBMA LONG
            TERMS, AND 21 FBMA RECENTS. ALL SUB-
            JECTS WERE BETWEEN THE AGES OF 18 AND
            30, WITH 54 WOMEN AND 77 MEN. EACH SUB-
            JECT WAS ADMINISTERED A QUESTIONNAIRE
            BY AN MA INTERVIEWER OF THE SAME SEX
            AND AGE. FACTOR SCORES WERE COMPUTED
            FOR STEREOTYPE ETHNOCENTRISM (SE)
            AMONG THE GROUPS. DATA INDICATE THAT
            NO DIFFERENCE EXISTS IN THE SE BETWEEN
            FBMA LONG-TERM AND NBMA SUBJECTS, WHILE
            A SIGNIFICANT DIFFERENCE EXISTS BETWEEN
            NBMA AND FBMA-RECENT SUBJECTS. EXAMI-
            NATION OF STEREOTYPES MENTIONED BY MA'S

TO DESCRIBE ANGLOS REVEALS THAT NBMA AND FBMA LONG-TERM SUBJECTS SELECT NEARLY IDENTICAL UNFAVORABLE STEREO-TYPES OF THE ANGLO. THE FBMA-RECENTS MENTION IMAGES THAT ARE FAVORABLE TO THE ANGLO. IT SEEMS THAT NATIONAL ORIGIN IS NOT THE VARIABLE WHICH ACCOUNTS FOR THE FBMA-NBMA DICHOTOMY FOUND IN A PREVIOUS STUDY. RATHER, THE RELATIVE AMOUNT OF TIME EACH GROUP HAS BEEN EX-POSED TO ANGLO DISCRIMINATION AND PREJUDICE (MEASURED BY LENGTH OF BAR-RIO RESIDENCE) IS THE ESSENTIAL COMPO-NENT. 8 REFERENCES.

ACCN   000410

488 AUTH   **DWORKIN, A. G.**
    TITL   THE PEOPLES OF LA RAZA: THE MEXICAN-AMERICANS OF LOS ANGELES.
    SRCE   *IN N. P. GIST & A. G. DWORKIN (EDS.), THE BLENDING OF RACES: MARGINALITY AND IDENTITY IN WORLD PERSPECTIVE. NEW YORK: WILEY-INTERSCIENCE, A DIVISION OF JOHN WILEY & SONS, INC., 1972, PP. 167-190.*
    INDX   MEXICAN AMERICAN, ESSAY, HISTORY, DIS-CRIMINATION, EDUCATION, ECONOMIC FAC-TORS, CULTURAL FACTORS, POLICE-COMMU-NITY RELATIONS, CHICANO MOVEMENT, SEX ROLES, FAMILY STRUCTURE, STEREOTYPES, URBAN, DEMOGRAPHIC, CALIFORNIA, SOUTH-WEST
    ABST   A PORTRAIT OF THE MEXICAN AMERICAN (MA) OF LOS ANGELES IS PRESENTED BY MEANS OF AN HISTORICAL, DEMOGRAPHIC, AND EXPERI-ENTIAL DESCRIPTION. IN TRACING VARIOUS LEVELS OF OPPRESSION, BY EARLY SPAN-IARDS AND LATER AMERICAN ANGLOS, PROB-LEMS FACING MA IN THE BARRIOS OF LOS AN-GELES   INCLUDE   DISCRIMINATION   IN EDUCATION (I.E., LACK OF CULTURAL SENSI-TIVITY AND RACISM), POLICE-INITIATED VIO-LENCE, AND POOR ECONOMIC RESOURCES FOR HOUSING, INSURANCE, AND CONSUMER-ISM. THOUGH MANY ISSUES ARE FREQUENTLY EXPLAINED BY THE DOMINANT CULTURE THROUGH CULTURAL "FOLK IMAGES, WHICH CONTRIBUTE TO STEREOTYPES OF THE MA, REAL DIFFERENCES SUCH AS USE OF SPANISH LANGUAGE, STRESS ON FAMILISM, AND EM-PHASIS ON LA RAZA CANNOT BE IGNORED. THOUGH A DICHOTOMY EXISTS BETWEEN THE HISPANO AND THE CHICANO BECAUSE OF SPANISH AND/OR INDIAN LINEAGE, MA ARE SEEN AS WORKING TOWARDS GREATER UNITY AND STRIVING FOR SIGNIFICANT CHANGES IN AN ANGLO SOCIETY. RELEVANT ISSUES ARE SEEN AS THE PREVALENCE OF STEREOTYPIC IMAGES AND THE NEED FOR AN ACCURATE PICTURE OF HISTORY WHICH INCLUDES THE MA. 14 REFERENCES.

ACCN   000411

489 AUTH   **DWORKIN, A. G.**
    TITL   STEROTYPES AND SELF-IMAGES HELD BY NA-TIVE-BORN AND FOREIGN-BORN MEXICAN AMERICANS.
    SRCE   *SOCIOLOGY AND SOCIAL RESEARCH, 1965, 49(2), 214-224.*

INDX   MEXICAN AMERICAN, STEREOTYPES, SELF CONCEPT, SES, COLLEGE STUDENTS, ADULTS, ETHNIC IDENTITY, ACCULTURATION, EMPIRI-CAL, SURVEY, SOUTHWEST, IMMIGRATION
ABST   STEREOTYPES OF THE ANGLO AND SELF-IM-AGES WERE OBTAINED FROM 280 U.S.-BORN AND MEXICAN-BORN MEXICAN AMERICAN STUDENTS AND COMMUNITY RESIDENTS. THE LOW-SOCIOECONOMIC INDIVIDUALS THAT DID NOT MEET THE CRITERIA FOR ASSIMILATION (OCCUPATIONAL ACHIEVEMENT, WEALTH, AND COMMAND OF ANGLO WAYS) WERE SELECTED FOR STUDY FROM THIS HETEROGENEOUS GROUP. STATISTICAL COMPARISONS INDICATE THAT SIGNIFICANTLY MORE FOREIGN-BORN SUBJECTS HOLD FAVORABLE STEREOTYPES AND SELF-IMAGES THAN DO NATIVE-BORN SUBJECTS. THE NATIVE-BORN SUBJECT MAY HAVE COMPARED THE ANGLOS' SOCIOECO-NOMIC CONDITION WITH HIS OWN AND NOTED HIS RELATIVE DISADVANTAGE. THE FOREIGN-BORN SUBJECT MAY HAVE COMPARED THE SO-CIOECONOMIC CONDITION OF HIS PEER GROUP IN MEXICO WITH HIS OWN AND NOTED HIS RELATIVE ADVANTAGE. IT IS SUGGESTED THAT THE NATIVE-BORN MEXICAN AMERICAN DE-VELOPS STRONG NEGATIVE STEREOTYPES OF THE ANGLO IN ORDER TO EXPLAIN THE AN-GLO'S RELATIVE SUPERIORITY AND TO JUSTIFY HIS OWN INFERIOR POSITION WITHIN SOCIETY. THE FOREIGN-BORN MEXICAN AMERICANS DE-VELOP POSITIVE STEREOTYPES IN ORDER TO JUSTIFY THEIR RECENT MOVE TO THE UNITED STATES; THEY HAVE DEVELOPED POSITIVE SELF-IMAGES TO EXPLAIN THEIR ASPIRATION AND DESIRE FOR IMPROVEMENT BY MAKING SUCH A MOVE. 13 REFERENCES.

ACCN   000412

490 AUTH   **EAST LOS ANGELES HEALTH SYSTEM, INC.**
    TITL   THE COMMUNITY FUNDS FLOW DATA SYSTEM: A STUDY OF PERSONAL HEALTH CARE EX-PENDITURES.
    SRCE   *LOS ANGELES: AUTHOR, JANUARY 1974. (AVAILABLE FROM AUTHOR, 1307 S. ATLANTIC BLVD., LOS ANGELES, CALIF., 90022.)*
    INDX   HEALTH, ECONOMIC FACTORS, HEALTH DELIV-ERY SYSTEMS, MEXICAN AMERICAN, FINANC-ING, SPANISH SURNAMED, URBAN, EMPIRICAL, CALIFORNIA, SOUTHWEST
    ABST   DESIGNED TO IDENTIFY THE METHODS OF FI-NANCING THE EXISTING HEALTH CARE DELIV-ERY SYSTEM IN THE GREATER EAST LOS AN-GELES AREA, THE COMMUNITY FUNDS FLOW DATA SYSTEM REPRESENTS AN INNOVATIVE USE OF EVALUATIVE METHODS. THIS REPORT BY THE SYSTEM (1) DESCRIBES THE STUDY AREA (EAST AND NORTHEAST LOS ANGELES), (2) DEFINES THE AREAS RELATIONSHIP TO EX-ISTING HEALTH SERVICES, (3) DETAILS THE GOALS, OBJECTIVES AND METHODOLOGY OF THE STUDY, (4) PRESENTS AN ANALYSIS AND GRAPHICAL SUMMARY OF THE FINDINGS, AND (5) MAKES RECOMMENDATIONS FOR FURTHER STUDY. 30 REFERENCES. (AUTHOR SUMMARY MODIFIED)

ACCN   000413

491 AUTH **EAST LOS ANGELES HEALTH SYSTEM, INC.**
TITL FOCUS ON PERSONAL HEALTH CARE EXPENDITURES.
SRCE *IN COMMUNITY HEALTH BULLETIN (SPECIAL REPORT NO. 1). LOS ANGELES: EAST LOS ANGELES HEALTH SYSTEM, INC., UNDATED.*
INDX HEALTH, MEXICAN AMERICAN, SPANISH SURNAMED, EMPIRICAL, ECONOMIC FACTORS, FINANCING, URBAN, HEALTH DELIVERY SYSTEMS, CALIFORNIA, SOUTHWEST
ABST DATA FROM THE EAST LOS ANGELES HEALTH SYSTEM'S COMMUNITY FUNDS FLOW DATA ANALYSIS PROJECT REVEALS THAT ANNUAL PER CAPITA HEALTH EXPENDITURES IN EAST AND NORTHEAST LOS ANGELES ARE NEARLY THE SAME AS THOSE NATIONALLY. DESPITE THIS FACT, STUDY AREA RESIDENTS HAVE SPECIAL PROBLEMS AND ARE CONFRONTED WITH REAL BARRIERS WHEN THEY TRY TO GET HEALTH CARE. A CLOSER LOOK AT THE DATA BREAKDOWN (PRESENTED IN TABULAR AND GRAPH FORM) INDICATES SIGNIFICANT DIFFERENCES IN SOURCE OF HEALTH CARE FUNDS AND PERCENTAGE DISTRIBUTION BY HEALTH SERVICE BETWEEN EAST LOS ANGELES RESIDENTS AND NATIONWIDE AVERAGES. RECOMMENDATIONS FOR A COUNTY-WIDE ANALYSIS OF HEALTH SERVICES AND THEIR FUNDING ARE PROPOSED. 1 REFERENCE.
ACCN 000414

492 AUTH **EAST LOS ANGELES HEALTH SYSTEM, INC.**
TITL A SUMMARY REPORT ON THE HOUSEHOLD INTERVIEW SURVEY.
SRCE *IN COMMUNITY HEALTH BULLETIN (SPECIAL REPORT NO. 2). LOS ANGELES: EAST LOS ANGELES HEALTH SYSTEM, INC., UNDATED.*
INDX HEALTH, EMPIRICAL, SURVEY, POVERTY, MEXICAN AMERICAN, SPANISH SURNAMED, HEALTH DELIVERY SYSTEMS, URBAN, CALIFORNIA, SOUTHWEST
ABST AS PART OF ITS RESPONSIBILITY TO PROMOTE THE DEVELOPMENT OF ALTERNATIVE WAYS OF COMBINING PUBLIC, PRIVATE, AND VOLUNTARY COMMUNITY HEALTH RESOURCES IN ORDER TO ACHIEVE EQUITY OF ACCESS, COST MODERATION AND IMPROVEMENT IN HEALTH SERVICES, THE EAST LOS ANGELES HEALTH SYSTEM UNDERTOOK A HOUSEHOLD INTERVIEW SURVEY. THIS REPORT SUMMARIZES THE SURVEY'S DATA ON COMMUNITY NEEDS AND UTILIZATION PATTERNS GATHERED FROM INTERVIEWS WITH 1,005 FAMILIES FROM EAST LOS ANGELES. FINDINGS ARE CATEGORIZED UNDER PHYSICIAN CARE, HOSPITALIZATION, DISABILITY, CHRONIC ILLNESS, SERVICE ACCESSIBILITY, AND HEALTH-RELATED FINDINGS. 2 REFERENCES.
ACCN 000415

493 AUTH **THE EAST LOS ANGELES HEALTH TASK FORCE.**
TITL STUDY OF CONSUMER PERCEPTIONS OF MENTAL HEALTH NEEDS AND RESOURCES IN THE EAST LOS ANGELES COMMUNITY.
SRCE *UNPUBLISHED MANUSCRIPT, SUBMITTED TO THE NATIONAL INSTITUTE OF MENTAL HEALTH, UNDATED. (AVAILABLE FROM AUTHOR, 1307 S. ATLANTIC BLVD., LOS ANGELES, CALIFORNIA 90022.)*
INDX MENTAL HEALTH, ATTITUDES, MEXICAN AMERICAN, COMMUNITY, SURVEY, EMPIRICAL, BILINGUAL-BICULTURAL PERSONNEL, HEALTH DELIVERY SYSTEMS, CALIFORNIA, SOUTHWEST
ABST TO DEVELOP AN APPROPRIATE MENTAL HEALTH MASTER PLAN FOR THE EAST LOS ANGELES AREA, A SURVEY OF CONSUMER PERCEPTIONS WAS CONDUCTED BY THE EAST LOS ANGELES (ELA) HEALTH TASK FORCE. THE SURVEY RESULTS INCLUDE: (1) CHARACTERISTICS OF THE CONSUMER POPULATION; (2) CONSUMER OPINIONS ABOUT THE QUALITY AND ACCESSIBILITY OF SERVICES; AND (3) IDENTIFICATION OF CULTURALLY RELEVANT ELEMENTS OF SERVICE DELIVERY. THE RESULTS ARE PRESENTED IN DESCRIPTIVE FORM ONLY, AND ARE DISCUSSED IN TERMS OF THE CRITICAL PATHS TO SERVICE UTILIZATION, SATISFACTION WITH SERVICES, AND COMMUNITY PARTICIPATION. 25 REFERENCES. (AUTHOR SUMMARY MODIFIED)
ACCN 000416

494 AUTH **EBERSTEIN, I. W., & FRISBIE, W. P.**
TITL DIFFERENCES IN MARITAL STABILITY AMONG MEXICAN AMERICANS, BLACKS, AND ANGLOS: 1960 AND 1970.
SRCE *SOCIAL PROBLEMS, 1976, 23(5), 609-621.*
INDX MARRIAGE, FAMILY STRUCTURE, MEXICAN AMERICAN, CROSS CULTURAL, MARITAL STABILITY, CULTURAL FACTORS, SES, EMPIRICAL, CENSUS
ABST A COMPARATIVE ANALYSIS OF DIFFERENCES IN MARITAL INSTABILITY, CARRIED OUT OVER TIME AS WELL AS CROSS-SECTIONALLY, INDICATES THAT THE RELATIVE FREQUENCY OF MARITAL DISRUPTION OF EVER-MARRIED WOMEN IS LOW AMONG MEXICAN AMERICANS, FOLLOWED BY ANGLOS AND BLACKS IN ASCENDING ORDER. INTRODUCTION OF CONTROLS FOR AGE, AGE AT FIRST MARRIAGE, AND OTHER POTENTIAL DETERMINANTS OF MARITAL SOLIDARITY DOES NOT ALTER THE RANKING BY ETHNICITY. THE RESULTS SUGGEST THAT CURRENT OPINIONS, BASED ON PREVIOUS RESEARCH THAT THE LEVEL OF MARITAL INSTABILITY CHARACTERISTIC OF MEXICAN AMERICANS IS HIGHER THAN THAT OF ANGLOS AND THAT THE TREND IN MARITAL INSTABILITY AMONG MEXICAN AMERICANS IS CONVERGING WITH THAT OF BLACKS, ARE IN NEED OF REVISION. 40 REFERENCES. (JOURNAL ABSTRACT)
ACCN 000417

495 AUTH **EDGERTON, R. B., KARNO, M., & FERNANDEZ, I.**
TITL CURANDERISMO IN THE METROPOLIS: THE DIMINISHING ROLE OF FOLK PSYCHIATRY AMONG LOS ANGELES MEXICAN-AMERICANS.
SRCE *AMERICAN JOURNAL OF PSYCHOTHERAPY, 1970, 24(1), 124-134.*
INDX MEXICAN AMERICAN, CURANDERISMO, FOLK MEDICINE, ADULTS, CASE STUDY, RESOURCE UTILIZATION, MENTAL HEALTH, REVIEW, CALIFORNIA, SOUTHWEST

ABST CURANDERISMO, MEXICAN AMERICAN (MA) FOLK PSYCHOTHERAPY, HAS BEEN REPORTED TO BE WIDESPREAD IN THE SOUTHWESTERN UNITED STATES. SOME RESEARCH HAS INDICATED THAT CURANDERISMO IS AN IMPORTANT MEANS FOR THE TREATMENT AND PREVENTION OF MENTAL ILLNESS AMONG MEXICAN AMERICANS. HOWEVER, RESEARCH AMONG EAST LOS ANGELES MA'S INDICATES THAT WHILE CURANDERISMO IS PRESENT IN THE COMMUNITY, ITS IMPORTANCE HAS DIMINISHED GREATLY. BOTH ETHNOGRAPHIC OBSERVATIONS AND FORMAL INTERVIEWS INDICATE THAT FOR MA'S IN EAST LOS ANGELES THE PREFERRED TREATMENT RESOURCE FOR MENTAL ILLNESS IS THE GENERAL PHYSICIAN AND NOT THE CURANDERO. THUS THE EVIDENCE SUGGESTS THAT THE REPORTED UNDERREPRESENTATION OF MEXICAN AMERICANS IN PSYCHIATRIC TREATMENT FACILITIES IS NOT DUE TO THE WIDESPREAD PRACTICE OF FOLK PSYCHOTHERAPY. 14 REFERENCES.

ACCN 000418

496 AUTH **EDGERTON, R. B., & KARNO, M.**
TITL COMMUNITY ATTITUDES TOWARD THE HOSPITAL CARE OF THE MR.
SRCE *MENTAL RETARDATION, 1972, 10(5), 3-5.*
INDX ACCULTURATION, ADULTS, COPING MECHANISMS, CROSS CULTURAL, CULTURAL FACTORS, MENTAL RETARDATION, EMPIRICAL, ENVIRONMENTAL FACTORS, ECONOMIC FACTORS, MENTAL HEALTH, MEXICAN AMERICAN, RESOURCE UTILIZATION, SES, URBAN, CALIFORNIA, SOUTHWEST, ATTITUDES
ABST WHEN ASKED TO CHOOSE BETWEEN HOME AND HOSPITAL CARE FOR A MODERATELY RETARDED BOY, MOST ANGLO AND MEXICAN AMERICAN RESPONDENTS FROM A LARGE CALIFORNIA URBAN AREA PREFERRED HOME CARE. ALTHOUGH MOST OF THE 667 RESPONDENTS REJECTED THE HOSPITAL IN FAVOR OF THE HOME FOR A MODERATELY RETARDED CHILD, THE ANGLO RESPONDENTS HAD THE HIGHEST PERCENTAGE OF "HOSPITAL ANSWERS, WHILE THE LEAST ACCULTURATED MEXICAN AMERICAN SAMPLE HAD THE LOWEST. MOREOVER, THE OLDER AND POORER THE ANGLO RESPONDENTS WERE, THE MORE LIKELY THEY WERE TO CHOOSE HOSPITAL CARE. CONVERSELY, THE MORE "MIDDLE CLASS MEXICAN AMERICANS WERE MORE LIKELY THAN LOW-SES MEXICAN AMERICANS TO CHOOSE HOSPITAL CARE. THE THREE BEST PREDICTORS OF HOME CARE CHOICE AMONG MEXICAN AMERICANS WERE: (1) RECENT ARRIVAL FROM MEXICO—WITHIN THE LAST 10 YEARS; (2) BELIEF THAT "MENTAL DISORDERS WERE STIGMATIZING; AND (3) EMBEDDEDNESS IN A NEIGHBORHOOD NETWORK (I.E., RESIDENCE CLOSE TO AND RELYING UPON A NEIGHBORHOOD CHURCH, STORE, DOCTOR AND KINSMEN). THE PRESENCE OF SUCH ATTITUDINAL DIVERSITY AMONG ETHNIC MINORITIES AND PERSONS OF LOW-SES IN A LARGE CITY MAY BE OF SIGNIFICANCE TO THOSE WHO PLAN OR PROVIDE RESIDENTIAL SERVICES FOR THE MENTALLY RETARDED. 8 REFERENCES.

ACCN 002076

497 AUTH **EDGERTON, R. B., & KARNO, M.**
TITL MEXICAN-AMERICAN BILINGUALISM AND THE PERCEPTION OF MENTAL ILLNESS.
SRCE *ARCHIVES OF GENERAL PSYCHIATRY, 1971, 24(6), 286-290.*
INDX PSYCHOPATHOLOGY, MEXICAN AMERICAN, ATTITUDES, RESOURCE UTILIZATION, MENTAL HEALTH, HEALTH DELIVERY SYSTEMS, BILINGUAL-BICULTURAL PERSONNEL, BILINGUAL, CROSS CULTURAL, SURVEY, CULTURAL FACTORS, BILINGUALISM, DEPRESSION, SCHIZOPHRENIA, EXTENDED FAMILY, CALIFORNIA, SOUTHWEST
ABST THE RELATIONSHIP BETWEEN BILINGUALISM AND ATTITUDES TOWARD MENTAL ILLNESS AMONG 444 MEXICAN AMERICAN (MA) ADULTS WAS EXPLORED BY MEANS OF A SURVEY INSTRUMENT HAVING 200 QUESTIONS INVOLVING BIOGRAPHICAL, DEMOGRAPHIC, AND ATTITUDINAL INFORMATION IN ADDITION TO MENTAL ILLNESS ITEMS. APPROXIMATELY 60 PERCENT OF THE MA'S TOOK THE HOUSEHOLD INTERVIEW IN SPANISH. RESULTS SHOW THAT 75 PERCENT OF THE RESPONSES BETWEEN SPANISH RESPONDENTS AND ENGLISH RESPONDENTS WERE NOT SIGNIFICANTLY DIFFERENT. HOWEVER, THE LANGUAGE IN WHICH THE RESPONDENT TOOK THE INTERVIEW WAS BY FAR THE BEST PREDICTOR OF RESPONSE TO MENTAL ILLNESS QUESTIONS. THE 260 MA'S WHO TOOK THE INTERVIEW IN SPANISH, DIFFERED FROM 184 MA'S WHO TOOK THE INTERVIEW IN ENGLISH IN SIX RESPONSE CATEGORIES: (1) DEPRESSION, (2) JUVENILE DELINQUENCY, (3) SCHIZOPHRENIA, (4) THE INHERITANCE OF MENTAL ILLNESS, (5) THE EFFECTIVENESS OF PRAYER, AND (6) FAMILISTIC ORIENTATION. THE DIFFERENCES SUGGEST THAT MA'S, AT LEAST IN EAST LOS ANGELES, WHO MAINLY OR ONLY SPEAK SPANISH, REFLECT THE COMMONLY DESCRIBED CULTURAL TRAITS OF FATALISM, FAMILISM, STRONG ATTACHMENT TO FORMAL RELIGIOUS VALUES, PATRIARCHAL AUTHORITARIANISM, AND CONSERVATIVE MORALITY REGARDING DEVIANT BEHAVIOR IN THE PERCEPTIONS OF MENTAL ILLNESS. THUS, LANGUAGE USAGE AND ATTITUDES TOWARD MENTAL ILLNESS ARE RELATED AND BOTH REFLECT CULTURAL DISTINCTIONS WITH DEEP PSYCHOLOGICAL INVOLVEMENTS. THERE IS A GREAT NEED FOR SPANISH-SPEAKING MENTAL HEALTH PROFESSIONALS WHO ARE SENSITIVE TO AND UNDERSTANDING OF THE MA CULTURE. 15 REFERENCES.

ACCN 000419

498 AUTH **EDINGER, J. D., BOGAN, J. B., HARRIGAN, P. H., & ELLIS, M. F.**
TITL ALTITUDE QUOTIENT-IQ DISCREPANCY AS AN INDEX OF PERSONALITY DISORGANIZATION AMONG DRUG OFFENDERS.
SRCE *JOURNAL OF CLINICAL PSYCHOLOGY, 1975, 31(3), 575-578.*
INDX DRUG ABUSE, MMPI, WISC, PUERTO RICAN-M, CROSS CULTURAL, INTELLIGENCE, PSY-

ABST CHOTHERAPY, EMPIRICAL, INSTITUTIONALIZA-
TION, PSYCHOPATHOLOGY, MENTAL HEALTH,
CRIMINOLOGY, VIRGINIA, SOUTH

ABST INVESTIGATORS ADMINISTERED THE MMPI AND
THE WAIS TO 1 PUERTO RICAN, 18 BLACK, AND
6 WHITE INMATES (AGES 20 TO 28) WHO WERE
RESIDENT PARTICIPANTS IN A FEDERAL REF-
ORMATORY DRUG ABUSE PROGRAM. THE FOL-
LOWING RATINGS WERE ALSO OBTAINED FOR
EACH SUBJECT: RESIDENT COUNSELOR RAT-
INGS, GROUP THERAPY RATINGS, DORMITORY
BEHAVIOR RATING, WORK PROGRESS RE-
PORTS, AND OVERALL ADJUSTMENT RATING.
INTERCORRELATIONS AMONG ATTITUDE QUO-
TIENT (AQ)-IQ DISCREPANCIES, MMPI SCALES,
AND BEHAVIORAL ADJUSTMENT RATING WERE
COMPUTED. RESULTS SUGGEST THAT THE AQ-
IQ DISCREPANCY IS OF QUESTIONABLE EFFI-
CACY AS AN INDEX OF PERSONALITY DISOR-
GANIZATION. 6 REFERENCES. (PASAR AB-
STRACT)

ACCN 000420

499 AUTH EISELEIN, E. B.
TITL TELEVISION AND THE MEXICAN-AMERICAN.
SRCE PUBLIC TELECOMMUNICATIONS REVIEW, 1974,
2(1), 13-18.
INDX MEXICAN AMERICAN, MASS MEDIA, SURVEY,
EMPIRICAL, SOUTHWEST
ABST THE TELETEMAS PROJECT FUNDED BY THE
CORPORATION FOR PUBLIC BROADCASTING
TO OBTAIN INFORMATION FOR TELEVISION
PRODUCERS, SURVEYED THE USE AND POTEN-
TIAL USE OF TELEVISION AMONG THE MEXI-
CAN AMERICAN POPULATION IN THE SOUTH-
WEST. THE FINDINGS INDICATE THAT MEXICAN
AMERICANS WANT A GREATER SCOPE OF PRO-
GRAMMING THAT IS SPANISH OR MEXICAN IN
CONTENT; NEWS THAT RELATES TO THE MEXI-
CAN AMERICAN COMMUNITY AND ABOUT
MEXICO AND LATIN AMERICA; AND TELEVISION
LANGUAGE REFLECTIVE OF THE LANGAUGE
USAGE WITHIN THE SPANISH-SPEAKING COM-
MUNITY.
ACCN 000421

500 AUTH ELINSON, J.
TITL THE PHYSICIAN'S DILEMMA IN PUERTO RICO.
SRCE JOURNAL OF HEALTH AND HUMAN BEHAVIOR,
1962, 3(1), 14-20.
INDX PHYSICIANS, PUERTO RICAN-I, PROFESSIONAL
TRAINING, MEDICAL STUDENTS, SOCIAL MO-
BILITY, ATTITUDES, SURVEY, EMPIRICAL
ABST TWO-THIRDS OF THE MEDICAL CARE IN PUERTO
RICO IS RENDERED UNDER GOVERNMENT
AUSPICES. THE PRIVATE PRACTICE OF MEDI-
CINE ALSO FLOURISHES, HOWEVER, AND AS A
RESULT PHYSICIANS FACE A SHARP DILEMMA
IN CHOICE OF CAREERS. THIS DILEMMA HAS
BECOME EVEN MORE ACUTE WITH THE IM-
PROVED ECONOMIC CONDITION OF PUERTO
RICO WHICH HAS INCREASED THE PROPOR-
TION OF THE PUBLIC ABLE TO AFFORD HEALTH
INSURANCE AND FEES FOR PRIVATE CARE. TO
DETERMINE WHAT INFLUENCE THIS DILEMMA
HAS ON PHYSICIANS' CHOICE OF GOVERN-
MENT VS. PRIVATE PRACTICE, A STUDY WAS
UNDERTAKEN IN 1959. OVER 500 PHYSICIANS

WERE INTERVIEWED AT LENGTH REGARDING
THEIR MEDICAL TRAINING, WORK EXPERI-
ENCE, AND ATTITUDES TOWARD PRIVATE AND
GOVERNMENT SERVICE. THREE VARIABLES
EMERGED AS HAVING A BEARING ON A PHYSI-
CIAN'S CHOICE OF PRIVATE OR GOVERNMENT
SERVICE: (1) THE PHYSICIAN'S SOCIAL ORIGINS,
ESPECIALLY FATHER'S OCCUPATION; (2) COUN-
TRY OF MEDICAL TRAINING; AND (3) "MORALE
OF THE PHYSICIAN IN GOVERNMENT SERVICE,
ESPECIALLY ATTITUDES TOWARD GOVERN-
MENT INTERFERENCE IN MEDICINE. 3 REFER-
ENCES.
ACCN 000422

501 AUTH ELIZONDO, V. P.
TITL ANTHROPOLOGICAL AND PSYCHOLOGICAL
CHARACTERISTICS OF THE MEXICAN AMERI-
CAN.
SRCE SAN ANTONIO, TEXAS: MEXICAN AMERICAN
CULTURAL CENTER, 1974.
INDX CULTURE, MEXICAN AMERICAN, SELF CON-
CEPT, FAMILY ROLES, FAMILY STRUCTURE, AC-
CULTURATION, JUDICIAL PROCESS, INTERPER-
SONAL RELATIONS, BILINGUALISM, DEATH,
RELIGION, ESSAY
ABST GENERAL CHARACTERISTICS OF MEXICAN
AMERICAN CULTURE ARE DESCRIBED TO AID
AN UNDERSTANDING OF THE CULTURAL AND
HISTORICAL DIFFERENCES BETWEEN THE
MEXICAN AMERICAN CULTURE AND THE DOMI-
NANT NORTH AMERICAN CULTURE (WHITE, AN-
GLO-SAXON, PROTESTANT). (1) LIFE VIEW OF
THE HISPANIC, (2) LA FAMILIA, (3) THE LAW, (4)
COMMUNICATION, (5) SUFFERING AND DEATH,
(6) TIME, AND (7) FIESTA ARE THE CULTURAL
FEATURES DISCUSSED IN THIS ESSAY. 3 REF-
ERENCES.
ACCN 000423

502 AUTH ELIZONDO, V. P.
TITL RELIGIOUS PRACTICES OF THE MEXICAN
AMERICAN AND CATECHESIS.
SRCE SAN ANTONIO, TEXAS: MEXICAN AMERICAN
CULTURAL CENTER, 1975.
INDX HISTORY, RELIGION, ESSAY, MEXICAN AMERI-
CAN, CULTURE
ABST RELIGIOUS PRACTICES BY MEXICAN AMERI-
CAN CATHOLICS HAVE THEIR HISTORICAL
ROOTS IN A CULTURE AND TRADITION THAT
ARE UNIQUE AND DISTINCT FROM NORTH
AMERICAN OR EUROPEAN ANCESTRY. PRE-
HISPANIC, INDIGENOUS AND SPANISH INFLU-
ENCES HAVE ALL STRONGLY INFLUENCED HOW
MEXICAN AMERICANS PRACTICE THEIR FAITH
TODAY. BY KNOWING THE HERITAGE OF THE
INDO-HISPANIC PEOPLE, TODAY'S MISSION-
ERS, PARISH PRIESTS AND SISTERS, CAN BET-
TER UNDERSTAND THE CONTEMPORARY RELI-
GIOUS LITURGY AND ITS PLACE IN
CATECHETICAL INSTRUCTION INSTEAD OF
PERCEIVING SOME PRACTICES AS PAGAN OR
SUPERSTITIOUS. UNDER THE GUIDELINES OF
THE SECOND VATICAN COUNCIL, THE MISSION
OF THE CHURCH HAS BEEN REDEFINED AND
EXPANDED TO INCLUDE ACCEPTANCE AND
USE OF THOSE CULTURAL, SOCIAL, NATIONAL
AND RELIGIOUS TRADITIONS WHICH MAY AS-

SIST THE CHURCH IN RELATING TO CHRISTIANS AND NON-CHRISTIANS. RELIGIOUS PRACTICES IN CONTEMPORARY MEXICAN AMERICAN CULTURE ARE DISCUSSED IN TERMS OF THEIR HISTORICAL DEVELOPMENT AND USEFULNESS IN CHURCH EDUCATION AND EVANGELIZATION EFFORTS. THE TRADITIONAL LITURGICAL CALENDAR IS ESPECIALLY EMPHASIZED AS A SOURCE OF SPECIAL RELIGIOUS EVENTS AROUND WHICH RELIGIOUS LEADERS CAN PLAN CATECHETICAL PROGRAMS.

ACCN 000424

503 AUTH **ELLING, R. H., & MARTIN, R. F.**
TITL HEALTH AND HEALTH CARE FOR THE URBAN POOR (NO. 5).
SRCE *NORTH HAVEN, CONN.: CONNECTICUT HEALTH SERVICES RESEARCH SERIES, 1974.*
INDX HEALTH, HEALTH DELIVERY SYSTEMS, URBAN, POVERTY, PUERTO RICAN-M, CROSS CULTURAL, DEMOGRAPHIC, SURVEY, DEATH, DISEASE, HOUSING, SES, ATTITUDES, BIRTH CONTROL, DEPRESSION, EMPIRICAL, COMMUNITY, COMMUNITY INVOLVEMENT, DISCRIMINATION, PERSONNEL, PHYSICIANS, CONNECTICUT, EAST
ABST CONCERN FOR THE POOR HEALTH AND INADEQUATE HEALTH CARE OF RESIDENTS OF THE NORTH END IN HARTFORD, CONNECTICUT, PROMPTED AN INVESTIGATION OF THE SOCIAL, CULTURAL AND ECONOMIC CHARACTERISTICS OF THIS POPULATION. INFORMATION FROM AN IN-DEPTH SURVEY CONDUCTED AMONG 457 RESIDENTS, MOSTLY BLACK AND PUERTO RICAN, LIVING IN THIS AREA IS PRESENTED IN DETAIL. DEMOGRAPHIC DATA OBTAINED FROM U.S. CENSUS AND OTHER SOURCES ARE CATEGORICALLY COMPARED TO DATA OBTAINED FROM THE RESPONDENTS IN THE SURVEY. THE STUDY FOCUSED ON HEALTH STATUS AND SOME DIMENSIONS OF HEALTH CARE INCLUDING BIOGRAPHICAL INFORMATION, RESOLUTION OF HEALTH PROBLEMS, PAYMENT OF CARE, REPORTS OF MORTALITY AND MORBIDITY, AND ENVIRONMENTAL AND LIFE CONDITIONS. THE FINDINGS INDICATE THAT THIS POPULATION REFLECTS CHARACTERISTICS SIMILAR TO OTHERS OF LOWER SOCIOECONOMIC STATUS LIVING IN THE INNER CITY, SUCH AS HIGH UNEMPLOYMENT, POOR HOUSING, HIGHER MORTALITY AND MORBIDITY RATE, AND OVERALL LOWER LEVELS OF HEALTH STATUS AND HEALTH CARE. SEVERAL ACTIONS ARE PROPOSED TO IMPROVE THESE CONDITIONS SUCH AS ADDITIONAL RESOURCE FUNDING, NEIGHBORHOOD ORIENTED CARE TEAMS AND COMMUNITY REPRESENTATION TO A REGIONAL BOARD WHICH WILL COORDINATE HEALTH DELIVERY SYSTEMS IN HARTFORD'S NORTH END. THIS REPORT INCLUDES 2 APPENDICES CONCERNING THE SURVEY DESIGN, SAMPLING, AND A COPY OF THE QUESTIONNAIRE USED IN THE STUDY.
ACCN 000425

504 AUTH **ELLIS, J. M.**
TITL SPANISH SURNAME MORTALITY DIFFERENCES IN SAN ANTONIO, TEXAS.

SRCE *JOURNAL OF HEALTH AND HUMAN BEHAVIOR, 1962, 3(2), 125-127.*
INDX DEATH, SPANISH SURNAMED, CENSUS, DEMOGRAPHIC, CROSS CULTURAL, SEX COMPARISON, DISEASE, TEXAS, SOUTHWEST, FEMALE, URBAN
ABST THE MORTALITY DATA FOR SAN ANTONIO SHOW THAT THE FAVORABLE MORTALITY EXPERIENCE OF WHITE WOMEN GENERALLY IS NOT SHARED TO ANY GREAT EXTENT BY SPANISH SURNAME WOMEN. THESE WOMEN HAVE HIGHER DEATH RATES THAN MEN IN A NUMBER OF AGE CATEGORIES, HAVE HIGHER RATES FOR SEVERAL OF THE LEADING CAUSES OF DEATH, AND HAVE A LIFE EXPECTANCY ONLY SLIGHTLY ABOVE THAT OF MEN. IN CONTRAST, OTHER WHITE WOMEN IN SAN ANTONIO ENJOY A MUCH MORE FAVORABLE MORTALITY RELATIVE TO MALES IN THEIR GROUP. 6 REFERENCES. (AUTHOR SUMMARY)
ACCN 000426

505 AUTH **ENGLISH, R. A., & SETTLE, T. J.**
TITL MINORITY STUDENTS IN HIGHER EDUCATION.
SRCE *INTEGRATED EDUCATION, 1976, 14(3), 3-6.*
INDX REPRESENTATION, EQUAL OPPORTUNITY, HIGHER EDUCATION, DEMOGRAPHIC, COLLEGE STUDENTS, CROSS CULTURAL, FINANCING, ESSAY
ABST TO ALLEVIATE THE PROBLEM OF UNDERREPRESENTATION OF MINORITIES IN PROFESSIONAL FIELDS, THE FEDERAL GOVERNMENT NEEDS TO DEVELOP PROGRAMS OF FINANCIAL ASSISTANCE FOR MINORITY STUDENTS ENTERING GRADUATE AND PROFESSIONAL SCHOOLS AND ALSO FINANCIAL SUPPORT TO UNIVERSITIES ENABLING THEM TO DEVELOP EFFECTIVE RECRUITING AND SUPPORT SYSTEMS FOR MINORITY STUDENTS. STATISTICS REVEAL THAT MINORITY STUDENTS RELY UPON FINANCIAL ASSISTANCE MORE THAN WHITES TO CONTINUE THEIR EDUCATION. THE ISSUE OF ADMISSIONS CRITERIA IS INTERLOCKED WITH FINANCIAL SUPPORT SYSTEMS SINCE EVEN IF MINORITIES ARE ADMITTED INTO HIGHER LEVELS OF EDUCATION THEY COULD NOT REMAIN IN THE EDUCATIONAL INSTITUTION WITHOUT SUBSTANTIAL AND CONTINUED FINANCIAL AID. 16 REFERENCES.
ACCN 000427

506 AUTH **EPSTEIN, E. H. (ED.)**
TITL POLITICS AND EDUCATION IN PUERTO RICO: A DOCUMENTARY SURVEY OF THE LANGUAGE ISSUE.
SRCE *METUCHEN, N.J.: THE SCARECROW PRESS, 1970.*
INDX PUERTO RICAN-M, BILINGUALISM, BILINGUAL-BICULTURAL EDUCATION, LANGUAGE LEARNING, SES, EDUCATION, POLITICS, POLITICAL POWER, CULTURAL PLURALISM, CULTURAL FACTORS, LEGISLATION, JUDICIAL PROCESS, HISTORY, ACCULTURATION, CULTURAL CHANGE, CULTURE, ESSAY, BOOK
ABST THE PURPOSE OF THIS VOLUME IS TO DEAL WITH THE ISSUES SURROUNDING PUERTO RICO'S TIES TO THE UNITED STATES AND THE CONFLICT THIS HAS CAUSED IN THE CUL-

TURAL VALUES, EDUCATION AND LANGUAGE OF ALL PUERTO RICANS. THE COMPILATION BRINGS TOGETHER ESSAYS AND DOCUMENTS REPRESENTING A WIDE VARIETY OF VIEWS OF THE LANGUAGE QUESTION, ESPECIALLY AS THAT ISSUE RELATES TO PROSPECTS FOR STATEHOOD AND INDEPENDENCE. PARTICULAR ATTENTION IS GIVEN TO THE IMPLICATIONS OF HAVING ENGLISH SERVE AS A MEDIUM OF INSTRUCTION IN SCHOOLS. DIVIDED INTO THEIR PARTS, THE BOOK FIRST PROVIDES A GENERAL OVERVIEW OF THE SCHOOL LANGUAGE ISSUE AND EVALUATES THE ROLE THAT NORTH AMERICAN LEADERS PLAY IN FOSTERING PUERTO RICO'S AMBIVALENT NATIONALITY. SECONDLY, IT FOCUSES ON THE SIGNIFICANCE OF HAVING ENGLISH AS THE PRINCIPAL MEDIUM OF INSTRUCTION IN MANY SCHOOLS. PART THREE PLACES PUERTO RICO'S SCHOOL LANGUAGE PROBLEMS IN A CROSS-CULTURAL PERSPECTIVE, ALLOWING US TO USE THE EXPERIENCES OF THE GROUPS TO ASSESS THE POTENTIAL CONSEQUENCES OF ALTERNATIVE LANGUAGE POLICIES. ABOUT HALF THE ARTICLES ARE IN SPANISH. (AUTHOR SUMMARY MODIFIED)

ACCN   000428

507 AUTH   **ESCARSEGA, Y. D., MONDACA, E. C., & TORRES, V. G.**

TITL   ATTITUDES OF CHICANA LESBIANS TOWARDS THERAPY.

SRCE   *UNPUBLISHED MASTER'S THESIS, DEPARTMENT OF SOCIAL WORK, UNIVERSITY OF SOUTHERN CALIFORNIA, LOS ANGELES, JUNE 1975.*

INDX   HOMOSEXUALITY, EMPIRICAL, MEXICAN AMERICAN, ATTITUDES, PSYCHOTHERAPY, FEMALE, SPANISH SURNAMED, SEXUAL BEHAVIOR, SOCIALIZATION, CALIFORNIA, SOUTHWEST, STRESS, PSYCHOTHERAPY OUTCOME

ABST   ALTHOUGH HOMOSEXUALITY IS NO LONGER CLASSIFIED AS A MENTAL ILLNESS, RESEARCHERS AND THERAPISTS NEGLECT TO EXAMINE SOCIAL FACTORS WHICH MAY INFLUENCE A PERSON'S SEXUAL PREFERENCE. THE CHICANA LESBIAN USUALLY EXPERIENCES GREATER OSTRACISM BY MEMBERS OF HER OWN CULTURE THAN THE ANGLO LESBIAN. TWENTY SPANISH SURNAMED LESBIANS WERE INTERVIEWED, OF WHICH TEN HAD PERSONAL THERAPY EXPERIENCES BECAUSE OF RELATIONSHIP PROBLEMS ASSOCIATED WITH SOCIETAL PRESSURE. ONLY FOUR WERE SATISFIED WITH THE THERAPY SESSIONS. THESE FEMALES HAD SOUGHT THERAPY FOR SUPPORT RATHER THAN TURNING TO THEIR FAMILIES BECAUSE OF POSSIBLE NEGATIVE REACTIONS. THOSE NOT LIVING WITH WOMEN INDICATED STRONGER FEELINGS OF ETHNIC RESTRICTIVENESS AND EXPECTED ADDITIONAL ETHNIC CONFLICT. RESPONDENTS VIEWED THERAPY AS A SUPPORT MECHANISM TO HELP DEAL WITH THEIR LESBIAN LIFE STYLE. 5 REFERENCES.

ACCN   000429

508 AUTH   **ESCOBAR LITSINGER, D.**

TITL   THE CHALLENGE OF TEACHING MEXICAN AMERICAN STUDENTS.

SRCE   *NEW YORK: AMERICAN BOOK CO., 1973.*

INDX   MEXICAN AMERICAN, CHILDREN, ADOLESCENTS, CULTURAL PLURALISM, EDUCATION, SCHOLASTIC ACHIEVEMENT, SES, LEGISLATION, BILINGUALISM, BILINGUAL-BICULTURAL EDUCATION, BILINGUAL-BICULTURAL PERSONNEL, HISTORY, CULTURAL CHANGE, IMMIGRATION, CURRICULUM, INSTRUCTIONAL TECHNIQUES, LANGUAGE LEARNING, TEACHERS, BOOK

ABST   THIS VOLUME DISCUSSES THE FOLLOWING ISSUES IN RELATION TO THE TEACHER'S ROLE IN THE EDUCATION OF MEXICAN AMERICAN STUDENTS. (1) THE TEACHER IS THE CRITICAL ELEMENT IN DEVELOPING STUDENTS' PERSONAL AND ACADEMIC COMPETENCIES. SCHOOLS, TO DATE, HAVE FAILED TO HELP THE MAJORITY OF MEXICAN AMERICAN STUDENTS ACHIEVE ACADEMIC SUCCESS AND ALL THE SOCIAL BENEFITS THAT ACCRUE FROM IT. (2) THE ROLE OF THE CHICANO COMMUNITY AND CHICANO STUDENTS IN BRINGING ABOUT INSTITUTIONAL AND SOCIAL CHANGE HAS EMERGED. (3) IMPROVED INSTRUMENTS AND TECHNIQUES OF EVALUATION, INNOVATIVE SCHOOL REORGANIZATION, CURRICULUM DESIGN AND TEACHING STRATEGIES WHICH FOCUS ON THE NEEDS OF MEXICAN AMERICAN STUDENTS MUST BE DESIGNED, EVALUATED AND IMPLEMENTED BEFORE REAL AND BENEFICIAL RESULTS WILL BE SEEN. (4) NONE OF THIS WILL OCCUR UNTIL INDIVIDUAL TEACHERS TAKE IT UPON THEMSELVES TO MAKE THESE CHANGES IN THEIR OWN TEACHING SITUATIONS WITH MEXICAN AMERICAN STUDENTS. (AUTHOR SUMMARY MODIFIED)

ACCN   000430

509 AUTH   **ESCOTET, M. A.**

TITL   A SURVEY OF THE VALUE HIERARCHIES OF ANGLO AND CHICANO STUDENTS.

SRCE   *INTERAMERICAN JOURNAL OF PSYCHOLOGY. 1976, 10, 7-12.*

INDX   MEXICAN AMERICAN, CROSS CULTURAL, CULTURE, ADOLESCENTS, EMPIRICAL, SEX COMPARISON, ACCULTURATION, COLORADO, SOUTHWEST, VALUES

ABST   THE CONCEPT OF VALUES HAS BECOME PREVALENT IN CROSS-CULTURAL RESEARCH. A VALUE HIERARCHY SCALE WAS UTILIZED IN A SAMPLE OF 155 ANGLO AND MEXICAN AMERICAN JUNIOR HIGH STUDENTS RANGING IN AGE FROM 12 TO 14 TO ASCERTAIN THE FOLLOWING: DO VALUES VARY BETWEEN ANGLO AND CHICANO MALE AND FEMALE STUDENTS?; WHAT ARE THE WITHIN AND BETWEEN GROUP DIFFERENCES AND SIMILARITIES AMONG THESE FOUR GROUPS? THE RESULTS INDICATED THAT: (1) LOVE RANKED HIGH FOR BOTH ANGLO FEMALES AND CHICANO MALES; (2) CHICANO FEMALES AND ANGLO MALES RANKED HEALTH AS NUMBER ONE; (3) ANGLOS RATED RELIGIOUS FAITH HIGHER THAN CHICANOS; (4) CHICANO FEMALES RANKED RESPECT HIGHER THAN THE OTHER GROUPS; AND (5) ALL FOUR GROUPS RANKED WEALTH

AT THE BOTTOM OF THE HIERARCHICAL SCALE. THE VALUE PATTERNS FOR BOTH CULTURAL GROUPS FOR THIS AGE GROUP APPEAR TO REFLECT A SIMILAR VALUE ORIENTATION. 19 REFERENCES.

ACCN   000431

510 AUTH   **ESPARZA, R.**
    TITL   THE VALUE OF CHILDREN AMONG LOWER CLASS MEXICAN, MEXICAN AMERICAN AND ANGLO COUPLES.
    SRCE   *UNPUBLISHED DOCTORAL DISSERTATION, DEPARTMENT OF PSYCHOLOGY, UNIVERSITY OF MICHIGAN, 1977.*
    INDX   ATTITUDES, FAMILY ROLES, FAMILY STRUCTURE, CROSS CULTURAL, MEXICAN AMERICAN, BIRTH CONTROL, ECONOMIC FACTORS, FERTILITY, EMPIRICAL, SURVEY, ADULTS, RELIGION, CHILDREN, MICHIGAN, MIDWEST, VALUES, FAMILY PLANNING
    ABST   THIS STUDY COMPARES CERTAIN MOTIVATIONS POSTULATED TO UNDERLIE FERTILITY BEHAVIOR IN FOUR CULTURAL GROUPS—MEXICAN CATHOLICS, MEXICAN AMERICAN CATHOLICS, ANGLO CATHOLICS, AND ANGLO PROTESTANTS—AS THEY ARE RELATED TO ETHNICITY AND RELIGION. USING THE THEORETICAL MODEL OF FERTILITY BEHAVIOR PROPOSED BY HOFFMAN AND HOFFMAN, THE GROUPS WERE COMPARED ON THE VALUES CONTRIBUTING TO (1) THE DECISION TO HAVE CHILDREN OR NOT, (2) FAMILY SIZE, AND (3) THE PREFERRED SEX OF CHILDREN. THIRTY COUPLES IN EACH OF THE FOUR GROUPS (TOTAL N = 240) WERE SELECTED FROM AMONG COUPLES ATTENDING A COMMUNITY HEALTH CLINIC IN DETROIT, MICHIGAN. A QUESTIONNAIRE INTERVIEW WAS USED TO COLLECT THE DATA ON THE VALUE OF CHILDREN, THE COSTS OF AND BARRIERS TO FERTILITY, AND FAMILY PLANNING AND DECISION-MAKING PROCESSES. THE RESPONDENTS VALUED CHILDREN FOR REASONS UNDER THE MAJOR HOFFMAN AND HOFFMAN (1973) CATEGORIES OF PRIMARY GROUP TIES, STIMULATION, EXPANSION OF SELF, ADULT STATUS AND ECONOMIC UTILITY. EACH GROUP DIFFERENTIATED ITS FAMILY PLANNING BEHAVIOR. DIFFERENCES WERE OBSERVED IN ATTITUDES, METHODS, USAGE AND DECISION-MAKING REGARDING BIRTH CONTROL. BOYS WERE PREFERRED OVER GIRLS BY ALL THE RESPONDENTS. THE CONCLUSION SUGGESTS THAT THE VALUES AND COSTS ASSOCIATED WITH HAVING CHILDREN DO DIFFER ACROSS THESE ETHNIC/RELIGIOUS GROUPS, BUT THAT THE MAJOR FACTOR IS A DIFFERENT ORDERING OF SIMILAR VALUES. CULTURAL BACKGROUND AND SOCIAL CHANGE ALSO APPEAR TO BE IMPORTANT FACTORS WHICH INFLUENCED INTENDED FAMILY SIZE AS WELL AS SEX OF CHILDREN PREFERENCES. 66 REFERENCES. (AUTHOR ABSTRACT)

ACCN   000432

511 AUTH   **EURESTE, B.**
    TITL   MIDWEST REPORT, SUMMER 1970.

SRCE   *UNPUBLISHED MANUSCRIPT, NATIONAL INSTITUTE OF MENTAL HEALTH, OFFICE OF PROGRAM LIAISON, 1970.*
    INDX   MEXICAN AMERICAN, COMMUNITY INVOLVEMENT, CASE STUDY, CHICANO MOVEMENT, POLICY, POLITICAL POWER, SOCIAL SERVICES, COMMUNITY, DRUG ABUSE, HOUSING, EDUCATION, SPANISH SURNAMED, PUERTO RICAN-M, FARM LABORERS, DEMOGRAPHIC, MIDWEST, OHIO, ILLINOIS, MICHIGAN
    ABST   TO ASSESS THE NEEDS OF THE SPANISH-SPEAKING COMMUNITIES IN THE MIDWEST THE OFFICE OF PROGRAM LIAISON, A FEDERAL AGENCY OF THE NATIONAL INSTITUTE OF MENTAL HEALTH, CONDUCTED VISITS TO FIVE MAJOR MIDWESTERN CITIES—TOLEDO, DETROIT, CHICAGO, SAGINAW, AND LANSING. REPORTS ON EACH OF THESE CITIES FOCUS ON THE FOLLOWING: (1) PHYSICAL DESCRIPTION OF THE CITY AND OF THE HISPANIC COMMUNITY WITH RESPECT TO THE SOCIAL, ECONOMIC, AND POLITICAL STRUCTURES; (2) IDENTIFICATION OF INFLUENTIAL HISPANIC LEADERS; AND (3) IDENTIFICATION OF VIABLE HISPANIC ORGANIZATIONS AND SOCIAL SERVICES AND THEIR RELATIONSHIPS TO THE MINORITY COMMUNITY. EACH REPORT REITERATES THAT THE NEEDS OF THE SPANISH-SPEAKING POPULATION ARE NOT BEING ADEQUATELY ADDRESSED AND LEADERS WITHIN THE HISPANIC COMMUNITIES HAVE BEEN UNABLE TO ACHIEVE POLITICAL POWER OR TO INFLUENCE THOSE HAVING POSITIONS OF POWER. IT IS ALSO NOTED THAT EVEN WHEN A SPANISH-SPEAKING PERSON BECOMES INFLUENTIAL, IT DOES NOT NECESSARILY FOLLOW THAT THIS PERSON UNDERSTANDS THE NEEDS OF THE SPANISH-SPEAKING POPULATION SINCE THEIR RESIDENCE IS NOT ALWAYS WITHIN THE COMMUNITY ITSELF.

ACCN   000433

512 AUTH   **EVANS, F. B., & ANDERSON, J. G.**
    TITL   THE PSYCHOCULTURAL ORIGINS OF ACHIEVEMENT AND ACHIEVEMENT MOTIVATION: THE MEXICAN-AMERICAN FAMILY.
    SRCE   *SOCIOLOGY OF EDUCATION, 1973, 46(4), 396-416.*
    INDX   ACHIEVEMENT MOTIVATION, SELF CONCEPT, SCHOLASTIC ASPIRATIONS, EMPIRICAL, MEXICAN AMERICAN, CROSS CULTURAL, SCHOLASTIC ACHIEVEMENT, CHILDREARING PRACTICES, AUTHORITARIANISM, FATALISM, POVERTY, TIME ORIENTATION, CHILDREN, SOCIALIZATION, ADOLESCENTS, NEW MEXICO, SOUTHWEST, VALUES
    ABST   THIS STUDY EXAMINES THE EFFECTS OF VARIATIONS IN SELF-CONCEPT OF ABILITY, ACHIEVEMENT MOTIVATION, VALUES, AND ASPIRATIONS AMONG MEXICAN AMERICAN AND ANGLO AMERICAN JUNIOR HIGH SCHOOL STUDENTS ON THEIR ACHIEVEMENT. ANALYSES OF DATA FROM A SAMPLE OF 87 MEXICAN AMERICAN AND 39 ANGLO AMERICAN STUDENTS INDICATED THAT MEXICAN AMERICAN STUDENTS, REGARDLESS OF THE AMOUNT OF ENGLISH SPOKEN IN THE HOME, HAD LOWER SELF-CONCEPTS OF ABILITY, EXPERIENCED

LESS DEMOCRATIC PARENTAL INDEPENDENCE TRAINING, HAD FATALISTIC, PRESENT-TIME ORIENTATIONS, HAD HIGH STRIVING ORIENTATION, AND HELD LOWER EDUCATIONAL ASPIRATIONS THAN THEIR ANGLO AMERICAN PEERS. THESE RESULTS SUGGEST THAT THE TYPICAL EXPLANATIONS GIVEN BY EDUCATORS FOR THE FAILURE OF MEXICAN AMERICAN STUDENTS ARE SERIOUSLY IN ERROR. CONTRARY TO THESE EXPLANATIONS, MEXICAN AMERICAN STUDENTS WERE FOUND TO COME FROM HOMES WHERE EDUCATION WAS STRESSED AND THE PARENTS ENCOURAGED THEIR CHILDREN TO DO WELL IN SCHOOL. THESE STUDENTS' DEPRESSED ACHIEVEMENT WAS FOUND TO BE RELATED TO VALUES AND EXPERIENCES ASSOCIATED WITH THE CULTURE OF POVERTY, SPECIFICALLY LOW SELF-CONCEPTS OF ABILITY, FATALISTIC, PRESENT-TIME ORIENTATION, AND NON-DEMOCRATIC CHILD REARING EXPERIENCES. 45 REFERENCES. (JOURNAL ABSTRACT)

ACCN   000434

513 AUTH   **EVANS, J. S.**
    TITL   WORD-PAIR DISCRIMINATION AND IMITATION ABILITIES OF PRESCHOOL SPANISH-SPEAKING CHILDREN.
    SRCE   *JOURNAL OF LEARNING DISABILITIES, 1974, 7(9), 573-580.*
    INDX   BILINGUALISM, CHILDREN, POVERTY, SPANISH SURNAMED, EMPIRICAL, BILINGUAL-BICULTURAL EDUCATION, CROSS CULTURAL, LANGUAGE ASSESSMENT, LINGUISTIC COMPETENCE, TEXAS, SOUTHWEST
    ABST   AUDITORY ABILITIES, MEASURED BY WORD-PAIR DISCRIMINATION AND SINGLE WORD IMITATION, OF ECONOMICALLY DISADVANTAGED NATIVE SPANISH-SPEAKING PRESCHOOL CHILDREN WERE INVESTIGATED IN TWO LANGUAGES, SPANISH AND ENGLISH. IN ORDER TO PROVIDE AGE-RELATED COMPARATIVE INFORMATION, A GROUP OF NONDISADVANTAGED, NATIVE ENGLISH SPEAKERS WERE EVALUATED ON THE SAME TASKS. IN SPITE OF THE DUAL PROBLEMS OF ECONOMIC DISADVANTAGE AND SECOND LANGUAGE LEARNING, THESE CHILDREN WERE NOT SIGNIFICANTLY DIFFERENT FROM THEIR ADVANTAGED ENGLISH-SPEAKING PEERS IN TOTAL PERFORMANCE ON THE FOUR TASKS. IN ADDITION, THE SPANISH SPEAKERS MADE LESS ERRORS IN THEIR NATIVE LANGUAGE THAN DID THE ENGLISH SPEAKERS. THUS, PREVIOUSLY HYPOTHESIZED NEGATIVE EFFECTS OF POVERTY OR OF LINGUISTIC INTERFERENCE DO NOT APPEAR TO BE DEPRESSING AUDITORY PERFORMANCE. A DESCRIPTIVE ANALYSIS OF ERRORS INDICATES DIRECTIONS FOR EDUCATIONAL PROGRAMS IN THE AREA OF AUDITORY TRAINING FOR PRESCHOOL BILINGUAL PROGRAMS. 16 REFERENCES. (JOURNAL ABSTRACT)

ACCN   000435

514 AUTH   **FABREGA, H., JR.**
    TITL   BEGGING IN A SOUTHEASTERN MEXICAN CITY.
    SRCE   *HUMAN ORGANIZATION: JOURNAL OF THE SOCIETY FOR APPLIED ANTHROPOLOGY, 1971, 30(3), 277-287.*
    INDX   POVERTY, MEXICAN, URBAN, EMPIRICAL, SEX COMPARISON, ECONOMIC FACTORS, MEXICO
    ABST   MODES OF BEGGING AND ATTITUDES OF PATRONS OR "CLIENTS" ARE EXAMINED IN THE CATHEDRAL CITY OF SAN CRISTOBAL, CHIAPAS, MEXICO. STATISTICS ARE GIVEN FOR ETHNIC COMPOSITION, AGE AND SEX DISTRIBUTION, AND PHYSICAL CONDITION OF SAN CRISTOBAL BEGGARS. INTERVIEWS IDENTIFIED FACTORS THAT CAUSE ONE TO ADOPT BEGGING: TEMPORARY UNEMPLOYMENT, PHYSICAL INCAPACITY, FAMILY POVERTY, LACK OF FAMILY, AND DISSATISFACTION WITH THE FEW EXISTING CHURCH AND CITY WELFARE AGENCIES. THE CITY'S TRADITION OF BENEVOLENCE AND LACK OF WELFARE INSTITUTIONS HAVE COMBINED TO ATTRACT BEGGARS FROM THE SURROUNDING HIGHLANDS. BUT WHILE ECONOMICALLY PROFITABLE, BEGGING ON THE STREET CAUSES EXTREME SOCIAL STIGMA. 26 REFERENCES. (JOURNAL ABSTRACT)

ACCN   000436

515 AUTH   **FABREGA, H., JR.**
    TITL   MEXICAN AMERICANS OF TEXAS: SOME SOCIAL PSYCHIATRIC FEATURES.
    SRCE   *IN E. G. BRODY (ED.), BEHAVIOR IN NEW ENVIRONMENTS: ADAPTATION OF MIGRANT POPULATIONS. BEVERLY HILLS, CALIF.: SAGE PUBLICATIONS, 1970, PP. 249-273.*
    INDX   MEXICAN AMERICAN, HISTORY, DEMOGRAPHIC, CULTURAL FACTORS, PSYCHOPATHOLOGY, SCHIZOPHRENIA, SYMPTOMATOLOGY, CROSS CULTURAL, SES, POVERTY, ACCULTURATION, EMPIRICAL, TEXAS, SOUTHWEST, PSYCHOSIS
    ABST   THE AUTHOR REVIEWS HIS EARLIER WORK ON THE MIGRATION-ACCULTURATION PROCESS OF THE MEXICAN AMERICAN (MA) AS RELATED TO PSYCHIATRIC PROBLEMS. THE REPORT BEGINS WITH A DESCRIPTION OF THE SOCIODEMOGRAPHIC AND CULTURAL CHARACTERISTICS OF MA'S. RESULTS FROM THE PSYCHIATRIC STUDIES REVIEWED SUGGEST THAT, COMPARED WITH PATIENTS, MA NONPATIENTS WHO ARE MORE SOCIALLY PRODUCTIVE AND ECONOMICALLY SUCCESSFUL ARE OVERREPRESENTED AT BOTH ENDS OF A VALUE SCALE WHICH MEASURES TRADITIONALISM; IN CONTRAST, MORE THAN THREE-QUARTERS OF THE PATIENTS ARE FOUND IN THE CENTRAL PART OF THE SCALE. THUS, BY RELYING EXCLUSIVELY ON EITHER MEXICAN OR ANGLO CHOICES, PSYCHOLOGICAL CONSISTENCY COULD BE MAINTAINED AND SOCIAL PRODUCTIVITY INCREASED. ANOTHER STUDY WHICH COMPARED MA, NEGRO, AND ANGLO AMERICAN SCHIZOPHRENICS SHOWS GREATER INDICES OF PSYCHOSIS AND REGRESSION IN MA PATIENTS. SIMILARLY, WHEN MA AND ANGLO OUTPATIENTS ARE COMPARED, THE MA GROUP TENDS TOWARD GREATER REGRESSION AND PSYCHOSIS. IN THIS REGARD, IT IS THE GROUP OF UNACCULTURATED MA PATIENTS WHICH SHOWS THE MOST PROMINENT CLINICAL DIFFERENCES. THESE RESULTS POINT TO UNDER-

LYING DIFFERENCES IN SUCH ISSUES AS THE DEFINITION OF ILLNESS, THE NEED FOR TREATMENT, AND TOLERANCE OF PSYCHIATRIC SYMPTOMS. 28 REFERENCES.

ACCN   000437

516 AUTH   **FABREGA, H., JR.**
    TITL   THE NEED FOR AN ETHNOMEDICAL SCIENCE.
    SRCE   *SCIENCE, 1975, 189, 969-975.*
    INDX   CROSS CULTURAL, DISEASE, FOLK MEDICINE, ESSAY, HEALTH, CULTURE
    ABST   ETHNOMEDICINE EMBRACES THEORETICAL CONCERNS THAT ARE RELEVANT TO BOTH THE SOCIAL AND BIOLOGICAL SCIENCES. THE RELATION WHICH EXISTS BETWEEN DISEASE, SOCIAL BEHAVIOR, AND HUMAN ADAPTATION CONSTITUTES THE PRIMARY SUBJECT MATTER OF ETHNOMEDICINE. THIS RELATION IS EXAMINED IN TERMS OF MAN'S UNIQUE CAPACITIES FOR SYMBOLIZATION AND CULTURE. SINCE ETHNOMEDICAL GENERALIZATIONS EXPLAIN HOW SOCIAL GROUPS DEAL WITH A GENERIC DISEASE, THEY CAN BE USED TO EXAMINE CONTEMPORARY PROBLEMS WHICH INVOLVE THE ORGANIZATION AND PRACTICE OF MEDICINE AS WELL AS PROBLEMS THAT STEM FROM RELATIONS OF THE MEDICAL SYSTEM WITH OTHER SUBSYSTEMS IN THE GROUP. RECASTING CONTEMPORARY SOCIAL PROBLEMS IN THIS WAY MAY HELP CLARIFY THEIR ROOTS AND SOURCES. IN FOCUSING ON FUNDAMENTAL PROPERTIES OF DISEASE IN MAN, ETHNOMEDICINE CAN ALSO HELP TO CLARIFY THE EFFECTS AND MEANINGS OF DISEASE AND THEREBY MAKE ITS CONTROL MORE RATIONAL. A THEORY OF DISEASE, AN ULTIMATE AIM OF ETHNOMEDICAL INQUIRY, WILL SERVE AS AN EXPLANATORY DEVICE WITH WIDE-RANGING APPLICATIONS. 58 REFERENCES. (AUTHOR SUMMARY)

ACCN   000438

517 AUTH   **FABREGA, H., JR., RUBEL, A. J., & WALLACE, C. A.**
    TITL   WORKING-CLASS MEXICAN PSYCHIATRIC OUTPATIENTS.
    SRCE   *ARCHIVES OF GENERAL PSYCHIATRY, 1967, 16(6), 704-712.*
    INDX   MEXICAN, SES, SYMPTOMATOLOGY, ADULTS, EMPIRICAL, SEX COMPARISON, MENTAL HEALTH, SEX ROLES, PSYCHOPATHOLOGY, GENDER IDENTITY, MALE, FEMALE, TEXAS, SOUTHWEST
    ABST   RESULTS OF A SOCIAL PSYCHIATRIC EVALUATION DEALING WITH DEMOGRAPHIC, CULTURAL AND CLINICAL FEATURES OF 30 WORKING-CLASS MEXICAN OUTPATIENTS ARE REPORTED. TWO HYPOTHESES ADVANCED BY THIS REPORT ENTAIL VIEWING THE PATIENTS FROM THE STANDPOINT OF THEIR GENDER IDENTITY AND THEIR VALUE ORIENTATION. THE PATIENTS WERE INTERVIEWED AND ADMINISTERED A FOUR-POINT QUESTIONNAIRE IN THEIR NATIVE LANGUAGE. RESULTS INDICATE THAT THERE ARE DEFINITE GENDER DIFFERENCES IN THE SYMBOLS USED TO EXPRESS ISSUES RELATED TO PSYCHIATRIC PROBLEMS. MEN TEND TO USE MEDICOSOMATIC DESCRIPTIONS, WHEREAS WOMEN ALLOW AFFECTIVE

AND PSYCHOSOCIAL CONSIDERATIONS TO INTERVENE. WOMEN REPORTED SIGNIFICANTLY MORE PSYCHIATRIC SYMPTOMS THAN MEN, AND THE GROUP AS A WHOLE HAD A VERY HIGH MEAN SCORE ON THE MIDTOWN-DEVELOPED INSTRUMENT. MEN WHO HELD VALUE POSITIONS AT THE ENDS OF THE TRADITIONALISM SCALE REPORTED MORE SYMPTOMS THAN MEN IN THE INTERMEDIATE REGION. NO SIGNIFICANT RESULTS IN SYMPTOM RESPONSES WHEN VALUE ORIENTATION WAS CONSIDERED AS AN ANALYTIC VARIABLE WERE SHOWN FOR WOMEN. SOCIAL, CULTURAL, AND PSYCHIATRIC IMPLICATIONS OF THESE RESULTS ARE DISCUSSED. 63 REFERENCES.

ACCN   000439

518 AUTH   **FABREGA, H., JR., SWARTZ, J. D., & WALLACE, C. A.**
    TITL   ETHNIC DIFFERENCES IN PSYCHOPATHOLOGY-I. CLINICAL CORRELATES UNDER VARYING CONDITIONS.
    SRCE   *ARCHIVES OF GENERAL PSYCHIATRY, 1968, 19(2), 218-226.*
    INDX   MEXICAN AMERICAN, PSYCHOPATHOLOGY, CULTURAL FACTORS, EMPIRICAL, ADULTS, SCHIZOPHRENIA, SES, SYMPTOMATOLOGY, PROJECTIVE TESTING, CROSS CULTURAL, TEXAS, SOUTHWEST
    ABST   AN EXAMINATION OF PSYCHOPATHOLOGY AND CORRELATES OF ETHNICITY IN ANGLO-, MEXICAN-, AND NEGRO-AMERICAN SCHIZOPHRENICS IS PRESENTED. THE STUDY ATTEMPTS TO COMPARE ETHNIC CLINICAL DIFFERENCES THAT MIGHT EXIST WHEN CONTROL OVER THE RELATED VARIABLES IS VARIED. THE THREE ETHNIC GROUPS WERE EVALUATED UNDER THREE CONDITIONS: (I) RANDOM, (II) WITH SOCIAL CLASS HELD CONSTANT, AND (III) WHEN INDIVIDUALS OF THE GROUPS WERE MATCHED ON AGE, SEX, IQ, NUMBER OF PREVIOUS PSYCHIATRIC HOSPITALIZATIONS, AND EDUCATION. DATA WERE OBTAINED FROM PSYCHIATRISTS' EVALUATIONS, NURSES' OBSERVATIONS, AND A PERSONALITY PROJECTIVE TEST. RESULTS INDICATE THAT THE DEGREE OF SIGNIFICANT DIFFERENCES BETWEEN GROUPS IN CONDITIONS I AND II DIMINISHED WHEN THE PATIENTS WERE MATCHED (CONDITION III). HOWEVER, SOME DIFFERENCES PERSISTED DESPITE THE MATCHING WHEN ETHNIC GROUPS WHICH DIFFER IN CULTURAL VALUES AND PATTERNS WERE COMPARED. METHODOLOGICAL ISSUES RELATED TO THIS STUDY ARE DISCUSSED. IT IS SUGGESTED THAT THE NATURE OF THE ASSOCIATION BETWEEN ETHNICITY AND SYMPTOMATIC BEHAVIOR IN SCHIZOPHRENIC PATIENTS DEPENDS ON THE DEGREE TO WHICH OTHER VARIABLES (SUCH AS SOCIAL CLASS, DEGREE OF EDUCATION, OR IQ) ARE CONTROLLED. 45 REFERENCES.

ACCN   000440

519 AUTH   **FABREGA, H., JR., SWARTZ, J. D., & WALLACE, C. A.**
    TITL   ETHNIC DIFFERENCES IN PSYCHOPATHOLOGY-II. SPECIFIC DIFFERENCES WITH EMPHASIS ON THE MEXICAN AMERICAN GROUP.

SRCE   *PSYCHIATRIC RESEARCH, 1968, 6(3), 221-235.*

INDX   MEXICAN AMERICAN, PSYCHOPATHOLOGY, CULTURAL FACTORS, EMPIRICAL, ADULTS, SCHIZOPHRENIA, SES, SYMPTOMATOLOGY, PROJECTIVE TESTING, ACCULTURATION, CROSS CULTURAL, TEXAS, SOUTHWEST

ABST   MEXICAN AMERICAN SCHIZOPHRENICS WERE COMPARED WITH NEGRO AND ANGLO SCHIZOPHRENICS. PATIENTS WERE MATCHED ON THE BASIS OF AGE, SEX, IQ ESTIMATE, EDUCATION, AND PRIOR PSYCHIATRIC HOSPITALIZATIONS. PSYCHIATRISTS' SCALED EVALUATIONS OF A PATIENT'S PSYCHOPATHOLOGY; THE NURSE'S OBSERVATION SCALE FOR INPATIENT EVALUATION AND THE HOLTZMAN INKBLOT TECHNIQUE WERE ALSO USED IN THIS SURVEY. THE DATA WERE ANALYZED IN ACCORDANCE WITH PREDICTIONS BASED ON A RATIONALE DEVELOPED FROM PSYCHOLOGICAL, ANTHROPOLOGICAL, AND EPIDEMIOLOGICAL INVESTIGATIONS OF MEXICAN AMERICANS. THE GENERAL TREND FOR GROSS IMPAIRMENT OR PATHOLOGY WAS FOUND TO BE GREATER IN MEXICAN AMERICAN SCHIZOPHRENICS. IT IS SUGGESTED THAT THE FAMILIES OF MEXICAN AMERICAN PATIENTS MAY BE MORE TOLERANT OF DEVIANT PSYCHOTIC BEHAVIOR THAN FAMILIES OF THE OTHER TWO GROUPS AND CONSEQUENTLY DELAY SEEKING HELP OR HOSPITALIZATION LONGER. PREDICTIONS BASED ON CULTURE-PSYCHODYNAMIC REASONS WERE NOT SUPPORTED. THE EVIDENCE INDICATES THAT THE MEXICAN AMERICAN SCHIZOPHRENICS WERE MORE CHRONIC, REGRESSED, AND DISORGANIZED. PROJECTIVE DATA DID NOT SHOW SIGNIFICANT DIFFERENCES BETWEEN GROUPS. THE IMPLICATIONS OF THE FINDINGS ARE ANALYZED. 66 REFERENCES.

ACCN   000441

520 AUTH   **FABREGA, H., JR., & METZGER, D.**

TITL   PSYCHIATRIC ILLNESS IN A SMALL LADINO COMMUNITY.

SRCE   *PSYCHIATRY, 1968, 31(4), 339-351.*

INDX   PSYCHOPATHOLOGY, MEXICAN, CULTURAL FACTORS, ATTITUDES, CASE STUDY, COMMUNITY INVOLVEMENT, FOLK MEDICINE, MENTAL HEALTH

ABST   SOCIAL AND CULTURAL ASPECTS OF PSYCHIATRIC ILLNESS IN A SMALL LADINO COMMUNITY IN THE HIGHLANDS OF CHIAPAS, MEXICO, ARE EXAMINED. THE STUDY PORTRAYS THE MEANING OF PSYCHIATRIC ILLNESS AND PSYCHIATRICALLY ILL PERSONS FROM THE POINT OF VIEW OF THE INHABITANTS THEMSELVES. MUCH OF THE DATA WERE OBTAINED BY MEANS OF INTERVIEWS USING AN ETHNOGRAPHIC INVESTIGATION TECHNIQUE. CONCEPTION, BELIEFS, DESCRIPTIVE FEATURES, AND ATTITUDES ABOUT PSYCHIATRIC ILLNESS AND THEIR CAUSES ARE EMPHASIZED. IT IS SHOWN THAT ILLNESS IS MADE A SOCIAL AFFAIR, AND THE CARE OF THE PSYCHIATRICALLY ILL IS INITIATED AND CARRIED OUT BY NEIGHBORS AND IMPORTANT LEADERS OF THE COMMUNITY USING MEASURES THAT HAVE LOCAL MEANING. INTERVENTION MEANS THE RESTO-

RATION OF SOCIAL FUNCTIONING AND THE ELIMINATION OF SOCIAL ISOLATION AND WITHDRAWAL. INTERVENTION HERE REFERS TO MEETING THE PHYSICAL AND PSYCHOSOCIAL NEEDS OF THE SICK PERSON. THIS HUMANISTIC PATTERN OF HELPING THE ILL PERSON PLAY AN IMPORTANT ROLE IN THE COMMUNITY STANDS IN CONTRAST TO THAT ADOPTED IN WESTERN CIVILIZATION. IT IS SUGGESTED THAT THE CURRENT EMPHASIS ON COMMUNITY MENTAL HEALTH IS NOT UNIQUE TO WESTERN MEDICINE. 45 REFERENCES.

ACCN   000442

521 AUTH   **FABREGA, H., JR., & ROBERTS, R. E.**

TITL   ETHNIC DIFFERENCES IN THE OUTPATIENT USE OF A PUBLIC CHARITY HOSPITAL.

SRCE   *AMERICAN JOURNAL OF PUBLIC HEALTH, 1972, 62, 936-941.*

INDX   HEALTH DELIVERY SYSTEMS, PHYSICIANS, HEALTH, CROSS CULTURAL, SES, POVERTY, DEMOGRAPHIC, RESOURCE UTILIZATION, ENVIRONMENTAL FACTORS, MEXICAN AMERICAN, ADULTS, EMPIRICAL, SOUTHWEST

ABST   THE DIFFERENTIAL USE MADE OF HEALTH SERVICES IN CONTEMPORARY AMERICAN SOCIETY, PARTICULARLY BY DISADVANTAGED SUBGROUPS, IS OF CONSIDERABLE CONCERN. THIS STUDY EXPLICATES THE DIFFERENCES IN PATTERN OF HOSPITAL USE BY THE THREE PRINCIPAL ETHNIC GROUPS IN THE SOUTHWEST (ANGLOS, BLACKS AND CHICANOS). THE 4200 CASES STUDIED WERE TAKEN FROM A HOSPITAL'S "MASTER FILE" WHICH PROVIDED INFORMATION ON AGE, SEX AND BLACK OR WHITE ETHNIC IDENTITY. MEXICAN AMERICAN OR CHICANO PATIENTS WERE DETERMINED BY THEIR SPANISH SURNAME. FINDINGS ARE PRESENTED IN TABULAR FORM AND DISCUSSED IN TERMS OF SEVERAL FACTORS; (1) SOCIO-ENVIRONMENTAL CHARACTERISTICS OF THE POPULATION SERVED BY THE HOSPITAL; (2) USE OF MEDICAL SERVICES OTHER THAN THE HOSPITAL BY SOCIAL AND ETHNIC STATUS; AND (3) PATTERN OF USE OF HOSPITAL FACILITIES ONLY BY SOCIAL AND ETHNIC STATUS. ALTHOUGH IT IS DIFFICULT TO MAKE GENERALIZATIONS ABOUT THE CHICANO GROUP SINCE THEIR NUMBER IN THE SAMPLE IS RELATIVELY SMALL (N=340), THE DATA SUGGEST THEY DO DIFFER FROM THE OTHER TWO ETHNIC GROUPS IN CERTAIN RESPECTS, REFLECTING THE ECONOMIC COMPOSITION AND GEOGRAPHIC DISTRIBUTION OF THE LARGER POPULATION WHICH GENERATED THE PATIENT SAMPLE. 25 REFERENCES. (AUTHOR SUMMARY MODIFIED)

ACCN   000443

522 AUTH   **FABREGA, H., JR., & WALLACE, C. A.**

TITL   ACCULTURATION AND PSYCHIATRIC TREATMENT: A STUDY INVOLVING MEXICAN-AMERICANS.

SRCE   *THE BRITISH JOURNAL OF SOCIAL PSYCHIATRY, 1970-1971, 4(2), 124-136.*

INDX   ACCULTURATION, SYMPTOMATOLOGY, MEXICAN AMERICAN, EMPIRICAL, ADULTS, CUL-

TURAL FACTORS, POVERTY, CROSS CULTURAL, PSYCHOPATHOLOGY, ATTITUDES, FOLK MEDICINE, RESOURCE UTILIZATION, TEXAS, SOUTHWEST

ABST AN ATTEMPT WAS MADE TO EXAMINE THE RELATIONSHIP BETWEEN SOCIOPSYCHOLOGICAL FACTORS RELATED TO ETHNIC IDENTITY AND PSYCHIATRIC SYMPTOMS. IN ORDER TO PAY SPECIFIC ATTENTION TO MEXICAN AMERICANS WHO ARE IN DIFFERENT STAGES OF ACCULTURATING TO ANGLO AMERICAN PATTERNS, THE SAMPLE, DRAWN FROM OUTPATIENTS ATTENDING A SOUTH TEXAS MENTAL HEALTH CLINIC, WAS LIMITED TO HOLLINGSHEAD'S SES CLASSES IV AND V. EACH MEXICAN AMERICAN SUBJECT WAS ASSIGNED AN ACCULTURATION SCORE BASED ON DEMOGRAPHIC, ATTITUDINAL AND BEHAVIORAL VARIABLES. ALL SUBJECTS WERE INTERVIEWED BY INTAKE WORKERS TO ASCERTAIN BELIEFS AND ATTITUDES ABOUT THEIR PROBLEMS AND SYMPTOMS, BY SOCIAL WORKERS TO COLLECT PERSONAL AND SOCIAL HISTORY AND TO BE RATED FOR FAMILY RELATIONS, AND BY A PSYCHIATRIST WHO COMPLETED A PSYCHIATRIC RATING SCALE AND A PSYCHOTICISM-REGRESSION SCALE. UNACCULTURATED MEXICAN AMERICANS, COMPARED TO THE ACCULTURATED AND THE ANGLOS, SHOWED GREATER RELIANCE ON FOLK MEDICAL CONCEPTIONS, LESS PROMINENT FAMILY CONFLICTS AND GREATER INDICES OF PSYCHOTICISM-REGRESSION. FINDINGS ARE BELIEVED TO BE CONCEPTUALLY LINKED AND TO INDICATE THAT CULTURAL FACTORS AFFECT MEXICAN AMERICANS SEEKING PSYCHIATRIC TREATMENT. IN ADDITION, RESULTS INDICATED THAT THE UNACCULTURATED, COMPARED TO THE OTHER SUB-GROUPS, WERE SEEN LESS FREQUENTLY DURING THEIR PERIOD OF TREATMENT AND MAINLY RECEIVED DRUG THERAPY. THE IMPLICATION OF THE RESULTS THAT WERE OBTAINED ARE DISCUSSED. 30 REFERENCES. (AUTHOR SUMMARY MODIFIED)

ACCN 000444

523 AUTH **FABREGA, H., JR., & WALLACE, C. A.**
TITL HOW PHYSICIANS JUDGE SYMPTOM STATEMENTS: A CROSS CULTURAL STUDY.
SRCE *THE JOURNAL OF NERVOUS AND MENTAL DISEASE, 1968, 145(6), 486-491.*
INDX PHYSICIANS, SYMPTOMATOLOGY, MEXICAN, CROSS CULTURAL, MENTAL HEALTH PROFESSION, EMPIRICAL, SEX COMPARISON, PSYCHOPATHOLOGY, CULTURAL FACTORS, SOUTHWEST
ABST PSYCHIATRISTS AND NONPSYCHIATRISTS FROM MEXICO AND THE UNITED STATES SCALED THE SERIOUSNESS OF THE SYMPTOM ITEMS THAT MAKE UP THE MIDTOWN MENTAL HEALTH QUESTIONNAIRE. EACH PHYSICIAN WAS ASKED TO ASSESS THE SYMPTOMS IN EITHER A MALE OR FEMALE PATIENT AND TO ASSUME THAT HE HAD ENCOUNTERED THE SYMPTOM DURING THE COURSE OF A CLINICAL EVALUATION. ALL THREE VARIABLES-PHYSICIAN TYPE, NATIONALITY AND GENDER-SHOWED SIGNIFICANT EFFECTS ON SOME SYMPTOMS, AND TWO CLEAR

TRENDS EMERGED. PSYCHIATRISTS OF EACH NATION JUDGED A NUMBER OF SYMPTOMS TO BE "MORE SERIOUS THAN DID NONPSYCHIATRISTS OF THE SAME NATION. THE TWO AMERICAN PHYSICIAN GROUPS SCALED SEVERAL ITEMS HIGHER THAN DID EQUIVALENT MEXICAN PHYSICIAN GROUPS. GENDER APPEARED TO BE A SIGNIFICANT VARIABLE IN THE MEXICAN PSYCHIATRY GROUP. A POSSIBLE GENDER DIFFERENCE WAS SUGGESTED IN THE AMERICAN NONPSYCHIATRY SUBGROUP. IN EACH CASE MALES RECEIVED HIGHER SYMPTOM SCORES. THIS STUDY ILLUSTRATES SOME OF THE CONCEPTUAL AND METHODOLOGICAL BIASES THAT MAY BE PRESENT IN CROSS-CULTURAL PSYCHIATRIC STUDIES THAT USE STRUCTURED SYMPTOM QUESTIONNAIRES. 17 REFERENCES. (AUTHOR SUMMARY)

ACCN 000445

524 AUTH **FABREGA, H., JR., & WALLACE, C. A.**
TITL VALUE IDENTIFICATION AND PSYCHIATRIC DISABILITY: AN ANALYSIS INVOLVING AMERICANS OF MEXICAN DESCENT.
SRCE *BEHAVIORAL SCIENCE, 1968, 13(5), 362-371.*
INDX MEXICAN AMERICAN, ACCULTURATION, PSYCHOPATHOLOGY, MARITAL STABILITY, EMPIRICAL, ADULTS, STRESS, SES, ATTITUDES, FOLK MEDICINE, SEX ROLES, CULTURE, TEXAS, SOUTHWEST, MENTAL HEALTH, VALUES
ABST THIS STUDY COMPARED DEMOGRAPHIC FEATURES AND VALUE IDENTIFICATIONS BETWEEN PSYCHIATRIC OUTPATIENTS AND NONPATIENTS OF MEXICAN DESCENT. BOTH GROUPS RESIDE IN A SETTING (BORDER REGIONS OF SOUTH TEXAS) CHARACTERIZED BY COMPETING CULTURAL SYSTEMS AND KNOWN TO BE UNDERGOING SOCIAL CHANGE. QUESTIONNAIRES WERE ADMINISTERED TO 76 HOSPITAL PATIENTS AND TO 48 NONPATIENTS WHO WERE SELECTED FROM A REPRESENTATIVE SMALL TOWN USING A PROBABILITY SAMPLING PLAN. THE FINDINGS SHOW THAT SOCIAL FUNCTIONING AND ECONOMIC ASSIMILATION ARE HIGHER IN THE NONPATIENT GROUP. THE NONPATIENT GROUP SHOWS HIGHER MEASURES ON THE VARIABLES OF EDUCATION, OCCUPATION, AND MARITAL STABILITY. ANSWERS TO THE VALUE IDENTIFICATION SCALE WHICH REFLECT EITHER TRADITIONALISM (MEXICAN) OR NONTRADITIONALISM (ANGLO) VALUE PREFERENCE SHOW THAT THERE IS NO SIGNIFICANT DIFFERENCE BETWEEN THE GROUPS IN DEGREE OF TRADITIONALISTIC EMPHASIS. THE DISTRIBUTION ACROSS THE VALUE CONTINUUM BETWEEN TRADITIONALISM AND NONTRADITIONALISM SHOWS A SIGNIFICANTLY LARGER PROPORTION OF NONPATIENTS WHO PREFER EITHER EXTREME OF THE CONTINUUM AS COMPARED TO THE PATIENTS. MORE THAN THREE-QUARTERS (78%) OF THE PATIENTS ARE FOUND IN THE CENTRAL PART OF THE SCALE. IT IS SUGGESTED THAT THE RESULTS INVOLVING THE DEMOGRAPHIC VARIABLES IMPLY GROUP DIFFERENCES IN SOCIAL PRODUCTIVITY AND ASSIMILATION. THESE DIFFERENCES MAY RELATE TO THE IMPLICATIONS OF THE DISTRIBUTIONAL PATTERNS OF THE GROUPS ON THE

VALUE SCALE RATHER THAN TO DIFFERENCES IN THE OVERALL EXTENT OF IDENTIFICATION WITH TRADITIONAL VALUES. 42 REFERENCES.

ACCN 000446

525 AUTH **FABREGAT, C. E.**

TITL FAMILIA Y MATRIMONIO EN MEXICO. (FAMILY AND MARRIAGE IN MEXICO.)

SRCE *REVISTA DE INDIAS, 1969, 29, 173-278. (SPANISH)*

INDX FAMILY STRUCTURE, MARRIAGE, MEXICAN, ESSAY, URBAN, RURAL, CULTURAL CHANGE, FAMILY ROLES

ABST AS THE RESULT OF BOTH HIS 17 YEARS OF RESIDENCE IN MEXICO AND THE ANALYSIS OF 88 QUESTIONNAIRES DISTRIBUTED TO AN UNSPECIFIED SAMPLE OF INDIVIDUALS SELECTED ACCORDING TO PROFESSION, ETHNIC ORIGIN, AND SEX, RESIDING IN THE STATES OF JALISCO, VERACRUZ, QUERETARO, PUEBLA, AND THE FEDERAL DISTRICT, THE AUTHOR DISCUSSES THE TRADITIONAL FAMILY AND MATRIMONIAL ROLES IN MEXICAN SOCIETY. NO MENTION IS MADE OF THE CRITERIA USED IN SELECTING INDIVIDUALS FOR THE SURVEY NOR OF THE SPECIFIC DATA OBTAINED. THE MEXICAN FAMILY IS SEEN AS AN EXTREMELY PATRIARCHAL UNIT IN WHICH THE FATHER FUNCTIONS BOTH AS BREAD WINNER AND DECISION-MAKER. MOREOVER, THE DIFFERENT SEXUAL VALUES APPLICABLE TO MEN AND WOMEN PLAY AN IMPORTANT ROLE IN MAINTAINING THIS STRUCTURE AND THE SUBORDINATE POSITION OF THE WIFE/MOTHER WITHIN THE FAMILY. THE LEVEL OF COHESION OF THE FAMILY UNIT IS SEEN AS INCREASING PROPORTIONATELY TO THE DEGREE OF DEPENDENCE OF FAMILY MEMBERS UPON THE FATHER. BECAUSE RURAL LIFE OFFERS FEWER CHANCES FOR EMPLOYMENT OUTSIDE OF THE IMMEDIATE FAMILY, THE ROLE AND IMPORTANCE OF THE FATHER IN THE RURAL FAMILY IS MUCH GREATER THAN IN THE URBAN FAMILY WHERE BOTH WOMEN AND CHILDREN HAVE GREATER OPPORTUNITIES OF FINDING JOBS. IT IS ALSO SEEN THAT IN THE ABSENCE OF A FATHER FIGURE, THE OLDEST MALE CHILD TENDS TO GRADUALLY ASSUME THE ECONOMIC AND DECISION-MAKING RESPONSIBILITIES OF THE HEAD OF THE HOUSEHOLD. IN RECENT YEARS, INCREASED OPPORTUNITIES FOR WOMEN AND THE WEAKENING OF THE MALE EGO THROUGH THE POSSIBILITY OF A WIFE EARNING MORE THAN HER HUSBAND HAVE LED TO GRADUAL CHANGES IN FAMILY AND MATRIMONIAL ROLES.

ACCN 000447

526 AUTH **FALLOWS, M.**

TITL THE MEXICAN AMERICAN LABORERS: A DIFFERENT DRUMMER?

SRCE *THE MASSACHUSETTS REVIEW, 1967, 8, 166-176.*

INDX MEXICAN AMERICAN, LABOR FORCE, ACCULTURATION, SES, BILINGUALISM, CULTURAL FACTORS, ESSAY, CULTURE, STEREOTYPES, LEADERSHIP, FARM LABORERS, RELIGION, POVERTY, RURAL, MIGRANTS, POLITICAL POWER, CALIFORNIA, SOUTHWEST, CHICANO MOVEMENT

ABST THE "GRAPE PICKER'S MOVEMENT" LED BY CESAR CHAVEZ TO ESTABLISH THE RIGHT TO BARGAIN AMONG MIGRANT FARM WORKERS HAD TREMENDOUS IMPACT ON PREVIOUSLY ACCEPTED STEREOTYPES HELD BY OUR SOCIETY REGARDING THE UNORGANIZABLE MEXICAN AMERICAN. SINCE THIS GROUP HAS REFUSED TO ASSIMILATE INTO THE AMERICAN MAINSTREAM, THEIR POVERTY HAS LONG BEEN CONSIDERED A PRODUCT OF THEIR CULTURAL HERITAGE. CHAVEZ HAS DEMONSTRATED IT IS POSSIBLE TO GAIN POLITICAL POWER WITHIN THE AMERICAN VALUE SYSTEM AND STILL MAINTAIN THE SOCIAL AND CULTURAL VALUES OF THE MEXICAN AMERICAN PEOPLE.

ACCN 000448

527 AUTH **FARBER, H., & MAYER, G. R.**

TITL BEHAVIOR CONSULTATION IN A BARRIO HIGH SCHOOL.

SRCE *PERSONNEL AND GUIDANCE JOURNAL, 1972, 51(4), 273-279.*

INDX BEHAVIOR MODIFICATION, ADOLESCENTS, EDUCATION, EDUCATIONAL COUNSELING, EMPIRICAL, TEACHERS, PROGRAM EVALUATION, PERFORMANCE EXPECTATIONS, URBAN, CALIFORNIA, SOUTHWEST

ABST EFFECTIVE USE OF BEHAVIOR MODIFICATION APPROACHES BY SECONDARY SCHOOL COUNSELORS, PARTICULARLY AS CONSULTANTS TO TEACHERS, IS NOT WIDELY DOCUMENTED IN THE LITERATURE. WITH THE INCREASING PROBLEMS OF INNER-CITY SCHOOLS IN PROVIDING MEANINGFUL EDUCATION TO DISENCHANTED STUDENTS, THE BEHAVIORAL APPROACH TO GUIDANCE AND COUNSELING SEEMS WORTHY OF TESTING IN THE CLASSROOM. THE STUDY DESCRIBES BEHAVIORAL CONSULTATION WITH A COUNSELOR WHO WAS, IN TURN, ASSISTING A 10TH GRADE ENGLISH TEACHER TO DEAL WITH HIS STUDENTS' "LACKADAISICAL ATTITUDE TOWARD COMPLETING ASSIGNMENTS. THE ENTIRE CONSULTATION PROCESS IS DESCRIBED: (1) THE BEHAVIOR CHANGE PROCEDURE; (2) DATA COLLECTION; (3) GOALS, CRITERION LEVEL AND BASELINE MEASURES; (4) PROJECT PHASES; AND (5) GRAPHIC PRESENTATION OF STUDENTS' ASSIGNMENT COMPLETION BEHAVIOR. IT IS CONCLUDED THAT THE BEHAVIORAL APPROACHES USED FACILITATED THE CHANGES THE TEACHER DESIRED AND THAT THE DATA COLLECTED PROVIDE APPROPRIATE MEASURES AND INCIDENTS FOR THE COUNSELOR TO REINFORCE THE TEACHER AND THE TEACHER TO PROVIDE AN ENVIRONMENT MORE CONDUCIVE TO STUDENT LEARNING. 15 REFERENCES.

ACCN 000449

528 AUTH **FARGE, E. J.**

TITL LA VIDA CHICANA: HEALTH CARE ATTITUDES AND BEHAVIORS OF HOUSTON CHICANOS.

SRCE *SAN FRANCISCO: R AND E RESEARCH ASSOCIATES, 1975.*

INDX HEALTH, HEALTH DELIVERY SYSTEMS, ACCUL-

TURATION, PERSONALITY, FOLK MEDICINE, DE-
MOGRAPHIC, SES, REVIEW, SURVEY, ATTI-
TUDES, THEORETICAL, ETHNIC IDENTITY,
EMPIRICAL, MEXICAN AMERICAN, URBAN,
TEXAS, SOUTHWEST

ABST DIFFERENCES IN MEXICAN AMERICAN HEALTH
CARE ATTITUDES AND BEHAVIORS WITHIN
SUBGROUPS OF CHICANOS WERE COMPARED
AMONG 150 HEADS OF HOUSEHOLD FROM
THREE AREAS OF HOUSTON, TEXAS. SUB-
JECTS WERE INTERVIEWED USING A RE-
SEARCH INSTRUMENT DESIGNED TO COM-
PARE A VARIETY OF SOCIAL, COGNITIVE AND
SOCIODEMOGRAPHIC VARIABLES. THREE MA-
JOR HYPOTHESES, DEVELOPED FROM AN EX-
TENSIVE REVIEW OF THE LITERATURE ON MEX-
ICAN AMERICAN HEALTH BELIEFS AND
PRACTICES, ARE TESTED. ALTHOUGH CON-
CLUSIONS DID NOT GENERALLY SUPPORT THE
PROPOSED FRAMEWORK FOR CHICANO
HEALTH CARE BEHAVIOR AS APPLIED TO MEX-
ICAN AMERICANS IN HOUSTON, IT DID SUP-
PORT THE USE OF INDICATORS SUCH AS SELF
DETERMINISM, AND MAINTENANCE OF MEXI-
CAN CULTURE IN PREDICTING CHICANO HEALTH
ATTITUDES AND BEHAVIOR. AN IN-DEPTH
THEORETICAL FRAMEWORK AND ANALYSIS OF
DATA IS INCLUDED ALONG WITH A REVIEW OF
CHICANO HEALTH CARE BEHAVIOR LITERA-
TURE. 101 REFERENCES.

ACCN 000450

529 AUTH **FARGE, E. J.**
TITL A REVIEW OF FINDINGS FROM "THREE GEN-
ERATIONS" OF CHICANO HEALTH CARE BEHAV-
IOR.
SRCE *SOCIAL SCIENCE QUARTERLY, 1977, 58(3), 407-
411.*
INDX ADULTS, MEXICAN AMERICAN, TEXAS, SOUTH-
WEST, URBAN, HEALTH, EMPIRICAL, SES, SUR-
VEY, RURAL, ATTITUDES, HEALTH DELIVERY
SYSTEMS, FOLK MEDICINE, CROSS GENERA-
TIONAL
ABST WEAVER'S (1973) HISTORICAL REVIEW OF THE
LITERATURE ON CHICANO HEALTH CARE
(DEALING PRIMARILY WITH RURAL AREAS DUR-
ING THE 1940'S AND UP THROUGH THE 1960'S)
IDENTIFIED GENERATION-LEVEL DIFFERENCES
AMONG CHICANOS WITH REGARD TO HEALTH
CARE PRACTICES. WEAVER'S HYPOTHESES
WERE TESTED IN THIS STUDY OF 150 CHICANO
HOUSEHOLD HEADS IN HOUSTON, TEXAS.
SUBJECTS WERE RANDOMLY SELECTED FROM
A METROPOLITAN TRACT AREA AND ADMINIS-
TERED A QUESTIONNAIRE WHICH ADDRESSED
NINE OF WEAVER'S HYPOTHESES. THE RE-
SULTS FOUND NO SUPPORT FOR SEVEN OF
THE NINE HYPOTHESES. THAT IS, OVERALL,
THE CHICANOS DID NOT ADHERE AS MUCH TO
FOLK MEDICAL BELIEFS NOR HAVE AS MUCH
RESISTANCE TO SCIENTIFIC MEDICAL PRAC-
TICES AS SUGGESTED BY WEAVER. HOWEVER,
TWO HYPOTHESES WERE SUPPORTED: (1) THE
BELIEF AND PRACTICE OF FOLK MEDICINE
VARIED INVERSELY WITH SES; AND (2) FOLK BE-
LIEFS DID NOT DETER CHICANOS FROM USING
CLINICAL SERVICES. IN GENERAL, THE SURVEY
DISCOVERED SOME MEASURE OF BELIEF IN

FOLK MEDICINE BUT DID NOT SUGGEST THAT
THIS CAUSES A LACK OF BELIEF IN MODERN
MEDICINE. DIFFERENCES IN THESE FINDINGS
FROM WEAVER'S ARE ATTRIBUTED TO RURAL-
URBAN DIFFERENCES AND THE LENGTH OF
TIME BETWEEN STUDIES. IT IS CONCLUDED
THAT A MORE VALID MODEL OF ETHNICITY
AND HEALTH CARE SHOULD INCLUDE RE-
SEARCH WHICH IS TRI-ETHNIC. 9 REFERENCES.
ACCN 002270

530 AUTH **FARRIS, B. E., & GLENN, N. D.**
TITL FATALISM AND FAMILIALISM AMONG ANGLOS
AND MEXICAN AMERICANS IN SAN ANTONIO.
SRCE *SOCIOLOGY AND SOCIAL RESEARCH, 1976, 60,
393-402.*
INDX CROSS CULTURAL, MEXICAN AMERICAN, AC-
CULTURATION, SCHOLASTIC ACHIEVEMENT,
FAMILY ROLES, FAMILY STRUCTURE, FATALISM,
SES, EMPIRICAL, TEXAS, SOUTHWEST
ABST A COMPARISON OF THE RESPONSES OF AN-
GLOS AND MEXICAN AMERICANS TO INTER-
VIEW ITEMS DESIGNED TO MEASURE FATALISM
AND FAMILISM SHOWS A MODERATE ETHNIC
DIFFERENCE IN FATALISM AND A LARGER DIF-
FERENCE IN FAMILISM. CONTROLS FOR EDU-
CATION LARGELY REMOVE THE DIFFERENCE IN
FATALISM, BUT AT EACH EDUCATIONAL LEVEL
THE MEXICAN AMERICANS APPEAR, AS A
WHOLE, TO HAVE BEEN DISTINCTLY MORE
FAMILISTIC THAN THE ANGLOS. SINCE FATAL-
ISM RATHER THAN FAMILISM IS EMPHASIZED IN
MOST "CULTURAL HANDICAP" EXPLANATIONS
FOR THE LOW SOCIOECONOMIC STATUS OF
MEXICAN AMERICANS, THE FINDINGS LEND
LITTLE SUPPORT TO THOSE EXPLANATIONS. 6
REFERENCES. (JOURNAL ABSTRACT)
ACCN 000451

531 AUTH **FARRIS, B., & BRYMER, R.**
TITL A FIVE-YEAR ENCOUNTER WITH A MEXICAN-
AMERICAN CONFLICT GANG: ITS IMPLICA-
TIONS FOR DELINQUENCY THEORY.
SRCE *PAPER PRESENTED AT THE ANNUAL SOUTH-
WESTERN SOCIOLOGICAL ASSOCIATION
MEETING, APRIL 1965.*
INDX CASE STUDY, REVIEW, THEORETICAL, ROLE EX-
PECTATIONS, GANGS, MEXICAN AMERICAN,
DELINQUENCY, ADOLESCENTS, TEXAS,
SOUTHWEST
ABST IN AN ATTEMPT TO STATE AND EXPLORE A
VIEW OF DELINQUENCY THAT BOTH INCLUDES
APPROPRIATE ASPECTS OF EXISTING THEO-
RIES AND EXPLAINS BEHAVIORS NOT COV-
ERED IN EXISTING THEORIES, A REVIEW AND
RECONCEPTUALIZATION OF CURRENT DELIN-
QUENCY LITERATURE IS PRESENTED. OBSER-
VATIONS OF BOTH DELINQUENTS AND GANG
WORKERS OVER A 5-YEAR PERIOD BY PARTICI-
PANTS IN THE WESLEY COMMUNITY CENTER,
SAN ANTONIO, PROVIDES THE BASIS FOR
CRITICISM OF PRESENT THEORY AND SUG-
GESTIONS FOR A MORE ADEQUATE EXPLANA-
TION OF DELINQUENCY AS WELL AS A FUNC-
TIONAL RATIONALE FOR GANG WORKERS'
ACTIONS. THE MAJOR REVISIONS PROPOSED
ARE: (1) THAT DELINQUENCY SHOULD BE PER-

CEIVED AS A MUTUAL DISAGREEMENT BE-
TWEEN THE BOY AND THE MIDDLE-CLASS IN-
STITUTION, NOT MERELY THE BOY'S REALIZA-
TION THAT HE CANNOT ACHIEVE MIDDLE-CLASS
VALUES; (2) THAT GANG MEMBERSHIP DOES
NOT APPEAR TO BE A REACTION TO ANYTHING
IN PARTICULAR, BUT MORE AS A CONSE-
QUENCE OF BEING A LOWER CLASS PERSON;
AND MOST IMPORTANTLY, (3) THAT SOME NO-
TION OF THE LIFE CYCLE MUST BE INCLUDED
IN A COMPREHENSIVE THEORY OF DELIN-
QUENCY. STATEMENTS ARE OFFERED AS HY-
POTHESES, DERIVED FROM EXPERIENCE AND
LITERATURE REVIEW, WITH THE CAUTION THAT
THEY REMAIN TO BE TESTED. 11 REFERENCES.

ACCN 000452

532 AUTH **FARRIS, B., & BRYMER, R. A.**
TITL DIFFERENTIAL SOCIALIZATION OF LATIN AND
ANGLO-AMERICAN YOUTH: AN EXPLORATORY
STUDY OF THE SELF CONCEPT.
SRCE *IN J. H. BURMA (ED.), MEXICAN-AMERICANS IN
THE U.S. NEW YORK: HARPER AND ROW INC.,
1970, PP. 411-426.*
INDX SELF CONCEPT, SOCIALIZATION, CHILDREN,
SPANISH SURNAMED, ADOLESCENTS, EMPIRI-
CAL, CROSS CULTURAL, INTERPERSONAL RE-
LATIONS, SCHOLASTIC ACHIEVEMENT, EDU-
CATION, PEER GROUP, SES, URBAN
ABST IN AN EFFORT TO EXPLORE CONCEPTS ABOUT
THE DIFFERENTIAL SOCIALIZATION OF LATIN
AND ANGLO-AMERICAN CHILDREN, A "SELF-
CONCEPT" INSTRUMENT WAS ADMINISTERED
TO SCHOOL CLASSES AT THREE GRADE LEV-
ELS-4, 8, 11. BASIC CONCEPTS EXPLORED
WERE: SCHOOL, FAMILY, PEER GROUPS, SEX
AND AGE GROUPS, RELIGIOUS GROUPS AND
ETHNIC STATEMENTS, AMBITIONS, INTERESTS,
LIKES, DISLIKES, ABILITIES, AND ACTIVITIES.
THE FINDINGS REVEAL THAT LATINS AND AN-
GLOS APPEAR TO BE APPROXIMATELY EQUAL
IN TERMS OF THEIR PARTICIPATION IN GROUPS
AT THE ELEMENTARY SCHOOL LEVEL. WITH
TIME, HOWEVER, A DIVERGENCE DEVELOPS,
SO THAT BY THE HIGH SCHOOL LEVEL, AN-
GLOS PERCEIVE THEMSELVES AS MORE AC-
TIVE IN SOCIAL GROUPS AND IN MORE SOCIAL
ROLES THAN DO LATINS. IN GENERAL IT ALSO
APPEARS THAT THERE ARE RELATIVELY DIS-
TINCT DIFFERENCES BETWEEN LATINS WHO
"MAKE IT" IN THE SCHOOL SYSTEM AND LATINS
WHO DON'T "MAKE IT." TWO EXPLANATIONS
OFFERED FOR THE DIFFERENCE BETWEEN THE
LATIN GROUPS ARE AS FOLLOWS: (1) THERE
ARE TWO TYPES OF LATINS FROM THE ELE-
MENTARY AGES, THE ALIENATED LATIN AND
THE INTEGRATED LATIN. THE ALIENATED LATIN
DROPS OUT AT JUNIOR HIGH SCHOOL
GRADUATION BECAUSE OF OUTSIDE PRES-
SURES AS WELL AS LOW ACADEMIC INTEREST.
(2) LATINS ARE ESSENTIALLY THE SAME WHEN
THEY ENTER ELEMENTARY SCHOOL, BUT OVER
THE YEARS SOME GET INVOLVED WITH THE
SCHOOL SYSTEM AND LITERALLY, "OUT ANGLO
THE ANGLOS", I.E., DEVELOP AN OVER-ABUN-
DANCE OF CHARACTERISTICS THAT GET THEM
THROUGH THE SCHOOL SYSTEM. ALTHOUGH
THERE ARE SOME DIFFERENCES BETWEEN

LATINS AND ANGLOS, THERE ARE NO STRONG
EXPLANATORY CONTEXTS IN WHICH TO PLACE
THEM. 13 REFERENCES.

ACCN 000453

533 AUTH **FARRIS, B., & HALE, W. M.**
TITL RESPONSIBLE WARDHEELERS: NEIGHBOR-
HOOD WORKERS AS MEDIATORS.
SRCE *PAPER PRESENTED AT THE NATIONAL CONFER-
ENCE OF SOCIAL WELFARE, CHICAGO, 1966.*
INDX COMMUNITY, PARAPROFESSIONALS, COMMU-
NITY INVOLVEMENT, SOCIAL SERVICES, ESSAY,
THEORETICAL
ABST "RESPONSIBLE WARDHEELERS" REFERS TO
WORKERS IN LOWER-CLASS NEIGHBOR-
HOODS WHO HAVE AN ETHICAL OUTLOOK EN-
ABLING THEM TO BE RESPONSIVE TO ALL AS-
PECTS OF PEOPLE INVOLVED IN SOCIAL
SERVICES. IN THIS MODEL THE "RESPONSIBLE
WARDHEELER" ACTS AS A MEDIATOR WHO
EQUALIZES THE POWER POSITIONS OF PAR-
TICIPANTS BEFORE RESOLVING THEIR CON-
FLICTING VIEWPOINTS. COMPARED TO THE
OTHER MODELS UTILIZED IN SOCIAL WORK
(CLINICAL AND SOCIAL ACTION), EMPLOYING
THE "WARDHEELER" PERSPECTIVE ENABLES
THE SOCIAL WORKER TO FUNCTION AT THE
NEIGHBORHOOD LEVEL AS WELL AS AT THE
COMMUNITY LEVEL IN PROVIDING SERVICES
TO CLIENTS. THIS MODEL PROVIDES A THEO-
RETICAL FRAMEWORK IN THAT THE SOCIAL
WORKER ACTING AS A MEDIATOR ASSUMES A
ROLE ALSO AS A PARTICIPANT. BY THUS BE-
COMING INVOLVED IN THE INTERACTION PRO-
CESS, THE SOCIAL WORKER IS NO LONGER
FUNCTIONING AS AN OUTSIDER TO THOSE
BEING PROVIDED SOCIAL SERVICES. 13 REF-
ERENCES.

ACCN 000454

534 AUTH **FEAGIN, J. R.**
TITL RACIAL AND ETHNIC RELATIONS.
SRCE *ENGLEWOOD CLIFFS, N.J.: PRENTICE-HALL, INC.,
1978.*
INDX IMMIGRATION, REVIEW, DISCRIMINATION, MEX-
ICAN AMERICAN, CROSS CULTURAL, CUL-
TURAL FACTORS, ECONOMIC FACTORS,
PREJUDICE, ACCULTURATION, SOCIAL MOBIL-
ITY, EDUCATION, RELIGION, STEREOTYPES,
HISTORY, POLITICAL POWER, BOOK
ABST GEARED PRIMARILY TOWARD UNDERGRADU-
ATE SOCIAL SCIENCE AND MINORITY/RACE RE-
LATIONS COURSES, THIS TEXT PROVIDES THE
STUDENT WITH A COMPREHENSIVE OVERVIEW
OF THE RAPIDLY GROWING RACIAL/ETHNIC
GROUP LITERATURE IN THE SOCIAL SCIENCES,
HISTORY, ECONOMICS, AND POLITICAL SCI-
ENCE. IN THE INTRODUCTORY CHAPTERS ON
INTERGROUP CONTACT, A THEORETICAL
FRAMEWORK IS POSITED WHICH CHARACTER-
IZES THE IMMIGRANT EXPERIENCE IN TERMS
OF ADAPTATION, STRATIFICATION, AND SO-
CIAL INEQUALITY. FOLLOWING ARE CHAPTERS
DEVOTED TO EACH OF EIGHT U.S. ETHNIC
GROUPS—ENGLISH, IRISH, ITALIAN, JEWISH,
BLACK, MEXICAN, JAPANESE, AND NATIVE
AMERICANS. EACH CHAPTER TRACES THE

ETHNIC GROUP'S (1) MIGRATION, (2) STEREO-TYPES, (3) POLITICAL INVOLVEMENT, (4) ECONOMIC MOBILITY, (5) EDUCATION, (6) RELIGION AND ARTS, AND (7) ASSIMILATION EXPERIENCES. IN THE CHAPTER ON MEXICAN AMERICANS, EXTENSIVE HISTORICAL DATA ON THEIR IMMIGRATION EXPERIENCE ARE PRESENTED, AND PARTICULAR ATTENTION IS GIVEN TO THE SIMILARITIES BETWEEN MEXICAN AMERICANS' AND BLACKS' STRUGGLES FOR POLITICAL AND ECONOMIC PARITY. BUT DESPITE THESE SIMILARITIES, IT IS NOTED THAT MEXICAN AMERICANS HAVE PROVEN TO BE LESS MILITANT ON SELECTED CIVIL RIGHTS ISSUES, THUS MAKING IT DIFFICULT FOR THE TWO GROUPS TO FORM COALITIONS AGAINST THE DOMINANT GROUP. IN THE CONCLUDING CHAPTER, THE AUTHOR CRITICIZES THE COMMONLY HELD NOTION THAT THE U.S. IS AN EGALITARIAN SOCIETY, AND HE EMPHASIZES THE FRUSTRATIONS WHICH SUCH A CONCEPT HAS IMPOSED ON RACIALLY OPPRESSED MINORITIES. 735 REFERENCES.

ACCN   001774

535   AUTH   **FEATHERMAN, D.**
      TITL   THE SOCIOECONOMIC ACHIEVEMENT OF WHITE RELIGIO-ETHNIC SUBGROUPS: SOCIAL AND PSYCHOLOGICAL EXPLANATIONS.
      SRCE   *AMERICAN SOCIOLOGICAL REVIEW, 1971, 36(20), 207-222.*
      INDX   SOCIAL MOBILITY, SES, RELIGION, CROSS CULTURAL, MEXICAN AMERICAN, DISCRIMINATION, ACHIEVEMENT MOTIVATION, MALE, ADULTS, EMPIRICAL, OCCUPATIONAL ASPIRATIONS, EDUCATION, URBAN, DEMOGRAPHIC
      ABST   LONGITUDINAL DATA WERE EXAMINED FOR THE DECADE 1957-1967 ON THE SOCIOECONOMIC ACHIEVEMENT OF 715 WHITE MALES FROM FIVE RELIGIOETHNIC BACKGROUNDS: 88 JEWISH; 121 ANGLO-SAXON PROTESTANT; 142 PROTESTANT, OTHER; 216 ROMAN CATHOLIC, EXCEPT ITALIAN AND MEXICAN; 100 ITALIAN AND MEXICAN ROMAN CATHOLICS; AND 48 NONE OR OTHER RELIGION. FINDINGS INDICATE THAT JEWS ATTAIN HIGHER LEVELS OF EDUCATION, OCCUPATION, AND INCOME THAN ALL OTHER SUBGROUPS, WHILE ROMAN CATHOLICS OF ITALIAN AND MEXICAN HERITAGE ACHIEVE THE LOWEST LEVELS. THERE IS NO EVIDENCE OF OCCUPATIONAL AND INCOME DISCRIMINATION ON PURELY RELIGIOUS OR ETHNIC GROUNDS. CONTRARY TO CURRENT EMPHASIS IN SOCIAL PSYCHOLOGY OF RELIGIOETHNIC ACHIEVEMENT, ACHIEVEMENT-RELATED WORK VALUES AND MOTIVATIONAL FACTORS (WORK ORIENTATION, MATERIALISTIC ORIENTATION, AND SUBJECTIVE ACHIEVEMENT EVALUATION) OF ADULTS ARE NEITHER KEY INTERVENING VARIABLES NOR DO THEY INFLUENCE THE PROCESS OF STRATIFICATION. THE MOST IMPORTANT VARIABLE IN EXPLAINING THE DIFFERENTIAL SOCIOECONOMIC ACHIEVEMENT OF THE RELIGIOETHNIC SUBGROUPS IS EDUCATION AFTER THE VARIATIONS OWING TO THE HANDICAPS AND BENEFITS OF SOCIAL ORIGINS HAVE BEEN REMOVED. 26 REFERENCES.

ACCN   000455

536   AUTH   **FELDMAN, C., & SHEN, M.**
      TITL   SOME LANGUAGE-RELATED COGNITIVE ADVANTAGES OF BILINGUAL FIVE-YEAR-OLDS.
      SRCE   *JOURNAL OF GENETIC PSYCHOLOGY, 1971, 118(2), 235-244.*
      INDX   BILINGUALISM, COGNITIVE DEVELOPMENT, CHILDREN, MEXICAN AMERICAN, EMPIRICAL, CROSS CULTURAL, LANGUAGE COMPREHENSION, LANGUAGE ASSESSMENT, SPANISH SURNAMED, EARLY CHILDHOOD EDUCATION, BILINGUAL
      ABST   FIFTEEN MONOLINGUAL AND 15 BILINGUAL (SPANISH-ENGLISH) HEADSTART CHILDREN WERE COMPARED IN THEIR ABILITY AT TASKS INVOLVING OBJECT CONSTANCY, NAMING, AND THE USE OF NAMES IN SENTENCES. THE THREE TASKS CONSTITUTE A NATURAL SEQUENCE OF LANGUAGE SKILLS. RESULTS INDICATE THAT BILINGUALS PERFORMED SIGNIFICANTLY BETTER THAN MONOLINGUALS IN ALL THREE TASKS. IN TASKS INVOLVING THE USE OF COMMON NAMES AND THE USE OF NONSENSE NAMES BOTH GROUPS OF SUBJECTS WERE EQUALLY COMPETENT. HOWEVER, THE BILINGUALS WERE BETTER THAN MONOLINGUALS IN THE USE OF THESE SAME NAMES IN RELATIONAL STATEMENTS. THE USE OF SWITCHED NAMES AS LABELS WAS ALSO SUPERIOR IN THE BILINGUALS, BUT THE KNOWLEDGE OF NAMES AND FACILITY FOR ACQUIRING NEW NAMES WAS EQUIVALENT IN BOTH GROUPS. IT IS SUGGESTED THAT YOUNG CHILDREN FIRST REGARD NAMES AS ATTRIBUTES OF THINGS THEY LABEL. LATER CHILDREN LEARN THAT NAMES REFER TO THE THINGS THEY LABEL BECAUSE SOMEONE SO USES THEM. HAVING A NOTION OF MEANING AS A FUNCTION OF USE MIGHT FACILITATE ACQUISITION OF THE ABILITY TO USE LABELS IN SENTENCES, AND IT IS CONCLUDED THAT THIS ABILITY IS GREATEST IN BILINGUAL CHILDREN. 7 REFERENCES.

ACCN   000456

537   AUTH   **FELDT, A. G., & WELLER, R. H.**
      TITL   THE BALANCE OF SOCIAL, ECONOMIC AND DEMOGRAPHIC CHANGE IN PUERTO RICO—1950-1960.
      SRCE   *DEMOGRAPHY, 1965, 2(4), 474-489.*
      INDX   DEMOGRAPHIC, POLITICS, ECONOMIC FACTORS, PUERTO RICAN-I, SOCIAL STRUCTURE, EMPIRICAL, MIGRATION, EMPLOYMENT, THEORETICAL, LABOR FORCE, FERTILITY, PHYSICIANS
      ABST   SOME RECENT STUDIES HAVE UTILIZED THE CONCEPTS OF BALANCE AND EQUILIBRIUM FOR INTERPRETING THE SOCIAL CHANGE THAT IS OBSERVED IN THE WAY SOCIETIES DEVELOP. THE VALIDITY OF THESE CONCEPTS WAS EXAMINED BY MEASURING CHANGES IN THE CHARACTERISTICS OF PUERTO RICO'S MUNICIPALITIES FROM 1950 TO 1960 AS TO THE FOLLOWING VARIABLES: FERTILITY, POPULATION, EMPLOYMENT RATIOS, DOCTORS PER CAPITA, AND WORK FORCE COMPOSITION. FINDINGS INDICATE THESE MUNICIPALITIES IN 1960 WERE RETURNING TO A HOMEOSTASIS

CONDITION. THIS SUPPORTS THE RESULTS OF PREVIOUS STUDIES REGARDING THE VALIDITY OF THE BALANCE AND DISEQUILIBRUIM CONCEPTS. 10 REFERENCES.

ACCN 000457

538 AUTH **FELICE, L. G.**

TITL MEXICAN AMERICAN SELF-CONCEPT AND EDUCATIONAL ACHIEVEMENT: THE EFFECTS OF ECONOMIC ISOLATION AND SOCIOECONOMIC DEPRIVATION.

SRCE *SOCIAL SCIENCE QUARTERLY, 1973, 53(4), 716-726.*

INDX SELF CONCEPT, SCHOLASTIC ACHIEVEMENT, MEXICAN AMERICAN, EDUCATION, EQUAL OPPORTUNITY, ADOLESCENTS, CROSS CULTURAL, SES, INTEGRATION, DISCRIMINATION, POVERTY, EMPIRICAL, ACHIEVEMENT MOTIVATION, AUTHORITARIANISM, DEMOGRAPHIC, TEXAS, SOUTHWEST

ABST MOST STUDIES IN EVALUATING SELF-CONCEPT AND EDUCATIONAL ACHIEVEMENT NEGLECT TO CONSIDER THE IMPORTANCE OF THE ETHNIC AND SOCIOECONOMIC (SES) COMPOSITION OF THE SCHOOL. THESE FACTORS WERE INCORPORATED IN A LONGITUDINAL PANEL STUDY WHICH EXAMINED EDUCATIONAL ACHIEVEMENT AND DROP OUT RATE AMONG 860 MALE AND FEMALE STUDENTS REGISTERED IN 9TH TO 12TH GRADE IN THE WACO, TEXAS, SCHOOL SYSTEM. THE RESULTS INDICATED THAT FOR MEXICAN AMERICANS EDUCATIONAL ACHIEVEMENT WAS SIGNIFICANTLY INFLUENCED BY SELF-CONCEPT AND THE SCHOOL'S RACIAL-ETHNIC COMPOSITION. IT WAS ALSO NOTED BY EXAMINING THE SCHOOL'S ETHNIC COMPOSITION THAT WHILE SEGREGATED SCHOOLS PROMOTE HIGHER ACHIEVEMENT FOR ANGLOS, THE OPPOSITE EFFECTS HOLD FOR BLACKS AND MEXICAN AMERICANS. IN EVALUATING A SCHOOL SYSTEM'S IMPACT ON MEXICAN AMERICANS, RESEARCHERS ALSO NEED TO TAKE INTO ACCOUNT THE DEGREE OF SOCIAL ISOLATION AND ECONOMIC LEVEL OF THE MEXICAN AMERICAN POPULATION WITH RESPECT TO THE GEOGRAPHICAL REGION UNDER INVESTIGATION. 28 REFERENCES.

ACCN 000458

539 AUTH **FELICE, L. G., & RICHARDSON, R. L.**

TITL THE EFFECTS OF BUSING AND SCHOOL DESEGREGATION ON MAJORITY AND MINORITY STUDENT DROPOUT RATES.

SRCE *JOURNAL OF EDUCATIONAL RESEARCH, 1977, 70(5), 242-246.*

INDX ADOLESCENTS, CROSS CULTURAL, EDUCATION, EMPIRICAL, INTEGRATION, MEXICAN AMERICAN, PERFORMANCE EXPECTATIONS, POLICY, SCHOLASTIC ASPIRATIONS, SOUTHWEST, TEACHERS, SCHOLASTIC ACHIEVEMENT

ABST THE EFFECTS OF SCHOOL DESEGREGATION BY COURT ORDERED BUSING ON THE SUBSEQUENT DROPOUT RATES OF MAJORITY AND MINORITY STUDENTS WERE STUDIED IN A SOUTHWESTERN COMMUNITY WITH A POPULATION WHICH IS APPROXIMATELY 65% ANGLO, 20% BLACK, AND 15% MEXICAN AMERI-CAN. USING BEFORE AND AFTER BUSING MEASURES OF DROPOUT RATES, SCHOOL RECORDS AND PERSONAL INTERVIEWS, THIS RESEARCH FOUND THAT MAJORITY 12TH GRADE DROPOUT RATES WERE NOT AFFECTED BY DESEGREGATION PROCEDURES. WHILE THE DROPOUT RATES OF BUSED MINORITY STUDENTS APPEARED TO BE IDENTICAL TO THOSE OF NONBUSED MINORITY STUDENTS, LARGE DISPARITIES BETWEEN MINORITY RATES IN VARIOUS BUSED SECTORS INDICATE HIGHLY UNEVEN EDUCATIONAL EXPERIENCES OF BUSED MINORITY STUDENTS. SCHOOL SOCIOECONOMIC COMPOSITION AND THE EXPECTATIONS OF TEACHERS CONCERNING STUDENT BEHAVIOR WERE USED TO ANALYZE THE DISPARITIES, WITH THE CONCLUSION THAT THE MORE FAVORABLE EXPECTATIONS OF TEACHERS AT HIGHER SOCIOECONOMIC CLIMATE SCHOOLS PRODUCE LOWER MINORITY STUDENT DROPOUT RATES. DESEGREGATION PRODUCES A POSITIVE BENEFIT FOR THIS MOST CRUCIAL DIMENSION OF MINORITY STUDENT EDUCATIONAL ACCOMPLISHMENT WHEN THE SCHOOL TO WHICH THE MINORITY STUDENT IS BUSED IS ONE WHERE TEACHERS' EXPECTATIONS ARE POSITIVE AND SUPPORTIVE. 7 REFERENCES. (NCHHI ABSTRACT)

ACCN 002077

540 AUTH **FERGUSON, G. D.**

TITL MOTHER-CHILD INTERACTIONS AS PREDICTORS OF SCHOOL BEHAVIOR (DOCTORAL DISSERTATION, UNIVERSITY OF CALIFORNIA, LOS ANGELES, 1971).

SRCE *DISSERTATION ABSTRACTS INTERNATIONAL, 1971, 31(8), 4034A. (UNIVERSITY MICROFILMS NO.71-04,869.)*

INDX MOTHER-CHILD INTERACTION, SCHOLASTIC ACHIEVEMENT, SOCIALIZATION, EMPIRICAL, CHILDREN, TEACHERS, PERFORMANCE EXPECTATIONS, PERSONALITY, CALIFORNIA, SOUTHWEST, EARLY CHILDHOOD EDUCATION

ABST THIRTY-TWO MOTHER-CHILD PAIRS FROM THE MEXICAN AMERICAN HEADSTART POVERTY POPULATION OF EAST LOS ANGELES WERE STUDIED IN ORDER TO ANALYZE THE RELATIONSHIP BETWEEN EMPATHETIC AND CONTROLLED MOTHER-CHILD INTERACTIONS AND TEACHER PREDICTIONS OF CHILDREN'S SCHOOL SUCCESS AND COPING BEHAVIORS. MULTIPLE STEPWISE REGRESSION ANALYSIS AND AN ANALYSIS OF VALIDATION BY A MULTI-TRAIT (EMPATHY AND CONTROL) MULTI-METHOD (PARENT AND TEACHER INTERVIEW, QUESTIONNAIRE AND OBSERVATION) MATRIX WERE USED IN TREATING THE DATA. FINDINGS INDICATE THAT IT IS POSSIBLE TO PREDICT CHILDREN'S SCHOOL BEHAVIOR FROM MOTHER-CHILD INTERACTION VARIABLES, BUT SCORES OBTAINED ARE INFLUENCED TO A GREAT DEGREE BY THE METHOD USED TO GATHER THE DATA. FINDINGS SUPPORTED THE HYPOTHESES THAT MOTHERS WHO SHOW A HIGH DEGREE OF EMPATHY, OR THE ABILITY TO SHARE AND ACCEPT THE CHILDS' FEELINGS, HAVE CHILDREN WHO, IN SCHOOL, ARE ABLE TO WORK IN GROUPS, SHARE, GET APPROPRI-

ATE HELP, AND ENGAGE IN PRODUCTIVE BE-
HAVIOR. ON THE OTHER HAND, THOSE MOTH-
ERS WHO TEND TO BE CRITICAL OR WITH-
DRAWN OR OPENLY REJECTING TEND TO HAVE
CHILDREN WHO ARE AGGRESSIVE, ENGAGE IN
NEGATIVE ATTENTION GETTING, OR ARE PAS-
SIVE OR WITHDRAWN. THE IMPLICATIONS OF
THESE FINDINGS, TO THE ROLE HEADSTART
PROGRAMS PLAY IN PREPARING MEXICAN
AMERICAN CHILDREN FOR SCHOOL ARE DIS-
CUSSED. 52 REFERENCES. (AUTHOR AB-
STRACT MODIFIED)

ACCN   000459

541 AUTH **FERNANDEZ-MARINA, R.**
     TITL THE PUERTO RICAN SYNDROME: ITS DYNAMIC
           AND CULTURAL DETERMINANTS.
     SRCE *PSYCHIATRY, 1961, 24(1), 79-82.*
     INDX PUERTO RICAN-I, ANXIETY, CULTURAL FAC-
           TORS, PSYCHOPATHOLOGY, SCHIZOPHRENIA,
           ESSAY, CHILDREARING PRACTICES, SYMP-
           TOMATOLOGY, VETERANS
     ABST CERTAIN BIZARRE PATTERNS, USUALLY PSY-
           CHOGENIC IN ORIGIN, SEEM TO BE IDENTIFIED
           AS "THE PUERTO RICAN SYNDROME BY MANY
           AMERICAN MEDICAL OFFICERS AND PSYCHIA-
           TRISTS. MANY PATIENTS TRANSFERRED FROM
           VA HOSPITALS TO THE PUERTO RICO INSTI-
           TUTE OF PSYCHIATRY HAD BEEN DIAGNOSED
           AS CASES OF ANXIETY OR CONVERSION RE-
           ACTION AND ASSUMED TO EXHIBIT THE PUERTO
           RICAN SYNDROME. SUFFICIENT EVIDENCE IS
           PRESENTED TO INDICATE THAT HYSTERICAL
           ATTACKS CAN ALSO FUNCTION AS EGO DE-
           FENSES AGAINST PSYCHOTIC BREAKS OR AS
           LIMITS TO EXTREME REGRESSION OR TOTAL
           DISORGANIZATION OF THE EGO. ENGLISH-
           SPEAKING U.S. ARMY PSYCHIATRISTS SEEMED
           TO HAVE FOUND A DECISIVE CLASSICAL SYMP-
           TOM AND NEGLECTED FURTHER INVESTIGA-
           TION. PUERTO RICAN CHILD-REARING PRAC-
           TICES THAT WOULD EXPLAIN THE PUERTO
           RICAN SYNDROME AND THE ABSENCE OF
           REGRESSION IN PUERTO RICAN SCHIZO-
           PHRENICS ARE DISCUSSED. 12 REFERENCES.

ACCN   000460

542 AUTH **FERNANDEZ-MARINA, R., MALDONADO-
           SIERRA, E. D., & TRENT, R. D.**
     TITL THREE BASIC THEMES IN MEXICAN AND PUERTO
           RICAN FAMILY VALUES.
     SRCE *JOURNAL OF SOCIAL PSYCHOLOGY, 1958, 48(1),
           167-181.*
     INDX FAMILY ROLES, AUTHORITARIANISM, FAMILY
           STRUCTURE, ADOLESCENTS, SEX ROLES, EM-
           PIRICAL, CROSS CULTURAL, CULTURE, SEX
           COMPARISON, MARRIAGE, CULTURAL CHANGE,
           MEXICAN, PUERTO RICAN-I, VALUES
     ABST AN INVESTIGATION OF THREE BASIC THEMES
           IN FAMILY VALUES IS PRESENTED. THE THEMES
           ARE FAMILY AFFECTIONAL PATTERNS, AU-
           THORITY PATTERNS, AND DIFFERENTIAL
           EVALUATION OF MALE AND FEMALE STATUS.
           THE PURPOSE OF THIS STUDY WAS TO DETER-
           MINE THE EXTENT TO WHICH FAMILY VALUES IN
           PUERTO RICO HAVE CHANGED FROM THOSE
           OF OTHER LATIN AMERICANS TO THOSE OF
           THE MAINLAND U.S. THE SUBJECTS, 494

PUERTO RICAN UNMARRIED HIGH SCHOOL
GRADUATES, WERE ADMINISTERED AN ADAP-
TATION AND EXTENSION OF A QUESTIONNAIRE
IN SPANISH DEVELOPED BY DIAZ-GUERRERO
TO SURVEY MEXICAN FAMILY VALUES. THE MA-
JOR RESULTS OF THE SURVEY INDICATED THE
FOLLOWING: (1) THE PUERTO RICAN MOTHER
APPEARS TO BE HELD IN HIGHER AFFEC-
TIONAL ESTEEM THAN DOES THE PUERTO RI-
CAN FATHER; (2) PUERTO RICANS STILL TEND
TO HOLD THE CONCEPT OF MALE SUPERIOR-
ITY AND DOMINANCE IN THE FAMILY AS IS
FOUND IN OTHER LATIN AMERICAN COUN-
TRIES; (3) IN PUERTO RICO THE MALE CHILD IS
ACCORDED GREATER STATUS THAN THE FE-
MALE CHILD; (4) THE CHARACTERISTICS UN-
DERLYING THE MIDDLE-CLASS PUERTO RICAN
FAMILY AT PRESENT TEND TO BE DISTINCTLY
MORE SIMILAR TO THOSE OF THE MEXICAN
THAN THOSE OF THE MAINLAND AMERICAN;
(5) THE CONFLICT OF LATIN AND AMERICAN
FAMILY VALUES IN PUERTO RICO INDICATES A
PROCESS OF CHANGE TOWARD AMERICANI-
ZATION OF BELIEFS; AND (6) IT WAS PRO-
POSED THAT THE POOR DEFINITION OF THE
MALE'S AUTHORITY AND INCREASING IMPOR-
TANCE OF THE ROLE OF WOMEN IN PUERTO
RICO THREATENS THE UNIQUE AUTHORITY OF
THE MALE THAT IS PROCLAIMED IN LATIN CUL-
TURES. DISCUSSION OF THE IMPLICATIONS OF
THE CHANGING VALUES AND THE EFFECT ON
MALE AND FEMALE ROLES IS PRESENTED. 29
REFERENCES.

ACCN   000461

543 AUTH **FERNANDEZ-MARINA, R., & VON ECKARDT, U.
           M.**
     TITL CULTURAL STRESSES AND SCHIZOPHRENO-
           GENESIS IN THE MOTHERING-ONE IN PUERTO
           RICO.
     SRCE *ANNALS OF THE NEW YORK ACADEMY OF SCI-
           ENCE, 1960, 84(17), 864-877.*
     INDX SCHIZOPHRENIA, PUERTO RICAN-I, MOTHER-
           CHILD INTERACTION, CULTURAL FACTORS,
           PSYCHOPATHOLOGY, THEORETICAL, COPING
           MECHANISMS, PSYCHOSOCIAL ADJUSTMENT,
           FEMALE
     ABST THE BIOLOGICAL, PSYCHOLOGICAL, AND SO-
           CIOLOGICAL FACTORS WHICH PREDISPOSE A
           MOTHER IN PUERTO RICO TOWARDS SCHIZO-
           PHRENOGENESIS ARE SPECIFIED IN A MATHE-
           MATICAL METALANGUAGE OF PROPOSITIONS
           AND RELATIONAL AXIOMS. IN THIS ANALYSIS
           THE INTENT IS TO FORMULATE THE DYNAMICS
           OF HUMAN INTERACTIONS OF THE PHENOME-
           NON OF SCHIZOPHRENOGENESIS WITH THE
           CLARITY AND PRECISION MADE POSSIBLE BY
           MATHEMATICALLY STRUCTURED STATEMENTS.
           CLINICAL EXPERIENCE IN PUERTO RICO RE-
           VEALS THE FOLLOWING CULTURAL FACTORS
           IN THE FAMILIES OF SCHIZOPHRENICS. (1) THE
           MOTHERING-ONE HAS A DEFORMED EGO BE-
           CAUSE SHE IS THE DAUGHTER OF A NARCIS-
           SISTIC AND SEDUCTIVE WOMAN AND AN ALOOF
           AND RIGID FATHER WHOSE STRONG SENSE OF
           MORALITY KEPT HIM IN THE HOME AND EN-
           COURAGED HIM TO PROTECT HIS WIFE. THE
           EGO DEFORMATIONS OF THE MOTHERING-ONE

SHADOW THOSE OF HER NARCISSISTIC MOTHER. (2) THE MOTHERING-ONE IS MARRIED TO A WEAK AND INEFFECTUAL MAN WHO THREATENS HER, AT THE MOMENT OF THE INFANT'S BIRTH, WITH LOSS OF LOVE AND LOSS OF PRESTIGE. THIS THREAT CONSTITUTES A SPECIFIC STRESS THAT BREAKS DOWN THE DEFORMED EGO OF THE MOTHERING-ONE. IT IS CONCLUDED THAT DIFFERENT PATTERNS OF SCHIZOPHRENOGENESIS MAY EXIST IN OTHER CULTURES. 13 REFERENCES.

ACCN   000462

544 AUTH   **FERRACUTI, F.**
TITL   LA DELINCUENCIA JUVENIL Y LOS CAMBIOS SOCIALES DE PUERTO RICO. (JUVENILE DELINQUENCY AND THE SOCIAL CHANGES OF PUERTO RICO.)
SRCE   *IN J. A. ROSSELLO (ED.), MANUAL DE PSIQUIATRIA SOCIAL. SPAIN: INDUSTRIAS GRAFICAS "DIARIO-DIA," 1968, PP. 565-571. (SPANISH)*
INDX   PUERTO RICAN-I, ESSAY, DELINQUENCY, CULTURAL CHANGE, URBAN, ADOLESCENTS, DEMOGRAPHIC
ABST   THE IMMIGRATION, URBANIZATION, AND AMERICANIZATION THAT PUERTO RICO HAS SEEN IN RECENT YEARS HAVE SUBJECTED THE ISLAND TO MANY OF THE SOCIAL PROBLEMS THAT ACCOMPANY RAPID SOCIAL CHANGE. ONE SUCH PROBLEM IS JUVENILE DELINQUENCY. BECAUSE ONLY 5.8% OF THE TOTAL POPULATION IS OVER 65 WHILE 48.1% AVERAGES 19 YEARS OF AGE, THIS PROBLEM IS OF PARTICULAR IMPORTANCE. BETWEEN 1956 AND 1963, THE NUMBER OF ARRESTS IN CASES REGARDING JUVENILE DELINQUENTS INCREASED BY 600, WITH 15,070 POLICE INTERVENTIONS IN 1963. MOST YOUTHFUL LAWBREAKERS FIRST ENCOUNTER PROBLEMS WITH THE POLICE DURING THE PRE-PUBERTY AND PUBERTY YEARS. MOREOVER, THEY USUALLY COME FROM RECENTLY URBANIZED FAMILIES—THOSE WHO MOST DIRECTLY SUFFER THE PROBLEMS BROUGHT ABOUT BY RAPID SOCIAL CHANGE. IT IS ALSO SHOWN THAT APPROXIMATELY 50% OF ALL PUERTO RICAN JUVENILE DELINQUENTS HAVE DEFECTS IN EITHER MENTAL ABILITY OR PERSONALITY WHICH ARE AGGRAVATED BY SOCIAL CONDITIONS. AS PREVENTION IS CONSIDERED TO BE MORE SOCIALLY AND ECONOMICALLY BENEFICIAL IN THE LONG RUN, IT IS SUGGESTED THAT A PLAN OF PREVENTION AGAINST JUVENILE DELINQUENCY BE INITIATED WHICH WOULD ENCOMPASS BOTH THE MASS MEDIA AND PUBLIC HEALTH AGENCIES. 19 REFERENCES.

ACCN   002271

545 AUTH   **FIELD, P. B., MALDONADO-SIERRA, E. D., WALLACE, S. E., BODARKY, C. J., & COEHLO, G. V.**
TITL   AN OTHER-DIRECTED FANTASY IN A PUERTO RICAN.
SRCE   *JOURNAL OF SOCIAL PSYCHOLOGY, 1962, 58, 43-60.*
INDX   ADOLESCENTS, PROJECTIVE TESTING, INTERPERSONAL RELATIONS, PUERTO RICAN-I, CULTURE, IMAGERY, AUTHORITARIANISM, AGGRESSION, CASE STUDY, FAMILY STRUCTURE, SEX ROLES, PEER GROUP, FATHER-CHILD INTERACTION, COLLEGE STUDENTS, MALE
ABST   AN ATTEMPT TO RELATE A PUERTO RICAN'S ACCEPTANCE OF AN OTHER-DIRECTED PEER GROUP INFLUENCE WITH HIS CULTURAL PATTERNS AND HIS PSYCHODYNAMICS IS ILLUSTRATED BY MEANS OF HIS PROJECTIVE FANTASIES. THIS CASE REPORT PRESENTS SOME OF THE PSYCHODYNAMIC MATERIAL OBTAINED THROUGH INTERVIEWS AND THE THEMATIC APPERCEPTION TEST (TAT). THE TAT STORIES WERE OBTAINED TWICE, ONCE DURING THE SENIOR YEAR OF HIGH SCHOOL AND ONCE DURING THE FRESHMAN YEAR IN COLLEGE. THE ANALYSIS WAS RELATED TO PUERTO RICAN CULTURAL THEMES WHICH INCLUDED FAMILISM, THE EXAGGERATED MASCULINE ROLE PRESCRIBED FOR MALES, AND THE PREFERENTIAL TREATMENT GIVEN THE OLDEST SON IN THE FAMILY. ALTHOUGH THERE IS A MULTIPLE DETERMINATION OF THE STUDENT'S OTHER-DIRECTED PEER GROUP DEPENDENCY, ONE MAJOR DETERMINING FACTOR IN HIS DEPENDENCY IS AN UNREWARDING, DISTANT RELATIONSHIP TO HIS FAMILY. THUS HE IS LED TO A SEARCH FOR COMPENSATING PERSONAL RELATIONSHIPS WITH OTHER SOCIAL GROUPS. THIS STUDENT'S UNSATISFYING FORMAL, HIERARCHICAL, AND IMPERSONAL FAMILY RELATIONSHIPS LEAD HIM TO SEEK INSTEAD THE INFORMAL, PERSONAL, LOOSELY ORGANIZED RELATIONSHIPS OF A PEER GROUP. HE TRIES TO ACHIEVE SUCCESS THROUGH DEPENDENCY, CONFORMITY, OBEDIENCE, AND CONCILIATION RATHER THAN THROUGH INDEPENDENT SELF-ASSERTION. 16 REFERENCES.

ACCN   000463

546 AUTH   **FIELD, P. B., MALDONADO-SIERRA, E. D., & COHELO, G. V.**
TITL   A STUDENT-TAT MEASURE OF COMPETENCE: A CROSS CULTURAL REPLICATION IN PUERTO RICO.
SRCE   *PERCEPTUAL AND MOTOR SKILLS, 1963, 16, 195-198.*
INDX   PROJECTIVE TESTING, ADOLESCENTS, PUERTO RICAN-I, TEST RELIABILITY, EMPIRICAL, CULTURAL FACTORS, COPING MECHANISMS, MENTAL HEALTH, COLLEGE STUDENTS, TAT
ABST   A SUCCESSFUL CROSS-CULTURAL REPLICATION OF A STUDENT-TAT STUDY OF ADOLESCENT COMPETENCE IN AMERICAN COLLEGE FRESHMEN WAS CONDUCTED WITH A PUERTO RICAN SAMPLE. THREE GROUPS OF PUERTO RICAN ADOLESCENTS WERE SCREENED INDEPENDENTLY TO PROVIDE SAMPLES COMPARABLE TO THOSE USED IN AN NIMH STUDY OF COMPETENT ADOLESCENT STUDENTS. STUDENT-TAT RESULTS SHOWED THAT FANTASIES OF ACTIVE MASTERY, DIRECTED STRIVING, AND OPTIMISM WERE MOST PROMINENT IN A HIGHLY COMPETENT GROUP OF PUERTO RICAN STUDENTS SELECTED FOR SUPERIOR ACADEMIC, SOCIAL, AND EXTRACURRICULAR ABILITIES, AND WERE LEAST PROMINENT IN A GROUP OF EMOTIONALLY DISTURBED COLLEGE STUDENTS. THIS RESULT CONFIRMS PREVIOUS

FINDINGS WITH AMERICAN STUDENTS. 8 REFERENCES.

ACCN 000464

---

547 AUTH **FIELDER, W. R., COHEN, R. D., & FEENEY, S.**
TITL AN ATTEMPT TO REPLICATE THE TEACHER EXPECTANCY EFFECT.
SRCE *PSYCHOLOGICAL REPORTS, 1971, 29(3), 1223-1228.*
INDX EDUCATION, PERFORMANCE EXPECTATIONS, TEACHERS, INTELLIGENCE, CHILDREN, EMPIRICAL, MEXICAN AMERICAN, CROSS CULTURAL, PERFORMANCE EXPECTATIONS, INTELLIGENCE TESTING, CALIFORNIA, SOUTHWEST
ABST THE DEMONSTRATION OF SIGNIFICANT TEACHER EXPECTANCY EFFECTS IN ONE SCHOOL SEMESTER AND THE DETERMINATION OF GRADE LEVEL, SEX, MINORITY GROUP MEMBERSHIP, OR SOCIAL CLASS IN RELATION TO THE EXPECTANCY EFFECT ARE INVESTIGATED. A SAMPLE OF 796 SUBJECTS IN 36 CLASSES FROM THREE ELEMENTARY SCHOOLS (GRADES ONE TO SIX) WERE ADMINISTERED THE TEST OF GENERAL ABILITY. TWO OF THREE SCHOOLS WERE PREDOMINANTLY MEXICAN AMERICAN (MA) AND THE OTHER ANGLO AMERICAN (AA) MIDDLE-CLASS. RESULTS INDICATE THAT NO SIGNIFICANT DIFFERENCES ARE EVIDENT FOR SCHOOLS WITH A PREDOMINANT MA POPULATION AND AN AA POPULATION. THERE ARE NO SIGNIFICANT DIFFERENCES IN TERMS OF THE "EXPECTANCY ADVANTAGE" OF THE MA GROUP AS MEASURED BY IQ GAIN P<.05 NOR ARE THERE ANY DISCERNIBLE POSITIVE OR NEGATIVE OVERALL TRENDS. IT IS SUGGESTED THAT PERHAPS EXPECTANCY EFFECTS DO NOT CONSISTENTLY APPEAR IN AS SHORT A PERIOD OF TIME AS ONE SEMESTER. IN CONCLUSION, THE FINDINGS APPEAR TO AGREE WITH BARBER'S (1969) STATEMENT THAT THE EXPECTANCY EFFECT IS NOT AS PERVASIVE AS SUGGESTED IN ROSENTHAL AND JACOBSON'S (1966) ORIGINAL STUDY. 7 REFERENCES.

ACCN 000465

---

548 AUTH **FIELDS, S.**
TITL FOLK HEALING FOR THE WOUNDED SPIRIT. I. STOREFRONT PSYCHOTHERAPY THROUGH SEANCE.
SRCE *INNOVATIONS, 1976, 3(1), 3-11.*
INDX FOLK MEDICINE, PUERTO RICAN-M, PROGRAM EVALUATION, CASE STUDY, ESSAY, ESPIRITISMO, MENTAL HEALTH, CULTURAL FACTORS, PSYCHOTHERAPY, COMMUNITY, NEW YORK, EAST
ABST THE OUTCOME OF A MENTAL HEALTH RESEARCH PROJECT IN NEW YORK CITY WHICH COMBINED THE TECHNIQUES OF PUERTO RICAN FOLK HEALERS WITH THOSE OF MENTAL HEALTH PROFESSIONALS IN COMMUNITY CENTERS IS DISCUSSED. THE PROJECT IS DESCRIBED IN STAGES: (1) FINDING OUT HOW THE COMMUNITY LOOKED AFTER ITSELF WITHOUT THE PROFESSIONALS, (2) LOCATING THE SITES WHERE FOLK HEALING WAS PRACTICED; (3) COMPARING THE NATURE OF COMMUNITY

MENTAL HEALTH CENTER PATIENTS' COMPLAINTS WITH THOSE OF THE FOLK HEALERS' PATIENTS; (4) INTERPRETING THE FOLK HEALERS' TREATMENT METHODS WITH PSYCHOTHERAPY; AND (5) DEFINING THE ADVANTAGES OF INTEGRATING TRADITIONAL AND NONTRADITIONAL METHODS OF MENTAL HEALTH TREATMENTS. A CASE REPORT AND DETAILED OBSERVATIONS OF SPIRITIST TREATMENT METHODS ARE INCLUDED. 2 REFERENCES.

ACCN 000466

---

549 AUTH **FIELDS, S.**
TITL PRIDE BEYOND THE BARRIOS.
SRCE *INNOVATIONS, 1975, 2(1), 3-11.*
INDX ESSAY, PARAPROFESSIONALS, COMMUNITY, URBAN, ADOLESCENTS, DELINQUENCY, SOCIAL SERVICES, PROFESSIONAL TRAINING, NEW MEXICO, SOUTHWEST
ABST BUILT ON THE PHILOSOPHY THAT CHICANOS CAN DEVELOP THE SKILLS NEEDED TO SOLVE THEIR OWN PROBLEMS AND THAT COMMUNITY PEOPLE MAKE BETTER MANAGERS THAN OUTSIDERS FOR COMMUNITY PROGRAMS, THE SANTA FE, NEW MEXICO, ORGANIZATION COPAS (CORPORACION ORGANIZADA PARA ACCION Y SERVIDORA) PROVIDES SERVICES TO DELINQUENT CHILDREN THROUGH ITS CHILD ADVOCACY PROGRAM. SEVERAL ASPECTS OF THE PROGRAM ARE DISCUSSED: (1) FUNDING AS A RESEARCH AND DEMONSTRATION PROJECT UNDER THE NATIONAL INSTITUTE OF MENTAL HEALTH; (2) TREATMENT PHILOSOPHY; (3) TRAINING CHICANO CHILD ADVOCATES; (4) COMMUNITY CONTACTS AND BOARD MEMBERS; AND (5) CORPORATE STRUCTURE AND FINANCIAL INDEPENDENCE. THE ORGANIZATION'S PROGRESS, SUCCESSES AND PROBLEMS ARE IDENTIFIED AND DISCUSSED.

ACCN 000467

---

550 AUTH **FIEVE, R.**
TITL PSYCHOPHARMACOLOGY HERE AND ABROAD: DIFFERENCES IN SIDE EFFECTS. A SUMMARY OF A PANEL DISCUSSION.
SRCE *IN E. R. PADILLA & A. M. PADILLA (EDS.), TRANSCULTURAL PSYCHIATRY: AN HISPANIC PERSPECTIVE (MONOGRAPH NO. 4). LOS ANGELES: UNIVERSITY OF CALIFORNIA, SPANISH SPEAKING MENTAL HEALTH RESEARCH CENTER, 1977, PP. 93-95.*
INDX PSYCHOPHARMACOLOGY, PSYCHOTHERAPY OUTCOME, CROSS CULTURAL, ESSAY, PROCEEDINGS, PUERTO RICAN-I
ABST PANELISTS AND PSYCHIATRISTS PARTICIPATING IN A JOINT MEETING OF THE PUERTO RICAN MEDICAL ASSOCIATION, THE CARIBBEAN PSYCHIATRIC ASSOCIATION, AND THE AMERICAN PSYCHIATRIC ASSOCIATION DISCUSSED WHETHER DIFFERENCES EXIST BETWEEN CULTURES IN PHARMACOLOGICAL, BEHAVIORAL AND PSYCHOLOGICAL ACTIONS OF THE FOLLOWING DRUGS: MAJOR AND MINOR TRANQUILIZERS, TRICYCLIC ANTIDEPRESSANTS, MAO INHIBITORS, LITHIUM, AND HYPNOTICS. THE PANEL WAS UNABLE TO DISCERN ANY MAJOR DIFFERENCES WITH RESPECT TO THE ACTION OF ANY OF THE DRUGS. HOWEVER, MINOR DIF-

FERENCES WERE DESCRIBED IN PHOTOSENSITIVITY, DISCLOSURE OF IMPOTENCE, WEIGHT GAIN, INTOLERANCE TO ANTICHOLINERGIC SYMPTOMS IN THE CARIBBEAN AT COMPARABLE DOSES OF THE SAME COMPOUND USED IN THE U.S. IN ADDITION, INCREASED LIKELIHOOD OF MILD LITHIUM SIDE EFFECTS IN TROPICAL AS COMPARED TO NORTHERN CLIMATES WAS DISCUSSED. THESE DIFFERENCES WERE DRAWN FROM THE PERSONAL EXPERIENCE OF THE PARTICIPANTS. TO VALIDATE CROSS-CULTURAL DIFFERENCES AND SIDE EFFECTS MORE PRECISE SCIENTIFIC STUDY IS REQUIRED.

ACCN   000468

551 AUTH   **FIGUEROA-TORRES, J., & PEARSON, R. E.**

TITL   EFFECTS OF STRUCTURED LEARNING THERAPY UPON SELF-CONTROL OF AGGRESSIVE PUERTO RICAN FATHERS.

SRCE   *HISPANIC JOURNAL OF BEHAVIORAL SCIENCES, 1979, 1(4), 345-354.*

INDX   AGGRESSION, MALE, PUERTO RICAN-I, BEHAVIOR THERAPY, EMPIRICAL, FAMILY ROLES, TAT, CULTURAL FACTORS

ABST   TO ASSESS THE EFFECTIVENESS OF STRUCTURED LEARNING THERAPY (SLT) FOR REDUCING FAMILY-DIRECTED AGGRESSION, 60 LOW-SES PUERTO RICAN FATHERS IN SAN JUAN WHO HAD DOCUMENTED HISTORIES OF SUCH AGGRESSION WERE STUDIED. THE COMPONENTS OF SLT ARE ROLE PLAYING, MODELING, SOCIAL REINFORCEMENT, AND TRANSFER OF TRAINING; THE OBJECTIVE IS TO REPLACE UNDESIRABLE WITH DESIRABLE BEHAVIOR. THE SUBJECTS WERE RANDOMLY ASSIGNED TO EXPERIMENTAL (SLT) AND CONTROL (NSLT) GROUPS. ON A PRE- AND POSTTEST BASIS, ALL SUBJECTS WERE ADMINISTERED THE FOLLOWING INSTRUMENTS: (1) BEHAVIORAL CHECKLIST; (2) THEMATIC APPERCEPTION TEST (TAT); (3) DIRECT SKILL MEASURE; (4) MINIMAL GENERALIZATION-OF-SKILL MEASURE; (5) EXTENDED GENERATIONALIZATION-OF-SKILL MEASURE; AND (6) BUSS-DURKEE INVENTORY. THE RESULTS DEMONSTRATED THAT SLT PRODUCED A SIGNIFICANT DIFFERENCE IN AGGRESSION ON THREE OF THE DEPENDENT VARIABLES—THE TAT, MINIMAL GENERALIZATION-OF-SKILL MEASURE, AND DIRECT SKILL MEASURE. NO SUCH REDUCTIONS WERE NOTED FOR THE CONTROL GROUP. INITIAL GROUP DIFFERENCES ON THE BUSS-DURKEE AND BEHAVIORAL CHECKLIST INSTRUMENTS NEGATED THE ASSUMPTION OF EQUIVALENCE ON THESE INSTRUMENTS AND PRECLUDED FURTHER INTERPRETATIONS OF RESULTS BASED ON THEM. NO DIFFERENCES WERE FOUND BETWEEN GROUPS ON THE EXTENDED GENERALIZATION-OF-SKILL MEASURE. WHILE THE GENERAL EFFECTIVENESS OF SLT AS A MEANS OF REDUCING AGGRESSION AMONG THIS POPULATION WAS GENERALLY SUSTAINED, THE SUGGESTION IS MADE THAT IT SHOULD BE USED IN CONJUNCTION WITH OTHER, BROADER APPROACHES AIMED AT AMELIORATING CULTURAL SUPPORT FOR MALE

AGGRESSION IN THE FAMILY CONTEXT. 30 REFERENCES. (JOURNAL ABSTRACT MODIFIED)

ACCN   001764

552 AUTH   **FISCHER, G.**

TITL   THE PERFORMANCE OF MALE PRISONERS ON THE MARLOWE-CROWNE SOCIAL DESIRABILITY SCALE: II. DIFFERENCES AS A FUNCTION OF RACE AND CRIME.

SRCE   *JOURNAL OF CLINICAL PSYCHOLOGY, 1967, 23(4), 473-475.*

INDX   PERSONALITY ASSESSMENT, CRIMINOLOGY, MALE, CROSS CULTURAL, MEXICAN AMERICAN, SCHOLASTIC ACHIEVEMENT, INTELLIGENCE, MMPI, ARMY GENERAL CLASSIFICATION TEST, CALIFORNIA ACHIEVEMENT TESTS, EMPIRICAL, CALIFORNIA, SOUTHWEST

ABST   THE RELATIONSHIP BETWEEN RACE, CRIMINAL OFFENSE, AGE, INTELLIGENCE, EDUCATIONAL ACHIEVEMENT LEVEL, 13 SCALES OF THE MINNESOTA MULTIPHASIC PERSONALITY INVENTORY (MMPI), AND THE MARLOWE-CROWNE SOCIAL DESIRABILITY SCALE (M-C) SCORE OF 782 MALE PRISONERS IS PRESENTED. A SAMPLE CONSISTING OF 492 WHITE, 108 MEXICAN AMERICAN (MA) AND 182 NEGRO MALE INMATES WAS GIVEN THE MMPI. THE M-C WAS GIVEN AS PART OF A LARGER TEST BATTERY. INTELLIGENCE WAS ASSESSED BY THE ARMY GENERAL CLASSIFICATION TEST (AGCT) AND EDUCATIONAL ACHIEVEMENT BY THE CALIFORNIA ACHIEVEMENT TESTS. THE DATA INDICATE THAT INTELLIGENCE AND EDUCATIONAL ACHIEVEMENT LEVEL ARE NEGATIVELY CORRELATED WITH THE M-C. MA'S AND NEGROES SCORED SIGNIFICANTLY HIGHER THAN WHITES ON THE MC, EVEN WHEN IQ DIFFERENCES WERE CONTROLLED. THREE MMPI VALIDITY SCALES CORRELATE WITH THE M-C. INTERPRETING THE M-C AS A MEASURE OF DEFENSIVENESS, CRIMINALS APPEAR TO BE MORE DEFENSIVE THAN NONCRIMINALS. NEGRO AND MEXICAN AMERICAN CRIMINALS ARE APPARENTLY EQUALLY DEFENSIVE, AND MORE DEFENSIVE THAN WHITE CRIMINALS. 8 REFERENCES.

ACCN   000469

553 AUTH   **FISHER, R. I.**

TITL   A STUDY OF NON-INTELLECTUAL ATTRIBUTES OF CHILDREN IN FIRST GRADE BILINGUAL-BICULTURAL PROGRAM.

SRCE   *JOURNAL OF EDUCATIONAL RESEARCH, 1974, 67(7), 323-328.*

INDX   BILINGUAL-BICULTURAL EDUCATION, CHILDREN, PROGRAM EVALUATION, MEXICAN AMERICAN, SCHOLASTIC ACHIEVEMENT, SELF CONCEPT, EMPIRICAL, SEX COMPARISON, CROSS CULTURAL, SES, COLORADO, SOUTHWEST

ABST   A STUDY OF A FIRST GRADE BILINGUAL-BICULTURAL PROGRAM WAS MADE TO DETERMINE THE EFFECT OF THE PROGRAM ON THREE NON-INTELLECTUAL/ATTRIBUTES OF CHILDREN: (1) SELF-CONCEPT, (2) SELF-DESCRIPTIONS, AND (3) STIMULUS SEEKING ACTIVITY. RESULTS INDICATE THAT THE BILINGUAL-BICULTURAL PROGRAM SIGNIFICANTLY EN-

HANCES THE SELF-CONCEPTS OF GIRLS BUT NOT BOYS. THE PRIMARY EFFECT OF THE PROGRAM ON SELF-DESCRIPTIONS APPEARS TO BE IN PROVIDING A SITUATION WHERE CHICANOS NO LONGER FEEL "PICKED ON" AND WHERE THEIR FEELINGS OF UNHAPPINESS AS EXPRESSED EARLIER IN THE PROGRAM ARE ALLEVIATED. IN TERMS OF CHANGES IN STIMULUS SEEKING ACTIVITY, I.E., OPENNESS TO ENVIRONMENTAL STIMULI, THERE SEEMS AGAIN TO BE A SEX DIFFERENCE WITH GIRLS SHOWING A SIGNIFICANT IMPROVEMENT AND BOYS SHOWING NO SIGNIFICANT CHANGE. THE CONTROL GROUP SHOWED NO SIGNIFICANT CHANGES IN SELF-CONCEPT OR IN STIMULUS SEEKING ACTIVITY FOR EITHER SEX. 8 REFERENCES. (JOURNAL ABSTRACT)

ACCN   000470

554 AUTH   **FISHMAN, J. A.**
     TITL   PUERTO RICAN INTELLECTUALS IN NEW YORK: SOME INTRAGROUP AND INTERGROUP CONTRASTS.
     SRCE   *CANADIAN JOURNAL OF BEHAVIORAL SCIENCE, 1969, 1(4), 215-226.*
     INDX   PUERTO RICAN-M, BILINGUALISM, ETHNIC IDENTITY, EMPIRICAL, SURVEY, ADULTS, NEW YORK, EAST
     ABST   A FACTOR ANALYSIS OF CODED INTERVIEW DATA ON 20 PUERTO RICAN INTELLECTUALS IN THE NEW YORK CITY AREA YIELDED FIVE ITEM-FACTORS (R) AND TWO PERSON-FACTORS (Q). THE R FACTORS DEALT WITH SPANISH LANGUAGE DOMINANCE, IDEOLOGICAL LANGUAGE MAINTENANCE, PUERTO RICAN CULTURAL EMPHASES, AMERICAN AWARENESS, AND SOCIOLINGUISTIC SOPHISTICATION. THE Q GROUPS DIFFERED MEANINGFULLY AND CONSISTENTLY ON THESE FIVE FACTORS AS WELL AS ON DEMOGRAPHIC BACKGROUND VARIABLES, PARTICULARLY WITH RESPECT TO IDEOLOGICAL VERSUS BEHAVIORAL PUERTO RICAN CULTURE AND LANGUAGE MAINTENANCE. IN ADDITION, INTELLECTUALS AS A GROUP WERE FOUND TO DIFFER GREATLY AND SYSTEMATICALLY FROM ORDINARY PUERTO RICAN MALES IN HAVING MORE IDEOLOGICAL POSITIONS WITH RESPECT TO PUERTO RICAN CULTURE AND SPANISH LANGUAGE MAINTENANCE IN NEW YORK. WHEREAS LANGUAGE CONSCIOUSNESS AND LANGUAGE LOYALTY ARE GENERALLY AT A RATHER LOW LEVEL AMONG ORDINARY PUERTO RICANS IN THE NEW YORK CITY AREA, THEY ARE HIGHER AMONG INTELLECTUALS. 9 REFERENCES.
     ACCN   000471

555 AUTH   **FISHMAN, J. A., & COOPER, R. L.**
     TITL   ALTERNATIVE MEASURES OF BILINGUALISM.
     SRCE   *JOURNAL OF VERBAL LEARNING AND VERBAL BEHAVIOR, 1969, 8(2), 276-282.*
     INDX   BILINGUALISM, EMPIRICAL, PUERTO RICAN-M, LINGUISTICS, LANGUAGE COMPREHENSION, RESEARCH METHODOLOGY, LANGUAGE ASSESSMENT, NEW JERSEY, EAST, BILINGUAL
     ABST   A VARIETY OF TECHNIQUES FOR THE MEASUREMENT AND DESCRIPTION OF BILINGUALISM DERIVED SEPARATELY FROM THE DISCI-

PLINES OF LINGUISTICS, PSYCHOLOGY, AND SOCIOLOGY WERE ADMINISTERED TO 48 SPANISH-ENGLISH BILINGUALS. THE INTENT WAS TO ASSESS THE RELATIONSHIP AMONG THESE MEASURES AND TO DETERMINE THEIR RELATIVE UTILITY AS PREDICTORS OF ACCENTEDNESS, ENGLISH REPERTOIRE RANGE, SPANISH REPERTOIRE RANGE, AND READING. A FACTOR ANALYSIS, PERFORMED ON THE INTERCORRELATIONS AMONG 124 SCORES, INDICATES AREAS OF INTERDISCIPLINARY OVERLAP AS WELL AS UNIQUENESS. THE BEST PREDICTORS ARE OBTAINED FROM RETROSPECTIVE REPORTS OF PROFICIENCY AND USAGE. HOWEVER, SCORES FROM OTHER LINGUISTIC, PSYCHOLOGICAL, AND SOCIOLOGICAL MEASUREMENTS OF BILINGUAL BEHAVIOR PROVIDE SIGNIFICANT INCREMENTS IN THE CUMULATIVE PREDICTION OF THE FORM PROFICIENCY CRITERIA—A VERY HIGH PROPORTION OF WHOSE VARIANCE IS EXPLAINED THROUGH MULTIPLE REGRESSION ANALYSIS. 11 REFERENCES.

ACCN   000472

556 AUTH   **FITZ-GERALD, J. D.**
     TITL   THE BILINGUAL-BIRACIAL PROBLEMS OF OUR BORDER STATES.
     SRCE   *HISPANIA, 1921, 4(1), 175-186.*
     INDX   ESSAY, BILINGUALISM, HISTORY, CHILDREN, EDUCATION, LEGISLATION, SPANISH SURNAMED, CROSS CULTURAL, NEW MEXICO, SOUTHWEST
     ABST   THE ADVANTAGES AND DISADVANTAGES OF TWO EUROPEAN SOLUTIONS TO BILINGUAL-BIRACIAL PROBLEMS ARE DISCUSSED WITH REGARD TO THE SPANISH- SPEAKING CHILDREN OF THE SOUTHWESTERN UNITED STATES. IT IS PROPOSED THAT THE FRENCH SYSTEM, IN WHICH CHILDREN ARE TAUGHT ALL CLASSWORK IN THE NATIONAL LANGUAGE BY BILINGUAL TEACHERS, IS MORE ADVANTAGEOUS TO BORDER STATE SCHOOLS THAN IS THE BRITISH METHOD, IN WHICH CHILDREN ARE TAUGHT IN THEIR HOME LANGUAGE FOR THE FIRST 3 YEARS OF SCHOOL WHILE ENGLISH IS BEING INTRODUCED AND THAN SWITCH COMPLETELY TO ENGLISH BY THE 4TH YEAR. THE BRITISH METHOD, ALTHOUGH SEEN AS BETTER THAN THE AMERICAN METHOD (NON-SPANISH-SPEAKING TEACHERS ATTEMPTING TO TEACH NON-ENGLISH-SPEAKING CHILDREN), CARRIES CERTAIN DANGERS THAT SHOULD BE AVOIDED. THESE DANGERS ARE (1) THAT THE HOME LANGUAGE WOULD BE PROMOTED PAST THE TIME NECESSARY TO LEARN ENGLISH, (2) THAT THIS DISCOURAGES RECOGNITION OF ONLY ONE LANGUAGE AS THE OFFICIAL LANGUAGE OF THE COUNTRY, AND (3) THAT NATIONAL SOLIDARITY IS DELAYED. THE FRENCH METHOD AS ADOPTED BY THE NEW MEXICO LEGISLATURE IN 1919 WILL OBTAIN ALL THE ADVANTAGES THAT CAN BE GAINED FROM THE BRITISH PRACTICE WITHOUT THE DANGERS INHERENT IN THE BRITISH METHOD. 1 REFERENCE.

ACCN   000473

557 AUTH **FITZGIBBONS, D. J.**
TITL SOCIAL CLASS DIFFERENCES IN PATIENTS' SELF-PERCEIVED TREATMENT NEEDS.
SRCE *PSYCHOLOGICAL REPORTS, 1972, 31, 987-997.*
INDX COPING MECHANISMS, CROSS CULTURAL, DEPRESSION, ANXIETY, EMPIRICAL, HEALTH, MENTAL HEALTH, PSYCHOPATHOLOGY, PUERTO RICAN-M, SES, URBAN, NEW YORK, EAST, SYMPTOMATOLOGY
ABST A COMPARISON WAS MADE OF THE FACTOR STRUCTURE OF SELF-PERCEIVED TREATMENT NEEDS BETWEEN PSYCHIATRIC PATIENTS OF LOW AND HIGH SOCIAL CLASS. DATA ON THE LOW SOCIAL CLASS SAMPLE (N = UNSPECIFIED) WERE COLLECTED AT A NEW YORK MEDICAL COLLEGE COMMUNITY MENTAL HEALTH CENTER WHICH SERVES THE INDIGENT FROM LARGE NEGRO AND PUERTO RICAN POPULATIONS. THE HIGH SOCIAL CLASS DATA WERE DERIVED FROM 163 PATIENTS AT THE INSTITUTE OF LIVING, A 413-BED PRIVATE NEW YORK PSYCHIATRIC HOSPITAL. BOTH SAMPLES WERE ADMINISTERED A VARIMAX TRANSFORMATION TEST, WITH SEVEN FACTORS REPRESENTING THE NEED FOR HELP WITH: (1) ANXIETY-DEPRESSION; (2) SUPEREGO; (3) GROSS PSYCHOTIC SYMPTOMS; (4) PHYSICAL SYMPTOMS THAT ARE FELT BY THE PATIENT TO BE RESPONSIBLE FOR EMOTIONAL PROBLEMS; (5) FEELINGS OF INADEQUACY; (6) ECONOMIC-VOCATIONAL COMPLAINTS; AND (7) MARITAL DIFFICULTIES. RESULTS WERE THAT THE TWO GROUPS REVEALED STRONG SIMILARITY ON SEVERAL FACTORS. REPORTS OF NEED FOR HELP WITH MARITAL AND ECONOMIC-VOCATIONAL DIFFICULTIES AND PSYCHOTIC SYMPTOMS WERE IDENTICAL. THE EXPERIENCE OF ANXIETY-DEPRESSION WAS INDISTINGUISHABLE, BUT HIGH SOCIAL CLASS PATIENTS EXPECTED RELIEF IN IMPROVED INTERPERSONAL RELATIONS, WHILE PATIENTS OF THE LOWER CLASS SOUGHT RELIEF IN ESCAPE. THE GROUPS, HOWEVER, DID DIFFER IN THEIR REPORTED FEELINGS OF INADEQUACY, AND ON ATTRIBUTION OF PROBLEMS TO PHYSICAL SYMPTOMS. GUILT APPEARED TO BE WITHOUT SPECIFIC REFERENCE IN THE LOWER CLASS GROUP BUT WAS ASSOCIATED WITH SPECIFIC BEHAVIORAL ACTS AMONG HIGHER CLASS PATIENTS. THE INFLUENCE OF PATIENTS' SELF-DEFINITION OF DISTURBANCE UPON CHOICE OF TREATMENT IS ALSO DISCUSSED. 16 REFERENCES.
ACCN 002078

558 AUTH **FITZGIBBONS, D. J., CUTLER, R., & COHEN, J.**
TITL PATIENTS' SELF-PERCEIVED TREATMENT NEEDS AND THEIR RELATIONSHIP TO BACKGROUND VARIABLES.
SRCE *JOURNAL OF CONSULTING AND CLINICAL PSYCHOLOGY, 1971, 37(2), 253-258.*
INDX PUERTO RICAN-M, CROSS CULTURAL, SYMPTOMATOLOGY, ADULTS, EMPIRICAL, SEX COMPARISON, RESEARCH METHODOLOGY, NEW YORK, EAST, MENTAL HEALTH
ABST A SCALE OF 93 ITEMS WAS DEVELOPED AND ADMINISTERED TO 118 FEMALE AND 114 MALE PSYCHIATRIC PATIENTS OF CAUCASIAN, PUERTO RICAN, AND NEGRO ETHNIC BACKGROUNDS. THE FACTOR CLUSTERS REPRESENT THE NEED FOR HELP WITH ANXIETY-DEPRESSION, SUPEREGO COMPLAINTS, GROSS PSYCHOTIC SYMPTOMS, PHYSICAL SYMPTOMS THAT ARE FELT BY THE PATIENT TO BE RESPONSIBLE FOR EMOTIONAL DIFFICULTIES, FEELINGS OF INADEQUACY, ECONOMIC VOCATIONAL COMPLAINTS, AND MARITAL DIFFICULTIES. A FURTHER ANALYSIS SHOWED THAT THESE SEVEN FACTORS HAVE ONLY A MINIMAL RELATIONSHIP TO THE BACKGROUND VARIABLES CHOSEN (SEX, AGE, AND ETHNIC BACKGROUND). THE FACTOR REPRESENTING ECONOMIC VOCATIONAL COMPLAINTS WAS ASSOCIATED WITH THE YOUNGER AGE GROUPS, FEMALES, AND THE RECENTLY ARRIVED IMMIGRANT GROUP. 11 REFERENCES.
ACCN 000474

559 AUTH **FITZPATRICK, F.**
TITL THE INTERMARRIAGE OF PUERTO RICANS IN NEW YORK CITY.
SRCE *AMERICAN JOURNAL OF SOCIOLOGY, 1966, 71, 395-406.*
INDX RELIGION, ACCULTURATION, PUERTO RICAN-M, PUERTO RICAN-I, NEW YORK, EAST, CROSS GENERATIONAL, IMMIGRATION, URBAN, MARRIAGE, SES, INTERMARRIAGE, SEX COMPARISON
ABST A STUDY OF OUT-GROUP MARRIAGES OF PUERTO RICANS, BASED ON ALL MARRIAGES IN WHICH ONE PARTNER WAS FIRST OR SECOND GENERATION PUERTO RICAN, INDICATES THAT ASSIMILATION IS TAKING PLACE RAPIDLY. INCREASES IN THE RATE OF OUT-GROUP MARRIAGE AMONG SECOND AS COMPARED TO FIRST GENERATION PUERTO RICANS IN 1949 AND 1959 WERE AS GREAT AS THOSE FOUND BY DRACHSLER FOR ALL IMMIGRANTS IN NEW YORK, 1908-12. OUT-GROUP MARRIAGE WAS POSITIVELY CORRELATED WITH HIGHER OCCUPATIONAL STATUS ONLY IN THE CASE OF BRIDES. AGE AT MARRIAGE DROPS IN THE SECOND GENERATION. CIVIL AND CATHOLIC CEREMONIES DROP IN NEW YORK IN CONTRAST TO PUERTO RICO; PROTESTANT CEREMONIES INCREASE. CATHOLIC CEREMONIES INCREASED IN 1959 OVER 1949 AND IN SECOND GENERATION OVER FIRST. 22 REFERENCES. (JOURNAL ABSTRACT MODIFIED)
ACCN 000475

560 AUTH **FITZPATRICK, J. P.**
TITL THE ADJUSTMENT OF PUERTO RICANS TO NEW YORK.
SRCE *THE JOURNAL OF INTERGROUP RELATIONS, 1959-60, 1(1), 43-51.*
INDX PSYCHOSOCIAL ADJUSTMENT, PUERTO RICAN-M, IMMIGRATION, CULTURAL FACTORS, INTEGRATION, PREJUDICE, DISCRIMINATION, ECONOMIC FACTORS, URBAN, COMMUNITY, ESSAY, ACCULTURATION, CULTURAL PLURALISM, NEW YORK, EAST
ABST TO EVALUATE THE ROLE OF PREJUDICE IN THE ADJUSTMENT OF PUERTO RICANS IN THE NEXT TEN YEARS, A NUMBER OF FACTORS AFFECTING THE LIFE OF PUERTO RICANS ON THE

MAINLAND MUST BE KEPT DISTINCT. CULTURAL INTEGRATION AND RACIAL INTEGRATION ARE DISCUSSED IN RELATION TO PREJUDICE WHICH PUERTO RICANS MUST FACE IN THEIR ADJUSTMENT TO NEW YORK CITY. CONFLICTS OF INTEREST AND CULTURE ARE EXPLORED AS THEY HAVE CAUSED PREJUDICE AND DISCRIMINATION AMONG "OLD" AND "NEW" NEW YORKERS AND RACIAL GROUPS. THE QUESTION OF COLOR AND CLASS AMONG PUERTO RICANS THEMSELVES AND HOPEFUL ASPECTS IN THE PRESENT MIGRATION, SUCH AS THE EMPHASIS ON CULTURAL PLURALISM BY PUBLIC OFFICIALS AND TEACHERS, ARE ALSO DISCUSSED. 12 REFERENCES. (AUTHOR SUMMARY MODIFIED)

ACCN   000476

561 AUTH   **FITZPATRICK, J. P.**
     TITL   PUERTO RICAN AMERICANS: THE MEANING OF MIGRATION TO THE MAINLAND.
     SRCE   *ENGLEWOOD CLIFFS, N.J.: PRENTICE-HALL, INC., 1971.*
     INDX   PUERTO RICAN-M, PUERTO RICAN-I, IMMIGRATION, ACCULTURATION, DEMOGRAPHIC, POVERTY, REVIEW, RELIGION, ETHNIC IDENTITY, SOCIAL SERVICES, DRUG ABUSE, MENTAL HEALTH, FAMILY ROLES, FAMILY STRUCTURE, POLITICAL POWER, EDUCATION, ECONOMIC FACTORS, CULTURE, DISCRIMINATION, COMMUNITY INVOLVEMENT, URBAN, NEW YORK, EAST, CULTURAL CHANGE, BOOK
     ABST   CALLING THIS VOLUME AN "INTERPRETIVE ESSAY" RATHER THAN A DESCRIPTIVE STUDY, THE AUTHOR (A CATHOLIC PRIEST) OFFERS A COLLEGE-LEVEL TEXT WHICH SUMMARIZES AND ASSESSES THE IMMIGRATION EXPERIENCE OF PUERTO RICANS—ESPECIALLY THOSE IN NEW YORK CITY. BASED ON AN EXTENSIVE REVIEW OF THE LITERATURE PLUS THE AUTHOR'S WORK EXPERIENCES IN THE PUERTO RICAN COMMUNITY, THE FOLLOWING ASPECTS OF PUERTO RICAN IMMIGRATION ARE EXAMINED: (1) CULTURAL ORIGINS; (2) THE DYNAMICS OF IMMIGRATION; (3) THE ISLAND BACKGROUND; (4) THE NEW YORK ENVIRONMENT; (5) THE ORGANIZATION OF THE PUERTO RICAN IMMIGRANT COMMUNITY; (6) THE PUERTO RICAN FAMILY; (7) COLOR DISCRIMINATION; (8) RELIGION; (9) EDUCATION IN NEW YORK CITY SCHOOLS; (10) WELFARE; (11) MENTAL ILLNESS AND DRUG ABUSE; AND (12) POLITICAL ACTIVISM AND ECONOMIC POWER. PARTICULAR EMPHASIS IS GIVEN TO PUERTO RICANS' QUEST FOR IDENTITY IN THE ASSIMILATION PROCESS, THE DISORGANIZATION IN THEIR COMMUNITY LIFE, AND THE NATURE OF COMMUNITY AGENCIES AND WELFARE PROGRAMS. DESPITE THE MANY PROBLEMS FACING THE PUERTO RICAN COMMUNITY, HOPE IS SEEN IN THEIR EMERGING POLITICAL ACTIVISM—PARTICULARLY AMONG SCOND-GENERATION PUERTO RICANS. FOR WITHIN PUERTO RICANS' PURSUIT OF GROUP INTERESTS REGARDING ANTIPOVERTY PROGRAMS, EDUCATION, AND PUBLIC WELFARE, ARE THE SEEDS OF COMMUNITY COHESIVENESS AND GROUP IDENTITY.

ACCN   001797

562 AUTH   **FITZPATRICK, J. P.**
     TITL   THE PUERTO RICAN FAMILY.
     SRCE   *IN C. H. MINDEL & R. W. HABENSTEIN (EDS.), ETHNIC FAMILIES IN AMERICA: PATTERNS AND VARIATIONS. NEW YORK: ELSEVIER SCIENTIFIC PUBLISHING CO., INC., 1976, PP. 192-217.*
     INDX   FAMILY STRUCTURE, FAMILY ROLES, ACCULTURATION, MIGRATION, PUERTO RICAN-I, PUERTO RICAN-M, ETHNIC IDENTITY, MARRIAGE, MARITAL STABILITY, CULTURAL FACTORS, HISTORY, EXTENDED FAMILY, ATTITUDES, ESSAY, STRESS, CULTURAL CHANGE, VALUES
     ABST   THE PUERTO RICAN FAMILY IS DISCUSSED FROM THE PERSPECTIVE OF MIGRATION BETWEEN THE ISLAND AND THE MAINLAND. A DESCRIPTION OF THE TRADITIONAL PUERTO RICAN FAMILY IS GIVEN, BEGINNING WITH THE HISTORICAL BACKGROUND OF THE SPANISH COLONIAL CULTURE, THE AMERICAN EDUCATIONAL AND RELIGIOUS SYSTEM, AND CONCLUDING WITH THE IMPACT OF PUERTO RICANS RETURNING HOME FROM THE MAINLAND. THE RANGE OF VALUES THAT DISTINGUISH THE FAMILY ON THE ISLAND—PERSONALISM, COMPADRAZGO, MACHISMO, FAMILY OBLIGATION, PRIMACY OF THE SPIRITUAL, FATALISM, AND A SENSE OF HIERARCHY—ARE CONTRASTED WITH THE PREDOMINANT MIDDLE-CLASS VALUES OF THE MAINLAND. IN THE PROCESS OF MIGRATION AND ADJUSTMENT TO THE U.S., THE FAMILY IS THE INSTITUTION THAT FACES THE MOST DIRECT SHOCK OF CULTURAL CHANGE, THOUGH IT ALSO PROVIDES THE MOST SUPPORT FOR ITS MEMBERS. MANY FEATURES OF THE TRADITIONAL FAMILY CONTINUE, BUT CHANGES CAN BE OBSERVED IN THE FAMILY STRUCTURE, RATE OF INTERMARRIAGE, FAMILY VALUES, RELIANCE ON THE EXTENDED FAMILY, AND THE REPLACEMENT OF PERSONALISTIC VALUES WITH THE IMPERSONAL NORMS OF THE AMERICAN SYSTEM. DIFFICULTIES OF ADJUSTMENT MAY RESULT IN DENIAL OF ETHNIC IDENTITY, WITHDRAWAL INTO THE OLD CULTURE, OR THE BUILDING OF A CULTURAL BRIDGE IN WHICH IDENTIFICATION WITH ONE'S CULTURAL HERITAGE IS INCLUDED IN THE ESTABLISHMENT OF A NEW WAY OF LIFE. 26 REFERENCES.

ACCN   002080

563 AUTH   **FITZPATRICK, J. P.**
     TITL   PUERTO RICANS IN PERSPECTIVE: THE MEANING OF MIGRATION TO THE MAINLAND.
     SRCE   *IN N. R. YETMAN & C. M. STEELE (EDS.), MAJORITY AND MINORITY: THE DYNAMICS OF RACIAL AND ETHNIC RELATIONS. BOSTON: ALLYN & BACON, 1975, PP. 297-304.*
     INDX   PUERTO RICAN-M, IMMIGRATION, STRESS, RURAL, URBAN, ACCULTURATION, RELIGION, POLITICS, POVERTY, CULTURAL CHANGE, ETHNIC IDENTITY, COMMUNITY INVOLVEMENT, ESSAY, NEW YORK, EAST
     ABST   LARGE-SCALE IMMIGRATION OF PUERTO RICANS TO THE UNITED STATES BEGAN AFTER WORLD WAR II. ALTHOUGH THE MOVEMENT BACK TO THE ISLAND HAS INCREASED, IT DOES NOT COMPARE WITH THE LARGE AND CONTINUOUS MOVEMENT TO THE MAINLAND. THE UNIQUE CHARACTERISTIC OF THIS MI-

THE UNIQUE CHARACTERISTIC OF THIS MIGRATION AS A LARGE-SCALE EXPERIENCE WITH PARTICULAR EMPHASIS ON THE PERSPECTIVE OF PUERTO RICANS IN NEW YORK CITY ARE EXPLORED. THE PROCESS OF ASSIMILATION IN RELATION TO THE SEARCH FOR IDENTITY WHICH PRESENTS A NUMBER OF SPECIAL PROBLEMS TO PUERTO RICANS IS STUDIED. ONE OF THESE IDENTITY PROBLEMS WHICH CONSISTS OF A SHIFT FROM AN EMPHASIS ON CULTURE TO AN EMPHASIS ON POWER AS THE BASIS FOR A STRONG PUERTO RICAN COMMUNITY IS ANALYZED. FINALLY, THE EXPERIENCE OF PUERTO RICANS AS PART OF THE HUMAN EFFORT AND SUFFERING INEVITABLY INVOLVED IN THE CONTINUING CREATIVE ACHIEVEMENT OF NEW YORK CITY IS EXPLORED. IT IS CONCLUDED THAT WITHIN THE HISTORICAL PERSPECTIVE OF PAST MIGRATIONS TO THE CITY, IT IS REASONABLE TO BE OPTIMISTIC ABOUT THE PRESENT MIGRATION. 3 REFERENCES. (AUTHOR SUMMARY MODIFIED)

ACCN   000477

564 AUTH   **FLORES, E. J., & ROMERO, P.**
     TITL   MENTAL HEALTH NEEDS ASSESSMENT: RECOMMENDING A DEMONSTRATION PROJECT IN EAST LOS ANGELES.
     SRCE   *UNPUBLISHED MANUSCRIPT, 1976. (AVAILABLE FROM E. J. FLORES, BRENTWOOD VETERAN'S ADMINISTRATION HOSPITAL, BRENTWOOD, CALIFORNIA.)*
     INDX   MENTAL HEALTH, SPANISH SURNAMED, BILINGUAL-BICULTURAL PERSONNEL, HEALTH DELIVERY SYSTEMS, RESOURCE UTILIZATION, EMPIRICAL, CALIFORNIA, SOUTHWEST, PROGRAM EVALUATION, VETERANS
     ABST   BASED ON CENSUS DATA AND BRENTWOOD, CALIFORNIA, VETERAN'S ADMINISTRATION HOSPITAL STATISTICS, THE MENTAL HEALTH NEEDS OF SPANISH SPEAKING/SPANISH SURNAMED (SS/SS) VETERANS ARE NOT BEING MET. MAJOR CAUSES ARE IDENTIFIED AS (1) OVERUTILIZATION OF AVAILABLE COMMUNITY MENTAL HEALTH SERVICES BY NON-VETERANS, (2) DISTANT LOCATION OF THE VETERAN'S HOSPITAL, AND (3) LACK OF ADEQUATE BICULTURAL-BILINGUAL MENTAL HEALTH SERVICES IN THE LOS ANGELES/LONG BEACH AREA WHERE THE SS/SS VETERAN POPULATION IS HIGH. RECOMMENDATIONS INCLUDE THE ESTABLISHMENT OF A TASK FORCE TO EXPLORE NEEDS AND GAIN FUNDING TO OPERATE A DEMONSTRATION PROGRAM. 3 REFERENCES.
     ACCN   000478

565 AUTH   **FLORES, J. M.**
     TITL   A STUDY OF MEXICAN AMERICAN CULTURAL CHARACTERISTICS AS PERCEIVED BY MEMBERS OF 100 IMPOVERISHED MEXICAN AMERICAN FAMILIES AND ITS EDUCATIONAL IMPLICATIONS.
     SRCE   *UNPUBLISHED DOCTORAL DISSERTATION, UNIVERSITY OF HOUSTON, 1972. (ERIC DOCUMENT REPRODUCTION SERVICE NO. ED 076 271)*
     INDX   MEXICAN AMERICAN, POVERTY, CULTURAL

FACTORS, EDUCATION, SCHOLASTIC ACHIEVEMENT, SES, ADULTS, ADOLESCENTS, FATALISM, ACHIEVEMENT MOTIVATION, SEX ROLES, TIME ORIENTATION, FAMILY STRUCTURE, TEXAS, SOUTHWEST
     ABST   TWO QUESTIONS WERE INVESTIGATED IN THIS STUDY: (1) DOES THE LOW-SOCIOECONOMIC MEXICAN AMERICAN PERCEIVE HIMSELF AS HE IS PORTRAYED IN LITERATURE?, AND (2) ARE THERE RELATIONSHIPS BETWEEN EDUCATIONAL ACHIEVEMENT, PERCEIVED CULTURAL CHARACTERISTICS, AND 7 SPECIFIC THEMES— (1) ETHNIC ISOLATION, (2) SPANISH LANGUAGE, (3) FATALISM, (4) PRESENT DAY ORIENTATION, (5) LIMITED ASPIRATIONS, (6) "MACHISMO, AND (7) FAMILY SOLIDARITY? A QUESTIONNAIRE WAS DEVELOPED FOR THE 100 NINTH-GRADE STUDENTS TESTED IN CORPUS CHRISTI, TEXAS, WHILE ANOTHER WAS ADMINISTERED TO THE 76 PARENTS. THE RESULTS INDICATED THAT MEXICAN AMERICAN CULTURAL CHARACTERISTICS AS PERCEIVED BY THE 100 LOW-SOCIOECONOMIC FAMILIES TESTED ARE NOT IN TOTAL ACCORD WITH THE LITERATURE. THE FINDINGS SHOW THE MEXICAN AMERICAN LIVING IN ISOLATION, MAINTAINING THE SPANISH LANGUAGE, AND HAVING STRONG FAMILY TIES. HE IS ALSO PRONE TO FUNCTION IN THE PRESENT RATHER THAN THE PAST OR FUTURE, BE NON-FATALISTIC, HAVE HIGH ASPIRATIONS, AND GENERALLY DISREGARD THE "MACHISMO CONCEPT. 83 REFERENCES. (RIE ABSTRACT MODIFIED)
     ACCN   000479

566 AUTH   **FLORES, Y. G.**
     TITL   CAREER AND ACADEMIC GUIDANCE FOR CHICANA ADOLESCENT GIRLS.
     SRCE   *UNPUBLISHED MASTER'S THESIS, CALIFORNIA STATE UNIVERSITY, LONG BEACH, 1975.*
     INDX   EDUCATIONAL COUNSELING, ADOLESCENTS, FEMALE, MEXICAN AMERICAN, PROGRAM EVALUATION, PSYCHOTHERAPY OUTCOME, ATTITUDES, EDUCATION, ACHIEVEMENT MOTIVATION, CALIFORNIA, SOUTHWEST, VOCATIONAL COUNSELING
     ABST   CAREER AND ACADEMIC GUIDANCE WAS PROVIDED TO NINE CHICANA ADOLESCENT GIRLS ON ACADEMIC PROBATION AT JUNIOR AND SENIOR HIGH SCHOOLS. A CONTROL GROUP OF NINE COMPARABLY SITUATED GIRLS, NOT INVOLVED IN THE PROGRAM, WAS SELECTED. THE PROGRAM ATTEMPTED TO IMPROVE THE GIRLS' SCHOOL ATTENDANCE AND GRADES, TO PROVIDE CAREER INFORMATION, AND TO DEVELOP CULTURAL AND COMMUNITY AWARENESS THROUGH THE USE OF COMMUNITY RESOURCES. THERE WERE TWO MEETINGS WEEKLY FOR EIGHT WEEKS. ONE INVOLVED ACADEMIC TUTORING AND SPEAKERS WHO PROVIDED CAREER INFORMATION. THE OTHER WAS A FIELD TRIP TO OBTAIN CAREER INFORMATION AND TO MEET CHICANA CAREER WOMEN WHO SERVED AS MODELS AND COUNSELORS. ONE EVALUATIVE TOOL WAS A PRE-POST ATTITUDINAL QUESTIONNAIRE DEVELOPED AND STANDARDIZED FOR THIS PROGRAM. THERE WERE NO SIGNIFICANT DIFFER-

ENCES BETWEEN THE PRE AND POST TEST SCORES FOR EITHER GROUP. SCHOOL ATTENDANCE AND GRADES WERE EXAMINED AND BOTH SHOWED A SIGNIFICANT IMPROVEMENT FOR THE EXPERIMENTAL GROUP. 7 REFERENCES. (AUTHOR ABSTRACT)

ACCN   000480

567 AUTH **FLOREZ, J.**
    TITL CHICANOS AND COALITIONS AS A FORCE FOR SOCIAL CHANGE.
    SRCE *IN M. M. MANGOLD (ED.), LA CAUSA CHICANA: THE MOVEMENT FOR JUSTICE. NEW YORK: FAMILY SERVICE ASSOCIATION OF AMERICA, PP. 78-86.*
    INDX MEXICAN AMERICAN, COMMUNITY INVOLVEMENT, POLITICAL POWER, CHICANO MOVEMENT, COMMUNITY, ESSAY, MENTAL HEALTH PROFESSION
    ABST AN EXAMINATION OF THE POLICIES OF LIBERALS, SOCIAL WORKERS, AND VARIOUS AGENCIES AS SOCIAL CHANGE AGENTS REVEALS THAT FAILURE TO CLOSELY ANALYZE THESE GROUPS RESULTS IN PURE RHETORIC AND NO POLITICAL ACTION. IT IS STATED THAT FOR TOO LONG CHICANOS HAVE MISSED OPPORTUNITIES TO RELATE DIRECTLY TO POWER BLOCKS AND INSTEAD HAVE DEALT WITH MIDDLEMEN. CHICANO COALITIONS, BASED ON A SELF-DETERMINATION PHILOSOPHY, COUPLED WITH THE DIVERSE SKILLS OF THE MEMBERS CAN SERVE AS CATALYSTS FOR SOCIAL CHANGE. THE COALITION PROCESS IS ONLY ONE METHOD OF INITIATING CHANGE, BUT IT IS ONE THAT NEEDS TO BE MORE FULLY EXPLORED. STRATEGIES, PRIORITIES, AND ALLIANCES FOR EFFECTING SOCIAL CHANGE MUST BE REEVALUATED AND REDEFINED.
    ACCN 000481

568 AUTH **FLYNN, P.**
    TITL MIGRANT HEALTH PROGRAMS: THE EXPERIENCE IN CALIFORNIA.
    SRCE *AGENDA, MARCH/APRIL 1977, 23-26.*
    INDX FARM LABORERS, HEALTH, HEALTH DELIVERY SYSTEMS, LEGISLATION, REVIEW, MIGRANTS, CALIFORNIA, SOUTHWEST, RURAL
    ABST THE MIGRANT HEALTH ACT, WHICH BECAME FEDERAL LAW IN 1962, IS REVIEWED. COMMUNITY HEALTH CLINICS AND CENTERS FUNDED BY THIS ACT CURRENTLY PROVIDE MEDICAL CARE TO OVER 450,000 PERSONS IN CALIFORNIA. MIGRANT HEALTH PROGRAMS HAVE STRUGGLED TO MAINTAIN THEIR SERVICES DESPITE OPPOSITION FROM TRADITIONAL MEDICAL INSTITUTIONS AND FUNDING DEFICITS. LEGISLATIVE CHANGES IN THE ACT SINCE 1962 HAVE HAD A BIG IMPACT ON THE DIRECTION OF THE PROGRAMS: (1) HOSPITAL CARE WAS ADDED AS A REQUIRED SERVICE IN 1965, (2) SEASONAL FARM WORKERS AND THEIR FAMILIES WERE EXTENDED COVERAGE IN 1970, AND (3) DIRECT CONSUMER INVOLVEMENT IN EVERY CENTER'S BOARD OF DIRECTORS WAS MANDATED IN 1970. OF CURRENT CONCERN TO RURAL CLINIC STAFF AND DIRECTORS IS THE CONTROVERSY AT THE FEDERAL LEVEL OVER THE RURAL HEALTH INITIATIVE (RHI). IF

THIS INITIATIVE WERE TO BECOME LAW, MIGRANT HEALTH PROGRAMS WOULD BE DEEMPHASIZED AND REPLACED BY A CATEGORICAL PROGRAM TO SERVE ALL PERSONS IN RURAL AREAS. MIGRANT HEALTH PROGRAM DIRECTORS ARGUE THAT THEIR CENTERS HAVE BEEN MANDATED TO AND CAN EFFECTIVELY PROVIDE SERVICES TO BOTH MIGRANT AND SEASONAL WORKERS.

ACCN   000482

569 AUTH **FOGEL, W.**
    TITL MEXICAN LABOR IN UNITED STATES LABOR MARKETS.
    SRCE *IN J. L. STERN & B. D. DENNIS (EDS.), INDUSTRIAL RELATIONS RESEARCH ASSOCIATION SERIES: PROCEEDINGS OF THE TWENTY-SEVENTH ANNUAL WINTER MEETING (VOL.9). MADISON, WISC.: INDUSTRIAL RELATIONS RESEARCH ASSOC., 1975, PP. 343-349.*
    INDX IMMIGRATION, EMPLOYMENT, MEXICAN, ECONOMIC FACTORS, UNDOCUMENTED WORKERS, POLICY, ESSAY, LABOR FORCE,
    ABST MEXICAN LABOR HAS BEEN VIEWED AS A MOBILE COMMODITY, MORE LIKE CAPITAL AND RAW MATERIAL RESOURCES THAN HUMAN LABOR. FIGURES CITED, ALTHOUGH ONLY ESTIMATES, SHOW THE RISE IN ILLEGAL IMMIGRATION, WHERE IMMIGRANTS ARE MAINLY CONCENTRATED, AND THE PERCENTAGE OF JOBS THEY OCCUPY. EDUCATIONAL DEFICIENCIES ARE BELIEVED TO BE THE DOMINANT CHARACTERISTIC CONFINING THE MEXICAN-BORN WORK FORCE TO LOW SKILL SECTORS OF MANUAL LABOR. THE IMPACT OF MEXICAN WORKERS ON THE U.S. LABOR MARKET HAS BEEN LOWER WAGES AND PRICES AND GREATER EMPLOYMENT AND OUTPUT THAN WOULD EXIST IN THEIR ABSENCE; THERE IS ALSO LESS UNIONIZATION AND GREATER INCOME EQUALITY. OVERALL, MEXICAN WORKERS PROVIDE ELASTIC INCREMENTS TO LABOR SUPPLY IN SECONDARY MARKET AND HELP TO MAINTAIN LOW WAGES. IT IS THIS "UNDECLARED POLICY" WHICH IS SEEN AS BENEFITING AMERICAN EMPLOYERS AND CONSUMERS MORE THAN EITHER THE MEXICAN OR AMERICAN POOR.
    ACCN 000483

570 AUTH **FOLAN, W. J., & WEIGARD, P. C.**
    TITL FICTIVE WIDOWHOOD IN RURAL AND URBAN MEXICO.
    SRCE *ANTHROPOLOGICA, 1968, 10(1), 119-128.*
    INDX MEXICO, ESSAY, SEX ROLES, MEXICAN, MARITAL STABILITY, SOCIAL STRUCTURE, MARRIAGE, FEMALE, SES, CULTURAL FACTORS
    ABST IN MEXICAN SOCIETY A FEMALE ACHIEVES STATUS THROUGH MARRIAGE AND CAN ONLY MAINTAIN HER SOCIAL POSITION BY REMAINING MARRIED AND HAVING CHILDREN. IF WIDOWED, SHE CAN STILL RETAIN HER STATUS, THOUGH SOCIAL DISAPPROVAL NOW EXISTS FOR HAVING CHILDREN. DIVORCED OR SEPARATED FEMALES SUFFER OSTRACISM FROM THE COMMUNITY AND THEREFORE TEND TO ASSUME THE ROLE OF FICTIVE WIDOWHOOD.

HER REAL STATUS IS USUALLY PROTECTED BY HER OR THE MALE MOVING TO A NEW TOWN. CULTURAL TRADITION ALSO INFLUENCES THE COMMUNITY TO LABEL THE DIVORCED OR SEPARATED FEMALE AS WIDOWED, EVEN WHEN KNOWLEDGE OF HER TRUE STATUS BECOMES KNOWN. THESE PARTICULAR ASPECTS WERE APPARENT IN THE CASE STUDIES OF FOUR FEMALES WHO HAVE BEEN EITHER DIVORCED OR SEPARATED. 3 REFERENCES.

ACCN   000484

571   AUTH   **FOLEY, A. R., ARCE, A., GREENBERG, I., & GORHAM, P.**

TITL   COLLABORATION BETWEEN PUBLIC AND PRIVATE AGENCIES IN DEVELOPING A COMMUNITY MENTAL HEALTH SERVICE.

SRCE   *HOSPITAL AND COMMUNITY PSYCHIATRY, 1971, 22(11), 337-340.*

INDX   COMMUNITY, MENTAL HEALTH, COMMUNITY INVOLVEMENT, ESSAY, PARAPROFESSIONALS, HEALTH DELIVERY SYSTEMS, PROGRAM EVALUATION, NEW YORK, EAST, HEALTH, SPANISH SURNAMED

ABST   MENTAL HEALTH SERVICES FOR A SPECIFIC POPULATION GROUP CAN BE PROVIDED IDEALLY THROUGH THE COLLABORATION OF PUBLIC AND PRIVATE AGENCIES, BUT EFFECTIVE COLLABORATION IS NOT ACHIEVED EASILY. THE SOUTH SHORE-ROCKAWAY MENTAL HEALTH SERVICES IN THE NEW YORK CITY AREA IS AN EXAMPLE OF AN EFFECTIVE PROGRAM BASED UPON COOPERATION BETWEEN A PUBLIC AND PRIVATE AGENCY WHICH PROVIDED SERVICES SOON AFTER INTENSIVE PLANNING. THE POPULATION OF THE AREA TOTALS 136,000 RESIDENTS, OF WHOM 77 PERCENT ARE WHITE, 20 PERCENT ARE BLACK, AND 3 PERCENT ARE SPANISH-SPEAKING. BEFORE THE INITIATION OF THE PROGRAM, GENERAL HEALTH CARE AND EMERGENCY PSYCHIATRIC CARE WERE NOT READILY AVAILABLE. EARLY IN THE PROGRAM, A SOCIAL WORKER WAS HIRED TO COORDINATE COMMUNITY AFFAIRS, AND THE FIRST FEW MONTHS OF COMMUNITY FIELD WORK WERE VERY PRODUCTIVE. MINOR PROBLEMS AROSE IN THE PROCESS OF STAFFING THE NEW SERVICE, BUT STAFF MEMBERS WERE ABLE TO MAKE THEIR OWN PERSONAL CONCERNS SUBORDINATE TO THE CREATION OF THE NEW FACILITY. PROGRAM ROLES FOR THE STAFF HAVE PURPOSELY BEEN KEPT FLEXIBLE IN ORDER TO MAINTAIN A HIGH DEGREE OF RELEVANCE OF THE PROGRAM TO THE RESIDENTS. THE BOARD MEMBERS OF THE FACILITY HELP TO IDENTIFY MENTAL HEALTH NEEDS, RECOMMEND PROGRAM CHANGES AND ADDITIONS, AND AID IN OBTAINING FINANCIAL AND OTHER SUPPORT FOR VARIOUS PROGRAMS. NO REFERENCES.

ACCN   000485

572   AUTH   **FORD, J. G., & GRAVES, J. R.**

TITL   DIFFERENCES BETWEEN MEXICAN-AMERICAN AND WHITE CHILDREN IN INTERPERSONAL DISTANCE AND SOCIAL TOUCHING.

SRCE   *PERCEPTUAL AND MOTOR SKILLS, 1977, 45, 779-785.*

INDX   CROSS CULTURAL, MEXICAN AMERICAN, SOUTHWEST, URBAN, CHILDREN, SEX COMPARISON, SOCIALIZATION, EMPIRICAL, INTERPERSONAL SPACING, FEMALE

ABST   TWO STUDIES IN A LARGE SOUTHWEST CITY EXAMINED DIFFERENCES IN CHILDREN'S SOCIAL IMMEDIACY TENDENCIES EXPRESSED THROUGH INTERPERSONAL DISTANCE AND TOUCHING. IT WAS PREDICTED THAT MEXICAN AMERICANS WOULD SPACE CLOSER AND TOUCH MORE FREQUENTLY THAN WHITES. STUDY 1 SHOWED AMONG 40 SECOND GRADERS THAT 20 MEXICAN AMERICAN DID SPACE SIGNIFICANTLY CLOSER THAN 20 WHITES. AMONG 40 EIGHTH GRADERS THE ETHNIC DIFFERENCE DISAPPEARED. STUDY 2 INDICATED AMONG SECOND GRADERS THAT THE GREATEST TACTUAL BEHAVIOR OCCURRED FOR MEXICAN AMERICAN FEMALES (16 BOYS, 16 GIRLS). EXTENSIVE MEASURES WERE TAKEN IN STUDY 1 TO AVOID A NUMBER OF CONFOUNDS THAT CHARACTERIZED PREVIOUS RESEARCH. RESULTS ARE DISCUSSED IN TERMS OF SOCIAL LEARNING AND ETHNIC SOCIALIZATION. 15 REFERENCES. (JOURNAL ABSTRACT MODIFIED)

ACCN   002274

573   AUTH   **FORM, W. H., & D'ANTONIO, W. V.**

TITL   INTEGRATION AND CLEAVAGE AMONG COMMUNITY INFLUENTIALS IN TWO BORDER CITIES.

SRCE   *AMERICAN SOCIOLOGICAL REVIEW, 1959, 24(6), 804-814.*

INDX   COMMUNITY, POLITICAL POWER, ECONOMIC FACTORS, MEXICO, CROSS CULTURAL, MEXICAN, TEXAS, SOUTHWEST

ABST   STUDIES OF COMMUNITY POWER STRUCTURE HAVE TENDED TO ASSUME THE EXISTENCE OF SINGLE, SOCIALLY INTEGRATED ELITE GROUPS DOMINATING THE DECISION-MAKING PROCESS. THE PRESENT STUDY WAS DESIGNED TO ASCERTAIN WHETHER OR NOT THOSE WHO WERE PRESUMED TO BE BUSINESS AND POLITICAL INFLUENTIALS ARE INDEED INTEGRATED. INTEGRATION WAS MEASURED IN FOUR WAYS: (1) EXTENT TO WHICH BUSINESSMEN AND POLITICOS WERE CHOSEN AS INFLUENTIAL BOTH IN BUSINESS AND POLITICS; (2) EXTENT OF COMMONALITY OF SOCIAL BACKGROUNDS AND PARTICIPATION IN SELECTED VOLUNTARY ASSOCIATIONS; (3) EXTENT OF PERCEPTUAL AGREEMENT OF BUSINESS AND GOVERNMENT PRACTICES; AND (4) AGREEMENT ON MAJOR PROBLEMS FACING THE COMMUNITY AND GROUPS WORKING FOR OR AGAINST THE SOLUTION OF THESE PROBLEMS. THE STUDY WAS CARRIED OUT IN A CROSS CULTURAL SETTING, USING TWIN BORDER CITIES. THE DATA SHOW GREATER INTEGRATION IN THE AMERICAN THAN IN THE MEXICAN CITY, WHERE INSTITUTIONAL BOUNDARIES ARE RATHER SHARPLY DELINEATED. IN NEITHER CASE DO THE DATA SUGGEST THE EXISTENCE OF A SINGLE POWER SYSTEM; POWER CONFLICTS MAY ARISE BETWEEN GROUPS WHICH OVERLAP INSTITUTIONAL BOUNDARIES IN AMERICAN COMMUNITIES, WHILE IN MEXI-

CAN COMMUNITIES CONFLICTS MAY ARISE BE-
TWEEN INSTITUTIONS. 18 REFERENCES.
(JOURNAL ABSTRACT)

ACCN 000486

574 AUTH **FORT, J. G., WATTS, J. C., & LESSER, G. S.**
TITL CULTURAL BACKGROUND AND LEARNING IN
YOUNG CHILDREN.
SRCE *PHI DELTA KAPPAN, 1969, 50(7), 386-388.*
INDX PUERTO RICAN-M, INTELLIGENCE, INTELLI-
GENCE TESTING, EMPIRICAL, EDUCATION, SES,
CULTURAL FACTORS, CHILDREARING PRAC-
TICES, CHILDREN, CROSS CULTURAL, COGNI-
TIVE DEVELOPMENT, ABILITY TESTING, NEW
YORK, EAST
ABST A 5-YEAR LONGITUDINAL STUDY EXAMINED
WHETHER DIFFERENT ETHNIC GROUPS DIS-
PLAY DIFFERENT PATTERNS OF MENTAL ABILI-
TIES. CHILDREN FROM LOWER- AND MIDDLE-
CLASS HOMES OF CHINESE, JEWISH, NEGRO,
AND PUERTO RICAN ORIGIN WERE ADMINIS-
TERED THE DIVERSE MENTAL ABILITIES TEST.
ALL CHILDREN WERE ABLE TO TAKE THE TEST
IN THEIR NATIVE DIALECT AND/OR IN ENGLISH.
THE RESULTS INDICATE THAT MIDDLE-CLASS
CHILDREN ARE BETTER ABLE TO PERFORM ON
ALL TASKS THAN ARE LOWER-CLASS CHIL-
DREN AND THAT THE CHILDREN SHOW DIFFER-
ENT CONSTELLATIONS OF ABILITIES AS WELL
AS DIFFERENT LEVELS OF PERFORMANCE FOR
VARIOUS TASKS. MIDDLE-CLASS CHILDREN
FROM DIFFERENT ETHNIC GROUPS IN GEN-
ERAL PERFORM MORE LIKE EACH OTHER THAN
DO LOWER-CLASS CHILDREN FROM DIFFER-
ENT ETHNIC GROUPS. OTHER FINDINGS ARE:
(1) CHINESE CHILDREN PERFORM SPATIAL
TASKS BETTER THAN ANY OTHER TASK, THEY
PERFORM POOREST ON VERBAL TASKS; (2)
JEWISH CHILDREN EVIDENCED THEIR GREAT-
EST PROFICIENCY IN THE VERBAL AREA, THEIR
SPATIAL ABILITIES WERE THE POOREST; (3) NE-
GRO CHILDREN SHOWED THEIR GREATEST
SKILL TO BE IN THE VERBAL AREA, THEY PER-
FORMED LEAST WELL IN THE NUMERICAL AREA;
AND (4) PUERTO RICAN CHILDREN EVIDENCED
THE LEAST DIFFERENCE AMONG THE FOUR
ABILITIES, THEIR BEST AREA WAS SPACE CON-
CEPTUALIZATION AND THEIR WORST WAS VER-
BAL CONCEPTS. THESE FACTS SUGGEST THAT
THE DEVELOPMENTAL ORIGINS OF THE DIF-
FERENT PATTERNS OF ABILITY PROBABLY LIE
IN TWO MAIN AREAS. THE FIRST IS OCCUPA-
TIONAL AND SOCIAL STRUCTURE OF AMERI-
CAN SOCIETY WHICH, HISTORICALLY, HAS
FORCED DIFFERENT ETHNIC GROUPS INTO
DIFFERENT OCCUPATIONS AND SOCIAL ROLES.
THE SECOND MAJOR DETERMINANT OF DIF-
FERENT PATTERNS OF MENTAL ABILITY MAY BE
MORE SUBTLE, INVOLVING DIFFERENCES IN
GENERAL STYLES OF CHILD-REARING AS THESE
VARY NOT WITH SOCIAL CLASS BUT WITH ETH-
NIC OR CULTURAL GROUP MEMBERSHIP. IT IS
CONCLUDED THAT SCHOOL INSTRUCTION
MUST BE DESIGNED AROUND THE ABILITY PAT-
TERNS OF THE CHILDREN INVOLVED.

ACCN 000487

575 AUTH **FORT, J. P., JR.**

TITL HEROIN ADDICTION AMONG YOUNG MEN.
SRCE *PSYCHIATRY, 1954, 17(3), 251-259.*
INDX DRUG ADDICTION, PUERTO RICAN-M, ADULTS,
ADOLESCENTS, CROSS CULTURAL, PSYCHO-
PATHOLOGY, MOTHER-CHILD INTERACTION,
CASE STUDY, MALE, KENTUCKY, SOUTH
ABST THIS STUDY OF OVER 100 YOUNG MALE HEROIN
ADDICTS, MOST OF THEM IN THEIR TEENS AND
TWENTIES, WAS CARRIED OUT DURING 1951
AND 1952 IN THE U.S. PUBLIC HEALTH SERVICE
HOSPITAL AT LEXINGTON, KENTUCKY. IT EX-
PLAINS SOME OF THE UNDERLYING PSYCHO-
DYNAMICS OF HEROIN USE FROM A PSYCHI-
ATRIC POINT OF VIEW. THE SUBJECTS WERE
PREDOMINANTLY NEGRO, WITH A FAIR AMOUNT
OF PUERTO RICANS. AMONG THE WHITES,
JEWS AND CATHOLICS OUTNUMBERED PROT-
ESTANTS, MANY OF THEM REARED IN A STRICT,
ORTHODOX FAMILY SETTING. THEY CAME FROM
VARYING BACKGROUNDS, FEW HAD KNOWN
REAL POVERTY, AND MOST HAD EXPERIENCED
SOME SORT OF TROUBLE AT SCHOOL, SHARED
"FAR-OUT GOALS, AND WERE NOT CONTENT
WITH NONWHITE-COLLAR JOBS. A HIGH NUM-
BER CONSISTED OF PROFESSIONAL JAZZ MU-
SICIANS. THE MAJORITY MANIFESTED PRO-
FOUND INTEREST IN MUSIC AND INTELLECTUAL
MATTERS, TENDED TO BE INTROVERTED, SEN-
SITIVE, AND QUIET, AND HAD BEEN REARED BY
OVERPROTECTIVE, DOMINANT, AND INDUL-
GENT MOTHERS. IN THE RARE INSTANCES
WHERE THERE HAD BEEN A MALE FIGURE THIS
WAS MOSTLY A STRICT, DOMINEERING PER-
SON. ALTHOUGH SEEMINGLY DEVOTED TO
THEIR MOTHER, CLOSER EXAMINATION AL-
MOST ALWAYS REVEALED VIOLENTLY HOSTILE
FEELINGS TOWARD THEM. MOST ADDICTS RE-
PORTED LOSS OF LIBIDO WHILE ADDICTED.
EVEN IN SEVERE CASES, WITHDRAWAL WAS
SELDOM ACCOMPANIED BY DEPRESSION. 19
REFERENCES.

ACCN 000488

576 AUTH **FOSTER, G. M.**
TITL RELATIONSHIPS BETWEEN SPANISH AND
SPANISH AMERICAN FOLK MEDICINE.
SRCE *JOURNAL OF AMERICAN FOLKLORE, 1953, 66,
201-217.*
INDX FOLK MEDICINE, HISTORY, SPANISH SUR-
NAMED, SOUTH AMERICA, ESSAY, CENTRAL
AMERICA, CURANDERISMO, CULTURE, DIS-
EASE, HEALTH
ABST DURING THE CONQUEST PERIOD, SPANISH
MEDICINE, BASED ON CLASSICAL GREEK AND
ROMAN PRACTICE WITH MODIFICATION BY
THE ARAB WORLD, BECAME INCORPORATED
INTO THE FOLK PRACTICES OF LATIN AMERICA.
A FLOURISHING BODY OF FOLK BELIEFS ABOUT
THE NATURE OF HEALTH, CAUSES OF ILLNESS,
AND CURING TECHNIQUES COMPOSED OF NA-
TIVE AMERICAN, SPANISH FOLK, AND CLASSI-
CAL MEDICAL ELEMENTS DEVELOPED IN THE
AMERICAS. A DESCRIPTION OF CLASSICAL
CONCEPTS IN SPANISH AMERICAN FOLK MEDI-
CINE, SUCH AS HUMORS AND HERB REME-
DIES, AND NONCLASSICAL RELATIONSHIPS OF
FOLK MEDICINE INCLUDING THE MAGICAL, SU-
PERNATURAL, PHYSIOLOGICAL, AND EMO-

TIONAL CAUSES OF ILLNESS AND THEIR SPECIAL CURES IS PRESENTED. IT IS CONCLUDED THAT THE MEDICAL PRACTICES OF CLASSICAL ANTIQUITY AND CONQUEST SPAIN SURVIVE TO A GREATER EXTENT IN THE AMERICAS THAN IN SPAIN. SPANISH AND SPANISH AMERICAN FOLK MEDICINE PLAYS A FUNCTIONAL PART IN THE LIFE OF PEOPLE AND OFFERS RESISTANCE TO THE ACCEPTANCE OF MODERN MEDICAL SCIENCE.

ACCN   000490

577 AUTH **FRANCESCA, S. M.**
     TITL VARIATIONS OF SELECTED CULTURAL PATTERNS AMONG THREE GENERATIONS OF MEXICANS IN SAN ANTONIO, TEXAS.
     SRCE *AMERICAN CATHOLIC SOCIOLOGICAL REVIEW, 1958, 19, 24-34.*
     INDX ACCULTURATION, CULTURE, MEXICAN AMERICAN, EMPIRICAL, ATTITUDES, CROSS GENERATIONAL, SEX ROLES, FAMILY STRUCTURE, SOCIALIZATION, FOLK MEDICINE, EDUCATION, MARRIAGE, TEXAS, SOUTHWEST, VALUES
     ABST ALTHOUGH IT IS FELT THAT MEXICAN AMERICANS PASS ON THEIR CULTURAL TRADITIONS FROM GENERATION TO GENERATION, IT IS HYPOTHESIZED THAT OVER A PERIOD OF 3 GENERATIONS THE DEGREE OF ACCULTURATION INCREASES AND TRADITIONAL VALUES BECOME LESS IMPORTANT. FORTY-FIVE PARISH FAMILIES, 15 EACH FROM THE 1ST, 2ND, AND 3RD GENERATION, IN SAN ANTONIO, TEXAS, WERE INTERVIEWED CONCERNING FAMILY ROLES AND STATUSES, COURTSHIP AND MARRIAGE, EDUCATION, AND MEDICAL ATTITUDES AND PRACTICES. FINDINGS SUGGEST THAT IN THE 3RD GENERATION THERE IS (1) A TREND AWAY FROM MALE DOMINANCE AND TOWARDS MORE EQUALITY BETWEEN THE SEXES IN THE HOME, (2) MORE PERMISSIVE ATTITUDES CONCERNING SELECTION OF MATE, DATING, LENGTH OF COURTSHIP, AND TOLERANCE OF INTERMARRIAGE, (3) SEX EQUALITY IN ACCESS TO FORMAL EDUCATION, AND (4) THE USE OF SCIENTIFIC MEDICINE OVER THE TREATMENT BY FOLK MEDICINE. IT IS CONCLUDED, HOWEVER, THAT CULTURAL CHANGE WITHIN THIS GROUP IS SOMEWHAT RETARDED DUE TO RESIDENTIAL ISOLATION. GREATER ACCESS TO EDUCATIONAL, SOCIAL, AND RELIGIOUS OPPORTUNITIES WOULD INCREASE THE RATE OF ACCULTURATION AMONG MEXICAN AMERICANS. 3 REFERENCES.
     ACCN 000492

578 AUTH **FRANK, S., & QUINLAN, D. M.**
     TITL EGO DEVELOPMENT AND FEMALE DELINQUENCY: A COGNITIVE-DEVELOPMENTAL APPROACH.
     SRCE *JOURNAL OF ABNORMAL PSYCHOLOGY, 1976, 85(5), 505-510.*
     INDX FEMALE, DELINQUENCY, PUERTO RICAN-M, CROSS CULTURAL, PERSONALITY, COGNITIVE DEVELOPMENT, SELF CONCEPT, DEVIANCE, ENVIRONMENTAL FACTORS, SES, EMPIRICAL, ADOLESCENTS, AGGRESSION, URBAN, EAST
     ABST THREE GROUPS OF BLACK AND PUERTO RICAN INNER CITY ADOLESCENT GIRLS, COM-

PRISED OF 25 DELINQUENTS IN A CITY INSTITUTION, 25 NONDELINQUENTS WHO WERE PARTICIPANTS IN A SETTLEMENT HOUSE RECREATIONAL PROGRAM, AND 16 MEMBERS OF THE SETTLEMENT'S LEADERSHIP TRAINING PROGRAM, WERE ADMINISTERED THE WASHINGTON UNIVERSITY SENTENCE COMPLETION TEST FOR MEASURING EGO DEVELOPMENT. DELINQUENT GIRLS FELL AT LOWER LEVELS OF EGO DEVELOPMENT THAN NONDELINQUENT GIRLS WHEN SCORES WERE COVARIED FOR INTELLIGENCE. DELINQUENT GIRLS WERE MORE LIKELY TO FALL AT THE IMPULSIVE STAGE THAN NONDELINQUENT GIRLS, WHEREAS MORE OF THE NONDELINQUENT GIRLS WERE ABOVE THE SELF-PROTECTIVE STAGE. AN EQUAL NUMBER OF DELINQUENT AND NONDELINQUENT GIRLS WERE AT THE SELF-PROTECTIVE STAGE. THE RELATIONS OF PARTICULAR STAGES OF DEVELOPMENT TO SPECIFIC BEHAVIORS WAS EXPLORED. FIGHTING, IN PARTICULAR, WAS RELATED TO EGO STAGE. 20 REFERENCES. (JOURNAL ABSTRACT)

ACCN   000493

579 AUTH **FREEDMAN, A.**
     TITL THE COMMUNITY MENTAL HEALTH CENTER IN THE INNER CITY: ISSUES FOR THE ADMINISTRATOR.
     SRCE *IN E. R. PADILLA & A. M. PADILLA (EDS.), TRANSCULTURAL PSYCHIATRY: AN HISPANIC PERSPECTIVE (MONOGRAPH NO. 4). LOS ANGELES: UNIVERSITY OF CALIFORNIA, SPANISH SPEAKING MENTAL HEALTH RESEARCH CENTER, 1977, PP. 21-24.*
     INDX ADMINISTRATORS, MENTAL HEALTH, COMMUNITY INVOLVEMENT, ESSAY, CONFLICT RESOLUTION, GROUP DYNAMICS, URBAN
     ABST SINCE 1963 WHEN THE COMMUNITY MENTAL HEALTH CENTER PROGRAM BEGAN, THE CENTERS ENCOUNTERING THE MOST DIFFICULTY HAVE BEEN THOSE IN THE CENTRAL CITY. THE LEADERSHIP OF SUCH CENTERS, PARTICULARLY ADMINISTRATORS AND DIRECTORS, SHOULD BE AWARE OF THE FOLLOWING ISSUES: (1) APPROACHES USED WITH INDIVIDUALS WHO INHABIT THE CATCHMENT AREA; (2) ATTITUDES TOWARD SHARING LEADERSHIP WITH COMMUNITY ORGANIZATIONS; (3) METHODS USED FOR PRIORITIZING COMMUNITY AND CENTER NEEDS; (4) GOALS FOR TRAINING AND SEVICE PROGRAMS; AND (5) METHODS OF PROGRAM DEVELOPMENT AND EVALUATION. SUGGESTIONS FOR DEALING WITH THESE ISSUES ARE DISCUSSED.

ACCN   000494

580 AUTH **FREEMAN, D. M.**
     TITL A NOTE ON INTERVIEWING MEXICAN-AMERICANS.
     SRCE *SOCIAL SCIENCE QUARTERLY, 1969, 49(4), 909-918.*
     INDX RESEARCH METHODOLOGY, MEXICAN AMERICAN, SURVEY, EMPIRICAL, CENSUS, ARIZONA, SOUTHWEST, POLITICAL POWER
     ABST .MEXICAN AMERICAN POLITICAL BEHAVIOR HAS NOT BEEN RESEARCHED BY SURVEY METHODS DUE TO SEVERAL PROBLEMS STATED BY

SOCIAL SCIENTISTS TO BE PECULIAR TO MEXICAN AMERICANS: (1) SPANISH LANGUAGE; (2) POPULATION CONCENTRATED IN MARGINAL COMMUNITIES; (3) CULTURAL DIFFERENCES MARKED AND DIFFICULT TO BRIDGE; (4) COMMUNITIES OFTEN CONTAIN SUBCULTURES REQUIRING SPECIAL SAMPLING TECHNIQUES; AND (5) BELIEF THAT NON-CITIZENS WILL NOT PARTICIPATE IN SURVEYS. THIS STUDY CONDUCTED IN SOUTH TUCSON, ARIZONA, IN 1966 DEMONSTRATES THAT MEXICAN AMERICAN POLITICAL BEHAVIOR CAN BE STUDIED BY SURVEY TECHNIQUES AND THAT THOSE REAL OR IMAGINED OBSTACLES MENTIONED ABOVE CAN BE OVERCOME. 23 REFERENCES. (AUTHOR SUMMARY MODIFIED)

ACCN 000495

581 AUTH **FREUDENBERGER, H. J.**
TITL DEVELOPING A PARAPROFESSIONAL STAFF ENRICHMENT PROGRAM IN AN ALTERNATIVE INSTITUTION AND THIRD GATHERING OF THE NATIONAL FREE CLINIC COUNCIL: WHERE WERE THE PSYCHOLOGISTS?
SRCE *PROFESSIONAL PSYCHOLOGY, 1973, 4(4), 429-433; 434-435.*
INDX ADOLESCENTS, ADULTS, CURRICULUM, DRUG ABUSE, EDUCATION, ESSAY, COMMUNITY INVOLVEMENT, GROUP DYNAMICS, HEALTH EDUCATION, INSTRUCTIONAL TECHNIQUES, MENTAL HEALTH, PARAPROFESSIONALS, PUERTO RICAN-M, SOCIAL SERVICES, THERAPEUTIC COMMUNITY, NEW YORK, EAST
ABST THIS ESSAY DESCRIBES THE FORMATION OF A PARAPROFESSIONAL TRAINING PROGRAM AT S.E.R.A.—A BILINGUAL PUERTO RICAN THERAPEUTIC COMMUNITY FOR DRUG ABUSERS IN THE SOUTH BRONX OF NEW YORK CITY. THE PROGRAM BEGAN INFORMALLY WITH A WEEKLY MEETING OF S.E.R.A. STAFF AND COMMUNITY MEMBERS TO DISCUSS COMMUNITY MATTERS. IN TIME, A BIWEEKLY CLASS SETTING DEVELOPED IN WHICH MEMBERS VOLUNTEERED TO RESEARCH AND TEACH ON A VARIETY OF DRUG, HUMAN SERVICES, AND THERAPEUTIC COMMUNITY-RELATED SUBJECTS. THIS EVOLVED INTO A STRUCTURED, SELF-DETERMINED TEACHING PROGRAM IN WHICH AN EDUCATION ENRICHMENT COMMITTEE DESIGNED A CURRICULUM OF ONE-MONTH CYCLES TAUGHT BY COMMUNITY-MEMBER PARAPROFESSIONALS. SUBJECTS RANGED FROM HUMAN GROWTH AND DEVELOPMENT TO EVALUATION, PLANNING, AND PROJECTION FOR THE FUTURE OF S.E.R.A. THOUGH CLASSES WERE INFORMAL, THERE WERE SPECIFIC REQUIREMENTS—READING LISTS AND INDIVIDUAL AND GROUP ASSIGNMENTS. ENTHUSIASM AND A PERCEPTION OF SUCCESS ON THE PART OF BOTH PARAPROFESSIONALS AND STUDENTS HAD SPECIFIC, POSITIVE RESULTS: MOST OF THE PARAPROFESSIONALS DEVELOPED FORMAL EDUCATIONAL GOALS AND THE STUDENTS APPLIED THEIR NEW LEARNING WITH S.E.R.A.'S YOUTH POPULATION, AS WELL AS WITH GANGS ON THE STREET. THE SUCCESS OF THIS PROGRAM ON A LARGELY SCHOOL DROP-OUT POPULATION POINTS TO

THE VALUE OF SUCH AN APPROACH IN SIMILAR SETTINGS.
ACCN 002081

582 AUTH **FREUDENBERGER, H. J.**
TITL THE DYNAMICS AND TREATMENT OF THE YOUNG DRUG ABUSER IN AN HISPANIC THERAPEUTIC COMMUNITY.
SRCE *JOURNAL OF PSYCHEDELIC DRUGS, 1975, 7(3), 273-280.*
INDX ADOLESCENTS, ANXIETY, ACCULTURATION, EMPIRICAL, COPING MECHANISMS, CULTURAL FACTORS, DELINQUENCY, DRUG ABUSE, FAMILY STRUCTURE, GANGS, MENTAL HEALTH, PEER GROUP, PROGRAM EVALUATION, PUERTO RICAN-M, REHABILITATION, ROLE EXPECTATIONS, SELF CONCEPT, SES, THERAPEUTIC COMMUNITY, URBAN, NEW YORK, EAST, PSYCHOTHERAPY, SEXUAL BEHAVIOR, DEPRESSION, FAMILY THERAPY, POLICY
ABST PERSONALITY DYNAMICS AND FAMILIAL RELATIONSHIPS OF YOUNG HISPANIC DRUG ABUSERS (AGES 12-18) WERE OBSERVED IN A NEW YORK CITY OUTREACH PROGRAM. INITIALLY AT S.E.R.A. (AN HISPANIC THERAPEUTIC COMMUNITY), RELIANCE WAS PLACED ON THE ENCOUNTER AS A TOOL OF TREATMENT INTERVENTION. HOWEVER, BECAUSE THE YOUNG COMMUNITY MEMBERS DID NOT EXHIBIT SUFFICIENT DEFENSE STRUCTURES TO WITHSTAND THE HARD LINE CONFRONTATION METHOD, A CASE CONFERENCE APPROACH WAS ADOPTED—INCLUDING RAP GROUPS, INDIVIDUAL THERAPY SESSIONS, AND FAMILY THERAPY SESSIONS. CHARACTERISTICS OF HISPANIC YOUTH IN SUCH A SETTING ARE NOTED, ALONG WITH THEIR ASSOCIATED MEDICAL AND PSYCHOLOGICAL PROBLEMS. BASED ON THE UNIQUE DYNAMICS AND TREATMENT APPROACH TAKEN AT S.E.R.A. WITH YOUNG HISPANIC DRUG ABUSERS, IT WAS DETERMINED THAT EACH ETHNIC GROUP HAS ITS OWN PERSONALITY TRAITS, FAMILIAL RELATIONSHIPS, AND CULTURAL, LINGUISTIC, EDUCATIONAL, AND ADJUSTMENT-MECHANISM PECULIARITIES TO BE TAKEN INTO CONSIDERATION. IT IS RECOMMENDED THAT A SENSE OF CULTURAL IDENTIFICATION, HISTORY, CUSTOMS, AND PERSONAL NATURE FOR ALL ETHNIC GROUPS BE INCORPORATED IN TREATMENT PROGRAMS FOR YOUNG DRUG ABUSERS. 4 REFERENCES. (NCMHI ABSTRACT MODIFIED)
ACCN 002082

583 AUTH **FRIEDMAN, H. H., & GOLDSTEIN, L.**
TITL EFFECT OF ETHNICITY OF SIGNATURE ON THE RATE OF RETURN AND CONTENT OF A MAIL QUESTIONNAIRE.
SRCE *JOURNAL OF APPLIED PSYCHOLOGY, 1975, 60(6), 770-771.*
INDX CROSS CULTURAL, DISCRIMINATION, EMPIRICAL, PREJUDICE, EAST, NEW YORK, STEREOTYPES, SPANISH SURNAMED, SURVEY
ABST 1,200 TRAVEL AGENTS WERE SENT A QUESTIONNAIRE DEALING WITH TOPICS OF CURRENT INTEREST TO THEM AND SIGNED BY EITHER A JEWISH, HISPANIC, OR ETHNICALLY UNIDENTIFIABLE NAME. (THE NAMES WERE

TESTED FOR ETHNIC IDENTIFICATION AMONG 100 UNDERGRADUATES AT TWO NEW YORK CITY UNIVERSITIES.) IT WAS HYPOTHESIZED THAT IF ETHNIC BIAS EXISTED IT WOULD BE REFLECTED IN SIGNIFICANTLY DIFFERENT RATES OF RETURN AND/OR BY SIGNIFICANTLY DIFFERENT RESPONSES. ANALYSIS OF THE DATA (1,193 RESPONDENTS) SUGGESTED THAT THE ETHNICITY OF THE SIGNATURE HAS NO SIGNIFICANT EFFECT EITHER ON THE RESPONDENTS' RETURNING OF THE QUESTIONNAIRE OR ON THE CONTENT OF THEIR RESPONSES. FUTURE STUDIES INVESTIGATING THE INTERACTION BETWEEN ETHNICITY OF SIGNATURE AND ETHNICITY OF RESPONDENT WOULD BE OF INTEREST, BUT LACK OF SUCH INTERACTIONS IN THE INTERVIEWER DOMAIN SUGGESTS THAT THEY MAY NOT BE OF ANY RECOGNIZABLE SIGNIFICANCE. 5 REFERENCES.

ACCN   002083

584 AUTH   **FRISBIE, P.**
     TITL   ILLEGAL MIGRATION FROM MEXICO TO THE UNITED STATES: A LONGITUDINAL ANALYSIS.
     SRCE   *INTERNATIONAL MIGRATION REVIEW, 1975, 9(1), 3-13.*
     INDX   UNDOCUMENTED WORKERS, IMMIGRATION, MEXICAN, ECONOMIC FACTORS, HISTORY, EMPIRICAL, FARM LABORERS
     ABST   THE RATE OF ILLEGAL IMMIGRATION FROM MEXICO TO THE UNITED STATES ENCOMPASSING THE YEARS 1946 THROUGH 1965 WAS CORRELATED WITH SIX ECONOMIC AND AGRICULTURAL VARIABLES: (1) MEXICAN FARM WAGES; (2) MEXICAN AGRICULTURAL PRODUCTIVITY; (3) AGRICULTURAL COMMODITY PRICES IN MEXICO; (4) U.S. FARM WAGES; (5) U.S. AGRICULTURAL PRODUCTIVITY; AND (6) RATE OF CAPITAL INVESTMENT IN THE U.S. IT IS HYPOTHESIZED THAT THESE ASPECTS OF MEXICAN AND U.S. AGRICULTURE AND ECONOMY ARE A DETERMINANT OF MIGRATION. AS PREDICTED, CHANGES IN MEXICAN FARM WAGES, AGRICULTURAL PRODUCTIVITY AND FARM PRICES ARE INVERSELY CORRELATED WITH CHANGES IN THE RATE OF ILLEGAL MIGRATION. IN ADDITION, THE POSITIVE RELATIONSHIPS BETWEEN MIGRATION AND U.S. FARM WAGES AND AGRICULTURAL PRODUCTION INDICES ARE IN LINE WITH THE HYPOTHESES PROPOSED. THE MOST SIGNIFICANT VARIABLES ARE CHANGES IN AGRICULTURAL PRODUCTIVITY AND PER DIEM WAGES IN BOTH MEXICO AND THE U.S. CLEARLY, THE EBB AND FLOW OF ILLEGAL ALIENS IS AFFECTED BY CHANGES IN THE RELATIVE VIGOR OF AGRICULTURAL ENTERPRISE IN THE TWO COUNTRIES. 15 REFERENCES. (AUTHOR SUMMARY MODIFIED)
     ACCN   000496

585 AUTH   **FRISBIE, P.**
     TITL   MILITANCY AMONG MEXICAN AMERICAN HIGH SCHOOL STUDENTS.
     SRCE   *SOCIAL SCIENCE QUARTERLY, 1973, 53(4), 865-883.*
     INDX   MEXICAN AMERICAN, ADOLESCENTS, CHICANO MOVEMENT, POLITICAL POWER, DIS-

CRIMINATION, PREJUDICE, EMPIRICAL, SES, SEX COMPARISON, SOUTHWEST, URBAN
     ABST   ONE OF THE MORE REMARKABLE ASPECTS OF THE MILITANT EXPRESSION OF DISCONTENT THAT HAS EMANATED FROM THE MEXICAN AMERICAN COMMUNITY SINCE THE STRIKES OF 1965, LED BY CESAR CHAVEZ, TO THE PRESENT, IS THE FACT THAT HIGH SCHOOL STUDENTS HAVE OFTEN BEEN THE VANGUARD. THIS RESEARCH ATTEMPTS TO IDENTIFY SOME OF THE VARIABLES WHICH DIFFERENTIATE MILITANT MEXICAN AMERICAN YOUTH FROM THEIR NON-MILITANT COUNTERPARTS. THE STUDY IS BASED ON QUESTIONNAIRE RESPONSES FROM OVER 2,000 MEXICAN AMERICAN STUDENTS IN TWO SOUTHWESTERN CITY HIGH SCHOOLS. FOUR FACTORS ARE FOUND TO BE SIGNIFICANTLY RELATED TO MILITANCY: (1) PERCEPTION OF ANGLO DISCRIMINATION, (2) EXPECTANCY OF SUCCESS OF MILITANT ACTION, (3) USE OF SPANISH, AND (4) SEX (MALES ARE MORE LIKELY TO DEMONSTRATE A MILITANT ORIENTATION THAN FEMALES). SEVERAL INTERACTION EFFECTS ARE ALSO DISCUSSED; ALL INVOLVE THE EXPECTATION THAT MILITANCY WILL BE EFFECTIVE. 44 REFERENCES. (AUTHOR SUMMARY MODIFIED)
     ACCN   000497

586 AUTH   **FRISBIE, W. P., & NEIDERT, L.**
     TITL   INEQUALITY AND THE RELATIVE SIZE OF MINORITY POPULATIONS: A COMPARATIVE ANALYSIS.
     SRCE   *AMERICAN JOURNAL OF SOCIOLOGY, 1977, 82(5), 1007-1030.*
     INDX   SES, MEXICAN AMERICAN, CROSS CULTURAL, DISCRIMINATION, MIGRATION, URBAN, EMPLOYMENT
     ABST   SOCIOECONOMIC DIFFERENTIALS SEPARATING WHITES AND BLACKS HAVE BEEN SHOWN TO CORRELATE POSITIVELY WITH THE PERCENTAGE OF BLACKS IN A POPULATION. HOWEVER, IN MULTIRACIAL OR MULTIETHNIC POPULATIONS, IT IS NECESSARY TO TAKE INTO ACCOUNT THE EFFECTS OF THE RELATIVE SIZE OF EACH MINORITY PRESENT IN NONNEGLIGIBLE NUMBERS. IN THE RESEARCH REPORTED HERE, THE RELATIONSHIP BETWEEN SOCIOECONOMIC INEQUALITY AND THE PROPORTION OF MEXICAN AMERICANS AND BLACKS IN THE POPULATION OF METROPOLITAN AREAS WAS DECOMPOSED THROUGH PATH-ANALYTIC TECHNIQUES. ANALYSIS OF A MODEL INCORPORATING THE IMPACT OF THE SIZE OF BOTH MINORITIES INDICATES THAT MINORITY INCOME LEVELS ARE INVERSELY RELATED TO MINORITY SIZE AND THAT DISPARITIES BETWEEN MAJORITY AND MINORITY INCOME AND OCCUPATION TEND TO GROW AS RELATIVE MINORITY SIZE INCREASES. MEXICAN AMERICAN OCCUPATIONAL LEVELS VARY POSITIVELY WITH THE PERCENTAGE OF BLACKS, BUT BLACK OCCUPATIONAL STATUS WAS FOUND TO BE VIRTUALLY UNRELATED TO THE PROPORTIONAL REPRESENTATION OF MEXICAN AMERICANS IN METROPOLITAN AREAS. OVERALL, THE POSITIVE RELATIONSHIP BETWEEN MINORITY PERCENTAGE IN THE POPULATION AND THE INE-

QUALITIES OF INCOME AND OCCUPATION PERSISTS IN SPITE OF CONTROLS FOR A NUMBER OF PLAUSIBLE ALTERNATIVE EXPLANATIONS. IT IS THEREFORE CONCLUDED THAT THE RELATIVE SIZE OF THE MINORITY POPULATION IS A SIGNIFICANT PREDICTOR OF INEQUALITY. 38 REFERENCES. (JOURNAL ABSTRACT MODIFIED)

ACCN   000498

587 AUTH   **FUENTES, J. A.**
     TITL   PLEASE DOCTOR, LISTEN TO ME!.
     SRCE   *UNPUBLISHED MANUSCRIPT, 1972. (AVAILABLE FROM AUTHOR, SCHOOL OF HEALTH, LOMA LINDA UNIVERSITY, LOMA LINDA, CALIF.)*
     INDX   PHYSICIANS, CULTURAL FACTORS, HEALTH DELIVERY SYSTEMS, INTERPERSONAL RELATIONS, HEALTH, FATALISM, SEX ROLES, FAMILY ROLES, FAMILY STRUCTURE, RELIGION, BIRTH CONTROL, TIME ORIENTATION, ESSAY, ACCULTURATION, MEXICAN AMERICAN
     ABST   IN AN EFFORT TO FAMILIARIZE DOCTORS WITH THE INFORMATION THEY NEED TO WORK MORE EFFECTIVELY WITH MEXICAN AND MEXICAN AMERICAN PATIENTS, THIS PAPER PRESENTS FOURTEEN CONCEPTS SELECTED FROM RELEVANT LITERATURE ON THE BEHAVIOR OF MEXICAN AMERICANS IN HEALTH AND ILLNESS. AMONG THE CONCEPTS DISCUSSED ARE: (1) DIFFERENCES IN DISEASE ETIOLOGY; (2) ATTITUDES TOWARD ILLNESS; (3) DECISION-MAKING IN ILLNESS SITUATIONS; (4) IMPORTANCE OF ELDERS, RELIGION AND RESPECT IN THE CULTURE; (5) IMPERSONALITY AND SPECIALIZATION IN ANGLO MEDICINE AS BARRIERS TO MEDICAL CARE; AND (6) HOSPITALIZATION AS A FAMILY AFFAIR. IT IS POSITED THAT MEDICAL SERVICES MUST CHANGE, PARTICULARLY IN THE AREAS OF PERCEPTION, COMMUNICATION AND EMPATHY BASED ON KNOWLEDGE AND UNDERSTANDING OF CULTURAL DIFFERENCES IF THEY ARE TO WORK SUCCESSFULLY AND MAKE SENSE TO MEXICAN AMERICAN RECIPIENTS. 17 REFERENCES.
     ACCN   000499

588 AUTH   **FUENTES, J. A.**
     TITL   SOCIO-CULTURAL BARRIERS RESPONSIBLE FOR THE LIMITED ACCEPTANCE AND UTILIZATION OF ANGLO HEALTH FACILITIES AND MEDICAL CARE BY MEXICAN AMERICANS.
     SRCE   *UNPUBLISHED MANUSCRIPT, LOMA LINDA UNIVERSITY, 1972.*
     INDX   ESSAY, RESOURCE UTILIZATION, MEXICAN AMERICAN, HEALTH DELIVERY SYSTEMS, RURAL, URBAN, FOLK MEDICINE, DISEASE, CURANDERISMO, INSTRUCTIONAL TECHNIQUES, HEALTH, CULTURAL FACTORS, POLICY
     ABST   ANGLO HEALTH PROGRAMS HAVE NOT BEEN SUCCESSFUL IN REACHING MEXICAN AMERICANS BECAUSE OF THEIR LACK OF AWARENESS AND UNDERSTANDING OF THIS MINORITYS' CULTURE AND SUBCULTURES. SEVERAL SUGGESTIONS FOR PLANNING AND IMPLEMENTING A PROGRAM FOR MEXICAN AMERICANS WHICH CONSIDERS THE IMPORTANCE OF CULTURAL RESPONSES AND ATTITUDES TOWARD ILLNESS AND TREATMENT ARE

PRESENTED. FACTORS IN BOTH ANGLO AND MEXICAN CULTURES WHICH AFFECT THE PLANNING AND USE OF MEDICAL SERVICES ARE DISCUSSED: (1) CONCEPTS OF HOT AND COLD FOODS IN PRESERVING HEALTH; (2) CATEGORIES OF ILLNESS; (3) SOCIAL AND ECONOMIC FACTORS INVOLVED IN MEDICAL CARE AND DISEASE PATTERN; (4) THE IMPORTANCE OF MODESTY IN TREATMENT; AND (5) A SUMMARY OF MEXICAN AMERICAN CONCEPTIONS OF HEALTH AND ILLNESS. TWENTY-THREE SUGGESTIONS FOR PLANNING A PRACTICAL AND EFFECTIVE PROGRAM ARE PRESENTED. 18 REFERENCES.

ACCN   000500

589 AUTH   **FUNK, S. G., HOROWITZ, A., LIPSHITZ, R., & YOUNG, F. W.**
     TITL   THE PERCEIVED STRUCTURE OF AMERICAN ETHNIC GROUPS: THE USE OF MULTIDIMENSIONAL SCALING IN STEREOTYPE RESEARCH.
     SRCE   *SOCIOMETRY, 1976, 39(2), 116-130.*
     INDX   STEREOTYPES, PUERTO RICAN-M, PERCEPTION, RESEARCH METHODOLOGY, EMPIRICAL, CROSS CULTURAL, MEXICAN AMERICAN, SOUTH
     ABST   ALTHOUGH STRUCTURE IS THE CENTRAL ASPECT OF STEREOTYPE RESEARCH, INVESTIGATORS FAIL TO FOCUS THEIR STUDIES ON THE STRUCTURAL ISSUE. A METHODOLOGY IN STEREOTYPE RESEARCH, INCLUDING AN EXPERIMENTAL PARADIGM AND AN ANALYTIC METHOD IS PRESENTED. THE PARADIGM INVOLVES THE COLLECTION OF THREE DIFFERENT TYPES OF SIMILARITIES DATA CONCERNING ETHNIC GROUPS AND RATING-SCALE ADJECTIVES. THE ANALYTIC TECHNIQUE INCLUDES THE USE AND INTERCOMPARISON OF SEVERAL MULTIDIMENSIONAL SCALING TECHNIQUES. A COMPUTER-ADMINISTERED EXPERIMENT DEALING WITH THE PERCEIVED SIMILARITIES OF SEVERAL ETHNIC SUBGROUPS OF THE AMERICAN CULTURE EXEMPLIFIES THIS APPROACH TO STEREOTYPE RESEARCH. THE RESULTS REVEAL THAT THE UNFOLDING TECHNIQUES YIELDED MORE RICHLY DETAILED CONFIGURATIONS THAN THE METRIC AND NON METRIC MULTIDIMENSIONAL SCALINGS. 32 REFERENCES. (JOURNAL ABSTRACT MODIFIED)

ACCN   000501

590 AUTH   **FURLONG, M. J., ATKINSON, D. R., & CASAS, J. M.**
     TITL   EFFECTS OF COUNSELOR ETHNICITY AND ATTITUDINAL SIMILARITY ON CHICANO STUDENTS' PERCEPTIONS OF COUNSELOR CREDIBILITY AND ATTRACTIVENESS.
     SRCE   *HISPANIC JOURNAL OF BEHAVIORAL SCIENCES, 1979, 1(1), 41-53.*
     INDX   MEXICAN AMERICAN, PSYCHOTHERAPISTS, ATTITUDES, EMPIRICAL, COLLEGE STUDENTS, CALIFORNIA, SOUTHWEST, CROSS CULTURAL, CULTURAL FACTORS, INTERPERSONAL ATTRACTION
     ABST   TWO AUDIO TAPES DEPICTING A COUNSELING SESSION WERE DEVELOPED IN ORDER TO MEASURE HISPANICS' PERCEPTIONS OF THERAPISTS. THE TAPES WERE IDENTICAL, EX-

CEPT THAT IN ONE THE COUNSELOR SUPPORTED CULTURAL ASSIMILATION WHILE IN THE OTHER THE COUNSELOR SUPPORTED CULTURAL PLURALISM. SEVENTY-NINE CHICANO STUDENTS, 55 FEMALES AND 24 MALES, ATTENDING THREE COMMUNITY COLLEGES IN SOUTHERN CALIFORNIA WERE RANDOMLY ASSIGNED TO ONE OF FOUR COUNSELOR INTRODUCTION AND ATTITUDE COMBINATIONS. THESE COMBINATIONS WERE GENERATED BY CROSSING THE TWO TAPE RECORDINGS WITH TWO INTRODUCTIONS—ONE BY AN ANGLO AND THE OTHER BY AN HISPANIC COUNSELOR. STUDENTS WHO PERCEIVED THEIR ATTITUDES AS SIMILAR TO THE COUNSELOR RATED THE COUNSELOR'S CREDIBILITY AND ATTRACTIVENESS MORE FAVORABLY THAN DID STUDENTS WHO PERCEIVED THEIR ATTITUDES AS NOT SIMILAR TO THE COUNSELOR'S. COUNSELOR ETHNICITY AND ATTITUDE ALONE WERE NOT FOUND TO BE RELATED TO THE RATINGS ASSIGNED THE COUNSELOR. 30 REFERENCES. (JOURNAL ABSTRACT MODIFIED)

ACCN   001765

591 AUTH   **GABET, Y. H.**
    TITL   BIRTH ORDER AND ACHIEVEMENT IN ANGLO, MEXICAN-AMERICAN AND BLACK AMERICANS (DOCTORAL DISSERTATION, UNIVERSITY OF TEXAS, AUSTIN, 1971).
    SRCE   *DISSERTATION ABSTRACTS INTERNATIONAL, 1972, 33(1), 190A. (UNIVERSITY MICROFILMS NO. 72-19,587.)*
    INDX   MEXICAN AMERICAN, CROSS CULTURAL, FAMILY STRUCTURE, ACHIEVEMENT TESTING, SEX COMPARISON, CHILDREN, ADOLESCENTS, SEX ROLES, TEXAS, SOUTHWEST, SCHOLASTIC ACHIEVEMENT
    ABST   THE MAJOR PURPOSE OF THIS STUDY WAS TO DETERMINE WHETHER THE TYPICAL "BIRTH ORDER EFFECT" OF HIGHER ACHIEVEMENT OF FIRST-BORN COMPARED WITH SECOND-BORN, FOUND IN ANGLO FAMILIES, WAS EVIDENT IN MEXICAN AMERICAN AND BLACK AMERICAN FAMILIES. THE SUBJECTS FOR THIS RESEARCH WERE 130 SIBLING PAIRS OF STUDENTS IN AN URBAN SCHOOL SYSTEM. THE DEMOGRAPHIC DATA AND ACHIEVEMENT MEASURES WERE AVAILABLE IN THE CUMULATIVE RECORDS OF THE STUDENTS. GRADE-EQUIVALENT SCORES ON THE IOWA TESTS OF BASIC SKILLS ADMINISTERED IN THE FOURTH-GRADE WERE USED AS A MEASURE OF ACHIEVEMENT. A 3X4X2 ANALYSIS OF VARIANCE COMPARED ACHIEVEMENT TEST SCORES OF FIRST-BORN MALES AND FEMALES WITH THE SAME OPPOSITE SEX SECOND-BORN SIBLINGS IN THREE ETHNIC GROUPS—ANGLO, MEXICAN AMERICAN, AND BLACK AMERICAN. AN INTERACTION OF ETHNICITY, SEX AND SEX OF SIBLING, AND BIRTH ORDER WAS SIGNIFICANT. THE "BIRTH ORDER EFFECT WAS EVIDENT IN THE SIGNIFICANTLY HIGHER ACHIEVEMENT OF FIRST-BORN ANGLO FEMALES WHEN COMPARED WITH SIBLINGS OF EITHER SEX. THE REVERSE WAS FOUND FOR FIRST-BORN ANGLO MALES WHEN COMPARED WITH MALE SIBLINGS. MEXICAN

AMERICAN FEMALE FIRST-BORN SCORED SIGNIFICANTLY HIGHER THAN MALE SIBLINGS, AND BLACK FEMALE FIRST-BORN SCORED SIGNIFICANTLY HIGHER THAN FEMALE SIBLINGS. DIFFERENCES BETWEEN OTHER SIBLING PAIRS WERE NOT SIGNIFICANT. IT IS SUGGESTED THAT THE INCONSISTENCY OF THE RESULTS MAY BE EXPLAINED IN TERMS OF CULTURAL DIFFERENCES IN THE SOCIAL ROLES OF EACH SEX. THE INTERACTION OF ORDINAL POSITION AND SEX SUPPORTS MACDONALD'S THEORY OF DIFFERENTIAL LEVELS OF SOCIALIZATION. 87 REFERENCES. (AUTHOR ABSTRACT)

ACCN   000502

592 AUTH   **GAEL, S., GRANT, D. L., & RITCHER, R. J.**
    TITL   EMPLOYMENT TEST VALIDATION FOR MINORITY AND NONMINORITY TELEPHONE OPERATORS.
    SRCE   *JOURNAL OF APPLIED PSYCHOLOGY, 1975, 60(4), 411-419.*
    INDX   JOB PERFORMANCE, EMPLOYMENT, SPANISH SURNAMED, CROSS CULTURAL, CULTURAL FACTORS, TEST VALIDITY, ABILITY TESTING
    ABST   TEN PENCIL-AND-PAPER TESTS WERE VALIDATED AGAINST TELEPHONE OPERATOR PROFICIENCY MEASURED IN SPECIALLY DEVELOPED JOB SIMULATIONS. JOB ANALYSIS INFORMATION PLUS PATTERNS OF VALIDITY COEFFICIENTS FOR A NATIONWIDE SAMPLE (N = 1,091) WORKING IN THREE DIFFERENT TELEPHONE OPERATOR JOBS INDICATED THAT A NUMBER OF BEHAVIORAL DIMENSIONS WERE COMMON TO ALL THREE JOBS. DATA, THEREFORE, WERE COMBINED ACROSS JOBS AND ANALYZED SEPARATELY FOR BLACK, SPANISH SURNAMED, AND WHITE OPERATORS. A COMPOSITE OF THE FOUR MAXIMALLY PREDICTIVE TESTS WAS SIGNIFICANTLY PREDICTIVE OF A COMPOSITE CRITERION FOR ALL ETHNIC GROUPS, BUT LESS SO FOR THE SPANISH SURNAMED. ETHNIC REGRESSION-LINE SLOPES AND INTERCEPTS DIFFERED SIGNIFICANTLY. THE COMMON REGRESSION EQUATION GENERALLY DID NOT UNDERPREDICT MINORITY OPERATOR PROFICIENCY, AND A COMPOSITE TEST CUTOFF, CONSIDERED FAIR FOR MINORITY AND NONMINORITY APPLICANTS, IS RECOMMENDED. 25 REFERENCES. (JOURNAL ABSTRACT)

ACCN   000503

593 AUTH   **GAEL, S., GRANT, D. L., & RITCHIE, R. J.**
    TITL   EMPLOYMENT TEST VALIDATION FOR MINORITY AND NONMINORITY CLERKS WITH WORK SAMPLE CRITERIA.
    SRCE   *JOURNAL OF APPLIED PSYCHOLOGY, 1975, 60(4), 420-426.*
    INDX   EMPLOYMENT, JOB PERFORMANCE, SPANISH SURNAMED, CROSS CULTURAL, CULTURAL FACTORS, TEST VALIDITY, ABILITY TESTING
    ABST   TEN TESTS OF INTELLECTUAL ABILITY AND PERCEPTUAL SPEED AND ACCURACY WERE VALIDATED AGAINST SPECIALLY DEVELOPED CLERICAL WORK SAMPLES WITH A NEWLY HIRED SAMPLE OF 143 BLACKS, 74 SPANISH SURNAMED, AND 195 WHITES. MOST VALIDITY

COEFFICIENTS WERE STATISTICALLY SIGNIFI-CANT, AND IN ONLY 2 OUT OF 36 COMPARI-SONS WERE ETHNIC SAMPLE VALIDITY COEF-FICIENTS SIGNIFICANTLY DIFFERENT. A COMBINATION OF FOUR TESTS WAS SIGNIFI-CANTLY PREDICTIVE OF CLERICAL PROFI-CIENCY FOR EACH ETHNIC SAMPLE AND FOR THE TOTAL COMBINED SAMPLE. COMPARI-SONS OF ETHNIC SAMPLE REGRESSION EQUA-TIONS INDICATED THAT THE SLOPES ARE ES-SENTIALLY THE SAME BUT THAT THE INTERCEPTS DIFFER SIGNIFICANTLY. THE TO-TAL SAMPLE REGRESSION EQUATION DOES NOT UNDERPREDICT PROSPECTIVE PROFI-CIENCY LEVELS FOR MINORITY CLERKS, AND A COMPOSITE PREDICTOR FOUND TO BE APPRO-PRIATE FOR MINORITY AND NONMINORITY AP-PLICANTS FOR CLERICAL JOBS IS RECOM-MENDED FOR EMPLOYMENT OFFICE USE. 17 REFERENCES. (JOURNAL ABSTRACT)

ACCN   000504

594 AUTH   **GALBIS, R.**
TITL   MENTAL HEALTH SERVICE IN A HISPANO COM-MUNITY.
SRCE   URBAN HEALTH, SEPTEMBER 1977, PP. 31; 33-35.
INDX   ACCULTURATION, ADULTS, ADOLESCENTS, AL-COHOLISM, AUTHORITARIANISM, COMMUNITY INVOLVEMENT, BILINGUAL-BICULTURAL PER-SONNEL, CULTURAL FACTORS, DRUG ABUSE, HEALTH DELIVERY SYSTEMS, MENTAL HEALTH, PSYCHOTHERAPY, RESOURCE UTILIZATION, TIME ORIENTATION, EAST, WASHINGTON D.C., ESSAY, PROGRAM EVALUATION, POLICY
ABST   BASED ON HIS EXPERIENCES AS DIRECTOR OF ANDROMEDA (A WASHINGTON, D.C., NEIGH-BORHOOD MENTAL HEALTH CENTER), THE AU-THOR OUTLINES ISSUES AND RECOMMENDA-TIONS FOR MEMBERS OF THE MEDICAL COMMUNITY WHO PROVIDE HEALTH SERVICES TO HISPANICS. FIRST, SPECIAL MENTAL HEALTH PROGRAMS FOR HISPANICS MUST TREAT PA-TIENTS ON THEIR OWN TERMS, AND THEY MUST HAVE A STAFF THAT NOT ONLY SPEAKS THE LANGUAGE FLUENTLY BUT IS WELL VERSED IN THE CULTURE. SECOND, GRASS ROOTS COMMUNITY FACILITIES SHOULD BE MAIN-TAINED AT ALL COSTS, BUT IT SHOULD BE REC-OGNIZED THAT TOO MUCH EGALITARIANISM CAN BREED CHAOS. THESE COMMUNITY SITES SHOULD OPERATE AS MEDICAL FACILITIES, WITH STAFF RESPONSIBILITIES CLEARLY DE-LINEATED AND STRUCTURE MAINTAINED IN RE-CORD-KEEPING AND STANDARD OF CARE. THIRD, SPECIFIC PROBLEMS FACED BY THE AUTHOR'S ANDROMEDA MENTAL HEALTH CEN-TER INCLUDE: (1) PATIENT LACK OF TRUST; (2) PRESENT AND ACTION ORIENTATION; (3) FEAR OF HOSPITALS; (4) THE ELDERLY; AND (5) CRI-SIS INTERVENTION. IT IS CONCLUDED THAT FU-TURE REPORTS ON OTHER ASPECTS OF HEALTH CARE FOR HISPANICS ARE BOTH NEEDED AND ANTICIPATED BY MEMBERS OF THE MEDICAL COMMUNITY CHARGED WITH SERVICE TO THIS PORTION OF THE POPULATION. 5 REFER-ENCES.
ACCN   002084

595 AUTH   **GALLARDO, M. J. (ED.)**
TITL   PROCEEDINGS OF THE CONFERENCE ON EDU-CATION OF PUERTO RICAN CHILDREN ON THE MAINLAND.
SRCE   NEW YORK: ARNO PRESS, 1975.
INDX   ACCULTURATION, BILINGUALISM, COMMUNITY, COMMUNITY INVOLVEMENT, CULTURAL CHANGE, CULTURAL FACTORS, CULTURAL PLURALISM, CULTURE, EDUCATION, EDUCA-TIONAL ASSESSMENT, EMPLOYMENT, ENVI-RONMENTAL FACTORS, EQUAL OPPORTUNITY, INTELLIGENCE TESTING, LANGUAGE COMPRE-HENSION, LEARNING, LANGUAGE LEARNING, PROCEEDINGS, SPECIAL EDUCATION, PUERTO RICAN-M, SCHOLASTIC APTITUDE TEST, SES, BOOK
ABST   ALL THE SESSIONS OF THE CONFERENCE ON EDUCATION OF PUERTO RICAN CHILDREN ON THE MAINLAND, HELD IN PUERTO RICO FROM OCTOBER 18 TO 21, 1970, ARE PRESENTED. THE CONFERENCE FOCUSED ON IDENTIFYING AND DISCUSSING THE PROBLEMS AND SOLU-TIONS OF THE NORTH AMERICAN EDUCA-TIONAL SYSTEMS HAVING LARGE PUERTO RI-CAN POPULATIONS WITH RESPECT TO: (1) THE TRAINING AND RECRUITMENT OF TEACHERS FOR BILINGUAL PROGRAMS; (2) THE TEACH-ING OF ENGLISH AS A SECOND LANGUAGE; AND (3) THE PREPARATION OF SUITABLE DI-DACTIC MATERIALS. 29 SPEAKERS AD-DRESSED THE FOLLOWING TOPICS: (1) CUL-TURAL BACKGROUND OF THE PUERTO RICAN CHILD; (2) TESTING AND PLACEMENT OF SPAN-ISH-SPEAKING CHILDREN; (3) VIEWS OF STATE-SIDE EDUCATORS; (4) OVERCOMING THE LAN-GUAGE BARRIER OF THE SPANISH-SPEAKING CHILD; (5) RECRUITMENT AND TRAINING OF TEACHERS OF ENGLISH FOR SPANISH-SPEAK-ING CHILDREN; (6) PREPARATION OF INSTRUC-TIONAL MATERIALS; AND (7) EFFECTIVE CO-OPERATION OF PUERTO RICAN AGENCIES.
ACCN   000505

596 AUTH   **GALLEGOS, L. L.**
TITL   A COMPARISON OF SOCIAL STUDIES CURRICU-LUM NEEDS AS PERCEIVED BY MEXICAN AMERICAN PARENTS, STUDENTS AND TEACH-ERS (DOCTORAL DISSERTATION, UNIVERSITY OF HOUSTON, 1974).
SRCE   DISSERTATION ABSTRACTS INTERNATIONAL, 1974, 35(12), 7608A. (UNIVERSITY MICROFILMS NO. 75-10,749.)
INDX   EDUCATION, CURRICULUM, ADULTS, TEACH-ERS, ATTITUDES, EMPIRICAL, SURVEY, POLICY, MEXICAN AMERICAN, CULTURAL FACTORS, TEST RELIABILITY, TEST VALIDITY, TEXAS, SOUTH-WEST, ADOLESCENTS
ABST   BASIC CONCEPTS WITHIN THE SOCIAL STUD-IES CURRICULUM CAN PROVIDE THE MEXICAN AMERICAN STUDENT AN OPPORTUNITY TO LEARN THE VARIOUS ACADEMIC AND SOCIAL SKILLS, PROPER CHANNELS, AND SPECIFIC PROCEDURES NECESSARY FOR EFFECTIVE CITIZENSHIP. TO ACCOMPLISH THIS GOAL THE COMPONENTS OF THE CURRICULUM MUST BE DESIGNED TO RELATE TO THE EDUCATIONAL NEEDS OF THE MEXICAN AMERICAN. THERE-FORE, THIS STUDY CONCERNS ITSELF WITH

THE FOLLOWING: (1) DEVELOPING AN INSTRU-MENT TO ASSESS THE PERCEPTION OF SOCIAL STUDIES CURRICULUM NEEDS AS VIEWED BY 9TH GRADE MEXICAN AMERICAN STUDENTS, THEIR PARENTS, AND THE CLASSROOM TEACHER; AND (2) TO COMPARE THE PER-CEIVED DIFFERENCES IN SOCIAL STUDIES CURRICULUM NEEDS AMONG THESE INDI-VIDUALS. A TOTAL OF 192 RESPONDENTS RE-SIDING IN CORPUS CHRISTI, TEXAS, WERE IN-TERVIEWED. SIGNIFICANT PERCEIVED DIFFERENCES AMONG THE RESPONDENTS WERE FOUND IN (1) CONCEPTS AND SKILLS DEALING WITH TIME, LOCATION, AND PLACE-MENT OF EVENTS, (2) ECONOMIC, HISTORICAL, AND POLITICAL CONCEPTS, (3) INTERPRETA-TION, ORGANIZATION, AND COMMUNICATION, AND (4) IDENTIFICATION OF PEOPLE'S SOCIAL AND CULTURAL NEEDS. IT IS SUGGESTED THAT THE PRESENT SOCIAL STUDIES CURRICULUM BE REVISED IN ACCORDANCE WITH THE NEEDS OF THE MEXICAN AMERICAN STUDENT. ALSO, FURTHER RESEARCH SHOULD BE CON-DUCTED TO DETERMINE IF THE RESULTS OF THIS STUDY CAN BE GENERALIZED TO OTHER MEXICAN AMERICAN COMMUNITIES. 54 REF-ERENCES.

ACCN   000506

597 AUTH   **GALLI, N.**
TITL   THE INFLUENCE OF CULTURAL HERITAGE ON THE HEALTH STATUS OF PUERTO RICANS.
SRCE   *JOURNAL OF SCHOOL HEALTH, 1975, 45(1), 10-16.*
INDX   CULTURAL FACTORS, HEALTH, PUERTO RICAN-M, ACCULTURATION, HISTORY, RELIGION, DIS-EASE, NUTRITION, FERTILITY, SEX ROLES, FAMILY ROLES, SEXUAL BEHAVIOR, ESSAY, ESPIRI-TISMO
ABST   THE PROBLEMS OF POOR HEALTH AMONG PUERTO RICANS TODAY ARE COMPOUNDED BY THEIR CULTURAL TRADITIONS. MANY PUERTO RICANS STILL RELY ON FOLK MEDI-CINE TO CURE THEIR ILLS. ASIDE FROM THE UNSOPHISTICATED HEALTH PRACTICES STEM-MING FROM A KNOWLEDGE OF PUERTO RICAN FOLK MEDICINE, THE CULTURAL PHENOME-NON OF SPIRITUALISM PLAYS A SIGNIFICANT ROLE IN RETARDING THE HEALTH STATUS OF THE PUERTO RICAN. PUERTO RICANS WHO VIEW ILLNESS AS POSSESSION BY EVIL SPIRITS WILL CONSULT A MEDIUM OR ESPIRITISTA FOR TREATMENT INSTEAD OF A PHYSICIAN. THE HOT AND COLD THEORY OF DISEASE HAS A PROFOUND INFLUENCE ON THE PUERTO RI-CANS' HEALTH STATUS. IN THE ATTEMPT TO ACHIEVE EQUILIBRIUM OF THE FOUR BODY HUMORS, PUERTO RICANS WILL OFTEN DIS-REGARD A PHYSICIAN'S ADVICE WHICH DOES NOT CONFORM TO THIS THEORY. ALSO, MACH-ISMO, THE CONCEPT OF MALE DOMINANCE AND SUPERIORITY LEADS TO SEXUAL PROM-ISCUITY, OVER-POPULATION, VENEREAL DIS-EASE, FAMILY BREAKDOWN, EARLY MARRIAGE, AND A VARIETY OF HEALTH-RELATED PROB-LEMS. 18 REFERENCES. (AUTHOR SUMMARY MODIFIED)
ACCN   000507

" 598 AUTH   **GALLOIS, C., & MARKEL, N. N.**
TITL   TURN TAKING: SOCIAL PERSONALITY AND CONVERSATIONAL STYLE.
SRCE   *JOURNAL OF PERSONALITY AND SOCIAL PSY-CHOLOGY, 1975, 31(6), 1134-1140.*
INDX   BILINGUALISM, BILINGUAL, INTERPERSONAL RELATIONS, COLLEGE STUDENTS, MODELING, ROLE EXPECTATIONS, CULTURAL FACTORS, CUBAN, FLORIDA, SOUTH, MALE, LINGUISTIC COMPETENCE
ABST   THE EFFECT OF LANGUAGE SPOKEN AND CONVERSATIONAL PHASE ON TEMPORAL AS-PECTS OF SPEAKING STYLE WERE EXAMINED. THIRTEEN MALE CUBAN BILINGUALS CON-VERSED ONCE IN SPANISH AND ONCE IN EN-GLISH; THEIR CONVERSATIONS WERE MONI-TORED TO DETERMINE FREQUENCY AND DURATION OF SPEECH. SUBJECTS SPOKE LONGER AND MORE FREQUENTLY PER TURN IN ENGLISH THAN IN SPANISH, WHICH IS INTER-PRETED AS REFLECTING THEIR IDENTIFI-CATION WITH TWO DIFFERENT SOCIAL GROUPS. RESULTS ALSO SHOWED THAT VARIATIONS IN TURN-TAKING BEHAVIOR, AS A FUNCTION OF CONVERSATIONAL PHASE, WERE THE SAME IN ENGLISH AND SPANISH, WHICH IS INTER-PRETED AS A MANIFESTATION OF LARGER CULTURAL NORMS REGULATING THE PHASES OF CONVERSATION. IN GENERAL TERMS, THE RESULTS INDICATE THAT MEASURES OF TURN-TAKING STYLE ARE POWERFUL TOOLS FOR EX-AMINING THE SOCIAL PSYCHOLOGY OF CON-VERSATION. 22 REFERENCES. (JOURNAL AB-STRACT)
ACCN   000508

599 AUTH   **GALVAN, R. R.**
TITL   BILINGUALISM AS IT RELATES TO INTELLI-GENCE TEST SCORES AND SCHOOL ACHIEVE-MENT AMONG CULTURALLY DEPRIVED SPAN-ISH-AMERICAN CHILDREN (DOCTORAL DISSERTATION, TEXAS TECH UNIVERSITY, 1967).
SRCE   *DISSERTATION ABSTRACTS, 1968, 28(8), 3021A. (UNIVERSITY MICROFILMS NO. 68-01,131.)*
INDX   BILINGUALISM, SPANISH SURNAMED, INTELLI-GENCE TESTING, SCHOLASTIC ACHIEVEMENT, EMPIRICAL, WISC, ACHIEVEMENT TESTING, UR-BAN, SEX COMPARISON, BILINGUAL, TEXAS, SOUTHWEST, CALIFORNIA ACHIEVEMENT TESTS, TEST VALIDITY
ABST   THE RESPONSE OF THE MONOLINGUAL SCHOOL TO SPANISH-SPEAKING MEXICAN AMERICAN CHILDREN IS TO CLASSIFY THEM AS MENTALLY RETARDED OR AS SLOW LEARN-ERS, BASED UPON SCORES ON INTELLIGENCE TESTS THAT ARE GIVEN IN ENGLISH. THIS STUDY INVESTIGATES THE RELATIONSHIP BE-TWEEN INTELLIGENCE SCORES AND SCHOOL ACHIEVEMENT TEST SCORES AS THEY RELATE TO BILINGUALISM AMONG MEXICAN AMERI-CAN CHILDREN. THE SAMPLE CONSISTED OF ONE HUNDRED MEXICAN AMERICAN CHIL-DREN BETWEEN THE AGES OF EIGHT AND TEN YEARS TEN MONTHS FROM THE SAME NEIGH-BORHOOD. THE CHILDREN WERE IN THE THIRD, FOURTH AND FIFTH GRADES OF A DALLAS, TEXAS, ELEMENTARY GRADE SCHOOL; SPAN-ISH WAS THE PRIMARY LANGUAGE IN THE

HOME. STUDENTS WERE ADMINISTERED THE WECHSLER INTELLIGENCE SCALE FOR CHILDREN (WISC) IN ENGLISH AND SPANISH. TEST SCORES FROM THE CALIFORNIA ACHIEVEMENT TEST FORM X WHICH INDICATES THE GRADE LEVEL OF ACHIEVEMENT IN READING, ARITHMETIC, AND LANGUAGE WERE OBTAINED FROM SCHOOL RECORDS. IN EXAMINING THE SCORES BETWEEN BOTH VERSIONS OF THE WISC AND THE CALIFORNIA ACHIEVEMENT TEST THE FINDINGS REVEALED THAT CHILDREN HAD HIGHER SCORES, ESPECIALLY IN THE VERBAL SECTION, WHEN THE TEST WAS ADMINISTERED IN SPANISH. IT IS CONCLUDED THAT ACHIEVEMENT TESTS FOR PREDICTING SCHOOL ACHIEVEMENT ARE NOT A VALID MEASURE FOR BILINGUAL CHILDREN AND PERHAPS NON-VERBAL TESTS OF INTELLIGENCE MIGHT PROVE TO BE A BETTER INDICATOR THAN VERBAL TESTS. 63 REFERENCES.

ACCN   000509

600   AUTH   **GALVIN, J. A. V., & LUDWIG, A. M.**
        TITL   A CASE OF WITCHCRAFT.
        SRCE   *JOURNAL OF NERVOUS AND MENTAL DISEASES, 1961, 133(2), 161-168.*
        INDX   SPANISH SURNAMED, PSYCHOPATHOLOGY, FEMALE, CASE STUDY, ADOLESCENTS, FAMILY THERAPY, COLORADO, SOUTHWEST, FOLK MEDICINE
        ABST   AN EXAMINATION OF THE PSYCHODYNAMICS INVOLVED IN A FAMILY CLAIMING TO BE "BEWITCHED" REVEALS THE UNDERLYING PSYCHOPATHOLOGY OF EACH MEMBER. THE "BEWITCHED" VICTIM IS A 17 YEAR-OLD SPANISH AMERICAN GIRL WHO WAS ADMITTED INTO THE HOSPITAL FOR TREATMENT. THE PATIENT WAS COMPLETELY AMNESIC AS TO WHAT TRANSPIRED DURING THE TRANCES SHE EXPERIENCED; THE INFORMATION WAS SUPPLIED BY HER MOTHER AND STEPFATHER. THE DAUGHTER'S "BEWITCHED BEHAVIOR CEASED WHEN THE VISITS OF THE PARENTS WERE TEMPORARILY STOPPED. INTERESTINGLY ENOUGH, A CLOSER EXAMINATION OF THE PARENTS' BEHAVIOR REVEALS THAT THEY TOO HAD BEEN TERRIFIED BY PECULIAR PERSONAL EXPERIENCES. THE FINDINGS INDICATE THAT FOR ALL PERSONS INVOLVED IN THIS FAMILY, THEIR BEWITCHMENT, WHICH IS SIMILAR TO OTHER HYSTERICAL SYMPTOMS, SERVED AS A SUBSTITUTE GRATIFICATION FOR THEIR INDIVIDUAL AND MUTUAL UNCONSCIOUS STRIVINGS. IN OTHER WORDS, THE BEWITCHMENT REPRESENTED FOR THE GIRL AND HER PARENTS BOTH THE EXPRESSION OF AN UNCONSCIOUS IMPULSE AND THE DEFENSE AGAINST IT. THE FAMILY'S OEDIPAL FEELINGS COULD NOT HAVE BEEN EXPRESSED IN THEIR MUTUAL BEWITCHMENT WITHOUT A FOURTH PERSON (THE AUNT) TO BLAME FOR THEIR UNCONSCIOUS IMPULSE. WITH THIS FAMILY'S BACKGROUND, BELIEFS, AND PSYCHOPATHOLOGY, EVEN IF A WITCH HAD NOT EXISTED, ONE WOULD HAVE HAD TO BE CREATED TO UNLOCK THEIR UNCONSCIOUS SEXUAL FEELINGS. 19 REFERENCES.

ACCN   000510

601   AUTH   **GAMIO, M.**
        TITL   MEXICAN IMMIGRATION TO THE UNITED STATES: A STUDY OF HUMAN MIGRATION AND ADJUSTMENT.
        SRCE   *NEW YORK: DOVER PUBLICATIONS, 1971.*
        INDX   UNDOCUMENTED WORKERS, IMMIGRATION, MEXICAN, DEMOGRAPHIC, EMPIRICAL, CASE STUDY, SES, CULTURE, CULTURAL FACTORS, ATTITUDES, CENSUS, DISCRIMINATION, ECONOMIC FACTORS, RELIGION, POLICY, ACCULTURATION, EMPLOYMENT, MEXICAN AMERICAN, HOUSING, LABOR FORCE, BOOK
        ABST   CONDUCTED IN 1926-27, DURING THE EARLY PHASE OF MEXICAN IMMIGRATION TO THE UNITED STATES, THIS STUDY ADDRESSED FIVE ISSUES: (1) THE NUMBER OF IMMIGRANTS; (2) THEIR SOCIAL CLASS; (3) THEIR PLACE OF ORIGIN IN MEXICO AND PLACE OF SETTLEMENT IN THE U.S.; (4) THEIR SOCIAL AND ECONOMIC CONDITION IN THE U.S.; AND (5) THEIR ASSIMILATION INTO U.S. SOCIETY. THE DATA WERE OBTAINED FROM IN-DEPTH INTERVIEWS WITH IMMIGRANTS PLUS AN EXAMINATION OF SUCH OFFICIAL RECORDS AS POSTAL MONEY ORDERS, IMMIGRATION OFFICE RECORDS, AND U.S. CENSUS REPORTS. INCLUDED ARE 25 TABLES AND 6 MAPS PROVIDING INFORMATION ON POPULATION CHARACTERISTICS AND SETTLEMENT PATTERNS. THE BOOK'S 14 CHAPTERS FOCUS ON THE IMMIGRANTS' INTERRACIAL RELATIONS, CULTURAL BACKGROUND (E.G., FOLKLORE, RELIGION, MUSIC), SOCIOECONOMIC CONDITION (E.G., FOOD, CLOTHING, DWELLINGS), AND ATTITUDES ABOUT THE IMMIGRATION EXPERIENCE. MOREOVER, 6 APPENDICIES OFFER GUIDELINES FOR FIELDWORKERS WHO WISH TO STUDY IMMIGRANTS, ISSUES OF IMMIGRANTS' REPATRIATION, AND A DISCUSSION OF MEXICAN SOCIAL ORGANIZATIONS IN THE UNITED STATES. THE STUDY CONCLUDES, OVERALL, THAT ALTHOUGH THERE ARE SOME ECONOMIC GAINS, THE MEXICAN FARES RATHER BADLY IN THE U.S.; AND EVEN WHEN THE IMMIGRANT BECOMES A CITIZEN, RACIAL PREJUDICE AGAINST HIM CONTINUES AND HIS SOCIAL CONDITION IS SCARCELY CHANGED. THEREFORE, THE AUTHOR FAVORS REPATRIATION OF MEXICAN IMMIGRANTS AND HE OFFERS SPECIFIC RECOMMENDATIONS ON HOW THIS CAN BE ACCOMPLISHED. 134 REFERENCES.

ACCN   001754

602   AUTH   **GANNON, T. M.**
        TITL   DIMENSIONS OF CURRENT GANG DELINQUENCY.
        SRCE   *IN M. E. WOLFGANG, L. SAVITZ, & N. JOHNSTON (EDS.), THE SOCIOLOGY OF CRIME AND DELINQUENCY. NEW YORK: JOHN WILEY AND SONS, 1970, PP. 340-350.*
        INDX   GANGS, ADOLESCENTS, PUERTO RICAN-M, DELINQUENCY, EMPIRICAL, SURVEY, NEW YORK, URBAN, EAST
        ABST   AN ANALYSIS OF DATA CONCERNING STREET CORNER GANGS, PROVIDED BY NEW YORK CITY YOUTH BOARD'S STREET WORKERS, IS PRESENTED. THE AVERAGE GROUP IS THE DEFENSIVE GANG OF ABOUT 35 MEMBERS, 10 OF

WHOM CAN BE CLASSIFIED AS HARDCORE. THE GROUP RANGES IN AGE FROM 13 TO 19 YEARS, IS EITHER PUERTO RICAN OR NEGRO, AND DISPLAYS A RATHER LOOSELY KNIT STRUCTURE, INFORMAL LEADERSHIP, AND SOME RELATIONSHIP TO AN OLDER OR OTHER GROUP. MORE BOYS ARE IN SCHOOL OR EMPLOYED THAN ARE DOING NOTHING. AGGRESSION AS A PRINCIPAL MECHANISM OF GROUP MAINTENANCE HAS CONSIDERABLY DECLINED. GROUP COHESION HAS LESSENED WHILE THE GROUP'S TOLERANCE FOR OTHER FORMS OF DEVIANT BEHAVIOR (E.G., USE OF NARCOTICS) HAS INCREASED. THE BOYS SEEM MOST CONCERNED WITH GETTING A JOB, GETTING AHEAD, OR A GIRL FRIEND'S PREGNANCY, AND EXPRESS A STRONGER DESIRE TO STAY AWAY FROM FIGHTING. GROUP CONFLICTS MOST OFTEN ARE DIRECTED TOWARD MEMBERS OF OTHER GROUPS. THESE ARE USUALLY PROVOKED BY DRINKING, GIRLS, AND NEIGHBORHOOD GROUP DIFFERENCES. AGGRESSIVE SKILLS CONTINUE TO RANK HIGH AS GROUP STATUS SYMBOLS. SIMILARLY, THE GROUPS DISPLAY EXTREME SENSITIVITY TO ANY KIND OF STATUS THREAT. 20 REFERENCES.

ACCN   000511

603 AUTH **GARCIA, A.**
     TITL   THE CHICANO AND SOCIAL WORK.
     SRCE   *SOCIAL CASEWORK, 1971, 52(5), 274-278. (REPRINTED IN M. M. MANGOLD (ED.), LA CAUSA CHICANA: THE MOVEMENT FOR JUSTICE. NEW YORK: FAMILY SERVICE ASSOCIATION OF AMERICA, 1971, PP. 106-114.)*
     INDX   MENTAL HEALTH PROFESSION, DISCRIMINATION, MEXICAN AMERICAN, ESSAY, PROFESSIONAL TRAINING, CULTURAL FACTORS, RELIGION, SOCIAL SERVICES, REPRESENTATION
     ABST   IT APPEARS THAT SOCIAL SERVICE AGENCIES HAVE REMAINED INSENSITIVE TO THE DIFFERENCES BETWEEN THE CHICANO AND ANGLO CULTURES. THE NEEDS, PROBLEMS AND CULTURAL DIFFERENCES OF THE CHICANO ARE DISCUSSED, AND THE CHICANO'S PLIGHT IN TERMS OF EDUCATION, RACIAL, AND CULTURAL STEREOTYPIC OBSTACLES AND PROBLEMS IS DESCRIBED. THE SOCIAL WORK PROFESSION HAS DONE LITTLE TO EASE THE CHICANO'S BURDEN. BILINGUALISM AMONG SOCIAL WORKERS GENERALLY IS NOT CONSIDERED AN ADVANTAGE. IT IS SHOWN HOW SOCIAL WORKERS WHO DO NOT SPEAK SPANISH MAKE THE CLIENT FEEL GUILTY AND INFERIOR FOR NOT KNOWING HOW TO SPEAK ENGLISH. AN EXAMINATION OF THE CHICANO LIFESTYLE IN A HOUSEHOLD REVEALS A PATRIARCHAL FAMILIAL RELATIONSHIP. THE SOCIETAL RACISM AND DISCRIMINATION CONFRONTED BY THE CHICANO MALE IS VIEWED IN THE CONTEXT OF HIS ROLE IN THE FAMILY. RECRUITMENT OF MORE CHICANO SOCIAL WORKERS, SPANISH CLASSES FOR SOCIAL WORKERS, AND REEVALUATION OF ENTRANCE REQUIREMENTS IN HIGHER EDUCATION INSTITUTIONS ARE SUGGESTED. IT IS CONCLUDED THAT IF THE SOCIAL WORK PROFESSION IS DETERMINED TO ERADICATE RACISM AND POV-

ERTY, IT MUST CRITICALLY EXAMINE ITS ROLE IN HELPING THE CHICANO WITH HIS PLIGHT. 1 REFERENCE.

ACCN   000512

604 AUTH **GARCIA, A. B., & ZIMMERMAN, B. J.**
     TITL   THE EFFECT OF EXAMINER ETHNICITY AND LANGUAGE ON THE PERFORMANCE OF BILINGUAL MEXICAN AMERICAN FIRST GRADERS.
     SRCE   *JOURNAL OF SOCIAL PSYCHOLOGY, 1972, 87(1), 3-11.*
     INDX   EXAMINER EFFECTS, CHILDREN, BILINGUAL, EMPIRICAL, MEXICAN AMERICAN, ARIZONA, SOUTHWEST
     ABST   THE INFLUENCE OF EXAMINER ETHNICITY AND LANGUAGE ON THE BAR-PRESSING BEHAVIOR OF 40 LOW SOCIOECONOMIC BILINGUAL MEXICAN AMERICAN (MA) FIRST-GRADE PUPILS IS INVESTIGATED. AN ANGLO AMERICAN (AA) AND AN MA FEMALE EXAMINER INDIVIDUALLY WORKED WITH TWO GROUPS OF CHILDREN, PRAISING THEM IN SPANISH AND THEN IN ENGLISH OR THE REVERSE ORDER DURING TWO EXPERIMENTAL PHASES. IT WAS HYPOTHESIZED THAT PRAISE FROM AN MA ADULT WOULD BE MORE REINFORCING TO AN MA CHILD THAN PRAISE FROM AN AA. FURTHERMORE, IT WAS HYPOTHESIZED THAT PRAISE IN SPANISH WOULD BE MORE REINFORCING TO AN MA CHILD THAN PRAISE DELIVERED IN ENGLISH. RESULTS SHOW THE ETHNICITY MAIN EFFECT AND ORDER BY LANGUAGE INTERACTION ATTAINED SIGNIFICANCE. MA PUPILS PRAISED BY THE MA EXAMINER EXHIBITED HIGHER RESPONSE LEVELS THAN THOSE PRAISED BY THE AA EXAMINER. WHILE EFFECTIVENESS OF SPANISH PRAISE WAS NOT AFFECTED BY ORDER, THAT OF ENGLISH INCREASED WHEN DISPENSED AFTER SPANISH. 31 REFERENCES.

ACCN   000514

605 AUTH **GARCIA, C. S.**
     TITL   ASPECTOS SOCIALES DE LA PSIQUIATRIA Y DEL TRABAJO SOCIAL PSIQUIATRICO. (SOCIAL ASPECTS OF PSYCHIATRY AND OF PSYCHIATRIC SOCIAL WORK.)
     SRCE   *IN J. A. ROSSELLO (ED.), MANUAL DE PSIQUIATRIA SOCIAL. SPAIN: INDUSTRIAS GRAFICAS "DIARIO-DIA", 1968, PP. 499-516. (SPANISH)*
     INDX   PUERTO RICAN-I, MENTAL HEALTH, COMMUNITY INVOLVEMENT, FAMILY THERAPY, CULTURAL CHANGE
     ABST   THE ROLE OF THE SOCIAL WORKER IN THE PUERTO RICAN PROGRAM FOR MENTAL HEALTH IS DISCUSSED IN RELATIONSHIP TO THE PATIENT, HIS FAMILY, AS WELL AS THE COMMUNITY AT LARGE. BECAUSE PUERTO RICO IS PRESENTLY UNDERGOING A PERIOD OF GREAT SOCIAL CHANGE THROUGH THE IMPLANTATION OF NORTH AMERICAN SOCIAL STRUCTURES AND ATTITUDES, IT IS HIGHLY POSSIBLE FOR THE INDIVIDUAL TO BE CONFRONTED WITH A CONFUSION OF ROLES AND CONTRADICTION IN EXPECTATIONS. CONSEQUENTLY, THE SOCIAL ASPECTS OF MENTAL HEALTH HAVE BEEN GIVEN PARTICULAR ATTENTION IN PUERTO RICO IN RECENT YEARS. AS ONE OF THE PRIMARY GOALS OF A MENTAL HEALTH

PROGRAM IS TO RETURN THE PATIENT TO A USEFUL AND ACTIVE ROLE IN SOCIETY, HE SHOULD BE SEPARATED AS LITTLE AS POSSIBLE AND FOR AS SHORT A TIME AS POSSIBLE FROM THE OUTSIDE WORLD. THE SOCIAL WORKER SERVES TO KEEP THE PATIENT INTEGRATED IN SOCIETY BY PROMOTING REHABILITATION PROGRAMS INVOLVING BOTH PROFESSIONALS AND MEMBERS OF THE COMMUNITY. SERVING AS A COUNSELOR FOR FAMILY MEMBERS, THE SOCIAL WORKER ASSURES COOPERATION AND PARTICIPATION OF THE FAMILY IN THE PATIENT'S THERAPY. OF UTMOST IMPORTANCE IS THE INITIATION OF PROGRAMS WHICH DEVELOP PUBLIC AWARENESS OF THE NATURE OF MENTAL ILLNESS. 32 REFERENCES.

ACCN   002275

606 AUTH **GARCIA, C. S.**
     TITL   INVESTIGACION CIENTIFICA EN ADICCION EN PUERTO RICO. (A SCIENTIFIC INVESTIGATION INTO ADDICTION IN PUERTO RICO.)
     SRCE   *IN E. TONGUE, R. T. LAMBO & B. BLAIR (EDS.), PROCEEDINGS OF THE INTERNATIONAL CONFERENCE ON ALCOHOLISM AND DRUG ABUSE, SAN JUAN, PUERTO RICO, 1973. LAUSANNE, SWITZERLAND: INTERNATIONAL COUNCIL ON ALCOHOL AND ADDICTION, 1975, PP. 335-338. (SPANISH)*
     INDX   PUERTO RICAN-I, DRUG ADDICTION, DRUG ABUSE, PROGRAM EVALUATION, ATTITUDES, EMPIRICAL, ADOLESCENTS, ADULTS
     ABST   A PERSONAL ACCOUNT OF THE AUTHOR'S FIVE YEARS IN DEALING WITH THE PROBLEM OF DRUG ADDICTION IN PUERTO RICO IS PRESENTED. IN ORDER TO MEET THE NEEDS FOR STATISTICAL DATA CONCERNING THE EXTENT OF THIS PROBLEM, INTERVIEWS WERE CONDUCTED IN 1968 WITH THE 84 AGENCIES THAT DEALT WITH THIS PROBLEM ON THE ISLAND. IT WAS ESTABLISHED THAT, AT THIS TIME, THERE WERE 6,794 KNOWN ADDICTS. AT THE SAME TIME, DATA WERE COLLECTED IN AN UNSPECIFIED MANNER CONCERNING ATTITUDES REGARDING ADDICTION AND THE GENERAL CHARACTERISTICS OF THE PUERTO RICAN ADDICT. YOUNG PEOPLE DEMONSTRATED GREAT CURIOSITY REGARDING DRUGS, WHILE ADULTS (PARTICULARLY PARENTS) DISPLAYED MUCH FEAR. GENERAL ATTITUDES CONSIDERED PUNITIVE METHODS THE BEST WAY OF DEALING WITH THE ADDICT AND PLACED RESPONSIBILITY AT THE LEVEL OF THE STATE RATHER THAN AT THAT OF THE FAMILY. A PROFILE OF THE TYPICAL DRUG ADDICT IN PUERTO RICO IN 1968 IS GIVEN. HIS AVERAGE AGE IS 25, HE IS SINGLE, HAS A SECONDARY LEVEL EDUCATION, IS USUALLY UNEMPLOYED, AND LIVES AT HOME. IN 1968, THE AVERAGE AGE FOR FIRST EXPERIMENTATION WITH DRUGS WAS 18, A FIGURE WHICH WAS LOWERED IN A 1973 SURVEY TO BETWEEN 14 AND 16. IN THE SAME WAY, WHILE THE ADDICT OF 1968 FIRST BEGAN HIS CONTACT WITH DRUGS THROUGH THE USE OF MARIJUANA, LSD, OR AMPHETAMINES, IN RECENT YEARS THE USE OF HEROIN AS AN INITIAL DRUG HAS STEADILY INCREASED. AN-

OTHER GENERAL CHARACTERISTIC IS THAT THE ADDICT WAS MUCH MORE PROTECTED AND ENCOUNTERED FEWER PROBLEMS DURING HIS EARLY CHILDHOOD THAN HIS OTHER SIBLINGS. THIS IS A POSSIBLE EXPLANATION OF THE INSECURITY HE ENCOUNTERED DURING HIS FIRST YEARS OF SCHOOL. IN DEALING WITH DRUG ADDICTION, IT HAS BEEN SEEN THAT FAMILIES TEND TO DENY THE FACT THAT THIS PROBLEM MAY STEM FROM SITUATIONS WITHIN THE HOME ENVIRONMENT. THEREFORE, THEY DO NOT TAKE PART IN TREATMENT NOR GIVE THE ADDICT MUCH ENCOURAGEMENT. THIS LEADS TO THE HIGH PROPORTION OF ADDICTS WHO BEGIN TREATMENT BUT DROP OUT AFTER A FEW WEEKS. 6 REFERENCES.

ACCN   002085

607 AUTH **GARCIA, E. E.**
     TITL   PRESCHOOL BILINGUALISM RESEARCH PROGRAM (QUARTERLY PROGRESS REPORT GRANT NO. 90-C-262).
     SRCE   *SALT LAKE CITY: UNIVERSITY OF UTAH, DEPARTMENT OF PSYCHOLOGY, NOVEMBER 1974.*
     INDX   EARLY CHILDHOOD EDUCATION, BILINGUAL-BICULTURAL EDUCATION, BILINGUAL-BICULTURAL PERSONNEL, BILINGUALISM, CULTURAL PLURALISM, PARENTAL INVOLVEMENT, PROGRAM EVALUATION, LANGUAGE COMPREHENSION, LINGUISTIC COMPETENCE, LANGUAGE ACQUISITION, LANGUAGE ASSESSMENT, MEXICAN AMERICAN, CHILDREN, UTAH, WEST, MOTHER-CHILD INTERACTION
     ABST   AS A QUARTERLY PROGRESS REPORT FOR AN OFFICE OF CHILD DEVELOPMENT RESEARCH PROJECT CONDUCTED AT A PRESCHOOL IN UTAH ON THE USE OF SPANISH AND ENGLISH BY YOUNG CHILDREN AND THEIR MOTHERS, THIS PAPER INCLUDES AN UPDATE ON THE PROJECTS' PERSONNEL, CONSULTANTS AND EQUIPMENT AND A SUMMARY OF THREE PARTS OF THE RESEARCH IN PROGRESS. THESE ARE: (1) AN INITIAL SPANISH-ENGLISH EVALUATION ON EACH CHILD ATTENDING THE PRESCHOOL USING THE AUDITORY COMPREHENSION TEST; (2) AN ASSESSMENT OF SPANISH-ENGLISH USAGE IN STRUCTURED VS. FREE PLAY SITUATIONS FOR MOTHERS AND CHILDREN; AND (3) HOME RECORDING OF MOTHER-CHILD INTERACTIONS. THE THEORETICAL FRAMEWORK AND LITERATURE REVIEW FOR THE RESEARCH ARE PRESENTED. THE MAJOR OBJECTIVES OF THE RESEARCH PROJECT ARE (1) TO DESCRIBE THE BILINGUAL REPERTOIRE OF THE CHILDREN, (2) TO IDENTIFY THE RELEVANT VARIABLES WHICH INFLUENCE A CHILD'S LEARNING SPANISH AND ENGLISH, AND (3) TO DO AN EXPERIMENTAL ANALYSIS OF THESE IDENTIFIED VARIABLES. SOME PRELIMINARY DESCRIPTIVE DATA ARE GIVEN, BUT ANALYSIS IS NOT INCLUDED. A PROGRAM FOR PRESCHOOL BILINGUAL CHILDREN WHICH DIRECTLY INVOLVES MOTHERS IN AN EARLY CHILDHOOD EDUCATION PROGRAM IS ALSO DESCRIBED.

ACCN   000515

608 AUTH **GARCIA, E. E.**
TITL THE STUDY OF EARLY CHILDHOOD BILINGUAL-ISM: STRATEGIES FOR LINGUISTIC TRANSFER RESEARCH.
SRCE *IN J. L. MARTINEZ, JR. (ED.), CHICANO PSY-CHOLOGY. NEW YORK: ACADEMIC PRESS, 1977, PP. 141-151.*
INDX RESEARCH METHODOLOGY, BILINGUALISM, GRAMMAR, PHONOLOGY, SEMANTICS, SYN-TAX, REVIEW, MEXICAN AMERICAN, CHILDREN, LINGUISTICS, LINGUISTIC COMPETENCE, CALI-FORNIA, SOUTHWEST
ABST THREE STRATEGIES FOR RESEARCH IN BILIN-GUAL TRANSFER ARE DISCUSSED: (1) LONGI-TUDINAL LANGUAGE ACQUISITION RESEARCH COMBINED WITH LINGUISTIC ERROR ANALY-SIS; (2) "NO DIFFERENCE" RESEARCH WHICH COMPARES MONOLINGUALS TO BILINGUALS WITHIN A SERIES OF LINGUISTIC TASKS; AND (3) "LANGUAGE MANIPULATION" RESEARCH WHICH CALLS FOR SPECIFIC LINGUISTIC MA-NIPULATION OF ONE LANGUAGE AND THE CONCOMITANT ASSESSMENT OF THE MANIPU-LATION ON A SECOND LANGUAGE. EXAMPLES OF THE "NO DIFFERENCE" AND "LANGUAGE MANIPULATION" RESEARCH ARE PRESENTED IN DETAIL. DATA GATHERED IN PHONEME AND SYNTAX TASKS WITH 60 BILINGUAL OR MONOLINGUAL CHILDREN AND IN A SYN-TAX SCREENING TEST WITH 3 BILINGUAL CHIL-DREN ARE ALSO PRESENTED. THE USE OF THESE APPROACHES SHOULD BE VALUABLE IN OBTAINING MUCH NEEDED INFORMATION DEALING WITH BILINGUAL ACQUISITION DUR-ING EARLY CHILDHOOD. 12 REFERENCES. (AU-THOR SUMMARY MODIFIED)
ACCN 000516

609 AUTH **GARCIA, E. E., TRUJILLO, A., & LEBLANC, L.**
TITL SPANISH-ENGLISH IMITATION AND COMPRE-HENSION IN SPANISH-ENGLISH BILINGUAL PRESCHOOL CHILDREN.
SRCE *UNPUBLISHED MANUSCRIPT, UNDATED. (AVAIL-ABLE FROM DR. E. E. GARCIA, DEPARTMENT OF PSYCHOLOGY, UNIVERSITY OF CALIFORNIA, SANTA BARBARA, CA.)*
INDX LINGUISTICS, LANGUAGE COMPREHENSION, LINGUISTIC COMPETENCE, PHONOLOGY, SYN-TAX, GRAMMAR, CHILDREN, MEXICAN AMERI-CAN, BILINGUALISM, EMPIRICAL, UTAH, SOUTHWEST, LANGUAGE ACQUISITION
ABST THREE LINGUISTIC TASKS—PHONEME, SYN-TAX AND AUDITORY COMPREHENSION—WERE INVESTIGATED TO MEASURE THE PARALLEL DEVELOPMENT OF SPANISH AND ENGLISH IN PRESCHOOL CHILDREN AT LA ESCUELITA IN UTAH. DESCRIPTIVE DATA INDICATE THAT THE CHILDREN UNDERSTAND MORE ENGLISH THAN SPANISH, ALTHOUGH SPANISH COMPREHEN-SION IS NOT AT ZERO LEVELS. IT IS CON-CLUDED THAT LANGUAGE DEVELOPMENT IS FAR MORE PRONOUNCED IN ENGLISH THAN SPANISH IN SYNTACTIC IMITATION AND COM-PREHENSION, ALTHOUGH THE ABILITY TO IMI-TATE PHONETIC STRUCTURES IS ABOUT EQUAL IN EACH LANGUAGE. THESE DATA WHEN COM-BINED WITH ACTUAL LINGUISTIC SAMPLES FROM TESE CHILDREN AND OTHERS FROM

DIFFERENT GEOGRAPHICAL POPULATIONS WILL BEGIN TO PROVIDE A BASIC UNDERSTANDING OF BILINGUAL DEVELOPMENT IN YOUNG CHIL-DREN. (AUTHOR SUMMARY MODIFIED)
ACCN 000517

610 AUTH **GARCIA, F. C.**
TITL THE POLITICAL WORLD OF THE CHICANO CHILD.
SRCE *PAPER PRESENTED AT THE ANNUAL MEETING OF THE AMERICAN POLITICAL SCIENCE ASSO-CIATION, NEW ORLEANS, LA., SEPTEMBER 1973. (ERIC DOCUMENT REPRODUCTION SERVICE NO. ED 101 905)*
INDX MEXICAN AMERICAN, POLITICS, CHILDREN, ESSAY, CROSS CULTURAL, COGNITIVE DEVEL-OPMENT, SELF CONCEPT, CULTURE
ABST CHICANOS COMPRISE BOTH THE OLDEST AND NEWEST MINORITY IN THE UNITED STATES, WITH THE LARGEST NUMBER BEING SECOND AND THIRD GENERATION. THEY ARE CHARAC-TERIZED BY GREAT INTRA-GROUP DIVERSITY ALONG GENERATIONAL, LOCATIONAL, SOCIO-ECONOMIC, AND ACCULTURATIONAL LINES. THERE IS ALSO EVIDENCE OF INCREASING DIF-FERENTIATION IN SOCIAL RELATIONS WITH NON-CHICANOS, IN FAMILY PATTERNS, AND IN THE MAINTENANCE OF CULTURAL DISTINC-TIVENESS. YET CHICANOS SHARE TO VARYING DEGREES SOME COMMON ELEMENTS OF HIS-TORY, CULTURE, "BLOOD," AND POSITION RELATIVE TO THE AMERICAN CORE CULTURE. THE POLITICAL EXPERIENCES OF A MEXICAN AMERICAN YOUNGSTER ARE DIFFERENT FROM THOSE OF HIS CORE CULTURE COUNTERPART. HIS POLITICAL WORLD IS MORE "LOCALLY CIR-CUMSCRIBED" THAN THAT OF CORE CULTURE CHILDREN. THE CHICANO'S POLITICAL DEVEL-OPMENT IS INFLUENCED BY THREE COMPLEX AND INTERRELATED PHENOMENA: (1) HIS CUL-TURAL VALUES: (2) HIS CONTACTS WITH THE DOMINANT CORE CULTURE; AND (3) HIS SO-CIETAL POSITION WHICH RESULTS FROM BOTH HIS CULTURAL VALUES AND HIS CONTACTS WITH THE DOMINANT CORE CULTURE. HIS PO-LITICAL DEVELOPMENT IS ALSO INFLUENCED BY COLONIALISM, HIS PHYSICAL DISTINCTIVE-NESS, HIS LANGUAGE, THE SCHOOL, THE LO-CAL COMMUNITY (BARRIO), AUTHORITY RELA-TIONS, AND HIS FAMILY. 51 REFERENCES. (RIE ABSTRACT)
ACCN 000518

611 AUTH **GARCIA, J.**
TITL INTELLIGENCE TESTING: QUOTIENTS, QUOTAS AND QUACKERY.
SRCE *IN J. L. MARTINEZ, JR. (ED.), CHICANO PSY-CHOLOGY. NEW YORK: ACADEMIC PRESS, 1977, PP. 197-212.*
INDX INTELLIGENCE TESTING, INTELLIGENCE, TEST VALIDITY, WISC, COGNITIVE DEVELOPMENT, SEX COMPARISON, PREJUDICE, DISCRIMINATION, CULTURAL FACTORS, PROFESSIONAL TRAIN-ING, EDUCATION, CULTURAL PLURALISM, CROSS CULTURAL, ESSAY, POLICY
ABST VARIOUS BIASES ARE REFLECTED IN THE NA-TURE OF TESTS THAT PROFESS TO REPRESENT VALID AND RELIABLE MEASURES OF INTELLI-GENCE. MODERN TESTING PROCEDURES AND

CRITERIA ARE BASED ON PREJUDICIAL AS-SUMPTIONS AND THEREFORE DO NOT REPRE-SENT VALID MEASUREMENTS FOR MEMBERS OF MINORITY GROUPS. THE FOLLOWING PREMISES ARE PRESENTED: (1) RACE AND IN-TELLIGENCE IS A POLEMIC, NOT A RESEARCH ISSUE; (2) ETHNIC DIFFERENCES IN IQ ARE NOT POSSIBLE; (3) INTELLIGENCE TESTS CHANGE OVER AGE AND TIME; (4) RACE IQ RESEARCH RESTS ON PREJUDICED ASSUMPTIONS; (5) IQ IS NOT AN INHERITED TRAIT; (6) INTELLIGENCE AND RACE IS A NUMBER GAME PLAYED FOR FAME AND PROFIT; AND (7) SINCE QUOTAS AL-READY EXIST IN ALL COLLEGES, GRADUATE SCHOOLS AND PROFESSIONS, A LOTTERY IS A MORE REASONABLE WAY TO SELECT CANDI-DATES. IT IS CONCLUDED THAT IN AN UNFAIR SOCIETY, TESTS THAT ARE UNFAIR ARE CON-SIDERED VALID. 22 REFERENCES.

ACCN   000519

612 AUTH   **GARCIA, J.**
     TITL   IQ: THE CONSPIRACY.
     SRCE   *PSYCHOLOGY TODAY, SEPTEMBER 1972, PP. 42-43; 92; 94.*
     INDX   INTELLIGENCE, INTELLIGENCE TESTING, ES-SAY, CROSS CULTURAL, RESEARCH METHOD-OLOGY, SEX COMPARISON, SEX ROLES, POLICY, TEST VALIDITY, STANFORD-BINET INTELLI-GENCE TEST
     ABST   EVOLUTION OF THE STANFORD-BINET TEST OF INTELLIGENCE AS A STANDARDIZED MEASURE OF "GENERAL INTELLIGENCE" IS EXAMINED. THE INTELLIGENCE QUOTIENT IS A SOCIAL CONTRACT BETWEEN EDUCATORS AND PSY-CHOMETRICIANS. THE RELATIVE INTELLI-GENCE OF DIFFERENT BIOSOCIAL GROUPS HAS GIVEN IQ A MEANING AND EXISTENCE THAT IGNORES THE VERY REAL LIMITS OF MENTAL MEASUREMENT TECHNIQUES. THAT IS, THE DESIGNERS OF IQ TESTS BUILT INTO THEM SOME INTRINSIC ASSUMPTIONS (BIASES AND LIMITATIONS) THAT MAKE THE TESTS USE-LESS FOR COMPARING THE INTELLIGENCE OF SOME BIOSOCIAL GROUPS (E.G., BLACKS AND CHICANOS). BINET CONCEPTUALIZED HIS TEST OF INTELLIGENCE ON THE ASSUMPTION OF A SINGLE "GENERAL INTELLIGENCE" FACTOR WHICH IMMEDIATELY AFFECTED THE CHOICE OF INDIVIDUAL ITEMS USED FOR QUESTIONS. THE STANFORD-BINET, HOWEVER, TESTS "SCHOLASTIC PERFORMANCE INTELLIGENCE" AND NOT "GENERAL INTELLIGENCE." THE STANDARDIZATION OF THE STANFORD-BINET TEST INCLUDED A SINGLE BIOSOCIAL GROUP OF WHITE ENGLISH-SPEAKING CHILDREN. THUS, THE STANFORD-BINET BECAME AN AN-GLOCENTRIC IQ TEST. THE PSYCHOMETRI-CIANS ALSO SUPPRESSED THE EFFECTS OF THE MATURING OF THE INTELLECT FACTOR. THE DESIGNERS ELIMINATED ANY ITEM THAT DID NOT SHOW A SIMPLE AGE-DEPENDENT PERFORMANCE IMPROVEMENT. EACH TIME THEY NARROWED THE RANGE OF ACCEPT-ABLE QUESTIONS THE CONCEPT OF INTELLI-GENCE DIMINISHED. THE NOTION THAT A SINGLE GENERAL INTELLIGENCE EXISTS INDE-PENDENT OF ENVIRONMENT IS INVALID. THE

USE OF IQ DATA FOR GROUP COMPARISONS CHANGES THE SOCIAL CONTRACT INTO A SO-CIAL CONSPIRACY THROUGH WHICH PARTICU-LAR GROUPS ARE LABELED INFERIOR, THEREBY PROPAGATING THE STATUS QUO. 10 REFER-ENCES.

ACCN   000520

613 AUTH   **GARCIA, J. A.**
     TITL   CHICANO VOTING PATTERNS IN SCHOOL BOARD ELECTIONS: BLOC VOTING AND INTERNAL LINES OF SUPPORT FOR CHICANO CANDI-DATES.
     SRCE   *ATISBOS: JOURNAL OF CHICANO RESEARCH, WINTER 1976-1977, PP. 1-14.*
     INDX   ECONOMIC FACTORS, EMPIRICAL, MEXICAN AMERICAN, POLITICAL POWER, POLITICS, SES, ARIZONA, SOUTHWEST
     ABST   CHICANO SCHOOL BOARD ELECTORAL BE-HAVIOR WAS EXAMINED IN THE TUCSON MET-ROPOLITAN AREA TO DOCUMENT THE PRES-ENCE OF BLOC VOTING BY CHICANO VOTERS FOR CHICANO CANDIDATES, AND WHETHER OR NOT BLOC VOTING REPRESENTED UNIFIED SUPPORT FOR CHICANO CANDIDATES. THE VOTING BEHAVIOR OF 18 CITY PRECINCTS EN-COMPASSING THE 25-30% CHICANO POPULA-TION OF TUCSON WAS EVALUATED. TO ILLUS-TRATE THE PRESENCE OF BLOC VOTING, THE 1972 AND 1974 SCHOOL BOARD ELECTORATE WAS ANALYZED BY FOUR SOCIOPOLITICAL VARIABLES: (1) SOCIOECONOMIC STATUS; (2) PERCENTAGE OF DEMOCRATS PER PRECINCT; (3) PERCENT SPANISH SURNAME; AND (4) TUR-NOUT RATE. ALTHOUGH BLOC VOTING DID EX-IST, THE NEGATIVE CORRELATIONS OF REGIS-TRATION AND TURNOUT WITH CHICANO PRECINCTS RAISED QUESTIONS ABOUT THE FULL EFFECTIVENESS OF BLOC VOTING. STEP-WISE REGRESSION WAS UTILIZED TO ASSESS THE RELATIVE STRENGTHS OF CLASS MEM-BERSHIP AND PARTISANSHIP ON VOTING BE-HAVIOR REGARDING TWO CHICANO CANDI-DATES. THE EXISTENCE OF INTERNAL VARIATION OF CHICANO SUPPORT OF VARIOUS CHICANO CANDIDATES INDICATES A NEED TO LOOK AT THE DIVERSITY OF CHICANO VOTERS WHEN SELECTING AMONG SEVERAL CHICANO CAN-DIDATES. 18 REFERENCES.

ACCN   002086

614 AUTH   **GARCIA, M., & LEGA, L. I.**
     TITL   DEVELOPMENT OF A CUBAN ETHNIC IDENTITY QUESTIONNAIRE.
     SRCE   *HISPANIC JOURNAL OF BEHAVIORAL SCI-ENCES, 1979, 1(3), 247-261.*
     INDX   CUBAN, ETHNIC IDENTITY, RESEARCH METH-ODOLOGY, FLORIDA, NEW JERSEY, SOUTH, EAST, SPANISH SURNAMED, TEST VALIDITY, TEST RELIABILITY, EMPIRICAL
     ABST   THE METHODOLOGICAL AND STATISTICAL PROCEDURES USED FOR DEVELOPING AN 8-ITEM CUBAN BEHAVIORAL IDENTITY QUES-TIONNAIRE (CBIQ) ARE REPORTED. THE ORIGI-NAL INSTRUMENT CONSISTED OF 38 ITEMS AND WAS ADMINISTERED IN TWO SCREENING PHASES TO 272 RESPONDENTS. THE FIRST SCREENING SAMPLE INCLUDED 106 CUBANS

IN FLORIDA AND NEW JERSEY AND 24 NON-CU-BAN HISPANICS IN NEW JERSEY. THE SECOND SCREENING SAMPLE INCLUDED 104 CUBANS IN FLORIDA AND NEW JERSEY AND 38 NON-CU-BAN HISPANICS IN NEW JERSEY. THE ITEMS WERE SUBJECTED TO A ONE-WAY MULTIVAR-IATE ANALYSIS OF VARIANCE (MANOVA). BY THIS MEANS, 8 ITEMS WERE IDENTIFIED WHICH ACCOUNTED FOR 68% OF THE VARIANCE IN SELF-REPORTED LEVEL OF "CUBANNESS" AND SUCCESSFULLY CLASSIFIED 94% OF THE CASES INTO CUBAN AND NON-CUBAN HISPANIC ETH-INIC GROUPS. THESE 8 ITMES ARE ANSWERA-BLE IN A 7-POINT, LIKERT-SCALE FORMAT, AND THEY PERTAIN TO (1) THE FREQUENCY WITH WHICH RESPONDENTS ENGAGE IN SEVERAL ETHNIC BEHAVIORS, AND (2) THE DEGREE TO WHICH THEY ARE FAMILIAR WITH CUBAN IDIO-MATIC EXPRESSIONS AND CUBAN ARTISTS/MUSICIANS. FACTORIALLY, THE ITEMS GROUP INTO A SINGLE INTERPRETABLE FACTOR WHICH ACCOUNTS FOR 89.5% OF THE COMMON FAC-TOR VARIANCE. AT THE SAME TIME, THE IN-STRUMENT DEMONSTRATES A HIGH DEGREE OF INTERNAL CONSISTENCY (ALPHA .84). A COPY OF THE 8-ITEM, FINAL VERSION OF THE CBIQ COMPLETES THE REPORT. 13 REFER-ENCES. (JOURNAL ABSTRACT MODIFIED)

ACCN   001766

615 AUTH   **GARCIA, R. L.**
     TITL   MEXICAN AMERICAN BILINGUALISM AND EN-GLISH LANGUAGE DEVELOPMENT.
     SRCE   *JOURNAL OF DEVELOPMENTAL READING, 1974, 17(6), 467-472.*
     INDX   BILINGUALISM, MEXICAN AMERICAN, LINGUIS-TICS, LINGUISTIC COMPETENCE, SCHOLASTIC ACHIEVEMENT, REVIEW
     ABST   THEORIES ON THE RELATIONSHIP BETWEEN LANGUAGE DEVELOPMENT AND BILINGUAL-ISM HAVE SUPPORTED TWO DIVERGENT THEMES. ONE PROPOSES THAT BILINGUALISM HAS A NEGATIVE EFFECT UPON LANGUAGE DEVELOPMENT TO THE EXTENT THAT BILIN-GUALISM IS BELIEVED TO CAUSE RETARDA-TION IN READING AND LANGUAGE ACHIEVE-MENT. THE OTHER THEME PROPOSES THAT BILINGUALISM HAS A POSITIVE EFFECT UPON LANGUAGE DEVELOPMENT AS IT ENHANCES READING AND LANGUAGE SKILLS IN THE BI-LINGUAL. RECENT RESEARCH REPORTS THAT BILINGUALISM DOES NOT HAVE A NEGATIVE EFFECT UPON LANGUAGE DEVELOPMENT WHEN SOCIO-ENVIRONMENTAL FACTORS ARE CONTROLLED OR ACCOUNTED. RESEARCH ON THE SYNTACTIC DEVELOPMENT OF BILINGUAL CHICANO YOUNGSTERS DOES NOT AFFECT THE CHICANO'S ENGLISH LANGUAGE DEVEL-OPMENT. ALTHOUGH GENERALIZATIONS ARE PREMATURE, IT CAN BE CONCLUDED THAT BI-LINGUALISM, PER SE, IS NOT DETRIMENTAL TO THE CHICANO'S ENGLISH LANGUAGE DEVEL-OPMENT AND THAT REASONS FOR THE CHI-CANO'S READING AND LANGUAGE DIFFICUL-TIES MUST BE SOUGHT AMONG OTHER FACTORS-PROBABLY SOCIO-ENVIRONMENTAL, CULTURAL OR MOTIVATIONAL. 11 REFER-ENCES. (AUTHOR SUMMARY MODIFIED)

ACCN   000521

616 AUTH   **GARCIA-BAHNE, B.**
     TITL   LA CHICANA AND THE CHICANO FAMILY.
     SRCE   *IN R. SANCHEZ & R. M. CRUZ (EDS.), ESSAYS ON LA MUJER, (ANTHOLOGY NO. 1). LOS ANGE-LES: UNIVERSITY OF CALIFORNIA, CHICANO STUDIES CENTER, 1977, PP. 30-47.*
     INDX   FEMALE, FAMILY STRUCTURE, FAMILY ROLES, SEX ROLES, ECONOMIC FACTORS, SES, SO-CIALIZATION, ESSAY, THEORETICAL, LABOR FORCE, CAPITALISM, STEREOTYPES, SOCIAL SCIENCES, MARXIAN THEORY, ATTITUDES, MEXICAN AMERICAN, CONFORMITY, CULTURAL FACTORS, SOCIAL MOBILITY, SOCIAL STRUC-TURE, AUTHORITARIANISM
     ABST   CONTEMPORARY LITERATURE CONTINUES TO FIND EXPLANATIONS FOR THE SOCIOECO-NOMIC CONDITIONS OF CHICANOS IN THE GROUP'S LIFE STYLE, CULTURAL VALUES, AND FAMILY STRUCTURE. THIS ARTICLE DEVELOPS A MORE INTERACTIONAL PERSPECTIVE BY FO-CUSING ON THE IMPACT OF SOCIAL STRATIFI-CATION AND LOWER SOCIOECONOMIC STA-TUS ON THE CHICANO FAMILY. SEVERAL CONSIDERATIONS ARE TAKEN INTO ACCOUNT: (1) THE FUNCTION AND DYNAMICS OF THE FAMILY AS THE MAIN VEHICLE OF GROUP AND PERSONAL IDENTITY; (2) THE FAMILY AS AN ECONOMIC UNIT WHOSE FUNCTION IS THE RE-PRODUCTION AND MAINTENANCE OF LABOR POWER; AND (3) THE FAMILY AS AN INSTRU-MENT OF SOCIAL CONTROL. ALTHOUGH IT HAS BEEN SUGGESTED THAT QUALITIES OF PATERNALISM, AUTHORITARIANISM, LOW LEV-ELS OF ASPIRATION, FATALISM, FEMALE PAS-SIVITY, AND MALE DOMINATION ARE INHERENT IN CHICANO CULTURE, THESE PATTERNS ARE LARGELY DETERMINED BY THE SOCIOECO-NOMIC POSITION OF THE FAMILY. SECONDLY, SUCH STEREOTYPIC CHARACTERISTICS MUST BE EXAMINED IN LIGHT OF BOTH THEIR POSI-TIVE AND NEGATIVE FUNCTIONAL ASPECTS. FI-NALLY, SPECIAL ATTENTION IS GIVEN TO THE ECONOMIC EXPLOITATION OF WOMEN AND THEIR RESULTING SOCIOECONOMIC VULNER-ABILITY. CHICANAS HAVE FEW ROLE MODELS FOR AN INDEPENDENT LIFE STYLE AND MUST STRUGGLE BETWEEN MEETING TRADITIONAL EXPECTATIONS AND DEVELOPMENT OF THEIR OWN CAPABILITIES. IT IS CONCLUDED THAT A FAMILY STRUCTURE WHICH FULFILLS THE BA-SIC NEEDS OF CHICANOS AND SIMULTANE-OUSLY PROMOTES INDEPENDENCE AND SO-CIOPOLITICAL AWARENESS WOULD PRODUCE ASSERTIVE, PARTICIPATORY INDIVIDUALS WHOSE EFFORTS COULD ALLEVIATE THE PRESENT SOCIOECONOMIC POSITION OF THE CHICANO. 8 REFERENCES.

ACCN   002087

617 AUTH   **GARCIA-ESTEVE, J., & SHAW, M. E.**
     TITL   RURAL AND URBAN PATTERNS OF RESPONSI-BILITY ATTRIBUTION IN PUERTO RICO.
     SRCE   *JOURNAL OF SOCIAL PSYCHOLOGY, 1968, 74(2), 143-149.*
     INDX   ATTRIBUTION OF RESPONSIBILITY, PUERTO RI-

CAN-I, CHILDREN, EMPIRICAL, URBAN, RURAL, ADOLESCENTS, FAMILY ROLES

ABST ATTRIBUTION OF RESPONSIBILITY (AR) STUDIED IN PUERTO RICAN SUBCULTURES WAS FOUND TO BE GREATER AMONG RURAL SUBJECTS THAN URBAN. THE 176 SUBJECTS WERE DIVIDED INTO FOUR AGE GROUPS, THE YOUNGEST OF WHICH (7 YEARS) WAS FOUND TO HAVE THE GREATEST AR. THREE CHARACTERISTICS OF AN OUTCOME SITUATION WERE PRESENTED: QUALITY, INTENSITY, AND LEVELS OF CAUSALITY. NO SIGNIFICANT DIFFERENCES WERE FOUND IN OUTCOME VARIABLES BETWEEN PUERTO RICAN AND AMERICAN URBAN POPULATIONS; DIFFERENCES SEEMED TO CORRESPOND TO DIFFERENT PRACTICES WITHIN THE FAMILY. 8 REFERENCES.

ACCN 000522

618 AUTH **GARCIA-MANZANEDO, H. B.**
TITL MOTHER, CHILD AND CULTURE: SELECTED PROBLEMS IN MATERNAL AND CHILD HEALTH IN A MEXICAN AMERICAN POPULATION (DOCTORAL DISSERTATION, UNIVERSITY OF CALIFORNIA, BERKELEY, 1967).
SRCE *DISSERTATION ABSTRACTS INTERNATIONAL, 1968, 29(1), 262B. (UNIVERSITY MICROFILMS NO. 68-10,446.)*
INDX HEALTH, ADULTS, CHILDREN, CULTURAL FACTORS, HEALTH DELIVERY SYSTEMS, ECONOMIC FACTORS, POLICY, EMPIRICAL, SES, FEMALE, MEXICAN AMERICAN, CALIFORNIA, SOUTHWEST
ABST AN ANTHROPOLOGICAL APPROACH WAS USED TO EXAMINE CENSUS DATA PERTAINING TO VARIOUS SOCIOCULTURAL FACTORS IN ALAMEDA COUNTY, CALIFORNIA, A PREDOMINANTLY MEXICAN AMERICAN COMMUNITY. IN ADDITION, UNSTRUCTURED INTERVIEWS WERE CONDUCTED WITH REPRESENTATIVES OF PUBLIC AND PRIVATE HEALTH AGENCIES AND 33 FAMILIES REGARDING THE RELATIONSHIP BETWEEN THE STATUS OF MATERNAL AND CHILD HEALTH WITH RESPECT TO LANGUAGE COMMUNICATION PROBLEMS, SOCIAL CLASS, STANDARD OF LIVING, INCOME, AND MIGRANT STATUS. THE CHANGES IN HEALTH BEHAVIOR BETWEEN THAT OF RURAL MEXICO AND CALIFORNIA SEEM TO BE RELATED TO TWO FACTORS: (1) EXPECTED BEHAVIOR AS A RESULT OF ACCEPTING MODERN MEDICAL PRACTICES SUCH AS PRENATAL CARE, AND (2) AVAILABILITY OR SCARCITY OF HEALTH SERVICES. THE LENGTH OF RESIDENCE, COMMAND OF THE ENGLISH LANGUAGE, AND INCOME ARE CONSIDERED TO BE SIGNIFICANTLY RELATED TO HEALTH CARE STATUS. FINDINGS SUGGEST THAT THE LONGER THE MEXICAN AMERICAN FAMILY HAS LIVED IN CALIFORNIA, THE GREATER THEIR AWARENESS OF AVAILABLE HEALTH SERVICES. THE FAMILY'S INCOME LEVEL ACTS AS AN AGENT WITH RESPECT TO WHERE THESE PEOPLE CAN ACQUIRE HEALTH CARE AS WELL AS THE TYPE OF HEALTH SERVICES PROVIDED FOR THEM. LANGUAGE CONTINUES TO BE RELATED TO UNDERUTILIZATION OF HEALTH FACILITIES. IT IS CONCLUDED THAT PUBLIC HEALTH AGENCIES NEED TO HIRE BILINGUAL PERSONNEL AND IMPLEMENT BILINGUAL-BICULTURAL PROGRAMS IN ORDER TO ADEQUATELY DEAL WITH MATERNAL AND CHILD HEALTH PROBLEMS OF THE NEWLY ARRIVED IMMIGRANTS AND THOSE WHO HAVE NOT ACQUIRED A COMMAND OF THE ENGLISH LANGUAGE. 58 REFERENCES.

ACCN 000523

619 AUTH **GARRETSON, O. K.**
TITL A STUDY OF CAUSES OF RETARDATION AMONG MEXICAN CHILDREN IN A SMALL PUBLIC SCHOOL SYSTEM IN ARIZONA.
SRCE *JOURNAL OF EDUCATIONAL PSYCHOLOGY, 1928, 19(1), 31-40.*
INDX MENTAL RETARDATION, MEXICAN AMERICAN, CHILDREN, EDUCATION, SCHOLASTIC ACHIEVEMENT, CROSS CULTURAL, EMPIRICAL, INTELLIGENCE TESTING, ACHIEVEMENT TESTING, ARIZONA, SOUTHWEST
ABST THREE SCALES MEASURED THE MENTAL ABILITY OF 197 ANGLO AMERICAN (AA) AND 117 MEXICAN AMERICAN (MA) PUPILS OF THREE DIFFERENT GRADE LEVELS: THE NATIONAL INTELLIGENCE TEST; THE PANTOMIME GROUP INTELLIGENCE TEST; AND THE PINTER-CUNNINGHAM PRIMARY MENTAL TEST. THE FOLLOWING FINDINGS ARE REPORTED: (1) BY ALL STANDARDS, THE MA PUPIL IS 10.53 MONTHS BEHIND HIS AA CLASSMATE; (2) 30.01% MORE MA'S FALL INTO THE CATEGORY OF RETARDED; (3) THE MA IS MORE IRREGULAR IN SCHOOL ATTENDANCE (THOUGH THIS DIFFERENCE IS QUESTIONABLE AS A FACTOR IN RETARDATION); (4) TRANSIENCY DOES NOT APPEAR TO BE A VALID EXPLANATION FOR THE GREATER RETARDATION OF THE MA GROUP; (5) ALTHOUGH MA'S IN GRADES ONE AND TWO SUFFER LANGUAGE DIFFICULTIES, THIS FACTOR IS OF LESS IMPORTANCE IN GRADES THREE TO EIGHT; AND (6) VERBAL TESTS ARE AS RELIABLE AS NONVERBAL TESTS FOR PUPILS GRADES THREE TO EIGHT. IT IS CONCLUDED THAT THE PRINCIPAL FACTOR GOVERNING THE RETARDATION OF THE MA CHILD IS HIS MENTAL ABILITY AS MEASURED BY THE GROUP TEST. 3 REFERENCES.

ACCN 000524

620 AUTH **GARRISON, V.**
TITL DOCTOR, ESPIRITISTA OR PSYCHIATRIST?: HEALTH-SEEKING BEHAVIOR IN A PUERTO RICAN NEIGHBORHOOD OF NEW YORK CITY.
SRCE *MEDICAL ANTHROPOLOGY, 1977, 1(2), 65-191.*
INDX FOLK MEDICINE, HEALTH, MENTAL HEALTH, PUERTO RICAN-M, ESPIRITISMO, RESOURCE UTILIZATION, MENTAL HEALTH PROFESSION , PHYSICIANS, PSYCHOTHERAPY, PSYCHOTHERAPISTS, DEMOGRAPHIC, SEX COMPARISON, COMMUNITY, NEW YORK, EAST, SES, HEALTH DELIVERY SYSTEMS, CULTURAL FACTORS, RELIGION, PSYCHOPATHOLOGY, ATTITUDES, ADULTS, EMPIRICAL
ABST TO ASSESS THE IMPACT OF FOLK HEALING UPON THE PHYSICAL AND MENTAL HEALTH OF A MODERN URBAN COMMUNITY, ETHNOGRAPHIC AND EPIDEMIOLOGICAL EVIDENCE

WAS GATHERED ON THE ROLE OF ESPIRITISMO IN A LOW-INCOME PUERTO RICAN NEIGHBORHOOD IN NEW YORK. RESULTS WERE DERIVED PRIMARILY FROM PARTICIPANT OBSERVATION OF 14 HEALING CULTS, INTERVIEWS WITH NINE CULT LEADERS, TRANSCRIPTS OF PUBLIC SESSIONS WITHIN ONE SPIRITUALIST CENTER, AND STATISTICAL DATA ON THE DEMOGRAPHIC AND SOCIOECONOMIC CHARACTERISTICS, HEALTH STATUS, AND RESOURCE UTILIZATION AMONG FOUR POPULATIONS. THE SAMPLE CONSISTED OF (1) A RANDOM SAMPLE OF NEIGHBORHOOD RESIDENTS (N = 115), (2) THE SPIRITIST CLIENTELE (N = 232), (3) LOCAL PSYCHIATRIC CLINIC OUTPATIENTS (N = 172), AND (4) LOCAL PSYCHIATRIC INPATIENTS (N = 34). IT WAS FOUND THAT SPIRITISM IS PRIMARILY A CRISIS HEALING CULT WHICH ATTRACTS PEOPLE IN TIMES OF PSYCHIC AND INTERPERSONAL STRESS, AND SUBSTITUTES IN MANY CASES FOR PROFESSIONAL MENTAL HEALTH CARE. IT IS FAMILIAR TO ALL COMMUNITY RESIDENTS AND IS UTILIZED EPISODICALLY BY ALL SEX, AGE, EDUCATIONAL, AND SOCIOECONOMIC GROUPS WITHIN THE POPULATION. THE BENEFICIAL OR DETRIMENTAL EFFECTS OF SPIRITISM REST WITH THE CLINICAL KNOWLEDGE AND ASTUTENESS OF THE INDIVIDUAL MEDIUM. SINCE THE GREATEST DANGER LIES IN THE FRAGMENTATION OF HEALTH SERVICES, A CLOSER INTEGRATION OF THE MEDICAL AND MENTAL HEALTH PROFESSIONS AND THE SPIRITISTS WOULD CLEARLY BENEFIT THE PUERTO RICAN COMMUNITY. 94 REFERENCES.

ACCN   002088

621   AUTH   **GARRISON, V.**

TITL   ESPIRITISMO: IMPLICATIONS FOR PROVISION OF MENTAL HEALTH SERVICES TO PUERTO RICAN POPULATIONS.

SRCE   *PAPER PRESENTED AT THE EIGHTH ANNUAL MEETING OF THE SOUTHERN ANTHROPOLOGICAL SOCIETY, COLUMBIA, MO., FEBRUARY 1972.*

INDX   ESPIRITISMO, HEALTH DELIVERY SYSTEMS, MENTAL HEALTH, RESOURCE UTILIZATION, FOLK MEDICINE, PRIMARY PREVENTION, PSYCHOTHERAPY, PUERTO RICAN-M, ESSAY, EMPIRICAL, NEW YORK, EAST

ABST   PRACTICES IN 14 SPIRITIST CENTERS LOCATED WITHIN THE CATCHMENT AREA OF A COMMUNITY MENTAL HEALTH CLINIC IN NEW YORK WERE STUDIED. ATTENTION IS GIVEN TO THE DIAGNOSTIC PROCESS, THE SPIRITIST TAXONOMY OF DISORDER, AND THE TREATMENT PROCESS AS IT IS VIEWED BY MEDIUMS AND PARTICIPANTS. THE PREVALENCE AND SPECIALIZED FUNCTIONS OF SPIRITIST CENTERS INDICATE THAT THIS FORM OF FOLK PSYCHOTHERAPY HAS MANY SIMILARITIES WITH GROUP PSYCHOTHERAPY AND PSYCHODRAMA. THE IMPLICATIONS FOR PROVISION OF MENTAL HEALTH SERVICES OF THIS ALTERNATIVE SYSTEM OF CARE ARE AS FOLLOWS: (1) THERE IS AN OVERLAP IN TREATMENT POPULATIONS, AS TWO-THIRDS OF THE CLINIC PATIENTS ADMIT TO HAVING SEEN ESPIRITISTAS WITH THE SAME OR SIMILAR PROBLEMS THAT BRING THEM TO THE CLINIC; (2) THE PARAL-

LELS IN THE TWO TREATMENT PROCESSES INDICATE THAT MENTAL HEALTH FACILITIES MUST ADOPT THOSE MODALITIES AND TECHNIQUES MOST ANALOGOUS TO SPIRITIST TREATMENT CENTERS (I.E., WALK-IN SERVICE, SHORT-TERM TREATMENT, USE OF PARAPROFESSIONALS); (3) THE EFFICACY OF ESPIRITISTA PRACTICES IN THE TOTAL COMMUNITY MENTAL HEALTH PICTURE PLAYS A SIGNIFICANT ROLE IN THE PUERTO RICAN COMMUNITIES WHETHER OR NOT THEY ARE DESIRED OR ACKNOWLEDGED BY THE PROFESSIONAL SERVICE AGENCIES; (4) THE EFFICACY OF PROFESSIONAL TREATMENT PRACTICES IS CONFOUNDED BY THE EXISTENCE OF THIS ALTERNATIVE SYSTEM OF MENTAL HEALTH; AND (5) FOR PROGRAM PLANNING IT IS NECESSARY TO HAVE A COLLABORATION OF EFFORTS FOR CONSULTATION AND REFERRALS IN PREVENTION PROGRAMS. 19 REFERENCES.

ACCN   000525

622   AUTH   **GARRISON, V.**

TITL   SECTARIANISM AND PSYCHOSOCIAL ADJUSTMENT: A CONTROLLED COMPARISON OF PUERTO RICAN PENTECOSTALS AND CATHOLICS.

SRCE   *IN I. I. ZARETSKY & M. P. LEONE (EDS.), RELIGIOUS MOVEMENTS IN CONTEMPORARY AMERICA. PRINCETON, N.J.: PRINCETON UNIVERSITY PRESS, 1974, PP. 298-329.*

INDX   RELIGION, PSYCHOSOCIAL ADJUSTMENT, PUERTO RICAN-M, EMPIRICAL, SURVEY, SES, ADULTS, ADOLESCENTS, ECONOMIC FACTORS, SOCIAL MOBILITY, MIGRATION, RURAL, URBAN, FAMILY STRUCTURE, EXTENDED FAMILY, INTERPERSONAL RELATIONS, SYMPTOMATOLOGY, MENTAL HEALTH, NEW YORK, EAST

ABST   DEMOGRAPHIC CHARACTERISTICS, SOCIOECONOMIC VARIABLES, MIGRATION HISTORY, FAMILY ORGANIZATION, PATTERNS OF SOCIAL PARTICIPATION, AND SEVERAL OTHER INDICES OF MENTAL HEALTH OF 398 PUERTO RICAN SUBJECTS WERE COMPARED TO DETERMINE: (1) WHAT DIFFERENCES, IF ANY, CHARACTERIZE THOSE WHO CHOOSE MINORITY RELIGIOUS GROUPS OVER THE MAJOR DENOMINATION; AND (2) WHAT EFFECTS MEMBERSHIP IN THE SECT HAS UPON THE INDIVIDUAL. FINDINGS INDICATE THAT THE PENTECOSTAL MINORITY DIFFERS VERY LITTLE FROM THE MAJOR CHURCH MEMBERS OF THE SAME SUBCULTURAL AND SOCIOECONOMIC SITUATION IN CHARACTERISTICS OTHER THAN THOSE RELATED TO THE RELIGIOUS LIFE. NO EVIDENCE WAS FOUND FOR INADEQUATE FUNCTIONING IN OCCUPATIONAL OR SOCIAL ROLES OR FOR EMOTIONAL DISTURBANCE. THE PUERTO RICAN PENTECOSTALS ARE NOT DRAWN DISPROPORTIONALLY FROM ANY SPECIFIC AGE GROUP, FROM THE LOWEST SOCIOECONOMIC STRATUM, FROM THE MOST RECENT MIGRANT POPULATION, OR FROM THOSE WHOSE FAMILY AND OTHER INTERPERSONAL RELATIONS SHOW DISORGANIZATION. THEY ARE NO LESS, AND POSSIBLY MORE, SOCIOECONOMICALLY MOBILE AS A GROUP AND ARE AS INVOLVED IN THE LIFE OF THE COMMUNITY AS THE CATHO-

LICS FROM THE SAME ENVIRONMENT. THEY SHOW NO GREATER AND POSSIBLY LESSER RATES OF PSYCHIATRIC DISTURBANCE. 38 REFERENCES.

ACCN 000526

623 AUTH **GARRISON, V.**
TITL SOCIAL NETWORKS AND SOCIAL CHANGE IN THE 'CULTURE OF POVERTY'.
SRCE *PAPER PRESENTED AT THE 138TH MEETING OF THE AMERICAN ASSOCIATION FOR THE AD-VANCEMENT OF SCIENCE, PHILADELPHIA, DE-CEMBER 28, 1971.*
INDX CULTURE, POVERTY, URBAN, COMMUNITY, EX-TENDED FAMILY, PUERTO RICAN-M, IMMIGRA-TION, MIGRATION, EMPIRICAL, SES, FAMILY STRUCTURE, FICTIVE KINSHIP, SOCIAL MOBIL-ITY, OCCUPATIONAL ASPIRATIONS, SEX ROLES, RELIGION, COMMUNITY INVOLVEMENT, ACCUL-TURATION, CASE STUDY, SURVEY, PSYCHOSO-CIAL ADJUSTMENT, ENVIRONMENTAL FAC-TORS, EMPLOYMENT, NEW YORK, EAST
ABST THE NATURE OF SOCIAL ORGANIZATION IN URBAN SLUM COMMUNITIES BEYOND THE NU-CLEAR AND EXTENDED FAMILY LEVELS, AND THE CHANGE IN THE TRAITS OF THE CONCEPT OF "CULTURE OF POVERTY" AS DELINEATED BY OSCAR LEWIS ARE EXAMINED. DATA WERE OB-TAINED FROM TWO RANDOM SAMPLES OF PUERTO RICANS LIVING IN A 10-CENSUS-TRACT AREA OF THE SOUTH BRONX AND FROM PAR-TICIPANT-OBSERVATIONS OVER A 3-YEAR PE-RIOD, 1966-1969. INFORMATION ON SOCIAL NETWORKS, FAMILY AND EMPLOYMENT HIS-TORIES, MIGRATION HISTORIES, AND OTHER SOCIAL AND PSYCHOLOGICAL VARIABLES WERE RECORDED. SUFFICIENT EVIDENCE OF CHANGE IN KEY TRAITS OF THE CULTURE OF POVERTY—ECONOMIC, SOCIAL, AND PSYCHO-LOGICAL—EVEN WITHIN THE LIFETIME OF THE FIRST GENERATION MIGRANT, HAVE BEEN SHOWN TO DEMAND A TOTAL REEXAMINATION OF THE QUESTION OF PERSISTENCE OR CHANGE IN THE SO-CALLED CULTURE OF POV-ERTY. THE SOUTH BRONX AREA DOES NOT LACK PATTERNS OF CONGREGATION AND DIS-PERSION OR ASSOCIATIONS OF INDIVIDUALS IN PAIRS AND IN GROUPS, OR VALUES AND NORMS SANCTIONING THESE INTERACTIONS. THIS SOCIAL ORGANIZATION RESEMBLES AN URBAN VILLAGE OR PEER GROUP SOCIETY. AS-SOCIATIONS ARE BASED ON SEX, AGE, ETHNI-CITY, AND TERRITORIALITY MORE THAN UPON CATEGORICAL NORMS OR OCCUPATIONAL, EDUCATIONAL, OR OTHER STATUSES AND FORMALIZED ROLES FAMILIAR TO THE MIDDLE CLASS.
ACCN 000527

624 AUTH **GARRISON, V.**
TITL SUPPORTING STRUCTURES IN A DISORGA-NIZED PUERTO RICAN MIGRANT COMMUNITY.
SRCE *PAPER PRESENTED AT THE 70TH ANNUAL MEETING OF THE AMERICAN ANTHROPOLOGI-CAL ASSOCIATION, NEW YORK, NOVEMBER 1971. (AVAILABLE FROM THE AUTHOR AT DE-PARTMENT OF PSYCHIATRY, NEW JERSEY, COL-LEGE OF MEDICINE AND DENTISTRY, 100 BER-GEN STREET, NEWARK, NJ 07103.)*
INDX COMMUNITY, PUERTO RICAN-M, COPING MECHANISMS, ESPIRITISMO, EXTENDED FAMILY, FICTIVE KINSHIP, FOLK MEDICINE, RELIGION, COMMUNITY INVOLVEMENT, EMPIRICAL, ADULTS, SURVEY, SEX COMPARISON, RE-SOURCE UTILIZATION, MENTAL HEALTH, HEALTH, HEALTH DELIVERY SYSTEMS, NEW YORK, EAST, URBAN, SOCIAL STRUCTURE
ABST IT IS HYPOTHESIZED THAT THE FOLLOWING SUPPORTIVE STRUCTURES FUNCTION TO RE-DUCE RATES OF PSYCHIATRIC TREATMENT AND EMOTIONAL DISTURBANCE AMONG PUERTO RICAN MIGRANTS: (1) THE EXTENDED FAMILY NETWORK; (2) THE FRIENDSHIP NETWORK AND INFORMAL GROUPS; (3) ESPIRITISMO AND SANTERIA CULTS; (4) CHURCHES, ESPECIALLY PENTECOSTAL SECTS; AND (5) SOCIAL CLUBS, COMMUNITY ACTION, POLITICAL, AND CIVIC ORGANIZATIONS. IT IS ALSO HYPOTHESIZED THAT IF THESE SYSTEMS FUNCTION TO PRE-VENT MENTAL ILLNESS AND/OR TO SUPPORT, MAINTAIN, OR REHABILITATE THE MENTALLY ILL, THE PARTICIPANTS WILL BE EITHER (1) UN-DERREPRESENTED IN THE PATIENT POPULA-TION OF PSYCHIATRIC CLINICS SERVING THE SAME AREA, OR (2) CHARACTERIZED BY DIS-PROPORTIONATE RATES OF THOSE SAME CHARACTERISTICS WHICH MOST STRONGLY DISTINGUISH PSYCHIATRIC CLINIC POPULA-TION FROM THE GENERAL POPULATION. RE-SULTS INDICATE THAT PARTICIPATION IN SOME OF THE SUPPORTIVE STRUCTURES (I.E., THE EXTENDED FAMILY NETWORK AND FRIENDSHIP NETWORK FOR FEMALES, AND THE "STREET CORNER GROUP" FOR MALES) IS UNDERRE-PRESENTED IN THE PSYCHIATRIC CLINIC POPULATION DRAWN FROM THE SAME AREA. OTHER GROUPS SUCH AS THE ESPIRITISTA CENTROS AND THE PENTECOSTAL CHURCHES SHOW AN UNDERREPRESENTATION BY PRO-PORTIONAL REPRESENTATION IN THE CLINIC SAMPLE. IT IS CONCLUDED THAT THE "DISOR-GANIZED" COMMUNITY HAS ITS OWN UNIQUE, INFORMAL ORGANIZATIONAL STRUCTURE WHICH IS AT LEAST AS EFFECTIVE IN MAIN-TAINING, TREATING, AND REHABILITATING ITS MEMBERS PSYCHOLOGICALLY AND SOCIALLY AS IS THE LIMITED AND DEFICIENT FORMAL AGENCY STRUCTURE. 34 REFERENCES.
ACCN 000528

625 AUTH **GARRISON, V.**
TITL THE "PUERTO RICAN SYNDROME" IN PSYCHIA-TRY AND ESPIRITISMO.
SRCE *IN V. CRAPANZANO & V. GARRISON (EDS.), CASE STUDIES IN SPIRIT POSSESSION. NEW YORK: JOHN WILEY AND SONS, 1977, PP. 383-449.*
INDX ESPIRITISMO, PUERTO RICAN-M, FOLK MEDI-CINE, MENTAL HEALTH, CASE STUDY, CULTURE, PSYCHOTHERAPISTS, NEW YORK, EAST, PSY-CHOPATHOLOGY, SYMPTOMATOLOGY, FEMALE
ABST MARIA, A 39 YEAR-OLD MARRIED PUERTO RI-CAN IN NEW YORK CITY, EXPERIENCES AN "ATAQUE DE NERVIOS" (NERVOUS ATTACK), WHICH IS INTERPRETED BY THE 'ESPIRITISTA' (FOLK HEALER) AS 'OBSESION' (POSSESSION)

BY THREE MISGUIDED SPIRITS. A DETAILED RECORD OF THE EVENTS MARIA UNDERGOES IN BEING TREATED IN A SPIRITIST CENTRO OVER A SIX-WEEK PERIOD ARE DESCRIBED TO PROVIDE AN UNDERSTANDING OF THE MEANING OF "SPIRIT POSSESSION" AS IT RELATES TO THE BIOLOGICAL, SOCIOCULTURAL, AND PSYCHOLOGICAL REALITIES OF MARIA'S LIFE. IT IS NOTED THAT THE TWO TYPES OF HEALERS (FOLK AND PROFESSIONAL) HAVE THE SAME TREATMENT GOALS AND SOMETIMES EVEN SIMILAR TREATMENT TECHNIQUES. HOWEVER, THEY ARE DIAMETRICALLY OPPOSED IN THAT LOCUS OF THE ILLNESS IS CONCEPTUALIZED INSIDE THE SELF BY THE MODERN PRACTIONER AND OUTSIDE THE SELF BY THE ESPIRITISTA. FOR MARIA AND OTHER MEMBERS OF HER ETHNIC GROUP WHOSE CULTURE IS DIFFERENT FROM THE MODERN, WESTERN, INDUSTRIAL SOCIETY OF THE UNITED STATES, THE PUERTO RICAN ESPIRITIST IS CONSIDERED TO REPRESENT A LEGITIMATE HEALER WHO IS MORE QUALIFIED THAN WESTERNIZED PROFESSIONALS TO TREAT HER ILLNESSES. 29 REFERENCES.

ACCN   000529

626 AUTH   **GARTH, T. R.**
    TITL   A COMPARISON OF THE INTELLIGENCE OF MEXICAN AND MIXED AND FULL BLOOD INDIAN CHILDREN.
    SRCE   *PSYCHOLOGICAL REVIEW, 1923, 30(5), 388-401.*
    INDX   CROSS CULTURAL, INTELLIGENCE, INTELLIGENCE TESTING, MEXICAN AMERICAN, EMPIRICAL, SCHOLASTIC ACHIEVEMENT, ACCULTURATION, INDIGENOUS POPULATIONS, OKLAHOMA, TEXAS, WEST, CHILDREN, SOUTHWEST, SES, NEW MEXICO, MIDWEST
    ABST   THE NATIONAL INTELLIGENCE TEST (NIT) WAS ADMINISTERED TO 307 MEXICAN AMERICAN, 126 MIXED-BLOOD INDIAN, AND 430 FULL-BLOOD INDIAN SCHOOL CHILDREN FROM NEW MEXICO, OKLAHOMA AND TEXAS. THE FULL-BLOOD INDIANS CONSISTED OF THREE GROUPS, TWO OF NOMADIC ANCESTRY: FIRST, A GROUP OF PLAINS AND SOUTHEASTERN INDIANS; SECOND, A GROUP OF NAVAJO AND APACHE INDIANS; THIRD, A GROUP OF PUEBLO INDIANS OF SEDENTARY ANCESTRY. THE MIXED-BLOOD INDIAN IS A MIXTURE OF WHITE AND BOTH PLAINS AND SOUTHEASTERN INDIAN BLOOD. NIT RESULTS INDICATE THE FOLLOWING. (1) WHEN SCORES ARE ARRANGED IN FREQUENCY DISTRIBUTIONS, EACH GROUP WHETHER MIXED OR FULL-BLOOD TENDS TO HAVE A SINGLE CENTRAL TENDENCY. (2) THE MEASURE OF INTELLIGENCE IN DECREASING ORDER INDICATES THE FOLLOWING SEQUENCE: MIXED-BLOOD INDIANS, MEXICAN AMERICANS, PLAINS AND SOUTHEASTERN INDIANS, PUEBLO INDIANS, AND NAVAJO AND APACHE INDIANS. (3) ESTIMATES OF SOCIAL STATUS INDICATE THE SAME SEQUENCE AS THE FOREGOING. (4) THE AVERAGE AMOUNT OF EDUCATION RUNS IN THE SAME SEQUENCE EXCEPT THAT THE PUEBLO INDIANS HAVE SLIGHTLY MORE THAN THE PLAINS AND SOUTHEASTERN INDIANS. (5) THE MIXED

BREEDS EXCEL THE PURE BREEDS IN INTELLIGENCE SCORES. (6) THE NOMADIC TRIBES EXCEL THOSE OF SEDENTARY TRIBES IN INTELLIGENCE SCORES. (7) IF THESE GROUPS MAY BE TAKEN AS REPRESENTATIVE OF THEIR RACIAL STOCKS, THE RESULTS INDICATE DIFFERENCES BETWEEN THEIR RACIAL STOCKS IN INTELLIGENCE. SINCE SOCIAL STATUS AND EDUCATION HAVE NOT BEEN CONTROLLED, ONE CANNOT POSITIVELY STATE THAT THESE DATA INDICATE INNATE RACIAL DIFFERENCES IN INTELLIGENCE. 3 REFERENCES.

ACCN   000530

627 AUTH   **GARTH, T. R.**
    TITL   THE INTELLIGENCE OF MEXICAN SCHOOL CHILDREN.
    SRCE   *SCHOOL AND SOCIETY, 1928, 27(705), 791-794.*
    INDX   INTELLIGENCE, MEXICAN AMERICAN, CHILDREN, SEX COMPARISON, INTELLIGENCE TESTING, SPECIAL EDUCATION, EMPIRICAL, SOUTHWEST, COLORADO, NEW MEXICO, TEXAS
    ABST   A TOTAL OF 1,004 MEXICAN AMERICAN SCHOOL CHILDREN FROM GRADES THREE TO EIGHT IN THE URBAN AND RURAL AREAS OF COLORADO, NEW MEXICO, AND TEXAS WERE TESTED ON THE NATIONAL INTELLIGENCE TEST (NIT). THE DATA REVEAL THE FOLLOWING. (1) THE MEDIAN NIT-IQ FOR THIS GROUP IS 78.1, WITH A VARIABILITY OF 22.6 IQ POINTS. SEX IS NOT A SIGNIFICANT FACTOR IN IQ SCORES. (2) THE IQ INCREASES FOR EACH SCHOOL GRADE BUT NOT IN REGULAR STEPS. (3) THE MEDIAN SCORE FOR EACH SCHOOL GRADE INCREASES WITH THE GRADE. ACCORDING TO MENTAL AGE EQUIVALENT THE MEXICAN CHILDREN ARE ON THE AVERAGE 11 YEARS MENTALLY YOUNGER THAN THE WHITE FOR THE CORRESPONDING SCHOOL GRADES. (4) THE INFLUENCE OF SCHOOL GRADE ON IQ SCORES FOR 498 ARTIFICIALLY SELECTED CASES IS HIGH IF AGE IS DISREGARDED. (5) THE INFLUENCE OF AGE ON IQ SCORE WHEN SCHOOL GRADE IS HELD CONSTANT IS NEGLIGIBLE. (6) THE RETARDATION OF THE MEXICAN AMERICAN CHILDREN IS 80.5 PERCENT ON THE AVERAGE. IT IS HIGHEST FOR BOYS IN THE LOWER GRADES. IT IS NOTED THAT THIS REPRESENTATIVE IQ IS LOWER THAN HAS BEEN PREVIOUSLY OBTAINED BY OTHER INVESTIGATORS. 6 REFERENCES.

ACCN   000531

628 AUTH   **GARTH, T. R. , & JOHNSON, H. D.**
    TITL   THE INTELLIGENCE AND ACHIEVEMENT OF MEXICAN CHILDREN IN THE UNITED STATES.
    SRCE   *JOURNAL OF ABNORMAL AND SOCIAL PSYCHOLOGY, 1934, 29(2), 222-229.*
    INDX   INTELLIGENCE, INTELLIGENCE TESTING, SCHOLASTIC ACHIEVEMENT, MEXICAN AMERICAN, CHILDREN, EMPIRICAL, CROSS CULTURAL, TEXAS, SOUTHWEST
    ABST   AN INVESTIGATION OF THE INFLUENCE OF EDUCATIONAL ACHIEVEMENT UPON THE INTELLIGENCE SCORES OF 683 MEXICAN AMERICAN CHILDREN IN GRADES FOUR TO NINE IS PRESENTED. THE OTIS CLASSIFICATION TEST,

COMPOSED OF AN ACHIEVEMENT AND AN IN-TELLIGENCE SECTION, WAS ADMINISTERED TO THE SUBJECTS. SOME PROPOSED QUESTIONS ARE: WHAT IS THE INDICATED MENTAL AND EDUCATIONAL GROWTH OF THE SUBJECTS? WHAT IS THEIR EDUCATIONAL RETARDATION? WHAT IS THEIR MENTAL (IQ) AND EDUCA-TIONAL AGE (EQ) FOR A SCHOOL GRADE? WHAT CAN BE ASCERTAINED REGARDING THE GROUP IQ AND EQ AND, LASTLY, THE ACCOM-PLISHMENT RATIO (AR)? ANALYSIS OF THE DATA REVEALS THE FOLLOWING. (1) MEXICAN AMERICAN CHILDREN ARE MORE LIKE THE AMERICAN WHITE AT THE EARLY AGES BUT LESS LIKE THEM IN BOTH ACHIEVEMENT AND INTELLIGENCE AS THEY GROW OLDER. (2) BOTH THE CHRONOLOGICAL AGE AND THE EXTENT OF EDUCATIONAL RETARDATION ARE HIGH. (3) THE MENTAL AND EDUCATIONAL AGES FOR A GRADE ARE BELOW THE AMERI-CAN WHITE NORMS, BUT THE EDUCATIONAL AGE IS SLIGHTLY ABOVE THE MENTAL AGE FOR A GRADE. (4) THE OTIS AND TERMAN GROUP IQ'S ARE, FOR THE TOTAL GROUP RESPEC-TIVELY, 83.02 AND 79.6. (5) THE MEDIAN EQ IS HIGHER THAN THE MEDIAN IQ. (6) THE AR IN-DICATES THAT, ON THE WHOLE, THE RATIO BE-TWEEN IQ AND EQ IS HIGHER THAN IT IS FOR THE AMERICAN WHITE. (7) THE HIGHEST COR-RELATION IS FOUND BETWEEN INTELLIGENCE AND ACHIEVEMENT, AND NEXT BETWEEN IN-TELLIGENCE AND SCHOOL GRADE. (8) A MUL-TIPLE CORRELATION OF .58 IS FOUND BE-TWEEN INTELLIGENCE AND THE FACTORS OF SCHOOL PLACEMENT AND EDUCATIONAL ACHIEVEMENT. (9) THE RELATIVE WEIGHTS AS-SIGNED TO SCHOOL PLACEMENT AND ACHIEVEMENT ARE 1.0 AND 3.7, SHOWING THE LATTER TO BE THE MORE INFLUENTIAL IN OB-TAINING AN INTELLIGENCE SCORE. 3 REFER-ENCES.

ACCN   000532

629   AUTH   **GARTH, T. R., ELSON, T. R. H., & MORTON, M. M.**
      TITL   THE ADMINISTRATION OF NON-LANGUAGE IN-TELLIGENCE TESTS TO MEXICANS.
      SRCE   *JOURNAL OF ABNORMAL AND SOCIAL PSY-CHOLOGY, 1936, 31(1), 53-58.*
      INDX   INTELLIGENCE, INTELLIGENCE TESTING, TEST VALIDITY, CROSS CULTURAL, EMPIRICAL, CHIL-DREN, ADOLESCENTS, MEXICAN AMERICAN
      ABST   AN INVESTIGATION TO SECURE A SATISFAC-TORY MEASURE OF THE INTELLIGENCE OF MEXICAN AMERICAN CHILDREN WITH A RELI-ABLE NONLANGUAGE TEST IS PRESENTED. THE OBJECTIVES WERE TO DETERMINE THE IN-FLUENCE OF LANGUAGE AND EDUCATION ON CHILDREN WHEN THEIR ABILITY ON A NON-LANGUAGE INTELLIGENCE TEST IS KNOWN AND TO ASCERTAIN HOW THE CHILDREN WOULD DO WHEN ADMINISTERED A VERBAL AND AN ACHIEVEMENT TEST. FOUR HUNDRED FIFTY-FIVE MEXICAN AMERICAN CHILDREN, AGES 8 TO 16 YEARS, WERE TESTED WITH THE PINTER NONLANGUAGE INTELLIGENCE TEST AND THE OTIS CLASSIFICATION TEST. ANALY-SIS OF THE DATA REVEALS THE FOLLOWING.

(1) AGE FOR AGE AND GRADE FOR GRADE, THE MEXICAN AMERICAN CHILDREN ARE IN-FERIOR TO AMERICAN WHITES IN VERBAL TEST RESULTS. (2) IN THE NONLANGUAGE TEST RE-SULTS, THE MEXICAN AMERICANS ARE PRAC-TICALLY EQUAL IN PERFORMANCE TO THE AMERICAN WHITES. (3) IQ'S DERIVED FROM THE NONLANGUAGE TESTS FOR THE MEXICAN AMERICANS ARE ON THE WHOLE ABOUT EQUAL TO THE AMERICAN WHITE IQ. (4) THIS STUDY POINTS TO THE POSSIBILITY THAT VERBAL TESTS ARE UNFAIR TO MEXICAN AMERICAN CHILDREN. 4 REFERENCES.

ACCN   000533

630   AUTH   **GARTH, T. R., HOLCOMB, W. M., & GESHE, I.**
      TITL   MENTAL FATIGUE OF MEXICAN SCHOOL CHIL-DREN.
      SRCE   *JOURNAL OF APPLIED PSYCHOLOGY, 1932, 16(6), 675-680.*
      INDX   MEXICAN AMERICAN, CROSS CULTURAL, CHIL-DREN, EMPIRICAL, SCHOLASTIC ACHIEVE-MENT, TEXAS, SOUTHWEST, ABILITY TESTING
      ABST   WORK EFFICIENCY AS MEASURED BY THE THORNDIKE ADDITION TEST WAS RECORDED FOR A GROUP OF 195 MEXICAN AMERICAN (MA) CHILDREN FROM THE THIRD, FOURTH, SEVENTH, AND EIGHTH GRADE LEVELS. THE DATA WERE HANDLED WITH REFERENCE TO TWO CATEGORIES-ATTEMPTED PERFORM-ANCE AND ACCURATE PERFORMANCE. THE FINDINGS SHOW THAT THE YOUNGER SUB-JECTS LOSE 15 PERCENT EFFICIENCY IN AT-TEMPTED PERFORMANCE AND 25.8 PERCENT IN ACCURATE PERFORMANCE OVER A PERIOD OF 28 MINUTES. THE YOUNGER CHILDREN ARE DISPOSED TO DO SLIGHTLY MORE THAN HALF OF THEIR WORK BY THE TIME HALF OF THE PE-RIOD IS FINISHED. THE OLDER SUBJECTS SHOW 1.9 PERCENT EFFICIENCY LOSS IN ATTEMPTED PERFORMANCE AND 15.4 PERCENT LOSS ON ACCURATE PERFORMANCE OVER A PERIOD OF 42 MINUTES. WHEN THE DATA ARE COMPARED WITH THE PERFORMANCE OF WHITE SUB-JECTS FROM A PREVIOUS STUDY, THE RESULTS SHOW THAT MA CHILDREN ARE MORE LIKE WHITES IN THEIR ACCURATE PERFORMANCE THAN THEY ARE IN ATTEMPTED PERFORM-ANCE. BUT THE SAME IS NOT CONSISTENTLY TRUE FOR THE OLDER MA STUDENTS. FAC-TORS WHICH MIGHT ACCOUNT FOR THE DIF-FERENCE BETWEEN THE WORK PERFORM-ANCE OF THE YOUNGER MA CHILDREN AND THE WHITE CHILDREN ARE: SELECTION PRO-CESS, TRAINING, AND NUTRITION. 4 REFER-ENCES.

ACCN   000534

631   AUTH   **GARTH, T. R., & CANDOR, E.**
      TITL   MUSICAL TALENT OF MEXICANS.
      SRCE   *AMERICAN JOURNAL OF PSYCHOLOGY, 1937, 49(2), 298-301.*
      INDX   CROSS CULTURAL, MEXICAN, MUSIC, ADOLES-CENTS, TEST RELIABILITY, EMPIRICAL, ABILITY TESTING
      ABST   IN AN EFFORT TO DETERMINE WHETHER MEX-ICAN (M) CHILDREN ARE MORE MUSICAL THAN OTHER ETHNIC CHILDREN, SIX SEASHORE

TESTS OF MUSICAL TALENT WERE GIVEN TO 665 MEXICANS. THE SUBJECTS WERE DRAWN FROM THE FIRST, SECOND, AND THIRD YEARS OF PUBLIC SECONDARY SCHOOLS IN MEXICO. RESULTS SHOW THAT: (1) THE RELIABILITY OF THE SEASHORE TESTS IS AS HIGH FOR THE M CHILDREN AS FOR OTHER ETHNIC GROUPS. (2) M CHILDREN'S PERFORMANCE IN PITCH, INTENSITY CONSONANCE, AND MEMORY IS INFERIOR TO THAT OF THE ANGLO-AMERICAN (AA). IT IS NOT KNOWN WHY M CHILDREN ARE NOT AS ADEPT AS AA'S IN THEIR PERFORMANCE ON THE TEST FOR PITCH. THE INEXPERIENCE OF TAKING TESTS IS SUGGESTED AS A POSSIBLE EXPLANATION FOR M'S PERFORMANCE. AS FOR RHYTHM, M'S DEMONSTRATE SUPERIOR PERFORMANCE OVER AA CHILDREN. THE DANCING EXPERIENCE OF M CHILDREN IS GIVEN AS THE REASON FOR SUPERIOR PERFORMANCE. IT IS CONCLUDED THAT DIFFERENCES BETWEEN THE TWO GROUPS ARE NOT DUE TO NATURE BUT TO NURTURE.

ACCN   000535

632 AUTH   **GARZA, R. T.**
     TITL   AFFECTIVE AND ASSOCIATIVE QUALITIES IN THE LEARNING STYLES OF CHICANOS AND ANGLOS.
     SRCE   *PSYCHOLOGY IN THE SCHOOLS, 1978, 15(1), 111-115.*
     INDX   TEXAS, SOUTHWEST, COLLEGE STUDENTS, CROSS CULTURAL, CULTURAL FACTORS, EMPIRICAL, LEARNING, MEXICAN AMERICAN
     ABST   THE ROLE OF AFFECTIVE AND ASSOCIATIVE MEANINGFULNESS IN THE LEARNING STYLES OF CHICANOS AND ANGLOS WAS EXAMINED IN THE PRESENT STUDY. SIXTY-FOUR CHICANO AND ANGLO UNDERGRADUATES WERE COMPARED ON THEIR LEARNING OF AFFECTIVELY AND ASSOCIATIVELY ASSESSED CONSONANT-VOWEL-CONSONANT TRIGRAMS. CHICANOS DID NOT DIFFER FROM ANGLOS IN THEIR RELIANCE ON THE AFFECTIVE RELATIVE TO THE ASSOCIATIVE DIMENSION OF MEANINGFULNESS IN THEIR LEARNING STYLE. HOWEVER, CHICANOS DIFFERED SIGNIFICANTLY FROM ANGLOS IN AFFECTIVE LEARNING STYLE, MANIFESTING A GREATER PROPENSITY TO LEARN THEIR LIKED MATERIALS MORE READILY THAN THEIR DISLIKED MATERIALS. IT WAS FURTHER FOUND THAT WHILE THE PERFORMANCE OF THE TWO ETHNIC GROUPS WAS COMPARABLE IN THE DISLIKED CONDITION, THE CHICANO SUBJECTS PERFORMED SIGNIFICANTLY BETTER THAN THE ANGLO SUBJECTS IN THE LIKED CONDITION. IT IS SUGGESTED THAT THE INTENSIFIED CHICANO SENSITIVITY TO AFFECTIVE MEANINGFULNESS IS CONSISTENT WITH THEIR CULTURAL CONCERNS. 12 REFERENCES. (AUTHOR ABSTRACT)
     ACCN   002089

633 AUTH   **GARZA, R. T., & ALVA, I. C.**
     TITL   LANGUAGE DOMINANCE AND SEMANTIC ORGANIZATION IN SPANISH-ENGLISH BILINGUAL CHILDREN.
     SRCE   *HISPANIC JOURNAL OF BEHAVIORAL SCIENCES, 1979, 1(1), 55-62.*
     INDX   CHILDREN, BILINGUAL, BILINGUALISM, MEXICAN AMERICAN, CALIFORNIA, SOUTHWEST, EMPIRICAL, LINGUISTICS, LANGUAGE ASSESSMENT, LINGUISTIC COMPETENCE, SEMANTICS
     ABST   AN EXAMINATION WAS CONDUCTED OF THE EFFECTS OF AGE AND LANGUAGE DOMINANCE ON THE RECALL OF BILINGUAL CHILDREN IN TWO SEMANTICALLY DIFFERENT MODES OF PRESENTATION. THE SUBJECTS WERE 72 SPANISH-ENGLISH BILINGUALS IN SOUTHERN CALIFORNIA, RANGING FROM PRESCHOOL TO SECOND GRADE, WITH SIX SUBJECTS IN EACH OF THE THREE LANGUAGE DOMINANCE CONDITIONS AT EACH GRADE LEVEL. COUNTERBALANCING FOR BETWEEN-SUBJECTS ORDER OF PRESENTATION, TWO RANDOMIZED LISTS WERE ADMINISTERED TO EACH CHILD. IN THE CONCORDANT CONDITION, ONE SEMANTIC CATEGORY WAS IN THE OTHER LANGUAGE. IN THE DISCORDANT CONDITION, LANGUAGE AND SEMANTIC CONTENT WERE CROSSED SO THAT HALF OF THE ITEMS IN EACH CATEGORY WERE IN ONE LANGUAGE AND HALF IN THE OTHER. THE FINDINGS INDICATE THAT ONLY OLDER CHILDREN WERE ABLE TO BENEFIT FROM THE ORGANIZATIONAL ADVANTAGE OF THE CONCORDANT MODE OF PRESENTATION—AS HAS BEEN PREVIOUSLY FOUND WITH ADULT SUBJECTS. THE FINDINGS ALSO REVEAL THAT BILINGUALS LEARN AND ORGANIZE LEXICAL INFORMATION IN TERMS OF ITS SEMANTIC FEATURES OR ASSOCIATIONS. THE RESULTS ARE DISCUSSED IN RELATION TO CONTEMPORARY THEORETICAL ISSUES IN THE FIELD OF BILINGUALISM, STRESSING THE NEED FOR INNOVATIVE, SEMANTICALLY-BASED THEORETICAL MODELS OF BILINGUAL FUNCTIONING. 11 REFERENCES. (JOURNAL ABSTRACT MODIFIED)
     ACCN   001767

634 AUTH   **GARZA, R. T., & AMES, R. E.**
     TITL   A COMPARISON OF ANGLO- AND MEXICAN-AMERICAN COLLEGE STUDENTS ON LOCUS OF CONTROL.
     SRCE   *JOURNAL OF CONSULTING AND CLINICAL PSYCHOLOGY, 1974, 42(6), 919.*
     INDX   ATTITUDES, ATTRIBUTION OF RESPONSIBILITY, COLLEGE STUDENTS, CROSS CULTURAL, CULTURAL FACTORS, EMPIRICAL, LOCUS OF CONTROL, SES, MIDWEST, MEXICAN AMERICAN, ROTTER INTERNAL-EXTERNAL SCALE, FATALISM
     ABST   STUDIES SUGGESTING THAT MEXICAN AMERICANS LACK FEELINGS OF PERSONAL CONTROL HAVE NOT ALWAYS TAKEN INTO ACCOUNT SOCIOECONOMIC FACTORS. THE TEST INSTRUMENT WAS ROTTER'S I-E SCALE, ADMINISTERED TO 47 ANGLO AMERICAN AND 47 MEXICAN AMERICAN COLLEGE STUDENTS MATCHED ON SOCIOECONOMIC BACKGROUND AND SEX. IN ADDITION TO THE ITEMS ON THE FULL I-E SCALE, DIFFERENCES WERE EXAMINED IN FIVE SUBCATEGORIES: (A) LUCK/FATE; (B) POLITICS; (C) RESPECT; (D) LEADERSHIP/SUCCESS; AND (E) ACADEMICS. RESULTS WERE THAT MEXICAN AMERICANS SCORED SIGNIFICANTLY LESS ON EXTERNAL CONTROL

THAN ANGLO AMERICANS ON THE FULL I-E SCALE, AND SIGNIFICANT DIFFERENCES WERE FOUND ON TWO OF THE FIVE DIMENSIONAL CATEGORIES—LUCK/FATE AND RESPECT. THESE FINDINGS ARE DISCUSSED IN TERMS OF CULTURAL VALUES OF MEXICAN AMERICANS: THE FAMILY-CENTERED ORIENTATION, AND THE PERENNIEL RESISTANCE TO ENCROACHMENTS ON CULTURE AND HERITAGE (A RESISTANCE TO EXTERNAL INFLUENCES). IT IS CONCLUDED THAT THE FINDINGS NOT ONLY CONTRADICT THE STEREOTYPE THAT MEXICAN AMERICANS ARE FATALISTIC BUT THEY SEEM TO SUGGEST THAT THEIR CULTURE CONTRIBUTES TO A GREATER PERCEPTION OF INTERNAL CONTROL. 3 REFERENCES.

ACCN   002659

635 AUTH **GARZA, R. T., & AMES, R. E., JR.**
     TITL A COMPARISON OF CHICANOS AND ANGLOS ON LOCUS OF CONTROL.
     SRCE *IN C. HERNANDEZ, M. J. HAUG & N. N. WAGNER (EDS.), CHICANOS: SOCIAL AND PSYCHOLOGICAL PERSPECTIVES. SAINT LOUIS: C. V. MOSBY COMPANY, 1976, PP. 133-135.*
     INDX MEXICAN AMERICAN, EMPIRICAL, FATALISM, SES, CROSS CULTURAL, STEREOTYPES, LOCUS OF CONTROL, ROTTER INTERNAL-EXTERNAL SCALE, COLLEGE STUDENTS, TEXAS, SOUTHWEST
     ABST THE ETHNIC PRIDE AND IMPORTANCE OF THE FAMILY EMBODIED WITHIN THE MEXICAN AMERICAN CULTURE SUGGESTS THAT THEY MIGHT HAVE GREATER INTERNAL LOCUS OF CONTROL SCORES THAN ANGLOS. TO TEST THIS HYPOTHESIS, ANGLO AND MEXICAN AMERICAN COLLEGE STUDENTS WERE MATCHED TO CONTROL FOR SEX AND SOCIO-ECONOMIC BACKGROUND DIFFERENCES AND GIVEN ROTTER'S INTERNAL-EXTERNAL LOCUS OF CONTROL SCALE. FINDINGS INDICATE THAT MEXICAN AMERICANS ARE SIGNIFICANTLY LESS EXTERNAL THAN ANGLOS ON THE TOTAL I-E SCALE SCORES. MEXICAN AMERICANS, CONTRARY TO THE STEREOTYPIC BELIEF THAT THEY ARE FATALISTIC, SCORED LESS EXTERNAL THAN ANGLOS ON LUCK AND FATE. RESULTS ALSO SUGGEST THAT THE MEXICAN AMERICAN CULTURE PROVIDES FOR A MORE INTERNAL PERCEPTION OF CONTROL. 14 REFERENCES.
     ACCN 000537

636 AUTH **GARZA, R. T., & NELSON, D. B.**
     TITL A COMPARISON OF MEXICAN- AND ANGLO-AMERICAN PERCEPTIONS OF THE UNIVERSITY ENVIRONMENT.
     SRCE *JOURNAL OF COLLEGE STUDENT PERSONNEL, 1973, 14(5), 399-401.*
     INDX COLLEGE STUDENTS, MEXICAN AMERICAN, CROSS CULTURAL, HIGHER EDUCATION, ATTITUDES, EMPIRICAL, TEXAS, SOUTHWEST, ESSAY
     ABST IN COMPARING PERCEPTIONS OF THE UNIVERSITY ENVIRONMENT, ANGLO AND MEXICAN AMERICAN COLLEGE STUDENTS WERE MATCHED ACCORDING TO AGE, SEX, MARITAL STATUS AND ACADEMIC ACHIEVEMENT AND

THEN GIVEN THE COLLEGE AND UNIVERSITY ENVIRONMENT SCALES (CUES, DEVELOPED BY THE EDUCATIONAL TESTING SERVICE). CUES REFLECTS SEVEN DIMENSIONS: PRACTICALITY, COMMUNITY, AWARENESS, PROPRIETY, SCHOLARSHIP, CAMPUS MORALE, AND THE QUALITY OF TEACHING AND FACULTY-STUDENT RELATIONSHIPS. THE FINDINGS INDICATE SIGNIFICANT DIFFERENCES BETWEEN THE TWO GROUPS ON THE PROPRIETY AND SCHOLARSHIP SCALES. THE MEXICAN AMERICANS PERCEIVED THE UNIVERSITY AS BEING MORE CONVENTIONAL AND PLACED A GREATER EMPHASIS ON ACADEMIC ACHIEVEMENT. THE ANGLOS WERE MORE COMFORTABLE IN THE UNIVERSITY SETTING AND TENDED TO FOCUS MORE ON THE PRACTICAL GAINS AND BENEFITS DERIVED FROM BEING A COLLEGE STUDENT. 7 REFERENCES.

ACCN   000538

637 AUTH **GARZA, R. T., & WIDLAK, F. W.**
     TITL ANTECEDENTS OF CHICANO AND ANGLO STUDENT PERCEPTIONS OF THE UNIVERSITY ENVIRONMENT.
     SRCE *JOURNAL OF COLLEGE STUDENT PERSONNEL, 1976, 17(4), 295-299.*
     INDX MEXICAN AMERICAN, ATTITUDES, SCHOLASTIC ACHIEVEMENT, CROSS CULTURAL, CULTURAL FACTORS, EMPIRICAL, COLLEGE STUDENTS, SES, HIGHER EDUCATION, SCHOLASTIC ASPIRATIONS, TEXAS, SOUTHWEST, VALUES
     ABST TO IDENTIFY SOCIOCULTURAL DETERMINANTS OF CHICANO AND ANGLO COLLEGE STUDENTS' PERCEPTIONS OF THE UNIVERSITY ENVIRONMENT, 145 ANGLO AND 79 MEXICAN AMERICAN STUDENTS AT A TEXAS UNIVERSITY WERE TESTED ON THE COLLEGE AND UNIVERSITY ENVIRONMENTAL SCALES (CUES). CONCERNING GROUP DIFFERENCES, ANGLOS HAD HIGHER LEVELS OF PARENTS' INCOME, PARENTS' EDUCATION, AND GPA. OF THE SEVEN CUES DIMENSIONS OF PERCEPTIONS, THE GROUPS DIFFERED ON ONLY TWO, WITH CHICANOS SCORING HIGHER ON PERCEPTIONS RELATING TO SCHOLARSHIP AND COMMUNITY. SUBSTANTIAL VARIATION IN PERCEPTUAL ANTECEDENTS WAS FOUND: ANGLOS WHO VIEWED THE COLLEGE ENVIRONMENT MORE FAVORABLY TENDED TO BE OLDER, HAVE A LOWER GPA, AND HAVE LESS WELL-EDUCATED FATHERS; WHILE THE CHICANOS WITH MORE FAVORABLE PERCEPTIONS OF THE UNIVERSITY TENDED TO BE MARRIED AND ENROLLED IN LIFE-RELATED AREAS OF STUDY. THESE DIFFERENCES IN PREDICTIVE VARIABLES ARE PRESUMED TO REFLECT DIFFERENCES IN CULTURAL VALUES (I.E., GREATER FAMILY-CENTERED ORIENTATION AMONG CHICANOS). IT IS CONCLUDED THAT SUCH CULTURAL VALUE DIFFERENCES SHOULD BE TAKEN INTO CONSIDERATION IN MAKING HIGHER EDUCATION MORE APPEALING AND RELEVANT TO THE CHICANO POPULATION. CHICANO STUDIES PROGRAMS AND RESPONSIVE CHICANO FACULTY MAY BE THE MOST EFFECTIVE WAY OF MEETING SUCH CULTURAL NEEDS. 10 REFERENCES.

ACCN   000536

638 AUTH   **GARZA, R. T., & WIDLAK, F. W.**
     TITL   THE VALIDITY OF LOCUS OF CONTROL DIMEN-
            SIONS FOR CHICANO POPULATIONS.
     SRCE   *JOURNAL OF PERSONALITY ASSESSMENT, 1977,*
            41(6), 635-643.
     INDX   COLLEGE STUDENTS, CROSS CULTURAL, EM-
            PIRICAL, LOCUS OF CONTROL, MEXICAN
            AMERICAN, TEXAS, SOUTHWEST, ROTTER IN-
            TERNAL-EXTERNAL SCALE
     ABST   THE MULTIDIMENSIONAL LOCUS OF CONTROL
            LITERATURE SUPPORTS THE TENABILITY OF
            FIVE FACTORIAL DIMENSIONS: (A) LUCK/FATE;
            (B) LEADERSHIP/SUCCESS; (C) ACADEMICS;
            (D) POLITICS; AND (E) RESPECT. CONTENDING
            THAT THE CONTRADICTORY LOCUS OF CON-
            TROL FINDINGS INVOLVING CHICANO POPU-
            LATIONS MAY BE DUE TO METHODOLOGICAL
            INADEQUACIES, THE PURPOSE OF THE PRES-
            ENT STUDY WAS TO EMPIRICALLY DETERMINE
            THE APPROPRIATENESS OF THE FIVE CATE-
            GORIES FOR COMPARING CHICANO AND AN-
            GLO POPULATIONS. THIS WAS DONE BY FAC-
            TOR ANALYZING THE RESPONSES OF 203
            ANGLO AND 244 CHICANO UNDERGRADUATES
            TO ROTTER'S (1966) I-E SCALE SEPARATELY,
            AND THEN COMPARING THE CORRESPONDING
            FACTOR PAIRS BY USING CLIFF'S (1966) CON-
            GRUENCE PROCEDURE. THE LUCK/FATE AND
            LEADERSHIP/SUCCESS FACTORS SHOW SUB-
            STANTIAL INVARIANCE ACROSS THE TWO
            SAMPLES, WHEREAS THE CULTURAL EQUIVA-
            LENCE OF THE REMAINING THREE FACTORS IS
            SOMEWHAT QUESTIONABLE. THE FINDINGS
            ARE DISCUSSED IN RELATION TO CURRENT
            KNOWLEDGE OF CROSS-CULTURAL DIFFER-
            ENCES BETWEEN ANGLO AND CHICANO
            POPULATIONS. 34 REFERENCES. (AUTHOR AB-
            STRACT)
     ACCN   002044

639 AUTH   **GAVIRA, M., VASQUEZ, A., HOLGUIN, P., GEN-**
            TILE, M., & TIRADO, J.
     TITL   A COMMUNITY MENTAL HEALTH PROGRAM
            FOR THE SPANISH SPEAKING POPULATION IN
            CHICAGO: EIGHT YEARS OF EVOLUTION.
     SRCE   *IN E. R. PADILLA & A. M. PADILLA (EDS.), TRAN-*
            SCULTURAL PSYCHIATRY: AN HISPANIC PER-
            SPECTIVE (MONOGRAPH NO. 4). LOS ANGE-
            LES: UNIVERSITY OF CALIFORNIA, SPANISH
            SPEAKING MENTAL HEALTH RESEARCH CEN-
            TER, 1977, PP. 35-43.
     INDX   PROGRAM EVALUATION, SPANISH SURNAMED,
            COMMUNITY INVOLVEMENT, COMMUNITY, HIS-
            TORY, MENTAL HEALTH, MENTAL HEALTH
            PROFESSION, PARAPROFESSIONALS, PRIMARY
            PREVENTION, FINANCING, HEALTH DELIVERY
            SYSTEMS, BILINGUAL-BICULTURAL PERSON-
            NEL, ILLINOIS, MIDWEST
     ABST   THE DEVELOPMENTAL HISTORY OF THE WEST-
            SIDE MEDICAL CENTER COMMUNITY MENTAL
            HEALTH PROGRAM IN CHICAGO FOR THE YEARS
            1967-1975 IS PRESENTED. OVER THIS EIGHT-
            YEAR PERIOD CHANGES IN THE POLITICAL CLI-
            MATE, COMMUNITY AWARENESS, FEDERAL
            SUPPORT, INSTITUTIONAL CONTROL AND ETH-

NIC DISTRIBUTION OF THE CATCHMENT AREA
BROUGHT ABOUT A METAMORPHOSIS. A PRO-
GRAM EMPHASIZING TRAINING AND RE-
SEARCH DEVELOPED INTO A COMMUNITY
PROGRAM SERVING A LARGE POPULATION OF
LATINO RESIDENTS. THE DISCUSSION IN-
CLUDES AN ANALYSIS OF THE SOCIAL AND PO-
LITICAL FORCES INVOLVED IN THE DEVELOP-
MENT OF EACH STAGE OF THE PROGRAM, THE
CONTRADICTIONS WHICH RESULTED, AND THE
REDEFINED GOALS AND NEW STRATEGIES
WHICH ALLOWED THE PROGRAM TO SURVIVE.
THIS PROCESS SHOULD BE HELPFUL TO OTH-
ERS DEVELOPING MENTAL HEALTH PROGRAMS
FOR SPANISH-SPEAKING POPULATIONS. MA-
JOR CHANGES DISCUSSED ARE: SHIFT IN THE
POPULATION TO BE SERVED; MOVE FROM A
HOSPITAL-CENTERED TO A COMMUNITY-CEN-
TERED PROGRAM; TRANSITION FROM ANGLO
PROFESSIONAL STAFF TO LATINO, BILINGUAL,
PARAPROFESSIONAL   AND   PROFESSIONAL
STAFF; ADDITION OF A COMMUNITY BOARD;
AND CHANGE FROM FEDERAL TO STATE FUND-
ING. 18 REFERENCES. (AUTHOR SUMMARY
MODIFIED)

     ACCN   000539

640 AUTH   **GAY, G.**
     TITL   TEACHERS' ACHIEVEMENT EXPECTATIONS OF
            AND INTERACTIONS WITH ETHNICALLY DIFFER-
            ENT STUDENTS.
     SRCE   *CONTEMPORARY EDUCATION, 1975, 46(3), 166-*
            172.
     INDX   REVIEW, TEACHERS, ATTITUDES, MEXICAN
            AMERICAN, CROSS CULTURAL, CHILDREN,
            EDUCATION, SCHOLASTIC ACHIEVEMENT, CUL-
            TURAL FACTORS, PERFORMANCE EXPECTA-
            TIONS, DISCRIMINATION
     ABST   RESEARCH STUDIES AVAILABLE ON TEACH-
            ERS' EXPECTATIONS AND BEHAVIOR WITH ETH-
            NICALLY DIFFERENT STUDENTS ARE REVIEWED
            AND DISCUSSED. ALTHOUGH THESE STUDIES
            ARE TOO FEW FOR THE FINDINGS TO BE CON-
            CLUSIVE, THEY STRONGLY SUGGEST THAT
            STUDENT ETHNICITY IS A MAJOR DETERMI-
            NANT OF TEACHERS' EXPECTATIONS AND IN-
            TERACTIONAL BEHAVIORS. THE STUDIES RE-
            VIEWED   SHOWED   THAT   TEACHERS
            CONSISTENTLY EXPECT LESS OF BLACKS, CHI-
            CANOS AND OTHER MINORITIES IN TERMS OF
            ACADEMIC SUBSTANCE AND QUALITY. THESE
            STUDENTS, IN TURN, BEHAVE IN WAYS CON-
            SONANT WITH THEIR TEACHERS' REDUCED EX-
            PECTATIONS. TEACHERS GIVE SUCH STU-
            DENTS FEWER OPPORTUNITIES AND LESS
            ENCOURAGEMENT TO PARTICIPATE IN CLASS-
            ROOM VERBAL INTERACTIONS, WHILE ANGLO
            STUDENTS GET MORE OPPORTUNITY TO PAR-
            TICIPATE, MORE PRAISE AND OTHER POSITIVE
            FEEDBACK. IF IT IS AGREED THAT THE HEART
            OF THE EDUCATIONAL PROCESS IS THE INTER-
            ACTION BETWEEN STUDENT AND TEACHER,
            AND THAT THIS INTERACTION IS A MAJOR DE-
            TERMINANT OF QUALITY EDUCATION, THEN
            THE DATA PRESENTED DEMONSTRATE THAT
            ETHNICALLY DIFFERENT STUDENTS ARE BEING
            DENIED OPPORTUNITIES FOR QUALITY EDU-
            CATION BECAUSE OF THE DISPARITIES IN

TEACHERS' EXPECTATIONS AND BEHAVIORS. 30 REFERENCES. (AUTHOR SUMMARY MODIFIED)

ACCN   000540

641   AUTH   **GECAS, V.**
      TITL   SELF-CONCEPTIONS OF MIGRANT AND SETTLED MEXICAN AMERICANS.
      SRCE   *SOCIAL SCIENCE QUARTERLY, 1973, 54(3), 579-595.*
      INDX   SELF CONCEPT, MEXICAN AMERICAN, FARM LABORERS, MIGRATION, MENTAL HEALTH, FAMILY ROLES, FAMILY STRUCTURE, ACCULTURATION, EMPIRICAL, URBAN, RURAL, ALTRUISM, SEX ROLES, MIGRANTS, WASHINGTON, WEST, ETHNIC IDENTITY
      ABST   TWO MAJOR DIMENSIONS OF EMPIRICAL RESEARCH ON SELF-CONCEPT HAVE BEEN THE EVALUATIVE AND THE SUBSTANTIVE. MOST OF THE RESEARCH ON THE SELF-CONCEPTIONS OF MEXICAN AMERICANS (MA) HAS STRESSED THE EVALUATIVE DIMENSION, WITH INCONCLUSIVE RESULTS. THIS STUDY IS AN EXPLORATION OF THE SELF-CONCEPTS OF POOR, RURAL, MIGRANT AND SETTLED MA'S IN TERMS OF THEIR SUBSTANTIVE IDENTITY PATTERNS AND SELF-EVALUATIONS. EIGHTY-FIVE FAMILIES FROM THE YAKIMA VALLEY AGRICULTURAL AREA OF WASHINGTON STATE (ABOUT HALF MIGRANT FAMILIES, THE OTHERS SETTLED IN THE AREA FOR AT LEAST ONE YEAR) WERE INTERVIEWED BY BILINGUAL RESEARCHERS USING A MODIFIED VERSION OF THE TWENTY STATEMENTS TEST TO MEASURE SELF-CONCEPT. WITHIN EACH FAMILY THE MOTHER, FATHER, AND TWO CHILDREN WERE INTERVIEWED. RESPONSES WERE CODED INTO SEVEN CATEGORIES: (1) ASCRIBED CHARACTERISTICS, (2) ROLES AND MEMBERSHIPS, (3) ABSTRACT IDENTIFICATION, (4) INTERESTS AND ACTIVITIES, (5) MATERIAL REFERENCES, (6) SENSES OF SELF, AND (7) PERSONAL CHARACTERISTICS. DIFFERENCES IN THE MIGRANT AND SETTLED FAMILIES SELF-CONCEPTS ARE DISCUSSED IN TERMS OF THE PROCESS OF ACCULTURATION, FAMILY BONDS, ETHNIC IDENTITY AND THE CHICANO MOVEMENT. SOME OF THE MOST SIGNIFICANT FINDINGS ARE THAT MIGRANTS APPEAR TO BE MORE FAMILY ROOTED IN STRUCTURAL SOURCES OF IDENTITY (I.E., FAMILY, RELIGION, WORK, ETHNICITY) THAN ARE THE SETTLED MA'S, AND THAT MIGRANTS HAVE A MORE POSITIVE VIEW OF THEMSELVES THAN THE SETTLED MA'S BOTH IN GENERAL EVALUATIONS OF SELF AND IN SPECIFIC REFERENCE TO MORAL WORTH, COMPETENCE, SELF-DETERMINATION AND ALTRUISM. 33 REFERENCES.
      ACCN   000541

642   AUTH   **GECAS, V., THOMAS, D. L., & WEIGERT, A. J.**
      TITL   SOCIAL IDENTITIES IN ANGLO AND LATIN ADOLESCENTS.
      SRCE   *SOCIAL FORCES, 1973, 51(4), 477-484.*
      INDX   PUERTO RICAN-I, GENDER IDENTITY, MEXICAN, CROSS CULTURAL, ADOLESCENTS, SELF CONCEPT, SEX COMPARISON, RELIGION, FAMILY ROLES, SEX ROLES, CULTURAL FACTORS, NEW YORK, EAST, MINNESOTA, MIDWEST
      ABST   SOCIAL IDENTITIES, CONCEPTUALIZED AS SELF-ATTITUDES AND MEASURED BY THE TWENTY STATEMENTS TEST (TST), ARE EXAMINED FOR SAMPLES OF PAROCHIAL HIGH SCHOOL STUDENTS IN THREE SOCIETIES: UNITED STATES, PUERTO RICO, AND MEXICO. FOUR IDENTITIES ARE EXPLORED IN TERMS OF SALIENCE, FREQUENCY AND VALENCE: (1) GENDER, (2) RELIGION, (3) FAMILY, AND (4) PEERS. A SECOND SAMPLE OF PROTESTANT, PUBLIC HIGH SCHOOL STUDENTS IN MINNEAPOLIS IS PRESENTED FOR COMPARATIVE AND GENERALIZATION PURPOSES. GENERAL FINDINGS ARE: (1) GENDER IS THE MOST PROMINENT IDENTITY FOR BOTH MALES AND FEMALES IN BOTH LATIN AND ANGLO CULTURES; (2) POSITIVE GENDER AND FAMILY IDENTITIES ARE MOST FREQUENT FOR LATIN ADOLESCENTS, WHILE PEER IDENTITIES ARE SLIGHTLY MORE COMMON FOR ANGLOS; AND (3) STRONGEST CULTURAL DIFFERENCE IS FOUND FOR NEGATIVE RELIGIOUS IDENTITIES AND THESE ARE SIGNIFICANTLY MORE FREQUENT FOR ANGLO ADOLESCENTS. SOCIAL AND CULTURAL DIFFERENCES BETWEEN ANGLO AND LATIN SOCIETIES ARE DISCUSSED AS EXPLANATIONS FOR VARIATIONS IN ADOLESCENT IDENTITY STRUCTURES. 20 REFERENCES. (AUTHOR ABSTRACT MODIFIED)
      ACCN   000542

643   AUTH   **GEIS, G., MUNNS, J., & BULLINGTON, B.**
      TITL   THE USE OF EX-ADDICTS IN A REHABILITATIVE AND EDUCATIONAL PROGRAM.
      SRCE   *IN C. WINICK (ED.), SOCIOLOGICAL ASPECTS OF DRUG DEPENDENCE. CLEVELAND, OHIO: CRC PRESS, 1974, PP. 239-252.*
      INDX   REHABILITATION, DRUG ADDICTION, PRIMARY PREVENTION, MEXICAN AMERICAN, PROGRAM EVALUATION, CROSS CULTURAL, SEX COMPARISON, SEX ROLES, EMPIRICAL, REVIEW, CASE STUDY, PARAPROFESSIONALS, CALIFORNIA, SOUTHWEST, SES, URBAN, PERSONNEL, FINANCING
      ABST   THE EMPLOYMENT OF EX-ADDICTS AS CASEWORKERS AND SOCIAL SERVICE PERSONNEL AT THE EAST LOS ANGELES NARCOTICS PREVENTION PROJECT WAS EVALUATED AS TO THE EFFECT ON BOTH ADDICT CLIENTS AND EX-ADDICT PERSONNEL. INVESTIGATION OF SUBSEQUENT DRUG USE AND INCARCERATION AMONG 36 EX-ADDICT CASEWORKERS OVER A 3-YEAR PERIOD DETERMINED THAT 13 WERE SUCCESSFULLY REHABILITATED (ABSTINENT AND STEADILY EMPLOYED), 12 WERE FAILURES (RE-ADDICTED OR INCARCERATED), AND 11 WERE MARGINAL. THE VARIABLES OF MARITAL STATUS, CRIMINAL BACKGROUND, EDUCATIONAL AND INCOME LEVEL, SEX, AND ETHNICITY DISCRIMINATED AMONG OUTCOME GROUPS. THE FAILURE OF FEMALE EX-ADDICTS IS GIVEN PARTICULAR ATTENTION IN A DISCUSSION OF SEX ROLES AND ADDICTION. A FOLLOW-UP EVALUATION OF 54 PREDOMINANTLY MEXICAN AMERICAN ADDICT CLIENTS REVEALED THAT 46% SHOWED IMPROVEMENT

IN AVOIDANCE OF INCARCERATION, 33% IN THEIR EMPLOYMENT RECORD, AND 46% IN ABSTAINING FROM DRUG USE. ALTHOUGH THE DATA PROVIDE ONLY QUALIFIED SUPPORT FOR ANY CONCLUSION REGARDING THE UTILITY OF USING EX-ADDICTS IN REHABILITATION, PROJECTS OF THIS NATURE APPEAR TO HAVE CONSIDERABLE POTENTIAL FOR SUCCESS. IT IS SUGGESTED THAT THE RELATIONSHIP BETWEEN EX-ADDICT TRAITS AND REHABILITATION OUTCOME BE CONSIDERED SO AS TO MAXIMIZE SUCCESS POTENTIAL IN HIRING. 35 REFERENCES.

ACCN   000543

644   AUTH   **GEISMAR, L. L., & KRISBERG, J.**
TITL   THE FORGOTTEN NEIGHBORHOOD: SITE OF AN EARLY SKIRMISH IN THE WAR ON POVERTY.

SRCE   *METUCHEN, N.J.: SCARECROW PRESS, 1967.*
INDX   PUERTO RICAN-M, SOCIAL SERVICES, JUDICIAL PROCESS, COMMUNITY, CHILDREN, ADULTS, EARLY CHILDHOOD EDUCATION, LANGUAGE LEARNING, POVERTY, ADOLESCENTS, ECONOMIC FACTORS, URBAN, CONNECTICUT, EAST
ABST   THE SPECIAL NEEDS OF THE PUERTO RICAN POPULATION OF FARNAM COURTS, NEW HAVEN, ARE DISCUSSED. ONE PROBLEM IS THE LANGUAGE BARRIER. THE PROGRAMS INSTITUTED FOR THIS MINORITY GROUP WERE FAMILY CENTERED CASEWORK, A PRESCHOOL NURSERY, AN ADULT ENGLISH CLASS, AND GROUP WORK WITH YOUTH. THE PROBLEMS CONFRONTING THESE FAMILIES SHOWED A PREDOMINANCE OF FINANCIAL DIFFICULTIES, FOLLOWED BY HEALTH PROBLEMS. THE PUERTO RICAN LABOR DEPARTMENT RECOMMENDED THAT LANGUAGE INSTRUCTION BE CONFINED TO TEACHERS WHO WERE ALSO CONVERSANT IN SPANISH, THAT THE RESIDENTIAL BUILDING PROVIDE A SITTER FOR THE CHILDREN, THAT FUNCTIONAL ENGLISH BE STRESSED, AND THAT HOME VISITING BE DONE BEFORE AND DURING THE PROGRAM. VARIOUS SUCCESSES AND OBSTACLES ARISING FROM THE PROGRAMS ARE DISCUSSED.

ACCN   000544

645   AUTH   **GEISMAR, L., & GERHART, V.**
TITL   SOCIAL CLASS, ETHNICITY, AND FAMILY FUNCTIONING: EXPLORING SOME ISSUES RAISED BY THE MOYNIHAN REPORT.
SRCE   *JOURNAL OF MARRIAGE AND THE FAMILY, 1968, 30(3), 480-487.*
INDX   SES, CROSS CULTURAL, FAMILY STRUCTURE, FAMILY ROLES, PUERTO RICAN-M, EMPIRICAL, SOCIAL MOBILITY, MIGRATION, CHILDREARING PRACTICES, NEW JERSEY, EAST
ABST   AN ATTEMPT TO ASSESS THE INFLUENCE OF SOCIAL CLASS ON THE WAY ETHNIC GROUP MEMBERSHIP AFFECTS FAMILY BEHAVIOR IS EXAMINED. A STRATIFIED RANDOM SAMPLE OF 133 CASES WAS DIVIDED INTO THREE GROUPS—50 NEGROES, 50 WHITES, AND 33 PUERTO RICANS. DATA FROM INTERVIEWS AND STRUCTURED QUESTIONNAIRES ON CHILDREARING ATTITUDES AND ALIENATION FROM

SOCIETY WERE OBTAINED. THE ST. PAUL SCALE OF FAMILY FUNCTIONING REVEALED SHARP CONTRASTS IN THE LEVEL OF FUNCTIONING AMONG THE GROUPS. SIXTY-SIX PERCENT OF THE NEGROES, 46 PERCENT OF THE PUERTO RICANS AND 16 PERCENT OF THE WHITES INDICATED PROBLEMATIC OR NEAR PROBLEMATIC FAMILY FUNCTIONING. ADEQUATE FUNCTIONING APPEARED TO BE CHARACTERISTIC OF 44 PERCENT OF THE WHITES, 21 PERCENT OF THE PUERTO RICANS, AND 12 PERCENT OF THE NEGRO FAMILIES. THE DATA SHOW THAT 82 PERCENT OF WHITES, 73 PERCENT OF PUERTO RICANS, AND 44 PERCENT OF NEGROES HAD A SUFFICIENT SOURCE OF INCOME. NEGRO AND PUERTO RICAN WAGE EARNERS HELD LOWER STATUS JOBS THAN WHITES. THE PUERTO RICAN HEAD OF THE FAMILY HAD LESS DIFFICULTY IN HOLDING A JOB THAN A NEGRO. IT IS SUGGESTED THAT IT IS A DELICATE INTERPLAY AMONG SOCIAL, ECONOMIC, AND PSYCHOLOGICAL FACTORS RATHER THAN THE OPERATION OF ANY ONE OF THEM WHICH DETERMINES THE SOCIAL FUNCTIONING OF FAMILIES IN THE VARIOUS ETHNIC GROUPS. 28 REFERENCES.

ACCN   000545

646   AUTH   **GEKOSKI, W. L.**
TITL   EFFECTS OF LANGUAGE ACQUISITION CONTEXTS ON SEMANTIC PROCESSING IN BILINGUALS.
SRCE   *PROCEEDINGS OF THE 78TH ANNUAL CONVENTION OF THE AMERICAN PSYCHOLOGICAL ASSOCIATION, 1970, 487-488.*
INDX   LINGUISTICS, BILINGUALISM, COMPOUND-COORDINATE DISTINCTION, LANGUAGE ACQUISITION, MICHIGAN, MIDWEST, BILINGUAL, EMPIRICAL
ABST   THE COMPOUND-COORDINATE DISTINCTION MAINTAINS THAT BILINGUALS DIFFER IN THE MANNER IN WHICH THEY STORE AND STRUCTURE THE SEMANTIC COMPONENT OF THEIR LINGUISTIC REPERTOIRES. THE BASIS OF THE DIFFERENCE IS SEEN AS DERIVING FROM THE CULTURAL AND LINGUISTIC CONTEXTS IN WHICH LANGUAGE ACQUISITION OCCURRED. SPANISH-ENGLISH BILINGUALS WERE ASKED TO GIVE INTRALINGUAL AND INTERLINGUAL WORD ASSOCIATIONS TO EQUIVALENT STIMULI FOR WHICH THE RESPONSES OF MONOLINGUAL SPANISH AND ENGLISH SPEAKERS WERE NOT EQUIVALENT. AS PREDICTED, COMPOUND BILINGUALS GAVE MORE TRANSLATION EQUIVALENT RESPONSES THAN DID COORDINATE BILINGUALS, THUS OFFERING SOME SUPPORT FOR THE COMPOUND-COORDINATE DISTINCTION.

ACCN   000546

647   AUTH   **GENTILE, L. M.**
TITL   EFFECT OF TUTOR SEX ON LEARNING TO READ.
SRCE   *READING TEACHER, 1975, 28(8), 726-730.*
INDX   READING, COGNITIVE DEVELOPMENT, PARAPROFESSIONALS, CHILDREN, MEXICAN AMERICAN, EDUCATIONAL COUNSELING, EXAMINER

EFFECTS, EMPIRICAL, ARIZONA, SOUTHWEST, MALE

ABST 60 MEXICAN AMERICAN BOYS FROM THE 2ND, 3RD, AND 4TH GRADES OF AN ARIZONA SCHOOL WERE TUTORED IN READING FOR ONE HOUR TWICE A WEEK FOR 8 WEEKS. ONE BOY FROM EACH GRADE WAS RANDOMLY AS-SIGNED TO EACH OF 10 MALE AND 10 FEMALE TUTORS (HALF OF WHOM WERE MEXICAN AMERICAN AND HALF ANGLO AMERICAN) WHO WERE SPECIALLY TRAINED FOR THE STUDY. THE GROUP AS A WHOLE MADE A SIGNIFICANT GAIN WITH THE TREATMENT, BUT IMPROVE-MENT VARIED IN THE DIFFERENT GRADES, 4TH-GRADE SUBJECTS TUTORED BY MALES SHOW-ING THE MOST GAIN. RESULTS ARE PRE-SENTED IN DETAIL AND ASPECTS NEEDING FURTHER INVESTIGATION ARE SPECIFIED. 15 REFERENCES. (PASAR ABSTRACT)

ACCN 000547

648 AUTH **GERARD, D. L., & KORNETSKY, C.**
TITL A SOCIAL AND PSYCHIATRIC STUDY OF ADO-LESCENT OPIATE ADDICTS.
SRCE *PSYCHIATRIC QUARTERLY, 1954, 28(1), 113-125.*
INDX PSYCHOSOCIAL ADJUSTMENT, DRUG ADDIC-TION, PROJECTIVE TESTING, RORSCHACH TEST, TAT, PUERTO RICAN-M, ADOLESCENTS, EMPIR-ICAL, CROSS CULTURAL, SCHIZOPHRENIA, KENTUCKY, SOUTH, PSYCHOPATHOLOGY

ABST THE SOCIAL AND PSYCHIATRIC CHARACTER-ISTICS OF 32 MINOR MALE OPIATE ADDICTS WERE STUDIED DURING THEIR STAY AT THE U.S. PUBLIC HEALTH SERVICE HOSPITAL AT LEXINGTON, KENTUCKY. THE MAJORITY WERE NEGRO AND PUERTO RICAN ADOLESCENTS FROM DEPRIVED COMMUNITIES IN NEW YORK CITY OR CHICAGO BUT THE WHITE ADDICTS HAD BEEN REARED IN ECONOMICALLY COM-FORTABLE, MIDDLE-CLASS FAMILIES. ALL AD-DICTS SHOWED MARKED DISTURBANCES IN ADJUSTMENT PRIOR TO DRUG USE. THESE WERE DIAGNOSED AS OVERT SCHIZOPHRE-NIA, INCIPIENT SCHIZOPHRENIA OR BORDER-LINE STATES, DELINQUENCY-DOMINATED CHARACTER DISORDERS, AND INADEQUATE PERSONALITIES. THEY ALL HAD DYSPHORIA, DISTURBANCES IN SEXUAL IDENTIFICATION, AND INTERPERSONAL RELATIONS CHARAC-TERIZED BY INABILITY TO FORM PROLONGED, CLOSE, OR FRIENDLY RELATIONSHIPS WITH PEERS OR ADULTS. EVIDENCE OBTAINED IN THE PROJECTIVE MATERIAL-RORSCHACH, THEMATIC APPERCEPTION TEST, AND DRAW-A-MAN TEST-CORROBORATED THE CLINICAL OB-SERVATIONS. OPIATE DRUG USE HELPED TREAT THE OVERT PSYCHIATRIC SYMPTOMS OF SOME ADDICTS, CONTROLLED THE ANXIETY AND STRAIN THE PATIENTS EXPERIENCED IN VARI-OUS INTERPERSONAL SITUATIONS, AND HELPED THEM COPE WITH LIFE.

ACCN 000548

649 AUTH **GERARD, H. B.**
TITL FACTORS CONTRIBUTING TO ADJUSTMENT AND ACHIEVEMENT (PROGRESS REPORT OF GRANT NO. PHS HD/02863).

SRCE *LOS ANGELES: DEPARTMENT OF PSYCHOLOGY, UNIVERSITY OF CALIFORNIA, MAY 1968.*
INDX EDUCATION, SCHOLASTIC ACHIEVEMENT, PSY-CHOSOCIAL ADJUSTMENT, INTEGRATION, CHILDREN, EMPIRICAL, SCHOLASTIC ASPIRA-TIONS, OCCUPATIONAL ASPIRATIONS, SELF CONCEPT, ANXIETY, PEABODY PICTURE-VO-CABULARY TEST, PREJUDICE, ETHNIC IDEN-TITY, MEXICAN AMERICAN, CROSS CULTURAL, INTELLIGENCE TESTING, LOCUS OF CONTROL, CALIFORNIA, SOUTHWEST

ABST THIS PROJECT WAS DESIGNED TO DETERMINE PRIOR AND MEDIATING FACTORS INVOLVED IN THE SUCCESSFUL OR UNSUCCESSFUL INTE-GRATION OF ANGLO, BLACK, AND MEXICAN AMERICAN CHILDREN IN A PUBLIC SCHOOL SYSTEM. THE TWO MAJOR DEPENDENT VARI-ABLES INVESTIGATED WERE ACADEMIC ACHIEVEMENT AND EMOTIONAL ADJUSTMENT. THE DATA COLLECTED REPRESENT FOUR DIF-FERENT PERSPECTIVES: THE CHILD'S PAR-ENTS, TEACHER, CLASSMATES, AND CHILD'S SELF-EVALUATION. THE INITIAL SAMPLE WAS COMPRISED OF ALL CHILDREN ATTENDING SEGREGATED MINORITY ELEMENTARY SCHOOLS AND A RANDOM SAMPLE OF ANGLO CHILDREN ATTENDING FORMERLY SEGRE-GATED ANGLO ELEMENTARY SCHOOLS IN THE RIVERSIDE UNIFIED SCHOOL DISTRICT, CALI-FORNIA, DURING THE SCHOOL YEAR 1965-66. FOR THE PREDESEGREGATION MEASURES EACH CHILD WAS TESTED EXTENSIVELY FOR TWO ONE HOUR SESSIONS REGARDING DE-LAYED GRATIFICATION, SELF-PERCEPTIONS, ATTITUDES TOWARDS DIFFERENT ETHNIC/RA-CIAL CHILDREN, FIELD INDEPENDENCE/DE-PENDENCE, DISSONANCE, VERBAL AND NON-VERBAL INTELLIGENCE TESTS, CONFORMITY, AND OTHER BEHAVIORAL DIMENSIONS. IN AD-DITION, INFORMATION WAS OBTAINED FROM PARENTAL INTERVIEWS, SOCIOMETRIC RAT-INGS OF EACH CLASSROOM, AND TEACHER RATINGS ON CHILD'S CLASSROOM BEHAVIOR. THE POSTMEASUREMENT DATA OBTAINED DURING 1967 WERE SIMILAR TO THE INITIAL STUDY EXCEPT THAT INTELLIGENCE AND DIS-SONANCE MEASURES WERE NOT REPEATED, A NEW DELAY OF GRATIFICATION VARIABLE WAS USED, AND ADDITIONAL MEASURES OF LOCUS OF CONTROL AND DESIRE FOR MASTERY WERE INTRODUCED. THE DATA REPORTED ARE IN THE EARLY STAGES OF ANALYSIS; SOME OF THE PREVIOUS FINDINGS ARE REPORTED. 25 REFERENCES.

ACCN 000549

650 AUTH **GERARD, H. B.**
TITL FACTORS CONTRIBUTING TO ADJUSTMENT AND ACHIEVEMENT (PROGRESS REPORT OF GRANT NO. PHS HD/02863).
SRCE *LOS ANGELES: DEPARTMENT OF PSYCHOLOGY, UNIVERSITY OF CALIFORNIA, MAY 1969.*
INDX EDUCATION, SCHOLASTIC ACHIEVEMENT, PSY-CHOSOCIAL ADJUSTMENT, INTEGRATION, CHILDREN, EMPIRICAL, SURVEY, RESEARCH METHODOLOGY, ATTITUDES, SCHOLASTIC AS-PIRATIONS, OCCUPATIONAL ASPIRATIONS, SELF CONCEPT, ANXIETY, PEABODY PICTURE-VO-

CABULARY TEST, PREJUDICE, ETHNIC IDENTITY, MEXICAN AMERICAN, CROSS CULTURAL, INTELLIGENCE TESTING, CALIFORNIA, SOUTHWEST

ABST THIS REPORT OF THE PROGRESS UNDER STUDY OF THE DESEGREGATION OF THE RIVERSIDE, CALIFORNIA UNIFIED SCHOOL DISTRICT FOCUSES ON ACHIEVEMENT RELATED ATTITUDES. ONGOING RESEARCH IS BEING CONDUCTED CONCERNING THE EFFECT OF FAMILY BACKGROUND CHARACTERISTICS ON THEIR ATTITUDES AND THE DEGREE TO WHICH THEIR ATTITUDES SUBSEQUENTLY AFFECT EMOTIONAL ADJUSTMENT AND ACHIEVEMENT IN THE RACIALLY MIXED CLASSROOMS AS WELL AS THE EFFECT THAT INTEGRATED CLASSROOMS HAVE ON ACHIEVEMENT RELATED ATTITUDES. IN THIS THIRD YEAR FOLLOW-UP STUDY 1305 CHILDREN OUT OF THE ORIGINAL TOTAL SAMPLE OF 1800 CHILDREN HAVE BEEN LOCATED. INSTRUMENTS USED IN THE EARLIER STUDIES ARE BEING UTILIZED ONCE AGAIN, SUCH AS THE CHILDREN'S APPERCEPTION TEST (CAT). PRELIMINARY FINDINGS FOR THE YEARS 1966 AND 1967 ARE REPORTED ON SOME OF THE VARIABLES. HOWEVER, FURTHER ANALYSIS IS PRESENTLY BEING PERFORMED REGARDING THE FOLLOWING FACTORS: DELAYED GRATIFICATION; DISSONANCE REDUCTION; FIELD DEPENDENCE-INDEPENDENCE; LEVELS OF ASPIRATION, NEEDS, FEARS, AND TRANSCENDENCE; SPEECH PARAPRAXES; DIALECT DANGERS; AND RESPONSIVENESS TO SOCIAL REINFORCEMENT. 6 REFERENCES.

ACCN 000550

651 AUTH **GERRY, M. H.**
TITL CULTURAL FREEDOM IN THE SCHOOLS: THE RIGHT OF MEXICAN AMERICAN CHILDREN TO SUCCEED.
SRCE *IN A. CASTANEDA, M. RAMIREZ, III, C. E. CORTES, & M. BARRERA (EDS.), MEXICAN AMERICANS AND EDUCATIONAL CHANGE. NEW YORK: ARNO PRESS, 1974, PP. 226-254.*
INDX LEGISLATION, JUDICIAL PROCESS, MEXICAN AMERICAN, EDUCATION, SCHOLASTIC ACHIEVEMENT, DISCRIMINATION, EQUAL OPPORTUNITY, REPRESENTATION, BILINGUAL-BICULTURAL EDUCATION, BILINGUAL-BICULTURAL PERSONNEL, BILINGUALISM, LEADERSHIP, ADMINISTRATORS, ACHIEVEMENT TESTING, PROGRAM EVALUATION, CULTURAL PLURALISM
ABST A REVIEW IS PRESENTED OF THE OFFICE ON CIVIL RIGHTS' (OCR) 1970 MEMORANDUM WHICH ENUMERATES FOUR MAIN AREAS OF CONCERN RELATING TO COMPLIANCE BY SCHOOL DISTRICTS WITH TITLE VI: (1) EXCLUSION OF MINORITY CHILDREN FROM EDUCATIONAL PROGRAMS DUE TO THEIR LACK OF ENGLISH-SPEAKING ABILITY; (2) ASSIGNMENT OF THESE CHILDREN TO CLASSES FOR THE MENTALLY RETARDED; (3) INAPPROPRIATE TRACKING SYSTEMS TO DEAL WITH SPECIAL LANGUAGE SKILLS; AND (4) NEGLIGENCE IN THE NOTIFICATION OF THESE CHILDREN'S PARENTS ABOUT SCHOOL ACTIVITIES. THE METHODS UNDERTAKEN TO PROVE SCHOOL

DISTRICTS' NONCOMPLIANCE IN THESE FOUR AREAS ARE OUTLINED IN FOUR SECTIONS. SECTION 1: A SERIES OF PILOT REVIEWS GATHERING DATA ON THE CULTURAL BACKGROUND OF MEXICAN AMERICAN CHILDREN UPON ENTERING THE SCHOOL SYSTEM, AND DATA ON THE ACADEMIC PERFORMANCE OF THESE CHILDREN UP THROUGH 8TH GRADE. SECTION 2: A REVIEW OF VERBAL IQ SCORES. SECTION 3: PILOT CASES OF RACIALLY DISCRIMINATORY ASSIGNMENT PRACTICES. SECTION 4: INTERVIEWS WITH PARENTS AND SCHOOL PERSONNEL. BASED ON THESE DATA-GATHERING STRATEGIES, A SET OF SIX RECOMMENDATIONS ARE OFFERED TO GUIDE EFFECTIVE IMPLEMENTATION OF THE OCR MEMORANDUM. 11 REFERENCES.

ACCN 000552

652 AUTH **GERRY, M. H.**
TITL CULTURAL MYOPIA: THE NEED FOR A CORRECTIVE LENS.
SRCE *JOURNAL OF SCHOOL PSYCHOLOGY, 1973, 11(4), 307-315.*
INDX DISCRIMINATION, EDUCATION, SES, INTELLIGENCE TESTING, TEST VALIDITY, MENTAL RETARDATION, SPECIAL EDUCATION, ESSAY, CHILDREN, MEXICAN AMERICAN, CROSS CULTURAL, BILINGUAL-BICULTURAL EDUCATION, POLICY
ABST THE OFFICE FOR CIVIL RIGHTS ON MAY 25, 1970, ISSUED A MEMORANDUM TO SCHOOL DISTRICTS IN ORDER TO PROHIBIT DISCRIMINATION AGAINST NATIONAL ORIGIN MINORITY CHILDREN. SUCH DISCRIMINATION RESULTS FROM A FAILURE BY SCHOOL DISTRICTS TO RECOGNIZE THE DIFFERING LINGUISTIC CHARACTERISTICS AND CULTURAL IDENTITY OF SUCH CHILDREN IN THE PLANNING AND OPERATION OF EDUCATION PROGRAMS. SPECIFICALLY, THE MEMORANDUM PROHIBITS THE ASSIGNMENT OF CHILDREN TO CLASSES FOR THE MENTALLY RETARDED ON THE BASIS OF CRITERIA WHICH ESSENTIALLY MEASURE OR EVALUATE ENGLISH LANGUAGE SKILLS. A TASK GROUP WAS APPOINTED BY THE SECRETARY OF HEW TO DEVELOP EDUCATIONAL POLICIES TO IMPLEMENT THIS ANTIDISCRIMINATION PROVISION. THIS TASK GROUP RECOMMENDED THAT ADDITIONAL POLICIES BE DEVELOPED BY THE OFFICE FOR CIVIL RIGHTS (1) TO NOTIFY SCHOOL DISTRICTS AND MEMBERS OF THE GENERAL PUBLIC OF THE TYPES OF DISCRIMINATORY PRACTICES THAT MIGHT BE OCCURRING, AND (2) TO SET FORTH MODEL PROCEDURES WHICH SCHOOL DISTRICTS COULD FOLLOW IN AN EFFORT TO ELIMINATE DISCRIMINATORY PRACTICES WHICH MIGHT CURRENTLY EXIST. THIS PAPER DISCUSSES THOSE PROCEDURES RECOMMENDED BY THE COMMITTEE. 4 REFERENCES. (NCMHI ABSTRACT MODIFIED)

ACCN 000553

653 AUTH **GHALI, S. B.**
TITL CULTURE SENSITIVITY AND THE PUERTO RICAN CLIENT.
SRCE *SOCIAL CASEWORK, 1977, 58(8), 459-466.*

INDX   PUERTO RICAN-M, MENTAL HEALTH, HEALTH DELIVERY SYSTEMS, CULTURAL FACTORS, POLICY, SOCIAL SERVICES, FAMILY STRUCTURE, FAMILY ROLES, IMMIGRATION, ACCULTURATION, ADOLESCENTS, ADULTS, ATTITUDES, RESOURCE UTILIZATION, ESSAY, FAMILY THERAPY, ECONOMIC FACTORS, PSYCHOTHERAPY

ABST   CULTURAL CONFLICTS, BREAKDOWN OF PARENTAL AUTHORITY, AND PROBLEMS OF UNEMPLOYMENT ARE SOME OF THE SERIOUS PROBLEMS SUFFERED BY PUERTO RICAN FAMILIES WHEN THEY ARE MAKING THE TRANSITION TO MAINLAND URBAN CENTERS. TO HELP SOLVE SUCH PROBLEMS, MENTAL HEALTH PERSONNEL MUST GO BEYOND THEIR CUSTOMARY DELIVERY STRATEGIES TO PROVIDE SERVICES THAT ARE CULTURALLY RELEVANT TO PUERTO RICAN IMMIGRANTS. IT IS SUGGESTED THAT THERAPISTS MAKE THEIR CLIENTS FEEL COMFORTABLE BY PROVIDING A HOME-LIKE ENVIRONMENT, BY EMPLOYING SPANISH-SPEAKING STAFF, AND BY COORDINATING AUXILIARY SOCIAL SERVICES TO ASSIST IN THE CLIENT'S ADAPTATION TO THE U.S. THEY SHOULD CLEARLY DEMONSTRATE THEIR ACCEPTANCE OF THE CLIENT'S CULTURE, COLOR, AND VALUES—EVEN ENCOURAGING, AT TIMES, PARTICIPATION IN THE FOLK-HEALING PROCESS. FAMILY COHESIVENESS SHOULD BE REINFORCED BY MEANS OF HOME VISITS AND IMPLEMENTATION OF FAMILY THERAPY. THE SPECIAL PROBLEMS OF PUERTO RICAN ADOLESCENTS HAVE TO BE RECOGNIZED—IN PARTICULAR, THEIR CULTURE CONFLICT INVOLVING THEIR PARENTS' TRADITIONAL EXPECTATIONS AND THOSE OF THE NEW SOCIETY. MOREOVER, THE THERAPIST SHOULD BEAR IN MIND THAT THE PUERTO RICAN FAMILY HAS WITHIN ITSELF THE RESOURCES AND STRENGTHS TO RESTORE HOMEOSTASIS. IN CONCLUSION, THE FUNDAMENTAL POINT IS THAT AN UNDERSTANDING OF PUERTO RICAN CULTURE IS ESSENTIAL FOR PROVIDING ACCEPTABLE RESOLUTIONS TO FAMILY OR PERSONAL PROBLEMS. THREE CASE STUDIES ARE PROVIDED AS ILLUSTRATIVE EXAMPLES. 4 REFERENCES.

ACCN   002090

654 AUTH   **GIBSON, G.**
TITL   AN APPROACH TO IDENTIFICATION AND PREVENTION FOR DEVELOPMENTAL DIFFICULTIES AMONG MEXICAN AMERICAN CHILDREN.
SRCE   *AMERICAN JOURNAL OF ORTHOPSYCHIATRY, 1978, 48(1), 96-113.*
INDX   BILINGUALISM, BILINGUAL-BICULTURAL PERSONNEL, CHILDREN, CULTURAL FACTORS, DISEASE, ESSAY, HEALTH, HEALTH DELIVERY SYSTEMS, IMPAIRMENT, LEARNING DISABILITIES, LEGISLATION, MENTAL HEALTH, MEXICAN AMERICAN, PHYSICAL DEVELOPMENT, POVERTY, PRIMARY PREVENTION, RESOURCE UTILIZATION, SES, PROGRAM EVALUATION
ABST   FOLLOWING A REVIEW OF THE LITERATURE REGARDING THE MEXICAN AMERICAN'S UNMET MENTAL HEALTH NEEDS, AN APPROACH FOR PROVIDING SCREENING AND REMEDIAL

SERVICES RESPONSIVE TO THE NEEDS OF CHICANOS IS OUTLINED. A WELL DOCUMENTED FACT IS THAT CHICANOS ARE UNDERREPRESENTED IN AVAILABLE HEALTH AND MENTAL HEALTH PROGRAMS. THEREFORE, THE EARLY AND PERIODIC SCREENING DIAGNOSIS AND TREATMENT (EPSDT) PROGRAM, LEGISLATED IN 1967, AUTHORIZED STATES TO SET UP DIAGNOSIS AND TREATMENT CLINICS FOR LOW-INCOME CHILDREN UNDER 21. BUT A POTENTIAL PITFALL OF SUCH PROGRAMS IS THE USE OF DIAGNOSTIC AND TREATMENT PROCEDURES THAT REINFORCE THE ALREADY ENTRENCHED STEREOTYPED THINKING ABOUT CHICANOS; THIS IS PARTICULARLY SIGNIFICANT WHEN USING TESTING INSTRUMENTS THAT ARE ETHNOCENTRIC AND IRRELEVANT TO THE CHICANO EXPERIENCE. THE PROJECTED BENEFIT OF A WELL-ADMINISTERED, CREATIVE PROGRAM FOR PREVENTING AND ALLEVIATING THE DEVELOPMENTAL PROBLEMS OF POOR MEXICAN AMERICANS IS TREMENDOUS. WHILE SCREENING FOR WHAT IS WRONG, AN ATTEMPT MAY BE MADE TO IDENTIFY THE STRENGTHS AND POSITIVE POTENTIALS OF CHILDREN. MOREOVER, A WELL-FUNDED PROGRAM WITH BILINGUAL-BICULTURAL STAFF SERVING AS ADVOCATES COULD BE INSTRUMENTAL IN PROMOTING SOCIAL CHANGE. EPSDT HAS THE INTENT AND PROMISE OF IDENTIFYING AND PREVENTING PROBLEMS AND PROMOTING A MORE HUMANE LIFE FOR MANY FAMILIES; AND IN THIS REGARD, A MODEL IMPLEMENTATION PLAN IS PROPOSED TO MAXIMIZE THIS POTENTIAL BENEFIT OF THE EPSDT PROGRAM FOR THE CHICANO COMMUNITY. 117 REFERENCES.
ACCN   002091

655 AUTH   **GIBSON, G.**
TITL   TRAINING ASPECTS IN WORKING WITH CHICANOS.
SRCE   *MANO A MANO. HOUSTON: CHICANO TRAINING CENTER, 1975, 4, 1-4.*
INDX   PROFESSIONAL TRAINING, PARAPROFESSIONALS, CULTURAL FACTORS, BILINGUAL-BICULTURAL PERSONNEL, ESSAY, DISCRIMINATION, MENTAL HEALTH, MEXICAN AMERICAN, HEALTH DELIVERY SYSTEMS, POLICY
ABST   TRAINING PROGRAMS FOR CHICANO MENTAL HEALTH PROFESSIONALS HAVE HAD SOME FAVORABLE RESULTS BUT A GREAT DEAL MORE NEEDS TO BE DONE. THIS PAPER DISCUSSES TRAINING ASPECTS THAT WILL: (1) PROMOTE UNDERSTANDING BETWEEN CHICANO MENTAL HEALTH WORKERS AND NON-CHICANO PROFESSIONALS; (2) CONTRIBUTE TO THE DEVELOPMENT OF INNOVATIVE TREATMENT APPROACHES FOR CHICANO CLIENTELE; AND (3) ULTIMATELY ENHANCE THE MENTAL HEALTH SERVICE DELIVERY IN THE BARRIO. THE CONCEPTS OF RACISM AND BILINGUALISM AS THEY INFLUENCE TRAINERS AND TRAINEES ARE DISCUSSED. THE FOLLOWING POINTS ARE EMPHASIZED: (1) A BETTER TEACHING CLIMATE EXISTS WHEN EQUAL STATUS BETWEEN TRAINERS AND TRAINEES EXISTS; (2) A CULTURALLY DEMOCRATIC LEARNING ENVIRONMENT THAT

RECOGNIZES THE TRAINEES' UNIQUE COGNITIVE AND RELATIONAL STYLE IS THE MOST PRODUCTIVE IN PREPARING BOTH CHICANOS AND ANGLOS TO WORK IN THE BARRIO; (3) THE STRENGTHS CHICANO MENTAL HEALTH WORKERS BRING TO THE LEARNING SITUATION ARE AN ASSET FOR TRAINING IN GROUPS AND WILL HELP NON-CHICANO STAFF TO ACQUIRE A DIFFERENT PERSPECTIVE FOR DIAGNOSIS AND TREATMENT OF CHICANOS; (4) CHICANO MENTAL HEALTH WORKERS CAN SERVE THE BARRIO MORE EFFICIENTLY IF THEY RETAIN THEIR SENSE OF THE BARRIO; (5) NON-CHICANO MENTAL HEALTH PROFESSIONALS WHO WORK WITH CHICANO TRAINEES MUST CHANGE CONDESCENDING AND DEMEANING BELIEFS ABOUT CHICANOS; AND (6) ALL MENTAL HEALTH PERSONNEL COMMITTED TO SERVING THE BARRIO SHOULD DEVELOP BILINGUAL SKILLS AND CULTURAL SENSITIVITY. 24 REFERENCES. (AUTHOR SUMMARY MODIFIED)

ACCN   000554

656 AUTH   **GIBSON, G., GOMEZ, E., & SANTOS, Y.**
    TITL   BILINGUAL-BICULTURAL SERVICE FOR THE BARRIO.
    SRCE   *SOCIAL WELFARE FORUM, 1973, 213-235.*
    INDX   ESSAY, MEXICAN AMERICAN, CULTURAL PLURALISM, MENTAL HEALTH PROFESSION, SOCIAL SERVICES, PROFESSIONAL TRAINING, BILINGUAL-BICULTURAL PERSONNEL, CULTURAL FACTORS, TEXAS, SOUTHWEST
    ABST   THIS PAPER OFFERS A RATIONALE FOR A BILINGUAL-BICULTURAL SOCIAL WORK MODEL BASED ON THE EDUCATION AND PRACTICE OF SOCIAL WORKERS AT THE CENTRO DEL BARRIO IN SAN ANTONIO, TEXAS. IT IS POSITED THAT SERVICES TO CHICANOS CAN BE RELEVANTLY AND EFFECTIVELY DEVELOPED WITHIN THE ESTABLISHED VALUE BASE OF SOCIAL WORK IF SOCIAL WORKERS ACKNOWLEDGE THE ROLE THESE VALUES PLAY IN THEIR PRACTICE AND IF THEY MINIMIZE THE INTRUSION OF THESE PERSONAL BIASES INTO THEIR PROFESSIONAL WORK. AS THE MODEL HAS EVOLVED, THE BILINGUAL-BICULTURAL SOCIAL WORKER HAS LEARNED TO ASSUME A VARIETY OF ROLES: OUTREACH WORKER, ADVOCATE, BEHAVIOR CHANGER, AND TEACHER. THE KNOWLEDGE, SKILLS AND ATTITUDES ESSENTIAL FOR BILINGUAL-BICULTURAL SOCIAL WORK PRACTICE ARE BEING IDENTIFIED AND REFINED. IMPLICATIONS FOR THE ACCEPTANCE AND USE OF THIS MODEL ON CHICANO SOCIAL WORK STUDENTS, SCHOOLS, AND AGENCIES ARE DISCUSSED. 22 REFERENCES.

ACCN   000555

657 AUTH   **GIBSON, R. W.**
    TITL   EVALUATION AND QUALITY CONTROL OF MENTAL HEALTH SERVICES.
    SRCE   *IN E. R. PADILLA & A. M. PADILLA (EDS.), TRANSCULTURAL PSYCHIATRY: AN HISPANIC PERSPECTIVE (MONOGRAPH NO. 4). LOS ANGELES: UNIVERSITY OF CALIFORNIA, SPANISH SPEAKING MENTAL HEALTH RESEARCH CENTER, 1977, PP. 13-20.*

    INDX   RESOURCE UTILIZATION, MENTAL HEALTH, COMMUNITY, PROGRAM EVALUATION, EQUAL OPPORTUNITY, MENTAL HEALTH PROFESSION, SPANISH SURNAMED, PROFESSIONAL TRAINING, PSYCHOTHERAPY, PSYCHOTHERAPY OUTCOME, ESSAY
    ABST   EVALUATION AND QUALITY CONTROL ARE TWO ESSENTIAL TOOLS FOR IMPROVING THERAPEUTIC METHODS IN HEALTH CARE. HOWEVER IN THE FIELD OF MENTAL HEALTH WHERE (1) OUTCOME STUDIES ARE INADEQUATE, (2) STANDARDS AND CRITERIA ARE NOT AS YET AVAILABLE, AND (3) IT IS DIFFICULT TO BALANCE HUMANISTIC CONCERNS AGAINST COST EFFECTIVENESS, THE TASK OF EVALUATION AND QUALITY CONTROL IS AN ESPECIALLY DIFFICULT ONE. WHEN MENTAL HEALTH SERVICES FOR MINORITY AND LOWER SOCIOECONOMIC GROUPS ARE CONSIDERED, THE PROBLEM BECOMES EVEN GREATER DUE TO THE DIFFICULTY OF DETERMINING THE APPROPRIATENESS AND EFFICACY OF TRADITIONAL TREATMENT WITH THESE POPULATIONS. FEDERAL, STATE AND COUNTY REGULATORY AGENCIES DEMAND EVER MORE EVIDENCE THAT HEALTH SERVICES ARE EFFECTIVE AND EFFICIENT BEFORE FUNDS ARE PROVIDED. THESE REGULATIONS ARE OFTEN UNREASONABLE AND EXCESSIVE

658 AUTH   **GILBERT, M. J.**
    TITL   INTERACTION AND EXCHANGE PATTERNS OF MEXICAN AMERICAN FAMILIES IN TWO SOUTHERN CALIFORNIA SETTINGS.
    SRCE   *PAPER PRESENTED AT THE ANNUAL MEETING OF THE SOUTHWESTERN ANTHROPOLOGICAL ASSOCIATION, SAN DIEGO, APRIL 1977.*
    INDX   MEXICAN AMERICAN, ADULTS, SURVEY, URBAN, RURAL, EMPIRICAL, SES, FAMILY STRUCTURE, FAMILY ROLES, MIGRATION, INTERPERSONAL RELATIONS, CALIFORNIA, SOUTHWEST
    ABST   FAMILY ACTIVITY PATTERNS IN A VARIETY OF SECOND GENERATION MEXICAN AMERICAN FAMILIES ARE STUDIED. THIS PRELIMINARY ANALYSIS OF RESEARCH FINDINGS DESCRIBES THE SAMPLE POPULATIONS, DIFFERENCES IN THE GEOGRAPHIC DISTRIBUTION OF THEIR KINSMEN, AND VARIATIONS IN THEIR INTERACTION AND EXCHANGE PATTERNS. THE GROUPS STUDIED ARE COMPRISED OF 119 SECOND GENERATION MEXICAN AMERICAN ADULTS FROM TWO SOUTHERN CALIFORNIA AREAS, ONE RURAL, THE OTHER URBAN. THE SAMPLES ARE FURTHER DIVIDED BY NEIGHBORHOOD COMPOSITION—PREDOMINANTLY ANGLO, MIXED, OR BARRIO. THE DIFFERENCES IN THE ECONOMIC, EDUCATIONAL, AND GENERAL CHARACTERISTICS OF THE PERSONS INTERVIEWED SHOW SEVERAL CORRELATIONS WITH VARIATION IN KINSHIP INTERACTION AND EXCHANGE PATTERNS. AMONG THESE ARE: (1) URBAN RESIDENTS HAVE A MUCH MORE LOCALIZED KIN STRUCTURE THAN DO RURAL RESIDENTS; (2) THE MORE KIN AVAILABLE FOR INTERACTION, THE SMALLER THE PERCENTAGE WITH WHOM THE RESPONDENT VISITS, IN-

DICATING A SELECTION PROCESS; (3) THE NUMBER OF BOTH PRIMARY AND SECONDARY KIN VISITED BY RESPONDENTS IS POSITIVELY RELATED TO THE NUMBER OF KIN LOCALLY AVAILABLE FOR BOTH URBAN AND RURAL RESIDENTS; (4) A HIGHER RANGE OF ACTIVITIES WITH PRIMARY KINSMEN IS ASSOCIATED WITH HIGHER INCOMES; (5) OVERALL, KINSMEN OUTSIDE THE PRIMARY GROUP PLAY A MINIMAL ROLE IN EXCHANGE PATTERNS FOR MOST OF THE RESPONDENTS. THESE FINDINGS SUGGEST THAT THE MAINTENANCE OF VIABLE AND STABLE INTERACTION AND EXCHANGE RELATIONSHIPS WITH THOSE MOST LIKELY TO BE OF HELP TO INDIVIDUALS, THEIR PRIMARY KINSMEN, IS DEPENDENT ON ACCESS TO OUTSIDE RESOURCES, A PROCESS SIMILAR TO DOMINANT SOCIETY FAMILIES IN THE U.S. 16 REFERENCES.

ACCN   000557

659 AUTH **GILBERT, M. J.**
TITL   QUALITATIVE ANALYSIS OF THE DRINKING PRACTICES AND ALCOHOL-RELATED PROBLEMS OF THE SPANISH SPEAKING IN THREE CALIFORNIA LOCALES.
SRCE   *ALHAMBRA, CALIF.: TECHNICAL SYSTEMS INSTITUTE, MARCH 1977.*
INDX   ALCOHOLISM, SPANISH SURNAMED, SURVEY, RURAL, URBAN, ATTITUDES, COMMUNITY, SEX ROLES, EMPIRICAL, FAMILY ROLES, INTERPERSONAL RELATIONS, ECONOMIC FACTORS, CROSS CULTURAL, MEXICAN AMERICAN, CENSUS, PROGRAM EVALUATION, CALIFORNIA, SOUTHWEST, MACHISMO
ABST   THE ALCOHOL PRACTICES AND PROBLEMS RELATED TO DRINKING ARE EXAMINED AMONG THE SPANISH-SPEAKING POPULATIONS RESIDING IN FRESNO COUNTY, EAST SAN JOSE, AND THE EAST LOS ANGELES-MONTEBELLO AREAS OF CALIFORNIA. THE INFORMATION PRESENTED IS DERIVED FROM INTERVIEWS WITH SELECTED COMMUNITY PERSONS IN EACH AREA AND OBSERVATIONS OF DRINKING SITES IN EACH LOCALE. SUPPLEMENTARY MATERIALS FROM THE 1970 U.S. CENSUS AND THE FRESNO COUNTY SPECIAL CENSUS ARE ALSO USED. EIGHT CHAPTERS COVER THE FOLLOWING: (1) METHODOLOGY AND APPROACH USED IN INTERVIEWING; (2) STRUCTURAL AND DEMOGRAPHIC DESCRIPTIONS OF EACH SETTING; (3) ETHNOGRAPHIC OBSERVATIONS OF EACH LOCALE; (4) RESPONDENT PERCEPTIONS OF ALCOHOL-RELATED BEHAVIORS AND PROBLEMS IN THE SPANISH-SPEAKING POPULATION OF EACH LOCALE; (5) RESPONDENT PERCEPTIONS CONCERNING THE FAMILY AND MACHISMO AS CULTURAL FACTORS IN THE SPANISH-SPEAKING DRINKING MILIEU; (6) RESPONDENT KNOWLEDGE ABOUT ALCOHOLISM SERVICES; AND (7) RESPONDENT EVALUATIONS OF ALCOHOL TREATMENT PROGRAMS. 7 REFERENCES. (AUTHOR SUMMARY MODIFIED)
ACCN   000558

660 AUTH **GILL, L. J., & SPILKA, B.**
TITL   SOME NONINTELLECTUAL CORRELATES OF ACADEMIC ACHIEVEMENT AMONG MEXICAN-AMERICAN SECONDARY SCHOOL CHILDREN.
SRCE   *JOURNAL OF EDUCATIONAL PSYCHOLOGY, 1962, 53(3), 144-149.*
INDX   SCHOLASTIC ACHIEVEMENT, MEXICAN AMERICAN, ADOLESCENTS, CONFORMITY, MOTHER-CHILD INTERACTION, CPI, SEX COMPARISON, EMPIRICAL, ANXIETY, CULTURAL FACTORS, ACHIEVEMENT MOTIVATION, COLORADO, SOUTHWEST, MALE, FEMALE
ABST   AN INVESTIGATION TO DETERMINE PERSONAL AND PARENTAL CORRELATES OF ACADEMIC ACHIEVEMENT AMONG MEXICAN AMERICAN (MA) SECONDARY SCHOOL STUDENTS IS PRESENTED. FOUR GROUPS (15 EACH) OF HIGH- AND LOW-ACHIEVING MALES AND FEMALES WERE EQUATED ON AGE, GRADE LEVEL, AND IQ SCORES. PARENTAL VARIABLES WERE EVALUATED BY A MODIFICATION OF THE SHOFEN'S PARENT ATTITUDE SURVEY AND IQ SCORES WERE ASSESSED BY THE OTIS SA TEST OF MENTAL ABILITY. IN ADDITION, THE CALIFORNIA PSYCHOLOGICAL INVENTORY AND THE SIEGAL MANIFEST HOSTILITY SCALE WERE EMPLOYED. STATISTICAL EVALUATION INDICATES THAT ACHIEVERS MANIFEST RELIABLY LESS HOSTILITY AND MORE SOCIAL MATURITY, INTELLECTUAL EFFICIENCY, AND CONFORMITY TO RULES THAN DO UNDERACHIEVERS. ACHIEVING GIRLS AND UNDERACHIEVING BOYS APPEAR TO COME FROM STRONG MOTHER-DOMINATED HOMES. SINCE THESE FINDINGS SEEM MEANINGFUL WITH RESPECT TO THIS SUBCULTURE, IT IS SUGGESTED THAT ADDITIONAL SPECIFICATION OF GROUP CUSTOMS AND MILIEU MAY SIMILARLY CONTRIBUTE TO FURTHER UNDERSTANDING OF NONINTELLECTUAL FACTORS ASSOCIATED WITH ACADEMIC ACHIEVEMENT. 19 REFERENCES.
ACCN   000559

661 AUTH **GILMAN, R. A.**
TITL   A SELECTIVE ANNOTATED BIBLIOGRAPHY OF BIBLIOGRAPHIES AND OTHER SOURCES OF INFORMATION AND RESOURCES POTENTIALLY USEFUL IN MEXICAN-AMERICAN BILINGUAL/BICULTURAL EDUCATION.
SRCE   *MLA FORUM ON BILINGUALISM; BIBLIOGRAPHIC AND INFORMATIONAL RESOURCES IN BILINGUALISM, SAN FRANCISCO, 1975.*
INDX   BIBLIOGRAPHY, BILINGUAL-BICULTURAL EDUCATION, BILINGUALISM, SPANISH SURNAMED, MEXICAN AMERICAN, EDUCATIONAL MATERIALS, LINGUISTICS, PROCEEDINGS
ABST   THIS BIBLIOGRAPHY COMPILES BIBLIOGRAPHIC AND INFORMATIONAL RESOURCES PERTINENT TO MEXICAN AMERICAN BILINGUAL-BICULTURAL EDUCATION. THE REFERENCE BOOK IS ORGANIZED INTO 5 SECTIONS: (1) GENERAL BIBLIOGRAPHIES AND RESOURCE GUIDES; (2) SPECIFIC GUIDES TO THE LITERATURE ON BILINGUAL EDUCATION; (3) SUGGESTED READINGS; (4) JOURNALS AND NEWSLETTERS; AND (5) CATALOGUES. ALMOST 100 ITEMS ARE ANNOTATED REGARDING THEIR USEFULNESS TO THE STUDY OF BILINGUAL/BICULTURAL EDUCATION FOR MEXICAN AMERICANS. THE SUGGESTED READINGS AND GUIDES

TO THE LITERATURE SECTIONS INCLUDE GOVERNMENT PUBLICATIONS, REVIEWS AND ANTHOLOGIES AS WELL AS TEXTS, RESEARCH AND CONFERENCE PROCEEDINGS RELATED TO BILINGUALISM.

ACCN   000560

662 AUTH   **GILMORE, G. M., & STALLINGS, W. M.**
    TITL   A COMMENT ON NEDLER AND SEBRA'S "INTERVENTION STRATEGIES FOR SPANISH SPEAKING PRESCHOOL CHILDREN."
    SRCE   *CHILD DEVELOPMENT, 1972, 43, 1035-1038.*
    INDX   RESEARCH METHODOLOGY, EARLY CHILDHOOD EDUCATION, CHILDREN, SPANISH SURNAMED, BILINGUALISM, PROGRAM EVALUATION, REVIEW
    ABST   THE RESULTS OF A RESEARCH STUDY BY NEDLER AND SEBERA (CHILD DEVELOPMENT, 1971, 42, 259-267) WHICH COMPARED THREE STRATEGIES OF EARLY INTERVENTION DESIGNED TO INCREASE THE LANGUAGE AND COMMUNICATION SKILLS OF DISADVANTAGED 3 YEAR-OLD MEXICAN AMERICAN CHILDREN ARE REVIEWED. SPECIFIC CRITICISMS FOCUS ON THE STUDY'S ERRORS OR WEAKNESSES IN THE AREAS OF: (1) EXPERIMENTAL DESIGN; (2) STATISTICAL ANALYSIS; AND (3) THE DATA REPORTED IN TABLE FORMAT. THE RESEARCH CONCLUDED THAT A PLANNED BILINGUAL EARLY CHILDHOOD EDUCATIONAL PROGRAM RESULTED IN SIGNIFICANTLY GREATER GAINS IN TEST CHILDREN THAN DID A PARENTAL INVOLVEMENT PROGRAM OR A TRADITIONAL DAY-CARE CENTER. THIS ARTICLE MAINTAINS THAT THE RESEARCH ANALYSES DO NOT SUPPORT THAT CONCLUSION AND THAT FURTHER EVALUATION OF THE PROGRAM IS INDICATED. 5 REFERENCES.
    ACCN   000561

663 AUTH   **GILMORE, G., CHANDY, J., & ANDERSON, T.**
    TITL   THE BENDER GESTALT AND THE MEXICAN AMERICAN STUDENT: A REPORT.
    SRCE   *PSYCHOLOGY IN THE SCHOOLS, 1975, 12(2), 172-175.*
    INDX   BENDER VISUAL-MOTOR GESTALT TEST, PERSONALITY ASSESSMENT, ADOLESCENTS, CHILDREN, CROSS CULTURAL, CULTURAL FACTORS, EMPIRICAL, MEXICAN AMERICAN, TEXAS, SOUTHWEST
    ABST   THE PERFORMANCE OF 64 MEXICAN AMERICAN STUDENTS IN 6 AGE GROUPS ON THE BENDER GESTALT WAS STUDIED. RESULTS SUGGEST THAT WITH THE EARLIER AGE GROUPS THERE WAS NO SIGNIFICANT DIFFERENCE BETWEEN THE MEAN SCORES OF THE MEXICAN AMERICAN SAMPLE AND THE KOPPITZ NORMATIVE GROUP. BEGINNING AT AGE 7 THERE WAS A TREND FOR THE SAMPLE TO MAKE MORE ERRORS ON THE TEST THAN THE NORMATIVE GROUP. 14 REFERENCES. (PASAR ABSTRACT)
    ACCN   000562

664 AUTH   **GINORIO, A. B., & BERRY, P. C.**
    TITL   MEASURING PUERTO RICANS PERCEPTIONS OF RACIAL CHARACTERISTICS.
    SRCE   *PROCEEDINGS OF THE 80TH ANNUAL CONVENTION OF THE AMERICAN PSYCHOLOGICAL ASSOCIATION, 1972, 7(1), 287-288.*
    INDX   ETHNIC IDENTITY, PUERTO RICAN-I, ADOLESCENTS, EMPIRICAL, SELF CONCEPT
    ABST   IN ORDER TO MEASURE HOW PUERTO RICANS CLASSIFY EACH OTHER INTO RACIAL GROUPS BY PHYSICAL APPEARANCE, A STIMULUS SET OF 60 FULL FACE AND PROFILE COLOR SLIDES OF VOLUNTEER STUDENTS FROM THE UNIVERSITY OF PUERTO RICO WERE PREPARED. THEIR CHARACTERISTICS RANGED FROM NORTHERN EUROPEAN TO WEST AFRICAN WITH THE GREATEST NUMBER SUGGESTING MEDITERRANEAN. OVER 200 HIGH SCHOOL STUDENTS THEN SORTED THESE PORTRAITS INTO GROUPS RANGING FROM "MORE WHITE" TO "MORE BLACK." EACH SUBJECT MADE THREE RATINGS OF HIMSELF AND OF EACH SLIDE. JUDGES ALSO RATED THE SUBJECTS AS TO THEIR COLOR. THE SUBJECTS EVALUATED THE PICTURES WITH AN EXTRAORDINARY CONSISTENCY AND ALSO REPORTED SELF-DESCRIPTIONS WHICH WERE IN CLOSE AGREEMENT WITH THOSE REPORTED BY THE JUDGES. LITTLE TENDENCY WAS FOUND FOR A SUBJECT'S OWN COLOR TO ALTER HIS PERCEPTION OF OTHERS, NOR DID THE SUBJECTS MAKE FINER DISTINCTION AMONG SLIDES WHOSE COLOR WAS NEAR THEIR OWN. INSTEAD THE SUBJECTS APPEARED TO GROUP TOGETHER A BROAD RANGE OF INTERMEDIATE CHARACTERISTICS. THIS PROCEDURE COULD BE USED TO STUDY THE EFFECTS OF CULTURAL CONTEXT ON RACIAL PERCEPTIONS. DETAILED ANTHROPOMETRIC MEASUREMENTS OF FEATURES DEPICTED IN THE SLIDES (I.E., HAIR TEXTURE, SKIN COLOR, WIDTH OF NOSE, FULLNESS OF MOUTH) WOULD PERMIT ONE TO STATE MORE PRECISELY WHICH PHYSICAL CHARACTERISTICS ARE CUES TO RACIAL CLASSIFICATION. 8 REFERENCES. (AUTHOR SUMMARY MODIFIED)
    ACCN   000563

665 AUTH   **GINSBERG, G. P., MCGINN, N. F., & HARBURG, E.**
    TITL   RECALLED PARENT-CHILD INTERACTION OF MEXICAN AND UNITED STATES MALES.
    SRCE   *JOURNAL OF CROSS-CULTURAL PSYCHOLOGY, 1970, 1(2), 139-152.*
    INDX   ADOLESCENTS, COLLEGE STUDENTS, CHILDREARING PRACTICES, MEXICAN, CROSS CULTURAL, FATHER-CHILD INTERACTION, MOTHER-CHILD INTERACTION, FAMILY ROLES, EMPIRICAL, MALE, CULTURE, MICHIGAN, MIDWEST
    ABST   DIMENSIONS OF RECALLED PARENT-CHILD INTERACTION, FROM THE VIEWPOINT OF THE CHILD, WERE OBTAINED BY MEANS OF A PARENT IMAGE DIFFERENTIAL (PID). PID DATA OF A NORTH AMERICAN GROUP AND A MEXICAN GROUP, ALL MALES, WERE FACTOR ANALYZED AND ANALYTICALLY COMPARED. A NUMBER OF HIGHLY STABLE DIMENSIONS EMERGED, SOME CULTURALLY SPECIFIC, SOME SPECIFIC TO SEX OF PARENT, BUT ALMOST ALL SPECIFIC TO A PARTICULAR CONTEXT OF PARENT-CHILD INTERACTION. CROSS-CULTURAL DIFFERENCES ARE DISCUSSED, AND REASONS FOR THE DIF-

FERENCE BETWEEN THESE RESULTS AND THOSE REPORTED BY OTHERS ARE OFFERED. IT IS SUGGESTED THAT TO PROFITABLY EXAMINE PRIMARY INTERACTIONS, INCLUDING PARENT-CHILD RELATIONS, AND TO GET THE MOST OUT OF CROSS-CULTURAL INVESTIGATIONS OF PRIMARY RELATIONS, SEPARATE INTERACTION CATEGORIES DEFINED AS CONTEXT-BY-PARTICIPANT SUBSETS SHOULD BE SAMPLED AND STUDIED. THE PID APPEARS TO BE ONE TECHNIQUE FOR APPROACHING THIS OBJECTIVE. 28 REFERENCES. (JOURNAL ABSTRACT MODIFIED)

ACCN   000564

666 AUTH   **GIORDANO, J., & GIORDANO, G. P.**

TITL   THE ETHNO-CULTURAL FACTOR IN MENTAL HEALTH: A LITERATURE REVIEW AND BIBLIOGRAPHY.

SRCE   *NEW YORK: INSTITUTE ON PLURALISM AND GROUP IDENTITY OF THE AMERICAN JEWISH COMMITTEE, 1977.*

INDX   BIBLIOGRAPHY, SPANISH SURNAMED, MENTAL HEALTH, PSYCHOTHERAPY, CULTURAL PLURALISM, REVIEW, CULTURAL FACTORS, FAMILY STRUCTURE, MIGRANTS, PSYCHOSOCIAL ADJUSTMENT, POLITICAL POWER, ETHNIC IDENTITY, RESOURCE UTILIZATION, HEALTH DELIVERY SYSTEMS, IMMIGRATION, ACCULTURATION

ABST   DRAWN FROM A CROSS-SECTION OF DISCIPLINES, THIS REVIEW AND BIBLIOGRAPHY ADDRESSES THE GROWING AWARENESS IN GOVERNMENT, EDUCATION, AND HEALTH FIELDS THAT THE U.S. IS A PLURALISTIC NATION HAVING NO SINGLE IDEAL FAMILY STRUCTURE OR MODE OF BEING. ETHNIC DIFFERENCES, ONCE VIEWED AS LIABILITIES, ARE INCREASINGLY BEING REGARDED AS POTENTIAL BASES FOR SELF-ESTEEM AND IMPROVED MENTAL HEALTH. SPECIFIC ASPECTS OF ETHNICITY AND MENTAL HEALTH DISCUSSED IN THIS REVIEW ARE: (1) THE NEW ETHNICITY AND THE NEW PLURALISM; (2) THE ETHNIC FACTOR IN PREVALENCE OF MENTAL ILLNESS; (3) IMMIGRATION, MIGRATION AND MENTAL HEALTH; (4) PERCEPTION OF ILLNESS AND UTILIZATION OF SERVICES; (5) CULTURAL BARRIERS IN TREATMENT; AND (6) STRENGTHENING AN ETHNIC GROUP'S NATURAL SUPPORT SYSTEMS. THE BIBLIOGRAPHY— CONTAINING ALMOST 500 ENTRIES AND INCLUDING A CROSS REFERENCE SUBJECT GUIDE—IS DESIGNED TO GIVE SPECIALISTS AS WELL AS THOSE ENTERING THIS AREA FOR THE FIRST TIME A BROAD PERSPECTIVE ON THE WORK THAT HAS BEEN DONE. AS THIS LITERATURE REVIEW INDICATES, MENTAL HEALTH PROFESSIONALS ARE BEGINNING TO RESPOND TO AMERICAN PLURALISM AND THERE ARE NUMEROUS EXAMPLES OF "CULTURALLY RESPONSIVE" SERVICES. HOWEVER, SIGNIFICANT GAPS EXIST IN THEORY AND KNOWLEDGE, AND METHODS FOR DEALING WITH THE REAL NEEDS OF THE PEOPLE REMAIN TO BE FOUND. THERE IS AN OBVIOUS NEED FOR FUTURE WORK IN THE DEVELOPMENT OF AN OVERALL CONCEPTUAL APPROACH THAT INTEGRATES CULTURAL FACTORS WITH ALL ASPECTS OF MENTAL HEALTH PRACTICES. 472 REFERENCES.

ACCN   002092

667 AUTH   **GIOVANNONI, J. M., & BILLINGSLEY, A.**

TITL   CHILD NEGLECT AMONG THE POOR: A STUDY OF PARENTAL ADEQUACY IN FAMILIES OF THREE ETHNIC GROUPS.

SRCE   *IN J. E. LEAVITT (ED.), THE BATTERED CHILD. MORRISTOWN, N.J.: GENERAL LEARNING PRESS, 1974, PP. 170-177.*

INDX   CHILD ABUSE, POVERTY, SPANISH SURNAMED, CHILDREARING PRACTICES, CROSS CULTURAL, EMPIRICAL, FAMILY STRUCTURE, MARITAL STABILITY, SES, URBAN, EXTENDED FAMILY, FICTIVE KINSHIP, FAMILY ROLES, CALIFORNIA, SOUTHWEST, FEMALE, MOTHER-CHILD INTERACTION

ABST   PREVIOUS RESEARCH IN THE AREA OF CHILD NEGLECT HAS HIGHLIGHTED THE HIGHER INCIDENCE OF THE PROBLEM AMONG LOWER SOCIOECONOMIC GROUPS. THIS STUDY ATTEMPTS TO ELUCIDATE ADDITIONAL FACTORS THAT DISTINGUISH NEGLECTFUL PARENTS FROM MORE ADEQUATE ONES WITHIN LOWER SES GROUPS. LOW-INCOME BLACK, ANGLO AND SPANISH-SPEAKING MOTHERS (N = 186) WERE INTERVIEWED ABOUT THEIR PAST AND CURRENT LIFE SITUATIONS. PREJUDGED BY PUBLIC HEALTH NURSES AS ADEQUATE OR POTENTIALLY NEGLECTFUL AND IDENTIFIED BY PROTECTIVE SERVICES AS NEGLECTFUL, THE MOTHERS WERE CATEGORIZED BY PARENTAL ADEQUACY AND ETHNICITY. INTERVIEW RESPONSES WERE COMPARED WITHIN AND ACROSS THESE GROUPS ON THE FOLLOWING INFORMATION CATEGORIES: (1) SOCIAL AND FAMILY BACKGROUND OF MOTHERS; (2) CURRENT SITUATIONAL FACTORS; (3) MOTHERS' SOCIAL FUNCTIONING IN FORMAL AND INFORMAL SOCIAL SYSTEMS; AND (4) CHILD-REARING PRACTICES. MAJOR FINDINGS ARE: (1) SOCIAL AND FAMILIAL BACKGROUND FACTORS DO NOT SIGNIFICANTLY DIFFERENTIATE NEGLECTFUL MOTHERS; (2) CURRENT LIFE SITUATIONS OF NEGLECTFUL MOTHERS ARE CONSIDERABLY MORE STRESSFULL THAN THAT OF ADEQUATE ONES; (3) NEGLECTFUL MOTHERS HAVE IMPOVERISHED RELATIONSHIPS WITH EXTENDED KIN, WHILE ADEQUATE MOTHERS HAVE FREQUENT, REWARDING CONTACTS WITH RELATIVES; (4) NEGLECTFUL MOTHERS DEVIATE FROM ADEQUATE ONES IN THEIR ACCEPTANCE OF AND MEETING DEPENDENCY NEEDS OF VERY YOUNG CHILDREN; AND (5) ETHNIC VARIATIONS ARE NOTED ESPECIALLY IN KINSHIP RELATIONS, FORMAL SOCIAL SYSTEMS AND CHILD-REARING PRACTICES. IMPLICATIONS ARE DISCUSSED IN TERMS OF SOCIAL AND COMMUNITY CONDITIONS AND CHANGES WITHIN THE CHILD WELFARE FIELD. 7 REFERENCES. (AUTHOR SUMMARY MODIFIED)

ACCN   000565

668 AUTH   **GIRALDO, O.**

TITL   EL MACHISMO COMO FENOMENO PSICOCULTURAL. (MACHISMO AS A PSYCHOCULTURAL PHENOMENON.)

SRCE   *REVISTA LATINOAMERICANA DE PSICOLOGIA, 1972, 4(3), 295-309. (SPANISH)*

INDX   ESSAY, SEX ROLES, SELF CONCEPT, CHILDREARING PRACTICES, SPANISH SURNAMED, FATHER-CHILD INTERACTION, CULTURE, MALE, MACHISMO

ABST   BASED ON OSCAR LEWIS'S ANTHROPOLOGICAL WORKS, THIS ARTICLE EXAMINES THE CULTURAL TRAITS OF "MACHISMO." TWO OF THESE TRAITS, HETEROSEXUALITY AND AGGRESSION, ARE COMMONLY EXAGGERATED AND MANIFESTED THROUGH THE MASTERY OVER WOMEN AND THE RECIPROCAL SUBMISSION TO MEN. OTHER TRAITS INCLUDE COURAGE, SEXUAL FREEDOM, AFFECTIVE DETACHMENT, PHYSICAL DOMINANCE, AND EXCESSIVE ALCOHOL CONSUMPTION. ACCORDING TO THE ADLERIAN THEORY, THESE TRAITS WOULD BE A COMPENSATION FOR INFERIORITY FEELINGS. THE ORIGINS OF THE INFERIORITY COMPLEX ARE FOUND IN PATTERNS OF CHILD-REARING AND THE FAMILY EDUCATION SYSTEM: (1) THE AFFECTIONLESS FATHER; (2) THE CHILD'S RESPECT FOR THE FATHER (BASED ON FEAR, SEPARATION, DISTANCE); (3) RUDENESS AND HOSTILITY IN FATHER-SON RELATIONS; (4) PRAISE OF MASCULINE TRAITS AND FEMININE SUBMISSION; AND (5) OBEDIENCE AND VIRGINITY. IT IS CONCLUDED THAT "MACHISMO" IS A CULTURAL TRAIT AIMED AT SATISFYING A PSYCHOLOGICAL NEED— NAMELY, THE INFERIORITY COMPLEX WHICH ORIGINATES IN CHILD-REARING PRACTICES. 17 REFERENCES. (JOURNAL ABSTRACT MODIFIED)

ACCN   000566

669 AUTH   **GLASER, D., INCIARDI, J., & BABST D.**
     TITL   LATER HEROIN USE BY ADOLESCENT MARIJUANA AND HEROIN USERS AND BY NONDRUG USING ADOLESCENT OFFENDERS.
     SRCE   *PROSECUTOR, 1969, 5(1), 10-13.*
     INDX   DRUG ADDICTION, ADOLESCENTS, EMPIRICAL, PUERTO RICAN-M, DRUG ABUSE, ADULTS, CROSS CULTURAL, MALE, NEW YORK, EAST
     ABST   THE EXTENT TO WHICH MARIJUANA USE LEADS TO HEROIN USE, THE EXTENT TO WHICH ADOLESCENT HEROIN USE IS CONTINUED IN ADULTHOOD, AND THE EXTENT TO WHICH ADOLESCENT NONDRUG DELINQUENCY IS FOLLOWED BY HEROIN ADDICTION IN ADULTHOOD WAS EXAMINED IN A 5- TO 10-YEAR FOLLOWUP STUDY OF ADOLESCENTS REFERRED TO THE NEW YORK CITY YOUTH COUNCIL BUREAU. DATA WERE OBTAINED BY SEARCHING THE CITY HEALTH DEPARTMENT'S NARCOTICS REGISTER FOR REPORTS OF HEROIN USE AFTER 1963 FOR 716 MALE OFFENDERS CHARGED WITH MARIJUANA OR HEROIN USE OR NONDRUG OFFENSES IN 1957 AND 1962. ANALYSIS OF THE DATA REVEALED SUBSEQUENT HEROIN RECORDS FOR APPROXIMATELY 50% OF THOSE REFERRED FOR MARIJUANA USAGE AND 15% FOR THOSE REFERRED FOR DELINQUENCY NOT INVOLVING ANY DRUG USE. EVEN HIGHER RATES OF SUBSEQUENT HEROIN USAGE WERE FOUND FOR THOSE NONDRUG-INVOLVED ADOLESCENT OFFENDERS WHO WERE NEGRO OR PUERTO RICAN, WHO HAD TWO OR MORE CODEFENDANTS, WHO HAD PRIOR REFERRALS TO COURT, OR WHO HAD DROPPED OUT OF SCHOOL. THESE CHARACTERISTICS DID NOT MARKEDLY AFFECT THE SUBSEQUENT HEROIN RATE FOR ADOLESCENT RECORD AND SUBSEQUENT HEROIN USE FOR ALL SUBJECTS. THE FACT THAT THESE RATES OF LATER HEROIN USE ARE HIGHER THAN THOSE FOUND IN THE FEW SOMEWHAT COMPARABLE STUDIES ELSEWHERE IS ASCRIBED TO THE HIGHER CONCENTRATION OF HEROIN USAGE IN NEW YORK CITY. 13 REFERENCES.

ACCN   000567

670 AUTH   **GLATT, K. M.**
     TITL   AN EVALUATION OF THE FRENCH, SPANISH, AND GERMAN TRANSLATIONS OF THE MMPI.
     SRCE   *ACTA PSYCHOLOGICA, 1969, 29(1), 65-84.*
     INDX   MMPI, EMPIRICAL, RESEARCH METHODOLOGY, PERSONALITY ASSESSMENT, CROSS CULTURAL, BILINGUAL, CULTURE-FAIR TESTS, TEST VALIDITY, MINNESOTA, MIDWEST
     ABST   A SAMPLE OF 77 COLLEGE AND NONCOLLEGE BILINGUAL SUBJECTS WERE ADMINISTERED BOTH THE ENGLISH MMPI AND THE FOREIGN LANGUAGE VERSION OF THE TEST TO DETERMINE THE ADEQUACY OF THE LANGUAGE TRANSLATION. IN COMPARING THE INDIVIDUAL PROFILES RESULTING FROM THE SPANISH AND GERMAN TRANSLATIONS WITH THEIR ENGLISH COUNTERPARTS, IT WAS FOUND THAT SCORES ON CERTAIN SCALES WERE ON THE AVERAGE SIGNIFICANTLY MORE ELEVATED IN THE FOREIGN LANGUAGE VERSION THAN IN THE ENGLISH VERSION. THESE DIFFERENCES TEND TO BE SMALL AND CLINICALLY NONSIGNIFICANT. FOR THE MOST PART, THE CLINICAL MEANING OF THE OVERALL SPANISH AND GERMAN PROFILE CONFIGURATIONS DID NOT DIFFER FROM THAT OF THE ENGLISH. IN COMPARING THE RESULTS OF THE FRENCH TRANSLATIONS WITH THOSE OF THE ENGLISH, THE FRENCH VERSION WAS FOUND TO BE UNRELIABLE. THE RESULTS LEND SUPPORT TO THE ADEQUACY AND CLINICAL UTILITY OF THE SPANISH AND GERMAN TRANSLATIONS AND ARE SUGGESTIVE OF GROSS DEFICIENCIES IN THE FRENCH TRANSLATION. 15 REFERENCES.

ACCN   000568

671 AUTH   **GOEBEL, J. B., & COLE, S. G.**
     TITL   MEXICAN-AMERICAN AND WHITE REACTIONS TO STIMULUS PERSONS OF SAME AND DIFFERENT RACE: SIMILARITY AND ATTRACTION AS A FUNCTION OF PREJUDICE.
     SRCE   *PSYCHOLOGICAL REPORTS, 1975, 36, 827-833.*
     INDX   PREJUDICE, ATTITUDES, ADOLESCENTS, MEXICAN AMERICAN, CROSS CULTURAL, EMPIRICAL, INTERPERSONAL RELATIONS, TEXAS, SOUTHWEST
     ABST   FORTY-FOUR MEXICAN AMERICAN AND FORTY-FOUR WHITE 9TH GRADERS RATED A WHITE AND A MEXICAN AMERICAN STIMULUS PERSON WHOSE BELIEFS WERE UNKNOWN ON A SIMILARITY, FRIENDLINESS, AND SOCIAL DISTANCE SCALE. HIGH AND LOW PREJUDICED SUBJECTS WERE IDENTIFIED BY SCORES ON

THE SOCIAL DISTANCE SCALE. THE HIGH PREJUDICED WHITES PERCEIVED THE WHITE STIMULUS PERSON AS SIGNIFICANTLY MORE SIMILAR TO THEMSELVES AND REPORTED THAT THEY WOULD BE SIGNIFICANTLY MORE FRIENDLY TOWARD THAT PERSON THAN TOWARD THE MEXICAN AMERICAN STIMULUS PERSON. NO SIGNIFICANT DIFFERENCE WAS OBTAINED FOR THE HIGH PREJUDICED MEXICAN AMERICANS' RATINGS OF THE MEXICAN AMERICAN AND WHITE STIMULUS PERSONS FOR EITHER SIMILARITY OR FRIENDLINESS OR FOR RATINGS OF LOW PREJUDICED SUBJECTS, EITHER WHITE OR MEXICAN AMERICAN. RATINGS ON SIMILARITY AND FRIENDLINESS WERE GENERALLY CORRELATED FOR BOTH MEXICAN AMERICAN AND WHITE SUBJECTS WHEN LEVEL OF PREJUDICE WAS IGNORED. WHEN LEVEL OF PREJUDICE WAS CONSIDERED, RATINGS WERE SIGNIFICANTLY CORRELATED FOR HIGH PREJUDICED SUBJECTS BUT NOT FOR LOW PREJUDICED SUBJECTS. 10 REFERENCES. (PASAR ABSTRACT)

ACCN 000569

672 AUTH **GOEBES, D. D., & SHORE, M. F.**
TITL SOME EFFECTS OF BICULTURAL AND MONOCULTURAL SCHOOL ENVIRONMENTS ON PERSONALITY DEVELOPMENT.
SRCE *AMERICAN JOURNAL OF ORTHOPSYCHIATRY, 1978, 48(3), 398-407.*
INDX PERSONALITY, CHILDREN, FEMALE, BILINGUAL-BICULTURAL EDUCATION, EDUCATION, EMPIRICAL, WASHINGTON D.C., EAST, URBAN, PREJUDICE, PEER GROUP, SELF CONCEPT, CROSS CULTURAL, BILINGUAL-BICULTURAL PERSONNEL, SPANISH SURNAMED, CULTURAL PLURALISM, INTEGRATION, SES, ENVIRONMENTAL FACTORS
ABST TO EXPLORE THE EFFECT OF BICULTURAL VS. MONOCULTURAL SCHOOL ENVIRONMENTS ON THE PERSONALITY DEVELOPMENT OF CHILDREN, 47 ANGLO AND LATINO GIRLS, 8 TO 12 YEARS-OLD, WERE COMPARED. 22 GIRLS WERE IN A BICULTURAL SCHOOL AND 25, MATCHED FOR AGE AND ETHNICITY, WERE IN A MONOCULTURAL SCHOOL. BOTH SCHOOLS WERE IN A MIXED LOWER AND MIDDLE CLASS, ENGLISH- AND SPANISH-SPEAKING AREA IN WASHINGTON, D.C. PEER GROUP ORGANIZATION WAS MEASURED BY LUNCH ROOM OBSERVATIONS AND THE GIRLS' SELECTION OF GAME PARTNERS. A MODIFIED SEMANTIC DIFFERENTIAL "ME, MEXICAN AMERICAN, ANGLO AMERICAN" TEST WAS USED TO ASSESS SELF-IMAGE AND ACCEPTANCE OF CULTURAL DIFFERENCES; AND ROLE-TAKING ABILITY WAS ALSO TESTED, USING A STORY-TELLING TASK. THE PREADOLESCENT GIRLS (10 TO 12 YEARS-OLD) IN THE BICULTURAL SCHOOL EXHIBITED A MORE HETEROCULTURAL PEER GROUP ORGANIZATION, BETTER SELF-IMAGE, AND GREATER ACCEPTANCE OF AN UNKNOWN CULTURAL GROUP THAN DID THE MONOCULTURAL SCHOOL STUDENTS. THESE DIFFERENCES WERE NOT FOUND, HOWEVER, AMONG YOUNGER CHILDREN IN THE TWO SCHOOLS. NO SIGNIFICANT DIFFERENCES APPEARED IN ROLE-TAKING ABILITY BETWEEN THE TWO GROUPS. THE RESULTS SUGGEST THAT A BICULTURAL SCHOOL ENVIRONMENT MAY HAVE IMPORTANT POSITIVE EFFECTS ON PERSONALITY DEVELOPMENT. THIS FACTOR IS ENHANCED AMONG CHILDREN EXPERIENCING A TRULY BICULTURAL TEACHING ENVIRONMENT WHEREIN THE BICULTURAL STAFF SHARE RESPONSIBILITY AND AUTHORITY. 19 REFERENCES.

ACCN 002093

673 AUTH **GOGGIN, J., & WICKENS, D. D.**
TITL PROACTIVE INTERFERENCE AND LANGUAGE CHANGE IN SHORT TERM MEMORY.
SRCE *JOURNAL OF VERBAL LEARNING AND VERBAL BEHAVIOR, 1971, 19(4), 453-458.*
INDX BILINGUALISM, MEMORY, COLLEGE STUDENTS, EMPIRICAL, TEXAS, SOUTHWEST
ABST BILINGUAL COLLEGE STUDENTS WHO VOLUNTEERED TO PARTICIPATE IN A WORD RECALL EXPERIMENT WERE PRESENTED CATEGORIZED WORDS IN A SERIES OF TESTS CONFORMING TO THE BROWN-PETERSON STM PARADIGM. DESIGNED TO INDICATE COGNITIVE ORGANIZATION, THIS PARADIGM IS BASED ON SEVERAL ASSUMPTIONS: (1) PERCEIVING A WORD INVOLVES ENCODING THE WORD INTO SEVERAL DIFFERENT CATEGORIES; (2) WHEN A SERIES OF ITEMS COMES FROM THE SAME CATEGORY THEY WILL INTERFERE WITH EACH OTHER AT RECALL; (3) IF A NEW ITEM SET IS ENCODED INTO DIFFERENT CATEGORIES, THERE WILL BE A REDUCTION IN INTERFERENCE AND A CORRESPONDING INCREASE AT RECALL. THEREFORE THE MORE DISSIMILAR THE WORD SETS ENCODING, THE MORE RELEASE FROM PROACTIVE INTERFERENCE (PI). IN TESTING BILINGUALS, IT WAS HYPOTHESIZED THAT A CHANGE IN LANGUAGE BETWEEN WORD SETS WOULD PRODUCE ALMOST COMPLETE RELEASE FROM INTERFERENCE IF THE TWO LANGUAGES HAVE SEPARATE MEMORY STORES; ALTERNATIVELY, IF THE TWO LANGUAGES HAVE THE SAME MEMORY STORE THE AMOUNT OF INTERFERENCE WOULD BE GREATER AND RECALL LESS. RESULTS INDICATE THAT RELEASE FROM PI DID OCCUR WHEN EITHER THE LANGUAGE OR THE TAXONOMIC CATEGORY OF THE WORD ITEMS WAS CHANGED. WITH A DOUBLE SHIFT OF BOTH LANGUAGE AND CATEGORY, THERE WAS A SLIGHTLY GREATER RELEASE THAN WITH A SINGLE SHIFT. DIFFERENCES BETWEEN FLUENT AND NONFLUENT BILINGUALS WERE FOUND AND INTERPRETED IN TERMS OF THE DIFFERENTIAL TENDENCY TO TRANSLATE ITEMS FROM THE NONPREFERRED INTO THE DOMINANT LANGUAGE. 9 REFERENCES. (JOURNAL ABSTRACT MODIFIED)

ACCN 000570

674 AUTH **GOLD, S. R., & COGHLAN, A. J.**
TITL THE EFFECT OF RESIDENTIAL TREATMENT ON ADOLESCENT DRUG ABUSERS: A PRELIMINARY REPORT.
SRCE *PROCEEDINGS OF THE 81ST ANNUAL CONVEN-*

TION OF THE AMERICAN PSYCHOLOGICAL AS-SOCIATION, 1973, 8, 397-398.

INDX INSTITUTIONALIZATION, ADOLESCENTS, DRUG ABUSE, SELF CONCEPT, CONFORMITY, ATTITUDES, SEX COMPARISON, CROSS CULTURAL, EMPIRICAL, SES, PERSONALITY, THERAPEUTIC COMMUNITY, REHABILITATION, PUERTO RICAN-M, ROTTER INTERNAL-EXTERNAL SCALE, NEW YORK, EAST

ABST PRELIMINARY DATA ARE PRESENTED ON SPECIFIED CHANGES IN RESIDENTS' ATTITUDES IN A COED RESIDENTIAL TREATMENT PROGRAM FOR ADOLESCENT DRUG ABUSERS, FOLLOWING 6 MONTHS OF TREATMENT. ROTTERS INTERNAL-EXTERNAL CONTROL SCALE AND THE SELF-ESTEEM SURVEY WERE ADMINISTERED TO 32 MALE AND 21 FEMALE PUERTO RICAN, NEGRO AND CAUCASIAN DRUG ABUSERS. THE THEORETICAL MODEL OF THE PROGRAM (COGNITIVE-AFFECTIVE-PHARAMACOGENIC CONTROL THEORY) IS RELATED TO THE DATA COLLECTED. RESULTS ON THE 2 MEASURES OF CHANGING ATTITUDE, LOCUS OF CONTROL AND SELF-ESTEEM, INDICATE MOVEMENT IN THE DESIRED DIRECTION, I.E., MORE INTERNAL CONTROL AND RAISED SELF-ESTEEM. A POSITIVE CORRELATION WAS FOUND BETWEEN EXTERNALITY IN FEMALES AND SELF-CUTTING ACTS. IN ADDITION, DIFFERENCES ON ROTTER'S SCALE WERE FOUND FOR BOYS VS. GIRLS WHO WENT AWOL. 24 REFERENCES. (PASAR ABSTRACT MODIFIED)

ACCN 000571

---

675 AUTH **GOLDMAN, R. D., & HARTIG, L. K.**

TITL THE WISC MAY NOT BE A VALID PREDICTOR OF SCHOOL PERFORMANCE FOR PRIMARY GRADE MINORITY CHILDREN.

SRCE *AMERICAN JOURNAL OF MENTAL DEFICIENCY, 1975, 80(6), 583-587.*

INDX WISC, INTELLIGENCE TESTING, SCHOLASTIC ACHIEVEMENT, MEXICAN AMERICAN, CHILDREN, CULTURAL FACTORS, SES, CROSS CULTURAL, EMPIRICAL, TEST VALIDITY, CALIFORNIA, SOUTHWEST

ABST STUDENTS FROM SEVERAL RIVERSIDE, CALIF., ELEMENTARY SCHOOLS (430 ANGLO, 320 BLACK, AND 201 MEXICAN AMERICAN) WERE GIVEN THE WISC AND RATED BY THEIR TEACHERS ON A COMPETENCE SCALE. IN ADDITION, SOCIAL AND ACADEMIC GRADE POINT AVERAGES WERE COMPUTED FOR EACH CHILD. FINDINGS INDICATE THAT THE VALIDITIES AMONG THESE CRITERIA AND WISC SCORES WHEN THE GROUPS ARE COMBINED ARE GOOD, BUT VALIDITIES FOR THE SEPARATE GROUPS DIFFER MARKEDLY. VALIDITIES ARE GOOD FOR THE ANGLO CHILDREN, BUT NEAR ZERO FOR THE BLACK AND MEXICAN AMERICAN CHILDREN. OVERALL, IT IS CONCLUDED THAT THE WISC IS NOT A VALID PREDICTOR OF MINORITY CHILDREN'S SCHOLASTIC PERFORMANCE AND, THEREFORE, SHOULD NOT BE USED. IMPLICATIONS FOR EDUCATIONAL PLACEMENT AND THE HEREDITY ENVIRONMENT CONTROVERSY ARE DISCUSSED. 10 REFERENCES.

ACCN 000572

---

676 AUTH **GOLDMAN, R. D., & HEWITT, B. N.**

TITL AN INVESTIGATION OF TEST BIAS FOR MEXICAN-AMERICAN COLLEGE STUDENTS.

SRCE *JOURNAL OF EDUCATIONAL MEASUREMENT, 1975, 12(3), 187-196.*

INDX ABILITY TESTING, COLLEGE STUDENTS, CROSS CULTURAL, EDUCATION, EDUCATIONAL ASSESSMENT, EMPIRICAL, HIGHER EDUCATION, MEXICAN AMERICAN, SPANISH SURNAMED, SOUTHWEST, TEST VALIDITY

ABST IN AN INVESTIGATION OF TEST BIAS FOR MEXICAN AMERICAN COLLEGE STUDENTS, HIGH SCHOOL GRADE POINT AVERAGE (HSGPA) AND THE VERBAL AND MATHEMATICAL SCALES OF THE SCHOLASTIC APTITUDE TESTS (SAT-V, SAT-M) WERE USED TO PREDICT COLLEGE GRADE POINT AVERAGE (GPA) FOR MEXICAN AMERICAN AND ANGLO AMERICAN COLLEGE STUDENTS. SUBJECTS (MEXICAN AMERICANS = 656, ANGLO AMERICANS = 11,553) WERE SELECTED FROM FOUR UNIVERSITIES WITHIN A WESTERN MULTI-CAMPUS STATE UNIVERSITY SYSTEM. RESULTS INDICATED (1) THAT REGRESSION SYSTEMS WERE ESSENTIALLY PARALLEL FOR BOTH GROUPS, WITH VIRTUALLY NO DIFFERENCE IN INTERCEPTS, (2) THAT PREDICTION OF GPA IS SLIGHTLY MORE ACCURATE FOR THE ANGLO AMERICAN SAMPLES, AND (3) THAT HSGPA, SAT-V, AND SAT-M ARE MORE HIGHLY INTERCORRELATED FOR THE MEXICAN AMERICAN SAMPLE. ALTHOUGH THERE WAS NO SYSTEMATIC UNDERPREDICTION OR OVERPREDICTION OF MEXICAN AMERICAN GPA'S, IT IS CONCLUDED THAT THERE IS PROBABLY A NEED FOR DISCRIMINATING ACADEMIC PREDICTORS FOR THIS GROUP—ESPECIALLY PREDICTORS WHICH CAN MEASURE UNCORRELATED ASPECTS OF ACADEMIC APTITUDE. 12 REFERENCES. (NCMHI ABSTRACT MODIFIED)

ACCN 002094

---

677 AUTH **GOLDMAN, R. D., & HEWITT, B. N.**

TITL PREDICTING THE SUCCESS OF BLACK, CHICANO, ORIENTAL AND WHITE COLLEGE STUDENTS.

SRCE *JOURNAL OF EDUCATIONAL MEASUREMENT, 1976, 13, 107-143.*

INDX ACHIEVEMENT TESTING, SCHOLASTIC ACHIEVEMENT, CROSS CULTURAL, HIGHER EDUCATION, COLLEGE STUDENTS, MEXICAN AMERICAN, TEST VALIDITY, EMPIRICAL, CALIFORNIA, SOUTHWEST

ABST STUDIES OF TEST BIAS HAVE GENERALLY FOCUSED ON BLACKS AND WHITES, AND THE FINDINGS ARE NOT NECESSARILY APPLICABLE TO OTHER ETHNIC GROUPS SUCH AS CHICANOS OR ASIAN AMERICANS. THEREFORE, THE FOLLOWING WAS EXAMINED: (1) SIMILARITY OF GRADE POINT AVERAGE (GPA) FOR BLACKS AND WHITES COMPARED TO OTHER MINORITY GROUPS; AND (2) ETHNIC DIFFERENCES IN TEST SCORES RESULTING FROM A PERSON'S FIELD OF STUDY. THE FINDINGS WERE SIMILAR AT FOUR DIFFERENT CAMPUSES OF THE UNIVERSITY OF CALIFORNIA. DUMMY CODING FOR ETHNICITY IN THE MULTIPLE REGRESSION EQUATION REVEALS THAT GPA IS INDEPENDENT OF ETHNIC DIFFERENCES IN CHOSEN

FIELDS. HIGH SCHOOL GRADE POINT AVERAGE COMBINED WITH BOTH SETS OF SAT SCORES WAS A MORE RELIABLE PREDICTOR OF GPA AT THE UNIVERSITY LEVEL FOR WHITES AND ASIANS, BUT NOT FOR BLACKS OR CHICANOS. IT IS RECOGNIZED THAT THE PREDICTORS AND CRITERIA IN THIS STUDY MAY BE REFLECTING THE SAME TYPE OF BIAS. WHILE THERE NEEDS TO BE CONSENSUS ON THE DEFINITION OF TEST BIAS, THE PROBLEM CANNOT BE RESOLVED WITHOUT DEVELOPING CONSTRUCTS THAT ARE VALID PREDICTORS FOR BLACKS AND CHICANOS. 15 REFERENCES.

ACCN   000573

678 AUTH   **GOLDMAN, R. D., & RICHARDS, R.**
      TITL   THE SAT PREDICTION OF GRADES FOR MEXICAN-AMERICAN VERSUS ANGLO-AMERICAN STUDENTS AT THE UNIVERSITY OF CALIFORNIA, RIVERSIDE.
      SRCE   *JOURNAL OF EDUCATIONAL MEASUREMENT, 1974, 11(2), 129-135.*
      INDX   SCHOLASTIC ACHIEVEMENT, SCHOLASTIC APTITUDE TEST, COLLEGE STUDENTS, MEXICAN AMERICAN, CROSS CULTURAL, ACHIEVEMENT TESTING, CALIFORNIA, SOUTHWEST, TEST VALIDITY
      ABST   THIS STUDY EXAMINES THE PREDICTABILITY OF SAT SCORES FOR MEXICAN AMERICAN AND ANGLO COLLEGE STUDENTS. THE GPA FOR FRESHMEN COMPLETING TWO QUARTERS AND THEIR RESPECTIVE SAT SCORES WERE OBTAINED FROM THE SCHOOL RECORDS AT THE UNIVERSITY OF CALIFORNIA AT RIVERSIDE (UCR). REGRESSION ANALYSIS INDICATED THAT THE TWO GROUPS DIFFERED SIGNIFICANTLY, AND USING THE REGRESSION EQUATION OF THE ANGLO SAMPLE IN PREDICTING GPA REVEALED AN OVER PREDICTION FOR THE MEXICAN AMERICANS. A FOLLOW-UP REPLICATION STUDY WITH A LARGER SAMPLE REVEALED A SIMILAR OUTCOME. IT IS CONCLUDED THAT THE STANDARDIZED REGRESSION WEIGHTS FOR GPA AND SAT DO NOT PREDICT ADEQUATELY THE GRADES FOR MEXICAN AMERICAN STUDENTS AS A GROUP. SINCE UCR IS A SMALL CAMPUS OF ABOUT 5,000 STUDENTS, IT MAY NOT BE REPRESENTATIVE OF OTHER UNIVERSITIES. THEREFORE, IT IS SUGGESTED THAT FURTHER INVESTIGATIONS IN ASSESSING THE RELIABILITY AND VALIDITY OF SAT SCORES AS A PREDICTOR OF GRADES FOR MEXICAN AMERICANS BE CONDUCTED AT OTHER INSTITUTIONS OF HIGHER LEARNING. 13 REFERENCES.
      ACCN   000574

679 AUTH   **GOLDMAN, R. D., & WIDAWSKI, M. H.**
      TITL   ERRORS IN THE SELECTION OF MINORITY COLLEGE STUDENTS.
      SRCE   *PAPER PRESENTED AT THE WESTERN PSYCHOLOGICAL ASSOCIATION ANNUAL MEETING, LOS ANGELES, APRIL 1976.*
      INDX   SCHOLASTIC APTITUDE TEST, HIGHER EDUCATION, MEXICAN AMERICAN, CROSS CULTURAL, REPRESENTATION, EQUAL OPPORTUNITY, TEST VALIDITY, EMPIRICAL, DISCRIMINATION, CALIFORNIA, SOUTHWEST
      ABST   THE DATA PRESENTED IN THIS REPORT PROJECT THE SELECTION ERRORS WHICH WOULD RESULT FROM THE USE OF THE SCHOLASTIC APTITUDE TEST (SAT) IN SELECTING BLACK AND MEXICAN AMERICAN COLLEGE STUDENTS. SEVERAL TABLES PRESENT DATA GATHERED ON 656 MEXICAN AMERICAN APPLICANTS TO FOUR UNIVERSITY OF CALIFORNIA CAMPUSES (UCLA, UCSD, UC IRVINE AND UC DAVIS). RESULTS, COMPARED WITH SAT DATA FOR ANGLOS AND BLACKS, INDICATE THAT THE SAT PRODUCED ONLY MINIMAL IMPROVEMENTS IN SELECTION ACCURACY FOR MINORITY STUDENTS. THESE WERE ACHIEVED BY DECREASING FALSE-POSITIVES SELECTION ERRORS WHILE INCREASING FALSE-NEGATIVE ERRORS. THE NET RESULT WAS THE ADMISSIBILITY OF FEWER MINORITY STUDENTS. (AUTHOR ABSTRACT MODIFIED)
      ACCN   000575

680 AUTH   **GOLDSTEIN, M. J., & PALMER, J. O.**
      TITL   THE EXPERIENCE OF ANXIETY: A CASE BOOK (2ND ED.).
      SRCE   *NEW YORK: OXFORD UNIVERSITY PRESS, 1975, PP. 106-120.*
      INDX   PSYCHOTHERAPY, SES, FAMILY STRUCTURE, INTERPERSONAL RELATIONS, AUTHORITARIANISM, ANXIETY, CASE STUDY, FAMILY ROLES, SYMPTOMATOLOGY, SEX ROLES, FAMILY THERAPY, CALIFORNIA, SOUTHWEST, SPANISH SURNAMED
      ABST   IN THIS CHAPTER, "THE CASE OF THE R. FAMILY: HOW TO BE A MAN," A MEXICAN AMERICAN FAMILY IS STUDIED VIA PRESENTATION OF MATERIAL FROM FAMILY THERAPY SESSIONS WITH A CLINICAL PSYCHOLOGIST AT A LOS ANGELES MENTAL HEALTH CLINIC. THE PRESENTING PROBLEM IS RAMON, AGE 15, ONE OF EIGHT CHILDREN. HE AND HIS PARENTS WERE REFERRED TO THE CLINIC BY A TEACHER, AFTER RAMON'S DETENTION FOR POSSESSION OF MARIJUANA. THE BACKGROUND OF THE FAMILY—MOTHER AND FATHER AND SEVERAL OF THE OLDER CHILDREN—IS DESCRIBED IN DETAIL. A BRIEF SUMMARY OF TREATMENT PROGRESS IS ALSO GIVEN. QUESTIONS FOR CONSIDERATION IN UNDERSTANDING THE DYNAMICS OF THIS FAMILY AND ITS MEMBERS AND HOW THEY ARE AFFECTED BY EVENTS WITHIN AND OUTSIDE OF THE FAMILY ARE LISTED. THE CASE STUDY IS PRESENTED IN THIS FORMAT AS A TEACHING GUIDE FOR DISCUSSION. 8 REFERENCES.
      ACCN   000576

681 AUTH   **GOMEZ, A. G.**
      TITL   SOME CONSIDERATIONS IN STRUCTURING HUMAN SERVICES FOR THE SPANISH SPEAKING POPULATION OF THE UNITED STATES.
      SRCE   *INTERNATIONAL JOURNAL OF MENTAL HEALTH, 1976, 5(2), 60-68.*
      INDX   PUERTO RICAN-M, PUERTO RICAN-I, MENTAL HEALTH, IMMIGRATION, REVIEW, HEALTH, POVERTY, SPANISH SURNAMED, ESPIRITISMO, HEALTH DELIVERY SYSTEMS, POLICY

ABST ADAPTED FROM A PAPER PRESENTED DURING PSYCHIATRIC GRAND ROUNDS AT TWO NEW YORK CITY MEDICAL CENTERS, THIS ARTICLE BRIEFLY DISCUSSES THE FOLLOWING: (1) SOCIOECONOMIC FACTORS FACED BY PUERTO RICANS ON BOTH THE NATIVE ISLAND AND THE MAINLAND; (2) SOCIAL AND ECONOMIC DEPRIVATION LEADING TO INEQUALITY OF OPPORTUNITY; (3) THE RELATIONSHIP OF HEALTH AND SOCIAL PROBLEMS; AND (4) DEFICITS AND NEEDS TO BE CONSIDERED IN PLANNING FOR AND DELIVERING SERVICES TO SPANISH-SPEAKING POPULATIONS. THE NEED FOR CHANGES IN PRESENT SERVICES ARE EMPHASIZED AS ARE THE METHODS FOR ACHIEVING CHANGE-SOCIAL ACTION, COMMUNITY CRISIS INTERVENTION, AND RECOGNITION OF OTHER THAN CONVENTIONAL HUMAN SERVICES PROFESSIONALS (E.G., ESPIRITISTAS). CHANGE WITHIN THE MENTAL HEALTH PROFESSIONS AND SERVICES CANNOT BE AVOIDED IF THE RECIPIENTS OF HUMAN SERVICES ARE TO TRULY BENEFIT.

ACCN 000577

682 AUTH **GOMEZ, R. J.**
TITL CONDICIONES ECONOMICAS DE LA FAMILIA MEXICANA DE LA CLASE MEDIA, DESPUES DE LA REVOLUCION. (ECONOMIC CONDITIONS OF THE MIDDLE CLASS MEXICAN FAMILY SINCE THE REVOLUTION.)
SRCE *REVISTA MEXICANA DE SOCIOLOGIA, 1959, 21, 127-134. (SPANISH)*
INDX MEXICAN, CULTURAL CHANGE, ECONOMIC FACTORS, ESSAY, FAMILY STRUCTURE, FAMILY ROLES, HISTORY, CULTURE, MEXICO, SES
ABST THE MEXICAN REVOLUTION HAS GENERATED IMPORTANT CHANGES IN THE SOCIAL AND ECONOMIC ORGANIZATION OF MEXICO. NEVERTHELESS, THE FACTS PRESENTED IN THIS STUDY—SUCH AS THE POOR DISTRIBUTION OF INCOME, EXPENSES BEING HIGHER THAN INCOME, INCOME BEING BARELY ENOUGH TO SATISFY NEEDS OF NUTRITION, MEDICAL EXPENSES, RENT AND CLOTHING—SHOW THAT FUNDAMENTALLY THE ECONOMIC CONDITIONS OF MIDDLE-CLASS MEXICAN FAMILIES HAVE NOT CHANGED.
ACCN 000578

683 AUTH **GOMEZ-QUINONES, J.**
TITL BAKKE AND THE MEXICAN COMMUNITY.
SRCE *EL MIRLO CANTA DE NOTICATLAN, 1976, 4(3-4), 1-3. (PUBLICATION OF CHICANO STUDIES DEPARTMENT, UNIVERSITY OF CALIFORNIA, LOS ANGELES.)*
INDX DISCRIMINATION, REPRESENTATION, EDUCATION, EQUAL OPPORTUNITY, ESSAY, JUDICIAL PROCESS, HIGHER EDUCATION, POLICY
ABST VARIOUS ASPECTS OF THE BAKKE CASE WITH RESPECT TO ITS POTENTIAL IMPACT ON THE MINORITY COMMUNITY ARE EXAMINED. THE UNIVERSITY'S DECISION TO APPEAL THE BAKKE CASE TO THE U.S. SUPREME COURT IS NOT CONSIDERED AS A STAND TO DEFEND THE SPECIAL ADMISSIONS PROGRAM, BUT RATHER TO SUPPORT THE RACIST MYTH THAT MINORITIES ARE LESS QUALIFIED. THE CALIFORNIA

SUPREME COURT RULING WAS AN ACT TO MAINTAIN HARMONY IN THE DOMINANT GROUP AND NOT TAKE INTO ACCOUNT THE NEEDS OR RIGHTS OF MINORITIES. THE BAKKE ISSUE REFLECTS THE INSTITUTIONAL RACISM WHICH HAS CONTINUALLY OPPRESSED THE MEXICAN PEOPLE. ONLY BY MOBILIZING AROUND BAKKE CAN THE MEXICAN COMMUNITY HOPE TO AWAKEN THE RATIONAL CONSCIENCE TO THE HISTORICAL DENIAL OF THEIR RIGHT TO HIGHER EDUCATION.

ACCN 000579

684 AUTH **GONZALES, A. S.**
TITL MINORITIES AND THE U.S. ECONOMY.
SRCE *SANTA BARBARA: UNIVERSITY OF CALIFORNIA, UNIVERSITY LIBRARY, 1974.*
INDX BIBLIOGRAPHY, MEXICAN AMERICAN, PUERTO RICAN-M, HISTORY, POLICY, EMPLOYMENT, DEMOGRAPHIC, SES, CAPITALISM, ECONOMIC FACTORS, EQUAL OPPORTUNITY, REPRESENTATION, HOUSING, INTEGRATION, POVERTY, URBAN, DISCRIMINATION, SOCIAL SERVICES, ACCULTURATION, LABOR FORCE, MIGRATION, IMMIGRATION, SOCIAL SCIENCES, FARM LABORERS, COMMUNITY INVOLVEMENT
ABST THIS ANNOTATED BIBLIOGRAPHY PROVIDES AN OVERVIEW OF THE PROGRESS AND DIRECTION OF MINORITY PARTICIPATION IN THE U.S. ECONOMY. 969 CITATIONS REPRESENT BOTH MAJORITY AND MINORITY VIEWS AND ARE DRAWN SUBSTANTIALLY FROM BUSINESS AND INDUSTRIAL LITERATURE AND INTERDISCIPLINARY SOURCES AVAILABLE AT THE UNIVERSITY OF CALIFORNIA AT SANTA BARBARA LIBRARY. PART I PROVIDES THE SOCIOECONOMIC BACKGROUND OF MINORITIES, EMPHASIZING THEIR ECONOMIC DEVELOPMENT AND ROLE IN THE HISTORY OF THE UNITED STATES. PART II INCLUDES MATERIALS DEALING WITH POLICY ISSUES, ECONOMIC ANALYSIS, AND THE IMPLICATIONS OF PROGRAMS FOR MINORITIES. PART III CITES MATERIALS IN MANPOWER DEVELOPMENT, EMPLOYMENT, AND PRODUCTIVITY. PART IV COVERS THE DEMOGRAPHIC PROFILE OF THE MINORITY MARKET, INCLUDING INCOME AND MARKET BEHAVIOR. PART V INCLUDES MATERIALS ON MINORITIES IN THE PROFESSIONS, SMALL BUSINESS, MANAGEMENT, AND CAPITAL AND CORPORATE DEVELOPMENT. PART VI DEALS WITH MINORITY HOUSING AND WELFARE. THE SUBJECT INDEX LISTS 24 ARTICLES UNDER THE HEADING "CHICANOS" AND 5 UNDER "PUERTO RICAN AMERICANS."

ACCN 002095

685 AUTH **GONZALES, E.**
TITL THE ROLE OF CHICANO FOLK BELIEFS AND PRACTICES IN MENTAL HEALTH.
SRCE *IN C. HERNANDEZ, M. J. HAUG & N. N. WAGNER (EDS.), CHICANOS: SOCIAL AND PSYCHOLOGICAL PERSPECTIVES. SAINT LOUIS: C. V. MOSBY COMPANY, 1976, PP. 263-281.*
INDX MEXICAN AMERICAN, MENTAL HEALTH, CURANDERISMO, REVIEW, FOLK MEDICINE, RESOURCE UTILIZATION, MENTAL HEALTH PROFESSION, DISEASE, CULTURAL FACTORS, PSYCHOTHERAPY, POLICY

ABST   THE LITERATURE PERTAINING TO THE PRAC-
TICE OF CURANDERISMO AS A METHOD OF
FOLK PSYCHIATRY AND COMMUNITY TREAT-
MENT FOR MEXICAN AMERICANS IS REVIEWED
WITH RESPECT TO THE FOLLOWING: (1) THE IS-
SUE OF FORMULATING MENTAL HEALTH SER-
VICES TO MEET THE NEEDS OF CHICANOS; (2)
THE VARIOUS CONCEPTS IMPLIED BY THE TERM
CURANDERISMO, I.E. MAL OJO, MAL DE SUSTO,
EMPACHO, MAL PUESTO (SORCERY), AND
CAIDA DE LA MOLLERA; (3) THE USE OF FOLK
BELIEFS AND PRACTICES RELATED TO CUR-
ANDEROS (FOLKHEALERS); AND (4) THEORETI-
CAL SPECULATIONS CONCERNING HOW AND
WHY CURANDERISMO FUNCTIONS AMONG
CHICANOS. THE IMPORTANCE OF INCORPO-
RATING CURANDERISMO INTO THE PRESENT
MENTAL HEALTH PRACTICE RELATES DIRECTLY
TO THE CHICANO PERCEPTION OF ILLNESS
AND HEALTH. CHICANO RELIGIOUS VIEWS, SO-
CIOLOGICAL VIEWS, SUPERNATURALISTIC
VIEWS, AND NATURALISTIC VIEWS SUGGEST
THAT AN ALTERNATIVE FORMAT SHOULD BE IM-
PLEMENTED IN NATIONAL MENTAL HEALTH
SERVICES. 36 REFERENCES.

ACCN   000580

686   AUTH   **GONZALES, J. D.**
TITL   EL CENTRO: AN NIMH PROGRAM REPORT.
(DHEW PUBLICATION NO. (ADM) 76-398.)
SRCE   *ROCKVILLE, MD.: NATIONAL INSTITUTE OF
MENTAL HEALTH, 1976.*
INDX   BILINGUAL-BICULTURAL PERSONNEL, COM-
MUNITY, CULTURAL FACTORS, CURRICULUM,
ECONOMIC FACTORS, EDUCATION, ESSAY,
HEALTH DELIVERY SYSTEMS, HIGHER EDUCA-
TION, MENTAL HEALTH, MENTAL HEALTH
PROFESSION, MEXICAN AMERICAN, PARA-
PROFESSIONALS, PROFESSIONAL TRAINING,
SES, SOCIAL SERVICES, CALIFORNIA, SOUTH-
WEST, URBAN
ABST   AT EL CENTRO (AN ACRONYM STANDING FOR
EAST LOS ANGELES CHICANO EDUCATION,
TRAINING, AND RESEARCH ORGANIZATION) A
COMPREHENSIVE PROGRAM OF RESEARCH,
TRAINING, AND SERVICE ACTIVITIES WAS ES-
TABLISHED IN 1971 TO RESPOND TO THE NEED
FOR TRAINED CHICANO MENTAL HEALTH
PROFESSIONALS. THE PROGRAM IS FUNDED
BY THE NATIONAL INSTITUTE OF MENTAL
HEALTH (NIMH) THROUGH ITS CENTER FOR MI-
NORITY GROUP MENTAL HEALTH PROGRAMS
AND SERVES THE ESTIMATED 500,000 RESI-
DENTS WITHIN THE 44 SQUARE MILE EAST LOS
ANGELES MEXICAN AMERICAN BARRIO. THIS
POPULATION IS REPORTED TO HAVE SPECIAL
NEEDS DUE TO LANGUAGE BARRIERS, HIGH
UNEMPLOYMENT, AND LOW SES. THE PRO-
GRAM WAS ORIGINALLY ESTABLISHED IN CO-
OPERATION WITH UCLA'S AND USC'S SCHOOLS
OF SOCIAL WORK AND THE TRABAJADORES
DE LA RAZA (NATIONAL ORGANIZATION OF
CHICANO SOCIAL WORKERS) AS A TRAINING
CENTER FOR SOCIAL WORKERS. THE TRAIN-
ING GRANT TERMINATED IN JUNE OF 1973, AT
WHICH TIME EL CENTRO WAS INCORPORATED
AS A NONPROFIT ORGANIZATION. WITH THE
ASSISTANCE OF NIMH'S CENTER FOR MI-

NORITY GROUP MENTAL HEALTH PROGRAMS,
A SERVICE PROGRAM WAS ESTABLISHED AS
AN ADJUNCT TO THE TRAINING PROGRAM.
THE CURRICULUM FOR THE 12 SOCIAL WORK
TRAINEES CONSISTS OF FORMAL LECTURES,
SEMINARS, AND CLIENT INTERACTION. IF
FUNDED IN THE FUTURE, EL CENTRO WILL
HIRE A PERMANENT STAFF TO OPERATE A LI-
CENSED PSYCHIATRIC CLINIC TO SERVE THE
URBAN CHICANO POPULATION.

ACCN   002096

687   AUTH   **GONZALEZ, A.**
TITL   THE STRUGGLE TO DEVELOP SELF-HELP INSTI-
TUTIONS.
SRCE   *SOCIAL CASEWORK, 1974, 55(2), 90-93.*
INDX   URBAN, ESSAY, BILINGUAL-BICULTURAL PER-
SONNEL, FINANCING, POLITICAL POWER,
HEALTH DELIVERY SYSTEMS, PREJUDICE, DIS-
CRIMINATION, SOCIAL SERVICES, COMMUNITY
INVOLVEMENT, PUERTO RICAN-M, EAST, NEW
YORK
ABST   THIS AUTOBIOGRAPHICAL SKETCH DE-
SCRIBES A PUERTO RICAN WHO CAME TO NEW
YORK CITY AND STRUGGLED TO CREATE EF-
FECTIVE MENTAL HEALTH PROGRAMS FOR
PUERTO RICANS. EVEN WITH A MASTER'S DE-
GREE IN SOCIAL WORK, GONZALEZ EXPERI-
ENCED MANY OF THE TRANSITIONAL PROB-
LEMS FACING OTHER PUERTO RICANS WHEN
THEY MIGRATE TO THE MAINLAND. AS A CASE-
WORKER, HE SOON REALIZED THAT THE LACK
OF BILINGUAL AND BICULTURAL COUNSELING
SERVICES WAS A MANIFESTATION OF THE RI-
GIDITY OF THE ANGLO INSTITUTIONS. THERE-
FORE, HE ARRIVED AT THE CONCLUSION THAT
UNLESS PUERTO RICANS DEVELOPED THEIR
OWN INSTITUTIONS, THEY WOULD HAVE NO
CHOICE BUT TO RESIGN THEMSELVES TO LIFE
IN THE GHETTO. WITH OTHERS SHARING HIS
CONCERN, THE LONG POLITICAL BATTLE TO
OBTAIN THE FUNDS NECESSARY TO SET UP A
SELF-HELP INSTITUTION HAS RESULTED IN THE
DEVELOPMENT OF SEVERAL MENTAL HEALTH
PROGRAMS FOR PUERTO RICANS. HOWEVER,
GONZALEZ POINTS OUT THAT THOSE WITHIN
THE POWER STRUCTURE ARE UNWILLING TO
PROVIDE FINANCIAL ASSISTANCE OR GIVE UP
THEIR POLITICAL POWER TO MINORITY GROUP.
THUS, IT IS UP TO LEADERS IN THE MINORITY
COMMUNITIES TO FIGHT, NOT ONLY FOR THE
NEEDS OF THEIR OWN PARTICULAR GROUP
BUT ALSO AGAINST THOSE WHO, BECAUSE OF
THEIR VESTED INTERESTS, ARE RELUCTANT TO
MEET THE NEEDS OF PEOPLE.

ACCN   000581

688   AUTH   **GONZALEZ, A., & ROMERO, S.**
TITL   INCLUSION OF PUERTO RICAN CURRICULUM
CONTENT IN SOCIAL WORK TRAINING.
SRCE   *SOCIAL WORK EDUCATION REPORTER, 1971,
19(1), 42-43.*
INDX   PUERTO RICAN-M, MENTAL HEALTH, MENTAL
HEALTH PROFESSION, PROFESSIONAL TRAIN-
ING, CURRICULUM, ESSAY, POLICY, NEW YORK,
EAST
ABST   A GREAT NUMBER OF PUERTO RICANS IN NEW
YORK CITY UTILIZE SOCIAL WELFARE AGEN-

CIES. SINCE MOST SOCIAL WORKERS ARE NON-PUERTO RICAN, THEY ARE UNABLE TO COMMUNICATE VERBALLY OR CULTURALLY WITH THEIR PUERTO RICAN CLIENTS. THE SOCIAL WORKERS ARE NOT TRAINED ADEQUATELY TO MEET THE NEEDS OF THEIR CLIENTS. IT IS RECOMMENDED THAT THIS PROBLEM BE ALLEVIATED BY INCORPORATING PUERTO RICAN CONTENT IN THE TRAINING OF SOCIAL WORKERS BY: (1) FIELD INSTRUCTION PLACEMENTS FOR BOTH PUERTO RICAN AND NON-PUERTO RICAN STUDENTS TO EXPERIENCE HOW PUERTO RICAN AGENCIES FUNCTION; (2) SPECIFIC COURSES DEALING WITH PUERTO RICAN ISSUES; (3) INTEGRATING PUERTO RICAN CONTENT INTO CASE STUDIES; AND (4) MAKING A CONCERTED EFFORT TO RECRUIT PUERTO RICAN STUDENTS AND FACULTY. IT IS ALSO RECOMMENDED THAT THE HUMAN RESOURCES OF OTHER PROFESSIONALS RESIDING WITHIN THE PUERTO RICAN COMMUNITY BE TAPPED AS A VEHICLE TO DEVELOP AND IMPLEMENT AN EFFECTIVE PROGRAM IN THE SCHOOLS OF SOCIAL WORK.

ACCN   000582

689 AUTH **GONZALEZ, G.**
     TITL THE IDENTIFICATION OF COMPETENCIES FOR CHILD DEVELOPMENT ASSOCIATES WORKING WITH CHICANO CHILDREN.
     SRCE *WASHINGTON, D.C.: CHILD DEVELOPMENT ASSOCIATE CONSORTIUM, RESEARCH AND DEVELOPMENT, 1974.*
     INDX PARAPROFESSIONALS, CULTURE, LINGUISTICS, MEXICAN AMERICAN, ESSAY, BILINGUALISM, CULTURAL PLURALISM, PSYCHOTHERAPY, BIBLIOGRAPHY, TEACHERS, PROFESSIONAL TRAINING
     ABST THE AIM OF A PROJECT CARRIED OUT BY THE CHILD DEVELOPMENT ASSOCIATES CONSORTIUM (CDAC) WAS TO IDENTIFY A SET OF TEACHER COMPETENCIES AND CORRESPONDING BEHAVIORAL REFERENTS FOR CHILD DEVELOPMENT ASSOCIATES (CDA) WORKING WITH CHICANO CHILDREN. THE RESULTING COMPETENCY REQUIREMENTS ARE INTENDED TO SUPPLEMENT THOSE COMPETENCIES TO BE REQUIRED OF ALL CDA. THE CDAC FRAMEWORK, EXAMINED FOR ITS ADEQUACY IN MEETING THE SPECIAL NEEDS OF CHICANO CHILDREN, WAS SEEN AS NEEDING THE AREAS OF CULTURE, SPANISH LANGUAGE AND COGNITIVE/AFFECTIVE INTERRELATION ADDED TO ITS EXISTING PROGRAM OF PLANNING, ORGANIZING, TEACHING/INTERACTING, EVALUATION AND KNOWLEDGE. AN ANALYSIS OF THE INSTRUMENTS DEVELOPED FOR USE IN ASSESSING COMPETENCIES, THE INTEGRATED COMPETING ASSESSMENT SCALE (ICAS) AND THE Q-SORT SELF-ASSESSMENT SCALE, IS PRESENTED. TO INSURE THAT THE COMPETENCIES REFLECT CURRENT THINKING IN THE FIELD, THE PROJECT INCLUDED A LITERATURE SEARCH COMPONENT. ABSTRACTS OF THESES, ARTICLES AND DISSERTATIONS THAT BEAR ON THE CHICANO PRE-SCHOOL CHILD ARE INCLUDED, ALONG WITH APPENDICES RELATING TO COMPETENCY DETERMINATION, CULTURE-

BASED CURRICULA AND INSTRUMENT ASSESSMENT. THE COMPETENCY STATEMENTS WERE REVIEWED BY A PANEL OF CHICANO PROFESSIONALS FROM THROUGHOUT THE COUNTRY; THE RESULTING COMPETENCY STATEMENTS REFLECT THEIR RECOMMENDATIONS. 45 REFERENCES.

ACCN   000583

690 AUTH **GONZALEZ, N. L.**
     TITL THE SPANISH-AMERICANS OF NEW MEXICO: A HERITAGE OF PRIDE.
     SRCE *ALBUQUERQUE: UNIVERSITY OF NEW MEXICO PRESS, 1969.*
     INDX HISTORY, CULTURE, SOCIAL STRUCTURE, NEW MEXICO, URBAN, ACCULTURATION, MEXICAN AMERICAN, SOUTHWEST, SES, EMPLOYMENT, FAMILY STRUCTURE, EDUCATION, INTERMARRIAGE, ADULTS, ADOLESCENTS, ECONOMIC FACTORS, RURAL, POLITICAL POWER, POLITICS, CULTURAL FACTORS, IMMIGRATION, ETHNIC IDENTITY, CULTURAL CHANGE, DEMOGRAPHIC, PREJUDICE, DISCRIMINATION, BOOK
     ABST THE SPANISH AMERICANS OF NEW MEXICO, COMPRISING ONE QUARTER OF THE STATE'S POPULATION, HAVE MAINTAINED THEIR IDENTITY, LANGUAGE, AND CUSTOMS TO A GREATER EXTENT THAN OTHER HISPANICS THROUGHOUT THE SOUTHWEST. STILL, A REVIEW OF THE STATE'S SOCIAL HISTORY, BY EMPHASIZING THOSE EVENTS MOLDING THE PRESENT SOCIOCULTURAL SITUATION, REVEALS THE TENSION BETWEEN THE TRADITIONAL SPANISH CULTURE AND THE ANGLO WAY OF LIFE. RECENT YEARS HAVE SEEN URBANIZATION, ANGLICIZATION, AND THE RAPID GROWTH OF POLITICAL ACTIVISM; AND THE QUESTION IS RAISED AS TO WHAT EXTENT THE HISPANOS OF NEW MEXICO DIFFER FROM MEXICAN AMERICANS IN OTHER PARTS OF THE NATION. SIMILARITIES DO EXIST IN THE CULTURE, THE PROBLEMS FACED BY THE PREDOMINANTLY SPANISH AMERICAN LOWER CLASS, AND THE PREJUDICE AND DISTRUST BETWEEN SPANISH AND ANGLO GROUPS. BUT THERE IS A SIGNIFICANT DIFFERENCE IN THE WAY IN WHICH SPANISH AMERICANS ARE ARTICULATED INTO THE LARGER SOCIETY. THE STATUS OF THE SPANISH AMERICAN MIDDLE AND UPPER CLASSES IN NEW MEXICO APPEARS CONSIDERABLY HIGHER THAN IN OTHER PARTS OF THE SOUTHWEST. MOREOVER, ANGLOS IN NEW MEXICO HAVE ADOPTED MANY SPANISH CULTURAL TRAITS AND ARE PROUD OF THE STATE'S SPANISH AND INDIAN HERITAGE. FINALLY, THE DISASSOCIATION FROM THE TERM "MEXICAN" CAN BE TRACED TO A DESIRE AMONG SPANISH AMERICANS TO PRESERVE THE DIGNITY AND PRESTIGE OF THEIR CULTURE DURING PERIODS OF HEAVY MEXICAN AND ANGLO MIGRATION. 240 REFERENCES.

ACCN   002097

691 AUTH **GONZALEZ-PABON, J. F.**
     TITL PATTERNS OF PSYCHOPATHOLOGY: CORRESPONDENCES AND DISTINCTIONS BETWEEN SAMPLES OF AMERICAN AND PUERTO RICAN

MENTAL HOSPITAL PATIENTS (DOCTORAL DISSERTATION, RUTGERS UNIVERSITY, 1971).

SRCE *DISSERTATION ABSTRACTS INTERNATIONAL, 1971, 31, 5439B. (UNIVERSITY MICROFILMS NO. 72-9624).*

INDX PSYCHOPATHOLOGY, PERSONALITY ASSESSMENT, PUERTO RICAN-I, MALE, SES, DEPRESSION, SCHIZOPHRENIA, SEXUAL BEHAVIOR, ANXIETY, TEST VALIDITY, CROSS CULTURAL, SEX ROLES, EMPIRICAL, ADULTS, DEVIANCE, SYMPTOMATOLOGY, HOMOSEXUALITY, NEW JERSEY, EAST

ABST AN INVESTIGATION OF SYMPTOM CLUSTERS AND THE FORMS OF MANIFESTED BEHAVIOR OF MENTAL HEALTH WAS CONDUCTED TO ASSESS CULTURAL DIFFERENCES AMONG 160 ANGLO PATIENTS AT A NEW JERSEY STATE HOSPITAL AND 165 PUERTO RICANS AT A PSYCHIATRIC HOSPITAL IN SAN JUAN, PUERTO RICO. PATIENTS WERE RATED BY TRAINED OBSERVERS USING THE WITTENBORN PSYCHIATRIC SCALE CONTAINING 72 SYMPTOMS OF MENTAL HEALTH ITEMS. RESULTS FROM FACTOR ANALYSES REVEALED THE FOLLOWING: (1) SYNDROMES OF DEPRESSIVE RETARDATION AND PARANOIA WERE MORE DESCRIPTIVE AND GENERALIZED IN THE POPULATION; (2) TWO FORMS OF PSYCHOTIC BELLIGERANCE WERE DISTRIBUTED IN THE SAMPLE, BUT ONLY 1 IN THE PUERTO RICAN SAMPLE; (3) SCHIZOPHRENIC EXCITEMENT INVOLVED MERE SYMPTOMS AMONG THE PUERTO RICANS; (4) HOMOSEXUAL AGGRESSION WAS DISTINCTIVE OF THE UNITED STATES PATIENTS; AND (5) SYNDROMES OF ANXIETY AND INTELLECTUAL IMPAIRMENT WERE ANALOGOUS IN BOTH SAMPLES. THE SYMPTOM CLUSTERS AMONG PUERTO RICANS WERE SUFFICIENTLY DIFFERENT TO SUGGEST THE NEED TO STANDARDIZE THE SCALE BASED ON PUERTO RICAN DATA. IT IS ALSO SUGGESTED THAT CULTURAL FACTORS MAY CONTRIBUTE TO DIFFERENCES IN PSYCHOPATHOLOGY REGARDING SYMPTOMS AND THEIR MANIFESTATION. FURTHER RESEARCH IS NEEDED AS WELL AS THE CONSTRUCTION OF MEASURES TO ASCERTAIN THE EFFECTS OF THE "MACHO" CONCEPT AND THE TRADITIONAL FAMILY ROLES WITH RESPECT TO THEIR RELATION TO PUERTO RICAN DISORDERS. 70 REFERENCES. (AUTHOR ABSTRACT MODIFIED)

ACCN 000585

692 AUTH **GOODENOUGH, F.**

TITL RACIAL DIFFERENCES IN THE INTELLIGENCE OF SCHOOL CHILDREN.

SRCE *JOURNAL OF EXPERIMENTAL PSYCHOLOGY, 1926, 9(5), 388-397.*

INDX INTELLIGENCE TESTING, MEXICAN AMERICAN, CHILDREN, CROSS CULTURAL, EMPIRICAL, INTELLIGENCE, GOODENOUGH DRAW-A-MAN TEST

ABST A SAMPLE OF 2,456 AMERICAN-BORN SCHOOL CHILDREN, IN GRADES ONE TO FOUR, OF FOREIGN PARENTAGE (ARMENIAN, ITALIAN, SPANISH MEXICAN, NEGRO, JEWISH, ASIAN, GERMAN, ENGLISH, PORTUGUESE, DANISH, AND ASSYRIAN STOCKS) WERE ADMINISTERED THE GOODENOUGH INTELLIGENCE TEST. RESULTS SHOW THAT THE SOUTHERN EUROPEAN AND NEGRO GROUPS RANK BELOW THE ANGLO-AMERICAN AND THOSE OF NORTHERN EUROPEAN STOCK. THE COEFFICIENT OF VARIABILITY IS HIGHEST FOR THE NEGROES AND LOWEST FOR THE JEWISH CHILDREN. CHILDREN OF DIFFERENT RACIAL STOCKS ARE FOUND TO DIFFER GREATLY AND THE RANK-ORDER OF THE VARIOUS GROUPS CORRESPOND VERY CLOSELY TO THE RESULTS OF OTHER INVESTIGATIONS USING VERBAL TESTS, THE GROUPS WITH LOWER MEDIAN IQ'S ARE THE FOLLOWING: SOUTHERN NEGRO 76.5, CALIFORNIA NEGRO 82.7, INDIAN 85.6, SPANISH MEXICAN 87.2, AND ITALIAN 87.5. THE JEWISH AND DANISH GROUPS HAVE THE HIGHEST MEDIAN IQ'S, 106.3 AND 104.5, RESPECTIVELY. 46 REFERENCES.

ACCN 000586

693 AUTH **GOODMAN, M. E., & BEMAN, A.**

TITL CHILD'S-EYE-VIEWS OF LIFE IN AN URBAN BARRIO.

SRCE *IN N. N. WAGNER, & M. J. HAUG (ED.), CHICANOS: SOCIAL AND PSYCHOLOGICAL PERSPECTIVES. SAINT LOUIS: C. V. MOSBY COMPANY, 1971, PP. 109-122.*

INDX ENVIRONMENTAL FACTORS, ACCULTURATION, INTERPERSONAL RELATIONS, DEVIANCE, FAMILY ROLES, FAMILY STRUCTURE, INTERPERSONAL SPACING, SEX ROLES, ATTITUDES, EDUCATION, MEXICAN AMERICAN, URBAN, POVERTY, EMPIRICAL, TEXAS, SOUTHWEST, VALUES

ABST PERCEPTIONS, LIFE STYLES, AND VALUES OF SCHOOL-AGE CHILDREN IN A MEXICAN AMERICAN POVERTY ENCLAVE ARE EXAMINED. THIRTY-FOUR CHILDREN IN GRADES ONE THROUGH SIX WERE INTERVIEWED AND ADMINISTERED A LENGTHY QUESTIONNAIRE. THE INTERVIEW CONTENT RANGED FROM FACTUAL ITEMS SUCH AS A LIST OF FAMILY MEMBERS TO VALUE JUDGMENTS ABOUT GOOD AND BAD PEOPLE. RESULTS REVEAL THAT THE CHILDREN GIVE EQUAL WEIGHT TO SCHOOL AND TELEVISION. THE MEXICAN CHILDREN ASPIRE MAINLY TO SIMPLE AND LOCALLY FAMILIAR WORK ROLES, AND PAY LITTLE ATTENTION TO THE GLAMOUR ROLES THEY SEE ON TELEVISION. THE CHILDREN ARE TRAINED AND DISCIPLINED TO RESPECT AND HELP OTHERS. MOST CHILDREN HAVE NUMEROUS RELATIVES WHO TAKE ACTIVE INTEREST IN THEM. ON THE AVERAGE, THE CHILDREN ASPIRE TO JOBS SOMEWHAT BETTER THAN THOSE THEIR ADULT RELATIVES HAVE. THEY HAVE A TENDENCY TO EVALUATE THEIR SITUATION AND THEIR LIFE CHANCES REALISTICALLY. IN GENERAL, THE LIFE STYLES AND VALUES OF THE BARRIO CHILDREN ARE CONDUCIVE TO MODEST SUCCESS IN THE CONTEMPORARY URBAN SOCIETY. THE CHILDREN ARE GROWING UP WITHOUT GREAT AMBITION BUT WITH SELF-RESPECT. 11 REFERENCES.

ACCN 000587

694 AUTH **GOODMAN, P. W., & BROOKS, B. S.**

TITL A COMPARISON OF ANGLO AND MEXICAN-

AMERICAN STUDENTS ATTENDING THE SAME UNIVERSITY.

SRCE *THE KANSAS JOURNAL OF SOCIOLOGY, 1974, 10(2), 181-203.*

INDX SES, CROSS CULTURAL, MEXICAN AMERICAN, COLLEGE STUDENTS, EMPIRICAL, BILINGUAL, BILINGUALISM, SES, LINGUISTIC COMPETENCE, LANGUAGE ASSESSMENT, HIGHER EDUCATION, POLICY, REPRESENTATION, EMPLOYMENT, FAMILY STRUCTURE, RELIGION, ECONOMIC FACTORS, TEXAS, SOUTHWEST

ABST LITTLE INFORMATION HAS BEEN OBTAINED ABOUT MEXICAN AMERICANS WHO ATTEND INSTITUTIONS OF HIGHER EDUCATION. THE DEVELOPMENT OF EFFECTIVE PROGRAMS TO MEET THE NEEDS OF THESE STUDENTS DEPENDS UPON ASCERTAINING THEIR NEEDS. A SURVEY WAS CONDUCTED AT THE UNIVERSITY OF TEXAS AT EL PASO WHERE 30% OF THE STUDENT POPULATION IS MEXICAN AMERICAN. A STRATIFIED RANDOM SAMPLE CONSISTED OF 148 MONOLINGUAL ANGLO AND 150 BILINGUAL MEXICAN AMERICAN STUDENTS. FINDINGS INDICATE THAT ANGLOS HAD HIGHER SOCIAL CLASS STANDING, RECEIVED HIGHER HOURLY WAGES, AND HAD FATHERS WHO RECEIVED HIGHER YEARLY SALARIES. MEXICAN AMERICAN STUDENTS WERE MORE FINANCIALLY AUTONOMOUS, HAD MORE SIBLINGS, AND USED MORE SPANISH IN ALL SETTINGS. SIMILARITIES INCLUDED AGE, LEVEL OF ASPIRATION, PERCENTAGE OF WORKING STUDENTS, NUMBER OF HOURS EMPLOYED, AND PERCENT IN RECEIPT OF LOANS, SCHOLARSHIPS AND GRANTS. 12 REFERENCES. (JOURNAL ABSTRACT MODIFIED)

ACCN 000588

695 AUTH **GORDON, M. W.**

TITL CULTURAL ASPECTS OF PUERTO RICO'S RACE PROBLEMS.

SRCE *AMERICAN SOCIOLOGICAL REVIEW, 1950, 15(3), 382-392.*

INDX PREJUDICE, HISTORY, ESSAY, DISCRIMINATION, PUERTO RICAN-I, CULTURAL CHANGE, POLICY, EDUCATION

ABST RACE PREJUDICE IN PUERTO RICO IS USUALLY CONSIDERED A RESULT OF THE UNITED STATES ACQUIRING POSSESSION OF THE ISLAND IN 1898. HOWEVER, PUERTO RICO HAS ITS OWN HISTORY OF SLAVERY, DISCRIMINATION, AND PREJUDICE WHICH DATES BACK TO THE PERIOD OF EARLY EUROPEAN COLONIALISM. PUERTO RICO'S POPULATION REPRESENTS A COMPOSITE OF SPANISH, AFRICAN, AND NATIVE INDIANS. THE HISTORICAL ASPECTS OF SPANISH COLONIALISM HAVE HAD A SIGNIFICANT IMPACT ON THE MODERN DAY PUERTO RICAN'S ATTITUDES OF RACE TOLERANCE, ESPECIALLY WITH RESPECT TO INTERRACIAL MARRIAGE, RESIDENTIAL PATTERNS, AND COLOR-CONSCIOUSNESS. THE UNITED STATES' POLICY WITH PUERTO RICO CONTINUES TO PERPETUATE THE ALREADY EXISTING RACE PROBLEMS. FOR EXAMPLE, THE EDUCATIONAL SYSTEM IN PUERTO RICO, PATTERNED AFTER UNITED STATES SCHOOLS, HAS PRODUCED CULTURAL CONFLICTS FOR MANY PUERTO RI-

CAN CHILDREN. PROGRAMS REFLECTING INTER-CULTURAL UNDERSTANDING NEED TO BE IMPLEMENTED IN PUERTO RICO'S EDUCATIONAL SYSTEM IN ORDER TO REDUCE SOME OF ITS CURRENT RACE PROBLEMS. 60 REFERENCES.

ACCN 000589

696 AUTH **GORDON, S. B.**

TITL ETHNIC AND SOCIOECONOMIC INFLUENCES ON THE HOME LANGUAGE EXPERIENCES OF CHILDREN.

SRCE *WASHINGTON, D.C.: OFFICE OF EDUCATION, DHEW, 1970. (ERIC DOCUMENT REPRODUCTION SERVICE NO. ED 043 377)*

INDX SES, CULTURAL FACTORS, COGNITIVE DEVELOPMENT, CHILDREN, BILINGUALISM, CROSS CULTURAL, MOTHER-CHILD INTERACTION, ITPA, LANGUAGE ACQUISITION, EARLY CHILDHOOD EDUCATION, ARIZONA, NEW MEXICO, SOUTHWEST, EMPIRICAL

ABST THE MAJOR HYPOTHESIS OF THIS STUDY IS THAT A SIGNIFICANT RELATIONSHIP EXISTS BETWEEN ENGLISH LANGUAGE ABILITY (AS MEASURED BY THE ILLINOIS TEST OF PSYCHOLINGUISTIC ABILITIES (ITPA) FULL SCALE SCORE) AND LANGUAGE MODELING BY THE MOTHER (AS MEASURED BY THE MOTHER-CHILD INTERACTION SCORE ON THE LANGUAGE MODEL MATRIX), AND BETWEEN ENGLISH LANGUAGE ABILITY AND TOTAL HOME LANGUAGE MODELING (AS MEASURED BY THE TOTAL INTERACTION SCORE ON THE LANGUAGE MODEL MATRIX). SUBHYPOTHESES STATE THAT ENGLISH LANGUAGE ABILITY, LANGUAGE MODELING BY THE MOTHER, AND TOTAL HOME LANGUAGE MODELING SIGNIFICANTLY DIFFER ACCORDING TO (1) ETHNICITY, (2) SOCIOECONOMIC STATUS, AND (3) LANGUAGE TYPE. THE SAMPLE CONSISTED OF 155 FIRST-GRADE CHILDREN: 50 NAVAJO INDIAN, 55 PUEBLO INDIAN, AND 50 RURAL SPANISH/AMERICAN. A LANGUAGE MODEL MATRIX WAS DESIGNED TO PROVIDE AN OPERATIONAL FRAMEWORK. TEST RESULTS SUPPORT THE MAJOR AND SUB-HYPOTHESES. AS ACCULTURATION AND SES INCREASE, SO DOES THE QUANTITY OF VERBAL INTERACTION IN THE HOME. PROGRAMS TO ALLEVIATE POVERTY AND TO TEACH MOTHERS HOW TO TEACH THEIR CHILDREN ARE OF VITAL IMPORTANCE IN THE ELIMINATION OF LINGUISTIC DISADVANTAGE. 21 REFERENCES. (RIE ABSTRACT)

ACCN 000590

697 AUTH **GORDON, S. B.**

TITL THE RELATIONSHIP BETWEEN ENGLISH LANGUAGE ABILITIES AND HOME LANGUAGE EXPERIENCES OF FIRST GRADE CHILDREN FROM THREE ETHNIC GROUPS OF VARYING SOCIOECONOMIC STATUS AND VARYING DEGREES OF BILINGUALISM.

SRCE *UNPUBLISHED DOCTORAL DISSERTATION, UNIVERSITY OF NEW MEXICO, 1969. (ERIC DOCUMENT REPRODUCTION SERVICE NO. ED 050 092)*

INDX BILINGUALISM, MEXICAN AMERICAN, COGNITIVE DEVELOPMENT, SES, CROSS CULTURAL,

CHILDREN, ARIZONA, NEW MEXICO, SOUTH-WEST, LANGUAGE ACQUISITION, ITPA, LINGUISTIC COMPETENCE, MOTHER-CHILD INTERACTION, INDIGENOUS POPULATIONS, MODELING, RURAL, EMPIRICAL

ABST THE RELATIONSHIP BETWEEN A VARIETY OF HOME LANGUAGE-MODELING SITUATIONS AND THE ENGLISH LANGUAGE ABILITIES OF CHILDREN IS EXAMINED WITH PARTICULAR EMPHASIS ON THE LANGUAGE MODELING OF THE MOTHER. THE INFLUENCE OF ETHNICITY, SES, AND LANGUAGE MODEL TYPE (DEGREE OF BILINGUALISM) ON ENGLISH LANGUAGE ABILITY, ON LANGUAGE-MODELING BY THE MOTHER, AND ON TOTAL LANGUAGE MODELING IS ALSO CONSIDERED. THE SAMPLE CONSISTED OF 55 PUEBLO INDIANS, 50 SPANISH AMERICANS FROM THE RURAL AREA OF BERNALILLO, NEW MEXICO, AND 50 NAVAJO INDIANS FROM THE RURAL TOWN OF SANDERS, ARIZONA. DATA GATHERING INSTRUMENTS INCLUDED THE ILLINOIS TEST OF PSYCHOLINGUISTIC ABILITIES (ITPA), THE WOLF HOME INTERVIEW QUESTIONNAIRE, AND A SPECIALLY DEVISED LANGUAGE MODEL MATRIX. THESE MEASURES ASSESSED PSYCHOLINGUISTIC ABILITIES, ASPECTS AND CONTEXTS OF HOME ENVIRONMENTS RELATED TO INTELLIGENCE, AND A QUANTIFICATION OF THE PARTICULAR COMBINATION OF LANGUAGE-MODELING SOURCE AND CONTEXT. RESULTS SHOW THAT LANGUAGE-MODELING VARIES WITH ETHNICITY, SES, AND LANGUAGE MODEL TYPE AND THAT THIS WAS RELATED TO AND PREDICTIVE OF ENGLISH LANGUAGE ABILITY. THE QUANTITY OF VERBAL INTERACTION INCREASED WITH ACCULTURATION AND SES, THUS APPROXIMATING MIDDLE-MAJORITY NORMS. RECOMMENDATIONS ARE MADE TO INCREASE THE QUANTITY AND QUALITY OF VERBAL INTERACTIONS IN NON-MIDDLE-MAJORITY HOMES. ADULT EDUCATION PROGRAMS STRESSING LEARNING-INDUCING DIALOGUES BETWEEN MOTHER AND CHILD NEED TO BE DESIGNED.

ACCN 000591

698 AUTH **GORDON, T. L., & DUBE, W. F.**
TITL MEDICAL STUDENT ENROLLMENT, 1971-72 THROUGH 1975-76.
SRCE *JOURNAL OF MEDICAL EDUCATION, 1976, 51(2), 144-146.*
INDX MEDICAL STUDENTS, EDUCATION, PROFESSIONAL TRAINING, MENTAL HEALTH PROFESSION, HEALTH, EMPIRICAL, OCCUPATIONAL ASPIRATIONS, MEXICAN AMERICAN, CROSS CULTURAL, PUERTO RICAN-M, CUBAN, REPRESENTATION
ABST FIRST YEAR AND TOTAL U.S. MEDICAL SCHOOL ENROLLMENTS FOR MEN, WOMEN, MINORITY AND FOREIGN STUDENTS ARE SUMMARIZED FROM THE DIVISION OF STUDENT STUDIES OF THE ASSOCIATION OF AMERICAN MEDICAL COLLEGES ANNUAL SURVEYS OF 1971-72 THROUGH 1975-76. MEXICAN AMERICAN PERCENTAGE OF ENROLLMENT WENT FROM .6% IN 1971-72 TO 1.3% IN 1975-76, WHEREAS MAINLAND PUERTO RICAN ENROLLMENT SLIGHTLY INCREASED FROM .2% TO .4%. DATA SHOW

VIRTUALLY NO CUBAN AMERICANS ENROLLED UNTIL 1975-76 WHEN THEY WERE .3% OF THE TOTAL U.S. MEDICAL SCHOOL ENROLLMENT. THE TOTAL HISPANIC (MEXICAN AMERICAN, CUBAN AMERICAN AND MAINLAND PUERTO RICAN) ENROLLMENT INCREASED FROM .8% IN 71-72 TO 2% IN 75-76. 2 REFERENCES.

ACCN 000149

699 AUTH **GORDON, T. L., & JOHNSON, D. G.**
TITL STUDY OF U.S. MEDICAL SCHOOL APPLICANTS, 1975-76.
SRCE *JOURNAL OF MEDICAL EDUCATION, 1977, 52(9), 707-730.*
INDX COLLEGE STUDENTS, DEMOGRAPHIC, EDUCATION, EMPIRICAL, EQUAL OPPORTUNITY, HIGHER EDUCATION, MEDICAL STUDENTS, MEXICAN AMERICAN, OCCUPATIONAL ASPIRATIONS, SEX COMPARISON, PROFESSIONAL TRAINING, PUERTO RICAN-M, SES, REPRESENTATION
ABST THE 1975-76 STUDY OF MEDICAL SCHOOL APPLICANTS PROVIDES A DESCRIPTION OF DEMOGRAPHIC AND BACKGROUND CHARACTERISTICS, ACADEMIC ABILITY, AND CAREER PLANS OF BOTH APPLICANTS AND ACCEPTEES TO U.S. MEDICAL SCHOOL FIRST-YEAR CLASSES. COMPARISON WITH THE PRECEDING YEAR'S APPLICANT POOL SHOWS A SLIGHT DECLINE IN THE SIZE OF THE POOL, A CONTINUED INCREASE IN THE NUMBER OF WOMEN APPLICANTS AND ACCEPTEES, AND A SLIGHTLY HIGHER ACCEPTANCE RATE FOR ALL APPLICANTS. APPLICANTS DESCRIBING THEMSELVES AS BELONGING TO VARIOUS MINORITY RACIAL/ETHNIC GROUPS NUMBERED 5,903 AND ACCOUNTED FOR 14% OF THE TOTAL APPLICANT POOL FOR 1975-76. THIS WAS AN INCREASE OVER 1974-75 OF 34 MINORITY APPLICANTS. THE RELATIVE PRESENCE OF UNDERREPRESENTED MINORITIES (BLACKS, AMERICAN INDIANS, MEXICAN AMERICANS, AND MAINLAND PUERTO RICANS) IN THE 1975-76 APPLICANT POOL SHOWED A SLIGHT DECLINE OVER 1974-75 FROM 7.4% TO 7.2%. THEIR REPRESENTATION AMONG ACCEPTEES (8.5%) WAS 0.8% LOWER THAN THE 9.3% REPORTED FOR 1974-75. THE ACCEPTANCE RATE FOR UNDERREPRESENTED MINORITY GROUP APPLICANTS AS A WHOLE (42.9%) CONTINUED TO BE ABOVE THE NATIONAL AVERAGE (36.3%) FOR 1975-76. A CONCLUSION OUTLINES THOSE ACTIVITIES OF THE ASSOCIATION OF AMERICAN MEDICAL COLLEGES OVER THE PAST YEAR THAT ARE RELATED TO THE MEDICAL SCHOOL ADMISSION PROCESS. 12 REFERENCES.

ACCN 002098

700 AUTH **GOSSETT, J. T., LEWIS, J. M., & PHILLIPS, V. A.**
TITL EXTENT AND PREVALENCE OF ILLICIT DRUG USE AS REPORTED BY 56,745 STUDENTS.
SRCE *JAMA: JOURNAL OF THE AMERICAN MEDICAL ASSOCIATION, 1971, 216, 1464-1470.*
INDX DRUG ABUSE, DEMOGRAPHIC, SEX COMPARISON, SURVEY, INHALANT ABUSE, ADOLESCENTS, SES, MEXICAN AMERICAN, EMPIRICAL,

URBAN, TEST RELIABILITY, TEST VALIDITY, ALCOHOLISM, TEXAS, SOUTHWEST

ABST IN RESPONSE TO THE NEED FOR DATA THAT ADEQUATELY ASSESS THE ACTUAL EXTENT AND PREVALENCE OF DRUG ABUSE, A SURVEY MEASURING FREQUENCY OF USE OF 61 DRUGS WAS CONDUCTED AMONG 56,745 JUNIOR AND SENIOR HIGH STUDENTS IN DALLAS, TEXAS. THE QUESTIONNAIRE HAD UNDERGONE SEVERAL PILOT TESTS TO ENSURE RELIABILITY AND VALIDITY. THE FOLLOWING RESULTS WERE OBTAINED: (1) 28% OF THE STUDENTS REPORTED TO HAVE USED AN ILLICIT DRUG; (2) 8% INDICATED USING A DRUG MORE THAN TEN TIMES; (3) 4% STATED CURRENT DRUG USE; (4) MALES HAD HIGHER RATES OF DRUG USE THAN FEMALES; (5) STUDENTS ATTENDING HIGHER SOCIOECONOMIC LEVEL SCHOOLS WHICH REFLECT A PREDOMINANTLY WHITE POPULATION WERE MORE APT TO HAVE USED DRUGS; AND (6) PEERS WERE THE LIKELY SOURCE FOR OBTAINING DRUGS. THE MOST COMMON USED DRUGS REPORTED BY THESE STUDENTS WERE ALCOHOL, TOBACCO, GLUE, MARIJUANA, SOLVENT INHALANTS, AND NONPRESCRIPTION STIMULANTS. THESE FINDINGS SHOULD BE UTILIZED WHEN DEVELOPING DRUG EDUCATION PROGRAMS. 5 REFERENCES.

ACCN 000592

701 AUTH **GOTTLIEB, D., & HEINSOHN, A. L. (EDS.)**
TITL AMERICA'S OTHER YOUTH: GROWING UP POOR.
SRCE *ENGLEWOOD CLIFFS, N. J.: PRENTICE-HALL, 1971.*
INDX POVERTY, SES, ETHNIC IDENTITY, RURAL, URBAN, CULTURAL FACTORS, MEXICAN AMERICAN, PUERTO RICAN-M, DISCRIMINATION, BOOK
ABST THIS READER CONSISTS OF A NUMBER OF EXCERPTS FROM VARIOUS ARTICLES REGARDING THE SOCIALIZATION AND LIFESTYLES OF POOR YOUTH FROM DIFFERENT ETHNIC BACKGROUNDS. THE MATERIAL PRESENTED IS DESIGNED TO PROVIDE A MORE DIRECT UNDERSTANDING OF POOR YOUTH. THE RANGE OF TOPICS COVERS ACCOUNTS OF URBAN LIFE AND POVERTY, SOCIALIZATION PROCESSES, DISCRIMINATION, SCHOOL EXPERIENCES AND THE INEQUITIES OF ECONOMICS, HOUSING AND HEALTH. SECTIONS DEALING WITH PUERTO RICAN, MEXICAN AMERICAN AND MIGRANT WORKER YOUTH INCLUDE THE FOLLOWING: (1) "TWO BLOCKS APART: JUAN GONZALES AND PETER QUINN" IS A NARRATIVE DESCRIBING SURVIVAL IN A PUERTO RICAN NEIGHBORHOOD IN NEW YORK, FOCUSING ON GANG ACTIVITY, POLICE HARASSMENT, NARCOTICS USE, AND TEACHER INSENSITIVITY IN THE SCHOOLS; (2) "UP FROM PUERTO RICO" IS A CASE STUDY OF THE RIOS FAMILY'S IMMIGRATION EXPERIENCE FROM PUERTO RICO TO NEW YORK; (3) SPANISH HARLEM "DIARY OF A RENT STRIKER" DOCUMENTS THE ONE-WEEK DIARY OF A STRIKING TENANT IN EAST HARLEM AND HER DAY-TO-DAY STRUGGLE TO MAINTAIN HER FAMILY AND MAKE THE STRIKE SUCCESSFUL; (4) "POVERTY ON THE LOWER EAST SIDE: 6 LIVE "HEAVY LIFE" ON $1 A DAY" EXAMINES THE

POVERTY FACED BY A PUERTO RICAN FAMILY IN NEW YORK WHO SURVIVE ON AN ANNUAL INCOME OF $2000; (5) "PEONAGE IN FLORIDA" ASSESSES THE BACKGROUNDS AND LIFESTYLES OF MIGRANT FARM WORKERS FROM DIFFERENT ETHNIC GROUPS IN FLORIDA; (6) "MEXICAN AMERICAN YOUTH: FORGOTTEN AT THE CROSSROADS" IS AN OVERVIEW OF MEXICAN AMERICAN YOUTH STRESSING LANGUAGE, FAMILY SIZE AND TRADITIONAL MEXICAN CULTURE AS BARRIERS TO ACCULTURATION AND UPWARD MOBILITY; (7) "SPANISH SPEAKING CHILDREN OF THE SOUTHWEST" EXPLORES SOCIAL PRESSURES AND RACIAL PREJUDICE IN SEVERAL NARRATIVES BY MEXICAN AMERICAN YOUTH; (8) "THORNS ON THE YELLOW ROSE OF TEXAS" DISCUSSES POVERTY, POLITICAL UNDERREPRESENTATION AND LOW EDUCATIONAL ATTAINMENT OF THE MEXICAN AMERICAN POPULATION IN TEXAS. OVERALL THIS READER PRESENTS A PORTRAYAL OF THE ASPIRATIONS, EXPECTATIONS, ATTITUDES, AND VALUES OF THE MAJORITY OF POOR YOUTH.

ACCN 000593

702 AUTH **GRACE, W. J.**
TITL ATAQUE.
SRCE *NEW YORK MEDICINE, 1959, 15(1), 12-13.*
INDX FOLK MEDICINE, PUERTO RICAN-M, STRESS, ESSAY, ESPIRITISMO, COPING MECHANISMS, PSYCHOPATHOLOGY, PSYCHOTHERAPY, PSYCHOTHERAPISTS, SYMPTOMATOLOGY
ABST THE CLINICAL PHENOMENON OF ATAQUE NERVIOSA IS DESCRIBED FOR PHYSICIANS NOT ACQUAINTED WITH PUERTO RICANS. AN EPISODE OF ATAQUE OCCURS SUDDENLY AND WITHOUT WARNING FOR THE PATIENT. THERE IS A SHORT CRY OR SCREAM, THE PATIENT FALLS, IS UNCOMMUNICATIVE, AND THEN BEGINS MOVING BOTH ARMS AND LEGS IN A PURPOSEFUL MANNER SUCH AS BEATING HIS FISTS ON THE FLOOR, STRIKING OUT AT PERSONS NEARBY, OR BANGING HIS HEAD ON THE FLOOR. THE ATAQUE CEASES AS ABRUPTLY AS IT BEGAN, LASTING USUALLY BETWEEN 5 AND 10 MINUTES. BOTH MEN AND WOMEN HAVE BEEN OBSERVED DURING AN ATAQUE. THE PHENOMENON OCCURS GENERALLY WHEN THE PATIENT IS CONFRONTED WITH AN OVERWHELMING CATASTROPHE (E.G., DEATH OF A LOVED ONE, ILLNESS IN A CHILD). IN SOME INSTANCES MORE THAN ONE PERSON IS OBSERVED DURING AN ATAQUE (E.G., AT FUNERALS). THE PHYSICIAN TREATING PUERTO RICANS SHOULD BE FAMILIAR WITH ATAQUE SINCE OFTEN THIS PHENOMENON WILL DOMINATE THE CLINICAL PICTURE OF AN ILL PERSON.

ACCN 000594

703 AUTH **GRAND, S., MARCOS, L. R., FREEDMAN, N., & BARROSO, F.**
TITL RELATION OF PSYCHOPATHOLOGY AND BILINGUALISM TO KINESIC ASPECTS OF INTERVIEW BEHAVIOR IN SCHIZOPHRENIA.
SRCE *JOURNAL OF ABNORMAL PSYCHOLOGY, 1977, 85(5), 492-500.*

INDX BILINGUAL, PSYCHOPATHOLOGY, SPANISH SURNAMED, STRESS, ADULTS, EMPIRICAL, SCHIZOPHRENIA, ADULTS, NEW YORK, EAST, BILINGUALISM, PSYCHOTHERAPY, LINGUISTIC COMPETENCE

ABST TEN BILINGUAL SCHIZOPHRENIC PATIENTS WERE INTERVIEWED IN BOTH THEIR NATIVE AND SECOND LANGUAGES BY MEANS OF A PRERECORDED AUDIOTAPE. HAND MOVEMENT BEHAVIOR OBSERVED DURING THE VIDEO-TAPED INTERVIEWS WAS SCORED AND RE-LATED TO RATINGS OF PSYCHOPATHOLOGY DERIVED FROM THE "BRIEF PSYCHIATRIC RAT-ING SCALE." DISCRETE SYMPTOM CLUSTERS WERE FOUND TO BE MEANINGFULLY RELATED TO VARIOUS TYPES OF KINESIC (HAND MOVE-MENT) BEHAVIOR DURING THE NONDOMI-NANT-LANGUAGE INTERVIEW. THESE PAT-TERNS OF CORRELATIONS PROVIDE SUPPORT FOR THE ASSUMPTION THAT KINESIC BEHAV-IOR IS RELATED TO COGNITIVE PROCESSING DYSFUNCTIONS AND LANGUAGE ENCODING STRESS IN A BILINGUAL PATIENT POPULATION. THE FINDINGS ARE DISCUSSED IN TERMS OF THE FUNCTION OF KINESIC BEHAVIOR IN MOD-ULATING STRESS AND IN TERMS OF PSYCHI-ATRIC EVALUATIONS OF BILINGUALS. 21 REF-ERENCES. (JOURNAL ABSTRACT MODIFIED)

ACCN 001827

704 AUTH **GRAVES, T. D.**
TITL ACCULTURATION, ACCESS, AND ALCOHOL IN A TRI-ETHNIC COMMUNITY.
SRCE *AMERICAN ANTHROPOLOGIST, 1967, 69(3-4), 306-321.*
INDX ACCULTURATION, ALCOHOLISM, CROSS CUL-TURAL, ADULTS, EMPIRICAL, DISCRIMINATION, PSYCHOSOCIAL ADJUSTMENT
ABST GROSS ETHNIC DIFFERENCES IN EXCESSIVE DRINKING AND OTHER FORMS OF SOCIAL PROBLEM BEHAVIOR AMONG INDIANS, SPAN-ISH AMERICANS, AND ANGLO-AMERICANS LIV-ING IN A SINGLE SOUTHWESTERN COMMUNITY ARE INVESTIGATED. TWO HUNDRED TWENTY-ONE ADULTS, COMPRISING A RANDOM, STRAT-IFIED SAMPLE, WERE INTERVIEWED USING A VARIETY OF STRUCTURED AND SEMISTRUC-TURED PROCEDURES. THE INDIAN AND SPAN-ISH-AMERICAN ETHNIC GROUPS SHOW DIF-FERENTIAL EFFECTS OF ACCULTURATION ON TWO CLASSES OF VARIABLES: SOCIAL AND PSYCHOLOGICAL PRESSURES FOR EXCESSIVE ALCOHOL CONSUMPTION, AND SOCIAL AND PSYCHOLOGICAL CONTROLS AGAINST SUCH BEHAVIOR. IT APPEARS THAT FOR THE SPAN-ISH-AMERICAN GROUP ACCULTURATION IS CONSISTENTLY ASSOCIATED WITH HIGHER RATES OF DRINKING AND DEVIANT BEHAVIOR, WHEREAS WITHIN THE INDIAN GROUP THE OP-POSITE IS TRUE. WITH THE UNACCULTURATED MEMBERS OF THE TWO ETHNIC GROUPS, THE SPANISH AMERICAN DOES NOT DISPLAY DE-VIANT BEHAVIOR WHEREAS THE INDIAN GROUP DOES. THE EXPLANATIONS OFFERED FOR THIS PARADOX ARE: (1) THE ACCULTURATED ETH-NIC MEMBERS HAVE LIMITED ECONOMIC AC-CESS TO THE REWARDS OF AMERICAN SOCI-ETY, THUS MAINTAINING STRONGER FEELINGS

OF RELATIVE DEPRIVATION, SIGNIFICANTLY GREATER ALIENATION, AND SIGNIFICANTLY MORE PSYCHOLOGICAL PROBLEM-SOLVING REASONS FOR DRINKING; (2) THE UNACCUL-TURATED SPANISH AMERICANS DISPLAY STRONG SOCIAL AND PSYCHOLOGICAL CON-TROLS (FROM FAMILY AND CHURCH) THAT ARE INTERNALIZED; (3) THE UNACCULTURATED IN-DIAN DISPLAYS WEAK SOCIAL AND PSYCHO-LOGICAL CONTROLS; AND (4) THE INFLUENCE OF FAMILY AND CHURCH BEGINS TO BREAK DOWN AS THE SPANISH AMERICANS MOVE TO-WARD THE MORE SECULAR AMERICAN NORM, WHEREAS THE INDIANS, WHOSE NONACCUL-TURATED BACKGROUND IS SOCIALLY ANOMIC, BECOME MAPPED INTO NEW CONTROL STRUCTURES. THESE STRUCTURAL CHANGES ARE PARALLELED BY PSYCHOLOGICAL CHANGES. THE IMPLICATION OF THE RESULTS FOR GENERAL ACCULTURATION THEORY IS THEN DRAWN. 41 REFERENCES.

ACCN 000595

705 AUTH **GRAVES, T. D.**
TITL PSYCHOLOGICAL ACCULTURATION IN A TRI-ETHNIC COMMUNITY.
SRCE *SOUTHWESTERN JOURNAL OF ANTHROPOL-OGY, 1967, 23, 337-350.*
INDX ACCULTURATION, ATTITUDES, FATALISM, TIME ORIENTATION, INTERPERSONAL RELATIONS, SOUTHWEST, SPANISH SURNAMED, CROSS CULTURAL, REVIEW, THEORETICAL, EMPIRICAL, COLORADO
ABST INVESTIGATION OF PSYCHOLOGICAL CORRE-LATES OF ACCULTURATION AMONG 221 MEM-BERS OF A TRI-ETHNIC SOUTHWESTERN COM-MUNITY SUGGESTS THAT CHANGES IN VALUE ORIENTATIONS AMONG MINORITY GROUPS PROBABLY OCCUR WITHIN SITUATIONS OF (1) HIGH EXPOSURE TO AND IDENTIFICATION WITH THE ANGLO GROUP AND (2) ECONOMIC AC-CESS TO THE RESOURCES AND REWARDS OF THE GREATER SOCIETY. 93 ANGLOS, 60 SPAN-ISH AMERICANS, AND 68 AMERICAN INDIANS WERE INTERVIEWED ON A 21-ITEM SCALE OF VARIOUS ASPECTS OF INTERPERSONAL RELA-TIONS, A 17-ITEM FORCED-CHOICE MEASURE OF FEELINGS OF FATALISM OR PERSONAL CONTROL, AND THE "LIFE SPACE SAMPLE" MEASURING FUTURE TIME PERSPECTIVE. ON ALL THREE MEASURES, THE SPANISH AMERI-CANS DIFFERED MOST FROM THE ANGLO NORM, WHILE THE AMERICAN INDIAN GROUP WAS ALWAYS SOMEWHAT INTERMEDIATE. THE RANGE OF INDIVIDUAL DIFFERENCES AMONG THE NON-ANGLOS WAS IMPRESSIVE. WHEN IDEATIONAL DIFFERENCES WERE COMPARED WITH MORE OVERT ASPECTS OF ACCULTURA-TION (I.E., FORMAL EDUCATION, OCCUPATION, AND OTHER BEHAVIORS SUCH AS OWNING A TV OR VOTING), ALL CORRELATIONS WERE IN THE EXPECTED DIRECTION. PSYCHOLOGICAL ACCULTURATION IS THUS DEMONSTRATED TO ACCOMPANY MORE OBSERVABLE ASPECTS OF BEHAVIORAL ACCULTURATION. ALTHOUGH THE CAUSAL DIRECTION IS UNCLEAR, THE RE-SULTS ILLUSTRATE THE HOMOGENIZATION OF THE INDIVIDUAL AND HIS ENVIRONMENT WITHIN

A MUTUALLY INTERACTING FEEDBACK SYSTEM. 34 REFERENCES.

ACCN   002099

706 AUTH   **GREBLER, L., MOORE, J. W., & GUZMAN, R. C.**
    TITL   THE MEXICAN-AMERICAN PEOPLE: THE NATION'S SECOND LARGEST MINORITY.
    SRCE   *NEW YORK: THE FREE PRESS, 1970.*
    INDX   INTERMARRIAGE, SEX COMPARISON, POLITICAL POWER, ETHNIC IDENTITY, CULTURE, EMPIRICAL, SURVEY, CALIFORNIA, SOUTHWEST, MEXICAN AMERICAN, TEXAS, IMMIGRATION, MIGRANTS, URBAN, RURAL, POVERTY, SES, CULTURAL FACTORS, RELIGION, ECONOMIC FACTORS, DISCRIMINATION, DEMOGRAPHIC, SCHOLASTIC ACHIEVEMENT, EMPLOYMENT, POLITICS, MALE, FEMALE, ACCULTURATION, HOUSING, SEX ROLES, MARRIAGE, FAMILY ROLES, EDUCATION, BOOK
    ABST   ADDRESSING THE ECONOMIC, SOCIAL, AND EDUCATIONAL CONDITIONS OF MEXICAN AMERICANS (MA) IN THE UNITED STATES, THIS CLASSIC WORK REPRESENTS THE EFFORTS OF 20 SCHOLARS AND A LARGE NUMBER OF STAFF AND STUDENTS, AND IT INCORPORATES MONOGRAPHS PRODUCED OVER A 4-YEAR PERIOD (1964-68) PLUS NUMEROUS SOCIOLOGICAL STUDIES. THE REPORT DRAWS UPON AN ARRAY OF RESEARCH MATERIALS, INCLUDING LITERATURE ON MA'S, CENSUS DATA, HOUSEHOLD SAMPLE SURVEYS IN LOS ANGELES AND SAN ANTONIO, INFORMAL INTERVIEWS WITH MA'S AND ANGLOS THROUGHOUT THE SOUTHWEST, AND THE AUTHORS' OBSERVATIONS ON FIELD TOURS. OPENING WITH AN HISTORICAL OVERVIEW OF MA'S EMERGENCE INTO THE U.S., THE STUDY PROCEEDS TO AN EXAMINATION OF THE MAJOR ASPECTS OF MA'S EXPERIENCE IN THIS COUNTRY, ESPECIALLY IN THE SOUTHWEST—E.G., ASSIMILATION; NATURALIZATION; EDUCATIONAL PATTERNS; JOB AND EARNING DIFFERENTIALS; HOUSING; THE FAMILY; THE ROLE OF THE CHURCH; CLASS STRUCTURE; AND POLITICS. IDENTIFIED AS THE MOST SIGNIFICANT PROBLEMS FACING MA'S ARE POVERTY, ACCULTURATION, SOCIAL AND ECONOMIC DISCRIMINATION, AND THE NEED FOR MORE ACTIVE PARTICIPATION IN GOVERNMENTAL DECISION-MAKING BODIES. REGARDING THE EDUCATIONAL AND ECONOMIC COMPARISON OF LOS ANGELES AND SAN ANTONIO, ON ALL SCALES THE SOCIAL ISOLATION AND POVERTY IN THE TEXAS CITY IS GREATER. NEVERTHELESS, THE CONTINUING STRUGGLES FOR SOCIAL, ECONOMIC, AND POLITICAL PARITY IN BOTH CITIES ARE ENCOURAGING, LEADING THE AUTHORS TO CONCLUDE ON A HOPEFUL NOTE REGARDING THE FUTURE OF MA'S IN THE UNITED STATES. 1,588 REFERENCES.
    ACCN   001781

707 AUTH   **GREEN, J. A.**
    TITL   RACIAL AWARENESS AND IDENTIFICATION IN YOUNG CHILDREN.
    SRCE   *PAPER PRESENTED AT THE MEETING OF THE AMERICAN PSYCHOLOGICAL ASSOCIATION, WASHINGTON, D.C., 1969.*

    INDX   CHILDREN, EDUCATION, INTEGRATION, SELF CONCEPT, ETHNIC IDENTITY, ATTITUDES, SEX COMPARISON, CROSS CULTURAL, EMPIRICAL, CALIFORNIA, SOUTHWEST
    ABST   PRELIMINARY FINDINGS ARE REPORTED ON THE EFFECT OF DESEGREGATION ON RACIAL IDENTITY AND RACIAL AWARENESS. DATA WERE COLLECTED FROM 3190 MEXICAN AMERICAN, ANGLO AND BLACK ELEMENTARY SCHOOL AGE CHILDREN (K THROUGH 6TH GRADE) OF THE RIVERSIDE SCHOOL SYSTEM BEFORE AND AFTER INTEGRATION. THE SUBJECTS WERE SHOWN 6 SAME-SEX PICTURES OF 2 ANGLO, 2 BLACK, AND 2 MEXICAN AMERICAN SCHOOL AGE CHILDREN AND ASKED QUESTIONS REGARDING ETHNIC IDENTIFICATION AND RACIAL STEREOTYPES BEFORE AND AFTER INTEGRATION OCCURRED. THE RESULTS INDICATE FEWER CROSS-GROUP CHOICES WITH INCREASING AGE, BUT THIS PATTERN WAS REVERSED FOR ANGLOS. BEFORE DESEGREGATION MINORITY CHILDREN USED ETHNIC GROUP CLASSIFICATION LESS THAN ANGLOS AND THIS TREND REPEATS ITSELF THE YEAR AFTER INTEGRATION. THE DATA ALSO REVEAL THAT ANGLO FEMALES AND TO A GREATER EXTENT MINORITY CHILDREN DECREASED IN THE SELECTION OF ANGLO FACES. ALTHOUGH THIS STUDY IS IN THE EARLY STAGES, IT APPEARS CHILDREN WHO SELECTED PICTURES OF THEIR OWN ETHNIC GROUP GAVE MORE POSITIVE RATINGS THAN CHILDREN WHO CHOSE PICTURES OTHER THAN THEIR OWN ETHNIC GROUP. 4 REFERENCES.
    ACCN   000596

708 AUTH   **GREEN, J. A., & GERARD, H. B.**
    TITL   SCHOOL DESEGREGATION AND ETHNIC ATTITUDES.
    SRCE   *IN H. L. FROMKIN & J. J. SHERWOOD (EDS.), INTEGRATING THE ORGANIZATION: A SOCIAL PSYCHOLOGICAL ANALYSIS. NEW YORK: FREE PRESS, 1974, PP. 291-311.*
    INDX   INTEGRATION, GROUP DYNAMICS, ETHNIC IDENTITY, DISCRIMINATION, MEXICAN AMERICAN, CHILDREN, CROSS CULTURAL, EDUCATION, ATTITUDES, EMPIRICAL, CALIFORNIA, SOUTHWEST
    ABST   TO STUDY THE EFFECTS OF DESEGREGATION, ANGLO, BLACK AND MEXICAN AMERICAN 1ST THROUGH 6TH GRADE CHILDREN WERE ADMINISTERED A PRE- AND POST-ETHNIC PICTURES TEST. THE CHILDREN WERE FIRST SHOWN SIX PICTURES OF ELEMENTARY SCHOOL BOYS, THEN SIX OF SAME AGE GIRLS, AND THEN THOSE OF THEIR OWN SEX AGAIN. TWO OF THE PICTURES WERE OF ANGLOS, TWO WERE OF BLACKS, AND TWO WERE OF MEXICAN AMERICANS. TO ASSESS RACIAL ATTITUDES, THE CHILDREN WERE ASKED TO RANK ORDER THE PICTURES ON FIVE DIMENSIONS: MOST KIND, HAPPIEST, STRONGEST, FASTEST, AND BEST GRADES. RACIAL AWARENESS AND IDENTITY WAS ASSESSED BY HAVING THEM INDICATE PREFERENCE FOR THE ONE MOST LIKE THEM, THE ONE THEY WOULD LIKE TO BE, AND THE MOST DESIRED AS A FRIEND. THE RESULTS FIND ANGLOS STEREO-

TYPED AS KINDER, HAPPIER, AND BETTER SCHOLASTICALLY WHILE THE MINORITIES ARE SEEN AS STRONGER AND FASTER. ALTHOUGH THERE IS SOME VARIATION OVER AGE, FOR THE MOST PART, STEREOTYPIC DIFFERENCES IN SCHOLASTIC PERFORMANCE BECAME MORE EXAGGERATED WITH AGE AND DESEGREGA- TION. TEACHER AND PARENTAL EXPECTATIONS AND A SELF-FULFILLING PROPHECY IS SUG- GESTED AS A POSSIBLE CAUSE. THE RACIAL AWARENESS AND IDENTITY RESULTS ARE VAR- IED BUT IT APPEARS THAT MINORITY CHIL- DREN CHOOSE THEIR OWN ETHNIC GROUP MORE OFTEN AFTER DESEGREGATION. 13 REF- ERENCES.

ACCN   000597

709 AUTH   **GREEN, J. M., TRANKINA, F. J., & CHAVEZ, N.**
     TITL   THERAPEUTIC INTERVENTION WITH MEXICAN AMERICAN CHILDREN.
     SRCE   *PSYCHIATRIC ANNALS, 1976, 6(5), 60-75.*
     INDX   PSYCHOTHERAPY, HEALTH DELIVERY SYS- TEMS, CHILDREN, MEXICAN AMERICAN, ESSAY, RESOURCE UTILIZATION, MENTAL HEALTH, CULTURAL FACTORS, PEER GROUP, DISCRIMI- NATION, SEX ROLES, CHILDREARING PRAC- TICES, REPRESENTATION
     ABST   SEVERAL ISSUES RELATING TO THERAPEUTIC INTERVENTION WITH MEXICAN AMERICAN CHILDREN ARE DISCUSSED. THE MEXICAN AMERICAN POPULATION IS UNDERREPRE- SENTED IN MENTAL HEALTH FACILITIES DUE TO POOR UTILIZATION OF SERVICES. WHILE SOME ARGUMENTS SUPPORT THE PROPOSITION THAT MEXICAN AMERICAN FAMILIES HAVE LESS NEED FOR MENTAL HEALTH SERVICES THAN OTH- ERS, THERE ARE MORE ARGUMENTS TO SUP- PORT THE VIEW THAT THEIR NEEDS ARE AS MUCH AS THOSE OF ANY OTHER ETHNIC GROUP. INDICES THAT DEFINE CHILDREN OR FAMILIES AT HIGH RISK ARE OFTEN FOUND IN THE BARRIO: POVERTY AND ITS CONCOMITANT POOR NUTRITION, LACK OF PRENATAL AND PE- DIATRIC CARE AND ABSENCE OF ADEQUATE INTELLECTUAL STIMULATION. SENSITIVITY TO CULTURAL DIFFERENCES IS ESSENTIAL FOR EFFECTIVE THERAPEUTIC INTERVENTION. WHEN DEALING WITH A MEXICAN AMERICAN, THE THERAPIST THAT DISREGARDS CULTURAL DIF- FERENCES WILL PROBABLY BE CONFRONTED WITH RESISTANCE AND A CLIENT WHO WILL PROBABLY DROP OUT EARLY IN THE PROCESS. RELEVANT FACTORS INCLUDE THE PRIVACY OF THE FAMILY OVER THE INDIVIDUAL, THE ROLE OF THE EXTENDED FAMILY, RESPECT TOWARDS AUTHORITY AND DIFFERENT EMPHASES ON CHILD-REARING. FINALLY THE THERAPEUTIC RELATION MUST BE EXPERIENCED AS CON- STRUCTIVE, ESPECIALLY IN VIEW OF THE VALUE THAT MEXICAN AMERICANS PLACE ON POSI- TIVE INTERPERSONAL RELATIONS.
     ACCN   000598

710 AUTH   **GREEN, R. F.**
     TITL   AGE-INTELLIGENCE RELATIONSHIP BETWEEN AGES SIXTEEN AND SIXTY-FOUR: A RISING TREND.

SRCE   *DEVELOPMENTAL PSYCHOLOGY, 1969, 1(5), 618- 627.*
INDX   INTELLIGENCE, INTELLIGENCE TESTING, ADULTS, PUERTO RICAN-I, WAIS, TEST VA- LIDITY, EMPIRICAL
ABST   DATA SUBSTANTIATING THAT INTELLIGENCE AS MEASURED BY THE WECHSLER ADULT IN- TELLIGENCE SCALE (WAIS) INCREASES UNTIL APPROXIMATELY AGE 65 IS OFFERED. IN ADDI- TION, THIS STUDY DEMONSTRATES THAT IF WECHSLER AND OTHER INVESTIGATORS HAD CONDUCTED A DIFFERENT TYPE OF DATA ANALYSIS, THEIR CONCLUSION WOULD HAVE BEEN DIFFERENT. FOUR STRATIFIED, RANDOM GROUPS, AGES 25-29, 35-39, 45-49, AND 55-64, WERE DRAWN FROM THE PUERTO RICAN POPULATION AND ADMINISTERED THE NEWLY ADAPTED SPANISH-LANGUAGE VERSION OF THE WAIS. THESE GROUPS WERE ALTERED TO MAKE THEIR EDUCATIONAL DISTRIBUTION NEARLY IDENTICAL. TWO SETS OF ANALYSES DEMONSTRATE THAT INTELLIGENCE AS MEA- SURED BY THE WAIS DOES NOT DECLINE IN THE PUERTO RICAN POPULATION BEFORE ABOUT AGE 65. SPECIFICALLY, THE FULL-SCALE SCORE MEANS RISE TO AGE 40 AND NEVER FALL; VERBAL TOTAL SCALED MEANS RISE TO AGE 50 AND NEVER FALL; PERFORMANCE TO- TAL SHOWS A SMALL DECLINE AFTER AGE 40. THE SAME CONCLUSION FOR THE UNITED STATES IS ALSO DEMONSTRATED. HAD WECHS- LER AND OTHERS CONTROLLED FOR EDUCA- TION WHEN DETERMINING AGE-INTELLIGENCE TRENDS BY ANALYSIS OF COVARIANCE THEIR CONCLUSION WOULD HAVE BEEN INVERTED. IT IS CONCLUDED THAT (A) MOST STUDIES IN THIS AREA ARE DEFICIENT IN THAT THEY HAVE TAKEN INADEQUATE ACCOUNT OF EDUCATION AS A CONCOMITANT OF INTELLIGENCE TEST PERFORMANCE, (B) MUCH REANALYSIS IS NEEDED TO CORRECT THE RECORD, AND (C) FUTURE RESEARCH MUST ACCOUNT FOR THIS VARIABLE. 25 REFERENCES.
ACCN   000599

711 AUTH   **GREEN, R. F.**
     TITL   DESARROLLO Y ESTANDARIZACION DE UNA ESCALA INDIVIDUAL DE INTELIGENCIA PARA ADULTOS EN ESPANOL. (DEVELOPMENT AND STANDARDIZATION IN SPANISH OF AN INDI- VIDUAL SCALE OF INTELLIGENCE FOR ADULTS.)
     SRCE   *REVISTA MEXICANA DE PSICOLOGIA, 1964, 1(3), 231-244. (SPANISH)*
     INDX   WAIS, PUERTO RICAN-I, TEST RELIABILITY, TEST VALIDITY, EMPIRICAL, RESEARCH METHOD- OLOGY, INTELLIGENCE TESTING, CULTURE-FAIR TESTS
     ABST   A DETAILED REVIEW OF THE PROCEDURES FOLLOWED IN THE DEVELOPMENT AND STAN- DARDIZATION OF A SPANISH FORM OF THE WECHSLER ADULT INTELLIGENCE SCALE (WAIS) IN PUERTO RICO IS REPORTED. EXISTING TESTS WHICH ARE SIMPLY TRANSLATIONS INTO SPAN- ISH OR PARTIAL ADAPTATIONS ARE UNSATIS- FACTORY FOR USE IN HISPANIC AMERICA. IN THE PUERTO RICO PROJECT, THE TRANSLATED FORM IS TO BE REVIEWED BY LINGUISTS FA- MILIAR WITH THE NATIONAL AND REGIONAL

USES OF THE SPANISH VERNACULAR TO ASSURE THAT THE VERBAL MATERIAL IS AS SIGNIFICANT AS POSSIBLE TO ALL HISPANIC AMERICAN SUBCULTURES. THE SOCIOCULTURAL ASPECTS ARE TO BE EXAMINED BY PSYCHOLOGISTS IN SEVERAL LATIN AMERICAN COUNTRIES WITH THE HOPE OF MAKING THE EIWA (WAIS IN SPANISH) APPLICABLE IN ALL OF LATIN AMERICA. SIMULTANEOUS WITH THE LINGUISTIC AND CULTURAL REVIEWS, PRETESTING OF A SAMPLE GROUP (250 SUBJECTS) IS TO BE CONDUCTED IN PUERTO RICO TO DETERMINE THE ORDER OF DIFFICULTY FOR EACH ITEM AND TO EVALUATE THE ENTIRE TEST IN ITS REVISED FORM. DURING FINAL EVALUATION, 1,800 SUBJECTS ARE TO BE ADDED TO THE PRETEST GROUP. A PROCEDURE HAS BEEN DEVELOPED WHICH SHOULD PERMIT AUTOMATIC CORRECTION FOR THE INCREASE IN IQ BECAUSE OF GENERAL CULTURAL ENRICHMENT OVER TIME. 1 REFERENCE.

ACCN   000600

712 AUTH   **GREEN, R. F.**
    TITL   ON THE CORRELATION BETWEEN I.Q. AND AMOUNT OF WHITE BLOOD.
    SRCE   *PROCEEDINGS OF THE ANNUAL CONVENTION OF THE AMERICAN PSYCHOLOGICAL ASSOCIATION, 1972, 7, 285-286.*
    INDX   INTELLIGENCE TESTING, PREJUDICE, ADOLESCENTS, ADULTS, ETHNIC IDENTITY, ATTITUDES, COGNITIVE DEVELOPMENT, PUERTO RICAN-I, SURVEY, EMPIRICAL, DISCRIMINATION, WAIS
    ABST   SEVERAL WRITERS IN RECENT YEARS HAVE DEFENDED THE THESIS OF GENETICALLY BASED CAUCASIAN COGNITIVE SUPERIORITY OVER NEGROES. SOME CLAIM THAT THE PERCENTAGE OF NEGRO ANCESTRY IS CORRELATED WITH IQ. PUERTO RICO PROVIDES AN IMPORTANT CONTRAST TO THE UNITED STATES. TO BE CALLED NEGRO IN PUERTO RICO ONE HAS TO BE ALMOST A FULL-BLOODED NEGRO. WHEREAS IN THE UNITED STATES, IF ONE HAS ANY NEGRO ANCESTRY AT ALL HE IS CALLED NEGRO. DATA FROM A STRATIFIED RANDOM SAMPLE OF 16 TO 64 YEAR-OLD PUERTO RICANS SHOW CLEARLY THAT IQ IS MUCH MORE CLOSELY CORRELATED WITH THE PREJUDICE LINE THAN WITH THE GENETIC LINE. 4 REFERENCES. (PASAR ABSTRACT)
    ACCN   000601

713 AUTH   **GREENBERG, S., & FORMANEK, R.**
    TITL   THE RELATIONAL JUDGMENTS OF PRE-SCHOOL CHILDREN.
    SRCE   *CHILD STUDY JOURNAL, 1973, 3(1), 1-27.*
    INDX   CHILDREN, EARLY CHILDHOOD EDUCATION, COGNITIVE DEVELOPMENT, SES, CROSS CULTURAL, INTELLIGENCE TESTING, PUERTO RICAN-M, EMPIRICAL, NEW YORK, EAST
    ABST   AS PART OF A LARGER PROJECT AIMED AT FINDING A NORMATIVE BASE FOR THE CONSTRUCTION OF A CURRICULUM FOR PRESCHOOL CHILDREN, ESPECIALLY CHILDREN WITH DISADVANTAGED BACKGROUNDS, THIS PAPER PRESENTS A STUDY OF PRESCHOOLERS' CONCEPTUAL DEVELOPMENT. USING MANUAL AND PAPER TESTS BASED ON BOLHME'S (1965) 18 RELATIONAL CONCEPTS, A LATERALITY TEST AND THE CALDWELL PRESCHOOL INVENTORY FOR MEASURING INTELLIGENCE, 151 CHILDREN, 4-5 YEARS-OLD, OF DIFFERENT ETHNIC AND SOCIOECONOMIC BACKGROUNDS WERE STUDIED. HYPOTHESIZED WAS THAT: (1) RELATIONAL JUDGMENTS MADE BY PRESCHOOLERS OF 3-DIMENSIONAL OBJECTS WOULD GIVE A DIFFERENT HIERARCHY OF CONCEPT DIFFICULTY THAN BOLHME FOUND WITH 5-7 YEAR-OLDS; (2) THERE IS A DEVELOPMENT REGULARITY TO THE ACQUISITION OF RELATIONAL CONCEPTS WHICH IS HEAVILY INFLUENCED BY SOCIAL CLASS; AND (3) CHILDREN WHO HAVE STABILIZED LATERALITY WOULD ACHIEVE HIGHER SCORES ON RELATIONAL CONCEPT TASKS. RESULTS SHOWED: (1) NO SIGNIFICANT DIFFERENCE BETWEEN MANUAL AND PAPER TEST RESULTS; (2) SIGNIFICANT AND POSITIVE RELATIONSHIPS BETWEEN CONCEPT AND INTELLIGENCE TEST RESULTS; (3) NO SIGNIFICANT DIFFERENCE IN SCORES OF CHILDREN WITH STABILIZED AS COMPARED TO MIXED LATERALITY; AND (4) MIDDLE CLASS SUBJECTS SCORING SIGNIFICANTLY HIGHER THAN LOWER CLASS SUBJECTS. IMPLICATIONS FOR THESE FINDINGS ON THE DEVELOPMENT OF PRESCHOOL CURRICULUM ARE DISCUSSED. 11 REFERENCES. (AUTHOR SUMMARY MODIFIED)

ACCN   000602

714 AUTH   **GREENE, J. F., & ZIRKEL, P. A.**
    TITL   THE USE OF PARALLEL TESTING OF AURAL ABILITY AS AN INDICATOR OF BILINGUAL DOMINANCE.
    SRCE   *PSYCHOLOGY IN THE SCHOOLS, 1974, 11(1), 51-55.*
    INDX   BILINGUALISM, LINGUISTIC COMPETENCE, CHILDREN, SPANISH SURNAMED, RESEARCH METHODOLOGY, LANGUAGE COMPREHENSION, EMPIRICAL, TEST RELIABILITY, CONNECTICUT, EAST
    ABST   THE INCREASE OF BILINGUAL EDUCATION HAS CREATED A DEMAND FOR MORE PRACTICAL MEANS TO SCREEN BILINGUAL STUDENTS AND TO EVALUATE THE EFFECTIVENESS OF BILINGUAL PROGRAMS. THIS STUDY FOCUSES ON THE DIFFERENCES OF 148 SPANISH-SPEAKING 1ST GRADE STUDENTS IN THEIR PERFORMANCES ON ALTERNATE FORMS OF THE ORAL VOCABULARY SUBTEST OF THE INTER-AMERICAN TEST OF GENERAL ABILITIES IN SPANISH AND ENGLISH AND WHETHER THE RESULTING DIFFERENCES MAY BE DUE TO PRACTICE EFFECT, LANGUAGE LEVEL, AND ERROR MEASUREMENT. THE SAMPLE WAS RANDOMLY DIVIDED INTO TWO GROUPS, THE FIRST RECEIVING THE TEST IN ENGLISH AND THEN SPANISH AND THE SECOND GROUP ADMINISTERED THE TESTS IN REVERSE ORDER. THE RESULTS INDICATE THAT REGARDLESS OF TEST ORDER THE SPANISH SCORES WERE HIGHER THAN THE ENGLISH SCORES. DIFFERENCES COULD BE DUE TO THE LOWER LEVEL OF DIFFICULTY OF THE SPANISH FORM OR THE HIGHER LEVEL OF LANGUAGE ABILITY OF THIS SAMPLE. THE FINDINGS SUGGEST THAT PARALLEL TESTS

OF ABILITY IN TWO LANGUAGES IS AN INDICATOR RATHER THAN A MEASURE OF LANGUAGE DOMINANCE. 23 REFERENCES.

ACCN 000603

715 AUTH **GREENE, R. L., & CLARK, J. R.**
TITL BIRTH ORDER AND COLLEGE ATTENDANCE IN A CROSS CULTURAL SETTING.
SRCE *JOURNAL OF SOCIAL PSYCHOLOGY, 1968, 75(2), 289-290.*
INDX FAMILY STRUCTURE, CROSS CULTURAL, SCHOLASTIC ACHIEVEMENT, SPANISH SURNAMED, COLLEGE STUDENTS, SES, NEW MEXICO, SOUTHWEST
ABST AN INVESTIGATION OF BIRTH ORDER AND COLLEGE ATTENDANCE IN A CROSS-CULTURAL SETTING IS PRESENTED. DATA ON LIVE BIRTH ORDER, ETHNIC GROUP, FAMILY SIZE, AND SOCIAL CLASS WERE COLLECTED FOR 168 ANGLO AMERICAN (AA) AND 180 SPANISH AMERICAN (SA) COLLEGE STUDENTS IN NEW MEXICO WHO WERE BORN IN THE YEARS 1946-1949. IN THE AA GROUP THERE IS A SIGNIFICANT OVERREPRESENTATION OF FIRST-BORNS IN COMPARISON WITH CENSUS DATA, WHILE IN THE SA GROUP THERE IS AN UNDERREPRESENTATION OF FIRST-BORNS, PRIMARILY AS A RESULT OF THE LARGE FAMILY SIZES WHICH ARE NOT REFLECTED IN THE CENSUS DATA. WHEN THE SUBJECTS' OBSERVED BIRTH ORDERS ARE COMPARED WITH THE EXPECTED BIRTH ORDERS BY OBSERVED FAMILY SIZES, THERE IS AN OVERREPRESENTATION OF FIRST-BORNS IN BOTH GROUPS, ALTHOUGH THE DIFFERENCE IS NOT STATISTICALLY SIGNIFICANT IN THE SA GROUP. THE COMPARISONS OF THE OBSERVED BIRTH ORDERS WITH THE EXPECTED BIRTH ORDERS, ADJUSTED FOR FAMILY SIZE WITHIN EACH SOCIAL CLASS, SHOWS THAT FIRST-BORNS ARE OVERREPRESENTED IN ALL SOCIAL CLASSES IN BOTH GROUPS. A TOTAL CHI-SQUARE FOR ALL FIVE SOCIAL CLASSES WAS STATISTICALLY SIGNIFICANT FOR THE AA GROUP AND APPROACHED SIGNIFICANCE IN THE SA GROUP. THE RESULTS SUPPORT THE FINDINGS OF AN OVERREPRESENTATION OF FIRST-BORNS IN THE COLLEGE POPULATION REPORTED BY OTHER INVESTIGATORS. EVEN WHEN THE VARIABLES OF FAMILY SIZE AND SOCIAL CLASS ARE CONTROLLED, THERE IS A SIGNIFICANT OVERREPRESENTATION OF FIRST-BORNS. 6 REFERENCES.

ACCN 000604

716 AUTH **GRIMMET, S. A.**
TITL THE INFLUENCE OF ETHNICITY AND AGE ON SOLVING TWENTY QUESTIONS.
SRCE *JOURNAL OF SOCIAL PSYCHOLOGY, 1971, 83(1), 143-144.*
INDX SES, MEXICAN AMERICAN, CHILDREN, SEX COMPARISON, CROSS CULTURAL, MEMORY, INTELLIGENCE, LEARNING, COGNITIVE DEVELOPMENT
ABST AN ETHNIC COMPARISON ON STRATEGY, CATEGORIZATION, AND CONCEPTUAL TEMPO DERIVED FROM MEASURES OF PERFORMANCE ON A PROBLEM-SOLVING TASK WAS CONDUCTED. THE SUBJECTS WERE 156 LOWER-

SOCIOECONOMIC STATUS MALES DISTRIBUTED AMONG MEXICAN AMERICAN, INDIAN AMERICAN, BLACK AMERICAN AND APPALACHIAN CAUCASIAN AMERICAN GROUPS. THESE GROUPS WERE COMPARED TO A MIDDLE-CLASS WHITE SAMPLE COMPOSED OF 40 MALES. EACH OF THE GROUPS WAS DIVIDED EQUALLY BETWEEN GRADES THREE AND SIX. THE FINDINGS SHOWED NO SIGNIFICANT ETHNIC DIFFERENCES FOR THE PROBLEM-SOLVING VARIABLES. THE HIGHER SOCIOECONOMIC STATUS GROUP, HOWEVER, OBTAINED A SIGNIFICANTLY GREATER MEAN FOR NOMINAL-FUNCTIONAL QUESTIONS. WHEN GRADE LEVELS WITHIN THE GROUPS WERE COMPARED FOR NOMINAL-FUNCTIONAL QUESTIONS, SIXTH-GRADE BOYS, EXCLUSIVE OF THE INDIAN AMERICANS, EARNED SIGNIFICANTLY HIGHER MEANS THAN THEIR YOUNGER COUNTERPARTS. CONCEPTUAL TEMPO WAS AFFECTED BY ETHNICITY, WITH THE APPALACHIAN AND INDIAN GROUPS, WHO DID NOT DIFFER, DELAYING SIGNIFICANTLY LONGER THAN THE OTHER GROUPS. IMPLICATIONS FROM THESE FINDINGS ARE THAT: (1) SOCIOECONOMIC STATUS FACTORS HAVE A STRONGER INFLUENCE THAN ETHNICITY ON LEVEL OF STRATEGY AND CATEGORIZATION; AND (2) PLACE OF RESIDENCE MORE THAN ETHNICITY FOSTERS DIFFERENT CONCEPTUAL TEMPO RATES. 3 REFERENCES.

ACCN 000606

717 AUTH **GRISWOLD, D. L.**
TITL AN ASSESSMENT OF THE CHILD-REARING INFORMATION NEEDS AND ATTITUDES OF ANGLO, BLACK AND MEXICAN AMERICAN MOTHERS (DOCTORAL DISSERTATION, ARIZONA STATE UNIVERSITY, 1975).
SRCE *DISSERTATION ABSTRACTS INTERNATIONAL, 1975, 35(10), 6529A. (UNIVERSITY MICROFILMS NO. 76-9157.)*
INDX EMPIRICAL, FEMALE, CHILDREARING PRACTICES, MOTHER-CHILD INTERACTION, MEXICAN AMERICAN, CROSS CULTURAL, PRIMARY PREVENTION, HEALTH EDUCATION
ABST MATERNAL CHILDREARING INFORMATION NEEDS AND ATTITUDES, AS A FUNCTION OF ETHNIC BACKGROUND AND SOCIOECONOMIC LEVEL, WERE INVESTIGATED IN 114 MOTHERS (52 ANGLO, 31 BLACK, 31 MEXICAN AMERICAN). THESE MOTHERS HAD INTACT FAMILIES AND A CHILD IN THE 2ND GRADE. TWO INTERVIEW INSTRUMENTS WERE ADMINISTERED: THE MATERNAL INFORMATION NEEDS AND ATTITUDES ASSESSMENT (MINAA), AND THE PARENT AS A TEACHER INVENTORY (PAAT). A NONSTATISTICAL ANALYSIS OF MINAA RESPONSES PROVIDED ONLY AN INDICATION OF SIMILARITIES AND DIFFERENCES RELATED TO ETHNICITY AND SES, WHEREAS STATISTICAL ANALYSIS OF PAAT RESPONSES LED TO MORE SIGNIFICANT RESULTS. SOME MAJOR CONCLUSIONS WERE: (1) ANGLOS AND MEXICAN AMERICANS EXPRESSED A GREATER NEED FOR CHILDREARING INFORMATION; (2) MEXICAN AMERICANS EXPRESSED GREATER CONCERN ABOUT THEIR CHILDREN'S SCHOOL EX-

PERIENCES; (3) BLACKS AND MEXICAN AMERICANS EXPRESSED GREATER PLEASURE THAN ANGLOS IN THEIR CHILDREN'S ACCOMPLISHMENTS; (4) MEXICAN AMERICANS WERE THE LEAST LIKELY TO CONSULT AGENCIES, SERVICES, AND PRINTED MATTER FOR HELP IN CHILDREARING; (5) NO SIGNIFICANT ETHNIC DIFFERENCES WERE FOUND ON THE CREATIVITY, CONTROL, PLAY, AND TEACHING-LEARNING PAAT SUBSCALES; (6) UPPER-CLASS MOTHERS EXPRESSED LESS CONCERN ABOUT SCHOOL PROBLEMS; AND (7) LOWER-CLASS MOTHERS, MORE THAN MIDDLE- AND UPPER-CLASS MOTHERS, EXPRESSED GREAT PRIDE IN THEIR CHILDREN'S RESPONSIBLE BEHAVIOR. RECOMMENDATIONS FOR FURTHER RESEARCH ARE DISCUSSED. 269 REFERENCES.

ACCN   000607

---

718   AUTH   **GROSSMAN, H.**
      TITL   NINE ROTTEN LOUSY KIDS.
      SRCE   *NEW YORK: HOLT, RINEHART & WINSTON, 1972.*
      INDX   PSYCHOSOCIAL ADJUSTMENT, DELINQUENCY, ADOLESCENTS, MENTAL HEALTH PROFESSION, FAMILY STRUCTURE, SOCIALIZATION, SCHOLASTIC ACHIEVEMENT, CASE STUDY, MALE, CURRICULUM, PUERTO RICAN-M, CROSS CULTURAL, BEHAVIOR MODIFICATION, PSYCHOTHERAPY OUTCOME, NEW YORK, EAST, BOOK
      ABST   THE PLANNING, DEVELOPMENT AND EVALUATION OF AN EXPERIMENTAL SCHOOL FOR MALE, ADOLESCENT DELINQUENTS IN NEW YORK'S EAST VILLAGE IS DESCRIBED THROUGH THE PARTICIPANT OBSERVATIONS OF ITS STAFF PSYCHOLOGISTS AND TEACHERS. THE NINE BOYS WHOSE CASE STUDIES ARE THE FOCUS OF THE VOLUME ARE OF SPANISH SURNAMED, BLACK AND ANGLO BACKGROUND. ALL OF THEM HAD BEEN THROUGH THE TRADITIONAL SCHOOL AND THERAPY PROGRAM FOR DELINQUENTS. THIS SPECIAL SCHOOL WAS THEIR LAST STOP BEFORE CORRECTIONAL PLACEMENT. THE BOOK'S DESCRIPTION OF THE SCHOOL'S FACILITIES AND CURRICULUM AND ITS STAFF'S BEHAVIORAL AND THERAPEUTIC APPROACHES WITH THE BOYS ARE BASED ON DAILY STAFF RECORDINGS OF ONE YEAR IN THE PROGRAM. IT IS THE VERY PERSONAL ACCOUNT OF SIX ADULTS WHO CHOSE TO BE RESPONSIBLE FOR YOUNGSTERS CONSIDERED HOPELESS BY THEIR PARENTS, THE COURTS AND MANY OTHERS.

ACCN   000608

---

719   AUTH   **GROUP FOR THE ADVANCEMENT OF PSYCHIATRY. THE COMMITTEE ON THE FAMILY.**
      TITL   CASE STUDY METHOD IN THE STUDY OF FAMILY PROCESS.
      SRCE   *GROUP FOR THE ADVANCEMENT OF PSYCHIATRY, 1970, VOL. 6, REPORT NO. 76, 237-380.*
      INDX   PUERTO RICAN-M, FAMILY STRUCTURE, FAMILY ROLES, CASE STUDY, ESSAY, EXTENDED FAMILY, MARRIAGE, SEX ROLES, RESEARCH METHODOLOGY, PSYCHOTHERAPY, FAMILY THERAPY
      ABST   A SYSTEMATIC APPROACH TO MODIFY THE TRADITIONAL PSYCHIATRIC CASE HISTORY FOR USE IN FAMILY DIAGNOSIS, TREATMENT, AND RESEARCH IS PRESENTED. THIS APPROACH IS A WORKING TOOL FOR THE PSYCHIATRIST, PROVIDING A DETAILED OUTLINE OF INFORMATION TO BE INCLUDED IN A FAMILY CASE HISTORY. IN ATTEMPTING TO MAINTAIN A BALANCE BETWEEN THE FAMILY AS A WHOLE AND ITS INDIVIDUAL MEMBERS, THE CASE HISTORY METHOD DESCRIBED UTILIZES DESIGNATED CATEGORIES OF DATA TO BE GATHERED AND REASSEMBLED IN A PRESCRIBED SEQUENCE FOR INDIVIDUAL FAMILY MEMBERS. THE USEFULNESS OF THIS METHOD IS DEMONSTRATED IN A STUDY OF A PUERTO RICAN FAMILY, UNDERTAKEN BY RESEARCHERS ACCORDING TO THE FAMILY CASE HISTORY OUTLINE AND RECORDED IN GREAT DETAIL. THIS METHOD OF ASSEMBLING A FAMILY CASE HISTORY TAKES INTO ACCOUNT CULTURAL, INTERPERSONAL, PSYCHOLOGICAL, AND BIOLOGICAL DETERMINANTS OF FAMILY FUNCTIONING. PARTICULAR EMPHASIS IS GIVEN TO THE CULTURAL DETERMINANTS OF FAMILY BEHAVIOR, AN AREA THAT HAS BEEN LARGELY IGNORED UP TO NOW. SOME OF THE DIFFICULTIES IN COLLECTING AND ORGANIZING FAMILY CASE HISTORIES ARE DISCUSSED. TWO DETAILED APPENDICES PROVIDE THE SUGGESTED OUTLINE TO BE FOLLOWED. 3 REFERENCES.

ACCN   000609

---

720   AUTH   **GROUP FOR THE ADVANCEMENT OF PSYCHIATRY. THE COMMITTEE ON THE FAMILY.**
      TITL   INTEGRATIONS AND MAL-INTEGRATIONS IN SPANISH AMERICAN FAMILY PATTERNS.
      SRCE   *GROUP FOR THE ADVANCEMENT OF PSYCHIATRY REPORTS AND SYMPOSIUMS, 1968, VOL. 6, REPORT NO. 27A, 959-966.*
      INDX   MEXICAN AMERICAN, EXTENDED FAMILY, FAMILY STRUCTURE, FAMILY ROLES, SEX ROLES, INTERPERSONAL RELATIONS, COMPETITION, COOPERATION, CULTURAL FACTORS
      ABST   AN EXPLORATION OF LIFE PATTERNS, CULTURAL VALUE ORIENTATIONS, AND EXTENDED SOCIAL SYSTEMS OF THE SPANISH AMERICAN IN THE SOUTHWEST IS PRESENTED. CONTRASTS BETWEEN THE SPANISH AMERICAN AND ANGLO AMERICAN FAMILY AND VALUE ORIENTATIONS ARE GIVEN. THE SPANISH AMERICANS ARE LINEAL, BEING, PRESENT, AND SUBJUGATION-TO-NATURE ORIENTED; THE ANGLO AMERICANS ARE INDIVIDUALISTIC, DOING, FUTURE, AND MASTERY-OVER-NATURE ORIENTED. INTERRELATIONSHIPS IN SPANISH-AMERICAN VILLAGES REFLECT CLOSE FAMILY TIES, EXTENSIVE AND WELL-DEFINED AUTHORITY LINES, AGE GRADING, SOCIAL STRATIFICATION, AND SEXUAL DIFFERENTIATION IN AUTHORITY. THE FEMININE ROLE, CONSTRICTED BY ANGLO AMERICAN STANDARDS, IS COMFORTABLE AND SUPPORTIVE FOR ITS SPANISH AMERICAN OCCUPANT. NOTICEABLE CHANGES IN SPANISH AMERICAN VALUE ORIENTATIONS HAVE TAKEN PLACE IN THE LAST TWO DECADES.

ACCN   000610

---

721   AUTH   **GUILFORD, J. S., & GUPTA, W.**

TITL   DEVELOPMENT OF THE VALUES INVENTORY FOR CHILDREN.

SRCE   *PROCEEDINGS OF THE 79TH ANNUAL CONVENTION OF THE AMERICAN PSYCHOLOGICAL ASSOCIATION, 1971, 6, 513-514.*

INDX   RESEARCH METHODOLOGY, PERSONALITY ASSESSMENT, MEXICAN AMERICAN, CHILDREN, CROSS CULTURAL, PROCEEDINGS, EMPIRICAL, TEST RELIABILITY, ATTITUDES, SELF CONCEPT, CONFORMITY, DEVIANCE, SEX ROLES, HEALTH, CALIFORNIA, SOUTHWEST, VALUES

ABST   THE RELATIONSHIP BETWEEN CHILDREN'S VALUES AND THEIR ACADEMIC ACHIEVEMENT IS ASSESSED. THE DEVELOPMENT OF A VALUES INVENTORY FOR CHILDREN IS DESCRIBED AS THE FIRST PHASE OF THE RESEARCH. A TOTAL OF 996 FIRST, SECOND, AND THIRD-GRADE CHILDREN OF FIVE ETHNIC GROUPS (MEXICAN AMERICAN, ORIENTAL, ANGLO, NEGRO, AND PAPAGO INDIAN CHILDREN) WERE ADMINISTERED THE FINAL VERSION OF THE VALUES INVENTORY SCALE. THE RESULTS INDICATE THAT CHILDREN IN MINORITY GROUPS (PARTICULARLY NEGROES AND MEXICAN AMERICANS) VALUE SCHOOL AND HEALTH HABITS MORE THAN DO CHILDREN OF THE MIDDLE-CLASS MAJORITY (ORIENTALS AND ANGLOS), BUT AT THE SAME TIME THEY ALSO VALUE NONCONFORMITY AND ASOCIAL BEHAVIOR MORE. THUS, THE MINORITY NEGRO AND MEXICAN AMERICAN CHILDREN HAVE A SET OF VALUES THAT IS IN ACCORD WITH THOSE OF THE EDUCATIONAL SYSTEM WHILE HOLDING TO ANOTHER SET OF VALUES THAT IS IN CONFLICT WITH THE SAME SYSTEM. SUCH VALUE CONFLICTS CAN BE EXPECTED TO HAVE SERIOUS IMPLICATIONS FOR ADJUSTMENT TO AND PROGRESS IN SCHOOL.

ACCN   000611

722   AUTH   **GUINN, R.**

TITL   ALCOHOL USE AMONG MEXICAN-AMERICAN YOUTH.

SRCE   *JOURNAL OF SCHOOL HEALTH, 1978, 48(2), 90-91.*

INDX   ATTITUDES, ADOLESCENTS, CULTURAL FACTORS, EMPIRICAL, FATHER-CHILD INTERACTION, MEXICAN AMERICAN, TEXAS, SOUTHWEST, FEMALE, MALE, SEX COMPARISON, RURAL, ECONOMIC FACTORS, SES, ALCOHOLISM

ABST   THIS STUDY INVESTIGATED SELECTED DEMOGRAPHIC, ATTITUDINAL, AND BEHAVIORAL VARIABLES WITH RESPECT TO ALCOHOL USE AMONG MEXICAN AMERICAN HIGH SCHOOL STUDENTS. A CHI-SQUARE TEST WAS PERFORMED BETWEEN ALCOHOL USE AND GRADE LEVEL AND SEX OF THE RESPONDENTS—937 MEXICAN AMERICAN HIGH SCHOOL STUDENTS FROM THE LOWER RIO GRANDE OF TEXAS. OF THESE, 518 WERE MALES AND 419 FEMALES, 308 WERE FRESHMEN, 185 SOPHOMORES, 286 JUNIORS, AND 158 SENIORS. A SIGNIFICANT RELATIONSHIP WAS FOUND FOR BOTH SEX AND GRADE LEVEL: (1) THE HIGHER THE GRADE LEVEL, THE GREATER THE ALCOHOL USE; (2) MALES WERE MORE LIKELY TO DRINK THAN FEMALES. CONTRARY TO THE FINDINGS OF MOST STUDIES, THERE WAS NO CLEAR CONNECTION BETWEEN SES AND ALCOHOL USE. HOWEVER, GRADE-POINT AVERAGE AND FREQUENCY OF SCHOOL ABSENCES SEEMED CAUSALLY LINKED: THE HIGHER THE GRADE-POINT AVERAGE, THE LESS FREQUENT THE USE; AND INCREASED CONSUMPTION LED TO INCREASED ABSENTEEISM. IN CONCLUSION, WHEN ASKED WHICH TYPE OF DRUG EDUCATION WOULD BE MOST EFFECTIVE IN SCHOOLS, MOST ALCOHOL USERS AND NON-USERS RATED LIVE PANELS WITH PROFESSIONALS AND FORMER USERS AS THE MOST EFFECTIVE, AND BOOKS OR READING MATERIAL AS THE LEAST. 1 REFERENCE.

ACCN   002360

723   AUTH   **GUINN, R.**

TITL   CHARACTERISTICS OF DRUG USE AMONG MEXICAN-AMERICAN STUDENTS.

SRCE   *JOURNAL OF DRUG EDUCATION, 1975, 5(3), 235-241.*

INDX   DRUG ABUSE, MEXICAN AMERICAN, ADOLESCENTS, SES, ATTITUDES, SURVEY, SCHOLASTIC ACHIEVEMENT, EMPIRICAL, SEX COMPARISON, TEXAS, SOUTHWEST, MALE, FEMALE

ABST   AN 88-ITEM QUESTIONNAIRE WAS ADMINISTERED TO 1,789 MEXICAN AMERICAN HIGH SCHOOL STUDENTS TO DETERMINE THE RELATIONSHIP OF DRUG USE TO SOCIOECONOMIC STATUS (SES), ATTITUDES TOWARD DRUGS, ACADEMIC ACHIEVEMENT, PARTICIPATION IN SCHOOL-RELATED ACTIVITES, AND DEMOGRAPHIC CHARACTERISTICS. 254 STUDENTS WERE IDENTIFIED AS DRUG USERS FROM THE TOTAL SAMPLE IN 1 JUNIOR AND 11 SENIOR HIGH SCHOOLS IN TEXAS. RESULTS SHOW THAT: (1) EDUCATIONAL LEVEL AND OCCUPATION OF THE DRUG USERS' FATHERS WERE SIGNIFICANTLY HIGHER THAN THAT OF THE TOTAL SAMPLE; (2) A HIGHER PERCENTAGE OF USERS THAN SS IN THE TOTAL SAMPLE FELT THAT DRUGS WERE USED TO EXPRESS FEELINGS MORE EASILY; AND (3) DRUG USERS HAD LOWER GRADE POINT AVERAGES, HIGHER RATES OF ABSENTEEISM, AND LOWER RATES OF CHURCH ATTENDANCE THAN THE TOTAL SAMPLE. OTHER FINDINGS SUGGEST THAT THE TYPICAL MEXICAN AMERICAN HIGH SCHOOL DRUG USER TENDS TO BE FROM A HIGHER SES LEVEL AND HAVE A RELATIVELY UNSTABLE FAMILY BACKGROUND. BOREDOM CREATED BY A LACK OF PARTICIPATION IN SCHOOL ACTIVITIES ALSO APPEARED TO BE A PRECIPITATING FACTOR IN DRUG USE. USE OF DRUGS BY MALES WAS TWICE THAT OF FEMALES. 8 REFERENCES. (PASAR ABSTRACT)

ACCN   000612

724   AUTH   **GUINN, R., & HURLEY, R. S.**

TITL   A COMPARISON OF DRUG USE AMONG HOUSTON AND LOWER RIO GRANDE VALLEY SECONDARY STUDENTS.

SRCE   *ADOLESCENCE, 1976, 6(43), 455-459.*

INDX   DRUG ABUSE, MEXICAN AMERICAN, ADOLESCENTS, CROSS CULTURAL, EMPIRICAL, INHALANT ABUSE, ALCOHOLISM, SEX COMPARISON, TEXAS, SOUTHWEST, URBAN, RURAL

ABST TO ASCERTAIN DIFFERENCES IN DRUG USE BETWEEN ANGLOS AND MEXICAN AMERICANS A SELF-REPORT SURVEY WAS CONDUCTED IN TEXAS AMONG 7,544 ADOLESCENT STUDENTS RESIDING EITHER IN AN URBAN (HOUSTON) OR RURAL (LOWER RIO GRANDE RIVER VALLEY) AREA; THE FORMER REPRESENTED VARIOUS ETHNIC GROUPS ENROLLED IN GRADES 7 THRU 12, WHILE THE LATTER REFLECTED A MEXICAN AMERICAN STUDENT POPULATION ENROLLED IN GRADES 9 THRU 12. THE RESULTS INDICATE THAT HOUSTON STUDENTS REPORT A HIGHER USE OF DRUGS AND DRUG-RELATED SUBSTANCES THAN THE VALLEY STUDENTS. IN COMPARISON TO USING OTHER DRUGS, THE HOUSTON SAMPLE REPORTS A HIGHER RATE OF ALCOHOL AND TOBACCO USE. THESE FINDINGS SUGGEST THAT THE INCIDENCE OF DRUG USE IS HIGHER AMONG ANGLOS THAN MEXICAN AMERICANS AND THAT ALCOHOL AND TOBACCO EDUCATION SHOULD BE INTEGRATED WITH SCHOOL DRUG EDUCATION PROGRAMS. 7 REFERENCES.

ACCN 000613

725 AUTH **GUMPERZ, J. J.**
TITL ON THE LINGUISTIC MARKERS OF BILINGUAL COMMUNICATION.
SRCE *JOURNAL OF SOCIAL ISSUES, 1967, 23(2), 48-57.*
INDX BILINGUALISM, CASE STUDY, CROSS CULTURAL, SPANISH SURNAMED, PHONOLOGY, SYNTAX, LINGUISTICS, NEW YORK, EAST, BILINGUAL
ABST OVERLAP AND LANGUAGE DISTANCE OF CONSTITUENT LINGUISTIC VARIETIES ARE DEMONSTRATED BY THE USE OF TRANSLATABILITY MEASURES. BILINGUAL SAMPLES CONSISTED OF HINDI-PUNJABI, KANNADA-MARATHI, AND SPANISH-ENGLISH SPEAKERS. TAPE RECORDED SPEECH SAMPLES IN TWO LANGUAGES WERE COLLECTED FROM BILINGUAL SPEAKERS INTERACTING IN NATURAL SETTINGS. TEXTS RECORDED IN LANGUAGE A WERE THEN RETOLD ORALLY IN LANGUAGE B BY OTHER NATIVE SPEAKERS, AND TEXTS RECORDED IN LANGUAGE B WERE RETOLD IN LANGUAGE A. THE OBJECTIVE WAS TO DETERMINE THE MINIMUM NUMBER OF DIFFERENCES NECESSARY FOR UTTERANCES TO BE PERCEIVED AS DISTINCT LANGUAGES BY THEIR SPEAKERS. FINDINGS SHOW THAT ALL REPERTOIRES MAINTAIN A LARGE NUMBER OF VARIANTS AT THE MORPHOPHONEMIC LEVEL. REGARDLESS OF THE NUMBER OF NONSHARED RULES, HOWEVER, DIFFERENCES IN THE PHONOLOGICAL REALIZATIONS OF MORPHEMES PLAY AN IMPORTANT PART. VARIANTS ARE SHOWN TOO IN CO-OCCURRENT PATTERNS AND NEVER IN ISOLATION. THE RIGIDITY OF SUCH CO-OCCURRENCE RULES REINFORCES THE PERCEPTUAL DISTINCTNESS OF CODES. IN SPITE OF THE UNDERLYING GRAMMATICAL SIMILARITIES, THE SHIFT BETWEEN CODES HAS A QUALITY OF ABRUPTNESS WHICH TO SOME EXTENT ACCOUNTS FOR THE SPEAKER'S VIEW OF THEM AS DISTINCT LANGUAGES. INTRALANGUAGE VARIA-

TION PLAYS AN IMPORTANT PART IN BILINGUAL BEHAVIOR, AND MEASURES OF BILINGUAL COMPETENCE MUST ACCOUNT FOR IT IF THEY ARE TO BE SOCIALLY REALISTIC. 22 REFERENCES.

ACCN 000614

726 AUTH **GUTIERREZ, A., & HIRSCH, H.**
TITL THE MILITANT CHALLENGE TO THE AMERICAN ETHOS: "CHICANOS" AND "MEXICAN AMERICANS."
SRCE *SOCIAL SCIENCE QUARTERLY, 1973, 53(4), 830-845. (REPRINTED IN C. HERNANDEZ, M. J. HAUG & N. N. WAGNER (EDS.), CHICANOS: SOCIAL AND PSYCHOLOGICAL PERSPECTIVES. SAINT LOUIS: C. V. MOSBY COMPANY, 1976, PP. 26-37.)*
INDX DISCRIMINATION, PREJUDICE, POLITICAL POWER, POLITICS, HISTORY, SURVEY, ETHNIC IDENTITY, ADOLESCENTS, MEXICAN AMERICAN, ACHIEVEMENT MOTIVATION, TEXAS, SOUTHWEST, CHICANO MOVEMENT
ABST SHORTLY AFTER THE MEXICAN AMERICAN COMMUNITY OF CRYSTAL CITY, SOUTH TEXAS, GAINED POLITICAL POWER AND CONTROL OF THE SCHOOL DISTRICT, A SURVEY WAS CONDUCTED AMONG 726 7TH TO 12TH GRADE STUDENTS RESIDING IN THIS GULF COAST TOWN. THE QUESTIONNAIRE WAS DESIGNED TO ASCERTAIN DIFFERENCES IN SOCIAL AND POLITICAL AWARENESS BETWEEN STUDENTS WHO CLASSIFIED THEMSELVES AS EITHER MEXICAN AMERICAN OR CHICANO. THE FINDINGS INDICATE THE FOLLOWING: (1) NO SIGNIFICANT DIFFERENCES REGARDING PERCEPTIONS OF SUCCESS; (2) CHICANOS SCORED HIGHER ON CIVIL LIBERTIES AND POLITICAL CYNICISM THAN THOSE IDENTIFYING THEMSELVES AS MEXICAN AMERICANS; (3) STUDENTS CONSIDERING THEMSELVES CHICANOS WERE MORE APT TO APPROVE OR ENGAGE IN COLLECTIVE POLITICAL ACTION; AND (4) CHICANO IDENTIFIERS APPEARED MORE AWARE OF THE SUBTLE INSTITUTIONAL FORMS OF DISCRIMINATION THAN THE OTHER GROUP. IT IS CONCLUDED THAT A STRONG IDENTIFICATION WITH ONE'S CULTURAL ETHNIC GROUP INCREASES POLITICAL AWARENESS WHICH WILL RESULT IN GREATER POLITICAL ACTIVITY AND THUS PROVIDE GREATER SUPPORT FOR THE CHICANO MOVEMENT. 20 REFERENCES.

ACCN 000615

727 AUTH **GUTIERREZ, E., & LUJAN, H. D.**
TITL THE KANSAS MIGRANT SURVEY: AN INTERPRETIVE PROFILE OF THE MEXICAN AMERICAN MIGRANT FAMILY.
SRCE *KANSAS COUNCIL OF AGRICULTURAL WORKERS AND LOW INCOME FAMILIES, GARDEN CITY, KANSAS, 1973. (ERIC DOCUMENT REPRODUCTION SERVICE NO. ED 107 419)*
INDX MIGRATION, RURAL, POVERTY, MEXICAN AMERICAN, FAMILY STRUCTURE, EMPIRICAL, DEMOGRAPHIC, FARM LABORERS, ATTITUDES, EMPLOYMENT, SOCIAL SERVICES, EDUCATION, RELIGION, CHILDREN, RESOURCE UTILIZATION, KANSAS, MIDWEST, MIGRANTS
ABST ORIGINALLY A FEDERALLY-FUNDED ORGANI-

ZATION CREATED TO SERVE MIGRANT FAMILIES IN THE 16 COUNTIES OF WESTERN KANSAS, THE KANSAS COUNCIL OF AGRICULTURAL WORKERS AND LOW-INCOME FAMILIES (KCAW-LIF) MARKED THE FIRST MAJOR EFFORT TO COPE WITH THE PROBLEMS OF MIGRANT LIFE BY PROVIDING BASIC SERVICES AT PUBLIC COST. A SURVEY OF 245 MIGRANT FAMILIES WAS CONDUCTED FROM JUNE THROUGH AUGUST 1972 IN 10 OF THE 16 COUNTIES SERVED BY KCAW-LIF. FARMWORKERS WERE CLASSIFIED AS SEASONAL, FARM, AND NONFARM RESIDENTS. THE ANALYSIS UNIT WAS THE FAMILY; THE FAMILY'S PRINCIPLE BREADWINNER WAS INTERVIEWED. SINCE CHICANOS COMPRISED THE LARGEST SEGMENT OF MIGRANTS, THOSE INTERVIEWED WERE MEXICAN AMERICAN. A QUESTIONNAIRE DESIGNED IN ENGLISH AND SPANISH WAS ADMINISTERED TO OBTAIN DATA CONCERNING: CITIZENSHIP, FAMILY SIZE, EDUCATION, LANGUAGE FACILITY, RELIGION, SETTLING OUT, LIVING AND WORKING CONDITIONS, SERVICE AVAILABILITY, AND BASIC MIGRANT ATTITUDES ABOUT SERVICES. INTERVIEWERS WERE 14 LOCAL BILINGUAL CHICANOS WITH EXPERIENCE AS FARMWORKERS IN THE SURVEY AREA. SOME FINDINGS WERE: (1) JOBS AND LEGAL SERVICES WERE MOST OFTEN CITED AS BEING NEEDED; (2) MORE FAMILIES KNEW OF THE AVAILABILITY OF SERVICES THAN HAD ACTUALLY USED THEM; AND (3) 57.9 PERCENT OF THE MIGRANT FAMILIES INDICATED THAT THEY WOULD SETTLE OUT IN KANSAS IF PERMANENT WORK WERE AVAILABLE, AND 37.7 PERCENT SAID THEY WOULD NOT SETTLE OUT IN KANSAS. (RIE ABSTRACT)

ACCN   000616

728 AUTH   **GUTIERREZ, L. P.**
    TITL   ATTITUDES TOWARDS BILINGUAL EDUCATION: A STUDY OF PARENTS WITH CHILDREN IN SELECTED BILINGUAL PROGRAMS.
    SRCE   *UNPUBLISHED DOCTORAL DISSERTATION, UNIVERSITY OF NEW MEXICO, 1972. (ERIC DOCUMENT REPRODUCTION SERVICE NO. ED 070 550)*
    INDX   EDUCATION, ATTITUDES, BILINGUAL-BICULTURAL EDUCATION, BILINGUAL, MEXICAN AMERICAN, EMPIRICAL, SES, LANGUAGE LEARNING, PARENTAL INVOLVEMENT, SOCIAL MOBILITY, SEX COMPARISON, ADULTS, NEW MEXICO, SOUTHWEST
    ABST   THE PURPOSE OF THIS STUDY WAS TO INVESTIGATE THE ATTITUDES TOWARD BILINGUAL EDUCATION OF PARENTS WHOSE CHILDREN WERE IN BILINGUAL PROGRAMS AND TO FIND IF ATTITUDE DIFFERENCES RELATED TO SEX, AGE, MOBILITY, AND EDUCATION EXISTED BETWEEN INCOME GROUPS. THE SAMPLE CONSISTED OF 110 PAIRS OF PARENTS WHOSE CHILDREN WERE IN BILINGUAL PROGRAMS IN 10 SCHOOLS IN THE ALBUQUERQUE PUBLIC SCHOOL SYSTEM. THE SAMPLE WAS DIVIDED INTO 2 SOCIOECONOMIC GROUPS BASED ON OCCUPATION AND SUBDIVIDED BY SEX, AGE, MOBILITY, AND EDUCATION. A 63-ITEM QUESTIONNAIRE WAS ADMINISTERED TO EACH PAIR

OF PARENTS BY A TRAINED SPANISH-SPEAKING INTERVIEWER. THE RESULTS INDICATED (1) A HOMOGENEOUS POSTITIVE ATTITUDE TOWARD BILINGUAL EDUCATION WITH FEW SIGNIFICANT DIFFERENCES BETWEEN SOCIOECONOMIC GROUPS, (2) THAT THOSE UNDER AGE 35 WERE MORE POSITIVE IN THEIR ATTITUDES THAN WERE THE OLDER GROUP, (3) THAT AMOUNT OF EDUCATION DID NOT SEEM TO ALTER ATTITUDES SIGNIFICANTLY, AND (4) THAT THE AMOUNT OF MOBILITY SIGNIFICANTLY AFFECTED THE RESPONSE TOWARD CERTAIN STATEMENTS. THE MAJOR CONCLUSION OF THE STUDY WAS THAT PARENTS ENTHUSIASTICALLY APPROVED OF THE ON-GOING BILINGUAL AND BICULTURAL PROGRAMS TO WHICH THEIR CHILDREN WERE BEING EXPOSED. (ERIC ABSTRACT)

ACCN   000617

729 AUTH   **GUTTMACHER, S., & ELISON, J.**
    TITL   ETHNO-RELIGIOUS VARIATION IN PERCEPTIONS OF ILLNESS: THE USE OF ILLNESS AS AN EXPLANATION FOR DEVIANT BEHAVIOR.
    SRCE   *SOCIAL SCIENCE AND MEDICINE, 1971, 5(2), 117-125.*
    INDX   DEVIANCE, CROSS CULTURAL, MENTAL HEALTH, PUERTO RICAN-M, ATTITUDES, PSYCHOPATHOLOGY, SYMPTOMATOLOGY, HEALTH, RELIGION, SES, NEW YORK, EAST, EMPIRICAL, SURVEY
    ABST   DIFFERENCES IN PERCEPTION OF BEHAVIOR AS SIGNS OF "MENTAL" ILLNESS AMONG EIGHT ETHNORELIGIOUS GROUPS WERE EXAMINED IN A STUDY OF OVER 2,000 REPRESENTATIVE NEW YORKERS. PERCEPTIONS OF 13 VIGNETTES DESCRIBING VARYING DEGREES OF DEVIANT OR PROBLEMATIC BEHAVIOR WERE ASCERTAINED AND 12 OF THESE WERE USED IN CONSTRUCTING A GUTTMAN ATTITUDE SCALE. ETHNORELIGIOUS DIFFERENCES WERE THEN CONSIDERED BY FREQUENCY OF DISTRIBUTION OF SCALE TYPES. THE PUERTO RICAN GROUP WAS FOUND TO HAVE THE MOST DISTINCTIVE DISTRIBUTION. 8 REFERENCES.

ACCN   000618

730 AUTH   **HABERMAN, P. W.**
    TITL   DENIAL OF DRINKING IN A HOUSEHOLD SURVEY.
    SRCE   *QUARTERLY JOURNAL OF STUDIES ON ALCOHOL, 1970, 31(3), 710-717.*
    INDX   ALCOHOLISM, CROSS CULTURAL, SURVEY, DEMOGRAPHIC, RESEARCH METHODOLOGY, ADULTS, EMPIRICAL, PUERTO RICAN-M, SES, SEX COMPARISON, MALE, FEMALE, NEW YORK, EAST
    ABST   A SURVEY OF NINE SELF-APPRAISAL QUESTIONS RELATED TO THE DENIAL OF DRINKING AMONG A SAMPLE OF 1,391 NEW YORK CITY RESIDENTS IS REPORTED. DATA REVEAL THAT ABOUT ONE-THIRD OF THE RESPONDENTS DID NOT DRINK AT ALL. THE FEMALE-MALE RATIO OF REPORTED NONDRINKERS IS 2.2:1. THERE IS MORE DENIAL OF DRINKING IN THE NEW YORK CITY SURVEY THAN HAS BEEN REPORTED FROM THE MIDDLE ATLANTIC REGION. DENIAL OF DRINKING IS DIRECTLY RELATED TO

AGE AND INVERSELY RELATED TO EDUCATION. PROPORTIONATELY MORE WIDOWED AND FEWER NEVER-MARRIED PERSONS INDICATE THAT THEY DO NOT DRINK. THE ETHNORELIGIOUS GROUPS WITH THE LARGEST PROPORTION OF REPORTED NONDRINKERS ARE THE PUERTO RICANS, JEWS, AND ITALIANS. THERE ARE RELATIVELY MORE NONDRINKERS AMONG BOTH MALES AND FEMALES IN THESE GROUPS WITH THE EXCEPTION OF PUERTO RICAN MEN. THREE-QUARTERS OF THE PUERTO RICAN WOMEN STATED THAT THEY DID NOT DRINK, SO THAT THE FEMALE-MALE RATIO OF REPORTED NONDRINKERS AMONG PUERTO RICANS IS 4.6:1, WHICH IS MUCH HIGHER THAN ANY OTHER ETHNORELIGIOUS GROUP. IT IS CONCLUDED THAT MORE DENIAL OF DRINKING IS FOUND AMONG OLDER THAN YOUNGER RESPONDENTS. 9 REFERENCES.

ACCN   000619

731 AUTH   **HABERMAN, P. W.**
    TITL   ETHNIC DIFFERENCES IN PSYCHIATRIC SYMPTOMS REPORTED IN COMMUNITY SURVEYS.
    SRCE   *PUBLIC HEALTH REPORTS, 1970, 85(6), 495-502.*
    INDX   CROSS CULTURAL, ADULTS, SES, SYMPTOMATOLOGY, DEMOGRAPHIC, PUERTO RICAN-M, EMPIRICAL, PSYCHOPATHOLOGY, MENTAL HEALTH, RESEARCH METHODOLOGY, SURVEY, NEW YORK, EAST
    ABST   REPRESENTATIVE SAMPLES OF 1,883 ADULT RESIDENTS OF THE WASHINGTON HEIGHTS HEALTH DISTRICT OF NEW YORK CITY AND 706 ADULT RESPONDENTS IN A CITYWIDE SAMPLE WERE ASKED QUESTIONS ABOUT SYMPTOMS USUALLY ASSOCIATED WITH PSYCHIATRIC IMPAIRMENT. THE SYMPTOMS ELICITED BY QUESTIONS INCLUDED ANXIETY, DEPRESSIVE STATES, AND INSOMNIA. THE ABSOLUTE AND RELATIVE PROPORTIONS GIVING SYMPTOMATIC RESPONSES TO THE MIDTOWN ITEMS IN THE TWO SURVEYS, BOTH OVERALL AND BY DEMOGRAPHIC SUBGROUPS, WERE SIMILAR. THE PROPORTIONS GIVING SYMPTOMATIC RESPONSES VARIED INVERSELY WITH SOCIAL CLASS, AS INDICATED BY EDUCATIONAL LEVEL AND FAMILY INCOME. WOMEN, PREVIOUSLY MARRIED PERSONS, AND, AMONG ETHNIC GROUPS, PUERTO RICANS REPORTED THE MOST PSYCHIATRIC SYMPTOMS. DIFFERENCES BETWEEN THE TWO SURVEYS, FOR THE MOST PART, WERE ATTRIBUTABLE TO DIFFERENCES IN WORDING OF QUESTIONS AND ETHNIC COMPOSITION OF THE SAMPLES, AS DISPROPORTIONATELY MORE IRISH IN WASHINGTON HEIGHTS REPORTED THE LEAST SYMPTOMS AND DISPROPORTIONATELY MORE ITALIANS IN NEW YORK CITY REPORTED A MODERATELY HIGH NUMBER OF SYMPTOMS. THE USE OF A SINGLE CUTTING POINT TO INDICATE IMPAIRMENT IN SURVEYS OF HETEROGENEOUS COMMUNITIES IS QUESTIONED. USING DIFFERENT CUTTING POINTS FOR VARIOUS ETHNIC GROUPS IS SUGGESTED AS A POSSIBLE MEANS OF COMPENSATING FOR VARIATION IN RESPONSE STYLE. 15 REFERENCES.
    ACCN   000620

732 AUTH   **HABERMAN, P. W.**
    TITL   PSYCHIATRIC SYMPTOMS AMONG PUERTO RICANS IN PUERTO RICO AND NEW YORK CITY.
    SRCE   *ETHNICITY, 1976, 3, 133-144.*
    INDX   ADULTS, ANXIETY, COPING MECHANISMS, DEPRESSION, EMPIRICAL, MENTAL HEALTH, PSYCHOPATHOLOGY, PSYCHOSOCIAL ADJUSTMENT, PUERTO RICAN-I, PUERTO RICAN-M, URBAN, NEW YORK, EAST, SYMPTOMATOLOGY
    ABST   IN FIELD STUDIES, PUERTO RICANS HAVE CONSISTENTLY TENDED TO REPORT MORE PSYCHIATRIC SYMPTOMS THAN HAVE OTHER ETHNIC/RACIAL GROUPS. MOREOVER, THE RATES OF REPORTED SYMPTOMS AMONG PUERTO RICANS HAVE REMAINED RELATIVELY HIGH AT ALL SOCIOECONOMIC CLASS LEVELS. TO INVESTIGATE THIS PHENOMENON, REPRESENTATIVE SAMPLES OF RESIDENTS OF PUERTO RICO AND PUERTO RICANS LIVING IN THE WASHINGTON HEIGHTS HEALTH DISTRICT AND IN THE FIVE BOROUGHS OF NEW YORK CITY WERE ASKED ABOUT PSYCHIATRIC SYMPTOMS IN A 22-ITEM SCREENING INSTRUMENT FROM THE MIDTOWN MANHATTAN STUDY. HIGHER SYMPTOM SCORES WERE REPORTED BY PUERTO RICANS LIVING IN PUERTO RICO THAN BY THOSE LIVING IN NEW YORK CITY AND THOSE LIVING IN THE CITY A SHORTER LENGTH OF TIME. THESE FINDINGS SUGGEST THAT THE CONSISTENTLY HIGH RATES OF SURVEY-REPORTED SYMPTOMS AMONG PUERTO RICAN RESPONDENTS DERIVE PRIMARILY FROM CULTURALLY PATTERNED DIFFERENCES IN MODES OF EXPRESSING DISTRESS. 12 REFERENCES. (AUTHOR ABSTRACT MODIFIED)
    ACCN   002278

733 AUTH   **HALL, D. C.**
    TITL   EXECUTIVE SUMMARY: A CRITICAL LITERATURE REVIEW OF THE PROBLEM DRINKING BEHAVIOR IN SPECIAL POPULATION GROUPS, VOL. I. (SRI PROJECT URU-5580)
    SRCE   *MENLO PARK, CA.: STANFORD RESEARCH INSTITUTE, 1977.*
    INDX   RESEARCH METHODOLOGY, SPANISH SURNAMED, ALCOHOLISM, BIBLIOGRAPHY, POLICY, HEALTH DELIVERY SYSTEMS, PRIMARY PREVENTION, DEMOGRAPHIC, CROSS CULTURAL
    ABST   THIS TWO-PHASE STUDY OF ALCOHOLISM BEGAN WITH A BROAD SURVEY OF THE RESEARCH-BASED LITERATURE ON THE RELATIONSHIP BETWEEN PROBLEM DRINKING AND SELECTED DEMOGRAPHIC VARIABLES. NEXT, A RESEARCH STRATEGY (ORGANIZED AS A SERIES OF NINE STEPS) WAS FORMULATED TO IMPROVE BOTH ALCOHOLISM TREATMENT AND PREVENTION SERVICES. IN THIS STRATEGY, THE INFORMATION ABOUT THE IDENTIFIABILITY OF A SPECIAL POPULATION GROUP IS GATHERED, AND THEN AN EXAMINATION IS MADE OF THE GROUP'S LOCATABILITY, THE EXTENT OF THEIR PROBLEM DRINKING, THE MEANS BY WHICH THEIR DRINKING PROBLEMS CAN BE TREATED OR PREVENTED, AND THE EXTENT TO WHICH THE GROUP NEEDS IMPROVED SERVICE DELIVERY. AS A CASE IN POINT, EXISTING INFORMATION ON THE PROB-

LEM DRINKING WITHIN THE SPANISH-SPEAK-ING POPULATION WAS COLLECTED AND OR-GANIZED IN ORDER TO IDENTIFY PRIORITIES FOR RESEARCH AND IMPROVEMENT OF SER-VICE DELIVERY. RESULTS INDICATE THAT THIS GROUP IS A PRIME TARGET FOR FUTURE RE-SEARCH.

ACCN   002101

734 AUTH   **HALL, D. C.**
    TITL   A RESEARCH STRATEGY FOR REVIEWING THE PROBLEM DRINKING BEHAVIOR LITERATURE ASSOCIATED WITH SPECIAL POPULATION GROUPS, VOL. II. (SRI PROJECT URU-5580)
    SRCE   *MENLO PARK, CA.: STANFORD RESEARCH IN-STITUTE, 1977.*
    INDX   ALCOHOLISM, ADULTS, REVIEW, DEMO-GRAPHIC, ENVIRONMENTAL FACTORS, HEALTH, HEALTH DELIVERY SYSTEMS, MENTAL HEALTH, PSYCHOSOCIAL ADJUSTMENT, SES, FEMALE, MALE, RESEARCH METHODOLOGY
    ABST   SECOND IN A FOUR-PART SERIES ON PROB-LEM DRINKING, THIS RESEARCH REPORT DE-SCRIBES AN APPROACH FOR ORGANIZING AND EVALUATING EXISTING INFORMATION ABOUT SPECIAL POPULATION GROUPS, THEIR ASSOCIATED DRINKING CHARACTERISTICS, AND THE NATURE OF TREATMENT OR PREVEN-TION SERVICES BEING RECEIVED BY GROUP MEMBERS. THE RESEARCH STRATEGY IS OR-GANIZED AS A SERIES OF NINE STEPS. IN THE FIRST FOUR STEPS, THE GROUPS ARE EXAM-INED ACCORDING TO (1) IDENTIFIABILITY, (2) LOCATABILITY, (3) EXTENT OF PROBLEM DRINKING, AND (4) EVIDENCE REGARDING HOW EASILY THE DRINKING PROBLEMS CAN BE TREATED OR PREVENTED. IN EACH OF THESE FOUR STAGES, THE QUALITY OF AVAILABLE IN-FORMATION ON EACH SPECIAL POPULATION GROUP IS RATED AS (1) HIGH, (2) LOW, (3) UN-SUITABLE, OR (4) UNDETERMINED. A DETERMI-NATION IS THEN MADE REGARDING EACH GROUP'S NEED FOR IMPROVED SERVICE DE-LIVERY OR FOR FURTHER RESEARCH BASED ON RATING COMBINATION PERMUTATIONS. PROCEDURES FOR THIS DETERMINATION ARE SPECIFIED IN STEPS 5 THROUGH 9. GROUPS CATEGORIZED AS "HIGH" ON ALL FACTORS RATED ARE DESIGNATED AS PRIME TARGETS FOR IMPROVED SERVICE DELIVERY. GROUPS CATEGORIZED AS "HIGH" ON THREE OF THE FOUR FACTORS AND "UNDETERMINED" ON ONE ARE DESIGNATED AS PRIME TARGETS FOR FURTHER RESEARCH. IN THE FINAL STAGES OF THE RESEARCH STRATEGY, PROCEDURES FOR SPECIFYING IMPROVED SERVICE DELIVERY AND RESEARCH PRIORITIES AMONG OTHER RATING COMBINATION PERMUTATIONS ARE DIS-CUSSED. (AUTHOR SUMMARY MODIFIED)
    ACCN   002102

735 AUTH   **HALL, D. C.**
    TITL   A REVIEW OF THE PROBLEM DRINKING BEHAV-IOR LITERATURE ASSOCIATED WITH THE SPAN-ISH-SPEAKING POPULATION GROUP, VOL. III. (SRI PROJECT URU-5580)
    SRCE   *MENLO PARK, CA.: STANFORD RESEARCH IN-STITUTE, 1977.*

    INDX   ALCOHOLISM, SPANISH SURNAMED, MEXICAN AMERICAN, PRIMARY PREVENTION, REVIEW, SES, STRESS, RESOURCE UTILIZATION, CUL-TURAL FACTORS, ENVIRONMENTAL FACTORS
    ABST   A CRITICAL LITERATURE REVIEW IS PRE-SENTED CONCERNING PROBLEM DRINKING AND ITS TREATMENT AND PREVENTION WITHIN THE U.S. SPANISH-SPEAKING POPULATION. STUDIES INDICATE THAT THE EXTENT OF PROBLEM DRINKING IS FAR GREATER AMONG THE SPANISH-SPEAKING THAN EITHER THE GENERAL POPULATION OR THE ANGLO POPU-LATION. HOWEVER, THE SPANISH-SPEAKING GROUP (COMPRISED OF MEXICAN AMERI-CANS, PUERTO RICANS, CUBANS, AND CEN-TRAL AND SOUTH AMERICANS) HAS SUBSTAN-TIAL INTERNAL HETEROGENEITY IN TRAITS AND CULTURE. AND DATA INDICATE THAT IT IS MEXICAN AMERICANS IN THE SOUTHWEST (PRIMARILY IN CALIFORNIA) WHO HAVE THE HIGHEST DEGREE OF PROBLEM DRINKING AMONG SPANISH-SPEAKING SUBGROUPS. THESE FINDINGS ARE LARGELY BASED UPON ALCOHOL-RELATED ARREST AND MORTALITY FIGURES. OTHER INDICATORS INCLUDE ABOVE-AVERAGE CONCENTRATIONS OF LIQUOR STORES IN THEIR COMMUNITIES AND HIGH RATES OF ALCOHOLISM. WITH REGARD TO TREATMENT AND PREVENTION, THERE IS EVI-DENCE THAT PSYCHOLOGICAL BARRIERS ARISING FROM CULTURAL AND ENVIRONMEN-TAL FACTORS MAY LIMIT THE USE OF ALCO-HOLISM TREATMENT SERVICES. MOREOVER, TREATMENT SERVICES WHICH ARE CULTUR-ALLY SENSITIVE FOR MEXICAN AMERICANS AND OTHER SPANISH-SPEAKING GROUPS ARE RARE. THE EXPANSION OF SUCH CULTURALLY RELEVANT ALCOHOLISM TREATMENT SER-VICES IS ADVOCATED. 84 REFERENCES.
    ACCN   002103

736 AUTH   **HALL, E. T.**
    TITL   THE SILENT LANGUAGE.
    SRCE   *IN R. O'BRIEN (ED.), READINGS IN GENERAL SOCIOLOGY, BOSTON: HOUGHTON MIFFLIN, 1969.*
    INDX   CROSS CULTURAL, SPANISH SURNAMED, BI-LINGUALISM, INTERPERSONAL RELATIONS, IN-TERPERSONAL SPACING, CULTURAL FACTORS, PERSONALITY, THEORETICAL, ESSAY
    ABST   SOME OF THE MAJOR OBSTACLES TO MUTUAL UNDERSTANDING AMONG PEOPLE IN NORTH AND SOUTH AMERICA ARE DISCUSSED. THE PROBLEM OFTEN CAN BE FOUND IN HIDDEN PSYCHOLOGICAL PATTERNS, SPECIFICALLY IN THE AREAS OF TIME CONCEPTS, SPACE CON-CEPTS, AND FRIENDSHIP PATTERNS. CON-CEPTS OF TIME AND PATTERNS OF PUNCTUAL-ITY DIFFER MARKEDLY. FOR EXAMPLE, THE NORTH AMERICAN BUSINESSMAN TRIES TO MAKE HIS POINT WITH NEATNESS AND DIS-PATCH-QUICKLY AND EFFICIENTLY WHILE THE LATIN AMERICAN PUTS EMPHASIS ON COUR-TESY RATHER THAN SPEED. THE DIFFERENCE IN THE TWO SYSTEMS LIES IN THE CONTROLS. ONE IS FORMAL, PERSONAL, AND DEPENDS UPON FAMILY AND FRIENDS. THE OTHER IS TECHNICAL-LEGAL, IMPERSONAL, AND DE-

PENDS UPON COURTS AND CONTRACTS. TO THE COLOMBIAN OR MEXICAN, THE NORTH AMERICAN MAY SEEM COLD AND WITHDRAWN BECAUSE HE TALKS FROM BEHIND A DESK OR AT A DISTANCE OF 2 FEET OR MORE—THE CUSTOM IN THE UNITED STATES, BUT DEFINED AS DETACHED AND SEPARATED IN THE CUSTOMS OF LATIN AMERICA. THE TRADITIONAL HOME OF THE LATIN AMERICAN IS BUILT AROUND A PATIO AND CLOSED FROM THE STREET WHICH OFTEN MAKES A NORTH AMERICAN FEEL ISOLATED SINCE HE IS ACCUSTOMED TO OPEN NEIGHBORHOODS. RECOGNITION OF THESE DIFFERING BEHAVIOR PATTERNS WILL PRODUCE EASIER COMMUNICATION BETWEEN INDIVIDUALS OF DIFFERENT CULTURES.

ACCN   000622

737 AUTH   **HALL, L. H.**

TITL   PERSONALITY VARIABLES OF ACHIEVING AND NON-ACHIEVING MEXICAN AMERICAN AND OTHER COMMUNITY COLLEGE FRESHMEN.

SRCE   *JOURNAL OF EDUCATIONAL RESEARCH, 1972, 65(5), 224-228.*

INDX   PERSONALITY, POVERTY, SES, SCHOLASTIC ACHIEVEMENT, MEXICAN AMERICAN, SELF CONCEPT, COLLEGE STUDENTS, CROSS CULTURAL, EMPIRICAL, TAT

ABST   AN INVESTIGATION OF PERSONALITY VARIABLES OF ACHIEVING AND NONACHIEVING COLLEGE STUDENTS OF DIFFERENT SOCIOECONOMIC STATUS (SES) IS PRESENTED. GROUPS CONSISTING OF 111 LOWER-SES MEXICAN AMERICAN (MA), 150 LOWER-SES ANGLO AMERICAN (AA), AND 207 MIDDLE-SES AA STUDENTS WERE MEASURED BY MCCLELLAND'S TAT OF NEED ACHIEVEMENT AND THE INVENTORY OF SELF APPRAISAL (ISA). ANALYSES OF VARIANCE BETWEEN SES GROUPS AND ACADEMICALLY ACHIEVING 'C' AVERAGE OR BETTER) AND NONACHIEVING MA'S WERE CALCULATED. ACADEMIC PROGRESS OVER A FIVE-SEMESTER PERIOD WAS OBSERVED. IN TERMS OF SCHOLASTIC ACHIEVEMENT, PERSISTENCE IN COLLEGE, COMPLETION OF GRADUATION REQUIREMENTS, AND TRANSFER TO 4-YEAR INSTITUTIONS OF HIGHER LEARNING, MIDDLE-SES SUBJECTS ARE MORE SUCCESSFUL THAN ARE LOW-SES STUDENTS. THE SIMILARITIES IN ACADEMIC ACHIEVEMENT AND PERSONALITY VARIABLES OF THE MA AND AA OF LOWER-SES SUGGEST THAT SOCIOECONOMIC STATUS, AND NOT ETHNICITY, IS THE MORE SIGNIFICANT DETERMINANT OF PERSONALITY TRAITS RELATED TO ACADEMIC SUCCESS. THE RELATIVELY HIGH NEED TO ACHIEVE SCORES OF BOTH LOWER-SES SUBGROUPS, VIEWED IN CONJUNCTION WITH THEIR LOW ACHIEVEMENT LEVELS, SUGGESTS THAT EITHER THE COLLEGE IS NOT PROVIDING CURRICULA WHICH MEET THE NEEDS OF THE STUDENTS OR THAT THE FACULTY AND ADMINISTRATION HAVE NOT DETERMINED HOW THEIR INSTITUTIONS MAY AFFECT THEIR ACCEPTED AIMS. A LARGE PROPORTION OF LOWER-SES COLLEGE FRESHMEN DID NOT SATISFY THEIR DESIRES TO SUCCEED IN THE ATTAINMENT OF HIGHER EDUCATIONAL GOALS. 13 REFERENCES.

ACCN   000623

738 AUTH   **HALLOWITZ, E., & REISSMAN, F.**

TITL   THE ROLE OF THE INDIGENOUS NONPROFESSIONAL IN A COMMUNITY MENTAL HEALTH NEIGHBORHOOD SERVICE CENTER.

SRCE   *AMERICAN JOURNAL OF ORTHOPSYCHIATRY, 1967, 37(4), 766-778.*

INDX   PARAPROFESSIONALS, PSYCHOTHERAPISTS, POVERTY, PUERTO RICAN-M, PRIMARY PREVENTION, CURRICULUM, ESSAY, PROGRAM EVALUATION, MENTAL HEALTH, NEW YORK, EAST, URBAN, CASE STUDY

ABST   METHODS FOR UTILIZING THE PARTICULAR SKILLS AND STYLES OF INDIGENOUS NONPROFESSIONALS OF THE LINCOLN HOSPITAL MENTAL HEALTH SERVICES PROGRAM, LOCATED IN A DISADVANTAGED URBAN AREA OF NEW YORK CITY, ARE DISCUSSED IN TERMS OF THE ROLE OF THE WORKER AS A NEIGHBORHOOD FRIEND, RATHER THAN AS A JUNIOR CASEWORKER OR JUNIOR COMMUNITY ORGANIZER. SEVERAL ISSUES AND PROBLEMS IN THE USE AND DEVELOPMENT OF NONPROFESSIONALS ARE PRESENTED. ILLUSTRATIONS OF HOW THE MENTAL HEALTH AIDES HAVE INTERVENED IN THE LIVES OF THEIR CLIENTS ARE GIVEN IN DETAIL FOR 2 PATIENT CASES. THE SELECTION AND TRAINING PROCESS FOR MENTAL HEALTH AIDES IS ALSO DESCRIBED. ALTHOUGH LIMITATIONS AND PROBLEMS ARE RECOGNIZED, IT IS BELIEVED THAT NONPROFESSIONAL MENTAL HEALTH WORKERS CAN AND DO MAKE VALUABLE CONTRIBUTIONS IN COMMUNITY MENTAL HEALTH PROGRAMS. 8 REFERENCES. (JOURNAL ABSTRACT MODIFIED)

ACCN   000624

739 AUTH   **HALPERN, S.**

TITL   THE RELATIONSHIP BETWEEN ETHNIC GROUP MEMBERSHIP AND SEX AND ASPECTS OF VOCATIONAL CHOICE IN PRE-COLLEGE BLACK AND PUERTO RICAN HIGH SCHOOL STUDENTS (DOCTORAL DISSERTATION, FORDHAM UNIVERSITY, 1972).

SRCE   *DISSERTATION ABSTRACTS INTERNATIONAL, 1972, 33(1), 190A. (UNIVERSITY MICROFILMS NO. 72-20,591.)*

INDX   ADOLESCENTS, SEX COMPARISON, OCCUPATIONAL ASPIRATIONS, PUERTO RICAN-M, CROSS CULTURAL, VOCATIONAL COUNSELING, EDUCATIONAL COUNSELING, ATTITUDES, EMPLOYMENT, NEW YORK, EAST, URBAN, EMPIRICAL

ABST   IN 1969 TWO MEASURES OF VOCATIONAL MATURITY AND ASPIRATIONS (THE VOCATIONAL DEVELOPMENT INVENTORY (VDI) AND THE VOCATIONAL ASPIRATION SCALE (VAS)) WERE ADMINISTERED TO 255 TENTH-GRADE STUDENTS FROM 3 NEW YORK CITY HIGH SCHOOLS ENROLLED IN A PRE-COLLEGE PROGRAM FOR POOR AND MINORITY YOUTH—57 PUERTO RICAN AND 198 BLACK. DATA ANALYSIS FOR 6 HYPOTHESES RELATING SEX AND/OR ETHNICITY AND THEIR INTERACTION TO VOCATIONAL MATURITY, ASPIRATIONS AND JOB VALUES INCLUDED REGRESSION ANALYSIS, PEARSON-R

AND DESCRIPTIVE TABLES. MAJOR FINDINGS WERE: (1) THE EFFECTS OF SEX AND ETHNICITY ON VOCATIONAL MATURITY WERE SIGNIFICANT, WITH BLACKS SCORING HIGHER THAN PUERTO RICANS, AND FEMALES HIGHER THAN MALES; (2) THE EFFECTS OF SEX ON VAS SCORES WERE SIGNIFICANT, WITH MALES TENDING TO SCORE HIGHER THAN FEMALES; (3) VAS DISCREPANCY SCORES SHOWED NO SIGNIFICANT DIFFERENCES FOR SEX; (4) IN NO INSTANCE WAS THE EFFECT OF INTERACTION BETWEEN ETHNICITY AND SEX FOUND SIGNIFICANT; AND (5) STATED JOB VALUES WERE RELATED TO SEX AND/OR ETHNICITY. IT IS HOPED THAT THIS AND RELATED RESEARCH WILL HELP IMPLEMENT PROGRAMS FOR POOR AND MINORITY STUDENTS BY IDENTIFYING THOSE FACTORS RELATED TO THEIR VOCATIONAL CHOICE, CHOICE PROCESS AND JOB VALUES. 106 REFERENCES. (AUTHOR SUMMARY MODIFIED)

ACCN   000625

740   AUTH   **HAMBURGER, S.**

TITL   PROFILE OF CURANDEROS: A STUDY OF MEXICAN FOLK PRACTITIONERS.

SRCE   *INTERNATIONAL JOURNAL OF SOCIAL PSYCHIATRY, 1978, 24(1), 19-25.*

INDX   CURANDERISMO, FOLK MEDICINE, CALIFORNIA, SOUTHWEST, EMPIRICAL, DEMOGRAPHIC, MENTAL HEALTH, MENTAL HEALTH PROFESSION, PARAPROFESSIONALS, HEALTH DELIVERY SYSTEMS, MEXICAN AMERICAN

ABST   ALLIED HEALTH PRACTITIONERS (I.E., DOCTOR'S ASSISTANTS) ARE BEING INCREASINGLY UTILIZED IN MODERN ANGLO MEDICINE. IT HAS BEEN SUGGESTED THAT SUCH PRACTITIONERS COULD PLAY AN ESPECIALLY IMPORTANT ROLE IN MINORITY COMMUNITIES. TO INVESTIGATE THIS POSSIBILITY, A STUDY OF CURANDEROS (MEXICAN FOLK MEDICINE PRACTITIONERS) WAS UNDERTAKEN IN A SMALL TOWN IN CALIFORNIA. THE FIRST METHOD FOR LOCATING CURANDEROS, QUESTIONING MEXICAN AMERICAN CLINIC PATIENTS ABOUT THEIR HEALTH PRACTICES AND PRACTITIONERS, FAILED TO PROVIDE SUCCESSFUL LEADS TO CURANDEROS. A SECOND APPROACH IN WHICH THE AUTHOR ESTABLISHED A SOCIAL RELATIONSHIP WITH THE LEAST ANGLICIZED MEXICAN AMERICANS LED TO THE IDENTIFICATION OF 17 CURANDEROS, OF WHOM 14 WERE SUCCESSFULLY INTERVIEWED. THE QUESTIONNAIRE COVERED SUCH DEMOGRAPHIC INFORMATION AS SEX, AGE, MARITAL STATUS, YEARS OF SCHOOLING, TYPE OF CURING PRACTICE, AND OTHER OCCUPATIONS. OTHER QUESTIONS DEALT WITH THE CURANDEROS' CONCEPTIONS OF ILLNESS AND ROLE CONCEPTIONS. THE FINDINGS, PRESENTED IN FOUR TABLES, LED TO THE DEVELOPMENT OF A COMPOSITE PROFILE AS WELL AS TO INDIVIDUAL PROFILES OF EACH CURANDERO. THE FINDINGS SUGGEST THAT AT LEAST SOME CURANDEROS MIGHT BE INCORPORATED AS ALLIED HEALTH PROFESSIONALS IN ANGLO MEDICAL CARE. POSSIBLE WAYS TO ACCOMPLISH THIS AND THE BENEFITS TO BE DERIVED ARE DISCUSSED. 7 REFERENCES. (JOURNAL ABSTRACT MODIFIED)

ACCN   002104

741   AUTH   **HAMILTON, A.**

TITL   THE OLD EQUALIZER.

SRCE   *AMERICAN EDUCATION, 1975, 11(2), 6-10.*

INDX   BILINGUALISM, BILINGUAL-BICULTURAL EDUCATION, ESSAY, INSTRUCTIONAL TECHNIQUES, HISTORY, MEXICAN AMERICAN, CUBAN, SCHOLASTIC ACHIEVEMENT, CURRICULUM, CASE STUDY, CALIFORNIA, SOUTHWEST, URBAN

ABST   BILINGUAL EDUCATION CAN BE UTILIZED TO IMPROVE THE SOCIOECONOMIC STATUS OF MINORITY, PARTICULARLY HISPANIC, YOUTH. THE BILINGUAL PROGRAM AT HUNTINGTON DRIVE ELEMENTARY SCHOOL IN EAST LOS ANGELES IS USED TO ILLUSTRATE HOW SUCH A PROGRAM CAN BE INITIATED AND MAINTAINED. FIVE ESSENTIAL ELEMENTS IN BILINGUAL-BICULTURAL EDUCATION AS DEVELOPED AT HUNTINGTON SCHOOL ARE: (1) READING INSTRUCTION IN THE CHILD'S DOMINANT LANGUAGE; (2) INSTRUCTION IN A SECOND LANGUAGE; (3) CONCURRENT INSTRUCTION IN BOTH LANGUAGES; (4) DEVELOPMENT OF CONFIDENCE AND SELF-ESTEEM; AND (5) DEVELOPMENT OF CULTURAL AWARENESS AND PRIDE IN THE HISTORY AND THE TRADITION OF THE CHILDS' ANCESTORS. BILINGUAL-BICULTURAL EDUCATION SERVES THE NEWLY ARRIVED IMMIGRANT CHILDREN'S NEED TO LEARN IN THEIR OWN LANGUAGE, PROVIDES THE ENGLISH-SPEAKING, THIRD GENERATION CHILDREN WITH AN OPPORTUNITY FOR EDUCATIONAL ENRICHMENT, AND ALLOWS THE BILINGUAL CHILDREN TO PERFECT AND RETAIN THEIR LANGUAGE ASSET. A TYPICAL DAY AT THE SCHOOL DEMONSTRATES HOW A BILINGUAL PROGRAM SHOULD BE STRUCTURED FOR BEST RESULTS: THE TWO LANGUAGES MUST BE USED AND TAUGHT CONCURRENTLY TO DEVELOP BASIC SKILLS. OTHER POINTS EMPHASIZED ARE THE RECRUITMENT OF BILINGUAL-BICULTURAL STAFF AND THE COOPERATION BETWEEN PARENTS AND SCHOOL STAFF.

ACCN   000626

742   AUTH   **HAMILTON, M. L.**

TITL   EVALUATION OF A PARENT AND CHILD CENTER PROGRAM.

SRCE   *UNPUBLISHED MANUSCRIPT, WASHINGTON STATE UNIVERSITY, 1970. (ERIC DOCUMENT REPRODUCTION SERVICE NO. ED 345 189)*

INDX   PROGRAM EVALUATION, PARENTAL INVOLVEMENT, COGNITIVE DEVELOPMENT, MEXICAN AMERICAN, EMPIRICAL, CHILDREARING PRACTICES, EARLY CHILDHOOD EDUCATION, CHILDREN, MENTAL RETARDATION, MIGRANTS, MOTHER-CHILD INTERACTION, LANGUAGE ACQUISITION, WASHINGTON, WEST

ABST   WITH PROGRAM EMPHASIS ON STIMULATING RETARDED DEVELOPMENT, CHILDREN UNDER 3 YEARS OF AGE WERE GIVEN A NURSERY SCHOOL TYPE OF EXPERIENCE FIVE DAYS A WEEK FOR EIGHT OR MORE HOURS A DAY. MOTHERS WERE GIVEN IN-SERVICE TRAINING

AVERAGING 3 HOURS PER WEEK, STRESSING DEVELOPMENT OF MOTHERS' SELF-CONCEPT, GENERAL HANDLING OF THE CHILD, LANGUAGE DEVELOPMENT OF THE CHILD, PHYSICAL CARE, AND DEVELOPMENT OF CHILD'S GROSS AND FINE MOTOR CONTROL. A MINIMUM OF 10 WEEKS OF PAID PARTICIPATION AS A TEACHER AIDE WAS AVAILABLE FOR EACH OF THE MOTHERS. DATA ARE REPORTED FOR AN 11-MONTH PERIOD ON 18 FAMILIES FROM TWO CENTERS THAT PRIMARILY SERVE CHICANO MIGRANT FAMILIES. CHILDREN WERE PRE- AND POSTTESTED ON MEASURES TO DETERMINE MOTOR, LANGUAGE, AND SOCIAL DEVELOPMENT AND, IN ADDITION, A TEST WAS GIVEN TO ASSESS THE STIMULATION POTENTIAL OF EACH CHILD'S HOME. CONCLUSIONS MUST BE TENTATIVE IN THE ABSENCE OF A CONTROL GROUP, BUT POSTTEST SCORES INDICATED A SIGNIFICANT IMPROVEMENT IN THE AMOUNT AND QUALITY OF DEVELOPMENTAL HOME STIMULATION. SUBTEST SCORES SHOWED THE GREATEST IMPROVEMENT IN THE AREAS OF LANGUAGE DEVELOPMENT AND DEVELOPMENTAL AND VOCAL STIMULATION. (RIE ABSTRACT MODIFIED)

ACCN 000627

743 AUTH **HAMMER, H. B., III.**
TITL A CROSS CULTURAL INVESTIGATION OF FOSTER'S IMAGE OF LIMITED GOOD.
SRCE *REVISTA INTERAMERICANA DE PSICOLOGIA, 1972, 6(3-4), 255-264.*
INDX COGNITIVE STYLE, CHILDREN, CONFORMITY, CROSS CULTURAL, ENVIRONMENTAL FACTORS, SES, SEX COMPARISON, EMPIRICAL, MEXICAN, CULTURAL FACTORS, TEXAS, SOUTHWEST
ABST THE COGNITIVE ORIENTATION OF REGARDING ONE'S OWN LOCALITY AS A CLOSED SYSTEM WITH LIMITED NATURAL AND SOCIAL RESOURCES HAS BEEN HYPOTHESIZED TO CHARACTERIZE MEXICAN PEASANTS. TWO OBJECTIONS TO THIS HAVE SUGGESTED THAT THIS IMAGE OF LIMITED GOOD IS PRESENT IN VARYING DEGREES IN ALL CULTURES AND THAT THERE HAS NOT BEEN INDEPENDENT VALIDATION. A QUESTIONNAIRE WAS CONSTRUCTED TO TEST FOSTER'S CONCEPT OF THE IMAGE OF LIMITED GOOD. STUDENTS IN TWO SIXTH-GRADE CLASSROOMS IN EACH OF TWO CULTURES, MEXICAN AND AMERICAN, WERE GIVEN THE QUESTIONNAIRE. THE MEXICAN SAMPLE SCORED SIGNIFICANTLY HIGHER THAN THE AMERICAN SAMPLE, SUPPORTING FOSTER'S CONCEPT. A MEASURE OF WILLINGNESS TO ADMIT NONCONFORMITY WAS ALSO OBTAINED. ALTHOUGH THE MAIN EFFECT OF CULTURE MEMBERSHIP UPON THE MEASURE DID NOT ATTAIN SIGNIFICANCE, GIRLS IN BOTH CULTURES SCORED SIGNIFICANTLY HIGHER ON THE NONCONFORMITY MEASURE. IT IS RECOMMENDED THAT FURTHER RESEARCH BE CONDUCTED AMONG CHILDREN RESIDING IN A MEXICAN VILLAGE SO AS TO PROVIDE ADDITIONAL EVIDENCE SUPPORTING THE CONTINUUM MODEL OF THE LIMITED GOOD CONCEPT.

6 REFERENCES. (JOURNAL ABSTRACT MODIFIED)
ACCN 000628

744 AUTH **HANDLIN, O.**
TITL THE NEWCOMERS: NEGROES AND PUERTO RICANS IN A CHANGING METROPOLIS.
SRCE *CAMBRIDGE, MASS.: HARVARD UNIVERSITY PRESS, 1971.*
INDX PUERTO RICAN-M, MIGRATION, PSYCHOSOCIAL ADJUSTMENT, HISTORY, ACCULTURATION, SES, POVERTY, LABOR FORCE, PREJUDICE, ETHNIC IDENTITY, URBAN, ECONOMIC FACTORS, EMPIRICAL, STRESS, CROSS CULTURAL, DEMOGRAPHIC, HOUSING, EDUCATION, EMPLOYMENT, SOCIAL MOBILITY, INTERPERSONAL SPACING, DISCRIMINATION, HEALTH, MENTAL HEALTH, EQUAL OPPORTUNITY, ENVIRONMENTAL FACTORS, NEW YORK, EAST, BOOK
ABST THIS THIRD VOLUME OF THE NEW YORK METROPOLITAN REGION STUDY, A PROJECT DESIGNED TO ANALYZE THE KEY ECONOMIC AND DEMOGRAPHIC CHARACTERISTICS OF 22 COUNTIES IN THE TRI-STATE REGION, FOCUSES ON THE CITY'S POPULATION IN TERMS OF ITS ETHNIC CHARACTERISTICS. AN HISTORICAL EXAMINATION OF THE INFLUX OF BLACKS AND PUERTO RICANS TO THE CITY IS DISCUSSED WITH RESPECT TO PATTERNS OF ADJUSTMENT. BLACKS, IT IS CONTENDED, HAVE GREATER OBSTACLES TO OVERCOME IN THEIR SOCIAL ADJUSTMENT. HOWEVER, BOTH BLACKS AND PUERTO RICANS EXPERIENCE RACIAL PREJUDICE AND DISCRIMINATION AS WELL AS SIMILAR SOCIAL AND ECONOMIC HANDICAPS. THE SOCIAL DISORDER WHICH CHARACTERIZES THEIR LIVES CAN BE RESOLVED THROUGH THE DEVELOPMENT OF COMMUNAL INSTITUTIONS, UNDER LEADERSHIP THAT WILL PROVIDE ORDER AND PURPOSE TO THEIR LIVES. EVIDENCE ALSO INDICATES THAT PUERTO RICANS AND BLACKS WILL CONTINUE TO LIVE IN COHESIVE CLUSTERS WITHIN THE CITY. IT IS CONCLUDED THAT PUERTO RICANS AND BLACKS WILL BECOME MORE DEPENDENT UPON GOVERNMENTAL SERVICES FOR EDUCATION AND WELFARE. HOWEVER, EDUCATION IS CONSIDERED THE KEY TO THEIR IMPROVEMENT IN ECONOMIC STATUS.
ACCN 000629

745 AUTH **HANEY, R., MICHAEL, M. & MARTOIS, J.**
TITL THE PREDICTION OF SUCCESS OF THREE ETHNIC SAMPLES ON A STATE BOARD CERTIFICATION EXAMINATION FOR NURSES FROM PERFORMANCE ON ACADEMIC COURSE VARIABLES AND ON STANDARDIZED ACHIEVEMENT AND STUDY SKILLS MEASURES.
SRCE *EDUCATIONAL AND PSYCHOLOGICAL MEASUREMENT, 1977, 37(4), 949-964.*
INDX MEXICAN AMERICAN, NURSING, HIGHER EDUCATION, ACHIEVEMENT TESTING, CROSS CULTURAL, EDUCATIONAL ASSESSMENT, EMPIRICAL, TEST VALIDITY, PROFESSIONAL TRAINING, SCHOLASTIC ACHIEVEMENT
ABST TO EXAMINE THE PROGNOSTIC CAPABILITY OF ACADEMIC COURSEWORK ACHIEVEMENT AND ACHIEVEMENT TEST SCORES FOR EACH OF

THREE SAMPLES OF 207 CAUCASIANS, 61 MEX-
ICAN AMERICANS, AND 53 NEGROES IN A
NURSING TRAINING PROGRAM AT A VERY
LARGE METROPOLITAN HOSPITAL, VALIDITY
COEFFICIENTS OF 15 PREDICTOR VARIABLES
AVAILABLE PRIOR TO TRAINING AND OF 13
PREDICTOR VARIABLES OBTAINED CONCUR-
RENTLY WITH TRAINING WERE CALCULATED
RELATIVE TO EACH OF FIVE SUBTESTS OF A
STATE BOARD CERTIFICATION EXAMINATION
FOR NURSES. IN ADDITION, STEPWISE MUL-
TIPLE REGRESSION ANALYSES RELATIVE TO
EACH OF THE SAME FIVE CRITERION MEA-
SURES AS WELL AS WITH RESPECT TO AN AV-
ERAGE SCORE ON THE FIVE SUBTESTS OF THE
CERTIFICATION EXAMINATION WERE CARRIED
OUT FOR SELECTED SETS OF PREDICTOR VARI-
ABLES IN EACH OF THE THREE SAMPLES.
STANDARDIZED TEST MEASURES INVOLVING
READING SKILLS WERE THE MOST VALID OF
THE PREDICTOR VARIABLES OBTAINED PRIOR
TO NURSING TRAINING, WHEREAS TOTAL
GRADE POINT AVERAGE IN PROGRAM COURSES
AS WELL AS SCORES ON THE NATIONAL
LEAGUE FOR NURSING ACHIEVEMENT TESTS
PROVIDED HIGHEST VALIDITY COEFFICIENTS
FOR EACH ETHNIC GROUP. IN TERMS OF THE
PREDICTOR VARIABLES SELECTED, THE STEP-
WISE MULTIPLE REGRESSION ANALYSES
SERVED ESSENTIALLY TO REINFORCE THE
OTHER CORRELATIONAL FINDINGS. 3 REFER-
ENCES. (NCHHI ABSTRACT)

ACCN   002541

746   AUTH   **HANSON, M.**
      TITL   CULTURAL DEMOCRACY, SCHOOL ORGANIZA-
             TION AND EDUCATIONAL CHANGE.
      SRCE   IN A. CASTANEDA, M. RAMIREZ III, C. E. CORTES
             & M. BARRERA (EDS.), MEXICAN AMERICANS
             AND EDUCATIONAL CHANGE. NEW YORK: ARNO
             PRESS, 1974, PP. 40-74.
      INDX   CULTURAL PLURALISM, EQUAL OPPORTUNITY,
             DISCRIMINATION, EDUCATION, CULTURAL FAC-
             TORS, SOCIAL STRUCTURE, HISTORY, BILIN-
             GUAL-BICULTURAL EDUCATION, ACCULTURA-
             TION, ETHNIC IDENTITY, CURRICULUM,
             INSTRUCTIONAL TECHNIQUES, MEXICAN
             AMERICAN, ESSAY
      ABST   EQUAL EDUCATIONAL OPPORTUNITY FOR SUCH
             GROUPS AS MEXICAN AMERICANS DEPENDS
             UPON EQUAL OPPORTUNITY TO LEARN AS
             WELL AS THE ABILITY OF STUDENTS TO RETAIN
             THEIR OWN CULTURAL IDENTITY. EMBODIED IN
             THIS IDEOLOGY IS THE CONCEPT OF A CUL-
             TURALLY DEMOCRATIC EDUCATIONAL CLASS-
             ROOM ENVIRONMENT WHICH IS IMPLICIT IN
             THE LIBERAL-PROGRESSIVE TRADITION. HOW-
             EVER, THOUGH THE DOMINANT CONSERVA-
             TIVE-ESSENTIALIST TRADITION EMPHASIZES A
             STRUCTURED LEARNING CURRICULUM, IT IG-
             NORES DIFFERENCES IN THE INDIVIDUAL'S
             LEARNING ENVIRONMENT AND THUS IS DIA-
             METRICALLY OPPOSED TO THE CONCEPT OF
             CULTURAL DEMOCRACY. THE CONSERVATIVE-
             ESSENTIALIST TRADITION REFLECTS THE FOL-
             LOWING CHARACTERISTICS: (1) PRINCIPLES
             OF DISCIPLINE AND RATIONAL INTELLECTUAL
             PROCEDURES; (2) TRANSMISSION OF DOMI-

NANT CULTURAL VALUES; (3) TEACHERS ACTS
AS THE TRANSMITTER OF KNOWLEDGE; (4)
CERTAIN KNOWLEDGE IS ESSENTIAL TO ALL
STUDENTS; AND (5) ASSIMILATION OF VARIOUS
CULTURES INTO THE DOMINANT ONE. IN CON-
TRAST, THE LIBERAL-PROGRESSIVE TRADI-
TION, ALTHOUGH LESS INFLUENTIAL, EX-
PRESSES THE FOLLOWING PRINCIPLES: (1)
THE MAJOR FUNCTION OF SCHOOL IS TO PRO-
MOTE SOCIAL CHANGE; (2) THERE IS NO SPE-
CIAL BODY OF KNOWLEDGE THAT NEEDS TO
BE PASSED FROM GENERATION TO GENERA-
TION; (3) THE LEARNING ENVIRONMENT IS
COMPOSED OF THE CHILD'S HOME, SCHOOL,
AND FRIENDSHIP PATTERNS; AND (4) CURRICU-
LUM SHOULD REFLECT RELEVANT ISSUES AND
NEEDS OF THE CHILD. THIS TRADITION EM-
PHASIZES THAT THE LEARNING PACKAGE
SHOULD NOT BE RIGID BUT RATHER BASED
UPON THE INDIVIDUAL'S LEARNING ENVIRON-
MENT. THERE APPEARS TO BE A GROWING
AWARENESS AMONG EDUCATORS THAT THE
DOMINANT TRADITION DOES NOT PROVIDE
VARIOUS CULTURAL GROUPS AND EQUAL OP-
PORTUNITY TO LEARN. AS THIS AWARENESS
GROWS, THE CONCEPT OF CULTURAL DEMOC-
RACY IN THE CLASSROOM CAN BECOME A RE-
ALITY.

ACCN   000630

747   AUTH   **HANSON, R. C., SIMMONS, O. G., & MCPHEE,
             W. N.**
      TITL   QUANTITATIVE ANALYSIS OF THE URBAN EX-
             PERIENCES OF SPANISH-AMERICAN MI-
             GRANTS.
      SRCE   IN J. HELM (ED.), SPANISH SPEAKING PEOPLE
             IN THE UNITED STATES, PROCEEDINGS OF THE
             1968 ANNUAL MEETING OF THE AMERICAN
             ETHNOLOGICAL SOCIETY. SEATTLE: UNIVER-
             SITY OF WASHINGTON PRESS, 1968, PP. 65-83.
      INDX   URBAN, MIGRATION, RESEARCH METHOD-
             OLOGY, SURVEY, DEMOGRAPHIC, SES, SPAN-
             ISH SURNAMED, EMPIRICAL, ECONOMIC
             FACTORS, OCCUPATIONAL ASPIRATIONS,
             THEORETICAL, COLORADO, SOUTHWEST, MI-
             GRANTS
      ABST   USING THE CASE HISTORY DATA OF 66 RURAL
             MIGRANTS IN DENVER, COLO., THE AUTHORS
             PRESENT A THEORETICAL MODEL FOR THEIR
             QUANTITATIVE DATA. THE USEFULNESS OF THE
             MODEL, DESIGNED TO SIMULATE URBANIZA-
             TION PROCESSES IN PREDICTING THE BEHAV-
             IOR OF RURAL MIGRANTS ENTERING AN UR-
             BAN ENVIRONMENT OVER TIME, IS DISCUSSED.
             GENERATION OF THE TIME SERIES DATA AND
             ITS ARRANGEMENT FOR TIME TREND ANALYSIS
             ARE EXPLAINED. A MAJOR ADVANTAGE OF
             THIS MODEL IS THAT IT INCREASES THE
             PROBABILITY OF DISCOVERING SIGNIFICANT
             SOCIAL PROCESSES NOT YET FORMALLY OR
             EXPLICITLY PRESENTED IN URBANIZATION LIT-
             ERATURE. SEVERAL TABLES AND GRAPHS ARE
             INCLUDED TO ILLUSTRATE HOW THE VARIABLE
             OF FINANCIAL INDEPENDENCE FOR THE 66 MI-
             GRANTS OVER A 48-MONTH TIME PERIOD IS
             ANALYZED WITHIN THE MODEL'S FRAMEWORK.
             9 REFERENCES.
      ACCN   000631

748 AUTH **HANSON, R. C., & SIMMONS, O. G.**
TITL DIFFERENTIAL EXPERIENCE PATHS IN RURAL MIGRANTS TO THE CITY.
SRCE *IN E. B. BRODY (ED.), BEHAVIOR IN NEW ENVIRONMENTS: ADAPTATION OF MIGRANT POPULATIONS. BEVERLY HILLS: SAGE PUBLICATIONS, 1970, PP. 145-166.*
INDX URBAN, MIGRATION, SES, EMPIRICAL, PSYCHOSOCIAL ADJUSTMENT, STRESS, ENVIRONMENTAL FACTORS, DEVIANCE, ALCOHOLISM, HEALTH, FAMILY STRUCTURE, SPANISH SURNAMED, SOCIAL SERVICES, THEORETICAL, MIGRANTS, COLORADO, SOUTHWEST
ABST THE CHARACTERISTIC ATTRIBUTES AND TRENDS OF FOUR RURAL MIGRANT GROUPS IN THE ADJUSTMENT PROCESS TO THE URBAN CITY ARE COMPARED. DETAILED CASE HISTORY INTERVIEWS WERE OBTAINED FROM 66 SPANISH-AMERICAN RURAL MIGRANTS. THE SUBJECTS WERE DIVIDED INTO HIGH- AND LOW-SOCIOECONOMIC (SES) GROUPS. MONTH-BY-MONTH DATA ON EACH MIGRANT WERE COMPUTED. DATA INDICATE THAT AMONG HIGH-SES MIGRANTS, UNSUCCESSFUL ADJUSTMENT BY PART OF THE GROUP CANNOT BE PREDICTED FROM ARRIVAL ATTRIBUTES BUT FROM EMERGENT PHENOMENA SUCH AS EMPLOYMENT AND MISFORTUNE EXPERIENCE (E.G., A FINE, LAWYER'S FEE). AMONG THE MIGRANTS WHO ARRIVE IN THE CITY WITH LOW-SES, TWO ARRIVAL ATTRIBUTES BEAR ON PROBABLE LATER UNSUCCESSFUL ADJUSTMENT: STATE OF HEALTH AND PHASE IN THE FAMILY CYCLE (E.G., INCREASE IN FAMILY SIZE). HEALTHY, SINGLE MEN OR WAGE EARNERS IN NEWLY FORMED FAMILIES ARE MORE LIKELY TO MAINTAIN FINANCIAL INDEPENDENCE THAN OLDER MIGRANTS WHO ARRIVE IN RELATIVELY POOR HEALTH WITH LARGE FAMILIES TO SUPPORT. THE HIGH PROBABILITY OF WELFARE ASSISTANCE FOR THE OLDER LOW-SES GROUPS IS EVIDENT. HEALTHY MIGRANTS WITH ABOVE-AVERAGE SKILLS AND EDUCATION ARE LIKELY TO INTEGRATE INTO THE CITY WITHIN A PERIOD OF ABOUT 6 TO 12 MONTHS. AN INTERPRETATION OF THE PROCESS OF RURAL MIGRANT ADJUSTMENT TO THE CITY IS PROVIDED. 7 REFERENCES.
ACCN 000632

749 AUTH **HARDYCK, C., GOLDMAN, R., & PETRINOVICH, L.**
TITL HANDEDNESS AND SEX, RACE, AND AGE.
SRCE *HUMAN BIOLOGY, 1975, 47(3), 369-375.*
INDX SEX COMPARISON, CROSS CULTURAL, CULTURAL FACTORS, MEXICAN AMERICAN, CONFORMITY, CHILDREN, CALIFORNIA, SOUTHWEST, EMPIRICAL, PHYSICAL DEVELOPMENT
ABST THE INCIDENCE OF RIGHT- AND LEFT-HANDEDNESS, AS MEASURED BY BEHAVIORAL TESTING IN 7,688 CALIFORNIA SCHOOL CHILDREN IN GRADES ONE THROUGH SIX, WAS EXAMINED FOR RELATIONSHIPS TO SEX, RACE, AND AGE. EACH CHILD WAS ASKED TO WRITE HIS NAME, PICK UP A PAIR OF SCISSORS AND CUT A CARD, AND THEN PICK UP A PAPER TUBE AND LOOK THROUGH IT. OVERALL, 10.5% OF THE BOYS AND 8.7% OF THE GIRLS WERE FOUND TO BE LEFT-HANDED. LEFT-HANDEDNESS WAS NOTED IN 10.2% OF THE WHITES (N = 3820), 9.5% OF THE BLACKS (N = 3178), 6.5% OF THE ORIENTALS (N = 538), AND 8.8% OF THE MEXICAN AMERICANS (N = 148). ALTHOUGH STATISTICALLY SIGNIFICANT RELATIONSHIPS WERE FOUND FOR RACE AND SEX, THESE WERE SO SLIGHT THAT IT IS CONCLUDED THAT THESE FACTORS HAVE LITTLE MEANINGFUL RELATIONSHIP TO THE INCIDENCE OF HANDEDNESS. DIFFERENCES PRESENT IN OTHER CULTURES AND IN DIFFERENT RACIAL GROUPS WITHIN THE SAME CULTURE ARE CONSIDERED TO BE PRIMARILY CULTURALLY DETERMINED. 17 REFERENCES.
ACCN 002105

750 AUTH **HARMON, G. C.**
TITL PARTICIPATION OF MEXICAN-AMERICAN PARENTS IN SCHOOL ACTIVITIES AT KINDERGARTEN LEVEL IN POVERTY AREAS OF LOS ANGELES (DOCTORAL DISSERTATION, UNIVERSITY OF SOUTHERN CALIFORNIA, 1971).
SRCE *DISSERTATION ABSTRACTS INTERNATIONAL, 1971, 32(3), 1659A. (UNIVERSITY MICROFILMS NO. 71-21,461.)*
INDX PARENTAL INVOLVEMENT, EDUCATION, POVERTY, MEXICAN AMERICAN, ATTITUDES, CHILDREN, COMMUNITY INVOLVEMENT, COMMUNITY, EMPIRICAL, TEACHERS, PROGRAM EVALUATION, EARLY CHILDHOOD EDUCATION, FAMILY ROLES, CALIFORNIA, SOUTHWEST,
ABST LEVELS OF MEXICAN AMERICAN PARENT PARTICIPATION IN PRESCHOOL- AND KINDERGARTEN-RELATED ACTIVITIES WERE INVESTIGATED TO DETERMINE (1) WHETHER ATTENDANCE AT PRESCHOOL FUNCTIONS AFFECTS PARENT PARTICIPATION IN THE FOLLOWING SCHOOL YEAR AND (2) WHETHER SELECTED DEMOGRAPHIC VARIABLES ARE RELATED TO FAVORABLE CIRCUMSTANCES THAT ENCOURAGE PARENTAL PARTICIPATION AND TO UNFAVORABLE CIRCUMSTANCES THAT RESTRICT IT. SIXTY PARENTS OF 30 PRESCHOOLERS AND 30 NON-PRESCHOOLERS ATTENDING KINDERGARTEN IN 10 EAST LOS ANGELES AND SAN FERNANDO VALLEY PUBLIC SCHOOLS WERE INTERVIEWED REGARDING DEMOGRAPHIC DATA, LEVEL OF SCHOOL PARTICIPATION, AND LISTING OF FAVORABLE AND UNFAVORABLE CIRCUMSTANCES INFLUENCING SCHOOL PARTICIPATION. CONCLUSIONS SUPPORTED BY THE STUDY FINDINGS ARE: (1) ACTION OF THE TEACHER IS THE CIRCUMSTANCE WHICH MOST INFLUENCED PARENTAL SCHOOL INVOLVEMENT ON A REGULAR BASIS; (2) DIFFERENCES BETWEEN PRESCHOOL- AND NON-PRESCHOOL PARENT PARTICIPATION IN KINDERGARTEN ACTIVITIES WAS NOT FOUND TO BE SIGNIFICANT, PROBABLY DUE TO INABILITY OF MANY PARENTS TO PARTICIPATE BECAUSE OF PERSONAL PROBLEMS AND FAMILY RESPONSIBILITIES; (3) LEVEL OF PARENTS' EDUCATION IS POSITIVELY RELATED TO SCHOOL PARTICIPATION; AND (4) RELATIONSHIP OF CONTINUED PARENT PARTICIPATION TO PRESCHOOL ATTENDANCE IS NOT SIGNIFICANT. RECOMMENDATIONS FOR INVOLVING LOW-INCOME

MEXICAN AMERICAN PARENTS IN THEIR CHILDREN'S EARLY SCHOOL YEARS ARE DISCUSSED. 52 REFERENCES.

ACCN   000633

751 AUTH   **HARO, C.**
     TITL   THE CALIFORNIA SCHOOL FINANCING CASE: SERRANO VS. PRIEST.
     SRCE   *EL MIRLO CANTA DE NOTICATLAN, 1977, 4(5-6), 1-4. (PUBLICATION OF CHICANO STUDIES DEPARTMENT, UNIVERSITY OF CALIFORNIA, LOS ANGELES.)*
     INDX   EDUCATION, EQUAL OPPORTUNITY, JUDICIAL PROCESS, DISCRIMINATION, MEXICAN AMERICAN, ECONOMIC FACTORS, REVIEW, FINANCING, POLICY, CALIFORNIA, SOUTHWEST, TEXAS
     ABST   THE HISTORY OF THE CALIFORNIA SCHOOL FINANCING CASE, SERRANO VS. PRIEST, IS SUMMARIZED AND MAJOR STATE AND FEDERAL ACTIONS RELEVANT TO THE CASE ARE DISCUSSED. THE LEGAL BATTLE BEGAN IN 1968 WHEN JOHN SERRANO, A MEXICAN AMERICAN AND FATHER OF SCHOOL-AGE CHILDREN, WAS ADVISED BY HIS LOCAL SCHOOL PRINCIPAL TO MOVE TO ANOTHER, BETTER FUNDED SCHOOL DISTRICT IF HE WANTED BETTER EDUCATION FOR HIS CHILDREN. THE SUIT FILED BY MR. SERRANO AGAINST THE LOCAL SCHOOL BOARD CLAIMED THAT THE WAY IN WHICH SCHOOLS ARE FINANCED IS UNCONSTITUTIONAL; THE SYSTEM OF CALIFORNIA SCHOOL FINANCING DEPRIVES RESIDENTS OF POORER DISTRICTS OF AN EQUAL PROTECTION OF THE LAWS UNDER THE 14TH AMENDMENT OF THE CONSTITUTION. THE FINAL DISPOSITION FOLLOWS FROM PREVIOUS FEDERAL-STATE CONFLICTS IN WHICH IT WAS DETERMINED THAT THE U.S. SUPREME COURT HAS FINAL AUTHORITY ON THE FEDERAL CONSTITUTION, BUT GENERALLY, A STATE SUPREME COURT IS THE ULTIMATE INTERPRETER OF A STATE CONSTITUTION. SOME STATISTICS DOCUMENTING THE PROBLEM OF LOCAL PROPERTY TAXES FOR SCHOOL FINANCING ARE PRESENTED.
     ACCN   000634

752 AUTH   **HARO, C. M.**
     TITL   MEXICAN/CHICANO CONCERNS AND SCHOOL DESEGREGATION IN LOS ANGELES (MONOGRAPH NO. 9).
     SRCE   *LOS ANGELES: UNIVERSITY OF CALIFORNIA, CHICANO STUDIES CENTER, 1977.*
     INDX   MEXICAN AMERICAN, EDUCATION, COMMUNITY, SCHOLASTIC ASPIRATIONS, SES, CROSS CULTURAL, JUDICIAL PROCESS, SPANISH SURNAMED, CULTURAL FACTORS, STEREOTYPES, CALIFORNIA, SOUTHWEST, URBAN, INTEGRATION, EQUAL OPPORTUNITY, HISTORY, SURVEY, ESSAY, ATTITUDES, DISCRIMINATION, ADULTS, BOOK
     ABST   ON JUNE 26, 1976, THE CALIFORNIA STATE SUPREME COURT AFFIRMED A 1970 LOWER COURT DECISION THAT THE LOS ANGELES CITY UNIFIED SCHOOL DISTRICT SHOULD BE DESEGREGATED. THIS DECISION NOT ONLY AFFECTS BLACK AND ANGLO POPULATIONS, BUT CHICANOS AS WELL. IT IS PROJECTED THAT BY 1980, BLACK YOUTHS WILL CONSTITUTE 26.0%

OF THE STUDENT ENROLLMENT, WHITE STUDENTS 32.5%, AND CHICANOS 35.9%—THE LARGEST ETHNIC/RACIAL GROUP IN THE DISTRICT. THIS REPORT FOCUSES ON THE DESEGREGATION CASE (CRAWFORD VS. BOARD OF EDUCATION OF THE CITY OF LOS ANGELES) THAT PRECIPITATED THE LANDMARK DECISION; SECONDLY, IT DISCUSSES THE CHICANO/MEXICANO PERCEPTIONS AND EXPECTATIONS REGARDING THAT MANDATED RACIAL/ETHNIC DESEGREGATION. CHAPTER 1 REVIEWS THE EDUCATIONAL ACHIEVEMENTS AND THE SCHOOLING EXPERIENCE OF THE CHICANO IN THIS COUNTRY. CHAPTER 2 PROVIDES A BRIEF INTRODUCTION TO THE INVOLVEMENT OF THE JUDICIARY IN THE PROVISION OF EQUAL EDUCATIONAL OPPORTUNITY, SPECIFICALLY WITH SCHOOL SEGREGATION. CHAPTER 3 CONSIDERS SCHOOL SEGREGATION IN LOS ANGELES, THE FINDINGS OF THE TRIAL COURT IN THE CRAWFORD DECISION, AND THE CALIFORNIA STATE SUPREME COURT DECISION ON THE CASE. IN THIS CHAPTER AND IN CHAPTER 5, THE IMPORTANCE OF SCHOOL DISTRICT DESEGREGATION FOR THE CHICANO IS ALSO CONSIDERED. THE FINAL PORTION OF THE MONOGRAPH PROVIDES THE CHICANO PERSPECTIVE. THE RECOMMENDATIONS OF CHICANO RESIDENTS AND LOCAL COMMUNITY LEADERS CONVEY A FEELING OF URGENCY REGARDING "QUALITY SCHOOLING" AND THE DESEGREGATION OF THE LOS ANGELES SCHOOL DISTRICT. 128 REFERENCES.

ACCN   002106

753 AUTH   **HARRIS, B. H.**
     TITL   FIELDWORK ASSIGNMENT: INNER CITY.
     SRCE   *ELEMENTARY SCHOOL GUIDANCE AND COUNSELING, 1972, 6(3), 180-185.*
     INDX   URBAN, SES, POVERTY, CHILDREN, EDUCATIONAL COUNSELING, PSYCHOTHERAPY, MEXICAN AMERICAN, PROFESSIONAL TRAINING, CROSS CULTURAL, CASE STUDY, CALIFORNIA, SOUTHWEST
     ABST   THE ESTABLISHMENT AND WORKINGS OF A 'RAP ROOM', A PLACE FOR THE FREE VENTILATION OF FRUSTRATIONS AND PROBLEMS IN AN ELEMENTARY SCHOOL WITH APPROXIMATELY 95% BLACK AND 5% MEXICAN AMERICAN STUDENTS ARE DESCRIBED. THE OBSERVATIONS AND DIARY ENTRIES OF THE GRADUATE COUNSELOR EDUCATION STUDENT WHO STAFFED THE ROOM ARE PRESENTED. THE SUCCESSES AND FAILURES OF THE PROJECT, INCLUDING DIFFICULTIES WITH THE ADMINISTRATION AND TEACHERS ARE DISCUSSED. THE THEORETICAL BASIS OF THE PROJECT WAS THAT THESE STUDENTS KNEW WHAT THEIR PROBLEMS WERE AND WOULD BE WILLING TO SHARE THEM WITH OTHERS. (PASAR ABSTRACT MODIFIED)
     ACCN   000635

754 AUTH   **HARRIS, M. B.**
     TITL   AGGRESSIVE REACTIONS TO A FRUSTRATING PHONE CALL.
     SRCE   *JOURNAL OF SOCIAL PSYCHOLOGY, 1974, 92(2), 193-198.*
     INDX   AGGRESSION, STRESS, ANXIETY, SEX COM-

PARISON, INTERPERSONAL RELATIONS, SPAN-ISH SURNAMED, CROSS CULTURAL, ETHNIC IDENTITY, EMPIRICAL, NEW MEXICO, SOUTH-WEST

ABST   NINETY MALES AND FEMALES WITH ANGLO OR SPANISH SURNAMES WERE RANDOMLY SE-LECTED FROM THE TELEPHONE BOOK TO TEST REACTIONS TO AGGRESSIVE AND NON-AG-GRESSIVE SITUATIONS. SUBJECTS WERE CALLED BY 6 EXPERIMENTERS WHO WERE EITHER POLITE OR AGGRESSIVE AND HAD EITHER PREVIOUSLY CALLED AND HUNG UP OR DID NOT PREVIOUSLY CALL. NO DIFFER-ENCES DUE TO SEX OR ETHNIC BACKGROUND OF SUBJECTS WERE FOUND, AND A PREVIOUS TELEPHONE RING HAD NO EFFECT. HOWEVER, SUBJECTS CALLED BY A MALE EXPERIMENTER OR BY AN AGGRESSIVE EXPERIMENTER WERE MORE AGGRESSIVE AS EVIDENCED BY THEIR TONE OF VOICE AT THE BEGINNING AND END OF THE CALL, THEIR COMMENTS, AND EXPER-IMENTER SUBJECT OVERALL IMPRESSION. PARTICULARLY IN THE AGGRESSIVE CONDI-TION, BUT EVEN IN THE POLITE ONE, SUB-JECTS INCREASED THE AGGRESSIVENESS OF THEIR TONE OF VOICE FROM THE BEGINNING TO THE END OF THE CALL. THE STUDY PRO-VIDES CONFIRMATION THAT AGGRESSIVE BE-HAVIOR OUTSIDE THE LABORATORY CAN BE AFFECTED SYSTEMATICALLY BY EXPERIMEN-TAL MANIPULATIONS. 4 REFERENCES. (PASAR ABSTRACT MODIFIED)

ACCN   000636

755 AUTH   **HARRIS, M. B., & BAUDIN, H.**
     TITL   THE LANGUAGE OF ALTRUISM: THE EFFECTS OF LANGUAGE, DRESS, AND ETHNIC GROUP.
     SRCE   *THE JOURNAL OF SOCIAL PSYCHOLOGY, 1973, 91, 37-41.*
     INDX   COOPERATION, SEX COMPARISON, CROSS CULTURAL, SPANISH SURNAMED, SES, ALTRU-ISM, INTERPERSONAL RELATIONS, EXAMINER EFFECTS, EMPIRICAL, DYADIC INTERACTION, NEW MEXICO, SOUTHWEST
     ABST   THE EFFECTS BETWEEN THE EXPERIMENTER'S ETHNICITY, LANGUAGE, TYPE OF DRESS, AND SEX AND THE SUBJECT'S SEX, LANGUAGE RE-SPONSE AND ALTRUISTIC RESPONSE WERE EX-AMINED. NINETY-SIX MALES AND FEMALES WERE SELECTED AT A STATE FAIR ON THE BA-SIS OF APPEARING TO BE SPANISH AMERICAN. THEY WERE ASKED BY EITHER AN ANGLO (MALE OR FEMALE) SPEAKING ENGLISH, AN HISPANIC SPEAKING ENGLISH (MALE OR FE-MALE), OR AN HISPANIC SPEAKING SPANISH IF THEY HAD CHANGE FOR A DIME. THE RESULTS INDICATE THAT THE SPANISH EXPERIMENTERS WERE HELPED THE MOST WHILE ANGLOS WERE HELPED THE LEAST. EXPERIMENTERS WERE ALSO HELPED MORE WHEN THEY WERE WELL DRESSED. ALTHOUGH THE LANGUAGE RE-SPONSE BY THE SUBJECTS WAS THE SAME AS USED BY THE EXPERIMENTERS, THERE AP-PEARED TO BE NO RELATION BETWEEN ALTRU-ISM AND THE LANGUAGE OF THE SUBJECTS. 9 REFERENCES.

     ACCN   000637

756 AUTH   **HARRIS, M. B., & HASSEMER, W. G.**
     TITL   SOME FACTORS AFFECTING THE COMPLEXITY OF CHILDREN'S SENTENCES: THE EFFECTS OF MODELING, AGE, SEX, AND BILINGUALISM.
     SRCE   *JOURNAL OF EXPERIMENTAL CHILD PSY-CHOLOGY, 1972, 13, 447-455.*
     INDX   CHILDREN, MODELING, EMPIRICAL, LAN-GUAGE LEARNING, BILINGUAL, MEXICAN AMERICAN, NEW MEXICO, SOUTHWEST
     ABST   THE EFFECTS OF THE COMPLEXITY OF THE SENTENCES SPOKEN BY A MODEL UPON THE LENGTH AND COMPLEXITY OF SENTENCES SPOKEN BY MONOLINGUAL CHILDREN HEAR-ING ENGLISH SENTENCES, BILINGUAL CHIL-DREN HEARING SPANISH AND BILINGUAL CHILDREN HEARING ENGLISH WERE AS-SESSED. SECOND AND FOURTH-GRADE BOYS AND GIRLS SERVED AS SUBJECTS. A CLEAR MODELING EFFECT WAS FOUND, AS WELL AS AN EFFECT OF GRADE LEVEL ON SENTENCE LENGTH. NO SIGNIFICANT EFFECTS OF SEX OR LANGUAGE WERE FOUND. THE RESULTS SUG-GEST THAT MODELING CAN INDEED AFFECT THE COMPLEXITY OF CHILDREN'S SENTENCES EVEN IN THE ABSENCE OF REINFORCEMENT OR INSTRUCTIONS TO IMITATE. 9 REFERENCES. (JOURNAL ABSTRACT)

     ACCN   000638

757 AUTH   **HARRIS, M. B., & KLINGBEIL, D. R.**
     TITL   THE EFFECTS OF ETHNICITY OF SUBJECT AND ACCENT AND DEPENDENCY OF CONFEDERATE ON AGGRESSIVENESS AND ALTRUISM.
     SRCE   *JOURNAL OF SOCIAL PSYCHOLOGY, 1976, 98, 47-53.*
     INDX   AGGRESSION, COOPERATION, CROSS CUL-TURAL, EMPIRICAL, DISCRIMINATION, ADULTS, SPANISH SURNAMED, NEW MEXICO, SOUTH-WEST
     ABST   IN ORDER TO ASSESS THE EFFECTS OF THE ACCENT AND NEED OF A CALLER UPON THE AGGRESSIVENESS AND HELPFULNESS OF SPANISH SURNAMED AND ANGLO SURNAMED SUBJECTS, 96 MALE AND FEMALE PERSONS PICKED AT RANDOM FROM THE TELEPHONE BOOK WERE CALLED BY SOMEONE WHO WANTED TO SPEAK TO A PHARMACY AND WHO HAD APPARENTLY REACHED A WRONG NUM-BER. NEED OF THE CALLER AND SURNAME OF THE SUBJECT WERE NOT DIRECTLY RELATED TO AGGRESSIVENESS, BUT SPANISH SUR-NAMED SUBJECTS WERE LESS AGGRESSIVE TO A DESPERATE CONFEDERATE (C) AND AN-GLO SUBJECTS TO A NONDESPERATE C. THERE WAS ALSO A TENDENCY FOR SUBJECTS TO BE MORE AGGRESSIVE TOWARD A CALLER WITH A SPANISH ACCENT AND TO BECOME LESS AG-GRESSIVE TO ANGLO CALLERS AS THE CALL PROGRESSED. NO SEX DIFFERENCES ON ANY MEASURES WERE FOUND, BUT MORE WOMEN IN THE SPANISH SURNAMED HOUSEHOLDS AND MORE MEN IN THE ANGLO HOUSEHOLDS ANSWERED THE PHONE. MOREOVER, ANGLO SURNAMED INDIVIDUALS REQUESTED TO LOOK UP A PHONE NUMBER WERE MORE LIKELY TO COMPLY WITH THE CALLER'S REQUEST THAN

SPANISH SURNAMED INDIVIDUALS. 10 REFER-
ENCES. (AUTHOR SUMMARY MODIFIED)
ACCN   000639

758 AUTH **HARTIGAN, R. R.**
TITL   A TEMPORAL-SPATIAL CONCEPT SCALE: A DE-
VELOPMENTAL STUDY.
SRCE   *JOURNAL OF CLINICAL PSYCHOLOGY, 1971,
27(2), 221-223.*
INDX   COGNITIVE DEVELOPMENT, BILINGUAL, MEXI-
CAN AMERICAN, CROSS CULTURAL, TEST RE-
LIABILITY, TEST VALIDITY, EMPIRICAL, RE-
SEARCH METHODOLOGY, PERCEPTION,
CHILDREN, MIDWEST, EAST, PUERTO RICAN-M,
URBAN
ABST   A REVISION OF THE TEMPORAL-SPATIAL CON-
CEPT SCALE WITH AN INCREASED NUMBER
AND RANGE OF QUESTIONS WAS ADMINIS-
TERED TO A SAMPLE OF 2,383 PAROCHIAL
SCHOOL CHILDREN. TWENTY-THREE PERCENT
OF THE SAMPLE WERE MEXICAN AMERICAN,
6.7 PERCENT PUERTO RICAN, .3 PERCENT
BLACK, AND 70 PERCENT ANGLO AMERICAN.
THE TEMPORAL-SPATIAL CONCEPT SCALE
YIELDS THREE SCORES: PART I, LATERALITY;
PART II, SPACE; AND PART III, TIME. NORMS FOR
GRADES 3 THROUGH 12 ARE PRESENTED. A
COMPARISON IS MADE OF THE PERFORM-
ANCES OF AN INNER CITY SAMPLE AND A SUB-
URBAN SAMPLE, OF A MONOLINGUAL AND A
BILINGUAL MEXICAN AMERICAN SAMPLE, AND
OF A MIDWESTERN AND AN EAST COAST
SAMPLE. 4 REFERENCES.
ACCN   000640

759 AUTH **HARWOOD, A.**
TITL   RX: SPIRITIST AS NEEDED. A STUDY OF A
PUERTO RICAN COMMUNITY MENTAL HEALTH
RESOURCE.
SRCE   *NEW YORK: JOHN WILEY & SONS, INC., 1977.*
INDX   ESPIRITISMO, PUERTO RICAN-M, EMPIRICAL,
DEMOGRAPHIC, CASE STUDY, FOLK MEDICINE,
ADULTS, PSYCHOTHERAPY, SURVEY, RE-
SOURCE UTILIZATION, ROLE EXPECTATIONS,
PSYCHOTHERAPY OUTCOME, NEW YORK, EAST,
URBAN, THEORETICAL, BOOK
ABST   THE ETIOLOGICAL AND NOSOLOGICAL SYS-
TEM UNDERLYING SPIRITIST THERAPY, THE
KINDS OF PROBLEMS BROUGHT TO ITS THERA-
PISTS, THEIR TREATMENT PROCEDURES, AND
OTHER INFORMATION PERTINENT TO THE UN-
DERSTANDING OF THEIR ACTIVITIES IN COM-
MUNITY HEALTH ARE EXAMINED. THE STUDY
WAS CONDUCTED IN A SECTOR OF NEW YORK
CITY HAVING A HIGH CONCENTRATION OF
PUERTO RICANS. THE INTENT OF THE INVESTI-
GATION WAS TO ASSIST PUERTO RICAN COM-
MUNITY LEADERS AND THOSE INVOLVED IN
COMMUNITY HEALTH PROGRAMS ASSESS EX-
ISTING RESOURCES AND ALSO PROVIDE A
SOURCE OF INFORMATION ESSENTIAL TO
PROFESSIONALS WORKING WITH PUERTO RI-
CAN PATIENTS. THE FIRST PART OF THE BOOK
PRESENTS GENERAL DEMOGRAPHIC DATA OF
THE AREA. THIS IS FOLLOWED BY THE CEN-
TRAL TOPIC WHICH PERTAINS TO THE IDE-
OLOGY, SOCIAL ORGANIZATION, AND RITUAL
PROCEDURES OF SPIRITISM, DISCUSSION OF

SPIRITIST DIAGNOSIS, TREATMENT OF PSY-
CHOLOGICAL AND SOCIAL PROBLEMS, AND
THE EVERYDAY USE OF SPIRITIST CONCEPTS
AND RITUALS BY PUERTO RICANS. THE CON-
CLUDING SECTION DEALS WITH TWO CRUCIAL
ISSUES: (1) THE PRACTICAL CONCERN WITH
THE POSSIBLE RELATIONSHIPS BETWEEN SPI-
RITISTS AND HEALTH FACILITIES; AND (2) THE
PHILOSOPHICAL PROBLEM OF THE NATURE OF
HEALING. THE APPENDIX DISCUSSES THE SE-
LECTION AND TRAINING OF COMMUNITY RE-
SEARCHERS WHO WORKED ON THIS PROJECT.
171 REFERENCES. (AUTHOR SUMMARY MODI-
FIED)
ACCN   000641

760 AUTH **HAUGHT, B. F.**
TITL   THE LANGUAGE DIFFICULTY OF SPANISH
AMERICAN CHILDREN.
SRCE   *JOURNAL OF APPLIED PSYCHOLOGY, 1931,
15(1), 92-95.*
INDX   INTELLIGENCE, INTELLIGENCE TESTING, SPAN-
ISH SURNAMED, BILINGUALISM, LINGUISTIC
COMPETENCE, CHILDREN, ADOLESCENTS, EM-
PIRICAL, NEW MEXICO, SOUTHWEST
ABST   THIS COMPARISON OF INTELLIGENCE QUO-
TIENTS ACROSS CHRONOLOGICAL AGE AT-
TEMPTS TO PROVIDE INFORMATION ON DE-
GREES OF LANGUAGE DIFFICULTY FOUND IN
SPANISH AMERICAN (SA) CHILDREN. ALL SA
CHILDREN WERE FROM FOUR SCHOOL SYS-
TEMS, RANGED IN AGE FROM 7 TO 19, AND
WERE IN GRADES 1 TO 12. THE PINTNER-CUN-
NINGHAM MENTAL TEST (PCMT) WAS USED IN
GRADES 1 TO 3, THE NATIONAL INTELLIGENCE
TEST (NIT) IN GRADES 4 TO 7, AND THE TER-
MAN GROUP TESTS OF MENTAL ABILITY
(TGTMA) IN GRADES 8 TO 12. IT WAS HYPOTHE-
SIZED THAT A LANGUAGE HANDICAP ENCOUN-
TERED IN TAKING AN IQ TEST SHOULD DE-
CREASE AS CHILDREN BECOME OLDER AND
BECOME BETTER ACQUAINTED WITH THE EN-
GLISH LANGUAGE. DATA INDICATE THAT THE
IQ OF SA CHILDREN DECREASED WITH
CHRONOLOGICAL AGE. THERE WAS A SUDDEN
DROP IN IQ SCORES AT ABOUT 10 YEARS OF
AGE. SINCE THE OLDER CHILDREN WERE
HANDICAPPED AS MUCH AS THE YOUNGER,
THERE SEEMED TO BE NO JUSTIFICATION FOR
ASSIGNING THE DIFFICULTY TO AN INABILITY
TO USE OR UNDERSTAND ENGLISH. UNTIL THE
EXISTENCE OF A LANGUAGE HANDICAP IN SA
CHILDREN IS DEMONSTRATED BY PROPERLY
CONTROLLED EXPERIMENTS, IT SEEMS SAFE
TO AVOID USING THE CONCEPT AS AN EX-
PLANATORY PRINCIPLE IN EDUCATIONAL
PROBLEMS.
ACCN   000642

761 AUTH **HAUSER, R. W., & FEATHERMAN, D.**
TITL   EQUALITY OF SCHOOLING: TRENDS AND
PROSPECTS.
SRCE   *SOCIOLOGY OF EDUCATION, 1976, 49(2), 99-
120.*
INDX   SES, EDUCATION, CROSS GENERATIONAL,
SPANISH SURNAMED, FAMILY STRUCTURE, DE-
MOGRAPHIC, EMPIRICAL, EMPLOYMENT, ENVI-
RONMENTAL FACTORS, ECONOMIC FACTORS

ABST DATA DRAWN FROM THE 1962 AND 1973 OCCUPATIONAL CHANGES IN A GENERATION SURVEYS INDICATE THAT AS EDUCATIONAL ATTAINMENT AMONG U.S. MEN BORN 1901-1951 INCREASED, ITS VARIABILITY HAS DECREASED AND THE LENGTH OF SCHOOLING HAS BECOME MORE EQUALLY DISTRIBUTED. THE SURVEYS, WHICH WERE CARRIED OUT IN CONJUNCTION WITH THE CURRENT POPULATION SURVEY, REVEAL THAT INTERGENERATIONAL DIFFERENCES IN SCHOOLING ARE LARGER THAN THREE YEARS IN SOME COHORTS, BUT THESE DIFFERENCES MAY BE DECLINING, AND THE PERIOD OF RAPID INCREASE IN LEVELS OF SCHOOLING APPEARS TO BE ENDING. THE DISADVANTAGES ASSOCIATED WITH FARM BACKGROUND, BROKEN FAMILIES, SOUTHERN BIRTH, BLACK SKIN, AND SPANISH ORIGIN APPEAR TO BE DECLINING AS FAR AS EDUCATIONAL ATTAINMENT IS CONCERNED, BUT FACTORS ASSOCIATED WITH POORLY EDUCATED OR LOW STATUS FATHERS AND WITH LARGE FAMILIES HAVE PERSISTED. FAMILY ORIGINS CONSISTENTLY EXPLAIN AT LEAST 55% OF THE VARIANCE IN SCHOOLING, AND PERHAPS AS MUCH AS 70%. SINCE THE END OF WORLD WAR II, SCHOOLING OF PARENTS HAS CONTINUED TO INCREASE, IMPLYING A CONTINUING DEMAND FOR INCREASED SCHOOLING IN FUTURE YEARS. 27 REFERENCES. (JOURNAL ABSTRACT MODIFIED)

ACCN 002108

762 AUTH **HAWKES, G. R., TAYLOR, M., & BASTIAN, B. E.**
TITL PATTERNS OF LIVING IN CALIFORNIA'S MIGRANT FAMILIES (RESEARCH MONOGRAPH NO. 12).
SRCE *UNIVERSITY OF CALIFORNIA AT DAVIS, DEPARTMENT OF APPLIED BEHAVIORAL SCIENCES, 1973. (ERIC DOCUMENT REPRODUCTION SERVICE NO. ED 107 359)*
INDX FAMILY STRUCTURE, MEXICAN AMERICAN, FARM LABORERS, MIGRATION, SES, FAMILY ROLES, POVERTY, CHILDREARING PRACTICES, FEMALE, MEXICAN, SURVEY, MIGRANTS, CALIFORNIA, SOUTHWEST, EMPIRICAL

ABST THIS REPORT PRESENTS A STUDY OF THE LIVING PATTERNS OF CALIFORNIA'S MIGRANT LABOR FAMILIES, ONE PART OF A NATIONAL STUDY ON THE IDENTIFICATION OF LIFE PATTERNS AMONG RELATIVELY DISADVANTAGED FAMILIES. DATA WERE COLLECTED FROM 169 INTERVIEWS WITH HOMEMAKERS RANDOMLY SELECTED FROM 12 STATE-OWNED MIGRANT CAMPS IN CALIFORNIA. THE INTERVIEWS CONSISTED OF FIXED ALTERNATIVE QUESTIONS IN THE FOLLOWING AREAS: (1) NEIGHBORING PRACTICES (SOCIAL INTERACTION); (2) INCOME INDEX; (3) STEADINESS OF INCOME; (4) KINSHIP ORIENTATION; (5) FAMILY ORIENTATION; (6) FAMILY COHESIVENESS; (7) PARENTAL PERMISSIVENESS; (8) MARITAL SATISFACTION; AND (9) VALUE ORIENTATIONS TO EDUCATION AND EMPLOYMENT. SOME GENERAL FINDINGS IN EACH OF THESE AREAS ARE EXAMINED. 3 REFERENCES. (RIE ABSTRACT)

ACCN 000643

763 AUTH **HAWKES, G. R., & TAYLOR, M.**
TITL POWER STRUCTURE IN MEXICAN AND MEXICAN-AMERICAN FARM LABOR FAMILIES.
SRCE *JOURNAL OF MARRIAGE AND THE FAMILY, 1975, 3(4), 807-811.*
INDX FAMILY ROLES, SEX ROLES, CULTURAL FACTORS, RURAL, FARM LABORERS, MIGRATION, ACCULTURATION, MEXICAN AMERICAN, EMPIRICAL, SURVEY, MEXICAN, MIGRANTS, CALIFORNIA, SOUTHWEST, FEMALE, AUTHORITARIANISM

ABST TO DETERMINE THE VALIDITY OF THE COMMONLY HELD VIEW OF HUSBAND DOMINANCE IN MEXICAN AND MEXICAN AMERICAN FAMILIES, STANDARDIZED INTERVIEWS WERE CONDUCTED WITH 76 MEXICAN AND MEXICAN AMERICAN FEMALES, AGES 16 TO 65. SUBJECTS RESIDED IN 12 CALIFORNIA STATE-OWNED AND OPERATED MIGRANT FAMILY CAMPS. RESULTS INDICATE THAT EGALITARIANISM WAS BY FAR THE MOST COMMOM MODE IN BOTH DECISION MAKING AND ACTION TAKING. FINDINGS SUGGEST EITHER THAT DOMINANCE-SUBMISSION PATTERNS ARE MUCH LESS UNIVERSAL THAN PREVIOUSLY ASSUMED, THAT THEY NEVER EXISTED BUT WERE AN IDEAL, OR THAT THESE PATTERNS ARE UNDERGOING RADICAL CHANGE. 9 REFERENCES. (PASAR ABSTRACT)

ACCN 000644

764 AUTH **HAYDEN, R. G.**
TITL SPANISH AMERICANS OF THE SOUTHWEST: LIFE STYLE PATTERNS AND THEIR IMPLICATIONS.
SRCE *WELFARE IN REVIEW, 1966, 4(10), 20.*
INDX FAMILY STRUCTURE, FAMILY ROLES, SPANISH SURNAMED, ESSAY, EQUAL OPPORTUNITY, BILINGUAL-BICULTURAL EDUCATION, BILINGUAL-BICULTURAL PERSONNEL, SOCIAL MOBILITY, POLICY, SOCIAL SERVICES, POVERTY, DISCRIMINATION, ETHNIC IDENTITY, CULTURAL PLURALISM, SOUTHWEST

ABST EQUAL OPPORTUNITY FOR SPANISH AMERICANS DEPENDS UPON THE EDUCATIONAL SYSTEM AND THE SOCIAL WELFARE SYSTEM BEING ABLE TO MEET THE NEEDS OF THIS POPULATION. SPANISH AMERICANS HAVE REFUSED TO ASSIMILATE INTO THE ANGLO AMERICAN MAINSTREAM AND HAVE THUS BEEN CONSISTENTLY DENIED ACCESS TO THE REWARDS CONSIDERED OBTAINABLE IN THE DOMINANT CULTURE. ANGLOS TEND TO IGNORE THE VALUE ORIENTATIONS OF THE SPANISH-SPEAKING PEOPLES IN THE SOUTHWEST WHO PLACE STRONG EMPHASIS ON LOYALTY TO THEIR CULTURAL HERITAGE AND LANGUAGE. UNLESS THE MEANS FOR SOCIOECONOMIC MOBILITY BECOME AVAILABLE TO THESE PEOPLE, THEY WILL CONTINUE THEIR LIFE OF POVERTY AND DISCRIMINATION. ONLY BY DEVELOPING PROGRAMS THAT REFLECT A BICULTURAL-BILINGUAL CHARACTERISTIC CAN ANGLOS BECOME BETTER SENSITIZED TO THE NEEDS OF THE HISPANIC COMMUNITY, THEREBY GENERATING EQUALITY OF OPPORTUNITY TO THIS GROWING MINORITY. 50 REFERENCES.

ACCN 000645

765 AUTH **HAYES-BAUTISTA, D. E.**

TITL MODIFYING THE TREATMENT: PATIENT COM-PLIANCE, PATIENT CONTROL AND MEDICAL CARE.

SRCE *SOCIAL SCIENCE AND MEDICINE, 1976, 10, 233-238.*

INDX ADULTS, CONFLICT RESOLUTION, FEMALE, HEALTH DELIVERY SYSTEMS, MEXICAN AMERI-CAN, PHYSICIANS, CALIFORNIA, SOUTHWEST, HEALTH, ESSAY, DYADIC INTERACTION, INTER-PERSONAL RELATIONS

ABST A THEORETICAL MODEL, GROUNDED IN THE EXPERIENCE OF ABOUT 200 SAN FRANCISCO BAY AREA CHICANO PATIENTS (PRIMARILY WOMEN), OF PATIENT NON-COMPLIANCE AS A MEANS OF ASSERTING CONTROL IN A PATIENT-PRACTITIONER RELATIONSHIP IN ORDER TO OBTAIN SATISFACTION WITH THE TREATMENT IS PRESENTED. THE NEED TO MODIFY THE TREATMENT ARISES WHEN IT APPEARS TO THE PATIENT THAT THE ORIGINAL TREATMENT IS NOT TOTALLY APPROPRIATE. THE PATIENT MAY RELY UPON CONVINCING TACTICS (THE DE-MAND, THE DISCLOSURE, THE SUGGESTION AND THE LEADING QUESTION) TO BRING HER CONCERN TO THE PRACTITIONER'S ATTEN-TION IN ORDER THAT HE MIGHT MODIFY THE TREATMENT. THE PATIENT MAY ALSO TAKE MATTERS INTO HER OWN HANDS AND USE COUNTERING TACTICS TO MODIFY THE TREAT-MENT HERSELF. THESE MAY BE OF THE AUG-MENTATION TYPE (SIMPLE AND ADDITIVE) OR OF THE DIMINISHMENT TYPE (SIMPLE AND SUBTRACTIVE). CONVINCING AND COUNTER-ING TACTICS MAY BE USED SEQUENTIALLY OR SIMULTANEOUSLY. WHEN A PRACTITIONER IS AWARE OF HER MODIFICATION ATTEMPTS, HE MAY BE PERCEIVED TO RESORT TO COUNTER-MANAGEMENT TACTICS TO NEUTRALIZE HER OWN ACTIONS. THESE TACTICS MAY BE THE OVERWHELMING KNOWLEDGE, THE MEDICAL THREAT, THE DIRECT DISCLOSURE, AND THE PERSONAL FRIEND. BARGAINING OCCURS, EITHER UNILATERALLY OR BILATERALLY, DUR-ING WHICH EACH PARTY TRIES FOR A SETTLE-MENT IN WHICH THE TREATMENT ACTION OF ONE IS AT LEAST HONORED, IF NOT ADOPTED OUTRIGHT, BY THE OTHER. IF THE BARGAINING ENDS TO THE SATISFACTION OF BOTH, A DE-SIRE TO MAINTAIN THE RELATIONSHIP DEVEL-OPS. IF EITHER OR BOTH PARTIES ARE DISSAT-ISFIED WITH THE RESULT OF THE BARGAINING, THE RELATIONSHIP BECOMES STRAINED AND TERMINATION BECOMES LIKELY. 41 REFER-ENCES. (AUTHOR ABSTRACT)

ACCN 002337

766 AUTH **HAYES-BAUTISTA, D. E.**

TITL THE RELATION BETWEEN CHICANO FREE CLIN-ICS AND THE LARGER HEALTH CARE MATRIX: THE MYTH OF THE 'FREE' CLINIC.

SRCE *IN J. L. SCHWARTZ (ED.), FREE MEDICAL CLIN-ICS: INNOVATIONS IN HEALTH CARE DELIVERY. WASHINGTON, D.C.: U.S. GOVERNMENT PRINT-ING OFFICE, 1973, PP. 12-21.*

INDX HEALTH DELIVERY SYSTEMS, COMMUNITY, MEXICAN AMERICAN, ESSAY, HEALTH, FINANC-ING, POLICY, PARAPROFESSIONALS, CALIFOR-NIA, SOUTHWEST, PROGRAM EVALUATION

ABST THE STRUCTURE OF FREE CLINICS AND THEIR RELATIONSHIPS TO THE LARGER HEALTH CARE SYSTEM ARE DISCUSSED. SINCE 1967 WHEN THE FIRST FREE CLINIC OPENED ITS DOORS, HUNDREDS OF FREE CLINICS HAVE OPERATED ACROSS THE COUNTRY. HOWEVER, MOST CLINICS HAVE NOT TAKEN THE TIME TO EVALU-ATE THEIR OWN STRUCTURE, THEIR PLACE IN THE OVERALL HEALTH DELIVERY SYSTEM OF THE COUNTRY, AND THE IMPLICATIONS OF BOTH FOR THE SURVIVAL OF FREE CLINICS. MAJOR POINTS EMPHASIZED ARE: (1) THE PARASITIC VS. SYMBIOTIC RELATIONSHIP OF FREE CLINICS TO THE LARGER HEALTH MA-TRIX; (2) THE FREE CLINIC'S LACK OF AUTON-OMY AND INDEPENDENCE; (3) THE ROLE OF FREE CLINICS IN POOR AND MINORITY COM-MUNITIES; (4) THE SOURCES OF MANPOWER, MATERIALS AND FINANCES FOR FREE CLINICS; AND (5) THE ROLE OF GOODWILL, PROFES-SIONAL VOLUNTEERS AND COMMUNITY VOL-UNTEERS IN CLINIC OPERATION. THE HISTORY OF CHICANO FREE CLINICS IN THE SAN FRAN-CISCO BAY AREA IS USED IN ILLUSTRATING THESE POINTS. ALTERNATIVES FOR STABILIZ-ING FREE CLINIC STAFF AND SERVICES WITH-OUT BECOMING "CARBON COPIES" OF THE IN-STITUTIONALIZED, BUREAUCRATIC HEALTH SYSTEM ARE SUGGESTED.

ACCN 000647

767 AUTH **HAYES-BAUTISTA, D. E.**

TITL TERMINATION OF THE PATIENT-PRACTIONER RELATIONSHIP: DIVORCE, PATIENT STYLE.

SRCE *JOURNAL OF HEALTH AND SOCIAL BEHAVIOR, 1976, 17(1), 12-21.*

INDX PSYCHOTHERAPY, MEXICAN AMERICAN, MEN-TAL HEALTH PROFESSION, SOCIAL SERVICES, PSYCHOSOCIAL ADJUSTMENT, ROLE EXPEC-TATIONS, PSYCHOTHERAPY OUTCOME, THEO-RETICAL, REVIEW, DYADIC INTERACTION

ABST THE EXPERIENCES OF ABOUT 200 URBAN CHI-CANO PATIENTS WERE ANALYZED WITH RE-SPECT TO THE TERMINATION OF THE RELA-TIONSHIP BETWEEN PATIENT AND PRACTITIONER. TERMINATION MAY BE PATIENT ORIGINATED, PRACTITIONER ORIGINATED, OR THE RESULT OF OVERRIDING CONDITIONS. EACH TERMINATION POSSESSES COMBINA-TIONS OF THE PROPERTIES OF DESIRABILITY, DURATION, CLOSURE, AND ANTICIPATION. PA-TIENT ORIGINATED TERMINATION RESULTS FROM ABSOLUTE PRACTITIONER INADE-QUACY, CHANGE IN PRACTITIONER'S COMPE-TENCY, AND/OR COMPARISON WITH ANOTHER PRACTITIONER'S COMPETENCY. PRACTI-TIONER ORIGINATED TERMINATION IS DUE TO THE PATIENT'S UNWILLINGNESS TO COMPLY WITH THE PRACTITIONER'S REGIMEN OR TO THE PRACTITIONER'S SELF-RECOGNIZED IN-ABILITY TO HANDLE AN EPISODE. TERMINA-TION ITSELF MAY BE ACHIEVED BY TACTICS SUCH AS MUTUAL WITHDRAWAL, CONFRON-TATION, OR FADE OUT. THE PARTY BEING TER-MINATED MAY RESORT TO PROLONGING TAC-TICS. OVERRIDING CONDITIONS MAY

FRUSTRATE THE TERMINATION OR MAKE IT IN-
EVITABLE. SOME HYPOTHESES RESULTING
FROM THE STUDY ARE OFFERED, BUT NOT
TESTED. 26 REFERENCES. (JOURNAL AB-
STRACT MODIFIED)

ACCN   000648

768 AUTH   **HAYNER, N. S.**
    TITL   THE FAMILY IN MEXICO.
    SRCE   *MARRIAGE AND FAMILY LIVING, 1954, 16, 369-373.*
    INDX   FAMILY STRUCTURE, FAMILY ROLES, EMPIRI-
            CAL, MEXICAN, MEXICO, SEXUAL BEHAVIOR,
            SEX ROLES, BIRTH CONTROL, SES, CULTURAL
            CHANGE, MARITAL STABILITY, RURAL, URBAN,
            MARRIAGE, CULTURAL FACTORS
    ABST   COURTSHIP AND MARITAL AND MATE SELEC-
            TION PRACTICES IN MEXICAN SOCIETY ARE
            DISCUSSED WITH REGARD TO RURAL, URBAN
            AND CLASS DIFFERENCES. STRICT RULES
            BASED ON RELIGIOUS AND CLASS STAN-
            DARDS GOVERN MALE-FEMALE PREMARITAL
            RELATIONS. BEGINNING WITH THE 1910 REVO-
            LUTION, HOWEVER, THERE HAVE BEEN SOME
            CHANGES IN WOMEN'S ROLES REGARDING
            COURTSHIP PRACTICES AND EMPLOYMENT
            OUTSIDE THE HOME; THE WOMEN'S BASIC IN-
            TERESTS, THOUGH, ARE STILL HOME AND
            CHILDREN. BECAUSE OF PREVAILING DOUBLE
            STANDARDS, THE MALE RETAINS HIS DOMI-
            NANT POSITION AS EVIDENCED BY THE CAS-
            UAL ATTITUDES TOWARDS HIS SEXUAL INFI-
            DELITIES. CHANGES OCCURRING IN MARRIAGE
            AND COURTSHIP ARE PRIMARILY AMONG THE
            MIDDLE CLASS. RURAL VILLAGERS, IN CON-
            TRAST TO URBAN POOR, HAVE A HIGHER PER-
            CENTAGE OF LEGAL MARRIAGES AND TRADI-
            TIONAL COURTSHIP PRACTICES. UPPER-CLASS
            MEXICANS REMAIN MORE TRADITIONAL THAN
            THE MIDDLE CLASS WHICH IS EXPERIENCING
            THE MOST CHANGES IN THIS REGARD. THE
            SMALL INCIDENCE OF DIVORCE IS EXPLAINED
            AS A REFLECTION OF MALE DOMINANCE, BOTH
            IN COURTS OF LAW AND THE FAMILY. CONTRA-
            CEPTIVE METHODS ARE BELIEVED TO BE UTI-
            LIZED, BUT MOSTLY AMONG THE HIGHER SO-
            CIAL CLASSES. FINALLY, URBAN CIVILIZATION
            IS SEEN AS HAVING POWERFUL INFLUENCE ON
            INCOMING RURAL MIGRANTS, LEADING TO IN-
            CREASED FAMILY MALADJUSTMENT. 2 REFER-
            ENCES.
    ACCN   000649

769 AUTH   **HAYNER, N. S.**
    TITL   NOTES ON THE CHANGING MEXICAN FAMILY.
    SRCE   *AMERICAN SOCIOLOGICAL REVIEW, 1942, 7, 489-497.*
    INDX   MEXICAN, FAMILY STRUCTURE, CULTURE, ES-
            SAY, SEX ROLES, SES, RURAL, URBAN, CUL-
            TURAL CHANGE, REVIEW, FAMILY ROLES
    ABST   MEXICO HAS A STRONG FAMILY TRADITION,
            AND ANYTHING THAT TENDS TO DESTROY THE
            BASIC PATTERN OF DOMESTIC RELATIONSHIP
            MEETS WITH OPPOSITION, ESPECIALLY IN THE
            RURAL DISTRICTS AND SMALL TOWNS. UNDER
            THE INFLUENCE OF INDUSTRIALIZATION, THE
            OPENING OF NEWLY PAVED HIGHWAYS, THE
            POPULARITY OF AMERICAN MOVIES, AND THE

EXPANSION OF PUBLIC EDUCATION, NEW
PROBLEMS ARE BEING CREATED. IN VIEW OF
THESE CHANGES, IT IS PREDICTED THAT MEXI-
CAN MARRIAGE AND FAMILY LIFE WILL BE-
COME LESS AUTHORITARIAN AND MORE
DEMOCRATIC. 13 REFERENCES. (AUTHOR
SUMMARY MODIFIED)

ACCN   000650

770 AUTH   **HEALEY, G. W., & DEBLASSIE, R. R.**
    TITL   A COMPARISON OF NEGRO, ANGLO AND SPAN-
            ISH-AMERICAN ADOLESCENT'S SELF CON-
            CEPTS.
    SRCE   *ADOLESCENCE, 1974, 9(33), 15-24.*
    INDX   SELF CONCEPT, CROSS CULTURAL, ADOLES-
            CENTS, SEX COMPARISON, SES, EMPIRICAL,
            SPANISH SURNAMED, NEW MEXICO, SOUTH-
            WEST
    ABST   IN ORDER TO DETERMINE (1) IF DIFFERENCES
            EXIST IN THE SELF-CONCEPT OF BLACK, AN-
            GLO AND SPANISH SURNAMED ADOLESCENTS
            AND (2) THE EXTENT TO WHICH DIFFERENCES
            ARE INFLUENCED BY ETHNICITY, SEX OR SO-
            CIOECONOMIC POSITION OR THE INTERAC-
            TION AMONG THESE VARIABLES, 607 ADOLES-
            CENTS WERE ADMINISTERED THE TENNESSEE
            SELF-CONCEPT SCALE (TSCS) AND A DEMO-
            GRAPHIC QUESTIONNAIRE. THE SUBJECTS' (425
            ANGLO, 40 BLACK AND 142 SPANISH AMERI-
            CAN 9TH GRADE STUDENTS FROM SOUTHCEN-
            TRAL NEW MEXICO) SCORES ON THE 14 TSCS
            MEASURES OF SELF-CONCEPT ARE ANALYZED
            BY A FIXED MODEL, THREE-WAY CLASSIFICA-
            TION OF VARIANCE. AN ETHNICITY X SEX X SES
            FACTORIAL DESIGN ANALYSIS INDICATED THAT
            SIX OF THE FOURTEEN MEASURES WERE SIG-
            NIFICANTLY INFLUENCED BY ONE OR MORE OF
            THE INDEPENDENT VARIABLES. THE EIGHT
            MEASURES NOT AFFECTED BY THE INDEPEN-
            DENT VARIABLES WERE TOTAL POSITIVE SCORE,
            IDENTITY, BEHAVIOR, PERSONAL SELF, FAMILY
            SELF, VARIABILITY SCORE, DISTRIBUTION
            SCORE AND TOTAL CONFLICT SCORE. SPAN-
            ISH AMERICAN STUDENTS HAD THE HIGHEST
            SCORES ON SELF-SATISFACTION, FOLLOWED
            BY BLACKS AND THEN ANGLOS. SPANISH
            AMERICANS ALSO HAD THE HIGHEST SCORES
            ON THE MORAL ETHICAL SELF SCALES, FOL-
            LOWED BY ANGLOS, THEN BLACKS. IT IS POS-
            ITED THAT THE BLACK AND SPANISH AMERI-
            CAN TOTAL POSITIVE SCORES WERE PROBABLY
            HIGHER THAN EXPECTED (NO SIGNIFICANT
            DIFFERENCE WITH ANGLOS) BECAUSE THE
            TWO ETHNIC GROUPS RESPONDED SIGNIFI-
            CANTLY HIGHER THAN ANGLOS ON THE DE-
            FENSIVE SCALE. SES WAS FOUND TO INFLU-
            ENCE SOCIAL SELF AND SELF-SATISFACTION
            SCALES. PHYSICAL SELF WAS SIGNIFICANTLY
            AFFECTED BY SEX DIFFERENCES. RESULTS DO
            NOT SUPPORT THE HYPOTHESIS THAT SELF-
            CONCEPT SCORES VARY ACROSS SES AND
            WITHIN ETHNIC GROUPS. 18 REFERENCES.
    ACCN   000651

771 AUTH   **HEATH, L. L., ROPER, B. S., & KING, C. D.**
    TITL   A RESEARCH NOTE ON CHILDREN VIEWED AS
            CONTRIBUTORS TO MARITAL STABILITY: THE

RELATIONSHIP TO BIRTH CONTROL USE, IDEAL AND EXPECTED FAMILY SIZE.

SRCE   *JOURNAL OF MARRIAGE AND THE FAMILY, 1974, 36(2), 304-306.*

INDX   MARITAL STABILITY, BIRTH CONTROL, MEXICAN AMERICAN, ATTITUDES, SEXUAL BEHAVIOR, CROSS CULTURAL, EMPIRICAL, SOUTHWEST, ADULTS, FERTILITY

ABST   A TRI-ETHNIC STUDY OF ANGLOS, BLACKS AND CHICANOS WAS CONDUCTED TO DETERMINE THE RELATIONSHIP BETWEEN THE PERCEIVED CONTRIBUTIONS OF CHILDREN TO MARITAL STABILITY, THE USE OF CONTRACEPTIVE TECHNIQUES, AND DESIRED AND EXPECTED FAMILY SIZE. ONE HUNDRED TWENTY RESPONDENTS WITH EQUAL REPRESENTATION FROM THE THREE ETHNIC GROUPS WERE INTERVIEWED. THE FINDINGS INDICATE THAT: (1) BLACKS AND CHICANOS RATED CHILDREN AS A SIGNIFICANTLY GREATER AID TO MARITAL STABILITY THAN ANGLOS; (2) BELIEF IN CHILDREN AS CONTRIBUTORS TO MARITAL STABILITY WAS SIGNIFICANTLY RELATED TO IDEAL AND EXPECTED FAMILY SIZE—THOSE WHO VIEWED CHILDREN AS A POSITIVE CONTRIBUTION TO THE MARRIAGE HAD SIGNIFICANTLY LARGER IDEAL AND EXPECTED FAMILY SIZES THAN THOSE WHO DID NOT; AND (3) CONTRACEPTIVE USE WAS NOT DIRECTLY RELATED TO THE RESPONDENTS' ATTITUDES ABOUT CHILDREN AND MARITAL STABILITY. IT IS SUGGESTED THAT THE DIFFERENCES IN FAMILY SIZE ORIENTATION ARE A STRONG INDICATION THAT ATTITUDES TOWARD CHILDREN DO PLAY A SIGNIFICANT ROLE IN DETERMINING FERTILITY OUTCOMES. A MORE EXTENSIVE STUDY IS RECOMMENDED TO EXAMINE THE RELATIONSHIP OF THESE ATTITUDINAL VARIABLES AS THEY RELATE TO FERTILITY. 4 REFERENCES.

ACCN   000652

772 AUTH   **HEIMAN, E. M.**
TITL   THE ROLE OF THE PSYCHIATRIST IN A NEIGHBORHOOD HEALTH CENTER.
SRCE   *HOSPITAL AND COMMUNITY PSYCHIATRY, 1974, 25(7), 470-472.*
INDX   PSYCHOTHERAPY, MENTAL HEALTH PROFESSION, MENTAL HEALTH, HEALTH DELIVERY SYSTEMS, PSYCHOTHERAPISTS, SES, MEXICAN AMERICAN, ESSAY, ARIZONA, SOUTHWEST, CASE STUDY, PROFESSIONAL TRAINING

ABST   A DESCRIPTION AND EVALUATION OF THE ROLE OF THE PSYCHIATRIST AT THE EL RIO SANTA CRUZ NEIGHBORHOOD HEALTH CENTER IN TUCSON IS PRESENTED. HIS ACTIVITIES CONSIST OF: (1) CONSULTATION TO THE CENTER'S HEALTH CARE TEAMS; (2) TEACHING OF MENTAL HEALTH CONCEPTS AND REVIEW OF CASES WITH PSYCHIATRIC ASPECTS AT THE CENTER; (3) INITIATION OF SEMINARS FOR CENTER STAFF MEMBERS AND OTHER COMMUNITY PROFESSIONALS ON ASPECTS OF MENTAL HEALTH SERVICES TO THE POOR; AND (4) PLANNING OF CENTER SERVICES. THE RELATIONSHIP OF THE PSYCHIATRIST AND MENTAL HEALTH SERVICES TO THE NEIGHBORHOOD HEALTH CENTER AND TO HEALTH MAINTENANCE ORGANIZATIONS IS ALSO DISCUSSED.

ACCN   000653

773 AUTH   **HEIMAN, E. M., BURRUEL, G., & CHAVEZ, N.**
TITL   FACTORS DETERMINING EFFECTIVE PSYCHIATRIC OUTPATIENT TREATMENT FOR MEXICAN-AMERICANS.
SRCE   *HOSPITAL AND COMMUNITY PSYCHIATRY, 1975, 26(8), 515-517.*
INDX   PRIMARY PREVENTION, ENVIRONMENTAL FACTORS, BILINGUAL-BICULTURAL PERSONNEL, HEALTH EDUCATION, MASS MEDIA, PSYCHOTHERAPY, RESOURCE UTILIZATION, ESSAY, MEXICAN AMERICAN, MENTAL HEALTH, PROGRAM EVALUATION, COMMUNITY INVOLVEMENT, HEALTH DELIVERY SYSTEMS, ARIZONA, SOUTHWEST, POLICY

ABST   LA FRONTERA, A MENTAL HEALTH OUTPATIENT CLINIC SERVING THE TUCSON AREA, OPERATES UNDER PATIENT ORIENTED GUIDELINES WHICH HAVE RESULTED IN INCREASED SERVICE TO THE MEXICAN AMERICAN (MA) POPULATION. FACTORS IDENTIFIED AS DETERMINANTS IN EFFECTIVE OUTPATIENT TREATMENT FOR MA'S ARE DISCUSSED. (1) THE MENTAL HEALTH CENTER SHOULD BE CENTRALLY LOCATED IN THE MA COMMUNITY. (2) IT SHOULD HAVE A BICULTURAL AND BILINGUAL STAFF. (3) AN INFORMAL ATMOSPHERE WITH A MINIMUM OF BUREAUCRATIC PROCEDURES IS MOST CONDUCIVE TO TREATMENT. (4) THE CENTER'S SERVICES SHOULD BE PUBLICIZED IN A WAY THAT MINIMIZES THE STIGMATIZATION OF MENTAL ILLNESS, PROMOTES PREVENTIVE CARE, AND DEMONSTRATES THAT STAFF UNDERSTOOD MA PROBLEMS. A CASE STUDY ILLUSTRATES THE TREATMENT APPROACH USED BY LA FRONTERA STAFF.

ACCN   000654

774 AUTH   **HEIMAN, E. M., & KAHN, M. W.**
TITL   MENTAL HEALTH PATIENTS IN A BARRIO HEALTH CENTER.
SRCE   *INTERNATIONAL JOURNAL OF SOCIAL PSYCHIATRY, 1976, 21(3), 197-204.*
INDX   SES, MEXICAN AMERICAN, POVERTY, MENTAL HEALTH, RESOURCE UTILIZATION, EMPIRICAL, COMMUNITY INVOLVEMENT, PSYCHOTHERAPY, SYMPTOMATOLOGY, ARIZONA, SOUTHWEST

ABST   UTILIZATION BY MEXICAN AMERICANS OF MENTAL HEALTH FACILITIES IN A BARRIO AREA NEIGHBORHOOD HEALTH CENTER IN TUCSON, ARIZONA, AND DEMOGRAPHIC AND SYMPTOM CHARACTERISTICS OF THIS POPULATION ARE INVESTIGATED. CONTRARY TO OTHER STUDIES, THIS DESCRIPTIVE SURVEY INDICATES (1) THAT THE MENTAL HEALTH PROGRAM IS ABLE TO REACH A HIGH RISK MEXICAN AMERICAN POPULATION FREQUENTLY MISSED BY MENTAL HEALTH PROGRAMS, AND (2) THAT THE MEXICAN AMERICAN PATIENTS COMING TO THIS MENTAL HEALTH PROGRAM ARE IN MANY WAYS SIMILAR TO GENERAL POPULATION USING NON-BARRIO CLINICS (I.E., MOST PATIENTS ARE FEMALES, AGES 20-40, WITH FAMILY PROBLEMS AND SYMPTOMS OF DEPRESSION). REASONS FOR THE MENTAL HEALTH PROGRAM'S SUC-

CESS ARE IDENTIFIED AS (1) ITS INTEGRATION WITHIN THE NEIGHBORHOOD HEALTH CARE SETTING, (2) ITS LARGE PROPORTION OF SPANISH-SPEAKING AND LOCAL PERSONNEL, AND (3) ITS OUTREACH EFFORTS. REASONS WHY THE PROGRAM IS FAILING TO REACH MEXICAN AMERICAN CHILDREN AND ADULT MALES ARE DISCUSSED. 18 REFERENCES. (AUTHOR ABSTRACT MODIFIED)

ACCN   000655

775 AUTH   **HEIMAN, E. M., & KAHN, M. W.**
    TITL   MEXICAN-AMERICAN & EUROPEAN-AMERICAN PSYCHOPATHOLOGY AND HOSPITAL COURSE.
    SRCE   *ARCHIVES OF GENERAL PSYCHIATRY, 1977, 34(2), 167-170.*
    INDX   PSYCHOPATHOLOGY, CULTURAL FACTORS, SEX COMPARISON, SES, CROSS CULTURAL, MEXICAN AMERICAN, DEMOGRAPHIC, EMPIRICAL, ARIZONA, SOUTHWEST
    ABST   DEMOGRAPHIC INFORMATION, REASON FOR ADMISSION, MENTAL STATUS ON ADMISSION, HOSPITAL COURSE VARIABLES, AND DISCHARGE DIAGNOSIS DATA WERE COLLECTED FOR 99 PATIENTS ADMITTED CONSECUTIVELY TO THE PSYCHIATRIC INPATIENT UNIT OF A COMMUNITY MENTAL HEALTH CENTER SERVING A LOW-INCOME POPULATION WITH A LARGE PROPORTION OF MEXICAN AMERICANS. PATIENT ETHNIC DISTRIBUTION REFLECTED THAT OF THE CATCHMENT AREA. ALTHOUGH ETHNICITY, SEX, AND SOCIAL CLASS EACH SHOWED DISTINCT CHARACTERISTICS, WHEN ANY TWO OF THE FACTORS WERE HELD CONSTANT, ONLY THREE VARIABLES MAINTAINED SIGNIFICANCE. THESE WERE (1) AGITATED MENTAL STATUS, (2) USE OF ANTI-DEPRESSANT MEDICATION DURING HOSPITALIZATION AND, (3) SPEAKING OPENLY DURING HOSPITAL TREATMENT. NONE OF THESE INDICATED SEVERE, FLAMBOYANT PSYCHOPATHOLOGY. THIS STUDY DOES NOT SUPPORT EARLIER REPORTS THAT HOSPITALIZED MEXICAN AMERICANS ARE MORE SEVERELY DISTURBED THAN OTHER ETHNIC GROUPS. 4 REFERENCES. (JOURNAL ABSTRACT)

ACCN   000656

776 AUTH   **HELLER, C. A.**
    TITL   REGIONAL PATTERNS OF DIETARY DEFICIENCY: SPANISH AMERICANS OF NEW MEXICO AND ARIZONA.
    SRCE   *AMERICAN ACADEMY OF POLITICAL AND SOCIAL SCIENCE, 1943, 225, 49-51.*
    INDX   NUTRITION, POVERTY, SES, PHYSICAL DEVELOPMENT, SPANISH SURNAMED, EMPIRICAL, NEW MEXICO, ARIZONA, SOUTHWEST, HEALTH, ECONOMIC FACTORS
    ABST   THE SPANISH AMERICANS OF NEW MEXICO AND ARIZONA ADHERE CLOSELY TO A LIMITED FOOD PATTERN WHICH DOES NOT MEET THEIR NUTRITIONAL REQUIREMENTS SATISFACTORILY. THE DIET IS LIMITED TO CORN, BEANS, CHILI PEPPERS, LARD, FLOUR, AND COFFEE. GREENS ARE USED IN SOME IRRIGATED AREAS, BUT ONLY DURING THE GROWING SEASON. THE ECONOMIC STATUS OF THE SPANISH AMERICAN TODAY DOES NOT ALLOW FOR AN EXTENSIVE NUTRITIONAL DIET. AN ANALYSIS OF MOST FREQUENTLY FOUND DIETS IN SPANISH AMERICAN HOMES SHOWS THE FOLLOWING: (1) THEY ARE LOW IN CALORIES; (2) THEY ARE LOW IN PROTEIN, BOTH IN KIND AND AMOUNT; (3) CALCIUM IS ALSO LOW; (4) THE DIET IS ADEQUATE IN IRON; AND (5) THE DIET LACKS IN VITAMINS A AND C BUT IS ADEQUATE IN VITAMIN B. IT IS NOT SURPRISING, THEREFORE, THAT NEW MEXICO AND ARIZONA WOULD HAVE INFANT MORTALITY RATES OF OVER 100 PER 100,000. THIS IS NEARLY TWICE THOSE OF THE SOUTHERN STATES. EDUCATION IN THE NEWER KNOWLEDGE OF NUTRITION AND FOOD PREPARATION IS UNDOUBTEDLY AN IMPORTANT FACTOR IN IMPROVING THE PRESENT-DAY DIET OF THE SPANISH PEOPLE OF THE SOUTHWEST. THE MOST IMPORTANT FACTOR, HOWEVER, IS INCOME. 3 REFERENCES.

ACCN   000657

777 AUTH   **HELM, J. (ED.)**
    TITL   SPANISH SPEAKING PEOPLE IN THE UNITED STATES. PROCEEDINGS OF THE 1968 ANNUAL MEETING OF THE AMERICAN ETHNOLOGICAL SOCIETY.
    SRCE   *SEATTLE: UNIVERSITY OF WASHINGTON PRESS, 1968.*
    INDX   PROCEEDINGS, MEXICAN AMERICAN, SES, ACCULTURATION, DEMOGRAPHIC, MIGRATION, URBAN, CHILDREN, FOLK MEDICINE, CORRECTIONS, POLITICAL POWER, POLITICS, COMMUNITY, SOCIAL SCIENCES, ECONOMIC FACTORS, SPANISH SURNAMED, BOOK
    ABST   A DIVERSE AND COMPREHENSIVE COLLECTION OF 13 PAPERS ON THE SPANISH-SPEAKING POPULATION OF THE UNITED STATES IS PRESENTED. INCLUDED ARE BOTH EMPIRICAL STUDIES AND ESSAYS WRITTEN BY RECOGNIZED AUTHORS AS WELL AS GRADUATE STUDENTS. TOPICS INCLUDE SAMPLING IN ANTHROPOLOGICAL RESEARCH, POLITICAL AND ECONOMIC REFORM IN NEW MEXICO, AND CHILDREN'S PERCEPTIONS OF LIFE IN URBAN BARRIOS. THESE PAPERS ILLUSTRATE THE RANGE AND DEPTH OF CURRENT ETHNOGRAPHIC STUDIES ON THE SPANISH-SPEAKING POPULATION IN THIS COUNTRY.

ACCN   000658

778 AUTH   **HELMS, L.**
    TITL   MEXICAN-AMERICANS.
    SRCE   *JOURNAL OF THE AMERICAN COLLEGE HEALTH ASSOCIATION, 1974, 22(4), 269-271.*
    INDX   MENTAL HEALTH, HEALTH, ATTITUDES, CULTURAL FACTORS, HEALTH DELIVERY SYSTEMS, ESSAY, PSYCHOTHERAPY, FOLK MEDICINE, CURANDERISMO, MEXICAN AMERICAN, PHYSICIANS, RESOURCE UTILIZATION
    ABST   MEXICAN AMERICAN ATTITUDES TOWARDS PHYSICAL AND MENTAL HEALTH ARE DISCUSSED. CULTURAL BELIEFS AND LACK OF ADEQUATE MEDICAL CARE DUE TO POVERTY CONTRIBUTE TO THE PRACTICE OF FAMILY TREATMENT. SOME ILLNESSES ARE PERCIEVED AS HAVING SUPERNATURAL ORIGINS, WHICH ARE OFTEN CURED BY FOLK HEALING METH-

ODS. WITCHCRAFT IS BELIEVED TO BE A MAJOR CAUSE OF MANY DISEASES. AMONG THE LOWER CLASS MEXICAN AMERICANS, THERE IS A TENDENCY TO MISTRUST PHYSICIANS AND RELY ON THE CURANDERO. AS CURANDEROS ARE UTILIZED WITH MORE CONFIDENCE THAN PHYSICIANS, FOLK HEALING METHODS ARE OFTEN MORE SUCCESSFUL IN THE TREATMENT OF MENTAL ILLNESS THAN PSYCHOTHERAPY. CULTURAL VALUES AND BELIEFS OF MEXICAN AMERICANS MUST BE UNDERSTOOD AND RESPECTED IN ORDER FOR SOCIETY TO EFFECTIVELY DEAL WITH THIS POPULATION.

ACCN   000659

779 AUTH   **HENDERSON, R. W.**
     TITL   ENVIRONMENTAL PREDICTORS OF ACADEMIC PERFORMANCE OF DISADVANTAGED MEXICAN-AMERICAN CHILDREN.
     SRCE   *JOURNAL OF CONSULTING AND CLINICAL PSYCHOLOGY, 1972, 38(2), 297.*
     INDX   ACHIEVEMENT TESTING, READING, BILINGUAL, ENVIRONMENTAL FACTORS, ACHIEVEMENT MOTIVATION, EDUCATIONAL COUNSELING, MODELING, EDUCATION, ATTITUDES, SCHOLASTIC ACHIEVEMENT, MEXICAN AMERICAN, CHILDREN, EMPIRICAL, RESEARCH METHODOLOGY, ARIZONA, SOUTHWEST
     ABST   TO DETERMINE INTERRELATIONSHIPS BETWEEN ENVIRONMENTAL PROCESS VARIABLES (EPV'S) AND ACADEMIC PERFORMANCE AMONG 35 MEXICAN AMERICAN (MA) THIRD-GRADE CHILDREN, SUBJECTS WERE ADMINISTERED THE CALIFORNIA READING TEST (CRT) AS A CRITERION MEASURE FOR ACADEMIC ACHIEVEMENT. SIGNIFICANT CORRELATIONS BETWEEN CRT SCORES AND THE EPV MEASURES ARE AS FOLLOWS: ACHIEVEMENT PRESS, LANGUAGE MODELS, ACADEMIC GUIDANCE, ACTIVENESS OF FAMILY, RANGE OF SOCIAL INTERACTION, INTELLECTUALITY IN THE HOME, IDENTIFICATION WITH MODELS, AND PERCEIVED VALUE OF EDUCATION. THE RELATIONSHIP BETWEEN CRT SCORES AND EPV WORK HABITS IN FAMILY DID NOT ACHIEVE SIGNIFICANCE. THESE RESULTS DEMONSTRATE THE PREDICTIVE RELATIONSHIP BETWEEN ENVIRONMENTAL MEASURES TAKEN WHEN A SAMPLE OF MA CHILDREN ENTERED THE FIRST GRADE AND THEIR PERFORMANCE ON A READING ACHIEVEMENT TEST AT THE END OF THIRD-GRADE. THE ENVIRONMENTAL MEASURES DEVELOPED IN THIS INVESTIGATION MAY PROVE PRACTICAL AND APPROPRIATE FOR USE BY PSYCHOLOGISTS ENGAGED IN FAMILY COUNSELING OR PARENTAL EDUCATION. 3 REFERENCES.
     ACCN   000660

780 AUTH   **HENDERSON, R. W.**
     TITL   ENVIRONMENTAL STIMULATION AND INTELLECTUAL DEVELOPMENT OF MEXICAN-AMERICAN CHILDREN: AN EXPLORATORY PROJECT.
     SRCE   *TUCSON: UNIVERSITY OF ARIZONA, 1966. (ERIC DOCUMENT REPRODUCTION SERVICE NO. ED 010 587)*
     INDX   EARLY CHILDHOOD EDUCATION, EDUCATION, COGNITIVE DEVELOPMENT, MEXICAN AMERICAN, CHILDREN, ENVIRONMENTAL FACTORS, PARENTAL INVOLVEMENT, EMPIRICAL, BILINGUAL, ARIZONA, SOUTHWEST
     ABST   THE RELATIONSHIP BETWEEN SPECIFIC ENVIRONMENTAL (SUBCULTURAL) FACTORS AND THE DEVELOPMENT OF INTELLECTUAL ABILITIES OF MEXICAN AMERICANS WAS STUDIED. THE SAMPLE CONSISTED OF 80 FIRST GRADERS AND THEIR FAMILIES. ASSIGNMENTS INTO EITHER A HIGH POTENTIAL GROUP OR A LOW POTENTIAL GROUP WERE MADE BY COMPOSITE SCORES OBTAINED ON THE VAN ALSTYNE PICTURE-VOCABULARY TEST AND THE GOODENOUGH-HARRIS DRAWING TEST. INTERVIEWS WERE THEN CONDUCTED WITH THE MOTHERS OF THE SUBJECTS AND TRANSCRIBED. RATING SCALES WERE USED TO MEASURE 33 CHARACTERISTICS, RELATING TO A SET OF NINE ENVIRONMENTAL PROCESS VARIABLES. AN INDEX OF STATUS CHARACTERISTICS WAS COMPUTED FOR EACH FAMILY, AND ENVIRONMENTAL RATINGS OF FAMILY LIFE WERE OBTAINED. THE CHILDREN IN THE HIGH POTENTIAL GROUP WERE FOUND TO COME FROM BACKGROUNDS THAT OFFERED A GREATER VARIETY OF STIMULATING EXPERIENCES THAN WERE AVAILABLE TO MOST CHILDREN IN THE LOW POTENTIAL GROUP. IN ADDITION, HIGH POTENTIAL CHILDREN SCORED SIGNIFICANTLY HIGHER ON VOCABULARY TESTS IN BOTH ENGLISH AND SPANISH. FURTHER RESEARCH WAS SUGGESTED TO BE BASED ON OBSERVATION RATHER THAN INTERVIEW REPORTS AND TO FOCUS IN GREATER DEPTH ON A NARROWER RANGE OF VARIABLES IN A STUDY OF INTELLECTUAL DEVELOPMENT. 56 REFERENCES. (RIE ABSTRACT MODIFIED)
     ACCN   000661

781 AUTH   **HENDERSON, R. W., BERGAN, J. R., & HURT, M. JR.**
     TITL   DEVELOPMENT AND VALIDATION OF THE HENDERSON ENVIROMENTAL LEARNING PROCESS SCALE.
     SRCE   *JOURNAL OF SOCIAL PSYCHOLOGY, 1972, 88(2), 185-196.*
     INDX   ENVIRONMENTAL FACTORS, RESEARCH METHODOLOGY, SES, POVERTY, CROSS CULTURAL, LINGUISTIC COMPETENCE, SCHOLASTIC ACHIEVEMENT, EDUCATION, ATTITUDES, STANFORD ACHIEVEMENT TEST
     ABST   THE HENDERSON ENVIRONMENTAL LEARNING PROCESS SCALE (HELPS) WAS DEVELOPED AS A MEASURE OF CHARACTERISTICS OF HOME ENVIRONMENTS. THE INSTRUMENT WAS ADMINISTERED TO THE MOTHERS OF 60 LOWER-SOCIOECONOMIC MEXICAN AMERICAN AND 66 MIDDLE-SOCIOECONOMIC ANGLO FIRST GRADERS. ITEMS WERE GENERATED TO ELICIT RESPONSES RELATING TO THE VARIABLES OF ASPIRATION LEVEL, ENVIRONMENTAL STIMULATION, MODELS, GUIDANCE, REINFORCEMENT, AND TOTAL SCORE. THE STANFORD EARLY ACHIEVEMENT TEST (SEAT) AND THE BOEHM TEST OF BASIC CONCEPTS (BTBC) WERE ADMINISTERED TO ALL CHILDREN TO DETERMINE THE PREDICTIVE VALIDITY OF THE HELPS. A FACTOR ANALYSIS OF THE HELPS IN-

DICATED THAT THE SCALE CONSISTED OF FIVE FACTORS: I, EXTENDED INTERESTS AND COMMUNITY INVOLVEMENT; II, VALUING LANGUAGE AND SCHOOL RELATED BEHAVIOR; III, INTELLECTUAL GUIDANCE; IV, PROVIDING A SUPPORTIVE ENVIRONMENT FOR SCHOOL LEARNING; AND V, ATTENTION. FURTHER ANALYSES WITH THE SEAT AND BTBC AS CRITERION VARIABLES INDICATED THAT FACTORS I, II, IV, AND V WERE SIGNIFICANTLY RELATED TO ACADEMIC ACHIEVEMENT. IT IS SUGGESTED THAT THERE IS A NEED TO MAKE MEMBERS OF LOWER-SOCIOECONOMIC GROUPS MORE AWARE OF THE POSSIBILITY OF EDUCATION AS A VEHICLE FOR ATTAINING THE REWARDS AVAILABLE IN SOCIETY. 22 REFERENCES.

ACCN   000662

782 AUTH   **HENDERSON, R. W., & GARCIA, A. B.**
     TITL   THE EFFECTS OF A PARENT TRAINING PROGRAM ON THE QUESTION-ASKING BEHAVIOR OF MEXICAN-AMERICAN CHILDREN.
     SRCE   *AMERICAN EDUCATIONAL RESEARCH JOURNAL, 1973, 10(3), 193-201.*
     INDX   PARENTAL INVOLVEMENT, MODELING, BEHAVIOR MODIFICATION, CLASSROOM BEHAVIOR, EMPIRICAL, MEXICAN AMERICAN, CHILDREN, MOTHER-CHILD INTERACTION, ARIZONA, SOUTHWEST
     ABST   MOTHERS OF MEXICAN AMERICAN FIRST GRADERS WERE DIVIDED INTO FOUR GROUPS ACCORDING TO THE SOLOMON DESIGN. EXPERIMENTAL MOTHERS WERE TRAINED TO USE MODELING, CUEING, AND REINFORCEMENT TO INFLUENCE THEIR FIRST GRADERS' QUESTION-ASKING; CONTROL MOTHERS WERE NOT. THE EFFECTS OF TREATMENT ON THE CHILD'S BASELINE QUESTION-ASKING LEVEL AND ABILITY TO LEARN FROM EXAMINER INSTRUCTION WERE EXAMINED BY ADMINISTERING A MEASURE TO THE CHILDREN, PRE- AND POST-PARENT TRAINING. THEIR QUESTION-ASKING WAS ASSESSED DURING THREE CONDITIONS: BASELINE, EXAMINER INSTRUCTION ON QUESTION-ASKING, AND GENERALIZATION. POST-TREATMENT ASSESSMENT REVEALED THAT THE QUESTION-ASKING OF BOTH EXPERIMENTAL AND CONTROL SUBJECTS INCREASED SIGNIFICANTLY IN RESPONSE TO INSTRUCTION PROVIDED BY AN EXAMINER WHO MODELED QUESTION-ASKING BEHAVIOR. EXPERIMENTAL SUBJECTS ASKED SIGNIFICANTLY MORE QUESTIONS THAN CONTROL SUBJECTS ACROSS ALL THREE POST-TREATMENT MEASUREMENT CONDITIONS (BASELINE, INSTRUCTION, AND GENERALIZATION). 19 REFERENCES. (JOURNAL ABSTRACT)

ACCN   000663

783 AUTH   **HENDERSON, R. W., & MERRITT, C. B.**
     TITL   ENVIRONMENTAL BACKGROUND OF MEXICAN AMERICAN CHILDREN WITH DIFFERENT POTENTIALS FOR SCHOOL SUCCESS.
     SRCE   *JOURNAL OF SOCIAL PSYCHOLOGY, 1968, 75(1), 101-106.*
     INDX   ENVIRONMENTAL FACTORS, SCHOLASTIC ACHIEVEMENT, SCHOLASTIC ASPIRATIONS,

CHILDREN, MEXICAN AMERICAN, EMPIRICAL, SES, ARIZONA, SOUTHWEST
     ABST   AN INVESTIGATION OF A WIDE RANGE OF ENVIRONMENTAL STIMULI IN THE BACKGROUND OF MEXICAN AMERICAN (MA) CHILDREN HAVING A HIGH OR LOW POTENTIAL FOR SUCCESS IN SCHOOL IS DESCRIBED. SUBJECTS WERE 38 HIGH-POTENTIAL AND 42 LOW-POTENTIAL MA FIRST-GRADE STUDENTS. HOME ENVIRONMENTS WERE STUDIED BY INTERVIEWING THE MOTHERS OF THE SUBJECTS. INTERVIEW TRANSCRIPTS WERE RATED ON NINE ENVIRONMENTAL VARIABLES, AND GROUP DIFFERENCES WERE TESTED FOR SIGNIFICANCE WITH A MULTIVARIATE ANALYSIS. IT WAS FOUND THAT CHILDREN IN THE HIGH-POTENTIAL GROUP CAME FROM BACKGROUNDS THAT OFFERED A GREATER VARIETY OF STIMULATING EXPERIENCES THAN WERE AVAILABLE TO THOSE CHILDREN IN THE LOW-POTENTIAL GROUP. LOW-POTENTIAL CHILDREN CAME FROM LARGER FAMILIES THAN DID HIGH-POTENTIAL CHILDREN. THE TWO GROUPS WERE ALSO COMPARED ON A SERIES OF SOCIOLOGICAL FACTORS THAT REVEALED SOME SIGNIFICANT SIMILARITIES AND DIFFERENCES BETWEEN THE GROUPS. FOR EXAMPLE, "PRESENCE OF EXTENDED FAMILY" SEEMS TO BE MOST TYPICAL OF MA FAMILIES REGARDLESS OF SOCIOECONOMIC LEVEL. RELATED SIMILARITIES WERE OBSERVED FOR "PREFER RELATIVES AS ASSOCIATES," TRAVEL TO VISIT KIN," AND "VALUE FAMILY LIFE." IT IS CONCLUDED THAT THE PRESCHOOL ENVIRONMENTS OF THE HIGH-POTENTIAL CHILDREN INCLUDE A GREATER VARIETY OF INTELLECTUALLY STIMULATING EXPERIENCES THAN DO THE PRESCHOOL ENVIRONMENTS OF THE LOW-POTENTIAL GROUP. 13 REFERENCES.

ACCN   000664

784 AUTH   **HENDERSON, R. W., & RANKIN, R. J.**
     TITL   WPPSI RELIABILITY AND PREDICTIVE VALIDITY WITH DISADVANTAGED MEXICAN-AMERICAN CHILDREN.
     SRCE   *JOURNAL OF SCHOOL PSYCHOLOGY, 1973, 11(1), 16-20.*
     INDX   INTELLIGENCE TESTING, EMPIRICAL, TEST RELIABILITY, TEST VALIDITY, CHILDREN, SCHOLASTIC ACHIEVEMENT, METROPOLITAN READING READINESS TEST, ARIZONA, SOUTHWEST, MEXICAN AMERICAN
     ABST   THE RELIABILITY AND PREDICTIVE VALIDITY OF THE WECHSLER PRESCHOOL AND PRIMARY SCALE OF INTELLIGENCE (WPPSI) WAS INVESTIGATED WITH 49 LOWER-SOCIOECONOMIC SCALE MEXICAN AMERICAN CHILDREN. RELIABILITY WAS DETERMINED USING SPLIT-HALF PROCEDURES PARALLEL TO THOSE REPORTED IN THE TEST MANUAL. PREDICTIVE VALIDITY WAS DETERMINED BY CORRELATING WPPSI SCORES WITH SCORES FROM THE METROPOLITAN READING TEST. RESULTS REVEAL THAT THE WPPSI HAS HIGH RELIABILITY AS DETERMINED BY INTERNAL CONSISTENCY PROCEDURES, BUT THAT VALIDITY COEFFICIENTS WERE NOT SIGNIFICANT. IT IS SUGGESTED

THAT THE WPPSI MAY BE INAPPROPRIATE FOR SPECIAL PROGRAM PLACEMENT PURPOSES WITH THIS POPULATION. 4 REFERENCES. (PASAR ABSTRACT MODIFIED)

ACCN   000665

785 AUTH   **HENGGELER, S. W., & TAVORMINA, J. B.**
    TITL   STABILITY OF PSYCHOLOGICAL ASSESSMENT MEASURES FOR CHILDREN OF MEXICAN AMERICAN MIGRANT WORKERS.
    SRCE   *HISPANIC JOURNAL OF BEHAVIORAL SCIENCES, 1979, 1(3), 263-270.*
    INDX   CHILDREN, MIGRANTS, VIRGINIA, SOUTH, EMPIRICAL, TEST VALIDITY, WISC, TEST RELIABILITY, INTELLIGENCE TESTING, PERSONALITY ASSESSMENT, LOCUS OF CONTROL, SELF CONCEPT, PEABODY PICTURE-VOCABULARY TEST, MEXICAN AMERICAN, ACHIEVEMENT TESTING, GOODENOUGH DRAW-A-MAN TEST
    ABST   THE ONE-YEAR STABILITIES OF SEVERAL WELL-STANDARDIZED INTELLECTUAL, EDUCATIONAL, AND PERSONALITY TESTS WERE EVALUATED ON A GROUP OF 15 CHILDREN OF MEXICAN AMERICAN MIGRANT FARM WORKERS LIVING IN VIRGINIA DURING THE FULL HARVEST SEASON. THE TESTS INCLUDED (1) THE WECHSLER INTELLIGENCE SCALE FOR CHILDREN—REVISED (WISC-R), (2) THE PEABODY PICTURE-VOCABULARY TEST (PPVT), (3) THE GOODENOUGH-HARRIS DRAW-A-PERSON TEST (DAP), (4) THE WIDE-RANGE ACHIEVEMENT TEST (WRAT), (5) THE PIERS-HARRIS CHILDREN'S SELF-CONCEPT SCALE, AND (6) THE LOCUS OF CONTROL SCALE FOR CHILDREN. THE TEST BATTERY WAS ADMINISTERED AND THEN READMINISTERED ONE YEAR LATER UNDER ALMOST IDENTICAL CONDITIONS. MOST OF THE STABILITY COEFFICIENTS OBSERVED FOR THE INTELLECTUAL INDICES (I.E., THE WISC-R, PPVT, DAP) WERE STATISTICALLY SIGNIFICANT AND WERE SIMILAR TO THOSE REPORTED FOR THEIR NORMATIVE SAMPLES. HOWEVER, THE STABILITY OF THE OTHER TESTS WAS VERY LOW. SUCH FINDINGS DEMONSTRATE THE IMPORTANCE OF ESTABLISHING TEST STABILITY BEFORE CONDUCTING VALIDATION STUDIES. IT IS RECOMMENDED THAT FURTHER EVALUATION OF THE VALIDITY OF THESE TESTS FOR SPANISH-SPEAKING/SURNAMED GROUPS BE CONDUCTED. 18 REFERENCES. (JOURNAL ABSTRACT MODIFIED)
    ACCN   001768

786 AUTH   **HENSEY, F.**
    TITL   GRAMMATICAL VARIABLES IN SOUTHWESTERN AMERICAN SPANISH.
    SRCE   *LINGUISTICS: AN INTERNATIONAL REVIEW, 1973, 108, 5-26.*
    INDX   MEXICAN AMERICAN, BILINGUALISM, GRAMMAR, EMPIRICAL, LINGUISTICS, RESEARCH METHODOLOGY, TEXAS, SOUTHWEST, COLLEGE STUDENTS
    ABST   LINGUISTIC STUDIES OF MEXICAN AMERICAN SPEECH COMMUNITIES TEND TO CONCENTRATE ON LEXICON, WITH EMPHASIS ON ARCHAISMS AND ANGLICISMS OR PHONOLOGY. GRAMMAR STUDIES, IN THE SENSE OF MORPHO-SYNTAX, ARE POORLY REPRESENTED IN SOCIOLINGUISTIC LITERATURE. THERE ARE SEVERAL REASONS WHY GRAMMATICAL STUDIES ARE RARE; ONE IS THE LACK OF A CLEAR-CUT NOTION OF HOW GRAMMATICAL VARIABLES CAN BE RECOGNIZED, COUNTED AND CORRELATED WITH OTHER LINGUISTIC OR SOCIOECONOMIC TRAITS OF THE INFORMANTS. THIS STUDY ATTEMPTS TO IDENTIFY GRAMMATICAL VARIABLES PERTINENT TO THE SPANISH OF EL PASO, TEXAS. A REPRESENTATIVE CROSS-SECTION OF GRAMMATICAL DEVIATIONS FOUND IN 365 ESSAYS WRITTEN BY INFORMANTS AT THE UNIVERSITY OF TEXAS AT EL PASO WERE ANALYZED. MOST OF THE INFORMANTS WERE YOUNG PEOPLE FROM THE CITY AND SURROUNDING AREAS WHO WERE CLASSIFIED AS MEXICAN AMERICAN OR CHICANO. DATA TREATMENT WAS LIMITED TO (1) ESTABLISHING A TAXONOMY OF INSTANCES OF USAGE WHICH WILL INCLUDE POTENTIAL GRAMMATICAL VARIABLES, AND (2) ANALYZING A FEW OF THE COMMONEST INSTANCES IN TERMS OF CURRENT LINGUISTIC THEORY. THE MOST COMMON DEVIATIONS FOUND WERE IN NOUN AND VERB PHRASES AND IN TRANSFORMATIONS. THE POSSIBLE USE OF THESE DEVIATIONS AS GRAMMATICAL VARIABLES IN FUTURE STUDIES IS DISCUSSED. 19 REFERENCES.

ACCN   000666

787 AUTH   **HERAS, I., & NELSON, K. E.**
    TITL   RETENTION OF SEMANTIC, SYNTACTIC, AND LANGUAGE INFORMATION BY YOUNG BILINGUAL CHILDREN.
    SRCE   *PSYCHONOMIC SCIENCE, 1972, 29(6B), 391-393.*
    INDX   BILINGUALISM, SYNTAX, SEMANTICS, LANGUAGE ACQUISITION, CHILDREN, SPANISH SURNAMED, EMPIRICAL, LINGUISTIC COMPETENCE, CALIFORNIA, SOUTHWEST
    ABST   TWENTY BILINGUAL 5 YEAR-OLDS WERE READ STORIES IN ENGLISH AND SPANISH. USING VARIANTS OF THE SECOND SENTENCE IN EACH STORY, RECOGNITION MEMORY WAS TESTED FOR SEMANTIC AND SYNTACTIC INFORMATION. THE CHILDREN WERE ALSO ASKED TO IDENTIFY THE LANGUAGE OF THE THIRD SENTENCE IN EACH STUDY. THE DATA INDICATE THAT THE CHILDREN SUCCESSFULLY CODED AND REMEMBERED SENTENCES IN TERMS OF MEANING BUT RAPIDLY FORGOT DETAILS OF SYNTACTIC FORM. CODING BY LANGUAGE (SPANISH OR ENGLISH) FOR THE THIRD SENTENCE WAS FORGOTTEN IF FOLLOWED BY MATERIAL IN THE ALTERNATE LANGUAGE. 9 REFERENCES.
    ACCN   000667

788 AUTH   **HERNANDEZ, D.**
    TITL   MEXICAN AMERICAN CHALLENGE TO A SACRED COW (MONOGRAPH NO. 1).
    SRCE   *LOS ANGELES: UNIVERSITY OF CALIFORNIA, AZTLAN PUBLICATIONS, 1970.*
    INDX   REVIEW, DISCRIMINATION, RESEARCH METHODOLOGY, CULTURE, CULTURAL FACTORS, EDUCATION, ATTITUDES, SCHOLASTIC ASPIRA-

TIONS, ACHIEVEMENT MOTIVATION, MEXICAN AMERICAN

ABST TWO RESEARCH STUDIES ARE CRITICALLY RE-VIEWED: THE FIRST BY A. J. SCHWARTZ, "COM-PARATIVE VALUES AND ACHIEVEMENT OF MEX-ICAN AMERICAN AND ANGLO PUPILS" (1969) AND THE SECOND BY C. W. GORDON AND A. J. SCHWARTZ, "EDUCATIONAL ACHIEVEMENT AND ASPIRATIONS OF MEXICAN AMERICAN YOUTH IN A METROPOLITON CONTEXT" (1968). IT IS EMPHASIZED THAT THE STUDIES ERR IN CAUSALLY RELATING CULTURAL VALUES OF MEXICAN AMERICAN PUPILS TO THEIR LOW ACADEMIC ACHIEVEMENT IN THE PUBLIC SCHOOLS. IF THESE STUDIES ARE ACCEPTED AT FACE VALUE THEY, ALONG WITH MANY PRE-VIOUS SIMILAR STUDIES ON MEXICAN AMERI-CAN STUDENTS, MAY ADVERSELY AFFECT EDU-CATIONAL ATTITUDES AND POLICIES. ARGUMENTS SUPPORTING THESE CONCLU-SIONS ARE MADE REGARDING THE STUDIES' (1) RESEARCH BIAS, (2) INADEQUATE AND IN-APPROPRIATE THEORETICAL FRAMEWORK, AND (3) INAPPROPRIATE AND SUBJECTIVE SURVEY TECHNIQUES. 42 REFERENCES.

ACCN 000668

789 AUTH **HERNANDEZ, J. L.**
TITL THE PERCEPTIONS OF STUDENTS AND PAR-ENTS TOWARD COLLEGE ADVISEMENT WITH IMPLICATIONS FOR MEXICAN AMERICANS (DOCTORAL DISSERTATION, UNIVERSITY OF SOUTHERN CALIFORNIA, 1973).
SRCE *DISSERTATION ABSTRACTS INTERNATIONAL, 1974, 34(9), 5660A. (UNIVERSITY MICROFILMS NO. 74-5864.)*
INDX EDUCATIONAL COUNSELING, CROSS CUL-TURAL, MEXICAN AMERICAN, ADULTS, PAREN-TAL INVOLVEMENT, SELF CONCEPT, ATTITUDES, CULTURAL FACTORS, EMPIRICAL, SCHOLASTIC ASPIRATIONS, HIGHER EDUCATION, CALIFOR-NIA, SOUTHWEST
ABST TO ASCERTAIN PERCEPTUAL DIFFERENCES OF COLLEGE ADVISEMENT BETWEEN MEXICAN AMERICANS AND NON-MEXICAN AMERICANS, A QUESTIONNAIRE WAS ADMINISTERED TO 100 NON-MEXICAN AMERICAN AND 30 MEXICAN AMERICAN HIGH SCHOOL STUDENTS AS WELL AS THE MEXICAN AMERICAN PARENTS IN SAN JOSE, CALIFORNIA. THE INSTRUMENT SCHED-ULE CONSISTED OF 35 ITEMS REGARDING ETHNICITY, SOCIOECONOMIC STATUS, ACCUL-TURATION, PARENTAL INFLUENCE, SELF-PER-CEPTION, AND COLLEGE ADVISEMENT. FIND-INGS WERE AS FOLLOWS: (1) MEXICAN AMERICAN STUDENTS PERCEIVED THE AD-VISEMENT PROCESS AS SATISFACTORY; (2) MEXICAN AMERICAN STUDENTS HAD A MORE POSITIVE ATTITUDE TOWARD ADVISEMENT THAN DID THEIR PARENTS OR NON-MEXICAN AMERI-CAN STUDENTS; (3) MEXICAN AMERICANS FELT THEY HAD FREER ACCESS TO COUNSELORS; (4) MEXICAN AMERICANS FELT THEIR MOTH-ERS WERE MORE INTERESTED IN THEIR EDU-CATION WHILE NON-MEXICAN AMERICAN STU-DENTS BELIEVED BOTH OF THEIR PARENTS WERE INTERESTED IN THEIR EDUCATION; AND (5) MEXICAN AMERICAN STUDENTS WERE MORE

INDECISIVE THAN THE OTHER STUDENTS ABOUT FUTURE PLANS CONCERNING COL-LEGE. IT IS RECOMMENDED THAT CONTINUING EDUCATION BE EXPANDED IN THE MEXICAN AMERICAN COMMUNITY, THAT AWARENESS OF SELF-IMAGE AS INFLUENCING EDUCATIONAL MOTIVATION MUST BECOME A CONCERN FOR TEACHERS, COUNSELORS, AND ADMINISTRA-TORS, AND A COMMUNITY SCHOOL CONCEPT SHOULD BE ENCOURAGED FOR THE MEXICAN AMERICAN POPULATION SO AS TO PROVIDE FAMILIARITY WITH THE EDUCATIONAL PRO-CESS. 116 REFERENCES. (AUTHOR ABSTRACT MODIFIED)

ACCN 000669

790 AUTH **HERNANDEZ, J., ESTRADA, L., & ALVIREZ, D.**
TITL CENSUS DATA AND THE PROBLEM OF CON-CEPTUALLY DEFINING THE MEXICAN AMERI-CAN POPULATION.
SRCE *SOCIAL SCIENCE QUARTERLY, 1973, 53(4), 671-687.*
INDX CENSUS, RESEARCH METHODOLOGY, SES, DE-MOGRAPHIC, ETHNIC IDENTITY, SPANISH SUR-NAMED, MEXICAN AMERICAN
ABST TO CLARIFY THE VARIOUS METHODS USED BY THE U.S. BUREAU OF THE CENSUS TO CON-CEPTUALIZE AND ENUMERATE THE MEXICAN AMERICAN POPULATION, TWO GENERIC WAYS OF DEFINING ETHNIC POPULATIONS AND THEIR USE BY THE BUREAU ARE EXPLAINED: (1) AN OBJECTIVE CRITERION SUCH AS SURNAME OR COUNTRY OF BIRTH, AND (2) A SUBJECTIVE RESPONSE OF SELF-IDENTIFICATION. PRIOR TO 1970, THE BUREAU RELIED ALMOST EXCLU-SIVELY ON OBJECTIVE CRITERIA. THE FOREIGN BIRTH OR FOREIGN PARENTAGE CONCEPT DATES FROM 1850 AND IS AVAILABLE FOR MEX-ICAN FOREIGN-BORN AND FOREIGN PARENT-AGE FOR THE 1940 THROUGH 1970 CENSUSES. SPANISH LANGUAGE OR MOTHER TONGUE CATEGORIES ARE IDENTIFIED IN THE 1910 TO 1970 CENSUSES, EXCLUDING 1950. AN EXPAN-SION OF THE SPANISH LANGUAGE DEFINITION IN 1970 RESULTED IN THE LARGEST POPULA-TION OF SPANISH HERITAGE EVER RECORDED IN THE U.S. THE SELF-IDENTIFICATION CON-CEPT HAS BEEN TRIED ON SMALL SAMPLES ONLY FOUR TIMES SINCE 1969. ALTHOUGH MANY RESEARCHERS BELIEVE THIS METHOD PROVIDES THE CLOSEST APPROXIMATION TO THE SOCIOLOGICAL CONCEPT OF ETHNIC GROUP IDENTITY OF ALL CENSUS METHODS CURRENTLY USED (RESPONDENTS CHECK ONE CATEGORY—MEXICAN, PUERTO RICAN, CU-BAN, CENTRAL OR SOUTH AMERICAN, OTHER SPANISH), THE INTERPRETATION OF THESE RE-SULTS FOR MEXICAN AMERICANS REMAINS COMPLICATED. PROBLEMS AND ADVANTAGES ASSOCIATED WITH THESE CENSUS CATE-GORIES AND THE COMPARABILITY OF THE MEASURES ARE DISCUSSED. TABLES SUMMA-RIZING THE USE OF THESE MEASURES FOR 1950, 1960 AND 1970 AND THE PRELIMINARY POPULATION TOTALS ACCORDING TO VARI-OUS ETHNIC MEASURES FOR 1970 ARE PRE-SENTED. 6 REFERENCES.

ACCN 000670

791 AUTH **HERNANDEZ, N. G.**
TITL ANOTHER LOOK AT MULTICULTURAL EDUCATION TODAY.
SRCE *JOURNAL OF RESEARCH AND DEVELOPMENT IN EDUCATION, 1977, 11(1), 4-9.*
INDX ESSAY, BILINGUAL-BICULTURAL EDUCATION, EDUCATION, EQUAL OPPORTUNITY, HIGHER EDUCATION, TEACHERS, POLICY, CULTURAL PLURALISM
ABST THIS ESSAY IDENTIFIES ARGUMENTS, PRO AND CON, CONCERNING THE CONTROVERSIAL PHENOMENON OF MULTICULTURAL EDUCATION. SPECIFIC ISSUES CURRENTLY BEING DEBATED ARE: (1) MANDATORY MULTICULTURAL COURSES TO BE INCLUDED IN ALL TEACHER EDUCATION—A QUESTION NOW BEING ARGUED WITHIN THE MEMBER RANKS OF THE NATIONAL COUNCIL OF ACCREDITATION OF TEACHER EDUCATION AND THE NATIONAL EDUCATIONAL ASSOCIATION; (2) BUSING; (3) BILINGUAL EDUCATION; (4) CULTURALLY RELEVANT CURRICULA; AND (5) EQUAL EDUCATIONAL OPPORTUNITY. THE CENTRAL THRUST OF OPPOSITION TO MULTICULTURAL EDUCATION IS THAT THESE INNOVATIONS WILL UNDERMINE THE TRADITIONAL GOAL OF PUBLIC EDUCATION—ACADEMIC EXCELLENCE. PROPONENTS ARGUE, ON THE OTHER HAND, THAT THIS KIND OF EXPANDED MULTICULTURAL APPROACH TO LEARNING WILL BETTER PREPARE STUDENTS FOR LIVING IN A NECESSARILY PLURALISTIC WORLD—A GOAL FAR MORE IMPORTANT THAN MERE SUBJECT MATTER ACHIEVEMENT. THE ESSAY CONCLUDES THAT FROM THESE ARGUMENTS THE FOLLOWING QUESTIONS EMERGE: ARE WE PREPARED TO GIVE UP STRICT SCHOLASTIC ACHIEVEMENT TO DEVELOP CURRICULA RESPONSIVE TO STUDENTS' TOTAL NEEDS? CAN WE SACRIFICE OUR BELIEF THAT THE "IDEAL CULTURE AND LANGUAGE" ARE THE ONLY CONDUITS TO SUCCESS? LOOKING AHEAD, WHAT HAPPENS TO OUR SOCIETY IN THE 1980'S DEPENDS IN LARGE MEASURE ON THE RESPONSES TAKEN NOW TO THESE QUESTIONS. 10 REFERENCES.
ACCN 002110

792 AUTH **HERNANDEZ, N. G.**
TITL VARIABLES AFFECTING ACHIEVEMENT OF MIDDLE SCHOOL MEXICAN-AMERICAN STUDENTS.
SRCE *REVIEW OF EDUCATIONAL RESEARCH, 1973, 43(1), 1-39.*
INDX MEXICAN AMERICAN, BILINGUAL-BICULTURAL EDUCATION, EDUCATIONAL MATERIALS, INSTRUCTIONAL TECHNIQUES, CURRICULUM, CULTURAL PLURALISM, EDUCATION, ATTITUDES, CULTURE, REVIEW, ADOLESCENTS, SCHOLASTIC ASPIRATIONS, SES, SELF CONCEPT, INTELLIGENCE, SCHOLASTIC ACHIEVEMENT, CHILDREN, ANXIETY
ABST A REVIEW OF THE LITERATURE PERTAINING TO VARIABLES WHICH MAY ACCOUNT FOR DIFFERENCES IN ACADEMIC ACHIEVEMENT OF MEXICAN AMERICAN STUDENTS IS PRESENTED. FACTORS IDENTIFIED ARE SELF-CONCEPT, EXPECTATIONS, ASPIRATIONS, MOTIVATION, ANXIETY, ALIENATION, INTELLIGENCE

MEASUREMENT, VALUE ORIENTATIONS, CULTURAL DIFFERENCES, LANGUAGE, AND POVERTY. THE WEIGHT OF EVIDENCE SUGGESTS THAT EDUCATIONAL SYSTEMS HAVE NOT BEEN RESPONSIVE TO THE NEEDS OF INDIVIDUALS IN GENERAL, AND OF MINORITY GROUPS IN PARTICULAR, WHO DEVIATE SIGNIFICANTLY FROM THE CHARACTERISTICS OF THE MODAL STUDENT FOR WHOM THE CURRICULUM IS DESIGNED. 227 REFERENCES. (PASAR ABSTRACT MODIFIED)
ACCN 000671

793 AUTH **HEROLD, P. L., RAMIREZ, M., III, & CASTANEDA, A.**
TITL NEW APPROACHES TO BILINGUAL, BICULTURAL EDUCATION. (MANUAL 5, FIELD SENSITIVE AND FIELD INDEPENDENT TEACHING STRATEGIES.)
SRCE *AUSTIN, TEXAS: DISSEMINATION AND ASSESSMENT CENTER FOR BILINGUAL EDUCATION, 1978, PP. 63-81.*
INDX COGNITIVE STYLE, BILINGUAL-BICULTURAL EDUCATION, COGNITIVE DEVELOPMENT, CHILDREN, INSTRUCTIONAL TECHNIQUES, FIELD DEPENDENCE-INDEPENDENCE
ABST FIFTH IN A SERIES OF SEVEN MANUALS AND SELF-ASSESSMENT UNITS DESIGNED AS TEACHER TRAINING MATERIALS FOR USE IN BILINGUAL-BICULTURAL PROJECTS, THIS MANUAL ACQUAINTS TEACHERS WITH BOTH FIELD SENSITIVE AND FIELD INDEPENDENT TEACHING STRATEGIES. INTENDED TO HELP TEACHERS ADJUST THEIR TEACHING STYLES TO THE LEARNING STYLES OF THEIR STUDENTS, THE MANUAL BEGINS WITH A NUMBER OF EXERCISES WHICH INDICATE HOW EASILY THE TWO STRATEGIES CAN BE MASTERED. INSTRUCTIONS FOR USING FIELD SENSITIVE AND FIELD INDEPENDENT TEACHING STRATEGIES ARE CAREFULLY EXPLAINED. A RATING FORM TO USE IN DETERMINING SUCCESS IN USING EITHER STRATEGY IS ALSO INCLUDED. FINALLY, A DISCUSSION OF CURRICULUM INDICATES HOW THE STYLE OF INSTRUCTIONAL MATERIALS CAN BE IDENTIFIED AND ALTERED FOR USE IN FIELD SENSITIVE OR FIELD INDEPENDENT TEACHING. (AUTHOR SUMMARY MODIFIED)
ACCN 000672

794 AUTH **HERR, S. E.**
TITL THE EFFECT OF PRE-FIRST-GRADE TRAINING UPON READING READINESS AND READING ACHIEVEMENT AMONG SPANISH-AMERICAN CHILDREN.
SRCE *JOURNAL OF EDUCATIONAL PSYCHOLOGY, 1946, 37, 87-102.*
INDX INTELLIGENCE TESTING, CHILDREN, SPANISH SURNAMED, EMPIRICAL, ACHIEVEMENT TESTING, METROPOLITAN READING READINESS TEST, BILINGUALISM, SCHOLASTIC ACHIEVEMENT, EARLY CHILDHOOD EDUCATION, NEW MEXICO, SOUTHWEST, PROGRAM EVALUATION, METROPOLITAN ACHIEVEMENT TEST
ABST READING READINESS AND ACHIEVEMENT OF SPANISH-SPEAKING CHILDREN WHO PARTICIPATED IN A 1-YEAR, PRE-FIRST-GRADE TRAIN-

ING PROGRAM ARE COMPARED TO A CONTROL GROUP WHO DID NOT PARTICIPATE IN THE SPECIAL PROGRAM. CHILDREN FROM NINE TOWNS IN NEW MEXICO PARTICIPATED IN THIS STUDY. THE TWO GROUPS WERE INITIALLY MATCHED ON THE PINTNER-CUNNINGHAM PRIMARY INTELLIGENCE TEST (PPIT) AND BY A SUBJECTIVE ANALYSIS OF VOCABULARY ABILITY AND HOME ENVIRONMENT. A YEAR LATER WHEN BOTH GROUPS BEGAN THE USUAL FIRST-GRADE PROGRAM THEY WERE GIVEN THE PPIT AND THE METROPOLITAN READING READINESS TEST (MRRT), FOLLOWED BY THE METROPOLITAN ACHIEVEMENT TEST (MAT) A FEW MONTHS THEREAFTER. RESULTS INDICATE THAT THE INITIAL IQ'S FOR THE TWO GROUPS WERE ALMOST PARALLEL. HOWEVER, A YEAR LATER THEIR IQ'S SHOWED A DIFFERENCE OF 17.46 POINTS IN FAVOR OF THE EXPERIMENTAL GROUP. SIMILARLY, THE SCORES FOR THE MRRT AND FOR THE METROPOLITAN READING ACHIEVEMENT TEST WERE HIGHER FOR THE EXPERIMENTAL GROUP. THE FINDINGS SUGGEST THAT SPANISH AMERICAN CHILDREN WITH PRE-FIRST-GRADE TRAINING HAVE A DECIDED ADVANTAGE OVER THE CHILDREN WHO DO NOT HAVE THE EXPERIENCE OF SUCH TRAINING.

ACCN   000673

795 AUTH   **HERRANS, L. L.**
    TITL   CULTURAL FACTORS IN THE STANDARDIZATION OF THE SPANISH WAIS OR EIWA AND THE ASSESSMENT OF SPANISH SPEAKING CHILDREN.
    SRCE   *SCHOOL PSYCHOLOGIST, 1973, 28(2), 27-34.*
    INDX   CULTURAL FACTORS, INTELLIGENCE TESTING, CULTURE-FAIR TESTS, SPANISH SURNAMED, PUERTO RICAN-I, BILINGUALISM, CHILDREN, WAIS, ESCALA DE INTELIGENCIA WECHSLER, TEST VALIDITY, TEST RELIABILITY
    ABST   THE TRANSLATION, ADAPTATION OF ITEMS, TRAINING OF TESTERS, AND ADMINISTRATION OF THE WECHSLER ADULT INTELLIGENCE SCALE FOR USE WITH A PUERTO RICAN POPULATION ARE DESCRIBED. PROBLEMS SPECIFIC TO ITS USE IN PUERTO RICO ARE DISCUSSED. 6 REFERENCES. (PASAR ABSTRACT MODIFIED)

ACCN   000674

796 AUTH   **HERRERA, A. E.**
    TITL   THERAPIST PREFERENCES OF BILINGUAL MEXICAN-AMERICAN PSYCHOTHERAPY CANDIDATES (DOCTORAL DISSERTATION, UNIVERSITY OF SOUTHERN CALIFORNIA, 1977).
    SRCE   *DISSERTATION ABSTRACTS INTERNATIONAL, 1978, 38, 5019B. (AVAILABLE FROM DOHENY LIBRARY, UNIVERSITY OF SOUTHERN CALIFORNIA, MICROFILM NO. 2467-D.)*
    INDX   PSYCHOTHERAPY, MEXICAN AMERICAN, EMPIRICAL, BILINGUAL, SES, PARAPROFESSIONALS, EXAMINER EFFECTS, INTERPERSONAL ATTRACTION, ATTITUDES, PSYCHOTHERAPISTS, BILINGUAL-BICULTURAL PERSONNEL
    ABST   THIS PSYCHOTHERAPY ANALOGUE WAS DESIGNED TO EXPLORE WHAT TYPES OF PATIENT-THERAPIST MATCHING MIGHT BE MOST CONDUCIVE TO ESTABLISHING A VIABLE THERAPEUTIC RELATIONSHIP. EIGHTY-EIGHT LOW-INCOME, BILINGUAL MEXICAN AMERICAN (MA) CLIENTS FROM A COMMUNITY HEALTH CENTER, PRIOR TO THEIR INTAKE INTERVIEW, WERE SHOWN VIDEOTAPES CONSISTING OF SIMULATED PSYCHOTHERAPY INTERVIEWS WITH AN ETHNICALLY SIMILAR AND DISSIMILAR THERAPIST, A MONOLINGUAL ENGLISH AND BILINGUAL SPANISH THERAPIST, AND A PROFESSIONAL AND PARAPROFESSIONAL THERAPIST. SUBJECTS WERE THEN ASKED TO INDICATE, ON A PROJECTIVE SELF-DISCLOSURE SCALE, WILLINGNESS TO SELF-DISCLOSE TO THE PARTICULAR THERAPIST SEEN. THERAPIST ETHNICITY-LANGUAGE INTERACTION—BASED ON ATTRACTION, PERCEIVED COMPETENCY, AND WILLINGNESS TO SELF-DISCLOSE—REVEAL THAT MA'S PREFER THERAPISTS WHO ARE BOTH ANGLO AND BILINGUAL AND THOSE WHO ARE MA'S BUT NOT BILINGUAL. PROFESSIONAL STATUS HAD NO SIGNIFICANCE. A LANGUAGE USAGE SURVEY REVEALED THAT BILINGUAL MA'S CHOSE SPANISH SUBSTANTIALLY LESS OFTEN THAN ENGLISH, DID NOT FEEL IT NECESSARY FOR THERAPISTS TO BE BILINGUAL, AND DID NOT PREFER SPANISH FOR THE DISCLOSURE OF EMOTIONAL MATERIAL. THE CRITICAL FACTORS DETERMINING THERAPIST PREFERENCES ARE SEEN AS A JOINT FUNCTION OF THERAPIST ETHNICITY AND LANGUAGE ORIENTATION. DELIVERY OF MENTAL HEALTH SERVICES AND RELEVANT PSYCHOTHERAPY FOR MA'S ARE ALSO DISCUSSED. 47 REFERENCES. (AUTHOR ABSTRACT MODIFIED)

ACCN   000676

797 AUTH   **HERRERA, A. E., & SANCHEZ, V. C.**
    TITL   BEHAVIORALLY ORIENTED GROUP THERAPY: A SUCCESSFUL APPLICATION IN THE TREATMENT OF LOW INCOME SPANISH SPEAKING CLIENTS.
    SRCE   *IN M. R. MIRANDA (ED.), PSYCHOTHERAPY WITH THE SPANISH SPEAKING: ISSUES IN RESEARCH AND SERVICE DELIVERY (MONOGRAPH NO. 3). LOS ANGELES: UNIVERSITY OF CALIFORNIA, SPANISH SPEAKING MENTAL HEALTH RESEARCH CENTER, 1976, PP. 73-84.*
    INDX   PSYCHOTHERAPY OUTCOME, PSYCHOTHERAPY, BEHAVIOR THERAPY, DEPRESSION, ANXIETY, PSYCHOPATHOLOGY, PSYCHOTHERAPISTS, CASE STUDY, MEXICAN AMERICAN, BILINGUAL-BICULTURAL PERSONNEL, PROGRAM EVALUATION, ASSERTIVENESS, CALIFORNIA, SOUTHWEST, SES
    ABST   THE UTILITY OF THE GROUP FORMAT AS AN EFFECTIVE TREATMENT MODALITY IN WORKING WITH LOW INCOME SPANISH-SPEAKING (SS) CLIENTS IS DISCUSSED AND DEMONSTRATED. A CASE STUDY OF 13 SS CLIENTS IN ONE THERAPY GROUP LED BY SS THERAPISTS INDICATES THAT A STRUCTURED-BEHAVIORAL APPROACH CAN BE VERY SUCCESSFUL IN DEALING WITH A WIDE VARIETY OF PROBLEMS INCLUDING SOMATIC COMPLAINTS, DEPRESSION, ANXIETY, MARITAL DISCORD, AND SUBASSERTIVENESS. THIS FINDING IS CONSISTENT WITH THOSE OF GOLDSTEIN (1973) AND SAR-

ASON (1971) WHO ARGUE FOR THE USE OF HIGHLY STRUCTURED, BEHAVIOR-CHANGE ORIENTED APPROACHES TO THE TREATMENT OF LOW-SES PATIENTS. BESIDES DEMONSTRATING THE VALUE OF CLASS-LINKED PSYCHOTHERAPY, THIS STUDY DEMONSTRATES THAT CULTURE-LINKED THERAPY IS A SIGNIFICANT COMPONENT IN OUTCOME SUCCESS. IT IS SUGGESTED THAT GREATER EFFORT BE DIRECTED TOWARD DEVISING TREATMENT PLANS THAT ARE TAILORED TO THE NEEDS OF TARGET POPULATIONS—I.E., ALLOWING DISCUSSION OF CURANDERISMO, FORMING SPECIAL GROUPS FOR SS CLIENTS ONLY, RECOGNIZING THAT SUB-ASSERTIVE BEHAVIORS ARE CONSEQUENCES OF DISCRIMINATION AND PREJUDICE. UNTIL THESE TREATMENT METHODS ARE USED AND EVALUATED, IT IS PREMATURE TO CLAIM THAT GROUP THERAPY CANNOT BE SUCCESSFUL WITH LOWER-CLASS MEXICAN AMERICANS. 27 REFERENCES. (AUTHOR SUMMARY MODIFIED)

ACCN   000677

798 AUTH   **HERRERA, J. J., MOLL, L. C., REZA-GRACE, R., RUEDA, R. S., & VASQUEZ, L. C.**

TITL   CHICANO MENTAL HEALTH IN AN URBAN COMMUNITY: A CASE STUDY OF AN EAST LOS ANGELES MENTAL HEALTH AGENCY.

SRCE   *UNPUBLISHED MASTER'S THESIS, SCHOOL OF SOCIAL WORK, UNIVERSITY OF SOUTHERN CALIFORNIA, 1974.*

INDX   SPANISH SURNAMED, MEXICAN AMERICAN, MENTAL HEALTH, RESOURCE UTILIZATION, HEALTH DELIVERY SYSTEMS, CULTURAL FACTORS, EMPIRICAL, ADULTS, COMMUNITY, SES, PSYCHOTHERAPY OUTCOME, BILINGUAL-BICULTURAL PERSONNEL, CALIFORNIA, SOUTHWEST, POLICY, PROGRAM EVALUATION

ABST   A DESCRIPTIVE STUDY OF THE PROVIDERS AND CONSUMERS AT THE EAST LOS ANGELES MENTAL HEALTH SERVICE (ELAMHS) IS PRESENTED TO ASSESS THE MENTAL HEALTH NEEDS AND RESOURCES AS PERCEIVED BY BOTH. THE RESEARCH FOCUSED ON 5 QUESTIONS: (1) WHAT IS THE ELAMHS CLIENT POPULATION PROFILE?; (2) WHAT ARE THE CLIENTS' PERCEPTIONS OF UNMET MENTAL HEALTH NEEDS AND OF EXISTING SERVICES?; (3) WHAT ARE THE CLIENTS' EVALUATIONS OF SERVICES RECEIVED AT ELAMHS?; (4) WHAT ARE THE PROVIDERS' PERCEPTIONS OF THE NEEDS AND SERVICES?; AND (5) WHAT ARE THE CLIENTS' PERCEPTIONS OF THE CAUSES OF MENTAL HEALTH PROBLEMS? SOME GENERAL FINDINGS ARE: (1) CONSUMERS DID NOT REFER TO THE AGENCYS' BILINGUAL-BICULTURAL SERVICES IN RESPONDING TO QUESTIONS ON EVALUATION, RATHER THEY EMPHASIZED ETHNICITY AND INTERPERSONAL RELATIONSHIPS; (2) INSTEAD OF LOOKING TO RESOURCES SUCH AS CHURCH, FAMILY AND FRIENDS, ALMOST HALF OF THE CONSUMERS INDICATED THEY WOULD USE A MENTAL HEALTH AGENCY WHEN HAVING A PERSONAL OR EMOTIONAL PROBLEM; (3) CONSUMERS WERE NOT AWARE OF THE VARIETY OF SERVICES AVAILABLE NOR OF THE OPPORTUNITY FOR COMMUNITY IN-

VOLVEMENT; (4) AGENCY REFERRAL ACCOUNTED FOR 70% OF THE CONSUMERS, ONLY 5% WERE SELF-REFERRED. RECOMMENDATIONS BASED ON THE STUDY'S FINDINGS INCLUDE USING MORE INNOVATIVE INTERVIEWING WITH CHICANO CLIENTS, EXPANDING OUTREACH AND ADVERTISING METHODS IN THE COMMUNITY AND OTHER AGENCIES, AND WORKING TO MAKE THE FAMILY AN INTEGRAL PART OF CLIENT TREATMENT PLANS. 10 REFERENCES. (AUTHOR SUMMARY MODIFIED)

ACCN   000678

799 AUTH   **HERTZIG, M. E.**

TITL   ASPECTS OF COGNITIVE STYLE IN YOUNG CHILDREN OF DIFFERING SOCIAL AND ETHNIC BACKGROUNDS.

SRCE   *IN J. HELLMUTH (ED.), COGNITIVE STUDIES: II. DEFICITS IN COGNITION. NEW YORK: BRUNNER/MAZEL, 1971, PP. 149-170.*

INDX   COGNITIVE STYLE, CHILDREN, ETHNIC IDENTITY, SES, CURRICULUM, COGNITIVE DEVELOPMENT, EDUCATIONAL MATERIALS, LINGUISTIC COMPETENCE, PUERTO RICAN-M, CROSS CULTURAL, CULTURAL FACTORS, REVIEW

ABST   STUDIES EXAMINING THE RELATIONSHIP BETWEEN SOCIAL DISADVANTAGE AND REDUCED LEVELS OF COGNITIVE FUNCTIONING IN CHILDREN GENERALLY FAIL TO IDENTIFY THE VARIOUS ASPECTS OF THE PROBLEM. THERE ARE FOUR BASIC LEVELS OF CONCERN: (1) DIFFERENCE IN COGNITIVE COMPETENCE BETWEEN THE RELATIVELY ADVANTAGED AND DISADVANTAGED; (2) RELATION OF COGNITIVE STYLE TO MEASURES OF COGNITIVE COMPETENCE; (3) FACTORS UNDERLYING STYLE AND COMPETENCE LEVELS; AND (4) IMPLICATIONS OF SOCIAL CLASS DIFFERENCES IN STYLE AND COMPETENCE FOR FORMAL LEARNING IN SOCIAL SETTINGS. FOR THE MOST PART, PRE-SCHOOL CHILDREN ARE NOT INCLUDED IN THE RESEARCH OF COGNITIVE STYLES. HOWEVER, RESULTS FROM A LONGITUDINAL STUDY INDICATE THAT PRE-SCHOOL CHILDREN WHO DIFFER FROM ONE ANOTHER WITH RESPECT TO SOCIAL AND ETHNIC BACKGROUND ALSO DIFFER IN THEIR RESPONSE TO DEMANDS FOR COGNITIVE FUNCTIONING. IF SCHOOLS ARE GOING TO BE SUCCESSFUL IN IMPROVING PERFORMANCE LEVELS THEY NEED TO DEVELOP PROGRAMS WHICH TAKE INTO ACCOUNT THE PARTICULAR CHARACTERISTICS OF THE CHILDREN. THIS MEANS THAT NOT ONLY THE GLOBAL DIFFERENCES BETWEEN CHILDREN FROM DIFFERENT POPULATION SUBGROUPS BUT ALSO INDIVIDUAL DIFFERENCES BETWEEN CHILDREN OF SIMILAR SOCIAL AND ETHNIC BACKGROUND NEED TO BE CONSIDERED. 48 REFERENCES. (AUTHOR SUMMARY MODIFIED)

ACCN   000679

800 AUTH   **HERTZIG, M. E., BIRCH, H. G., THOMAS, A., & MENDEZ, O. A.**

TITL   CLASS AND ETHNIC DIFFERENCES IN THE RESPONSIVENESS OF PRE-SCHOOL CHILDREN TO COGNITIVE DEMANDS.

SRCE MONOGRAPH OF SOCIETY FOR RESEARCH IN CHILD DEVELOPMENT, 1968, 33(1), 1-69.

INDX STANFORD-BINET INTELLIGENCE TEST, SES, CROSS CULTURAL, MEXICAN AMERICAN, COGNITIVE STYLE, PUERTO RICAN-M, POVERTY, COGNITIVE DEVELOPMENT, FAMILY STRUCTURE, INTELLIGENCE, LINGUISTIC COMPETENCE, LANGUAGE ACQUISITION, EMPIRICAL

ABST THE STYLE OF RESPONSIVENESS TO DEMANDS FOR COGNITIVE FUNCTIONING IN PRESCHOOL CHILDREN FROM DIFFERENT SOCIAL AND ETHNIC GROUPS IS EXAMINED. THE SUBJECTS WERE 116 MIDDLE-CLASS AMERICAN CHILDREN WITH A MEAN AGE OF 3 YEARS, 4 MONTHS, AND 60 PUERTO RICAN CHILDREN WITH A MEAN AGE OF 3 YEARS, 6 MONTHS. THE MIDDLE-CLASS CHILDREN COME FROM NATIVE-BORN PROFESSIONAL FAMILIES, AND THE PUERTO RICAN CHILDREN COME FROM PREDOMINANTLY SPANISH-SPEAKING, WORKING-CLASS FAMILIES LIVING IN PUBLIC HOUSING PROJECTS. THE BEHAVIORAL INFORMATION ON RESPONSE STYLE TO COGNITIVE DEMANDS WAS OBTAINED BY OBSERVATION OF THE BEHAVIOR AND RECORDING OF THE VERBALIZATIONS OF THE CHILD IN THE COURSE OF STANFORD-BINET INTELLIGENCE TESTING. THE FINDINGS CLEARLY DEMONSTRATE THAT THE TWO GROUPS DIFFER FROM EACH OTHER IN THE BEHAVIORAL STYLES WITH WHICH THEY RESPOND TO DEMANDS FOR COGNITIVE FUNCTIONING. THE TWO GROUPS SHOW DIFFERENCES IN: (1) THE PROPORTION OF TIMES THE CHILD ATTEMPTED TO DO WHAT WAS ASKED OF HIM (I.E., WORK RESPONSE); (2) THE TENDENCY TO MAKE WORK RESPONSES AFTER AN INITIAL NOT-WORK RESPONSE; (3) THE PROPORTION OF VERBALLY EXPRESSED RESPONSES; (4) THE STYLE OF MAKING NOT-WORK RESPONSES; (5) THE KINDS OF VERBALIZATIONS THAT ACCOMPANY NOT-WORK RESPONSES; (6) THE TENDENCY TO MAKE SPONTANEOUS WORK EXTENSIONS; (7) THE FREQUENCY WITH WHICH SUCH SPONTANEOUS EXTENSIONS ARE VERBALLY EXPRESSED; AND (8) THE DEGREE TO WHICH WORK RESPONSES ARE MADE TO VERBAL AND NONVERBAL COGNITIVE TASKS, RESPECTIVELY. EACH OF THESE DIFFERENCES IN STYLE WAS SUSTAINED WHEN IQ WAS HELD CONSTANT AND WHEN BIRTH ORDER WAS CONTROLLED. FAMILY INSTABILITY, LACK OF MATERNAL CARE, AND EXAMINER BIAS WERE ALSO REJECTED AS POSSIBLE CONTRIBUTING FACTORS TO THE DIFFERENCES BETWEEN GROUPS. IT IS CONCLUDED THAT CHILDREARING PRACTICES AND LIFESTYLES OF THE PUERTO RICAN GROUP DIFFER FROM THOSE OF THE MIDDLE-CLASS IN WAYS THAT RESULT IN THE DEVELOPMENT OF THE BEHAVIORAL DIFFERENCES FOUND. 68 REFERENCES.

ACCN 000680

801 AUTH **HERTZIG, M. E., & BIRCH, H. G.**
TITL LONGITUDINAL COURSE OF MEASURED INTELLIGENCE IN PRESCHOOL CHILDREN OF DIFFERENT SOCIAL AND ETHNIC BACKGROUNDS.

SRCE AMERICAN JOURNAL OF ORTHOPSYCHIATRY, 1971, 47(3), 416-425.

INDX PUERTO RICAN-M, STANFORD-BINET INTELLIGENCE TEST, BILINGUALISM, COGNITIVE STYLE, CROSS CULTURAL, EMPIRICAL, SES, COGNITIVE DEVELOPMENT, INTELLIGENCE

ABST WHITE MIDDLE-CLASS AND PUERTO RICAN WORKING-CLASS CHILDREN IN THE PRESCHOOL YEARS PROVIDE THE OPPORTUNITY TO COMPARE THE COURSE OF MEASURED INTELLIGENCE BY A LONGITUDINAL STUDY. SIXTY PUERTO RICAN AND 116 WHITE CHILDREN WERE ADMINISTERED THE STANFORD BINET AT 3 YEARS OF AGE. PRACTICALLY ALL THE SAME CHILDREN WERE EXAMINED AT 6 YEARS OF AGE. THE DATA SHOW NO INCREASE IN IQ BETWEEN 3 AND 6 YEARS OF AGE FOR CHILDREN OF EITHER SOCIOECONOMIC GROUP. IN FACT, THE FINDINGS SUGGEST THAT THE MEASURED INTELLIGENCE IS RELATIVELY STABLE OVER THE PRESCHOOL YEARS AND THAT FOR BOTH GROUPS OF CHILDREN THE GENERAL TREND IS TOWARD A SMALL INCREASE IN SCORE. THE PUERTO RICAN CHILDREN WERE SIGNIFICANTLY MORE STABLE IN IQ OVER THE AGE RANGE STUDIED THAN THE WHITE CHILDREN. IT IS CONCLUDED THAT FOR THE DISADVANTAGED GROUP, IQ LEVEL IS ALREADY WELL ESTABLISHED BY 3 YEARS OF AGE AND TENDS TO REMAIN REMARKABLY STABLE THEREAFTER. FAILURE OF THE MIDDLE-CLASS CHILD TO ATTAIN AN IQ SCORE AT 3 YEARS OF AGE IS IDIOSYNCRATIC AND NOT SIGNIFICANT, WHILE FOR THE PUERTO RICAN CHILD IT MAY WELL BE REFLECTIVE OF A PATTERN OF FUNCTIONING. IT IS SUGGESTED THAT FOR PUERTO RICAN CHILDREN INTERVENTION MIGHT BE EFFECTIVE IN MODIFYING BEHAVIOR STYLE AND PRODUCING SIGNIFICANT CHANGES IN LEVELS OF INTELLIGENCE. 13 REFERENCES.

ACCN 000681

802 AUTH **HESSLER, R. M.**
TITL CITIZEN PARTICIPATION, SOCIAL ORGANIZATION, AND CULTURE: A NEIGHBORHOOD HEALTH CENTER FOR CHICANOS.

SRCE HUMAN ORGANIZATION, 1977, 36(2), 124-134.

INDX HEALTH DELIVERY SYSTEMS, URBAN, SOUTHWEST, COMMUNITY INVOLVEMENT, CULTURAL FACTORS, POLITICAL POWER, ADMINISTRATORS, MEXICAN AMERICAN, ESSAY, LEADERSHIP, POLITICS, PROGRAM EVALUATION, POLICY, HEALTH

ABST THE FITFUL EVOLUTION OF A BARRIO COMMUNITY HEALTH CENTER (CHC) IN A SOUTHWESTERN CITY REVEALS THAT IS IS IMPERATIVE TO HAVE INPUT FROM COMMUNITY MEMBERS FROM THE BEGINNING. THE CHC EXAMINED IN THIS STUDY WAS INITIALLY DEVELOPED BY ANGLO MEDICAL ADMINISTRATORS WHO WANTED AN ON-SITE TRAINING FACILITY FOR MEDICAL STUDENTS, AND THEY CONSIDERED CITIZENS' CONTRIBUTIONS TO THE PROGRAM AS SUBORDINATE AND ANTITHETICAL TO THEIR GOAL. THIS ATTITUDE, COMBINED WITH THE AMBIGUITY OF HEW GUIDELINES AND THE LACK OF PROVIDER EXPERIENCE WITH EITHER THE CULTURE OR THE

BARRIO, LED TO GENERAL CONFUSION. A DOWNWARD TWO-YEAR SPIRAL ENSUED IN WHICH THE CHC FLOUNDERED, THE RELATIONSHIP WITH A MODEL CITIES PROGRAM COLLAPSED, OTHER HEALTH CARE INSTITUTIONS BEGAN TO PULL OUT THEIR FINANCIAL AND POLITICAL SUPPORT, AND THE AUTHORITY OF THE CHC DEGENERATED INTO A POWER STRUGGLE BETWEEN CONSUMERS AND PROVIDERS. SLOWLY, HOWEVER, THE CONSUMERS LINKED THE CHC TO GENERIC CHICANO CULTURAL PROCESSES THROUGH PRESSURE AT CHC MEETINGS; AND GRADUALLY, THE BARRIO PARTICIPANTS MOVED FROM AN ADVISORY STATUS TO A CONTROL BOARD. THE CHC IS NOW UNDER THE TOTAL CONTROL OF A BARRIO ORGANIZATION AND FUNCTIONING EFFECTIVELY. 19 REFERENCES.

ACCN   002111

803 AUTH **HEWES, G. W.**
     TITL MEXICANS IN SEARCH OF THE MEXICAN: NOTES ON MEXICAN NATIONAL CHARACTER STUDIES.
     SRCE *THE AMERICAN JOURNAL OF ECONOMICS AND SOCIOLOGY, 1953-54, 13(1-4), 209-224.*
     INDX MEXICAN, PERSONALITY, CULTURE, REVIEW, SOCIAL SCIENCES
     ABST NATIONAL CHARACTER STUDIES, WITH A LONG LITERARY AND PHILOSOPHICAL PAST, HAVE RECENTLY BECOME A SUBJECT OF SCIENTIFIC RESEARCH, PRINCIPALLY BY ANTHROPOLOGISTS. MODERN APPROACHES TO THE SUBJECT ARE FROM THE POINT OF VIEW OF LEARNING AND PERSONALITY THEORY; RACIAL OR GENETIC FACTORS ARE NO LONGER CONSIDERED IMPORTANT IN THE FORMATION OF PERSONALITY PATTERNS COMMON TO MEMBERS OF GIVEN CULTURAL GROUPS. IN THIS PAPER, THE CONTRIBUTIONS OF MEXICAN WRITERS TO MEXICAN NATIONAL CHARACTER STUDIES ARE SUMMARIZED. WITH FEW EXCEPTIONS, THEIR WORK HAS BEEN IMPRESSIONISTIC, INTUITIVE, OR SPECULATIVE. THERE HAS BEEN, HOWEVER, SOME INFLUENCE FROM MODERN PSYCHOLOGY AND FROM PSYCHOANALYSIS IN PARTICULAR, AS WELL AS FROM SOCIOLOGICAL AND ANTHROPOLOGICAL FIELD STUDIES SUCH AS THOSE OF GAMIO, REDFIELD, PARSONS, BEALS, FOSTER, LEWIS, KELLY, PALERM, AND OTHERS. THE OUTSTANDING EARLIER MEXICAN CONTRIBUTORS WERE CHAVEZ (1928) AND RAMOS (1934). USEFUL LEADS WERE PROVIDED BY VELASCO GIL (1944) IN HIS SINARQUISTA STUDY. RECENT WRITERS HAVE BEEN ZEA, URANGA, CORDOVA, SANDOVAL, AND TAVERA, ALONG WITH THE REVIEW CHAPTER IN ITURRIAGA'S BOOK. THE SECOND PORTION OF THE PAPER IS A COMPOSITE DESCRIPTION OF THE MODAL MEXICAN PERSONALITY, BASED ON THE IDEAS OF THE FOREGOING WRITERS. IT IS EMPHASIZED THAT THESE IDEAS ARE QUITE INCONCLUSIVE, AND THAT A GREAT DEAL OF SCIENTIFIC FIELDWORK IS REQUIRED. THE NOTIONS SO FAR PRESENTED ARE AT BEST ONLY CLUES OR LEADS FOR FUTURE INVESTIGATIONS OF A MORE RIGOROUS CHARACTER. 34 REFERENCES. (AUTHOR SUMMARY MODIFIED)

ACCN   000682

804 AUTH **HICKEY, T.**
     TITL BILINGUALISM AND THE MEASUREMENT OF INTELLIGENCE AND VERBAL LEARNING ABILITY.
     SRCE *EXCEPTIONAL CHILDREN, 1972, 39(1), 24-28.*
     INDX BILINGUALISM, BILINGUAL, INTELLIGENCE TESTING, LEARNING, COGNITIVE DEVELOPMENT, CHILDREN, MEXICAN AMERICAN, EARLY CHILDHOOD EDUCATION, LINGUISTIC COMPETENCE, EDUCATIONAL ASSESSMENT, EDUCATION, PEABODY PICTURE-VOCABULARY TEST, CALIFORNIA, SOUTHWEST, EMPIRICAL
     ABST SOME OF THE PROBLEMS OF MEASURING INTELLIGENCE AND VERBAL LEARNING ABILITY AMONG MEXICAN AMERICAN PRESCHOOLERS ARE ANALYZED. THE 160 BILINGUAL MEXICAN AMERICAN HEADSTART SUBJECTS ENCOUNTERED GREATER DIFFICULTY IN CORRECTLY IDENTIFYING VERBAL NOUN CONCEPTS ON THE PEABODY PICTURE VOCABULARY TEST THAN THE 160 MONOLINGUAL ENGLISH-SPEAKING SUBJECTS. STRUCTURAL AND IDIOMATIC DIFFERENCES BETWEEN THE ENGLISH AND SPANISH LANGUAGES ARE CONSIDERED AS THE SOURCE OF THE DIFFICULTY. THE DANGERS OF RELIANCE UPON METHODS OF EVALUATION AND PREDICTION WHICH ARE NOT ANALOGOUS TO THE CONTEXT OF THE PARTICULAR LEARNING HANDICAP ARE EMPHASIZED. 8 REFERENCES. (PASAR ABSTRACT)

ACCN   000683

805 AUTH **HIDALGO, H. A., & CHRISTENSEN, E. H.**
     TITL THE PUERTO RICAN LESBIAN AND THE PUERTO RICAN COMMUNITY.
     SRCE *JOURNAL OF HOMOSEXUALITY, 1976-77, 2(2), 109-121.*
     INDX HOMOSEXUALITY, PUERTO RICAN-M, FEMALE, SEX ROLES, CULTURAL FACTORS, EMPIRICAL, ATTITUDES
     ABST THE FEELINGS AND PERCEPTIONS OF 264 MEMBERS OF THE PUERTO RICAN COMMUNITY AND 61 PUERTO RICAN LESBIANS IN RELATION TO LESBIANISM WERE EXAMINED. LESBIANS INTERVIEWED WERE BETWEEN 18 AND 55 YEARS OF AGE AND INCLUDED STUDENTS, PROFESSIONALS, AND WORKING-CLASS WOMEN. THIS STUDY CONFIRMS THE GAY WOMEN'S FEAR OF BEING REJECTED BY THE PUERTO RICAN STRAIGHT COMMUNITY. THE MOST DIFFICULT AREA OF CONCERN FOR THE GAYS IS THE QUESTION OF EMPLOYMENT. THE COMMUNITY RESPONSES SUGGEST AN ACCEPTANCE OF LESBIANS IN "LONE" OR NON-SOCIAL-INFLUENCE POSITIONS, BUT NOT IN SOCIAL SERVICE AND "GUIDING" PROFESSIONS. IF SOCIETY IS TO ACCEPT AND UNDERSTAND THE GAYS' REALITY, THE RESPONSIBILITY RESTS ON GAYS TO FIGHT FOR THEIR RIGHTS. THE PUERTO RICAN GAY LIVING IN THE UNITED STATES EXPERIENCES A DOUBLE OPPRESSION AS A PUERTO RICAN AND AS A LESBIAN. THE STRUGGLE FOR PUERTO RICAN GAY LIBERATION AND PUERTO RICAN LIBERATION IS BOTH A STRUGGLE FOR IDENTITY AND AGAINST OPPRESSION. 4 REFERENCES.

ACCN   000684

806 AUTH **HILL, W. H., & FOX, W. M.**
TITL BLACK AND WHITE MARINE SQUAD LEADERS' PERCEPTIONS.
SRCE *ACADEMY OF MANAGEMENT JOURNAL, 1973, 16(4), 680-686.*
INDX INTEGRATION, CROSS CULTURAL, LEADERSHIP, ATTITUDES, PREJUDICE, PERFORMANCE EXPECTATIONS, DISCRIMINATION, GROUP DYNAMICS, PUERTO RICAN-M, SOUTH, MALE, MILITARY
ABST A QUESTIONNAIRE WAS ADMINISTERED TO 7 BLACK AND 22 WHITE U.S. MARINE CORPS SQUAD LEADERS CONCERNING THEIR ATTITUDES AND ACTIONS TOWARD 87 WHITE, 35 BLACK, AND 16 PUERTO RICAN MEMBERS OF THEIR SQUADS. NON-TASK-PRESCRIBED DIMENSIONS (E.G., UNCERTAINTY, AVOIDANCE OF FAILURE, ADMINISTRATION OF REPRIMANDS AND PRAISE, AND EVALUATION OF SUBORDINATES) WERE MEASURED. RESULTS INDICATE THAT WHITE SQUAD LEADERS REPORTED PROPORTIONATELY MORE REPRIMANDS TO THEIR WHITE SUBORDINATES AND BETTER PERFORMANCE RATINGS TO THEIR BLACK SUBORDINATES THAN DID THE BLACK SQUAD LEADERS. THEY ALSO GAVE MORE PRAISE TO THE PUERTO RICANS. BLACKS REPORTED BETTER RELATIONS WITH WHITE SUBORDINATES THAN DID WHITES. IT IS CONCLUDED THAT RECENT EMPHASIS ON RACIAL HARMONY IN THE ARMED FORCES HAS RESULTED IN (1) WHITE LEADERS TREATING THEIR BLACK SUBORDINATES WITH SPECIAL CARE, AND (2) BLACK LEADERS WORKING TO MAKE THEIR INTERRACIAL RELATIONS FREE OF DISCRIMINATION. 8 REFERENCES. (PASAR ABSTRACT MODIFIED)
ACCN 000685

807 AUTH **HINDELANG, M. J.**
TITL EDUCATIONAL AND OCCUPATIONAL ASPIRATIONS AMONG WORKING-CLASS NEGRO, MEXICAN AMERICAN AND WHITE ELEMENTARY SCHOOL CHILDREN.
SRCE *JOURNAL OF NEGRO EDUCATION, 1970, 39(4), 351-353.*
INDX OCCUPATIONAL ASPIRATIONS, SCHOLASTIC ASPIRATIONS, CROSS CULTURAL, SES, POVERTY, CHILDREN, MEXICAN AMERICAN, EMPIRICAL, WEST
ABST AN INVESTIGATION OF EDUCATIONAL AND OCCUPATIONAL ASPIRATIONS AMONG WORKING-CLASS NEGRO (N), MEXICAN AMERICAN (MA), AND WHITE (W) ELEMENTARY SCHOOL CHILDREN IS PRESENTED. A PRETESTED INTERVIEW SCHEDULE WAS USED IN INTERVIEWING 187 FOURTH, FIFTH, AND SIXTH-GRADE PUPILS. THE RACIAL COMPOSITION OF THE SUBJECTS WAS 68 N, 74 MA, AND 45 W, AND THE INTERVIEWERS WERE ETHNICALLY MATCHED TO THE SAMPLE. IT IS SHOWN THAT, EVEN AMONG ELEMENTARY PUPILS, DIFFERENCES IN EDUCATIONAL AND OCCUPATIONAL ASPIRATIONS OF THE N, MA, AND W GROUPS EXIST. THE N SUBSAMPLE HAD THE HIGHEST EDUCATIONAL ASPIRATIONS, FOLLOWED BY W, AND FINALLY THE MA SUBSAMPLE. WHEN EDUCATIONAL ASPIRATION WAS HELD CONSTANT, W AND MA PU-

PILS WERE FOUND TO ASPIRE TO HIGHER OCCUPATIONAL CATEGORIES. IT IS SUGGESTED THAT THE LATTER DIFFERENCE MAY BE RELATED TO THE FACT THAT ONLY N CHILDREN FELT THAT TEACHERS WERE PREJUDICED AGAINST THEM, AND CONSEQUENTLY N STUDENTS MAY HAVE BEEN PREPARING THEMSELVES FOR JOB DISCRIMINATION IN THE FUTURE. 8 REFERENCES.
ACCN 000686

808 AUTH **HISHIKI, P. C.**
TITL SELF-CONCEPTS OF SIXTH-GRADE GIRLS OF MEXICAN-AMERICAN DESCENT.
SRCE *CALIFORNIA JOURNAL OF EDUCATIONAL RESEARCH, 1969, 20(2), 56-62.*
INDX SELF CONCEPT, MEXICAN AMERICAN, SCHOLASTIC ACHIEVEMENT, INTELLIGENCE TESTING, CROSS CULTURAL, EMPIRICAL, CHILDREN, ACHIEVEMENT TESTING, FEMALE, CALIFORNIA, SOUTHWEST, GEORGIA, SOUTH, STANFORD ACHIEVEMENT TEST
ABST TO DETERMINE THE RELATIONSHIPS AMONG SELF-CONCEPT, ACADEMIC ACHIEVEMENT, INTELLIGENCE, AND INTERESTS, THE SELF-CONCEPT SCALE (SCS) AND THE CHILD SELF-DESCRIPTION SCALE (CSS) WERE ADMINISTERED TO 65 CALIFORNIA SIXTH-GRADE GIRLS OF MEXICAN AMERICAN (MA) DESCENT. SCHOLASTIC CHARACTERISTICS WERE DEFINED BY THE LORGE-THORNDIKE INTELLIGENCE TEST SCORES AND BY THE STANFORD ACHIEVEMENT TEST SCORES. THE RESULTS OBTAINED WERE COMPARED WITH THE RESULTS FROM A SIMILAR STUDY OF WHITE SIXTH-GRADE GIRLS IN GEORGIA. THE COMPARISON BETWEEN GROUPS REVEALED THAT THE MEAN CONCEPT SCORES FOR BOTH SELF AND IDEAL SELF WERE HIGHER FOR THE GEORGIA GROUP THAN THE MA GROUP. THERE WAS A SIGNIIFCANT POSITIVE RELATIONSHIP BETWEEN SELF-CONCEPT AND FACTORS OF INTELLIGENCE AND ACADEMIC ACHIEVEMENT FOR THE MA GROUP. MEAN GRADE PLACEMENTS ON THE ACHIEVEMENT TEST FOR THE MA GROUP WERE TWO GRADE LEVELS LOWER THAN ACTUAL GRADE. FURTHER, THE FINDINGS SHOW THAT BOTH GROUPS OF GIRLS ASSIGNED THEMSELVES SIMILAR PATTERNS OF SELF-DESCRIPTION. HOWEVER, THE MA SIXTH-GRADE GIRL WITH A HIGH SELF-CONCEPT HAD MORE SUCCESS IN ACADEMIC ACHIEVEMENT THAN DID THE SIXTH-GRADER OF A SIMILAR BACKGROUND WITH A LOW SELF-CONCEPT. IN VIEW OF THE RESULTS OF INTELLIGENCE AND ACHIEVEMENT TESTING, THE GROUP OF GIRLS FROM GEORGIA WOULD HAVE A BETTER CHANCE OF ENTERING AND SUCCEEDING IN COLLEGE. 9 REFERENCES.
ACCN 000687

809 AUTH **HOCKER, P. N., & MULLER, D.**
TITL STIMULUS DISCRIMINATION LEARNING AND TRANSPOSITION IN BILINGUAL CHILDREN.
SRCE *PERCEPTUAL AND MOTOR SKILLS, 1976, 42(1), 55-62.*
INDX ABILITY TESTING, BILINGUAL, CHILDREN, CROSS CULTURAL, EMPIRICAL, LANGUAGE ASSESS-

MENT, LINGUISTIC COMPETENCE, MEXICAN AMERICAN, NEW MEXICO, SOUTHWEST, LEARNING

ABST AN ATTEMPT WAS MADE TO DETERMINE WHETHER THE SPANISH/ENGLISH-SPEAKING CHILD'S ABILITY TO LEARN A DISCRIMINATION TASK AND TO DEMONSTRATE A MORE MATURE TRANSPOSITION WAS GREATER WHEN SPANISH WAS USED AS THE LANGUAGE OF INSTRUCTION AND VERBALIZATION. A TWO-STIMULUS SIZE DISCRIMINATION AND TRANSPOSITION TASK WAS ADMINISTERED TO 120 NEW MEXICAN, NATIVE SPANISH-SPEAKING, BILINGUAL FIRST-, SECOND-, AND THIRD-GRADE SUBEJECTS FROM BILINGUAL AND ENGLISH-ONLY INSTRUCTION CLASSROOMS. HALF OF THE SUBEJECTS LEARNED THE TASK AND VERBALIZED STIMULUS SELECTION RESPONSES IN SPANISH, AND HALF DID SO IN ENGLISH. RESULTS SUGGEST THAT THESE BILINGUAL SUBEJECTS LEARNED THE INITIAL DISCRIMINATION TASK MORE RAPIDLY WHEN THEY VERBALIZED IN SPANISH. ENGLISH-ONLY CLASSROOM STUDENTS TENDED TO TRANSPOSE MORE WHEN THEY HAD VERBALIZED SELECTION RESPONSES IN SPANISH; BILINGUAL CLASSROOM STUDENTS TRANSPOSED MORE WHEN THEY HAD VERBALIZED IN ENGLISH. NO SIGNIFICANT DIFFERENCES IN RATE OF DISCRIMINATION TASK LEARNING WERE OBSERVED BETWEEN THE TWO INSTRUCTIONAL PROGRAMS. 4 REFERENCES. (NCMHI ABSTRACT)

ACCN 002112

810 AUTH **HOFFMAN, G., & FISHMAN, J. A.**

TITL LIFE IN THE NEIGHBORHOOD: A FACTOR ANALYTIC STUDY OF PUERTO RICAN MALES IN THE NEW YORK CITY AREA.

SRCE *INTERNATIONAL JOURNAL OF COMPARATIVE SOCIOLOGY, 1971, 12(2), 85-100.*

INDX PUERTO RICAN-M, URBAN, INTERPERSONAL RELATIONS, ACCULTURATION, RESEARCH METHODOLOGY, SES, EDUCATION, FAMILY STRUCTURE, FAMILY ROLES, BILINGUAL, NEW YORK, EAST, MALE, VALUES

ABST THIS FACTOR ANALYTIC STUDY OF PUERTO RICAN MALES IN THE NEW YORK CITY AREA ATTEMPTED TO CLARIFY THOSE OBSERVED BEHAVIORS IN BILINGUAL PERSONS WHICH SEEM MOST CLEARLY TO REFLECT PUERTO RICAN AND AMERICAN VALUES. AN ANALYSIS OF EXTENSIVE INTERVIEW DATA DISPROVED THE FALLACY THAT CONTACT WITH A DOMINANT CULTURE RESULTS IN THE DISINTEGRATION OF TRADITIONAL SOCIAL AND CULTURAL PATTERNS. FURTHER, ACCULTURATION NEED NOT BE DISRUPTIVE, NOR DOES CONTACT RESULT IN ACCULTURATION. RESPONDENTS VIEWED DAILY BEHAVIORS AS BEING CLOSELY RELATED TO PUERTO RICAN ACTIVITIES, AND EDUCATION AND MOBILITY AS RELATED TO MORE AMERICAN ACTIVITIES. EVEN FOR A WORKING-CLASS POPULATION, HIGH CULTURE ACTIVITIES ARE VIEWED WITH SUFFICIENT CLARITY TO CLUSTER TOGETHER IN ONE FACTOR. THE ANALYSIS PROVIDED FURTHER UNDERSTANDING OF THE CULTURAL VALUES THAT THE SUB-

JECTS ATTACHED TO THE VARIOUS ACTIVITIES COVERED. EDUCATION AND HOME ARE THE DOMAINS WHICH HAVE EMERGED MOST CLEARLY. IN ADDITION, SOLIDARITY OF THE MAINLAND SUGGESTS A DOMAIN WHICH TOUCHES UPON INTERACTIONS WITH PUERTO RICANS OTHER THAN THOSE IN THE IMMEDIATE FAMILY. IT IS THIS FEELING OF SOLIDARITY WITH OTHER PUERTO RICANS THAT MAKES LIFE IN THE NEIGHBORHOOD A BICULTURAL EXPERIENCE. IT TRANSCENDS THE FAMILY BUT IT DOES NOT CAPITULATE TO THE LURES OF EDUCATION AND MOBILITY. 3 REFERENCES.

ACCN 000688

811 AUTH **HOGAN-GARCIA, M. H., MARTINEZ, J. L., JR., & MARTINEZ, S.**

TITL THE SEMANTIC DIFFERENTIAL: A TRI-ETHNIC COMPARISON OF SEX AND FAMILIAL CONCEPTS.

SRCE *HISPANIC JOURNAL OF BEHAVIORAL SCIENCES, 1979, 1(2), 135-149.*

INDX COLLEGE STUDENTS, EMPIRICAL, CALIFORNIA, SOUTHWEST, EMPIRICAL, SEX ROLES, MEXICAN AMERICAN, CROSS CULTURAL, SEX COMPARISON, FAMILY ROLES, ATTITUDES, CULTURAL FACTORS

ABST IN FOUR SOUTHERN CALIFORNIA COLLEGES, A SEMANTIC DIFFERENTIAL SCALE WAS ADMINISTERED TO A TRI-ETHNIC SAMPLE OF 201 SUBJECTS—35 CHICANOS, 70 BLACKS, AND 96 ANGLOS. THE SCALE CONSISTED OF 15 BIPOLAR ADJECTIVES REPRESENTING THE DIMENSIONS OF EVALUATION, POTENCY, AND ACTIVITY. THE FIVE CONCEPTS MEASURED WERE MALE, FEMALE, SELF, MOTHER, AND FATHER. THERE WERE THREE MAIN ANALYSES OF THE UNTRANSFORMED DATA: (1) A MULTIVARIATE ANALYSIS OF VARIANCE (MANOVA) FOR THE SOCIOCULTURAL DATA; (2) A MANOVA FOR THE SEMANTIC DATA; AND (3) A DISCRIMINANT ANALYSIS FOR THE SEMANTIC AND SOCIOCULTURAL VARIABLES. THE RESULTS DEMONSTRATED THE UTILITY OF USING THE SEMANTIC DIFFERENTIAL IN CONJUNCTION WITH QUESTIONS RELATED TO SOCIOCULTURAL STATUS, SINCE NOT ALL ETHNIC DIFFERENCES ON THE SEMANTIC DIFFERENTIAL ARE RELATED TO SOCIOCULTURAL DIFFERENTIATION. FURTHERMORE, THE SCALE REVEALED SUBCULTURAL DIFFERENCES AMONG GROUPS THAT SPEAK THE SAME LANGUAGE. GENERALLY, THE DIFFERENCES OBSERVED IN SEMANTIC DIFFERENTIAL RESPONSES WERE GREATEST, OR MORE POLAR, BETWEEN BLACKS AND ANGLOS. NO EXTREME RESPONSE DIFFERENCES WERE OBSERVED BETWEEN CHICANOS AND BLACKS, BUT WERE ALWAYS OBSERVED BETWEEN CHICANOS AND ANGLOS OR BETWEEN BLACKS AND ANGLOS. THE OVERALL PATTERN OF RESULTS SUGGESTS THAT MINORITY EXPERIENCE IS MORE IMPORTANT THAN CULTURAL EXPERIENCE IN PRODUCING THE OBSERVED DIFFERENCES. IN ADDITION, THERE ARE SEX DIFFERENCES WHICH CROSS-CUT ETHNIC LINES, AS THE RESULTS INDICATE THAT THE MALES ARE MORE STEREOTYPIC IN THEIR

RESPONSES THAN FEMALES. 27 REFERENCES. (JOURNAL ABSTRACT MODIFIED)

ACCN   001769

812 AUTH   **HOLLAND, W. R.**
     TITL   LANGUAGE BARRIER AS AN EDUCATIONAL PROBLEM OF SPANISH SPEAKING CHILDREN.
     SRCE   *EXCEPTIONAL CHILDREN, 1960, 27(1), 42-50.*
     INDX   CHILDREN, BILINGUALISM, LANGUAGE COMPREHENSION, SES, SCHOLASTIC ACHIEVEMENT, SPANISH SURNAMED, INTELLIGENCE TESTING, EDUCATION, EMPIRICAL, ARIZONA, SOUTHWEST, WISC, BILINGUAL
     ABST   AN ATTEMPT WAS MADE TO DEFINE AND ANALYZE THE SOCIAL AND CULTURAL BACKGROUND OF THE EDUCATIONAL PROBLEMS OF 36 SPANISH-SPEAKING CHILDREN. THESE CHILDREN FROM GRADE 1C (A FIRST GRADE CLASS SPECIALLY DESIGNED TO TEACH ENGLISH TO UNACCULTURATED SPANISH-SPEAKING CHILDREN) THROUGH GRADE 5 WERE TESTED BILINGUALLY WITH A SPECIAL SPANISH-ENGLISH ADAPTATION OF THE WISC. RESULTS SHOW THAT ALL BUT THREE OF THE CHILDREN HAD SOME LANGUAGE BARRIER. LACK OF ENGLISH COMPREHENSION WAS A SERIOUS HANDICAP TO THE EDUCATIONAL ADJUSTMENT OF OVER 40% OF THIS GROUP. THE LANGUAGE BARRIER WAS GREATEST AMONG GRADE 1C CHILDREN, DECREASED STEADILY WITH ADDED SCHOOLING, BUT WAS STILL PRESENT AMONG FIFTH-GRADE STUDENTS. A LANGUAGE BARRIER IS THE RESULT OF A LACK OF ACCULTURATION. HOWEVER, THE GENERALLY LOW VERBAL DEVELOPMENT IN BOTH SPANISH AND ENGLISH IS MORE LIKELY THE CONSEQUENCE OF BILINGUALISM IN AN UNDERPRIVILEGED ETHNIC GROUP. IT IS SUGGESTED THAT BILINGUAL EDUCATION FOR BILINGUAL CHILDREN MIGHT PROVE TO BE A WORTHWHILE EXPERIMENT. TEACHERS CAPABLE OF SUPPLEMENTING THE LANGUAGE OF THE CLASSROOM WITH THE LANGUAGE OF THE HOME MIGHT ACHIEVE MORE OPTIMAL RESULTS THAN CLASSROOM INSTRUCTION CONDUCTED EXCLUSIVELY IN ENGLISH. 6 REFERENCES.

ACCN   000689

813 AUTH   **HOLLINGSHEAD, A. B., & ROGLER, L. H.**
     TITL   LOWER SOCIOECONOMIC STATUS AND MENTAL ILLNESS.
     SRCE   *SOCIOLOGY AND SOCIAL RESEARCH, 1962, 46, 387-396.*
     INDX   SCHIZOPHRENIA, MENTAL HEALTH, PUERTO RICAN-I, SES, RESEARCH METHODOLOGY, CULTURAL FACTORS, POVERTY, BILINGUAL-BICULTURAL PERSONNEL, ADULTS, EMPIRICAL, PSYCHOPATHOLOGY
     ABST   FOCUSING UPON SCHIZOPHRENIA IN THE LOWEST SOCIOECONOMIC CLASS, THIS STUDY EXAMINED 40 FAMILIES IN SAN JUAN, PUERTO RICO. IN 20 FAMILIES ONE SPOUSE SUFFERED FROM SCHIZOPHRENIA, WHILE IN THE OTHER 20 FAMILIES BOTH SPOUSES WERE MENTALLY HEALTHY. COMPARABLE DATA WERE OBTAINED FOR BOTH TYPES OF FAMILIES, AND RESULTS REVEAL THAT MORE MENTAL ILLNESS WAS EV-

IDENT IN THOSE FAMILIES WITH ONE SCHIZOPHRENIC SPOUSE THAN IN THE NON-PSYCHOTIC GROUP. THIS REPORT PROVIDES NEW INSIGHTS INTO SCHIZOPHRENIA IN LOW-SES GROUPS; AND FURTHER STUDIES WILL BE REPORTED ANSWERING QUESTIONS OF HOW, WHERE, AND TO WHAT EXTENT SCHIZOPHRENICS ARE ABLE TO MAINTAIN MEANINGFUL CONTACTS WITHIN THE SOCIOCULTURAL REALITY WHICH SURROUNDS THEM. (JOURNAL ABSTRACT MODIFIED)

ACCN   000690

814 AUTH   **HOLTZ, J. A.**
     TITL   THE "LOW-RIDERS: PORTRAIT OF AN URBAN YOUTH SUBCULTURE.
     SRCE   *YOUTH AND SOCIETY, 1975, 6(4), 495-508.*
     INDX   ADOLESCENTS, URBAN, GANGS, DELINQUENCY, CASE STUDY, CALIFORNIA, SOUTHWEST, CULTURE, POVERTY, MEXICAN AMERICAN
     ABST   A DISCUSSION ON LOW-RIDERS, AN URBAN YOUTH SUBCULTURE, IS PRESENTED, BASED UPON TAPE RECORDED CONVERSATIONS AND FIELD OBSERVATIONS OF YOUTH IN PUBLIC AND PRIVATE SETTINGS FROM THE EAST LOS ANGELES COMMUNITY. PARTICIPANTS IN THE LOW-RIDER SUBCULTURE ARE MAINLY MALE CHICANOS IN THEIR LATE TEENS; MOST OF THEM COME FROM POOR FAMILIES AND ARE LIFE-TIME RESIDENTS OF THE BARRIO. BEING A LOW-RIDER CONSTITUTES AN IDENTITY THAT IS ACHIEVED BY THE ACQUISITION OF A SPECIAL KIND OF CAR. FOR THE LOW-RIDERS THE AUTOMOBILE IS THE PRIMARY VEHICLE OF SELF-EXPRESSION AND THE BASIS FOR SOCIAL GATHERINGS. THE AUTOMOBILE IS MODIFIED TO COMMUNICATE THE MOTIONS OF SLEEKNESS, CLEANLINESS AND LUXURY. AN ANALOGY IS OFTEN DRAWN BETWEEN ONE'S WOMAN AND ONE'S CAR, IN WHICH IT IS IMPLIED THAT THE WOMAN HAS A SECONDARY IMPORTANCE. THIS DISTINCTIVE PATTERN OF SOCIABILITY, KNOWN AS CRUISING THE BOULEVARD OR CRUISING FOR ACTION, IS HIGHLY VISIBLE IN THE BARRIO. IT IS AS IF THE FACTORS OF POVERTY FEED A MEDIA-ENGENDERED FANTASY OF AFFLUENT LEISURE THAT THE LOW-RIDER YOUTH MATERIALLY ENACT.

ACCN   000691

815 AUTH   **HOLTZMAN, W. H.**
     TITL   CROSS CULTURAL AND LONGITUDINAL COMPARISONS OF COGNITIVE, PERCEPTUAL AND PERSONALITY MEASURES IN MEXICO AND THE UNITED STATES.
     SRCE   *PAPER PRESENTED AT THE MEETING OF THE AMERICAN EDUCATIONAL RESEARCH ASSOCIATION, NEW ORLEANS, 1973. (ERIC DOCUMENT REPRODUCTION SERVICE NO. ED 079-183)*
     INDX   CROSS CULTURAL, COGNITIVE STYLE, RESEARCH METHODOLOGY, MEXICAN, EMPIRICAL, PERSONALITY ASSESSMENT, WISC, WAIS, PROJECTIVE TESTING, COGNITIVE DEVELOPMENT, CULTURAL FACTORS, CHILDREN, ADOLESCENTS, TEXAS, SOUTHWEST, SES
     ABST   INSIGHT CAN BE GAINED INTO THE ROLE OF

SPECIFIED CULTURAL VARIABLES IN HUMAN DEVELOPMENT IF CARE IS TAKEN (1) TO INCLUDE SUBCULTURAL VARIATIONS WHICH CAN BE MATCHED CROSS-CULTURALLY, (2) TO EMPLOY WELL TRAINED NATIVE EXAMINERS WHO HAVE BEEN CALIBRATED CROSS-CULTURALLY, (3) TO USE TECHNIQUES WHICH CAN BE DEFENDED, AND (4) TO INVOLVE THE CLOSE AND CONTINUAL COLLABORATION OF INVESTIGATORS SENSITIVE TO THE ABOVE ISSUES. THIS PAPER REPORTS FINDINGS FROM SIX YEARS OF REPEATED TESTING OF CHILDREN FROM TEXAS AND MEXICO WHO WERE SELECTED TO REPRESENT A BROAD RANGE OF WORKING CLASS, BUSINESS, AND PROFESSIONAL FAMILIES. A COMPLEX ANALYSIS OF VARIANCE DESIGN WAS CONSTRUCTED WITH FIVE MAIN FACTORS: (1) SOCIOECONOMIC STATUS; (2) SEX; (3) AGE GROUP WHEN TESTED INITIALLY; (4) CULTURE, MEXICAN OR AMERICAN; AND (5) YEAR OF REPEATED TESTING OR TRIAL. THE MAIN EFFECTS FOR CULTURE PROVED HIGHLY SIGNIFICANT, REVEALING IMPORTANT DIFFERENCES IN DEVELOPMENTAL TRENDS FOR THE ENTIRE AGE SPAN OF 6-17 YEARS IN MEXICAN AND AMERICAN CHILDREN. THIS STUDY REPORTS ONLY HIGHLIGHTS OF A MUCH LARGER RESEARCH PROGRAM INVOLVING HUNDREDS OF CHILDREN AND THEIR FAMILIES. ADDITIONAL STUDIES ARE AIMED AT GAINING GREATER INSIGHT INTO THE COMPLEX RELATIONSHIPS BETWEEN COGNITIVE, PERCEPTUAL AND PERSONALITY MEASURES ON THE ONE HAND AND FAMILY LIFE-STYLE, HOME ENVIRONMENT AND SCHOOL PERFORMANCE VARIABLES AS THESE ASPECTS OF PERSONALITY DEVELOPMENT CHANGE OVER TIME IN THE TWO CULTURES. 5 REFERENCES. (RIE ABSTRACT MODIFIED)

ACCN 000692

816 AUTH **HOLTZMAN, W. H.**
TITL MENTAL HEALTH AND PERSONALITY DEVELOPMENT IN THE BORDER STATES.
SRCE *TEXAS PSYCHOLOGIST, 1975, 27(1), 56-61.*
INDX FIELD DEPENDENCE-INDEPENDENCE, MENTAL HEALTH, CROSS CULTURAL, SES, PERSONALITY, SEX COMPARISON, EMPIRICAL, CHILDREN, CULTURAL CHANGE, ADOLESCENTS, COGNITIVE STYLE, FAMILY ROLES, COOPERATION, COMPETITION, TEXAS, SOUTHWEST, URBAN, MEXICAN
ABST THE HIGHLIGHTS OF A CROSS-CULTURAL LONGITUDINAL STUDY OF OVER 400 AMERICAN CHILDREN IN AUSTIN, TEXAS, AND A COMPARABLE NUMBER IN MEXICO CITY ARE DISCUSSED IN RELATION TO PREVIOUS STUDIES. ALTHOUGH STATISTICAL DATA ARE NOT GIVEN, MAJOR SIMILARITIES AND DIFFERENCES ARE PRESENTED. CLEAR AND UNIFORM DIFFERENCES WERE FOUND ACROSS THE TWO CULTURES FOR MANY OF THE PSYCHOLOGICAL DIMENSIONS, REGARDLESS OF THE SEX, AGE, OR SES OF THE CHILD. IN OTHER INSTANCES, THE SIGNIFICANT DIFFERENCES BETWEEN MEXICANS AND ANGLO AMERICANS MUST BE QUALIFIED SINCE THEY WERE NOT UNIFORMLY PRESENT FOR BOTH BOYS AND GIRLS, FOR

ALL AGES, OR FOR BOTH UPPER AND LOWER SOCIAL CLASSES. THESE QUALIFICATIONS ARE DISCUSSED IN TERMS OF: (1) DEVELOPMENT OF MENTAL ABILITIES; (2) ACTIVE VERSUS PASSIVE COPING STYLE; (3) FIELD DEPENDENCY AND SOCIALIZATION; (4) SOCIAL CLASS AND SEX DIFFERENCES; AND (5) MENTAL HEALTH AND SOCIAL CHANGE. IT IS POSITED THAT THE MEXICANS AND NORTH AMERICANS LIVING IN THE BORDERLANDS ARE BECOMING MORE ALIKE DUE TO CULTURAL INTERACTION AND DIFFUSION. 8 REFERENCES.

ACCN 000693

817 AUTH **HOLTZMAN, W. H.**
TITL PERSONALITY DEVELOPMENT AND MENTAL HEALTH OF PEOPLE IN THE BORDER STATES.
SRCE *IN S. R. ROSS, (ED.), VIEWS ACROSS THE BORDER: THE UNITED STATES AND MEXICO. ALBUQUERQUE: UNIVERSITY OF NEW MEXICO PRESS, 1978, PP. 308-329.*
INDX CHILDREARING PRACTICES, CHILDREN, COGNITIVE DEVELOPMENT, COMPETITION, SES, COOPERATION, COPING MECHANISMS, CROSS CULTURAL, CROSS GENERATIONAL, ECONOMIC FACTORS, EDUCATION, FIELD DEPENDENCE-INDEPENDENCE, HISTORY, MENTAL HEALTH, MEXICAN, MEXICAN AMERICAN, PERSONALITY, REVIEW, SOUTHWEST
ABST A REVIEW OF STUDIES ON ANGLO AND MEXICAN AMERICAN POPULATIONS IN THE SOUTHWESTERN BORDER STATES PROVIDES AN INSIGHT INTO ISSUES OF CROSS-CULTURAL PSYCHOLOGY. FIRST, A MAJOR LONGITUDINAL STUDY INVOLVING EXTENSIVE ANNUAL PSYCHOLOGICAL TESTING OF ANGLO AMERICAN CHILDREN FROM A BORDER STATE AND MEXICAN CHILDREN FROM MEXICO CITY REVEALED CLEAR AND UNIFORM DIFFERENCES IN PERSONALITY AND IN COGNITIVE AND PERCEPTUAL DEVELOPMENT, REGARDLESS OF SEX, AGE, OR SES. SECOND, DIFFERENCES IN FAMILY CHARACTERISTICS, PARENTAL ATTITUDES, AND LIFE STYLE APPEAR TO INFLUENCE COGNITIVE DEVELOPMENT OF CHILDREN. THE ANGLO CHILD, REGARDLESS OF SOCIAL CLASS, SEEMS TO BE ENCOURAGED TOWARD INDEPENDENT THINKING AND AN ACHIEVEMENT ORIENTATION TO A GREATER EXTENT THAN THE MEXICAN CHILD. AND BASED ON THE WITKIN EMBEDDED FIGURES TEST, MEXICAN CHILDREN HAVE BEEN FOUND TO BE MORE FIELD DEPENDENT THAN THEIR ANGLO PEERS. THIRD, RECENT STUDIES DEMONSTRATE THAT MEXICAN AMERICAN CHILDREN DO AS WELL IN CONCEPT LEARNING TASKS AS ANGLO AMERICAN CHILDREN WHEN GIVEN EQUAL FACILITATIVE CONDITIONS PRIOR TO TESTING. FINALLY, MANY OF THE DIFFERENCES BETWEEN MEXICAN AND ANGLO AMERICAN CHILDREN ARE ATTRIBUTABLE TO DIFFERENT COPING STYLES. THE MEXICANS TEND TO HAVE A COPING STYLE BASED ON PASSIVE OBEDIENCE WHILE THE ANGLO CHILD HAS AN ACTIVE COPING STYLE. DIFFERENCES IN COPING STYLES MAY ACCOUNT FOR THE LOWER INCIDENCE OF MENTAL ILLNESS FOR MEXICAN AMERICANS. HOWEVER, INADEQUATE FACILITIES FOR THIS

GROUP'S NEEDS MAY ALSO ACCOUNT FOR THE APPARENT DIFFERENCE. 32 REFERENCES.

ACCN   002113

818 AUTH   **HOLTZMAN, W. H., DIAZ-GUERRERO, R., SWARTZ, J. D., & TAPIA, L. L.**
     TITL   CROSS-CULTURAL LONGITUDINAL RESEARCH ON CHILD DEVELOPMENT: STUDIES OF AMERICAN AND MEXICAN SCHOOL CHILDREN.
     SRCE   *IN J. P. HILL (ED.), MINNESOTA SYMPOSIA ON CHILD PSYCHOLOGY (VOL. 2). MINNEAPOLIS: UNIVERSITY OF MINNESOTA PRESS, 1968, PP. 125-159.*
     INDX   COGNITIVE DEVELOPMENT, CHILDREN, CROSS CULTURAL, EMPIRICAL, PERSONALITY, PERSONALITY ASSESSMENT, CULTURE, TAT, WISC, ANXIETY, WAIS, SES, FAMILY STRUCTURE, CHILDREARING PRACTICES, MEXICAN, TEXAS, SOUTHWEST, PROJECTIVE TESTING
     ABST   A LONGITUDINAL STUDY OF COGNITIVE, PERCEPTUAL, AND PERSONALITY DEVELOPMENT OF 4117 ANGLO-AMERICAN (AA) AND 443 MEXICAN (M) CHILDREN IS DESCRIBED. IN ADDITION TO THE HOLTZMAN INKBLOT TECHNIQUE, THE BASIC TEST BATTERY INCLUDED SELECTED COGNITIVE, PERCEPTUAL, AND PERSONALITY TESTS GIVEN INDIVIDUALLY TO EACH CHILD ONCE A YEAR FOR 6 YEARS. PRELIMINARY FINDINGS ARE INTERPRETED FROM AN ACTIVE-PASSIVE PERSPECTIVE IN WHICH AA CHILDREN WERE FOUND TO BE MORE ACTIVE IN COPING WITH STRESS THAN M CHILDREN. THE M CHILD IN A TESTING SITUATION WOULD COOPERATE TO PLEASE THE EXAMINER WHILE THE AA CHILD WOULD VIEW THE TESTING SITUATION AS A CHALLENGE TO BE MASTERED. RESULTS FROM THE INKBLOT SCORES INDICATE THAT THE AA CHILD PRODUCES FASTER REACTION TIMES, USES LARGER PORTIONS OF THE INKBLOTS IN GIVING HIS RESPONSES, GIVES MORE DEFINITE FORM TO HIS RESPONSES, AND IS ABLE TO INTEGRATE MORE PARTS OF THE INKBLOT. IN ADDITION, THE AA CHILD INCORPORATES OTHER STIMULUS PROPERTIES OF THE INKBLOT, SUCH AS COLOR AND SHADING, INTO HIS RESPONSES MORE OFTEN THAN DOES THE M CHILD. IN ATTEMPTING TO DEAL WITH ALL ASPECTS OF THE INKBLOTS IN SUCH AN ACTIVE FASHION, THE AA CHILD FAILS MORE OFTEN THAN THE M CHILD. THIS FAILURE IS INDICATED BY SUCH VARIABLES AS FORM APPROPRIATENESS, PATHOGNOMIC VERBALIZATION, ANXIETY, AND HOSTILITY. THE M CHILD GIVES RESPONSES WITH BETTER FORM AND FEWER RESPONSES THAT SHOW DEVIANT THINKING, ANXIOUSNESS, AND HOSTILE CONTENT. THE AA CHILD TRIES TO DEAL WITH THE TESTING SITUATION IN A MUCH MORE ACTIVE FASHION THAN THE M CHILD EVEN WHEN HE IS UNABLE TO DO SO SUCCESSFULLY. DEFINITE CONCLUSIONS MUST AWAIT COMPLETION OF THE OVERALL LONGITUDINAL DESIGN. 37 REFERENCES.

     ACCN   000694

819 AUTH   **HOPPE, C. M., KAGAN, S. M., & ZAHN, G. L.**
     TITL   CONFLICT RESOLUTION AMONG FIELD-INDEPENDENT AND FIELD-DEPENDENT ANGLO-

AMERICAN AND MEXICAN-AMERICAN CHILDREN AND THEIR MOTHERS.

     SRCE   *DEVELOPMENTAL PSYCHOLOGY, 1977, 13(6), 591-598.*
     INDX   CONFLICT RESOLUTION, MEXICAN AMERICAN, CROSS CULTURAL, EMPIRICAL, COGNITIVE STYLE, CHILDREN, SEX COMPARISON, MOTHER-CHILD INTERACTION, FIELD DEPENDENCE-INDEPENDENCE, CALIFORNIA, SOUTHWEST
     ABST   THIRTY-TWO ANGLO AMERICAN AND MEXICAN AMERICAN BOYS AND GIRLS, SELECTED FOR THEIR EXTREME FIELD INDEPENDENCE OR DEPENDENCE, INTERACTED WITH THEIR MOTHERS IN THREE ROLE PLAYS DESIGNED TO PROVOKE CONFLICT OVER ISSUES OF MATERNAL AUTHORITY AND CHILDREN'S INDEPENDENCE. THE MOTHER-CHILD INTERACTIONS WERE RECORDED, TRANSCRIBED, AND CONTENT ANALYZED. CONSISTENT WITH PREVIOUS BEHAVIORAL STUDIES, ANGLO AMERICAN AND TO SOME EXTENT MALE CHILDREN, MORE OFTEN THAN MEXICAN AMERICAN AND FEMALE CHILDREN, ENTERED AND PERSISTED IN DIRECT CONFLICT AS INDICATED BY A NUMBER OF VARIABLES SUCH AS DISAGREEMENT AND JUSTIFICATION OF THEIR OWN WILL. MOTHERS OF THE TWO CULTURAL GROUPS TENDED NOT TO DIFFER. FIELD INDEPENDENCE AMONG BOYS AND FIELD DEPENDENCE AMONG GIRLS WERE ASSOCIATED WITH MORE ASSERTIVE BEHAVIORS. MOTHERS OF FIELD INDEPENDENT CHILDREN USED A MORE ELABORATE VERBAL CODE. THE STUDY INDICATES CULTURAL DIFFERENCES IN MOTHER-CHILD INTERACTION PATTERNS, BUT THESE DIFFERENCES ARE NOT CONSISTENTLY RELATED TO COGNITIVE STYLE. FURTHERMORE, COGNITIVE STYLE HAD DIFFERENT CORRELATES FOR BOYS AND GIRLS. 43 REFERENCES. (AUTHOR ABSTRACT MODIFIED)

     ACCN   000695

820 AUTH   **HOPPE, S. K., & HELLER, P. L.**
     TITL   ALIENATION, FAMILISM AND THE UTILIZATION OF HEALTH SERVICES BY MEXICAN AMERICANS.
     SRCE   *JOURNAL OF HEALTH AND SOCIAL BEHAVIOR, 1975, 16(3), 304-314.*
     INDX   RESOURCE UTILIZATION, ANOMIE, SES, POVERTY, DEPRESSION, MEXICAN AMERICAN, EMPIRICAL, FAMILY STRUCTURE, PSYCHOPATHOLOGY, MENTAL HEALTH, TEXAS, SOUTHWEST, HEALTH, THEORETICAL
     ABST   THE INFLUENCE OF FAMILISM AND OCCUPATIONAL STABILITY ON ALIENATION AND HEALTH CARE UTILIZATION AMONG LOWER-CLASS MEXICAN AMERICANS WAS EXAMINED AMONG 197 MEXICAN AMERICAN MOTHERS OF A SAN ANTONIO BARRIO. FAMILIES WERE INTERVIEWED REGARDING THEIR HUSBANDS' CURRENT AND PAST EMPLOYMENT, FAMILY HEALTH CARE PRACTICES, FAMILISM AND ALIENATION. ANALYSIS INDICATED THAT FAMILISM AND OCCUPATIONAL STABILITY WERE POSITIVELY CORRELATED TO TIMING OF PRENATAL CARE, BUT NEGATIVELY CORRELATED TO CONSULTING A PHYSICIAN WHEN ILL. POWERLESSNESS WAS NEGATIVELY RELATED TO TIMING OF PRE-

NATAL CARE AND POSITIVELY RELATED TO CONSULTING WHEN ILL. THE RESULTS SUGGEST IT IS IMPORTANT TO DISTINGUISH BETWEEN PREVENTIVE AND CURATIVE COMPONENTS OF HEALTH CARE BEHAVIOR WHEN MEASURING RESOURCE UTILIZATION. IN ADDITION, THE ROLE OF FAMILISM SHOULD BE CONSIDERED IN THE COMPLEX RELATIONSHIP BETWEEN ALIENATION AND HEALTH CARE UTILIZATION. A THEORETICAL FRAMEWORK EXPLAINING THIS ROLE IS DISCUSSED. 41 REFERENCES. (JOURNAL ABSTRACT MODIFIED)

ACCN   000696

821 AUTH   **HOPPE, S. K., & LEON, R. L.**
    TITL   COPING IN THE BARRIO: CASE STUDIES OF MEXICAN-AMERICAN FAMILIES.
    SRCE   *CHILD PSYCHIATRY AND HUMAN DEVELOPMENT, 1977, 7(4), 264-275.*
    INDX   MEXICAN AMERICAN, CHILDREN, ADULTS, CHILDREARING PRACTICES, MOTHER-CHILD INTERACTION, FATHER-CHILD INTERACTION, EMPIRICAL, TEXAS, SOUTHWEST, COPING MECHANISMS, SES, TIME ORIENTATION, MENTAL HEALTH, ATTITUDES, SCHOLASTIC ASPIRATIONS, OCCUPATIONAL ASPIRATIONS, HEALTH, PERSONALITY
    ABST   TO IDENTIFY FACTORS RELATED TO ADAPTIVE OR COPING BEHAVIOR, EIGHT LOWER-CLASS MEXICAN AMERICAN FAMILIES WERE INTERVIEWED ON BACKGROUND, MARITAL HISTORY, EMPLOYMENT HISTORY, AND CHILDREARING ATTITUDES AND BEHAVIORS. A COMPLEX OF FACTORS DIFFERENTIATED FAMILIES WHO WERE JUDGED TO BE DEALING EFFECTIVELY WITH THEIR ENVIRONMENT (COPERS) FROM THOSE WHO WERE NOT (NONCOPERS). DIFFERENCES IN THE HEALTH STATUS OF THE CHILDREN IN COPING AND NONCOPING FAMILIES WERE APPARENT. PARENTS WHO WERE COPERS SHOWED MORE CONCERN ABOUT THEIR CHILDREN'S INTERESTS AND ACTIVITIES, HAD HIGHER EDUCATIONAL AND OCCUPATIONAL ASPIRATIONS FOR THEM, AND RECOGNIZED THE IMPORTANCE OF LOVE AND AFFECTION. NONCOPERS EXPRESSED MORE CONCERN WITH THEIR OWN PROBLEMS AND EMPHASIZED BOTH THE CHILDREN'S BASIC NEEDS (FOOD AND SHELTER) AND THE IMPORTANCE OF CLEANLINESS. ALTHOUGH THE OLDER CHILDREN OF NONCOPERS APPEARED MATURE FOR THEIR AGE, THE YOUNGER CHILDREN EXHIBITED FEWER THAN EXPECTED AGE-APPROPRIATE BEHAVIORS. NONCOPING PARENTS ALSO WERE MORE DISORGANIZED AND LESS ABLE TO TAKE A LEADERSHIP ROLE. IN PARTICULAR, NONCOPERS SEEMED UNABLE TO CONCEPTUALIZE AFFECTIONATE EMOTIONAL RELATIONSHIPS OR TO CONCEPTUALIZE AND ORGANIZE TIME, AND A POSSIBLE RELATIONSHIP BETWEEN THESE TWO CHARACTERISTICS HAS IMPLICATIONS FOR MENTAL HEALTH PLANNING. 9 REFERENCES.

ACCN   002114

822 AUTH   **HORN, J. M., & TURNER, R. G.**
    TITL   PERSONALITY CORRELATES OF DIFFERENTIAL

ABILITIES IN A SAMPLE OF LOWER THAN AVERAGE ABILITY.

SRCE   *PSYCHOLOGICAL REPORTS, 1974, 35(3), 1211-1220.*
INDX   PERSONALITY, INTELLIGENCE, INTELLIGENCE TESTING, SEX COMPARISON, MEXICAN AMERICAN, LINGUISTIC COMPETENCE, MATHEMATICS, SCHOLASTIC ACHIEVEMENT, COLLEGE STUDENTS, TEXAS, SOUTHWEST, REVIEW
ABST   CRITICS OF IQ TESTS OFTEN EMPHASIZE THE IMPORTANCE OF NON-INTELLECTUAL COMPONENTS OF INTELLIGENT BEHAVIOR. PREVIOUS RESEARCH HAS IDENTIFIED MASCULINITY-FEMININITY AS ONE FACTOR CONTRIBUTING TO THE DIFFERENTIATION OF PEOPLE ALONG A DIMENSION OF HIGH VERBAL ABILITY AT ONE END AND HIGH MATHEMATICAL (OR OTHER "PRACTICAL") ABILITY AT THE OTHER. HOWEVER, ALMOST ALL OF THIS INFORMATION WAS DERIVED FROM THE STUDY OF GROUPS WHOSE OVER-ALL ABILITY WAS ABOUT 1 SD ABOVE THE POPULATION MEAN. TO TEST THE GENERALIZABILITY OF THESE FINDINGS, THE GUILFORD-ZIMMERMAN PERSONALITY CORRELATES OF DIFFERENTIAL ABILITIES WERE INVESTIGATED IN A LOWER THAN AVERAGE ABILITY GROUP COMPRISED OF 405 COLLEGE STUDENTS ENROLLED IN A PSYCHOLOGY CLASS IN SAN ANTONIO, TEXAS. MASCULINITY WAS RELATED TO THE HIGH MATHEMATICAL-LOW VERBAL ABILITY COMPLEX FOR FEMALES BUT NOT FOR MALES. THE IMPORTANCE OF STUDYING THE INTERACTION OF SEX AND TYPE OF ABILITY IS DISCUSSED. 22 REFERENCES. (JOURNAL ABSTRACT MODIFIED)

ACCN   000697

823 AUTH   **HOROWITZ, R., & SCHWARTZ, G.**
    TITL   HONOR, NORMATIVE AMBIGUITY AND GANG VIOLENCE.
    SRCE   *AMERICAN SOCIOLOGICAL REVIEW, 1974, 39(2), 238-251.*
    INDX   GANGS, ROLE EXPECTATIONS, MODELING, SELF CONCEPT, ADOLESCENTS, MEXICAN AMERICAN, INTERPERSONAL SPACING, AGGRESSION, SOCIALIZATION, COMMUNITY, CRIMINOLOGY, INTERPERSONAL RELATIONS, ILLINOIS, MIDWEST
    ABST   THE SOCIAL CONTEXT IN WHICH GANG VIOLENCE OCCURRED AMONG 31 ACTIVE CHICANO GANG MEMBERS, AGES 16-20, IS EXAMINED, WITH EMPHASIS ON HOW ADHERENCE TO A CODE OF PERSONAL HONOR SHAPES RESPONSES TO A PERCEIVED INSULT. DATA CONSISTED OF APPROXIMATELY 50 EPISODES OF INTERGANG VIOLENCE INVOLVING ONE OR MORE MEMBERS WHO WERE OBSERVED AND WHO GAVE PARTICIPANT REPORTS. HYPOTHESIZED WAS THAT GANG VIOLENCE ARISES IN SITUATIONS WHERE ONE PARTY IMPUGNS THE HONOR OF HIS ADVERSARY, THUS VIOLATING THE NORMS OF INTERPERSONAL ETIQUETTE AND CONSTITUTING A VIOLATION OF PERSONAL SPACE. IN THE ABSENCE OF HIGHER-ORDER RULES FOR RECONCILING CONTRADICTIONS BETWEEN CONFLICTING CODES OF CONDUCT, NORMATIVE AMBIGUITY OCCURS. GANG VIOLENCE OCCURS WHEN HONOR BE-

COMES A PRESSING ISSUE IN INTERPERSONAL RELATIONS, AND PARTICIPANTS FEEL THEY CANNOT TALK THEIR WAY OUT OF A SITUATION. ON THE WHOLE, CHICANO GANG MEMBERS WERE ADEPT IN ASSUMING ROLES CONGRUENT WITH THE DEMANDS OF DIVERSE SOCIAL SITUATIONS IN AN URBAN SOCIETY. AS THEY GROW OLDER, THEY LEARN TO DEAL MORE EFFECTIVELY IN THE ADULT WORLD. IT IS CONCLUDED THAT CHICANO GANG MEMBERSHIP IS A RESULT OF SOCIAL MARGINALITY IN THE LARGER SOCIETY WHICH IMPOSES RESTRICTIONS ON THEIR ASPIRATIONS. 17 REFERENCES.

ACCN 000698

824 AUTH **HOSFORD, R. E., & BOWLES, S. A.**
TITL DETERMINING CULTURALLY APPROPRIATE REINFORCERS FOR ANGLO AND CHICANO STUDENTS.
SRCE *ELEMENTARY SCHOOL GUIDANCE AND COUNSELING, 1974, 8(4), 290-300.*
INDX MEXICAN AMERICAN, READING, EDUCATIONAL COUNSELING, CURRICULUM, MENTAL HEALTH, BEHAVIOR MODIFICATION, CULTURAL FACTORS, EMPIRICAL
ABST THE OBJECTIVES, IMPLEMENTATION, OBSERVATIONS AND RESULTS OF A READING PROGRAM USING CULTURALLY APPROPRIATE BEHAVIORAL REINFORCEMENTS ARE DESCRIBED IN DETAIL. ONE HUNDRED THIRTY-SIX ANGLO AND CHICANO 4TH, 5TH AND 6TH GRADERS ATTENDING SUMMER SCHOOL WERE ASSIGNED TO EITHER THE SPECIAL PROGRAM OR THE REGULAR READING PROGRAM. READING ABILITIES WERE MATCHED, WHILE ETHNICITY, SEX, AND GRADE LEVEL WERE VARIED RANDOMLY FOR EACH READING GROUP. RESULTS INDICATE THAT: (1) BETWEEN THE FIRST AND LAST WEEK'S PROGRAM OBSERVATIONS, THE EXPERIMENTAL GROUP SHOWED A SIGNIFICANT INCREASE IN THEIR READING BEHAVIOR, AND (2) NUMBER OF DAYS ABSENT WAS SIGNIFICANTLY LOWER FOR THE SPECIAL READING GROUP. IT IS POSITED THAT THESE STRONG DIFFERENCES OCCURRING IN SO SHORT A TIME (5 WEEKS) DEMONSTRATE THAT PROVIDING STUDENTS WITH THE OPPORTUNITY TO SELECT THEIR OWN REINFORCERS IS A POTENT TECHNIQUE FOR TEACHERS AND COUNSELORS TO HELP STUDENTS MODIFY A VARIETY OF BEHAVIORS. 2 REFERENCES. (AUTHOR SUMMARY MODIFIED)

ACCN 000699

825 AUTH **HOUTS, P. L.**
TITL AN INTERVIEW WITH GEORGE I. SANCHEZ.
SRCE *THE NATIONAL ELEMENTARY PRINCIPAL, 1970, 50(2), 102-104.*
INDX EDUCATION, EQUAL OPPORTUNITY, CHICANO MOVEMENT, MEXICAN AMERICAN, POLITICAL POWER, HEALTH, BILINGUAL-BICULTURAL EDUCATION, TEXAS, ESSAY, SOUTHWEST, POLICY, POLITICAL POWER
ABST IN THIS PARTIAL WRITE-UP OF A LONGER INTERVIEW, GEORGE I. SANCHEZ, PROFESSOR OF LATIN AMERICAN EDUCATION AT THE UNIVERSITY OF TEXAS IN AUSTIN, DISCUSSES SEV-

ERAL FACTORS IMPORTANT TO CHICANOS AND EDUCATION. SOME OF THESE ARE: (1) CHANGES IN THE CONCEPT OF EQUAL OPPORTUNITY; (2) THE ROLE OF THE FEDERAL GOVERNMENT AND COMMUNITY IN BRINGING ABOUT CHANGE IN EDUCATION; (3) THE EFFECT OF CHICANO YOUTH MOVEMENTS ON ANGLO INSTITUTIONS; (4) POLITICAL POTENTIAL OF CHICANOS IN ATTAINING REFORM; (5) DIFFERENCES BETWEEN CHICANOS AND PUERTO RICANS OR CUBANS; AND (6) OTHER HIGH PRIORITY NEEDS OF THE CHICANO POPULATION IN THE SOUTHWEST.

ACCN 000700

826 AUTH **HOUTS, P. L.**
TITL AN INTERVIEW WITH JULIAN SAMORA.
SRCE *THE NATIONAL ELEMENTARY PRINCIPAL, 1970, 50(2), 98-101.*
INDX EDUCATION, EQUAL OPPORTUNITY, MEXICAN AMERICAN, COMMUNITY INVOLVEMENT, CHICANO MOVEMENT, PARENTAL INVOLVEMENT, POLITICS, ESSAY
ABST THIS PARTIAL WRITE-UP OF A LONGER INTERVIEW WITH JULIAN SAMORA, PROFESSOR OF SOCIOLOGY AT THE UNIVERSITY OF NOTRE DAME, DISCUSSES THE FOLLOWING FACTORS RELEVANT TO MEXICAN AMERICANS AND EDUCATION: (1) THE EFFECTS OF ORGANIZATION ON MEXICAN AMERICAN COMMUNITIES; (2) AN EVALUATION OF THE GOAL OF EQUAL EDUCATIONAL OPPORTUNITIES FOR SPANISH-SPEAKING AMERICANS; (3) THE RESPONSIBILITY OF LOCAL COMMUNITIES IN EDUCATIONAL CHANGE; (4) THE EFFECT OF CHICANO YOUTH MOVEMENTS ON SCHOOL SYSTEMS; (5) SOME PROBLEMS WITH PLANNING MEXICAN AMERICAN STUDIES PROGRAMS; (6) THE ROLE OF CONFRONTATION IN PROMOTING CHANGE; (7) THE FUTURE ROLE OF COALITIONS AMONG MINORITY POPULATIONS TO PROMOTE CHANGE; (8) THE EFFECT OF TITLE VII, MIGRANCY AND ISOLATED SCHOOL DISTRICTS; AND (9) THE NEED FOR MEXICAN AMERICAN PARENTS TO BECOME INVOLVED IN SCHOOL PTA ORGANIZATIONS.

ACCN 000701

827 AUTH **HOUTS, P. L.**
TITL AN INTERVIEW WITH THOMAS P. CARTER.
SRCE *THE NATIONAL ELEMENTARY PRINCIPAL, 1970, 50(2), 94-97.*
INDX EDUCATION, CHICANO MOVEMENT, MEXICAN AMERICAN, TEACHERS, DISCRIMINATION, EQUAL OPPORTUNITY, TEXAS, SOUTHWEST, ATTITUDES, ADMINISTRATORS, COMMUNITY INVOLVEMENT
ABST IN THIS PARTIAL WRITE-UP OF A LONGER INTERVIEW, DR. CARTER, PROFESSOR OF EDUCATION AND SOCIOLOGY AT THE UNIVERSITY OF TEXAS, EL PASO, DISCUSSES SEVERAL FACTORS RELEVANT TO CHICANOS AND EDUCATION. AMONG THESE ARE: (1) CHANGES IN THE ATTITUDES OF EDUCATORS; (2) THE ROLE OF TEACHER TRAINING, THE FEDERAL GOVERNMENT, AND POLITICIANS IN BRINGING ABOUT CHANGES IN THE EDUCATIONAL SYSTEM; (3) THE RESPONSIBILITIES OF THE ELEMENTARY

SCHOOL PRINCIPAL IN BEING MORE RESPONSIVE TO HIS CONSTITUENCY; (4) COMMUNITY INVOLVEMENT; (5) THE DIRECTION AND PURPOSE OF CHICANO AND OTHER CULTURAL STUDIES; AND (6) THE PURSUIT OF OPPORTUNITIES BY YOUNG CHICANOS.

ACCN   000702

828 AUTH   **HOUTS, P. L. (ED.)**
     TITL   EDUCATION FOR THE SPANISH SPEAKING.
     SRCE   *THE NATIONAL ELEMENTARY PRINCIPAL, 1970, 50(WHOLE ISSUE NO. 2).*
     INDX   EDUCATION, MEXICAN AMERICAN, PUERTO RICAN-M, SPANISH SURNAMED, SCHOLASTIC ACHIEVEMENT, HISTORY, BILINGUAL-BICULTURAL EDUCATION, COMMUNITY INVOLVEMENT, MIGRATION, FARM LABORERS, CHILDREN, CULTURAL PLURALISM, CURRICULUM, PROFESSIONAL TRAINING, DISCRIMINATION, PREJUDICE, READING, ADULT EDUCATION, LEGISLATION, EQUAL OPPORTUNITY, BOOK
     ABST   THIS ISSUE, DEDICATED ENTIRELY TO THE TOPIC OF EDUCATION FOR THE SPANISH-SPEAKING PEOPLE OF THE U.S., CONTAINS 23 ARTICLES AND ONE BOOK REVIEW. SOME OF THE TOPICS ADDRESSED INCLUDE: (1) MIGRANT CHILDREN, (2) CULTURAL DEMOCRACY, (3) ADULT EDUCATION, (4) TEACHER PREPARATION FOR BILINGUAL PROGRAMS, (6) PROGRESS AND STATISTICAL REPORTS FROM THE U.S. COMMISSION ON CIVIL RIGHTS, AND (7) NEW READING AND TEACHING PROGRAMS AND CURRICULUM DEVELOPMENT. THOMAS P. CARTER'S BOOK, "MEXICAN AMERICANS IN SCHOOL: A HISTORY OF EDUCATIONAL NEGLECT," IS REVIEWED. THE JOURNAL ALSO CONTAINS SEVERAL ILLUSTRATIONS OF ORIGINAL ART DONE ESPECIALLY FOR THE JOURNAL. ANOTHER FEATURE INCLUDES SUMMARIES OF INTERVIEWS WITH THREE LEADERS IN MEXICAN AMERICAN EDUCATION—THOMAS P. CARTER, JULIAN SAMORA, AND GEORGE I. SANCHEZ.
     ACCN   000703

829 AUTH   **HUET, Y. J.**
     TITL   RELATIVE INFLUENCE OF BILINGUALISM AND INTELLECTUAL STIMULATION WITHIN THE HOME UPON ACADEMIC ACHIEVEMENT OF ECONOMICALLY DEPRIVED CHICANO ELEMENTARY SCHOOL CHILDREN.
     SRCE   *UNPUBLISHED MASTER'S THESIS, DEPARTMENT OF PSYCHOLOGY, UNIVERSITY OF MISSOURI, KANSAS CITY, 1976.*
     INDX   MEXICAN AMERICAN, EMPIRICAL, BILINGUALISM, SES, CROSS CULTURAL, SCHOLASTIC ACHIEVEMENT, SOCIALIZATION, CHILDREN, MISSOURI, MIDWEST
     ABST   THIRTY-SEVEN MEXICAN AMERICAN PARENTS AND THIRTY-SEVEN CHILDREN WERE SELECTED TO EXAMINE THE RELATIVE INFLUENCE OF PARENTAL BILINGUALISM AND INTELLECTUAL STIMULATION WITHIN THE HOME UPON THE ACADEMIC ACHIEVEMENT OF THIRD AND SIXTH-GRADE CHILDREN FROM A LOW SOCIOECONOMIC BACKGROUND. A MODIFIED FORM OF THE REACTION TIME TEST OF BILINGUALISM WAS EMPLOYED TO MEASURE DE-

GREE OF PARENTAL LANGUAGE DOMINANCE. INTELLECTUAL STIMULATION WITHIN THE HOME WAS MEASURED BY WHO READS TO THE CHILD, AT WHAT AGE DID READING TO THE CHILD BEGIN, AND WHETHER REFERENCE BOOKS AND PERIODICALS WERE FOUND IN THE HOME. MEASURES OF ACADEMIC ACHIEVEMENT INCLUDED TEACHERS' GRADES (IN READING, ENGLISH, SPELLING, ARITHMETIC, SOCIAL STUDIES) AND GRADE EQUIVALENT SCORES ON THE IOWA TEST OF BASIC SKILLS. ANALYSES OF VARIANCE WERE USED TO TEST GROUP DIFFERENCES. RESULTS SHOWED PATTERNS OF WEAK RELATIONSHIPS. INTELLECTUAL STIMULATION AND PARENT'S READING TO CHILD WERE FOUND TO HAVE A SIGNIFICANT INCREASING EFFECT UPON CHILDREN'S READING ACHIEVEMENT. THE INTERACTION OF PARENTAL LANGUAGE DOMINANCE AND A DAILY NEWSPAPER AT HOME WERE FOUND TO HAVE SIGNIFICANT INFLUENCE ON SPELLING SCORES. IT WAS ALSO FOUND THAT A SIGNIFICANT RELATIONSHIP EXISTED BETWEEN CHILDREN'S ENGLISH ACHIEVEMENT AND PARENTAL ENGLISH DOMINANCE AND BILINGUALISM. THIS STUDY FAILS TO SUPPORT THE ASSUMPTION THAT THE COMBINATION OF BILINGUALISM AND INTELLECTUAL STIMULATION IN THE HOME MAY BE MORE IMPORTANT THAN BILINGUALISM ALONE. IT IS SUGGESTED THAT THIS SUDY BE REPLICATED USING PARENTS WITH GREATER EXTREMES OF ENGLISH AND SPANISH DOMINANCE AND/OR WITH A LARGER SUBSAMPLE TO FACILITATE ATTAINMENT OF LARGER VARIATION WITHIN INTELLECTUALLY STIMULATING VARIABLES. 36 REFERENCES. (AUTHOR ABSTRACT MODIFIED)

ACCN   000704

830 AUTH   **HUMPHREY, N. D.**
     TITL   FAMILY PATTERNS IN A MEXICAN MIDDLETOWN.
     SRCE   *SOCIAL SERVICE REVIEW, 1952, 26, 195-201.*
     INDX   FAMILY STRUCTURE, MEXICAN, CASE STUDY, FAMILY ROLES, MARRIAGE, CHILDREARING PRACTICES, EXTENDED FAMILY, SEX ROLES, INFANCY, CULTURE, FICTIVE KINSHIP
     ABST   AN ETHNOGRAPHIC DESCRIPTION OF FAMILY PATTERNS IS PRESENTED. FAMILY IS REGARDED AS BOTH A MICROCOSM OF THE SOCIETY AND THE MAJOR CONTROL AGENT FOR THE TRANSMISSION OF THE CULTURE. THE FATHER IS THE HEAD OF THE FAMILY, HIS WORD HAS TO BE OBEYED, AND HIS OBLIGATION IS TO PROVIDE FOR HIS WIFE AND CHILDREN. THE WIFE IS RESPONSIBLE FOR TAKING CARE OF THE CHILDREN AND THE HOUSEHOLD DUTIES AND RARELY QUESTIONS HER SUBORDINATE ROLE. IN THE HIGHER CLASS GROUPS, MORE EQUAL FAMILY ROLES ARE FOUND. CHILDREN ARE DESIRED BY BOTH PARENTS AND ARE A PROOF OF A MAN'S VIRILITY. BOYS ACQUIRE THEIR SKILLS MAINLY BY WORKING WITH THE FATHER, AND GIRLS BY IMITATING THEIR MOTHER'S HOUSEHOLD TASKS. CHILDREN ARE FREE FROM ADULT SUPERVISION IN THEIR PLAY, ALTHOUGH SEX SEGREGATION IS STRONGLY FORMALIZED BY SCHOOL AGE. THE

RELATION BETWEEN GRANDPARENT AND GRANDCHILD IS STRONG AND ONE OF PRO-NOUNCED RESPECT ON THE PART OF THE CHILD. THE RELIGIOUS PADRINO AND MAD-RINA CARRY OUT CHURCH-PRESCRIBED AND CUSTOMARY OBLIGATIONS, SUCH AS CLOTH-ING AND EDUCATION. THE MADRINA AND PAD-RINO OF MARRIAGE, NORMALLY A MARRIED COUPLE, PREPARE THE NEW COUPLE FOR THEIR ROLE AS MARRIAGE PARTNERS.

ACCN   000705

831 AUTH   **HUMPHREY, N. D.**
    TITL   ON ASSIMILATION AND ACCULTURATION.
    SRCE   *PSYCHIATRY, 1943, 6(4), 343-345.*
    INDX   ACCULTURATION, ESSAY, MEXICAN AMERICAN, URBAN, MICHIGAN, THEORETICAL, CULTURAL CHANGE, MIDWEST, CULTURE
    ABST   THE RELATIONSHIP BETWEEN ASSIMILATION AND ACCULTURATION WITHIN AN IMMIGRANT MEXICAN GROUP IN DETROIT IS PRESENTED. ASSIMILATION IS BASICALLY A SOCIOPSY-CHOLOGICAL PHENOMENON. IT HAS ITS ROOTS IN THE PERSON, ENCUMBERED BY SENTI-MENTS AND BELIEFS WROUGHT INTO HIM AS HE GROWS IN A CULTURE. WHEN THE PERSON INJECTS HIMSELF INTO A SECOND CULTURE, HE CONFRONTS THE EMOTIONAL PULLS, AL-IEN MEANINGS, AND NEW MEANS OF EXPRES-SION ASSOCIATED WITH THE PROCESS OF AS-SIMILATION. ONE ASSIMILATES A NEW CULTURE LARGELY THROUGH THE PERCEPTION AND IM-ITATION OF EXAMPLES. THE MEANINGS AC-QUIRED FROM THE SECOND CULTURE SUP-PLANT OR MODIFY MEANINGS LEARNED IN THE FIRST CULTURE. ACCULTURATION IS A PROCESS IN WHICH CULTURAL ELEMENTS IN CONTACT WITH ANOTHER CULTURE MERGE AND FUSE. THE ASSIMILATION OF AMERICAN CULTURE BY MEXICANS IN DETROIT HAS LED TO CONSIDERABLE FUSION OF AMERICAN ELEMENTS INTO THE RETAINED CULTURE AS IS EVIDENCED IN THE STRUCTURE OF THE FAMILY. RELATIVELY LITTLE MEXICAN CULTURE HAS BEEN TAKEN ON BY AMERICANS, AND FEW MEXICAN CULTURAL ELEMENTS HAVE BEEN IN-CORPORATED INTO AMERICAN CULTURE. IT IS CONCLUDED THAT MEXICAN CULTURE AS A FUNCTIONAL UNITY WILL PROBABLY BE EX-PUNGED BY THE THIRD GENERATION. (AU-THOR ABSTRACT MODIFIED)
    ACCN   000706

832 AUTH   **HUMPHREY, N. D.**
    TITL   SOME MARRIAGE PROBLEMS OF DETROIT MEXICANS.
    SRCE   *APPLIED ANTHROPOLOGY, 1943, 3, 13-15.*
    INDX   MARITAL STABILITY, MARRIAGE, MEXICAN AMERICAN, URBAN, EMPIRICAL, INTERMAR-RIAGE, PERFORMANCE EXPECTATIONS, SEX-UAL BEHAVIOR, MICHIGAN, MIDWEST, CROSS GENERATIONAL, MEXICAN, SEX ROLES
    ABST   A CASE DIGEST EXAMINING MARITAL DISCORD IN UNIONS OF MEXICAN MEN AND AMERICAN WOMEN IN DETROIT IS PRESENTED. CONFLICT IN SUCH UNIONS WHEN THE AMERICAN WOMEN DO NOT CONFORM IN THEIR CONDUCT TO MEXICAN NORMS AND EXPECTATIONS AND

THE MEXICAN MEN DO NOT BEHAVE AS THEIR CONSORTS WOULD EXPECT AMERICAN MEN TO BEHAVE. IN MANY CASES OF INTERMAR-RIAGES, NO FORMAL LEGAL MARRIAGE IS CONTRACTED. IN THE SECOND GENERATION THE PROPORTION OF INTERMARRIAGES AP-PEARS TO INCREASE. YOUNG MEN APPEAR TO MARRY OUTSIDE OF THE GROUP TO A GREATER EXTENT THAN YOUNG WOMEN. SOME ILLEGI-TIMACY IS REPORTED FOR SECOND GENERA-TION GIRLS OF MEXICAN DESCENT, BUT WITH LESS FREQUENCY THAN YOUNG SOUTHWEST MEXICANS. ALTHOUGH A LARGE PROPORTION OF IMMIGRANT UNIONS ARE NOT FORMAL-IZED, VOLUNTARY SEPARATION AND DESER-TION OCCUR MORE THAN DIVORCE. THE CUL-TURALLY SENSITIVE SOCIAL WORKER SHOULD USE CASE WORK SKILLS TO BRING ABOUT AN UNDERSTANDING OF THE SITUATION IN TERMS OF AMERICAN NORMS. FACTORS OF DISOR-GANIZATION ARE SEEN AS DERIVING FROM RE-TENTION OF MEXICAN NORMS, ALTHOUGH SECOND GENERATION MEXICANS ARE BE-LIEVED TO BE MORE ACCULTURATED TO AMERICAN VALUES. 1 REFERENCE.

ACCN   000707

833 AUTH   **HUMPHREY, N. D.**
    TITL   THE STEREOTYPE AND THE SOCIAL TYPES OF MEXICAN AMERICAN YOUTHS.
    SRCE   *JOURNAL OF SOCIAL PSYCHOLOGY, 1945, 22(1), 69-78.*
    INDX   STEREOTYPES, MEXICAN AMERICAN, CASE STUDY, ADOLESCENTS, MICHIGAN, MIDWEST, CULTURAL FACTORS, ACCULTURATION, PER-SONALITY
    ABST   A DISCUSSION OF THE STEREOTYPE AND THE SOCIAL TYPES OF MEXICAN AMERICAN YOUTHS IS PRESENTED THROUGH AN EXAMINATION OF FIVE GENERAL CASE STUDY OBSERVATIONS BY SOCIAL WORKERS IN DETROIT. THE FIRST TYPE IS CHARACTERIZED BY THE MEXICAN IM-MIGRANT WHO IDENTIFIES WITH HIS NATIVE CULTURE. HE IS SUBSERVIENT TO AUTHORITY AND ASSOCIATES WITH OTHER MEXICAN INDI-VIDUALS. THE SECOND TYPE HAS BEEN EX-POSED TO MEXICAN AND AMERICAN CUL-TURES AND FINDS CONFLICTS WITH THE FORMER'S CUSTOMS. HE MINGLES WITH NON-MEXICAN INDIVIDUALS. THE THIRD TYPE IS THE MEXICAN YOUTH WHOSE MAIN CONCERN IS TO DIVORCE HIMSELF FROM THE CONNOTA-TION OF THE WORD "MEXICAN. BY HIS CHOICE, HIS PEERS ARE NON-MEXICAN AMERICANS. THE FOURTH TYPE, AMERICAN-BORN MEXICAN AMERICAN, IS MODEST AND UNAGGRESSIVE AND RARELY REBELS AGAINST PARENTAL AU-THORITY. THE FIFTH TYPE IS THE SON OF MEX-ICAN PARENTS WHO BECAUSE OF LIGHT SKIN COLOR, ATHLETIC ABILITY, AND SAVOIR-FAIRE WITH GIRLS, FINDS HIMSELF ACCEPTABLE TO MIDDLE-CLASS AMERICANS AND TENDS ULTI-MATELY TO ASSIMILATE COMPLETELY. DISCUS-SION OF ROLES OF EACH OF THE FIVE TYPES FOR MALE AND FEMALE YOUTHS IS PRE-SENTED. IT IS CONCLUDED THAT DIVERGENT TYPES OF PERSONALITIES SEEMINGLY ARE CONSEQUENCES OF DIFFERING DEGREES AND

LEVELS OF PARTICIPATION IN THE CULTURE. A SOCIAL TYPE IS MOLDED INTO A PARTICULAR ROLE BY THE FORCES IN THE SOCIAL FIELD WITHIN WHICH HE OPERATES.

ACCN   000708

834 AUTH   **HUNT, I. F., OSTERGARD, N. J., CARROLL, L. P., HSIEH, B., BROWN, R., & GLADNEY, V.**

TITL   IRON, THIAMIN, RIBOFLAVIN, AND NIACIN CONTENT OF CORN TORTILLAS MADE IN LOS ANGELES, CALIFORNIA.

SRCE   *ECOLOGY OF FOOD AND NUTRITION, 1978, 7,* 37-39.

INDX   EMPIRICAL, MEXICAN AMERICAN, FEMALE, CALIFORNIA, SOUTHWEST, URBAN, NUTRITION, HEALTH

ABST   BECAUSE CORN TORTILLAS ARE A STAPLE FOOD IN THE DIET OF PEOPLE OF MEXICAN DESCENT WHO LIVE IN THE LOS ANGELES AREA, A STUDY WAS UNDERTAKEN TO ASCERTAIN THEIR NUTRITIONAL VALUE. SAMPLES OF CORN TORTILLAS AND CORN PRODUCTS WHICH INCLUDED WHOLE DRY WHITE CORN, "NIXTAMAL (CORN COOKED WITH LIME), AND "MASA (DOUGH) WERE OBTAINED FROM TEN LOCAL TORTILLERIAS. THE TORTILLAS AND CORN PRODUCTS WERE SUBSEQUENTLY SHIPPED TO QUAKER OATS COMPANY IN ILLINOIS WHERE AN ANALYSIS OF THE IRON, THIAMIN, RIBOFLAVIN, AND NIACIN CONTENT WAS PERFORMED. ON A WEIGHT BASIS, CORN TORTILLAS CONTAIN LESS IRON, THIAMIN, RIBOFLAVIN, AND NIACIN THAN ENRICHED WHITE BREAD. MOREOVER, THE MEAN INTAKE OF IRON, THIAMIN, AND RIBOFLAVIN IS BELOW TWO-THIRDS OF THE RDA FOR AN IMPORTANT SEGMENT OF THE POPULATION CONSUMING THIS PRODUCT. THE AUTHORS CONCLUDE THAT THE ADDITION OF THESE NUTRIENTS TO CORN TORTILLAS MADE IN LOS ANGELES WOULD BE AN EFFECTIVE MEANS OF INCREASING IRON AND VITAMIN INTAKE. 9 REFERENCES. (JOURNAL ABSTRACT MODIFIED)

ACCN   002372

835 AUTH   **HYMAN, M. M.**

TITL   THE SOCIAL CHARACTERISTICS OF PERSONS ARRESTED FOR DRIVING WHILE INTOXICATED.

SRCE   *QUARTERLY JOURNAL OF STUDIES ON ALCOHOL, 1968, (SUPPLEMENT NO. 4), 138-177.*

INDX   ADULTS, ALCOHOLISM, ANOMIE, CORRECTIONS, CROSS CULTURAL, CULTURAL FACTORS, DELINQUENCY, DEMOGRAPHIC, DEVIANCE, ECONOMIC FACTORS, EMPIRICAL, MENTAL HEALTH, MEXICAN AMERICAN, SES, SEX COMPARISON, SPANISH SURNAMED, OHIO, CALIFORNIA, MIDWEST, SOUTHWEST, POLICE-COMMUNITY RELATIONS

ABST   THE SOCIAL CHARACTERISTICS OF DRUNK DRIVERS WERE ANALYZED IN PERSONS ARRESTED IN THE FIRST 6 MONTHS OF 1962 IN TWO AREAS—SANTA CLARA COUNTY, CALIF. (1147 ARRESTS) AND COLUMBUS, OHIO (575 ARRESTS). THESE TWO JURISDICTIONS WERE CHOSEN FOR INVESTIGATION BECAUSE BOTH POLICE DEPARTMENTS PRACTICE CHEMICAL TESTING FOR BLOOD ALCOHOL CONCENTRATION AND THE POLICE REPORTS WERE MADE ACCESSABLE BY THE CHIEF ADMINISTRATORS. ARRESTS FOR DRIVING WHILE INTOXICATED (ADWI) USUALLY RESULT FROM DRIVING WHICH ATTRACTS THE ATTENTION OF LAW ENFORCEMENT OFFICIALS (ACCIDENT OR A VIOLATION) AND/OR BLOOD ALCOHOL CONCENTRATIONS WHICH ARE ABOVE NORAML LIMITS. VULNERABILITY TO ARREST OF RESIDENTS OF SANTA CLARA WAS HIGHEST AMONG MEN AGED 21-54, AND AMONG MEN AGED 25-54 IN THE COLUMBUS METROPOLITAN AREA. MEN FROM DISADVANTAGED ETHNIC GROUPS (SPANISH AMERICANS IN SANTA CLARA AND BLACKS IN COLUMBUS) WERE AT LEAST TWICE AS VULNERABLE TO ARREST AS OTHER MEN. HOWEVER, POLICE ETHNIC AND/OR RACIAL BIAS WAS CONSIDERED NEGLIGIBLE IN BOTH JURISDICTIONS. IT IS CONCLUDED THAT THOSE ARRESTED FOR DRUNKEN DRIVING DIFFER IN DEMOGRAPHIC CHARACTERISTICS FROM THE GENERAL POPULATION. THE CONCEPT OF ALIENATION OR ANOMIE MAY AID IN THE INTERPRETATION OF DIFFERENTIAL ARREST RATES. SUCH CHARACTERISTICS AS LOW SES, LOW ETHNIC PRESTIGE, SOCIAL SEGREGATION, INCOMPLETENESS AND AND INSTABILITY OF FAMILY LIFE, AND NOT OWNING ONE'S HOME ARE ALL STRONGLY ASSOCIATED WITH ALIENATION FROM SOCIETAL REGULATIONS. OTHER STUDIES WHICH SHOW THAT MANY DRUNK DRIVERS ARE ALCOHOLICS ARE DISCUSSED, AND THE AGE, ECONOMIC AND FAMILIAL CHARACTERISTICS OF PROBLEM DRINKERS IN DIFFERENT REPORTED CONTEXTS ARE COMPARED. 69 REFERENCES.

ACCN   002115

836 AUTH   **HYNES, K., & WERBIN, J.**

TITL   GROUP PSYCHOTHERAPY FOR SPANISH-SPEAKING WOMEN.

SRCE   *PSYCHIATRIC ANNALS, 1977, 7(12), 52-63.*

INDX   ESSAY, FEMALE, MENTAL HEALTH, CULTURAL FACTORS, ANXIETY, MEXICAN AMERICAN, BILINGUAL, CENTRAL AMERICA, COMPETITION, CULTURAL FACTORS, DEPRESSION, GROUP DYNAMICS, SELF CONCEPT, SEX ROLES, PSYCHOTHERAPY, PSYCHOTHERAPISTS, PSYCHOTHERAPY OUTCOME, PSYCHOSOCIAL ADJUSTMENT, SYMPTOMATOLOGY, ADULTS, CALIFORNIA, SOUTHWEST

ABST   THE PHENOMENON OF 10 SPANISH-SPEAKING WOMEN IN A NORTHERN CALIFORNIA SUBURB INTERACTING IN A GROUP THERAPY SETTING IS EXAMINED AND EVALUATED. GROUP SESSIONS, CONDUCTED IN SPANISH, WERE LED BY AN ANGLO, SPANISH-SPEAKING PUBLIC HEALTH NURSE AND A PSYCHIATRIST BORN AND EDUCATED IN CUBA. THE 10 MEMBERS OF THE GROUP INCLUDED 6 MEXICAN AMERICANS (ONE BORN IN TEXAS AND THE OTHER 5 IN MEXICO), WHILE THE REMAINING MEMBERS WERE NATIVES OF NICARAGUA AND EL SALVADOR. AGES RANGED FROM 35 TO 68, WITH MOST OF THE WOMEN IN THEIR 40'S. PRESENTING PROBLEMS INCLUDED LONELINESS—SOME EVEN DISPLAYING ISOLATION-RELATED DELUSIONAL STATES—SACRIFICIAL AND OBSESSIONAL ATTITUDES TOWARD CHILDREN, AND

WIDESPREAD AND SEVERE SOMATIC COM-
PLAINTS. IN THE PROGRAM'S INITIAL STAGES
THERE WAS LACK OF GROUP COHESIVENESS,
AND GENERAL NONPRODUCTIVE COMPETI-
TION FOR THE ATTENTION OF THE PSYCHIA-
TRIST IN THE FORM OF LONG RECITALS OF
PHYSICAL ILLS. SUCH PERSONAL ACCOUNTS
OF PHYSICAL SYMPTOMS WERE SO PRO-
TRACTED THAT THE GROUP DUBBED THEM-
SELVES "LAS AFLIGIDAS" (THE ANGUISHED
ONES). HOWEVER, WITH THE PASSAGE OF
TIME THE WOMEN SEEMED ABLE TO WORK
THROUGH THEIR INITIAL PROBLEMS OF SO-
CIAL ISOLATION AND FEELINGS OF PHYSICAL
ILLNESS. A SENSE OF GROUP IDENTITY AND
MUTUAL SUPPORT EMERGED, RESULTING IN
THE SPONTANEOUS RENAMING OF THE GROUP
AS "LAS COMPANERAS" (THE COMPANIONS).
THE MANY POSITIVE CHANGES THAT TOOK
PLACE IN THESE 10 WOMEN INDICATE THAT
COUNTER TO MISGIVINGS EXPRESSED IN THE
LITERATURE, SPANISH-SPEAKING WOMEN IN
THE UNITED STATES CAN BENEFIT FROM GROUP
PSYCHOTHERAPY EXPERIENCE AND CAN BE-
COME DYNAMICALLY INVOLVED IN IT—EVEN
WHEN THE THERAPISTS COME FROM DIS-
TINCTLY DIFFERENT CULTURES THAN THE
GROUP MEMBERS. 1 REFERENCE.

ACCN   002116

837 AUTH   **IIYAMA, P., SETSUKO, M., & JOHNSON, B. D.**
     TITL   DRUG USE AND ABUSE AMONG U.S. MINORI-
             TIES.
     SRCE   *NEW YORK: PRAEGAR PUBLISHERS, 1976.*
     INDX   BIBLIOGRAPHY, REVIEW, ESSAY, RESEARCH
             METHODOLOGY, DRUG ABUSE, STEREOTYPES,
             MEXICAN AMERICAN, PUERTO RICAN-M, POLICY,
             THEORETICAL, ATTITUDES, DEMOGRAPHIC,
             ADULTS, ADOLESCENTS, PROGRAM EVALUA-
             TION, CRIMINOLOGY, PREJUDICE, DISCRIMI-
             NATION, DRUG ADDICTION

     ABST   THIS BIBLIOGRAPHY ON DRUG USE AND ABUSE
             AMONG ASIAN AMERICANS, BLACKS, MEXICAN
             AMERICANS, NATIVE AMERICANS, AND PUERTO
             RICANS, CONSISTS PRIMARILY OF RESEARCH
             MATERIALS ON OPIATE ADDICTION (OMITTING,
             FOR THE MOST PART, MATERIAL ON THE USE
             OF MARIJUANA, HALLUCINOGENS, AMPHETA-
             MINES, AND BARBITURATES). AN INTRODUC-
             TORY ESSAY REVIEWS THE LITERATURE (112
             REFERENCES) AND THE HISTORY OF OFFICIAL
             POLICY AND PUBLIC ATTITUDES TOWARD DRUG
             USE AMONG RACIAL MINORITIES. DRUG ABUSE
             AS A SOCIOPOLITICAL PROBLEM IS LINKED
             HISTORICALLY TO AMERICA'S TREATMENT OF
             ETHNIC GROUPS AND THE PERPETUATION OF
             RACIST STEREOTYPES. THIS IS REFLECTED IN
             GOVERNMENTAL APPROACHES TO DRUG ADD-
             ICTION, PROBLEMS WITH STATISTICS ON DRUG
             USE, AND THE MISCONSTRUCTION OF RE-
             SEARCH TO FURTHER RACIST VIEWS. CRIMIN-
             ALIZATION OF ADDICTION, PSYCHOLOGICAL
             AND SOCIOLOGICAL MODELS OF ADDICTION,
             DRUG TREATMENT PROGRAMS, AND RE-
             SEARCH METHODOLOGY ARE DISCUSSED. CI-
             TATIONS ARE LISTED ACCORDING TO MI-
             NORITY GROUP, AND INCLUDE 88 ARTICLES

ON PUERTO RICAN AND 39 ON MEXICAN
AMERICAN DRUG ABUSE.

ACCN   002117

838 AUTH   **INNISS, J.**
     TITL   COUNSELING THE CULTURALLY DISRUPTED
             CHILD.
     SRCE   *ELEMENTARY SCHOOL GUIDANCE AND COUN-
             SELING, 1977, 2(3), 229-235.*
     INDX   ACCULTURATION, BEHAVIOR MODIFICATION,
             CASE STUDY, CHILDREN, CLASSROOM BEHAV-
             IOR, EDUCATIONAL COUNSELING, LANGUAGE
             LEARNING, PSYCHOSOCIAL ADJUSTMENT,
             PUERTO RICAN-M, SOCIALIZATION, PENNSYL-
             VANIA, EAST, STRESS, CULTURAL FACTORS, BE-
             HAVIOR THERAPY, ESSAY

     ABST   THE CASES OF THREE PUERTO RICAN CHIL-
             DREN ENTERING KINDERGARTEN IN A PENN-
             SYLVANIA ELEMENTARY SCHOOL IN WHICH IN-
             ABILITY TO COMMUNICATE IN A NEW
             LANGUAGE LED TO INTROVERSION AND RE-
             FUSAL TO VERBALIZE ARE DESCRIBED. THE
             SOURCE OF THE CHILDREN'S BEHAVIORS WAS
             FOUND IN PSYCHOCULTURAL FACTORS WHICH
             WERE MANIFESTED IN LINGUISTIC AND SOCIAL
             DIFFICULTIES. THE SCHOOL COUNSELOR DE-
             VELOPED A PROGRAM INVOLVING A SPANISH-
             SPEAKING TUTOR OF ENGLISH AND MATTER-
             OF-FACT BEHAVIOR BY TEACHERS WHICH DID
             NOT REINFORCE REFUSAL TO SPEAK. THE
             SPEAKING DIFFICULTIES OF THE CHILDREN
             AND THEIR ASOCIAL BEHAVIOR WERE RE-
             SOLVED BY THE TIME THEY ENTERED FIRST
             GRADE, WITHOUT NEED OF EXTRAORDINARY
             PSYCHOLOGICAL INTERVENTION. 6 REFER-
             ENCES. (NCMHI ABSTRACT)

     ACCN   002118

839 AUTH   **IOWA ADVISORY COMMITTEE TO THE U.S.
             COMMISSION ON CIVIL RIGHTS.**
     TITL   HOW FAR HAVE WE COME? MIGRANT FARM LA-
             BOR IN IOWA: 1975.
     SRCE   *WASHINGTON, D.C.: U.S. GOVERNMENT PRINT-
             ING OFFICE, 1976.*
     INDX   POLICY, ADMINISTRATORS, CULTURAL FAC-
             TORS, RURAL, BILINGUAL-BICULTURAL EDU-
             CATION, EDUCATION, CHILDREN, COMMUNITY,
             DEMOGRAPHIC, DISEASE, EMPIRICAL, EQUAL
             OPPORTUNITY, FARM LABORERS, HEALTH,
             HEALTH DELIVERY SYSTEMS, HOUSING, JUDI-
             CIAL PROCESS, LABOR FORCE, IOWA, MID-
             WEST, MENTAL HEALTH, SES, MEXICAN AMERI-
             CAN, MIGRANTS, SOCIAL SERVICES

     ABST   CONDITIONS AFFECTING MEXICAN AMERICAN
             FARMWORKERS IN EASTERN IOWA WERE THE
             SUBJECT OF A 1970 INVESTIGATION BY THE
             CIVIL RIGHTS COMMISSION'S IOWA ADVISORY
             COMMITTEE. FOCUSING ON ACTIVITY IN THE
             COMMUNITY OF MUSCANTINE, INFORMATION
             ON PUBLIC PROGRAMS FOR MIGRANT LABOR-
             ERS AND "SETTLED OUT FARM WORKERS—
             THOSE WHO HAVE LEFT THE MIGRANT STREAM
             SEEKING BETTER, MORE PERMANENT EM-
             PLOYMENT—ARE DETAILED. THE STUDY EX-
             AMINED THE MIGRANTS' INTERACTION WITH
             THE COMMUNITY-AT-LARGE, SCHOOLS, THE
             CRIMINAL JUSTICE SYSTEM, HEALTH CARE,
             SOCIAL AND ADVOCACY AGENCIES, AND IN-

CLUDES STATEMENTS BY GOVERNMENT OFFI-CIALS, COMMUNITY LEADERS, GROWERS, AND MIGRANT ADVOCATES. THE REPORT ALSO IN-CLUDES STATISTICS AND PROGRAM INFOR-MATION SUPPLIED BY THESE SAME CORRE-SPONDENTS, AS WELL AS AVAILABLE NATIONAL DATA. FROM THEIR FINDINGS, A PROFILE EMERGES OF AN IMPOVERISHED MIGRANT WORKER, POORLY EDUCATED AND POORLY HOUSED, OFTEN SUFFERING FROM COMPLEX HEALTH PROBLEMS, AND MORE IN NEED OF SUPPORT SERVICES THAN MOST. HOWEVER, ACCESS TO THESE SERVICES IS FREQUENTLY COMPLICATED BY INTERAGENCY RIVALRY AND BY THE MIGRANTS' INABILITY TO MAKE THEIR NEEDS FELT. FOUR RECOMMENDATIONS ARE OFFERED. (1) HOUSING: TIGHTENING OF IN-SPECTION PROCEDURES TO IMPROVE "DE-PLORABLE CONDITIONS. (2) EDUCATION: BI-LINGUAL-BICULTURAL EDUCATION FOR MIGRANTS NEEDS SUPPORT AT ALL LEVELS. (3) AGENCIES: LOCAL AGENCIES SHOULD MAKE CLEAR WHICH AGENCY WILL PROVIDE SER-VICES TO MIGRANTS; ALSO, A SEPARATE STATE COMMISSION SHOULD BE ESTABLISHED TO ASSUME RESPONSIBILITY FOR ALL SERVICE TO MIGRANTS. (4) EDUCATION: A SINGLE AGENCY SHOULD ASSUME RESPONSIBILITY FOR THE PLACEMENT OF MIGRANTS SEEKING PERMA-NENT EMPLOYMENT. 144 REFERENCES.

ACCN 002119

840 AUTH **IWAMOTO, C. K., KAPLAN, M., & ANILOFF, L.**
TITL HIGH SCHOOL DROPOUTS: EFFECTS OF HIS-PANIC BACKGROUND AND PREVIOUS SCHOOL ACHIEVEMENT.
SRCE *URBAN EDUCATION, 1976, 11(1), 23-30.*
INDX SCHOLASTIC ACHIEVEMENT, ETHNIC IDENTITY, ADOLESCENTS, CROSS CULTURAL, EDUCA-TION, SEX COMPARISON, SPANISH SURNAMED, EMPIRICAL, PENNSYLVANIA, EAST, URBAN
ABST SCHOOL RECORDS WERE OBTAINED ON 108 SPANISH SURNAMED EIGHTH-GRADE GRADU-ATES OF TITLE 1 PAROCHIAL SCHOOLS AND 108 NON-SPANISH SURNAMED EIGHTH-GRADE GRADUATES OF PUBLIC SCHOOLS IN PHILA-DELPHIA. STUDENTS WERE MATCHED AC-CORDING TO GRADUATION YEAR, SEX, SCHOOL, AND GRADE POINT AVERAGE TO AS-CERTAIN IF SPANISH SURNAMED PUPILS HAD A HIGHER HIGH SCHOOL DROPOUT RATE AND IF SCHOOL ACHIEVEMENT AFFECTED PUPILS' DROPOUT RATE. FINDINGS INDICATED NO SIG-NIFICANT RELATIONSHIP BETWEEN SPANISH SURNAME AND DROPOUT RATE AMONG STU-DENTS OF COMPARABLE ABILITY. PREVIOUS ACADEMIC ACHIEVEMENT TENDED TO INFLU-ENCE DROPOUT RATE; AND SINCE HIGH ACA-DEMIC ACHIEVEMENT STUDENTS TEND TO EN-TER NON-PUBLIC SCHOOLS, THIS TYPE OF SCHOOL HAD A LOWER DROPOUT RATE. 5 REFERENCES.
ACCN 000709

841 AUTH **JACKSON, G., & COSCA, C.**
TITL THE INEQUALITY OF EDUCATIONAL OPPORTU-

NITY IN THE SOUTHWEST: AN OBSERVATIONAL STUDY OF ETHNICALLY MIXED CLASSROOMS.
SRCE *AMERICAN EDUCATIONAL RESEARCH JOUR-NAL, 1974, 11(3), 219-229.*
INDX EDUCATION, ETHNIC IDENTITY, SOCIAL SCI-ENCES, INTERPERSONAL RELATIONS, CUL-TURAL FACTORS, EDUCATIONAL MATERIALS, TEACHERS, CHILDREN, MEXICAN AMERICAN, CROSS CULTURAL, CLASSROOM BEHAVIOR, EMPIRICAL, EQUAL OPPORTUNITY
ABST AN ASSESSMENT IS MADE OF TEACHER BE-HAVIORS AS A FACTOR IN THE QUALITY OF EDUCATIONAL OPPORTUNITY AFFORDED TO MEXICAN AMERICANS AND ANGLOS WITHIN SCHOOLS OF THE SOUTHWEST. FIFTY-TWO SCHOOLS WERE RANDOMLY SAMPLED FROM 430 ELIGIBLE SCHOOLS IN SELECTED AREAS IN THE STATES OF CALIFORNIA, TEXAS, AND NEW MEXICO. IN SUM, 494 CLASSROOMS WERE VISITED IN WHICH COMPLETE DATA WERE STUDIED FOR 429 CLASSROOMS. OBSERVERS USED A SLIGHTLY MODIFIED FLANDERS INTER-ACTION CODING SYSTEM TO CODE TEACHER VERBAL BEHAVIORS WITH REFERENCE TO THE ETHNICITY OF THE STUDENT TO WHOM EACH BEHAVIOR WAS DIRECTED. THE RESULTS SHOW SUBSTANTIAL AND STATISTICALLY SIGNIFI-CANT DIFFERENCES BETWEEN MEXICAN AMERICAN AND ANGLO STUDENTS IN THE FOLLOWING INTERACTIONS: TEACHER PRAISE OR ENCOURAGEMENT OF STUDENTS, TEACHER ACCEPTANCE OR USE OF STUDENTS' IDEAS; TEACHER QUESTIONING; THE TEACHERS' GIV-ING OF POSITIVE FEED BACK; ALL NON-CRITI-CIZING TEACHER TALK; AND ALL STUDENT SPEAKING. A NUMBER OF TEACHER, STUDENT, CLASSROOM, AND SCHOOL CHARACTERIS-TICS WERE ALSO INVESTIGATED FOR POS-SIBLE ASSOCIATION WITH THESE DISPARITIES AND A FEW SIGNIFICANT RELATIONSHIPS WERE FOUND. BASED ON PREVIOUS RESEARCH THAT HAS CONSISTENTLY DEMONSTRATED A RELA-TIONSHIP BETWEEN STUDENT ACHIEVEMENT AND TEACHERS' BEHAVIOR, IT IS ARGUED THAT THE BEHAVIORS OF TEACHERS IN THE SOUTHWEST ARE AT LEAST PARTLY CONTRIB-UTING TO THE POOR ACADEMIC ACHIEVEMENT OF MANY MEXICAN AMERICAN STUDENTS. OTHER REASONS FOR MEXICAN AMERICANS' LOW ACADEMIC PERFORMANCE ARE DIS-CUSSED. IT IS RECOMMENDED THAT THE IN-STRUCTIONAL PROCESS IN THE CLASSROOMS OF THE SOUTHWEST MUST BE CHANGED IF MEXICAN AMERICAN YOUTH ARE TO BE GIVEN EDUCATIONAL OPPORTUNITIES EQUAL TO THOSE AVAILABLE TO ANGLO STUDENTS. 11 REFERENCES. (JOURNAL ABSTRACT MODI-FIED)
ACCN 000710

842 AUTH **JACKSON, S. R., & KUVLESKY, W. P.**
TITL INFLUENCES OF FAMILY DISABILITY ON SOCIAL ORIENTATIONS OF HOMEMAKERS AMONG DIF-FERENT ETHNIC POPULATIONS: SOUTHERN BLACK, WESTERN MEXICAN FARM MIGRANT AND EASTERN WHITE RURAL FAMILIES.
SRCE *UNPUBLISHED MANUSCRIPT, WASHINGTON, D.C., COOPERATIVE STATE RESEARCH SER-*

VICE, DEPARTMENT OF AGRICULTURE. (ERIC DOCUMENT REPRODUCTION SERVICE NO. ED 085 168)

INDX HOUSING, PSYCHOSOCIAL ADJUSTMENT, SURVEY, EMPIRICAL, FAMILY STRUCTURE, FAMILY ROLES, HEALTH, CROSS CULTURAL, MEXICAN AMERICAN, SES, POVERTY, ENVIRONMENTAL FACTORS, MIGRANTS, CALIFORNIA, TEXAS, SOUTHWEST, VERMONT, EAST, RURAL

ABST THE RESEARCH EXPLORED WHETHER THE OCCURRENCE AND DEGREE OF FAMILY DISABILITY PRODUCED A DISTINGUISHABLE PATTERNED SET OF SOCIAL LIFE VIEWS AMONG HOMEMAKERS AND TO WHAT EXTENT THE PATTERNS ARE GENERAL TO DIFFERENT POPULATIONS. DISABILITY WAS DEFINED AS THE INABILITY TO ASSUME EXPECTED ROLES. THE TOTAL NUMBER OF RESPONDENTS WAS 643, OF WHICH THE DISABLED FAMILIES CONSTITUTED SEVEN MEXICAN AMERICAN MIGRANT WORKERS IN CALIFORNIA, 75 SMALL TOWN BLACKS IN EAST TEXAS, AND 37 RURAL WHITES IN VERMONT. THE SOCIAL LIFE ORIENTATION VARIABLES EMPLOYED IN THIS STUDY WERE EVALUATION OF LIFE SITUATION (RELATIVE TO PARENTS), IMPROVEMENT OF LIFE CONDITIONS (OVER LAST 5 YEARS), LIFE SATISFACTION, HOUSING SATISFACTION, AND MARITAL SATISFACTION. MAJOR CONCLUSIONS WERE: (1) THE OCCURRENCE OF MEMBERSHIP DISABILITY HAS A TENDENCY TO NEGATIVELY INFLUENCE, TO A VERY LIMITED EXTENT, EVALUATIONS OF LEVELS OF POSITIVE EVALUATION OF IMPROVING LIFE CIRCUMSTANCES; (2) THE OCCURRENCE OF MEMBERSHIP DISABILITY DOES NOT PRODUCE A NEGATIVE IMPACT ON PERCEIVED LIFE SATISFACTIONS; AND (3) THE LEVEL OF DISABILITY AMONG DISABLED FAMILIES DOES NOT INFLUENCE THE VIEWS HOMEMAKERS HAVE OF LIFE PROGRESS AND SOCIAL SATISFACTIONS. 14 REFERENCES. (RIE ABSTRACT MODIFIED)

ACCN 000711

843 AUTH **JACO, E. G.**
TITL MENTAL HEALTH OF THE SPANISH-AMERICAN IN TEXAS.
SRCE IN M. K. OPLER (ED.), CULTURE AND MENTAL HEALTH: CROSS-CULTURAL STUDIES. NEW YORK: MACMILLAN COMPANY, 1959, PP. 467-485.
INDX MEXICAN AMERICAN, PSYCHOPATHOLOGY, CULTURAL FACTORS, SURVEY, MENTAL HEALTH, DEMOGRAPHIC, PSYCHOSIS, RESOURCE UTILIZATION, DEPRESSION, ANXIETY, SYMPTOMATOLOGY, SES, POVERTY, ACCULTURATION, TEXAS, SOUTHWEST, SEX COMPARISON, URBAN, RURAL
ABST MAJOR MENTAL DISORDERS AMONG THE SPANISH SURNAMED (SS), ANGLO AMERICAN (AA), AND NONWHITE (NW) POPULATIONS OF TEXAS ARE COMPARED. THE PRINCIPAL HYPOTHESIS WAS THAT THE SS POPULATION WOULD EXHIBIT SIGNIFICANT DIFFERENCES IN BOTH FORM AND FREQUENCY OF MAJOR MENTAL DISORDERS FROM THE OTHER GROUPS. DATA ON DIAGNOSED PSYCHOTIC

CASES FOR THE SS GROUP WERE OBTAINED FROM A SURVEY DEALING WITH THE INCIDENCE OF MENTAL DISORDERS DURING 1951-1952. CASES WERE AVERAGED INTO AN ANNUAL RATE AND COMPUTED FOR THE 27 ECONOMIC SUBREGIONS OF THE STATE. MENTAL DISORDER RATES WERE ADJUSTED FOR AGE, SEX, AND ETHNIC COMPOSITION. FROM THE TOTAL NUMBER OF 11,298 PSYCHOTIC CASES THERE WERE 648 (6%) SS, 9,557 (84.6%) AA, AND 1,057 (9.4%) NW. THE RESULTS INDICATE THAT: (1) THE INCIDENCE RATE OF TOTAL PSYCHOSES FOR THE SS IS CONSIDERABLY LOWER THAN FOR THE OTHER GROUPS; (2) THE ECOLOGICAL DISTRIBUTION OF INCIDENCE RATES FOR THE SUBGROUPS DIFFER SIGNIFICANTLY; (3) AVAILABILITY OF PSYCHIATRIC TREATMENT FACILITIES ARE NOT SIGNIFICANTLY RELATED TO THE INCIDENCE RATES FOR SUBREGIONS; (4) THE INCIDENCE RATES OF PSYCHOSES FOR THE SS MALE TEND TO INCREASE WITH ADVANCING AGE; (5) THE INCIDENCE OF FUNCTIONAL, OLD AGE, AND ORGANIC PSYCHOSES IS LOWER FOR SS; (6) URBAN RATES ARE HIGHER THAN RURAL RATES FOR ALL GROUPS; (7) BIRTH PLACE IS NOT RELATED TO THE INCIDENCE OF PSYCHOSES FOR ANY SUBGROUP; (8) DIFFERENCES IN RATES FOR THE THREE SUBGROUPS ARE FOUND FOR FIVE FORMS OF MARITAL STATUS AND BETWEEN SEXES; (9) OCCUPATIONAL DIFFERENCES IN INCIDENCE RATES ARE FOUND AMONG THE SUBGROUPS AND BY SEX; AND (10) EDUCATION IS CORRELATED WITH INCIDENCE RATE FOR ONLY THE SS SUBGROUP. THESE FINDINGS GENERALLY SUPPORT THE HYPOTHESIS THAT THE SS EXHIBIT DIFFERENCES IN THE INCIDENCE AND TYPES OF MENTAL DISORDERS FROM THE OTHER SUBGROUPS WITH A LOWER RATE OF INCIDENCE. 8 REFERENCES. (AUTHOR SUMMARY MODIFIED)

ACCN 000712

844 AUTH **JACO, E. G.**
TITL SOCIAL FACTORS IN MENTAL DISORDERS IN TEXAS.
SRCE SOCIAL PROBLEMS, 1957, 4(4), 322-328.
INDX PSYCHOPATHOLOGY, SES, POVERTY, SEX COMPARISON, RURAL, URBAN, DEMOGRAPHIC, EMPIRICAL, CULTURAL FACTORS, PSYCHOSIS, ACCULTURATION, TEXAS, SOUTHWEST, CROSS CULTURAL, MEXICAN AMERICAN
ABST AN EXAMINATION OF THE SOCIAL AND CULTURAL FORCES INVOLVED IN THE INCIDENCE OF MENTAL DISORDERS IN TEXAS IS PRESENTED. THE STUDY WAS DESIGNED TO INCLUDE ALL TEXAS RESIDENTS WHO SOUGHT PSYCHIATRIC TREATMENT FOR PSYCHOSIS FOR THE FIRST TIME DURING THE 2-YEAR PERIOD OF 1951-1952. DATA WERE OBTAINED FROM PSYCHIATRISTS IN PRIVATE PRACTICE, VETERANS HOSPITALS, AND CITY-COUNTY AND STATE MENTAL HOSPITALS THROUGHOUT THE STATE. THE MAJOR HYPOTHESES TESTED WERE: (1) THE PROBABILITY OF ACQUIRING A PSYCHOSIS IS NOT RANDOM OR EQUAL AMONG SUBGROUPS OF THE POPULATION; (2) INHABITANTS OF DIFFERENT AREAS EXHIBIT DIFFER-

ENT INCIDENCES OF PSYCHOSIS; AND (3) PERSONS WITH DIFFERENT SOCIAL ATTRIBUTES OF AFFILIATION HAVE DIFFERENT INCIDENCES OF PSYCHOSIS. CASES FOR THE 2-YEAR PERIOD WERE AVERAGED INTO AN ANNUAL RATE AND COMPUTED FOR THE 27 SUBREGIONS OF THE STATE. ALL RATES WERE ADJUSTED FOR AGE, SEX, AND ETHNIC COMPOSITION OF EACH SUBREGION. FINDINGS INDICATE THAT HIGHEST INCIDENCE RATES ARE FOUND IN THE GULF COAST REGION AND THE LOWEST RATES IN WEST TEXAS. AGE IS POSITIVELY CORRELATED WITH THE INCIDENCE OF PSYCHOSIS. FEMALES HAVE HIGHER PSYCHOSIS RATES THAN MALES. ANGLO AMERICANS EXHIBIT THE HIGHEST PSYCHOSIS RATES AND THE SPANISH AMERICANS THE LOWEST. SPANISH AMERICANS HAVE A HIGHER INCIDENCE OF MANIC DEPRESSIVE AND INDIVIDUAL PSYCHOSES THAN DO THE NONWHITES. THESE RESULTS ARE CONSIDERABLY DIFFERENT FROM THOSE YIELDED BY OTHER SURVEYS. THE FINDINGS SUPPORT THE THREE MAJOR HYPOTHESES OF THE STUDY. 15 REFERENCES.

ACCN   000713

845 AUTH   **JACOBS, S. H., & PIERCE-JONES, J.**
     TITL   PARENT INVOLVEMENT IN PROJECT HEAD START, PART OF THE FINAL REPORT ON HEAD START EVALUATION AND RESEARCH: 1968-1969.
     SRCE   *WASHINGTON, D.C.: OFFICE OF ECONOMIC OPPORTUNITY. (ERIC DOCUMENT REPRODUCTION NO. ED 037 244)*
     INDX   PARENTAL INVOLVEMENT, EARLY CHILDHOOD EDUCATION, PROGRAM EVALUATION, MEXICAN AMERICAN, COMMUNITY, PRIMARY PREVENTION, CROSS CULTURAL, TEXAS, SOUTHWEST, EMPIRICAL
     ABST   THE PRESENT STUDY WAS AN ATTEMPT TO ASSESS THE IMPACT OF PROJECT HEAD START UPON THE PARENTS OF CHILDREN WHO PARTICIPATED IN A 6-MONTH HEAD START INTERVENTION PROGRAM IN AUSTIN, TEXAS. THE SAMPLE WAS COMPRISED OF 57 NEGRO AND 51 LATIN AMERICAN PARENTS. FROM THE PARENT INTERVIEW, WHICH WAS ADMINISTERED TO THE FEMALE CARETAKER (USUALLY THE MOTHER) OF EACH CHILD ENROLLED IN THE HEAD START PROGRAM BOTH BEFORE AND AFTER THE INTERVENTION HAD TAKEN PLACE, SCALES WERE CONSTRUCTED TO MEASURE THE LEVEL OF GENERAL OPTIMISM REPORTED BY EACH PARENT AND THE ASPIRATION LEVEL FOR THE PARTICIPATING CHILD REPORTED BY EACH PARENT. IT WAS HYPOTHESIZED THAT PRIOR PARENTAL EXPERIENCE WITH PROJECT HEAD START, CURRENT PARENTAL EXPERIENCE WITH THE PROGRAM, AND ACTIVE PARENTAL PARTICIPATION IN THE PROGRAM WOULD INCREASE PARENTAL SCORES ON THE TWO SCALES. NONE OF THESE HYPOTHESES WAS CONFIRMED. IT WAS FURTHER PREDICTED THAT CHILDREN OF PARENTS WHO SHOWED FAVORABLE CHANGES ON A SCALE WOULD GAIN MORE FROM THEIR OWN HEAD START EXPERIENCES, IN TERMS OF CHANGES IN THE SCORES ON THE TESTS ADMINISTERED TO THEM BOTH BEFORE AND AFTER THE PRO-

GRAM, THAN CHILDREN OF PARENTS WHO SHOWED UNFAVORABLE CHANGES ON THAT SCALE. THIS PREDICTION WAS NOT CONFIRMED. IT WAS ALSO HYPOTHESIZED THAT LATIN AMERICAN PARENTS WOULD SHOW MORE FAVORABLE CHANGE ON THE SCALES THAN NEGRO PARENTS; THIS HYPOTHESIS WAS NOT CONFIRMED. 41 REFERENCES. (RIE ABSTRACT)

ACCN   000714

846 AUTH   **JACOBSON, B., & KENDRICK, J.**
     TITL   EDUCATION: SOCIAL FACT OR SOCIAL PROCESS?
     SRCE   *AMERICAN BEHAVIORAL SCIENTIST, 1970, 14(2), 255-272.*
     INDX   PROGRAM EVALUATION, EDUCATION, RESEARCH METHODOLOGY, SURVEY, SCHOLASTIC ACHIEVEMENT, PUERTO RICAN-I, SES, THEORETICAL, SOCIAL MOBILITY, SCHOLASTIC ASPIRATIONS, LABOR FORCE
     ABST   AN ATTEMPT IS MADE TO INTEGRATE INFERENCES FROM "PEOPLE PROCESSING" RESEARCH WITH OTHER INFERENCES FROM WHAT MIGHT LOOSELY BE TERMED "MACRO THEORY" THROUGH THE USE OF PANEL SURVEY RESEARCH DATA. ATTENTION IS GIVEN TO THE APPROPRIATE WAY IN WHICH TO CONCEIVE OF THE RELATIONSHIP BETWEEN ORGANIZATIONS AND THEIR CLIENTELE. A DISCUSSION FOLLOWS IN WHICH THE FRAGILITY OF TWO CONVENTIONAL ASSUMPTIONS REGARDING RESEARCH AND THEORETICAL ANALYSES ACCOMPLISHED UNDER THE GUIDELINES OF MACRO THEORY IS EXAMINED. SPECIFICALLY, THE LIKELY AGREEMENT OF THE MEANING AND INDEX OF EDUCATION ACROSS UNITS AND THEIR STABILITY ACROSS TIME IN A SOCIAL SETTING OF RAPID TECHNOLOGICAL AND DEMOGRAPHIC CHANGE IS EXAMINED, AND SOME BROADER IMPLICATIONS OF THE ROLE OF EDUCATION IN THE SOCIALIZATION PROCESS ARE NOTED. TO DEMONSTRATE THE BASIC DIFFERENCES FOUND, AN EXAMINATION OF A SET OF DATA FROM A PANEL SURVEY RESEARCH PROJECT ON THE PUERTO RICAN LABOR FORCE IS INCLUDED, FOLLOWED BY SOME GENERAL CONCLUSIONS AND SUGGESTIONS FOR IMPROVING RESEARCH METHODS IN THE FIELD OF SOCIAL ORGANIZATION. 12 REFERENCES.

ACCN   000715

847 AUTH   **JACOBSON, C. K.**
     TITL   SEPARATISM, INTEGRATIONISM, AND AVOIDANCE AMONG BLACK, WHITE, AND LATIN ADOLESCENTS.
     SRCE   *SOCIAL FORCES, 1977, 55(4), 1011-1027.*
     INDX   INTEGRATION, ACCULTURATION, CROSS CULTURAL, INTERPERSONAL RELATIONS, ADOLESCENTS, SPANISH SURNAMED, INTERPERSONAL ATTRACTION, CHILDREN, EMPIRICAL, WISCONSIN, MIDWEST
     ABST   ALTHOUGH MANY STUDIES HAVE EXAMINED SUPPORT FOR INTEGRATION OR SEPARATISM AMONG RACIAL OR ETHNIC GROUPS, MOST HAVE IGNORED OTHER REACTIONS TO INTERGROUP CONTACT SUCH AS AVOIDANCE. THE

RESPONSES OF JUNIOR AND SENIOR HIGH SCHOOL ADOLESCENTS TO A SERIES OF ATTITUDE ITEMS ARE EXAMINED IN A FACTOR ANALYSIS. TWO CLEAR AND DISTINCT RESPONSE TENDENCIES EMERGED: AN INTEGRATION-SEPARATISM DIMENSION AND AN APPROACH-AVOIDANCE DIMENSION. THE SOCIAL CORRELATES OF BOTH DIMENSIONS ARE PRESENTED AND THE IMPLICATIONS OF THE TWO DIMENSIONS FOR CONTINUED RESEARCH ON RACE AND ETHNIC RELATIONS ARE BRIEFLY DISCUSSED. 31 REFERENCES. (JOURNAL ABSTRACT MODIFIED)

ACCN   000716

848   AUTH   **JARECKE, W. H.**
TITL   IDENTIFYING THE VOCATIONAL POTENTIAL OF A DISADVANTAGED POPULATION.
SRCE   *VOCATIONAL EVALUATION AND WORK ADJUSTMENT BULLETIN, 1973, 6(2), 29-32.*
INDX   VOCATIONAL COUNSELING, MEXICAN AMERICAN, PUERTO RICAN-M, WAIS, RAVEN PROGRESSIVE MATRICES, STANFORD-BINET INTELLIGENCE TEST, INTELLIGENCE TESTING, EMPIRICAL, CROSS CULTURAL, TEST VALIDITY
ABST   WHEN ASSESSING VOCATIONAL POTENTIAL AMONG A DISADVANTAGED POPULATION THE SOCIAL, EDUCATIONAL, AND ECONOMIC CHARACTERISTICS SPECIFIC TO THIS GROUP MUST BE CONSIDERED. THE USUAL MEASURES USED TO IDENTIFY AND EVALUATE VOCATIONAL POTENTIAL WILL NOT PRODUCE THE DESIRED RESULTS WHEN APPLIED TO THE DISADVANTAGED. INSTEAD OF DESIGNING A NEW TEST FOR THIS GROUP, NORMS SPECIFIC TO THIS POPULATION WERE DEVELOPED FOR ALREADY STANDARDIZED INSTRUMENTS. A TOTAL OF 422 17-60 YEAR-OLD MALES AND FEMALES, RANGING IN EDUCATION FROM GRADE 1 TO HIGH SCHOOL GRADUATES, AND CONSISTING OF AMERICAN-BORN NEGROES, MEXICANS, AMERICANS, PUERTO RICANS, AND JAMAICANS WERE TESTED. TESTS ADMINISTERED WERE THE REVISED STANFORD-BINET FORM L-M, RAVEN PROGRESSIVE MATRICES, ARTHUR POINT SCALES OF PERFORMANCE FORM 1, COLUMBIA MENTAL MATURITY TEST (2ND EDITION), AND THE WAIS. THE LATTER TWO WERE FOUND TO BE THE MOST USEFUL. A NUMBER OF THOSE IDENTIFIED AS HIGH POTENTIAL SUBJECTS HAD ADVANCED THEIR JOB POSITIONS WITHIN SIX MONTHS. IT IS SUGGESTED THAT ALTHOUGH THE COLUMBIA MENTAL MATURITY TEST IDENTIFIES POTENTIAL, ADDITIONAL VOCATIONAL ORIENTATION AND TRAINING WAS NECESSARY FOR SUCCESS TO OCCUR. (PASAR ABSTRACT MODIFIED)
ACCN   000717

849   AUTH   **JENKINS, S., & MORRISON, B.**
TITL   ETHNICITY AND SERVICE DELIVERY.
SRCE   *AMERICAN JOURNAL OF ORTHOPSYCHIATRY, 1978, 48(1), 160-165.*
INDX   MEXICAN AMERICAN, PUERTO RICAN-M, ETHNIC IDENTITY, CULTURAL PLURALISM, SOCIAL SERVICES, ATTITUDES, CROSS CULTURAL, POLICY, EMPIRICAL, SURVEY, RESEARCH METHODOLOGY, TEST VALIDITY, TEST RELIABILITY, HEALTH DELIVERY SYSTEMS, PROGRAM EVALUATION, PERSONNEL, CULTURAL FACTORS
ABST   TO OPERATIONALIZE ETHNIC ISSUES IN SERVICE DELIVERY, AN ETHNIC COMMITMENT ATTITUDE SCALE WAS DEVELOPED AND ADMINISTERED TO A NATIONAL SAMPLE OF 1,606 SOCIAL WORKERS IN TRADITIONAL CHILD WELFARE SETTINGS AND 583 MINORITY WORKERS (ASIAN AMERICANS, BLACKS, MEXICAN AMERICANS, NATIVE AMERICANS, AND PUERTO RICANS) IN INNOVATIVE ETHNIC SETTINGS. IT WAS HYPOTHESIZED THAT SIGNIFICANT DIFFERENCES BETWEEN WORKERS IN TRADITIONAL AND INNOVATIVE AGENCIES WOULD BE FOUND. THE INSTRUMENT REQUIRED CHOICES ON A SERIES OF 30 ALTERNATIVES TO SERVICE ISSUES, FOCUSING ON CULTURAL CONTENT OF PROGRAMS, MIXING VERSUS MATCHING ALONG ETHNIC LINES, AND ISSUES OF DECISION-MAKING IN POLICY FORMULATION. THE VARIABLES OF AGE, SAMPLE, ETHNICITY, AND AGENCY TYPE EMERGED AS SIGNIFICANT PREDICTORS OF ETHNIC COMMITMENT. WORKERS IN ETHNIC AGENCIES SHOWED GREATER ETHNIC COMMITMENT THAN RESPONDENTS ON THE NATIONAL SAMPLE. ITEMS DEALING WITH CULTURAL CONTENT DID NOT DISCRIMINATE AS STRONGLY AS DID MIXING-MATCHING ITEMS. ANALYSIS OF INTER-ETHNIC DIFFERENCES INDICATED THAT THE RESPONSES RELATED TO SPECIFIC ISSUES EXPERIENCED BY THE GROUP IN QUESTION. INTER-ETHNIC AGREEMENT WAS HIGHEST ON MIXING-MATCHING ITEMS, VERY LOW ON CULTURAL ITEMS, AND ABSENT ON DECISION-POWER ITEMS. IT IS CONCLUDED THAT, ALTHOUGH CULTURAL ISSUES ARE DIFFUSE, THE ETHNIC COMMITMENT SCALE IDENTIFIES ISSUES RELEVANT TO THE ETHNIC IDENTITY-ETHNIC OPPORTUNITY DILEMMA. 4 REFERENCES.
ACCN   002120

850   AUTH   **JENSEN, A. R.**
TITL   DO SCHOOLS CHEAT MINORITY CHILDREN?
SRCE   *EDUCATIONAL RESEARCH, 1971, 14(1), 3-28.*
INDX   MEXICAN AMERICAN, CHILDREN, INTELLIGENCE, SCHOLASTIC ACHIEVEMENT, PERSONALITY, SES, ENVIRONMENTAL FACTORS, CULTURAL FACTORS, ACHIEVEMENT TESTING, CROSS CULTURAL, EMPIRICAL
ABST   LARGE REPRESENTATIVE SAMPLES OF NEGRO AND MEXICAN AMERICAN CHILDREN FROM KINDERGARTEN TO EIGHTH GRADE IN LARGELY DE FACTO SEGREGATED SCHOOLS WERE COMPARED WITH WHITE CHILDREN IN THE SAME CALIFORNIA SCHOOL DISTRICT ON A COMPREHENSIVE BATTERY OF TESTS OF MENTAL ABILITIES AND OF SCHOLASTIC ACHIEVEMENT, IN ADDITION TO PERSONALITY INVENTORIES AND INDICES OF SOCIO-ECONOMIC AND CULTURAL DISADVANTAGE. IT WAS FOUND THAT WHEN CERTAIN ABILITY AND BACKGROUND FACTORS, OVER WHICH THE SCHOOLS HAVE LITTLE OR NO INFLUENCE, ARE STATISTICALLY CONTROLLED, THERE ARE NO APPRECIABLE DIFFERENCES BETWEEN THE

SCHOLASTIC ACHIEVEMENTS (AS MEASURED BY THE STANFORD ACHIEVEMENT TESTS) OF MINORITY AND MAJORITY PUPILS. MOREOVER, THERE WAS NO EVIDENCE OF A 'CUMULATIVE DEFICIT' (AN INCREASING GAP FROM LOWER TO HIGHER GRADE LEVELS BETWEEN THE MEAN ACHIEVEMENTS OF MINORITY AND MAJORITY PUPILS), WHEN THE MAJORITY-MINORITY DIFFERENCES WERE MEASURED IN STANDARD DEVIATION UNITS. IT IS CONCLUDED THAT SCHOOLS IN THE DISTRICT UNDER CONSIDERATION DO NOT CHEAT MINORITY STUDENTS IN TERMS OF CONVENTIONAL EDUCATIONAL CRITERIA. BUT IT MIGHT BE CONCLUDED THAT MINORITY CHILDREN ARE, IN FACT, CHEATED IF IT WERE SHOWN THAT THEIR ABILITY PATTERNS REQUIRE DIFFERENT INSTRUCTIONAL APPROACHES TO OPTIMIZE THEIR SCHOLASTIC LEARNING. MARKED DIFFERENCES, NOT ONLY IN OVERALL LEVEL OF ABILITY BUT ALSO IN THE PATTERN OF ABILITIES, WERE FOUND BETWEEN ALL THREE OF THE ETHNIC GROUPS IN THIS STUDY. 19 REFERENCES. (JOURNAL ABSTRACT)

ACCN   000718

851 AUTH   **JENSEN, A. R.**
     TITL   ETHNICITY & SCHOLASTIC ACHIEVEMENT.
     SRCE   *PSYCHOLOGICAL REPORTS, 1974, 34(2), 659-668.*
     INDX   CROSS CULTURAL, SCHOLASTIC ACHIEVEMENT, SES, CULTURAL FACTORS, PERSONALITY, MEXICAN AMERICAN, CHILDREN, EMPIRICAL, SEX COMPARISON, MEMORY, LEARNING, ENVIRONMENTAL FACTORS, RAVEN PROGRESSIVE MATRICES, INTELLIGENCE, STANFORD ACHIEVEMENT TEST, ACHIEVEMENT TESTING, CALIFORNIA, SOUTHWEST
     ABST   SCORES ON TESTS IN 8 AREAS OF SCHOLASTIC ACHIEVEMENT WERE PREDICTED BY MULTIPLE REGRESSION FROM 7 NONSCHOLASTIC TESTS OF ABILITY, A PERSONALITY INVENTORY, AND ITEMS OF PERSONAL BACKGROUND DATA IN SOME SIX THOUSAND WHITE, NEGRO, AND MEXICAN AMERICAN CALIFORNIA SCHOOL CHILDREN IN GRADES 1 TO 8. AVERAGED OVER GRADES, THE MULTIPLE CORRELATION (R) BETWEEN THE PREDICTOR VARIABLES AND ACHIEVEMENT SCORES RANGED FROM .60 TO .80 FOR VARIOUS SCHOOL SUBJECTS. ETHNICITY MADE NO SIGNIFICANT CONTRIBUTION TO THE MULTIPLE R INDEPENDENTLY OF THE SEVERAL PREDICTOR VARIABLES. 4 REFERENCES. (JOURNAL ABSTRACT)
     ACCN   000719

852 AUTH   **JENSEN, A. R.**
     TITL   HOW BIASED ARE CULTURE-LOADED TESTS?
     SRCE   *GENETIC PSYCHOLOGY MONGRAPHS, 1974, 90(2), 185-244.*
     INDX   INTELLIGENCE TESTING, CULTURE-FAIR TESTS, CHILDREN, PEABODY PICTURE-VOCABULARY TEST, RAVEN PROGRESSIVE MATRICES, MEXICAN AMERICAN, CROSS CULTURAL, ADOLESCENTS, INTELLIGENCE, SEX COMPARISON, EMPIRICAL, TEST RELIABILITY, TEST VALIDITY, CALIFORNIA, SOUTHWEST

ABST   THE CULTURE-LOADED PEABODY PICTURE-VOCABULARY TEST (PPVT) AND THE CULTURE REDUCED RAVEN'S PROGRESSIVE MATRICES (COLORED AND STANDARD FORMS) WERE EXAMINED AND COMPARED IN TERMS OF VARIOUS INTERNAL CRITERIA OF CULTURE BIAS IN LARGE REPRESENTATIVE SAMPLES OF WHITE, BLACK, AND MEXICAN AMERICAN SCHOOL CHILDREN, FROM KINDERGARTEN THROUGH EIGHTH GRADE, IN THREE CALIFORNIA SCHOOL DISTRICTS. ON BOTH THE PPVT AND THE RAVEN THE THREE ETHNIC GROUPS, WHICH SHOW LARGE MEAN DIFFERENCES, SHOWED VERY LITTLE DIFFERENCE IN THE RANK ORDER OF ITEM DIFFICULTIES, THE RELATIVE DIFFICULTY OF ADJACENT ITEMS, THE LOADINGS OF ITEMS ON THE FIRST PRINCIPAL COMPONENT, AND THE CHOICE OF DISTRACTORS FOR INCORRECT RESPONSES. ANALYSIS OF VARIANCE REVEALED VERY SMALL ETHNIC GROUP X ITEMS INTERACTION; BUT A SENSITIVE INDEX OF ITEM BIAS DERIVED FROM ANOVA INDICATES THAT THE RAVEN IS CONSIDERABLY LESS BIASED THAN THE PPVT, ESPECIALLY IN THE MEXICAN GROUP. THE GROUPS X ITEMS INTERACTION WAS SHOWN TO BE ATTRIBUTABLE LARGELY TO DIFFERENCES IN MENTAL MATURITY. ON BOTH TESTS GROUPS OF CULTURALLY HOMOGENEOUS YOUNGER AND OLDER WHITE CHILDREN (SEPARATED BY TWO YEARS) PERFECTLY SIMULATED THE WHITE-BLACK DIFFERENCES IN GROUP X ITEM INTERACTIONS AND CHOICE OF ERROR DISTRACTORS IN THE RAVEN. CERTAIN EXPECTATIONS FROM A CULTURE BIAS HYPOTHESIS WERE BORNE OUT ONLY FOR THE PPVT IN THE MEXICAN GROUP. UNLESS THE UNLIKELY AND EMPIRICALLY UNSUBSTANTIATED ASSUMPTION IS MADE THAT CULTURE BIAS AFFECTS ALL KINDS OF TEST ITEMS ABOUT EQUALLY, THE VARIOUS ITEM ANALYSES OF THE PRESENT STUDIES LEND NO SUPPORT TO THE PROPOSITION THAT EITHER THE PPVT OR THE RAVEN IS A CULTURALLY BIASED TEST FOR BLACKS. THE EVIDENCE REGARDING CULTURAL OR LANGUAGE BIAS IN THE MEXICAN AMERICAN GROUP IS LESS CLEAR. 16 REFERENCES. (JOURNAL ABSTRACT MODIFIED)

ACCN   000720

853 AUTH   **JENSEN, A. R.**
     TITL   INTELLIGENCE, LEARNING ABILITY AND SOCIO-ECONOMIC STATUS.
     SRCE   *JOURNAL OF SPECIAL EDUCATION, 1969, 3(1), 23-35.*
     INDX   INTELLIGENCE, INTELLIGENCE TESTING, STANFORD-BINET INTELLIGENCE TEST, EMPIRICAL, SES, CULTURAL FACTORS, LEARNING, MEXICAN AMERICAN, CROSS CULTURAL, LEARNING DISABILITIES, CALIFORNIA, SOUTHWEST
     ABST   THE INTERACTION OF IQ, ASSOCIATIVE LEARNING ABILITY, AND SOCIOECONOMIC STATUS (SES) IN GROUPS OF CHILDREN FROM CAUCASIAN, MEXICAN AMERICAN, AND NEGRO POPULATIONS IS INVESTIGATED. FINDINGS INDICATE THAT LOW-SES CHILDREN OF LOW MEASURED IQ'S (60 TO 80) ARE GENERALLY SUPERIOR TO THEIR MIDDLE-CLASS COUNTERPARTS IN IQ ON TESTS OF ASSOCIATIVE

LEARNING ABILITY: FREE RECALL, SERIAL LEARNING, PAIRED-ASSOCIATIVE LEARNING, AND DIGIT SPAN. LOW-SES CHILDREN OF AVERAGE IQ OR ABOVE, ON THE OTHER HAND, DO NOT DIFFER FROM THEIR MIDDLE-CLASS COUNTERPARTS ON THESE ASSOCIATIVE LEARNING TASKS. THE RESULTS ARE INTERPRETED IN TERMS OF A HIERARCHIC MODEL OF MENTAL ABILITIES, RANGING FROM ASSOCIATIVE LEARNING TO CONCEPTUAL THINKING, IN WHICH THE DEVELOPMENT OF LOWER LEVELS IN THE HIERARCHY IS NECESSARY BUT NOT SUFFICIENT FOR THE DEVELOPMENT OF HIGHER LEVELS. THE FINDINGS HELP LOCALIZE THE NATURE OF THE INTELLECTUAL DEFICIT OF CULTURALLY DISADVANTAGED CHILDREN AND SHOW THAT ENVIRONMENTAL DEPRIVATION DOES NOT HAVE AN EQUAL EFFECT ON ALL MENTAL ABILITIES. THE NEED FOR STANDARD TESTS TO ASSESS A BROADER SPECTRUM OF MENTAL ABILITIES THAN IS SAMPLED BY CURRENT TESTS OF INTELLIGENCE IS DISCUSSED. 27 REFERENCES.

ACCN   000721

854 AUTH   **JENSEN, A. R.**
    TITL   LEARNING ABILITIES IN MEXICAN AMERICAN AND ANGLO AMERICAN CHILDREN.
    SRCE   *CALIFORNIA JOURNAL OF EDUCATIONAL RESEARCH, 1961, 12(4), 147-159.*
    INDX   MEXICAN AMERICAN, CHILDREN, CROSS CULTURAL, INTELLIGENCE, SCHOLASTIC ACHIEVEMENT, INTELLIGENCE TESTING, CULTURAL FACTORS, ENVIRONMENTAL FACTORS, LEARNING DISABILITIES, CALIFORNIA, SOUTHWEST, EMPIRICAL
    ABST   GROUPS OF FOURTH- AND SIXTH-GRADE MEXICAN AMERICAN AND ANGLO CHILDREN, OF DIFFERENT IQ LEVELS RANGING FROM 60 TO 120 OR ABOVE, WERE COMPARED ON A NUMBER OF LEARNING TASKS CONSISTING OF IMMEDIATE RECALL, SERIAL LEARNING, PAIRED-ASSOCIATES, AND LEARNING OF FAMILIAR AND ABSTRACT OBJECTS. THE MAIN FINDING WAS THAT ON THE DIRECT MEASURES OF LEARNING ABILITY USED IN THIS STUDY, ANGLO AMERICAN CHILDREN OF LOW IQ ARE SLOW LEARNERS AS COMPARED WITH MEXICAN AMERICANS OF THE SAME IQ. MEXICAN AMERICANS OF ABOVE-AVERAGE IQ DO NOT DIFFER SIGNIFICANTLY IN LEARNING ABILITY FROM ANGLO AMERICANS OF THE SAME IQ. HIGH IQ'S ARE RARE AMONG THE MEXICAN AMERICAN POPULATION AND IT IS NOTED THAT THE MAJORITY OF MEXICAN AMERICANS WITH LOW IQ'S, AS MEASURED BY THE CALIFORNIA TEST OF MENTAL MATURITY, ARE ACTUALLY QUITE NORMAL IN BASIC LEARNING ABILITY THOUGH THEY MAY BE POOR IN SCHOLASTIC PERFORMANCE. IT IS SUGGESTED THAT MOST OF THE LOW IQ MEXICAN AMERICANS, NOT BEING BASICALLY SLOW LEARNERS, SHOULD NOT BE PLACED IN CLASS WITH ANGLO AMERICANS OF LOW IQ WHO ARE SLOW LEARNERS; INSTEAD, DIFFERENT METHODS OF TEACHING SHOULD BE REQUIRED. DISCUSSION OF PERTINENT QUESTIONS RELATING TO THE IQ OF THE MEXICAN AMERICAN IS PRESENTED. THE

DEVELOPMENT OF A COMPLETE BATTERY OF DIRECT LEARNING TESTS WOULD SEEM TO HAVE CONSIDERABLE PROMISE FOR IMPROVING THE DIAGNOSIS OF EDUCATIONAL DISABILITIES, ESPECIALLY IN ETHNIC AND CULTURAL GROUPS FOR WHOM THE IQ TESTS ARE NOT HIGHLY APPROPRIATE. 12 REFERENCES.

ACCN   000722

855 AUTH   **JENSEN, A. R.**
    TITL   LEVEL I & LEVEL II ABILITIES IN THREE ETHNIC GROUPS.
    SRCE   *AMERICAN EDUCATIONAL RESEARCH JOURNAL, 1973, 10(4), 263-276.*
    INDX   INTELLIGENCE, INTELLIGENCE TESTING, SCHOLASTIC ACHIEVEMENT, MEMORY, CHILDREN, MEXICAN AMERICAN, CROSS CULTURAL, EMPIRICAL, STANFORD ACHIEVEMENT TEST, RAVEN PROGRESSIVE MATRICES, SES, RURAL, CALIFORNIA, SOUTHWEST, RURAL
    ABST   A LARGE BATTERY OF TESTS OF INTELLIGENCE, SCHOLASTIC ACHIEVEMENT, AND SHORT-TERM MEMORY WAS ADMINISTERED TO 700 WHITE, 556 BLACK, AND 668 MEXICAN AMERICAN PUPILS IN GRADES, 4, 5, AND 6 IN A LARGELY AGRICULTURAL SCHOOL DISTRICT IN THE CENTRAL VALLEY OF CALIFORNIA. THE THREE GRADES WERE USED AS SEPARATE REPLICATIONS OF THE STUDY. FACTOR ANALYSIS WITH OBLIQUE ROTATION YIELDED THREE MAIN FACTORS, IDENTIFIED AS FLUID (GF) AND CRYSTALIZED (GC) INTELLIGENCE (BOTH ARE ASPECTS OF LEVEL II ABILITY IN JENSEN'S THEORY) AND A MEMORY FACTOR (A LEVEL I ABILITY). MEAN FACTOR SCORES FOR THE THREE ETHNIC GROUPS DIFFERED SIGNIFICANTLY AND SHOWED SIGNIFICANT INTERACTIONS WITH ETHNICITY LARGELY IN ACCORD WITH EXPECTATIONS FROM JENSEN'S TWO LEVEL THEORY OF ABILITIES. THE WHITE AND BLACK GROUPS DIFFERED MARKEDLY IN GC AND GF BUT NOT IN MEMORY; THE WHITE AND MEXICAN AMERICAN GROUPS DIFFERED MARKEDLY IN GC, AND MUCH LESS IN GF AND MEMORY. THE BLACK AND MEXICAN AMERICAN GROUPS DIFFERED THE MOST IN GF BUT ONLY SLIGHTLY IN GC. THERE WERE ALSO SYSTEMATIC ETHNIC GROUP DIFFERENCES IN THE PATTERN OF INTERCORRELATIONS AMONG FACTOR SCORES, AND IN THE CORRELATIONS OF THE FACTOR SCORES WITH AN INDEX OF SOCIOECONOMIC STATUS. THE RESULTS ARE DISCUSSED IN RELATION TO JENSEN'S TWO LEVEL THEORY OF MENTAL ABILITIES AND CATTELL'S THEORY OF FLUID AND CRYSTALLIZED INTELLIGENCE. 14 REFERENCES. (JOURNAL ABSTRACT)

ACCN   000723

856 AUTH   **JENSEN, A. R.**
    TITL   PERSONALITY & SCHOLASTIC ACHIEVEMENT IN THREE ETHNIC GROUPS.
    SRCE   *BRITISH JOURNAL OF EDUCATIONAL RESEARCH, 1973, 43(2), 115-125.*
    INDX   PERSONALITY, SCHOLASTIC ACHIEVEMENT, MEXICAN AMERICAN, STANFORD ACHIEVEMENT TEST, CROSS CULTURAL, SES, INTELLIGENCE, INTELLIGENCE TESTING, CULTURAL

FACTORS, RAVEN PROGRESSIVE MATRICES, SEX COMPARISON, CHILDREN, RURAL, EMPIRICAL, CALIFORNIA, SOUTHWEST

ABST   SCORES ON THE JUNIOR EYSENCK PERSONALITY INVENTORY (JEPI) OF 720 WHITE, 733 BLACK, AND 758 MEXICAN AMERICAN SCHOOL CHILDREN, AGES 9 TO 13, WERE EXAMINED IN RELATION TO MEASURES OF INTELLIGENCE AND HOME ENVIRONMENT AS PREDICTORS OF SCHOLASTIC ACHIEVEMENT. THE JEPI SCALES SHOWED QUITE LOW, BUT SIGNIFICANT AND SYSTEMATIC, CORRELATIONS WITH ACHIEVEMENT; EXTRAVERSION (E) CORRELATED POSITIVELY AND NEUROTICISM (N) AND THE LIE (L) SCALE CORRELATED NEGATIVELY WITH ACHIEVEMENT. THE INDEPENDENT CONTRIBUTIONS SEPARATELY OF E, N, AND L TO ACHIEVEMENT VARIANCE OVER THE VARIANCE ACCOUNTED FOR BY THE ABILITY AND BACKGROUND MEASURES ARE NEGLIGIBLE, BUT THE THREE JEPI SCALES COMBINED IN A MULTIPLE REGRESSION EQUATION ALONG WITH MEASURES OF INTELLIGENCE AND HOME BACKGROUND INDEPENDENTLY CONTRIBUTE A SMALL SHARE OF THE PREDICTED PART OF THE SCHOLASTIC ACHIEVEMENT VARIANCE. IN THIS NEITHER THE THREE ETHNIC GROUPS NOR THE AGE GROUPS DIFFER APPRECIABLY OR SYSTEMATICALLY, ALTHOUGH THERE ARE SIGNIFICANT AND SYSTEMATIC AGE AND ETHNIC GROUP DIFFERENCES IN MEAN SCORES ON THE JEPI SCALES. 18 REFERENCES. (JOURNAL ABSTRACT MODIFIED)

ACCN   000724

857 AUTH   **JESSOR, R., GRAVES, T. D., HANSON, R. C., & JESSOR, S. L.**

TITL   SOCIETY, PERSONALITY, AND DEVIANT BEHAVIOR. A STUDY OF A TRI-ETHNIC COMMUNITY.

SRCE   *NEW YORK: HOLT, RINEHART & WINSTON, 1968.*

INDX   DEVIANCE, ALCOHOLISM, PSYCHOPATHOLOGY, DISCRIMINATION, PREJUDICE, FAMILY ROLES, SOCIALIZATION, CONFORMITY, ANOMIE, DELINQUENCY, CULTURAL FACTORS, SEX COMPARISON, ATTITUDES, GANGS, PEER GROUP, ROLE EXPECTATIONS, RESEARCH METHODOLOGY, SURVEY, ADULTS, ADOLESCENTS, RURAL, EMPIRICAL, SPANISH SURNAMED, CROSS CULTURAL, COLORADO, SOUTHWEST, THEORETICAL, SOCIAL SCIENCES, BOOK

ABST   AN INTERDISCIPLINARY THEORY OF DEVIANT BEHAVIOR WAS TESTED IN A SMALL, RURAL COMMUNITY IN SOUTHWESTERN COLORADO, USING HEAVY ALCOHOL DRINKING AS AN EXAMPLE OF SUCH BEHAVIOR. THE RESEARCH BEGAN WITH THE TASK OF ACCOUNTING FOR DIFFERENTIAL RATES OF OCCURRENCE OF HEAVY ALCOHOL USE AMONG THREE ETHNIC GROUPS: ANGLO AMERICANS (DEFINED AS WHITES, WHETHER ENGLISH, GERMAN, OR ITALIAN), SPANISH AMERICANS, AND INDIANS. THREE MAJOR CONVERGING INVESTIGATIONS WERE MADE BY A FIELD THEORY APPROACH IN AN ATTEMPT TO SHOW THAT THE BEHAVIOR EXAMINED WAS A CONSEQUENCE OF THE INTERACTION OF FACTORS IN THE PERSONALITY AND IN THE SOCIOCULTURAL ENVIRONMENT.

TREATING DEVIANT BEHAVIOR AS LEARNED, PURPOSIVE, GOAL ORIENTED, AND ADAPTIVE, THE PROBLEM BECAME ONE OF ACCOUNTING FOR SELECTION AMONG POSSIBLE ADAPTIVE ALTERNATIVES. A COMMUNITY SURVEY WAS CONDUCTED TO ASSESS THE APPLICABILITY OF THE THEORY OF DEVIANCE TO THE ADULT POPULATION. SUBJECTS WERE CHOSEN BY STRATIFIED RANDOM SAMPLING FROM A COMPLETE CENSUS LIST, AND DATA WERE OBTAINED BY INTERVIEWS CROSS-CHECKED WITH COURT RECORDS. A SECOND STUDY USED THE ENTIRE COMMUNITY SENIOR HIGH SCHOOL BODY AND DERIVED DATA BY GROUP-ADMINISTERED QUESTIONNAIRES OR TESTS. FINALLY, A SOCIALIZATION STUDY, DONE BY INTERVIEWS WITH PARENTS, FOCUSED ON THE PROCESSES WHICH ANTEDATE THE PERSONALITY AND BEHAVIOR SYSTEMS AND MEDIATE THE RELATION OF THE LATTER TO THE SOCIOCULTURAL ENVIRONMENT. IT WAS DEMONSTRATED IN ALL THREE STUDIES THAT EXCESSIVE ALCOHOL USE IS RELATED TO DIFFERENTIAL PRESSURES AND CONTROLS, BOTH SOCIOCULTURAL AND PERSONAL. THE RESEARCH SUGGESTS THAT A LACK OF NORMATIVE CONSENSUS WITHIN A GROUP MAY BE RELEVANT TO DEVIANCE AND THAT DIFFERENCES IN ACHIEVEMENT EXPECTATIONS CRUCIALLY INFLUENCE RATES OF DEVIANCE AMONG GROUPS. 200 REFERENCES.

ACCN   000725

858 AUTH   **JIMENEZ, R. L.**

TITL   AN EXPERIMENTAL PROJECT IN TRAINING NEIGHBORHOOD MENTAL HEALTH PRACTITIONERS IN THE RESOLUTION OF INTERGROUP CONFLICT.

SRCE   *IN L. B. MACHT, D. J. SCHERL & S. SHARFSTEIN (EDS.), NEIGHBORHOOD PSYCHIATRY. LEXINGTON, MASS.: D.C. HEATH AND COMPANY, 1977, PP. 191-201.*

INDX   ESSAY, CONFLICT RESOLUTION, CROSS CULTURAL, GROUP DYNAMICS, INTERPERSONAL RELATIONS, MENTAL HEALTH, PARAPROFESSIONALS, ROLE EXPECTATIONS, SES, SPANISH SURNAMED, BILINGUAL-BICULTURAL PERSONNEL, PUERTO RICAN-M, ADULTS, MASSACHUSETTS, EAST, PSYCHOTHERAPY, PSYCHOTHERAPY OUTCOME

ABST   A GROUP EXPERIMENT DESIGNED TO RESOLVE ONGOING CONFLICTS BETWEEN HISPANIC NEIGHBORHOOD WORKERS AND NON-SPANISH-SPEAKING SOCIAL SERVICE STAFF MEMBERS IN A NEIGHBORHOOD HEALTH CENTER IN THE BOSTON AREA IS DISCUSSED. TWENTY HUMAN SERVICE PROFESSIONALS AND NEIGHBORHOOD WORKERS PARTICIPATED—5 BILINGUAL PROFESSIONALS; 5 NON-SPANISH-SPEAKING PROFESSIONALS; 2 NATIVE, SPANISH-SPEAKING HUMAN SERVICE PROFESSIONALS; 4 HISPANIC COMMUNITY WORKERS; AND 4 HISPANIC NEIGHBORHOOD WORKERS FROM OTHER CENTERS. THE BASIC FORMAT WAS THAT OF A TASK-ORIENTED TRAINING GROUP, DESIGNED TO EXPLORE SYSTEMATICALLY THE ISSUES INVOLVED IN PRACTICING MENTAL HEALTH SKILLS IN THE SPANISH-SPEAKING

COMMUNITY—AND IN THE PROCESS, EN-
COUNTER CONFLICTS AND DYNAMICS WHICH
SUCH PERSONNEL FACE DAILY IN THEIR WORK.
THE GROUP MET ONCE EACH WEEK FOR A
YEAR AT BOSTON UNIVERSITY (FOR COLLEGE
CREDIT IF DESIRED). THE GROUP UNDERWENT
VARIOUS CHANGES, FROM INITIAL ENTHUSI-
ASM ABOUT DISCUSSING PRESSING PROB-
LEMS IN THE HISPANIC COMMUNITY, TO GROUP
DIVISIONS AND HOSTILITIES, AND FINALLY, VIA
GUIDANCE AND GROUP STRUCTURE, TO A PE-
RIOD OF FREE EXPRESSION, TRUST, AND
SHARING. IT IS CONCLUDED THAT THE PROJ-
ECT PROVED SUCCESSFUL IN RECREATING
THE EMOTIONS AND STRESSES INHERENT IN
SUCH PHENOMENA AS CULTURE CONFLICTS,
MIGRATION, AND THE EFFECTS OF SOCIAL
CLASS MOBILITY ON PROFESSIONAL IDENTITY.
IT IS SUGGESTED THAT SUCH GROUP CROSS-
CULTURAL TRAINING PROGRAMS IN NEIGH-
BORHOOD MENTAL HEALTH WORK CAN PRO-
VIDE AN EXCELLENT MEANS OF PROVIDING
PRACTITIONERS WITH UNDERSTANDING AND
PRACTICE IN RESOLVING INTERGROUP CON-
FLICT. 15 REFERENCES.

ACCN   002121

859 AUTH   **JOHANSEN, S.**
     TITL   FAMILY ORGANIZATION IN A SPANISH AMERI-
            CAN CULTURE AREA.
     SRCE   *SOCIOLOGY AND SOCIAL RESEARCH, 1943, 28,*
            123-131.
     INDX   FAMILY STRUCTURE, FAMILY ROLES, SPANISH
            SURNAMED, EMPIRICAL, CULTURAL CHANGE,
            RURAL, CASE STUDY, NEW MEXICO, SOUTH-
            WEST, MARITAL STABILITY
     ABST   THE ROLE OF THE FAMILY IN THE SOCIAL OR-
            GANIZATION OF EIGHT SPANISH AMERICAN
            VILLAGES IN DONA ANA COUNTY, NEW MEXICO,
            IS DISCUSSED. THE FAMILY ASSUMES GREAT
            IMPORTANCE IN THIS AREA DUE TO THE MINOR
            IMPORTANCE OR ABSENCE OF OTHER SOCIAL
            OR SPECIAL INTEREST GROUPS. THE STRONG
            INFLUENCE OF THE FAMILY IS DISCUSSED IN
            TERMS OF FAMILY INTERRELATIONSHIPS
            (NEARLY 3/4THS OF THE SPANISH AMERICAN
            HOUSEHOLD HEADS ARE RELATED TO SOME
            OTHER HEAD) AND SOCIAL CONTROL (NONE
            OF THE CENTERS HAS A LOCAL GOVERN-
            MENT). CHANGING ASPECTS OF THE FAMILY
            ARE ALSO DISCUSSED. ALTHOUGH THE VIL-
            LAGES REMAIN RELATIVELY ISOLATED, THIS
            ISOLATION IS BREAKING DOWN, ESPECIALLY
            FOR THE YOUNGER FAMILY MEMBERS. OUT-
            SIDE CONTACTS THROUGH SCHOOL, RECREA-
            TION, AND EMPLOYMENT ACTIVITIES HAVE IN-
            CREASED. NEW IDEAS AND ATTITUDES HAVE
            FOUND THEIR WAY INTO THE AREA AND AF-
            FECTED FAMILY LIFE. SOCIAL CHANGE HAS
            LED TO A BREAKDOWN IN FAMILY MORES AND
            SOCIAL CONTROL, AND IN MANY CASES TO
            FAMILY DISINTEGRATION. THE CHIEF REASON
            FAMILY SOLIDARITY HAS REMAINED AS STRONG
            AS IT HAS AND THAT MORE PEOPLE HAVE NOT
            LEFT THE AREA IS THAT OUTSIDE OPPORTUNI-
            TIES ARE SCARCE. (AUTHOR SUMMARY MODI-
            FIED)

ACCN   000726

860 AUTH   **JOHNSON, A. S.**
     TITL   AN ASSESSMENT OF MEXICAN-AMERICAN PAR-
            ENT CHILDREARING FEELINGS AND BEHAV-
            IORS (DOCTORAL DISSERTATION, ARIZONA
            STATE UNIVERSITY, 1975).
     SRCE   *DISSERTATION ABSTRACTS INTERNATIONAL,*
            1975, 36(5), 2614A. (UNIVERSITY MICROFILMS
            NO. 75-25,374.)
     INDX   CHILDREARING PRACTICES, CHILDREN,
            MOTHER-CHILD INTERACTION, FATHER-CHILD
            INTERACTION, ATTITUDES, MEXICAN AMERI-
            CAN, EMPIRICAL, ARIZONA, SOUTHWEST
     ABST   CHILD-REARING FEELINGS AND BEHAVIORS
            OF MEXICAN AMERICAN (MA) PARENTS WERE
            EXAMINED ON THE BASIS OF (1) THEIR RE-
            SPONSES TO THE PARENT AS A TEACHER IN-
            VENTORY (PAAT) AND (2) CONSISTENCY IN
            CHILD-PARENT INTERACTIONS OBSERVED
            DURING HOME VISITS. TO IDENTIFY COMMON
            FEATURES ACROSS INCOME-LEVELS AND DIF-
            FERENCES WITH THE MA SUBJECT GROUP AS
            A FUNCTION OF INCOME-LEVEL, SEX, EDUCA-
            TION, FAMILY SIZE, PARENTAL ACCESSIBILITY,
            AND CONSISTENCY IN OBSERVED BEHAVIORS,
            30 INTACT MA FAMILIES WITH A PRESCHOOL
            SON IN PHOENIX, ARIZONA, WERE SAMPLED.
            THE INFLUENCE OF EACH OF THE FIVE CLAS-
            SIFICATION VARIABLES ON PAAT SCORES WAS
            EXAMINED BY ANALYSIS OF VARIANCE OF THE
            FIVE PAAT SUBSCALES (CREATIVITY, FRUSTRA-
            TION, CONTROL, PLAY AND LEARNING). THE
            CONTROL SUBSCALE TENDED TO DISCRIMI-
            NATE MORE BETWEEN PARENTS THAN THE
            OTHER SUBSCALES. PARENT RESPONSES TO
            CONTROL ITEMS VARIED SIGNIFICANTLY WITH
            RESPECT TO FAMILY INCOME, EDUCATION, SIZE,
            AND PARENTAL ACCESSIBILITY. POVERTY IN-
            COME-LEVEL PARENTS EXPRESSED HIGHEST
            NEED FOR CONTROL, AS DID THOSE WITH
            LESS THAN A NINTH-GRADE EDUCATION AND
            WHO SPENT LESS THAN TWO HOURS WEEKLY
            WITH THEIR CHILD. PARENTS WHO SPENT MORE
            THAN TWO HOURS PER WEEK WITH THEIR
            CHILD SHOWED DISTINCT ADVANTAGE IN THE
            CREATIVITY, CONTROL, AND TOTAL SCORES.
            CONTRARY TO POPULAR VIEW, LEVEL OF PAR-
            ENT EDUCATION DID NOT HAVE A SIGNIFICANT
            EFFECT ON THE TEACHING-LEARNING SUBS-
            CALE. PARENTS WHO SPENT MORE TIME WITH
            THEIR CHILD SHOWED GREATER CONSIS-
            TENCY BETWEEN EXPRESSED FEELINGS AND
            OBSERVED BEHAVIORS. 128 REFERENCES.
            (AUTHOR ABSTRACT MODIFIED)

ACCN   000727

861 AUTH   **JOHNSON, C. A.**
     TITL   MEXICAN-AMERICAN WOMEN IN THE LABOR
            FORCE AND LOWERED FERTILITY.
     SRCE   *AMERICAN JOURNAL OF PUBLIC HEALTH, 1976,*
            66(12), 1186-1188.
     INDX   DEMOGRAPHIC, MEXICAN AMERICAN, FE-
            MALE, FERTILITY, SOUTHWEST, URBAN, SES,
            BIRTH CONTROL, HEALTH EDUCATION, CUL-
            TURAL CHANGE, FAMILY STRUCTURE, LABOR
            FORCE, ADULTS, ADOLESCENTS, EMPLOY-
            MENT

ABST EVIDENCE FROM THE 1970 CENSUS SUGGESTS A BREAK IN THE TRADITIONAL PATTERN OF SUSTAINED AND FREQUENT CHILDBEARING AMONG MEXICAN AMERICAN WOMEN 15 TO 49 YEARS OF AGE (BASED ON A SAMPLE OF 7,659 SOUTHWEST URBAN HOUSEHOLDS). USING THE DICHOTOMIZED CHARACTERISTICS OF EDUCATION, LABOR FORCE PARTICIPATION, AND LANGUAGE, SEVERAL PATTERNS OF CHILDBEARING WERE IDENTIFIED WITHIN THIS SINGLE ETHNIC GROUP. LABOR FORCE PARTICIPATION WAS ASSOCIATED WITH LOWER FERTILITY IN BOTH HIGH AND LOW EDUCATION CATEGORIES AND AMONG SPANISH AND ENGLISH SPEAKING WOMEN. THE EFFECT OF LABOR FORCE PARTICIPATION IS ENHANCED BY EDUCATIONAL ACHIEVEMENT AND ASSOCIATED WITH FERTILITY REDUCTION EVEN IN THE ABSENCE OF EDUCATION BEYOND THE EIGHTH GRADE. AGE DISTRIBUTION TENDED TO ENHANCE THE EFFECT OF BOTH EDUCATIONAL ACHIEVEMENT AND LABOR FORCE PARTICIPATION, WITH THE RELATION OF EDUCATION TO FERTILITY BEING STRONGEST IN WOMEN UNDER 20 YEARS OF AGE, AND THE GROUP MOST LIKELY TO ACHIEVE A CONTROLLED FERTILITY PATTERN BEING WOMEN IN THE LABOR FORCE AGED 20-34 YEARS. IT IS SUGGESTED (1) THAT CHILDBEARING CAREER PERSPECTIVES MAY BE A STRATEGIC ASPECT OF HIGH SCHOOL HEALTH EDUCATION, AND (2) THAT MORE ATTENTION SHOULD BE PAID TO THE CAREERS OF MINORITY WOMEN, BY LOCATING FAMILY PLANNING AND OTHER WOMEN'S HEALTH SERVICES AT THE WORKPLACE. 8 REFERENCES.

ACCN 002122

862 AUTH **JOHNSON, D. G., SMITH, V. C., JR., & TARNOFF, S. L.**

TITL RECRUITMENT AND PROGRESS OF MINORITY MEDICAL SCHOOL ENTRANTS, 1970-1972.

SRCE *JOURNAL OF MEDICAL EDUCATION, 1975, 50(7), 711-755.*

INDX MEDICAL STUDENTS, REPRESENTATION, EQUAL OPPORTUNITY, PROFESSIONAL TRAINING, MENTAL HEALTH PROFESSION, DEMOGRAPHIC, CROSS CULTURAL, HIGHER EDUCATION, EMPIRICAL, SES, SPANISH SURNAMED, MEXICAN AMERICAN, PUERTO RICAN-M

ABST A NATIONAL STUDY OF MINORITY GROUP APPLICANTS AND ENTRANTS TO THE U.S. MEDICAL COLLEGES, 1970-1972, WAS CONDUCTED TO IDENTIFY FACTORS INVOLVED IN INCREASING MINORITY REPRESENTATION. DATA FROM THE ASSOCIATION OF AMERICAN MEDICAL COLLEGE WERE USED TO EXAMINE CHARACTERISTICS OF SUCCESSFUL AND UNSUCCESSFUL MINORITY APPLICANTS. SOCIOECONOMIC, PERSONAL, INSTITUTIONAL, AND GEOGRAPHICAL FACTORS WERE ANALYZED, EVALUATED, AND COMPARED WITH CHARACTERISTICS OF MAJORITY GROUP STUDENTS. IT WAS FOUND THAT: (1) THE RACIAL CHARACTERIZATIONS REPORTED BY MEDICAL SCHOOL APPLICANTS HAVE A HIGH DEGREE OF COMPLETENESS; (2) THE ENROLLMENT OF LOW-INCOME MEDICAL STUDENTS HAS INCREASED, MOSTLY DUE TO THE INCREASE IN MINORITY

GROUP STUDENTS; (3) A GREATER PROPORTION OF MINORITY MEDICAL STUDENTS ARE FEMALE, OLDER, AND MARRIED; AND (4) PARTLY DUE TO THEIR DIVERSITY IN SOCIOECONOMIC AND EDUCATIONAL BACKGROUNDS, MINORITY GROUP STUDENTS HAVE A SLIGHTLY LOWER MEDICAL SCHOOL RETENTION RATE. 12 TABLES SUMMARIZE THESE AND OTHER DATA. (AUTHOR SUMMARY MODIFIED)

ACCN 000728

863 AUTH **JOHNSON, D. L., KAHN, A. J., & LELER, H.**

TITL HOUSTON PARENT-CHILD DEVELOPMENT CENTER (FINAL REPORT, GRANT NO. DHEW 90-C-379).

SRCE *HOUSTON: UNIVERSITY OF HOUSTON, DEPARTMENT OF PSYCHOLOGY, AUGUST 1976.*

INDX PARENTAL INVOLVEMENT, PARAPROFESSIONALS, EDUCATION, PRIMARY PREVENTION, EARLY CHILDHOOD EDUCATION, ATTITUDES, FAMILY ROLES, CHILDREARING PRACTICES, CHILDREN, MEXICAN AMERICAN, PROGRAM EVALUATION, INSTRUCTIONAL TECHNIQUES, MOTHER-CHILD INTERACTION, EMPIRICAL, TEXAS, SOUTHWEST

ABST THIS REPORT DESCRIBES THE DEVELOPMENT AND EVALUATION OF A PARENT EDUCATION PROGRAM CARRIED OUT AT THE HOUSTON PARENT-CHILD DEVELOPMENT CENTER. THE RATIONALE FOR THE PROGRAM WAS A CONCERN FOR IMPROVING THE EDUCATIONAL FUTURE OF YOUNG CHILDREN OF LOW-INCOME MINORITY BACKGROUND. THE ULTIMATE GOAL OF THE PROGRAM WAS TO TRAIN PARENTS SO THEY COULD HELP THEIR CHILDREN OPTIMIZE THEIR SCHOOL PERFORMANCE. EACH FAMILY WAS ENROLLED IN THE PROGRAM WHEN THE CHILD WAS ONE YEAR OF AGE AND CONTINUED TO PARTICIPATE IN A HOME AND CENTER BASED PROGRAM UNTIL THE CHILD WAS 3 YEARS-OLD. EVALUATION RESULTS ARE BASED ON COHORT AND TIME ANALYSES. THE REPORT CONCLUDES THAT ALTHOUGH THE PROGRAM HAS OBTAINED THE IMMEDIATE GOALS OF PREPARING CHILDREN FOR SCHOOL, THE EFFECTIVENESS OF THE PROGRAM CAN ONLY BE DETERMINED BY A FOLLOW-UP STUDY. 91 REFERENCES. (AUTHOR ABSTRACT MODIFIED)

ACCN 000729

864 AUTH **JOHNSON, D. L., LELER, H., RIOS, L., BRANDT, L., KAHN, A. J., MAZEIKA, E., FREDE, M., & BISSET, B.**

TITL THE HOUSTON PARENT-CHILD DEVELOPMENT CENTER: A PARENT EDUCATION PROGRAM FOR MEXICAN-AMERICAN FAMILIES.

SRCE *AMERICAN JOURNAL OF ORTHOPSYCHIATRY, 1974, 44(1), 121-128.*

INDX PARENTAL INVOLVEMENT, CHILDREN, MEXICAN AMERICAN, EARLY CHILDHOOD EDUCATION, STANFORD-BINET INTELLIGENCE TEST, COGNITIVE DEVELOPMENT, MOTHER-CHILD INTERACTION, EMPIRICAL, BILINGUAL-BICULTURAL EDUCATION, PROGRAM EVALUATION, CHILDREARING PRACTICES, PHYSICAL DEVELOPMENT, TEXAS, SOUTHWEST

ABST A TWO-YEAR PARENT EDUCATION PROGRAM DESIGNED TO INVOLVE THE ENTIRE FAMILY IN

PREPARATION OF THE CHILD FOR SCHOOL IS DESCRIBED AND EVALUATED. THE PROGRAM BEGINS WHEN THE CHILD IS 1 YEAR-OLD AND INCLUDES IN-HOME TRAINING OF THE MOTHER, PLUS SEVERAL WEEKEND SESSIONS FOR THE ENTIRE FAMILY. IN THE 2ND YEAR, THE MOTHER AND CHILD PARTICIPATE IN A NURSERY SCHOOL SETTING AND THE FATHER IS INVOLVED IN EVENING MEETINGS. BILINGUAL TRAINING IS EMPHASIZED THROUGHOUT. SIGNIFICANT IMPROVEMENTS ON THE MENTAL SUBSCALE OF THE BAYLEY SCALES OF INFANT DEVELOPMENT WERE FOUND FOR 32 MEXICAN AMERICAN CHILDREN PARTICIPATING IN THE FIRST-YEAR PROGRAM. STANFORD-BINET IQ'S AT 30 MONTHS OF AGE WERE SIGNIFICANTLY HIGHER FOR CHILDREN IN THE PROGRAM THAN FOR A CONTROL GROUP. IMPROVEMENT ON MEASURES OF MATERNAL INVOLVEMENT WITH THE CHILD AND HOME ENVIRONMENT WERE IN THE EXPECTED DIRECTION. CAUTIONS IN INTERPRETING THE RESULTS ARE DISCUSSED. 6 REFERENCES. (PASAR ABSTRACT MODIFIED)

ACCN   000730

865 AUTH   **JOHNSON, D. L., & SIKES, M. P.**
    TITL   RORSCHACH AND TAT RESPONSES OF NEGRO, MEXICAN AMERICAN, AND ANGLO PSYCHIATRIC PATIENTS.
    SRCE   *JOURNAL OF PROJECTIVE TECHNIQUES, 1965, 29(2), 183-188.*
    INDX   RORSCHACH TEST, TAT, PERSONALITY ASSESSMENT, CULTURAL FACTORS, FAMILY ROLES, PROJECTIVE TESTING, MEXICAN AMERICAN, EMPIRICAL, ADULTS, CROSS CULTURAL, MALE, TEXAS, SOUTHWEST
    ABST   A COMPARISON OF THE RORSCHACH AND THEMATIC APPERCEPTION PROJECTIVE TEST (TAT) RESPONSES OF 75 ANGLO, NEGRO, AND MEXICAN AMERICAN (MA) PATIENTS IS PRESENTED. THE SUBJECTS WERE A RANDOM SAMPLE OF NONPSYCHOTIC MALE VETERANS WHOSE AGES, EDUCATIONAL BACKGROUNDS, AND OCCUPATIONAL LEVELS WERE QUITE SIMILAR. A NUMBER OF STATISTICALLY SIGNIFICANT DIFFERENCES WERE FOUND BETWEEN GROUPS, WITH MOST DISTINCT DIFFERENCES ON THE RORSCHACH APPEARING ON THE MEASURE OF HOSTILITY. THE TAT REVEALED DIFFERENCES BETWEEN THE MA'S AND THE OTHER TWO GROUPS IN THEMES OF FAMILY UNIT, PARTICULARLY IN FATHER-SON AND MOTHER-SON RELATIONSHIPS. THIS TAT FINDING POSSIBLY DEMONSTRATES THE PERSISTENCE OF MA CULTURAL VALUES REGARDING INTERPERSONAL RELATIONSHIPS WITHIN THE FAMILY. A TENDENCY FOR MA AND NEGRO GROUPS TO SHOW MORE ACHIEVEMENT IS NOTED. THE THEMES OF FRUSTRATION TEND TO APPEAR MOST FREQUENTLY IN THE NEGRO AND MA GROUP. RESULTS OF THIS STUDY SUGGEST THE UTILITY OF PROJECTIVE MEASURES IN THE FORMULATION OF CULTURE AND PERSONALITY THEORIES. 5 REFERENCES.
    ACCN   000731

866 AUTH   **JOHNSON, G. B.**
    TITL   BILIGUALISM AS MEASURED BY A REACTION-

TIME TECHNIQUE AND THE RELATIONSHIP BETWEEN A LANGUAGE AND NON-LANGUAGE INTELLIGENCE QUOTIENT.
    SRCE   *JOURNAL OF GENETIC PSYCHOLOGY, 1953, 82(1), 3-9.*
    INDX   BILINGUALISM, TEST RELIABILITY, INTELLIGENCE TESTING, GOODENOUGH DRAW-A-MAN TEST, SPANISH SURNAMED, EMPIRICAL, CHILDREN, TEST VALIDITY, SOUTHWEST
    ABST   THE EFFECTS OF BILINGUALISM, AS MEASURED BY A REACTION-TIME TECHNIQUE, UPON THE MEASUREMENT OF INTELLIGENCE ARE ILLUSTRATED THROUGH THE UTILIZATION OF A LANGUAGE AND NONLANGUAGE INTELLIGENCE TEST. THE REACTION-TIME TEST OF BILINGUALISM, THE HOFFMAN TEST OF BILINGUALISM, THE OTIS TEST OF MENTAL ABILITY (OTMA), AND THE GOODENOUGH DRAW-A-MAN TEST (GDMT) WERE ALL ADMINISTERED TO A GROUP OF 30 SPANISH AMERICAN BOYS FROM THE SOUTHWEST. THE RESULTS SHOWED A NEGATIVE RELATIONSHIP BETWEEN PERFORMANCE ON THE OTMA AND THE DEGREE OF BILINGUALISM. HOWEVER, THE RELATIONSHIP BETWEEN THE TESTS OF BILINGUALISM AND THE GDMT INDICATED THAT THE DEGREE OF BILINGUALISM IS ASSOCIATED WITH SUPERIOR RESPONSE ON THIS PERFORMANCE TEST OF INTELLIGENCE. THE RELATIONSHIP BETWEEN THE TWO MEASURES OF INTELLIGENCE WAS FOUND TO BE INSIGNIFICANT, INDICATING THAT THEY ARE PROBABLY TESTS OF SEPARATE FACTORS. OTHER FINDINGS WERE THAT GREATER KNOWLEDGE OF ENGLISH IN COMPARISON WITH KNOWLEDGE OF SPANISH IS ASSOCIATED WITH LESS DISCREPANCY BETWEEN THE OTMA AND THE GDMT INTELLIGENCE QUOTIENT SCORES. THE OTMA RESULTS MOST NEARLY APPROACHED GDMT RESULTS IN THOSE INDIVIDUALS WITH FEWEST SPANISH RESPONSES ON THE REACTION-TIME TEST. BECAUSE OF THE COMPLEXITY OF MEASURING THE INTELLIGENCE OF BILINGUALS, BOTH THE OTMA AND GDMT MAY BE INVALID INSTRUMENTS FOR THIS GROUP. 17 REFERENCES.
    ACCN   000732

867 AUTH   **JOHNSON, G. B.**
    TITL   THE ORIGIN AND DEVELOPMENT OF THE SPANISH ATTITUDE TOWARD THE ANGLO AND THE ANGLO ATTITUDE TOWARD THE SPANISH.
    SRCE   *JOURNAL OF EDUCATIONAL PSYCHOLOGY, 1950, 41(7), 428-439.*
    INDX   PROJECTIVE TESTING, CROSS CULTURAL, CHILDREN, ADOLESCENTS, SPANISH SURNAMED, PREJUDICE, STEREOTYPES, EMPIRICAL, TEXAS, SOUTHWEST
    ABST   AN INVESTIGATION OF THE ORIGIN AND DEVELOPMENT OF THE DEGREE OF PREJUDICE IN RACIAL ATTITUDES AMONG SPANISH AMERICAN AND ANGLO AMERICAN CHILDREN IS PRESENTED. A SAMPLE OF 90 SPANISH AMERICAN MALES AND 90 ANGLOS, AGES 4, 8, AND 12, WERE ADMINISTERED THE PROJECTIVE TEST OF RACIAL ATTITUDES WHICH CONTAINS SIX PICTURES RELEVANT TO ATTITUDES. DATA INDICATED THAT BOTH GROUPS MANIFESTED A CLEAR PICTURE OF DEVELOPMENT OF RA-

CIAL ATTITUDES FROM THE YOUNGER AGE LEVELS TO THE OLDER. THE SPANISH AMERICANS AT THE 4-YEAR LEVEL APPEAR LESS PREJUDICED THAN THE ANGLOS OF THE SAME AGE, BUT DURING THE ENSUING 4 YEARS A NEGATIVE ATTITUDE DEVELOPS TO A LEVEL APPROXIMATING THAT OF THE 12 YEAR-OLDS OF THAT ETHNIC GROUP. THE ANGLO ATTITUDE DEVELOPS LITTLE BETWEEN THE FOURTH AND EIGHTH YEARS. HOWEVER, RAPID ACCELERATION DURING THE NEXT 4 YEARS PUTS THE ANGLO AT THE HIGHEST LEVEL OF PREJUDICE OF ALL GROUPS AND AGES STUDIED. IN ADDITION, IT IS REVEALED THAT THE ANGLOS ARE LESS OPTIMISTIC ABOUT THE SPANISH-ANGLO RELATIONSHIP THAN ARE THE SPANISH AMERICANS. THE ANGLOS APPEAR TO BE THE AGGRESSORS, WHILE THE SPANISH AMERICANS MERELY ATTEMPT TO ADJUST TO THIS AGGRESSION. THE EARLY DEVELOPMENT OF ANGLO PREJUDICE AND DIFFERENT RATES OF PREJUDICE DEVELOPMENT INDICATE HOW THE ATTITUDES OF ONE GROUP MAY CONTRIBUTE TOWARD THE ATTITUDINAL DEVELOPMENT OF THE OTHER. THE DATA SUGGEST THAT THE ORIGIN OF PREJUDICE TOWARD THE SPANISH AMERICAN APPEARS AT ABOUT THE 3 1/2-YEAR LEVEL WHILE THE GENESIS OF PREJUDICE TOWARD THE ANGLO APPEARS SOMETIME AFTER 3 1/2 YEARS. 1 REFERENCE.

ACCN   000733

868 AUTH **JOHNSON, H. S.**
     TITL MENTAL HEALTH NEEDS OF MEXICAN AMERICANS.
     SRCE *SAN FERNANDO, CALIFORNIA: MONTAL EDUCATIONAL ASSOCIATES, 1972.*
     INDX MENTAL HEALTH, PSYCHOTHERAPY, RESOURCE UTILIZATION, FOLK MEDICINE, CULTURAL FACTORS, MEXICAN AMERICAN, REVIEW, SOUTHWEST, CURANDERISMO, THEORETICAL, ESSAY, PSYCHOPATHOLOGY, PROFESSIONAL TRAINING, PSYCHOTHERAPISTS, VALUES
     ABST THIS PAPER EXAMINES THE HISTORICAL EVOLUTION OF MEXICAN AMERICAN MENTAL HEALTH NEEDS AND EVALUATES MODES OF TREATMENT CURRENTLY OFFERED. CURRENT THERAPEUTIC STRATEGIES BASED ON THE MEDICAL MODEL DENY THE SPIRITUALITY OF THE SELF. CURANDERISMO IS DESCRIBED AS A VIABLE AND SOCIALLY RELEVANT THERAPEUTIC METHOD WHOSE BASIC TENETS CAN BE INTEGRATED INTO A NEW THEORETICAL APPROACH—TRANSCENDENTAL REALISM. THIS MODEL INCORPORATES THE BASIC CONCEPTS OF CURANDERISMO, CHICANISMO, AND CARNALISMO. IT IS SUGGESTED THAT CONTEMPORARY THERAPISTS MODIFY THEIR PRESENT APPROACHES AND THAT MORE MENTAL HEALTH SPECIALISTS BECOME AWARE OF MEXICAN AMERICAN VALUES AND ATTITUDES. 42 REFERENCES.

ACCN   000734

869 AUTH **JOHNSON, L. W.**
     TITL A COMPARISON OF THE VOCABULARIES OF ANGLO AMERICAN AND SPANISH AMERICAN HIGH SCHOOL PUPILS.
     SRCE *JOURNAL OF EDUCATIONAL PSYCHOLOGY, 1938, 29(2), 135-144.*
     INDX SPANISH SURNAMED, ADOLESCENTS, ABILITY TESTING, EMPIRICAL, CROSS CULTURAL, LANGUAGE ASSESSMENT, NEW MEXICO, SOUTHWEST
     ABST SPANISH AMERICAN (SA) AND ANGLO AMERICAN (AA) HIGH SCHOOL STUDENTS FROM NEW MEXICO WERE ADMINISTERED THE INGLIS TESTS OF ENGLISH VOCABULARY (TITEV). ADDITIONALLY, FOUR OTHER VOCABULARY TESTS WERE CONSTRUCTED AND GIVEN TO THE SUBJECTS. THE RESULTS INDICATE THAT: (1) SA HIGH SCHOOL PUPILS SUFFER FROM A DEFINITE VOCABULARY HANDICAP IN COMPARISON TO BOTH AA'S IN THE SAME SCHOOLS AND WITH THE NORMS FOR TITEV; (2) SA HIGH SCHOOL PUPILS ARE 7 TO 12 MONTHS BELOW GRADE LEVEL AS COMPARED WITH AA PUPILS; (3) THOUGH THE SCHOOL CENSUS SHOWS A POTENTIAL SA SCHOOL POPULATION AS GREAT AS THAT OF AA'S, THE AA'S OUTNUMBER THE SA'S IN HIGH SCHOOL BY A RATIO OF 3 TO 1; AND (4) SA SOPHOMORES, JUNIORS AND SENIORS, AND AA JUNIORS AND SENIORS WERE APPRECIABLY BELOW THE NORMS OF TITEV. IT IS SUGGESTED THAT FREQUENT TESTING WHEREBY THE PUPILS CAN CHECK AND COMPARE THEIR PROGRESS BE IMPLEMENTED AS A MEANS OF STIMULATION. FURTHERMORE, A MODIFIED CURRICULUM TO INCLUDE MORE ETHNIC CUSTOMS AND IDEALS OF THE SA PEOPLE IS RECOMMENDED.

ACCN   000735

870 AUTH **JOHNSTON, K. D., & KROVETZ, M. L.**
     TITL LEVELS OF AGGRESSION IN A TRADITIONAL AND A PLURALISTIC SCHOOL.
     SRCE *EDUCATIONAL RESEARCH, 1976, 18(2), 146-151.*
     INDX AGGRESSION, CULTURAL PLURALISM, EDUCATION, CHILDREN, MEXICAN AMERICAN, EMPIRICAL, CROSS CULTURAL, INTERPERSONAL RELATIONS, CALIFORNIA, SOUTHWEST
     ABST GIVEN THAT FRUSTRATION IS OFTEN AN INSTIGATION TO AGGRESSION AND THAT SCHOOLS ARE FRUSTRATING ENVIRONMENTS FOR MANY STUDENTS, IT WAS HYPOTHESIZED THAT THE LEARNING ENVIRONMENT IN WHICH THE STUDENT WAS PLACED WOULD INFLUENCE AGGRESSION ON THE PLAYGROUND. IT WAS FELT THAT STUDENTS WOULD DISPLAY LESS AGGRESSION ON THE PLAYGROUND OF A PLURALISTIC SCHOOL, WHICH OFFERS SEVERAL DISTINCT LEARNING ENVIRONMENTS AND ATTEMPTS TO PLACE STUDENTS APPROPRIATELY, THAN ON THE PLAYGROUND OF A TRADITIONAL SCHOOL. FIRST, SECOND, AND THIRD GRADERS WERE OBSERVED USING A TECHNIQUE DEVELOPED BY WALTERS ET AL. (1957). RESULTS INDICATED THAT SIGNIFICANTLY LESS PHYSICAL AND VERBAL AGGRESSION OCCURRED ON THE PLAYGROUND AT THE PLURALISTIC SCHOOL. ALTHOUGH METHODOLOGICAL AND SAMPLE SELECTION CONCERNS TEMPER CONCLUSIONS, IT IS SUGGESTED THAT PLURALISTIC SCHOOLS ATTEMPT TO MEET

THE PSYCHOLOGICAL AND INTELLECTUAL NEEDS OF THE CHILDREN. THE ROLE OF FRUSTRATION IN INCREASING LEVEL OF AGGRESSION IS DISCUSSED BRIEFLY AND FURTHER RESEARCH IS RECOMMENDED. 12 REFERENCES. (AUTHOR SUMMARY)

ACCN   000736

871 AUTH   **JONES, B. D., & SHORTER, R.**
TITL   THE RATIO MEASUREMENT OF SOCIAL STATUS: SOME CROSS-CULTURAL COMPARISONS.
SRCE   *SOCIAL FORCES, 1972, 50(4), 499-511.*
INDX   SES, CROSS CULTURAL, MEXICAN AMERICAN, EMPIRICAL, TEST VALIDITY, RESEARCH METHODOLOGY,THEORETICAL, TEXAS, SOUTHWEST, COLLEGE STUDENTS
ABST   SOCIAL SCIENTISTS HAVE RECENTLY FOUND THE SCALE CONSTRUCTION TECHNIQUES DEVELOPED IN PSYCHOPHYSICS TO BE RELEVANT TO THE MEASUREMENT PROBLEM IN SOCIAL SCIENCE. THIS PAPER REPORTS SOME EFFORTS AT THE RATIO MEASUREMENT OF SOCIAL STATUS, AND SOME ATTEMPTS AT FITTING FUNCTIONAL FORMS TO THE RELATION BETWEEN VALUED SOCIAL CHARACTERISTICS (E.G., EDUCATION AND INCOME) AND THE STATUS ACCORDED VARIOUS LEVELS OF THESE VARIABLES BY 49 COLLEGE STUDENTS FROM THREE DISTINCT CULTURAL GROUPS (MEXICAN AMERICAN 20, ANGLO 20, BLACK 9) ATTENDING COLLEGES IN HOUSTON, TEXAS. RESULTS ARE PRESENTED AND DISCUSSED IN TERMS OF THEIR AGREEMENT WITH PREVIOUSLY DETERMINED MATHEMATICAL EQUATIONS USED TO PREDICT THE RELATIONSHIP BETWEEN VALUED SOCIAL CHARACTERISTICS AND SOCIAL STATUS. THE AUTHORS DISAGREE WITH SOME OF THE FORMS FITTED BY EARLIER RESEARCHERS. 8 REFERENCES. (JOURNAL ABSTRACT MODIFIED)

ACCN   000737

872 AUTH   **JONES, L., & CALVO, E.**
TITL   THE BARSIT AS A GENERAL ABILITY SCREENING TEST FOR SPANISH-SPEAKING ADULTS IN NEW YORK.
SRCE   *PERSONNEL PSYCHOLOGY, 1970, 23(4), 513-519.*
INDX   INTELLIGENCE TESTING, LINGUISTIC COMPETENCE, ADULTS, PUERTO RICAN-M, EMPIRICAL, VOCATIONAL COUNSELING, ABILITY TESTING, TEST VALIDITY, NEW YORK, EAST, TEST RELIABILITY
ABST   THE UTILIZATION OF THE BARRANQUILLA RAPID SURVEY INTELLIGENCE TEST (BARSIT) PROVIDES A SET OF NORMS OF GENERAL MENTAL ABILITY FOR SPANISH-SPEAKING ADULTS IN NEW YORK. THE BARSIT WAS ORIGINALLY DEVELOPED IN VENEZUELA AND COLOMBIA TO BE USED AS A 10-MINUTE GROUP TEST WITH APPLICANTS HAVING SIXTH-GRADE EDUCATION OR LESS. A GROUP OF ADULTS WHO ENTERED IN A SPECIAL TRAINING PROGRAM WERE SEPARATED INTO EITHER A BASIC ENGLISH COURSE OR A CLERICAL AND BOOKKEEPING COURSE BY MEANS OF THEIR SCORE ON THE GATES READING SURVEY (GRS). BOTH OF THESE GROUPS WERE ADMINISTERED THE BARSIT. TEACHERS WERE ASKED TO RATE THE STUDENTS AT THE END OF THE COURSE ON A 7-POINT SCALE FROM "VERY BRIGHT" TO "VERY SLOW." THE FINDINGS SHOW THAT THE CORRELATIONS BETWEEN COURSE GRADES AND TEACHERS' RATINGS WERE LOW —.33 AND .24 FOR THE BASIC ENGLISH AND CLERICAL GROUPS, RESPECTIVELY. THE BARSIT SCORES AND THE TEACHERS' RATINGS, HOWEVER, WERE SIGNIFICANTLY RELATED TO ONE ANOTHER IN EACH OF THE TWO GROUPS—.62 AND .48 FOR THE BASIC ENGLISH AND CLERICAL GROUPS, RESPECTIVELY. THE HIGH DEGREE OF CORRELATION IS QUITE SUFFICIENT TO SUPPORT THE USEFULNESS OF BARSIT AS A SCREENING DEVICE. HOWEVER, SINCE IT IS A HIGHLY SPEEDED TEST, IT CAN BE EXPECTED TO YIELD ONLY A ROUGH ESTIMATE OF AN EXAMINEE'S MENTAL ABILITY. 1 REFERENCE.

ACCN   000738

873 AUTH   **JONES, R. C.**
TITL   ETHNIC FAMILY PATTERNS: THE MEXICAN AMERICAN FAMILY IN THE UNITED STATES.
SRCE   *AMERICAN JOURNAL OF SOCIOLOGY, 1948, 53(6), 450-452.*
INDX   MEXICAN AMERICAN, FAMILY STRUCTURE, ACCULTURATION, ECONOMIC FACTORS, DISCRIMINATION, STEREOTYPES, POVERTY, ESSAY, CROSS GENERATIONAL, REVIEW, FICTIVE KINSHIP, FAMILY ROLES, SEX ROLES
ABST   GENERALIZATIONS ON THE CHARACTERISTICS OF THE MEXICAN AMERICAN BASED ON CASE RECORDS AND INTENSIVE FIELD OBSERVATIONS ARE REPORTED. IT IS POINTED OUT THAT THE MAJORITY HAVE COME FROM A SIMPLE ECONOMY AND CULTURE IN WHICH CUSTOM AND TRADITION DOMINATE. HOME COMMUNITIES ARE CLOSELY INTEGRATED BY TRADITION AND PERSONAL TIES, SO THAT FAMILY LIFE IS CONTROLLED BY THE VILLAGE. FAMILY AUTHORITY IS USUALLY VESTED IN THE PRINCIPAL WAGE EARNER, WHO IS TYPICALLY THE FATHER OR THE OLDEST MALE SIBLING. IN COURTSHIP AND MARRIAGE THE INTEREST OF THE LARGER FAMILY IS CLOSELY FOLLOWED. DIVORCE IS ALMOST IMPOSSIBLE. SEX ROLES ARE SHARPLY DEFINED. IT IS NOT CONSIDERED PROPER FOR WOMEN TO WORK OUTSIDE THE HOME OR FOR MEN TO ENGAGE IN HOUSEHOLD ACTIVITIES. IN RELATION TO THE SECOND GENERATION MEXICAN AMERICANS, CONSIDERABLE ATTENTION HAS BEEN GIVEN TO CULTURAL CONFLICT AND DELINQUENCY. THE PERCENTAGE OF YOUNG PEOPLE IS LARGE AMONG THE SECOND GENERATION GROUP. OTHER FACTORS SUCH AS FARM WORK, POOR LIVING CONDITIONS, HIGH MOBILITY RATE, RACE DISCRIMINATION, AND RESTRICTED SOCIAL CONTACTS CONTRIBUTE TO THE FAMILY LIFESTYLE OF THE MEXICAN AMERICAN. IT IS RECOMMENDED THAT FUTURE RESEARCH ON THE MEXICAN AMERICAN BE SUPPORTED FINANCIALLY IN ORDER TO PROVIDE A BETTER UNDERSTANDING OF THE MEXICAN IMMIGRANT.

ACCN   000739

874 AUTH **JONES, S. E.**
  TITL A COMPARATIVE PROXEMICS ANALYSIS OF DYADIC INTERACTION IN SELECTED SUBCULTURES OF NEW YORK CITY.
  SRCE *JOURNAL OF SOCIAL PSYCHOLOGY, 1971, 84(1), 35-44.*
  INDX INTERPERSONAL RELATIONS, SEX COMPARISON, POVERTY, SES, PUERTO RICAN-M, CROSS CULTURAL, EMPIRICAL, DYADIC INTERACTION, INTERPERSONAL SPACING, NEW YORK, EAST
  ABST SUBCULTURAL AND SEX DIFFERENCES IN SPATIAL ORIENTATION BEHAVIOR WERE INVESTIGATED AMONG BLACK, CHINESE, ITALIAN, AND PUERTO RICAN SUBJECTS. TWO-PERSON GROUPS OF ADULTS IN FOUR SEPARATE POVERTY SUBCULTURES WERE OBSERVED ENGAGING IN SOCIAL INTERACTION ON PUBLIC STREETS OF NEW YORK CITY. TRAINED JUDGES MADE ESTIMATES OF THE INTERPERSONAL DISTANCE AND MUTUAL SHOULDER ORIENTATION OF EACH DYAD. REGARDLESS OF SUBCULTURAL GROUP MEMBERSHIP, WOMEN WERE FOUND TO BE MORE DIRECT IN SHOULDER ORIENTATION THAN MEN, AN OUTCOME WHICH APPEARS TO PARALLEL THE FINDINGS OF PREVIOUS STUDIES OF EYE-CONTACT BEHAVIOR. BLACK MALES APPEARED LESS DIRECT THAN MALES IN OTHER MINORITY GROUPS, ALTHOUGH THIS RESULT DID NOT APPROACH STATISTICAL SIGNIFICANCE. CONTRARY TO EXPECTATION, THE INTERACTION DISTANCE WAS STRIKINGLY SIMILAR IN ALL OF THE SUBCULTURES STUDIED. THIS LAST FINDING SUGGESTS THAT POVERTY GROUPS ARE RATHER HOMOGENEOUS IN THE STRUCTURING OF INTERPERSONAL DISTANCE. 12 REFERENCES.
  ACCN 000740

875 AUTH **JORSTAD, D.**
  TITL PSYCHOLINGUISTIC LEARNING DISABILITIES IN 20 MEXICAN AMERICAN STUDENTS.
  SRCE *JOURNAL OF LEARNING DISABILITIES, 1971, 4(3), 26-32.*
  INDX ITPA, GRAMMAR, PHONOLOGY, SYNTAX, CURRICULUM, INSTRUCTIONAL TECHNIQUES, SES, PROGRAM EVALUATION, RURAL, MEXICAN AMERICAN, CHILDREN, EMPIRICAL, LEARNING DISABILITIES, LANGUAGE ASSESSMENT, PERCEPTION, CALIFORNIA, SOUTHWEST
  ABST COMPOSITE PROFILES ON THE ILLINOIS TEST OF PSYCHOLINGUISTIC ABILITIES WERE MADE FOR 20 MEXICAN AMERICAN (MA) STUDENTS' DIFFERENTIAL ABILITIES. RESULTS INDICATE THAT HALF OF THEIR DIFFERENTIAL PSYCHOLINGUISTIC ABILITIES FALL IN THE BROAD "AVERAGE" RANGE OF ONE STANDARD DEVIATION (LISTED IN ORDER OF LEARNING POTENTIAL): VISUAL MEMORY, VERBAL EXPRESSION, VISUAL ASSOCIATION, MANUAL EXPRESSION, AND VISUAL CLOSURE. FURTHER INSPECTION OF THE COMPOSITE PROFILES SHOWS THAT ALL THE POINTS FALLING BELOW THE AVERAGE OF ALL MEAN SCORES ARE IN AUDITORY AREAS (LISTED IN ORDER OF DISABILITY): GRAMMATIC CLOSURE, AUDITORY ASSOCIATION, AUDITORY RECEPTION, AND AUDITORY MEMORY. FINDINGS REINFORCE THE THEORY THAT FOR YOUNG STUDENTS ADEQUATE ORAL LANGUAGE MUST BE DEVELOPED BEFORE ACTUAL READING CAN BE ACCOMPLISHED. THE NEXT STEP FOR SCHOOL PERSONNEL IN THE EDUCATION OF THE DISADVANTAGED IS TO GO INTO THE HOMES OF PRESCHOOL CHILDREN TO TRAIN THE PARENTS ON THE SPECIAL LINGUISTIC NEEDS OF THEIR CHILDREN. 7 REFERENCES.
  ACCN 000741

876 AUTH **JURALEWICZ, R. S.**
  TITL AN EXPERIMENT ON PARTICIPATION IN A LATIN AMERICAN FACTORY.
  SRCE *HUMAN RELATIONS, 1974, 27(7), 627-637.*
  INDX JOB PERFORMANCE, FEMALE, PUERTO RICAN-I, EMPLOYMENT, CROSS CULTURAL, ACHIEVEMENT MOTIVATION, ATTITUDES
  ABST IN A FIELD EXPERIMENT THE EXTENT OF PSYCHOLOGICAL PARTICIPATION WAS MANIPULATED FOR THREE GROUPS OF WOMEN OPERATORS IN THE GARMENT INDUSTRY IN PUERTO RICO. IT WAS FOUND THAT A MODERATE LEVEL OF PARTICIPATION THROUGH REPRESENTATIVES LED TO GREATER INCREASES IN PRODUCTIVITY THAN EITHER A HIGHER LEVEL OF DIRECT PARTICIPATION OR A LOWER LEVEL OF INDIRECT PARTICIPATION, AGAIN THROUGH REPRESENTATIVES. THIS RESULT IS COMPARED WITH THE STUDY OF COCH AND FRENCH (1948), WHO FOUND THAT DIRECT PARTICIPATION WAS MORE EFFECTIVE THAN PARTICIPATION THROUGH REPRESENTATION. NO CLEAR DIFFERENCES WERE FOUND BETWEEN THE GROUPS ON OTHER DEPENDENT VARIABLES OR IN THE EFFECT OF CONDITIONING VARIABLES. BOTH THE MAIN RESULT AND THE TRENDS IN THE DATA SUGGEST THAT THE EFFECTS OF PARTICIPATION VARY CROSS-CULTURALLY. 9 REFERENCES. (JOURNAL ABSTRACT MODIFIED)
  ACCN 000742

877 AUTH **JUSTIN, N.**
  TITL MEXICAN-AMERICAN ACHIEVEMENT HINDERED BY CULTURE CONFLICT.
  SRCE *SOCIOLOGY & SOCIAL RESEARCH, 1972, 56(4), 471-479.*
  INDX SCHOLASTIC ACHIEVEMENT, ATTITUDES, TIME ORIENTATION, FATALISM, CROSS CULTURAL, CULTURE, DISCRIMINATION, CULTURAL CHANGE, ADOLESCENTS, MEXICAN AMERICAN, EMPIRICAL, ARIZONA, SOUTHWEST, ACCULTURATION, CROSS GENERATIONAL
  ABST ONE HUNDRED SIXTY-EIGHT MEXICAN AMERICAN HIGH SCHOOL STUDENTS FROM 4 HIGH SCHOOLS LOCATED IN TUCSON, ARIZONA, WERE ADMINISTERED A QUESTIONNAIRE WHICH FOCUSSED ON 2 ANGLO SOCIOCULTURAL FACTORS AND 2 FACTORS RELATING LEVEL OF ACCULTURATION TO ACADEMIC ACHIEVEMENT. THE DOMINANT CULTURE VARIABLES UNDER INVESTIGATION WERE DELAYED GRATIFICATION AND FEELINGS OF PERSONAL CONTROL. ACCESS TO REWARDS AND EXPOSURE TO THE DOMINANT CULTURE WERE EXAMINED WITH RESPECT TO CULTURAL CHANGE. FINDINGS INDICATE THAT MEXICAN AMERICAN MALES' FEELINGS OF PERSONAL CONTROL

WERE RELATED TO DELAY OF GRATIFICATION, AND ACCESS TO REWARDS IN THE DOMINANT CULTURE WERE RELATED TO ACADEMIC ACHIEVEMENT. IT IS CONCLUDED THAT THOSE STUDENTS WHO ARE 3RD AND 4TH GENERATION MEXICAN AMERICANS ARE SLOWLY CHANGING FROM THE TRADITIONAL MEXICAN PRESENT-TIME ORIENTATION AND FATALISM TO THE DELAYED GRATIFICATION AND PERSONAL CONTROL REFLECTED IN THE ANGLO CULTURE. 18 REFERENCES.

ACCN   000743

878 AUTH   **JUSTIN, N.**
     TITL   MEXICAN-AMERICAN READING HABITS AND THEIR CULTURAL BASIS.
     SRCE   *JOURNAL OF READING, 1973, 16(6), 467-473.*
     INDX   READING, LEARNING DISABILITIES, CROSS CULTURAL, MEXICAN AMERICAN, ADOLESCENTS, CULTURAL FACTORS, EMPIRICAL, TIME ORIENTATION, FATALISM, CULTURE, URBAN, MASS MEDIA, ARIZONA, SOUTHWEST, VALUES
     ABST   PREVIOUS STUDIES INDICATE THAT THE SPANISH-SPEAKING PEOPLE ARE VERBALLY ORIENTED AND PLACE LITTLE EMPHASIS UPON READING. THE PRESENT STUDY EXAMINED READING MEDIA HABITS AMONG 209 ANGLO AND 168 MEXICAN AMERICAN MALE SENIOR HIGH SCHOOL STUDENTS IN TUCSON, ARIZONA. RESULTS FROM A QUESTIONNAIRE INDICATED A SIGNIFICANT RELATIONSHIP BETWEEN ETHNICITY AND READING MEDIA HABITS. AS THIS IS PART OF A LARGER STUDY WHOSE MAJOR FOCUS IS VARIOUS CULTURAL VALUES (TIME ORIENTATION, DELAYED GRATIFICATION, AND FATALISM), THESE VALUES ARE DISCUSSED ALONG WITH THE SOCIO-HISTORICAL BACKGROUND OF MEXICAN AMERICANS. IT IS CONCLUDED THAT SINCE MEXICAN AMERICANS ARE MORE APT TO WATCH TELEVISION THAN ANGLOS, VIDEO PROGRAMS SHOULD BE DEVELOPED TO PROVIDE EFFECTIVE EDUCATIONAL INSTRUCTION WHICH WOULD IMPROVE THE SCHOOL WORK OF MEXICAN AMERICAN STUDENTS. 8 REFERENCES.

ACCN   000744

879 AUTH   **KAESTNER, E., ROSEN, L., & APPEL, P.**
     TITL   PATTERNS OF DRUG ABUSE: RELATIONSHIPS WITH ETHNICITY, SENSATION SEEKING, AND ANXIETY.
     SRCE   *JOURNAL OF CONSULTING AND CLINICAL PSYCHOLOGY, 1977, 45(3), 462-468.*
     INDX   DRUG ABUSE, PUERTO RICAN-M, CROSS CULTURAL, ANXIETY, EMPIRICAL, MALE, CULTURAL FACTORS, INHALANT ABUSE, ALCOHOLISM, NEW YORK, EAST
     ABST   THE SENSATION-SEEKING SCALE AND THE STATE-TRAIT ANXIETY INVENTORY WERE ADMINISTERED TO 30 WHITE, 30 BLACK, AND 30 HISPANIC MALE NARCOTIC DRUG ABUSERS IN RESIDENTIAL TREATMENT. INDIVIDUAL DRUG ABUSE HISTORIES WERE ASSESSED IN SEMI-STRUCTURED INTERVIEWS. BASICALLY, THERE WERE THREE FINDINGS OF THE STUDY. (1) WHITE SUBJECTS SCORED SIGNIFICANTLY HIGHER ON THE FIVE SENSATION-SEEKING

SUBSCALES THAN DID EITHER BLACK OR HISPANIC SUBJECTS. NO SIGNIFICANT DIFFERENCES WERE OBTAINED BETWEEN ETHNIC GROUPS ON STATE OR TRAIT ANXIETY. (2) EVEN THOUGH THE PREVALENCE OF THE USE OF ALCOHOL, CANNABIS, STREET METHODONE, AND COCAINE WAS SIMILAR IN THE THREE ETHNIC GROUPS, SIGNIFICANTLY MORE WHITE SUBJECTS HAD USED AMPHETAMINES, BARBITURATES, TRANQUILIZERS, METHAQUALONE, AND PSYCHEDELICS. (3) MEASURES OF SENSATION-SEEKING AND ANXIETY CORRELATED SIGNIFICANTLY WITH THE NUMBER OF DIFFERENT DRUGS USED BY WHITES, ALTHOUGH THE MEASURES WERE VIRTUALLY UNRELATED TO DRUG USE AMONG NONWHITES. THE FREQUENCY OF USE OF STIMULANT, DEPRESSANT, OR HALLUCINOGENIC DRUGS WAS UNRELATED TO THE USER'S LEVEL OF SENSATION-SEEKING OR ANXIETY. AMONG INDIVIDUALS WITH EXTENSIVE HISTORIES OF DRUG ABUSE, ETHNICITY APPEARED TO BE MORE CLOSELY RELATED TO DRUG USE PATTERNS THAN MOTIVATIONAL VARIABLES SUCH AS SENSATION-SEEKING AND ANXIETY. 8 REFERENCES. (JOURNAL ABSTRACT)

ACCN   000745

880 AUTH   **KAGAN, S.**
     TITL   FIELD DEPENDENCE AND CONFORMITY OF RURAL MEXICAN AND URBAN ANGLO-AMERICAN CHILDREN.
     SRCE   *CHILD DEVELOPMENT, 1974, 45(3), 765-771.*
     INDX   COOPERATION, COMPETITION, COGNITIVE STYLE, PERSONALITY, URBAN, CONFORMITY, PEER GROUP, SEX COMPARISON, EMPIRICAL, CHILDREN, ACHIEVEMENT MOTIVATION, CHILDREARING PRACTICES, RURAL, MEXICAN, FIELD DEPENDENCE-INDEPENDENCE, CALIFORNIA, SOUTHWEST, CROSS CULTURAL
     ABST   A NUMBER OF THEORETICAL WORKS SUPPORT THE HYPOTHESIS THAT RURAL MEXICAN CHILDREN ARE MORE PASSIVE AND COMPLIANT THAN URBAN ANGLO AMERICAN CHILDREN. BASED ON THAT HYPOTHESIS IT WAS PREDICTED THAT RURAL MEXICAN CHILDREN WOULD BE MORE FIELD DEPENDENT AND CONFORMING IN SITUATIONS TRADITIONALLY USED TO MEASURE THOSE VARIABLES. IN A PORTABLE ROD AND FRAME EXPERIMENT, RURAL CHILDREN ERRED FROM THE TRUE UPRIGHT BY ALMOST TWICE AS MANY DEGREES AS URBAN ANGLO AMERICAN CHILDREN. IN ADDITION, RURAL MEXICAN CHILDREN WERE FOUND TO BE MORE CONFORMING AND MORE OFTEN EXPRESSED BELIEF IN THEIR MISLEADING PEERS THAN DID URBAN ANGLO AMERICAN CHILDREN. RESULTS WERE RELATED TO CULTURAL DIFFERENCES IN PRESS SENSITIVITY, NEED FOR ACHIEVEMENT, AND CHILD-REARING PRACTICES. 37 REFERENCES. (JOURNAL ABSTRACT MODIFIED)

ACCN   000747

881 AUTH   **KAGAN, S.**
     TITL   FIELD DEPENDENCE, DEVELOPMENT OF COGNITIVE ABILITIES AND ACCULTURATION AMONG

ANGLO AMERICAN AND MEXICAN AMERICAN CHILDREN: A SYMPOSIUM.

SRCE   *PAPER PRESENTED AT THE WESTERN PSYCHO-LOGICAL ASSOCIATION ANNUAL MEETING, LOS ANGELES, APRIL 1976.*

INDX   COGNITIVE STYLE, COGNITIVE DEVELOPMENT, SCHOLASTIC ACHIEVEMENT, READING, MATHEMATICS, MOTHER-CHILD INTERACTION, CULTURAL FACTORS, ACCULTURATION, MEXICAN AMERICAN, CHILDREN, PROCEEDINGS, SCHOLASTIC ASPIRATIONS, INTERPERSONAL RELATIONS, CONFLICT RESOLUTION

ABST   THE PRESENT INVESTIGATIONS WERE DESIGNED TO TEST THE CONCLUSIONS OF RECENT RESEARCH INDICATING THAT FIELD INDEPENDENCE EXPLAINS THE SCHOOL ACHIEVEMENT GAP BETWEEN ANGLO AMERICAN AND MEXICAN AMERICAN CHILDREN. THE FIRST STUDY EXAMINED THE RELATIONSHIP OF THREE MEASURES OF FIELD INDEPENDENCE TO THE READING AND MATH ACHIEVEMENT OF MEXICAN AMERICAN AND ANGLO AMERICAN CHILDREN. THE SECOND EXPERIMENT EXAMINED THE RELATIONSHIP OF FIELD INDEPENDENCE TO THE READING AND MATH GAIN SCORES OF ANGLO AMERICAN AND MEXICAN AMERICAN CHILDREN. THE THIRD STUDY EXAMINED THE RELATIONSHIP OF FIELD INDEPENDENCE TO ROLE TAKING ABILITY AMONG ANGLO AMERICAN AND MEXICAN AMERICAN CHILDREN. THE FOURTH INVESTIGATION ANALYZED THE RELATIONSHIP OF MATERNAL REWARD, PUNISHMENT, AND CONTINGENCY TO THE DEVELOPMENT OF FIELD INDEPENDENCE, READING, AND MATH ABILITY. THE FINAL PAPER ANALYZED RECENT FINDINGS THAT THIRD GENERATION MEXICAN AMERICAN CHILDREN ARE MOSTLY FIELD DEPENDENT. IN SUM, THE PRESENT FINDINGS CHALLENGE PREVIOUS CONCLUSIONS THAT (1) FIELD DEPENDENCE EXPLAINS THE ANGLO AMERICAN-MEXICAN AMERICAN SCHOOL ACHIEVEMENT GAP, (2) THAT MEXICAN AMERICAN CHILDREN ARE GENERALLY MORE FIELD DEPENDENT THAN ANGLO AMERICAN CHILDREN, AND (3) THAT FIELD DEPENDENCE AMONG MEXICAN AMERICANS IS A FUNCTION OF THEIR CLOSENESS TO TRADITIONAL MEXICAN CULTURE. (AUTHOR SUMMARY MODIFIED)

ACCN   000748

882 AUTH   **KAGAN, S.**

TITL   PREFERENCE FOR CONTROL IN RURAL MEXICAN AND URBAN ANGLO AMERICAN CHILDREN.

SRCE   *INTERAMERICAN JOURNAL OF PSYCHOLOGY, 1976, 10, 51-59.*

INDX   SEX COMPARISON, MEXICAN, CROSS CULTURAL, ATTITUDES, LOCUS OF CONTROL, EMPIRICAL, CHILDREN, CHILDREARING PRACTICES, CONFLICT RESOLUTION, CALIFORNIA, SOUTHWEST, RURAL, URBAN, ATTRIBUTION OF RESPONSIBILITY

ABST   URBAN UNITED STATES AND RURAL MEXICAN BOYS AND GIRLS WERE INDIVIDUALLY PRESENTED WITH A NOVEL BEHAVIORAL MEASURE, THE PREFERENCE FOR CONTROL WHEEL, TO ASSESS BOTH THEIR PREFERENCE FOR

CONTROL AND THEIR PERCEPTION OF LOCUS OF CONTROL. DUE TO AN ILLUSION, ALMOST ALL CHILDREN HAD AN INTERNAL PERCEPTION OF LOCUS OF CONTROL. NEVERTHELESS, URBAN UNITED STATES CHILDREN SIGNIFICANTLY MORE THAN RURAL MEXICAN CHILDREN ATTEMPTED TO CONTROL THE WHEEL OF CHANCE. BOYS OF BOTH CULTURES ATTEMPTED TO CONTROL THE WHEEL MORE THAN GIRLS, BUT THAT DIFFERENCE DID NOT REACH SIGNIFICANCE. RESULTS WERE RELATED TO ROTTER'S SOCIAL LEARNING THEORY, FESTINGER'S DISSONANCE THEORY, AND CULTURAL COMPARISONS OF CHILD-REARING PRACTICES. 40 REFERENCES. (JOURNAL ABSTRACT)

ACCN   000749

883 AUTH   **KAGAN, S.**

TITL   PSYCHOLOGICAL RESEARCH APPROACHES TO THE MEXICAN AMERICAN FAMILY: BRIEF OVERVIEW AND RESEARCH IMPLICATIONS.

SRCE   *REVISTA INTERAMERICANA DE PSICOLOGIA, 1977, 11(1), 27-32.*

INDX   RESEARCH METHODOLOGY, MEXICAN AMERICAN, FAMILY STRUCTURE, CULTURE, REVIEW, FAMILY ROLES, MOTHER-CHILD INTERACTION, STEREOTYPES

ABST   THIS OVERVIEW FOCUSES ON FOUR PSYCHOLOGICAL RESEARCH APPROACHES THAT HAVE BEEN UTILIZED IN ATTEMPTS TO UNDERSTAND THE MEXICAN AMERICAN FAMILY. THESE FOUR BASIC PERSPECTIVES—IMPRESSIONISTIC, INFERENTIAL, SURVEY, AND EXPERIMENTAL/OBSERVATIONAL—ARE DISCUSSED WITH RESPECT TO SOME OF THEIR LIMITATIONS. IMPRESSIONISTIC RESEARCH TENDS TO BE SPECULATIVE IN NATURE IN THAT IT BASES GENERALIZATIONS FROM NONEMPIRICAL STUDIES THAT USUALLY REFLECT STEREOTYPIC CONCEPTS OF THE MEXICAN AMERICAN FAMILY. INFERENTIAL RESEARCH EXHIBITS SEVERAL METHODOLOGICAL PROBLEMS OF BIAS IN ITS ENDEAVOR TO EXPLAIN MEXICAN AMERICAN FAMILY PATTERNS FROM SCORES ON SCALE ITEMS BELIEVED TO BE RELATED TO FAMILY DYNAMICS. ALTHOUGH SURVEY RESEARCH IS ESSENTIAL IN SUPPORTING GENERALIZATIONS OF THE MEXICAN FAMILY, THE VERY FEW THAT HAVE BEEN CONDUCTED REPRESENT SPECIFIC GEOGRAPHICAL AREAS. EXPERIMENTAL/OBSERVATIONAL RESEARCH FOCUSES USUALLY ON MOTHER-CHILD INTERACTION AND WHILE THEY PROVIDE FOR CONTROL IN MEASURING RESPONSES TO STIMULI, GENERALIZATIONS OF THE FINDINGS ARE NARROW IN SCOPE, SINCE THEY ARE CONDUCTED IN ARTIFICIAL RATHER THAN REAL LIFE SETTINGS. RECOGNIZING THE LIMITATIONS OF THESE RESEARCH PERSPECTIVES, IT IS SUGGESTED THAT A COMPREHENSIVE RESEARCH PROGRAM REFLECTING A MULTI-METHOD MODEL BE USED TO CONCEPTUALIZE FAMILY VARIABLES AS MEDIATING ASPECTS INFLUENCED BY EXTERNAL FACTORS WHICH IN TURN INFLUENCE THE CHILD'S DEVELOPMENT. 21 REFERENCES.

ACCN   000750

884 AUTH **KAGAN, S.**
TITL SOCIAL MOTIVES AND BEHAVIORS OF MEXI-CAN-AMERICAN AND ANGLO-AMERICAN CHILDREN.
SRCE *IN J. L. MARTINEZ (ED.), CHICANO PSYCHOLOGY. NEW YORK: ACADEMIC PRESS, 1977, PP. 45-86.*
INDX COMPETITION, COOPERATION, INTERPERSONAL RELATIONS, ALTRUISM, GROUP DYNAMICS, ACHIEVEMENT MOTIVATION, CULTURE, CULTURAL FACTORS, SES, CROSS CULTURAL, ECONOMIC FACTORS, RESEARCH METHODOLOGY, PERSONALITY, REVIEW, CHILDREN
ABST A CONCEPTUAL FRAMEWORK BY WHICH TO ANALYZE THE SOCIAL MOTIVE MATRIX OF MEXICAN AMERICAN (MA) CHILDREN IS PRESENTED. MA CHILDREN MAINTAIN MORE COOPERATIVE MOTIVES, ESPECIALLY GROUP ENHANCEMENT AND ALTRUISM, WHICH REFLECT DIFFERENCES IN CROSS MOTIVATIONAL ORIENTATIONS. THIS IS INFERRED FROM: (1) EXPERIMENTAL GAMES; (2) VERBAL ROLE PLAYS; (3) PROJECTIVE TECHNIQUES; AND (4) VERBAL QUESTIONS. THIS OBSERVED COOPERATIVENESS OCCURS ACROSS A VARIETY OF MA POPULATIONS. FINDINGS SUGGEST THAT COMMUNITY CHARACTERISTICS, SOCIALIZATION PRACTICES, AND CULTURAL BACKGROUND—RATHER THAN ECONOMIC CLASS, URBANIZATION LEVEL, MINORITY STATUS, OR COGNITIVE STYLES—ARE CAUSAL DETERMINANTS FOR THIS BEHAVIOR. IT IS CONCLUDED THAT DEFINING THE NATURE AND CAUSES OF SOCIAL MOTIVATION AND BEHAVIOR DEVELOPMENT OF MA CHILDREN IS NECESSARY NOT ONLY FOR A GREATER UNDERSTANDING OF HOW A CULTURAL GROUP MAINTAINS SOCIAL VALUES BUT IN PROVIDING A BASIS FOR MORE RESPONSIVE AND LESS DISCRIMINATORY PUBLIC INSTITUTIONS FOR THIS POPULATION. 86 REFERENCES.
ACCN 000751

885 AUTH **KAGAN, S.**
TITL SOCIAL MOTIVES AND CONFLICT RESOLUTION OF ANGLO AMERICAN, MEXICAN CHILDREN AND THEIR MOTHERS: A SYMPOSIUM.
SRCE *PAPER PRESENTED AT THE WESTERN PSYCHOLOGICAL ASSOCIATION ANNUAL MEETING, LOS ANGELES, APRIL 1976.*
INDX COMPETITION, COOPERATION, INTERPERSONAL RELATIONS, COGNITIVE STYLE, RESEARCH METHODOLOGY, PROJECTIVE TESTING, CHILDREN, MEXICAN AMERICAN, MEXICAN, CROSS CULTURAL, ALTRUISM, SEX COMPARISON, SES, ECONOMIC FACTORS, PROCEEDINGS, EMPIRICAL, CONFLICT RESOLUTION, PERSONALITY, MOTHER-CHILD INTERACTION
ABST PREVIOUS RESEARCH USING BEHAVIORAL CHOICES IN GAME SITUATIONS INDICATES GREATER COMPETITIVENESS AMONG ANGLO AMERICAN THAN MEXICAN AMERICAN AND RURAL MEXICAN CHILDREN. THE PAPERS PRESENTED AT THIS SYMPOSIUM USED VERBAL QUESTIONS, PROJECTIVE TESTS, CONTENT ANALYSIS OF VERBAL INTERACTIONS, AS WELL AS NOVEL BEHAVIORAL CHOICES TO TEST THE GENERALITY OF PAST FINDINGS AND TO DETERMINE THE RELATIONSHIP OF COMPETITIVENESS TO COGNITIVE ABILITIES, ECONOMIC CLASS, AND MOTHER-CHILD INTERACTION. THE FIRST STUDY USED CHOICE CARDS TO STUDY RIVALROUS BEHAVIOR OF 230 ANGLO AMERICAN AND MEXICAN AMERICAN CHILDREN OF FOUR AGES. THE SECOND PAPER DESCRIBES THE DEVELOPMENT AND VALIDATION OF A NEW SOCIAL BEHAVIOR SCALE GIVEN TO 197 ANGLO AND MEXICAN AMERICAN CHILDREN. THE THIRD STUDY EMPLOYED A NEW VERBAL TEST OF CONFLICT RESOLUTION TO STUDY 259 ANGLO AND MEXICAN AMERICAN AND MEXICAN CHILDREN OF THREE AGES. THE FOURTH PAPER USED PROJECTIVE TESTS TO EXAMINE MOTIVES FOR ACHIEVEMENT, AFFILIATION, AND POWER AMONG 194 ANGLO AND MEXICAN AMERICAN CHILDREN. THE FINAL PAPER, BY MEANS OF CONTENT ANALYSIS, INVESTIGATED VERBAL INTERACTIONS OF ANGLO AMERICAN AND MEXICAN AMERICAN CHILDREN AND THEIR MOTHERS IN THREE CONFLICT SITUATIONS. OVERALL, THESE PAPERS DOCUMENT SIMILAR CULTURE, CLASS, AND SEX DIFFERENCES ACROSS A VARIETY OF MEASUREMENT TECHNIQUES. (AUTHOR ABSTRACT MODIFIED)
ACCN 000752

886 AUTH **KAGAN, S., ZAHN, G. L., & GEALY, J.**
TITL COMPETITION AND SCHOOL ACHIEVEMENT AMONG ANGLO AMERICAN AND MEXICAN AMERICAN CHILDREN.
SRCE *JOURNAL OF EDUCATIONAL PSYCHOLOGY, 1977, 69(4), 432-441.*
INDX COMPETITION, SCHOLASTIC ACHIEVEMENT, MEXICAN AMERICAN, CROSS CULTURAL, EMPIRICAL, COGNITIVE STYLE, SEX COMPARISON, CHILDREN, FIELD DEPENDENCE-INDEPENDENCE, CALIFORNIA, SOUTHWEST
ABST THE HYPOTHESIS THAT THE LESS COMPETITIVE ORIENTATION OF MEXICAN AMERICAN CHILDREN IS RELATED TO THEIR LOWER SCHOOL ACHIEVEMENT WAS TESTED. A SAMPLE OF 144 ANGLO AMERICAN AND 86 MEXICAN AMERICAN CHILDREN ATTENDING GRADES K-2, 4, AND 6 OF A SEMI-RURAL LOW-INCOME SCHOOL WERE ADMINISTERED INDIVIDUAL MEASURES OF COMPETITION, INDIVIDUALISM, FIELD INDEPENDENCE, AND SCHOOL ACHIEVEMENT. RESULTS INDICATED SIGNIFICANT EFFECTS OF CULTURE, SEX, AND AGE, BUT COMPETITION AND INDIVIDUALISM WERE NOT SIGNIFICANTLY CORRELATED AND WERE NOT CONSISTENTLY RELATED TO FIELD INDEPENDENCE AND SCHOOL ACHIEVEMENT. RESULTS SUPPORT THE GENERAL CONCLUSION THAT THE LESS COMPETITIVE SOCIAL ORIENTATION OF MEXICAN AMERICAN CHILDREN AS MEASURED BY EXPERIMENTAL GAMES IS NOT NECESSARILY A DISADVANTAGE WITH REGARD TO SCHOOL ACHIEVEMENT. 24 REFERENCES. (AUTHOR ABSTRACT MODIFIED)
ACCN 000753

887 AUTH **KAGAN, S., & CARLSON, H.**

TITL DEVELOPMENT OF ADAPTIVE ASSERTIVENESS IN MEXICAN AND UNITED STATES CHILDREN.

SRCE *DEVELOPMENTAL PSYCHOLOGY, 1975, 11(1), 71-78.*

INDX COOPERATION, COMPETITION, CROSS CULTURAL, MEXICAN AMERICAN, MEXICAN, RURAL, URBAN, SEX COMPARISON, PERSONALITY, CHILDREN, EMPIRICAL, CONFLICT RESOLUTION, INTERPERSONAL RELATIONS, CALIFORNIA, SOUTHWEST

ABST A NOVEL BEHAVIORAL TASK, THE ASSERTIVENESS PULL SCALE, AND UNOBTRUSIVE MEASURES (E.G., THE NUMBER OF QUESTIONS ASKED OF THE EXPERIMENTER) WERE USED TO ASSESS THE DEVELOPMENT OF ASSERTIVENESS OF 154 BOYS AND GIRLS OF 3 AGE GROUPS (5-6, 7-9 AND 10-12 YRS) IN 4 POPULATIONS. URBAN MIDDLE-CLASS ANGLO AMERICAN CHILDREN WERE SIGNIFICANTLY MORE ASSERTIVE THAN SEMI-RURAL POOR ANGLO AMERICAN AND MEXICAN AMERICAN CHILDREN, WHO DID NOT DIFFER FROM EACH OTHER BUT WHO WERE BOTH SIGNIFICANTLY MORE ASSERTIVE THAN RURAL POOR MEXICAN CHILDREN. ASSERTIVENESS INCREASED WITH AGE FOR ALL GROUPS, BUT AT A SLOWER RATE AMONG RURAL MEXICAN THAN AMONG U.S. CHILDREN. NO SIGNIFICANT EFFECTS DUE TO SEX WERE OBSERVED. RESULTS PARALLEL POPULATION AND AGE FINDINGS OF PREVIOUS STUDIES OF COMPETITIVENESS. 26 REFERENCES. (PASAR ABSTRACT MODIFIED)

ACCN 000754

888 AUTH **KAGAN, S., & ENDER, P. B.**

TITL MATERNAL RESPONSE TO SUCCESS AND FAILURE OF ANGLO AMERICAN, MEXICAN-AMERICAN, AND MEXICAN CHILDREN.

SRCE *CHILD DEVELOPMENT, 1975, 46, 452-458.*

INDX MOTHER-CHILD INTERACTION, CROSS CULTURAL, ACHIEVEMENT MOTIVATION, COMPETITION, LOCUS OF CONTROL, EMPIRICAL, CHILDREN, CHILDREARING PRACTICES, MEXICAN AMERICAN, MEXICAN, SES, SEX COMPARISON, CALIFORNIA, SOUTHWEST, RURAL, FEMALE

ABST LITERATURE SUPPORTS THE HYPOTHESIS THAT USE OF PUNISHMENT AND NONCONTINGENT REINFORCEMENT ARE CRITICAL IN THE SOCIALIZATION OF COMPLIANCE, LOW ACHIEVEMENT MOTIVATION, AND A SENSE OF EXTERNAL CONTROL. A NOVEL BEHAVIORAL MEASURE WAS DESIGNED TO OBSERVE THE REACTIONS OF ANGLO AMERICAN, MEXICAN AMERICAN, AND RURAL MEXICAN MOTHERS TO THE SUCCESSES AND FAILURES OF THEIR CHILDREN. RESULTS INDICATED THAT UNITED STATES BUT NOT RURAL MEXICAN MOTHERS GAVE CONTINGENTLY BASED ON THEIR CHILD'S SUCCESS OR FAILURE. RURAL MEXICAN MOTHERS, HOWEVER, UNLIKE UNITED STATES MOTHERS, GAVE MORE TO BOYS THAN GIRLS. PUNISHMENT WAS RARE IN ALL 3 CULTURAL GROUPS, BUT USE OF BOTH PUNISHMENT AND NONCONTINGENT REINFORCEMENT TENDED TO BE MORE COMMOM AMONG LOWER-INCOME MOTHERS. THESE FINDINGS ARE POTENTIAL EXPLANATIONS OF CULTURAL AND ECONOMIC CLASS DIFFERENCES IN ACHIEVE-MENT MOTIVATION, COMPETITIVENESS, AND LOCUS OF CONTROL. 33 REFERENCES. (JOURNAL ABSTRACT)

ACCN 000755

889 AUTH **KAGAN, S., & MADSEN, M. C.**

TITL COOPERATION AND COMPETITION OF MEXICAN, MEXICAN AMERICAN, AND ANGLO AMERICAN CHILDREN OF TWO AGES UNDER FOUR INSTRUCTIONAL SETS.

SRCE *DEVELOPMENTAL PSYCHOLOGY, 1971, 5(1), 32-39.*

INDX COOPERATION, COMPETITION, MEXICAN, MEXICAN AMERICAN, CHILDREN, ACCULTURATION, CROSS CULTURAL, EMPIRICAL, RESEARCH METHODOLOGY, CONFLICT RESOLUTION, INTERPERSONAL RELATIONS, PERSONALITY, CALIFORNIA, SOUTHWEST, SEX COMPARISON

ABST AN ATTEMPT TO ASSESS THE DEGREE TO WHICH CHILDREN OF TWO AGES AND THREE SUBCULTURES DIFFER IN AMOUNT OF COOPERATIVE AND COMPETITIVE BEHAVIOR IS EXAMINED. A GAME MEASURING COOPERATION AND COMPETITION WAS PLAYED WITH PAIRS OF 4 TO 5 YEAR-OLD ANGLO AMERICANS (AA) AND MEXICAN AMERICANS (MA) AND WITH 7 TO 9 YEAR-OLD AA, MA, AND MEXICANS (M). COOPERATIVE PLAY ALLOWED BOTH PAIR MEMBERS TO RECEIVE AWARDS; COMPETITIVE PLAY WAS IRRATIONAL, ALLOWING NO SUBJECT TO REACH HIS GOAL. THE NUMBER OF MOVES THAT PAIRS TOOK TO REACH A GOAL INDICATES THAT 4 TO 5 YEAR-OLDS ARE MORE COOPERATIVE THAN THE OLDER SUBJECTS (P .001). AMONG THE 7 TO 9 YEAR-OLD CHILDREN, M ARE MOST COOPERATIVE, MA THE NEXT MOST, AND AA THE LEAST COOPERATIVE (P.001). AMONG THE OLDER CHILDREN, INSTRUCTIONAL SETS DESIGNED TO CREATE AN "I" ORIENTATION INCREASED COMPETITION, WHEREAS, SETS STRESSING A "WE" ORIENTATION INCREASED COOPERATION (P.001). WHILE QUALITATIVE DIFFERENCES BETWEEN PATTERNS OF PLAY ARE NOTED FOR THE CULTURAL AND AGE GROUP, SEX DIFFERENCES ARE NOT FOUND. 8 REFERENCES.

ACCN 000756

890 AUTH **KAGAN, S., & MADSEN, M. C.**

TITL EXPERIMENTAL ANALYSES OF COOPERATION AND COMPETITION AMONG ANGLO-AMERICAN AND MEXICAN CHILDREN.

SRCE *DEVELOPMENTAL PSYCHOLOGY, 1972, 6(1), 49-59.*

INDX EMPIRICAL, COOPERATION, COMPETITION, MEXICAN, MEXICAN AMERICAN, RURAL, URBAN, CROSS CULTURAL, INTERPERSONAL RELATIONS, CONFLICT RESOLUTION, CALIFORNIA, SOUTHWEST

ABST FOUR EXPERIMENTS WERE CONDUCTED TO ANALYZE COOPERATIVE AND COMPETITIVE BEHAVIOR OF ANGLO AMERICAN AND MEXICAN RURAL CHILDREN. RESULTS OF EXPERIMENT I FAILED TO SUPPORT THE HYPOTHESIS OF A CULTURAL DIFFERENCE IN MOTIVATION AND ABILITY TO COOPERATE. IN EXPERIMENT II, BOTH ANGLO AND MEXICAN CHILDREN APPEARED STRONGLY MOTIVATED TO TAKE A TOY

AWAY FROM A PEER WHEN THEY COULD KEEP IT FOR THEMSELVES. ANGLO CHILDREN, HOWEVER, WERE MORE MOTIVATED THAN MEXICANS TO LOWER ANOTHER CHILD'S OUTCOMES WHEN THEY COULD OBTAIN NO GAIN THEMSELVES. IN EXPERIMENT III, ANGLOS MORE THAN MEXICAN CHILDREN RESPONDED WITH CONFLICT TO A PEER'S RIVALROUS INTENTS IN AN INTERPERSONAL INTERACTION SITUATION; MEXICAN CHILDREN WERE MORE SUBMISSIVE. IN EXPERIMENT IV, MEXICAN CHILDREN WERE MORE AVOIDANT OF CONFLICT THAN ANGLO AMERICAN CHILDREN. THE IRRATIONAL REACTION TO CONFLICT OF BOTH ANGLO AMERICAN AND MEXICAN CHILDREN IS DISCUSSED. 5 REFERENCES. (JOURNAL ABSTRACT)

ACCN   000757

891 AUTH   **KAGAN, S., & MADSEN, M. C.**
     TITL   RIVALRY IN ANGLO-AMERICAN AND MEXICAN CHILDREN OF TWO AGES.
     SRCE   *JOURNAL OF PERSONALITY AND SOCIAL PSYCHOLOGY, 1972, 24(2), 214-220.*
     INDX   CHILDREN, COOPERATION, COMPETITION, EMPIRICAL, CROSS CULTURAL, MEXICAN, INTERPERSONAL RELATIONS, CONFLICT RESOLUTION, CALIFORNIA, SOUTHWEST
     ABST   AN EXPERIMENT DESIGNED TO TRACE THE DEVELOPMENT OF RIVALRY (BEHAVIOR INTENDED TO MINIMIZE GAINS OF A PEER) IN ANGLO-AMERICAN (AA) AND RURAL MEXICAN (M) CHILDREN IS PRESENTED. RIVALRY WAS MEASURED BY FOUR CHOICE CONDITIONS ADMINISTERED TO 48 CHILDREN FROM EACH CULTURE, SIX MALE PAIRS AND SIX FEMALE PAIRS AT AGES 5 TO 6, AND 8 TO 10. DATA WERE ANALYZED BY A FACTORIAL ANALYSIS OF VARIANCE. OLDER CHILDREN WERE SIGNIFICANTLY MORE RIVALROUS THAN YOUNGER CHILDREN. AA CHILDREN WERE SIGNIFICANTLY MORE RIVALROUS THAN M CHILDREN AND THE CULTURAL DIFFERENCE TENDED TO INCREASE WITH AGE. THE EFFECT OF CONDITIONS WAS SIGNIFICANT, WHICH INDICATES THAT FOR ALL GROUPS RIVALRY IS GREATEST WHEN ACCOMPANIED BY BOTH RELATIVE AND ABSOLUTE GAINS. THE OPPORTUNITY TO AVOID A SMALL RELATIVE LOSS INCREASED RIVALRY MORE THAN OPPORTUNITY TO ACCRUE A SMALL ABSOLUTE GAIN. THE DEVELOPMENT WITH AGE OF GREATER RIVALRY IN MALES THAN FEMALES WAS PRESENT FOR THE AA BUT NOT THE M CHILDREN. IT IS SUGGESTED THAT FOR CHILDREN IN AA AND M CULTURES, RIVALRY IS SIMILAR TO INTERPERSONAL CONFLICT. M CHILDREN AVOID CONFLICT AND AA CHILDREN ENTER CONFLICT EVEN WHEN TO DO SO IS IRRATIONAL IN TERMS OF THEIR GOALS. CHILD-REARING PRACTICES MAY ACCOUNT FOR THE SOURCE OF OBSERVED CULTURAL DIFFERENCES. 7 REFERENCES.

ACCN   000758

892 AUTH   **KAGAN, S., & ROMERO, C.**
     TITL   NON-ADAPTIVE ASSERTIVENESS OF ANGLO AMERICAN AND MEXICAN AMERICAN CHILDREN OF TWO AGES.
     SRCE   *INTERAMERICAN JOURNAL OF PSYCHOLOGY, 1977, 11, 27-32.*
     INDX   COMPETITION, CROSS CULTURAL, MEXICAN AMERICAN, CHILDREN, CULTURAL FACTORS, PSYCHOSOCIAL ADJUSTMENT, EMPIRICAL, CALIFORNIA, SOUTHWEST
     ABST   A NOVEL BEHAVIORAL MEASURE, THE ASSERTIVENESS PULL SCALE, WAS DEVELOPED TO TEST THE NONADAPTIVE ASSERTIVENESS AND PASSIVITY OF 48 SEMI-RURAL, LOW-INCOME ANGLO AMERICAN AND MEXICAN AMERICAN BOYS AND GIRLS OF 5-7 AND 8-9 YEARS. CONTRARY TO PREVIOUS RESULTS, CHILDREN WERE OFTEN TOO ASSERTIVE TO MAXIMIZE THEIR OUTCOMES. MORE ANGLO AMERICAN, MALE, AND YOUNGER CHILDREN WERE NONADAPTIVELY ASSERTIVE THAN THEIR MEXICAN AMERICAN, FEMALE, AND OLDER COUNTERPARTS. THE CULTURAL DIFFERENCE IS CONSISTENT WITH PREVIOUS RESEARCH INDICATING GREATER NONADAPTIVE COMPETITIVENESS AMONG ANGLO AMERICAN CHILDREN COMPARED TO MEXICAN AMERICAN CHILDREN. 22 REFERENCES. (AUTHOR ABSTRACT)

ACCN   000759

893 AUTH   **KAGAN, S., & ZAHN, G. L.**
     TITL   FIELD DEPENDENCE AND THE SCHOOL ACHIEVEMENT GAP BETWEEN ANGLO-AMERICAN AND MEXICAN AMERICAN CHILDREN.
     SRCE   *JOURNAL OF EDUCATIONAL PSYCHOLOGY, 1975, 67(5), 643-650.*
     INDX   COGNITIVE STYLE, CHILDREN, CROSS CULTURAL, CULTURAL FACTORS, EDUCATION, MEXICAN AMERICAN, SCHOLASTIC ACHIEVEMENT, EMPIRICAL, READING, MATHEMATICS, FIELD DEPENDENCE-INDEPENDENCE, CALIFORNIA ACHIEVEMENT TESTS, CALIFORNIA, SOUTHWEST, ACHIEVEMENT TESTING
     ABST   RESEARCH SUPPORTS THE HYPOTHESIS THAT FIELD DEPENDENCE EXPLAINS THE POORER SCHOOL ACHIEVEMENT OF MEXICAN AMERICAN CHILDREN COMPARED TO ANGLO AMERICAN CHILDREN. TO TEST THAT HYPOTHESIS, MULTIPLE REGRESSION AND PATH ANALYSES WERE USED TO INTERPRET THE RELATIONSHIPS AMONG CULTURE, FIELD DEPENDENCE, AND SCHOOL ACHIEVEMENT AMONG SECOND-, FOURTH-, AND SIXTH-GRADE ANGLO AMERICAN AND MEXICAN AMERICAN CHILDREN. FIELD DEPENDENCE WAS MEASURED BY THE MAN IN THE FRAME BOX, WHEREAS SCHOLASTIC ACHIEVEMENT WAS MEASURED BY THE CALIFORNIA-MANDATED ACHIEVEMENT TESTS. RESULTS INDICATE THAT: (1) MEXICAN AMERICANS WERE SIGNIFICANTLY BELOW ANGLO AMERICANS IN READING AND MATH ACHIEVEMENT; (2) FIELD INDEPENDENCE WAS SIGNIFICANTLY CORRELATED WITH BOTH READING AND MATH ACHIEVEMENT; (3) MEXICAN AMERICANS WERE SIGNIFICANTLY MORE FIELD DEPENDENT; AND (4) FIELD DEPENDENCE EXPLAINED THE CULTURAL DIFFERENCE IN MATH ACHIEVEMENT BUT DID NOT FULLY EXPLAIN THE CULTURAL DIFFERENCE IN READING ACHIEVEMENT. THE IMPLICATIONS OF THESE RESULTS FOR UNDERSTANDING BOTH FIELD DEPENDENCE AND THE

NATURE OF THE OBSERVED CULTURAL DIFFERENCES ARE DISCUSSED. 32 REFERENCES. (JOURNAL ABSTRACT MODIFIED)

ACCN   000760

894 AUTH   **KAHN, M. W., & HEIMAN, E. M.**
    TITL   FACTORS ASSOCIATED WITH LENGTH OF STAY IN TREATMENT OF PATIENTS FROM A BARRIO NEIGHBORHOOD MENTAL HEALTH SERVICE: A CROSS VALIDATION.
    SRCE   *UNPUBLISHED MANUSCRIPT, 1977. (AVAILABLE FROM THE PRIMARY AUTHOR, DEPARTMENT OF PSYCHOLOGY, UNIVERSITY OF ARIZONA, TUCSON, ARIZONA.)*
    INDX   SEX COMPARISON, PSYCHOTHERAPY, PSYCHOTHERAPISTS, PSYCHOTHERAPY OUTCOME, CROSS CULTURAL, DEMOGRAPHIC, MENTAL HEALTH, HEALTH DELIVERY SYSTEMS, EMPIRICAL, SOUTHWEST
    ABST   TO CROSS-VALIDATE FINDINGS OF AN EARLIER INVESTIGATION OF FACTORS RELATED TO THE LENGTH OF THERAPY AMONG A LOWER SOCIOECONOMIC, PREDOMINATELY MEXICAN AMERICAN, POPULATION, A STUDY WAS CONDUCTED AMONG 488 PATIENTS SEEN DURING A 4-MONTH PERIOD AT A NEIGHBORHOOD MENTAL HEALTH CLINIC. THE PROCEDURE FOLLOWED IN THIS STUDY WAS THE SAME AS IN THE ORIGINAL STUDY. THERAPISTS WERE GIVEN A 19-ITEM FORM AT THE END OF EACH SESSION PERTAINING TO NEW PATIENTS' SOCIODEMOGRAPHIC DATA AS WELL AS INFORMATION RELATED TO TREATMENT, SUCH AS REFERRAL SOURCE, MAJOR PSYCHIATRIC AND SOCIAL PROBLEMS, TYPE OF SERVICES PROVIDED, AND IMPROVEMENT EXPECTATIONS. THE FINDINGS IN THIS AND THE PREVIOUS STUDY INDICATE THAT AGE AND MARITAL STATUS ARE RELATED TO LENGTH OF THERAPY AND THAT SEX AND UNEMPLOYMENT DO NOT APPEAR TO BE RELATED. IN CONTRAST TO EARLIER FINDINGS, THE INCREASED PROPORTION OF CAUCASIANS HAVING LONGER THERAPY WAS NOT FOUND TO BE SIGNIFICANT IN THIS SAMPLE. THIS MAY BE DUE TO THE FACT THAT IN THIS STUDY SOCIAL CLASS WAS HELD CONSTANT AND WAS FOUND NOT TO DIFFERENTIATE BETWEEN THE VARIOUS ETHNIC POPULATIONS. ALTHOUGH THE THERAPIST'S ESTIMATE OF IMPROVEMENT WAS NOT SIGNIFICANT IN THE CROSS-VALIDATION, THE OTHER VARIABLES RELATED TO TREATMENT, ESPECIALLY SOURCE OF REFERRAL, WERE AGAIN ASSOCIATED WITH LENGTH OF PSYCHOTHERAPY. IT IS SUGGESTED THAT EMOTIONAL DISTRESS AND SELF-HELP SEEKING ARE THE PRIMARY DETERMINANTS EFFECTING LENGTH OF TREATMENT. 17 REFERENCES.
    ACCN   000761

895 AUTH   **KAHN, M. W., & HEIMAN, E. M.**
    TITL   FACTORS ASSOCIATED WITH NUMBER OF TREATMENT CONTACTS IN A BARRIO NEIGHBORHOOD MENTAL HEALTH SERVICE.
    SRCE   *INTERNATIONAL JOURNAL OF SOCIAL PSYCHIATRY, 1978, 24(4), 259-262.*
    INDX   SEX COMPARISON, PSYCHOTHERAPY, PSYCHOTHERAPISTS, PSYCHOTHERAPY OUTCOME, CROSS CULTURAL, DEMOGRAPHIC, MENTAL HEALTH, HEALTH DELIVERY SYSTEMS, EMPIRICAL, SOUTHWEST
    ABST   THE IMPORTANCE OF IDENTIFYING FACTORS RELATED TO THE NUMBER OF TREATMENT CONTACTS AMONG A LOWER SOCIOECONOMIC, PREDOMINATELY MEXICAN AMERICAN, POPULATION IS CRUCIAL IN DEVELOPING APPROPRIATE MENTAL HEALTH TREATMENT PROGRAMS. A STUDY WAS CONDUCTED IN A SOUTHWESTERN CITY AMONG 356 PATIENTS SEEN DURING A FOUR-MONTH PERIOD AT A NEIGHBORHOOD MENTAL HEALTH CLINIC. THERAPISTS WERE INTERVIEWED AT THE END OF EACH SESSION REGARDING EACH NEW PATIENT TO OBTAIN SOCIODEMOGRAPHIC DATA AS WELL AS INFORMATION RELATED TO THEIR TREATMENT, SUCH AS REFERRAL SOURCE, MAJOR PSYCHIATRIC AND SOCIAL PROBLEMS, AND TYPE OF SERVICES PROVIDED. THE FINDINGS REVEAL THE FOLLOWING: (1) SELF-REFERRAL PATIENTS WERE MORE APT TO HAVE LONG-TERM THERAPY THAN PHYSICIAN REFERRALS; (2) SHORT-TERM CASES WERE CHARACTERISTIC OF SOCIAL SERVICE AND FINANCIAL PROBLEMS RATHER THAN PSYCHOLOGICAL ONES; (3) CAUCASIANS HAD LONGER TERM THERAPY THAN MEXICAN AMERICANS OR BLACKS; (4) AGE AND MARITAL STATUS WERE ASSOCIATED WITH LENGTH OF STAY IN THERAPY. THESE FINDINGS SUGGEST THAT PATIENTS NEED TO BE EDUCATED BY MENTAL HEALTH AGENCIES AND THERAPISTS ON HOW TO USE TREATMENT. IT IS ALSO POINTED OUT THAT EVEN THOUGH THE CLINIC WAS LOCATED IN A BARRIO AND DESIGNED TO PROVIDE SERVICES TO MEXICAN AMERICANS, THE OVERREPRESENTATION OF ANGLOS MAY BE REFLECTING A CULTURALLY RELATED FACTOR. 5 REFERENCES.
    ACCN   000762

896 AUTH   **KALISH, R. A., & REYNOLDS, D. K.**
    TITL   DEATH AND ETHNICITY: A PSYCHOCULTURAL STUDY.
    SRCE   *LOS ANGELES: ETHEL PERCY ANDRUS GERONTOLOGY CENTER, UNIVERSITY OF SOUTHERN CALIFORNIA, 1976.*
    INDX   CALIFORNIA, SOUTHWEST, CROSS CULTURAL, ATTITUDES, ADULTS, GERONTOLOGY, DEATH, ETHNIC IDENTITY, MEXICAN AMERICAN, CULTURAL CHANGE, DEMOGRAPHIC, SURVEY, EMPIRICAL, RELIGION, CULTURE, FAMILY STRUCTURE, SES, BOOK
    ABST   THIS BOOK, STUDYING THE ATTITUDES AND EFFECTS OF DEATH ON THREE CULTURES (BLACK AMERICANS, JAPANESE AMERICANS, AND MEXICAN AMERICANS), HAS TWO CENTRAL FOCI: (1) HOW DO ETHNIC GROUPS VERBALIZE THEIR THINKING ABOUT DEATH, DYING, AND GRIEVING?; AND (2) HOW DO THEY BEHAVE IN THE FACE OF ACUTAL DEATH? THE 14-PAGE CHAPTER ON MEXICAN AMERICANS REPORTS ON A SAMPLE OF 114 LOW- AND MIDDLE-INCOME MEXICAN AMERICAN ADULTS WHO WERE INTERVIEWED. THESE LOS ANGELES BARRIO RESIDENTS WERE SEEN TO BE BOTH FAMILY-CENTERED AND CHURCH-INFLU-

ENCED—KEY CONSTRUCTS IN THEIR OVERALL IDEOLOGY OF DEATH. IN THIS ETHNIC POPULATION, DEATH IS PECULIARLY A FAMILY EVENT. SIGNIFICANTLY, MORE THAN THE OTHERS, MA'S EXPRESSED A DESIRE TO SPEND THEIR DYING DAYS WITH LOVED ONES AND TO HAVE FUNERALS WHICH INCLUDED LOTS OF FAMILY AND FRIENDS. SECONDLY, NINETY PERCENT OF THE SAMPLE IDENTIFIED THEMSELVES AS ROMAN CATHOLICS. SIGNIFICANTLY MORE THAN THE OTHER GROUPS, MA'S RESPONDED THAT THEY WOULD CALL FOR A PRIEST OR MINISTER ON THEIR DEATHBED, AND THAT THE TIME OF DEATH IS SOLELY IN GOD'S HANDS. A THIRD FACTOR IS THAT MEXICAN AMERICANS SEEM TO ACCEPT DEATH READILY AS AN ABSTRACT CONCEPT, WHILE ADMITTING THEIR WISH TO AVOID THE THOUGHT OF DEATH FOR THEMSELVES AND LOVED ONES. NONETHELESS, DEATH SEEMS HIGHLY PERVASIVE IN THE MA'S THOUGHTS AND DREAMS. IT APPEARS THAT HE COPES WITH THIS BY RITUALISTIC ACTS WHICH INTEGRATE THE CONCEPT OF DEATH INTO LIFE—I.E., DEATH IS EMBRACED IN SONGS, HOLIDAYS AND CELEBRATIONS, AND IN PAINTINGS AND RELIGION. IN FUNERALS, DEATH IS ALSO PROVIDED A SETTING FOR DRAMATIC EXPRESSIONS OF GRIEF AND ANGUISH. DEATH IS ALSO DISCUSSED OPENLY WITH ONE'S FAMILY AND FRIENDS. ALTHOUGH MEXICAN AMERICAN RESPONDENTS HAVE NOT UNIFORMLY SAID SO, THERE SEEMS A CONSENSUS THAT ONE SHOULD ACQUAINT ONESELF WITH DEATH AS THOROUGHLY AS POSSIBLE. UNLIKE THEIR ANGLO AMERICAN COUNTERPARTS WHO TRY DELICATELY TO KEEP DEATH AT ARM'S LENGTH, MEXICAN AMERICANS SEEM TO FEEL THAT ONE SHOULD TACKLE DEATH AND DYING HEAD ON—AND HENCE GROW STRONG FROM THE EXPERIENCE. 112 REFERENCES.

ACCN   000763

897 AUTH   **KALISH, R. A., & REYNOLDS, D. K.**
    TITL   PHENOMENOLOGICAL REALITY AND POST-DEATH CONTACT.
    SRCE   *JOURNAL FOR THE SCIENTIFIC STUDY OF RELIGION, 1973, 12(2), 209-221.*
    INDX   DEATH, MEXICAN AMERICAN, CROSS CULTURAL, CULTURAL FACTORS, IMAGERY, MENTAL HEALTH, SURVEY, RELIGION, EMPIRICAL, URBAN, ADULTS, DREAMS, SYMPTOMATOLOGY, PSYCHOPATHOLOGY, CALIFORNIA, SOUTHWEST
    ABST   INDIVIDUAL REALITIES OF PERSONS CLAIMING TO HAVE HAD ENCOUNTERS WITH OTHERS KNOWN TO BE DEAD OFTEN MARK THE EXPERIENCING INDIVIDUAL AS PATHOLOGICAL. NONETHELESS, A SURVEY OF THE AVAILABLE LITERATURE SHOWS THAT THE EXPERIENCE IS COMMON BOTH IN PRELITERATE COMMUNITIES AND AMONG THE RECENTLY BEREAVED; SOME AUTHORS HAVE INDICATED THAT IT IS MORE COMMON AMONG CONTEMPORARY AMERICANS THAN IS NORMALLY PRESUMED. THE PRESENT STUDY QUERIED 434 RESPONDENTS IN GREATER LOS ANGELES, DIVIDED APPROXIMATELY EQUALLY AMONG BLACK, JAPANESE, MEXICAN AND EUROPEAN ORIGINS,

WHETHER THEY HAD EXPERIENCED SUCH AN ENCOUNTER. APPROXIMATELY 44 PERCENT RESPONDED POSITIVELY, WITH OVER 25 PERCENT OF THESE PERSONS INDICATING THAT THE DEAD PERSON ACTUALLY VISITED OR WAS SEEN AT A SEANCE, WHILE OVER 60 PERCENT OF THE INCIDENTS INVOLVED A DREAM. A SUFFICIENTLY LARGE PROPORTION OF ALL POPULATION CATEGORIES HAVE EXPERIENCED THE PRESENCE OF A DEAD PERSON TO MAKE THIS PHENOMENON WORTHY OF FURTHER INVESTIGATION. 26 REFERENCES. (JOURNAL ABSTRACT MODIFIED)

ACCN   000764

898 AUTH   **KANDELL, A. S.**
    TITL   HARLEM CHILDREN'S STORIES: A STUDY OF EXPECTATIONS OF NEGRO AND PUERTO RICAN BOYS IN TWO READING-LEVEL GROUPS (DOCTORAL DISSERTATION, HARVARD UNIVERSITY, 1967).
    SRCE   *DISSERTATION ABSTRACTS, 1967, 28(6), 2338A. (UNIVERSITY MICROFILMS NO. 67-16,117.)*
    INDX   PUERTO RICAN-M, SCHOLASTIC ACHIEVEMENT, SCHOLASTIC ASPIRATIONS, OCCUPATIONAL ASPIRATIONS, EMPIRICAL, POVERTY, CROSS CULTURAL, CHILDREN, PROJECTIVE TESTING, READING, NEW YORK, EAST, URBAN, PERFORMANCE EXPECTATIONS
    ABST   A COMPARISON OF THE SCHOOL AND GENERAL LIFE EXPECTATIONS OF A GROUP OF LOWER SOCIOECONOMIC CLASS AMERICAN NEGRO AND PUERTO RICAN HARLEM BOYS IS REPORTED. THIRTY AMERICAN NEGRO BOYS AND 30 PUERTO RICAN BOYS WERE STUDIED WITH A PROJECTIVE TEST TECHNIQUE COMBINED WITH A DIRECT QUESTIONNAIRE. SUBJECTS WERE BOTH HIGH AND LOW ACHIEVERS. CONTENT ANALYSIS OF THEIR STORIES REVEALED MORE NEGATIVE EXPECTATIONS FROM THE NEGROES IN THE AREA OF SCHOOL. HIGH ACHIEVING NEGRO BOYS APPEARED TO HAVE MORE POSITIVE EXPECTATIONS IN TERMS OF MASTERY WHEN THEY BECAME FREE OF THE SCHOOL MILIEU. APATHY AND RESIGNATION WERE ALSO APPARENT. PUERTO RICAN BOYS WERE MORE CONFIDENT OF THEIR ABILITY TO ACHIEVE THROUGH DILIGENCE, A SENSE OF INDEPENDENCE, AND AN OPTIMISTIC VIEW OF THEIR ENVIRONMENT. STUDY FINDINGS ARE ALSO CONSIDERED IN TERMS OF THEIR IMPLICATIONS FOR EDUCATIONAL PROBLEMS. 123 REFERENCES.
    ACCN   000765

899 AUTH   **KAPLAN, B.**
    TITL   REFLECTIONS OF THE ACCULTURATION PROCESS IN THE RORSCHARCH TEST.
    SRCE   *JOURNAL OF PROJECTIVE TECHNIQUES, 1955, 19(1), 30-35.*
    INDX   PROJECTIVE TESTING, RORSCHACH TEST, ACCULTURATION, PERSONALITY ASSESSMENT, SPANISH SURNAMED, CROSS CULTURAL, PERSONALITY, MALE, INDIGENOUS POPULATIONS, NEW MEXICO, SOUTHWEST, VETERANS
    ABST   THE EFFECT OF THE ACCULTURATION PROCESS ON PERFORMANCE ON THE RORSCHACH

AMONG FOUR CULTURAL GROUPS IS EXAM-INED. THE 116 SUBJECTS—52 ZUNI, 20 SPAN-ISH AMERICAN, 20 MORMON, AND 24 NAVAJO MALES—WERE BETWEEN THE AGES OF 18 AND 42, AND IN EACH GROUP WERE DIVIDED INTO A VETERAN-NONVETERAN STATUS. BY MEANS OF AN ANALYSIS OF VARIANCE, SCORES ON EIGHT MAJOR RORSCHACH VARIABLES—W, F%, A%, M, R, FC, CF, AND T/R—WERE COM-PARED FOR VETERANS AND NONVETERANS IN ALL FOUR GROUPS. THE VETERAN-NONVET-ERAN VARIANCE REACHED THE .05 LEVEL OF SIGNIFICANCE IN TWO CASES, M AND FC. THE VARIANCE ON THREE OTHER VARIABLES—R, CF, AND T/R—APPROACHED THE .05 LEVEL CLOSELY, WHILE FOR W, A% AND F% THERE WAS NO CONSISTENT DIFFERENCE. IT IS CON-CLUDED THAT THE ACCULTURATION PROCESS HAS EFFECTED CHANGES WHICH ARE RE-FLECTED IN THE RORSCHACH PERFORMANCE. THESE CHANGES ARE IN THE NUMBER OF FORM COLOR RESPONSES. SINCE THE CF OR COLOR FORM VARIABLE ALSO SHOWS CHANGE WHICH APPROACHES SIGNIFICANCE, IT IS SUGGESTED THAT BOTH MOVEMENT AND COLOR RESPONSES ARE INCREASED SIGNIFI-CANTLY IN THE VETERAN GROUP. THIS DIFFER-ENCE OCCURRED IN EACH OF THE FOUR CUL-TURAL GROUPS. A DISCUSSION OF THE FINDINGS POINTS TO THE ATTITUDINAL LEVEL OF THE VETERAN AS A MAJOR FACTOR IN THE TEST PERFORMANCE. 8 REFERENCES.

ACCN   000766

900 AUTH   **KAPLAN, B., RICKERS-OVSIANKINA, M. A., & JOSEPH, A.**

TITL   AN ATTEMPT TO SORT RORSCHACH RECORDS FROM FOUR CULTURES.

SRCE   *JOURNAL OF PROJECTIVE TECHNIQUES, 1956, 20(2), 172-180.*

INDX   PROJECTIVE TESTING, RORSCHACH TEST, CROSS CULTURAL, EMPIRICAL, SPANISH SUR-NAMED, PERSONALITY ASSESSMENT, CUL-TURE, PERSONALITY, INDIGENOUS POPULA-TIONS, NEW MEXICO, SOUTHWEST

ABST   THE APPLICABILITY OF THE MODAL PERSON-ALITY HYPOTHESIS WAS INVESTIGATED BY AD-MINISTERING THREE SORTING AND MATCHING PROCEDURES OF RORSCHACH TESTS TO FOUR CULTURAL GROUPS. TWENTY-FOUR ROR-SCHACH RECORDS WERE SELECTED, SIX FROM EACH OF FOUR CULTURES: MORMON, SPANISH AMERICAN, ZUNI, AND NAVAJO. IN THE FIRST EXPERIMENT, A JUDGE WAS NOT TOLD ANY-THING ABOUT THE RORSCHACHS BEYOND THE FACT THAT FOUR CULTURAL GROUPS WERE REPRESENTED. THE TASK WAS TO SORT THE 24 RECORDS INTO FOUR HOMOGENEOUS GROUPS. IN THE SECOND EXPERIMENT, A JUDGE FAMILIAR WITH THE FOUR CULTURES WAS ASKED TO PERFORM THE SAME SORTING TASK AS THE JUDGE IN THE FIRST EXPERI-MENT. IN A THIRD SORTING TEST, A STATISTI-CAL TECHNIQUE BASED ON THE "DISCRIMI-NANT FUNCTION" WAS USED TO SORT A TOTAL OF 116 RORSCHACH RECORDS INTO ALL POS-SIBLE COMBINATIONS OF CULTURE PAIRS. RE-SULTS INDICATE THAT THE JUDGE IN THE FIRST

EXPERIMENT WAS UNSUCCESSFUL IN SORT-ING THE RECORDS INTO HOMOGENEOUS GROUPS. THE JUDGE IN THE SECOND EXPERI-MENT, ON THE OTHER HAND, ACHIEVED CON-SIDERABLE SUCCESS IN THE SORTING TASK (13 OUT OF 24 RORSCHACHS CORRECTLY SORTED IN THE INITIAL GROUPING AND 8 OUT OF 12 IN THE SECOND). THE RESULTS OF THE "DISCRIMINANT FUNCTION" TEST SHOWS THAT IN TWO PAIRS, NAVAJO VS. MORMON AND NA-VAJO VS. SPANISH AMERICAN, THE CULTURES ARE DISTINGUISHABLE, WITH ALMOST 85 PER-CENT OF THE RECORDS LABELED CORRECTLY. THE FINDINGS SUGGEST THAT RORSCHACH TESTS FROM THE FOUR CULTURES ARE DIF-FERENT AND CAN BE SORTED WITH CONSID-ERABLE SUCCESS. THE SIGNIFICANCE OF THE FINDINGS IS THAT THERE IS A STRONG PRE-SUMPTION THAT CERTAIN PERSONALITY CHARACTERISTICS OF INDIVIDUALS IN THE FOUR CULTURES ARE DIFFERENT, WHICH SUP-PORTS THE "MODAL PERSONALITY" HYPOTHE-SIS. 13 REFERENCES.

ACCN   000767

901 AUTH   **KAPLAN, H. R.**

TITL   THE MEANING OF WORK AMONG THE HARD-CORE UNEMPLOYED (DOCTORAL DISSERTA-TION, UNIVERSITY OF MASSACHUSETTS, 1971).

SRCE   *DISSERTATION ABSTRACTS INTERNATIONAL, 1971, 32(1), 566A. (UNIVERSITY MICROFILMS NO. 71-16,518.)*

INDX   LABOR FORCE, POVERTY, OCCUPATIONAL AS-PIRATIONS, PUERTO RICAN-M, CROSS CUL-TURAL, ADULTS, EMPIRICAL, SEX COMPARI-SON, VALUES

ABST   THE MEANING OF WORK AMONG AN EX-TREMELY DISADVANTAGED SEGMENT OF MALE AND FEMALE HARD-CORE UNEMPLOYED PER-SONS UNDER-GOING JOB TRAINING WAS IN-VESTIGATED. A TOTAL OF 86 PERCENT OF THE RESPONDENTS WERE BLACKS AND PUERTO RICANS. THE QUESTIONS WERE DESIGNED TO ELICIT THE WORK VALUES OF THE RESPON-DENTS BY ASKING THEM WHY THEY WANTED TO WORK, WHAT WAS IMPORTANT ABOUT HAV-ING A JOB, WHAT THEY LOOKED FOR IN THEIR WORK, AND THE TYPE OF JOB THEY WERE MOST INTERESTED IN HAVING. A TYPOLOGY OF MEANINGS OF WORK WAS CONSTRUCTED FOR ANALYTICAL PURPOSES. THE FINDINGS INDICATE THE PERVASIVE INFLUENCE THAT POVERTY HAD UPON THE RESPONDENTS' WORK VALUES. THE EXTREME ECONOMIC DEPRIVA-TION WHICH THEY WERE EXPERIENCING LED THEM TO VIEW THEIR WORK IN TOTALLY IN-STRUMENTAL TERMS. THERE WERE NO CON-SISTENT SIGNIFICANT DIFFERENCES BETWEEN THE VARIOUS RACIAL, ETHNIC, AGE, AND SEX GROUPS. HOWEVER, THERE WAS STRONG COMMITMENT TO WORK WHICH WAS EVI-DENCED BY THE FACT THAT 80 PERCENT OF THEM WOULD CONTINUE TO WORK EVEN IF THERE WAS NO ECONOMIC NECESSITY FOR DOING SO. FURTHERMORE, SOME SUBJECTS EVIDENCED ALTERNATIVE VALUE ORIENTA-TIONS TO WORK, VIEWING IT AS AN ACTIVITY THAT SHOULD PROVIDE THE INDIVIDUAL WITH

PSYCHOLOGICAL REWARDS SUCH AS SELF-ACTUALIZATION. IT IS CONCLUDED THAT WHILE SUBSTANTIAL EVIDENCE EXISTED SUPPORTING THE CONTENTION THAT THERE ARE INDEED CLASS DIFFERENTIATED VALUE SYSTEMS IN SOCIETY, THERE APPEARED TO BE SOME EVIDENCE SUPPORTING HYMAN RODMAN'S HYPOTHESIS OF THE VALUE STRETCH. 143 REFERENCES.

ACCN   000768

902 AUTH   **KAPLAN, R. M., & GOLDMAN, R. D.**
TITL   INTERRACIAL PERCEPTION AMONG BLACK, WHITE AND MEXICAN-AMERICAN HIGH SCHOOL STUDENTS.
SRCE   *JOURNAL OF PERSONALITY AND SOCIAL PSYCHOLOGY, 1973, 28(3), 383-389.*
INDX   MEXICAN AMERICAN, CROSS CULTURAL, ADOLESCENTS, EMPIRICAL, ETHNIC IDENTITY, INTERPERSONAL RELATIONS, GROUP DYNAMICS, CALIFORNIA, SOUTHWEST
ABST   THIRTY-THREE BLACK, 35 MEXICAN AMERICAN, AND 65 WHITE HIGH SCHOOL STUDENTS PARTICIPATED IN A STUDY OF PERCEIVED BELIEF SIMILARITY AND ACCURACY OF SOCIAL PERCEPTION. ONE-THIRD OF THE SUBJECTS WITHIN EACH ETHNIC GROUP RESPONDED TO A 20-ITEM QUESTIONNAIRE AS THEY THOUGHT A BLACK STUDENT WOULD RESPOND; ONE-THIRD RESPONDED AS THEY THOUGHT A MEXICAN AMERICAN STUDENT WOULD RESPOND; AND ONE-THIRD RESPONDED AS THEY THOUGHT A WHITE STUDENT WOULD RESPOND. THE BLACK SUBJECTS PERCEIVED BOTH THEIR WHITE AND MEXICAN AMERICAN CLASSMATES AS BEING DISSIMILAR TO THEMSELVES, BUT THE MEXICAN AMERICANS DID NOT DEMONSTRATE DIFFERENTIAL PERCEPTION BETWEEN THEMSELVES AND THE OTHER TWO GROUPS. ALL THREE GROUPS HAD RELATIVELY VERIDICAL PERCEPTION OF HOW BLACK AND MEXICAN AMERICAN STUDENTS WOULD RESPOND TO THE QUESTIONNAIRE. BLACKS AND MEXICAN AMERICANS WERE SUBSTANTIALLY INACCURATE IN THEIR PERCEPTION OF WHITES. THESE DATA SUGGEST THAT BLACKS AND MEXICAN AMERICANS ARE MORE AWARE OF EACH OTHER'S PERSONALITY CHARACTERISTICS THAN THEY ARE OF THE CHARACTERISTICS OF WHITE STUDENTS. 28 REFERENCES. (AUTHOR ABSTRACT)

ACCN   000769

903 AUTH   **KARNES, M. B., ZEHRBACH, R. R., & JONES, G. R.**
TITL   THE CULTURALLY DISADVANTAGED STUDENT AND GUIDANCE (MONOGRAPH NO. 5: GUIDANCE AND THE EXCEPTIONAL STUDENT).
SRCE   *BOSTON: HOUGHTON MIFFLIN, 1971.*
INDX   CULTURAL FACTORS, SES, ADOLESCENTS, CHILDREN, TEACHERS, ROLE EXPECTATIONS, EDUCATIONAL COUNSELING, CROSS CULTURAL, EDUCATION, ESSAY, CURRICULUM, MEXICAN AMERICAN, PUERTO RICAN-M, FINANCING, ADMINISTRATORS, PARAPROFESSIONALS, COMMUNITY INVOLVEMENT, PARENTAL INVOLVEMENT, SPECIAL EDUCATION, PROGRAM EVALUATION, BOOK

ABST   THE GOAL OF THIS VOLUME IS TO STIMULATE GUIDANCE COUNSELORS AND OTHER SCHOOL PERSONNEL TO (1) BETTER UNDERSTAND CULTURALLY DISADVANTAGED STUDENTS AND (2) DEVELOP EDUCATIONAL PROGRAMS AND SERVICES THAT MEET THE NEEDS OF THESE STUDENTS. THE LABEL "CULTURALLY DISADVANTAGED" IS APPLIED TO INDIVIDUALS IN THE UNITED STATES, SUCH AS APPALACHIAN WHITES, MEXICAN AMERICANS, PUERTO RICANS, BLACKS, AND NATIVE AMERICANS, WHO BY NOT REFLECTING THE MIDDLE-CLASS ORIENTATION HAVE BEEN PENALIZED IN THEIR EDUCATIONAL, VOCATIONAL, SOCIAL AND PERSONAL DEVELOPMENT. RECOGNIZING THE IMPORTANCE OF IDENTIFYING THE DISADVANTAGED STUDENT, THE MAJOR CHARACTERISTICS AMONG THE VARIOUS SUBGROUPS ARE EXAMINED. TO FACILITATE IMPROVED PROGRAMMING THAT WOULD MORE ADEQUATELY MEET THE NEEDS OF THESE SUBGROUPS, PREVIOUSLY USED APPROACHES THAT HAVE SOUGHT TO ACHIEVE CHANGES IN THEIR BEHAVIOR AND ATTITUDE ARE COMPARED AND EVALUATED. WITHIN THIS SAME CONTEXT THE TRADITIONAL ROLES OF SCHOOL PERSONNEL ARE REVIEWED AND SUGGESTIONS ARE PRESENTED REGARDING BOTH THE NECESSITY TO REDEFINE EXISTING ROLES AND CREATING NEW ROLES IN THE EDUCATIONAL STRUCTURE. FLEXIBILITY IN PROGRAMMING, CLASSROOM ORGANIZATION, DESIGN, USE OF THE SCHOOL PLANT, ROLE OF STAFF AND STAFFING PATTERNS, AND PARENTAL INVOLVEMENT IS VIEWED AS THE KEY FACTOR IN PROVIDING EDUCATION THAT WILL SUCCESSFULLY MEET THE NEEDS OF THE CULTURALLY DISADVANTAGED STUDENT.

ACCN   000770

904 AUTH   **KARNO, M.**
TITL   THE ENIGMA IN ETHNICITY IN A PSYCHIATRIC CLINIC.
SRCE   *ARCHIVES OF GENERAL PSYCHIATRY, 1966, 14(5), 516-520.*
INDX   CULTURAL FACTORS, PSYCHOTHERAPY, MEXICAN AMERICAN, MENTAL HEALTH, PSYCHOTHERAPISTS, ACCULTURATION, EMPIRICAL, CROSS CULTURAL, PERSONNEL, PROGRAM EVALUATION, POLICY, CULTURAL PLURALISM, HEALTH DELIVERY SYSTEMS
ABST   ETHNIC CLINICAL PATIENTS AND THE RELATIONSHIP BETWEEN THEIR CULTURAL CHARACTERISTICS AND TREATMENT RECEIVED MAY BE A SOURCE OF CONFUSION AND THERAPEUTIC FAILURE IN AN OUTPATIENT PSYCHIATRIC CLINIC. NEGROES, MEXICAN AMERICANS, AND THIRD GENERATION AMERICAN-BORN CAUCASIAN PATIENTS WERE ANALYZED AND COMPARED WITH RESPECT TO SOCIAL CLASS CHARACTERISTICS, TYPE OF TREATMENT, AND LENGTH OF TREATMENT. RESULTS SHOW THAT NONETHNIC PATIENTS ARE ACCEPTED INTO PSYCHOTHERAPY TO A SIGNIFICANTLY GREATER DEGREE THAN ETHNIC PATIENTS OF THE SAME SOCIAL CLASS. MOREOVER, ETHNIC PATIENTS WHO ARE ACCEPTED FOR TREATMENT RECEIVE LESS AND SHORTER PSY-

CHOTHERAPY THAN DO NONETHNIC PATIENTS OF THE SAME SOCIAL CLASS. PART OF THE PROBLEM IS EXPLAINED AS LYING WITH THE BEHAVIOR OF THE ETHNIC PATIENT HIMSELF. OF GREATER CONCERN ARE THE ATTITUDES AND ACTIONS OF CLINIC PERSONNEL. THERE IS A LACK OF DIRECT ATTENTION GIVEN TO ETHNICITY, RACE, SUBCULTURAL IDENTITY, AND BILINGUALISM BY CLINIC PERSONNEL. IN ADDITION TO THE AVOIDANCE OF ETHNICITY, THERE IS A PERVASIVE DEPENDENCE UPON THE PSYCHIATRIC MEDICAL INTERVIEW MODEL WHICH TENDS TO EXCLUDE SOCIOCULTURAL FACTORS THAT MAY BE IMPORTANT TO DIAGNOSIS AND TREATMENT. IT IS SUGGESTED THAT MENTAL HEALTH PERSONNEL LEARN TO UNDERSTAND AND RESPOND TO ETHNICITY AS AN INTEGRAL ASPECT OF THE ETHNIC PATIENT AND HIS LIFE PROBLEMS. 9 REFERENCES.

ACCN   000771

905 AUTH **KARNO, M., ROSS, R. N., & CAPER, R. A.**
     TITL MENTAL HEALTH ROLES OF PHYSICIANS IN A MEXICAN AMERICAN COMMUNITY.
     SRCE *COMMUNITY MENTAL HEALTH JOURNAL, 1969, 5(1), 62-69.*
     INDX MENTAL HEALTH, PSYCHOTHERAPY, PHYSICIANS, URBAN, ROLE EXPECTATIONS, EMPIRICAL, PSYCHOTHERAPISTS, SURVEY, CALIFORNIA, SOUTHWEST, RESOURCE UTILIZATION
     ABST FAMILY PHYSICIANS WHO PRACTICE IN LOS ANGELES BARRIO COMMUNITIES WERE INTERVIEWED AND ADMINISTERED QUESTIONNAIRES CONCERNING THEIR ATTITUDES, OPINIONS, AND EXPERIENCES WITH REGARD TO MENTAL ILLNESS AND PSYCHIATRY. OF THE 82 PHYSICIANS WHO COMPLETED THE QUESTIONNAIRE, HALF WERE FOREIGN BORN AND REPRESENTED MANY NON-SPANISH NATIONALITIES. THE RESULTS INDICATE THAT THE PHYSICIANS HAVE A VARIED, BUT OFTEN HIGH REGARD FOR PSYCHIATRY, AND A VERY DIVERSE DEGREE OF SENSITIVITY TO AND RECOGNITION OF EMOTIONAL DISORDERS IN OFFICE PRACTICE. THE MAJORITY REFUSED ADDITIONAL PSYCHIATRIC EDUCATION, CONSULTATION, AND RESOURCES. IT IS CONCLUDED THAT FAMILY PHYSICIANS SEEM TO SERVE AS THE MOST ACTIVE AND AVAILABLE MENTAL HEALTH SERVICE IN THIS PARTICULAR LOW-INCOME, ETHNIC-BASED COMMUNITY WITH ITS INADEQUATE FORMAL PSYCHIATRIC FACILITIES. 8 REFERENCES. (JOURNAL ABSTRACT MODIFIED)
     ACCN 000773

906 AUTH **KARNO, M., & EDGERTON, R. B.**
     TITL PERCEPTION OF MENTAL ILLNESS IN A MEXICAN AMERICAN COMMUNITY.
     SRCE *ARCHIVES OF GENERAL PSYCHIATRY, 1969, 20(2), 233-238.*
     INDX POVERTY, MEXICAN AMERICAN, CROSS CULTURAL, URBAN, RESOURCE UTILIZATION, PHYSICIANS, COMMUNITY, LINGUISTIC COMPETENCE, ROLE EXPECTATIONS, MENTAL HEALTH, PSYCHOPATHOLOGY, ATTITUDES, SURVEY, EMPIRICAL, CALIFORNIA, SOUTHWEST
     ABST THIS INITIAL INVESTIGATION OF AN EXTENSIVE STUDY OF MENTAL ILLNESS EXAMINES WHETHER OR NOT DIFFERENCES EXIST IN THE PERCEPTIONS AND DEFINITIONS OF MENTAL ILLNESS BETWEEN MEXICAN AMERICANS (MA) AND ANGLO AMERICANS (AA), AND IF ANY PERCEPTUAL DIFFERENCES MIGHT ACCOUNT FOR THE MA UNDERUTILIZATION OF MENTAL HEALTH FACILITIES. THESE TWO GROUPS WERE OF SIMILAR SOCIOECONOMIC STATUS AND LIVING IN THE SAME COMMUNITY AT THE SAME TIME. BIOGRAPHICAL, DEMOGRAPHIC, AND OTHER INFORMATION CONCERNING MENTAL ILLNESS WAS OBTAINED BY A SURVEY INTERVIEW IN EAST LOS ANGELES FROM 668 ADULTS—444 MA AND 224 AA. RESULTS SHOWED NO SIGNIFICANT DIFFERENCE BETWEEN THE TWO GROUPS IN THE PERCEPTION AND DEFINITION OF MENTAL ILLNESS. THE CULTURAL TRADITION OF THE MA DOES NOT ACCOUNT FOR A LOWER RATE OF INCIDENCE OF MENTAL HEALTH DISEASE AS SUSPECTED FROM THEIR LOW UTILIZATION OF TREATMENT FACILITIES. MORE IMPORTANT FACTORS WHICH INFLUENCE THE UNDERREPRESENTATION OF MA'S IN PSYCHIATRIC TREATMENT FACILITIES ARE: A FORMIDABLE LANGUAGE BARRIER; THE SIGNIFICANT MENTAL HEALTH ROLE OF THE ACTIVE FAMILY PHYSICIAN; THE SELF-ESTEEM REDUCING NATURE OF AGENCY-CLIENT CONTACTS EXPERIENCED BY MA'S; AND THE LACK OF MENTAL HEALTH FACILITIES IN THE MA COMMUNITIES. 28 REFERENCES.

ACCN   000774

907 AUTH **KARNO, M., & EDGERTON, R. B.**
     TITL SOME FOLK BELIEFS ABOUT MENTAL ILLNESS: A RECONSIDERATION.
     SRCE *INTERNATIONAL JOURNAL OF SOCIAL PSYCHIATRY, 1974, 20(3-4), 292-296.*
     INDX FOLK MEDICINE, CURANDERISMO, CULTURAL FACTORS, URBAN, ENVIRONMENTAL FACTORS, ATTITUDES, MENTAL HEALTH, MEXICAN AMERICAN, SYMPTOMATOLOGY, CROSS CULTURAL, SURVEY, CALIFORNIA, SOUTHWEST, RURAL
     ABST A SURVEY WAS CONDUCTED OF BELIEFS ABOUT MENTAL ILLNESS AMONG 444 MEXICAN AMERICAN AND 224 ANGLO AMERICAN RESIDENTS OF EAST LOS ANGELES. MEXICAN AMERICANS, AND ANGLO AMERICANS OF RURAL AND SMALL-TOWN BACKGROUND, WERE MORE LIKELY THAN URBAN-BORN AND RAISED ANGLO AMERICANS TO IDENTIFY THE SYMPTOMS OF DEPRESSION AS REPRESENTING ILLNESS, AND MORE LIKELY TO BELIEVE IN THE HERITABILITY OF MENTAL ILLNESS. SUCH FOLK NOTIONS MAY REPRESENT AN ACCUMULATION OF ACCURATE OBSERVATIONS MORE THAN AN ACCUMULATION OF MYTH BUILT ON IGNORANCE. 15 REFERENCES. (PASAR ABSTRACT)
     ACCN 000775

908 AUTH **KARNO, M., & MORALES, A.**
     TITL A COMMUNITY MENTAL HEALTH SERVICE FOR MEXICAN AMERICANS IN A METROPOLIS.
     SRCE *COMPREHENSIVE PSYCHIATRY, 1971, 12(2), 116-121. (ALSO IN N. N. WAGNER & M. J. HAUG. (EDS.), CHICANOS: SOCIAL AND PSYCHOLOGI-*

CAL PERSPECTIVES. SAINT LOUIS: C. V. MOSBY COMPANY, 1971, PP. 237-241.)

INDX PSYCHOTHERAPY, HEALTH DELIVERY SYSTEMS, BILINGUALISM, RESOURCE UTILIZATION,BILINGUAL-BICULTURAL PERSONNEL, CALIFORNIA, SOUTHWEST, COMMUNITY, MEXICAN AMERICAN, COMMUNITY INVOLVEMENT, PARAPROFESSIONALS, MENTAL HEALTH PROFESSION, ESSAY

ABST THE DEVELOPMENT OF A COMMUNITY MENTAL HEALTH SERVICE FOR MEXICAN AMERICANS IN EAST LOS ANGELES IN 1967 IS DESCRIBED. THIS PROGRAM REQUIRED A LARGE PERCENTAGE OF SPANISH-SPEAKING PERSONNEL WHO WERE COMMITTED TO A SOCIAL, PERSONAL, AND PROFESSIONAL INVOLVEMENT IN THE COMMUNITY. THE PREVENTIVE SERVICE PROGRAM EMPHASIZED PROFESSIONAL MENTAL HEALTH CONSULTATION TO A WIDE VARIETY OF COMMUNITY SERVICE AGENCIES, PUBLIC AND PRIVATE SCHOOLS, HEALTH AGENCIES, PROFESSIONALS, LAW ENFORCEMENT AGENCIES, AND OTHERS. IN ADDITION, SHORT-TERM, CRISIS ORIENTED TREATMENT WAS PROVIDED, AND PATIENTS REFERRED TO THE CENTER WERE ACCEPTED AND TREATED. A CLIENT-CENTERED CONSULTATION WAS STRONGLY EMPHASIZED. IN-SERVICE TRAINING REGARDING MENTAL HEALTH CONSULTATION CONSISTED MAINLY OF APPRENTICESHIP. PATIENTS' CHARACTERISTICS ARE DISCUSSED. IT IS CONCLUDED THAT MEXICAN AMERICAN PATIENTS RESPOND AS WELL AS ANGLOS WHEN THEY ARE OFFERED PROFESSIONALLY EXPERT TREATMENT IN A CONTEXT OF CULTURAL AND LINGUISTIC FAMILIARITY AND ACCEPTANCE.

ACCN 000776

909 AUTH **KASSCHAU, P. L.**
TITL AGE AND RACE DISCRIMINATION REPORTED BY MIDDLE-AGED AND OLDER PERSONS.
SRCE *SOCIAL FORCES, 1977, 55(3), 728-742.*
INDX DISCRIMINATION, ADULTS, GERONTOLOGY, MEXICAN AMERICAN, SURVEY, CROSS CULTURAL, CALIFORNIA, SOUTHWEST, URBAN
ABST A PROBABILITY SAMPLE OF 398 BLACK, 373 MEXICAN AMERICAN, AND 373 WHITE RESIDENTS OF LOS ANGELES COUNTY AGED 45-74 WERE ASKED ABOUT THEIR EXPERIENCES WITH RACE AND AGE DISCRIMINATION IN FINDING OR STAYING ON THE JOB. THE OVERWHELMING MAJORITY (60%-88%) OF EACH ETHNIC SAMPLE IDENTIFIED BOTH RACE AND AGE DISCRIMINATION AS COMMON IN THE COUNTRY TODAY. SMALLER PERCENTAGES OF EACH ETHNIC SUBSAMPLE (20%-45%) REPORTED THAT THEIR OWN FRIENDS AND ACQUAINTANCES HAD EXPERIENCED RACE OR AGE DISCRIMINATION. RESPECTIVELY SMALLER PERCENTAGES OF EACH GROUP (8%-34%) DIRECTLY IDENTIFIED PERSONAL EXPERIENCES WITH RACE AND AGE DISCRIMINATION. BLACKS WERE CONSIDERABLY MORE LIKELY TO ASSERT THE EXISTENCE OF RACE DISCRIMINATION AT EACH OF THESE THREE LEVELS OF OBSERVATION THAN WERE MEXICAN AMERICANS WHO, IN TURN, WERE MODERATELY MORE LIKELY TO REPORT RACE DIS-

CRIMINATION AT EACH LEVEL THAN WERE WHITES. DIFFERENCES AMONG THE ETHNIC SAMPLES WERE LESS DRAMATIC AND LESS CONSISTENT FOR REPORTED EXPERIENCES WITH AGE DISCRIMINATION AT THE THREE LEVELS OF OBSERVATION, ALTHOUGH BLACK RESPONDENTS STILL TENDED TO REPORT GREATER EXPOSURE TO AGE DISCRIMINATION THAN THE OTHER ETHNIC GROUPS. 28 REFERENCES. (JOURNAL ABSTRACT MODIFIED)

ACCN 000778

910 AUTH **KATATSKY, M. E.**
TITL A REVIEW OF ALCOHOLISM ACTIVITIES IN LATIN AMERICA.
SRCE *ALCOHOLISM: CLINICAL AND EXPERIMENTAL RESEARCH, 1977, 1(4), 355-358.*
INDX SOUTH AMERICA, CENTRAL AMERICA, ALCOHOLISM, REVIEW, POLICY, HEALTH DELIVERY SYSTEMS, PRIMARY PREVENTION, SOCIAL SERVICES, MENTAL HEALTH, CULTURAL FACTORS, DEMOGRAPHIC
ABST THE MAJOR TRENDS IN THE DEVELOPMENT OF ALCOHOLISM TREATMENT IN LATIN AMERICA ARE DESCRIBED AND ANALYZED. A BRIEF LOOK AT THE EXTENT OF ALCOHOLISM IN LATIN AMERICA IS PROVIDED; AND IN THAT CONNECTION, THE PRIMARY OBJECTIVES OF THE TEN-YEAR HEALTH PLAN FOR THE AMERICAS ADOPTED BY THE REGIONAL MINISTERS OF HEALTH ARE ELABORATED. IN AN EFFORT TO PLACE THE COUNTRIES ON A CONTINUUM IN THE DEVELOPMENT OF ALCOHOLISM PROGRAMS, FOUR STAGES OF DEVELOPMENT ARE IDENTIFIED: (1) LACK OF RECOGNITION BY TECHNICIANS, SCIENTISTS, LAY PUBLIC, OR POLITICIANS OF ALCOHOLISM AS A PUBLIC HEALTH OR SOCIAL PROBLEM (BOLIVIA, HAITI, PARAGUAY, ECUADOR); (2) SOME RECOGNITION OF THE PROBLEM (COLOMBIA, DOMINICAN REPUBLIC, PERU, EL SALVADOR); (3) SUFFICIENT RECOGNITION SO THAT SOME EPIDEMIOLOGICAL STUDIES HAVE BEEN CONDUCTED AND SOME ISOLATED ACTION HAS BEEN TAKEN BY THE GOVERNMENT AND PRIVATE ENTERPRISE (ARGENTINA, SEVERAL STATES IN BRAZIL, JAMAICA); AND (4) REALIZATION OF THE PROBLEM SO THAT SEVERAL EPIDEMIOLOGICAL AND OTHER STUDIES HAVE BEEN COMPLETED, THERE ARE SCIENTISTS DEDICATED TO THE STUDY OF THE PROBLEM, AND THERE ARE IDENTIFIABLE GOVERNMENT PROGRAMS, POLICIES, AND PRIORITIES (CHILE AND COSTA RICA). IN CONCLUSION, THE ROLE OF PAHO/WHO IS DESCRIBED—AN ORGANIZATION BY AND FOR THE GOVERNMENTS OF THE REGION OF THE AMERICAS, DEVOTED TO THE DETECTION, PREVENTION, AND MANAGEMENT OF ALCOHOLISM. 11 REFERENCES. (NCAI ABSTRACT MODIFIED)

ACCN 002123

911 AUTH **KATZ, J. M., GOLD, D. E., & JONES, E. T.**
TITL EQUALITY OF OPPORTUNITY IN A DEMOCRATIC INSTITUTION: THE PUBLIC JUNIOR COLLEGE.
SRCE *EDUCATION AND URBAN SOCIETY, 1973, 5(3), 261-276.*

INDX EQUAL OPPORTUNITY, MEXICAN AMERICAN, COLLEGE STUDENTS, DISCRIMINATION, EMPIRICAL, SCHOLASTIC ACHIEVEMENT, REPRESENTATION, COMMUNITY, HIGHER EDUCATION, SES, ACHIEVEMENT TESTING, CALIFORNIA, SOUTHWEST

ABST IT IS GENERALLY BELIEVED THAT EQUALITY OF OPPORTUNITY IS BEING ACHIEVED IN THE PUBLIC JUNIOR COLLEGE IN TWO BASIC WAYS: (1) BY KEEPING TUITION FEES TO A MINIMUM AND BEING LOCATED CLOSE TO THE HOMES OF POTENTIAL STUDENTS; AND (2) BY MAINTAINING AN OPEN DOOR POLICY FOR ADMISSIONS. THIS STUDY OF APPROXIMATELY 100 STUDENTS WHO ATTENDED GOLDEN CITY JUNIOR COLLEGE IN CALIFORNIA IN THE FALL OF 1960 INDICATES THAT THE "OPEN DOOR" POLICY DOES NOT ADMIT ALL MEMBERS OF THE COMMUNITY ON A REPRESENTATIVE BASIS. BY COMPARING THE COMMUNITY POPULATION CHARACTERISTICS (IN PARTICULAR, ETHNICITY AND INCOME) WITH THOSE OF THE STUDENTS, IT WAS FOUND THAT THE JUNIOR COLLEGE RECRUITED A PROPORTIONATELY LARGE NUMBER OF MIDDLE-INCOME, ANGLO STUDENTS. BLACKS, 9% OF THE COMMUNITY POPULATION, REPRESENTED A NEGLIGIBLE NUMBER OF THE JUNIOR COLLEGE STUDENTS. CHICANOS MADE UP 18% OF THE COMMUNITY BUT ONLY 7.9% OF THE STUDENT POPULATION. NO MINORITY STUDENT IN THE STUDY WAS FROM A FAMILY LIVING IN POVERTY. VERBAL APTITUDE TEST SCORES INDICATED THAT STUDENTS FROM DEPRIVED AND POVERTY INCOMES HAD HIGHER APTITUDES THAN STUDENTS FROM HIGHER INCOME LEVELS WHO ATTEND JUNIOR COLLEGE. WHEN QUANTITATIVE TEST SCORES AND FATHERS INCOME WERE RELATED, THIS CORRELATION WAS AGAIN SUBSTANTIATED. FOR THESE STUDENTS, AS INCOME INCREASES, APTITUDE DECREASES. APPARENTLY THIS JUNIOR COLLEGE, RATHER THAN PROVIDING A CHANNEL OF MOBILITY FOR THE ENTIRE COMMUNITY, GIVES LOW ABILITY STUDENTS FROM MIDDLE-INCOME FAMILIES THE OPPORTUNITY TO MAINTAIN THEIR FOOTHOLD IN THE CLASS STRUCTURE. ATTEMPTS TO OVERCOME DISADVANTAGES ACCRUING TO LOWER-INCOME MINORITY STUDENTS HAVE NOT BEEN NOTABLY SUCCESSFUL AND SOME PROJECTS, SUCH AS THE OPEN DOOR COLLEGES, HAVE ONLY FURTHER ADVANCED THE MIDDLE STRATA OPPORTUNITIES AT THE EXPENSE OF THOSE WHOM THEY WERE DESIGNED TO SERVE. 17 REFERENCES. (AUTHOR SUMMARY MODIFIED)

ACCN 000779

912 AUTH **KATZMAN, M. T.**

TITL DISCRIMINATION, SUBCULTURE, AND THE ECONOMIC PERFORMANCE OF NEGROS, PUERTO RICANS, AND MEXICAN AMERICANS.

SRCE *AMERICAN JOURNAL OF ECONOMICS AND SOCIOLOGY, 1968, 27(4), 371-375.*

INDX ECONOMIC FACTORS, CROSS CULTURAL, DISCRIMINATION, SES, EQUAL OPPORTUNITY, CULTURAL FACTORS, ACCULTURATION, THEORETICAL, SURVEY, PUERTO RICAN-M, MEXICAN AMERICAN, EMPIRICAL, NEW YORK, EAST, VALUES

ABST ECONOMIC UNDERACHIEVEMENT AMONG NEGROES, PUERTO RICANS AND MEXICAN AMERICANS, IN TERMS OF SUBCULTURAL VALUES AND DISCRIMINATION AGAINST THESE SUBCULTURES, IS EXAMINED. TO TEST THE RELATION BETWEEN RACIAL DISCRIMINATION (COLOR) AND ECONOMIC ACHIEVEMENT, SURVEYS WERE CONDUCTED OF NEGRO AND WHITE PUERTO RICANS. THE RESULTS WERE INCONCLUSIVE. TO TEST THE EFFECTS OF SUBCULTURAL VALUES ON ECONOMIC ACHIEVEMENT, SURVEYS WERE TAKEN OF NONPUERTO RICAN (ANGLO) AND PUERTO RICAN NEGROES, THUS HOLDING COLOR CONSTANT. THE PUERTO RICANS HAD MORE WHITE-COLLAR JOBS, WHILE ANGLOS HAD HIGHER MEDIAN INCOME AND EMPLOYMENT RATES. SURVEYS TAKEN OF WEST INDIAN AND NATIVE NEGROES SHOWED THE WEST INDIAN GROUP TO BE HIGHER ON ALL INDICES OF SUCCESS. IN SURVEYS TAKEN OF IMMIGRANT PUERTO RICANS AND MEXICANS, THE SECOND GENERATION PUERTO RICANS SHOWED A GENERAL IMPROVEMENT IN ECONOMIC STATUS OVER THEIR MEXICAN COUNTERPARTS. THE FINDINGS TEND TO EMPHASIZE SUBCULTURAL VALUES AND CLASS DISCRIMINATION OVER RACIAL DISCRIMINATION AS THE MAJOR CAUSAL FACTORS FOR INTERSUBCULTURAL ECONOMIC UNDERACHIEVEMENT. 5 REFERENCES.

ACCN 000780

913 AUTH **KATZMAN, M. T.**

TITL URBAN RACIAL MINORITIES AND IMMIGRANT GROUPS: SOME ECONOMIC COMPARISONS.

SRCE *AMERICAN JOURNAL OF ECONOMICS AND SOCIOLOGY, 1971, 30(1), 15-25.*

INDX SES, ACCULTURATION, CROSS CULTURAL, IMMIGRATION, EMPIRICAL, MIGRATION, URBAN, MEXICAN AMERICAN, SOCIAL MOBILITY, ECONOMIC FACTORS, POVERTY, THEORETICAL, RESEARCH METHODOLOGY, OCCUPATIONAL ASPIRATIONS, PUERTO RICAN-M

ABST A PREVIOUSLY DEVELOPED MODEL EXPLAINING DIFFERENCES IN ECONOMIC PERFORMANCE OF SEVERAL PREDOMINANTLY WHITE URBAN IMMIGRANT GROUPS IS EXTENDED TO SIX RACIALLY DISTINCTIVE MINORITIES. THE GROUPS, ALL WITH RELATIVELY SEVERE ECONOMIC PROBLEMS, WERE NEGROES, MEXICANS, PUERTO RICANS, CHINESE, FILIPINOS, AND JAPANESE. THE ECONOMIC PERFORMANCE OF THE MINORITIES DIVERGED MARKEDLY FROM PREDICTIONS BASED ON THE IMMIGRANT MODEL. THE THREE ORIENTAL GROUPS SHOWED A SPECTACULAR RISE FROM UNDERACHIEVEMENT BETWEEN 1950 AND 1960, WHILE MEXICAN AMERICANS AND NEGROES WERE STILL THE MOST SEVERE UNDERACHIEVERS. THIS UNDERACHIEVEMENT CANNOT BE EXPLAINED SOLELY BY PREJUDICE. IT MUST BE EXPLAINED ALSO IN TERMS OF SUBCULTURAL TRAITS—I.E., ATTITUDES TOWARD WORK, SAVING, EDUCATION, AND FERTILITY. 23 REFERENCES.

ACCN 000781

914 AUTH **KAUFERT, J., MARTINEZ, C., JR., & QUESADA, G.**

TITL A PRELIMINARY STUDY OF MEXICAN-AMERICAN MEDICAL STUDENTS.

SRCE *JOURNAL OF MEDICAL EDUCATION, 1975, 50(9), 856-866.*

INDX MEXICAN AMERICAN, DEMOGRAPHIC, SURVEY, COLLEGE STUDENTS, SES, EMPIRICAL, MEDICAL STUDENTS, ETHNIC IDENTITY, REPRESENTATION

ABST THE RESULTS OF A 1973 MAIL QUESTIONNAIRE SURVEY OF 230 CHICANO MEDICAL STUDENTS ARE REPORTED. 114 RESPONDED, INCLUDING 12 WOMEN. THE RESULTS INDICATE THAT THIS GROUP OF MEDICAL STUDENTS IS SIMILAR TO THE MAJORITY OF MEDICAL STUDENTS IN TERMS OF AGE, SEX, MARITAL STATUS AND ORDINAL POSITION IN THE FAMILY. HOWEVER, THEY DIVERGE WIDELY IN OTHER AREAS SUCH AS RELIGION, FIRST LANGUAGE AND SOCIOECONOMIC STATUS. DIFFERENCES IN ETHNIC IDENTIFICATION WITHIN THE GROUP WERE ALSO FOUND. CALIFORNIA AND TEXAS ARE EDUCATING THE MAJORITY OF CHICANO STUDENTS SURVEYED. AS WITH OTHER MEDICAL STUDENTS, THEY OVERWHELMINGLY SEE THEMSELVES AS FUTURE GENERAL PRACTITIONERS DURING THEIR EARLY MEDICAL EDUCATION, BUT CHANGE TO A MORE SPECIALIZED AREA NEAR GRADUATION. STUDENT RESPONSES TO MINORITY RECRUITMENT PROGRAMS, SPECIAL EDUCATION PROGRAMS AT THE PRE-MEDICAL SCHOOL LEVEL AND MEDICAL SCHOOL ADMISSIONS POLICIES ARE ALSO PRESENTED. 6 REFERENCES. (JOURNAL ABSTRACT MODIFIED)

ACCN 000782

915 AUTH **KEARNS, B. J.**

TITL CHILDREARING PRACTICES AMONG SELECTED CULTURALLY DEPRIVED MINORITIES.

SRCE *JOURNAL OF GENETIC PSYCHOLOGY, 1970, 116(2), 149-155.*

INDX CHILDREARING PRACTICES, POVERTY, CROSS CULTURAL, MEXICAN AMERICAN, AGGRESSION, FAMILY ROLES, COMPETITION, INTERPERSONAL RELATIONS, CONFLICT RESOLUTION, EMPIRICAL, INDIGENOUS POPULATIONS, CULTURAL FACTORS, ARIZONA, SOUTHWEST, FEMALE, VALUES

ABST AN INVESTIGATION OF CHILD-REARING PRACTICES AMONG SELECTED CULTURALLY DEPRIVED INDIANS, MEXICAN AMERICANS, AND ANGLOS IS PRESENTED. A COMPARISON OF THESE GROUPS WAS MADE IN TERMS OF WHETHER VALUES RELATED TO CHILD-REARING INDICATE CULTURAL DISSIMILARITIES. THE SUBJECTS, 50 PAPAGO INDIAN, 50 MEXICAN AMERICAN AND 50 ANGLO MOTHERS, WERE INTERVIEWED BY TRAINED INTERVIEWERS, REPRESENTATIVE OF EACH CULTURAL GROUP, WHO USED AN ADAPTED FORM OF THE INTERVIEW SCALE DEVELOPED BY SEARS, MACCOBY, AND LEVIN. RESULTS OF THE INVESTIGATION REVEALED THAT SIGNIFICANT DIFFERENCES DO EXIST AMONG THE PAPAGO, MEXICAN AMERICAN, AND ANGLO CHILDREARING PRACTICES. THE MEXICAN AMERICAN AND PAPAGO CHILD-REARING PATTERNS APPEAR TO BE GOVERNED TO A LARGE EXTENT BY TRADITIONAL VALUES AND PRACTICES. IN COMPARISON, THE BONDS WITH TRADITION APPEAR TO BE WEAKER WITHIN THE ANGLO GROUP. THE PATTERNS OF CHILD-REARING WITHIN EACH CULTURAL GROUP APPEAR TO BE ENCOURAGED BY CERTAIN COMMON CONDITIONS BASIC TO ALL THREE GROUPS—THE LACK OF ECONOMIC OPPORTUNITY, THE PRESENCE OF CLASS DISTINCTION, AND THE LACK OF EDUCATION. IT IS CONCLUDED THAT SIGNIFICANT DIFFERENCES EXIST IN CHILD-REARING PRACTICES, AND IT IS RECOMMENDED THAT EDUCATORS NEED TO REEXAMINE EARLY CHILDHOOD EDUCATION PROGRAMS, REEVALUATE THE BASIC CONCEPTS TAUGHT IN HOME ECONOMICS CLASSES, AND REDEFINE THE PRACTICAL APPROACHES WHICH HAVE BEEN DESIGNED TO INTEREST THESE CULTURAL GROUPS IN LEARNING. 7 REFERENCES.

ACCN 000783

916 AUTH **KEE, D. W., & ROHWER, W. D.**

TITL NOUN-PAIR LEARNING IN FOUR ETHNIC GROUPS: CONDITIONS OF PRESENTATION AND RESPONSE.

SRCE *JOURNAL OF EDUCATIONAL PSYCHOLOGY, 1973, 65(2), 226-232.*

INDX LEARNING, LINGUISTICS, GRAMMAR, SES, URBAN, MEXICAN AMERICAN, CHILDREN, CROSS CULTURAL, CULTURAL FACTORS, PERFORMANCE EXPECTATIONS, EMPIRICAL, BILINGUALISM, CALIFORNIA, SOUTHWEST

ABST NOUN-PAIR LEARNING EFFICIENCY WAS ASSESSED AMONG 4 LOW SOCIOECONOMIC STATUS ETHNIC GROUPS (BLACK, CHINESE AMERICAN, SPANISH AMERICAN, AND WHITE) AS A FUNCTION OF PRESENTATION CONDITIONS AND METHOD OF MEASUREMENT (VERBAL RECALL VS PICTORIAL RECOGNITION). A MIXED-LIST PAIRED-ASSOCIATE TASK WAS ADMINISTERED INDIVIDUALLY TO 40 SECOND-GRADE CHILDREN FROM EACH GROUP. THE RESULTS REVEALED SUBSTANTIAL EFFECTS FOR PRESENTATION CONDITIONS BUT NOT FOR ETHNIC GROUPS. IN ADDITION, SIMILAR PATTERNS OF CONDITION EFFECTS EMERGED ACROSS RESPONSE MODES FOR ALL ETHNIC GROUPS. THE RESULTS WERE TAKEN AS EVIDENCE OF THE GENERALITY OF PRESENTATION CONDITION EFFECTS IN NOUN-PAIR LEARNING AND AS AN EMPIRICAL DEMONSTRATION OF PARITY IN LEARNING ABILITY FOR CHILDREN FROM DIFFERENT ETHNIC BACKGROUNDS. 7 REFERENCES. (JOURNAL ABSTRACT)

ACCN 000784

917 AUTH **KEE, J. W.**

TITL SOME FEATURES OF GENERAL HOSPITAL UTILIZATION BY PEOPLE WITH SPANISH SURNAMES: A COMPARATIVE STUDY IN LOS ANGELES COUNTY (DOCTORAL DISSERTATION, UNIVERSITY OF CALIFORNIA, LOS ANGELES, 1970).

SRCE *DISSERTATION ABSTRACTS INTERNATIONAL, 1970, 31(5), 2794B. (UNIVERSITY MICROFILMS NO. 70-19,860).*

INDX SEX ROLES, FERTILITY, RESOURCE UTILIZATION, MEXICAN AMERICAN, CROSS CULTURAL, DEMOGRAPHIC, SES, CULTURAL FACTORS, HEALTH, HEALTH DELIVERY SYSTEMS, EMPIRICAL, CALIFORNIA, SOUTHWEST, URBAN

ABST RECENT LITERATURE SUGGESTS THAT MEXICAN AMERICANS, FOR A NUMBER OF CULTURAL REASONS, TEND TO AVOID USING MODERN MEDICAL SERVICES, PARTICULARLY HOSPITALS. SEVERAL ASPECTS OF THIS PROBLEM ARE PRESENTED IN THIS STUDY UTILIZING LOS ANGELES COUNTY BIRTH AND HOSPITAL RECORDS. TWO MAJOR HYPOTHESES ARE DISCUSSED: (1) SPANISH SURNAMED WOMEN ARE OVERREPRESENTED IN THE POPULATION OF MOTHERS WHO GAVE BIRTH OUT OF HOSPITAL; AND (2) WHEN MEXICAN AMERICANS DO USE A HOSPITAL, THEY ARE HOSPITALIZED FOR LONGER PERIODS AND HAVE A HIGHER IN HOSPITAL DEATH RATE THAN ANGLOS OR BLACKS. ANALYSIS OF OVER 120,000 BIRTH CERTIFICATES FOR THE YEAR 1966 LEADS TO REJECTION OF THE FIRST HYPOTHESIS. NEGRO WOMEN WERE FOUND TO BE OVERREPRESENTED IN TH OUT OF HOSPITAL DELIVERY GROUP, ALTHOUGH THE SIGNIFICANCE OF THE DIFFERENCE DIMINISHES GREATLY WHEN ONLY INTENTIONAL DELIVERIES ARE CONSIDERED. MEXICAN BORN WOMEN ARE OVERREPRESENTED AMONG SPANISH SURNAME WOMEN WHO GIVE BIRTH OUTSIDE THE HOSPITAL, REFLECTING TRADITIONAL RURAL MEXICAN PRACTICES. ANALYSIS OF HOSPITAL RECORDS DOES NOT SUPPORT THE SECOND HYPOTHESIS EITHER. ALTHOUGH MEXICAN AMERICANS DO NOT USE MEDICAL SERVICES AT A RATE EQUIVALENT TO POPULATION PARITY, IT WAS NOT FOUND THAT WHEN THEY DO THAT THEY ARE MORE SEVERELY ILL OR HAVE A HIGHER DEATH RATE IN HOSPITAL. TRADITIONAL VIEWS ABOUT MEXICAN AMERICANS HEALTH ATTITUDES AND PRACTICES ARE CHALLENGED BY THESE FINDINGS. IN EFFECT, MEMBERSHIP IN THE LOWEST SOCIOECONOMIC CLASS, RATHER THAN IN ANY ETHNIC OR CULTURE GROUP MOST INFLUENCES MEDICAL CARE UTILIZATION. IMPLICATIONS FOR PUBLIC HEALTH POLICY AND PROGRAM PLANNING ARE DISCUSSED. 25 REFERENCES. (AUTHOR ABSTRACT MODIFIED)

ACCN 000785

918 AUTH **KEEFE, J. A., & NASH, R.**

TITL RELIGION AND EDUCATION IN THE PUERTO RICAN CULTURE.

SRCE *JOURNAL OF EDUCATION, 1967, 150(2), 23-34.*

INDX RELIGION, EDUCATION, PUERTO RICAN-I, CULTURE, CULTURAL CHANGE, DEATH, ESPIRITISMO, EMPIRICAL

ABST INCONGRUITIES BETWEEN THE EXPLICIT AND IMPLICIT CULTURE OF PUERTO RICO AND THE ISLANDS' TWO MAJOR RELIGIOUS SECTS (CATHOLICISM AND PROTESTANTISM) ARE DISCUSSED. PRIMARY CONCERNS ARE: (1) THE WAYS IN WHICH THE PUERTO RICAN PEOPLE ARE OR ARE NOT CONSONANT WITH THE RELIGIOUS CONFIGURATION OF THEIR CULTURE; AND (2) THE DEGREE TO WHICH PUERTO RICAN PERSONALITIES ARE ABLE TO FUNCTION HARMONIOUSLY WITH THEIR EXPLICIT RELIGIOUS BEHAVIORS. INFORMATION GATHERED FROM THE GRASS-ROOTS, PROFESSIONAL AND LEADERSHIP LEVELS OF PUERTO RICAN RELIGIOUS ORGANIZATIONS, AS WELL AS FROM MANY INFORMAL DISCUSSIONS WITH PUERTO RICANS OF ALMOST EVERY SOCIAL CLASS, IS PRESENTED UNDER THESE FOUR AREAS OF DISCUSSION: (1) THE SAINT CULT; (2) SPIRITUALISM-SPIRITISM PRACTICES; (3) THE ROLE AND FUNCTION OF PROTESTANTISM AND CATHOLICISM IN PUERTO RICO IN TERMS OF "SOCIAL ACTION; AND (4) THE INTER-RELATIONSHIP OF RELIGION AND EDUCATION. 8 REFERENCES.

ACCN 000786

919 AUTH **KEEFE, S. E.**

TITL MENTAL HEALTH AND CULTURAL CONTEXT: IMPLICATIONS FOR USE OF MENTAL HEALTH CLINICS BY MEXICAN AMERICANS.

SRCE *IN J. M. CASAS & S. E. KEEFE (EDS.), FAMILY AND MENTAL HEALTH IN THE MEXICAN AMERICAN COMMUNITY (MONOGRAPH NO. 7). LOS ANGELES: UNIVERSITY OF CALIFORNIA, SPANISH SPEAKING MENTAL HEALTH RESEARCH CENTER, 1978, PP. 91-10.*

INDX MEXICAN AMERICAN, RESOURCE UTILIZATION, CULTURAL FACTORS, MENTAL HEALTH, HEALTH DELIVERY SYSTEMS, SURVEY, EMPIRICAL, CURANDERISMO, MARITAL STABILITY, ACCULTURATION, SES, EXTENDED FAMILY, CROSS GENERATIONAL, CALIFORNIA, SOUTHWEST, URBAN

ABST A SURVEY OF THE MENTAL HEALTH SERVICES UTILIZATION PATTERN OF 666 MEXICAN AMERICAN (MA) RESIDENTS OF THREE SOUTHERN CALIFORNIA URBAN AREAS IS DISCUSSED. CONCLUDED IS THAT THERE IS NO SIGNIFICANT RELATIONSHIP BETWEEN CONTACT WITH MENTAL HEALTH CLINICS BY MA'S AND THE FOLLOWING FACTORS: (1) SES; (2) THE PRESENCE OF AN INTEGRATED EXTENDED FAMILY; (3) RELIANCE ON RELATIVES, DOCTORS, CLERGYMEN, MEXICAN AMERICAN COMMUNITY WORKERS OR CURANDEROS FOR EMOTIONAL SUPPORT; (4) COMMITMENT TO FOLK MEDICAL SYSTEM; OR (5) ATTITUDES TOWARD MENTAL HEALTH SERVICES. OF ALL THE CULTURAL VARIABLES CONSIDERED, ONLY ENGLISH SPEAKING CORRELATES SIGNIFICANTLY WITH USE OF MENTAL HEALTH CLINICS. ACCULTURATION LEVEL ALONE IS THEREFORE RELATIVELY UNIMPORTANT IN EXPLAINING UNDERUTILIZATION BY MA'S. THE HIGH CORRELATION BETWEEN USE OF PRIVATE PSYCHIATRIC HELP AND USE OF PUBLIC MENTAL HEALTH CLINICS INDICATES THAT PERCEPTIONS OF MENTAL ILLNESS AND ITS TREATMENT ARE THE KEY TO UNDERSTANDING CLINIC UTILIZATION BY THE MA. THERAPY IS CONSIDERED A SIGN OF PERSONAL WEAKNESS BY MA'S, WHO CONSIDER PROFESSIONAL TREATMENT ONLY AFTER EVERY OTHER RECOURSE. IT IS SUGGESTED THAT FUTURE RESEARCH TAKE THIS POTENTIAL ETH-

NIC DIFFERENCE IN PERCEPTION OF MENTAL ILLNESS AND UTILIZATION RATES INTO CONSIDERATION. 36 REFERENCES. (AUTHOR SUMMARY MODIFIED)

ACCN 000787

920 AUTH **KEEFE, S. E.**

TITL MEXICAN AMERICANS' UNDERUTILIZATION OF MENTAL HEALTH CLINICS: AN EVALUATION OF SUGGESTED EXPLANATIONS.

SRCE *HISPANIC JOURNAL OF BEHAVIORAL SCIENCES, 1979, 1(2), 93-115.*

INDX MEXICAN AMERICAN, RESOURCE UTILIZATION, REVIEW, MENTAL HEALTH, EMPIRICAL, SOUTHWEST, CALIFORNIA, SURVEY, SES, EXTENDED FAMILY, ATTITUDES, FAMILY STRUCTURE, HEALTH DELIVERY SYSTEMS, CULTURAL FACTORS

ABST REASONS PROPOSED BY RESEARCHERS TO ACCOUNT FOR THE UNDERUTILIZATION OF PUBLIC MENTAL HEALTH CLINICS BY MEXICAN AMERICANS ARE SUMMARIZED AND THEN TESTED USING DATA FROM A SURVEY OF 666 MEXICAN AMERICANS IN THREE SOUTHERN CALIFORNIA COMMUNITIES. NO SIGNIFICANT RELATIONSHIP IS DEMONSTRATED BETWEEN MENTAL HEALTH CLINIC CONTACT AND SOCIOECONOMIC STATUS, EXTENDED FAMILY TIES, COMMITMENT TO THE FOLK MEDICAL SYSTEM, OR RELIANCE ON COMPADRES, DOCTORS, CLERGYMEN, COMMUNITY WORKERS, OR FOLK HEALERS FOR HELP WITH EMOTIONAL PROBLEMS. MOST SIGNIFICANT IS THE RELATIONSHIP BETWEEN MENTAL HEALTH CLINIC CONTACT AND THE USE OF PRIVATE THERAPISTS. IT IS SUGGESTED THAT ETHNIC PERCEPTIONS OF EMOTIONAL PROBLEMS ARE MOST IMPORTANT IN DETERMINING MENTAL HEALTH CLINIC UTILIZATION. 47 REFERENCES. (JOURNAL ABSTRACT)

ACCN 001770

921 AUTH **KEEFE, S. E.**

TITL SEX AND ETHNICITY IN POLITICS: A MINORITY GROUP MODEL OF POLITICAL INTERVENTION.

SRCE *WESTERN CANADIAN JOURNAL OF ANTHROPOLOGY, 1976, 6(3), 213-241.*

INDX MEXICAN AMERICAN, FEMALE, POLITICAL POWER, POLITICS, ETHNIC IDENTITY, CALIFORNIA, SOUTHWEST, EMPIRICAL

ABST WOMEN IN COMMUNITY LEADERSHIP POSITIONS IN TWO CALIFORNIA CITIES (34 MEXICAN AMERICANS, 98 ANGLOS) WERE INTERVIEWED TO DETERMINE (1) RESOURCES WHICH ALLOW THEM TO HAVE SOME EFFECT ON POLICY MAKING, (2) THEIR PARTICIPATION IN POLITICAL AFFAIRS WITHIN AND WITHOUT THE MAJORITY ETHNIC AND SEX GROUP, AND (3) THE POLITICAL NETWORK ESTABLISHED WITHIN THE COMMUNITY BY FEMALE LEADERS. SOME OBSERVATIONS MADE ARE: (1) WOMEN OF BOTH ETHNIC GROUPS BECOME COMMUNITY LEADERS WITH THE SUPPORT OF A FEMALE CONSTITUENCY; (2) ANGLO WOMEN GAIN INFLUENCE THROUGH INVOLVEMENT IN FEMALE VOLUNTARY ORGANIZATIONS CONCERNED WITH PUBLIC AFFAIRS, WHILE MEXICAN AMERICAN WOMEN DEPEND ON SUPPORT FROM INFORMAL SOLIDARITY GROUPS OF WOMEN WHO BELONG TO CIVIC ORGANIZATIONS WITH BOTH MALE AND FEMALE MEMBERS, AND FROM EGO-CENTRIC NETWORKS OF FEMALE CONTACTS; AND (3) WHEN INTER-ETHNIC POLITICAL ACTIVITIES OCCUR, CONTACT BETWEEN LEADERS OF THE TWO ETHNIC GROUPS IS LIMITED BY SEX. EXPLANATIONS FOR THESE PATTERNS OF SEX-LINKED POLITICAL BEHAVIOR ARE DISCUSSED IN TERMS OF (1) THE SEX ROLE DIFFERENTIATION FOUND IN EVERY SOCIETY WHICH RESULTS IN TWO SYSTEMS OF RESOURCE ACQUISITION AND DISTRIBUTION, ONE FOR MEN AND ANOTHER FOR WOMEN AND (2) THE ROLE OF VOLUNTEERISM IN THE DEVELOPMENT OF FEMALE LEADERS. IT IS CONCLUDED THAT WOMEN'S PARTICIPATION IN POLICY-MAKING IS DESTINED TO OCCUR AS PART OF A FEMALE MINORITY GROUP. CHANGES IN THE FUNDAMENTAL SOCIAL AND ECONOMIC INSTITUTIONS AND PATTERNS OF PERSONAL RELATIONS BETWEEN MEN AND WOMEN ARE REQUIRED TO DO OTHERWISE. 61 REFERENCES. (AUTHOR SUMMARY MODIFIED)

ACCN 000788

922 AUTH **KEEFE, S. E., CARLOS, M. L., & PADILLA, A. M.**

TITL THE MEXICAN AMERICAN EXTENDED FAMILY: A MENTAL HEALTH RESOURCE.

SRCE *PAPER PRESENTED AT THE SOUTHWESTERN ANTHROPOLOGICAL ASSOCIATION ANNUAL MEETING, SAN FRANCISCO, APRIL 1976.*

INDX EXTENDED FAMILY, MENTAL HEALTH, FAMILY STRUCTURE, MEXICAN AMERICAN, CULTURAL PLURALISM, FICTIVE KINSHIP, RESOURCE UTILIZATION, EMPIRICAL, PSYCHOTHERAPY, COPING MECHANISMS, SURVEY, CALIFORNIA, SOUTHWEST

ABST THE IMPORTANCE OF THE EXTENDED FAMILY AS COMPARED TO MENTAL HEALTH FACILITIES AND CURANDERISMO AS EXPLANATIONS FOR LOWER MENTAL HEALTH CLINIC USAGE BY MEXICAN AMERICANS IS DISCUSSED. SIX HUNDRED SIXTY-SIX MEXICAN AMERICAN (MA) FAMILIES, RESIDENTS OF URBAN AREAS IN THE SOUTHERN CALIFORNIA COUNTIES OF SANTA BARBARA AND VENTURA, WERE INTERVIEWED TO DETERMINE THEIR EXTENDED FAMILY CHARACTERISTICS AND USE OF MENTAL HEALTH RESOURCES. INTERPRETATION OF THE DESCRIPTIVE DATA SUPPORTS THE FOLLOWING CONCLUSIONS. (1) NATIVE MA (BORN IN U.S.) BEST FIT THE DESCRIPTION OF THE MA FAMILY SYSTEM FOUND IN THE LITERATURE— THEY HAVE MANY RELATIVES CLOSE BY WITH WHOM THEY VISIT FREQUENTLY AND RECIPROCALLY EXCHANGE GOODS AND SERVICES. WHILE IMMIGRANT MA'S (BORN IN MEXICO) ALSO HAVE RELATIVES NEARBY WHOM THEY VISIT OFTEN, THE AMOUNT OF KIN AND RECIPROCITY IS LOWER. (2) THERE IS A CLEAR PREFERENCE FOR INFORMAL METHODS OF DEALING WITH STRESS RATHER THAN RELIANCE ON PUBLIC AGENCIES BY MA FAMILIES. ALTHOUGH BOTH SEGMENTS OF THE MA POPULATION, NATIVE AND IMMIGRANT, APPEAR KNOWLEDGEABLE ABOUT LOCAL MENTAL HEALTH SOURCES AND THEIR LOCATION AND HAVE A POSITIVE ATTITUDE TOWARD THEIR

UTILIZATION, THEY PREFER OTHER SOURCES OF HELP DURING EMOTIONAL STRESS. (3) THE FAMILY DOCTOR AND A RELATIVE OR COMPADRE ARE SELECTED BY ALMOST HALF OF THE RESPONDENTS AS THE FIRST SOURCE FOR EMOTIONAL HELP. (4) IMMIGRANT MA'S, BECAUSE OF FEWER FAMILY SUPPORTS AND LACK OF TRADITIONAL CULTURAL RESOURCES, ARE THE MOST IN NEED OF AN EXPANSION OF MENTAL HEALTH TREATMENT ALTERNATIVES. SEVEN TABLES SUMMARIZE THE INTERVIEW DATA. 13 REFERENCES.

ACCN   000789

923 AUTH   **KEEFE, S. E., PADILLA, A. M., & CARLOS, M. L.**
    TITL   EMOTIONAL SUPPORT SYSTEMS IN TWO CULTURES: A COMPARISON OF MEXICAN AMERICANS AND ANGLO AMERICANS (OCCASIONAL PAPER NO. 7).
    SRCE   *LOS ANGELES: UNIVERSITY OF CALIFORNIA, SPANISH SPEAKING MENTAL HEALTH RESEARCH CENTER, 1978.*
    INDX   COMMUNITY, MENTAL HEALTH, MEXICAN AMERICAN, CROSS CULTURAL, EXTENDED FAMILY, ETHNIC IDENTITY, CULTURAL FACTORS, CURANDERISMO, HEALTH DELIVERY SYSTEMS, SURVEY, EMPIRICAL, CROSS GENERATIONAL, CALIFORNIA, SOUTHWEST, URBAN, RESOURCE UTILIZATION
    ABST   A SURVEY OF 1,006 ADULT RESIDENTS (666 MEXICAN AMERICANS AND 340 ANGLOS) OF THREE SOUTHERN CALIFORNIA CITIES REGARDING THEIR EMOTIONAL SUPPORT SYSTEMS IS PRESENTED. IN GENERAL, IT WAS FOUND THAT MEXICAN AMERICANS (MA) HAVE A PATTERN OF SEEKING MENTAL HEALTH CARE WHICH IS DIFFERENT FROM THAT OF ANGLOS AND WHICH IS MAINTAINED FROM GENERATION TO GENERATION. MA RELY PRIMARILY UPON THE EXTENDED FAMILY AMONG ALL SOURCES OF EMOTIONAL SUPPORT. KIN NETWORKS ESTABLISHED BY IMMIGRANTS ARE ENLARGED AND BECOME MORE INTEGRATED IN SUBSEQUENT GENERATIONS. IN CONTRAST, ANGLOS TEND TO RECOMMEND FRIENDS AS THE IDEAL SOURCE OF HELP FOR AN EMOTIONAL PROBLEM AND TEND TO TURN TO FRIENDS WHEN ACTUALLY CONFRONTED WITH A PROBLEM THEMSELVES. RELATIVES RANK HIGH, ESPECIALLY FOR ANGLOS WHO HAVE KIN NEARBY, BUT THEY NEVER SURPASS FRIENDS AS AN EMOTIONAL SUPPORT. BOTH MA AND ANGLOS PREFER TO EXHAUST THE POTENTIAL OF RELATIVES, FRIENDS, FAMILY PHYSICIAN, CLERGYMAN AND OTHERS BEFORE TURNING TO A MENTAL HEALTH CLINIC OR A PRIVATE THERAPIST. THIS DOES NOT APPEAR DUE TO LACK OF KNOWLEDGE OR CRITICISM OF MENTAL HEALTH SERVICES. DESPITE A SIMILAR PREFERENCE AND TENDENCY TO SEEK HELP ELSEWHERE, ANGLOS MAKE SIGNIFICANTLY GREATER USE OF MENTAL HEALTH CLINICS THAN MA. LACKING DATA SUPPORTING OTHER EXPLANATIONS, THIS APPEARS TO BE MAINLY THE RESULT OF INSTITUTIONAL POLICIES WHICH MAKE IT DIFFICULT FOR MA TO OBTAIN SERVICES. CHANGES IN THE LOCATION AND POLICIES OF MENTAL HEALTH

CENTERS SHOULD FACILITATE THEIR USE BY MEXICAN AMERICANS. 19 REFERENCES. (AUTHOR SUMMARY MODIFIED)

ACCN   000790

924 AUTH   **KEEFE, S. E., PADILLA, A. M., & CARLOS, M. L.**
    TITL   THE MEXICAN-AMERICAN EXTENDED FAMILY AS AN EMOTIONAL SUPPORT SYSTEM.
    SRCE   *HUMAN ORGANIZATION, 1979, 38(2), 144-152.*
    INDX   MEXICAN AMERICAN, MENTAL HEALTH, EXTENDED FAMILY, CALIFORNIA, SOUTHWEST, SURVEY, EMPIRICAL, FAMILY STRUCTURE, RESOURCE UTILIZATION, STRESS, COPING MECHANISMS, CULTURAL FACTORS, CROSS CULTURAL, ATTITUDES
    ABST   A THREE-YEAR SURVEY (1975-77) IN THREE SOUTHERN CALIFORNIA COMMUNITIES WAS CONDUCTED TO INVESTIGATE THE RELATIONSHIP BETWEEN FAMILY SUPPORT AND MENTAL HEALTH AMONG MEXICAN AMERICANS (MA) AND ANGLOS. THE RESULTS REVEALED A FUNDAMENTAL DIFFERENCE IN MA'S AND ANGLOS' FAMILY STRUCTURES. MA'S WERE MUCH MORE LIKELY TO HAVE A LARGE NUMBER OF KIN IN TOWN AND TO HAVE A WELL-INTEGRATED KIN GROUP ENCOMPASSING THREE OR MORE GENERATIONS. ANGLOS TENDED TO LIVE APART FROM THEIR EXTENDED FAMILIES. NEVERTHELESS, THIS DIFFERENCE DID NOT APPEAR TO HAVE MUCH EFFECT ON THE RESPONDENTS' SEEKING OF EMOTIONAL SUPPORT, FOR BOTH MA'S AND ANGLOS TENDED TO TURN TO RELATIVES FOR SUCH SUPPORT. WHAT PROVED TO BE SIGNIFICANT WAS ANGLOS' GREATER TENDENCY TO ALSO SEEK EMOTIONAL SUPPORT OUTSIDE THE FAMILY, WHILE MA'S TENDED TO RELY ON THE FAMILY AS THE ONLY SOURCE OF SUPPORT. THIS CLEARLY SUGGESTS THAN AN ABSENCE OR MALFUNCTION OF EXTENDED FAMILY SUPPORT IS PROBABLY MUCH MORE DISTRESSING TO MA'S THAN TO ANGLOS IN SIMILAR CIRCUMSTANCES. IT IS THEREFORE RECOMMENDED THAT THE ISOLATION AND STRESS EXPERIENCED BY MA'S WHO LACK SUPPORTIVE FAMILIES BE KEPT IN MIND WHEN TREATMENT IS NEEDED. 15 REFERENCES.

ACCN   001732

925 AUTH   **KELLER, A. B.**
    TITL   PSYCHOLOGICAL DETERMINANTS OF FAMILY SIZE IN A MEXICAN VILLAGE.
    SRCE   *MERRILL-PALMER QUARTERLY: BEHAVIOR AND DEVELOPMENT, 1973, 19(4), 289-299.*
    INDX   BIRTH CONTROL, FAMILY STRUCTURE, CULTURE, TAT, SEXUAL BEHAVIOR, FERTILITY, ACHIEVEMENT MOTIVATION, SEX ROLES, MEXICAN, MEXICO, EMPIRICAL, PERSONALITY ASSESSMENT, MALE, FEMALE
    ABST   DATA FROM INTERVIEWS AND PSYCHOLOGICAL TESTING WITH 65 COUPLES (22 COUPLES USED CONTRACEPTIVES; 43 DID NOT) LIVING IN A VILLAGE IN OAXACA, MEXICO, REVEALED PERSONALITY DIFFERENCES BETWEEN CONTRACEPTIVE USERS AND NONUSERS. INSTRUMENTS USED TO DIFFERENTIATE PERSONALITY CHARACTERISTICS WERE: (1) SEVERAL TRUE/FALSE ITEMS FROM THE SPANISH VERSION OF THE CALIFORNIA PSYCHOLOGICAL INVEN-

TORY, (2) TAT CARDS, AND (3) A CARD DRAW-ING SHOWING A MAN AND WOMAN EMBRAC-ING IN A VERTICAL POSITION. THE DEPENDENT MEASURES INCLUDED: (1) NEED FOR ACHIEVE-MENT, (2) EFFICACY, (3) NEED FOR EMOTIONAL SUPPORT, (4) SEXUAL RELATIONS, (5) PERCEP-TIONS OF OPPOSITE SEX, AND (6) IMPULSIVITY. RESULTS INDICATE: (1) BOTH MALE AND FE-MALE USERS HAD HIGHER SCORES ON FEEL-INGS OF EFFICACY AND ACHIEVEMENT NEED THAN NONUSERS; (2) FEMALE NONUSERS SCORED HIGHER IN NEED FOR EMOTIONAL CONTACT, WITH NO DIFFERENCE FOR MALES; (3) MALE USERS OBTAINED SIGNIFICANTLY HIGHER SCORES ON IMPULSIVITY THAN NON-USERS, A SURPRISING FINDING, WHILE FE-MALES SHOWED A SLIGHT OPPOSITE TREND; AND (4) FINDINGS ON ATTITUDES TOWARD SEXUAL RELATIONS AND EXPECTATIONS OF THE OPPOSITE SEX WERE NOT SIGNIFICANT. FINDINGS DO NOT SUPPORT THE OVERALL HY-POTHESIS THAT THE STRONGEST DIFFER-ENCES WOULD BE BETWEEN USERS WITH FEW CHILDREN AND NONUSERS WITH MANY CHIL-DREN WHILE THE TOTAL USER AND NONUSER GROUP DIFFERENCES WOULD BE WEAKER. EX-PLANATIONS FOR THESE UNEXPECTED FIND-INGS ARE PRESENTED. 14 REFERENCES.

ACCN   000791

926 AUTH   **KELLER, G. D.**
     TITL   THE SYSTEMATIC EXCLUSION OF THE LAN-GUAGE AND CULTURE OF BORICUAS, CHICA-NOS AND OTHER U.S. HISPANOS IN ELEMEN-TRY SPANISH GRAMMAR TEXTBOOKS PUBLISHED IN THE UNITED STATES.
     SRCE   *THE BILINGUAL REVIEW/LA REVISTA BILINGUE, 1974, 1(3), 227-235.*
     INDX   DISCRIMINATION, GRAMMAR, CULTURAL PLU-RALISM, EDUCATIONAL MATERIALS, CURRICU-LUM, BILINGUALISM, MEXICAN AMERICAN, PUERTO RICAN-M, REVIEW, ESSAY, LANGUAGE LEARNING, SPANISH SURNAMED
     ABST   A REVIEW OF TEN SPANISH GRAMMAR TEXT-BOOKS PUBLISHED BETWEEN 1967 AND 1974 EMPHASIZES THESE POINTS: (1) THE DIA-LOGUES AND READINGS IN THESE SPANISH GRAMMAR TEXTBOOKS DO NOT REFLECT THE EXISTENCE OF AN HISPANIC COMMUNITY IN THE U.S.; (2) THE VOCABULARY LISTS ARE GENERALLY EXCLUSIVE OF LEXICAL ITEMS COMMON TO SPANISH AS USED IN THE U.S.; (3) SYNTACTIC FORMS COMMONLY USED BY U.S. SPANISH SPEAKERS ARE GENERALLY NOT IN-CLUDED, RATHER EMPHASIS IS PLACED ON GRAMMARS CHARACTERISTIC ONLY OF CER-TAIN REGIONS OF THE SPANISH PENINSULA; AND (4) DIALOGUES TEND TO DEAL WITH SUB-JECT MATTER IRRELEVANT OR UNINTERESTING TO MOST CHICANO, BORICUA, OTHER HIS-PANIC, AND ANGLO STUDENTS. IT IS POSITED THAT MILLIONS OF AMERICAN STUDENTS HAVE BEEN INSTRUCTED IN SPANISH WITHOUT RE-ALIZING THAT THIS LANGUAGE IS THE MOTHER TONGUE OF OVER TEN MILLION FELLOW CITI-ZENS. SUGGESTIONS FOR CHANGE INCLUDE PROVIDING NEGATIVE FEEDBACK TO PUBLISH-ERS, INCREASING AWARENESS OF BILINGUAL-

ISM AS OFFICIAL POLICY IN MANY AREAS OF THE COUNTRY, AND MOST IMPORTANTLY, CHI-CANO AND BORICUA INVOLVEMNT IN WRITING SPANISH TEXTBOOKS RELEVANT TO THE UNITED STATES AND ITS SPANISH-SPEAKING POPULA-TION. 10 REFERENCES.

ACCN   000792

927 AUTH   **KELLER, G. D., & VAN HOOFT, K. S.**
     TITL   BILINGUALISM AND BILINGUAL EDUCATION IN THE UNITED STATES: A CHRONOLOGY FROM THE COLONIAL PERIOD TO 1976.
     SRCE   *JAMAICA, NEW YORK: BILINGUAL PRESS/EDI-TORIAL BILINGUE, 1976.*
     INDX   BILINGUALISM, BILINGUAL-BICULTURAL EDU-CATION, BILINGUAL-BICULTURAL PERSONNEL, EDUCATION, HISTORY, ESSAY, MEXICAN AMERI-CAN, SPANISH SURNAMED, FINANCING
     ABST   THE HISTORY OF BILINGUAL EDUCATION IN THE UNITED STATES IS DESCRIBED IN TERMS OF FIVE MAJOR PERIODS FROM THE COLONIAL PERIOD TO THE YEAR 1976. SPECIFIC LAWS, COURT DECISIONS, AND OTHER IMPORTANT EVENTS RELATED TO BILINGUAL EDUCATION AND ITS FINANCING ARE PRESENTED. THE CHRONOLOGY PROVIDES A SUCCINCT COM-PILATION OF THE SIGNIFICANT TRENDS AND EVENTS IN THE HISTORY OF BILINGUAL EDU-CATION IN THE U.S. EMPHASIZED ARE THE CHANGES WHICH CAUSED WIDESPREAD BI-LINGUAL EDUCATION IN THE COLONIAL PE-RIOD TO BE ALMOST COMPLETELY ABAN-DONED BY THE YEAR 1900, THE RENEWED INTEREST IN FOREIGN LANGUAGES IN THE 1950'S, AND THE INITIATION OF NEW BILIN-GUAL PROGRAMS IN THE 1960'S. 9 REFER-ENCES.

ACCN   000793

928 AUTH   **KELLY, E. T., & SPERANZA, K. A.**
     TITL   AN EXAMINATION OF SPANISH SPEAKING PA-TIENTS' SOURCES OF OVER-THE-COUNTER DRUG INFORMATION.
     SRCE   *DRUG INTELLIGENCE AND CLINICAL PHAR-MACY, 1978, 12, 169-171.*
     INDX   ADULTS, ATTITUDES, BILINGUAL, ECONOMIC FACTORS, EMPIRICAL, HEALTH, HEALTH EDU-CATION, PHYSICIANS, SES, URBAN, RURAL, EAST, PUERTO RICAN-M, MASS MEDIA
     ABST   TO INVESTIGATE OVER-THE-COUNTER DRUG INFORMATION SOURCES IN A LOW-INCOME SPANISH-SPEAKING URBAN POPULATION, A QUESTIONNAIRE SOUGHT SPANISH-SPEAKING PEOPLE'S PERCEPTIONS OF: (1) THE CREDI-BILITY AND ACCESSIBILITY OF HEALTH PROFESSIONALS AS DRUG INFORMATION SOURCES; AND (2) THE DESIRABILITY OF VARI-OUS MASS MEDIA FOR DRUG INFORMATION. THE SAMPLE CONSISTED OF 42 PUERTO RICAN RESPONDENTS IN A LARGE METROPOLITAN AREA AND A RURAL INDUSTRIAL POCKET IN THE NORTHEAST. THE QUESTIONNAIRES WERE CODED AND ANALYZED VIA KENDALL'S COEF-FICIENT OF CONCORDANCE. WITH A RANKING OF "1" INDICATING THE MOST DESIRABLE SOURCE OF INFORMATION, PROFESSIONALS WERE RANKED AS: PHYSICIANS = 1, NURSES = 2.5, AND PHARMACISTS = 2.5. RE-

SPONDENTS' MEAN RANKING OF ADVERTISING MEDIA WAS: TELEVISION = 1.6, RADIO = 2.2, NEWSPAPERS = 3.6, MAGAZINES = 3.7, AND BOOKS = 3.8. THE HIGH RANKING OF PHYSICIANS AS SOURCES OF DRUG INFORMATION IS TRACED TO THE WELFARE STATUS OF THE RESPONDENTS AND THE PRESENCE OF A HOSPITAL EMERGENCY ROOM IN ONE OF THE CENTRAL NEIGHBORHOODS. REGARDING MEDIA SOURCES, LOW RANKINGS FOR WRITTEN MEDIA ARE ATTRIBUTED TO THE SPANISH-SPEAKING PREFERENCE OF RESPONDENTS. IT IS CONCLUDED THAT THE MOST EFFICIENT APPROACH FOR PROVIDING DRUG INFORMATION TO THIS POPULATION VIA MEDIA WOULD BE TO RELY PRIMARILY ON RADIO AND TELEVISION. 6 REFERENCES.

ACCN   002379

929   AUTH   **KELLY, L. M.**
      TITL   COMMUNITY IDENTIFICATION AMONG SECOND GENERATION PUERTO RICANS: ITS RELATION TO OCCUPATIONAL SUCCESS (DOCTORAL DISSERTATION, FORDHAM UNIVERSITY, 1971).
      SRCE   *DISSERTATION ABSTRACTS INTERNATIONAL, 1971, 32(4), 2223A. (UNIVERSITY MICROFILMS NO. 71-26,977.)*
      INDX   EMPIRICAL, COMMUNITY, ETHNIC IDENTITY, ACCULTURATION, SES, JOB PERFORMANCE, OCCUPATIONAL ASPIRATIONS, SOCIAL MOBILITY, PUERTO RICAN-M, CROSS GENERATIONAL, MALE, NEW YORK, EAST, LABOR FORCE, CULTURAL CHANGE
      ABST   TO IDENTIFY FACTORS RELATED TO VARYING DEGREES OF OCCUPATIONAL SUCCESS AND TO GUIDE THOSE WHO DETERMINE POLICY AND PROGRAMS ASSISTING THE MOBILITY OF 1ST AND 2ND GENERATION PUERTO RICANS, AN EXPLORATORY STUDY WAS CONDUCTED AMONG 30 MARRIED PUERTO RICAN MEN RESIDING IN BROOKLYN. THE SUBJECTS REPRESENTED THREE LEVELS OF OCCUPATIONAL SUCCESS: SUCCESSFUL, STABLE, AND UNSUCCESSFUL. THE EVIDENCE SUGGESTS THAT OCCUPATIONAL SUCESS DOES NOT NECESSIATE A BREAK WITH ONE'S ETHNIC COMMUNITY. AMONG THE 2ND GENERATION, THE SUCCESSFUL ARE LIKELY TO RETAIN A CLOSE RELATIONSHIP WITH THE PUERTO RICAN COMMUNITY, TO EXPRESS PRIDE IN THEIR PUERTO RICAN IDENTITY, AND TO SEEK TO PERPETUATE IT IN THEIR CHILDREN. AS THE OCCUPATIONALLY STABLE ACQUIRE SKILLS FOR FUTURE MOBILITY, THEY BEGIN TO FOLLOW THIS SAME PATTERN. THE RESULTS FURTHER SUGGEST THAT MUCH OF WHAT HAS BEEN WRITTEN IN INDUSTRIAL SOCIOLOGY IS RELEVANT FOR UNDERSTANDING THE PUERTO RICANS IN THE WORK FORCE. AS ETHNIC IDENTITY CONTINUES INTO THE 2ND GENERATION, IT CEASES TO BE IDENTIFIED WITH A SPECIFIC GEOGRAPHICAL LOCALITY. INSTEAD, IT EVOLVES INTO A STRONG SENSE OF IDENTITY WITH PUERTO RICAN INTERESTS, MAINTAINED THROUGH SOCIAL CONTACTS WITH OTHER PUERTO RICANS AND AN APPRECIATION FOR CERTAIN ASPECTS OF ONE'S CULTURAL HERITAGE. 126 REFERENCES.

ACCN   000795

930   AUTH   **KENT, J., & RUIZ, R. A.**
      TITL   IQ AND READING SCORES AMONG ANGLO, BLACK, AND CHICANO THIRD- AND SIX-GRADE CHILDREN.
      SRCE   *HISPANIC JOURNAL OF BEHAVIORAL SCIENCES, 1979, 1(3), 271-277.*
      INDX   MEXICAN AMERICAN, CROSS CULTURAL, CHILDREN, EMPIRICAL, KANSAS, MIDWEST, SES, SCHOLASTIC ACHIEVEMENT, INTELLIGENCE TESTING, READING, ACHIEVEMENT TESTING, EDUCATIONAL ASSESSMENT, URBAN
      ABST   THIS STUDY EXAMINED THE RELATIONSHIP BETWEEN MEAN IQ SCORES AND MEAN SCHOLASTIC ACHIEVEMENT SCORES AS MEASURED BY GRADE-LEVEL EQUIVALENTS IN READING AMONG 137 ANGLO, BLACK, AND CHICANO ELEMENTARY SCHOOL CHILDREN IN A MIDWESTERN METROPOLIS. ALL CHILDREN BELONGED TO THE LOWEST SOCIOECONOMIC CLASS, RESIDED IN THE SAME INNER-CITY NEIGHBORHOOD, AND ATTENDED THE SAME PAROCHIAL SCHOOL SYSTEM. THE DATA SUGGEST THAT FROM THE THIRD TO THE SIXTH GRADE, THERE IS A PROCESS OF INTELLECTUAL DECLINE AMONG BLACKS AND A GRADUAL EROSION OF READING ABILITY AMONG BOTH, BLACKS AND CHICANOS. THE MAJOR FINDING WAS THAT IQ PREDICTS ACHIEVEMENT BEST FOR ANGLOS (R .65), FAIRLY WELL FOR BLACKS (R .57), BUT NOT AT ALL FOR CHICANOS (R .29 TO .09, NS). THEREFORE, CAUTION SHOULD BE EXERCISED IN MAKING EDUCATIONAL DECISIONS FOR CHICANOS ON THESE OR SIMILAR GROUP-ADMINISTERED, PAPER-AND-PENCIL TESTS OF INTELLIGENCE AND ACHIEVEMENT. 28 REFERENCES. (JOURNAL ABSTRACT MODIFIED)

ACCN   001771

931   AUTH   **KERNAN, J. B., & SCHKADE, L. L.**
      TITL   A CROSS CULTURAL ANALYSIS OF STIMULUS SAMPLING.
      SRCE   *ADMINISTRATIVE SCIENCE QUARTERLY, 1972, 17(3), 351-358.*
      INDX   CROSS CULTURAL, COGNITIVE STYLE, MEXICAN, COLLEGE STUDENTS, EMPIRICAL, PERSONALITY, PERSONALITY ASSESSMENT
      ABST   THIS EXPERIMENTAL STUDY INVESTIGATED THE AMOUNT OF INFORMATION USED BY 32 ANGLO AMERICAN AND 61 MEXICAN COLLEGE STUDENTS IN MAKING DECISIONS. BASED ON INFORMATION THEORY AND THE SHANNON-WEAVER MEASURE OF INFORMATION TOOL, THE SEARCH BEHAVIORS OF THE SUBJECTS WERE COMPARED THROUGH AN ANALYSIS OF THE ABSOLUTE AND RELATIVE AMOUNT OF INFORMATION SAMPLED, THE EFFECTIVENESS OF SEARCH HEURISTICS, AND SEARCH EFFICIENCY. SIGNIFICANT DIFFERENCES WERE FOUND, SUGGESTING THE MEDIATING EFFECT OF CULTURE ON SEARCH STYLE. CROSS CULTURAL PERSONALITY DIFFERENCES WERE ALSO MEASURED AND FOUND TO BE CONSISTENT WITH THE SUBJECTS' RESEARCH STYLE. SOME

FINDINGS WERE: (1) THE TENDENCY OF MEXI-CANS TO USE A SMALLER AMOUNT OF INFOR-MATION THAN NORTH AMERICANS; (2) THE GREATER RELIANCE OF MEXICANS ON THEIR INFERENTIAL ABILITY AND INFORMATION HAN-DLING HEURISTICS THAN NORTH AMERICANS; AND (3) THE MEXICANS' GREATER EFFICIENCY IN INFORMATION SAMPLING AS COMPLEXITY OF THE SEARCH ENVIRONMENT INCREASED. THE IMPLICATIONS OF THESE FINDINGS ON THE INTERACTION BETWEEN PERSONS OF DIF-FERENT CULTURES, ESPECIALLY IN BUSINESS, POLICY MAKING, AND RESEARCH, ARE DIS-CUSSED. 16 REFERENCES.

ACCN   000796

932 AUTH   **KERSHNER, J. R.**
    TITL   ETHNIC GROUP DIFFERENCES IN CHILDREN'S ABILITY TO REPRODUCE DIRECTION AND ORI-ENTATION.
    SRCE   *JOURNAL OF SOCIAL PSYCHOLOGY, 1972, 88(1), 3-13.*
    INDX   CROSS CULTURAL, COGNITIVE DEVELOPMENT, MEXICAN AMERICAN, CHILDREN, LANGUAGE COMPREHENSION, LINGUISTIC COMPETENCE, CALIFORNIA, SOUTHWEST, EMPIRICAL, COG-NITIVE STYLE
    ABST   ETHNOGRAPHIC OBSERVATIONS OF CHICANO AND ANGLO CHILDREN INDICATE THAT THE TWO GROUPS DIFFER QUALITATIVELY IN THEIR ADAPTIVE RESPONSES TO SOCIAL SITUA-TIONS. THE CHICANO CHILDREN SHOW AN IN-TEREST IN THE DETAILS AND ORGANIZATION OF THEIR SPATIAL SURROUNDINGS, WHEREAS THE BEHAVIOR OF THE ANGLOS IS CHARAC-TERIZED BY SPATIAL REMOTENESS AND THE TENDENCY TO SEEK OUT VERBAL INTERAC-TIONS WITH PEOPLE RATHER THAN ISOLATED PLAY. IT IS HYPOTHESIZED THAT CHICANO CHILDREN ARE BETTER THAN ANGLO CHIL-DREN IN CONSERVING MULTIPLE SPATIAL RE-LATIONS AND THAT THEIR SUPERIORITY IN DEALING WITH SPATIAL RELATIONS CAN BE EX-PLAINED AS A FORM OF FUNCTIONAL COM-PENSATION FOR RELATIVELY LOWER ACHIEVE-MENT IN LANGUAGE. EIGHT CHICANO AND EIGHT ANGLO CHILDREN WERE COMPARED IN SPATIAL AND LANGUAGE ABILITIES. THE CHIL-DREN LIVE IN THE SAME COMMUNITY, ATTEND THE SAME SCHOOL, REPRESENT A SIMILAR SOCIAL CLASS, AND COME FROM FAMILIES WHO PROVIDE AN EQUAL AMOUNT OF STIMU-LATION AND OPPORTUNITY FOR FREE SELF-DI-RECTED MOVEMENT EXPERIENCES. RESULTS INDICATE THAT THE CHICANO CHILDREN WERE BETTER IN SPATIAL ABILITY AND POORER IN LANGUAGE COMPREHENSION, SUPPORTING THE CATEGORIZATION OF THE CHICANOS AS "ANALYTIC-SPATIAL" AND THE ANGLOS AS "GLOBAL-VERBAL" IN COGNITIVE STYLE. THE FINDINGS WERE INTERPRETED AS DEMON-STRATING ETHNIC GROUP DIFFERENCES IN IN-FORMATION PROCESSING STRATEGIES AND THE POLARITY OF VERBAL AND SPATIAL SKILLS IN SOME CHILDREN. THE POSSIBLE INFLU-ENCE OF INNATE AND EXPERIENTIAL FACTORS IN PRODUCING THE RESULTS IS DISCUSSED. 13 REFERENCES.

ACCN   000797

933 AUTH   **KESTON, M. J., & JIMENEZ, C.**
    TITL   A STUDY OF THE PERFORMANCE ON ENGLISH AND SPANISH EDITIONS OF THE STANFORD BI-NET INTELLIGENCE TEST BY SPANISH-AMERI-CAN CHILDREN.
    SRCE   *JOURNAL OF GENETIC PSYCHOLOGY, 1954, 85(2), 263-269.*
    INDX   TEST RELIABILITY, TEST VALIDITY, STANFORD-BINET INTELLIGENCE TEST, LINGUISTIC COM-PETENCE, GRAMMAR, SEMANTICS, ACCULTUR-ATION, SCHOLASTIC ACHIEVEMENT, CULTURAL FACTORS, EMPIRICAL, CHILDREN, MEXICAN AMERICAN, INTELLIGENCE TESTING, BILIN-GUALISM, BILINGUAL, NEW MEXICO, SOUTH-WEST
    ABST   THE ENGLISH AND SPANISH TRANSLATIONS OF THE STANFORD-BINET INTELLIGENCE TEST WERE ADMINISTERED TO 50 BILINGUAL CHIL-DREN IN AN EFFORT TO DETERMINE THE MOST ACCURATE IQ TEST MEASURE FOR THESE CHILDREN. THE SUBJECTS WERE COMPOSED OF SPANISH AMERICAN CHILDREN IN THE FOURTH GRADE, DRAWN FROM FIVE SCHOOLS IN ALBUQUERQUE, NEW MEXICO. ONE FORM OF THE TEST WAS TRANSLATED INTO SPANISH BY A PROFESSOR FROM SPAIN. THE FINDINGS INDICATE THAT: (1) IF THE STANFORD-BINET TEST IS GOING TO BE USED, THE ENGLISH VERSION GIVES A FAIRER AND MORE ACCU-RATE ASSESSMENT THAN THE SPANISH VER-SION; (2) BILINGUAL CHILDREN ARE ABLE TO PERFORM BETTER IN THE LANGUAGE IN WHICH THEY HAVE HAD FORMAL INSTRUCTION; (3) THE DEVELOPMENT IN THE USE OF THE SPAN-ISH LANGUAGE BY THESE CHILDREN CEASED WHEN THEY ENTERED GRADE SCHOOL AND BEGAN THEIR FORMAL EDUCATION; (4) THE RANGE AND VARIABILITY OF ENGLISH SCORES ARE GREATER THAN THE RANGE AND VARI-ABILITY OF SPANISH SCORES; (5) BECAUSE OF THE SPANISH DIALECT OF THESE CHILDREN, THE SPANISH VERSION, AS TRANSLATED BY A SPANIARD, IS AN UNFAIR MEASURE OF THEIR INTELLECTUAL ABILITIES; (6) THE ENGLISH VERSION OF THE TEST IS ALSO UNFAIR BE-CAUSE OF ITS PRESENT LANGUAGE DIFFICUL-TIES; (7) THE CORRELATION BETWEEN SCHOOL GRADES AND IQ IS HIGHER FOR THE ENGLISH VERSION THAN FOR THE SPANISH VERSION OF THE TESTS; AND (8) BEFORE EFFECTIVE RE-SEARCH IN THIS AREA MAY PROCEED, A TRANSLATION OF THE STANFORD-BINET TEST THAT IS ADAPTED TO THIS REGION, OR THE DE-VELOPMENT OF A VALID INTELLIGENCE TEST FOR THESE CHILDREN, IS NECESSARY. 15 REF-ERENCES.

ACCN   000798

934 AUTH   **KHATON, O. M., & CARRIERA, R. P.**
    TITL   AN ATTITUDE STUDY OF MINORITY ADOLES-CENTS TOWARD MENTAL HEALTH.
    SRCE   *JOURNAL OF YOUTH AND ADOLESCENCE, 1972, 1(2), 131-141.*
    INDX   MENTAL HEALTH, PSYCHOPATHOLOGY, RE-SOURCE UTILIZATION, DEVIANCE, CROSS CUL-TURAL, MEXICAN AMERICAN, ADOLESCENTS,

EMPIRICAL, ATTITUDES, MALE, FEMALE, INDIANA, MIDWEST, SEX COMPARISON

ABST THE RESULTS OF AN ATTITUDINAL SURVEY ON MENTAL HEALTH SERVICES AND MENTAL ILLNESS AMONG 103 JUNIOR AND SENIOR INDIANA HIGH SCHOOL STUDENTS ARE PRESENTED. OVERALL FINDINGS INDICATED THAT PSYCHIATRIC KNOWLEDGE EXISTS AT A RELATIVELY HIGH LEVEL OF SOPHISTICATION IN THE BLACK AND SPANISH SURNAME POPULATION. MORE SPECIFIC FINDINGS WERE: (1) BLACK STUDENTS WERE MODERATELY SOPHISTICATED AND MORE KNOWLEDGEABLE THAN THEIR SPANISH COUNTERPARTS; (2) FEMALES RESPOND MORE INSIGHTFULLY THAN MALES; (3) OLDER BLACK FEMALES APPEAR MOST INSIGHTFUL; AND (4) SPANISH MALES SEEM LEAST KNOWLEDGEABLE ABOUT MENTAL HEALTH SERVICES. IN GENERAL, MEMBERSHIP IN A MINORITY GROUP HAS NO SIGNIFICANT RELATIONSHIP TO MENTAL HEALTH ATTITUDES WHEN KNOWLEDGE IS AVAILABLE. THE FINDINGS SEEM TO INDICATE THAT INSIGHT AND THE CAPACITY TO UTILIZE PSYCHIATRIC TREATMENT PROBABLY DEPEND MORE ON THE INDIVIDUAL THAN ON CULTURAL FACTORS. IT IS POSITED THAT MENTAL HEALTH SERVICES WOULD BE WELCOMED AND UTILIZED IF MADE AVAILABLE TO MINORITY GROUP ADOLESCENTS. 12 REFERENCES. (AUTHOR SUMMARY MODIFIED)

ACCN 000799

935 AUTH **KIEV, A.**

TITL CURANDERISMO: MEXICAN-AMERICAN FOLK PSYCHIATRY.

SRCE *NEW YORK: FREE PRESS, 1968.*

INDX FOLK MEDICINE, CURANDERISMO, PSYCHOTHERAPY, MEXICAN AMERICAN, PSYCHOPATHOLOGY, HISTORY, REVIEW, TEXAS, SOUTHWEST, RELIGION, BOOK

ABST CURANDERISMO IS A FORM OF FOLK PSYCHIATRY THAT INCORPORATES ELEMENTS FROM BOTH SIXTEENTH CENTURY EUROPEAN AND MAYAN-AZTEC MEDICINE. INTERVIEWS WITH FOUR CURANDEROS IN SAN ANTONIO, TEXAS, CONCERNING THEIR PRACTICES AND CLIENTS REVEAL THAT CULTURAL FACTORS FREQUENTLY DETERMINE THE ROLE OF THE SICK PERSON, THE NATURE OF ILLNESS, AND THE MODALITIES OF TREATMENT. TO THE MEXICAN AMERICAN, ILLNESS IS RELATED TO THE PATIENT'S LIFE, HIS INTERPERSONAL RELATIONSHIPS, HIS COMMUNITY, AND HIS RELIGION. ILLNESS IS NOT CONSIDERED A CHANCE EVENT, AS IT IS IN ANGLO AMERICAN CULTURE. CURANDERISMO IS A TRADITIONAL FORM OF PSYCHOLOGY WHICH SHARES MANY STRIKING SIMILARITIES WITH CONTEMPORARY PSYCHOTHERAPY. FOLK DISEASES SUCH AS SUSTO (FRIGHT), EMBRUJADO (BEWITCHMENT), AND MAL OJO (EVIL EYE) STEM EITHER FROM PHYSICAL CAUSES OR FROM PSYCHOLOGICAL CONFLICTS AND ARE TREATED BY THE CURANDERO WHO PERMITS CONFESSION, ENCOURAGES ACCEPTANCE OF SUFFERING, AND PRESCRIBES VARIOUS MEDICINAL HERBS AND OTHER THERAPEUTIC AIDS. CURANDERISMO IS SUCCESSFUL IN MEXICAN AMERICAN SOCI-

ETY BECAUSE IT OFFERS SECURITY THROUGH ADHERENCE TO TRADITIONAL VALUES, REDUCTION OF ANXIETY THROUGH CONFESSION, AND ACTIVE INVOLVEMENT IN THE THERAPEUTIC PROCESS. 103 REFERENCES.

ACCN 000800

936 AUTH **KIEV, A.**

TITL PRIMITIVE RELIGIOUS RITES AND BEHAVIOR: CLINICAL CONSIDERATIONS.

SRCE *INTERNATIONAL PSYCHIATRY CLINICS, 1969, 5(4), 119-131.*

INDX RELIGION, ROLE EXPECTATIONS, CURANDERISMO, FOLK MEDICINE, ESSAY, MEXICAN AMERICAN, PSYCHOTHERAPY, PSYCHOPATHOLOGY, STRESS, CULTURAL FACTORS

ABST PARTICIPATION IN RELIGIOUS GROUPS SUCH AS THE AMERICAN INDIAN PEYOTE CULTS AND THE PENTECOSTAL SECTS PROVIDES A FORM OF SOCIAL INTEGRATION FOR INDIVIDUALS IN ANOMIC, STRESSFUL, AND CHANGING SITUATIONS. THESE GROUPS PERMIT SOCIAL ACCEPTANCE FOR EVERYONE AND AFFORD SOCIALLY ACCEPTABLE METHODS FOR RELEASING SUPPRESSED EMOTIONS AND FRUSTRATIONS. A DISCUSSION OF THE PSYCHIATRIC CLASSIFICATION OF NORMAL AND ABNORMAL BEHAVIOR SUGGESTS THAT TO AVOID MISINTERPRETATION, THE PSYCHIATRIST MUST EXAMINE THE BELIEFS OF NONPATIENTS OF THE SAME CULTURAL BACKGROUND. SPIRIT POSSESSIONS, PSYCHONOXIOUS PROCESSES, AND FOLK SYNDROMES SUCH AS BEWITCHMENT, FRIGHT, SORCERY, ANGRY SPIRITS, AND EVIL EYE ARE EXAMINED. IT IS CONCLUDED THAT PARTICIPATION IN PRIMITIVE RELIGIOUS RITES DERIVES FROM A VARIETY OF MOTIVES AND MAY HAVE MANY BENEFICIAL EFFECTS. PARTICIPATION IN THESE RITUALS IS PROBABLY MOST HELPFUL FOR NEUROTIC PATIENTS, FOR THOSE IN BORDERLINE STATES, AND PERHAPS FOR PATIENTS WHO ARE SUFFERING FROM CHRONIC SCHIZOPHRENIC ILLNESSES AND WHO THEREFORE BENEFIT FROM THE INTEGRATION INTO GROUP ACTIVITIES. IT IS NOT AS BENEFICIAL FOR PEOPLE WITH ACUTE PSYCHOTIC ILLNESSES OR ACUTE ORGANIC ILLNESSES WHEN THE ILLNESS IS NOT RECOGNIZED BY THE MEMBERS OF THE GROUPS. 24 REFERENCES.

ACCN 000801

937 AUTH **KIEV, A.**

TITL TRANSCULTURAL PSYCHIATRY.

SRCE *NEW YORK: FREE PRESS, 1972.*

INDX PSYCHOPATHOLOGY, PSYCHOSIS, NEUROSIS, DEPRESSION, ANXIETY, ACCULTURATION, STRESS, PSYCHOSOCIAL ADJUSTMENT, CULTURAL FACTORS, MIGRATION, URBAN, CULTURE, IMAGERY, SCHIZOPHRENIA, FOLK MEDICINE, MENTAL HEALTH, HEALTH, CURANDERISMO, RESEARCH METHODOLOGY, THEORETICAL, ESSAY, BOOK

ABST FORMULATING THE BOUNDARIES OF TRANSCULTURAL PSYCHIATRY, ASSESSING THE CURRENT STATE OF KNOWLEDGE IN THIS FIELD, OUTLINING FEASIBLE AREAS OF FURTHER RE-

SEARCH, AND SPECIFYING PRIORITIES AND NEEDS IN THE DEVELOPING WORLD ARE THE PRIMARY OBJECTIVES OF THIS BOOK. THE FOLLOWING TOPICS ARE DISCUSSED: (1) THEORETICAL CONSIDERATIONS; (2) THE PROBLEM OF NORMALCY AND ABNORMALCY; (3) THE EFFECT OF CULTURE ON PSYCHIATRIC DISORDERS; (4) CULTURE-BOUND DISORDERS; (5) PRE-SCIENTIFIC MEDICINE AND PSYCHIATRY; (6) THE EPIDEMIOLOGY OF PSYCHIATRIC DISORDER IN DEVELOPING COUNTRIES; AND (7) INTRODUCING PSYCHIATRIC PROGRAMS TO DEVELOPING COUNTRIES. IT IS CONCLUDED THAT CERTAIN GUIDELINES NEED TO BE FOLLOWED IN FORMULATING PSYCHIATRIC PROGRAMS IN WHICH THE TREATMENT GOALS MUST BE FORMULATED WITHIN THE CONTEXT OF CULTURAL EXPECTATIONS OF THE HOST COUNTRY.

ACCN   000802

938 AUTH   **KILLIAN, L. R.**

TITL   WISC, ILLINOIS TEST OF PSYCHOLINGUISTIC ABILITIES AND BENDER VISUAL-MOTOR GESTALT TEST PERFORMANCE OF SPANISH AMERICAN KINDERGARTEN AND FIRST GRADE SCHOOL CHILDREN.

SRCE   *JOURNAL OF CONSULTING AND CLINICAL PSYCHOLOGY, 1971, 37(1), 38-43.*

INDX   WISC, ITPA, BENDER VISUAL-MOTOR GESTALT TEST, CROSS CULTURAL, CHILDREN, BILINGUALISM, SPANISH SURNAMED, INTELLIGENCE TESTING, LEARNING DISABILITIES, LINGUISTIC COMPETENCE, COGNITIVE STYLE, SCHOLASTIC ACHIEVEMENT

ABST   TO EXPLORE FOR COGNITIVE DEFICITS WHICH MIGHT ACCOUNT FOR THE POOR SCHOLASTIC PERFORMANCE OF SPANISH AMERICAN (SA) CHILDREN, 84 STUDENTS (INCLUDING ANGLO AMERICAN (AA) MONOLINGUALS AND SA MONOLINGUALS AND BILINGUALS) WERE ADMINISTERED A BATTERY OF THREE TESTS: THE WISC, ILLINOIS TEST OF PSYCHOLINGUISTIC ABILITIES, AND BENDER VISUAL-MOTOR GESTALT TEST. THE COMPARISON OF TEST RESULTS FOR THE TWO SA LANGUAGE GROUPS SUGGESTS THAT BILINGUALISM PER SE MAY NOT BE A GREAT FACTOR IN CAUSING POOR TEST PERFORMANCE. PROBABLY OF MORE IMPORTANCE ARE POVERTY, RESTRICTION OF EXPERIENCE, AND DIFFERENT VALUE SYSTEMS. IT IS SUGGESTED THAT REMEDIAL PROGRAMS FOR SA PRIMARY SCHOOL CHILDREN NEED TO EMPHASIZE COMPREHENSION OF MEANINGFUL MATERIAL PRESENTED SEQUENTIALLY THROUGH BOTH AUDITORY AND VISUAL CHANNELS. IT IS FURTHER SUGGESTED THAT PERHAPS THE SOURCE OF VARIANCE IN THE ACHIEVEMENT OF SA CHILDREN RESIDES IN THE ATTITUDINAL, MOTIVATION, AND/OR PERSONALITY REALM. 11 REFERENCES.

ACCN   000803

939 AUTH   **KIMBALL, W. L.**

TITL   PARENT AND FAMILY INFLUENCES ON ACADEMIC ACHIEVEMENT AMONG MEXICAN-AMERICAN STUDENTS (DOCTORAL DISSERTATION, UNIVERSITY OF CALIFORNIA, LOS ANGELES, 1968).

SRCE   *DISSERTATION ABSTRACTS INTERNATIONAL, 1968, 29(6), 1965A. (UNIVERSITY MICROFILMS NO. 68-16,550.)*

INDX   SCHOLASTIC ACHIEVEMENT, MEXICAN AMERICAN, CHILDREN, ADOLESCENTS, CHILDREARING PRACTICES, ROLE EXPECTATIONS, EDUCATION, ATTITUDES, URBAN, CROSS CULTURAL, PARENTAL INVOLVEMENT, ADOLESCENTS, SES, CULTURAL FACTORS, FAMILY STRUCTURE, SCHOLASTIC ASPIRATIONS, EMPIRICAL

ABST   MEXICAN AMERICANS (MA) AS A GROUP HAVE CONSIDERABLE DIFFICULTIES WITH SCHOOL ACHIEVEMENT, AND NOT ENOUGH IS KNOWN ABOUT THE DETERMINANTS OF SCHOOL PERFORMANCE OF THESE STUDENTS. THIS STUDY CONTRIBUTES TO THE UNDERSTANDING OF SCHOOL ACHIEVEMENT IN THIS GROUP BY INVESTIGATING HOW THE SCHOOL ACHIEVEMENT OF 1,457 URBAN NINTH-GRADE STUDENTS FROM EIGHT CALIFORNIA JUNIOR HIGH SCHOOLS (899 MEXICAN AMERICAN, 558 ANGLOS) IS DIFFERENTIATED BY SEVERAL INDEPENDENT VARIABLES: PARENTAL INFLUENCES SUCH AS TALK ABOUT SCHOOL; PARENTAL EDUCATION AND FAMILY MOBILITY; CULTURAL STATUS; AND PERCENT OF ANGLO STUDENTS AT SCHOOL. THE DEPENDENT VARIABLES WERE VARIOUS MEASURES OF ACADEMIC ACHIEVEMENT: SCHOOL GRADES AT END OF LAST SEMESTER, AND PERFORMANCE ON STANDARDIZED READING COMPREHENSION AND GENERAL ABILITY (IQ) TESTS. FINDINGS PROVIDED CONSIDERABLE SUPPORT FOR THE PREDICTION OF DIRECT PARENTAL INFLUENCES ON ACHIEVEMENT, PRIMARILY THROUGH PARENTAL EDUCATIONAL ASPIRATIONS FOR THEIR CHILD. THIS VARIABLE HAD THE STRONGEST RELATIONSHIPS TO STUDENT ACHIEVEMENT IN COMPARISON WITH PERSONAL IDENTITY, BACKGROUND, FAMILY STRUCTURE, SOCIAL STATUS AND ETHNICITY. AN UNEXPECTED FINDING WAS THE RELATIVELY HIGH ACHIEVEMENT OF THE MA STUDENTS BORN IN MEXICO. LITTLE RELATIONSHIP WITH SCHOOL ACHIEVEMENT WAS FOUND FOR SEX, AGE, BIRTH ORDER IN FAMILY, AND FAMILY SIZE. 122 REFERENCES. (AUTHOR ABSTRACT MODIFIED)

ACCN   000804

940 AUTH   **KING, L. W., COTLER, S. B., & PATTERSON, K.**

TITL   BEHAVIOR MODIFICATION CONSULTATION IN A MEXICAN AMERICAN SCHOOL: A CASE STUDY.

SRCE   *AMERICAN JOURNAL OF COMMUNITY PSYCHOLOGY, 1975, 3(3), 229-235.*

INDX   BEHAVIOR MODIFICATION, CHILDREN, CULTURAL FACTORS, EDUCATION, EMPIRICAL, MEXICAN AMERICAN, PROGRAM EVALUATION, SES, SPANISH SURNAMED, CALIFORNIA, SOUTHWEST, EDUCATIONAL COUNSELING

ABST   FOLLOWING CONSULTATION BY TWO PSYCHOLOGISTS IN AN ELEMENTARY SCHOOL POPULATED PRIMARILY BY MEXICAN AMERICAN STUDENTS, ABSENTEEISM WAS CHOSEN AS THE FIRST PROBLEM AREA REQUIRING IMPROVEMENT. THE SUBJECTS WERE 75 STU-

DENTS, GRADES 1 THROUGH 6, SELECTED ON THE BASIS OF THEIR FIRST-SEMESTER ATTENDANCE RECORD. THE 50 MOST FREQUENT NON-ATTENDERS WERE INCLUDED IN THE SAMPLE. A BETWEEN-GROUPS EXPERIMENTAL DESIGN, INVOLVING BOTH THE SAMPLE STUDENTS AND THEIR PARENTS, WAS USED TO EVALUATE THE EFFECT OF CONTINGENT REWARDS ON THE STUDENTS' ATTENDANCE. ANALYSIS OF THE DATA SHOWED THAT ALTHOUGH BOTH STUDENTS AND PARENTS RECEIVED SELECTIVE REWARDS, THERE WAS NO IMPROVEMENT IN ATTENDANCE. THESE RESULTS ARE DISCUSSED IN TERMS OF (1) A MORE THOROUGH BEHAVIOR ANALYSIS OF THE ABSENTEEISM PROBLEM, (2) METHODOLOGICAL RESTRAINTS OF A BETWEEN-GROUPS EXPERIMENTAL DESIGN, (3) THE NEED FOR CONSULTANTS TO BE MORE FAMILIAR WITH THE COMMUNITY IN WHICH THEY WORK, AND (4) THE SUCCESS OF THE LOCAL SCHOOL PSYCHOLOGIST IN IMPLEMENTING BEHAVIOR MODIFICATION PROGRAMS. 10 REFERENCES. (JOURNAL ABSTRACT MODIFIED)

ACCN   002670

941 AUTH   **KIRK, S. A.**
     TITL   ETHNIC DIFFERENCES IN PSYCHOLINGUISTIC ABILITIES.
     SRCE   *EXCEPTIONAL CHILDREN, 1972, 39(2), 112-118.*
     INDX   LINGUISTICS, COGNITIVE DEVELOPMENT, LANGUAGE ASSESSMENT, CROSS CULTURAL, CULTURAL FACTORS, MEMORY, CHILDREN, PERCEPTION, LINGUISTIC COMPETENCE, REVIEW, ITPA, MEXICAN AMERICAN, CHILDREARING PRACTICES
     ABST   THE RESULTS OF SEVERAL RESEARCH STUDIES ON THE PSYCHOLINGUISTIC ABILITIES, AS MEASURED BY THE ILLINOIS TEST OF PSYCHOLINGUISTIC ABILITIES OF BLACKS, INDIANS, AND MEXICAN AMERICANS ARE SUMMARIZED. BLACK CHILDREN APPEARED TO HAVE SUPERIOR ABILITY (AS COMPARED TO THEIR OTHER ABILITIES AND TO OTHER ETHNIC GROUPS) IN SHORT-TERM AUDITORY SEQUENTIAL MEMORY, WHILE INDIAN AND MEXICAN AMERICAN CHILDREN APPEARED TO HAVE SUPERIOR ABILITY IN SHORT-TERM VISUAL SEQUENTIAL MEMORY. IT IS HYPOTHESIZED THAT ETHNIC GROUP DIFFERENCES MAY BE ACCOUNTED FOR BY DIFFERENT CHILD-REARING PRACTICES AMONG THE ETHNIC GROUPS. 9 REFERENCES. (JOURNAL ABSTRACT MODIFIED)
     ACCN   000805

942 AUTH   **KIRK, S. A., VON ISSER, A., & ELKINS, J.**
     TITL   ETHNIC DIFFERENCES IN HEADSTART CHILDREN.
     SRCE   *JOURNAL OF CLINICAL CHILD PSYCHOLOGY, 1977, 6, 91-92.*
     INDX   CHILDREN, EARLY CHILDHOOD EDUCATION, MEXICAN AMERICAN, PROGRAM EVALUATION, ABILITY TESTING, ITPA, PERCEPTION, MEMORY, CROSS CULTURAL
     ABST   THE PURPOSE OF THIS STUDY WAS TO DETERMINE (A) ETHNIC DIFFERENCES IN PSYCHOLINGUISTIC ABILITIES AMONG HEADSTART CHILDREN AND (B) THE LEVEL OF FUNCTIONING OF THESE CHILDREN AFTER ATTENDING

HEADSTART FOR SEVEN MONTHS. ALTHOUGH EARLIER STUDIES FOUND HEADSTART CHILDREN TO SCORE BELOW THE AVERAGE ON THE ILLINOIS TEST OF PSYCHOLINGUISTIC ABILITY, THE PRESENT STUDY'S SAMPLE OF 101 PARTICIPANTS (36 ANGLOS, 24 BLACKS, 38 MEXICAN AMERICANS, AND 5 INDIANS OR ASIATICS) DID NOT SCORE BELOW AVERAGE. ALL ETHNIC GROUPS SCORED WITHIN THE AVERAGE RANGE AFTER ATTENDING THE PROGRAM ALTHOUGH BLACKS AND MEXICAN AMERICANS OBTAINED THE SAME SCORES AS ANGLOS ON ALL TESTS UTILIZING VISUAL MOTOR CHANNELS, ANGLOS STILL WERE SIGNIFICANTLY SUPERIOR ON TESTS OF VERBAL EXPRESSION AND TESTS UTILIZING THE AUDITORY-VOCAL CHANNEL AT THE REPRESENTATIONAL LEVEL. THESE FINDINGS MAY BE EXPLAINED BY THE FACT THAT CURRENT HEADSTART PROGRAMS ARE OBTAINING BETTER TEACHERS, BETTER INSTRUCTIONAL MATERIAL, AND ARE BETTER ORGANIZED. IT IS SUGGESTED THAT FUTURE RESEARCH INVESTIGATE THE KINDS OF PROGRAMS PRODUCING ACCELERATED DEVELOPMENT IN HEADSTART CHILDREN. 13 REFERENCES. (JOURNAL SUMMARY MODIFIED)

ACCN   002124

943 AUTH   **KITTELL, J. E.**
     TITL   INTELLIGENCE-TEST PERFORMANCE OF CHILDREN FROM BILINGUAL ENVIRONMENTS.
     SRCE   *ELEMENTARY SCHOOL JOURNAL, 1963, 64, 76-83.*
     INDX   BILINGUALISM, INTELLIGENCE TESTING, CHILDREN, BILINGUAL, CALIFORNIA TEST OF MENTAL MATURITY, SEX COMPARISON, ENVIRONMENTAL FACTORS, SES, SPANISH SURNAMED, EMPIRICAL, CALIFORNIA, SOUTHWEST, MALE, READING, FEMALE, COGNITIVE DEVELOPMENT
     ABST   THIS STUDY PROVIDES EVIDENCE THAT SUPPORTS PREVIOUS RESEARCH IN THESE AREAS: (1) BILINGUAL CHILDREN IN ELEMENTARY SCHOOL SUFFER FROM A LANGUAGE HANDICAP WHEN INTELLIGENCE IS MEASURED BY VERBAL TESTS; AND (2) THE LANGUAGE HANDICAP DECREASES AS THE CHILDREN PROGRESS THROUGH SCHOOL. IT ALSO INTRODUCES THE POSSIBILITY THAT A BILINGUAL ENVIRONMENT MAY BE AN ASSET TO VERBAL PROFICIENCY IN THE INTERMEDIATE GRADES. CHILDREN WHO ATTENDED BOTH THIRD AND FIFTH GRADES IN A BERKELEY, CA., ELEMENTARY SCHOOL (37 MALE AND 29 FEMALE) WERE CATEGORIZED AS UNILINGUAL VS. BILINGUAL (33 IN EACH GROUP). AMONG THE BILINGUAL SUBJECTS, 15 DIFFERENT LANGUAGES WERE FOUND IN THEIR HOME ENVIRONMENTS. ALL SUBJECTS WERE ADMINISTERED THE CALIFORNIA SHORT-FORM TEST OF MENTAL MATURITY AND THE CALIFORNIA READING TEST IN BOTH THE THIRD AND FIFTH GRADES. THESE TESTS SUPPLIED DATA ON CHRONOLOGICAL AND MENTAL AGE, LANGUAGE AND NON-LANGUAGE MENTAL AGE, AND READING AGE. COMPARISON WAS MADE

BETWEEN AND AMONG THE GROUPS BASED ON PARENTS' OCCUPATION AND BIRTHPLACE, LANGUAGE USE IN THE HOME, AND CHILD'S SEX AND AGE. IT WAS FOUND THAT: (1) THE CHILDREN, PARTICULARLY GIRLS, FROM BILINGUAL ENVIRONMENTS SHOW A PERFORMANCE HANDICAP IN THE LANGUAGE SECTION OF THE MENTAL MATURITY TEST GIVEN IN THIRD-GRADE; (2) THE TRUE POTENTIAL LANGUAGE MENTAL AND READING ABILITY OF THE CHILDREN, PARTICULARLY GIRLS, FROM A BILINGUAL ENVIRONMENT ARE NOT APPARENT IN THIRD-GRADE TESTS; (3) THE HANDICAP INDICATED IN THIRD-GRADE IS SIGNIFICANTLY LESS EFFECTIVE, IF STILL PRESENT, BY THE FIFTH GRADE TESTING FOR CHILDREN FROM A BILINGUAL ENVIRONMENT REGARDLESS OF PARENTAL OCCUPATION; AND (4) CHILDREN FROM A BILINGUAL ENVIRONMENT SHOW SUPERIOR TEST PERFORMANCE BY THE FIFTH GRADE. 6 REFERENCES. (AUTHOR SUMMARY MODIFIED)

ACCN   000806

---

944 AUTH **KLAPP, O. E.**
TITL MEXICAN SOCIAL TYPES.
SRCE *AMERICAN JOURNAL OF SOCIOLOGY, 1964, 69(4), 404-414.*
INDX MEXICAN, CULTURE, STEREOTYPES, PERSONALITY, EMPIRICAL, MACHISMO
ABST IN AN EXPLORATORY INVESTIGATION, SOCIAL TYPES DERIVED FROM SLANG NAME CLASSIFICATIONS (E.G., A COOL CAT, UN BATO CHINGON) WERE DIVIDED INTO POSITIVE AND NEGATIVE TYPES BY 119 MEXICAN SUBJECTS. IN ADDITION, SUBJECTS WERE GIVEN LISTS OF ANGLO AMERICAN SOCIAL TYPES AND WERE INSTRUCTED TO LIST MEXICAN EQUIVALENTS. HERO MODELS SUCH AS MUY MACHO (A REAL MAN), UN CABALLERO (A MAN WITH REAL CLASS), AND EL JEFE (THE BOSS) EXPRESSED POSITIVE THEMES OF THE MEXICAN ETHOS. ANOTHER SAMPLE OF 81 MEXICANS MATCHED THE FOLLOWING IMAGES TO FIVE ADMIRED FIGURES: PANCHO VILLA, REVOLUCIONARIO (REVOLUTIONARY); MIGUEL ALEMAN, POLITICO (POLITICIAN); BENITO JUAREZ, MUY MORAL (A VERY GOOD MAN); DON QUIXOTE, UN CABALLERO (A MAN WITH CLASS); AND UN TORERO, MACHO, VALIENTE (VALIANT). ON THE NEGATIVE SIDE OF THE MODEL SYSTEM, SOME SOCIAL TYPES ARE: ABUSON (THE BULLY); PELEONERO (THE TROUBLEMAKER); AND ESTAFADOR (THE CON MAN). WHILE THIS STUDY DOES NOT DRAW CONCLUSIONS ABOUT NATIONAL CHARACTER, IT IS IMPLIED THAT SOCIAL TYPES SHOULD BE TAKEN INTO ACCOUNT AND MAY OFFER A BASIS FOR COMPARATIVE STUDY. 12 REFERENCES.

ACCN   000808

---

945 AUTH **KLEINER, R. J., TUCKMAN, J., & LAVALL, M.**
TITL MENTAL DISORDER AND STATUS BASED ON RACE.
SRCE *PSYCHIATRY, 1960, 23, 271-274.*
INDX SES, CROSS CULTURAL, DEMOGRAPHIC, MENTAL HEALTH, PSYCHOPATHOLOGY, PSY-

CHOSIS, SCHIZOPHRENIA, EMPIRICAL, PENNSYLVANIA, EAST
ABST THE MENTAL BREAKDOWN PATTERNS OF A WHITE GROUP (N = 2,059), DESIGNATED AS HIGH STATUS, AND A NON-WHITE GROUP (N = 901), DESIGNATED AS LOW STATUS, WERE EXAMINED. ALL SUBJECTS WERE RESIDENTS OF PHILADELPHIA WHO HAD FIRST TIME ADMISSIONS TO ANY PENNSYLVANIA STATE MENTAL HOSPITAL DURING THE YEARS 1951-1956. TWO HYPOTHESES WERE TESTED: (1) THE PATTERN OF MENTAL DISORDER WILL SHOW A GREATER PREVALENCE OF SEVERE DISORDER (I.E. SCHIZOPHRENIA) FOR THE LOW STATUS THAN FOR THE HIGH STATUS GROUP; (2) THE LOW STATUS GROUP WILL SHOW AN EARLIER ONSET OF MENTAL ILLNESS THAN THE HIGH STATUS GROUP. DATA INCLUDED ETHNICITY, AGE, SEX, OCCUPATION, MARITAL STATUS AND PSYCHIATRIC DIAGNOSIS OBTAINED FROM HOSPITAL RECORDS. FINDINGS SUPPORT THE HYPOTHESES. THE CONCENTRATION OF THE LOW STATUS GROUP IN PARANOID AND OTHER SCHIZOPHRENIC REACTIONS DID NOT APPEAR TO BE CHANCE OCCURRENCE. THESE DISORDERS ARE REACTIONS TRIGGERED BY A HOSTILE, FRUSTRATING ENVIRONMENT. THE LOWER MEDIAN AGE FOR ONSET OF ALL CATEGORIES OF MENTAL DISORDER BY THE LOW STATUS GROUP INDICATES THAT ITS FRUSTRATION TOLERANCE IS IMPAIRED EARLIER AND MORE FREQUENTLY. GREATER ATTENTION NEEDS TO BE GIVEN TO PATIENTS' EXPERIENCES RESULTING FROM LOW-STATUS GROUP MEMBERSHIP AND THE ACCOMPANYING SOCIAL PRESSURES AND FRUSTRATIONS. 4 REFERENCES.

ACCN   000809

---

946 AUTH **KLEINMAN, P. H., & DAVID, D. S.**
TITL VICTIMIZATION AND THE PERCEPTION OF CRIME IN A GHETTO COMMUNITY.
SRCE *CRIMINOLOGY: AN INTERDISCIPLINARY JOURNAL, 1973, 11(3), 307-343.*
INDX ATTRIBUTION OF RESPONSIBILITY, CRIMINOLOGY, POVERTY, URBAN, ATTITUDES, PUERTO RICAN-M, CROSS CULTURAL, SES, COMMUNITY INVOLVEMENT, AGGRESSION, ADULTS, NEW YORK, EAST, SURVEY
ABST TO INVESTIGATE COMMUNITY MEMBERS' EXPERIENCES WITH AND ATTITUDES TOWARDS CRIME, 275 BLACK, 101 PUERTO RICAN, 89 ANGLO AND 145 BRITISH WEST INDIAN ADULTS FROM GHETTO AREAS IN NEW YORK CITY WERE INTERVIEWED. REVIEWS OF 7 PRIOR FIELD STUDIES RELATING TO SOCIAL CHARACTERISTICS OF VICTIMS AND PERCEPTIONS OF CRIME ARE PRESENTED. IT WAS HYPOTHESIZED THAT BEING SEEN AND KNOWN TO OTHERS IN THE COMMUNITY, THUS HAVING MORE CONTACT WITH OTHERS, LEADS TO VICTIMIZATION. A SET OF NINE VARIABLES WERE EMPLOYED: ETHNICITY, SEX, AGE, SES, LENGTH OF RESIDENCE, ORGANIZATION MEMBERSHIP, HAVING OFFERED STOLEN GOODS, FREQUENCY OF CHURCH ATTENDANCE, AND RELATIVES IN THE AREA. THE RESULTS REVEAL THAT: (1) RESPONDENTS OF EACH ETHNIC GROUP, AS WELL AS MALES AND FEMALES, RE-

PORT APPROXIMATELY THE SAME RATES OF VICTIMIZATION AND ARE SIMILAR IN THEIR PERCEPTIONS OF HIGH CRIME IN THEIR AREA; (2) AMONG BLACKS AND ANGLOS, LARGER PROPORTIONS OF OLD THAN YOUNG PEOPLE PERCEIVE CRIME AS HIGH, BUT THERE IS NO DIFFERENCE BY AGE AMONG BRITISH WEST INDIANS AND PUERTO RICANS; (3) INDIVIDUALS OF HIGHER SES, LONG-TERM RESIDENTS OF THE COMMUNITY, ORGANIZATION MEMBERS, OR THOSE WHO HAD BEEN OFFERED STOLEN GOODS ARE LIKELY TO BE VICTIMIZED IN ALL GROUPS; (4) PUERTO RICANS WHO ATTEND CHURCH AND HAVE MANY RELATIVES IN THE AREA ARE MORE LIKELY TO BE VICTIMIZED; (5) ANGLOS WHO ATTEND CHURCH AND HAVE MANY RELATIVES IN THE AREA PERCEIVE CRIME IN THE AREA AS LOWER THAN ANGLOS WHO DO NOT ; AND (6) ANGLOS AND PUERTO RICANS WHO HAD BEEN OFFERED STOLEN GOODS SEE CRIME AS HIGH IN THEIR AREA. 21 REFERENCES.

ACCN   000810

947 AUTH   **KLINE, F., ACOSTA, F. X., AUSTIN, W., & JOHNSON, J. G.**

TITL   SUBTLE BIAS IN THE TREATMENT OF THE SPANISH SPEAKING PATIENT.

SRCE   *IN E. R. PADILLA & A. M. PADILLA (EDS.), TRANSCULTURAL PSYCHIATRY: AN HISPANIC PERSPECTIVE (MONOGRAPH NO. 4). LOS ANGELES: UNIVERSITY OF CALIFORNIA, SPANISH SPEAKING MENTAL HEALTH RESEARCH CENTER, 1977, PP. 73-77.*

INDX   PSYCHOTHERAPY, RESOURCE UTILIZATION, PSYCHOTHERAPY OUTCOME, SPANISH SURNAMED, ROLE EXPECTATIONS, MENTAL HEALTH PROFESSION, BILINGUAL-BICULTURAL PERSONNEL, EMPIRICAL, CALIFORNIA, SOUTHWEST, PHYSICIANS, LANGUAGE COMPREHENSION

ABST   A STUDY OF 62 MEXICAN AMERICAN PATIENTS (21 SPANISH-SPEAKING AND 41 ENGLISH-SPEAKING) EVALUATED BY 19 ENGLISH-SPEAKING PSYCHIATRIC RESIDENTS IN A MENTAL HEALTH SETTING INVESTIGATED THE PATIENTS' AND PSYCHIATRIC RESIDENTS' SATISFACTION WITH SERVICES. RESULTS INDICATE THAT BOTH SPANISH SURNAMED PATIENT GROUPS, THOSE WHO WERE INTERVIEWED THROUGH AN INTERPRETER AND THOSE WHO WERE INTERVIEWED DIRECTLY IN ENGLISH, APPEARED IN GENERAL TO BE SATISFIED WITH SERVICES. HOWEVER, THE ENGLISH-SPEAKING PATIENTS WERE NOTICEABLY LESS PLEASED WITH THE DOCTORS' SPECIFIC ADVICE AND WITH HELP IN DEVELOPING SELF-UNDERSTANDING. PATIENTS INTERVIEWED VIA INTERPRETERS FOUND UNDERSTANDING AND SPECIFIC DIRECTION MORE HELPFUL THAN DID ENGLISH-SPEAKING LATINOS. BOTH GROUPS GOT MEDICATION MORE OFTEN THAN "AVERAGE" PATIENTS, BUT FOUND IT LESS HELPFUL THAN THE "AVERAGE" PATIENTS. THE RESIDENT PSYCHIATRISTS CONSISTENTLY MISINTERPRETED THEIR VALUE TO THE SPANISH-SPEAKING PATIENTS AND WERE NOT COMFORTABLE SEEING PATIENTS WHO REQUIRED AN INTERPRETER

BEYOND THE FIRST INTERVIEW. WHILE IT IS RECOGNIZED THAT MANY MORE BICULTURAL-BILINGUAL MENTAL HEALTH PROFESSIONALS ARE NEEDED, THE CONFIDENCE OF PATIENTS IN EXISTING THERAPISTS SHOULD NOT BE UNDERMINED. 5 REFERENCES.

ACCN   000811

948 AUTH   **KLINE, L. Y.**

TITL   SOME FACTORS IN THE PSYCHIATRIC TREATMENT OF SPANISH-AMERICANS.

SRCE   *AMERICAN JOURNAL OF PSYCHIATRY, 1969, 125(12), 1674-1681.*

INDX   STEREOTYPES, RESOURCE UTILIZATION, PSYCHOTHERAPY, PSYCHOTHERAPISTS, ATTITUDES, MENTAL HEALTH, HEALTH DELIVERY SYSTEMS, SPANISH SURNAMED, CASE STUDY, COLORADO, SOUTHWEST

ABST   SOCIOCULTURAL FACTORS IN THE PSYCHIATRIC TREATMENT OF SPANISH AMERICANS (SA) IN COLORADO RESULT IN AN UNDERUTILIZATION OF AVAILABLE PSYCHIATRIC SERVICES AND CREATE SPECIAL PROBLEMS IN THE TREATMENT OF THOSE WHO DO SEEK HELP. CASE STUDIES OF THREE SA INDIVIDUALS, ONE FEMALE AND TWO MALES, PROVIDE INSIGHT INTO THEIR ATTITUDES CONCERNING EMOTIONAL STRESS AND PSYCHIATRIC TREATMENT. THE ETIOLOGY OF PSYCHIATRIC DISORDERS AMONG SA PATIENTS IS ILLUSTRATED IN THE FIRST CASE STUDY. ROLES WITHIN THE LATIN AMERICAN FAMILY STRUCTURE AND THE EFFECT OF ACCULTURATION IN PRODUCING NEUROSIS ARE DISCUSSED. ANOTHER CASE STUDY DISCLOSES THE IMPORTANCE OF EMPATHY IN ANGLO-SPANISH RELATIONS IN TREATMENT SESSIONS. CULTURAL CONFLICT AND INTERRACIAL PROBLEMS ENCOUNTERED IN GROUP THERAPY BY A SA MALE ARE PRESENTED IN THE LAST CASE STUDY. PSYCHIATRIC TREATMENT IS PERCEIVED BY SA'S AS "ANGLO" AND NOT AS A POSSIBLE SOURCE OF UNDERSTANDING AND SUPPORT. A SOLUTION TO SA RESISTANCE TO PSYCHIATRIC TREATMENT IS THE DEVELOPMENT OF SERVICES UTILIZING THE PARTICIPATION OF COMMUNITY LEADERS AND TRADITIONAL HEALERS OR CURANDEROS. PSYCHIATRIC TREATMENT MAY BE MADE MORE EFFECTIVE THROUGH AN OPEN DISCUSSION BY THE SA OF HIS FEELINGS ABOUT ANGLOS WITHOUT FEAR OF RETALIATION BY THE THERAPIST. 28 REFERENCES.

ACCN   000812

949 AUTH   **KLOVEKORN, M. R., MADERA, M., & NARDONE, S.**

TITL   COUNSELING THE CUBAN CHILD.

SRCE   *ELEMENTARY SCHOOL GUIDANCE AND COUNSELING, 1974, 8(4), 255-260.*

INDX   EDUCATIONAL COUNSELING, PSYCHOSOCIAL ADJUSTMENT, CUBAN, CHILDREN, PSYCHOTHERAPY, CULTURAL FACTORS, CURRICULUM, LINGUISTIC COMPETENCE, EDUCATION, ESSAY, MENTAL HEALTH, FLORIDA, SOUTHWEST

ABST   THE NEEDS OF IMMIGRANT CUBAN CHILDREN ATTENDING AMERICAN SCHOOLS IN FLORIDA ARE DISCUSSED WITH REGARD TO SOME COUNSELING METHODS FOR EASING BOTH

THE TRANSITION BETWEEN FAMILY AND SCHOOL AND THE CONFLICTS BETWEEN CHILD AND TEACHER. THE COUNSELOR'S ROLE IS SEEN AS VITAL TO HELPING THE CHILD, HIS FAMILY, AND THE TEACHER UNDERSTAND THE SIMILARITIES AND DIFFERENCES BETWEEN THE TWO CULTURES. 3 REFERENCES.

ACCN   000813

950   AUTH   **KNAPP, R. R.**

TITL   THE EFFECTS OF TIME LIMITS ON THE INTELLIGENCE TEST PERFORMANCE OF MEXICAN AND AMERICAN SUBJECTS.

SRCE   *JOURNAL OF EDUCATIONAL PSYCHOLOGY, 1960, 51(1), 14-20.*

INDX   CATTELL CULTURE-FREE INTELLIGENCE TEST, MEXICAN, CROSS CULTURAL, TEST RELIABILITY, INTELLIGENCE TESTING, EMPIRICAL, EXAMINER EFFECTS, CALIFORNIA, SOUTHWEST, ADULTS

ABST   AN INVESTIGATION OF THE EFFECTS OF TIME LIMITS ON THE INTELLIGENCE TEST PERFORMANCE OF 100 MEXICAN AND 100 AMERICAN SUBJECTS IS PRESENTED. SUBJECTS WERE GIVEN THE CATTELL CULTURE FREE INTELLIGENCE TEST, FORMS 2A AND 2B, UNDER TWO TESTING CONDITIONS, POWER AND SPEED. THE TEST SCORES WERE SUBJECTED TO AN ANALYSIS OF VARIANCE. THE RESULTS INDICATE THAT WHILE BOTH THE MEXICAN AND AMERICAN SUBJECTS SCORED HIGHER UNDER POWER CONDITIONS, THE DIFFERENCE WAS SIGNIFICANTLY GREATER FOR THE MEXICANS THAN FOR THE AMERICANS. MOREOVER, THE MEXICAN SAMPLE SCORED SIGNIFICANTLY LOWER THAN THE AMERICAN SAMPLE IN TERMS OF OVERALL MEAN SCORES. THE POSSIBILITY THAT THE DIFFERENTIAL EFFECT OF TEST CONDITIONS WAS PRODUCED BY DIFFERENCES IN INTELLECTUAL LEVELS BETWEEN THE TWO SAMPLES, RATHER THAN BY CULTURAL DIFFERENCES, IS NOT SUPPORTED BY THE DATA. THERE WAS A SIGNIFICANT INCREASE IN TEST SCORES FROM THE FIRST TO THE SECOND ADMINISTRATION OF THE TEST, WHICH IS NOT SIGNIFICANTLY GREATER FOR THE MEXICAN THAN FOR THE AMERICAN SUBJECTS. THIS INDICATES THAT THE DIFFERENTIAL EFFECTS OF TEST CONDITIONS WERE PROBABLY NOT DUE TO DIFFERENCES IN TEST SOPHISTICATION. IT IS NOTED THAT SCORES WERE SIGNIFICANTLY HIGHER IN THE POWER-SPEED ORDER OF PRESENTATION THAN IN THE SPEED-POWER ORDER, WHICH SUGGESTS THAT THE FORMER TEST SEQUENCE PUTS BOTH MEXICAN AND AMERICAN SUBJECTS AT A DISADVANTAGE. 11 REFERENCES.

ACCN   000814

951   AUTH   **KNAPSTEIN, J. W.**

TITL   A CROSS CULTURAL STUDY OF CERTAIN PERSONALITY FEATURES OF TUBERCULOUS ALCOHOLIC PATIENTS (DOCTORAL DISSERTATION, TEXAS TECH. UNIVERSITY, 1971).

SRCE   *DISSERTATION ABSTRACTS INTERNATIONAL, 1971, 31(10), 6260B. (UNIVERSITY MICROFILMS NO. 71-9619.)*

INDX   CROSS CULTURAL, PERSONALITY, ALCOHOLISM, EMPIRICAL, SPANISH SURNAMED, HEALTH, PSYCHOPATHOLOGY, MENTAL HEALTH, SES, POVERTY

ABST   PERSONALITY VARIABLES WERE INVESTIGATED AMONG TUBERCULOUS, ALCOHOLIC, AND TUBERCULOUS ALCOHOLIC PATIENTS OF SPANISH AND ANGLO DESCENT. SEVERAL HYPOTHESES WERE GENERATED AND SUBMITTED TO DETAILED ANALYSIS. IT WAS FOUND THAT: (1) TUBERCULOUS ALCOHOLIC PATIENTS APPEAR TO BE MORE LIKE ALCOHOLIC PATIENTS THAN LIKE TUBERCULOUS PATIENTS; (2) THE ALCOHOLIC PATIENTS APPEAR TO BE VERY SIMILAR TO ALCOHOLIC PATIENTS IN PREVIOUS STUDIES; (3) ALL 3 GROUPS WERE MORE ANXIOUS AND INTROVERTED THAN THE NORMAL CONTROL GROUP; (4) TUBERCULOUS ALCOHOLIC PATIENTS WERE MORE TENDER MINDED, BOHEMIAN, AND IMPULSIVE THAN TUBERCULOUS PATIENTS; (5) TUBERCULOUS ALCOHOLIC PATIENTS AND ALCOHOLIC PATIENTS SEEM TO HAVE GREATER STATUS NEEDS THAN TUBERCULOUS PATIENTS; (6) THE HOSPITALIZED GROUPS WERE MORE THREAT-SENSITIVE THAN THE NORMAL CONTROL GROUP; (7) SPANISH AMERICAN SUBJECTS HAD LOWER SOCIOECONOMIC STANDING AND WERE MORE UNSOPHISTICATED, EXPEDIENT, AND IMPULSIVE THAN ANGLO AMERICAN SUBJECTS; AND (8) THE YOUNGER AGE GROUP WAS NOT MORE TENDER MINDED AND LIBERAL MINDED THAN THE OLDER AGE GROUP.

ACCN   000815

952   AUTH   **KNIGHT, G. P., KAGAN, S., NELSON, W., & GUMBINER, J.**

TITL   ACCULTURATION OF SECOND- AND THIRD-GENERATION MEXICAN AMERICAN CHILDREN: FIELD INDEPENDENCE, LOCUS OF CONTROL, SELF-ESTEEM, AND SCHOOL ACHIEVEMENT.

SRCE   *JOURNAL OF CROSS-CULTURAL PSYCHOLOGY, 1978, 9(1), 87-97.*

INDX   MEXICAN AMERICAN, CROSS CULTURAL, CROSS GENERATIONAL, CHILDREN, CALIFORNIA, SOUTHWEST, EMPIRICAL, LOCUS OF CONTROL, SELF CONCEPT, ACCULTURATION, SCHOLASTIC ACHIEVEMENT, FIELD DEPENDENCE-INDEPENDENCE, READING

ABST   THE RELATIONSHIP OF EDUCATIONAL ACHIEVEMENT, ACCULTURATION, AND SEVERAL MEASURES OF PSYCHOLOGICAL DIFFERENTIATION (I.E., FIELD INDEPENDENCE, LOCUS OF CONTROL, AND SELF-ESTEEM) WAS STUDIED IN A "TRADITIONAL" MEXICAN AMERICAN COMMUNITY IN SOUTHERN CALIFORNIA. THE SUBJECTS WERE 144 ANGLO AND MEXICAN AMERICAN (MA) ELEMENTARY SCHOOL CHILDREN; THE MA SUBJECTS INCLUDED 42 SECOND-GENERATION AND 58 THIRD-GENERATION CHILDREN. FROM SECOND- TO THIRD-GENERATIONS, MA CHILDREN INCREASINGLY APPROACHED ANGLO NORMS WITH RESPECT TO FIELD-INDEPENDENCE, READING ACHIEVEMENT, AND MATH ACHIEVEMENT. OPPOSITE TRENDS WERE OBTAINED WITH REGARD TO SELF-ESTEEM. NO SIGNIFICANT EFFECTS OF GENERATIONAL LEVEL WERE FOUND REGARDING LOCUS OF CONTROL. SEVERAL POSSIBLE

EXPLANATIONS ARE OFFERED CONCERNING THE APPARENT PARADOX OF DECREASING SELF-ESTEEM ALONGSIDE INCREASING ACHIEVEMENT LEVELS WITH GENERATION. 18 REFERENCES. (JOURNAL ABSTRACT MODIFIED)

ACCN 001734

953 AUTH **KNIGHT, G. P., & KAGAN, S.**
TITL ACCULTURATION OF PROSOCIAL AND COMPETITIVE BEHAVIORS AMONG SECOND- AND THIRD-GENERATION MEXICAN-AMERICAN CHILDREN.
SRCE *JOURNAL OF CROSS-CULTURAL PSYCHOLOGY, 1977, 8(3), 273-284.*
INDX MEXICAN AMERICAN, CHILDREN, ACCULTURATION, CROSS CULTURAL, COOPERATION, COMPETITION, CROSS GENERATIONAL, EMPIRICAL, CALIFORNIA, SOUTHWEST, SEX COMPARISON
ABST TO DETERMINE THE DIRECTION OF ACCULTURATION OF PROSOCIAL AND COMPETITIVE BEHAVIORS IN MEXICAN AMERICAN (MA) CHILDREN, AN EXPERIMENT USING BEHAVIORAL CHOICE CARDS WAS CONDUCTED IN A SOUTHERN CALIFORNIA ELEMENTARY SCHOOL. THE 143 SUBJECTS INCLUDED 44 ANGLOS, AND 41 SECOND-GENERATION AND 58 THIRD-GENERATION MA'S. INCREASING GENERATION LEVEL WAS ASSOCIATED WITH (1) A DECREASING FREQUENCY OF ALTRUISM/GROUP-ENHANCEMENT AND EQUALITY CHOICES, AND (2) AN INCREASING FREQUENCY OF RIVALRY/SUPERIORITY CHOICES. THESE RESULTS SUPPORT AN ACCULTURATION TO THE MAJORITY RATHER THAN AN ACCULTURATION TO THE BARRIO MODEL. 35 REFERENCES. (JOURNAL ABSTRACT MODIFIED)
ACCN 001735

954 AUTH **KNIGHT, G. P., & KAGAN, S.**
TITL DEVELOPMENT OF PROSOCIAL AND COMPETITIVE BEHAVIORS IN ANGLO AMERICAN AND MEXICAN AMERICAN CHILDREN.
SRCE *CHILD DEVELOPMENT, 1977, 48(4), 1385-1394.*
INDX MEXICAN AMERICAN, CROSS CULTURAL, SES, COMPETITION, INTERPERSONAL RELATIONS, COOPERATION, CHILDREN, URBAN, SEX COMPARISON, ALTRUISM, EMPIRICAL, CALIFORNIA, SOUTHWEST, MALE, FEMALE
ABST A NOVEL BEHAVIORAL CHOICE CARD DESIGNED TO DISTINGUISH FOUR SOCIAL BEHAVIORS (ALTRUISM/GROUP-ENHANCEMENT, EQUALITY, SUPERIORITY AND RIVALRY/SUPERIORITY) WAS ADMINISTERED TO 197 5-6 AND 7-9 YEAR-OLD CHILDREN FROM THREE POPULATIONS: 120 UPPER-MIDDLE SES ANGLO AMERICANS; 39 LOWER SES ANGLO AMERICANS; AND 38 LOWER SES MEXICAN AMERICANS. COMPARISON OF THE TWO LOWER SES GROUPS REVEALED AN ETHNIC DIFFERENCE IN THE DEVELOPMENT OF SOCIAL BEHAVIORS: WITH AGE, MEXICAN AMERICAN CHILDREN TENDED TO BE SOMEWHAT MORE PROSOCIAL IN CONTRAST TO ANGLO AMERICAN CHILDREN WHO WERE INCREASINGLY COMPETITIVE. COMPARISON OF THE TWO ANGLO AMERICAN GROUPS INDICATED LOWER SES CHILDREN MAKE MORE PROSOCIAL CHOICES

THAN UPPER-MIDDLE SES CHILDREN. BOYS MADE SIGNIFICANTLY MORE RIVALRY/SUPERIORITY AND LESS EQUALITY CHOICES THAN GIRLS ACROSS BOTH AGES IN ALL POPULATIONS AND CONDITIONS. USE OF CONDITIONS WHICH VARIED THE PRESENCE AND ACTIVITY LEVEL OF THE PEER REVEALED THAT TYPE OF COMPETITION WAS SOMEWHAT MORE INTENSE IN THE MOST ACTIVE PEER CONDITION AND THAT BEHAVIOR IN THE PEER ABSENT CONDITION WAS HIGHLY CORRELATED WITH BEHAVIOR IN THE PEER PRESENT CONDITIONS. FURTHER, SUPERIORITY AND EQUALITY APPEARED TO BE STRONG SOCIAL MOTIVES, RIVALRY AND ALTRUISM APPEARED TO BE INTERMEDIATE IN STRENGTH, AND GROUP-ENHANCEMENT WAS A VERY WEAK MOTIVE. 21 REFERENCES. (AUTHOR ABSTRACT MODIFIED)

ACCN 000817

955 AUTH **KNOLL, F. R.**
TITL CASEWORK SERVICES FOR MEXICAN AMERICANS.
SRCE *SOCIAL CASEWORK, 1971, 52(5), 279-284.*
INDX MENTAL HEALTH PROFESSION, MEXICAN AMERICAN, ESSAY, PSYCHOTHERAPY, PSYCHOTHERAPISTS, MENTAL HEALTH, FAMILY STRUCTURE, CASE STUDY, FAMILY THERAPY, MICHIGAN, MIDWEST, SOCIAL SERVICES, ESSAY, REVIEW, URBAN
ABST THE ROLE OF FAMILY SERVICE AGENCIES IN OFFERING CASEWORK SERVICES TO A MEXICAN AMERICAN (MA) BARRIO POPULATION IS EXAMINED. A DESCRIPTION OF THE DETROIT MA BARRIO REVEALS THE LACK OF SCIENTIFICALLY TRAINED MEDICAL PERSONNEL AND A DEPENDENCE ON THE CURANDERA. THREE CASES ILLUSTRATE: (1) THE NEED FOR TANGIBLE RATHER THAN INTANGIBLE SERVICES; (2) THE MANNER OF HANDLING PARENT-CHILD RELATIONSHIPS, AND THE EFFECTS OF THE EXTENDED FAMILY; AND (3) THE COMPLEX MANNER IN WHICH CULTURAL STRESS AND PERSONALITY PATHOLOGY ARE COMBINED. IT IS SUGGESTED THAT THERE IS A DEFINITE NEED FOR SOCIAL SERVICE AGENCIES TO EXTEND CONCRETE COUNSELING SERVICES WITH AN EFFECTIVE CLIENT FOLLOW-UP PROCEDURE TO THE BARRIO COMMUNITY. SOCIAL WORKERS MUST BE ABLE TO INTERPRET SPECIAL PROBLEMS OF THE FAMILY TO AUTHORITIES AND TO SERVE AS LINKS BETWEEN ALIENATED FAMILIES AND INSTITUTIONS. IT IS CONCLUDED THAT, ALTHOUGH THERE ARE CULTURAL DISSIMILARITIES, THE STRENGTHS AND PATHOLOGIES IN MA FAMILIES ARE NO DIFFERENT FROM THOSE OF OTHER FAMILIES WHO SEEK HELP FROM FAMILY SERVICES. IT IS SUGGESTED THAT SOCIAL WORKERS MUST GIVE TOP PRIORITY TO EDUCATING THE COMMUNITY REGARDING SOCIAL SERVICES.

ACCN 000818

956 AUTH **KNOWLTON, C. S.**
TITL CHANGES IN THE STRUCTURE AND ROLES OF SPANISH-AMERICAN FAMILIES OF NORTHERN NEW MEXICO.

SRCE   *PROCEEDINGS OF THE SOUTHWESTERN SO-CIOLOGICAL ASSOCIATION, 1965, 15, 38-48.*

INDX   FAMILY STRUCTURE, FAMILY ROLES, MEXICAN AMERICAN, ACCULTURATION, RURAL, EXTENDED FAMILY, FICTIVE KINSHIP, MIGRATION, CULTURAL CHANGE, EMPIRICAL, SEX ROLES, SES, EMPLOYMENT, CONFLICT RESOLUTION, NEW MEXICO, SOUTHWEST

ABST   DATA FOR THIS PAPER WERE OBTAINED FROM EXAMINATION OF AVAILABLE LITERATURE AND FROM FIELD WORK IN SAN MIGUEL AND MORA COUNTIES OF NORTHERN NEW MEXICO. THE EXTENDED PATRIARCHAL FAMILY WAS THE PRIMARY SOCIAL SYSTEM AMONG THE SPANISH AMERICANS, OFTEN CONSISTING OF MEMBERS OF THREE OR FOUR GENERATIONS HEADED BY THE GRANDFATHER. THIS FAMILY COOPERATED AS A SINGLE, TIGHTLY KNIT, POLITICAL, ECONOMIC, AND SOCIAL UNIT. DOMINANCE AND AUTHORITY WERE RELATED TO SEX AND AGE—THE MALES WERE DOMINANT OVER FEMALES AND THE OLDER MEMBERS HAD AUTHORITY OVER THE YOUNGER FAMILY MEMBERS. THE PRESSURES OF URBANIZATION, INDUSTRIALIZATION, AND LAND LOSSES HAVE BROKEN THIS TRADITIONAL FAMILY PATTERN IN ALL BUT THE MOST REMOTE VILLAGES. THE ADJUSTMENT OF THE LOWER-CLASS SPANISH AMERICAN FAMILY TO URBAN LIVING DEPENDS UPON THE HUSBAND'S SALARY. IF IT IS NOT ADEQUATE THEN THE WIFE MUST SEEK EMPLOYMENT, THUS STRENGTHENING HER ROLE AND DIMINISHING THE HUSBAND'S ROLE. THE MORE EDUCATED AND ACCULTURATED SPANISH AMERICAN FAMILIES TEND TO EMULATE THE NUCLEAR FAMILY MODEL OF THE ANGLO AMERICAN. (RIE ABSTRACT)

ACCN   000819

957 AUTH   **KNOWLTON, C. S.**

TITL   CHANGING SPANISH-AMERICAN VILLAGES OF NORTHERN NEW MEXICO.

SRCE   *SOCIOLOGY AND SOCIAL RESEARCH, 1969, 53(4), 455-474.*

INDX   CULTURE, MIGRATION, HISTORY, FAMILY STRUCTURE, FAMILY ROLES, RURAL, MEXICAN AMERICAN, FICTIVE KINSHIP, CULTURAL CHANGE, ACCULTURATION, ESSAY, RELIGION, ECONOMIC FACTORS, COMMUNITY, REVIEW, NEW MEXICO, COLORADO, SOUTHWEST, STRESS

ABST   THE SPANISH AMERICANS OF NORTHERN NEW MEXICO AND SOUTHERN COLORADO, LIVING IN ISOLATION FROM OTHER EUROPEAN GROUPS FOR ALMOST THREE HUNDRED YEARS, DEVELOPED A UNIQUE RURAL FARM VILLAGE CULTURE BASED UPON SUBSISTENCE AGRICULTURE, PASTORAL ACTIVITIES, BARTER, HANDICRAFTS, AND TRADE WITH THE INDIANS. UNTIL VERY RECENTLY EACH VILLAGE WAS A SMALL, ISOLATED, SELF-SUFFICIENT, AUTONOMOUS SOCIAL CELL. THE SOCIAL STRUCTURE OF THE VILLAGE WAS BASED UPON FOUR INTERRELATED SOCIAL SYSTEMS: (1) THE VILLAGE COMMUNITY; (2) THE PATRIARCHAL EXTENDED FAMILY; (3) THE PATRON SYSTEM; AND (4) FOLK CATHOLICISM. THE EXTENSION OF

AMERICAN CONTROL, THE MASSIVE LOSS OF RANGE AND FARMING LAND, THE EMIGRATION OF YOUNG ADULTS, INCREASING ACCULTURATIONAL AND SOCIAL DIFFERENCES, AND FINALLY THE BREAKDOWN AND MALFUNCTIONING OF THE TRADITIONAL SOCIAL SYSTEMS HAVE CREATED A LARGE APATHETIC POVERTY-STRICKEN VILLAGE POPULATION UNABLE TO LIVE IN THE TRADITIONAL MANNER OR TO DEVELOP THE NECESSARY SOCIAL MECHANISMS TO ADJUST TO THE DOMINANT ANGLO AMERICAN SOCIETY. 38 REFERENCES. (JOURNAL ABSTRACT)

ACCN   000821

958 AUTH   **KNUDSON, K. H. M., & KAGAN, S.**

TITL   VISUAL PERSPECTIVE ROLE-TAKING AND FIELD DEPENDENCE AMONG ANGLO AMERICAN AND MEXICAN AMERICAN CHILDREN OF TWO AGES.

SRCE   *JOURNAL OF GENETIC PSYCHOLOGY, 1977, 131, 243-253.*

INDX   COGNITIVE STYLE, CHILDREN, CROSS CULTURAL, MEXICAN AMERICAN, SEX COMPARISON, EMPIRICAL, FIELD DEPENDENCE-INDEPENDENCE, PERCEPTION, CALIFORNIA, SOUTHWEST

ABST   THE ABILITY TO TAKE THE PERSPECTIVE OF ANOTHER WAS STUDIED AMONG NINETY-SEVEN 5-6 AND 7-9 YEAR-OLD ANGLO AMERICAN AND MEXICAN AMERICAN BOYS AND GIRLS. THESE CHILDREN WERE ADMINISTERED SEVEN PERCEPTUAL ROLE TAKING TASKS AND THE "CHILDREN'S EMBEDDED FIGURES TEST" OF FIELD INDEPENDENCE. RESULTS INDICATED NO SIGNIFICANT CULTURAL DIFFERENCES. RESULTS WERE CONTRARY TO PREVIOUS FINDINGS IN THREE RESPECTS: (1) CHILDREN WERE ABLE TO TAKE THE ROLE OF ANOTHER AT A YOUNGER AGE THAN ORIGINALLY THEORIZED BY PIAGET; (2) ROLE TAKING AND FIELD INDEPENDENCE WERE NOT SIGNIFICANTLY RELATED WHEN AGE WAS CONTROLLED; AND (3) LOW AND INCONSISTENT CORRELATIONS AMONG THE VISUAL PERSPECTIVE ROLE TAKING TASKS INDICATE THAT VISUAL PERSPECTIVE ROLE TAKING IS NOT AN ESTABLISHED UNIDIMENSIONAL CONSTRUCT. 23 REFERENCES. (AUTHOR ABSTRACT MODIFIED)

ACCN   000822

959 AUTH   **KOLE, D. M.**

TITL   A CROSS-CULTURAL STUDY OF MEDICAL-PSYCHIATRIC SYMPTOMS.

SRCE   *JOURNAL OF HEALTH AND HUMAN BEHAVIOR, 1966, 7(3), 162-174.*

INDX   SYMPTOMATOLOGY, CROSS CULTURAL, EMPIRICAL, SPANISH SURNAMED, CENTRAL AMERICA, DEPRESSION, AGGRESSION, PSYCHOPATHOLOGY, CULTURAL FACTORS, SES, POVERTY, COPING MECHANISMS, SEX COMPARISON, HEALTH, DISEASE

ABST   THE DISSIMILARITIES IN THE NUMBER AND PATTERN OF MEDICAL AND PSYCHIATRIC SYMPTOMS BETWEEN 255 NORTH AMERICAN (NA) AND 155 LATIN AMERICAN (LA) PATIENTS AT GORGAS HOSPITAL IN THE CANAL ZONE WERE STUDIED. THE 195-ITEM SELF-ADMINIS-

TERED CORNELL MEDICAL INDEX (CMI), CONSISTING OF 144 GENERAL MEDICAL SYMPTOM QUESTIONS AND 51 PSYCHIATRIC SYMPTOM QUESTIONS, WAS USED. IT WAS FOUND THAT WOMEN HAD SIGNIFICANTLY MORE SYMPTOMS THAN MEN. PSYCHIATRIC PATIENTS SHOWED SIGNIFICANTLY MORE SYMPTOMS THAN MEDICAL PATIENTS OF THE SAME SEX. IN ADDITION, LA'S LISTED MORE SYMPTOMS THAN NA'S OF THE SAME SEX. THE RELATIVE INCIDENCE OF INDIVIDUAL SYMPTOMS IN THE CMI BETWEEN NA AND LA MEDICAL PATIENTS REVEALS A HIGHER INCIDENCE OF PERSONAL INADEQUACY, HYPERSENSITIVITY, AND HOSTILITY AMONG THE LA'S OF BOTH SEXES. OTHER DIFFERENCES FOUND APPEAR TO BE RELATED TO PHYSICAL ENVIRONMENT AND THE AVAILABILITY AND ADEQUACY OF MEDICAL FACILITIES FOR THE TWO GROUPS. 9 REFERENCES. (JOURNAL ABSTRACT MODIFIED)

ACCN   000823

960 AUTH   **KOMAROFF, A. L., MASUDA, M., & HOLMES, T. H.**
     TITL   THE SOCIAL READJUSTMENT RATING SCALE: A COMPARATIVE STUDY OF NEGRO, MEXICAN, AND WHITE AMERICANS.
     SRCE   *JOURNAL OF PSYCHOSOMATIC RESEARCH, 1968, 12(2), 121-128.*
     INDX   MEXICAN AMERICAN, CROSS CULTURAL, STRESS, PSYCHOSOCIAL ADJUSTMENT, EMPIRICAL, COPING MECHANISMS, SURVEY, CALIFORNIA, SOUTHWEST, MARRIAGE
     ABST   SIXTY-FOUR URBAN NEGROES AND 78 MEXICAN AMERICANS FROM POVERTY AREAS OF LOS ANGELES WERE ADMINISTERED THE SOCIAL READJUSTMENT RATING SCALE. THIS SCALE IS A LIST OF 43 EVENTS WHICH MIGHT CHANGE AN INDIVIDUAL'S LIFE. SUBJECTS WERE INSTRUCTED TO ASSIGN POINTS TO AN EVENT ACCORDING TO WHETHER IT WOULD CHANGE THEIR LIVES (E.G., MARRIAGE—500 POINTS). RESULTS INDICATED THAT IN THE MAJORITY OF LIFE-CHANGE ITEMS, THE NUMERICAL RESPONSES OF THE TWO SUBCULTURE GROUPS AND THE RESPONSES OF A PREVIOUSLY EXAMINED WHITE AMERICAN MIDDLE-CLASS GROUP DIFFERED SIGNIFICANTLY. THE SUBCULTURAL GROUPS REGARDED FOURTEEN LIFE-CHANGE EVENT ITEMS, RELATED TO THE AREA OF LABOR AND INCOME, AS ITEMS REQUIRING MORE OF A READJUSTMENT THAN DID THE WHITE AMERICANS. A LOW RESPONSE TO THE ITEM "DEATH OF SPOUSE" BY THE MA GROUP INDICATED THAT THE SECURITY OF THE EXTENDED FAMILY CUSHIONS THE ADJUSTMENT REQUIRED WHEN ILL HEALTH OR DEATH OCCURS IN A CLOSE FAMILY MEMBER. BOTH SUBCULTURE GROUPS REGARDED THE ITEM "PREGNANCY" AS REQUIRING MORE ADJUSTMENT THAN DID WHITE AMERICANS. IN ADDITION, THE SUBCULTURE GROUPS REGARDED "DIVORCE" AS REQUIRING LESS ADJUSTMENT THAN DID WHITE AMERICANS. THE MA GROUP THOUGHT NO ITEMS REQUIRED AS MUCH CHANGE AS DID MARRIAGE, WHILE NEGROES THOUGHT THAT OTHER LIFE-CHANGE ITEMS REQUIRED MORE ADJUSTMENT THAN

MARRIAGE. IT IS CONCLUDED THAT ALL THREE GROUPS RANKED ITEMS IN A VERY SIMILAR FASHION, THOUGH THE CORRELATION COEFFICIENTS INDICATE THAT THE TWO SUBGROUPS WERE MORE CLOSELY RELATED TO EACH OTHER THAN TO THE WHITE AMERICAN MIDDLE-CLASS INCOME GROUP. 4 REFERENCES.

ACCN   000824

961 AUTH   **KORMAN, M., TRIMBOLI, F., & SEMLER, I.**
     TITL   A PSYCHIATRIC EMERGENCY ROOM STUDY OF INHALANT USE.
     SRCE   *UNPUBLISHED MANUSCRIPT, 1976. (AVAILABLE FROM DR. M. KORMAN, DEPARTMENT OF PSYCHOLOGY, UNIVERSITY OF TEXAS HEALTH SCIENCE CENTER AT DALLAS, DALLAS, TEXAS.)*
     INDX   INHALANT ABUSE, DRUG ABUSE, ADOLESCENTS, MEXICAN AMERICAN, CROSS CULTURAL, PSYCHOPATHOLOGY, SYMPTOMATOLOGY, FAMILY ROLES, FAMILY STRUCTURE, JUDICIAL PROCESS, DELINQUENCY, ANXIETY, DEPRESSION, SUICIDE, AGGRESSION, INTELLIGENCE, TEXAS, SOUTHWEST
     ABST   CONCERN HAS RECENTLY BEEN EXPRESSED REGARDING CLINICAL EFFECTS, PARTICULARLY THE BEHAVIORAL CONSEQUENCES, OF VOLUNTARY INHALATION OF VOLATILE SOLVENTS. THIS STUDY EXAMINES THE DIFFERENCES BETWEEN 3 GROUPS—INHALANT USERS, POLYDRUG USERS, AND NON-INHALANT/NONPOLYDRUG USERS—WITH RESPECT TO EMOTIONAL DYSCONTROL, BEHAVIORAL DYSCONTROL, COGNITIVE DEFECTS, FAMILY BACKGROUND AND SOCIAL DISORGANIZATION, AGE, SEX AND ETHNICITY FACTORS, INTELLIGENCE, AND SIGNS OF SELF-DETERIORATION. INFORMATION WAS OBTAINED FROM THE PSYCHIATRIC INTERVIEW RECORD (PIR) GIVEN TO PATIENTS WHO SOUGHT TREATMENT DURING A 12-MONTH PERIOD AT A COUNTY TEACHING HOSPITAL'S EMERGENCY PSYCHIATRIC ROOM. THE TOTAL SAMPLE CAME TO 273, OF WHICH 91 WERE INHALANT USERS. THE GROUPS WERE MATCHED FOR SEX, AGE, AND ETHNICITY. THE FINDINGS INDICATE THE INHALANT GROUP APPEARS TO SHOW MORE SELF- AND OTHER-DIRECTED AGGRESSIVE BEHAVIOR AND A WIDER RANGE OF COGNITIVE DEFICITS AND SOCIAL DISRUPTION THAN THE OTHER TWO GROUPS. NO DIFFERENCE WAS FOUND BETWEEN THE GROUPS AS TO EMOTIONAL DYSCONTROL OR INTELLIGENCE. A CLOSER EXAMINATION OF THE INHALANT GROUP REVEALED THAT THOSE WHO WERE HEAVY USERS WERE MORE APT TO HAVE POOR HYGIENE, INAPPROPRIATE DRESS, FLATTENED AFFECT, AND SOFT AND MONOTONIC SPEECH. 27 REFERENCES.

ACCN   000825

962 AUTH   **KOSS, J. D.**
     TITL   ARTISTIC EXPRESSION AND CREATIVE PROCESS IN CARIBBEAN POSSESSION CULT RITUALS.
     SRCE   *IN J. CORDWELL (ED.), THE VISUAL ARTS: GRAPHIC AND PLASTIC. THE HAGUE: MOUTON, 1979.*

INDX ART, ESPIRITISMO, ESSAY, PUERTO RICAN-I, FOLK MEDICINE, CARIBBEAN

ABST THE AESTHETIC ASPECTS OF ARTISTIC EXPRESSIONS AND INSTRUMENTAL GOALS OF RITUALS PERFORMED BY SMALL CULT GROUPS WITH A MINIMUM OF RITUALISTIC PARAPHERNALIA ARE EXAMINED. IT IS SUGGESTED THAT RITUALS ARE IMPORTANT SINCE THEY APPEAR TO SATISFY AESTHETIC GOALS AND ARE FASCINATING AS EXPRESSIVE MEDIA FOR OBSERVERS AND PARTICIPANTS. NOT ONLY DO THE RITUALS CONTAIN A SOURCE OF ENTERTAINMENT, THESE DRAMAS PROVIDE A CREATIVE FORUM BY WHICH ORDINARY PEOPLE CAN EXPRESS IDEAS ABOUT HOW THEY FEEL, THINK, AND MOVE. ALTHOUGH THE PRIMARY FUNCTION OF THE SPIRITIST SESSIONS IS VIEWED AS A HEALING, DIVINING AND VALUE INTENSIFYING RITE, THE COMPLEMENTARY ASPECTS OF INDIVIDUAL SELF-EXPRESSION AND CREATIVITY ALSO REPRESENT SIGNIFICANT COMPONENTS OF THE RITUAL. IT IS CONCLUDED THAT SINCE THESE RITUAL DRAMAS MOVE OUT OF THE REALM OF THE MUNDANE THEY PROVIDE A STAGE FOR SPONTANEOUS ARTISTIC CREATIVITY TO TAKE PLACE. 26 REFERENCES.

ACCN 000826

963 AUTH **KOSS, J. D.**

TITL SPIRITS AS SOCIALIZING AGENTS: THE CASE STUDY OF A PUERTO RICAN GIRL REARED IN A MATRICENTRIC FAMILY.

SRCE IN V. CRAPANZANO & V. GARRISON (EDS.), CASE STUDIES IN SPIRIT POSSESSION. NEW YORK: WILEY & SONS, 1976, PP. 365-382.

INDX CASE STUDY, FOLK MEDICINE, FATHER-CHILD INTERACTION, ESPIRITISMO, PUERTO RICAN-I, RELIGION, PSYCHOTHERAPISTS, ATTITUDES, SEXUAL BEHAVIOR, MARRIAGE, FAMILY ROLES, FAMILY STRUCTURE, CULTURAL FACTORS, DEVIANCE, MOTHER-CHILD INTERACTION, SOCIALIZATION, CHILDREARING PRACTICES, MENTAL HEALTH, PERSONALITY

ABST IN PUERTO RICO, SPIRIT BELIEFS FUNCTION TO CONVEY, INTERPRET, AND REINFORCE MORAL INJUNCTIONS, PARTICULARLY WITH REFERENCE TO INTIMATE FAMILY RELATIONSHIPS. THIS CASE STUDY DESCRIBES A YOUNG PUERTO RICAN WOMAN REARED BY FIVE MAIDEN AUNTS WHOSE NEED FOR MALE AUTHORITY WAS FULFILLED BY CALLING UPON THEIR DECEASED FATHER AT REGULAR FAMILY SEANCES. THE GIRL DID NOT MEET HER BIOLOGICAL FATHER UNTIL SHE WAS 21 YEARS-OLD; SOON AFTER THEIR REUNION SHE BEGAN LIVING WITH HIM IN A CONJUGAL RELATIONSHIP. DATA OBTAINED FROM THE CALIFORNIA PERSONALITY INVENTORY INDICATED THAT BOTH THE DAUGHTER AND THE FATHER WERE WELL-ADJUSTED AND SOCIALLY EFFECTIVE INDIVIDUALS. ALTHOUGH AN ANALYSIS ACCORDING TO THE BASIC ASSUMPTIONS OF FREUDIAN AND NEO-FREUDIAN PSYCHODYNAMIC THEORY IS PRESENTED, ANOTHER INTERPRETATION MORE FAITHFUL TO A PUERTO RICAN CULTURALLY CONSTITUTED REALITY IS OFFERED AS WELL. IT IS SUGGESTED THAT THE WOMAN'S CHOICE OF LOVERS RELATED TO THE KIND OF "FATHER FIGURE" SHE EXPERIENCED AS A CHILD. HER SPIRIT GRANDFATHER TOOK ON AN OBJECTIVE EXISTENCE AS A PRINCIPAL SOCIALIZING AGENT AND BECAME INTERNALIZED AS A FATHER FIGURE NOT CHARACTERIZED BY PHYSICAL LOVE AND INTIMACY. THE MAN WITH WHOM SHE WAS LIVING THUS HAD NONE OF THE "FATHER" ATTRIBUTES SHE HAD EXPERIENCED AND NO SIGNIFICANCE AS A PSYCHOLOGICAL FATHER. 10 REFERENCES.

ACCN 000827

964 AUTH **KOSS, J. D.**

TITL TERAPEUTICA DEL SISTEMA DE UNA SECTA EN PUERTO RICO. (THERAPEUTICS OF THE SYSTEM IN A SECT IN PUERTO RICO.)

SRCE REVISTA DE CIENCIAS SOCIALES, 1970, 14(2), 259-278. (SPANISH)

INDX FOLK MEDICINE, PSYCHOTHERAPY, RELIGION, ESSAY, PUERTO RICAN-I, ESPIRITISMO, PSYCHOTHERAPISTS

ABST BASED UPON A PREVIOUS STUDY OF SPIRITIST CULTS AND CENTROS (CHURCHES) IN PUERTO RICO, THE AUTHOR DISCUSSES THE RELATIONSHIP BETWEEN THE SOCIAL ORGANIZATION OF THESE CULTS AND THE PSYCHOTHERAPY THEY PROVIDE. ALTHOUGH THE SPECIFIC PROBLEMS WHICH LEAD PEOPLE TO FIRST SEEK HELP FROM A SPIRITIST CULT ARE NOT EXAMINED IN DETAIL, IT IS SUGGESTED THAT MANY INVOLVE POOR RELATIONSHIPS WITH RELATIVES AND FRIENDS. CONCERNING PARTICIPATION, A NEW MEMBER'S TASKS AND FUNCTIONS WITHIN THE CULT INCREASE IN PROPORTION TO HIS CONFIDENCE IN THE "DIRECTOR" OF THE CENTRO. AT FIRST HE IS ONLY REQUESTED TO PRAY AND TO EXAMINE HIMSELF INWARDLY; BUT AS THE DIRECTOR GAINS GREATER DOMINION OVER HIM, HE IS ORDERED TO ENTER INTO TRANCES AND TRANSMIT MESSAGES RECEIVED FROM A SPIRIT. THEREBY, THE MEMBER ATTAINS THE RANK OF MEDIUM. WITH REGARD TO THERAPEUTIC EFFECTS, THESE ARE A PRODUCT OF THE DIRECTOR'S CONTROL OVER THE MEDIUM, AND THEY RESULT FROM CONTRADICTIONS IN THE MEDIUM'S BEHAVIOR. THAT IS, THE DIRECTOR ISSUES THE MEDIUM CONTRADICTORY COMMANDS WHICH ARE DESIGNED TO MAKE THE MEDIUM OBEY AGAINST HIS CONSCIOUS WILL. IN OBEYING THESE COMMANDS, THE MEDIUM IS FORCED TO DO THINGS WHICH HE WOULD NORMALLY CONSIDER HIMSELF INCAPABLE OF DOING; MOREOVER, HE BELIEVES THAT HIS ACTIONS ARE NOT HIS OWN AND THAT HE IS BUT THE PASSIVE AGENT OF A MORE POWERFUL AGENT (I.E., A SPIRIT). BY THIS MEANS, THE MEDIUM OFFERS SOLUTIONS TO THE PROBLEMS OF OTHERS, AND SIMULTANEOUSLY HE IMPROVES HIS OWN ABILITY TO RELATE TO AND DEAL WITH OTHER PEOPLE. WITHIN THE TEXT, PORTIONS OF AN ACTUAL SPIRITIST MEETING ARE REPRODUCED. 13 REFERENCES.

ACCN 000828

965 AUTH **KOSS, J. D.**
TITL THERAPEUTIC ASPECTS OF PUERTO RICAN CULT PRACTICES.
SRCE *PSYCHIATRY, 1975, 38(2), 160-171.*
INDX PUERTO RICAN-I, FOLK MEDICINE, RELIGION, ESPIRITISMO, ESSAY, PSYCHOTHERAPY, PSYCHOTHERAPISTS, INTERPERSONAL RELATIONS, SOCIAL STRUCTURE
ABST THE PHENOMENON OF POSSESSION TRANCE IN THE RITUAL CONTEXT IS ANALYZED AS AN ACTIVE AND PERHAPS NECESSARY COMPONENT IN THE DEVELOPMENT OF SIGNIFICANT PERSONAL RELATIONSHIPS BASIC TO THE ORGANIZATION AND GOALS OF SOME RELIGIOUS CULTS. THIS VIEW IS SUGGESTED BY DATA GATHERED IN A STUDY OF SOCIAL PROCESS IN PUERTO RICAN SPIRITIST CULTS IN WHICH THE RELATIONSHIP BETWEEN PATTERNS OF CULT SOCIAL ORGANIZATION AND THE CULT EXECUTION OF A CULTURALLY PATTERNED PSYCHOTHERAPEUTIC PROCESS FOR COMMITTED ADHERENTS WAS EXAMINED. EMOTIONAL PROBLEMS ARE DIAGNOSED BY CULT HEALERS AS MANIFESTATIONS OF DEVELOPING FACULTIES FOR COMMUNICATION WITH THE SPIRIT WORLD. 15 REFERENCES. (PASAR ABSTRACT MODIFIED)
ACCN 000829

966 AUTH **KOZOLL, R.**
TITL ASPECTOS PREVENTIVOS DEL SISTEMA RURAL DE ATENCION DE SALUD EN EL AREA "TABLERO DE DAMAS" DE NUEVO MEXICO. (PREVENTIVE ASPECTS OF RURAL HEALTH CARE DELIVERY: THE "CHECKERBOARD AREA" HEALTH SYSTEM OF NEW MEXICO.)
SRCE *BOLETIN DE LA OFICINA SANITARIA PANAMERICANA, 1978, 84(6), 481-490. (SPANISH)*
INDX ESSAY, HEALTH DELIVERY SYSTEMS, MEXICAN AMERICAN, RURAL, HEALTH, DEMOGRAPHIC, PRIMARY PREVENTION, NEW MEXICO, SOUTHWEST
ABST THE HEALTH CARE SYSTEM OF THE SO-CALLED "CHECKERBOARD AREA" OF NORTHERN NEW MEXICO WAS DESIGNED TO DEAL WITH THE OBSTACLES CONFRONTING THE DELIVERY OF SERVICES IN NEEDY RURAL AREAS WITH A TRIPLE-CULTURE POPULATION (MEXICAN AMERICAN, NAVAJO, AND ANGLO). THE MAJORITY OF OBSTACLES INCLUDE ISOLATION, POVERTY, AND THE ETHNIC GROUPS' DIFFERING PERCEPTIONS OF HEALTH CARE. THE SYSTEM COMPRISES 10 PREVENTIVE MEDICAL SERVICES, AND THERE ARE ALSO SUCH INNOVATIVE PROGRAMS AS (1) SATELLITE MEDICAL CONSULTATION OFFICES, (2) THE INTEGRATION OF "NON-CLINICAL" SERVICES, (3) AN INFORMATION CIRCULATION SYSTEM, AND (4) THE "MIXTURE" OF HUMAN RESOURCES. 3 REFERENCES. (AUTHOR SUMMARY MODIFIED)
ACCN 002311

967 AUTH **KREISMAN, J. J.**
TITL THE CURANDERO'S APPRENTICE: A THERAPEUTIC INTEGRATION OF FOLK AND MEDICAL HEALING.
SRCE *THE AMERICAN JOURNAL OF PSYCHIATRY, 1975, 132(1), 81-83.*
INDX CURANDERISMO, FOLK MEDICINE, MENTAL HEALTH, PSYCHOTHERAPY, FEMALE, MEXICAN AMERICAN, CASE STUDY, COLORADO, SOUTHWEST, POLICY
ABST ALTERNATIVE METHODS FOR DEALING WITH FOLK ILLNESS IN PSYCHOTHERAPY ARE DISCUSSED. TWO CASE REPORTS ARE PRESENTED THAT DESCRIBE PSYCHOTIC MEXICAN AMERICAN FEMALES WITH WHOM CONVENTIONAL THERAPY WAS UNSUCCESSFUL BUT WHOSE MENTAL HEALTH STATUS IMPROVED WHEN THE TREATMENT WAS INTEGRATED WITH CURANDERISMO. MODERN MENTAL HEALTH THERAPY IGNORES THE CULTURAL DIFFERENCE IN THE WAY ILLNESS IS PERCEIVED BY MEXICAN AMERICANS. THE HISPANIC CONCEPT OF ILLNESS IS THAT IT IS DUE TO EXTERNAL FACTORS AND HEALING CAN ONLY BE ACCOMPLISHED BY A CURANDERO. THREE ALTERNATIVES ARE PRESENTED: (1) IGNORE THE PATIENT'S CONCEPT OF DISEASE; (2) ACKNOWLEDGE THE PATIENT'S CONCEPT OF ILLNESS WITHOUT INCORPORATING IT INTO THE THERAPY; OR (3) ACCEPT THE PATIENT'S CONCEPT OF ILLNESS AND EMPLOY THE USE OF A CURANDERO IN THE TREATMENT OF THE PATIENT. BY UTILIZING THE 3RD APPROACH IN THE TREATMENT OF MENTAL HEALTH PROBLEMS OF MEXICAN AMERICANS, SUCCESSFUL THERAPY IS MORE LIKELY TO OCCUR. WITH RESPECT TO THE ETHICAL ISSUES RAISED BY INCORPORATING FOLK HEALING INTO SCIENTIFIC MEDICINE, IT IS NOT IMPLIED THAT THE THERAPISTS MUST NECESSARILY BELIEVE IN THE FOLK CONCEPT OF ILLNESS BUT SHOULD RATHER UTILIZE IT TO PROVIDE THE PATIENT WITH APPROPRIATE THERAPY. 7 REFERENCES.
ACCN 000830

968 AUTH **KRUGER, D.**
TITL THE RELATIONSHIP OF ETHNICITY TO UTILIZATION OF COMMUNITY MENTAL HEALTH CENTERS (DOCTORAL DISSERTATION, UNIVERSITY OF TEXAS AT AUSTIN, 1974).
SRCE *DISSERTATION ABSTRACTS INTERNATIONAL, 1974, 35, 1295A. (UNIVERSITY MICROFILMS NO. 74-24,887).*
INDX HEALTH DELIVERY SYSTEMS, POVERTY, SES, ACCULTURATION, PSYCHOTHERAPY, PSYCHOTHERAPISTS, ADMINISTRATORS, PARAPROFESSIONALS, REPRESENTATION, CROSS CULTURAL, MEXICAN AMERICAN, RURAL, URBAN, SEX COMPARISON, EDUCATION, RESOURCE UTILIZATION, TEXAS, SOUTHWEST
ABST THE DIFFERENTIAL USE OF 24 LOCALLY AUTONOMOUS TEXAS COMMUNITY MENTAL HEALTH CENTERS DURING 1972 BY 59,706 BLACKS, ANGLOS AND MEXICAN AMERICANS IS ANALYZED. THE TYPE OF SERVICE AND SERVICE PROVIDER ARE ANALYZED BY CLIENT ETHNICITY, AGE, SEX, EDUCATION, AND INCOME. BLACKS AND MEXICAN AMERICANS, IN THAT ORDER, COME TO TEXAS MENTAL HEALTH CENTERS IN HIGHER PROPORTIONS THAN WHITES, BUT RECEIVE LESS TRADITIONAL, LOWER STATUS TREATMENT (INCLUDING BOTH SERVICE AND PROVIDER TYPES). THESE ETHNIC TREATMENT PATTERNS ARE PARTIALLY IN-

DEPENDENT OF THE EFFECTS OF INCOME, SEX, AGE AND EDUCATION. ALL ARE MOST PRONOUNCED WHERE MINORITY CONCENTRATIONS ARE HIGHEST. THE LARGE AND OFTEN OPPOSING RESULTS FOR THE DIFFERENT CENTERS IN UTILIZATION AND TREATMENT WARRANT FURTHER STUDY OF: (1) THE TRUE PREVALENCE OF MENTAL ILLNESS AMONG THE ETHNIC GROUPS; (2) THE ETHNIC COMPOSITION AND ATTITUDES OF THE STAFF, DIRECTOR AND BOARD; (3) THE CENTERS' SETTING—URBAN, RURAL, COMMERCIAL, ETC.; AND (4) THE RELATIONSHIP OF THE CENTERS TO THEIR COMMUNITIES. 45 REFERENCES. (AUTHOR ABSTRACT MODIFIED)

ACCN   000831

969 AUTH   **KUTNER, N. G.**
    TITL   THE POOR VS. THE NON-POOR: AN ETHNIC AND METROPOLITAN-NONMETROPOLITAN COMPARISON.
    SRCE   *THE SOCIOLOGICAL QUARTERLY, 1975, 16(2), 250-263.*
    INDX   CROSS CULTURAL, MEXICAN AMERICAN, RURAL, URBAN, POVERTY, EMPIRICAL, FAMILY STRUCTURE, DEMOGRAPHIC, CULTURE, ENVIRONMENTAL FACTORS, ATTITUDES, ANOMIE, FATALISM, MEXICAN AMERICAN, MIGRATION, SPANISH SURNAMED
    ABST   INDICATORS OF OSCAR LEWIS POVERTY TRAITS WERE EXAMINED TO SEE IF POOR AND NONPOOR FAMILIES DIFFERED SIGNIFICANTLY IN FREQUENCY OF DEMONSTRATING THE TRAITS. FAMILIES REPRESENTING SIX ETHNIC/RESIDENCE POPULATION TYPES WERE CONSIDERED: METROPOLITAN WHITE, NONMETROPOLITAN WHITE, METROPOLITAN BLACK, NONMETROPOLITAN BLACK, METROPOLITAN SPANISH-SPEAKING, AND NONMETROPOLITAN SPANISH-SPEAKING. OF THE 29 TRAITS INVESTIGATED, FOR 24 TRAITS A SIGNIFICANT DIFFERENCE WAS FOUND BETWEEN POOR AND NONPOOR IN AT LEAST ONE ETHNIC/RESIDENCE GROUP. SIGNIFICANT DIFFERENCES BETWEEN POOR AND NONPOOR IN THE TWO SPANISH-SPEAKING GROUPS EXISTED ON CONSIDERABLY FEWER TRAITS THAN IN THE CASE OF THE TWO BLACK OR THE TWO WHITE GROUPS, SUGGESTING THAT THE TRAITS EXAMINED MAY BE MORE BROADLY BASED IN SPANISH CULTURE. 12 REFERENCES. (JOURNAL ABSTRACT)

ACCN   000832

970 AUTH   **KUVLESKY, W. P., WRIGHT, D., & JUAREZ, R. Z.**
    TITL   STATUS PROJECTIONS AND ETHNICITY: A COMPARISON OF MEXICAN AMERICAN, NEGRO, AND ANGLO YOUTH.
    SRCE   *JOURNAL OF VOCATIONAL BEHAVIOR, 1971, 1(2), 137-151.*
    INDX   SELF CONCEPT, CROSS CULTURAL, PERSONALITY, OCCUPATIONAL ASPIRATIONS, SCHOLASTIC ASPIRATIONS, RURAL, EMPIRICAL, SOCIAL MOBILITY, TEXAS, SOUTHWEST, SEX COMPARISON
    ABST   ETHNIC GROUP DIFFERENCES IN ADOLESCENTS' PROJECTED FRAMES OF STATUS REFERENCE ARE DISCUSSED. UTILIZING DATA OBTAINED FROM NEGRO, MEXICAN AMERICAN, AND ANGLO YOUTH RESIDING IN NONMETROPOLITAN AREAS OF TEXAS, ETHNIC COMPARISONS WERE MADE BY SEX ON SEVERAL DIMENSIONS OF OCCUPATIONAL AND EDUCATIONAL STATUS PROJECTIONS: LEVELS OF ASPIRATION AND EXPECTATION, ANTICIPATORY GOAL DEFLECTION, INTENSITY OF ASPIRATION, AND CERTAINTY OF EXPECTATION. THE FINDINGS INDICATED THAT THE THREE ETHNIC GROUPS WERE GENERALLY SIMILAR, EXCEPT WITH REFERENCE TO STATUS EXPECTATIONS AND INTENSITY OF ASPIRATION—I.E., NEGRO YOUTH MAINTAINED HIGHER LEVEL EXPECTATIONS AND MEXICAN AMERICAN YOUTH MAINTAINED STRONGER INTENSITY OF ASPIRATION. SEVERAL OTHER CONSISTENT BUT LESS SUBSTANTIAL PATTERNS OF ETHNIC VARIABILITY WERE NOTED: MEXICAN AMERICAN YOUTH FELT LEAST CERTAIN OF ATTAINING THEIR EXPECTATIONS, NEGRO YOUTH HELD HIGHER EDUCATIONAL GOALS, AND ANGLO YOUTH EXPERIENCED THE LEAST ANTICIPATORY DEFLECTION. IMPLICATIONS ARE DRAWN FOR THEORY AND FUTURE RESEARCH. 23 REFERENCES. (JOURNAL ABSTRACT MODIFIED)

ACCN   000833

971 AUTH   **KUVLESKY, W. P., & PATELLA, V. M.**
    TITL   DEGREE OF ETHNICITY AND ASPIRATIONS FOR UPWARD SOCIAL MOBILITY AMONG MEXICAN AMERICAN YOUTH.
    SRCE   *JOURNAL OF VOCATIONAL BEHAVIOR, 1971, 1(3), 231-244.*
    INDX   ETHNIC IDENTITY, SES, SEX COMPARISON, ROLE EXPECTATIONS, SOCIAL MOBILITY, MEXICAN AMERICAN, ADOLESCENTS, SCHOLASTIC ASPIRATIONS, OCCUPATIONAL ASPIRATIONS, EMPIRICAL, RURAL, SURVEY, PERCEPTION, MASS MEDIA, TEXAS, SOUTHWEST
    ABST   THE HYPOTHESIS THAT DEGREE OF IDENTIFICATION WITH THE MEXICAN AMERICAN SUBCULTURE AMONG ADOLESCENTS IS INVERSELY RELATED TO DESIRE FOR UPWARD SOCIAL MOBILITY WAS TESTED USING DATA FROM A 1967 STUDY OF OVER 500 MEXICAN AMERICAN HIGH SCHOOL SOPHOMORES IN SOUTH TEXAS. ETHNIC IDENTIFICATION WAS INDICATED BY AN INDEX OF THE USE OF SPANISH IN A VARIETY OF SITUATIONS. ASPIRATION FOR INTERGENERATIONAL MOBILITY WAS MEASURED THROUGH CROSS CLASSIFICATION OF THE RESPONDENTS' OCCUPATIONAL ASPIRATIONS WITH THE JOB OF THE MAIN BREADWINNER IN THE FAMILY. COMPARATIVE ANALYSIS OF UPWARDLY MOBILE AND NONMOBILE RESPONDENTS BY ETHNICITY, SOCIOECONOMIC STATUS (SES), AND SEX, AND COMPARISON OF ETHNICITY SCORES BY DEGREE OF MOBILITY PROJECTED FOR EACH SES TYPE DID NOT SUPPORT THE HYPOTHESIS. RELEVANT THEORETICAL IMPLICATIONS ARE DRAWN AND SUGGESTIONS ARE PROVIDED FOR FUTURE RESEARCH. 19 REFERENCES.

ACCN   000834

972 AUTH   **KUZMA, K. J., & STERN, C.**
    TITL   THE EFFECTS OF THREE PRESCHOOL INTER-

VENTION PROGRAMS ON THE DEVELOPMENT OF AUTONOMY IN MEXICAN-AMERICAN AND NEGRO CHILDREN.

SRCE   *JOURNAL OF SPECIAL EDUCATION, 1972, 6(3), 197-205.*

INDX   SELF CONCEPT, CHILDREN, COGNITIVE DEVELOPMENT, CURRICULUM, INSTRUCTIONAL TECHNIQUES, PROGRAM EVALUATION, EARLY CHILDHOOD EDUCATION, MEXICAN AMERICAN, CROSS CULTURAL, LINGUISTIC COMPETENCE, CALIFORNIA, SOUTHWEST, INTELLIGENCE, PEABODY PICTURE-VOCABULARY TEST

ABST   PREVIOUS RESEARCH INDICATES DISADVANTAGED CHILDREN SCORE SIGNIFICANTLY LOWER THAN MIDDLE-CLASS CHILDREN ON INTELLIGENCE TESTS, LANGUAGE AND REASONING DEVELOPMENT WHEN THEY BEGIN SCHOOL. TO ACCESS THE EFFECTS OF THE LEARNING ENVIRONMENT, THIS STUDY ASSIGNED 42 MEXICAN AMERICAN AND 35 BLACK CHILDREN IN 9 HEADSTART CLASSES TO EITHER AN AUTONOMY, LANGUAGE, OR CONTROL GROUP TO DETERMINE (1) THE EFFECTS OF A 7-WEEK SUMMER PROGRAM UPON THE DEVELOPMENT OF AUTONOMY, AND (2) WHETHER THE INSTRUCTIONAL TREATMENTS PRODUCED SIGNIFICANTLY DIFFERENT CHANGES IN AUTONOMY OR COGNITIVE ABILITY AS A FUNCTION OF ETHNICITY. SCORES ON THE CINCINNATI AUTONOMY TEST BATTERY INCREASED FOR ALL CHILDREN, WITH MEXICAN AMERICAN CHILDREN SHOWING SIGNIFICANT GAINS ON 9 AND BLACK CHILDREN ON 5 OF THE 11 AUTONOMY MEASURES. USING THE PEABODY PICTURE-VOCABULARY TEST AS A MEASURE OF MENTAL FUNCTIONING, RESULTS INDICATE THAT IQ SCORES INCREASED SIGNIFICANTLY FOR CHILDREN RECEIVING EITHER THE LANGUAGE OR AUTONOMY CURRICULUM. IT IS CONCLUDED THAT MAJOR CHANGES IN PSYCHOLOGICAL PATTERNS CANNOT BE PRODUCED BY A RELATIVELY SHORT TRAINING PERIOD, BUT THE SIGNIFICANT INCREASES BY THE MEXICAN AMERICAN CHILDREN STRONGLY SUGGEST THE USE OF MORE FOCUSED INTERVENTIONS AS PART OF THE HEADSTART PROGRAM. 14 REFERENCES. (PASAR ABSTRACT MODIFIED)

ACCN   000835

973 AUTH **LA BARRE, W.**
TITL   THE PEYOTE CULT: ENLARGED EDITION.
SRCE   *NEW YORK: SCHOKEN, 1969.*
INDX   DRUG ABUSE, CULTURAL FACTORS, MEXICAN, CROSS CULTURAL, ESSAY, RELIGION, MEXICO, INDIGENOUS POPULATIONS, FOLK MEDICINE, LEGISLATION, HISTORY, REVIEW, EMPIRICAL, BOOK

ABST   THIS CLASSICAL STUDY WHICH BEGAN IN THE MID-1930'S UTILIZES AN ANTHROPOLOGICAL APPROACH TO INVESTIGATE THE MEXICAN AND AMERICAN INDIAN RITUALISTIC USE OF THE PEYOTE PLANT. IT PROVIDES A COMPARATIVE ANALYSIS OF PEYOTISM AND AN EXTENSIVE REVIEW AND CRITIQUE OF THE LITERATURE PERTAINING TO PEYOTE STUDIES. INCLUDED IN THIS ENLARGED EDITION IS AN APPRAISAL OF THE USE OF ARTIFICAL PSY-

CHEDELIC DRUGS AS INSTRUMENTS OF REVOLT. AN ETHNOLOGY IS PRESENTED DESCRIBING THE FOLLOWING ASPECTS OF PEYOTISM: (1) NONRITUALISTIC USE OF THE PEYOTE; (2) ITS RITUALISTIC USE AMONG THE HUICHOL, TARAHUMARI, MESCALERO-APACHE, KIOWA-COMANCHE, AND THE AMERICAN INDIAN TRIBES; AND (3) A COMPARISON OF THE PEYOTE RITUALS IN MEXICO. THE BOTANICAL, PHYSIOLOGICAL, AND PSYCHOLOGICAL ASPECTS OF PEYOTE ARE ALSO DISCUSSED.

ACCN   000836

974 AUTH **LA BELLE, T. J.**
TITL   DIFFERENTIAL PERCEPTIONS OF ELEMENTARY SCHOOL CHILDREN REPRESENTING DISTINCT SOCIO-CULTURAL BACKGROUNDS.
SRCE   *JOURNAL OF CROSS-CULTURAL PSYCHOLOGY, 1971, 2(2), 145-156.*
INDX   SES, SEX COMPARISON, CHILDREN, SPANISH SURNAMED, EDUCATION, SCHOLASTIC ACHIEVEMENT, READING, TEACHERS, EMPIRICAL, ATTITUDES, CROSS CULTURAL, PERCEPTION, SELF CONCEPT, CALIFORNIA, SOUTHWEST

ABST   THE DIFFERENCE IN MEANING OF TEN SCHOOL-RELATED CONCEPTS FOR 882 FIFTH-GRADE STUDENTS REPRESENTING THREE SES LEVELS, TWO ETHNIC GROUPS, TWO SEX GROUPS, AND THREE LEVELS OF ACHIEVEMENT WAS STUDIED THROUGH THE USE OF THE SEMANTIC DIFFERENTIAL TECHNIQUE. SUBJECTS, 387 SPANISH AMERICANS AND 495 ANGLO AMERICANS, RESPONDED TO THE FOLLOWING TEN CONCEPTS: TEACHERS, SCHOOL, READING, STUDENTS WHO GET POOR GRADES, STUDENTS WHO GET GOOD GRADES, MY SCHOOL WORK, PERSON I WOULD LIKE TO BE, FOLLOWING RULES, ME, AND TAKING TESTS. FINDINGS INDICATE THAT HIGH ACHIEVERS DO NOT NECESSARILY PERCEIVE SCHOOL-RELATED CONCEPTS MORE POSITIVELY, POTENTLY, OR ACTIVELY THAN DO MIDDLE AND LOW ACHIEVERS. ANGLO AND SPANISH AMERICAN FIFTH GRADERS PERCEIVE SCHOOL-RELATED CONCEPTS MORE SIMILARLY THAN DIFFERENTLY. MIDDLE- AND HIGH-SES LEVEL STUDENTS PERCEIVE SCHOOL-RELATED CONCEPTS MORE POSITIVELY, POTENTLY, AND ACTIVELY THAN DO LOW-SES LEVEL STUDENTS. FEMALES (473) VIEW SCHOOL-RELATED CONCEPTS MORE POSITIVELY THAN DO MALES (445), BUT MALES TEND TO VIEW CONCEPTS RELATING TO SELF-IDENTITY MORE POTENTLY AND ACTIVELY. 15 REFERENCES.

ACCN   000837

975 AUTH **LA GRA, J. L., & BARKLEY, P. W.**
TITL   INCOME AND EXPENSE RECORDS OF 17 MEXICAN AMERICAN FAMILIES (REPORT NO. AES-C-526).
SRCE   *WASHINGTON, D.C.: U.S. DEPARTMENT OF AGRICULTURE, 1970. (ERIC DOCUMENT REPRODUCTION SERVICE NO. ED 055 715)*
INDX   ECONOMIC FACTORS, MEXICAN AMERICAN, FAMILY STRUCTURE, EMPIRICAL, SES, EMPLOYMENT, FARM LABORERS, MIGRANTS, WASHINGTON, WEST

ABST   A SELECTED GROUP OF 17 MEXICAN AMERI-
CAN FAMILIES WHO WENT TO THE OTHELLO,
WASHINGTON, AREA AS MIGRANT AGRICUL-
TURAL WORKERS AND TRIED TO BECOME A
PART OF THE RESIDENT POPULATION WERE
STUDIED TO LEARN SOMETHING OF THE EARN-
INGS AND SPENDING HABITS OF EX-MIGRANT
MEXICAN AMERICAN FAMILIES. TO OBTAIN AC-
CURATE DATA ON INCOME AND EXPENSES, A
DETAILED RECORD BOOK WAS PLACED IN
EACH PARTICIPATING HOME. IN ADDITION, AN
INTERVIEW SCHEDULE YIELDED DATA ON ES-
TIMATED INCOMES AND EXPENSES OF THE
FAMILIES DURING THE 1968 CALENDAR YEAR.
THE RECORD BOOK YIELDED DAY-TO-DAY IN-
FORMATION DURING A 2-MONTH PERIOD. THE
DECISION MAKERS IN THE FAMILIES STUDIED
WERE FOUND TO HAVE DESIRES AND MOTIVES
MUCH LIKE THOSE OF OTHER MIDDLE-CLASS
OR LOWER-MIDDLE-CLASS FAMILIES. THE MOST
SIGNIFICANT DIFFERENCE WAS THAT THE
FAMILIES STUDIED DEPENDED UPON INCOME
FROM HIGHLY VARIABLE SOURCES. ALTHOUGH
FAMILY INCOME WAS QUITE ACCEPTABLE OR
EVEN QUITE HIGH DURING A GIVEN PERIOD,
THE ACCUMULATION OF DEBTS FROM PAST
PERIODS OR THE ANTICIPATION OF FUTURE
PERIODS OF LOW INCOME OFTEN REQUIRED
THAT THE FAMILY LIVE AT A LEVEL INCOMMEN-
SURATE WITH CURRENT INCOME. (RIE AB-
STRACT MODIFIED)

ACCN   000838
cf5,7,9

976 AUTH   **LABOVITZ, E. M.**
      TITL   RACE, SES CONTEXTS AND FULFILLMENT OF
COLLEGE ASPIRATIONS.
      SRCE   *THE SOCIOLOGICAL QUARTERLY, 1975, 16(2),*
241-249.
      INDX   ENVIRONMENTAL FACTORS, SCHOLASTIC
ACHIEVEMENT, SCHOLASTIC ASPIRATIONS,
PERSONALITY, CROSS CULTURAL, MEXICAN
AMERICAN, SES, EDUCATION, SOCIAL MOBIL-
ITY,ADOLESCENTS, RESEARCH METHOD-
OLOGY, CENSUS, SURVEY, HIGHER EDUCA-
TION, CALIFORNIA, SOUTHWEST
      ABST   THE DIFFERENTIAL EFFECTS OF SOCIAL CON-
TEXTS AND RACE ON EDUCATIONAL BEHAVIOR
WERE EXAMINED IN TERMS OF A CAUSAL PRO-
CESS MODEL. BASED ON SEVERAL SOURCES
OF DATA (PRE- AND POST-HIGH SCHOOL
GRADUATION SURVEY OF COLLEGE ASPIRA-
TIONS AND CAREER GOALS, HIGH SCHOOL
TRANSCRIPTS, CENSUS TRACT INFORMATION
AND SCORES ON STANDARDIZED INTELLI-
GENCE TESTS) FOR 6,294 METROPOLITAN SAN
DIEGO HIGH SCHOOL STUDENTS, THE ROLE
OF SOCIOECONOMIC FACTORS WERE FOUND
TO AFFECT PERSONAL CHARACTERISTICS
WHICH, IN TURN, INFLUENCE EDUCATIONAL
ASPIRATIONS AND ATTAINMENT. UTILIZING
BOTH CORRELATIONAL AND TABULAR TECH-
NIQUES, THE BASIC MODEL HELD FOR ALL
ETHNIC GROUPS STUDIED (ANGLO, BLACK,
MEXICAN AMERICAN AND ORIENTAL AMERI-
CAN). ETHNICITY WAS FOUND TO AFFECT THE
LEVEL OF THE INDIVIDUAL VARIABLES (ASPI-
RATIONS, GPA AND COLLEGE ATTENDANCE).

FINDINGS SUGGEST THAT THE IMPORTANCE
OF SES CONTEXTS ARE MEDIATED BY ETHNI-
CITY AND CONTINGENT UPON THE COMMON
RELATIONS OF THESE CONTEXTS AND EDU-
CATIONAL BEHAVIOR TO INDIVIDUAL CHARAC-
TERISTICS. 20 REFERENCES. (JOURNAL AB-
STRACT MODIFIED)
      ACCN   000839

977 AUTH   **LACALLE, J. J.**
      TITL   GROUP PSYCHOTHERAPY WITH MEXICAN
AMERICAN DRUG ADDICTS (DOCTORAL DIS-
SERTATION, UNITED STATES INTERNATIONAL
UNIVERSITY, 1973).
      SRCE   *DISSERTATION ABSTRACTS INTERNATIONAL,*
1974, 34, 1753B. (UNIVERSITY MICROFILMS NO.
73-22,675).
      INDX   DRUG ADDICTION, PSYCHOTHERAPY OUT-
COME, PSYCHOTHERAPY, MALE, MEXICAN
AMERICAN, ADULTS, CROSS CULTURAL, EM-
PIRICAL, CPI, METHADONE MAINTENANCE, SELF
CONCEPT, PSYCHOSOCIAL ADJUSTMENT,
AGGRESSION, CRIMINOLOGY, CALIFORNIA,
SOUTHWEST
      ABST   GROUP PSYCHOTHERAPY (GP) WAS TESTED
FOR ITS EFFECTIVENESS IN INDUCING BEHAV-
IORAL CHANGES IN MEXICAN AMERICAN (MA)
DRUG ADDICTS AT A SAN DIEGO NARCOTICS
TREATMENT PROGRAM. ALL 138 OUT-PATIENTS
(60 MA'S) HAD BEEN RECEIVING TREATMENT
FOR AT LEAST 3 MONTHS AND WERE AS-
SIGNED TO ONE OF FOUR GROUPS: (1) MA RE-
CEIVING METHADONE ONLY; (2) MA RECEIVING
METHADONE PLUS GP; (3) NON-MA RECEIVING
METHADONE ONLY; AND (4) NON-MA RECEIV-
ING METHADONE PLUS GP. A SPECIALLY DE-
SIGNED BEHAVIORAL QUESTIONNAIRE AND
SELECTED SCALES OF THE CALIFORNIA PER-
SONALITY INVENTORY WERE USED TO MEA-
SURE BEHAVIORAL AND ATTITUDINAL CHANGES
AT 3- AND 6-MONTH INTERVALS AS COMPARED
WITH PRETEST RESPONSES GIVEN DURING
THE FIRST WEEK OF TREATMENT. FINDINGS
SHOW THAT MA'S UNDERGOING METHADONE
TREATMENT CHANGE THEIR SOCIAL BEHAVIOR
POSITIVELY AND SIGNIFICANTLY, WHILE MA'S
UNDER METHADONE PLUS GP FAIL TO PRO-
DUCE ANY SIGNIFICANT CHANGE IN THEIR SO-
CIAL BEHAVIOR. NO SIGNIFICANT DIFFERENCE
WAS FOUND BETWEEN THE BEHAVIORAL
CHANGES IN MA'S UNDER METHADONE PLUS
GP AND NON-MA'S UNDER THE SAME TREAT-
MENTS. THE BEHAVIORAL CHANGES OB-
SERVED IN MA'S UNDER METHADONE ONLY
WERE SIGNIFICANTLY DIFFERENT FROM THOSE
OBSERVED IN NON-MA'S UNDER METHADONE
ONLY. THE MAIN IMPLICATION—I.E., THAT GP
AS PRACTICED IN THIS PROGRAM IS NOT AN
EFFECTIVE THERAPEUTIC TOOL IN THESE SUB-
JECTS—IS DISCUSSED IN TERMS OF THE
TREATMENT'S DISREGARD FOR THE ETHNIC
CHARACTERISTICS OF PATIENTS. 83 REFER-
ENCES. (AUTHOR SUMMARY MODIFIED)
      ACCN   000840

978 AUTH   **LADNER, R. A., & LADNER, S.**
      TITL   SUBSTANCE ABUSE AND PATTERNS OF SER-
VICE UTILIZATION AMONG SINGLE- AND POLY-

DRUG ABUSING MALES AND FEMALES: A TRI-ETHNIC LOG-LINEAR ANALYSIS.

SRCE *UNPUBLISHED MANUSCRIPT, 1976. (AVAILABLE FROM AUTHORS, BEHAVIORAL SCIENCE RE-SEARCH CORP., 929 MAJORCA AVE., CORAL GABLES, FLORIDA 33134.)*

INDX DRUG ABUSE, CROSS CULTURAL, SEX COMPARISON, SPANISH SURNAMED, RESOURCE UTILIZATION, EMPIRICAL, RESEARCH METHODOLOGY, FLORIDA, SOUTH

ABST TREATMENT RECORDS OF A POPULATION OF 4,620 VOLUNTARILY ADMITTED DRUG ABUSING MALES AND FEMALES WERE SUBJECTED TO LOG LINEAR MODELING TO DETERMINE THE UNDERLYING RELATIONSHIPS AMONG PATIENT SEX, ETHNICITY, DRUG OF CHOICE, SINGLE VS. POLYDRUG INVOLVEMENT, AND CHOICE OF SERVICE SITE. SEPARATE MODELS FOR EACH ETHNIC GROUP SHOWED THE ANGLO DRUG POPULATION TO BE THE MOST COMPLEX AND THE SPANISH POPULATION TO BE SIMPLEST IN THE INTERRELATIONSHIPS AMONG THESE FACTORS. LOG LINEAR COEFFICIENTS INDICATED THAT SEVERAL ASSOCIATIONS OBSERVABLE IN THE RAW DATA WERE ARTIFACTS OF CORRELATIONS AMONG PATIENT DEMOGRAPHY, SITUATIONAL RISK AND SERVICE UTILIZATION FACTORS, AND MOST NOTABLY THE RELATIONSHIP BETWEEN SEX AND HOSPITAL UTILIZATION. THE IMPLICATIONS OF THESE MODELS FOR THE DEVELOPMENT OF TREATMENT STRATEGIES ARE DISCUSSED, WITH AN EMPHASIS ON THE USE OF LOG LINEAR ANALYSIS TO CONTROL FOR UTILIZATION BIAS IN THE INTERPRETATION OF TREATMENT RECORD STATISTICS. 41 REFERENCES. (AUTHOR ABSTRACT)

ACCN 000841

979 AUTH **LADNER, R., PAGE, W. F., & LEE, M. L.**

TITL ETHNIC AND SEX EFFECTS ON EMERGENCY WARD UTILIZATION FOR DRUG-RELATED PROBLEMS: A LINEAR MODEL ANALYSIS.

SRCE *JOURNAL OF HEALTH AND SOCIAL BEHAVIOR, 1975, 16(SEPTEMBER), 315-325.*

INDX DRUG ABUSE, RESOURCE UTILIZATION, SEX COMPARISON, CROSS CULTURAL, SPANISH SURNAMED, SUICIDE, CULTURAL FACTORS, MENTAL HEALTH, EMPIRICAL, RESEARCH METHODOLOGY, CUBAN, URBAN, DRUG ADDICTION, FLORIDA, SOUTH

ABST THE RATES FOR FIVE DRUG-RELATED COMPLAINTS (OVERDOSES, SUICIDE ATTEMPTS, ACUTE PSYCHIATRIC PROBLEMS, ADDICTION SYMPTOMS AND MEDICAL PROBLEMS) AT ADMISSION TO THE EMERGENCY ROOM OF A LARGE METROPOLITAN HOSPITAL WERE ANALYZED BY PATIENT SEX AND ETHNICITY IN ORDER TO DETERMINE THE POPULATIONS AT RISK FOR INDIVIDUAL COMPLAINTS. MEDICAL RECORDS FOR A ONE-YEAR PERIOD BETWEEN JULY 1973 AND JUNE 1974 WERE REVIEWED FOR 1,288 ANGLOS, 667 BLACKS AND 255 CUBAN AMERICANS. MATHEMATICAL MODELS OF THE DEMOGRAPHIC COMPOSITION OF THESE COMPLAINT POPULATIONS SHOWED REMARKABLE DIFFERENCES, SUGGESTING THAT THE PHENOMENON OF DRUG ABUSE IS DIFFEREN-

TIALLY EXPERIENCED ACROSS THESE ETHNIC AND SEX SUBGROUPS. FOR EXAMPLE, ALTHOUGH THE PRINCIPAL COMPLAINT FOR BOTH MEN AND WOMEN DRUG PATIENTS WAS OVERDOSE, SUICIDE ATTEMPTS WERE MUCH MORE COMMON AMONG FEMALES, WHEREAS PSYCHIATRIC AND ADDICTION PROBLEMS WERE MORE COMMON AMONG MALES. OVERDOSES WERE THE MOST COMMON ADMISSION COMPLAINT FOR PERSONS OF ALL ETHNIC GROUPS, BUT SUICIDE ATTEMPTS WERE MORE FREQUENT AMONG SPANISH PATIENTS. ADDICTION PROBLEMS WERE MORE FREQUENT AMONG ANGLOS, AND MEDICAL PROBLEMS WERE MORE FREQUENT AMONG BLACKS. LINEAR ANALYSIS IS RECOMMENDED AS THE ANALYSIS OF CHOICE FOR DETERMINING COMBINED SEX AND ETHNICITY EFFECTS. THE IMPLICATIONS OF THESE DIFFERENCES FOR THE DELIVERY OF SERVICES AND THE ANALYSIS OF OTHER EPIDEMIOLOGICAL DATA ARE DISCUSSED. 54 REFERENCES. (JOURNAL ABSTRACT MODIFIED)

ACCN 000842

980 AUTH **LAMANNA, R. A., & SAMORA, J.**

TITL MEXICAN AMERICANS IN A MIDWEST METROPOLIS: A STUDY OF EAST CHICAGO (MEXICAN AMERICAN STUDY PROJECT, ADVANCE REPORT NO. 8).

SRCE *UNPUBLISHED MANUSCRIPT, UNIVERSITY OF CALIFORNIA AT LOS ANGELES, DIVISION OF RESEARCH, GRADUATE SCHOOL OF BUSINESS ADMINISTRATION, 1967.*

INDX MEXICAN AMERICAN, FAMILY STRUCTURE, DEMOGRAPHIC, REVIEW, EMPIRICAL, ACCULTURATION, HISTORY, COMMUNITY, RELIGION, EDUCATION, MIGRATION, SOCIAL MOBILITY, EMPLOYMENT, PSYCHOSOCIAL ADJUSTMENT, SES, ILLINOIS, MIDWEST

ABST MEXICAN AMERICANS WHO HAVE MIGRATED TO THE INDUSTRIAL COMPLEX OF EAST CHICAGO ARE ANALYZED TO DETERMINE THE VALIDITY OF A HYPOTHESIS THAT THIS GROUP WAS PROVIDED OPPORTUNITIES NOT AVAILABLE TO THEIR COUNTERPARTS IN THE SOUTHWEST FOR ASSIMILATION INTO THE COMMUNITY. A CONCISE REPORT ON THE HISTORY OF THE MEXICAN AMERICAN COLONY IN EAST CHICAGO, ITS GROWTH INTO A COMMUNITY, FAMILY TRADITIONS, AND CHURCH RELATIONS IS INCLUDED. EDUCATION AND ITS EFFECTS, PATTERNS OF EMPLOYMENT AND OCCUPATIONAL STATUS, INTERNAL COHESION AND POLITICAL INFLUENCE, AND PERSONAL AND SOCIAL ADJUSTMENT STUDIES ARE SUPPORTED BY GRAPHS, CHARTS, AND TABLES. IT WAS DETERMINED THAT THE HYPOTHESIS WAS NOT VALID AND THAT GEOGRAPHIC DISPERSION BEYOND THE SOUTHWEST DID NOT NECESSARILY RESULT IN CONSPICUOUS STATUS BENEFITS UNOBTAINABLE IN THE SOUTHWEST. THE REPORT CONCLUDES THAT THERE IS VERY LITTLE VARIATION IN SOCIOECONOMIC POSITION BY MEXICAN AMERICANS MIGRATING TO AN INDUSTRIAL COMPLEX, IN REFERENCE TO GROUP ASSIMILATION, COMPARED TO THEIR

SOUTHWESTERN NEIGHBORS. (SOCIOLOGICAL ABSTRACT)

ACCN 000843

981 AUTH **LAMB, E. D.**
TITL RACIAL DIFFERENCES IN BI-MANUAL DEXTERITY OF LATIN AND AMERICAN CHILDREN.
SRCE *CHILD DEVELOPMENT, 1930, 1(3), 204-231.*
INDX PHYSICAL DEVELOPMENT, MEXICAN AMERICAN, CROSS CULTURAL, EMPIRICAL, ABILITY TESTING, CALIFORNIA, SOUTHWEST, GOODENOUGH DRAW-A-MAN TEST
ABST A COMPARATIVE STUDY OF RACIAL DIFFERENCES IN MANUAL DEXTERITY AMONG ITALIAN AMERICAN (IA), MEXICAN AMERICAN (MA), AND TWO ANGLO AMERICAN (AA) GROUPS IS REPORTED. 212 CHILDREN BETWEEN THE AGES OF 4 AND 7 (ALMOST EVENLY DISTRIBUTED AMONG THE RACIAL GROUPS) WERE EVALUATED WITH THE FOLLOWING TESTS: PEGBOARD, GOODENOUGH DRAWING TEST, TYING OF BOW, GODDARD FORMBOARD, NUT AND BOLT, BUTTONING OF BELT IN BACK, PEGBOARD COLORS, THREADING OF NEEDLES, MOTOR COORDINATION, PICTURE PUZZLES, AND STRINGING BUTTONS. DATA INDICAE THAT 77 PERCENT OF THE MA'S, 60 PERCENT OF AA GROUP I, 58 PERCENT OF THE IA'S, AND 56 PERCENT OF THE AA GROUP II HAD INTELLIGENCE QUOTIENTS ON THE GOODENOUGH DRAWING TEST WHICH WERE THE NORM. THE MA'S RANKED HIGHEST IN EIGHT OF THE MANIPULATION TESTS. THE MA'S WERE CLEARLY SUPERIOR TO AA CHILDREN IN THE QUICKNESS AND ACCURACY OF MANIPULATION. IT APPEARS THEN THAT RACIAL GROUPS DEVELOP MANIPULATIVE ABILITY AT DIFFERENTIAL RATES. 15 REFERENCES.
ACCN 000844

982 AUTH **LAMONT, J., & GOTTLIEB, H.**
TITL CONVERGENT RECALL OF PARENTAL BEHAVIORS IN DEPRESSED STUDENTS OF DIFFERENT RACIAL GROUPS.
SRCE *JOURNAL OF CLINICAL PSYCHOLOGY, 1975, 31(1), 9-11.*
INDX DEPRESSION, CHILDREARING PRACTICES, FATHER-CHILD INTERACTION, MOTHER-CHILD INTERACTION, CROSS CULTURAL, MEXICAN AMERICAN, PSYCHOPATHOLOGY, MENTAL HEALTH
ABST FORTY-THREE CHINESE AMERICAN, 81 MEXICAN AMERICAN AND 243 WHITE COLLEGE STUDENTS WERE ADMINISTERED A MEASURE OF DEPRESSION AND A MEASURE OF RECALL OF PARENTAL BEHAVIOR. DEPRESSION SCORES WERE CORRELATED WITH ITEM ENDORSEMENT ON THE RECALL OF PARENTAL BEHAVIOR FOR EACH ETHNIC GROUP. SEVEN PARENTAL BEHAVIOR ITEMS THAT PRODUCED SIGNIFICANT CORRELATIONS WITH DEPRESSION ACROSS ETHNIC GROUPS WERE IDENTIFIED, INDICATING THAT DEPRESSED SUBJECTS RECALLED THEIR MOTHERS AS LESS POSITIVELY INVOLVED WITH THEM, AS MORE CRITICAL, AND AS MORE GUILT-INDUCING. THE RESULTS PROVIDE CROSS-CULTURAL CONFIRMATION OF PRIOR FINDINGS IN THIS AREA. ISSUES OF CULTURAL BIAS AND VALIDITY IN GENERALIZATIONS FROM ONE CULTURAL GROUP TO ANOTHER ARE BRIEFLY DISCUSSED. 3 REFERENCES. (AUTHOR SUMMARY MODIFIED)
ACCN 000845

983 AUTH **LAMPE, P. E.**
TITL A COMPARATIVE STUDY OF ASSIMILATION OF MEXICAN AMERICAN PAROCHIAL VERSUS PUBLIC SCHOOLS.
SRCE *SAN FRANCISCO: R AND E RESEARCH ASSOCIATES, 1975.*
INDX ACCULTURATION, ADOLESCENTS, TEXAS, SOUTHWEST, RELIGION, EMPIRICAL, MEXICAN AMERICAN, ATTITUDES, ETHNIC IDENTITY, CROSS CULTURAL
ABST TO DISCOVER TO WHAT EXTENT THE MEXICAN AMERICAN STUDENT HAS BEEN ASSIMILATED INTO THE ANGLO AMERICAN SOCIETY AND WHETHER THIS SOCIAL PROCESS IS MORE OR LESS PRONOUNCED IN THE PUBLIC AS COMPARED TO THE PAROCHIAL SCHOOL SYSTEM, EIGHT HYPOTHESES WERE TESTED. IT WAS PREDICTED THAT THERE WOULD BE NO RELATIONSHIP BETWEEN SEVEN TYPES OR ASPECTS OF ASSIMILATION (ACCULTURATION, STRUCTURAL, AMALGAMATION, IDENTIFICATIONAL, BEHAVIOR RECEPTIONAL, ATTITUDE RECEPTIONAL, AND CIVIC ASSIMILATION) AND PUBLIC OR PAROCHIAL SCHOOL ATTENDANCE, AND NO DIFFERENCE IN THE DEGREE OF OVERALL ASSIMILATION BETWEEN STUDENTS AT THE TWO TYPES OF SCHOOLS. THE SAMPLE CONSISTED OF 383 EIGHTH-GRADE MEXICAN AMERICAN STUDENTS, 168 FROM NINE PUBLIC SCHOOLS AND 215 FROM NINE PAROCHIAL SCHOOLS IN SAN ANTONIO, TEXAS. DEGREE OF ASSIMILATION WAS MEASURED BY MEANS OF A SEVEN-PART QUESTIONNAIRE DESIGNED BY THE INVESTIGATOR. A SIGNIFICANT DIFFERENCE IN OVERALL ASSIMILATION WAS FOUND BETWEEN PUBLIC AND PAROCHIAL SCHOOL STUDENTS. PAROCHIAL SCHOOL STUDENTS REVEALED A GREATER DEGREE OF ACCULTURATION, STRUCTURAL ASSIMILATION, FAVORABLE ATTITUDE TOWARD AMALGAMATION, ATTITUDINAL ASSIMILATION, AND CIVIC ASSIMILATION; PUBLIC SCHOOL STUDENTS SHOWED MORE IDENTIFICATION AND ASSIMILATION. IT IS SUGGESTED THAT, ALTHOUGH ALMOST THE ENTIRE SAMPLE WAS CATHOLIC, RELIGIOUS SCHOOLING MAY DIRECTLY OR INDIRECTLY BE RESPONSIBLE FOR MANY OF THESE DIFFERENCES. 83 REFERENCES. (AUTHOR ABSTRACT MODIFIED)
ACCN 000846

984 AUTH **LAMPE, P. E.**
TITL MEXICAN AMERICAN SELF-IDENTITY AND ETHNIC PREJUDICE.
SRCE *CORNELL JOURNAL OF SOCIAL RELATIONS, 1975, 10(2), 223-237.*
INDX SELF CONCEPT, ETHNIC IDENTITY, MEXICAN AMERICAN, DISCRIMINATION, CULTURAL FACTORS, CHILDREN, CROSS CULTURAL, EMPIRICAL, PREJUDICE, TEXAS, SOUTHWEST

ABST THE RELATIONSHIP BETWEEN AN INDIVIDUAL'S CHOICE OF AN ETHNIC, SELF-IDENTIFYING TERM AND PREJUDICE TOWARD OTHER SPECIFIC ETHNIC GROUPS WAS STUDIED IN 369 EIGHTH-GRADE MEXICAN AMERICAN STUDENTS ATTENDING PUBLIC AND PAROCHIAL SCHOOLS IN SAN ANTONIO, TEXAS. THE QUESTIONNAIRE DIRECTED STUDENTS TO RANK IN ORDER OF PREFERENCE THE FOLLOWING ETHNIC GROUPS: ANGLO, MEXICAN AMERICAN, JEW, NEGRO AND ORIENTAL. SUBJECTS WERE ALSO DIRECTED TO RANK THE SAME GROUPS ACCORDING TO INFERIORITY. LASTLY, SUBJECTS CIRCLED THE TERM BY WHICH THEY PREFERRED TO BE KNOWN OR REFERRED: AMERICAN, MEXICAN AMERICAN, CHICANO, SPANISH AMERICAN OR ANGLO AMERICAN. THE FINDINGS INDICATED: (1) THE MAJORITY OF STUDENTS PREFERRED TO BE CALLED MEXICAN AMERICAN, FOLLOWED BY AMERICAN, CHICANO AND SPANISH AMERICAN; (2) PUBLIC SCHOOL AND MIDDLE-CLASS RESPONDENTS CHOSE THE TERM CHICANO MORE FREQUENTLY THAN THE TERM AMERICAN; (3) AMONG ALL GROUPS THE TERM MEXICAN AMERICAN WAS PREFERRED; (4) THE GREATEST INCIDENCE OF POSITIVE PREJUDICE WAS SHOWN TOWARD THE RESPONDENTS' OWN ETHNIC GROUP; (5) BOTH MIDDLE-CLASS AND PAROCHIAL SCHOOL CHICANOS, WHILE EXPRESSING A PREFERENCE FOR BLACKS OVER ANGLOS, INDICATED THE BELIEF THAT BLACKS WERE EQUAL OR INFERIOR TO ANGLOS; AND (6) CHICANO WORKING-CLASS RESPONDENTS RANKED ANGLOS LAST, MIDDLE-CLASS CHICANOS RANKED ANGLOS OVER BLACKS. IT IS CONCLUDED THAT THERE IS SOME RELATIONSHIP BETWEEN THE ETHNIC SELF-IDENTIFYING TERM SELECTED BY AN INDIVIDUAL AND HIS BIASES, BOTH POSITIVE AND NEGATIVE, TOWARD DIFFERENT ETHNIC GROUPS. 25 REFERENCES.

ACCN 000847

985 AUTH **LAMPKIN, L. C.**
TITL ALIENATION AS A COPING MECHANISM: "OUT WHERE THE ACTION IS."
SRCE *IN E. PAVENSTEDT & V. W. BERNARD (EDS.), CRISES OF FAMILY DISORGANIZATION: PROGRAMS TO SOFTEN THEIR IMPACT ON CHILDREN. NEW YORK: BEHAVIORAL PUBLICATIONS, 1971, PP. 43-50.*
INDX ADOLESCENTS, ANOMIE, FAMILY STRUCTURE, CULTURAL FACTORS, EDUCATION, CULTURAL PLURALISM, ENVIRONMENTAL FACTORS, POVERTY, ESSAY, PUERTO RICAN-M, SES, PEER GROUP, URBAN, CROSS CULTURAL, NEW YORK, EAST
ABST THE CONSEQUENCES OF STRESSES AND STRAINS CREATED BY SOCIAL INSTITUTIONS TO MEMBERS OF MINORITY AND LOW-SES GROUPS ARE DISCUSSED BY A SOCIAL WORKER PRACTICING IN NEW YORK CITY. ALIENATION, DEVIANCE, AND ACTING OUT ARE CONSIDERED AS POSSIBLY MEANINGFUL AND CONFORMING ADAPTATIONS TO MANY AN INDIVIDUAL'S REALITY. ALIENATION RESULTS FROM THE ACCEPTANCE OF PRESSING REALITIES OF LOWER-CLASS LIFE IN AN AFFLUENT SOCIETY RATHER THAN FROM REJECTION OF MAJORITY VALUES OR CULTURE. IF THE TIDE OF THE CRISIS IN DISORGANIZATION AMONG LOWER-CLASS FAMILIES IS TO BE ARRESTED, THE SOCIAL CONDITIONS IN WHICH THE FAMILY LIVES MUST BE AMELIORATED. IMPROVEMENT OF SOCIAL INSTITUTIONS UPON WHICH THESE FAMILIES DEPEND, WITH AN EMPHASIS ON PREVENTION, IS RECOMMENDED. 3 REFERENCES.

ACCN 000848

986 AUTH **THE LANCET.**
TITL DRUG ADDICTION IN ADOLESCENTS.
SRCE *THE LANCET, MARCH 29, 1952, NO. 6709, PP. 654-655.*
INDX DRUG ADDICTION, ADOLESCENTS, PUERTO RICAN-M, NEW YORK, EAST, REVIEW, DEMOGRAPHIC, PERSONALITY
ABST A GENERAL REVIEW OF DRUG ADDICTION IN ADOLESCENTS IN THE UNITED STATES PRIOR TO 1952 IS PRESENTED. IT IS ESTIMATED THAT THERE WERE BETWEEN 48,000 AND 100,000 ADDICTS IN THE UNITED STATES IN 1951. ONE STUDY INDICATED FROM 45,000 TO 90,000 IN NEW YORK CITY ALONE. FBI FIGURES FOR THE FIRST HALF OF 1951 SHOW THAT ALMOST HALF THE NARCOTICS OFFENDERS WERE UNDER 25 YEARS OF AGE. NO CASES OF HEROIN OR MORPHINE ADDICTS UNDER 21 YEARS OF AGE WERE REPORTED IN BELLEVUE HOSPITAL, NEW YORK CITY, BETWEEN 1940 AND 1948; IN 1949 THERE WAS ONE CASE, AND IN 1950, 11 CASES. IN THE FIRST 7 MONTHS OF 1951, 260 OF THESE YOUNGSTERS WERE ADMITTED, THEIR AGES RANGING FROM 14 TO 20. MOST WERE NEGRO OR PUERTO RICAN, AND ALL WERE FROM HARLEM, WHERE YOUNG PEOPLE SUFFER FROM DISCRIMINATION AGAINST THEIR RACIAL GROUPS, AND THE RATE OF CRIME AND DISEASE IS HIGHER THAN ANYWHERE ELSE IN NEW YORK. INVESTIGATORS FOUND THAT THESE ADOLESCENTS WERE NONAGGRESSIVE AND PASSIVE, WITH WEAK AND SUPERFICIAL SOCIAL RELATIONSHIPS, BUT HAVING CLOSE EMPATHETIC RELATIONSHIPS WITH THEIR MOTHERS. THEY LIVE A FANTASY LIFE, WITH GRANDIOSE DAYDREAMS, BECOMING INCREASINGLY ISOLATED AND WITHDRAWN FROM SOCIAL CONTACTS AND FROM THE REAL WORLD IN WHICH THEY FEEL INFERIOR AND INSECURE. 7 REFERENCES.
ACCN 000057

987 AUTH **LANDER, B., & LANDER, N.**
TITL A CROSS-CULTURAL STUDY OF NARCOTIC ADDICTION IN NEW YORK.
SRCE *IN INSTITUTE ON NEW DEVELOPMENTS IN THE TREATMENT OF THE NARCOTIC ADDICT (ED.), REHABILITATING THE NARCOTIC ADDICT. NEW YORK: ARNO PRESS, 1967, PP. 359-369.*
INDX REHABILITATION, ENVIRONMENTAL FACTORS, SES, POVERTY, CRIMINOLOGY, DRUG ADDICTION, SEXUAL BEHAVIOR, AGGRESSION, FAMILY STRUCTURE, JOB PERFORMANCE, OCCUPATIONAL ASPIRATIONS, EMPIRICAL, NEW YORK, EAST, URBAN, PUERTO RICAN-M

ABST   A PROJECT IS DESCRIBED WHICH WAS UNDER-
TAKEN TO PROVIDE A COMPREHENSIVE DE-
SCRIPTION AND EXPLANATION OF THE SOCIAL,
CULTURAL, AND PSYCHOLOGICAL FACTORS
RELATED TO NARCOTICS USE IN A PREDOMI-
NANTLY PUERTO RICAN SLUM BLOCK IN NEW
YORK CITY. THIS STUDY IS BEING PARALLELED
IN A NEGRO AREA IN WASHINGTON, D.C., AND
A SOUTHERN WHITE NEIGHBORHOOD IN CHI-
CAGO; THE LATTER AREAS, HOWEVER, WERE
SELECTED ON THE BASIS OF DELINQUENCY
RATHER THAN ON A HISTORY OF DRUG USE.
INTERVIEWS WERE CARRIED OUT WITH RESI-
DENT ADDICTS, NONRESIDENT ADDICTS WHO
REGULARLY VISIT THE BLOCK, FORMER AD-
DICTS WHO HAVE NOT USED NARCOTICS FOR
AT LEAST 1 YEAR, USERS OF OTHER DRUGS
SUCH AS MARIJUANA AND AMPHETAMINES,
AND RESIDENTS OF THE BLOCK WHO DO NOT
USE DRUGS, ESPECIALLY NONUSING SIBLINGS
OF INDIVIDUALS WHO DO USE DRUGS. DATA
HAVE BEEN COMPILED ON THE SOCIOECO-
NOMIC CHARACTERISTICS OF THE FAMILIES
RESIDING IN THE BLOCK AND ON THE HISTORY
AND ETHNOGRAPHY OF THE BLOCK. PRELIMI-
NARY FINDINGS ARE REPORTED ON THE DIS-
TRIBUTION AND MARKETING OF HEROIN, THE
QUALITY AND KINDS OF DRUGS USED, HEROIN
USE AND SEX DRIVE, HEROIN USE AND VIO-
LENCE, FAMILY PATTERNS, THE ADDICT SOCI-
ETY, THE PERSONALITY OF THE ADDICT, NAR-
COTICS ADDICTION AND THE SLUMS, AND
VOCATIONAL EXPERIENCE AND DRUG ADDIC-
TION.

ACCN   000849

988 AUTH   **LANE, A.**
TITL   SEVERE READING DISABILITY AND THE INITIAL
TEACHING ALPHABET.
SRCE   *JOURNAL OF LEARNING DISABILITIES, 1974,
7(8), 479-483.*
INDX   READING, SPECIAL EDUCATION, EDUCA-
TIONAL ASSESSMENT, EMPIRICAL, SCHOLAS-
TIC ACHIEVEMENT, INSTRUCTIONAL TECH-
NIQUES, CHILDREN, PUERTO RICAN-M, CROSS
CULTURAL, CULTURAL FACTORS
ABST   A PILOT STUDY WAS CONDUCTED TO DETER-
MINE WHETHER THE INITIAL TEACHING ALPHA-
BET (I.T.A.) CAN SERVE AS A REMEDIATION
TOOL THAT WOULD SIGNIFICANTLY IMPROVE
THE READING ACHIEVEMENT LEVEL OF 6TH
GRADE CHILDREN WITH A SEVERE READING
DISABILITY. DOING THE GRAY ORAL READING
TEST IN A PUBLIC ELEMENTARY SCHOOL, 11
BOYS AND 3 GIRLS, 9 OF WHICH WERE PUERTO
RICAN AND 3 BLACK, WERE IDENTIFIED AS
READING AT OR BELOW THE 2ND GRADE
READING LEVEL. A PRESCRIBED TRAINING
PROGRAM WITH I.T.A. WAS FOLLOWED FOR 100
SCHOOL DAYS. THE GRAY TEST WAS AGAIN
ADMINISTERED AND READING LEVELS WERE
FOUND TO BE SIGNIFICANTLY IMPROVED. THE
POSITIVE RESULTS PROVIDE EVIDENCE THAT
I.T.A. IS A TOOL WHICH CAN HELP REMEDIATE
THE SEVERELY DISABLED READERS IN THE
UNITED STATES. SINCE THIS STUDY REPRE-
SENTS ONLY A PILOT, FURTHER RESEARCH IS
NEEDED TO DEVELOP NEW READING MATE-

RIAL IN THE I.T.A. APPROPRIATE FOR THE RE-
MEDIAL READING STUDENTS IN 6TH TO 10TH
GRADE. ALSO, THE LENGTH OF OPTIMAL TIME
A STUDENT SHOULD SPEND WITH THE I.T.A.
NEEDS TO BE ESTABLISHED. 12 REFERENCES.
(AUTHOR ABSTRACT MODIFIED)

ACCN   000850

989 AUTH   **LANGGULUNG, H., & TORRANCE, R. P.**
TITL   THE DEVELOPMENT OF CAUSAL THINKING OF
CHILDREN IN MEXICO AND THE UNITED STATES.
SRCE   *JOURNAL OF CROSS CULTURAL PSYCHOLOGY,
1972, 3(3), 315-320.*
INDX   MEXICAN, CHILDREN, EMPIRICAL, CROSS CUL-
TURAL, COGNITIVE DEVELOPMENT, SEX COM-
PARISON, COGNITIVE STYLE, GEORGIA, SOUTH,
URBAN
ABST   160 4TH AND 6TH GRADE METROPOLITAN
MEXICAN AND AMERICAN CHILDREN, DIVIDED
EQUALLY BY GRADE, SEX, AND SOCIOECO-
NOMIC STATUS, HAD THEIR RESPONSES TO
THE GUESS CAUSES TEST OF THE TORRANCE
TESTS OF CREATIVE THINKING ANALYZED FOR
CAUSAL THINKING. IT WAS FOUND THAT
AMERICAN SUBJECTS, 6TH GRADERS, AND
THE ECONOMICALLY ADVANTAGED WERE MORE
CAUSALLY ORIENTED THAN THEIR OPPOSITES.
NO SEX DIFFERENCES WERE FOUND IN EITHER
CULTURE. 15 REFERENCES. (PASAR ABSTRACT
MODIFIED)

ACCN   000851

990 AUTH   **LANGNER, T. S.**
TITL   PSYCHOPHYSIOLOGICAL SYMPTOMS AND THE
STATUS OF WOMEN IN TWO MEXICAN COM-
MUNITIES.
SRCE   *IN J. M. MURPHY & A. H. LEIGHTON (EDS.), AP-
PROACHES TO CROSS-CULTURAL PSYCHIATRY.
NEW YORK: CORNELL UNIVERSITY PRESS, 1965,
PP. 360-392.*
INDX   SYMPTOMATOLOGY, HEALTH, SES, POVERTY,
MEXICAN, CULTURE, FEMALE, EMPIRICAL,
COPING MECHANISMS, SEX ROLES, PSY-
CHOTHERAPY, URBAN, RURAL
ABST   AN EXAMINATION OF PSYCHOPHYSIOLOGICAL
SYMPTOMS AND THE STATUS OF WOMEN IN
TWO MEXICAN COMMUNITIES IS PRESENTED.
LOWER-, MIDDLE- AND UPPER-CLASS MEN AND
WOMEN WERE ADMINISTERED A QUESTION-
NAIRE DEALING WITH PSYCHOPHYSIOLOGI-
CAL SYMPTOMS WHICH ARE HIGHLY INDICA-
TIVE   OF   IMPAIRMENT   DUE   TO
PSYCHONEUROTIC DISORDERS. FINDINGS IN-
DICATE: (1) IN A COMMUNITY WHERE WOMEN'S
PRESTIGE STATUS APPROACHES THAT OF MEN,
WOMEN REPORT SLIGHTLY MORE SYMPTOMS
THAN MEN, WHILE IN A COMMUNITY WHERE
WOMEN'S STATUS IS LOW, WOMEN REPORT
CONSIDERABLY MORE SYMPTOMS THAN MEN;
(2) THE LOWER THE INCOME LEVEL, THE
GREATER THE AVERAGE NUMBER OF SYMP-
TOMS REPORTED; (3) CROSS-CULTURAL COM-
PARISONS OF SYMPTOMATOLOGY ARE DIFFI-
CULT TO INTERPRET; (4) WOMEN GENERALLY
REPORT   MORE   PSYCHOPHYSIOLOGICAL
SYMPTOMS THAN MEN; AND (5) WOMEN'S AT-
TITUDES FAVORING SEXUAL EQUALITY ARE
NOT RELATED TO THEIR SEXUAL STATUS OR TO

THE NUMBER OF THEIR SYMPTOMS. THE HIGHER SOCIOECONOMIC STATUS WOMEN OF MEXICO CITY TEND, HOWEVER, TO VOICE EGALITARIAN ATTITUDES. IN GENERAL, METROPOLITAN RESIDENTS TEND TO REPORT MORE SYMPTOMS THAN PROVINCIAL RESIDENTS WHO MAINTAIN THEIR TRADITIONAL CUSTOMS AND LANGUAGE. 19 REFERENCES.

ACCN   000852

991 AUTH   **LANGNER, T. S., GERSTEN, J. C., & EISENBERG, J. G.**

TITL   APPROACHES TO MEASUREMENT AND DEFINITION IN THE EPIDEMIOLOGY OF BEHAVIOR DISORDERS: ETHNIC BACKGROUND AND CHILD BEHAVIOR.

SRCE   *INTERNATIONAL JOURNAL OF HEALTH SERVICES, 1974, 4(3), 483-501.*

INDX   STRESS, CHILDREN, SURVEY, SPANISH SURNAMED, CROSS CULTURAL, MARITAL STABILITY, MENTAL HEALTH, SES, NEW YORK, EAST

ABST   THIS PAPER PRESENTS METHODS OF APPROACHING MENTAL ILLNESS WHICH REPRESENT ALTERNATIVES TO THE MEDICAL MODEL AND THE CURRENT DIAGNOSTIC SYSTEM. IT ALSO POINTS TO NEW WAYS OF HANDLING SUCH COMPLEX INDEPENDENT VARIABLES AS RACE AND CLASS TO MORE CLEARLY DELINEATE THE CRITICAL COMPONENTS OF THOSE CONSTRUCTS FOR OBSERVED RELATIONSHIPS. THESE APPROACHES ARE BRIEFLY DISCUSSED AND THEN EXEMPLIFIED IN THE CONTEXT OF A STUDY WHICH INVESTIGATED THE TYPES AND LEVELS OF STRESS TO WHICH CHILDREN OF DIFFERENT ETHNICITY WERE EXPOSED AND THE CONGRUENCE BETWEEN IMPAIRMENT LEVELS AND STRESS EXPOSURE. DIFFERENTIAL BEHAVIOR PATTERNS BY ETHNICITY WERE DETERMINED, AS WERE THE RELATIVE ROLES OF CLASS VERSUS ETHNICITY IN CHILDREN'S DISTURBED BEHAVIORS. MEASURES WERE DEVELOPED FROM QUESTIONNAIRE DATA COLLECTED FROM 1034 RANDOMLY SELECTED MANHATTAN MOTHERS. WHITE CHILDREN WERE LEAST EXPOSED TO SOCIAL STRESS, HISPANIC MOST EXPOSED TO MARITAL-PARENTAL STRESS, AND BLACK MOST EXPOSED TO STRESSFUL PARENTAL PRACTICES. WHILE THE ESTIMATED IMPAIRMENT RANK-ORDER WAS WHITE, HISPANIC, AND BLACK, BOTH MINORITY GROUPS OF CHILDREN WERE SIGNIFICANTLY HIGHER THAN WHITES BUT SIMILAR TO EACH OTHER IN IMPAIRMENT LEVEL. ANALYSES SHOWED STRONG DIFFERENCES IN BEHAVIOR PATTERNS BY ETHNICITY AND INDICATED THAT RACE MADE A STRONGER CONTRIBUTION THAN CLASS TO DISTURBED BEHAVIORS. 23 REFERENCES. (JOURNAL ABSTRACT)

ACCN   000853

992 AUTH   **LANGNESS, L. L.**

TITL   HYSTERICAL PSYCHOSIS: THE CROSS CULTURAL EVIDENCE.

SRCE   *AMERICAN JOURNAL OF PSYCHIATRY, 1967, 124, 143-152.*

INDX   PSYCHOSIS, PSYCHOPATHOLOGY, CROSS CULTURAL, SYMPTOMATOLOGY, PUERTO RI-

CAN-I, AGGRESSION, SCHIZOPHRENIA, REVIEW, INDIGENOUS POPULATIONS

ABST   "HYSTERICAL PSYCHOSIS" HAS BEEN USED IN THE LITERATURE ON CROSS CULTURAL PSYCHOPATHOLOGY, AT LEAST IN PART, BECAUSE OF THE DIFFICULTIES INVOLVED IN APPLYING STANDARD NOSOLOGICAL CATEGORIES. UPON REVIEWING THE LITERATURE IN ANTHROPOLOGY AND PSYCHIATRY RELATED TO THIS TOPIC, IT NOW APPEARS THAT THERE MAY BE A WIDELY DISTRIBUTED TYPE OF ABNORMAL BEHAVIOR TO WHICH THE TERM COULD BE LEGITIMATELY APPLIED. INCIDENTS OF HYSTERICAL PSYCHOSIS DRAWN FROM THE RESEARCH OF SEVERAL AUTHORS WHO WORKED WITH (1) THE BENA BENA PEOPLES OF NEW GUINEA, (2) THE MOJAVE INDIANS OF ARIZONA AND CALIFORNIA AND (3) NATIVE PUERTO RICANS ARE PRESENTED. SEVERAL NON-WESTERN ILLNESSES, ALSO REPORTED IN THE LITERATURE, ARE DISCUSSED REGARDING THEIR SIMILAR ONSET AND RESOLUTION PATTERNS. AMONG THESE ARE: (1) AMOK AND LATAH, FIRST REPORTED IN MALAYA; (2) WHITIKA, WHICH OCCURS MAINLY AMONG THE OJIBWA INDIANS OF NORTHEASTERN U.S. AND CANADA; (3) PIBLOKTOQ, ALSO CALLED ARTIC PSYCHOSIS, AND (4) IMU, A DISEASE OCCURRING AMONG THE AINU OF JAPAN. CROSS-CULTURALLY, HYSTERICAL PSYCHOSES OCCUR IN MALES AND FEMALES, ARE NON-ORGANIC IN ORIGIN, ARE RELATED TO CROSS-CULTURALLY DEFINED STRESSFUL EVENTS AND ARE TRANSIENT. ALTHOUGH SOCIAL RESPONSES VARY FROM CULTURE TO CULTURE, THE BEHAVIOR DURING ATTACKS IS STEREOTYPED, APPEARS TO BE SHAPED AND DIRECTED BY THE PARTICULAR CULTURE AND IS, THEREFORE, LEARNED. THE PERSONALITY CHARACTERISTICS WHICH MIGHT BE SHARED CROSS-CULTURALLY BY VICTIMS OF HYSTERICAL PSYCHOSES ARE SUGGESTIBILITY, NONSCIENTIFIC MODES OF THINKING, AND PERHAPS AN OVERSENSITIVITY IN RESPONDING TO CUES. 37 REFERENCES. (AUTHOR SUMMARY MODIFIED)

ACCN   000854

993 AUTH   **LANGROD, J.**

TITL   SECONDARY DRUG USE AMONG HEROIN USERS.

SRCE   *INTERNATIONAL JOURNAL OF THE ADDICTIONS, 1970, 5(4), 611-635.*

INDX   DRUG ADDICTION, DRUG ABUSE, REHABILITATION, PUERTO RICAN-M, MALE, CROSS CULTURAL, EMPIRICAL, NEW YORK, EAST

ABST   THE PRESENCE OF EXTENSIVE SECONDARY DRUG ABUSE BY HEROIN ADDICTS IS A FACTOR IN DETERMINING ELIGIBILITY FOR ADMITTANCE TO TREATMENT PROGRAMS LIKE METHADONE MAINTENANCE BECAUSE THE METHADONE BLOCKAGE SUCCESSFULLY ELIMINATES ONLY THE HEROIN CRAVING AND THE "HIGH." INTERVIEWS WITH 422 MALE HEROIN USERS IN 6 DIFFERENT TREATMENT FACILITIES REVEALED THAT 77% USED MARIJUANA BEFORE HEROIN, WITH THE USE OF ALL OTHER DRUGS OCCURRING AFTER INITIAL HEROIN USE. OVER ONE-THIRD OF ALL AD-

DICTS SURVEYED REPORTED HAVING USED DRUGS SUCH AS COCAINE, AMPHETAMINES, AND BARBITURATES. THE MEAN NUMBER OF DRUGS USED, OTHER THAN HEROIN, WAS 3.4 PER ADDICT. ETHNICITY IS CLOSELY RELATED TO BOTH THE NUMBER AND TYPE OF SECONDARY DRUG ABUSE, WITH WHITES BEING MORE LIKELY THAN EITHER PUERTO RICANS OR BLACKS TO ABUSE A LARGER NUMBER OF SECONDARY DRUGS MORE THAN 6 TIMES. COCAINE WAS THE ONLY SECONDARY DRUG BLACKS WERE MORE LIKELY TO USE. THOSE RESPONDENTS WHO REPORTED AN ABSTENTION FROM HEROIN OF 3 MONTHS OR MORE WERE MORE LIKELY TO SUBSTITUTE OTHER DRUGS DURING THE PERIOD IF THEY HAD A PRIOR HISTORY OF SECONDARY DRUG USE. 28 REFERENCES.

ACCN   000855

994 AUTH   **LAOSA, L. M.**
    TITL   BILINGUALISM IN THREE UNITED STATES HISPANIC GROUPS: CONTEXTUAL USE OF LANGUAGE BY CHILDREN AND ADULTS IN THEIR FAMILIES.
    SRCE   *JOURNAL OF EDUCATIONAL PSYCHOLOGY, 1975, 67(5), 617-627.*
    INDX   BILINGUALISM, CUBAN, CROSS CULTURAL, SES, MEXICAN AMERICAN, URBAN, TEXAS, FLORIDA, CHILDREN, PUERTO RICAN-M, LINGUISTICS, ADULTS, BILINGUAL, MEXICAN AMERICAN, NEW YORK, EAST, SOUTH, SOUTHWEST
    ABST   THE USE OF LANGUAGE PATTERNS WAS STUDIED IN DIFFERENT SOCIAL CONTEXTS AMONG CENTRAL TEXAS MEXICAN AMERICAN, MIAMI CUBAN AMERICAN, AND NEW YORK PUERTO RICAN CHILDREN AND ADULTS IN THEIR FAMILIES. DATA WERE COLLECTED THROUGH STRUCTURED INTERVIEWS WITH 295 FAMILIES. CHILDREN WERE 1ST, 2ND, AND 3RD GRADERS, APPROXIMATELY EQUALLY DIVIDED BY SEX. RESULTS INDICATE THAT EVEN WITHIN SUBCULTURAL COMMUNITIES THERE IS SIGNIFICANT VARIABILITY IN THE LANGUAGE PATTERNS USED IN VARIOUS SOCIAL CONTEXTS. THE CENTRAL TEXAS MEXICAN AMERICAN EVIDENCED THE GREATEST DEGREE OF DISPLACEMENT OF MOTHER TONGUE. THERE WERE SIGNIFICANT CHILD-ADULT DIFFERENCES IN LANGUAGE USE AMONG THE MEXICAN AMERICAN AND CUBAN AMERICAN FAMILIES. RESULTS ARE DISCUSSED IN LIGHT OF FACTORS THAT MAY AFFECT LANGUAGE MAINTENANCE. 27 REFERENCES. (PASAR ABSTRACT MODIFIED)
    ACCN   000856

995 AUTH   **LAOSA, L. M.**
    TITL   CHILD CARE AND THE CULTURALLY DIFFERENT CHILD.
    SRCE   *CHILD CARE QUARTERLY, 1974, 3(4), 214-224.*
    INDX   ACCULTURATION, ATTITUDES, BILINGUAL-BICULTURAL PERSONNEL, CHILDREN, CLASSROOM BEHAVIOR, COGNITIVE DEVELOPMENT, COMMUNITY INVOLVEMENT, CULTURAL FACTORS, CULTURE, ENVIRONMENTAL FACTORS, ESSAY, INSTRUCTIONAL TECHNIQUES, MEXI-

CAN AMERICAN, POVERTY, PROFESSIONAL TRAINING, TEACHERS, VALUES
    ABST   TWO TOPICS ARE DISCUSSED IN AN ESSAY ON CHILD CARE FOR NATIONAL-ORIGIN MINORITY CHILDREN: (1) THE IMPORTANCE OF TAKING INTO ACCOUNT THE CULTURAL, LINGUISTIC, AND SES CHARACTERISTICS OF CHILDREN IN CHILD CARE PROGRAMS; AND (2) MAJOR AREAS OF COMPETENCY NEEDED FOR QUALIFIED CHILD CARE PERSONNEL TO WORK WITH NATIONAL-ORIGIN MINORITY CHILDREN IN THE U.S., SPECIFICALLY THOSE FROM SPANISH-SPEAKING BACKGROUNDS. MINORITY GROUP CHILDREN, PARTICULARLY THOSE THAT SHARE THE CULTURE OF POVERTY, FREQUENTLY DISPLAY SUCH CHARACTERISTICS AS LACK OF RESPONSE TO CONVENTIONAL APPROACHES BECAUSE THESE APPROACHES ARE MISUNDERSTOOD. THE COMPETENT CHILD CARE WORKER MUST COMPREHEND THESE BEHAVIORS WITHIN THEIR CULTURAL CONTEXT AND NOT LIMIT STUDENT EXPECTATIONS. A CHILD CARE WORKER MUST ALSO BE CAPABLE OF PROVIDING SITUATIONS AND TASKS IN WHICH THE CHILD CAN REALISTICALLY SUCCEED AND DEVELOP A POSITIVE SELF-IMAGE. CHILDREN WHO FIND THEIR VALUES AND LEARNING STYLES IGNORED BY THE INSTRUCTOR MAY BECOME ALIENATED; CONSEQUENTLY, CHILD CARE PERSONNEL MUST RECOGNIZE AND INCORPORATE THE CHILD'S CULTURAL VALUES AND PREFERRED RELATIONAL AND LEARNING STYLES. ACTIVE RECRUITMENT OF MINORITY GROUP TRAINEES IS NECESSARY AND MORE CROSS-CULTURAL SYSTEMATIC RESEARCH IN CHILD DEVELOPMENT AND CHILD CARE ARE NEEDED TO IMPROVE STANDARDS OF NATIONAL-ORIGIN MINORITY CHILD CARE. 16 REFERENCES.
    ACCN   002127

996 AUTH   **LAOSA, L. M.**
    TITL   COGNITIVE STYLES AND LEARNING STRATEGIES RESEARCH: SOME OF THE AREAS IN WHICH PSYCHOLOGY CAN CONTRIBUTE TO PERSONALIZED INSTRUCTION IN MULTICULTURAL EDUCATION.
    SRCE   *JOURNAL OF TEACHER EDUCATION, 1977, 28(3), 26-30.*
    INDX   BILINGUAL-BICULTURAL EDUCATION, CHILDREARING PRACTICES, CHILDREN, COGNITIVE DEVELOPMENT, COGNITIVE STYLE, EDUCATION, ESSAY, FIELD DEPENDENCE-INDEPENDENCE, INSTRUCTIONAL TECHNIQUES, MEXICAN AMERICAN, MOTHER-CHILD INTERACTION
    ABST   RESEARCH ON COGNITIVE STYLES AND LEARNING STRATEGIES CAN CONTRIBUTE TO PERSONALIZED INSTRUCTION IN MULTICULTURAL EDUCATION. COGNITIVE STYLE IS THE SELF-CONSISTENT WAY OF PROCESSING INFORMATION, WHILE A LEARNING STRATEGY IS THE PROCESS THAT TAKES PLACE AS A PERSON ATTEMPTS TO LEARN A TASK OR SOLVE A PROBLEM. CHILDREN'S LEARNING PREFERENCES APPEAR TO BE UNIQUE AND SPECIFIC TO THEIR CULTURAL GROUPS, AS INDIVIDUALS FROM CERTAIN CULTURES TEND TO FALL TOWARD ONE OR THE OTHER POLE OF ONE COG-

NITIVE STYLE CONTINUUM—FIELD DEPEN-
DENCE-INDEPENDENCE. THESE DIFFERENCES
ARE OFTEN ATTRIBUTED TO GROUP DIFFER-
ENCES IN HOW CHILDREN ARE SOCIALIZED. A
LINE OF RESEARCH HOLDING PROMISE FOR
MULTICULTURAL EDUCATION IS THE INVESTI-
GATION OF THE STRATEGIES THAT MOTHERS
EMPLOY TO TEACH THEIR CHILDREN. THESE
STRATEGIES USED IN THE SOCIOCULTURAL
CONTEXT OF THE HOME MAY BE INCORPO-
RATED INTO THE SCHOOL TO LESSEN THE AB-
RUPT DISCONTINUITY THAT TYPICALLY OC-
CURS FOR THE MINORITY CHILD. AN
UNDERSTANDING OF THE DEVELOPMENT OF
COGNITIVE STYLES AND LEARNING STRATE-
GIES WILL FACILITATE EDUCATIONAL IM-
PROVEMENTS AND CROSS-CULTURAL UNDER-
STANDING. 34 REFERENCES.

ACCN   002128

997 AUTH   **LAOSA, L. M.**
    TITL   CROSS-CULTURAL AND SUBCULTURAL RE-
            SEARCH IN PSYCHOLOGY AND EDUCATION.
    SRCE   *INTERAMERICAN JOURNAL OF PSYCHOLOGY,*
            1973, 7(3-4), 241-248.
    INDX   EDUCATION, CULTURE, RESEARCH METHOD-
            OLOGY, CROSS CULTURAL, CULTURAL FAC-
            TORS, REVIEW, CULTURE-FAIR TESTS, BILIN-
            GUAL-BICULTURAL PERSONNEL, TEST VALIDITY,
            TEST RELIABILITY, THEORETICAL
    ABST   CONCEPTUAL AND METHODOLOGICAL IS-
            SUES REGARDING THE TASK OF CONSTRICT-
            ING AND ADOPTING INSTRUMENTS, RE-
            SEARCH DESIGNS, AND DEVELOPING
            PROGRAMS FOR COMPARABLE USE ACROSS
            MULTIPLE CULTURAL AND LINGUISTIC GROUPS
            ARE EXAMINED. THE ABSENCE OF BICULTURAL
            AND BILINGUAL SPECIALISTS WHO CAN FUNC-
            TION IN TWO OR MORE CULTURAL-LINGUISTIC
            SETTINGS AND ARE SENSITIVE TO THE RELE-
            VANT ASPECTS IN THESE CULTURES HAS LED
            TO THE LACK OF GENERALIZABILITY IN THE
            FINDINGS. UNFORTUNATELY, DATA COLLECTED
            USUALLY REFLECT UNSYSTEMATIC REPLICA-
            TIONS OF PROGRAMS DEVELOPED IN AN-
            OTHER SOCIETY. RESEARCHERS HAVE GENER-
            ALLY IGNORED THE PROBLEMS OF SAMPLING,
            LINGUISTIC EQUIVALENCE OF MEANING, EX-
            AMINER VARIABILITY, AND CULTURAL VARIA-
            TION IN THE RESPONSE SET WHICH MAY IN
            FACT VARY CONCEPTUALLY BETWEEN CROSS-
            NATIONAL, CROSS-LANGUAGE, AND CROSS-
            SUBCULTURAL GROUPS. NEGLECTING THESE
            CRUCIAL ISSUES HAS CREATED SEVERAL
            METHODOLOGICAL PROBLEMS: CONFOUND-
            ING CULTURAL VARIABLES, LACK OF SEMAN-
            TIC EQUIVALENCE IN MEASUREMENT INSTRU-
            MENTS, AND METHODS OF COLLECTING DATA.
            ALTHOUGH THERE HAVE BEEN ATTEMPTS TO
            CONSTRUCT "CULTURE-FREE" TESTS, THESE
            TESTS TEND TO IGNORE OTHER CULTURAL
            FACTORS SUCH AS COGNITIVE STYLE AND
            WORKING HABITS WITH RESPECT TO TIME LIM-
            ITS. CONSIDERING THE POLITICAL, ECO-
            NOMIC, AND EDUCATIONAL IMPLICATIONS OF
            CROSS-CULTURAL AND SUBCULTURAL INVES-
            TIGATIONS IT IS SUGGESTED THAT MORE EM-
            PHASIS IS NEEDED IN THE FOLLOWING AREAS:

(1) NEW TECHNIQUES OF SCALING; (2) TEST
THEORY; (3) DEVELOPING MULTIVARIATE RE-
SEARCH DESIGNS; AND (4) TRAINING PER-
SONS WHO CAN ADEQUATELY FUNCTION AND
ARE SENSITIVE TO THE VARIOUS ISSUES IN
TWO OR MORE CULTURAL-LINGUISTIC SET-
TINGS. 13 REFERENCES.

ACCN   000857

998 AUTH   **LAOSA, L. M.**
    TITL   SOCIALIZATION, EDUCATION, AND CONTI-
            NUITY: THE IMPORTANCE OF THE SOCIOCUL-
            TURAL CONTEXT.
    SRCE   *YOUNG CHILDREN, 1977, 32(5), 21-27.*
    INDX   ACCULTURATION, BILINGUAL-BICULTURAL
            EDUCATION, CHILDREN, COGNITIVE STYLE,
            CROSS CULTURAL, CUBAN, DYADIC INTERAC-
            TION, EDUCATION, EMPIRICAL, MEXICAN
            AMERICAN, MOTHER-CHILD INTERACTION,
            PUERTO RICAN-M, SES, TEXAS, FLORIDA, NEW
            YORK, SOUTHWEST, EAST, SOUTH, INSTRUC-
            TIONAL TECHNIQUES
    ABST   TWO FACTORS AFFECTING THE TRANSITION
            WHICH CHILDREN MUST MAKE BETWEEN THE
            SOCIOCULTURAL CONTEXT OF THE FAMILY
            AND THE SCHOOL ARE (1) MATERNAL TEACH-
            ING STRATEGIES AND (2) LANGUAGE PAT-
            TERNS AT HOME. THE RESULTS OF TWO STUD-
            IES ON THIS SUBJECT ARE REPORTED. IN THE
            FIRST STUDY OF MATERNAL TEACHING
            STRATEGIES, 40 MEXICAN AMERICAN AND AN-
            GLO MOTHERS WERE OBSERVED BY TRAINED
            BILINGUAL MEXICAN AMERICANS. WHILE THE
            TOTAL NUMBER OF TEACHING BEHAVIORS WAS
            THE SAME FOR BOTH MEXICAN AMERICAN
            AND ANGLO MOTHERS, THE INTERACTIONS
            WHICH MEXICAN AMERICAN CHILDREN HAD
            WITH THEIR MOTHERS WERE MORE OFTEN
            NONVERBAL. ANGLO MOTHERS WERE VERBAL
            AND ASKED MORE QUESTIONS WHILE TEACH-
            ING THEIR CHILDREN. IT IS CONCLUDED THAT
            MEXICAN AMERICAN AND ANGLO AMERICAN
            CHILDREN FROM SIMILAR SES BACKGROUNDS
            ARE EXPOSED TO DIFFERENT ADULT-CHILD IN-
            TERACTION STYLES AND INSTRUCTIONAL
            STRATEGIES IN THE HOME. THE SECOND EM-
            PIRICAL STUDY EXAMINED FAMILIAL USE OF
            LANGUAGE AMONG CHILDREN AND ADULTS IN
            THREE DIFFERENT HISPANIC URBAN GROUPS
            IN THE U.S.: CENTRAL-TEXAS MEXICAN AMERI-
            CANS, NEW YORK PUERTO RICANS, AND MIAMI
            CUBAN-AMERICANS. FINDINGS INDICATE THAT
            THERE ARE DIFFERENCES IN THE LANGUAGE
            ENVIRONMENTS TO WHICH HISPANIC AMERI-
            CAN CHILDREN ARE EXPOSED IN THEIR HOMES.
            EXCEPT FOR SOME PUERTO RICAN CHILDREN,
            THERE WERE ABRUPT DISCONTINUITIES FOR
            MANY OF THE CHILDREN BETWEEN THE LIN-
            GUISTIC ENVIRONMENT EXPERIENCED AT HOME
            AND AT SCHOOL. DISCONTINUITY IN THE TO-
            TAL SOCIOCULTURAL CONTEXT, COM-
            POUNDED BY ISSUES RELATED TO ATTITUDES
            AND BEHAVIORS FROM INDIVIDUALS REPRE-
            SENTING THE TWO SOCIOCULTURAL CON-
            TEXTS, MAY BE AT THE ROOT OF PROBLEMS
            AFFECTING MINORITY CHILDREN'S ACADEMIC
            DEVELOPMENT. STUDY RESULTS RAISE SERI-
            OUS QUESTIONS CONCERNING WHETHER EN-

VIRONMENTS WHICH ARE IMPOSED ON CHILDREN PROVIDE SUFFICIENT ARTICULATED CONTINUITY WITH THE EARLY AND ONGOING SOCIOCULTURAL ENVIRONMENT OF THE HOME. 20 REFERENCES.

ACCN   002129

999 AUTH   **LAOSA, L. M.**
TITL   VIEWING BILINGUAL MULTICULTURAL EDUCATIONAL TELEVISION: AN EMPIRICAL ANALYSIS OF CHILDREN'S BEHAVIORS DURING TELEVISION VIEWING.
SRCE   *JOURNAL OF EDUCATIONAL PSYCHOLOGY, 1976, 68(2), 133-142.*
INDX   RESEARCH METHODOLOGY, CHILDREN, CROSS CULTURAL, MASS MEDIA, SES, COGNITIVE DEVELOPMENT, COGNITIVE STYLE, SEX COMPARISON, BILINGUAL-BICULTURAL EDUCATION, MEXICAN AMERICAN, PUERTO RICAN-M, CUBAN, ETHNIC IDENTITY, EMPIRICAL, BILINGUAL, EXAMINER EFFECTS, TEXAS, SOUTHWEST
ABST   A METHODOLOGY FOR RELIABLY OBSERVING AND RECORDING CHILDREN'S BEHAVIORS DURING TELEVISION VIEWING IS DESCRIBED. THE SUBJECTS WERE 385 ELEMENTARY SCHOOL CHILDREN—MEXICAN AMERICAN, PUERTO RICAN, CUBAN AMERICAN, AND ANGLO AMERICAN. THEY VIEWED 2 CARRASCOLENDAS PILOT PROGRAMS, AND THEIR VISUAL ATTENTION, FACIAL EXPRESSIONS OF MIRTH, VERBAL AND NONVERBAL IMITATIONS, AND PROGRAM- AND NONPROGRAM-RELATED VERBALIZATIONS WERE MEASURED. DATA ANALYSIS FOCUSED ON THE RELATIONSHIPS OF THESE BEHAVIORS TO EACH OTHER, TO PERCEPTUAL COGNITIVE ABILITY, TO LANGUAGE USED IN THE HOME, AND TO FAMILY SOCIOECONOMIC AND EDUCATIONAL STATUS. MOREOVER, THE STABILITY OF THE BEHAVIORS OVER TIME AND ACROSS PROGRAMS AS WELL AS THE EFFECTS AND INTERACTIONS OF ETHNIC GROUP MEMBERSHIP, GRADE LEVEL, AND SEX ON BEHAVIOR WERE EXAMINED. FINDINGS OF ETHNIC DIFFERENCES MAY BE RELATED TO EITHER (1) DIFFERENTIAL UNDERSTANDING OF PORTIONS OF THE PROGRAMS DUE TO THE LANGUAGE SPOKEN, (2) DIFFERENTIAL APPEAL OF THE MATERIAL, (3) CULTURALLY DETERMINED DIFFERENCES IN THE DEGREE, FREQUENCY, AND PATTERN IN WHICH THE BEHAVIORS STUDIED ARE PRODUCED IN EACH OF THE ETHNIC GROUPS, OR (4) CULTURAL DIFFERENCES IN THE OBSERVERS. 17 REFERENCES. (PASAR ABSTRACT MODIFIED)
ACCN   000858

1000 AUTH   **LAOSA, L. M., LARA-TAPIA, L., & SWARTZ, J. D.**
TITL   PATHOGNOMIC VERBALIZATIONS, ANXIETY, AND HOSTILITY IN NORMAL MEXICAN AND UNITED STATES ANGLO-AMERICAN CHILDREN'S FANTASIES: A LONGITUDINAL STUDY.
SRCE   *JOURNAL OF CONSULTING AND CLINICAL PSYCHOLOGY, 1974, 42(1), 73-78.*
INDX   ANXIETY, CHILDREN, COGNITIVE DEVELOPMENT, CROSS CULTURAL, CULTURAL FACTORS, EMPIRICAL, FAMILY STRUCTURE, COPING MECHANISMS, SES, MENTAL HEALTH,

MEXICAN, PSYCHOPATHOLOGY, PSYCHOSOCIAL ADJUSTMENT, SEX COMPARISON, PROJECTIVE TESTING, TEXAS, SOUTHWEST
ABST   THE EFFECTS OF CULTURE ON THE DEVELOPMENT OF LOGICAL THINKING AND DEGREE OF EMOTIONAL DISTURBANCE IN NORMAL CHILDREN WERE INVESTIGATED. A TOTAL OF 392 MEXICAN AND UNITED STATES ANGLO AMERICAN SCHOOL CHILDREN, CLOSELY PAIRED ON SEX, AGE, AND SOCIOECONOMIC STATUS, WERE EMPLOYED AS SUBJECTS IN AN OVERLAPPING LONGITUDINAL DESIGN COVERING A SPAN OF 12 YEARS IN ONLY 6 YEARS OF REPEATED TESTING. INITIAL TESTING WAS DONE AT AGES 6.7, 9.7, AND 12.7 YEARS FOR EACH OF THREE AGE GROUPS, RESPECTIVELY. A COMPLEX ANALYSIS OF VARIANCE DESIGN WAS CONSTRUCTED WITH FIVE MAIN FACTORS: CULTURE, SOCIOECONOMIC STATUS, SEX, AGE GROUP, AND TRIAL. THE MAIN EFFECT AS WELL AS INTERACTIONS INVOLVING CULTURE WERE INVESTIGATED ON THREE DEPENDENT VARIABLES: HOLTZMAN INKBLOT TECHNIQUE PATHOGNOMIC VERBALIZATION, ANXIETY, AND HOSTILITY. RESULTS SHOWED SIGNIFICANTLY HIGHER AMOUNTS OF DISTURBED THINKING AND ANXIOUS AND HOSTILE RESPONSE CONTENT IN ANGLO AMERICAN THAN IN MEXICAN CHILDREN. RESULTS ARE INTERPRETED IN LIGHT OF CULTURAL DIFFERENCES IN FAMILY STRUCTURE AND STYLES OF COPING. 15 REFERENCES. (JOURNAL ABSTRACT)
ACCN   002130

1001 AUTH   **LAOSA, L. M., SWARTZ, J. D., & DIAZ-GUERRERO, R.**
TITL   PERCEPTUAL-COGNITIVE AND PERSONALITY DEVELOPMENT OF MEXICAN AND ANGLO-AMERICAN CHILDREN AS MEASURED BY HUMAN FIGURE DRAWING.
SRCE   *DEVELOPMENTAL PSYCHOLOGY, 1974, 10(1), 131-139.*
INDX   PROJECTIVE TESTING, MEXICAN, MEXICAN AMERICAN, CHILDREN, CROSS CULTURAL, GOODENOUGH DRAW-A-MAN TEST, EMPIRICAL, SEX COMPARISON, CULTURAL FACTORS, PERSONALITY, PERSONALITY ASSESSMENT, COGNITIVE DEVELOPMENT, ADOLESCENTS, MALE, FEMALE, TEXAS, SOUTHWEST
ABST   LONGITUDINAL AND CROSS SECTIONAL HUMAN FIGURE DRAWING DATA ARE PRESENTED FOR 394 MEXICAN AND UNITED STATES ANGLO AMERICAN SCHOOL CHILDREN, AGES 8.7 THROUGH 17.7. THE FACTORS OF SEX, AGE, SOCIOECONOMIC STATUS, CULTURE, AND YEAR OF REPEATED TESTING WERE INVESTIGATED IN 2X3X2X2X4 COMPLEX ANALYSES OF VARIANCE FOR GOODENOUGH-HARRIS SCORES IN THE FIRST AND SECOND FIGURES DRAWN. PERCENTAGES OF CHILDREN DRAWING SELF-SEX FIGURES FIRST ARE PRESENTED. THE IMPORTANCE OF CULTURAL VARIABLES AS DETERMINANTS OF THE BEHAVIORS INVOLVED IN PERFORMANCE ON THESE MEASURES WAS EVIDENT FROM THE SIGNIFICANT MAIN EFFECTS AND COMPLEX INTERACTIONS OBTAINED. CULTURAL DIFFERENCES IN REARING PRACTICES LINKED WITH SEX OF CHILD WERE REFLECTED

IN THE POORER DEGREE OF SEXUAL DIFFER-
ENTIATION IN THE DRAWINGS OF ANGLO
AMERICAN, AS COMPARED WITH MEXICAN,
CHILDREN. IMPORTANT METHODOLOGICAL
AND INTERPRETATIVE ISSUES IN CROSS CUL-
TURAL RESEARCH AND CLINICAL APPLICA-
TION, SUCH AS THOSE INVOLVED IN EMPLOY-
ING UNICULTURALLY DEVELOPED INSTRU-
MENTS WITH CULTURALLY DIFFERENT
POPULATIONS, ARE DISCUSSED. 17 REFER-
ENCES. (JOURNAL ABSTRACT)

ACCN   000859

1002 AUTH   **LAOSA, L. M., SWARTZ, J. D., & DIAZ-GUE-
RRERO, R.**
TITL   SEMANTIC ANALYSES OF FREE-WORD ASSO-
CIATIONS OF MEXICAN AND AMERICAN CHIL-
DREN AT AGES NINE, TWELVE, AND FIFTEEN.
SRCE   *PROCEEDINGS OF THE 78TH ANNUAL CON-
VENTION OF THE AMERICAN PSYCHOLOGICAL
ASSOCIATION, 1970, 5, 305-306.*
INDX   CHILDREN, CROSS CULTURAL, EMPIRICAL, LIN-
GUISTICS, ADOLESCENTS, ADULTS, SOUTH-
WEST, TEXAS, LANGUAGE ASSESSMENT, UR-
BAN, MEXICAN, COGNITIVE STYLE
ABST   AN IDIODYNAMIC ASSOCIATIVE SET IS AN IN-
DIVIDUAL'S TENDENCY TO PREDOMINANTLY
CHOOSE ONE CATEGORY OF ASSOCIATION IN
A FREE-WORD ASSOCIATION EVALUATION (I.E.,
PERCEPTUAL, REFERENT, OBJECT REFERENT,
CONCEPT REFERENT, OR DIMENSION REFER-
ENT). TO DISCOVER IF IDIODYNAMIC ASSOCIA-
TIVE SETS VARY ACROSS CULTURES AND/OR
AGE GROUPS, TWO GROUPS OF CHILDREN
WERE STUDIED: 205 MEXICAN, MIDDLE-CLASS
CHILDREN IN MEXICO CITY, AND 203 ENGLISH-
SPEAKING CHILDREN IN AUSTIN, TEXAS. THE
TWO GROUPS WERE MATCHED BY SEX AND
SES, AND DIVIDED INTO THREE AGE GROUPS
(9.7, 12.7, & 15.7 YEARS). IN ADDITION, THE
FINDINGS FROM THESE CHILDREN WERE COM-
PARED TO THOSE FROM A PREVIOUS STUDY
OF MEXICAN AND JAPANESE ADULTS. THE
STUDY'S METHODOLOGY CONSISTED OF AD-
MINISTERING AN ENGLISH OR SPANISH VER-
SION OF AN 80-WORD ASSOCIATION LIST TO
THE CHILDREN; THEN SIX VARIABLES WERE
SCORED (SYNONYM; SUPERORDINATE; CON-
TRAST; COORDINATE; AND SENSORY AND
NONSENSORY PREDICATE). IT WAS FOUND
THAT NO SIGNIFICANT DIFFERENCES OB-
TAINED BETWEEN THE AMERICAN AND MEXI-
CAN CHILDREN, NOR BETWEEN THE CHILDREN
AND THE ADULTS. IT IS THEREFORE CON-
CLUDED THAT THESE LINGUISTIC HABITS ARE
NOT A FUNCTION OF CULTURE, BUT INSTEAD
REFLECT FUNDAMENTAL ASSOCIATION
STRUCTURES COMMON TO LANGUAGE USAGE
ACROSS CULTURES. 5 REFERENCES.
ACCN   002131

1003 AUTH   **LAOSA, L. M., SWARTZ, J. D., & MORAN L. J.**
TITL   WORD ASSOCIATION STRUCTURES AMONG
MEXICAN AND AMERICAN CHILDREN.
SRCE   *JOURNAL OF SOCIAL PSYCHOLOGY, 1971, 85,
7-15.*
INDX   COGNITIVE DEVELOPMENT, GRAMMAR, LIN-
GUISTICS, EMPIRICAL, CROSS CULTURAL,
MEXICAN, URBAN, CHILDREN, ADOLESCENTS,
SEMANTICS, TEXAS, SOUTHWEST
ABST   WORD ASSOCIATION STRUCTURES AMONG
MEXICAN AND AMERICAN CHILDREN WERE
STUDIED IN 408 URBAN SUBJECTS. BOTH EN-
GLISH- AND SPANISH-SPEAKING CHILDREN'S
WORD ASSOCIATION RESPONSES WERE FOUND
TO HAVE THE SAME FACTOR STRUCTURE
CLEARLY REPRESENTING THE SAME THREE IDI-
ODYNAMIC ASSOCIATIVE MODES: SYNONYM-
SUPERORDINATE (CONCEPT REFERENT SET),
CONTRAST-COORDINATE (DIMENSION REFER-
ENT SET), AND SENSORY AND NONSENSORY
PREDICATES (PERCEPTUAL REFERENT SET).
THE GENERAL HYPOTHESIS THAT THESE LIN-
GUISTIC HABITS REFLECT FUNDAMENTAL AS-
SOCIATION STRUCTURES COMMON TO LAN-
GUAGE USERS THUS GAINS IN CREDIBILITY.
THE INTERPRETABILITY OF THESE FINDINGS IN
TERMS OF UNIVERSALS IN COGNITION AMONG
HUMANS RESTS UPON FURTHER CROSS-CUL-
TURAL RESEARCH. ANALYSES OF THE GRAM-
MATICAL VARIABLES ACROSS THE SIX AGE-
CULTURE GROUPS INDICATED A CLOSE SIMI-
LARITY BETWEEN THE MEXICAN AND U.S.
SAMPLES. IN ADDITION, ORTHOGONAL NOUN
AND VERB-ADJECTIVE FACTORS IN THE
SAMPLES SUGGESTED THAT THE PARADIG-
MATIC SHIFT IS NOT A UNITARY PHENOMENON,
BUT RATHER TWO SEPARATE AND INDEPEN-
DENT SHIFTS. 12 REFERENCES.
ACCN   000860

1004 AUTH   **LARA-BRAUD, J.**
TITL   THE STATUS OF RELIGION AMONG MEXICAN
AMERICANS.
SRCE   *IN M. M. MANGOLD (ED.), LA CAUSA CHICANA:
THE MOVEMENT FOR JUSTICE. NEW YORK:
FAMILY SERVICE ASSOCIATION OF AMERICA,
1971, PP. 87-94.*
INDX   RELIGION, MEXICAN AMERICAN, HISTORY, ES-
SAY
ABST   THE STATUS OF RELIGION AMONG MEXICAN
AMERICANS TODAY IS DESCRIBED AS FLUC-
TUATING BETWEEN ROUTINE AND RENAIS-
SANCE. THE ROUTINE ROLE OF BOTH CATHO-
LIC AND PROTESTANT CHURCHES IN THE
HISTORY OF MEXICAN AMERICANS IS ONE OF
SPIRITUAL MINISTRATION AND ALSO DELIBER-
ATE AMERICANIZATION. A MAJOR DIFFERENCE
BETWEEN THE EXPERIENCES OF OTHER
CATHOLIC ETHNIC COMMUNITIES (IRISH, GER-
MAN, POLISH AND ITALIAN) AND THE MEXICAN
AMERICANS' EXPERIENCE IS THAT OTHER ETH-
NIC GROUPS HAD THEIR OWN INDIGENOUS
RELIGIONS LEADERS WHILE MEXICAN AMERI-
CANS HAD VERY FEW IF ANY IN MOST OF THEIR
PARISHES. ONLY RECENTLY HAS THE CATHO-
LIC CHURCH RECRUITED MORE MEXICAN
AMERICAN PRIESTS. THE PROTESTANT LEAD-
ERSHIP STILL LIES IN THE HANDS OF ANGLOS
EVEN THOUGH MANY LOCAL MINISTERS ARE
INDIGENOUS. THE DIFFERENCES BETWEEN
CATHOLIC AND PROTESTANT APPROACHES TO
BOTH SPIRITUAL MINISTRATION AND AMERI-
CANIZATION ARE DISCUSSED. IT IS POSITED
THAT BOTH CHURCHES HAVE SUCCEEEDED IN
MINISTERING BUT, FORTUNATELY, NOT IN

AMERICANIZING THE MEXICAN COMMUNITY. THE RENAISSANCE OF RELIGION FOR MEXICAN AMERICANS INVOLVES THEIR RENEWED QUEST FOR MORE INDIGENOUS FORMS OF WITNESS AND SERVICE RELEVANT TO THEIR OWN ETHNICITY AND ECUMENICAL SOLIDARITY. 1 REFERENCE.

ACCN   000861

1005 AUTH   **LARKIN, R. W.**
TITL   CLASS, RACE, SEX AND PREADOLESCENT ATTITUDES.
SRCE   *CALIFORNIA JOURNAL OF EDUCATIONAL RESEARCH, 1972, 23(5), 213-223.*
INDX   SES, SEX COMPARISON, MEXICAN AMERICAN, CHILDREN, ATTITUDES, CROSS CULTURAL, EMPIRICAL, SOCIAL MOBILITY, EDUCATION, OCCUPATIONAL ASPIRATIONS, SELF CONCEPT, FAMILY ROLES, CALIFORNIA, SOUTHWEST
ABST   TO TEST WHETHER LOWER-CLASS CHILDREN FAIL IN SCHOOL DUE TO ATTITUDINAL DEFICITS (POOR SELF-CONCEPT, NEGATIVE ATTITUDE TOWARDS SCHOOL, LACK OF PARENTAL CONTROL AND OPENNESS TO PEER INFLUENCE), 1067 ANGLO (A), 350 BLACK (B), 298 MEXICAN AMERICAN (MA) AND 35 ASIAN AMERICAN (AA) CALIFORNIA PUBLIC SCHOOL STUDENTS, GRADES 4 TO 6, WERE TESTED. FOUR ATTITUDES SURVEYED WERE SELF-ESTEEM, SCHOOL ORIENTATION, PEER GROUP ORIENTATION AND ORIENTATION TO FAMILY AUTHORITY. INTERNAL CONSISTENCY WAS ASSESSED THROUGH THE USE OF COEFFICIENT ALPHA, AND A PRETEST CONFIRMED THE CONCURRENT VALIDITY OF THE FOUR ATTITUDE SCALES. THE RESULTS INDICATED NO SIGNIFICANT RELATIONSHIPS BETWEEN SES AND ANY OF THE FOUR ATTITUDES. CONTROLLING FOR ETHNICITY, A SMALL RELATIONSHIP BETWEEN SES AND FAMILY AUTHORITY ORIENTATION WAS FOUND AMONG B AND MA CHILDREN, WITH THE MIDDLE-CLASS MORE FAMILY ORIENTED THAN LOWER-CLASS. THE HIGHER THE SOCIAL STATUS OF AA CHILDREN, THE LOWER THE FAMILY AUTHORITY ORIENTATION. THERE WERE SIGNIFICANT DIFFERENCES BETWEEN ETHNIC GROUPS ON SELF-ESTEEM AND INDEPENDENCE FROM FAMILY AUTHORITY, WITH AA HAVING THE HIGHEST SELF-ESTEEM FOLLOWED BY B, A AND MA, IN THAT ORDER. MINORITY GROUP CHILDREN REPORTED THAT THEIR FAMILIES HAD GREATER LATITUDES OF LEGITIMATE AUTHORITY OVER THEIR BEHAVIOR, THAN A CHILDREN. FINALLY, SEX WAS FAR MORE IMPORTANT IN RELATION TO INFLUENCES ON PREADOLESCENT ATTITUDES THAN WERE ETHNICITY OR SOCIAL STATUS, WITH THE GREATEST DIFFERENCE BEING BETWEEN LOWER-CLASS AND UPPER-MIDDLE-CLASS BOYS AND GIRLS. IN FAMILIES IN WHICH BOYS WERE GIVEN HIGHER STATUS THAN GIRLS, THE GIRLS' SELF-ESTEEM WAS NEGATIVELY AFFECTED; AND GIRLS WERE MORE FAMILY ORIENTED OVER ALL ETHNIC GROUPS AND SES LEVELS. 11 REFERENCES.

ACCN   000862

1006 AUTH   **LARNED, D. T., & MULLER, D.**

TITL   DEVELOPMENT OF SELF-CONCEPT IN MEXICAN AMERICAN AND ANGLO STUDENTS.
SRCE   *HISPANIC JOURNAL OF BEHAVIORAL SCIENCES, 1979, 1(3), 279-285.*
INDX   MEXICAN AMERICAN, CROSS CULTURAL, CHILDREN, NEW MEXICO, SOUTHWEST, RURAL, SELF CONCEPT, EMPIRICAL, SCHOLASTIC ACHIEVEMENT
ABST   THE SELF-CONCEPT AND SELF-ESTEEM OF MEXICAN AMERICAN AND ANGLO STUDENTS IN GRADES THREE THROUGH EIGHT IN A NEW MEXICO SCHOOL DISTRICT WERE COMPARED. STUDENTS WITH SPANISH SURNAMES WERE CLASSIFIED AS MEXICAN AMERICAN (N = 175) WHILE THOSE WHO WERE NEITHER BLACK NOR NATIVE AMERICAN WERE CLASSIFIED AS ANGLO (N = 268). THE POSITIVENESS OF SELF-CONCEPT AND SELF-ESTEEM WAS ASSESSED IN FOUR AREAS: PHYSICAL MATURITY; PEER RELATIONS; ACADEMIC SUCCESS; AND SCHOOL ADAPTIVENESS. THE RESULTS INDICATE THAT THE CHILDREN'S PHYSICAL MATURITY SELF-CONCEPTS TENDED TO INCREASE ACROSS GRADES, WHILE THE ACADEMIC SUCCESS AND SCHOOL ADAPTIVENESS SELF-CONCEPTS SHOWED A DRAMATIC DECLINE IN POSITIVENESS ACROSS GRADES. ACADEMIC SUCCESS AND SCHOOL ADAPTIVENESS SELF-ESTEEM ALSO TENDED TO DECLINE, THOUGH ONLY MODERATELY, ACROSS GRADES. THERE WAS NO EVIDENCE THAT THE MEXICAN AMERICAN AND ANGLO CHILDREN'S SELF-CONCEPTS WERE DIFFERENTIALLY AFFECTED BY THE SCHOOL EXPERIENCE. IN GENERAL, THE RESULTS FAIL TO DEMONSTRATE A NEED FOR DIFFERENTIAL SELF-CONCEPT REMEDIATION EXPERIENCES FOR MEXICAN AMERICAN AND ANGLO CHILDREN; THEY ALSO RAISE QUESTIONS ABOUT THE APPROPRIATENESS OF SELF-CONCEPT AS AN EXPLANATORY VARIABLE IN THE LOW ACADEMIC ACHIEVEMENT OF MEXICAN AMERICAN CHILDREN. IT IS CONCLUDED THAT POSITIVENESS OF SELF-CONCEPT SHOULD PROBABLY BE OF ONLY SECONDARY CONCERN TO EDUCATORS SINCE THERE IS VIRTUALLY NO EMPIRICAL DOCUMENTATION SHOWING THAT LOW SELF-CONCEPT IMPEDES CLASSROOM LEARNING. 9 REFERENCES. (JOURNAL ABSTRACT MODIFIED)

ACCN   001772

1007 AUTH   **LARRALDE, C.**
TITL   MEXICAN AMERICAN MOVEMENTS AND LEADERS.
SRCE   *LOS ALAMITOS, CA.: HWONG PUBLISHING CO., 1976.*
INDX   REVIEW, HISTORY, CHICANO MOVEMENT, DISCRIMINATION, POLITICAL POWER, BOOK, ECONOMIC FACTORS, MEXICAN AMERICAN, SOUTHWEST, CASE STUDY, CULTURE, POLITICS
ABST   TO DOCUMENT THAT CHICANO STRUGGLES ARE NOT NEW BUT HAVE EXISTED THROUGHOUT AMERICAN HISTORY UNDER DIFFERENT NAMES AND PLACES, A SERIES OF BIOGRAPHICAL SKETCHES OF CHICANO LEADERS SINCE THE MID-1980'S ARE PRESENTED. USING SUCH DOCUMENTS AS NEWSPAPERS, OFFICIAL RECORDS, ORAL ACCOUNTS, AND HIS OWN

FAMILY'S PAPERS AND MEMOIRS, THE AUTHOR DESCRIBES IN CHRONOLOGICAL ORDER FOUR CHICANO MOVEMENTS AND 19 OF THEIR LEADING FIGURES: (1) THE CORTINISTA MOVEMENT (1846-48), LED BY JUAN CORTINA; (2) THE TERESITA MOVEMENT (1888-1905), LED BY SANTA TERESA URREA; (3) THE MANGONISTA MOVEMENT (1904-14), LED BY RICARDO AND ENRIQUE MAGON; AND (4) THE CHICANO ACTIVISTS (1920-PRESENT), INCLUDING OCTAVIANO LARRAZOLO AND MANY OTHERS. IN STUDYING THESE PERSONALITIES AND POLITICAL MOVEMENTS, IT IS OBSERVED THAT THEY SHAPED MUCH OF CHICANO LIFE AND IDEOLOGY UP TO THE PRESENT DAY. FOR EXAMPLE, THE ROOTS OF CESAR CHAVEZ'S CURRENT STRUGGLES CAN BE TRACED TO THE PHILOSOPHY AND STRATEGIES OF THE CORTINISTA MOVEMENT OF ONE HUNDRED YEARS AGO. BUT DESPITE THIS FINE HISTORY OF POLITICAL ENDEAVORS AND ACHIEVEMENTS, THE AUTHOR CONCLUDES WITH PESSIMISM BY NOTING THAT CHICANOS STILL FACE BITTER STRUGGLES AGAINST DISCRIMINATION, REPRESSION, AND POLITICAL TYRANNY IN MANY FORMS. OF PARTICULAR INTEREST IN THIS VOLUME IS THE INCLUSION OF MANY OLD PHOTOGRAPHS OF CHICANO HISTORICAL INCIDENTS AND PERSONALITIES. 465 REFERENCES.

ACCN   001844

1008 AUTH   **LARSON, L. B., DODDS, J. M., MASSOTH, D. M., & CHASE, H. P.**

TITL   NUTRITIONAL STATUS OF CHILDREN OF MEXICAN-AMERICAN MIGRANT PARENTS.

SRCE   *JOURNAL OF AMERICAN DIET ASSOCIATION, 1974, 64(1), 29-35.*

INDX   NUTRITION, MEXICAN AMERICAN, CHILDREN, FARM LABORERS, RURAL, POVERTY, EMPIRICAL, SES, TEXAS, HEALTH, MIGRANTS, SOUTHWEST

ABST   AN INVESTIGATION TO DETERMINE THE DIETARY AND NUTRITIONAL STATUS OF CHILDREN FROM 149 MEXICAN AMERICAN MIGRANT FAMILIES BY EVALUATING THE DIETARY, BIOCHEMICAL, CLINICAL, AND SOCIOCULTURAL FACTORS WAS CONDUCTED OVER A THREE-YEAR PERIOD. THE SAMPLE CONSISTED OF CHILDREN WHO HAD BEEN ATTENDING THE FREE NEIGHBORHOOD CLINICS LOCATED IN THE LOWER RIO GRANDE VALLEY OF TEXAS. SOCIODEMOGRAPHIC DATA, HOUSING CONDITIONS, MEDICAL HISTORY, AND DIETARY INFORMATION WERE OBTAINED FROM THE PARENTS. IN ADDITION, THE CHILDREN UNDERWENT A THOROUGH PHYSICAL EXAMINATION. THE FINDINGS WERE AS FOLLOWS: (1) WHILE AN ADEQUATE DIETARY INTAKE OF VITAMIN A WAS REPORTED, BIOCHEMICAL AND CLINICAL EVIDENCE REVEALED THAT MANY CHILDREN HAD VITAMIN A DEFICIENCY; (2) VITAMIN D DEFICIENCY WAS PRESENT AMONG THE CHILDREN; (3) CONSUMPTION OF FOODS FROM THE FRUIT, VEGETABLE, AND MILK GROUPS WAS LOW; AND (4) IRON INTAKE WAS LOW, BUT PROTEIN INTAKE WAS ALMOST TWICE THE RECOMMENDED ALLOW-

ANCES. THE LOW HEIGHT AND WEIGHT ATTAINMENT SUGGESTS COMMON NUTRITIONAL PROBLEMS AMONG THE CHILDREN. EVEN THOUGH NUTRITIONAL AIDES WERE EMPLOYED TO WORK WITH FAMILIES IN THIS PROJECT, THE DATA REVEALED THAT OVER THE THREE-YEAR PERIOD ONLY SOME IMPROVEMENTS IN NUTRITIONAL STATUS WERE ATTAINED—AND THESE IMPROVEMENTS WERE NOT STATISTICALLY SIGNIFICANT. IT IS SUGGESTED THAT RESOLVING THE NUTRITIONAL PROBLEMS WILL REQUIRE AN INTEGRATED APPROACH, INCLUDING ECONOMICS, FOOD AVAILABILITY, HEALTH CARE, ENVIRONMENTAL CONDITIONS, AND EDUCATION. 17 REFERENCES.

ACCN   000863

1009 AUTH   **LASKOWITZ, D., & EINSTEIN, S.**

TITL   PERSONALITY CHARACTERISTICS OF ADOLESCENT ADDICTS: MANIFEST RIGIDITY.

SRCE   *CORRECTIVE PSYCHIATRY AND JOURNAL OF SOCIAL THERAPY, 1963, 9(4), 215-218.*

INDX   PERSONALITY, ADOLESCENTS, DRUG ADDICTION, PUERTO RICAN-M, CROSS CULTURAL, EMPIRICAL, CORRECTIONS, DRUG ABUSE, NEW YORK, EAST

ABST   A LARGE SAMPLE OF ADOLESCENT ADDICTS WAS STUDIED TO DETERMINE THE FREQUENCY WITH WHICH RIGIDITY OCCURS AS A PERSONALITY TRAIT. THE METCALF MANIFEST RIGIDITY SCALE WAS ADMINISTERED TO 126 NEWLY ADMITTED RIVERSIDE HOSPITAL PATIENTS. NO SIGNIFICANT SEX DIFFERENCE WAS DISCOVERED. HOWEVER, ETHNICITY AND LENGTH OF DRUG USE EMERGED AS SIGNIFICANT VARIABLES, WITH PUERTO RICANS BEING MOST RIGID, NEGROES NEXT, AND WHITES LEAST. PATIENTS INVOLVED IN DRUG USE FOR A SHORTER PERIOD OF TIME WERE SIGNIFICANTLY MORE RIGID. THE FINDINGS ON RIGIDITY FOR ADDICTS OF DIFFERENT ETHNIC BACKGROUNDS PARALLEL THOSE ON AUTHORITARIAN ATTITUDES. 7 REFERENCES.

ACCN   000864

1010 AUTH   **LAURIA, A., JR.**

TITL   "RESPETO," "RELAJO" AND INTERPERSONAL RELATIONS IN PUERTO RICO.

SRCE   *ANTHROPOLOGICAL QUARTERLY, 1964, 37(2), 53-67.*

INDX   PUERTO RICAN-I, INTERPERSONAL RELATIONS, AGGRESSION, CULTURE, FAMILY STRUCTURE, EXTENDED FAMILY, FICTIVE KINSHIP, REVIEW, SOCIAL STRUCTURE, THEORETICAL

ABST   RESPETO AND RELAJO ARE DISCUSSED AS COMPOSING A SYMBOLIC IDIOM THAT SERVES TO INTEGRATE PUERTO RICAN SOCIETY. THE RELATION OF THE TERM RELAJO TO THE CRUCIAL SELF-PROPERTY OF RESPETO IS DEMONSTRATED. THIS INCLUDES SHOWING WHY PUERTO RICANS USE RELAJO TO DESIGNATE THOSE BEHAVIORS TO WHICH IT REFERS. IT IS POSSIBLE TO OPERATIONALIZE AT LEAST SOME ASPECTS OF THE NOTION OF NATIONAL CHARACTER BY ORDERING DATA IN SUCH A WAY AS TO DELINEATE THE KINDS OF MESSAGES WHICH CONSTITUTE THE UNIVERSAL COMPONENTS

OF THE CIRCULATION OF SYMBOLS AND SELF-PRESENTATIONS THROUGH A COMPLEX SOCIETY. ON THE BASIS OF ANTHROPOLOGICAL OBSERVATIONS, A UNIQUELY PUERTO RICAN SYMBOLIC IDIOM (I.E., RESPETO AND RELAJO) IS POSTULATED. UNTIL ADDITIONAL COMPARATIVE STUDIES OF SUFFICIENT RIGOR ARE CONDUCTED, IT IS NOT POSSIBLE TO SPECIFY WITH CERTAINTY THE DEGREE TO WHICH THE IDIOM IS UNIQUE IN PUERTO RICAN SOCIETY. 41 REFERENCES.

ACCN   000865

1011 AUTH   **LEAVITT, R. R.**
TITL   THE PUERTO RICAN: CULTURE CHANGE AND LANGUAGE DEVIANCE.
SRCE   *TUCSON, ARIZ.: UNIVERSITY OF ARIZONA PRESS, 1974.*
INDX   CULTURAL CHANGE, LINGUISTICS, LINGUISTIC COMPETENCE, PHONOLOGY, CULTURAL FACTORS, PUERTO RICAN-M, ATTITUDES, EMPIRICAL, HISTORY, CULTURE, IMMIGRATION, SES, POVERTY, EDUCATION, EMPLOYMENT, DISCRIMINATION, SOCIAL STRUCTURE, SEX COMPARISON, FAMILY ROLES, SOCIALIZATION, HOUSING, SOCIAL MOBILITY, NEW YORK, EAST, VALUES
ABST   TO DETERINE WHETHER SOCIOCULTURAL FACTORS CONTRIBUTE TO THE ETIOLOGY OF STUTTERING AMONG PUERTO RICAN RURAL MIGRANTS LIVING IN THE TWO DIFFERENT CULTURAL MILIEUS OF NEW YORK CITY AND SAN JUAN, PUERTO RICO, THE FOLLOWING FACTORS WERE INVESTIGATED: (1) THE WORLDWIDE PREVALENCE OF STUTTERING; (2) THE RELATIONSHIP BETWEEN STUTTERING AND BILINGUALISM; (3) DIFFERENCES BETWEEN MALE AND FEMALE STUTTERING INCIDENCES; AND (4) STUTTERING RATES IN THE DIFFERENT SOCIOECONOMIC CLASSES. TO ASCERTAIN THE SOCIOCULTURAL CHARACTERISTICS ASSOCIATED WITH STUTTERING, COMPOSITE PROFILES WERE MADE OF CULTURES HAVING A HIGH INCIDENCE OF STUTTERING. THE CULTURAL VARIATIONS AND SIMILARITIES AMONG THE RURAL MIGRANTS WERE INVESTIGATED TO DETERMINE WHAT THEIR VALUES AND LIFE PATTERNS WERE BEFORE AND AFTER THEY MOVED TO THE TWO CITIES. THE DATA SUGGEST THAT THE PREVALENCE OF STUTTERING DEPENDS PARTIALLY ON THE DOMINANT VALUES OF A CULTURE, ESPECIALLY IN ITS ATTITUDE TOWARDS LANGUAGE.

ACCN   000866

1012 AUTH   **LECORGNE, L. L., & LAOSA, L. M.**
TITL   FATHER ABSENCE IN LOW-INCOME MEXICAN AMERICAN FAMILIES: CHILDREN'S SOCIAL ADJUSTMENT AND CONCEPTUAL DIFFERENTIATION OF SEX ROLE ATTTIBUTES.
SRCE   *DEVELOPMENTAL PSYCHOLOGY, 1976, 12(5), 470-471.*
INDX   FATHER-CHILD INTERACTION, INTERPERSONAL RELATIONS, SES, MEXICAN AMERICAN, SEX ROLES, CHILDREN, RAVEN PROGRESSIVE MATRICES, BENDER VISUAL-MOTOR GESTALT TEST, PSYCHOSOCIAL ADJUSTMENT, GOODENOUGH DRAW-A-MAN TEST, TEACHERS, SELF CONCEPT, GENDER IDENTITY, EMPIRICAL, PERSONALITY ASSESSMENT, PROJECTIVE TESTING, SEX COMPARISON, TEXAS, SOUTHWEST
ABST   THE EFFECTS OF PATERNAL DEPRIVATION ON 248 4TH GRADE MEXICAN AMERICAN STUDENTS WERE INVESTIGATED. DRAWINGS OF THE HUMAN FIGURE (1 MALE AND 1 FEMALE) WERE OBTAINED FROM EACH SUBJECT, FOLLOWING THE PROCEDURES OF THE GOODENOUGH-HARRIS DRAWING TEST. SUBJECTS WERE ALSO ADMINISTERED RAVEN'S PROGRESSIVE MATRICES AND THE BENDER GESTALT TEST. EACH SUBJECT WAS RATED ON DEGREE OF PERSONAL ADJUSTMENT BY HIS/HER CLASSROOM TEACHER ON A 4-POINT SCALE, RANGING FROM WELL ADJUSTED, NO PROBLEMS IN RELATING TO OTHERS, TO SERIOUS MALADJUSTMENT. RESULTS SHOW THAT FATHER-PRESENT SUBJECTS OBTAINED SIGNIFICANTLY HIGHER GOODENOUGH-HARRIS SCORES THAN FATHER-ABSENT SUBJECTS ON BOTH THE MALE AND THE FEMALE FIGURES DRAWN. THE FEMALE FIGURES DRAWN BY THE FATHER-ABSENT SUBJECTS HAD SIGNIFICANTLY FEWER FEMININE ATTRIBUTES THAN THOSE DRAWN BY FATHER-PRESENT SUBJECTS. WHEREAS TEACHERS FOUND FATHER-PRESENT MALES AND FEMALES AND FATHER-ABSENT FEMALES FAIRLY WELL ADJUSTED, FATHER-ABSENT MALES SHOWED SIGNIFICANTLY MORE SIGNS OF SOCIAL AND EMOTIONAL MALADJUSTMENT. 9 REFERENCES. (PASAR ABSTRACT)

ACCN   000867

1013 AUTH   **LEE, I. C.**
TITL   MEDICAL CARE IN A MEXICAN AMERICAN COMMUNITY.
SRCE   *LOS ALAMITOS, CA.: HWONG PUBLISHING CO., 1976. (ALSO AVAILABLE AS DOCTORAL DISSERTATION, UNIVERSITY OF CALIFORNIA, LOS ANGELES, 1972. SEE, DISSERTATION ABSTRACTS INTERNATIONAL, 1972, 33, 302B. UNIVERSITY MICROFILMS NO. 70-20,463.)*
INDX   HEALTH DELIVERY SYSTEMS, CULTURAL FACTORS, ACCULTURATION, ATTITUDES, BIRTH CONTROL, COMMUNITY, CULTURE, CROSS CULTURAL, MEXICAN AMERICAN, ADULTS, EMPIRICAL, PARAPROFESSIONALS, PROFESSIONAL TRAINING, RESOURCE UTILIZATION, SES, CALIFORNIA, SOUTHWEST, FAMILY PLANNING
ABST   A SIX-MONTH FIELD SURVEY OF 416 MEXICAN-BORN, SPANISH-SPEAKING AND AMERICAN-BORN, ENGLISH-SPEAKING MEXICAN AMERICAN PATIENT AND NONPATIENT FAMILIES WAS CONDUCTED TO ASSESS THE PATTERNS OF ENTRY INTO THE HEALTH CARE SYSTEM AND THE PATTERN OF MEDICAL CARE USE. IT IS HYPOTHESIZED THAT THE PATTERN OF ENTRY INTO THE HEALTH CARE SYSTEM WILL BE CLOSELY ASSOCIATED WITH THE PATIENTS' SOCIOCULTURAL ORIENTATION AND THAT THE PATTERN OF MEDICAL CARE USE WILL BE ASSOCIATED WITH THE FAMILY SOCIOECONOMIC STATUS, THE EMPLOYMENT OF LOCAL RESIDENTS AT THE HEALTH CENTER, AND THE SOCIOCULTURAL ATTRIBUTES OF THE FAMILY. RESULTS INDICATE NO CORRELATION BETWEEN

THE LEVEL OF FAMILY INCOME AND THE PATTERN OF MEDICAL CARE USE IN THE MEXICAN AMERICAN FAMILIES. THE INFLUENCE OF SOCIOCULTURAL ATTITUDES IS FOUND TO BE STRONGER THAN FAMILY INCOME. AMERICAN-BORN PATIENTS TEND TO ENTER THE CLINIC VIA PROFESSIONAL AND SOCIAL AGENCY REFERRAL, WHILE THE MEXICAN-BORN PATIENTS TEND TO ENTER THROUGH THE INFLUENCE OF RELATIVES AND FRIENDS. THE EFFECTIVE USE OF INDIGENOUS COMMUNITY HEALTH AIDES CONTRIBUTES TO INCREASED PATIENT ATTENDANCE AND ACCEPTANCE OF SERVICES. AMERICAN-BORN PATIENTS TEND TO BE MORE LIBERAL ABOUT FAMILY PLANNING, ABORTION AND CONTRACEPTION FOR UNWED TEENAGERS; THEY ARE ALSO MORE SOPHISTICATED THAN THE MEXICAN-BORN PATIENTS IN THEIR SELECTION OF MEDICAL CARE FACILITIES AND EVALUATION OF MEDICAL SERVICES. CONCLUSIONS AND RECOMMENDATIONS FOR IMPROVED HEALTH SERVICES AND HEALTH AIDE TRAINING ARE DISCUSSED. 67 REFERENCES. (AUTHOR ABSTRACT MODIFIED)

ACCN   000868

1014 AUTH   **LEFLEY, H. P.**
TITL   APPROACHES TO COMMUNITY MENTAL HEALTH: THE MIAMI MODEL.
SRCE   *PSYCHIATRIC ANNALS, 1975, 5(8), 26-32.*
INDX   COMMUNITY, COMMUNITY INVOLVEMENT, CROSS CULTURAL, CUBAN, CULTURAL FACTORS, CULTURAL PLURALISM, ESSAY, HEALTH DELIVERY SYSTEMS, MENTAL HEALTH, MENTAL HEALTH PROFESSION, PRIMARY PREVENTION, PROGRAM EVALUATION, PUERTO RICAN-M, SOCIAL SERVICES, FLORIDA, SOUTH, URBAN, POLICY, CARIBBEAN
ABST   THE MIAMI, FLORIDA, JACKSON MEMORIAL HOSPITAL COMMUNITY MENTAL HEALTH CARE MODEL EVOLVED FROM THE FINDINGS OF A 3-YEAR STUDY OF THE HEALTH SYSTEMS, BELIEFS, AND BEHAVIORS IN THE FIVE MAJOR ETHNIC GROUPS OF THEIR CATCHMENT AREA—BAHAMIANS, CUBANS, HAITIANS, PUERTO RICANS, AND BLACKS. THE FINDINGS INDICATE CULTURALLY PATTERNED DIFFERENCES IN (1) THE CLUSTERING OF SYMPTOMS, (2) CULTURE-BOUND SYNDROMES NOT RECOGNIZED BY THE ORTHODOX MEDICAL PROFESSION, AND (3) PERCEPTIONS OF PREVENTION, CAUSATION, AND TREATMENT OF ILLNESS. IT WAS DETERMINED THAT CULTURALLY SPECIFIC THERAPEUTIC INTERVENTIONS WERE NEEDED TO DEAL WITH ETHNIC VARIABLES. TEAMS ACTING AS RESOURCE SPECIALISTS LINK CONSUMERS WITH APPROPRIATE SERVICE AGENCIES, AND THEY SERVE AS CATALYSTS IN MOBILIZING NEIGHBORHOOD RESOURCES TO DEAL WITH A VARIETY OF COMMUNITY MENTAL HEALTH PROBLEMS. THE SIX SOURCES OF DATA IN THE PROJECTED EVALUATION MODEL ARE DISCUSSED. ANTICIPATED IS A REDUCTION IN HOSPITAL RECIDIVISM AND IMPROVEMENT IN NEIGHBORHOOD SOCIAL INDICATORS OVER TIME. 25 REFERENCES.

ACCN   002132

1015 AUTH   **LEFLEY, H. P.**
TITL   COMMUNITY MENTAL HEALTH IN SIX ETHNIC COMMUNITIES: THE MIAMI MODEL.
SRCE   *PAPER PRESENTED AT THE 83RD ANNUAL CONVENTION OF THE AMERICAN PSYCHOLOGICAL ASSOCIATION, CHICAGO, AUGUST 30-SEPTEMBER 3, 1975.*
INDX   HEALTH DELIVERY SYSTEMS, MENTAL HEALTH, COMMUNITY, SES, CULTURAL FACTORS, PSYCHOTHERAPY, GERONTOLOGY, PUERTO RICAN-M, CUBAN, ESSAY, COMMUNITY INVOLVEMENT, CROSS CULTURAL, FLORIDA, SOUTH
ABST   THE DEVELOPMENTAL HISTORY AND CONCEPTUAL FRAMEWORK OF THE JACKSON MEMORIAL HOSPITAL COMMUNITY MENTAL HEALTH PROGRAM (MIAMI, FLORIDA) ARE DESCRIBED. A MOST IMPORTANT PART OF THE PROGRAM IS THE STUDY OF THE HEALTH BELIEFS AND BEHAVIORS OF THE ETHNIC COMMUNITIES IN THE AREA (BAHAMIAN, PUERTO RICAN, CUBAN, AND NATIVE BLACK AMERICAN). THE PROGRAM FOCUSES ON DEVELOPING AN INTEGRATED THERAPEUTIC APPROACH TO MULTIPLE COMMUNITIES WITH MULTIPLE NEEDS. THEREFORE, KNOWLEDGE AND ASSESSMENT OF THE CULTURAL, ECONOMIC, AND POLITICAL CHARACTERISTICS OF THESE COMMUNITIES, THE RANGE AND PRIORITIES OF THEIR SELF-DEFINED NEEDS, THE STRESSORS, ADAPTIVE MECHANISMS AND RESOURCES AVAILABLE TO THESE COMMUNITIES ARE ALL REQUIRED TO PROVIDE EFFECTIVE MENTAL HEALTH SERVICES. SPECIFIC METHODS FOR ATTAINING PROGRAM OBJECTIVES ARE EXPLAINED IN TERMS OF STAFFING PATTERNS, TEAM FUNCTIONS, COMMUNITY INVOLVEMENT, AND SERVICES ORGANIZATION. OVERALL, THIS APPROACH TO COMMUNITY MENTAL HEALTH, WHICH STRESSES SOCIAL SYSTEMS MODIFICATION AND ETHNIC ACCOUNTABILITY, HAS PROVIDED DECENTRALIZED SERVICES, PERMITTED THE TYPE OF SOCIAL SYSTEMS CHANGE THAT THE COMMUNITIES THEMSELVES DEFINE AS RELEVANT TO THE MAINTENANCE OF MENTAL HEALTH, AND HAS FACILITATED AN ONGOING BEHAVIORAL SCIENCE PERSPECTIVE IN THE CONCEPTUALIZATION AND DELIVERY OF MENTAL HEALTH CARE. 26 REFERENCES. (AUTHOR SUMMARY MODIFIED)

ACCN   000870

1016 AUTH   **LEFLEY, H. P.**
TITL   ETHNIC PATIENTS AND ANGLO HEALERS: AN OVERVIEW OF THE PROBLEM IN MENTAL HEALTH CARE.
SRCE   *PRESENTED AT THE NINTH ANNUAL MEETING OF THE SOUTHERN ANTHROPOLOGICAL SOCIETY, BLACKSBURG, VIRGINIA, APRIL 4-6, 1974.*
INDX   PSYCHOTHERAPY, MEXICAN AMERICAN, HEALTH DELIVERY SYSTEMS, PREJUDICE, DISCRIMINATION, PSYCHOPATHOLOGY, EMPIRICAL, PROCEEDINGS, MENTAL HEALTH, PSYCHOTHERAPISTS, ESSAY, CROSS CULTURAL, PUERTO RICAN-M
ABST   RESEARCH ON PSYCHOPATHOLOGY ACROSS CULTURES HAS YIELDED A "HODGEPODGE OF OBSERVATIONS," LITTLE OF WHICH HAS BEEN INTEGRATED INTO AN OVERALL FRAMEWORK

OF CROSS-CULTURAL MENTAL HEALTH, AND EVEN LESS HAS BEEN APPLIED TOWARD IMPROVING PSYCHIATRIC CARE. UNTIL RECENTLY, WHEN COMMUNITY MENTAL HEALTH PROGRAMS WERE DEVELOPED, THIS ISSUE WAS NOT OF MONUMENTAL IMPORTANCE. HOWEVER, THE EXPANSION AND SUBSIDIZATION OF THE MENTAL HEALTH DELIVERY SYSTEM HAS RESULTED IN AN INCREASING NUMBER OF ETHNIC AND LOWER INCOME PATIENTS WHOSE CULTURE AND EXPERIENCE ARE DIFFERENT FROM THAT OF MOST MENTAL HEALTH PROFESSIONALS. THE CULTURAL GAP BETWEEN ETHNIC PATIENT AND ANGLO HEALER HAS TWO MAJOR ASPECTS: (1) THE CLIENTS MAY HAVE VERY DIFFERENT CONCEPTIONS OF APPROPRIATE REMEDIES FOR THEIR PROBLEMS; AND (2) THERAPISTS OFTEN DO NOT PERCEIVE THESE PATIENTS AS BENEFITING FROM THEIR SERVICES. THE LITERATURE SUPPORTING THESE ASSUMPTIONS HAS GROWN, AND THIS PAPER ATTEMPTS TO SUMMARIZE THE MAJOR PROBLEMS DERIVING FROM THE SOCIAL, CULTURAL AND COGNITIVE DIFFERENCES BETWEEN THESE TWO GROUPS. THE PROBLEMS DISCUSSED ARE: (1) DIFFERENCES IN REPORTED EPIDEMIOLOGY OF MENTAL DISORDERS AMONG CULTURAL GROUPS IN THE UNITED STATES; (2) POTENTIAL AREAS OF MISDIAGNOSIS THAT MAY GENERATE DIFFERENTIAL STATISTICS; (3) THE INTERACTION OF (1) AND (2) WITH THE DISPOSITION OF CASES AND SELECTION OF EFFECTIVE TREATMENT MODELS; AND (4) THE PROBLEM OF PSYCHIATRIC ETHNOCENTRISM AND CULTURAL MISUNDERSTANDING THAT MAY ARISE IN PSYCHOTHERAPY. 69 REFERENCES. (AUTHOR SUMMARY MODIFIED)

ACCN   000871

1017 AUTH   **LEHMANN, S.**
TITL   SELECTED SELF HELP: A STUDY OF CLIENTS OF A COMMUNITY SOCIAL PSYCHIATRY SERVICE.
SRCE   *AMERICAN JOURNAL OF PSYCHIATRY, 1970, 126(10), 1444-1454.*
INDX   PRIMARY PREVENTION, COMMUNITY, COMMUNITY INVOLVEMENT, PUERTO RICAN-M, PSYCHOTHERAPY, PROGRAM EVALUATION, MENTAL HEALTH, HEALTH DELIVERY SYSTEMS, NEW YORK, EAST
ABST   THREE COMMUNITY SOCIAL PSYCHIATRIC SERVICES CENTERS SET UP IN A DISADVANTAGED AREA IN NEW YORK CITY WERE ASSESSED IN TERMS OF WHO USED THE CENTERS AND WHY. CLIENTS OF THE CENTERS WERE INTERVIEWED 3 MONTHS AFTER THEIR VISITS AND COMPARED WITH THE REST OF THE COMMUNITY. PEOPLE IN THE COMMUNITY WITH THE MOST PROBLEMS HAD HIGHER UTILIZATION RATES, AND THEIR PROBLEMS WERE REPRESENTATIVE OF THOSE IN THE COMMUNITY. CLIENT FAMILIES WERE MORE APT TO BE FATHERLESS, NEWER TO THE AREA, LOWER IN OCCUPATIONAL LEVEL AND EDUCATION, AND POSSESS A LANGUAGE HANDICAP IF PUERTO RICAN. THE CLIENTS CAME ALMOST EXCLUSIVELY FROM WITHIN A FIVE-BLOCK RADIUS OF THE CENTERS. IT APPEARS THEN THAT PROBLEMS AND PROXIMITY ARE THE KEYS TO THE SELF-SELECTION OF CLIENTS. FINALLY, PSYCHIATRIC PROBLEMS WERE SELDOM PRESENTED, BUT PEOPLE WITH HISTORIES OF PSYCHIATRIC ILLNESS WERE THE MOST LIKELY TO VISIT THE CENTERS. 13 REFERENCES.

ACCN   000872

1018 AUTH   **LEI, T. J., BUTLER, E. W., & SABAGH, G.**
TITL   FAMILY SOCIOCULTURAL BACKGROUND AND BEHAVIORAL RETARDATION OF CHILDREN.
SRCE   *JOURNAL OF HEALTH AND SOCIAL BEHAVIOR, 1972, 13(3), 318-326.*
INDX   LEARNING DISABILITIES, MENTAL RETARDATION, SES, ENVIRONMENTAL FACTORS, SPANISH SURNAMED, EMPIRICAL, ACCULTURATION, IMPAIRMENT, SPECIAL EDUCATION, CALIFORNIA, SOUTHWEST
ABST   AN EXAMINATION OF BEHAVIORAL RETARDATION (I.E., THE INABILITY OF INDIVIDUALS TO PERFORM SOCIAL ROLES PRESCRIBED BY THE DOMINANT CULTURE) AMONG ANGLO AMERICAN (AA) AND MEXICAN AMERICAN (MA) CHILDREN ANALYZED ITS RELATION TO SOCIAL STATUS, COMMUNITY OF ORIGIN, AND RESIDENTIAL MOBILITY. IT WAS HYPOTHESIZED THAT THERE WOULD BE AN INCREASED LIKELIHOOD OF BEHAVIORALLY RETARDED CHILDREN FROM MINORITY CULTURES, OF LOW SOCIOECONOMIC STATUS, WHO COME FROM A DISTANT COMMUNITY, WHO MOVE FREQUENTLY, AND WHO HAVE LIVED IN THE LOCAL COMMUNITY A SHORTER PERIOD OF TIME. THE STRATIFIED RANDOM SAMPLE CONSISTED OF 1,065 AA AND 110 MA FAMILIES FROM A SOUTHERN CALIFORNIA CITY. OF A TOTAL OF 2,305 AA CHILDREN AND 336 MA CHILDREN IN THE FAMILIES, 360 AA AND 76 MA WERE IDENTIFIED AS BEHAVIORALLY RETARDED. THE FINDINGS SHOW THAT THE MOTHER'S EDUCATION HAS THE GREATEST EFFECT ON RETARDATION OF AA AND MA CHILDREN, THE FATHER'S EDUCATION AND OCCUPATION HAVING LESS IMPORTANCE. GENERALLY, MA FAMILIES WITH A BEHAVIORALLY RETARDED CHILD ARE MORE LIKELY TO BE FROM LARGER COMMUNITIES, EXPERIENCE FREQUENT MOVING, AND BE AFFECTED BY THE SIZE OF THE COMMUNITY OF ORIGIN. THERE IS NO STATISTICAL SIGNIFICANCE AS TO SOCIOCULTURAL AREA OF ORIGIN AND LENGTH OF RESIDENCE. FOR THE AA, COMMUNITY OF ORIGIN AND LENGTH OF RESIDENCE HAVE NO STATISTICAL SIGNIFICANCE. OVERALL THE DATA STRONGLY SUGGEST THERE IS MORE OF A RELATIONSHIP BETWEEN FAMILY SOCIOCULTURAL FACTORS AND BEHAVIORAL RETARDATION OF MA CHILDREN THAN OF AA CHILDREN. FURTHERMORE, MA FAMILIES WITH RETARDED CHILDREN ARE SEEN AS MORE CULTURALLY DEPRIVED AND LESS INTEGRATED INTO THE DOMINANT CULTURE. 21 REFERENCES.

ACCN   000873

1019 AUTH   **LEI, T., BUTLER, E. W., ROWITZ, L., & MCALLISTER, R. J.**
TITL   AGENCY-LABELED MENTALLY RETARDED PER-

SONS IN A METROPOLITAN AREA: AN ECO-
LOGICAL STUDY.

SRCE *AMERICAN JOURNAL OF MENTAL DEFICIENCY,
1974, 79(1), 22-31.*

INDX CALIFORNIA, URBAN, DISCRIMINATION, CHIL-
DREN, DEMOGRAPHIC, EDUCATION, EMPIRI-
CAL, ENVIRONMENTAL FACTORS, HEALTH DE-
LIVERY SYSTEMS, SOUTHWEST, MENTAL
RETARDATION, MEXICAN AMERICAN, CROSS
CULTURAL, RESOURCE UTILIZATION, SURVEY

ABST THIS STUDY IN A MODERATE SIZED CITY IN
CALIFORNIA, HYPOTHESIZED THAT THERE
WOULD BE ECOLOGICAL DIFFERENCES IN
RATES OF LABELED MENTAL RETARDATION (1)
BECAUSE OF VARYING REFERRAL SOURCES
THAT ARE USED BY THE POPULATIONS LIVING
IN DIFFERENT AREAS OF THE CITY, AND (2) BE-
CAUSE EACH AGENCY HAS ITS OWN UNIQUE
OPERATIONAL DEFINITION OF RETARDATION. A
SURVEY WAS CONDUCTED OF 241 AGENCIES
PROVIDING SERVICES FOR MENTALLY RE-
TARDED PERSONS IN 1963-1964, AND A TOTAL
OF 835 MENTALLY RETARDED PERSONS WERE
IDENTIFIED. IT WAS EVIDENT THAT THE PUBLIC
SCHOOL SYSTEM OPERATED AS THE MAJOR
IDENTIFIER AND LABELER. THE BASIC CON-
CLUSION WAS THAT REGARDLESS OF GEO-
GRAPHIC PROXIMITY TO AN AGENCY, PER-
SONS LABELED MENTALLY RETARDED BY
PUBLIC AGENCIES WERE PREDOMINANTLY THE
POOR AND/OR ETHNIC-MINORITIES WHO LIVED
IN AREAS OF DETERIORATED AND OLDER
HOUSING. SPECIFICALLY, THE HIGHEST RATES
OF LABELED MENTALLY RETARDED BY PUBLIC
SCHOOLS AND OTHER PUBLIC AGENCIES WERE
IN AREAS OF MAJOR CONCENTRATIONS OF
CHICANO AND BLACK POPULATIONS. PER-
SONS LABELED MENTALLY RETARDED BY PRI-
VATE CLINICAL AGENCIES WERE PREDOMI-
NANTLY ANGLO, MIDDLE- AND UPPER-CLASS,
AND RESIDED IN AREAS OF BETTER HOUSING
AND NEIGHBORHOOD QUALITY. PRIVATE NON-
CLINICAL AGENCIES WERE AN ANOMALY, HAV-
ING A LABELING PATTERN THAT DID NOT LEND
ITSELF TO EITHER OF THESE DESCRIPTIONS. IN
THE ACTUAL LABELING PROCESS, CHICANO
CHILDREN WERE DISPROPORTIONATELY LA-
BELED RETARDED, WHILE ANGLO CHILDREN
WITH THE SAME LOWER-LEVEL INTELLECTUAL
ABILITY WERE MORE LIKELY THAN CHICANO
OR BLACK CHILDREN TO BE LABELED "EDU-
CATIONALLY HANDICAPPED." 17 REFERENCES.
(AUTHOR ABSTRACT MODIFIED)

ACCN 002653

1020 AUTH **LEIFER, A.**
TITL ETHNIC PATTERNS IN COGNITIVE TASKS.
SRCE *PROCEEDINGS OF THE ANNUAL CONVENTION
OF THE AMERICAN PSYCHOLOGICAL ASSO-
CIATION, 1972, 7(PT. 1), 73-74.*
INDX COGNITIVE DEVELOPMENT, SES, POVERTY,
CHILDREN, ETHNIC IDENTITY, PUERTO RICAN-
M, CROSS CULTURAL, ACHIEVEMENT TESTING,
CULTURAL FACTORS, EMPIRICAL, EARLY
CHILDHOOD EDUCATION, NEW YORK, EAST
ABST THE CONSTRUCTIONAL ABILITY, UNDER-
STANDING OF BODY PARTS, ABILITY TO COPY

GEOMETRIC SHAPES, AND VERBAL FLUENCY
OF 80 ECONOMICALLY DISADVANTAGED PRES-
CHOOLERS (20 EACH CHINESE, ITALIAN, BLACK,
AND PUERTO RICAN) ATTENDING HEADSTART
AND DAY-CARE CENTERS IN MANHATTAN,
BROOKLYN AND LONG ISLAND, NEW YORK,
WERE COMPARED. THE INVESTIGATORS AT-
TEMPTED TO DETERMINE WHAT EDUCATION-
ALLY RELEVANT, CULTURALLY REINFORCED
ABILITIES THE MINORITY CHILD BRINGS TO
THE CLASSROOM SO THAT COMPENSATORY
EDUCATION PROGRAMS CAN BE MORE EFFEC-
TIVELY DEVELOPED. USING A ONE-WAY ANALY-
SIS OF VARIANCE TEST, SIGNIFICANT DIFFER-
ENCES WERE FOUND IN 3 OF THE 4 ABILITIES
TESTED. CHINESE CHILDREN EXCEEDED THE
OTHER GROUPS IN CONSTRUCTIONAL ABILITY
AND IN BODY UNDERSTANDING. ITALIAN, BLACK
AND PUERTO RICAN SUBJECTS SURPASSED
THE CHINESE IN VERBAL IDEATIONAL FLUENCY.
NO DISCERNIBLE DIFFERENCES WERE FOUND
IN ABILITY TO COPY GEOMETRIC SHAPES.
THESE FINDINGS ARE DISCUSSED IN TERMS
OF THE CULTURAL PRACTICES AND INTERAC-
TIONS WHICH MAY REINFORCE THE ABILITIES
DEMONSTRATED. THIS RESEARCH ARGUES
THAT THE MINORITY CHILD'S DOMINANT ABILI-
TIES SHOULD BE RECOGNIZED AND EN-
HANCED IN THE CLASSROOM, WHILE USING
THEM TO DEVELOP OTHER SKILLS. 22 REFER-
ENCES.

ACCN 000874

1021 AUTH **LEININGER, M.**
TITL WITCHCRAFT PRACTICES AND PSYCHOCUL-
TURAL THERAPY WITH URBAN U.S. FAMILIES.
SRCE *HUMAN ORGANIZATION, 1973, 32(1), 73-83.*
INDX FOLK MEDICINE, EMPIRICAL, SPANISH SUR-
NAMED, CROSS CULTURAL, EXTENDED FAMILY,
ACCULTURATION, URBAN, PSYCHOTHERAPY,
CASE STUDY, FAMILY STRUCTURE, FAMILY
THERAPY, MENTAL HEALTH PROFESSION,
THEORETICAL, POLICY
ABST A THEORETICAL FRAMEWORK, BASED UPON
EMPIRICAL DATA GATHERED WHILE WORKING
WITH OVER 200 FAMILIES, REGARDING WITCH-
CRAFT BEHAVIOR AND ITS FUNCTIONS IN UR-
BAN U.S. FAMILIES IS PRESENTED. A DESCRIP-
TIVE ANALYSIS OF SIX FAMILIES, FOUR SPANISH-
SPEAKING AND TWO ANGLO AMERICAN, DIS-
CLOSED THAT PSYCHOCULTURAL NURSING
THERAPY CAN BE EFFECTIVE IN HELPING THE
BEWITCHED VICTIMS AND THEIR FAMILIES.
THREE MAJOR PHASES IN THE THEORETICAL
MODEL SERVE AS IMPORTANT GUIDELINES IN
DETERMINING THE PSYCHOCULTURAL AND
SOCIAL MECHANISMS USED BY THE FAMILIES
TO COPE WITH ACCULTURATION, ECONOMIC,
AND SOCIAL STRESSES. THERAPY IS LARGELY
SUPPORTIVE AND EXPRESSIVE IN FORM IN-
VOLVING THE USE OF CULTURAL VALUE ORI-
ENTATIONS ADAPTED TO THE LIFE AND ENVI-
RONMENTAL SITUATION OF THE FAMILIES. THE
REPORTED INCREASE OF INTEREST IN WITCH-
CRAFT IN THIS COUNTRY AND THE INCREASE
OF BEWITCHED VICTIMS SEEKING HELP MAKE
IT IMPERATIVE THAT PROFESSIONAL STAFF, ES-
PECIALLY MENTAL HEALTH PERSONNEL, BE-

COME MORE KNOWLEDGEABLE OF THE WITCHCRAFT PHENOMENON AND EXPLORE WAYS TO WORK WITH VICTIMS AND THEIR FAMILIES. 4 REFERENCES. (AUTHOR SUMMARY MODIFIED)

ACCN   000875

1022 AUTH   **LEMAN, K. A.**
TITL   PARENTAL ATTITUDES TOWARDS HIGHER EDUCATION AND ACADEMIC SUCCESS AMONG MEXICAN-AMERICAN, BLACK AND ANGLO ECONOMICALLY DISADVANTAGED COLLEGE STUDENTS (DOCTORAL DISSERTATION, UNIVERSITY OF ARIZONA, 1974).
SRCE   *DISSERTATION ABSTRACTS INTERNATIONAL, 1974, 35(4), 2010A. (UNIVERSITY MICROFILMS NO. 74-21,126.)*
INDX   SCHOLASTIC ASPIRATIONS, SCHOLASTIC ACHIEVEMENT, CROSS CULTURAL, SES, MEXICAN AMERICAN, POVERTY, EDUCATION, ATTITUDES, EMPIRICAL, ARIZONA, SOUTHWEST, HIGHER EDUCATION, COLLEGE STUDENTS
ABST   THREE GROUPS OF 30 ECONOMICALLY DISADVANTAGED BLACK, MEXICAN AMERICAN AND ANGLO COLLEGE STUDENTS WERE RANDOMLY SELECTED FROM A POPULATION OF 400 ECONOMICALLY DISADVANTAGED STUDENTS. THE THREE GROUPS WERE ADMINISTERED THE LEMAN ATTITUDE SCALE TOWARD HIGHER EDUCATION (LASTHE), AN ADAPTATION OF AN EARLIER SCALE, TO DETERMINE PERCEIVED PARENTAL ATTITUDES TOWARD HIGHER EDUCATION. THE TEST-RETEST RELIABILITY FOR THE LASTHE WAS .974. THE PARTIAL CORRELATION COEFFICIENT FOR EACH ETHNIC GROUP REQUIRED THE COMPUTATION OF PEARSON PRODUCT MOMENT CORRELATION COEFFICIENTS BETWEEN PERCEIVED PARENTAL ATTITUDES AND GRADE POINT AVERAGE, PERCEIVED PARENTAL ATTITUDES AND ACT SCORE AND GRADE POINT AVERAGE AND ACT SCORE. THIS REPRESENTED THE CORRELATION OF PERCEIVED PARENTAL ATTITUDES AND GRADE POINT AVERAGES WITH THE INFLUENCE OF ACT SCORES ELIMINATED. THE HYPOTHESIS THAT THERE IS NO SIGNIFICANT DIFFERENCE IN THE RELATIONSHIP BETWEEN PERCEIVED PARENTAL ATTITUDES TOWARD HIGHER EDUCATION AND ACADEMIC SUCCESS AMONG MEXICAN AMERICAN, BLACK AND ANGLO ECONOMICALLY DISADVANTAGED COLLEGE STUDENTS WAS REJECTED. A SIGNIFICANT RELATIONSHIP BETWEEN PERCEIVED PARENTAL ATTITUDES AND GRADE POINT AVERAGE FOR MEXICAN AMERICAN STUDENTS WAS FOUND. THERE WERE NO SIGNIFICANT DIFFERENCES FOR EITHER THE ANGLO OR BLACK GROUP, ALTHOUGH A POSITIVE TREND EXISTED. 95 REFERENCES. (AUTHOR ABSTRACT MODIFIED)
ACCN   000876

1023 AUTH   **LEON, C. A.**
TITL   PSYCHIATRY IN LATIN AMERICA.
SRCE   *BRITISH JOURNAL OF PSYCHIATRY, 1972, 121(561), 121-136.*
INDX   MENTAL HEALTH PROFESSION, SOUTH AMERICA, PSYCHOTHERAPY, POVERTY, HISTORY, PROFESSIONAL TRAINING, CENTRAL AMERICA, REVIEW, DEMOGRAPHIC, HEALTH DELIVERY SYSTEMS
ABST   AN OVERVIEW OF PSYCHIATRY IN LATIN AMERICA IS PRESENTED, BASED UPON INFORMATION GATHERED AT THE 1968 CONFERENCE ON MENTAL HEALTH IN THE AMERICAS. THE OVERVIEW COVERS THE FOLLOWING AREAS: (1) LATIN AMERICA AND ITS PEOPLE, PER CAPITA INCOME AND POPULATION BY COUNTRY; (2) HEALTH SERVICES AND EPIDEMIOLOGICAL DATA; (3) SUMMARY OF THE HISTORICAL DEVELOPMENT OF PSYCHIATRY IN LATIN AMERICA INCLUDING FOLK MEDICINE, ESTABLISHMENT OF HOSPITALS AND PROFESSIONAL ORGANIZATIONS; (4) DATA ON THE NUMBER, PROFESSIONAL ACTIVITY AND SCIENTIFIC ORIENTATION OF LATIN AMERICAN PSYCHIATRISTS FOR THE YEARS 1966-1967, AND DISTRIBUTION OF PUBLIC PSYCHIATRIC HOSPITALS AND OTHER SERVICES; (5) EDUCATIONAL FACILITIES FOR TRAINING PSYCHIATRISTS, TYPES OF PROGRAMS, NUMBER OF DEPARTMENTS OF PSYCHIATRY, JOURNALS AND PROFESSIONAL SOCIETIES; AND (6) RECOMMENDATIONS FOR DEALING WITH MENTAL HEALTH PROBLEMS IN LATIN AMERICA. 83 REFERENCES.
ACCN   000877

1024 AUTH   **LEON, D. J.**
TITL   CHICANO COLLEGE DROPOUTS AND THE EDUCATIONAL OPPORTUNITY PROGRAM: FAILURE AFTER HIGH SCHOOL?
SRCE   *HIGH SCHOOL BEHAVIORAL SCIENCE, 1975, 3(1), 6-11.*
INDX   COLLEGE STUDENTS, CULTURAL FACTORS, EDUCATION, EDUCATIONAL COUNSELING, HIGHER EDUCATION, INTEGRATION, MEXICAN AMERICAN, PROGRAM EVALUATION, PSYCHOSOCIAL ADJUSTMENT, SCHOLASTIC ASPIRATIONS, SOCIALIZATION, CALIFORNIA, SOUTHWEST, EMPIRICAL, POLICY, SCHOLASTIC ACHIEVEMENT
ABST   INTENSIVE INTERVIEWS WITH 15 CHICANO STUDENTS WHO RECENTLY WITHDREW FROM A COLLEGE EDUCATIONAL OPPORTUNITY PROGRAM ARE EXAMINED TO DETERMINE CAUSES OF WITHDRAWAL AND POTENTIAL SOLUTIONS. FINDINGS ARE EXAMINED FROM AN ETHNOMETHODOLOGICAL PERSPECTIVE AND SUGGEST THAT THE CHICANOS DID NOT ACQUIRE A "CONTEXTUAL UNDERSTANDING" OF THE UNIVERSITY NOR A FAMILIARITY WITH EVERYDAY ROUTINES OF THE INSTITUTION. IMPLICATIONS FOR PROGRAMS WHICH MEET THE NEEDS OF STUDENTS FROM MINORITY OR RURAL GROUPS INCLUDE: (1) INFORMAL SUPPLEMENTS TO STRUCTURED SUPPORTIVE SERVICES, SUCH AS PAIRING OF MINORITY STUDENTS WITH OLDER STUDENTS FROM THE SAME MINORITY GROUP; AND (2) PREPARATION OF STUDENTS FOR UNIVERSITY LIFE AS AN INTEGRAL PART OF HIGH SCHOOL EDUCATION, PERHAPS IN THE CONTEXT OF SOCIAL SCIENCE COURSES. 12 REFERENCES. (NCMHI ABSTRACT)
ACCN   002133

1025 AUTH **LEON, G. R.**
TITL MARIA VALDEZ—A LIFETIME EXPOSURE TO AL-COHOL.
SRCE *IN G. R. LEON, CASE HISTORIES OF DEVIANT BEHAVIOR: A SOCIAL LEARNING ANALYSIS. BOSTON: HOLBROOK PRESS, INC., 1974, PP. 162-180.*
INDX ALCOHOLISM, POVERTY, MEXICAN AMERICAN, CASE STUDY, PSYCHOPATHOLOGY, DEVIANCE, INSTITUTIONALIZATION, PROGRAM EVALUATION, PSYCHOTHERAPY OUTCOME, FEMALE, ADULTS
ABST A CASE STUDY OF A 40 YEAR-OLD, FEMALE MEXICAN AMERICAN WHO VOLUNTARILY SOUGHT TREATMENT FOR ALCOHOL IS PRESENTED. THE STUDY INCLUDES AN IN-DEPTH DESCRIPTION OF HER CHILDHOOD AND YOUNG ADULTHOOD. THE PATIENT'S MARRIAGE IS EMPHASIZED IN THE TREATMENT HISTORY AND PSYCHOLOGICAL EVALUATION. THIS CASE ILLUSTRATES THE IMPORTANCE OF SOCIAL AND FAMILY FACTORS IN THE DEVELOPMENT OF A PARTICULAR DRINKING PATTERN. EVALUATION OF THE HOSPITAL TREATMENT EMPHASIZES THE UTILITY OF GROUP THERAPY AND ANTABUSE (A DRUG WHICH SUPPRESSES ALCOHOL CONSUMPTION) FOR THIS PATIENT. 15 REFERENCES.
ACCN 000878

1026 AUTH **LEON, G. R.**
TITL PARANOID SCHIZOPHRENIA—THE CASE OF CARLOS RIVERA.
SRCE *IN G. R. LEON (ED.), CASE HISTORIES OF DEVIANT BEHAVIOR: A SOCIAL LEARNING ANALYSIS. BOSTON: HOLBROOK PRESS, INC., 1974, PP. 258-277.*
INDX SCHIZOPHRENIA, CASE STUDY, MEXICAN AMERICAN
ABST A 47 YEAR-OLD MEXICAN AMERICAN PATIENT'S SOCIAL HISTORY, EDUCATIONAL BACKGROUND, DELINQUENCY RECORD, MARITAL HISTORY AND RELIGION ARE DISCUSSED IN RELATION TO HIS DIAGNOSIS OF PARANOID SCHIZOPHRENIA. HIS PSYCHIATRIC AND PSYCHOLOGICAL EVALUATIONS, WARD BEHAVIOR AND COURSE OF THERAPY ARE ALSO DESCRIBED. SOCIAL AND ENVIRONMENTAL FACTORS INFLUENCING HIS LIFE COURSE AND MENTAL HEALTH ARE EMPHASIZED IN EXPLAINING THE ILLNESS AND ITS TREATMENT IN THIS PATIENT. 17 REFERENCES.
ACCN 000879

1027 AUTH **LEON, G. R.**
TITL PERSONALITY CHANGE IN THE SPECIALLY ADMITTED DISADVANTAGED STUDENT AFTER ONE YEAR IN COLLEGE.
SRCE *JOURNAL OF CLINICAL PSYCHOLOGY, 1974, 30(4), 522-528.*
INDX PERSONALITY, SCHOLASTIC ACHIEVEMENT, ACHIEVEMENT MOTIVATION, COLLEGE STUDENTS, POVERTY, SES, CULTURAL FACTORS, INTERPERSONAL RELATIONS, PUERTO RICAN-M, CROSS CULTURAL, ROTTER INTERNAL-EXTERNAL SCALE, ATTRIBUTION OF RESPONSIBILITY
ABST THE PROCESS OF PERSONALITY CHANGE IN

COLLEGE STUDENTS OVER THE COURSE OF THEIR FRESHMEN YEAR IS EVALUATED. EIGHTY-SEVEN DISADVANTAGED STUDENTS ADMITTED TO AN EASTERN UNIVERSITY THROUGH A SPECIAL ENTRANCE PROGRAM (MOSTLY BLACK AND PUERTO RICAN) AND 36 CONTROL GROUP STUDENTS, VOLUNTEERS FROM AN INTRODUCTORY PSYCHOLOGY CLASS (MOSTLY ANGLO) WERE ADMINISTERED THE FOLLOWING TESTS AT THE BEGINNING AND AGAIN AT THE END OF THEIR FIRST YEAR IN COLLEGE: (1) INTERPERSONAL TRUST SCALE (ITS); (2) ITERNAL-EXTERNAL CONTROL OF REINFORCEMENT SCALE (I-E); AND (3) SELECTED PARTS OF THE OPINION, ATTITUDE AND INTERESTS SURVEY (OAIS). GRADE POINT AVERAGE (GPA) DATA AT THE END OF THE FIRST AND SECOND SEMESTERS WERE USED AS THE MEASURE OF ACADEMIC SUCCESS. FINDINGS INCLUDED: (1) NO SIGNIFICANT DIFFERENCE WAS FOUND BETWEEN THE EXPERIMENTAL AND CONTROL GROUPS ON THE I-E OR ITS SCALES BY SEX; AND (2) NO SIGNIFICANT DIFFERENCES WERE FOUND BETWEEN THE TWO GROUPS ON ANY OF THE PERSONALITY SCORES ON EITHER THE FIRST OR SECOND TESTING. FINDINGS SUPPORTED THESE CONCLUSIONS: (1) FOR THE CONTROL GROUP A POSITIVE RELATIONSHIP EXISTED BETWEEN HIGHER GRADES AND AN INCREASED AMOUNT OF INTERPERSONAL TRUST AT THE END OF THE COLLEGE YEAR; (2) FOR DISADVANTAGED STUDENTS THIS RELATIONSHIP WAS INVERSE; AND (3) FOR SPECIAL ENTRANCE STUDENTS, FEELINGS OF PERSONAL CONTROL SHOWED AN IMPORTANT RELATIONSHIP TO GPA. IMPLICATIONS OF THIS STUDY FOR THOSE WHO COUNSEL DISADVANTAGED STUDENTS ARE DISCUSSED. DATA ILLUSTRATING THE GENERAL DECLINE IN INTERPERSONAL TRUST AND THE TREND TOWARD A GREATER EXTERNAL CONTROL ORIENTATION IN COLLEGE STUDENTS OVER THE PAST DECADE ARE ALSO DISCUSSED. 9 REFERENCES.
ACCN 000880

1028 AUTH **LEON, J. J.**
TITL SEX-ETHNIC MARRIAGE IN HAWAII: A NONMETRIC MULTIDIMENSIONAL ANALYSIS.
SRCE *JOURNAL OF MARRIAGE AND THE FAMILY, 1975, 37(4), 775-781.*
INDX MARRIAGE, INTERMARRIAGE, CULTURAL FACTORS, PUERTO RICAN-M, SEX COMPARISON, DEMOGRAPHIC, HAWAII, WEST
ABST HIGH ETHNIC INTERMARRIAGE RATES HAVE LONG BEEN CHARACTERISTIC OF HAWAII AND HAVE BEEN POINTED TO AS AN INDICATOR OF ASSIMILATION IN THESE ISLANDS. THIS ANALYSIS EXPLORES THE DIMENSIONS OF ETHNIC INTERMARRIAGE FOR TWO TIME PERIODS: 1948-1953 AND 1965-1969. THE COMMON ELEMENTS THAT PREDISPOSE MALES AND FEMALES TO MARRY IN AND OUT OF THEIR ETHNIC GROUPS WERE INVESTIGATED. UTILIZING A MAPPING SENTENCE AND NONMETRIC MULTIDIMENSIONAL ANALYSIS, SEX AND ETHNICITY OF THE MARRIAGE PARTNERS WERE MAPPED INTO THE SAME STRUCTURAL SPACE FOR EACH TIME PERIOD. THE FINDINGS, DEPICTED SPA-

TIALLY, SHOW TWO GENERAL CLUSTERS. ONE CLUSTER CONSISTS OF JAPANESE, CHINESE AND KOREAN MALES AND FEMALES. THE OTHER CLUSTER CONSISTS OF CAUCASIAN, PART-HAWAIIAN, FILIPINO, AND PUERTO RICAN MALES AND FEMALES. THESE CLUSTERS ARE TERMED EAST AND WEST, RESPECTIVELY. THE FINDINGS SUGGEST THAT THE EAST CLUSTER ETHNIC GROUPS, REGARDLESS OF SEX, PREFER OTHER EAST CLUSTER ETHNIC GROUPS AND VICE VERSA. IN GENERAL, THIS INTERPRETATION LENDS SUPPORT TO THE IDEA OF SOCIAL HOMOGAMY ON A BROADER LEVEL THAN ETHNICITY. 20 REFERENCES. (JOURNAL ABSTRACT MODIFIED)

ACCN 000881

1029 AUTH **LEONARD, O. E., & JOHNSON, H. W.**

TITL LOW INCOME FAMILIES IN THE SPANISH SURNAMED POPULATION OF THE SOUTHWEST (REPORT NO. AER-112).

SRCE *WASHINGTON, D.C.: ECONOMIC RESEARCH SERVICE, DEPARTMENT OF AGRICULTURE, 1967. (ERIC DOCUMENT REPRODUCTION SERVICE NO. ED 036 384)*

INDX POVERTY, SES, ECONOMIC FACTORS, DEMOGRAPHIC, MEXICAN AMERICAN, EMPIRICAL, PSYCHOPATHOLOGY, DEVIANCE, INSTITUTIONALIZATION, SPANISH SURNAMED, FERTILITY, SOCIAL MOBILITY, CENSUS, SOUTHWEST, CULTURAL FACTORS

ABST DATA FROM THE SPECIAL CENSUS REPORTS FOR 1950 AND 1960 WERE ANALYZED TO IDENTIFY CHARACTERISTICS OF SPANISH SURNAME FAMILIES IN THE SOUTHWESTERN UNITED STATES AND TO RELATE THESE CHARACTERISTICS TO THEIR SOCIAL AND ECONOMIC PROBLEMS. RESULTS OF THE ANALYSES INDICATE THAT THE SPANISH SURNAME POPULATION HAD HIGHER MOBILITY AND HIGHER FERTILITY RATES THAN OTHER WHITE POPULATIONS OF THE SOUTHWEST. IN ADDITION, OVER ONE-HALF OF THE RURAL SPANISH SURNAME FAMILIES AND ONE-THIRD OF THE URBAN SPANISH SURNAME FAMILIES HAD INCOMES OF LESS THAN $3,000 IN 1959. HOWEVER, THE PROPORTIONS OF THE SPANISH SURNAME LABOR FORCE IN PROFESSIONAL, CLERICAL, CRAFTS, AND SERVICE OCCUPATIONS INCREASED, AND THE PROPORTIONS IN FARM AND NONFARM LABOR DECLINED BETWEEN 1950 AND 1960. EDUCATIONAL ACHIEVEMENT IMPROVED BETWEEN 1950 AND 1960 BUT REMAINED BELOW THE NATIONAL MEDIAN. CULTURAL FACTORS CONTRIBUTING TO THE DISADVANTAGED POSITION OF THE SPANISH SURNAME POPULATION WERE USE OF SPANISH AS THE PRIMARY LANGUAGE AND CONTINUED CULTURAL ISOLATION FROM ANGLO SOCIETY. 16 REFERENCES. (RIE ABSTRACT MODIFIED)

ACCN 000882

1030 AUTH **LESSER, G. S., FIFER, G., & CLARK, D. H.**

TITL MENTAL ABILITIES OF CHILDREN FROM DIFFERENT SOCIAL-CLASS AND CULTURAL GROUPS.

SRCE *MONOGRAPHS OF THE SOCIETY FOR RE-*

SEARCH IN CHILD DEVELOPMENT, 1965, 30(7), 1-115.

INDX SES, CULTURE, INTELLIGENCE, PUERTO RICAN-M, CHILDREN, CROSS CULTURAL, EMPIRICAL, INTELLIGENCE TESTING, POVERTY

ABST AN EXAMINATION OF MENTAL ABILITIES IN 6 AND 7 YEAR-OLD CHILDREN FROM DIFFERENT SOCIAL CLASSES AND CULTURAL BACKGROUNDS IS PRESENTED. THE EFFECTS OF SOCIAL CLASS AND ETHNIC AFFILIATION UPON FOUR MENTAL ABILITIES (VERBAL, REASONING, NUMBER FACILITY, AND SPACE CONCEPTUALIZATION) WERE STUDIED IN 320 FIRST GRADE CHILDREN FROM FOUR ETHNIC GROUPS (CHINESE, JEWISH, NEGRO, AND PUERTO RICAN) WITH EACH GROUP DIVIDED INTO MIDDLE-CLASS AND LOWER-CLASS GROUPS. A 4X4X2 ANALYSIS OF COVARIANCE RESULTED IN THREE MAJOR FINDINGS. (1) DIFFERENCES IN SOCIAL CLASS PLACEMENT DO PRODUCE SIGNIFICANT DIFFERENCES IN THE ABSOLUTE LEVEL OF EACH MENTAL ABILITY BUT DO NOT PRODUCE SIGNIFICANT DIFFERENCES IN THE PATTERNS AMONG THESE ABILITIES. (2) DIFFERENCES IN ETHNIC GROUP MEMBERSHIP DO PRODUCE SIGNIFICANT DIFFERENCES IN BOTH THE ABSOLUTE LEVEL OF EACH MENTAL ABILITY AND THE PATTERNS AMONG THESE ABILITIES. (3) SOCIAL CLASS AND ETHNICITY DO INTERACT TO AFFECT THE ABSOLUTE LEVEL OF EACH MENTAL ABILITY BUT DO NOT INTERACT TO AFFECT THE PATTERNS AMONG THESE ABILITIES. IT WAS ALSO FOUND THAT MIDDLE-CLASS CHILDREN WERE SIGNIFICANTLY SUPERIOR TO LOWER-CLASS CHILDREN IN ALL THE SCALES AND SUBTESTS. DISCUSSIONS ARE PRESENTED ON ETHNIC GROUP EFFECTS UPON MENTAL ABILITIES, SEX DIFFERENCES, AND THE INTERACTION OF SOCIAL CLASS AND ETHNICITY. IT SEEMS THAT DIFFERENT SOCIAL CLASSES AND ETHNIC GROUPS DIFFER IN THEIR RELATIVE STANDING ON DIFFERENT FUNCTIONS. HOWEVER, THE ETHNIC GROUPS DO FOSTER THE DEVELOPMENT OF A DIFFERENT PATTERN OF ABILITIES, WHILE SOCIAL CLASS DIFFERENCES DO NOT MODIFY THE BASIC ORGANIZATION ASSOCIATED WITH ETHNIC GROUP CONDITIONS. 189 REFERENCES.

ACCN 000883

1031 AUTH **LEUTZ, W. N.**

TITL THE INFORMAL COMMUNITY CAREGIVER: A LINK BETWEEN THE HEALTH CARE SYSTEM AND LOCAL RESIDENTS.

SRCE *AMERICAN JOURNAL OF ORTHOPSYCHIATRY, 1976, 46(4), 678-688.*

INDX ALCOHOLISM, COMMUNITY, CULTURAL FACTORS, DEMOGRAPHIC, DRUG ABUSE, CROSS CULTURAL, EMPIRICAL, HEALTH DELIVERY SYSTEMS, MENTAL HEALTH, PARAPROFESSIONALS, PUERTO RICAN-M, RESOURCE UTILIZATION, SOCIAL STRUCTURE, URBAN, NEW YORK, EAST, POLICY, COMMUNITY INVOLVEMENT, ADULTS, ADOLESCENTS

ABST A GROUP OF INFORMAL CAREGIVERS—LOCAL PEOPLE TO WHOM RESIDENTS TURN FOR INFORMATION AND ADVICE ABOUT DRUG AND

ALCOHOL ABUSE—WAS IDENTIFIED IN EAST HARLEM AND ENLISTED IN A PARTICIPANT-OBSERVATION STUDY. THE CAREGIVERS INCLUDED 7 CLERGYMEN, 6 SOCIAL CLUB OWNERS, 4 SPIRITUALISTS, AND 12 MERCHANTS. DURING THE TWO-MONTH PERIOD OF THE STUDY, CAREGIVERS COMPLETED A SIMPLE, ONE-PAGE CHECKLIST FOR EACH CONTACT HE OR SHE HAD WITH A PERSON SEEKING HELP WITH DRUG OR ALCOHOL PROBLEMS FOR HIM OR HERSELF, A FAMILY MEMBER, OR A FRIEND. THE CAREGIVERS RECORDED THE TYPE OF PROBLEM, THE CAREGIVER'S RESPONSE (INCLUDING SPECIFIC REFERRAL TO A FORMAL SERVICE AGENCY), AND SOME DEMOGRAPHIC CHARACTERISTICS OF THE PERSON SEEKING HELP. THE 29 CAREGIVERS RECORDED A TOTAL OF 61 VISITS WITH PEOPLE RANGING IN AGE FROM 15 TO 50—NEARLY HALF WERE IN THEIR TWENTIES, AND 72% WERE HISPANIC, 16% BLACK, 12% WHITE. DRUGS WERE MORE FREQUENTLY CITED AS A PROBLEM THAN ALCOHOL. INDIVIDUALS TURNED TO THE CAREGIVER FOR HELP WITH THEIR OWN PROBLEM IN 44% OF THE CASES, FOR A FAMILY MEMBER IN 41% OF THE CASES, AND FOR A FRIEND IN 15%. THE FINDINGS CONFIRM THE EXISTENCE OF INFORMAL COMMUNITY NETWORKS AND SUGGEST THAT FORMAL HUMAN SERVICES AGENCIES AND THEIR INTENDED CLIENTELE WOULD BENEFIT BY INCREASED EFFORTS TO LOCATE AND WORK WITH THESE COMMUNITY CAREGIVERS. 11 REFERENCES.

ACCN   002135

1032 AUTH   **LEVI, M., & SEBORG, M.**
TITL   THE STUDY OF IQ SCORES ON VERBAL VS. NONVERBAL TESTS AND VS. ACADEMIC ACHIEVEMENT AMONG DRUG ADDICTS FROM DIFFERENT RACIAL AND ETHNIC GROUPS.
SRCE   *INTERNATIONAL JOURNAL OF THE ADDICTIONS, 1972, 7(3), 581-584.*
INDX   INTELLIGENCE TESTING, DRUG ADDICTION, CULTURE-FAIR TESTS, CALIFORNIA ACHIEVEMENT TESTS, RAVEN PROGRESSIVE MATRICES, MEXICAN AMERICAN, CROSS CULTURAL, EMPIRICAL, FEMALE, TEST VALIDITY, TEST RELIABILITY
ABST   THE REVISED ARMY ALPHA EXAMINATION, RAVEN'S PROGRESSIVE MATRICES, AND CALIFORNIA ACHIEVEMENT TESTS WERE ADMINISTERED TO 200 WHITE, 67 MEXICAN AND 6 BLACK WOMEN IN A STATE INSTITUTION FOR WOMEN DRUG ADDICTS. AN ADDITIONAL GROUP OF 79 ILLITERATES (14 WHITE, 28 BLACK, AND 37 MEXICAN) WAS GIVEN THE REVISED ARMY BETA EXAMINATION AND RAVEN'S PROGRESSIVE MATRICES. WHITES SCORED HIGHEST ON ALL THREE MEASURES. THE REVISED ALPHA DID NOT APPEAR TO RELIABLY MEASURE THE IQ OF THE BLACKS AND MEXICANS, WHO DID MUCH BETTER ON THE NONVERBAL TESTS. HOWEVER, BLACKS AND MEXICANS SCORED SIGNIFICANTLY LOWER THAN THE WHITES EVEN ON THE NONVERBAL TESTS, SUGGESTING A CULTURAL LOADING IN TEST CONTENT. IMPLICATIONS FOR THE ASSESSMENT OF IQ IN MINORITY GROUPS, VOCA-

TIONAL REHABILITATION PROGRAMS, SCHOOL COUNSELORS AND RESEARCHERS ARE DISCUSSED. (PASAR ABSTRACT)

ACCN   000884

1033 AUTH   **LEVINE, E. S.**
TITL   ETHNIC ESTEEM AMONG ANGLO, BLACK, AND CHICANO CHILDREN.
SRCE   *SAN FRANCISCO: R AND E RESEARCH ASSOCIATES, 1976.*
INDX   CHILDREN, MEXICAN AMERICAN, CROSS CULTURAL, EMPIRICAL, KANSAS, MIDWEST, ETHNIC IDENTITY, SELF CONCEPT, SEX COMPARISON, EXAMINER EFFECTS, BOOK, RESEARCH METHODOLOGY, INTERPERSONAL ATTRACTION
ABST   ETHNIC ESTEEM WAS STUDIED AMONG 50 ANGLO, 36 BLACK, AND 44 CHICANO SECOND AND FIFTH GRADERS IN A KANSAS CITY SCHOOL. THE SUBECTS WERE ASKED BY ANGLO, BLACK, AND CHICANO EXPERIMENTERS TO ASSIGN TEN ESTEEM-RELATED STATEMENTS TO TWO SETS OF STIMULI: (1) PHOTOS OF ANGLO, BLACK, AND CHICANO CHILDREN (THE PHOTOGRAPHIC DIFFERENTIAL); AND (2) THE NAMES OF THEIR CLASSMATES (THE SOCIOMETRIC DIFFERENTIAL). THE RESULTS REVEALED, FIRST OF ALL, THAT THE PHOTOGRAPHIC AND SOCIOMETRIC DIFFERENTIALS WERE EFFECTIVE IN THE DISCRIMINATION OF PATTERNS OF OWN-GROUP PREFERENCES. SECOND, AMONG THE THREE ETHNIC GROUPS, BLACKS HAD THE HIGHEST OWN-GROUP PREFERENCES WHILE CHICANOS HAD THE SECOND HIGHEST. THIRD, ESTEEM-RELATED STATEMENTS WERE ASSIGNED SELECTIVELY TO ETHNIC GROUPS—I.E., ANGLO STIMULI WERE SELECTED MOST FREQUENTLY ON STATEMENTS OF COMPETENCE, BLACK STIMULI ON STATEMENTS OF SIGNIFICANCE AND POWER, AND CHICANO STIMULI ON STATEMENTS OF VIRTUE AND COMPETENCE. FOURTH, A HIGHER FEMALE THAN MALE OWN-GROUP PREFERENCE WAS ELICITED WITH THE SECOND GRADERS, BUT THIS SEX DIFFERENCE WAS REVERSED AMONG THE FIFTH GRADERS. FIFTH, PATTERNS OF ETHNIC SELF-ESTEEM VARIED SIGNIFICANTLY WITH THE ETHNICITY OF THE EXAMINER. THE IMPLICATIONS OF THESE AND OTHER FINDINGS ARE DISCUSSED—IN PARTICULAR, THE NEED FOR MORE STUDIES OF SELF-ESTEEM AND EXAMINER EFFECTS, AS THESE MAY BE RELATED TO CLIENT-COUNSELOR ETHNICITY MATCHES IN THERAPY. 196 REFERENCES.

ACCN   001841

1034 AUTH   **LEVINE, E. S., & BARTZ, K. W.**
TITL   COMPARATIVE CHILD-REARING ATTITUDES AMONG CHICANO, ANGLO, AND BLACK PARENTS.
SRCE   *HISPANIC JOURNAL OF BEHAVIORAL SCIENCES, 1979, 1(2), 165-178.*
INDX   MEXICAN AMERICAN, CROSS CULTURAL, MISSOURI, MIDWEST, ADULTS, ATTITUDES, CHILD-REARING PRACTICES, EMPIRICAL, SEX COMPARISON, FAMILY ROLES, SES
ABST   THE CHILD-REARING ATTITUDES OF 152 CHI-

CANO MOTHERS AND FATHERS WERE COMPARED TO THOSE OF 143 ANGLO AND 160 BLACK PARENTS IN A SEMI-ENCLOSED, LOW SOCIOECONOMIC URBAN COMMUNITY IN MISSOURI. PARTICIPANTS RESPONDED TO A 25-ITEM ORAL INTERVIEW. FACTOR ANALYSIS REVEALED SEVEN MAIN ATTITUDE CLUSTERS, WITH CHICANOS DIFFERING FROM ANGLOS AND/OR BLACKS IN SIX CATEGORIES. CHICANOS ARE CHARACTERIZED AS EMPHASIZING EARLY ASSUMPTION OF RESPONSIBILITY; IN CONTRAST, BLACKS EXPRESS LESS SUPPORT AND CONTROL ATTITUDES. IN GENERAL, CHICANOS ARE LESS EGALITARIAN IN CHILD-REARING ATTITUDES THAN EITHER ANGLOS OR BLACKS. ALTHOUGH ATTITUDES OF CHICANO MOTHERS AND FATHERS ARE NOT SIGNIFICANTLY DIFFERENT FROM ONE ANOTHER, CROSS-ETHNIC DIFFERENCES ARE MORE ATTRIBUTABLE TO CHICANO FATHERS THAN MOTHERS. COMPARISONS AND CONTRASTS TO THE WIDELY HELD ASSUMPTIONS ABOUT THE HISPANIC FAMILY ARE DRAWN, AND QUESTIONS ABOUT THE EFFECTS OF THESE CHILD-REARING ATTITUDES UPON THE BEHAVIOR OF HISPANIC CHILDREN ARE POSED. 24 REFERENCES. (JOURNAL ABSTRACT MODIFIED)

ACCN 001773

1035 AUTH **LEVINE, E. S., & RUIZ, R. A.**
TITL AN EXPLORATION OF MULTICORRELATES OF ETHNIC GROUP CHOICE.
SRCE *JOURNAL OF CROSS-CULTURAL PSYCHOLOGY, 1978, 9(2), 179-189.*
INDX CROSS CULTURAL, EXAMINER EFFECTS, SEX COMPARISON, CROSS CULTURAL, EMPIRICAL, MIDWEST, CHILDREN, MEXICAN AMERICAN, SELF CONCEPT, ETHNIC IDENTITY
ABST AN IMPORTANT SOCIOCULTURAL QUESTION TODAY IS "UNDER WHAT EXPERIMENTAL AND ENVIRONMENTAL CONDITIONS DO ETHNIC SUBJECTS SELECT STIMULI OF THEIR OWN GROUP?" TO ASSESS PATTERNS OF ETHNIC CHOICE, AN UNSPECIFIED NUMBER OF MIDWESTERN ANGLO, BLACK, AND CHICANO 2ND AND 5TH GRADE CHILDREN WERE ASKED TO RELATE 12 STATEMENTS TO ETHNIC CUES PRESENTED IN A PHOTOGRAPHIC AND SOCIOMETRIC MODALITY. PATTERNS OF ETHNIC CHOICE WERE INFLUENCED BY AGE AND SEX OF THE CHILDREN AND ETHNICITY OF THE EXAMINER. AFTER SEX AND ETHNICITY OF EXAMINERS, RELATIVE ATTRACTIVENESS OF PHOTOGRAPHS USED, AND SEX, AGE, AND SOCIOECONOMIC LEVEL OF SUBJECTS WERE CONTROLLED, RESULTS INDICATED THAT BLACKS HAD THE HIGHEST OWN-GROUP CHOICE ON STATEMENTS MEASURING FAMILIAL AND PERSONAL ETHNIC IDENTITY. OWN-GROUP PREFERENCE WAS GREATER AMONG BLACKS AND CHICANOS THAN AMONG ANGLOS ON THE SOCIOMETRIC INSTRUMENT. WITH THE SOCIOMETRIC MODALITY, OWN-GROUP CHOICE WAS HIGHER AMONG BLACKS AND CHICANOS WITH THE ANGLO EXAMINER THAN WITH EXAMINERS OF MATCHED ETHNICITY. PARALLEL DEVELOPMENT OF PATTERNS ON CHOICE SUGGEST THAT THE TWO INSTRUMENTS TAP SOME CON-

SISTENT PATTERNS AND DEMONSTRATE THE NEED FOR MULTI-INSTRUMENTATION IN ETHNIC CHOICE RESEARCH. 23 REFERENCES.

ACCN 002136

1036 AUTH **LEVINE, E. S., & RUIZ, R. A.**
TITL PREFERENCE STUDY BASED ON "LIKE BEST" CHOICES FOR PHOTOGRAPHIC SLIDES OF ANGLO, BLACK, AND CHICANO CHILDREN.
SRCE *PERCEPTUAL AND MOTOR SKILLS, 1977, 44(2), 511-518.*
INDX ATTITUDES, CHILDREN, CROSS CULTURAL, CULTURAL FACTORS, EDUCATION, MEXICAN AMERICAN, SELF CONCEPT, SPANISH SURNAMED, ETHNIC IDENTITY, MIDWEST, MISSOURI
ABST A STUDY OF 216 THIRD AND SIXTH GRADE ANGLO, BLACK, AND CHICANO SCHOOLCHILDREN INDICATED PREFERENCES FOR PHOTOGRAPHIC SLIDES OF UNFAMILIAR BOYS AND GIRLS FROM THE SAME GRADE LEVELS AND ETHNICITIES. TWO SLIDES WERE PRESENTED TO EACH GROUP OF SUBJECTS: ONE SLIDE SHOWING ONLY MALES OF ONE ETHNICITY AND FROM THE SAME APPROXIMATE GRADE LEVEL AS THE SUBJECTS, AND THE SECOND SLIDE SHOWING ONLY FEMALES OF ONE ETHNICITY AND SAME APPROXIMATE GRADE. THE SUBJECTS, ALL OF WHOM HAD BEEN TESTED ON A PREVIOUS STUDY FOR ABILITY TO IDENTIFY ETHNICITY VIA PHOTOGRAPHS, WERE THEN ASKED TO SELECT "LIKE BEST" PICTURES FROM EACH SLIDE. PATTERNS OF CHOICE EMERGED, AS PHOTOGRAPHS OF SOME CHILDREN WERE PREFERRED SIGNIFICANTLY MORE THAN OTHERS, REGARDLESS OF THE ETHNICITY OF THE RESPONDENT. SINCE PATTERN OF CHOICE WAS INDEPENDENT OF ETHNICITY OF SUBJECTS, IT WAS CONCLUDED THAT ATTRACTIVENESS OF PHOTOGRAPHIC STIMULI IS NOT UNIQUELY DIFFERENT AMONG CHILDREN OF THESE ETHNICITIES. 18 REFERENCES. (AUTHOR ABSTRACT MODIFIED)

ACCN 002305

1037 AUTH **LEVINE, H. G., WILLIAMS, L. B., & BRUHN, J. G.**
TITL SIX YEARS OF EXPERIENCE WITH A SUMMER PROGRAM FOR MINORITY STUDENTS.
SRCE *JOURNAL OF MEDICAL EDUCATION, 1976, 51, 735-742.*
INDX COLLEGE STUDENTS, EDUCATION, EMPIRICAL, HEALTH EDUCATION, HIGHER EDUCATION, MEDICAL STUDENTS, MEXICAN AMERICAN, OCCUPATIONAL ASPIRATIONS, SCHOLASTIC ASPIRATIONS, REPRESENTATION, TEXAS, SOUTHWEST, PROGRAM EVALUATION
ABST THIS ARTICLE SUMMARIZES SIX YEARS OF EXPERIENCE OF THE UNIVERSITY OF TEXAS MEDICAL BRANCH AT GALVESTON (UTMB) WITH A SUMMER PROGRAM FOR THE RECRUITMENT OF MINORITY STUDENTS. DURING THE SIX YEARS, UTMB CONDUCTED SIX SUMMER EXPERIENCES FOR 112 MEXICAN AMERICAN AND BLACK PREMEDICAL STUDENTS AND MADE NUMEROUS CONTACTS WITH UNDERGRADUATE COLLEGE FACULTY AND ADMINISTRATIVE STAFF FOR THE PURPOSE OF INCREASING MINORITY STUDENT ENROLLMENT IN MEDICAL SCHOOLS IN GENERAL AND IN UTMB IN PAR-

TICULAR. THE PROGRAM, WHICH EMPHASIZED EXPERIENCES WHICH WOULD INCREASE THE POTENTIAL STUDENT'S MOTIVATIONS, INFORMATION, AND ACADEMIC SKILLS, HAS RESULTED IN NUMEROUS MINORITY STUDENTS ENTERING MEDICAL SCHOOL; BUT THE IMPACT ON UTMB ENROLLMENTS HAS BEEN DISAPPOINTING. IMPLICATIONS OF THE RESULTS OF THE PROGRAM ON FUTURE EFFORTS TO RECRUIT MINORITY STUDENTS ARE DISCUSSED. 7 REFERENCES. (AUTHOR ABSTRACT)

ACCN 002137

1038 AUTH **LEWIS, H. D.**
TITL TO TRAIN OR NOT TO TRAIN TEACHERS FOR SPANISH SPEAKING COMMUNITIES.
SRCE *VIEWPOINTS, 1973, 49(4), 15-29.*
INDX PROFESSIONAL TRAINING, TEACHERS, INSTRUCTIONAL TECHNIQUES, CURRICULUM, BILINGUAL-BICULTURAL EDUCATION, BILINGUAL-BICULTURAL PERSONNEL, ESSAY, SPANISH SURNAMED
ABST THE NEED FOR TEACHERS TRAINED TO WORK WITH SPANISH-SPEAKING COMMUNITIES IS DISCUSSED. DEFICIENCIES IN THE AMERICAN SCHOOL SYSTEM AND THE INSTITUTIONS WHICH TRAIN TEACHERS THAT RESULT IN LITTLE OR NO EDUCATION FOR THE MAJORITY OF U.S. LATINOS ARE EMPHASIZED. RECOMMENDATIONS ADDRESSING THESE PROBLEMS ARE: (1) RECRUIT AND TRAIN LATINOS TO TEACH IN BARRIO SCHOOLS TO PROVIDE MODELS FOR LATINO CHILDREN; (2) INCLUDE LATINO HISTORY, SPANISH AND METHODS OF TEACHING IN THE BARRIO SCHOOLS IN TEACHERS' CURRICULUMS AND REQUIRE A FIELD TEACHING INTERNSHIP AND SPANISH LANGUAGE EXAM BEFORE ASSIGNMENT TO LATIN STUDENTS; (3) INCLUDE POSITIVE LATINO WRITINGS IN LATINO STUDENTS' CURRICULUMS AND RECOGNIZE THE CONTRIBUTIONS OF LATIN AMERICANS IN ALL COURSES; AND (4) FAMILIARIZE TEACHERS WITH THE CULTURAL PATTERNS OF LATINO PARENTS AND TRADITIONS WHICH AFFECT THEIR CHILDRENS' EDUCATION. TEACHER TRAINING PROGRAMS SHOULD PREPARE TEACHERS TO DEAL WITH MANY CULTURES AND TO BE SENSITIVE TO ALL STUDENTS. 25 REFERENCES.

ACCN 000885

1039 AUTH **LEWIS, H. P., & LEWIS, E. R.**
TITL WRITTEN LANGUAGE PERFORMANCE OF SIXTH GRADE CHILDREN OF LOW SOCIO-ECONOMIC STATUS FROM BILINGUAL AND MONOLINGUAL BACKGROUNDS.
SRCE *JOURNAL OF EXPERIMENTAL EDUCATION, 1965, 33(3), 237-242.*
INDX BILINGUALISM, GRAMMAR, SYNTAX, SEMANTICS, READING, CHILDREN, SEX COMPARISON, SES, POVERTY, INTELLIGENCE, SPANISH SURNAMED, EMPIRICAL, CROSS CULTURAL
ABST DIFFERENCES IN WRITTEN LANGUAGE PERFORMANCE OF 114 SUBJECTS (61 BOYS, 53 GIRLS) IN A MONOLINGUAL GROUP AND 98 SUBJECTS (55 BOYS, 43 GIRLS) IN A BILINGUAL GROUP ARE PRESENTED. CHINESE BILINGUALS (CB) NUMBERED 56 (30 BOYS, 26 GIRLS),

AND THE SPANISH BILINGUALS (SB) TOTALED 42 (25 BOYS, 17 GIRLS). A SAMPLE OF EACH SUBJECT'S WRITTEN LANGUAGE WAS OBTAINED UNDER UNIFORM CONDITIONS WHERE A STIMULUS WAS PROVIDED IN THE FORM OF A SILENT FILM ENTITLED "NEIGHBORS." IMMEDIATELY THEREAFTER SUBJECTS WERE GIVEN 20 MINUTES TO WRITE A COMPOSITION ABOUT THE FILM. A COMPARISON OF WRITTEN LANGUAGE PERFORMANCE OF SUBJECTS MATCHED BY IQ AND SIMILAR SCHOLASTIC BACKGROUND REVEALED THAT FOR CB FEMALES THE INCIDENCE OF MISSPELLED WORDS WAS SIGNIFICANTLY LOWER AND THE INCIDENCE OF GRAMMATICAL ERRORS WAS SIGNIFICANTLY HIGHER THAN FOR OTHER SUBJECTS. SIGNIFICANT SEX DIFFERENCES IN WRITTEN LANGUAGE PERFORMANCE FAVORING THE GIRLS IN THE MONOLINGUAL AND CB GROUPS DISAPPEARED WHEN GROUPS WERE MATCHED BY IQ. THE RELATIONSHIP BETWEEN THE EXTENT OF BILINGUAL BACKGROUND AND THE WRITTEN LANGUAGE PERFORMANCE WAS SLIGHT IN ALL GROUPS. IT IS CONCLUDED THAT BILINGUALISM DOES NOT APPEAR TO HAVE AN ADVERSE EFFECT UPON THE WRITTEN LANGUAGE PERFORMANCE OF THE SUBJECTS.

ACCN 000886

1040 AUTH **LEWIS, O.**
TITL A DAY IN THE LIFE OF A MEXICAN PEASANT FAMILY.
SRCE *MARRIAGE AND FAMILY LIVING, 1956, 18, 3-13.*
INDX MEXICAN, POVERTY, RURAL, CASE STUDY, FAMILY ROLES, FATHER-CHILD INTERACTION, MOTHER-CHILD INTERACTION, CULTURE
ABST THIS ETHNOGRAPHIC STUDY FOCUSES ON ONE FAMILY IN A MEXICAN VILLAGE AND, BASED UPON OBSERVATION AND AUTOBIOGRAPHICAL ACCOUNTS, DESCRIBES THE FAMILY EVENTS OCCURRING DURING A SINGLE DAY. THE 5 CHILDREN RANGE FROM AGES 7 TO 20; THE FATHER IS A CONVERTED PROTESTANT AND A RECOGNIZED LEADER OF 80 TLACOLOLEROS FAMILIES WHO FARM COMMUNAL LANDS. THE FATHER AND THE YOUNGEST SON SPEND THE DAY WORKING IN THE CORNFIELDS. THE FEMALES OF THE FAMILY CONCERN THEMSELVES WITH PREPARING MEALS AND TRYING TO BORROW MONEY TO OBTAIN ENOUGH FOOD TO FEED THE FAMILY. THE OLDER SONS WORK FOR A NEARBY FARMER. OTHER CONCERNS ARE THE FUTURE OF THE OLDEST DAUGHTER LIVING NEARBY WHOSE SON WAS BORN OUT OF WEDLOCK, AND THE YOUNGEST DAUGHTER WANTING TO GET MARRIED BUT HER FATHER DOES NOT WANT THE EXPENSE OF A WEDDING AND HER MOTHER DOES NOT WANT TO LOSE HER LABOR. 3 REFERENCES.

ACCN 000888

1041 AUTH **LEWIS, O.**
TITL THE EXTENDED FAMILY IN MEXICO.
SRCE *IN W. GOODE (ED.), READINGS IN FAMILY AND*

INDX   *SOCIETY. ENGLEWOOD CLIFFS, NEW JERSEY: PRENTICE-HALL, 1964.*

INDX   FAMILY STRUCTURE, EXTENDED FAMILY, FICTIVE KINSHIP, MEXICO, CULTURE, ESSAY, MEXICAN, CASE STUDY, ECONOMIC FACTORS

ABST   AN INVESTIGATION OF EXTENDED KIN TIES IN TEPOZTLAN, A SMALL, ANCIENT TOWN NOT FAR FROM MEXICO CITY, IS PRESENTED. FOR MARRIED COUPLES, THE GRANDMOTHER, ON EITHER SIDE OF THE FAMILY, IS SEEN AS THE CLOSEST KINSHIP TIE FOR REASON OF A MOTHER SUBSTITUTE. AUNTS, UNCLES AND COUSINS HAVE SPECIAL AFFECTIONATE RELATIONSHIPS WITH THE MARRIED INDIVIDUALS AND THEIR CHILDREN, AND OFTEN DO FAVORS OR GIVE GIFTS TO EACH OTHER. BECAUSE OF PATRILOCAL RESIDENCE, THE MOTHER AND DAUGHTER-IN-LAW RELATIONSHIP IS THE MOST IMPORTANT, USUALLY REQUIRING THE HUSBAND'S WIFE TO ASSUME A DAUGHTER ROLE AND DO WORK ASSIGNMENTS FOR THE MOTHER-IN-LAW. RELATIONS BETWEEN THE FATHER AND SON-IN-LAW DEPEND MORE ON PERSONAL FACTORS (E.G., TREATMENT OF WIFE) THAN ON FORMAL OBLIGATIONS. THE "COMPADRAZGO" SYSTEM, A FORMAL RELATIONSHIP BETWEEN GODPARENTS (PADRINOS) AND GODCHILDREN (AHIJADOS), AND GODPARENTS AND PARENTS (COMPADRES), IS DISCUSSED. THOUGH THE PURPOSE OF THE SYSTEM IS TO PROVIDE SECURITY FOR THE GODCHILD, THE COMPADRE RELATIONSHIP IS VIEWED AS MORE FUNCTIONAL AND IMPORTANT. THOUGH DIFFERENT GODPARENTS ARE USUALLY CHOSEN JUST FOR THE OCCASIONS OF BAPTISM, CONFIRMATION AND MARRIAGE, THE SYSTEM HAS BEEN EXTENDED BEYOND THE ORIGINAL CATHOLIC FORM TO INCLUDE OTHER EXPERIENCES. FINALLY, SOME FAMILIES ARE SEEN AS BASING THEIR SELECTION OF GODPARENTS ON THOSE WHO CAN PROVIDE FAMILIAL AND ECONOMIC SUPPORT.

ACCN   000889

1042 AUTH **LEWIS, O.**
TITL   FAMILY DYNAMICS IN A MEXICAN VILLAGE.
SRCE   *MARRIAGE AND FAMILY LIVING, 1959, 21, 218-226.*
INDX   MEXICO, MEXICAN, FAMILY ROLES, SES, POVERTY, RURAL, CASE STUDY, FAMILY STRUCTURE, CULTURE, FATHER-CHILD INTERACTION, MOTHER-CHILD INTERACTION, PERSONALITY, CULTURAL FACTORS, ECONOMIC FACTORS
ABST   THE INTERNAL STRUCTURE, PSYCHODYNAMICS, AND PERSONALITY DEVELOPMENT OF TWO FAMILIES LIVING IN THE VILLAGE OF AZTECA LOCATED IN THE HIGHLANDS 60 MILES SOUTH OF MEXICO CITY ARE DESCRIBED AND COMPARED. ONE FAMILY IS REPRESENTATIVE OF THE POORER LANDLESS FARMERS WHILE THE OTHER IS CONSIDERED TO BE IN THE UPPER ECONOMIC GROUP OF THE VILLAGE. BOTH FAMILIES ARE STRONG, COHESIVE UNITS REFLECTING THE TRADITIONAL BONDS OF FAMILY LOYALTY AND PARENTAL AUTHORITY. BOTH HAVE COMMON ECONOMIC STRIVINGS AND MUTUAL DEPENDENCE SINCE NEITHER HAVE EXTERNAL SUPPORT SYSTEMS OTHER THAN THE IMMEDIATE FAMILY. IT IS SUGGESTED THAT BY FOCUSING ON THE WHOLE FAMILY UNIT THE RESEARCHER CAN DETECT VARIATIONS IN PERSONALITY WITHIN THE CULTURE THAT OTHERWISE WOULD BE DIFFICULT TO EXAMINE. 8 REFERENCES.

ACCN   000890

1043 AUTH **LEWIS, O.**
TITL   FROM A STUDY OF SLUM CULTURE: BACKGROUNDS FOR LA VIDA.
SRCE   *IN J. C. STONE & D. P. DENEVI (EDS.), TEACHING MULTICULTURAL POPULATIONS: FIVE HERITAGES. NEW YORK: VAN NOSTRAND, 1971, PP. 111-117.*
INDX   PUERTO RICAN-M, URBAN, POVERTY, STRESS, FAMILY STRUCTURE, ECONOMIC FACTORS, BILINGUAL, EMPLOYMENT, EDUCATION, SCHOLASTIC ACHIEVEMENT, EMPIRICAL, PUERTO RICAN-I, IMMIGRATION, CULTURAL CHANGE, NEW YORK, EAST
ABST   A SUMMARY OF THE AUTHOR'S STUDY OF PUERTO RICAN FAMILIES LIVING IN NEW YORK AND SAN JUAN SLUMS IS PRESENTED. IN GENERAL, SPENDING AND SAVING PATTERNS TENDED TO REMAIN THE SAME IN NEW YORK AS THEY HAD BEEN IN THE ISLAND'S MAIN CITY, SAN JUAN, WHERE MOST OF THE MIGRANTS HAD LIVED BEFORE MOVING TO NEW YORK. THE MIGRANTS BELIEVED THEY HAD CHANGED LITTLE SINCE LIVING IN NEW YORK; THE QUESTIONNAIRE DATA TENDED TO CORROBORATE THIS. CERTAIN TRAITS OF THE CULTURE OF POVERTY—I.E., UNSTABLE MARRIAGES, MATRIFOCALITY, FREE UNIONS AND ILLEGITIMACY—WERE EQUALLY PRESENT IN NEW YORK AND PUERTO RICO. ALTHOUGH THE NEW YORK SAMPLE OF FAMILIES HAD IMPROVED THEIR STANDARD OF LIVING (MEDIAN INCOME IN NEW YORK WAS $3,678, IN PUERTO RICO $1,703), THEIR SENSE OF MARGINALITY TO THE LARGER SOCIETY WAS GREATER THAN IN PUERTO RICO. DATA ON FAMILY STRUCTURE, TYPE OF HOUSEHOLD, EDUCATION, EMPLOYMENT AND SPENDING PATTERNS OF THE NEW YORK AND PUERTO RICAN FAMILIES ARE ALSO INCLUDED.

ACCN   000891

1044 AUTH **LEWIS, O.**
TITL   HUSBANDS AND WIVES IN A MEXICAN VILLAGE: A STUDY OF ROLE CONFLICT.
SRCE   *AMERICAN ANTHROPOLOGIST, 1949, 51, 602-610.*
INDX   MEXICO, MEXICAN, FAMILY ROLES, SES, POVERTY, SEX ROLES, CULTURAL CHANGE, CONFLICT RESOLUTION, RURAL, AUTHORITARIANISM, MARRIAGE, SOCIAL STRUCTURE, FAMILY STRUCTURE, ROLE EXPECTATIONS, EMPIRICAL
ABST   THE EXPRESSED IDEAL PATTERNS FOR HUSBAND AND WIFE RELATIONS IN TEPOZTLAN, MEXICO, ARE CONTRASTED WITH THE ACTUAL BEHAVIOR THAT OCCURS BETWEEN HUSBAND AND WIFE. ACCORDING TO THE IDEAL MODEL, THE HUSBAND IS VIEWED AS AN AUTHORITARIAN, PATRIARCHAL FIGURE HAVING THE HIGHEST STATUS IN THE FAMILY. HE IS EXPECTED TO BE OBEYED, MAKE ALL THE IMPOR-

TANT DECISIONS, AND BE RESPONSIBLE FOR SUPPORTING THE FAMILY. THE WIFE IS EXPECTED, ON THE OTHER HAND, TO BE SUBMISSIVE, FAITHFUL, RESPECTFUL TO HER HUSBAND, AND TO SEEK HIS ADVICE AND PERMISSION IN ALL BUT HER ASSIGNED MENIAL TASKS. SHE IS ALSO SUPPOSED TO BE INDUSTRIOUS AND FRUGAL. HOWEVER, IN MOST HOMES THE HUSBAND DOES NOT TOTALLY CONTROL HIS FAMILY AND MOST MARRIAGES REFLECT CONFLICT OVER THE QUESTION OF AUTHORITY AND FAMILY ROLES. IT APPEARS THE STANDARDS OF BEHAVIOR ARE INFLUENCED MORE BY THE INDIVIDUAL'S OWN NEEDS AND EXPERIENCES WHICH ARE NOT ALWAYS CONSISTENT WITH THE IDEAL ROLES. WOMEN SEEM, HOWEVER, TO BE IN MORE CONFLICT WITH TRADITIONAL WAYS THAN ARE MEN. IN CONCLUSION, THE NOTED DISCREPANCY BETWEEN THE IDEAL ROLES AND ACTUAL BEHAVIOR AFFECTED IN THIS STUDY IS CONSIDERED TO BE A RESULT OF OBSERVING ACTUAL FAMILY SITUATIONS RATHER THAN RELYING UPON INFORMANTS. 3 REFERENCES.

ACCN   000892

1045 AUTH   **LEWIS, O.**
TITL   LA VIDA: A PUERTO RICAN FAMILY IN THE CULTURE OF POVERTY—SAN JUAN AND NEW YORK.
SRCE   *NEW YORK: RANDOM HOUSE, 1966.*
INDX   POVERTY, PUERTO RICAN-I, PUERTO RICAN-M, SES, FAMILY ROLES, FAMILY STRUCTURE, SOCIALIZATION, CHILDREARING PRACTICES, MOTHER-CHILD INTERACTION, FATHER-CHILD INTERACTION, ACCULTURATION, AGGRESSION, SCHOLASTIC ACHIEVEMENT, OCCUPATIONAL ASPIRATIONS, SCHOLASTIC ASPIRATIONS, INTERPERSONAL RELATIONS, URBAN, CASE STUDY, MARRIAGE, MARITAL STABILITY, FICTIVE KINSHIP, MIGRATION, FOLK MEDICINE, BILINGUALISM, STEREOTYPES, EMPIRICAL, NEW YORK, EAST, CULTURE
ABST   THIS BOOK, FIRST IN A SERIES OF VOLUMES BASED ON THE STUDY OF ONE HUNDRED PUERTO RICAN FAMILIES FROM FOUR SLUMS OF GREATER SAN JUAN AND OF THEIR RELATIVES IN NEW YORK CITY, DESCRIBES THE RIOS FAMILY. THE FAMILY, COMPRISED OF FIVE HOUSEHOLDS, 3 IN THE URBAN SLUMS OF SAN JUAN AND 2 IN THE BARRIOS OF NEW YORK, WERE EXTENSIVELY INTERVIEWED AND CLOSELY OBSERVED, AS WERE SEVERAL OTHER EXTENDED FAMILY MEMBERS. IN ALL, 16 PUERTO RICANS, RANGING IN AGES FROM 7 TO 64 YEARS AND REPRESENTING FOUR GENERATIONS, TELL THEIR LIFE STORIES. THESE CASE HISTORIES AND THE DETAILED OBSERVATIONS OF TYPICAL DAYS IN THE LIVES OF SEVERAL FAMILY MEMBERS ARE INTERPRETED WITHIN THE MAJOR OBJECTIVES OF THE OVERALL STUDY: (1) TO DEVELOP A COMPARATIVE LITERATURE ON INTENSIVE FAMILY CASE STUDIES; (2) TO DEVISE NEW FIELD METHODS AND NEW WAYS OF ORGANIZING AND PRESENTING FAMILY DATA; AND (3) TO TEST AND REFINE THE CONCEPT OF CULTURE OF POVERTY BY A COMPARISON OF MEXICAN AND PUERTO RICAN DATA.

ACCN   000893

1046 AUTH   **LEWIS, T. H.**
TITL   THERAPEUTIC TECHNIQUES OF HUICHOLE CURANDEROS WITH A CASE REPORT OF CROSS CULTURAL PSYCHOTHERAPY (MEXICO).
SRCE   *ANTHROPOS, 1977, 72(5/6), 709-716.*
INDX   CASE STUDY, FOLK MEDICINE, MEXICAN, CURANDERISMO, INDIGENOUS POPULATIONS, MEXICO, HEALTH, RURAL, ANXIETY
ABST   DURING 1956-1957, OBSERVATIONS WERE MADE OF THE HUICHOLE INDIANS—A CONSERVATIVE, ISOLATED TRIBE WHO LIVE IN AN ALMOST INACCESSIBLE PART OF RURAL MEXICO. AN ANKLE INJURY SUSTAINED BY ONE OF THE MEMBERS OF A RESEARCH TEAM WAS TREATED BY A LOCAL CURANDERO AND THIS CASE IS REPORTED FROM INTAKE TO CONVALESCENCE. IMPRESSIONS OF FOUR OBSERVERS OF THE TREATMENT, INCLUDING THE PATIENT, ARE PRESENTED BRIEFLY. AN EXAMPLE OF A REFERRAL, DESCRIPTION OF OTHER CURERS, PHOTOGRAPHS, AND A RURAL COMMENTARY ON THE NATURE OF ANXIETY ARE INCLUDED. 10 REFERENCES.

ACCN   002590

1047 AUTH   **LEYVA, R.**
TITL   EDUCATIONAL ASPIRATIONS AND EXPECTATIONS OF CHICANOS, NON-CHICANOS AND ANGLO-AMERICANS.
SRCE   *CALIFORNIA JOURNAL OF EDUCATIONAL RESEARCH, 1975, 26(1), 27-39.*
INDX   SCHOLASTIC ACHIEVEMENT, ACHIEVEMENT MOTIVATION, MEXICAN AMERICAN, CROSS CULTURAL, ETHNIC IDENTITY, ADOLESCENTS, CHICANO MOVEMENT, EMPIRICAL, COLLEGE STUDENTS, SCHOLASTIC ASPIRATIONS, CALIFORNIA, SOUTHWEST
ABST   BASED ON THE HYPOTHESIS THAT MEXICAN AMERICANS (MA) WHO IDENTIFY WITH THE IDEOLOGY OF CHICANISMO HAVE HIGHER EDUCATIONAL ASPIRATIONS AND EXPECTATIONS THAN COMPARABLE GROUPS OF ANGLOS AND NON-CHICANO MA'S, 39 CHICANO, 42 ANGLO, AND 49 NON-CHICANO EAST LOS ANGELES HIGH SCHOOL AND COLLEGE STUDENTS WERE SURVEYED. THE MA SAMPLE WAS DIFFERENTIATED ACCORDING TO DEGREE OF IDENTIFICATION WITH CHICANISMO, CONCEPTUALIZED ALONG DIMENSIONS OF CURRENT ACTIVISM, WILLINGNESS TO BECOME ACTIVELY INVOLVED, AND SELF VERSUS COLLECTIVE BETTERMENT. SIGNIFICANT DIFFERENCES WERE FOUND IN EACH OF THE THREE LEVELS OF DATA ANALYSIS. FIRST, CONSIDERING THE SUBJECTS AS A WHOLE, THE HYPOTHESIS DID RECEIVE SUPPORT: THE CHICANOS HAD HIGHER COLLEGE ASPIRATIONS AND EXPECTATIONS THAN ANGLOS AND NON-CHICANOS. SECOND, CONTROLLING FOR AGE, IT WAS FOUND THAT AMONG THOSE UNDER AGE 23 THE CHICANOS HAD HIGHER ASPIRATIONS AND EXPECTATIONS; HOWEVER, AMONG THOSE OVER AGE 23, AGE APPEARED TO HAVE ONLY A SLIGHT EFFECT. THIRD, CONTROLLING FOR EDUCATION, THE HYPOTHESIS WAS SUPPORTED BY THOSE WITH ONLY HIGH SCHOOL

EDUCATION BUT NOT BY THOSE WITH SOME COLLEGE EDUCATION. AMONG THOSE WHO HAD AT LEAST SOME COLLEGE, THE NON-CHICANOS HAD THE HIGHEST COLLEGE EXPECTATIONS AND POST-COLLEGE ASPIRATIONS. STILL, FOR THOSE WHO ONLY HAD A HIGH SCHOOL EDUCATION, CHICANISMO SEEMS TO PLAY A SIGNIFICANT ROLE IN COLLEGE ASPIRATIONS BY PROVIDING A FERTILE MEDIUM FOR AN EXPRESSION OF UPWARD MOBILITY. IT IS CONCLUDED THAT BEFORE THESE FINDINGS CAN BE GENERALIZED, FURTHER RESEARCH MUST BE CONDUCTED AMONG OTHER MA POPULATIONS THROUGHOUT THE U.S. 22 REFERENCES.

ACCN   000895

1048 AUTH   **LIEBLER, R.**
TITL   READING INTERESTS OF BLACK AND PUERTO RICAN, INNER CITY, HIGH SCHOOL STUDENTS.
SRCE   *GRADUATE RESEARCH IN EDUCATION AND RELATED DISCIPLINES, 1973, 6(2), 23-43.*
INDX   READING, ADOLESCENTS, PUERTO RICAN-M, SEX COMPARISON, URBAN, EDUCATION, CROSS CULTURAL, EMPIRICAL, NEW YORK, EAST
ABST   READING INTERESTS OF 74 BLACK (B) AND 96 PUERTO RICAN (PR) INNER CITY HIGH SCHOOL STUDENTS IN NEW YORK CITY WERE INVESTIGATED TO DETERMINE DIFFERENCES IN READING PREFERENCES BY SEX AND BY ETHNIC GROUPS AS WELL AS THE SIMILARITIES WITHIN THE TOTAL SAMPLE. A READING QUESTIONNAIRE WAS ADMINISTERED TO 14 CLASSES OF ELEVENTH AND TWELFTH GRADE ACADEMIC AND COLLEGE BOUND STUDENTS. ALL OF THESE STUDENTS HAD SCORED AT LEAST AT THE EIGHTH GRADE READING LEVEL ON THE METROPOLITAN ACHIEVEMENT ADVANCED READING TEST. THE QUESTIONNAIRE ASKED STUDENTS TO INDICATE WHICH ELEVEN AREAS THEY ENJOYED READING ABOUT AND WHICH 3 BOOKS "WERE MOST IMPORTANT TO YOU" AND WHY. FINDINGS REVEALED THAT A MAJORITY OF MALE PR STUDENTS WERE INTERESTED IN: (1) DETECTIVE AND MYSTERY; (2) ADVENTURE, WAR, AND SEA; (3) HUMOR; AND (4) SPORTS. A MAJORITY OF FEMALE PR STUDENTS PREFERRED: (1) LOVE AND ROMANCE; AND (2) HUMOR. EXCEPT FOR HUMOROUS BOOKS, MALE AND FEMALE PR STUDENTS DIFFERED IN THEIR READING PREFERENCE. FEMALE B STUDENTS DEMONSTRATED INTEREST IN ROMANCE, LOVE, HUMOR AND BIOGRAPHY; HOWEVER, MALE B STUDENTS WERE UNPREDICTABLE IN THEIR RESPONSES EXCEPT IN THEIR PREFERENCE FOR READING BIOGRAPHIES. GENERALLY PR READING INTERESTS WERE BASED MORE ON PERSONAL MATTERS WHILE B READING INTERESTS FOCUSED ON POLITICAL AND SOCIAL MATTERS. BOTH PR AND B STUDENTS CONSIDERED THE MOST IMPORTANT BOOKS TO BE RECENT AMERICAN PUBLICATIONS, BIOGRAPHICAL WITH PR OR B CHARACTERS. FINDINGS ALSO REVEALED THAT CERTAIN GROUPS OF INDIVIDUALS HAVE SIMILAR INTERESTS AND THAT DIFFERENCES ARE ATTRIBUTED MORE TO SEX RATHER THAN ETH-

NICITY. 14 REFERENCES. (AUTHOR ABSTRACT MODIFIED)
ACCN   000896

1049 AUTH   **LINDHOLM, B. W., & TOULIATOS, J.**
TITL   COMPARISON OF CHILDREN IN REGULAR AND SPECIAL EDUCATION CLASSES ON THE BEHAVIOR PROBLEM CHECKLIST.
SRCE   *PSYCHOLOGICAL REPORTS, 1976, 3(8), 451-458.*
INDX   CHILDREN, EARLY CHILDHOOD EDUCATION, CLASSROOM BEHAVIOR, TEST VALIDITY, EMPIRICAL, SPECIAL EDUCATION, TEXAS, SOUTHWEST, DEVIANCE
ABST   TO ESTABLISH THE VALIDITY OF THE BEHAVIOR PROBLEM CHECKLIST, USING THE METHOD OF CONTRASTED GROUPS, 1,999 ANGLO AND 192 MEXICAN AMERICAN CHILDREN IN REGULAR CLASSES (KINDERGARTEN TO 5TH GRADE) AND 192 ANGLO AND 17 MEXICAN AMERICAN CHILDREN IN SPECIAL EDUCATION CLASSES (KINDERGARTEN TO 5TH GRADE) ARE TESTED. TEACHERS PROVIDED GENERAL INFORMATION AND CHECKLIST RATINGS. MULTIPLE CORRELATIONS AND MULTIPLE REGRESSION ANALYSES OF VARIANCE WERE USED. CHILDREN IN REGULAR CLASSES HAD FEWER PROBLEMS ON ALL FOUR OF THE CHECKLIST FACTORS (CONDUCT DISORDER, PERSONALITY DISORDER, INADEQUACY-IMMATURITY AND SOCIALIZED DELINQUENCY) THAN THE CHILDREN IN SPECIAL EDUCATION CLASSES. ON THE BASIS OF THESE RESULTS AND A REVIEW OF PREVIOUS RESEARCH USING THE CONTRASTED GROUPS METHOD, IT IS CONCLUDED THAT ALL FOUR OF THE CHECKLIST FACTORS ARE VALID. 11 REFERENCES. (JOURNAL SUMMARY MODIFIED)
ACCN   000897

1050 AUTH   **LINDHOLM, K. J., PADILLA, A. M., & ROMERO, A.**
TITL   COMPREHENSION OF RELATIONAL CONCEPTS: USE OF BILINGUAL CHILDREN TO SEPARATE COGNITIVE AND LINGUISTIC FACTORS.
SRCE   *HISPANIC JOURNAL OF BEHAVIORAL SCIENCES, 1979, 1(4), 327-343.*
INDX   CHILDREN, LANGUAGE COMPREHENSION, LANGUAGE ACQUISITION, BILINGUAL, COGNITIVE DEVELOPMENT, LINGUISTICS, LEARNING, EMPIRICAL, MEXICAN AMERICAN, URBAN, CALIFORNIA, SOUTHWEST, RESEARCH METHODOLOGY
ABST   SPANISH/ENGLISH BILINGUAL CHILDREN'S COMPREHENSION OF 26 RELATIONAL CONCEPTS IN THEIR TWO LANGUAGES WAS STUDIED TO SEPARATE SOME COGNITIVE AND LINGUISTIC FACTORS IN RELATIONAL CONCEPT ACQUISITION. SUBJECTS WERE 120 MEXICAN AMERICAN CHILDREN (60 MALES, 60 FEMALES) IN LOS ANGELES PUBLIC SCHOOLS; THEY WERE EVENLY DIVIDED BETWEEN PRESCHOOL, KINDERGARTEN, AND FIRST GRADE, AND HALF WERE SPANISH-DOMINANT SPEAKERS WHILE HALF WERE ENGLISH-DOMINANT. A MONOLINGUAL-ENGLISH COMPARISON GROUP OF 24 ANGLO KINDERGARTENERS AND FIRST GRAD-

ERS (12 MALES, 12 FEMALES) WAS ALSO STUDIED. TESTING MATERIALS WERE 10 STIMULUS CARDS ILLUSTRATING 13 ANTONYM PAIRS—E.G., TALL/SHORT, WIDE/NARROW. THE MEXICAN AMERICAN CHILDREN WERE TESTED TWICE, ONCE IN SPANISH AND ONCE IN ENGLISH; THE ANGLOS WERE TESTED ONCE IN ENGLISH. THE RESULTS REVEALED THE FOLLOWING OPERATING PRINCIPLES: (1) THE ORDER IN WHICH CONCEPTS ARE ACQUIRED PROGRESSES FROM THE GENERAL TO THE SPECIFIC, FROM THOSE CONCEPTS WITH POSITIVE POLARITY TO THOSE WITH NEGATIVE POLARITY, AND FROM THOSE WHICH ARE MORPHOLOGICALLY RELATED TO THOSE WHICH ARE LEXICALLY DISTINCT; (2) TERMS ARE ACQUIRED IN IDENTICAL ORDER IN THE TWO LANGUAGES WHEN COGNITIVE COMPLEXITY IS EQUIVALENT; AND (3) WHEN TWO CONCEPTS HAVE EQUIVALENT COGNITIVE COMPLEXITY, THE TERM WITH A HIGHER FREQUENCY OF USAGE WILL BE ACQUIRED BEFORE THE ONE WITH A LOWER USAGE FREQUENCY. IT IS CONCLUDED THAT A METHODOLOGY WHICH TAKES ADVANTAGE OF THE TWO LINGUISTIC SYSTEMS OF BILINGUAL CHILDREN PROVIDES MORE INFORMATION ON THE SEPARATION OF COGNITIVE AND LINGUISTIC FACTORS UNDERLYING LANGUAGE ACQUISITION. 19 REFERENCES. (AUTHOR ABSTRACT MODIFIED)

ACCN 001794

1051 AUTH **LINDHOLM, K. J., & PADILLA, A. M.**
TITL CHILD BILINGUALISM: REPORT ON LANGUAGE MIXING, SWITCHING AND TRANSLATIONS.
SRCE *LINGUISTICS, 1978, 211, 23-44.*
INDX CHILDREN, MEXICAN AMERICAN, EMPIRICAL, BILINGUAL, BILINGUALISM, LANGUAGE ACQUISITION, LINGUISTIC COMPETENCE, CALIFORNIA, SOUTHWEST
ABST TO DETERMINE IF BILINGUAL CHILDREN ARE ABLE TO DISTINGUISH BETWEEN THEIR TWO LANGUAGE SYSTEMS, SPONTANEOUS LANGUAGE SAMPLES WERE OBTAINED FROM 18 SPANISH-ENGLISH BILINGUAL CHILDREN IN LOS ANGELES. SUBJECTS WERE U.S.-BORN, SECOND-GENERATION MEXICAN AMERICANS, AGES 2 TO 6. TEN OF THE CHILDREN HAD LEARNED SPANISH AND ENGLISH SIMULTANEOUSLY AT HOME, WHILE EIGHT ONLY LEARNED ENGLISH UPON ENTERING SCHOOL. THE DATA-GATHERING PROCESS CONSISTED OF EACH CHILD INTERACTING WITH A PAIR OF FEMALE EXPERIMENTS. ONE EXPERIMENTER ONLY SPOKE SPANISH, THE OTHER ONLY ENGLISH, AND THE CHILD SERVED AS A "MEDIATOR" BETWEEN THE TWO. EACH CHILD'S SPEECH WAS TAPE RECORDED IN THE HOME, AND THE TRANSCRIPTIONS WERE ANALYZED FOR THE INCIDENCE OF TYPES OF LINGUISTIC INTERACTION. OF THE 17,864 UTTERANCES RECORDED, ONLY 538 (3%) COULD BE CLASSIFIED AS MIXED UTTERANCES—WITH THE MAJORITY OCCURRING AS ENGLISH WORDS (MOSTLY NAMES OF ANIMALS) INSERTED INTO SPANISH ENVIRONMENTS. PHRASAL MIXES OCCURRED FAR LESS FREQUENTLY AND APPEARED TO HAVE BEEN ORIGINALLY INTENDED

AS LEXICAL MIXES. LANGUAGE SWITCHING WAS OBSERVED IN ONLY A FEW CHILDREN AND ACCOUNTED FOR 1% OF THE TOTAL SPEECH SAMPLES. SEVERAL BEHAVIORAL, ENVIRONMENTAL, AND LINGUISTIC REASONS ARE POSITED FOR THE CHILDREN'S OCCASIONAL MIXING AND SWITCHING—MOST OF WHICH POINT TO EVIDENCE OF SELECTIVE AND DELIBERATE DISCRIMINATIONS BY THE CHILDREN. IT IS THEREFORE CONCLUDED THAT, FROM AN EARLY AGE, BILINGUAL CHILDREN ARE ABLE TO DISTINGUISH BETWEEN THEIR TWO LANGUAGE SYSTEMS. 19 REFERENCES.

ACCN 001742

1052 AUTH **LINDHOLM, K. J., & PADILLA, A. M.**
TITL LANGUAGE MIXING IN BILINGUAL CHILDREN.
SRCE *JOURNAL OF CHILD LANGUAGE, 1977, 5, 327-335.*
INDX BILINGUALISM, EMPIRICAL, CHILDREN, MEXICAN AMERICAN, LINGUISTIC COMPETENCE, LANGUAGE ACQUISITION, BILINGUAL, CALIFORNIA, SOUTHWEST
ABST LANGUAGE SAMPLES OF FIVE SPANISH/ENGLISH BILINGUAL CHILDREN WERE EXAMINED FOR THE PREVALENCE OF LANGUAGE MIXES. THE CHILDREN (3 BOYS, 2 GIRLS) WERE BETWEEN THE AGES OF 2;6 AND 6;2 AND THEY ALL WERE U.S.-BORN, SECOND-GENERATION MEXICAN AMERICANS. LANGUAGE SAMPLES WERE OBTAINED BY A PAIR OF FEMALE EXPERIMENTERS; ONE SPOKE ONLY SPANISH, THE OTHER ONLY ENGLISH, WHILE THE CHILD DURING THE EXPERIMENTAL SETTING FUNCTIONED AS AN "INTERPRETER" BETWEEN THE TWO. THE CHILDREN'S SPONTANEOUS SPEECH WAS TAPE RECORDED IN THEIR HOME SETTING AND LATER TRANSCRIBED. A TOTAL OF 5,177 SEPARATE LANGUAGE UTTERANCES WERE PRODUCED BY THE CHILDREN, AND OF THESE ONLY 2% WERE FOUND TO CONTAIN MIXES. THE MOST COMMON TYPE OF MIX INVOLVED THE INSERTION OF SINGLE LEXICAL ENTRIES—MOSTLY ENGLISH NOUNS INTO SPANISH SENTENCES. VERY FEW PHRASAL MIXES WERE OBSERVED. IT IS CONCLUDED THAT LANGUAGE MIXES DO NOT CONSTITUTE A MAJOR INTERFERENCE IN THE ACQUISITION OF BILINGUALISM SINCE CHILDREN APPEAR CAPABLE OF DIFFERENTIATING BETWEEN THEIR TWO LANGUAGE SYSTEMS FROM AN EARLY AGE. 7 REFERENCES. (AUTHOR ABSTRACT MODIFIED)

ACCN 001741

1053 AUTH **LINN, G. B.**
TITL LINGUISTIC FUNCTIONS OF BILINGUAL MEXICAN-AMERICAN CHILDREN.
SRCE *JOURNAL OF GENETIC PSYCHOLOGY, 1967, 3(2), 183-193.*
INDX BILINGUALISM, LINGUISTICS, SES, SEX COMPARISON, READING, PHONOLOGY, SYNTAX, LINGUISTIC COMPETENCE, EMPIRICAL, MEXICAN AMERICAN, CROSS CULTURAL, READING
ABST MONOLINGUAL ENGLISH-SPEAKING ANGLO AMERICAN AND MEXICAN AMERICAN CHILDREN WERE COMPARED WITH SPANISH-ENGLISH BILINGUAL MEXICAN AMERICANS ON CERTAIN LINGUISTIC FUNCTIONS. THE GROUPS

WERE SEVENTH AND EIGHTH GRADE STUDENTS MATCHED IN NONLANGUAGE IQ, CHRONOLOGICAL AGE, GRADE, SEX, AND SOCIOECONOMIC STATUS. VARIOUS MEASURES WERE USED TO OBTAIN DATA REGARDING THE LINGUISTIC FUNCTIONING OF THE SUBJECTS. FINDINGS INDICATE THAT THERE WERE NO SIGNIFICANT DIFFERENCES BETWEEN THE GROUPS IN SILENT READING VOCABULARY, TOTAL SILENT READING, SPELLING, OR PHONETIC DISCRIMINATION. THERE WERE SIGNIFICANT DIFFERENCES IN FAVOR OF THE MONOLINGUAL SUBJECTS, BOTH MEXICAN AMERICAN AND ANGLO AMERICAN, IN SILENT READING COMPREHENSION, ORAL READING ACCURACY AND COMPREHENSION, INFLECTION, AND GENERAL LANGUAGE DEVELOPMENT. THE MONOLINGUAL SUBJECTS MADE FEWER ERRORS IN CONSONANT ARTICULATION. IN THE ACOUSTIC MEASUREMENTS OF CERTAIN VOWELS, THE BILINGUAL MEXICAN AMERICAN SUBJECTS DIFFERED SIGNIFICANTLY FROM THE OTHER GROUPS. THE MONOLINGUAL MEXICAN AMERICANS DIFFERED FROM OTHER GROUPS IN THE MEASUREMENT OF CERTAIN VOWELS. EDUCATIONAL AND RESEARCH IMPLICATIONS OF THE FINDINGS ARE PROVIDED. 12 REFERENCES.

ACCN   000900

1054 AUTH   **LINN, G. B.**
TITL   A STUDY OF SEVERAL LINGUISTIC FUNCTIONS OF MEXICAN-AMERICAN CHILDREN IN A TWO LANGUAGE ENVIRONMENT.
SRCE   *SAN FRANCISCO: R AND E RESEARCH ASSOCIATES, PUBLISHERS AND DISTRIBUTORS OF ETHNIC STUDIES, 1971. (REPRINTED FROM UNIVERSITY OF SOUTHERN CALIFORNIA, JUNE 1965.)*
INDX   EMPIRICAL, LINGUISTICS, MEXICAN AMERICAN, CHILDREN, BILINGUALISM, INTELLIGENCE TESTING, ACHIEVEMENT TESTING, CROSS CULTURAL, LANGUAGE ASSESSMENT, LANGUAGE COMPREHENSION, LINGUISTIC COMPETENCE, CALIFORNIA, SOUTHWEST, CALIFORNIA TEST OF MENTAL MATURITY, CALIFORNIA ACHIEVEMENT TESTS
ABST   AN EX-POST FACTO ANALYSIS TO ASSESS LINGUISTIC COMPONENTS AND THEIR VARIATIONS WAS CONDUCTED AMONG 7TH AND 8TH GRADE STUDENTS RESIDING IN SOUTHERN CALIFORNIA. THE STUDENTS REPRESENTED 3 GROUPS: (1) MEXICAN AMERICANS WHO SPOKE BOTH ENGLISH AND SPANISH WHEN THEY FIRST STARTED SCHOOL; (2) MEXICAN AMERICANS WHO SPOKE ONLY ENGLISH UPON ENTERING SCHOOL; AND (3) ANGLOS WHO SPOKE ONLY ENGLISH AT THE TIME THEY ENTERED SCHOOL. SCHOOL RECORDS WERE USED TO OBTAIN SCORES FROM VARIOUS TESTS MEASURING LANGUAGE ASSESSMENT, SUCH AS THE CALIFORNIA ACHIEVEMENT TEST, THE GRAY ORAL READING TEST, AND THE WEPMAN AUDITORY DISCRIMINATION TEST. NONLANGUAGE IQ WAS MEASURED FROM SCORES ON THE CALIFORNIA TEST OF MENTAL MATURITY. THE THREE GROUPS WERE APPROXIMATELY MATCHED ACCORDING TO SEX, AGE, GRADE,

AND SOCIOECONOMIC STATUS. THE RESULTS WERE AS FOLLOWS: (1) CHILDREN TAUGHT ONLY ENGLISH BEFORE ENTERING SCHOOL HAD HIGHER SCORES IN OVERALL READING COMPREHENSION, MECHANICS, AND GENERAL LANGUAGE DEVELOPMENT; (2) CHILDREN TAUGHT BOTH ENGLISH AND SPANISH BEFORE ENTERING KINDERGARTEN HAD DEFECTIVE ARTICULATION AND DIFFERENT INFLECTION THAN ENGLISH-ONLY SPEAKING CHILDREN; AND (3) THERE WERE DIFFERENCES IN A FEW ENGLISH VOWELS BETWEEN THE TWO GROUPS OF MEXICAN AMERICAN CHILDREN. SEVERAL RECOMMENDATIONS ARE SUGGESTED: (1) ALERTING SCHOOL PERSONNEL TO SPECIAL LANGUAGE PROBLEMS OF MEXICAN AMERICANS; (2) ESTABLISHING SPECIAL PROGRAMS FOR CHILDREN MANIFESTING A LANGUAGE HANDICAP; (3) IMPLEMENTING EARLY LANGUAGE CORRECTION; AND (4) TELLING MEXICAN AMERICAN PARENTS NOT TO TEACH THEIR CHILDREN SPANISH UNTIL THEY HAVE COMPLETED THE EARLY ELEMENTARY GRADES. 44 REFERENCES.

ACCN   000901

1055 AUTH   **LINN, L. S., & LAWRENCE, G. D.**
TITL   REQUESTS MADE IN COMMUNITY PHARMACIES.
SRCE   *AMERICAN JOURNAL OF PUBLIC HEALTH, 1978, 68(5), 492-493.*
INDX   CROSS CULTURAL, CULTURAL FACTORS, DYADIC INTERACTION, EMPIRICAL, HEALTH, HEALTH DELIVERY SYSTEMS, HEALTH EDUCATION, MEXICAN AMERICAN, PARAPROFESSIONALS, RESOURCE UTILIZATION, SEX COMPARISON, CALIFORNIA, SOUTHWEST, URBAN
ABST   AT 129 PHARMACIES IN LOS ANGELES, 2,580 PHARMACIST-CLIENT INTERACTIONS WERE OBSERVED (1) TO IDENTIFY AND DESCRIBE THE CONTENT OF QUESTIONS ASKED BY PHARMACY PATRONS, AND (2) TO EXPLORE WHETHER THE TYPES OF QUESTIONS ASKED WERE RELATED TO OBSERVABLE CHARACTERISTICS OF PATRONS. ALTHOUGH THE PHARMACIES WERE NOT RANDOMLY SELECTED, DIFFERENT TYPES OF PHARMACIES WERE WELL REPRESENTED IN THE SAMPLE. THREE CHARACTERISTICS OF THE PHARMACY PATRON WERE OBSERVED: SEX, RACE, AND LANGUAGE (ENGLISH, BROKEN ENGLISH, OR FOREIGN). THE 2,580 PATRON REQUESTS WERE CLASSIFIED BY CONTENT INTO ONE OF 25 CATEGORIES; AND OF THESE, REQUESTS FOR INFORMATION WERE CATEGORIZED AS PROFESSIONAL QUESTIONS (17%), PROFESSIONAL-CLERICAL QUESTIONS (62%), AND CLERICAL QUESTIONS (21%). A SIGNIFICANT RELATIONSHIP WAS FOUND BETWEEN RACE, ABILITY TO SPEAK ENGLISH, AND TYPE OF REQUEST. ASIANS, SPANISH, AND NON-WHITES WERE MORE LIKELY THAN BLACKS AND CAUCASIANS TO ASK FOR PROFESSIONAL ADVISE. IT WAS ALSO FOUND THAT PATRONS SPEAKING BROKEN ENGLISH OR FOREIGN LANGUAGES WERE MORE LIKELY TO ASK FOR PROFESSIONAL ADVISE. IN CONCLUSION, IT IS HYPOTHESIZED THAT ASIAN AND SPANISH MINORITY CLIENTS' RELIANCE

ON THE PHARMACY AS A PLACE FOR SEEKING ADVISE REFLECTS THEIR CULTURAL BACKGROUNDS SINCE THE ROLE OF THE PHARMACIST IN THESE CULTURES HAS TRADITIONALLY BEEN MORE ACTIVE WITH REGARDS TO ADVISE AND PROBLEM SOLVING. 5 REFERENCES.

ACCN   002138

1056 AUTH   **LINN, M. W., GUREL, L., CARMICHAEL, J., & WEED, P.**

TITL   CULTURAL COMPARISONS OF MOTHERS WITH LARGE AND SMALL FAMILIES.

SRCE   *JOURNAL OF BIOSOCIOLOGICAL SCIENCE, 1976, 8, 293-302.*

INDX   ADULTS, BIRTH CONTROL, CHILDREN, CROSS CULTURAL, CUBAN, ATTITUDES, EMPIRICAL, FAMILY STRUCTURE, FEMALE, FERTILITY, MEXICAN AMERICAN, RELIGION, SES, FLORIDA, SOUTH

ABST   CONTRACEPTIVE KNOWLEDGE AND BEHAVIOUR OF MOTHERS OF LARGE (FIVE OR MORE CHILDREN) AND SMALL (LESS THAN THREE CHILDREN) FAMILIES IN FOUR SUBCULTURES WERE COMPARED WITH WHITE PROTESTANTS. THE SAMPLE COMPRISED 449 ANGLO, BLACK, CUBAN, CHICANO, AND INDIAN MOTHERS, AGES 35 TO 45. WITH SOCIAL CLASS, KNOWLEDGE OF BIRTH CONTROL, AND DEGREE OF RELIGIOSITY HELD CONSTANT, THE BEST PREDICTORS OF FAMILY SIZE WERE THE MOTHER'S DESIRED FAMILY SIZE (EXPRESSED AS DESIRED MINUS ACTUAL CHILDREN), AGE AT CHILDBIRTH, AND AGE AT MARRIAGE. DATA SUGGEST THAT FAMILY SIZE IS NOT PURELY A FUNCTION OF BIRTH CONTROL KNOWLEDGE BUT RELATED TO EARLY MARRIAGE AND PREGNANCY AND IN KEEPING WITH ATTITUDES ABOUT AN IDEAL FAMILY SIZE. IN GENERAL, FACTORS RELATED TO SIZE WERE STRONGER IN THE WHITE GROUP THAN IN THE SUBCULTURES, AND IN A FEW INSTANCES CERTAIN CULTURES WERE NOT CONSISTENT WITH OTHERS IN OVERALL TRENDS. 20 REFERENCES. (AUTHOR SUMMARY)

ACCN   002139

1057 AUTH   **LIPTON, J. P., & GARZA, R. T.**

TITL   RESPONSIBILITY ATTRIBUTION AMONG MEXICAN-AMERICAN, BLACK, AND ANGLO ADOLESCENTS AND ADULTS.

SRCE   *JOURNAL OF CROSS-CULTURAL PSYCHOLOGY, 1977, 8(3), 259-272.*

INDX   ADOLESCENTS, ATTRIBUTION OF RESPONSIBILITY, ATTRIBUTION THEORY, CROSS CULTURAL, CULTURAL FACTORS, EMPIRICAL, ENVIRONMENTAL FACTORS, FATALISM, LOCUS OF CONTROL, MALE, FEMALE, MEXICAN AMERICAN, COLLEGE STUDENTS, REVIEW, SPANISH SURNAMED, CALIFORNIA, TEXAS, SOUTHWEST, ADULTS, ATTITUDES

ABST   ALTHOUGH THE LITERATURE DEALING WITH ATTRIBUTION OF RESPONSIBILITY (AR) IS EXTENSIVE, CROSS-CULTURAL PERSPECTIVES HAVE NOT BEEN FULLY EXPLORED. THIS STUDY INVESTIGATES AR IN A RIGOROUS FACTORIAL DESIGN INVOLVING 343 SUBJECTS—132 MEXICAN AMERICANS, 96 BLACKS, 115 ANGLOS; 146 MALES, 197 FEMALES; 166 ADULTS, 177

ADOLESCENTS. THE ADULTS WERE UNDERGRADUATES AT A CALIFORNIA AND A TEXAS UNIVERSITY; THE ADOLESCENTS WERE CALIFORNIA JUNIOR HIGH SCHOOL STUDENTS. THE INSTRUMENT WAS A 12-ITEM VERSION OF THE AR QUESTIONNAIRE DESCRIBING THE BEHAVIOR OF A FICTIONAL STIMULUS PERSON NAMED "PERRY." SUBJECTS RECORDED THEIR RESPONSES ON A 5-POINT SCALE, INDICATING THE DEGREE OF RESPONSIBILITY ATTRIBUTED TO THE STIMULUS PERSON RANGING FROM "NOT AT ALL RESPONSIBLE" TO "COMPLETELY RESPONSIBLE." OVERALL, THE CULTURAL FACTOR WAS HIGHLY SIGNIFICANT BOTH AS A MAIN EFFECT AND IN INTERACTION WITH OTHER COMBINATIONS OF VARIABLES. IT IS CONCLUDED THAT "CLASSIC" THEORIES OF AR DO NOT ALWAYS HAVE UNIVERSAL APPLICABILITY, AND IN FACT MAY ONLY BE VALID AMONG ANGLOS. EXPLANATIONS FOR THESE STRONG FINDINGS ARE SUGGESTED IN TERMS OF DIFFERENT FAMILY STRUCTURES AND INTERNALIZED ATTITUDES AMONG MINORITY GROUPS—PARTICULARLY MEXICAN AMERICANS—AS WELL AS THEIR "SUBORDINATE" STATUS WITHIN THE UNITED STATES. 29 REFERENCES.

ACCN   002140

1058 AUTH   **LIPTON, J. P., & GARZA, R. T.**

TITL   A SOCIOCULTURAL ANALYSIS OF VOLUNTEER WORK AMONG CHICANO AND ANGLO COLLEGE STUDENTS.

SRCE   *JOURNAL OF COLLEGE STUDENT PERSONNEL, 1978, 19(3), 268-274.*

INDX   ATTITUDES, COLLEGE STUDENTS, CROSS CULTURAL, CULTURAL FACTORS, EMPIRICAL, FEMALE, MALE, SOUTHWEST, MEXICAN AMERICAN, SES, SEX COMPARISON, CALIFORNIA, ALTRUISM, COMMUNITY INVOLVEMENT

ABST   THIS STUDY ASKS: WHAT PROMPTS CHICANO AND ANGLO UNIVERSITY STUDENTS TO PERFORM VOLUNTEER WORK? DO MOTIVATIONS AND ANTECEDENTS DIFFER? A TOTAL OF 147 LOS ANGELES COLLEGE STUDENTS—ALL WHO VOLUNTEER IN HELPING AGENCIES—WERE THE SUBJECTS. VIA A PERSONAL INFORMATION PRE-TEST, INFORMATION WAS TRANSFORMED INTO PREDICTOR VARIABLES, INCLUDING POLITICAL IDEOLOGY, DRUG USE, HOUSING, MARITAL STATUS, FAMILY INCOME, SEX, AND NUMBER OF SIBLINGS. CRITERION VARIABLES WERE: (1) HOURS A MONTH DEDICATED TO VOLUNTEERING, AND (2) THE ALTRUISM-SELFISHNESS INDEX (ASI). MULTIPLE REGRESSION ANALYSES OF ASI FINDINGS AND PREDICTOR AND CRITERION VARIABLES REVEALED THAT FOR ANGLOS, NUMBER OF CHILDREN, NUMBER OF SIBLINGS, AND FAMILY INCOME PROVED SIGNIFICANT. THE MORE CHILDREN OR THE MORE SIBLINGS THEY HAD, THE LESS TIME THEY PUT INTO VOLUNTEERING AND THE MORE "SELFISH" THE REASONS FOR VOLUNTEERING. FEMALES AND/OR POLITICAL LIBERALS WERE MORE LIKELY TO HAVE ALTRUISTIC MOTIVES. FOR CHICANOS, THE STRONG CORRELATION WAS BETWEEN ASI AND THE NUMBER OF HOURS A MONTH VOLUNTEERED—I.E., THE MORE TIME CHICANOS

VOLUNTEER, THE MORE LIKELY THEY HAVE AN ALTRUISTIC MOTIVATION (A RELATIONSHIP THAT DID NOT HOLD FOR THE ANGLO GROUP). THE AUTHORS CONCLUDE THAT EVEN THOUGH THE ANTECEDENTS AND SPECIFIC REASONS DIFFER, BOTH GROUPS PERFORM VOLUNTEER WORK FOR ESSENTIALLY ALTRUISTIC REASONS. 17 REFERENCES.

ACCN   002280

1059 AUTH   **LITTLE, J., & RAMIREZ, A.**
TITL   ETHNICITY OF SUBJECT AND TEST ADMINISTRATOR: THEIR EFFECT ON SELF-ESTEEM.
SRCE   *JOURNAL OF SOCIAL PSYCHOLOGY, 1976, 99(1), 149-150.*
INDX   ETHNIC IDENTITY, SELF CONCEPT, MEXICAN AMERICAN, CROSS CULTURAL, EXAMINER EFFECTS, CHILDREN, EMPIRICAL, PERSONALITY ASSESSMENT, TEST VALIDITY, ADOLESCENTS
ABST   THE RELATIONSHIP BETWEEN SELF-ESTEEM AND THE ETHNICITY OF THE SUBJECT WITH RESPECT TO THE ETHNICITY OF THE TESTER WAS EXAMINED AMONG 68 ANGLOS AND 68 CHICANOS WHO WERE MATCHED ACCORDING TO SEX, AGE, AND GRADE LEVEL. HALF OF THE SUBJECTS WERE IN THE 5TH AND 6TH GRADE AND THE OTHER HALF WERE IN THE 7TH AND 8TH GRADE. AN 18 SCALE SEMANTIC DIFFERENTIAL MEASURING SELF-ESTEEM WAS ADMINISTERED TO 4 GROUPS—2 GROUPS BY A MALE ANGLO EXAMINER AND THE OTHER 2 GROUPS BY A MALE CHICANO EXAMINER. THE RESULTS INDICATE THE SELF-ESTEEM OF THE CHICANOS WAS NO DIFFERENT FROM THE ANGLOS BUT THAT THE SCORES WERE INFLUENCED BY THE ETHNICITY OF THE TESTER. HOWEVER, WHILE THE ELEMENTARY STUDENTS WERE NOT INFLUENCED BY THE TESTER'S ETHNICITY, JUNIOR HIGH STUDENTS REFLECTED A MORE POSITIVE SELF-ESTEEM WHEN TESTED BY AN ANGLO. IT IS SUGGESTED THAT THESE FINDINGS DEMONSTRATE THAT OLDER STUDENTS PERCEIVE ANGLOS AS HAVING MORE AUTHORITY IN SOCIETY THAN CHICANOS, BUT FURTHER RESEARCH IS NEEDED TO INVESTIGATE OTHER POSSIBLE INTERPRETATIONS. 2 REFERENCES.
ACCN   000902

1060 AUTH   **LITTLEFIELD, R. P.**
TITL   SELF-DISCLOSURE AMONG SOME NEGRO, WHITE, AND MEXICAN AMERICAN ADOLESCENTS.
SRCE   *JOURNAL OF COUNSELING PSYCHOLOGY, 1974, 21(2), 133-136.*
INDX   PERSONALITY, PERSONALITY ASSESSMENT, FAMILY ROLES, FAMILY STRUCTURE, SEX COMPARISON, FATHER-CHILD INTERACTION, MOTHER-CHILD INTERACTION, ADOLESCENTS, CROSS CULTURAL, SELF CONCEPT, EMPIRICAL
ABST   SELF-DISCLOSURE RATINGS WERE TESTED FOR THE EFFECTS OF SEX, ETHNICITY, AND THE DIRECTION OF DISCLOSURE (I.E., TO WHOM ONE DISCLOSES). RIVERBARK'S REVISION OF JOURARDS'S SELF-DISCLOSURE QUESTIONNAIRE WAS ADMINISTERED TO 100 ANGLO, 100 BLACK, AND 100 MEXICAN AMERICAN 9TH GRADE STU-

DENTS IN THE RURAL SOUTH AND SOUTHWEST. EACH GROUP WAS COMPOSED OF AN EQUAL NUMBER OF MALES AND FEMALES. THE FINDINGS INDICATE THAT: (1) FEMALES IN ALL GROUPS REPORTED MORE DISCLOSURE THAN MALES; (2) WHEN SEXES WERE COMBINED, THE ANGLO SUBJECTS REPORTED THE GREATEST AMOUNT OF DISCLOSURE, WHILE THE MEXICAN AMERICAN REPORTED THE LEAST; (3) OF ALL SAMPLES, MEXICAN AMERICAN MALES REPORTED THE LEAST AMOUNT OF DISCLOSURE; AND (4) MALES FAVORED THE MOTHER AS THE TARGET OF MOST DISCLOSURE, WHEREAS FOR ALL GROUPS THE LEAST FAVORED TARGET OF SELF-DISCLOSURE WAS THE FATHER. 6 REFERENCES. (JOURNAL ABSTRACT MODIFIED)

ACCN   000903

1061 AUTH   **LOCASCIO, R., NESSELROTH, J., & THOMAS, M.**
TITL   THE CAREER DEVELOPMENT INVENTORY: USE AND FINDINGS WITH INNER CITY DROPOUTS.
SRCE   *JOURNAL OF VOCATIONAL BEHAVIOR, 1976, 8(3), 285-292.*
INDX   ADULTS, OCCUPATIONAL ASPIRATIONS, EMPLOYMENT, SEX COMPARISON, INTELLIGENCE, READING, MATHEMATICS, CROSS CULTURAL, DEVIANCE, ADOLESCENTS, EMPIRICAL, PUERTO RICAN-M, URBAN, TEST RELIABILITY, TEST VALIDITY
ABST   THE CAREER DEVELOPMENT INVENTORY WAS ADMINISTERED TO 107 BLACK, PUERTO RICAN, AND WHITE INNER CITY SCHOOL DROPOUTS TO EXAMINE ITS SUITABILITY FOR SUCH POPULATIONS. ALSO INVESTIGATED WERE THE INTERRELATIONSHIPS AMONG SEX, AGE, ETHNICITY, INTELLIGENCE, READING ACHIEVEMENT, ARITHMETIC ACHIEVEMENT, AND INVENTORY SCALES B (RESOURCES FOR EXPLORATION) AND C (INFORMATION AND DECISION MAKING). THE FINDINGS WERE: (1) SCALE A (PLANNING ORIENTATION) WAS UNSUITABLE FOR DROPOUTS DUE TO EXTENSIVE IN-SCHOOL REFERENCES; (2) SCALE B AND SCALE C WERE NOT SIGNIFICANTLY CORRELATED, RAISING QUESTIONS OF EITHER LOW SCALE B RELIABILITY OR AN UNSATISFACTORY LACK OF COMMUNALITY BETWEEN THE SCALES; (3) CONSISTENT WITH PREVIOUS FINDINGS AND THEORY, SEX AND AGE WERE UNRELATED TO SCALE B, SEX WAS UNRELATED TO SCALE C, AND AGE WAS RELATED TO SCALE C ONLY MARGINALLY; (4) IN CONTRAST TO PREVIOUS FINDINGS, INTELLIGENCE WAS NOT RELATED TO SCORES ON SCALES B AND C; (5) INITIAL ANALYSIS YIELDED NO SIGNIFICANT RELATIONSHIPS BETWEEN ETHNICITY AND SCALES B AND C, BUT A SECONDARY ANALYSIS INCLUDING BLACKS AND WHITES AND EXCLUDING PUERTO RICANS YIELDED A SIGNIFICANT CORRELATION BETWEEN ETHNICITY AND RESOURCES FOR EXPLORATION, BLACKS SCORING HIGHER, SUGGESTING THE NEED FOR FURTHER RESEARCH; AND (6) WHITES SCORED HIGHER THAN THE COMBINED BLACK AND PUERTO RICAN GROUPS ON INTELLIGENCE, READING, AND

ARTHMETIC ACHIEVEMENT. 7 REFERENCES. (JOURNAL ABSTRACT MODIFIED)

ACCN 000904

1062 AUTH **LOGAN, D. M.**
TITL NEED AFFILIATION OF MEXICAN-AMERICANS AND ANGLO-AMERICANS OF SOUTH TEXAS (DOCTORAL DISSERTATION, TEXAS TECH UNIVERSITY, 1971).
SRCE *DISSERTATION ABSTRACTS INTERNATIONAL, 1972, 33(1), 444B. (UNIVERSITY MICROFILMS NO. 72-20,298.)*
INDX MEXICAN AMERICAN, CROSS CULTURAL, EMPIRICAL, PERSONALITY, ACCULTURATION, SEX COMPARISON, URBAN, RURAL, SES, COLLEGE STUDENTS, TAT, ACHIEVEMENT MOTIVATION, TEXAS, SOUTHWEST, VOCATIONAL COUNSELING
ABST THE EFFECT OF CULTURAL DIFFERENCES ON NEED-AFFILIATION WAS INVESTIGATED IN A SAMPLE OF 162 MEXICAN AMERICAN AND ANGLO AMERICAN STUDENTS FROM A SOUTH TEXAS UNIVERSITY. THEMATIC APPERCEPTION IMAGERY WAS SCORED FOR POSITIVE, NEGATIVE AND MIXED (AMBIVALENT) NEED-AFFILIATION. A SIGNIFICANT DIFFERENCE IN POSITIVE NEED-AFFILIATION WAS FOUND BETWEEN MEXICAN AMERICANS AND ANGLO AMERICANS. MEXICAN AMERICANS SHOWED A TREND TOWARD HIGHER POSITIVE NEED-AFFILIATION. SEX DIFFERENCES, ORDINAL POSITION IN THE FAMILY, DISTANCE FROM THE MEXICAN BORDER, LENGTH OF TIME IN THE UNITED STATES, POPULATION OF THE HOME TOWN, AND SOCIOECONOMIC LEVEL WERE SHOWN NOT TO BE SIGNIFICANT FACTORS IN NEED-AFFILIATION. HOSTILE AND WITHDRAWN EXPRESSIONS OF NEGATIVE NEED-AFFILIATION WERE ALSO ANALYZED AND FOUND NOT TO BE SIGNIFICANTLY RELATED TO ETHNIC GROUP MEMBERSHIP. THE RESULTS ARE DISCUSSED IN RELATION TO VOCATIONAL COUNSELING AND PSYCHOTHERAPY WITH MEXICAN AMERICANS. AREAS FOR FURTHER RESEARCH ARE SUGGESTED. 46 REFERENCES. (AUTHOR SUMMARY MODIFIED)

ACCN 000905

1063 AUTH **LOMBARD, T. J., & HARNEY, B. J.**
TITL AUDITORY DISCRIMINATION AS A PREDICTOR OF READING FOR BILINGUAL MEXICAN-AMERICAN MIGRANT CHILDREN.
SRCE *PERCEPTUAL AND MOTOR SKILLS, 1977, 45, 479-484.*
INDX ABILITY TESTING, BILINGUAL, CHILDREN, EDUCATIONAL ASSESSMENT, EMPIRICAL, MEXICAN AMERICAN, PERCEPTION, TEST VALIDITY, MINNESOTA, MIDWEST, READING
ABST THE PERFORMANCE OF 61 BILINGUAL MEXICAN AMERICAN MIGRANT CHILDREN, AGES 8 TO 14 YEARS, WAS COMPARED FOR SPANISH AND ENGLISH FORMATS OF THE WEPMAN AUDITORY DISCRIMINATION TEST. THE TWO FORMATS CORRELATED SIGNIFICANTLY WITH EACH OTHER, AND BOTH WERE PREDICTIVE OF READING RECOGNITION AS MEASURED BY THE PEABODY INDIVIDUAL ACHIEVEMENT TEST. THE DATA SUGGEST THAT AUDITORY DISCRIMI-

NATION AS MEASURED BY THE POPULAR WEPMAN TEST MAY NOT BE A PURE PERCEPTUAL SKILL BUT MAY BE LANGUAGE BOUND. CONSEQUENTLY, AUDITORY DISCRIMINATION AS A PURE PERCEPTUAL SKILL MAY NOT BE ACCURATELY ASSESSED IN BILINGUAL OR MONOLINGUAL SPANISH-SPEAKING CHILDREN IF THE WEPMAN TEST IS USED IN ITS PUBLISHED FORMAT. A SPANISH-BASED ALTERNATIVE IS SUGGESTED FOR ASSESSING AUDITORY DISCRIMINATION FOR USES OTHER THAN READING PREDICTION. 12 REFERENCES. (AUTHOR ABSTRACT)

ACCN 002301

1064 AUTH **LOMBILLO, J. R., & GERAGHTY, M.**
TITL ETHNIC ACCOUNTABILITY IN MENTAL HEALTH PROGRAMS FOR MEXICAN-AMERICAN COMMUNITIES.
SRCE *PAPER PRESENTED AT THE ANNUAL MEETING OF THE SOCIETY FOR APPLIED ANTHROPOLOGY, TUCSON, APRIL 14, 1973.*
INDX MEXICAN AMERICAN, MENTAL HEALTH, COMMUNITY, HEALTH DELIVERY SYSTEMS, RURAL, FARM LABORERS, MIGRATION, CULTURE, BILINGUAL-BICULTURAL PERSONNEL, FLORIDA, SOUTH, COMMUNITY INVOLVEMENT, ESSAY, FOLK MEDICINE, CURANDERISMO, POVERTY, POLICY
ABST THE PROBLEMS AND APPROACHES OF A COMMUNITY MENTAL HEALTH CLINIC IN DEVELOPING SERVICE PROGRAMS FOR MEXICAN AMERICANS IN A RURAL AGRICULTURAL AREA IN SOUTHWEST FLORIDA ARE EXAMINED. IN THE ASSESSMENT OF RESOURCES, TRADITIONAL MEASURES IGNORE NOT ONLY LANGUAGE DIFFERENCES BUT REFLECT LITTLE UNDERSTANDING OF MEXICAN AMERICAN HEALTH PRACTICES AND BELIEFS. HEALTH DELIVERY SYSTEMS WOULD BETTER MEET THE NEEDS OF THIS POPULATION IF THEY UTILIZED THE EXISTING NETWORK OF FOLK HEALERS WITHIN THE COMMUNITY. TWO EXAMPLES ARE DESCRIBED WHICH DEMONSTRATE THE EFFECTIVENESS OF FOLK HEALERS IN THE TREATMENT OF MENTAL HEALTH PROBLEMS. IT IS SUGGESTED THAT THE SUCCESS OF A MENTAL HEALTH PROGRAM DEPENDS UPON DEVELOPING MEANINGFUL MENTAL HEALTH STATUS INDICATORS, MUTUAL TRUST BETWEEN AGENCIES AND THE MEXICAN AMERICAN COMMUNITY, DEVELOPING EDUCATIONAL AND TRAINING PROGRAMS, AND THE UTILIZATION OF FOLK HEALERS IN THE DELIVERY OF MENTAL HEALTH SERVICES. 38 REFERENCES.

ACCN 000906

1065 AUTH **LONG, E. G., HOERL, R., & RADINSKY, T.**
TITL SOME DIAGNOSTIC AND PROGNOSTIC SURPRISES IN SPANISH AMERICAN PATIENTS IN COLORADO.
SRCE *IN E. R. PADILLA & A. M. PADILLA (EDS.), TRANSCULTURAL PSYCHIATRY: AN HISPANIC PERSPECTIVE (MONOGRAPH NO. 4). LOS ANGELES: UNIVERSITY OF CALIFORNIA, SPANISH SPEAKING MENTAL HEALTH RESEARCH CENTER, 1977, PP. 51-54.*
INDX RESOURCE UTILIZATION, DEMOGRAPHIC, PSY-

CHOSIS, FAMILY STRUCTURE, SCHIZOPHRE-NIA, ALCOHOLISM, PSYCHOTHERAPY OUT-COME, SPANISH SURNAMED, PROGRAM EVALUATION, EMPIRICAL, COLORADO, SOUTH-WEST, COMMUNITY

ABST THE NORTHWEST DENVER COMMUNITY MEN-TAL HEALTH CENTER WHICH HAS A HIGHLY DE-VELOPED RESEARCH AND EVALUATION COM-PONENT HAS BEEN ABLE TO EXAMINE ITS CATCHMENT AREA WITH RESPECT TO DIFFER-ENCES IN UTILIZATION, DIAGNOSIS, AND TREATMENT CAREERS AND OUTCOMES AMONG THE VARIOUS ETHNIC GROUPS. WHILE IT AP-PEARS THAT UTILIZATION OF THE CENTER BY SPANISH SURNAMED PERSONS IS REPRESEN-TATIVE OF THE CATCHMENT'S AREA POPULA-TION, THIS IS NOT THE CASE WITH RESPECT TO THE TYPE OF TREATMENT. PRELIMINARY DATA ANALYSIS INDICATES THAT THE SPANISH SUR-NAMED ACCOUNT FOR 30% OF THE OUTPA-TIENTS BUT ONLY 20% OF THE INPATIENTS. THEIR LENGTH OF TREATMENT IS SHORTER, BUT THIS MAY BE A RESULT OF GREATER STA-BILITY OF THEIR FAMILY STRUCTURE. CASE RECORDS REVEAL THE MOST COMMON PROB-LEM AMONG SPANISH AMERICANS IS ALCO-HOLISM. SPANISH-SPEAKING MALES HAVE A BETTER FOLLOW-UP THAN THEIR FEMALE COUNTERPARTS, PARTICULARLY IF THEY HAVE BEEN DIAGNOSED AS ALCOHOLICS.

ACCN 000907

1066 AUTH **LONGRES, J. F., JR.**
TITL RACISM AND ITS EFFECTS ON PUERTO RICAN CONTINENTALS.
SRCE *SOCIAL CASEWORK, 1974, 55(2), 67-75.*
INDX PREJUDICE, DISCRIMINATION, ACCULTURA-TION, HISTORY, MIGRATION, CULTURE, PSY-CHOTHERAPY, PUERTO RICAN-I, PUERTO RI-CAN-M, POVERTY, MENTAL HEALTH, ETHNIC IDENTITY, POLICY, MARRIAGE
ABST THE DIFFERENCES IN RACIAL PREJUDICE AS IT EXISTS IN PUERTO RICO AND IN THE UNITED STATES ARE DISCUSSED. IN PUERTO RICO THE PRIMARY SOURCE OF SELF-IDENTITY IS CUL-TURE OR CLASS, NOT COLOR. HOWEVER, PUERTO RICANS DO USE RACIAL TERMS TO CHARACTERIZE EACH OTHER. ALTHOUGH PUERTO RICANS PLACE A POSITIVE VALUE ON WHITENESS, DARK SKINNED INDIVIDUALS ARE NOT CONSIDERED INFERIOR AND INTERRA-CIAL MARRIAGES ARE COMMONPLACE. WHEN PUERTO RICANS MIGRATE TO THE MAINLAND THEY NOT ONLY EXPERIENCE CULTURAL SHOCK RELATED TO LANGUAGE AND CUSTOMS, BUT IF THEY POSSESS ANY OVERT NEGROID FEA-TURES THEY ARE STIGMATIZED AS BLACK. AL-THOUGH IT HAS BEEN SUGGESTED THAT PUERTO RICANS SHOULD IDENTIFY THEM-SELVES AS "RAINBOW" PEOPLE, PERHAPS THE FOCUS SHOULD LIE IN EMPHASIZING PUERTO RICAN CULTURAL IDENTITY. 12 REFERENCES.
ACCN 000908

1067 AUTH **LONGSTRETH, L. E., LONGSTRETH, G. V., RA-MIREZ, C., & FERNANDEZ, G.**
TITL THE UBIQUITY OF BIG BROTHER.
SRCE *CHILD DEVELOPMENT, 1975, 46, 769-772.*

INDX MEXICAN AMERICAN, CHILDREN, CROSS CUL-TURAL, SEX COMPARISON, SEX ROLES, SES, PERSONALITY, FAMILY STRUCTURE, SOCIALI-ZATION, EMPIRICAL, ASSERTIVENESS, CALI-FORNIA, SOUTHWEST, URBAN, COLLEGE STU-DENTS
ABST THE INFLUENCE OF HAVING AN OLDER BROTHER WITH RESPECT TO MASCULINITY, CONFORMITY, AGGRESSIVENESS AND PHYSI-CALNESS WAS EXAMINED IN 4 LOS ANGELES ELEMENTARY SCHOOLS. TEACHERS FROM GRADES K THROUGH 6 NOMINATED THE MOST PHYSICALLY ACTIVE AND MOST PHYSICALLY PASSIVE STUDENTS FROM EACH SEX. HALF THE SCHOOLS WERE ATTENDED MAINLY BY LOW SES MEXICAN AMERICAN STUDENTS AND HALF BY UPPER MIDDLE SES CAUCASIAN STU-DENTS. THE MAIN FINDING WAS THAT PHYSI-CALLY ACTIVE STUDENTS WERE MORE LIKELY TO HAVE AN OLDER BROTHER THAN WERE PHYSICALLY PASSIVE STUDENTS. THIS EFFECT WAS INDEPENDENT OF SEX, GRADE LEVEL, RACE, SES, AND OTHER SIBLING COMBINA-TIONS. A SECOND STUDY CONFIRMED THIS RELATIONSHIP WHEN COLLEGE STUDENTS RATED THEMSELVES ON THE SAME ACTIVE-PASSIVE DIMENSION. 13 REFERENCES. (JOUR-NAL ABSTRACT MODIFIED)
ACCN 000909

1068 AUTH **LOOMIS, C. P.**
TITL A BACKWARD GLANCE AT SELF-IDENTIFI-CATION OF BLACKS AND CHICANOS.
SRCE *RURAL SOCIOLOGY, 1974, 39(1), 96.*
INDX ETHNIC IDENTITY, MEXICAN AMERICAN, CROSS CULTURAL, CULTURAL FACTORS, REVIEW
ABST THE INCREASED EMPHASIS ON ETHNICITY IN THE SELF-IDENTIFICATION OF MEXICAN AMERICANS IN THE LAST DECADE IS COM-MENTED UPON. STUDIES USING THE TWENTY STATEMENTS TEST IN 1954, 1966 AND 1973 TO COMPARE CHICANOS AND BLACKS ARE CITED TO SUPPORT THIS OBSERVATION. 3 REFER-ENCES.
ACCN 000910

1069 AUTH **LOPEZ, D. E.**
TITL LANGUAGE LOYALTY AND THE SOCIAL MOBIL-ITY OF CHICANOS.
SRCE *PAPER PRESENTED AT THE 71ST ANNUAL MEETING OF THE AMERICAN SOCIOLOGICAL ASSOCIATION, NEW YORK, AUGUST-SEPTEM-BER 1976.*
INDX BILINGUALISM, SOCIAL MOBILITY, OCCUPA-TIONAL ASPIRATIONS, SCHOLASTIC ASPIRA-TIONS, LABOR FORCE, SES, ETHNIC IDENTITY, SURVEY, EMPIRICAL, MEXICAN AMERICAN, CALIFORNIA, SOUTHWEST
ABST PREVIOUS RESEARCH HAS IMPLIED BUT NOT DEMONSTRATED THAT AMONG CHICANOS AND OTHER SPEAKERS OF A SUBORDINATE-TONGUE LANGUAGE, APOSTASY IS A REQUISITE FOR UPWARD MOBILITY. A CONSIDERATION OF THE SOCIAL CAUSES AND CONSEQUENCES OF LANGUAGE LOYALTY SUGGESTS THAT SPAN-ISH UPBRINGING AND CONTINUED USE SHOULD RETARD MOBILITY INTO THE MIDDLE CLASS BUT NOT WITHIN THE WORKING CLASS.

DATA FROM A RECENT LOS ANGELES SURVEY SHOW THAT IN FACT BOTH LOYALTY TO AND UPBRINGING IN SPANISH ARE POSITIVE SOCIOMETRIC AIDS FOR WORKING-CLASS MOBILITY AND DO NOT IMPEDE MOVEMENT INTO THE MIDDLE CLASS, EVEN THOUGH BOTH ARE NEGATIVELY RELATED TO EDUCATIONAL ATTAINMENT. 40 REFERENCES. (AUTHOR ABSTRACT)

ACCN   000911

1070 AUTH   **LOPEZ, D. E.**
     TITL   THE SOCIAL CONSEQUENCES OF CHICANO HOME-SCHOOL BILINGUALISM.
     SRCE   *SOCIAL PROBLEMS, 1976, 24(2), 234-246.*
     INDX   MEXICAN AMERICAN, BILINGUALISM, SES, EDUCATION, INSTRUCTIONAL TECHNIQUES, DISCRIMINATION, STEREOTYPES, EMPIRICAL, SCHOLASTIC ACHIEVEMENT, EMPLOYMENT, CALIFORNIA, SOUTHWEST
     ABST   A REVIEW OF THE LITERATURE ON THE SCHOLASTIC CONSEQUENCES OF BEING BILINGUAL SUGGESTS THAT THE NEGATIVE EFFECTS OF CHICANO HOME/SCHOOL BILINGUALISM STEM FROM EXTRINSIC FACTORS, PARTICULARLY THE REACTIONS OF OTHERS TO ETHNIC STIGMA, RATHER THAN FROM ANYTHING INTRINSIC TO BILINGUALISM. FOUR MODELS RELATING HOME/SCHOOL BILINGUALISM TO SUBSEQUENT ATTAINMENTS ARE PRESENTED. CONTRARY TO EXPECTATIONS, A MODEL OF BALANCED EFFECTS, IN WHICH NEGATIVE EFFECTS ON EDUCATIONAL ATTAINMENT ARE CANCELLED OUT BY THE SUBSEQUENT POSITIVE SOCIOMETRIC ADVANTAGE OF KNOWING SPANISH, IS BEST SUPPORTED BY RECENT DATA FROM LOS ANGELES. HOWEVER, IN MIDDLE CLASS CHICANO HOMES THE PATTERN OF EFFECTS IS REVERSED. 40 REFERENCES. (JOURNAL ABSTRACT MODIFIED)

ACCN   000912

1071 AUTH   **LOPEZ, D. E., & SABAGH, G.**
     TITL   UNTANGLING STRUCTURAL AND NORMATIVE ASPECTS OF THE MINORITY STATUS-FERTILITY HYPOTHESIS.
     SRCE   *AMERICAN JOURNAL OF SOCIOLOGY, 1978, 83(6), 1491-1497.*
     INDX   FERTILITY, SEXUAL BEHAVIOR, FAMILY STRUCTURE, MEXICAN AMERICAN, ACCULTURATION, ETHNIC IDENTITY, SES, POVERTY, HOUSING, EMPIRICAL, CALIFORNIA, SOUTHWEST, SURVEY
     ABST   SINCE THE RESIDUAL DIFFERENTIAL FERTILITY OF RACIAL AND ETHNIC MINORITIES CAN BE EXPLAINED IN THEORETICALLY OPPOSED WAYS, EFFECTS DUE TO SUBCULTURAL NORMS CAN BE ESTABLISHED ONLY BY DIRECT MEASUREMENT. DATA FROM A 1973 SURVEY OF LOS ANGELES COUNTY CHICANO COUPLES INDICATED THAT WITHIN THIS HIGH FERTILITY MINORITY GROUP SOCIOCULTURAL DIFFERENCES MAY ACTUALLY RESULT IN REDUCED FERTILITY. THAT FINDING IS INTERPRETED TO SUPPORT THE HYPOTHESIS (GOLDSCHEIDER AND UHLENBERG, 1969) THAT MINORITY STATUS PRODUCES REDUCED FERTILITY AS A REACTION TO EXTERNAL PRESSURE, AND SUG-

GESTS THAT ETHNIC INTEGRITY IS ONE ASPECT OF THAT REACTION. THIS REVIEW OF THE 1973 SURVEY DATA, HOWEVER, PUTS IN DOUBT THE NORMATIVE INCREASE FERTILITY EFFECT GOLDSCHEIDER AND UHLENBERG POSTULATED FOR "PRO-NATALIST" MINORITIES. DATA ANALYSIS SUGGESTS THAT THE HIGH FERTILITY OF CHICANOS AND OTHER LOW STATUS MINORITIES IS INSTEAD THE RESULT OF SOCIOECONOMIC DISPARITIES AND GHETTOIZATION. MORE GENERALLY, THE FINDINGS CONSTITUTE A RARE EXAMPLE OF A DIRECT CONFIRMATION OF THE SUPERIORITY OF STRUCTURAL OVER CULTURAL FERTILITY THEORIES. 8 REFERENCES. (JOURNAL ABSTRACT MODIFIED)

ACCN   000913

1072 AUTH   **LOPEZ, M.**
     TITL   BILINGUAL MEMORY RESEARCH: IMPLICATIONS FOR BILINGUAL EDUCATION.
     SRCE   *IN J. L. MARTINEZ (ED.), CHICANO PSYCHOLOGY. NEW YORK: ACADEMIC PRESS, 1977, PP. 127-140.*
     INDX   MEMORY, BILINGUALISM, BILINGUAL-BICULTURAL EDUCATION, GRAMMAR, SEMANTICS, COGNITIVE DEVELOPMENT, COMPOUND-COORDINATE DISTINCTION, MEXICAN AMERICAN, THEORETICAL, REVIEW
     ABST   THE RAPIDLY GROWING POPULARITY OF BILINGUAL EDUCATION HAS PRIMARILY FOCUSED ON PRACTICAL PROBLEMS AND PRAGMATIC SOLUTIONS AND THEREBY HAS FAILED TO ADDRESS SOME OF THE MAJOR ASPECTS OF BILINGUALISM. THUS, A MODERN CONCEPTUALIZATION OF BILINGUAL SEMANTIC MEMORY TO HELP RESOLVE CURRENT THEORETICAL PROBLEMS IN THE AREA OF BILINGUAL MEMORY IS PROPOSED. THE LITERATURE ON COMPOUND-COORDINATE BILINGUALISM IS REVIEWED AND ITS THEORETICAL AND EMPIRICAL WEAKNESSES DISCUSSED. PROBLEMS RESULTING FROM ITS USE IN BILINGUAL EDUCATION PROGRAMS ARE IDENTIFIED. AN ALTERNATIVE THEORY RECENTLY DEVELOPED IN PSYCHOLOGICAL RESEARCH ON SEMANTIC MEMORY AND THE IMPLICATIONS OF THIS NEW CONCEPTUALIZATION OF BILINGUAL MEMORY ON THE EDUCATION OF CHICANO BILINGUALS ARE ALSO DISCUSSED. 44 REFERENCES.

ACCN   000915

1073 AUTH   **LOPEZ, M., HICKS, R. E., & YOUNG, R. K.**
     TITL   RETROACTIVE INHIBITION IN A BILINGUAL A-B, A-B' PARADIGM.
     SRCE   *JOURNAL OF EXPERIMENTAL PSYCHOLOGY. 1974, 103(1), 85-90.*
     INDX   MEMORY, BILINGUALISM, LEARNING, MEXICAN AMERICAN, COLLEGE STUDENTS, EMPIRICAL, SEMANTICS, LANGUAGE ASSESSMENT, TEXAS, SOUTHWEST, COMPOUND-COORDINATE DISTINCTION
     ABST   AN EXPERIMENT DESIGNED TO INVESTIGATE BILINGUAL TRANSFER OF TRAINING AND RETROACTIVE INHIBITION IN A SITUATION THAT PROVIDED NO CONTEXTUAL CUES FOR THE RECODING OF SPECIFIC ITEMS INTO ONE LANGUAGE OR THE OTHER IS DESCRIBED. SUB-

JECTS WERE 32 BILINGUAL MEXICAN AMERI-
CAN COLLEGE STUDENTS WHO VOLUN-
TEERED TO PARTICIPATE IN MEMORIZING EN-
GLISH-SPANISH WORD PAIRS. THE DESIGN IS
SUMMARIZED AS A 2X4 FACTORIAL WITH TWO
EXPERIMENTORS AND FOUR CONDITIONS OF
TRANSFER. THE SUBJECTS APPEARED TO BE
COMPOUND BILINGUALS WHO ARE ENGLISH
DOMINANT. ANALYSIS OF THE NUMBER OF
CORRECT RESPONSES PER TRIAL AND CONDI-
TION IN SPANISH AND ENGLISH SUPPORTS AN
INTERDEPENDENCE HYPOTHESIS OF BILIN-
GUAL ORGANIZATION OF MEMORY. THE FIND-
ING OF NEGATIVE TRANSFER AND RETROAC-
TIVE INHIBITION IN AN A-B AND A-B' PARADIGM
IS TAKEN AS EVIDENCE THAT BILINGUALS
STORE WORDS IN MEMORY IN TERMS OF THE
SEMANTIC REPRESENTATION OF THOSE
WORDS, WITH THE PRESENTATION OF A WORD
AND ITS TRANSLATION RESULTING IN THE AC-
TIVATION OF THE SAME SEMANTIC REPRESEN-
TATION IN MEMORY. 13 REFERENCES.

ACCN   000917

1074 AUTH **LOPEZ, M., & YOUNG, R. K.**
TITL   THE LINGUISTIC INTERDEPENDENCE OF BILIN-
        GUALS.
SRCE   *JOURNAL OF EXPERIMENTAL PSYCHOLOGY,*
        1974, 102(6), 981-983.
INDX   COMPOUND-COORDINATE DISTINCTION, BI-
        LINGUALISM, COGNITIVE DEVELOPMENT,
        LEARNING, MEMORY, MEXICAN AMERICAN,
        EMPIRICAL, ADOLESCENTS
ABST   AN EXPERIMENT TO TEST THE INTERDEPEND-
        ENCE TRANSLATION HYPOTHESIS IN BILIN-
        GUALS IS DESCRIBED. SIXTY-FOUR SPANISH-
        ENGLISH BILINGUALS (JUNIOR AND SENIOR
        HIGH SCHOOL STUDENTS) WERE FIRST FAMIL-
        IARIZED WITH A LIST OF SPANISH OR ENGLISH
        WORDS. NEXT, THEY LEARNED A SPANISH OR
        AN ENGLISH LIST CONSISTING OF WORDS
        THAT WERE THE SAME AS (TRANSLATED) OR
        DIFFERENT FROM THOSE IN THE FAMILIARIZA-
        TION LIST. FAMILIARIZATION TECHNIQUES WERE
        UNIFORM BOTH BETWEEN AND WITHIN LAN-
        GUAGES IN THAT THE AMOUNT OF POSITIVE
        TRANSFER OBTAINED WAS THE SAME FOR ALL
        GROUPS. THE DATA WERE INTERPRETED AS
        SUPPORTIVE OF THE LANGUAGE INTERDEP-
        ENDENCE HYPOTHESIS. 6 REFERENCES.
        (JOURNAL ABSTRACT MODIFIED)
ACCN   000918

1075 AUTH **LOPEZ, R. E.**
TITL   ANXIETY, ACCULTURATION AND THE URBAN
        CHICANO.
SRCE   *BERKELEY, CALIF.: CALIFORNIA BOOK CO., LTD.,*
        1970
INDX   ANXIETY, ACCULTURATION, URBAN, MEXICAN
        AMERICAN, EMPIRICAL, CALIFORNIA, SOUTH-
        WEST, COLLEGE STUDENTS, POLICY
ABST   THIS STUDY EXPLORED THE RELATIONSHIP
        BETWEEN STAGES OF ACCULTURATION AND
        ANXIETY LEVEL OF CHICANOS. THE UCA (UR-
        BAN CHICANO ACCULTURATION) SCALE AND
        THE IPAT (INSTITUTE FOR PERSONALITY AND
        ABILITY TESTING) ANXIETY SCALE WERE THE
        INSTRUMENTS UTILIZED TO MEASURE ACCUL-

TURATION AND ANXIETY. TWO HYPOTHESES
WERE INVESTIGATED: (1) MEXICAN AMERICAN
COLLEGE FRESHMEN WHO ARE MODERATELY
ACCULTURATED INTO ANGLO CULTURE WILL
BE MORE ANXIOUS THAN MEXICAN AMERICAN
FRESHMEN WHO ARE EITHER HIGHLY ACCUL-
TURATED OR WHO ARE LOW IN ACCULTURA-
TION; AND (2) MEXICAN AMERICAN FRESHMEN
WHO ARE MOST HIGHLY ACCULTURATED INTO
ANGLO CULTURE WILL BE MORE ANXIOUS
THAN MEXICAN AMERICAN FRESHMEN WHO
ARE LOW IN ACCULTURATION. A TOTAL OF 67
CHICANO EOP (ECONOMIC OPPORTUNITY
PROGRAM) FRESHMEN ATTENDING SAN JOSE
STATE COLLEGE DURING THE FALL SEMESTER,
1969, WERE USED AS SUBJECTS. THE RESULTS
DID NOT SUPPORT THE TWO HYPOTHESES.
THE RESULTS SUGGEST THAT CHICANO EOP
FRESHMEN AT SAN JOSE STATE COLLEGE ARE
AT MANY STAGES OF ACCULTURATION AND
THAT ANXIETY LEVEL SEEMS TO BE HIGHEST
AMONG THOSE CHICANOS UNWILLING OR UN-
ABLE TO ATTEMPT CULTURAL TRANSFER. THE
SUGGESTION IS MADE THAT COLLEGES DE-
VELOP AND MAINTAIN PROGRAMS OFFERING
THE CHICANO STUDENT THE ALTERNATIVE OF
NOT HAVING TO EMULATE ANGLOS TO SUC-
CEED. 29 REFERENCES. (AUTHOR SUMMARY
MODIFIED)
ACCN   000919

1076 AUTH **LOPEZ, R. W., MADRID-BARELA, A., & FLORES
        MACIAS, R.**
TITL   CHICANOS IN HIGHER EDUCATION: STATUS
        AND ISSUES (MONOGRAPH NO. 7).
SRCE   *LOS ANGELES: CHICANO STUDIES CENTER*
        PUBLICATIONS, UNIVERSITY OF CALIFORNIA,
        1976.
INDX   MEXICAN AMERICAN, SCHOLASTIC ACHIEVE-
        MENT, HIGHER EDUCATION, REPRESENTATION,
        EQUAL OPPORTUNITY, DISCRIMINATION,
        PROFESSIONAL TRAINING, EMPIRICAL, BIBLI-
        OGRAPHY, PROCEEDINGS, BOOK
ABST   THIS REPORT, PREPARED AS A RESOURCE
        DOCUMENT FOR THE SYMPOSIUM ON THE
        STATUS OF CHICANOS IN HIGHER EDUCATION
        WHICH WAS HELD IN LOS ANGELES IN MAY
        1975, (1) PRESENTS A GENERAL CONTEXT FOR
        THE STUDY OF CHICANOS IN HIGHER EDUCA-
        TION, (2) DESCRIBES THE EXISTING DATA BASE,
        (3) ADDRESSES SOME OF THE DATA COLLEC-
        TION PROBLEMS INVOLVED IN MAKING SUCH A
        STUDY, (4) PROVIDES A PROFILE OF CHICANOS
        IN HIGHER EDUCATION WITH PARTICULAR EM-
        PHASIS ON ENROLLMENT PATTERNS, AND (5)
        INCLUDES AN EXTENSIVE SELECTED BIBLIOG-
        RAPHY ON THE SUBJECT. THE REPORT CON-
        TAINS OVER FIFTY TABLES SUMMARIZING DATA
        COLLECTED FROM BUREAU OF THE CENSUS
        AND OFFICE OF CIVIL RIGHTS SOURCES. MOST
        OF THE DATA ARE FOR 1970, WITH SOME PRE-
        SENTED FROM THE YEARS BEFORE AND AFTER
        TO INDICATE PATTERNS AND TRENDS IN EN-
        ROLLMENT OF CHICANOS AT UNDERGRADU-
        ATE AND GRADUATE LEVELS AS WELL AS DIS-
        TRIBUTION OF STUDENTS BY ACADEMIC FIELD
        AND GEOGRAPHIC AREA. 181 REFERENCES.
ACCN   000920

1077 AUTH **LOPEZ, R. W., & ENOS, D. D.**

TITL CHICANOS AND PUBLIC HIGHER EDUCATION IN CALIFORNIA.

SRCE *PAPER PREPARED FOR THE JOINT COMMITTEE ON THE MASTER PLAN FOR HIGHER EDUCATION, CALIFORNIA LEGISLATURE, SACRAMENTO, 1972.*

INDX MEXICAN AMERICAN, HIGHER EDUCATION, REPRESENTATION, EQUAL OPPORTUNITY, SCHOLASTIC ACHIEVEMENT, SES, EDUCATIONAL COUNSELING, PEER GROUP, PROFESSIONAL TRAINING, ADMINISTRATORS, ADOLESCENTS, COLLEGE STUDENTS, POLICY, SURVEY, CALIFORNIA, SOUTHWEST

ABST AN OVERVIEW OF CHICANOS IN PUBLIC HIGHER EDUCATION IN CALIFORNIA IS PRESENTED. QUALITATIVE AND QUANTITATIVE DATA ARE PRESENTED DESCRIBING EDUCATION AND ITS AFFECT ON CHICANOS AND THE CHARACTERISTICS OF CHICANOS IN THIS STATE'S COLLEGE AND UNIVERSITY SYSTEM. THE FOLLOWING SOURCES WERE USED TO OBTAIN THE DATA: (1) QUESTIONNAIRES MAILED TO SPANISH SURNAMED STUDENTS—MORE THAN 1,000 HIGH SCHOOL SENIORS AND 1,000 STUDENTS WHO HAD COMPLETED APPROXIMATELY ONE YEAR OF COLLEGE; (2) SITE VISITATIONS, CORRESPONDENCE, AND INTERVIEWS WITH STUDENTS AND SCHOOL OFFICIALS AT SELECTED HIGH SCHOOLS, PUBLIC COLLEGES, AND UNIVERSITIES; (3) INTERVIEWS WITH RELEVANT STAFF AT THE STATE DEPARTMENT OF EDUCATION AND WITH AT LEAST 5 TOP ADMINISTRATORS IN EACH OF THE STATE'S THREE PUBLIC HIGHER EDUCATION SYSTEMS; AND (4) A MAILED QUESTIONNAIRE TO THE CHIEF ADMINISTRATORS OF ALL PUBLIC COLLEGES AND UNIVERSITIES IN THE STATE. POLICY RECOMMENDATIONS ARE OFFERED TO IMPROVE THE STATUS OF CHICANOS IN HIGHER EDUCATION IN CALIFORNIA. APPENDICES INCLUDE REPORTS ON ACCESS TO HIGHER EDUCATION, IMPLEMENTATION OF AFFIRMATIVE ACTION PROGRAMS, ETHNIC GROUP IDENTIFICATION, AND COMMENTS FROM HIGH SCHOOL AND COLLEGE STUDENTS. 33 REFERENCES.

ACCN 000921

1078 AUTH **LOPEZ, S.**

TITL CLINICAL STEREOTYPES OF THE MEXICAN AMERICAN.

SRCE *IN J. L. MARTINEZ (ED.), CHICANO PSYCHOLOGY. NEW YORK: ACADEMIC PRESS, 1977, PP. 263-275.*

INDX STEREOTYPES, PSYCHOTHERAPISTS, ACCULTURATION, RELIGION, MENTAL HEALTH, CULTURAL FACTORS, COPING MECHANISMS, MEXICAN AMERICAN, EMPIRICAL, SOUTHWEST, CALIFORNIA, ARIZONA

ABST TO INVESTIGATE MENTAL HEALTH PROFESSIONALS' STEREOTYPES OF MEXICAN AMERICANS, 59 CLINICIANS IN TUCSON, POMONA, EAST LOS ANGELES, AND LOS ANGELES WERE ASKED TO RATE A NORMAL, HEALTHY MEXICAN AMERICAN, A NORMAL, HEALTHY ANGLO, AND ANOTHER NORMAL ADULT (ETHNICITY UNSPECIFIED) ON FIVE DIFFERENT SCALES: (1) EMOTIONALITY, (2) DOMINANCE, (3) RESPON-

SIBILITY, (4) RELIGIOSITY, AND (5) STEREOTYPIC CHARACTERISTICS. THE RESPONDENTS (20 MEXICAN AMERICAN, 32 ANGLO, 4 LATIN AMERICAN AND 3 "OTHER") WERE CATEGORIZED BY ETHNICITY, SEX, FAMILIARITY WITH MEXICAN AMERICAN CULTURE, PROFESSIONAL EXPERIENCE WITH CHICANOS, USE OF SPANISH WITH CLIENTS, AND PERCENTAGE OF MEXICAN AMERICAN CLIENTELE. MULTIVARIATE ANALYSIS OF VARIANCE PERFORMED ON THE CLINICIANS' RATINGS OF MENTAL HEALTH FOR THE THREE CATEGORIES INDICATED: (1) NO SIGNIFICANT MAIN EFFECTS FOR SEX OR FOR THE CULTURAL FAMILIARITY VARIABLES OF ETHNICITY, PROFESSIONAL EXPERIENCE, PERCENTAGE OF CHICANO CLIENTELE, AND SPANISH-SPEAKING ABILITY; AND (2) SIGNIFICANT DIFFERENCES FOR THE 3 CONCEPTS OF MENTAL HEALTH ON ALL FIVE SCALES, BUT NOT ALWAYS IN THE DIRECTION PREDICTED. OVERALL FINDINGS SUGGEST: (1) THAT CLINICIANS VIEW THE HEALTHY MEXICAN AMERICAN AS CLOSER TO THE HEALTHY ADULT THAN THE HEALTHY ANGLO; (2) THE SAMPLED THERAPISTS, NO MATTER WHAT THEIR ETHNICITY OR SPANISH-SPEAKING ABILITY, DO NOT DIFFER SIGNIFICANTLY IN THEIR VIEWS OF THE HEALTHY MEXICAN AMERICAN, ANGLO, AND ADULT; AND (3) ALL SAMPLED THERAPISTS STEREOTYPE MEXICAN AMERICANS EQUALLY. EXPLANATIONS FOR THESE UNEXPECTED FINDINGS ARE DISCUSSED. 26 REFERENCES.

ACCN 000922

1079 AUTH **LOWMAN, R. P., & SPUCK, D. W.**

TITL PREDICTORS OF COLLEGE SUCCESS FOR THE DISADVANTAGED MEXICAN-AMERICAN.

SRCE *JOURNAL OF COLLEGE STUDENT PERSONNEL, 1975, 16(1), 40-48.*

INDX SCHOLASTIC ACHIEVEMENT, SES, POVERTY, COLLEGE STUDENTS, INTELLIGENCE, INTELLIGENCE TESTING, CULTURAL FACTORS, LINGUISTIC COMPETENCE, ACHIEVEMENT MOTIVATION, MEXICAN AMERICAN, SCHOLASTIC APTITUDE TEST, PROGRAM EVALUATION, TEST VALIDITY, CALIFORNIA, SOUTHWEST

ABST IN PROVIDING GREATER ACCESS TO CULTURALLY DIFFERENT STUDENTS, THE CLAREMONT COLLEGES IN CALIFORNIA HAVE DEVELOPED A PROGRAM DESIGNED TO IDENTIFY AND RECRUIT STUDENTS FROM DISADVANTAGED BACKGROUNDS AND TO PREPARE THEM TO COMPETE EQUALLY WITH STUDENTS WHO MEET THE TRADITIONAL ADMISSIONS CRITERIA. AN EVALUATION OF THE PROGRAM OF SPECIAL DIRECTED STUDIES FOR TRANSITION TO COLLEGE FOR 32 FEMALE AND 43 MALE MEXICAN AMERICAN STUDENTS WHO PARTICIPATED IN THE PROGRAM IS PRESENTED. MULTIPLE REGRESSION ANALYSIS REVEALED THAT NONTRADITIONAL PREDICTORS SUCH AS LOW INCOME, ENGLISH DIFFICULTY, BEING DENIED REGULAR COLLEGE ADMISSIONS, AND HIGH SCHOOL UNDERACHIEVEMENT WITH HIGH IQ ACCOUNTED FOR MORE VARIANCE IN 1ST YEAR COLLEGE SUCCESS THAN DID THE TRADITIONAL PREDICTORS OF THE SCHOLASTIC APTITUDE TEST AND HIGH SCHOOL GRADE AV-

ERAGES. 14 REFERENCES. (PASAR ABSTRACT MODIFIED)

ACCN   000923

1080 AUTH **LOYA, F.**
TITL   INCREASES IN CHICANO SUICIDE, DENVER, COLORADO: 1960-1975. WHAT CAN BE DONE?
SRCE   *PAPER PRESENTED AT THE ANNUAL MEETING OF THE AMERICAN ASSOCIATION OF SUICIDOLOGY, LOS ANGELES, 1976.*
INDX   MEXICAN AMERICAN, SUICIDE, CROSS CULTURAL, EMPIRICAL, SEX COMPARISON, ECONOMIC FACTORS, PSYCHOTHERAPY, COLORADO, SOUTHWEST, DEMOGRAPHIC
ABST   DEATHS CERTIFIED AS SUICIDE FOR THE CITY AND COUNTY OF DENVER, COLORADO, BETWEEN THE YEARS OF 1960 TO 1975 WERE EXAMINED WITH RESPECT TO ETHNICITY, SEX, AND AGE. THE SUICIDE RATE CALCULATED PER 100,000 FOR DENVER WAS ABOUT 20.1 FOR THE YEARS 1960 THRU 1969. HOWEVER, DURING 1970-75 THE RATE INCREASED TO 24.2 PERSONS WHICH WAS OVER DOUBLE THE TOTAL U.S. RATE OF SUICIDE INCREASE. DURING THE PERIOD BETWEEN 1960 TO 1975, CHICANO AND BLACK SUICIDE RATES HAVE BEEN INCREASING WHILE ANGLO SUICIDE RATES HAVE BEEN ON THE DECLINE. THE DENVER STATISTICS ALSO REVEALED THAT SUICIDE IS PREVALENT AMONG YOUNG CHICANOS AND BLACKS, MALES AND FEMALES. THESE RESULTS INDICATE ETHNICITY, AGE, AND SEX ARE IMPORTANT FACTORS IN THE SUICIDE RATE AND THAT PERHAPS BY TRAINING MORE CHICANOS IN THE AREA OF MENTAL HEALTH, SUICIDE PREVENTION CENTERS WOULD MORE ADEQUATELY DEAL WITH THE SERIOUSNESS OF THIS PROBLEM. 26 REFERENCES.

ACCN   000924

1081 AUTH **LOYA, F.**
TITL   SUICIDE RATE AMONG CHICANO YOUTHS IN DENVER, COLORADO: A STATISTICAL AND CULTURAL COMPARISON.
SRCE   *PAPER PRESENTED AT THE AMERICAN ASSOCIATION OF SUICIDOLOGY MEETING IN HOUSTON, TEXAS, 1973.*
INDX   SUICIDE, EMPIRICAL, MEXICAN AMERICAN, CROSS CULTURAL, SEX COMPARISON, CULTURAL FACTORS, FAMILY ROLES, TIME ORIENTATION, URBAN, ADOLESCENTS, ADULTS, DEMOGRAPHIC, CULTURAL CHANGE, COLORADO, SOUTHWEST, ACCULTURATION, STRESS
ABST   IN RESPONSE TO THE ALARMING RISE OF SUICIDE AMONG CHICANO YOUTHS, A STUDY EXAMINING THE DIFFERENCES OF SUICIDE RATES BETWEEN CHICANOS, ANGLOS AND BLACKS WAS CONDUCTED IN DENVER, COLORADO, FOR THE YEARS 1965 THROUGH 1972. THE DATA INDICATE THAT MALES COMMITTED MORE SUICIDES THAN FEMALES. DURING THE LAST PART OF THE 1960'S THE CHICANO RATE OF SUICIDE IN DENVER WAS 10.1 PERSONS PER 100,000 WHICH WAS COMPARABLE TO THE NATIONAL RATE. HOWEVER, DURING THE EARLY 1970'S THERE HAS BEEN AN INCREASE IN THE CHICANO SUICIDE RATE OF ABOUT 42 PERCENT, AN INCREASE WHICH FAR EXCEEDS

THAT RECORDED FOR ANGLOS AND BLACKS DURING THE SAME TIME PERIOD. WHAT APPEARS TO BE SIGNIFICANT IS THAT WHILE 70 PERCENT OF ALL CHICANO SUICIDES OCCURRED DURING THE YOUTHFUL YEARS, THE OCCURRENCE OF ANGLO SUICIDES FOR THE SAME AGE PERIOD WAS 30 PERCENT. SEVERAL SOCIOCULTURAL FACTORS SEEM TO BE RESPONSIBLE FOR THIS SUDDEN INCREASE OF SUICIDE RATES AMONG CHICANOS: (1) MORE MIGRATION OCCURRING FROM RURAL TO AN URBAN AREA; (2) MINORITY GROUP STATUS AND LANGUAGE BARRIERS; AND (3) CULTURAL DIFFERENCES WITH RESPECT TO FAMILY, TIME ORIENTATION, EDUCATION, AND BUSINESS ATTITUDES. IT IS CONCLUDED THAT THESE FACTORS CONTRIBUTE SIGNIFICANTLY TO A CULTURAL CONFLICT IN WHICH THE PSYCHOLOGICAL PRESSURES OF LIVING WITHIN TWO SETS OF VALUES AND WITHIN TWO SETS OF ROLE EXPECTATIONS ARE MORE SEVERE DURING ADOLESCENCE AND YOUNG ADULTHOOD AND THEREBY PROVIDE AN EXPLANATION TO THE INCREASE IN SUICIDE AMONG YOUNG CHICANOS. 5 REFERENCES.

ACCN   000925

1082 AUTH **LOYA, F.**
TITL   VICTIM-PRECIPITATED HOMICIDE: AN ALTERNATE METHOD OF SUICIDE AMONG BLACKS AND CHICANOS?
SRCE   *PAPER PRESENTED AT THE ANNUAL MEETING OF THE AMERICAN ASSOCIATION OF SUICIDOLOGY, JACKSONVILLE, FLORIDA, 1975.*
INDX   SUICIDE, MEXICAN AMERICAN, CROSS CULTURAL, CRIMINOLOGY, EMPIRICAL, DEMOGRAPHIC, CALIFORNIA, SOUTHWEST
ABST   WOLFGANG'S "VICTIM-PRECIPITATED HOMICIDE" HYPOTHESIS IS INDICATIVE OF A VICTIM ACTUALLY COMMITTING SUICIDE BY PROVOKING ANOTHER TO PERPETRATE THE KILLING. WHILE WOLFGANG DID NOT EXAMINE ETHNICITY INDEPENDENTLY, THIS STUDY GATHERED DATA ON ANGLOS, BLACKS, AND CHICANOS FROM THE LOS ANGELES COUNTY DISTRICT ATTORNEY'S OFFICE, PROBATION DEPARTMENT, AND THE CORORNER'S FILES. TO TEST THE HYPOTHESIS THAT PERSONS WHO INITIATE THEIR OWN HOMICIDE ARE SUICIDAL, AN INSTRUMENT WAS CONSTRUCTED OF DEMOGRAPHIC AND LIFE HISTORY ITEMS TO MEASURE SUICIDE RISK BETWEEN VICTIM-PRECIPITATED HOMICIDE VICTIMS, NON-VICTIM-PRECIPITATED HOMICIDE VICTIMS, AND SUICIDE VICTIMS. THE RESULTS FAILED TO SUPPORT WOLFGANG'S HYPOTHESIS. IT IS SUGGESTED THAT "VICTIM-PRECIPITATED HOMICIDE" MAY IN FACT RESIDE IN THE SUBCULTURE OF VIOLENCE AND NOT AS AN ETHNIC CHARACTERISTIC. 9 REFERENCES.

ACCN   000926

1083 AUTH **LUBCHANSKY, I., ERGI, G., & STOKES, J.**
TITL   PUERTO RICAN SPIRITUALISTS VIEW MENTAL ILLNESS: THE FAITH HEALER AS A PARAPROFESSIONAL.
SRCE   *AMERICAN JOURNAL OF PSYCHIATRY, 1970, 127(3), 312-321.*
INDX   MENTAL HEALTH, PSYCHOTHERAPY, PSYCHO-

INDX MENTAL HEALTH, PSYCHOTHERAPY, PSYCHO-
PATHOLOGY, FOLK MEDICINE, CASE STUDY,
PARAPROFESSIONALS, PUERTO RICAN-M, NEW
YORK, EAST, SURVEY, ATTITUDES, ESPIRITISMO

ABST AN EXAMINATION OF THE ATTITUDES AND BE-
LIEFS ABOUT MENTAL ILLNESS OF 20 PUERTO
RICAN FAITH HEALERS IN NEW YORK CITY IS
PRESENTED. TWENTY PRESIDENTS OF PUERTO
RICAN SPIRITUALIST TEMPLES IN THE BRONX
WERE INTERVIEWED USING A SEMISTRUC-
TURED INTERVIEW THAT FOCUSED ON ATTI-
TUDES TOWARD MENTAL ILLNESS AND THE
MENTALLY ILL. FOR COMPARISON, A SAMPLE
OF SPANISH-SPEAKING COMMUNITY LEADERS
AND A PROBABILITY SAMPLE THAT PROVIDED
A CROSS SECTION OF MALE PUERTO RICANS
AND THEIR WIVES WERE USED. DATA INDICATE
THAT PUERTO RICAN SPIRITUALISTS HAVE A
BROADER VIEW OF THE RANGE OF MENTAL
ILLNESS THAN DO COMMUNITY LEADERS AND
COMMUNITY RESIDENTS. SPIRITUALISTS TEND
TO RECOMMEND THEIR OWN SERVICES MORE
FREQUENTLY THAN THOSE OF OTHER PROFES-
SIONALS. NONE OF THE SPIRITUALISTS INTER-
VIEWED HAD COMPLETED HIGH SCHOOL,
WHEREAS 34 PERCENT OF THE PUERTO RICAN
CROSS SECTION RESPONDENTS HAD. SPIRI-
TUALISTS DESCRIBED EPISODES OF SEVERE
MENTAL STRESS THAT THEY HAD UNDERGONE
AND THE INSIGHT RESULTING FROM SUCH EX-
PERIENCES DIFFERENTIATED THEM FROM MOST
CROSS SECTION RESPONDENTS. IN ADDITION,
SPIRITUALISTS HAVE HIGHLY IDIOSYNCRATIC
CONCEPTIONS OF MENTAL ILLNESS. THEY ARE
ORIENTED TOWARD THE POSSIBILITY OF
CHANGE IN THE ILLNESS OVER TIME AND TO
THE POSSIBILITY OF INTERVENTION AND THE
AVOIDANCE OF CHRONICITY. CASE REPORTS
ARE PRESENTED TO ILLUSTRATE HOW SPIRI-
TUALISTS HANDLE THEIR CASES. SPIRITUAL-
ISTS SEEM TO APPROACH A PSYCHIATRIC MODE
OF THINKING TO A CONSIDERABLY GREATER
DEGREE THAN OTHER HEALERS. IN PRACTICE,
THERE ARE SIMILARITIES BETWEEN PROFES-
SIONAL PSYCHIATRIC TREATMENT AND SPIRI-
TUALISTS. 25 REFERENCES.

ACCN 000927

1084 AUTH **LUCKER, G. W., ROSENFIELD, D., SIKES, J., &
ARONSON, E.**

TITL PERFORMANCE IN THE INTERDEPENDENT
CLASSROOM: A FIELD STUDY.

SRCE *AMERICAN EDUCATIONAL RESEARCH JOUR-
NAL, 1976, 13(2), 115-123.*

INDX CHILDREN, CLASSROOM BEHAVIOR, CROSS
CULTURAL, EDUCATION, EDUCATIONAL AS-
SESSMENT, EMPIRICAL, INSTRUCTIONAL
TECHNIQUES, LEARNING, MEXICAN AMERI-
CAN, TEXAS, SOUTHWEST, COOPERATION

ABST TO COMPARE THE PERFORMANCES OF AN-
GLOS, BLACKS, AND MEXICAN AMERICANS
WORKING IN SMALL INTERDEPENDENT LEARN-
ING GROUPS WITH THEIR PERFORMANCE IN
TRADITIONAL, TEACHER FOCUSED CLASS-
ROOMS, 303 STUDENTS IN THE 5TH AND 6TH
GRADES WERE STUDIED BY PLACING HALF IN
TRADITIONAL CLASSROOM LEARNING SITUA-
TIONS AND THE OTHER HALF IN INTERDEPEN-

DENT JIGSAW GROUPS. IN A JIGSAW GROUP,
EACH STUDENT LEARNS A PORTION OF THE
MATERIAL AND THEN TEACHES HIS PORTION
TO FELLOW GROUP MEMBERS WHILE LEARN-
ING THE REMAINDER FROM THEM. A COVARI-
ANCE ANALYSIS INDICATES THAT WHILE AN-
GLOS PERFORM EQUALLY WELL IN BOTH
INTERDEPENDENT AND TRADITIONAL CLASSES,
MINORITIES PERFORM SIGNIFICANTLY BETTER
IN THE INTERDEPENDENT CLASSES THAN IN
TRADITIONAL CLASSES. IT IS SUGGESTED THAT
THROUGH THE JIGSAW GROUPS, THE MINORI-
TIES MAY HAVE GAINED SKILLS AND MOTIVA-
TIONS BY WORKING CLOSELY WITH ANGLOS,
AND THAT THE NEWLY LEARNED SKILLS MAY
ACCOUNT FOR THE IMPROVED PERFORM-
ANCE. 23 REFERENCES. (NCHHI ABSTRACT)

ACCN 002142

1085 AUTH **LUERA, L. D., & KAHN, M. W.**

TITL LIFE STRESS IN A BARRIO AREA POPULATION
AS RELATED TO CULTURAL CONTACT AND SE-
RIOUSNESS OF ILLNESS.

SRCE *UNPUBLISHED MANUSCRIPT, UNDATED. (AVAIL-
ABLE FROM DR. M. W. KAHN, DEPARTMENT OF
PSYCHOLOGY, UNIVERSITY OF ARIZONA, TUC-
SON, ARIZONA.)*

INDX ADULTS, BILINGUAL, CULTURAL FACTORS, DE-
MOGRAPHIC, EMPIRICAL, HEALTH, MEXICAN
AMERICAN, POVERTY, SES, URBAN, ARIZONA,
SOUTHWEST, STRESS, NEUROSIS, PSYCHOSO-
CIAL ADJUSTMENT

ABST LIFE STRESS EVENTS IN RELATIONSHIP TO
CULTURE AND ILLNESS WERE INVESTIGATED
IN PATIENTS AT A BARRIO NEIGHBORHOOD
HEALTH CENTER WHICH SERVES AN IMPOVER-
ISHED, PREDOMINATELY MEXICAN AMERICAN
POPULATION. THE 64 VOLUNTEER SUBJECTS,
ALL LOW-INCOME PATIENTS WITH SOMATIC
DISORDERS AND AGE 19 AND OVER, WERE
ASKED TO COMPLETE A QUESTIONNAIRE (19
DEMOGRAPHIC ITEMS PLUS 42 ITEMS OF THE
HOLMES-RAHE LIFE STRESS QUESTIONNAIRE)
AND INSTRUCTED TO INDICATE WHETHER EACH
STRESSFUL EVENT LISTED OCCURRED DUR-
ING THE PAST TWO YEARS. THE MEDICAL DI-
AGNOSIS FOR THAT DAY'S VISIT WAS SCALED
AND WEIGHTED ACCORDING TO THE SERIOUS-
NESS OF ILLNESS SCALE (WYLER) AND COR-
RELATED WITH THE LIFE STRESS SCORES.
BASED ON ALL 64 CASES, THE MEAN LIFE
STRESS SCORE OVER THE PRIOR 2 YEARS WAS
314.50—SUGGESTING THAT STRESS LEVELS
OF THIS TYPE POPULATION MAY BE HIGHER
THAN FOR OTHER GROUPS. THE STUDY FUR-
THER SUGGESTS THAT IT MAY BE THOSE MEM-
BERS OF THE LOWER SOCIOECONOMIC, PRE-
DOMINATELY MEXICAN AMERICAN GROUP WITH
THE MOST INTERACTION WITH THE PREDOMI-
NATE CULTURE WHO EXPERIENCE THE GREAT-
EST DEGREE OF LIFE STRESS. FINALLY, NO SIG-
NIFICANT RELATIONSHIP BETWEEN STRESS AND
THE SERIOUSNESS OF ILLNESS WAS FOUND,
THOUGH THIS MAY HAVE BEEN DUE PRIMARILY
TO THE RESTRICTED RANGE OF ILLNESSES
BEING TREATED. 12 REFERENCES.

ACCN 002143

1086 AUTH **LUETGERT, M. J., & GOLDBERG, L. H.**

TITL THE EXISTENTIAL RESOLUTION OF BI-CUL-TURAL CONFLICT: A CASE STUDY.

SRCE *PAPER PRESENTED AT THE XV INTERAMERICAN CONGRESS OF PSYCHOLOGY, BOGOTA, CO-LUMBIA, DECEMBER 14-19, 1974.*

INDX CASE STUDY, ACCULTURATION, PSYCHOTHER-APY, SELF CONCEPT, MALE, SPANISH SUR-NAMED, COLLEGE STUDENTS, MIDWEST, SEX ROLES, PERSONALITY, PSYCHOTHERAPY OUT-COME, STRESS

ABST THE CASE STUDY OF A MALE, SPANISH SUR-NAMED FIRST-YEAR COLLEGE STUDENT AT A MIDWESTERN UNIVERSITY IS PRESENTED. THE THERAPEUTIC MODEL, EXISTENTIAL PSY-CHOTHERAPY, WAS EVALUATED AS EXTREMELY SUCCESSFUL IN TREATING THIS YOUNG ADULT WHO DEMONSTRATED THESE PROBLEM AREAS: (1) NEED TO ACHIEVE UNREALISTICALLY HIGH GOALS; (2) CONCERNS ABOUT TRUSTING OTH-ERS AND ANXIETIES OVER SEXUAL IDENTITY, ADEQUACY AND PERFORMANCE; AND (3) NEED TO SEPARATE FROM FAMILY RESTRAINTS AND INTRUSIONS AND TO BECOME AN INDEPEN-DENTLY FUNCTIONING ADULT. THESE PROB-LEMS ARE DISCUSSED IN TERMS OF (1) THE PA-TIENTS' BICULTURAL CONFLICTS, (2) NORMAL ADOLESCENT DEVELOPMENT, AND (3) THE GOALS OF EXISTENTIAL THERAPY. EMPHA-SIZED IS THE PATIENT'S PERCEPTION OF "MACHISMO" AND THE THERAPEUTIC PRO-CESS INVOLVING THIS SELF-CONCEPT. THE EX-ISTENTIAL APPROACH TO THERAPY, WHICH FOCUSES ON CHOICES, ALTERNATIVES, AND PERSONAL RESPONSIBILITY, IS RECOM-MENDED FOR ASSISTING PERSONS WHOSE IDENTITY IS IN CONFLICT BETWEEN CULTURAL VALUE SYSTEMS, WHETHER THEY BE ETHNIC, SOCIOECONOMIC OR RELIGIOUS.

ACCN 000928

1087 AUTH **LUJAN, S. S., & ALEMAN, R.**

TITL EL CHAVALO DE LOS HIJOS DE MACEP. (THE GRANDCHILD OF MACEP.)

SRCE *TEXAS PERSONNEL AND GUIDANCE ASSOCIA-TION JOURNAL, 1973, 2(1), 23-30.*

INDX EDUCATIONAL COUNSELING, PROFESSIONAL TRAINING, BILINGUAL-BICULTURAL PERSON-NEL, CHILDREN, ADOLESCENTS, CURRICU-LUM, VOCATIONAL COUNSELING, MEXICAN AMERICAN, PROGRAM EVALUATION, RURAL, TEXAS, SOUTHWEST, ESSAY

ABST A ONE SEMESTER GUIDANCE AND COUNSEL-ING PROGRAM IN THE RURAL AREAS OF HI-DALGO COUNTY, TEXAS, IS EVALUATED. THE PROGRAM WAS CONDUCTED BY THE AU-THORS AFTER THEY HAD BEEN TRAINED AT THE FEDERALLY FUNDED MEXICAN AMERICAN COUNSELOR EDUCATION PROGRAM (MACEP) AND WAS DESIGNED TO PROVIDE EXPERI-ENCED BILINGUAL-BICULTURAL TEACHER-COUNSELORS TO SMALL RURAL SCHOOLS, WITH LARGE CONCENTRATIONS OF MEXICAN AMERICAN STUDENTS, THAT COULD NOT INDI-VIDUALLY AFFORD FULL-TIME COUNSELING AND GUIDANCE SERVICES. EACH AUTHOR WAS ASSIGNED TO 3 SCHOOLS INVOLVING A TOTAL OF 87 TEACHERS AND 2,200 CHILDREN IN KIN-DERGARTEN THROUGH 8TH GRADE. DIFFICUL-

TIES ENCOUNTERED ARE DISCUSSED. THE AU-THORS' APPRECIATION OF THE BICULTURAL CONFLICTS FELT BY THE STUDENTS IS EMPHA-SIZED. THE EVALUATION OF THIS PROGRAM SHOULD BE HELPFUL IN PLANNING OTHER COOPERATIVE COUNSELING PROGRAMS.

ACCN 000929

1088 AUTH **LUKENS, E.**

TITL FACTORS AFFECTING UTILIZATION OF MENTAL HEALTH SERVICES BY MEXICAN-AMERICANS (WORKING PAPER NO. 47).

SRCE *LOS ANGELES: WELFARE PLANNING COUNCIL, LOS ANGELES REGION, JUNE 1963.*

INDX HEALTH DELIVERY SYSTEMS, MENTAL HEALTH, MEXICAN AMERICAN, RESOURCE UTILIZATION, ACCULTURATION, EMPIRICAL, EXTENDED FAMILY, CALIFORNIA, SOUTHWEST, CULTURAL FACTORS

ABST TO IDENTIFY FACTORS WHICH OBSTRUCT OR AID THE MEXICAN AMERICAN IN USING MEN-TAL HEALTH SERVICES, 23 CASES INVOLVING MEXICAN AMERICAN CLIENTS RECEIVING SOME KIND OF SERVICES FROM 7 EAST LOS ANGE-LES COMMUNITY AGENCIES ARE REVIEWED. DATA WERE OBTAINED FROM INTERVIEWS WITH NURSES AND SOCIAL WORKERS WHO PER-CEIVED THAT THESE CLIENTS OR THEIR FAMILY MEMBERS NEEDED MENTAL HEALTH SER-VICES. SINCE THE STUDY WAS EXPLORATORY IN NATURE, DESCRIPTIVE STATISTICS WERE USED TO ANALYZE THE DATA. CLUES TO THE IDENTIFICATION OF UTILIZATION FACTORS FOUND IN THE STUDY WERE: (1) PATIENTS WHO UTILIZED MENTAL HEALTH SERVICES HAD BEEN BORN IN THE U.S. AND HAD RELATIVES WHO LIVED IN THE COUNTRY FOR LIFE OR MANY YEARS, WHILE PATIENTS BORN IN MEXICO WERE PREDOMINANTLY UNABLE TO ACCEPT THESE SERVICES; (2) PATIENTS WHO USED MENTAL HEALTH SERVICES HAD POSITIVE AT-TITUDES TOWARD GETTING HELP, WHILE UN-SUCCESSFUL CASES WERE CHARACTERIZED BY ATTITUDES REFLECTING NO AWARENESS OF THE SERIOUSNESS OF THEIR BEHAVIOR OR BELIEF THAT MEDICAL CARE WOULD RELIEVE THE SYMPTOMS; (3) SUCCESSFUL CASES TENDED TO HAVE HIGHER INCOMES AND MORE EDUCATION IN THE U.S.; (4) SUCCESSFUL CASES UNIFORMLY HAD ACTIVE ASSISTANCE, WHILE IN UNSUCCESSFUL CASES THE PATIENT WAS FREQUENTLY TOLD WHERE TO APPLY BUT FORMAL REFERRALS WERE NOT MADE, LAN-GUAGE PROBLEMS WERE NOT WORKED OUT, AND RELATIVES NOT INCLUDED IN THE PLAN-NING; AND (5) PROCEDURES AND PRACTICES OF THE AGENCIES WERE FOUND TO PLAY A PART IN OBSTRUCTING SUCCESSFUL USE OF MENTAL HEALTH SERVICES. SEVERAL SUG-GESTIONS FOR FURTHER RESEARCH AND CHANGES IN PRESENT AGENCY SERVICES ARE DISCUSSED. 28 REFERENCES.

ACCN 000930

1089 AUTH **LURIE, H. J., & LAWRENCE, G. L.**

TITL COMMUNICATION PROBLEMS BETWEEN RU-RAL MEXICAN-AMERICAN PATIENTS AND THEIR PHYSICIANS: DESCRIPTION OF A SOLUTION.

SRCE   *AMERICAN JOURNAL OF ORTHOPSYCHIATRY, 1972, 42(5), 777-783.*

INDX   PHYSICIANS, HEALTH DELIVERY SYSTEMS, RURAL, HEALTH, CULTURAL FACTORS, ROLE EXPECTATIONS, RELIGION, BILINGUAL-BICULTURAL PERSONNEL, ATTITUDES, WASHINGTON, WEST, NURSING, MEXICAN AMERICAN, REVIEW

ABST   POINTS OF CONFLICT BETWEEN MEXICAN AMERICAN (MA) PATIENTS AND THEIR PHYSICIANS INCLUDE: (1) THE HESITANCY OF MA'S TO REVEAL THEIR DEFICIENCIES IN ENGLISH; (2) THE DESIRE OF OLDER MA'S TO RETURN TO MEXICO IN CASE OF A SERIOUS ILLNESS; (3) THE RELUCTANCE OF MA HUSBANDS TO LEAVE THE EXAMINING ROOM DURING THEIR WIVES' OBSTETRICAL AND UROGENITAL EXAMINATIONS; (4) FREQUENT VISITING BY THE PATIENT'S FAMILY; AND (5) HESITANCY TO CONSULT A PHYSICIAN ABOUT EMOTIONAL PROBLEMS. THE LIMITED ATTENTION GIVEN BY PHYSICIANS TO HOSPITALIZED MA'S IS OFTEN INTERPRETED AS LACK OF INTEREST AND POSSIBLY PREJUDICE. TO BRIDGE THE GAP BETWEEN CULTURAL AND LANGUAGE DIFFERENCES, A GROUP OF PHYSICIANS IN THE YAKIMA VALLEY IN WASHINGTON STATE HAVE ENLISTED THE SERVICES OF AN MA TRANSLATOR-NURSE. THE ROLES OF THE TRANSLATOR-NURSE ARE: (1) TO ASSIST THE PATIENTS IN UNDERSTANDING THE TREATMENT PLAN; (2) TO SERVE AS A TRANSLATOR DURING PHYSICAL EXAMINATIONS; (3) TO LESSEN THE HUSBAND'S CONCERN ABOUT HIS WIFE'S OBSTETRICAL OR UROGENITAL EXAMINATION AND TO FACILITATE THE PHYSICIAN'S EXAMINATION; (4) TO PREPARE THE PATIENT AND FAMILY FOR HOSPITALIZATION OR POSSIBLE SURGICAL PROCEDURES; AND (5) TO ARRANGE PAYMENT FOR MEDICAL SERVICES. 4 REFERENCES.

ACCN   000931

1090 AUTH   **MACCOBY, M.**

TITL   ON MEXICAN NATIONAL CHARACTER.

SRCE   *IN N. N. WAGNER & M. J. HAUG (EDS.), CHICANOS: SOCIAL AND PSYCHOLOGICAL PERSPECTIVES. SAINT LOUIS: C. V. MOSBY COMPANY, 1971, PP. 123-131.*

INDX   MEXICO, MEXICAN, PERSONALITY, CULTURE, ADULTS, ESSAY, SEX ROLES, CULTURAL CHANGE, CULTURAL FACTORS, MACHISMO

ABST   MEXICAN AUTHORS HAVE LIMITED THEIR DESCRIPTION OF THE MEXICAN NATIONAL CHARACTER TO THE MESTIZO POPULATION OF THE CENTRAL PLATEAU. THEIR ANALYSES ARE OVERBURDENED WITH A SELF-DENIGRATIVE VIEW OF MEXICAN NATIONAL CHARACTER, STRESSING INFERIORITY FEELINGS STAMPED BY THE CONQUEST. MORE RECENTLY, MEXICAN PSYCHOANALYSTS HAVE FOCUSED ON THE CONQUEST AND SUBSEQUENT REVOLUTIONARY UPHEAVALS AS GENERATORS OF CONFLICT BETWEEN THE SEXES, WHICH THEY SEE AS THE MOST CRUCIAL DETERMINANT OF MEXICAN PSYCHOPATHOLOGY. THE MEXICAN MALE TRIES TO IMPOSE A PATRIARCHAL IDEAL, BUT HE IS CONSTANTLY UNDERMINED BY RESENTFUL WOMEN. ATTEMPTING TO ACT WITH AN AUTHORITY HE DOES NOT FEEL, THE MALE ASSUMES AN EXAGGERATED ROLE OF MASCULINITY (MACHISMO), BUT THE FEMALE, ESPECIALLY THE MOTHER, HOLDS THE REAL POWER IN THE FAMILY. ALTHOUGH EMPIRICAL STUDY CONFIRMS THE EXISTENCE OF THIS PATTERN, IT ALSO SHOWS THAT THESE WRITERS IGNORE THE LARGE PERCENTAGE OF MEXICANS WHO ARE WELL ADAPTED TO THEIR SOCIETY AND HAVE CHARACTER TRAITS COMMON TO PEASANTS THROUGHOUT THE WORLD. FURTHERMORE, SOCIOECONOMIC FACTORS WHICH CONTRIBUTE TO MALADAPTIVE CHARACTER STRUCTURES ARE UNDERPLAYED. IN MEXICO, THE CLASH BETWEEN HIGH IDEALS AND THE REALITY OF A DEVELOPING SOCIETY INTENSIFIES FEELINGS OF INFERIORITY WITH THE RESULT THAT MEXICANS UNDERVALUE THEIR CREATIVE ASPECTS AND THE PROGRESS THEY HAVE MADE SINCE THE SEMIFEUDAL SOCIETY CRUMBLED WITH THE 1910 REVOLUTION. 26 REFERENCES. (JOURNAL ABSTRACT)

ACCN   000932

1091 AUTH   **MACCOBY, M., MODIANO, N., & LANDER, P.**

TITL   GAMES AND SOCIAL CHARACTER IN A MEXICAN VILLAGE.

SRCE   *PSYCHIATRY, 1964, 27(2), 150-162.*

INDX   COOPERATION, COMPETITION, PERSONALITY, MEXICAN, COGNITIVE DEVELOPMENT, CHILDREN, EMPIRICAL, INTERPERSONAL RELATIONS, RURAL, CULTURE, SEX COMPARISON, MEXICO, MALE, FEMALE

ABST   IN AN EFFORT TO UNDERSTAND HOW SOCIAL CHARACTER IS FORMED IN A MEXICAN VILLAGE, BELIEFS AND ATTITUDES EXPRESSED AND REINFORCED THROUGH PLAY ARE ANALYZED. THE THREE METHODS USED TO INVESTIGATE GAMES WERE OBSERVATIONS, QUESTIONNAIRES, AND THE INTRODUCTION OF NEW GAMES. THE RESULTS ARE ANALYZED IN TERMS OF AGE, SEX, AND CULTURAL DIFFERENCES IN GAMES PLAYED. THE AGE VARIABLE SHOWS THAT AS THE CHILD GROWS UP, HE PROCEEDS FROM DRAMATIC PLAY, TO CENTRAL-PERSON GAMES, TO TEAM SPORTS. THE CENTRAL-PERSON GAMES DIFFER SIGNIFICANTLY IN CONTENT FROM THE WAY THEY ARE PLAYED IN INDUSTRIAL SOCIETIES. THE TEAM SPORTS ARE INNOVATIONS PLAYED ONLY BY PARTICULAR VILLAGERS. THE CENTRAL-PERSON GAMES OF BOYS LACK STRUCTURE, THEY ARE MORE VIOLENT AND THEY CONCEIVE OF AUTHORITY ONLY AS AN IRRATIONAL PUNISHING FORCE. GIRLS' GAMES USUALLY DEMAND A CIRCLE; THEY ARE MORE STRUCTURED AND ORDERLY THAN THOSE PLAYED BY BOYS. THE GIRLS TAKE TURNS BEING LEADER, THE NONLEADER PARTICIPANTS ACCEPT AUTHORITY BY NEITHER REBELING NOR FLEEING FROM THE SITUATION. THE CONTENT OF MOST GAMES FOR GIRLS REFERS TO DANGER FROM THE MALE WORLD. IN THE MEXICAN VILLAGE STUDIED, BOTH GAMES AND SOCIAL CHARACTER REFLECT CONSERVATION, AUTHORITY RELATIONS BRANDED BY THE FEUDAL PAST AND SEMIFEUDAL PRESENT, AND THE DISTRUST OF ALL INDIVIDUALISM AS A THREAT TO THE STA-

TUS QUO. IN RELATION TO THE NEW GAME IN-
TRODUCED, BOTH BOYS AND GIRLS DIS-
TORTED THE GAME TO CONFORM TO THEIR
ATTITUDES TOWARD AUTHORITY AND TO THE
FORMAL STRUCTURE OF THE CENTRAL-PER-
SON GAMES THEY NORMALLY PLAY. THUS IT
APPEARS THAT NEW GAMES WILL NOT RE-
FORM CHARACTER AND SOCIETY, BUT THEY
DO SUPPORT THE PROCESS OF CULTURE
CHANGE. 21 REFERENCES.

ACCN   000933

1092 AUTH   **MACIAS, R. F.**
TITL   U.S. HISPANICS IN 2000 A. D.—PROJECTING
THE NUMBER.
SRCE   *AGENDA, MAY/JUNE 1977, PP. 16-19.*
INDX   SPANISH SURNAMED, CENSUS, DEMO-
GRAPHIC, FERTILITY, IMMIGRATION, REVIEW,
MEXICAN, MEXICAN AMERICAN, PUERTO RI-
CAN-M, UNDOCUMENTED WORKERS, CALI-
FORNIA, NEW YORK, TEXAS, ILLINOIS, NEW
JERSEY, FLORIDA, NEW MEXICO, COLORADO,
ARIZONA, SOUTH, SOUTHWEST, MIDWEST, EAST
ABST   FACTORS INFLUENCING THE GROWTH OF THE
U.S. LATINO POPULATION AND THE IMPLICA-
TIONS OF THAT GROWTH ARE CONSIDERED IN
A REVIEW OF DEMOGRAPHIC PROJECTIONS
OF THE LATINO POPULATION FOR THE YEAR
2000. REGARDING POPULATION ESTIMATES AT
PRESENT FOR LATINOS, FIGURES RANGE BE-
TWEEN 11.2 AND 23.4 MILLION. THIS LARGE
VARIATION IS DUE TO UNCERTAINTY CON-
CERNING THE NUMBER OF LATINO UNDOCU-
MENTED IMMIGRANTS AS WELL AS DEFICIEN-
CIES IN THE CENSUS BUREAU'S IDENTIFICATION
OF THE LATINO POPULATION. NOT UNTIL 1980
WILL THE CENSUS BUREAU MAKE, FOR THE
FIRST TIME, A DIRECT COUNT OF THE SPANISH
ORIGIN POPULATION. REGARDING THE PRO-
JECTED GROWTH OF THE LATINO POPULA-
TION, THE FACT THAT LATINO FAMILY SIZE IS
LARGER THAN THE NATIONAL AVERAGE AND
THAT THE LATINO MEDIAN AGE IS EIGHT YEARS
LOWER THAN THE NATIONAL AVERAGE MEANS
THAT THERE IS A PROPORTIONALLY LARGER
NUMBER OF LATINOS WHO WILL HAVE LARGER
FAMILIES OVER THE NEXT DECADE. BY THE
YEAR 2000 IT IS ESTIMATED THAT THERE WILL
BE AT LEAST 17.5 MILLION AND PERHAPS AS
MANY AS 55.3 MILLION LATINOS IN THE U.S.
(GROWTH RATES OF 6.7% AND 21% ANNUALLY,
RESPECTIVELY). THESE PROJECTIONS, HOW-
EVER, MUST BE ACCEPTED WITH CAUTION BE-
CAUSE THEY ASSUME (1) A CONSTANT RATE
OF NATURAL INCREASE, (2) NO ADDITIONAL IN
OR OUT MIGRATION OF LATINOS, AND (3) NO
SIGNIFICANT ADDITIONS TO THE TOTAL U.S.
POPULATION. IN CONCLUSION, THE CHANGES
IMPLIED BY THE GROWTH OF THE U.S. LATINO
POPULATION CAN BE EXPECTED TO PRO-
FOUNDLY AFFECT THE SOCIAL FABRIC OF THE
COUNTRY. 4 REFERENCES.

ACCN   002144

1093 AUTH   **MACIAS, R. F., FLORES, G. V., FIGUEROA, D.,
& ARAGON, L.**
TITL   A STUDY OF UNINCORPORATED EAST LOS AN-
GELES (MONOGRAPH NO. 3).

SRCE   *LOS ANGELES: AZTLAN PUBLICATIONS, UNI-
VERSITY OF CALIFORNIA, 1973.*
INDX   MEXICAN AMERICAN, URBAN, POLITICS, PO-
LITICAL POWER, COMMUNITY INVOLVEMENT,
HOUSING, SES, POVERTY, EMPIRICAL, ENVI-
RONMENTAL FACTORS, SCHOLASTIC ACHIEVE-
MENT, DELINQUENCY, CALIFORNIA, SOUTH-
WEST, BOOK
ABST   GENERAL DATA AND PRINTED MATERIALS ON
AND FROM THE AREAS OF UNINCORPORATED
EAST LOS ANGELES (ELA) AND OF CONTIG-
UOUS, PREDOMINANTLY CHICANO NEIGHBOR-
HOODS ARE PRESENTED IN ORDER TO DETER-
MINE THE FEASIBILITY OF THE INCORPORATION
OF ANY OR ALL OF THE STUDY AREA. DATA
WERE GATHERED THROUGH THE 1960 U.S.
CENSUS, THE 1965 SPECIAL CENSUS ON ELA,
REPORTS ON PRIOR INCORPORATION AT-
TEMPTS, AND PERSONAL INTERVIEWS WITH
POLITICAL FIGURES FOR AND AGAINST INCOR-
PORATION. AN EXAMINATION OF THE LOCAL
AGENCY FORMATION COMMISSION (LAFCO) IS
PROVIDED IN ORDER TO DESCRIBE THE IN-
CORPORATION PROCESS; LEGAL PROCE-
DURES ARE OUTLINED. SOCIO-DEMOGRAPHIC
DATA ARE PROVIDED ON SIZE OF THE POPU-
LATION, HOUSING CHARACTERISTICS, LAND
USE, TAX STRUCTURE, EDUCATION, POLITICAL
JURISDICTIONS, HEALTH NEEDS, AND VOTER
REGISTRATION. INCORPORATION OF ELA AS A
CITY WITHIN THE COUNTY IS SEEN AS A BET-
TER ALTERNATIVE THAN ANNEXATION TO A
SURROUNDING CITY. IMPLICATIONS OF INCOR-
PORATION AND RECOMMENDATION FOR ITS
IMPLEMENTATION ARE DISCUSSED THRO-
ROUGHLY. 39 REFERENCES.

ACCN   000934

1094 AUTH   **MACIEL, D. R., & PADILLA, A. M.**
TITL   THE NATIONAL CHARACTER OF MEXICO: MYTH
OR REALITY.
SRCE   *THE PACIFIC COAST COUNCIL OF LATIN AMERI-
CAN STUDIES PROCEEDINGS, SAN DIEGO, 1974,
3, 9-18.*
INDX   PERSONALITY, CULTURE, MEXICO, MEXICAN,
RESEARCH METHODOLOGY, ESSAY, MALE, HIS-
TORY, SEX ROLES, PROCEEDINGS, CULTURAL
FACTORS, REVIEW
ABST   SEVERAL ASPECTS OF MEXICAN NATIONAL
CHARACTER STUDIES ARE ADDRESSED: (1)
HOW MEXICAN WRITERS HAVE TREATED THE
QUESTION OF THEIR NATIONAL CHARACTER;
(2) ANALYSES OF METHODOLOGIES USED IN
THE STUDY OF MEXICAN NATIONAL CHARAC-
TER; AND (3) A LITERATURE REVIEW DIRECTED
AT THE QUESTION "IS MEXICAN NATIONAL
CHARACTER A MYTH OR REALITY?" THE LIT-
ERATURE REVEALS A GENERAL TENDENCY TO
DESCRIBE A STEREOTYPE MEXICANO MALE AS
POSSESSING A LATENT CAPACITY FOR VIO-
LENCE, A NEED TO MANIFEST MALE SUPERI-
ORITY AND DOMINANCE THROUGH SEXUAL
CONQUEST, AND HYPERSENSITIVITY TO IN-
SULT. METHODOLOGICAL STUDIES USUALLY
CONCLUDE THAT HISTORICAL FACTORS HAVE
CONTRIBUTED TO THE UNPRODUCTIVE-RE-
CEPTIVE CHARACTER OF THE MEXICAN MALE.
HOWEVER, THESE STUDIES CONTAIN NUMER-

OUS METHODOLOGICAL WEAKNESSES AND THEREFORE LEAVE THEMSELVES OPEN TO CRITICISMS OF BIAS. IT IS CONCLUDED THAT THE FAILURE TO DEMONSTRATE THE EXISTENCE OF A UNITARY SET OF CHARACTER TRAITS TO DESCRIBE THE MEXICAN STEMS FROM PROBLEMS OF GENERALIZATION, SPECULATION, LIMITED SCOPE, AND DEFINITION. MEXICO REPRESENTS A COMPLEX HETEROGENOUS SOCIETY AND THEREFORE IT BECOMES DIFFICULT TO ACCOUNT FOR ALL THE FACTORS INVOLVED IN ASCERTAINING THE NATIONAL CHARACTER. IT IS FELT THAT PERHAPS REGIONAL STUDIES WILL PROVIDE NEW INFORMATION ON EL MEXICANO. 18 REFERENCES.

ACCN   000935

1095 AUTH   **MACMILLAN, R. W.**
TITL   A STUDY ON THE EFFECT OF SOCIOECONOMIC FACTORS ON THE SCHOOL ACHIEVEMENT OF SPANISH SPEAKING SCHOOL BEGINNERS (DOCTORAL DISSERTATION, UNIVERSITY OF TEXAS AT AUSTIN, 1966).
SRCE   *DISSERTATION ABSTRACTS, 1967, 27(10), 3229A. (UNIVERSITY MICROFILMS NO. 67-03327.)*
INDX   SES, BILINGUALISM, CHILDREN, SCHOLASTIC ACHIEVEMENT, EDUCATION, FAMILY ROLES, EMPIRICAL, GOODENOUGH DRAW-A-MAN TEST, ENVIRONMENTAL FACTORS, CROSS CULTURAL, INTELLIGENCE, TEXAS, SOUTHWEST
ABST   A MODEL OF INQUIRY WAS DESIGNED TO TEST THE CORRELATION BETWEEN CERTAIN SOCIOECONOMIC VARIABLES AND SCHOOL ACHIEVEMENT OF SPANISH-SPEAKING 1ST GRADERS IN SAN ANTONIO, TEXAS. FOR ANALYSES OF THESE VARIABLES AS PREDICTORS OF ACHIEVEMENT AND ATTENDANCE, 305 MEXICAN CHILDREN WERE USED; 5 MEXICAN AMERICAN, 4 NEGRO, AND 3 ANGLO SCHOOLS WERE ALSO USED IN TESTING THE CORRELATION BETWEEN ETHNIC GROUP MEMBERSHIP AND ATTENDANCE. RESULTS OF ANALYSES, USING MULTIPLE LINEAR REGRESSION TECHNIQUES, WERE (1) THAT INDEPENDENT VARIABLES OF PARENT'S OCCUPATION, CHILD'S SCHOOL ATTENDANCE, PRESCHOOL EXPERIENCE, IQ, AND PRETEST SCORES WERE SIGNIFICANT ACHIEVEMENT PREDICTORS AND THAT, COMBINED, THE VARIABLES OF PARENT'S OCCUPATION, FAMILY SIZE AND ORGANIZATION, PRESCHOOL EXPERIENCE, PUPIL'S SEX, AND SCHOOL ATTENDANCE WERE MORE SIGNIFICANT ACHIEVEMENT PREDICTORS THAN WAS IQ; (2) THAT NONE OF THE FOREGOING INDEPENDENT VARIABLES WAS A SIGNIFICANT ATTENDANCE PREDICTOR; AND (3) THAT ANALYSIS OF ATTENDANCE IN RELATION TO ETHNIC GROUP MEMBERSHIP, USING TEMPERATURE AND PRECIPITATION AS CONCOMITANT VARIABLES, INDICATED THAT WEATHER HAS A MORE NEGATIVE EFFECT ON ATTENDANCE OF MEXICAN AMERICANS AND NEGROES THAN OF ANGLOS—PROBABLY DUE TO LACK OF PROPER CLOTHING AND MEDICAL CARE. ADDITIONALLY, A DEMOGRAPHIC STUDY WAS DONE ON SPANISH SURNAMED FAMILIES IN THE SOUTHWEST. RESULTS INDICATED MEXICAN AMERI-

CANS TO BE SOCIOECONOMICALLY BELOW ANGLOS AND NEGROES AND IN DANGER OF FALLING FURTHER BEHIND. 70 REFERENCES. (RIE ABSTRACT)

ACCN   000936

1096 AUTH   **MACPHERSON, D. P.**
TITL   THE ROLE OF NEW CAREERISTS.
SRCE   *YOUTH AUTHORITY QUARTERLY, 1970, 23(3), 31-35.*
INDX   CORRECTIONS, PRIMARY PREVENTION, CRIMINOLOGY, ADOLESCENTS, ADULTS, MEXICAN AMERICAN, ESSAY, COMMUNITY, COMMUNITY INVOLVEMENT, PERSONNEL, CALIFORNIA, SOUTHWEST, EMPLOYMENT, JOB PERFORMANCE, REHABILITATION, PROGRAM EVALUATION
ABST   ONE OF THE LARGEST NEW CAREER PROGRAMS IN ANY CORRECTIONAL AGENCY IS ADMINISTERED BY THE LOS ANGELES COUNTY PROBATION DEPARTMENT. ALMOST 100 AIDES FROM THE NEIGHBORHOOD ADULT PARTICIPATION PROJECT WERE TRANSFERRED TO WORK IN PERMANENT NEW CAREER POSITIONS WITHIN THE CIVIL SERVICE SYSTEM AS COMMUNITY WORKERS. THEY PERFORM A WIDE VARIETY OF FUNCTIONS AND TASKS, FROM TRANSPORTING CHILDREN AND FAMILIES TO JUVENILE COURT TO MORE COMPLEX RESPONSIBILITIES SUCH AS SERVING AS CO-LEADER WITH THE PROFESSIONAL PROBATION OFFICER IN FAMILY OR PEER GROUP COUNSELING SESSIONS. THE FACT THAT MANY OF THE NEW CAREERISTS ARE THEMSELVES EX-OFFENDERS CONTRIBUTES TO THEIR ABILITY TO RELATE EFFECTIVELY WITH PROBATION CLIENTS. MOREOVER, A SPECIAL MANPOWER PROGRAM IN THE MEXICAN AMERICAN COMMUNITY OF LOS ANGELES HAS PROVIDED A MUCH NEEDED MANPOWER RESOURCE TO THE DEPARTMENT. ALL OF THIS PROMISING WORK IN RECRUITING, SELECTING, TRAINING, ASSIGNING, AND COORDINATING THE WORK OF THE NEW CAREERISTS IS THE RESPONSIBILITY OF A SMALL GROUP OF PROFESSIONAL STAFF IN THE MANPOWER DEVELOPMENT UNIT.

ACCN   000937

1097 AUTH   **MADSEN, M. C.**
TITL   DEVELOPMENTAL AND CROSS-CULTURAL DIFFERENCES IN THE COOPERATIVE AND COMPETITION BEHAVIOR OF YOUNG CHILDREN.
SRCE   *JOURNAL OF CROSS-CULTURAL PSYCHOLOGY, 1971, 2(4), 365-371.*
INDX   COOPERATION, COMPETITION, INTERPERSONAL RELATIONS, CROSS CULTURAL, EMPIRICAL, MEXICAN, COGNITIVE DEVELOPMENT, CHILDREN, CALIFORNIA, SOUTHWEST
ABST   A TWO-PERSON EXPERIMENTAL TASK DEVELOPED FOR USE IN THE STUDY OF AGE AND CULTURAL DIFFERENCES IN THE COOPERATIVE-COMPETITIVE BEHAVIOR OF CHILDREN IS DESCRIBED. ONE HUNDRED TWELVE CHILDREN, 40 FROM A SMALL MEXICAN TOWN AND 72 FROM LOS ANGELES, CA., AGED 4-11 YEARS, WERE TOLD TO PLAY A GAME IN WHICH THEY CAN GET MARBLES (MARBLE-PULL GAME).

THE NUMBER OF MARBLES OBTAINED PROVIDED A MEASURE OF COOPERATIVE OR COMPETITIVE BEHAVIOR. THE RESULTS INDICATE A HIGHER LEVEL OF COOPERATION AMONG MEXICAN THAN ANGLO AMERICAN CHILDREN AND AN INCREASE IN NONADAPTIVE COMPETITION WITH AGE AMONG THE ANGLO CHILDREN. FINDINGS ARE DISCUSSED IN TERMS OF PIAGETIAN DEVELOPMENT. 7 REFERENCES. (JOURNAL ABSTRACT MODIFIED)

ACCN   000938

1098 AUTH **MADSEN, M. C., & SHAPIRA, A.**
TITL   COOPERATIVE AND COMPETITIVE BEHAVIOR OF URBAN AFRO-AMERICAN, ANGLO-AMERICAN, MEXICAN-AMERICAN, AND MEXICAN VILLAGE CHILDREN.
SRCE   *DEVELOPMENTAL PSYCHOLOGY, 1970, 3(1), 16-20.*
INDX   COOPERATION, COMPETITION, INTERPERSONAL RELATIONS, CROSS CULTURAL, EMPIRICAL, RURAL, URBAN, MEXICAN AMERICAN, SEX COMPARISON, MEXICAN, CHILDREN, ENVIRONMENTAL FACTORS, CALIFORNIA, SOUTHWEST
ABST   CHILDREN OF THREE CALIFORNIA ETHNIC GROUPS EQUALLY REPRESENTED WITH 48 SUBJECTS (24 OF EACH SEX, AGES 7 TO 9) PARTICIPATED IN THREE EXPERIMENTS ON THE COOPERATION BOARD DEVELOPED BY MADSEN. IN EXPERIMENT I, MEXICAN AMERICAN (MA) MALES WERE FOUND TO BE LESS COMPETITIVE THAN MA FEMALES AND AFRO AND ANGLO AMERICANS OF BOTH SEXES. IN EXPERIMENT II, ALL THREE ETHNIC GROUPS BEHAVED IN A HIGHLY COMPETITIVE MANNER. IN EXPERIMENT III, A SAMPLE OF 40 MEXICAN VILLAGE CHILDREN AGES 7 TO 9 BEHAVED COOPERATIVELY WHILE SUBJECTS FROM EXPERIMENTS I AND II BEHAVED IN A NONADAPTIVE MANNER. THE RESULTS IN EXPERIMENT III INDICATE A DRAMATIC DIFFERENCE BETWEEN THE UNITED STATES AND MEXICAN VILLAGE CHILDREN. THE OFTEN AGGRESSIVE, WILD SHOUTING MATCHES AMONG CHILDREN IN THE UNITED STATES WERE IN TOTAL CONTRAST TO THE RATHER SLOW, QUIET, AND DELIBERATELY COOPERATIVE BEHAVIOR OF THE MEXICAN CHILDREN. IT IS NOTED THAT IN AN EARLIER STUDY, URBAN CHILDREN IN MEXICO PERFORMED ON THE COOPERATION BOARD IN MUCH THE SAME MANNER AS THE COMPETITIVE GROUPS IN THE UNITED STATES. THE COOPERATIVE BEHAVIOR OF MEXICAN VILLAGE CHILDREN REPRESENTS A SPECIFIC SUBCULTURAL RATHER THAN A BROAD NATIONAL CHARACTERISTIC. 5 REFERENCES. (JOURNAL ABSTRACT MODIFIED)
ACCN   000939

1099 AUTH **MADSEN, W.**
TITL   THE ALCOHOLIC AGRINGADO.
SRCE   *AMERICAN ANTHROPOLOGIST, 1964, 66(2), 355-361.*
INDX   ALCOHOLISM, ACCULTURATION, MEXICAN AMERICAN, ADULTS, EMPIRICAL, PSYCHOPATHOLOGY, CULTURAL FACTORS, TEXAS, SOUTHWEST

ABST   A SOCIOCULTURAL ENVIRONMENT WHICH TENDS TO PRODUCE A HIGH PROPORTION OF PROBLEM DRINKERS AMONG THE AGRINGADOS (AN ACCULTURATED MEXICAN AMERICAN) OF SOUTH TEXAS IS ANALYZED. THE ANALYSIS WAS BASED ON DATA COLLECTED BY THE RESEARCH STAFF OF THE HIDALGO PROJECT ON DIFFERENTIAL CULTURE CHANGE AND MENTAL HEALTH. THE CULTURAL SETTING OF THE AGRINGADO INVOLVES VALUE CONFLICTS RESULTING IN LOSS OF IDENTITY AND COMMUNITY—A LOSS WHICH SEEMS TO FOSTER ALCOHOLISM. THIS IS PARTICULARLY TRUE WHEN THE INDIVIDUAL HAS BEEN EXPOSED TO THE TRADITION THAT ALCOHOL MAY FUNCTION AS AN ESCAPE MECHANISM. IT IS POSSIBLE THAT IN MANY OF THESE ALCOHOLICS THERE IS EITHER A CONSCIOUS OR AN UNCONSCIOUS REALIZATION THAT THE MEANS ARE LACKING TO ACHIEVE DESIRED GOALS. THE ALCOHOLIC PERSONALITY FREQUENTLY LACKS INTEGRATION AND A RATIONAL ORIENTATION TO SOCIAL REALITY. ANY THERAPY THAT IS CONCERNED WITH ALCOHOLICS WHO HAVE VALUE CONFLICTS MUST TAKE INTO ACCOUNT THE SOCIOCULTURAL VARIABLES INVOLVED. UNFORTUNATELY, SUCH THERAPY RARELY EXISTS FOR THE CONSERVATIVE MEXICAN AMERICAN OR THE AGRINGADO. 1 REFERENCE.
ACCN   000940

1100 AUTH **MADSEN, W.**
TITL   ANXIETY AND WITCHCRAFT IN MEXICAN AMERICAN ACCULTURATION.
SRCE   *ANTHROPOLOGY QUARTERLY, 1966, 39(2), 110-127.*
INDX   CURANDERISMO, FOLK MEDICINE, ACCULTURATION, MEXICAN AMERICAN, ANXIETY, ESSAY, PSYCHOPATHOLOGY, MENTAL HEALTH, CULTURAL FACTORS, TEXAS, SOUTHWEST, THEORETICAL, STRESS, VALUES
ABST   THE PREVALENCE OF WITCHCRAFT FEAR APPEARS TO BE ONE INDEX OF THE EMOTIONAL STRESS ACCOMPANYING ACCULTURATION AMONG THE MEXICAN AMERICANS (MA) IN SOUTH TEXAS. ANALYSIS OF THREE CASE STUDIES, INVOLVING INDIVIDUALS OF VARYING DEGREES OF ACCULTURATION IN HIDALGO COUNTY, INDICATES THAT WITCHCRAFT BELIEF PERFORMS THE FOLLOWING FUNCTIONS: (1) IT PROVIDES SOCIAL SANCTIONS AGAINST THE ADOPTION OF ANGLO VALUES, GOALS, AND BEHAVIORAL PATTERNS WHICH THREATEN COHESION OF MA FOLK SOCIETY; (2) IT PROVIDES THE DEVIANT MEMBER OF THE FOLK SOCIETY WITH A SOCIALLY ACCEPTED EXPLANATION FOR HIS FAILURE TO UPHOLD THE STANDARDS OF LA RAZA; AND (3) IT PROVIDES THE INGLESADO (ANGLICIZED MA) WITH A RATIONALIZATION FOR HIS FAILURE IN THE ANGLO WORLD AND A MEANS OF REENTRY INTO FOLK SOCIETY. THESE INTERPRETATIONS ARE RESTATED IN TERMS OF DISSONANCE THEORY. COGNITIVE DISSONANCE ARISES WHEN THE MA PURSUES THE ANGLO GOALS OF ECONOMIC ADVANCEMENT, CONSPICUOUS CON-

SUMPTION, AND SELF-BETTERMENT WITHOUT REFERENCE TO FAMILY OR FOLK TRADITION. THE DISSONANCE BETWEEN ANGLICIZED BEHAVIOR AND MA VALUES PRODUCES ANXIETY AND A FEAR OF RETALIATION BY WITCHCRAFT. DISSONANCE IS REDUCED WHEN THE DEVIANT MEMBER CHANGES HIS BEHAVIOR TO CONFORM TO TRADITIONAL MA CONCEPTS OF PROPRIETY OR WHEN A RATIONALIZATION FOR PSYCHIC STRESS CAN BE FOUND IN THE LATINO THEORY OF WITCHCRAFT. FURTHER REDUCTION OF DISSONANCE IS ACHIEVED BY SEEKING THE SOCIAL SUPPORT WHICH ACCOMPANIES TREATMENT FOR BEWITCHMENT BY A FOLK CURER. BY ADMITTING BELIEF IN WITCHCRAFT AND CONSULTING A CURANDERO, THE INDIVIDUAL EXHIBITS BEHAVIOR CONSONANT WITH MA VALUES. 9 REFERENCES.

ACCN   000941

1101 AUTH   **MADSEN, W.**
TITL   THE MEXICAN-AMERICANS OF SOUTH TEXAS. (2ND ED.)
SRCE   *NEW YORK: HOLT, RINEHART & WINSTON, 1973.*
INDX   MEXICAN AMERICAN, CULTURE, ACCULTURATION, TEXAS, SOUTHWEST, RURAL, URBAN, ECONOMIC FACTORS, CULTURAL FACTORS, MENTAL HEALTH, FAMILY STRUCTURE, FAMILY ROLES, RELIGION, HEALTH, CURANDERISMO, EMPIRICAL, MARRIAGE, POLITICS, SES, PREJUDICE, FARM LABORERS, FOLK MEDICINE, PSYCHOTHERAPY, SOCIAL STRUCTURE, SOCIAL MOBILITY, VALUES
ABST   PARTICIPANT-OBSERVATION FIELDWORK FROM 1957 TO 1960 IN FOUR COMMUNITIES IN SOUTH TEXAS (RANGING FROM RURAL TO URBAN) PROVIDED THE BASIS FOR THIS ETHNOGRAPHIC ACCOUNT OF MEXICAN AMERICANS' (MA) LIFESTYLE, ACCULTURATION, AND MENTAL HEALTH. THE SET OF 12 CHAPTERS BEGINS WITH AN HISTORICAL AND ECONOMIC OVERVIEW OF THE REGION, AN ANALYSIS OF THE CULTURE CONFLICT BETWEEN THE MA AND ANGLO POPULATIONS, AND THEN A DESCRIPTION OF THE MA'S WORLD VIEW. NEXT, A DISTINCTION IS MADE BETWEEN THREE MA SUBGROUPS, VARYING BY SES AND LEVEL OF ACCULTURATION: (1) THE LOWER CLASS, STEEPED IN MEXICAN FOLK CULTURE; (2) THE MIDDLE CLASS, CAUGHT UP IN A VALUE CONFLICT BETWEEN TWO CULTURES; AND (3) THE UPPER CLASS, ACHIEVING STATUS AND AND SUCCESS IN THE DOMINANT, ENGLISH-SPEAKING SOCIETY. DETAILED DESCRIPTIONS OF THESE THREE SUBGROUPS INCLUDE CASE HISTORIES OF TYPICAL INDIVIDUALS, RANGING FROM THE NEWLY ARRIVED BRACERO TO MEMBERS OF THE ELITIST UPPER CLASS. THE SUBSEQUENT CHAPTERS ATTEND TO (1) MA FAMILY STRUCTURE, ROLES, AND VALUES, (2) RELIGION, (3) HEALTH, INCLUDING FOLK MEDICINE BELIEFS, (4) WITCHCRAFT, (5) CURANDERISMO, (6) FOLK PSYCHOTHERAPY, AND (7) EDUCATION AND POLITICS. THE CONCLUDING MESSAGE IS THAT DISCRIMINATION AND VALUE CONFLICTS HAVE HAD DELETERIOUS EFFECTS ON THE MENTAL HEALTH OF THE MA POPULA-

TION, YET THERE IS HOPE IN THEIR NEW, POSITIVE IDENTITY AS "LA RAZA" AND THEIR EMERGING POLITICAL ACTIVISM. 8 REFERENCES.

ACCN   001747

1102 AUTH   **MADSEN, W.**
TITL   SOCIETY AND HEALTH IN THE LOWER RIO GRANDE VALLEY.
SRCE   *AUSTIN: HOGG FOUNDATION FOR MENTAL HEALTH, 1961.*
INDX   STEREOTYPES, PSYCHOPATHOLOGY, ACCULTURATION, PERSONALITY, SEX ROLES, SOCIALIZATION, SES, FAMILY ROLES, FAMILY STRUCTURE, FICTIVE KINSHIP, HEALTH, MENTAL HEALTH, FOLK MEDICINE, PHYSICIANS, CURANDERISMO, ESSAY, TEXAS, SOUTHWEST, HEALTH DELIVERY SYSTEMS, POLICY
ABST   AN INVESTIGATION OF THE FOLK CUSTOMS, SOCIAL ORGANIZATION, MEDICAL PRACTICES, AND BELIEFS OF THE MEXICAN AMERICAN (MA) IN SOUTH TEXAS SHEDS CONSIDERABLE LIGHT UPON THE PROBLEMS OF MENTAL HEALTH AND ILLNESS. IMPROVEMENT OF HEALTH FACILITIES AND PRACTICES PRESENTS THE TWOFOLD PROBLEM OF GAINING MA ACCEPTANCE OF SCIENTIFIC MEDICINE WITHOUT DISRUPTING THE SOCIAL ORGANIZATION AND CREATING UNNECESSARY TENSION. SPECIFIC RECOMMENDATIONS FOR AN INTEGRATED PROGRAM OF HEALTH SERVICE AMONG THE MA POPULATION ARE LISTED AS FOLLOWS: (1) IMPROVE COMMUNICATION BETWEEN HEALTH WORKERS AND MA PATIENTS BY MAKING A CONCERTED EFFORT TO OVERCOME THE LANGUAGE BARRIER; (2) INCREASE KNOWLEDGE AND UNDERSTANDING OF MA FOLK CULTURE AMONG HEALTH AND WELFARE PERSONNEL; (3) IMPROVE THE PHYSICAL APPEARANCE OF THE CLINICS, MAKING THEM MORE ATTRACTIVE TO MA'S SO THAT THEY WILL ASSOCIATE MODERN HEALTH SERVICES WITH PLEASANT SURROUNDINGS; (4) SHOW RESPECT FOR MA BELIEFS ABOUT HEALTH INSTEAD OF RIDICULING THEM AS "SUPERSTITIOUS; (5) COMBAT THE NOTION THAT CLINIC PATIENTS ARE ACCEPTING CHARITY; (6) ESTABLISH FRIENDLY DOCTOR-PATIENT AND NURSE-PATIENT RELATIONSHIPS IN PLACE OF THE AUTHORITARIAN RELATIONSHIP THAT NOW EXISTS; (7) DEAL WITH THE FAMILY AS WELL AS THE PATIENT; (8) PROTECT THE MA PATIENT'S STRONG SENSE OF MODESTY; (9) PUBLICIZE THE ADVANTAGES OF SCIENTIFIC MEDICINE; (10) ADD AN MA BILINGUAL INTERVIEWER TO THE STAFF AT EACH CLINIC OR HOSPITAL; AND (11) IMPROVE RELATIONS BETWEEN MEDICAL PERSONNEL AND CURANDEROS.

ACCN   000942

1103 AUTH   **MADSEN, W.**
TITL   VALUE CONFLICTS AND FOLK PSYCHIATRY IN SOUTH TEXAS.
SRCE   *IN A. KIEV (ED.), MAGIC, FAITH AND HEALING. NEW YORK: FREE PRESS, 1964, PP. 420-440.*
INDX   CURANDERISMO, FOLK MEDICINE, HEALTH, MENTAL HEALTH, ROLE EXPECTATIONS, AC-

CULTURATION, PHYSICIANS, HEALTH DELIVERY SYSTEMS, TEXAS, SOUTHWEST, CASE STUDY

ABST THE ETHNOCENTRIC ORIENTATION OF MODERN MEDICINE AND PSYCHIATRY HAS IMPEDED THE ACCULTURATION OF THE MEXICAN AMERICAN (MA) POPULATION IN SOUTH TEXAS. THE INTOLERANCE OF MEDICAL SCIENCE TOWARDS OTHER CURING TRADITIONS HAS HINDERED ITS ACCEPTANCE IN FOLK SOCIETIES. IT HAS ALSO RETARDED MEDICAL RECOGNITION OF THE ACTUAL THERAPEUTIC VALUE OF MANY FOLK CURING TECHNIQUES. HIDALGO COUNTY REGISTERS A HIGH PERCENTAGE MA POPULATION (75%), WHICH IS MOSTLY OF LOWER SOCIOECONOMIC STATUS. AN INCREASED RATE OF ACCULTURATION HAS RESULTED IN A THREAT TO MA SOCIAL AND CULTURAL TRADITIONS, WHICH HAS PRODUCED PSYCHOLOGICAL STRESS AND HIGH LEVELS OF ANXIETY. WHILE ONE MIGHT EXPECT TO FIND A HEAVY RELIANCE BY MA'S ON MEDICAL PSYCHIATRIC RESOURCES, MOST MA'S SEEK THE SERVICES OF THE CURANDERO, OR FOLK CURER. THE HIGH DEGREE OF SUCCESS IN TREATING MA PATIENTS BY CURANDEROS IS EXAMINED. SIX CASE STUDIES PROVIDE AN ILLUSTRATION OF THE CULTURE CONFLICT AND VALUE CONFLICT ENCOUNTERED IN THE PROCESS OF ACCULTURATION. THE INABILITY OF A PSYCHIATRIST OR PHYSICIAN TO COMMUNICATE LINGUISTICALLY OR CULTURALLY WITH THE MA GROUP IS DISCUSSED. 11 REFERENCES.

ACCN 000943

1104 AUTH **MADURO, R.**

TITL JOURNEY DREAMS IN LATINO GROUP PSYCHOTHERAPY.

SRCE *PSYCHOTHERAPY: THEORY, RESEARCH AND PRACTICE, 1976, 13(2), 148-155.*

INDX PSYCHOTHERAPY, BILINGUAL-BICULTURAL PERSONNEL, DREAMS, ACCULTURATION, PREJUDICE, CASE STUDY, ESSAY, MEXICAN AMERICAN, CULTURAL FACTORS, ADULTS, PSYCHOTHERAPY OUTCOME, MENTAL HEALTH

ABST THE IMPACT OF CULTURAL FACTORS ON THE SYMBOLIC FORM AND CONTENT OF A PARTICULAR TYPE OF DREAM REPORTED BY LATINO PATIENTS, ESPECIALLY THOSE WITH A STRONG INVESTMENT IN THE CONTEMPORARY CHICANO MOVEMENT OR STRONG ATTACHMENTS TO MEXICO, IS DISCUSSED. FOUR CASE STUDIES ARE PRESENTED TO ILLUSTRATE THE KIND OF THEMES USUALLY ENCOUNTERED IN THESE "JOURNEY DREAMS." IN GROUP AND INDIVIDUAL BILINGUAL THERAPY EXPERIENCES WITH OVER 200 LATINOS, IT IS FOUND THAT SERIOUS EXPLORATION OF THE JOURNEY MOTIF IN DREAM WORK HAS FREQUENTLY REVEALED A NEED FOR THE DREAMER TO MAKE CONTACT WITH REPRESSED FEELINGS, MEMORIES, ATTITUDES AND POTENTIALITIES FOR FURTHER GROWTH AND DEVELOPMENT WHICH ARE STRONGLY ASSOCIATED WITH ETHNIC ORIGINS AND ROOTS. THE VALUE AND EFFECTIVENESS OF ALL LATINO GROUPS WITH LATINO THERAPISTS IS EMPHASIZED IN THIS TYPE OF ANALYTICAL THERAPY. 22 REFERENCES. (AUTHOR SUMMARY MODIFIED)

ACCN 000944

1105 AUTH **MADURO, R., & MARTINEZ, C. F.**

TITL LATINO DREAM ANALYSIS: OPPORTUNITY FOR CONFRONTATION.

SRCE *SOCIAL CASEWORK, 1974, 55(OCTOBER), 461-469.*

INDX DREAMS, CULTURAL FACTORS, CASE STUDY, SPANISH SURNAMED, PSYCHOTHERAPY, MENTAL HEALTH, ESSAY, ADULTS, PSYCHOTHERAPY OUTCOME

ABST THE EFFECTIVENESS OF DREAM ANALYSIS AS A THERAPEUTIC TOOL IN PROVIDING MENTAL HEALTH SERVICES TO THE LATINO COMMUNITY IS DISCUSSED. THREE CASE STUDIES OF TWO MALES AND ONE FEMALE—SPANISH SURNAMED PARTICIPANTS IN ALL-LATINO PSYCHOTHERAPY GROUPS—ILLUSTRATE HOW DREAM MATERIAL CAN BE USED TO HELP PATIENTS EXPLORE THE PSYCHOSOCIAL CONFLICTS RESULTING FROM THEIR BICULTURALITY. IT IS POSITED THAT DREAMS SHOW CLEARLY THAT BICULTURALISM IS NOT A PSYCHOLOGICAL LIABILITY, BUT AN ASSET WHICH NEEDS TO BE RECOGNIZED AND CONFRONTED IN ORDER FOR PERSONAL GROWTH AND LIFE SATISFACTION TO OCCUR. 11 REFERENCES.

ACCN 000945

1106 AUTH **MAES, W. R., & RINALDI, J. R.**

TITL COUNSELING THE CHICANO CHILD.

SRCE *ELEMENTARY SCHOOL GUIDANCE AND COUNSELING, 1974, 8(4), 279-284.*

INDX MEXICAN AMERICAN, CHILDREN, EDUCATIONAL COUNSELING, LINGUISTIC COMPETENCE, BEHAVIOR MODIFICATION, CULTURAL FACTORS, BILINGUAL-BICULTURAL PERSONNEL, READING, LINGUISTICS, BILINGUALISM, ESSAY, VALUES

ABST NECESSARY CHARACTERISTICS AND PRIORITIES OF COUNSELORS WORKING WITH CHICANO SCHOOL CHILDREN ARE PRESENTED. THE FOUR MOST IMPORTANT PRIORITIES FOR PROVIDING ASSISTANCE AS COUNSELORS ARE: (1) LANGUAGE AND COGNITIVE SKILL DEVELOPMENT; (2) EXPANSION OF CAREER OPTIONS; (3) PERSONAL RESPECT AND PRIDE IN THE CHICANO CULTURE; AND (4) EXPLORATION AND CLARIFICATION OF PERSONAL VALUES. IN ADDITION TO THESE PRIORITIES, THE COUNSELOR OF CHICANO CHILDREN MUST HAVE: (1) THE ABILITY TO SPEAK SPANISH AND ENGLISH FLUENTLY; (2) AN UNDERSTANDING OF THE VALUES, GOALS AND BEHAVIOR OF CHICANO CHILDREN; (3) A LARGE REPERTOIRE OF COUNSELING TECHNIQUES, ESPECIALLY GEARED TOWARDS THE FAMILY AND ENVIRONMENTAL FACTORS; AND (4) HELPING CHARACTERISTICS SUCH AS EMPATHY, POSITIVE REGARD AND AUTHENTICITY. TO ASSIST THE CHICANO CHILD TO TAKE ADVANTAGE OF OPPORTUNITIES, THE COUNSELOR'S TASK REQUIRES THAT THE CHILD'S SKILLS AND ATTITUDES BE ENHANCED. 3 REFERENCES.

ACCN 000946

1107 AUTH **MAESTAS, A. L.**

TITL A SURVEY TO DETERMINE THE ATTITUDES AND OPINIONS OF RESIDENTS OF THE SAN LUIS VALLEY CONCERNING MENTAL HEALTH CONCEPTS AND SERVICES.

SRCE *UNPUBLISHED MANUSCRIPT, SAN LUIS VALLEY COMPREHENSIVE COMMUNITY MENTAL HEALTH CENTER, 1975.*

INDX HEALTH DELIVERY SYSTEMS, MENTAL HEALTH, ATTITUDES, CULTURAL FACTORS, SURVEY, FOLK MEDICINE, HEALTH, COMMUNITY, RURAL, EMPIRICAL, MEXICAN AMERICAN, COLORADO, SOUTHWEST, URBAN

ABST THE RESULTS OF A SURVEY DESIGNED TO ASCERTAIN THE OPINIONS AND ATTITUDES OF SAN LUIS VALLEY, COLORADO, RESIDENTS REGARDING MENTAL HEALTH CONCEPTS AND LOCAL MENTAL HEALTH CENTER SERVICES ARE PRESENTED. 200 INTERVIEWS WERE CONDUCTED WITH A RANDOM SAMPLING OF THE VALLEY'S TOTAL POPULATION OF 39,095. THE SAMPLE CONSISTED OF 98 MEXICAN AMERICANS, 102 ANGLOS, 80 MEN AND 120 WOMEN. RESPONSES TO THE 27-ITEM QUESTIONNAIRE, AVAILABLE IN SPANISH AND ENGLISH, WERE COMPARED BY SUBJECTS' ETHNICITY, SEX, RURAL VS. URBAN RESIDENCE AND COUNTY USING DESCRIPTIVE STATISTICS AND ZERO ORDER CORRELATIONS. GENERAL FINDINGS WERE: (1) ANGLOS APPEAR MORE INFORMED ABOUT MENTAL HEALTH SERVICES AND CONCEPTS THAN CHICANOS; (2) BY PERCENTAGES, MALES AND ANGLOS ARE MORE AWARE OF SERVICES PROVIDED THAN FEMALES AND CHICANOS; AND (3) RESIDENTS LIVING IN THE BUSINESS AND EDUCATIONAL CENTERS SEEM MORE INFORMED ABOUT MENTAL HEALTH AND DISPLAY MORE LIBERAL ATTITUDES TOWARD TREATMENT OF THE MENTALLY ILL. RECOMMENDATIONS INCLUDE INCREASING THE MENTAL HEALTH EDUCATION PROGRAM FOR VALLEY RESIDENTS—ESPECIALLY FOR THE LEAST INFORMED RESIDENTS OF ONE RURAL COUNTY—AND DEVELOPING A DRUG ABUSE CLINIC REQUESTED BY RESPONDENTS.

ACCN 000947

1108 AUTH **MAGNUS, R. E., WITT, J. W., & GOMEZ, A.**

TITL ATTITUDINAL TESTING: A TOOL FOR EFFECTIVE LAW ENFORCEMENT MANAGEMENT.

SRCE *JOURNAL OF POLICE SCIENCE AND ADMINISTRATION, 1977, 5(1), 74-78.*

INDX ATTITUDES, CORRECTIONS, CROSS CULTURAL, EMPIRICAL, EMPLOYMENT, INTERPERSONAL RELATIONS, PERSONNEL, SPANISH SURNAMED, NEW MEXICO, SOUTHWEST, JOB PERFORMANCE

ABST TO DETERMINE THE VALIDITY OF AN ATTITUDINAL CHANGE INSTRUMENT STILL UNDER DEVELOPMENT BY THE MARQUETTE UNIVERSITY CENTER FOR CRIMINAL JUSTICE AGENCY ORGANIZATION AND MINORITY EMPLOYMENT OPPORTUNITIES, THE INSTRUMENT WAS ADMINISTERED TO 63 MEMBERS OF MIXED ETHNIC AND RACIAL BACKGROUNDS OF THE LAS CRUCES, NEW MEXICO, POLICE DEPARTMENT. ANALYSIS OF DATA INDICATED THAT OVERALL JOB SATISFACTION WAS HIGH, BUT THAT AN IMPROVED CAREER DEVELOPMENT PROGRAM WAS DESIRED. THE BLACK RESPONDENTS DISCERNED NEGATIVE ASPECTS OF INTERPERSONAL RELATIONSHIPS WITHIN THE DEPARTMENT, WHILE SPANISH AMERICAN AND AMERICAN INDIAN RESPONDENTS DISCERNED COMMUNICATION DIFFICULTIES. IT IS CONCLUDED THAT THIS INSTRUMENT COULD PROVIDE VALUABLE MANAGERIAL DECISION-MAKING INFORMATION IN MATTERS REGARDING OVERALL JOB SATISFACTION AND POLICY IMPACT ON MINORITY GROUP ATTITUDES. (NCHHI ABSTRACT)

ACCN 002145

1109 AUTH **MAHAKIAN, C.**

TITL MEASURING INTELLIGENCE AND READING CAPACITY OF SPANISH-SPEAKING CHILDREN.

SRCE *ELEMENTARY SCHOOL JOURNAL, 1939, 39(10), 760-768.*

INDX INTELLIGENCE TESTING, ACHIEVEMENT TESTING, READING, MEXICAN AMERICAN, BILINGUALISM, EMPIRICAL, POLICY, CULTURAL PLURALISM

ABST INTELLIGENCE TESTS WERE ADMINISTERED TO SPANISH-SPEAKING CHILDREN FOR THE PURPOSE OF DETERMINING THEIR VALIDITY AND TO DISCOVER THE GRADE IN WHICH ENGLISH BECOMES THE DOMINANT LANGUAGE FOR THESE CHILDREN. THE OTIS GROUP INTELLIGENCE SCALE AND THE DURRELL-SULLIVAN READING CAPACITY TEST WERE ADMINISTERED TO 210 STUDENTS IN SPANISH AND IN ENGLISH USING A COUNTER-BALANCE DESIGN. THE FINDINGS SHOW THAT IN THE PRIMARY AND ATYPICAL GRADES THE AVERAGE PUPIL SCORED 7.6 POINTS HIGHER IN THE SPANISH INTELLIGENCE TEST. THE COMPREHENSION OF THE SPANISH VOCABULARY IS SIGNIFICANTLY GREATER IN THE FOURTH TO SEVENTH GRADES. ENGLISH IS FOUND TO BE THE DOMINANT LANGUAGE, AS FAR AS UNDERSTANDING OF PARAGRAPHS, FROM THE FIFTH GRADE ON. THE TOTAL SCORE IN READING CAPACITY FAVORS SPANISH IN THE FOURTH TO THE SEVENTH GRADES. THESE FINDINGS POINT TO THE FOLLOWING CONCLUSIONS AND RECOMMENDATIONS. (1) INTELLIGENCE TESTS ADMINISTERED IN ENGLISH TO SPANISH-SPEAKING CHILDREN ARE NOT VALID IN THE FIRST THREE GRADES AND IN ATYPICAL CLASSES AND SHOULD NOT BE USED AS A MEANS OF COMPARISON BETWEEN ENGLISH-SPEAKING AND SPANISH-SPEAKING CHILDREN. (2) THERE SHOULD BE NO RIGID CLASSIFICATION BASED ON INTELLIGENCE QUOTIENT. (3) ORAL LANGUAGE SHOULD BE USED EXTENSIVELY WITH THE OBJECTIVE OF INCREASING THE ENGLISH VOCABULARY. (4) NATIVE TRAITS AND CULTURE SHOULD BE ASSIMILATED WITH AMERICAN CULTURE AS A MEANS OF ENRICHING THE VOCABULARY. (5) INSTRUCTION IN FORMAL READING SHOULD BE POSTPONED UNTIL THE PUPIL HAS AN ADEQUATE UNDERSTANDING OF THE ENGLISH LANGUAGE. (6) SCHOOLS WITH LARGE PROPORTIONS OF BILINGUAL PUPILS SHOULD HAVE SPECIAL TESTING PROGRAMS. (7) ONLY

TEACHERS WITH AN UNDERSTANDING OF A BILINGUAL GROUP SHOULD BE EMPLOYED IN SCHOOLS WITH PREDOMINANTLY BILINGUAL CHILDREN. 2 REFERENCES.

ACCN   000949

1110 AUTH   **MALCOM, S. M., COWNIE, J., & BROWN, J. W. (EDS.)**

TITL   PROGRAMS IN SCIENCE FOR MINORITY STUDENTS: 1960-1975. (AAAS REPORT NO. 76-R-10.)

SRCE   *WASHINGTON, D.C.: AMERICAN ASSOCIATION FOR THE ADVANCEMENT OF SCIENCE, 1976.*

INDX   SURVEY, CURRICULUM, EDUCATION, EMPIRICAL, EQUAL OPPORTUNITY, HEALTH EDUCATION, SOCIAL SCIENCES, INSTRUCTIONAL TECHNIQUES, MEXICAN AMERICAN, PROFESSIONAL TRAINING, PUERTO RICAN-M, BIBLIOGRAPHY

ABST   AN INVENTORY OF 355 SCIENCE EDUCATION PROJECTS FOR MINORITIES IN EFFECT FROM 1960-1976 WAS COMPILED BY THE AMERICAN ASSOCIATION FOR THE ADVANCEMENT OF SCIENCE, OFFICE OF OPPORTUNITIES IN SCIENCE. THE MINORITY GROUPS CONSIDERED WERE BLACKS, CHICANOS, NATIVE AMERICANS, AND PUERTO RICANS. A SURVEY SOLICITING INFORMATION ON SCIENCE EDUCATIONAL PROGRAMS WAS SENT TO OVER 2000 PROFESSIONAL ORGANIZATIONS, COLLEGES AND UNIVERSITIES, STATE SUPERVISORS OF SCIENCE AND ENVIRONMENTAL EDUCATION, AND OTHER POTENTIAL INFORMANTS. ALL LEVELS OF SCIENCE EDUCATION WERE SURVEYED AND PROGRAMS IN SCIENCE WERE BROADLY DEFINED TO INCLUDE PHYSICAL AND BIOLOGICAL SCIENCES, ENGINEERING AND TECHNICAL FIELDS, HEALTH SCIENCES, AGRICULTURAL SCIENCE, AND SOME SOCIAL SCIENCES SUCH AS ANTHROPOLOGY, PSYCHOLOGY AND GEOGRAPHY. THE INVENTORY INCLUDES MANY TYPES OF EDUCATIONAL PROJECTS FOR MINORITIES INCLUDING CURRICULUM INNOVATIONS, EXPERIMENTAL TEACHING METHODS, MOTIVATIONAL PROGRAMS, SUMMER PROGRAMS, TEACHER IMPROVEMENT PROJECTS, AND RECRUITMENT EFFORTS. AN EXAMINATION OF THE BREAKDOWN OF PROJECTS ACCORDING TO TARGETED GROUPS REVEALS AN UNEVEN DISTRIBUTION. APPROXIMATELY 25% OF THE PROJECTS WERE LISTED FOR ALL MINORITIES, 35% FOR BLACKS, 7% FOR NATIVE AMERICANS, 4% FOR CHICANOS, AND THE REMAINDER FOR VARIOUS COMBINATIONS OF RACIAL/ETHNIC MINORITY GROUPS. AN ANNOTATED BIBLIOGRAPHY OF OTHER PROGRAM INVENTORIES IS INCLUDED IN THIS REPORT.

ACCN   002146

1111 AUTH   **MALDONADO, A. M. P.**

TITL   CONTROVERSIAS EN LA INVESTIGACION CIENTIFICA SOBRE LOS EFECTOS DEL USO DE LA MARIHUANA. (CONTROVERSIES IN THE SCIENTIFIC INVESTIGATION OF THE EFFECTS OF THE USAGE OF MARIHUANA.)

SRCE   *REVISTA DE CIENCIAS SOCIALES, 1975, 19(4), 395-422. (SPANISH)*

INDX   PUERTO RICAN-I, ESSAY, DRUG ABUSE, LEGISLATION, POLICY

ABST   STUDIES OF THE EFFECTS OF MARIJUANA HAVE LED TO CONTROVERSIES IN PUERTO RICO, WITH RESPECT TO BOTH LEGAL AND SCIENTIFIC ISSUES. PROBLEMS PERTAINING TO LABORATORY RESEARCH ARE DISCUSSED, AND INCLUDE THE VARIANCE IN MARIJUANA DOSES ACROSS EXPERIMENTS, THE ARTIFICIAL ENVIRONMENT OF THE LABORATORY, AND THE PARADOX THAT MOST MARIJUANA RESEARCH IS FUNDED BY GOVERNMENTAL GROUPS WHICH STRONGLY OPPOSE MARIJUANA USE. WITH REGARD TO LEGAL ISSUES, THE AUTHOR QUESTIONS THE WISDOM OF THE SEVERE PENALTIES DESIGNED TO DO AWAY WITH MARIJUANA USE. THE SAME ATTITUDE IS ASSUMED TOWARDS SCIENTISTS WHO HAVE PRETENDED TO MAKE INVESTIGATIONS BASED ON THE FICTION OF SCIENCE AS AN OBJECTIVE TASK (FREE OF VALUES). EVEN THOUGH A MORE SYSTEMATIC KNOWLEDGE OF DRUG SUBSTANCES IS URGENTLY NEEDED, IT IS PERHAPS MORE IMPORTANT FOR SCIENTISTS TO STOP BEING INDIFFERENT TO THE LEGAL SYSTEM'S SEVERE PUNISHMENT FOR THE POSSESSION OF MARIJUANA. 71 REFERENCES. (AUTHOR ABSTRACT MODIFIED)

ACCN   002147

1112 AUTH   **MALDONADO, B. B.**

TITL   THE IMPACT OF SKIN COLOR BY SEX ON SELF CONCEPT OF LOW SOCIOECONOMIC LEVEL MEXICAN-AMERICAN HIGH SCHOOL STUDENTS (DOCTORAL DISSERTATION, NEW MEXICO STATE UNIVERSITY, 1972.)

SRCE   *DISSERTATION ABSTRACTS INTERNATIONAL, 1972, 33(6), 2716A-2717A. (UNIVERSITY MICROFILMS NO. 72-31,647.)*

INDX   MEXICAN AMERICAN, ETHNIC IDENTITY, SES, POVERTY, ADOLESCENTS, EMPIRICAL, SELF CONCEPT, NEW MEXICO, SOUTHWEST

ABST   IN ORDER TO DETERMINE (1) IF SELF-CONCEPT IS AFFECTED BY THE INDEPENDENT CONDITIONS OF SKIN COLOR AND SEX, AND (2) IF SELF-CONCEPT IS AFFECTED BY THE INTERACTIONS RESULTING FROM THE VARIABLES OF SKIN COLOR AND SEX, 174 MEXICAN AMERICAN HIGH SCHOOL STUDENTS, CLASSIFIED BY SKIN COLOR AND SEX, WERE ADMINISTERED THE TENNESSEE SELF CONCEPT SCALE (TSCS). ALL SUBJECTS WERE FROM LOWER SOCIOECONOMIC LEVEL (SES) FAMILIES AS MEASURED BY HOLLINGSHEAD'S TWO-FACTOR INDEX OF SOCIAL POSITION. SKIN COLOR WAS DETERMINED BY THREE JUDGES' RATING OF A COLOR SLIDE OF EACH SUBJECT COMPARED AGAINST A SKIN COLOR CHART. THE DATA WERE ANALYZED BY MEANS OF A TWO-WAY ANALYSIS OF VARIANCE TO DETERMINE IF SEX AND SKIN COLOR HAVE A SIGNIFICANT INFLUENCE ON THE FOURTEEN MEASURES OF SELF-CONCEPT OF THE TSCS. FINDINGS REVEAL THAT SEX IS SIGNIFICANTLY RELATED TO 4 OF THE SELF-CONCEPT MEASURES: SELF-SATISFACTION, PHYSICAL SELF, VARIABILITY, AND OFFENSIVE POSITIVE SCORES. THE INDEPENDENT VARIABLE OF SKIN COLOR

AFFECTED THE SELF CRITICISM, TOTAL CONFLICT AND PHYSICAL SELF SCORES. THE ANALYSES ALSO REVEALED THAT INTERACTION EFFECTS WERE INSIGNIFICANT. SEX AND SKIN COLOR TOGETHER ONLY SLIGHTLY AFFECTED THE SUBJECTS' PERCEPTIONS OF THEIR PERSONAL WORTH, TO WHAT DEGREE THEY LIKED THEMSELVES, AND OF THEIR SELF CONFIDENCE. IT IS ALSO CONCLUDED THAT THESE LOWER SOCIOECONOMIC STUDENTS DID NOT EXHIBIT A SENSE OF INFERIORITY AND WORTHLESSNESS TO THE DEGREE GENERALLY ATTRIBUTED TO THEIR SOCIAL CLASS. IMPLICATIONS FOR EDUCATORS OF MEXICAN AMERICAN STUDENTS ARE DISCUSSED. 126 REFERENCES. (AUTHOR ABSTRACT MODIFIED)

ACCN   000950

1113 AUTH **MALDONADO, D., JR.**
TITL   THE CHICANO AGED.
SRCE   *SOCIAL WORK, 1975, 20(3), 213-216.*
INDX   GERONTOLOGY, MEXICAN AMERICAN, CULTURAL CHANGE, ESSAY, EXTENDED FAMILY, SOCIAL SERVICES, POLICY
ABST   SOCIOLOGISTS HAVE THEORIZED THAT AGED MEXICAN AMERICANS ARE ADEQUATELY CARED FOR THROUGH THE EXTENDED FAMILY PATTERNS COMMON TO THEIR CULTURE. THIS POPULAR VIEWPOINT, BASED ON EMPIRICAL DATA AND HISTORICAL OBSERVATION, IS NOW BEING QUESTIONED. SOCIAL AND ECONOMIC CHANGES SINCE WW II HAVE BEEN REFLECTED IN THE ADJUSTMENTS IN INDIVIDUAL, FAMILY AND COMMUNITY LIFE STYLES BY MEXICAN AMERICANS. LIKE THE LARGER ANGLO SOCIETY, THE BASIC STRUCTURE OF THE EXTENDED FAMILY HAS GRADUALLY BEEN REDUCED WHILE THE NUCLEAR FAMILY STRUCTURE HAS DEVELOPED AND STRENGTHENED. THESE CHANGES AND ADJUSTMENTS IN CHICANO FAMILY PATTERNS HAVE NOT BEEN RECOGNIZED OR ACTED UPON BY SOCIAL AGENCIES MANDATED TO PROVIDE FOR THE ELDERLY. WHILE SOCIAL SERVICES CONTINUE BELIEVING THE OUTDATED MYTH THAT MEXICAN AMERICAN ELDERLY HAVE FEW PHYSICAL OR EMOTIONAL NEEDS, A SERIOUS SHORTAGE OF SERVICES FOR THE MEXICAN AMERICAN ELDERLY HAS DEVELOPED. 7 REFERENCES.

ACCN   000951

1114 AUTH **MALDONADO, D., JR.**
TITL   ETHNIC SELF-IDENTITY AND SELF-UNDERSTANDING.
SRCE   *SOCIAL CASEWORK, 1975, 56(10), 618-622.*
INDX   ESSAY, MEXICAN AMERICAN, ETHNIC IDENTITY, SELF CONCEPT, ACCULTURATION, PERSONALITY ASSESSMENT, RESEARCH METHODOLOGY, CULTURE, SES, ENVIRONMENTAL FACTORS
ABST   SEVERAL FACTORS WHICH TEND TO BIAS STUDIES PERTAINING TO MINORITIES, ESPECIALLY CHICANOS, ARE DISCUSSED. THE NEGATIVE FINDINGS CONCERNING THE SELF-IDENTITY OF MINORITIES AND THEIR COMMUNITIES ARE CONSIDERED A RESULT OF STUDIES IN WHICH: (1) PERSONALITY TESTS MEASURING SELF-IDENTITY OF MINORITY GROUPS REFLECT ANGLO DEFINITIONS OF SELF-IDEN-

TITY; (2) PSYCHOLOGICAL TESTS ARE DEVELOPED WITH SPURIOUS ASSUMPTIONS, ESPECIALLY WITH RESPECT TO ACCULTURATION AND ASSIMILATION; (3) PERSONALITY THEORIES ARE BASED ON NONSCIENTIFIC MODELS; AND (4) PERSONALITY TESTS FAIL TO ADEQUATELY MEASURE ETHNIC SELF-IDENTITY. THE TRADITIONAL USE OF NONSCIENTIFIC MODELS IN THE EXAMINATION OF SELF-CONCEPTS OF MINORITIES HAS FOCUSED ON THE INNER PERSON. THE INFLUENCE OF THE EXTERNAL FACTORS OF NONASSIMILATION, PARTIAL ACCULTURATION, AND ETHNIC IDENTITY HAVE BEEN LARGELY IGNORED. 7 REFERENCES. (AUTHOR SUMMARY MODIFIED)

ACCN   000952

1115 AUTH **MALDONADO-DENIS, M.**
TITL   THE PUERTO RICANS: PROTEST OR SUBMISSION?
SRCE   *ANNALS OF THE NEW YORK ACADEMY OF POLITICAL AND SOCIAL SCIENCE, 1969, 382, 26-31.*
INDX   URBAN, HISTORY, SES, POVERTY, IMMIGRATION, ECONOMIC FACTORS, POLITICS, POLITICAL POWER, ACCULTURATION, PREJUDICE, POLICY, DISCRIMINATION, HISTORY, COMMUNITY INVOLVEMENT, ESSAY, PUERTO RICAN-I, PUERTO RICAN-M
ABST   THE RECENT MASS EXODUS OF PUERTO RICANS TO NEW YORK CITY IS LARGELY COMPOSED OF IMMIGRANTS FROM 15 TO 39 YEARS OF AGE WHO HAVE ENCOUNTERED PREJUDICES AND HARDSHIPS CHARACTERISTIC OF A NONWHITE GROUP IN A RACIST SOCIETY. THE PUERTO RICAN SITUATION IN THE UNITED STATES MUST BE CONSIDERED SIMILAR TO THOSE LIVING IN PUERTO RICO SINCE THE FORMER IS ONLY A MAGNIFICATION OF COLONIALISTIC PROBLEMS RELATED TO THE QUESTIONS OF IDENTITY, LANGUAGE AND ACHIEVING REPRESENTATIVE POLITICAL POWER. PUERTO RICO HAS BEEN A COLONY OF THE UNITED STATES SINCE 1898 AND THE MOST PERSUASIVE CHARACTERISTIC OF ITS POPULATION, BOTH IN THE ISLAND AND IN THE MAINLAND, TENDS TO BE THE SUBMISSIVE AND ACQUIESCENT ATTITUDE REFLECTED BY A COLONIZED PEOPLE. THE ONLY FORCES IN PUERTO RICO THAT REPRESENT THE PUERTO RICAN PROTEST AGAINST THE PERPETUATION OF THIS COLONIALISM ARE THE PROINDEPENDENCE GROUPS. THEIR GOAL IS CONSIDERED SIMILAR TO THAT OF THE BLACK POWER ADVOCATES IN THE UNITED STATES IN THEIR DESIRE TO COMBAT MINORITY GROUP ASSIMILATION INTO THE DOMINANT UNITED STATES SOCIETY. ONLY WHEN PUERTO RICANS HAVE ACHIEVED DECOLONIZATION, BOTH PSYCHOLOGICALLY AND POLITICALLY, WILL THEY BE ABLE TO COME OF AGE. IF THIS IS NOT ACCOMPLISHED, THEY RISK BOTH TOTAL DESTRUCTION OF PUERTO RICAN NATIONALITY AND CULTURAL ASSIMILATION BY THE UNITED STATES. 2 REFERENCES. (JOURNAL ABSTRACT MODIFIED)

ACCN   000953

1116 AUTH **MALDONADO-SIERRA, E. D.**
TITL A GROUP METHOD FOR TRAINING PUERTO RI-CAN PSYCHIATRIC RESIDENTS.
SRCE *PSYCHIATRIC QUARTERLY SUPPLEMENT, 1962, 36(1), 35-43.*
INDX PROFESSIONAL TRAINING, MENTAL HEALTH PROFESSION, GROUP DYNAMICS, INTERPER-SONAL RELATIONS, PSYCHOTHERAPY, PSY-CHOTHERAPISTS, ADULTS, CULTURAL FAC-TORS, PUERTO RICAN-I, CASE STUDY
ABST A GROUP METHOD USED TO CLARIFY UNCON-SCIOUS ATTITUDES TOWARD AUTHORITY AND TO FACILITATE INDIVIDUAL KNOWLEDGE OF PSYCHIATRIC CONCEPTS WITH EIGHT PUERTO RICAN PSYCHIATRIC RESIDENTS IS REPORTED. SUBJECTS MET WITH A GROUP LEADER ONCE A WEEK FOR A NINETY-MINUTE SESSION FOR A PERIOD OF A YEAR. THE CONCEPT OF "UN-EARNED AUTHORITY" (THE DECISIONS AND REGULATIONS TO WHICH THE INDIVIDUAL MUST CONFORM WITHOUT ANY VOICE IN THE DECI-SION-MAKING PROCESS) WAS DRAMATIZED BY THE BEHAVIOR OF THE FIRST SESSION'S LEADER, WHO WOULD SPEAK IN A LOUD VOICE, POUND THE TABLE, ASSERT AUTHORITY, AND DEMAND CONFORMITY. EACH SESSION THERE-AFTER WAS SUMMARIZED WITHOUT REFER-RING BACK TO THE RECORD FOR CONTENT AND PROCESS. VERBALIZATIONS OF SYMP-TOMS, INDICATIONS OF ANXIETY AND ITS MAN-IFESTATIONS, UNCONSCIOUS BEHAVIOR, AND DEFENSE MECHANISMS WERE OBSERVED AND EXPLAINED IN THE SESSIONS. THE FORMATION OF THE GROUP'S EGO AND ITS EVOLUTION WERE OBSERVED AND ENCOURAGED BY THE LEADER. THE METHOD, PROCEDURE, AND GOALS OF THE GROUP WERE NOT TO BE EX-POSED UNTIL THE RESIDENTS ACHIEVED CON-SCIOUS AWARENESS OF THE PROCESSES IN-VOLVED. A RADICAL CHANGE IN THE SUBJECTS' PERCEPTIONS AND RELATIONS CONCERNING THE LEADER OF THE GROUP WAS NOTED. A TWO-PART EVALUATION CONSISTING OF A 5-ITEM OPEN INTERVIEW AND A CONTENT ANALY-SIS OF THE FIRST AND LAST THREE SESSIONS INDICATED THAT THE PURPOSE OF THE GROUP EXPERIENCE WAS BASICALLY DIDACTIC IN NA-TURE.
ACCN 000954

1117 AUTH **MALDONADO-SIERRA, E. D., TRENT, R. D., FERNANDEZ-MARINA, R., FLORES-GAL-LARDO, A., VIGOREAUX-RIVERA, J., & DE CO-LON, L. S.**
TITL CULTURAL FACTORS IN THE GROUP PSY-CHOTHERAPEUTIC PROCESS FOR PUERTO RI-CAN SCHIZOPHRENICS.
SRCE *INTERNATIONAL JOURNAL OF GROUP PSY-CHOTHERAPY, 1960, 10(4), 373-382.*
INDX PSYCHOTHERAPY, SCHIZOPHRENIA, PUERTO RICAN-I, ADULTS, CULTURAL FACTORS, FAMILY ROLES, FAMILY STRUCTURE, MALE
ABST THIS STUDY REPORTS A PRELIMINARY INVES-TIGATION ON INTENSIVE GROUP PSYCHOTH-ERAPY WITH REGRESSED MALE PUERTO RI-CAN SCHIZOPHRENICS EMPLOYING A CULTURALLY RELEVANT "ADAPTED" GROUP PSYCHOTHERAPEUTIC METHOD. CERTAIN FEA-

TURES OF THE TRADITIONAL CHILD-REARING PATTERNS OF THE PATIENTS' FAMILIES, AS WELL AS SPECIFIC CHARACTERISTICS OF SCHIZOPHRENIC REACTIONS IN THIS CUL-TURAL MILIEU, ARE EXPLORED AND INCORPO-RATED INTO THE ADAPTED PSYCHOTHERA-PEUTIC PROCESS. THE ADAPTED GROUP TREATMENT METHOD IS DIFFERENTIATED FROM THE TRADITIONAL GROUP PSYCHOTHERAPY METHOD BY: (1) GREATER EMPHASIS UPON THE CREATION OF A THERAPY TEAM REPRE-SENTING THE SIGNIFICANT MEMBERS OF A HEALTHY FAMILY—THE FATHER, THE MOTHER, AND THE OLDER BROTHER; (2) GREATER EM-PHASIS UPON THE CLARIFICATION OF THE PA-TIENTS' BLURRED PERCEPTIONS OF OTHERS AS THE MAIN TASK OF THE THERAPY TEAM; AND (3) EMPHASIS UPON THE SIBLING FIGURE, AND THE CLARIFICATION OF THE ROLES OF MOTHER AND FATHER THROUGH INTERAC-TIONS BETWEEN HEALTHY SIBLING FIGURES AND THE PATIENTS, WHO REPRESENT YOUNGER DEPENDENT FIGURES. 22 REFERENCES.
ACCN 000955

1118 AUTH **MALDONADO-SIERRA, E. D., TRENT, R. D., & FERNANDEZ-MARINA, R.**
TITL NEUROSIS AND TRADITIONAL FAMILY BELIEFS IN PUERTO RICO.
SRCE *INTERNATIONAL JOURNAL OF SOCIAL PSY-CHIATRY, 1960, 6(3-4), 237-246.*
INDX FAMILY ROLES, FAMILY STRUCTURE, NEU-ROSIS, CULTURE, ACCULTURATION, PUERTO RICAN-I, COLLEGE STUDENTS, EMPIRICAL
ABST AN EXPERIMENTAL TEST OF A HYPOTHESIS, PREVIOUSLY CORROBORATED WITH MEXICAN SUBJECTS, OF THE RELATIONSHIP BETWEEN THE ACCEPTANCE OF TRADITIONAL LATIN AMERICAN FAMILY BELIEFS AND PSYCHOPATH-OLOGY AMONG 48 PUERTO RICAN SUBJECTS IS REPORTED. SIXTEEN SUBJECTS IN THE EX-PERIMENTAL GROUP WERE SUFFERING FROM NEUROTIC DISORDERS AND 32 SUBJECTS IN THE CONTROL GROUP WERE MENTALLY HEALTHIER. SUBJECTS WERE MATCHED ON THE BASIS OF 11 CRITERIA WHICH WERE PREDICATED TO BE CLOSELY RELATED TO THE ACCEPTANCE OF A FAMILY BELIEF SYSTEM. AN ADJECTIVE CHECK-LIST WAS EMPLOYED TO DIFFERENTIATE BETWEEN HEALTHY AND NEU-ROTIC SUBJECTS. TRADITIONAL LATIN AMERI-CAN FAMILY BELIEFS WERE OPERATIONALLY DEFINED IN TERMS OF THE SUBJECTS' RE-SPONSES TO A 32-ITEM SUBSCALE. THE MAIN FINDING OF THE STUDY WAS THAT THE PUERTO RICAN NONNEUROTICS WERE SIGNIFICANTLY MORE ACCEPTING OF TRADITIONAL LATIN AMERICAN FAMILY BELIEFS THAN WERE THE PUERTO RICAN NEUROTICS. THE CONVERSE RESULTS BETWEEN MEXICAN AND PUERTO RI-CAN SUBJECTS MAY BE ATTRIBUTABLE TO SAMPLE SELECTION PROCEDURES, TO VARIA-TIONS IN THE PROCESS OF SOCIOCULTURAL CHANGES OCCURRING WITH TWO CULTURES, AND TO THE KINDS OF EGO DEFENSES WHICH HAVE DEVELOPED TO COPE WITH ACCELER-ATED SOCIETAL CHANGE. 25 REFERENCES.
ACCN 000956

1119 AUTH **MALDONADO-SIERRA, E. D., & TRENT, R. D.**
TITL THE SIBLING RELATIONSHIP IN GROUP PSY-CHOTHERAPY WITH PUERTO RICAN SCHIZO-PHRENICS.
SRCE *AMERICAN JOURNAL OF PSYCHIATRY, 1960, 117(3), 239-244.*
INDX PSYCHOTHERAPY, FAMILY STRUCTURE, SCHIZOPHRENIA, ADULTS, MENTAL HEALTH, PUERTO RICAN-I, FAMILY ROLES, CULTURAL FACTORS
ABST PROPOSED IS THE INCLUSION OF THE SIBLING AS A MEMBER OF THE THERAPY TEAM FOR PUERTO RICAN AND OTHER LATIN AMERICAN SCHIZOPHRENICS. A DETAILED DESCRIPTION OF PUERTO RICAN FAMILY DYNAMICS IS PRESENTED. IT IS BELIEVED THAT CHILDREN DEVELOP UNCONSCIOUS RESENTMENT TOWARD MALE AUTHORITY FIGURES BECAUSE OF THE DOMINANT AND AUTHORITARIAN ROLE THAT THE PUERTO RICAN FATHER EXERCISES. THUS, WHEN THE CHILDREN FACE A PERSONAL PROBLEM THEY WILL TEND TO RELATE IN A MORE SPONTANEOUS AND CONFIDENTIAL MANNER WITH AN OLDER SIBLING OR PEER THAN WITH PATERNAL FIGURES. IN THE THERAPY PROPOSED HERE, A PSYCHIATRIC RESIDENT WHO REPRESENTS AN OLDER SIBLING ENGAGES IN PLAY ACTIVITIES WITH THE PATIENTS FOR 3 TO 4 WEEKS. ACTIVITIES INCLUDE GAMES, CLOSE-CONTACT SPORTS, PICNICS, SWIMMING, TRIPS OFF THE HOSPITAL GROUNDS, ETC. THE GOALS ARE: (1) TO GET CLOSER TO THE PATIENTS TO ESTABLISH CONTACT AND COMMUNICATION; (2) TO GAIN SOME INSIGHT INTO THE UNCONSCIOUS OF THE PATIENTS SO THAT THE RESIDENT MAY LATER ACT AS THEIR SPOKESMAN OR ALTER-EGO; AND (3) TO INTRODUCE THE PARENTS INTO THE THERAPY GROUP IN A WAY CONSISTENT WITH THE TRADITIONAL PATERNAL AND MATERNAL ROLES OF THIS CULTURE. THIS PSYCHOTHERAPEUTIC PROCESS USING THE PUERTO RICAN FAMILY PHENOMENON (THE CLOSENESS OF SIBLINGS) IS CULTURALLY RELEVANT FOR SCHIZOPHRENICS OF LATIN DESCENT. 41 REFERENCES.
ACCN 000957

1120 AUTH **MALLORY, S. G.**
TITL EFFECT OF STIMULUS PRESENTATION ON FREE RECALL OF REFLECTIVE AND IMPULSIVE MEXICAN AMERICAN CHILDREN.
SRCE *JOURNAL OF PSYCHOLOGY, 1970, 76(2), 193-198.*
INDX MEMORY, LEARNING, MEXICAN AMERICAN, CHILDREN, PERSONALITY, PEABODY PICTURE-VOCABULARY TEST, SES, EMPIRICAL, ARIZONA, SOUTHWEST
ABST TO STUDY THE EFFECT OF TACTUAL AND AUDITORY INTEGRATION OF FREE LEARNING COMBINED WITH THE INDEPENDENT VARIABLE OF REFLEXIVITY-IMPULSIVITY, 38 SECOND GRADERS WERE DIVIDED INTO A REFLECTIVE GROUP OF 10 MALES AND 9 FEMALES AND AN IMPULSIVE GROUP WITH 11 MALES AND 8 FEMALES. SUBJECTS WERE THEN RANDOMLY ASSIGNED TO AUDITORY OR AUDIOTACTUAL STIMULATION CONDITIONS. FOR BOTH CON-DITIONS A LIST OF 12 NOUNS CONTAINING SIX CONCEPTUALLY-RELATED WORDS WERE SCORED IN THE ORDER IN WHICH WORDS WERE RECALLED. IT WAS FOUND THAT AUDIOTACTUAL STIMULATION RESULTED IN SIGNIFICANTLY BETTER RECALL FOR TOTAL WORDS, CONCEPT WORDS, AND CLUSTERING. AUDITORY STIMULATION RESULTED IN MORE INTRUSIVE ERRORS. SINCE MANY OF THE ERRORS COULD BE ACCOUNTED FOR, IT WAS SUGGESTED THAT AUDIOTACTUAL STIMULATION INDUCES GREATER ATTENDING BEHAVIOR DURING FREE RECALL TEST PRESENTATION. 8 REFERENCES.
ACCN 000958

1121 AUTH **MALONEY, T.**
TITL FACTIONALISM AND FUTILITY: A CASE STUDY OF POLITICAL AND ECONOMIC REFORM IN NEW MEXICO.
SRCE *IN J. HELM (ED.), SPANISH-SPEAKING PEOPLE IN THE UNITED STATES, PROCEEDINGS OF THE 1968 ANNUAL SPRING MEETING OF THE AMERICAN ETHNOLOGICAL SOCIETY. SEATTLE: UNIVERSITY OF WASHINGTON PRESS, 1968, PP. 154-161.*
INDX POLITICS, POLITICAL POWER, MEXICAN AMERICAN, COMMUNITY INVOLVEMENT, LEADERSHIP, CULTURE, COMMUNITY, SES, POVERTY, ECONOMIC FACTORS, HISTORY, ESSAY, NEW MEXICO, SOUTHWEST
ABST THE ACTIVITIES OF THE DEMOCRATIC PARTY FROM 1964-1967 IN SAN MIGUEL COUNTY, NEW MEXICO, ARE RECOUNTED AND ANALYZED. THE MAJOR POLITICAL DEVELOPMENTS AROUND WHICH FACTIONALISM EVOLVED IN THOSE YEARS WERE: (1) PRIMARY CONTEST FOR THE DEMOCRATIC NOMINATION FOR THE CONGRESSIONAL SEAT VACATED BY JOSEPH MONTOYA WHEN HE RAN FOR THE U.S. SENATE IN 1964; (2) ATTEMPTS TO CONSOLIDATE THE TOWN AND CITY OF LAS VEGAS IN SAN MIGUEL COUNTY; (3) CONTROL OF THE COMMUNITY ACTION PROGRAM IN THE COUNTY; (4) PRIMARY CONTESTS FOR THE DEMOCRATIC NOMINATION FOR GOVERNOR AND OTHER STATE OFFICES IN 1966; AND (5) CONTROL OF THE MUNICIPAL COUNCIL OF THE CITY OF LAS VEGAS IN 1966. ALL OF THESE ISSUES PLUS THE OVERALL CONTROL OF THE COUNTY DEMOCRATIC ORGANIZATION, ARE DISCUSSED IN TERMS OF THE COUNTY'S MEXICAN AMERICAN POPULATION (68%) AND THE GRASSROOTS MOVEMENT (A GROUP OF ANGLO LIBERALS SUPPORTING HISPANIC ISSUES). IT IS CONCLUDED THAT FACTIONALISM WILL CONTINUE IN NORTHERN NEW MEXICO AND THAT ANY CHANGES IN THE POLITICAL ORDER TOWARD GREATER DEMOCRATIC CONTROL OR IN THE ECONOMIC ORDER TOWARD ADEQUATE INCOME AND LIVING CONDITIONS WILL CONTINUE TO BE SLOW. THERE IS NO UNITY AMONG HISPANICS IN THESE POLITICAL OR ECONOMIC EFFORTS, AS FACTIONALISM AND INDIVIDUALISM REMAIN IMPORTANT ASPECTS OF THE REGION RETARDING REFORM AND UNITY. ALTHOUGH THE HISPANO PEOPLE OF NORTHERN NEW MEXICO HAVE SHOWN MUCH PATIENCE

THROUGH A HUNDRED YEARS OF ANGLO EX-PLOITATION, ABETTED BY ASSIMILATED HISPANO LOCAL LEADERS, THE SITUATION IS RIPE FOR CHANGE. 1 REFERENCE.

ACCN   000959

1122 AUTH **MALZBERG, B.**
TITL   MENTAL DISEASE AMONG THE PUERTO RICAN POPULATION OF NEW YORK STATE 1960-1961.
SRCE   *ALBANY, NEW YORK: RESEARCH FOUNDATION FOR MENTAL HYGIENE, INC., 1965.*
INDX   MENTAL HEALTH, SCHIZOPHRENIA, SES, DEMOGRAPHIC, CROSS CULTURAL, ACCULTURATION, ALCOHOLISM, DEPRESSION, PSYCHOSIS, GERONTOLOGY, SURVEY, EMPIRICAL, PUERTO RICAN-M, URBAN, POVERTY, CHILDREN, ADOLESCENTS, ADULTS, SEX COMPARISON, CULTURAL FACTORS, NEW YORK, EAST
ABST   THE INCIDENCE OF MENTAL DISEASE AMONG PUERTO RICANS IN THE STATE OF NEW YORK FROM 1960 TO 1961 IS EXAMINED. A BRIEF HISTORY OF THE MIGRATION OF THE PUERTO RICAN TO THE CONTINENTAL UNITED STATES AND OF SOME OF THE BARRIERS WHICH IMPEDE HIS SOCIAL AND ECONOMIC ADVANCEMENT ARE PRESENTED. MENTAL HEALTH IS FOUND TO BE ASSOCIATED WITH AN INDIVIDUAL'S SOCIAL CONDITION. PUERTO RICAN MALES FROM 1960 TO 1961 HAD A HIGHER STANDARDIZED RATE OF FIRST ADMISSIONS THAN NON-PUERTO RICANS IN THE FOLLOWING MENTAL DISORDERS: (1) DEMENTIA PRAECOX; (2) GENERAL PARESIS; (3) ALCOHOLIC PSYCHOSES; (4) PSYCHOSES WITH CEREBRAL ARTERIOSCLEROSIS; (5) SENILE PSYCHOSES; AND (6) INVOLUTIONAL PSYCHOSES. THE ONLY MAJOR MENTAL DISORDER FOR WHICH PUERTO RICANS RATED LOWER THAN NON-PUERTO RICANS IS MANIC-DEPRESSIVE PSYCHOSES. FEMALE PUERTO RICANS HAD LOWER RATES OF GENERAL PARESIS, ALCOHOLIC PSYCHOSES AND MANIC-DEPRESSION THAN NON-PUERTO RICAN FEMALES. THERE WERE NO DATA SUGGESTING THAT THE HIGH INCIDENCE OF MENTAL DISEASE AMONG PUERTO RICANS IS A CONSEQUENCE OF GENETIC HANDICAPS. HOWEVER, THERE WERE DATA THAT SHOW THIS ETHNIC GROUP TO DIFFER WITH RESPECT TO SOCIAL CHARACTERISTICS. CLEARLY, THE PUERTO RICAN MIGRANTS TO THE UNITED STATES HAVE MARKED HANDICAPS WITH RESPECT TO EDUCATIONAL LEVEL, AND OCCUPATIONAL AND ECONOMIC STATUS. THESE HANDICAPS RESULT IN SEGREGATING PUERTO RICANS IN SUBSTANDARD AREAS WHICH OFFER SERIOUS IMPEDIMENTS TO THE ATTAINMENT OF GOOD PHYSICAL AND MENTAL HEALTH. 8 REFERENCES.

ACCN   000961

1123 AUTH **MALZBERG, B.**
TITL   MENTAL DISEASE AMONG THE PUERTO RICANS IN NEW YORK CITY 1949-1951.
SRCE   *JOURNAL OF NERVOUS AND MENTAL DISEASE, 1956, 123(3), 262-269.*
INDX   MENTAL HEALTH, SCHIZOPHRENIA, SES, DEMOGRAPHIC, CROSS CULTURAL, ACCULTURATION, ALCOHOLISM, DEPRESSION, PSY-

CHOSIS, NEUROSIS, GERONTOLOGY, SURVEY, EMPIRICAL, PUERTO RICAN-M, URBAN, POVERTY, CHILDREN, ADOLESCENTS, ADULTS, SEX COMPARISON, NEW YORK, EAST
ABST   AN EXAMINATION OF MENTAL DISEASE AMONG PUERTO RICANS IN NEW YORK FROM 1949 TO 1951 REVEALS AN EXTREMELY HIGH RATE OF INCIDENCE. THE PUERTO RICAN MIGRATION TO NEW YORK CITY HAS GROWN TO CONSIDERABLE PROPORTIONS AND HAS BEEN INFLUENCED BY ECONOMIC AND LANGUAGE FACTORS. AS A RESULT, PUERTO RICANS HAVE BEEN SEGREGATED TO AREAS WHICH ARE SUBSTANDARD WITH RESPECT TO HOUSING AND HEALTH. STATISTICS SHOW THAT PUERTO RICANS ARE ADMITTED TO MENTAL HOSPITALS IN NEW YORK CITY AT AN AVERAGE ANNUAL RATE OF 157.7 PER 100,000 AS OPPOSED TO 144.5 FOR THE REMAINDER OF THE POPULATION IN NEW YORK CITY. THIS DISCREPANCY IS EVEN GREATER (239.3 FOR PUERTO RICANS AND 185.5 FOR THE OTHERS) WHEN THE PUERTO RICAN POPULATION IS COMPARED BY AGE AND SEX ADJUSTED RATES. THE HOSPITALIZED PUERTO RICAN POPULATION HAS A LARGE PROPORTION OF DEMENTIA PRAECOX AND A SMALL PROPORTION OF PSYCHOSES OF OLD AGE DUE TO ITS YOUTHFUL AGE DISTRIBUTION. THE HIGHER RATE OF FIRST ADMISSIONS TO MENTAL HOSPITALS AMONG PUERTO RICANS IS ASSOCIATED WITH LOWER STANDARDS OF LIVING AND WITH A BIASED MIGRATORY SAMPLE FROM THE TOTAL POPULATION. MENTAL DISEASE IS EXPECTED TO RISE TO APPROXIMATELY 100 PER 1,000 IN THE NEAR FUTURE FOR THE PUERTO RICAN POPULATION. A PERSON OF PUERTO RICAN ORIGIN HAS A GREATER PROBABILITY OF DEVELOPING A MENTAL DISEASE DURING HIS OR HER LIFETIME THAN AN AVERAGE MEMBER OF THE ENTIRE POPULATION. 5 REFERENCES.

ACCN   000960

1124 AUTH **MANASTER, G. J., & AHUMADA, I.**
TITL   CULTURAL VALUES IN LATIN AND NORTH AMERICAN CITIES.
SRCE   *JOURNAL OF CROSS-CULTURAL PSYCHOLOGY, 1971, 2(2), 197-202.*
INDX   CULTURE, PUERTO RICAN-I, CROSS CULTURAL, ADOLESCENTS, EMPIRICAL, ACCULTURATION, ATTRIBUTION OF RESPONSIBILITY, PERSONALITY, RESEARCH METHODOLOGY, SOUTH AMERICA, ILLINOIS, MIDWEST, VALUES
ABST   A COMPARISON OF THE CULTURAL VALUES OF 13 AND 16 YEAR-OLD UPPER-LOWER AND UPPER-MIDDLE CLASS ADOLESCENTS IN BUENOS AIRES (BA) AND CHICAGO (C) WITH AN EQUIVALENT SAMPLE OF YOUTHS FROM SAN JUAN (SJ), PUERTO RICO, IS PRESENTED. THE USES TEST, WHICH IS COMPOSED OF 50 ITEMS, WAS USED TO MEASURE THE CULTURAL VALUES OF THE GROUPS. THE RESPONSE OF EACH ITEM WAS SCORED BY PLACING IT IN ONE OF THE FOLLOWING CATEGORIES: INSTRUMENTAL, BENEVOLENT, MALEVOLENT, HEDONISTIC, ESTHETIC, RELIGIOUS, STATUS, AND INTELLECTUAL. THE THREE-COUNTRY SAMPLES PRODUCED THE SAME RANK-ORDER

OF MEANS OF RESPONSE CATEGORIES. DATA INDICATE THAT THE SJ GROUP IS SIGNIFICANTLY HIGHER THAN THE OTHER TWO GROUPS IN INSTRUMENTAL AND MALEVOLENT RESPONSES, WHILE THE C GROUP GIVES MORE STATUS AND ESTHETIC RESPONSES. THE LOWEST MEANS ARE IN THE INTELLECTUAL AND RELIGIOUS RESPONSE CATEGORIES WHERE NO DIFFERENCE EXISTS BETWEEN THE THREE COUNTRIES. THE SJ GROUP IS THE LOWEST OF ALL GROUPS ON HEDONISTIC AND BENEVOLENT RESPONSES. THE SJ SAMPLE DOES NOT FIT INTO EITHER PATTERN USED TO DESCRIBE THE OTHER GROUPS. RATHER, THE SJ SAMPLE IS SAID TO EXHIBIT A HIGHLY INSTRUMENTAL AND ALSO A SOMEWHAT NEGATIVE PERSONAL, SUBJECTIVE ORIENTATION. IT IS CONCLUDED THAT THE SJ GROUPS ORIENTATION APPEARS TO BE AT A MIDPOINT BETWEEN THE CULTURAL ORIENTATIONS OF NORTH AND SOUTH AMERICA. 2 REFERENCES.

ACCN   000962

1125 AUTH   **MANGOLD, M. M. (ED.)**
TITL   LA CAUSA CHICANA: THE MOVEMENT FOR JUSTICE.
SRCE   *NEW YORK: FAMILY SERVICE ASSOCIATION OF AMERICA, 1972.*
INDX   MENTAL HEALTH PROFESSION, CHICANO MOVEMENT, POLITICS, POLITICAL POWER, MEXICAN AMERICAN, ESSAY, COMMUNITY INVOLVEMENT, BOOK
ABST   THIS VOLUME IS INTENDED TO PRESENT INFORMATION ABOUT CHICANOS TO SOCIAL WORKERS AND MEMBERS OF OTHER HELPING PROFESSIONS SO THEY MAY BECOME INVOLVED IN THE MOVEMENT TO REDUCE PREJUDICE AND IGNORANCE ABOUT CHICANOS. TWENTY-ONE CHICANO AUTHORS REFLECT THE PERSPECTIVES OF WORK IN VARIOUS SETTINGS AND GEOGRAPHICAL REGIONS, AS WELL AS THE DISCIPLINES OF LAW, EDUCATION, PSYCHOLOGY, THE MINISTRY, AND SOCIAL WORK. SOME ARTICULATE THEIR CONCERNS ABOUT SOCIAL CHANGE AND SOCIAL SERVICE, WHILE OTHERS PROVIDE PROFILES ABOUT THE CHICANO FAMILY AND COMMUNITY. NINE OF THE ARTICLES WERE PREVIOUSLY PUBLISHED IN SOCIAL CASEWORK, 1972, VOL. 52 (WHOLE ISSUE NO. 5).
ACCN   001724

1126 AUTH   **MANGOLD, M. M. (ED.)**
TITL   LA CAUSA CHICANA: THE MOVEMENT FOR JUSTICE.
SRCE   *SOCIAL CASEWORK, 1971, 52(WHOLE ISSUE NO. 5).*
INDX   MENTAL HEALTH PROFESSION, CHICANO MOVEMENT, POLITICS, POLITICAL POWER, MEXICAN AMERICAN, ESSAY, COMMUNITY INVOLVEMENT
ABST   THE PREMISE WHICH UNIFIES THE NINE ESSAYS COMPILED IN THIS ISSUE IS THAT THE CHICANO HAS CERTAIN UNIQUE CHARACTERISTICS THAT MUST BE UNDERSTOOD BEFORE ADEQUATE SOCIAL SERVICES CAN BE PLANNED. THE AUTHORS, ALL CHICANOS, WORK IN THE DISCIPLINES OF LAW, EDUCA-

TION, PSYCHOLOGY, AND SOCIAL WORK. THE ESSAYS MAY BE CATEGORIZED INTO FOUR SUBJECT AREAS: (1) SOCIAL CHANGE AND SOCIAL SERVICES AS THEY AFFECT CHICANOS; (2) CULTURAL PERSPECTIVES FOR AN UNDERSTANDING OF THE CHICANO FAMILY; (3) THE PORTRAYAL OF THE CHICANO IN THE MASS MEDIA; AND (4) PSYCHOLOGICAL CONSIDERATIONS IN UNDERSTANDING THE CHICANO.

ACCN   000963

1127 AUTH   **MANGUM, M. E., JR.**
TITL   FAMILIAL IDENTIFICATION IN BLACK, ANGLO AND CHICANO MENTALLY RETARDED CHILDREN USING KINETIC FAMILY DRAWING (DOCTORAL DISSERTATION, UNIVERSITY OF NORTHERN COLORADO, 1975).
SRCE   *DISSERTATION ABSTRACTS INTERNATIONAL, 1975, 36(11), 7343A. (UNIVERSITY MICROFILMS NO. 76-19,908.)*
INDX   FAMILY ROLES, FAMILY STRUCTURE, PROJECTIVE TESTING, SPECIAL EDUCATION, INTELLIGENCE, INTELLIGENCE TESTING, CROSS CULTURAL, MEXICAN AMERICAN, CHILDREN, EMPIRICAL, WASHINGTON, WEST, MENTAL RETARDATION, GOODENOUGH DRAW-A-MAN TEST
ABST   TO DETERMINE (1) HOW MENTALLY RETARDED CHILDREN PERCEIVE FAMILY MEMBERS AND (2) IF SEX AND ETHNICITY INFLUENCE THEIR PERCEPTIONS, THE KINETIC FAMILY DRAWING AND GOODENOUGH DRAW-A-PERSON TEST WAS ADMINISTERED TO 90 EDUCABLE MENTALLY RETARDED CHILDREN (30 EACH MEXICAN AMERICAN, BLACK AND ANGLO), AGES 10-12, ENROLLED IN INTERMEDIATE LEVEL SPECIAL EDUCATION CLASSES IN THREE WASHINGTON STATE SCHOOL DISTRICTS. ALL SUBJECTS HAD WISC SCORES BETWEEN 50-80. THE FOLLOWING CONCLUSIONS WERE MADE: (1) THE MENTALLY RETARDED CHILDREN OF ALL THREE ETHNIC GROUPS DO IDENTIFY WITH SPECIFIC FAMILY MEMBERS; (2) THEY DO NOT DIFFER SIGNIFICANTLY IN SPECIFIC FAMILY MEMBER IDENTIFICATION BY ETHNICITY; (3) THEY DO NOT DEMONSTRATE SIGNIFICANT SEXUAL DIFFERENCES IN SPECIFIC FAMILY MEMBER IDENTIFICATION; AND (4) THE KINETIC FAMILY DRAWING TECHNIQUE IS A RESPONSIVE INSTRUMENT FOR USE WITH EDUCABLE MENTALLY RETARDED CHILDREN AGE 10-12. IMPLICATIONS OF THESE FINDINGS FOR THE SCHOOL AS WELL AS THE HOME IN PLANNING A COMPLETE PROGRAM FOR EDUCABLE MENTALLY RETARDED CHILDREN ARE DISCUSSED. 67 REFERENCES. (AUTHOR ABSTRACT MODIFIED)
ACCN   000948

1128 AUTH   **MANNING, B. A., PIERCE-JONES, J., & PARELMAN, R. L.**
TITL   COOPERATIVE, TRUSTING BEHAVIOR IN A "CULTURALLY DEPRIVED," MIXED ETHNIC-GROUP POPULATION.
SRCE   *THE JOURNAL OF SOCIAL PSYCHOLOGY, 1974, 92(1), 133-141.*
INDX   MEXICAN AMERICAN, CHILDREN, CROSS CULTURAL, COOPERATION, COMPETITION, SEX

COMPARISON, INTERPERSONAL RELATIONS, TEXAS, SOUTHWEST, EMPIRICAL

ABST COOPERATIVE, TRUSTING BEHAVIOR OF CHILDREN REPRESENTING 3 ETHNIC GROUPS FROM A CULTURALLY DEPRIVED POPULATION IS EXAMINED. ONE HUNDRED FORTY-FOUR MEXICAN AMERICAN, BLACK, AND ANGLO AMERICAN, FIVE AND SIX YEAR-OLD "HEAD START" CHILDREN TOOK PART IN A TWO-PERSON, TWO-CHOICE GAME IN WHICH THEY COULD COOPERATE OR COMPETE WITH ANOTHER CHILD. THE 72 MALES AND 72 FEMALES WERE DIVIDED INTO SIMILAR AND DISSIMILAR ETHNIC GROUP PAIRS,AND IMMEDIATE AND DELAYED REWARD GROUPS. THE RESULTS OF A SERIES OF ANALYSES OF VARIANCE INDICATED THAT: (1) FOR FEMALES, SIMILAR ETHNIC PAIRS COOPERATED SIGNIFICANTLY MORE THAN DISSIMILAR PAIRS, WITH THE EXCEPTION OF MEXICAN AMERICAN/BLACK PAIRS WHO MAINTAINED A HIGH LEVEL OF COOPERATION; (2) FEMALES IN THE THREE ETHNIC GROUPS DIFFERED SIGNIFICANTLY IN THEIR AMOUNT OF COOPERATIVE BEHAVIOR, WITH ANGLO AMERICANS COMPETING THE MOST; AND (3) COOPERATIVE BEHAVIOR WAS NOT DIFFERENTIALLY AFFECTED BY THE TYPE OF REINFORCEMENT USED, NOR DID IT INCREASE AS A FUNCTION OF TRIALS. 13 REFERENCES. (JOURNAL ABSTRACT MODIFIED)

ACCN 000964

1129 AUTH **MANUEL, H. T.**
TITL A COMPARISON OF SPANISH-SPEAKING AND ENGLISH-SPEAKING CHILDREN IN READING AND ARITHMETIC.
SRCE *JOURNAL OF APPLIED PSYCHOLOGY, 1935, 19(1), 189-202.*
INDX SCHOLASTIC ACHIEVEMENT, READING, MATHEMATICS, BILINGUALISM, CROSS CULTURAL, MEXICAN AMERICAN, CHILDREN, SES, TEXAS, SOUTHWEST, ACHIEVEMENT TESTING
ABST THE NEW STANFORD READING AND ARITHMETIC TESTS WERE GIVEN IN THE FALL AND SPRING TO SPANISH-SPEAKING (SS) AND ENGLISH-SPEAKING (ES) CHILDREN IN GRADES TWO TO EIGHT IN A NUMBER OF SCHOOLS OF THE LOWER RIO GRANDE VALLEY IN TEXAS. FINDINGS FROM THE FALL TESTS REVEALED THAT THE SS PUPILS WERE FROM 1.6 YEARS TO 2.9 YEARS OLDER THAN THE ES PUPILS, AND THAT THE SS CHILDREN WERE ON THE AVERAGE ABOUT A YEAR LOWER IN READING THAN IN ARITHMETIC. THIS CONDITION IS INTERPRETED AS EVIDENCE OF A SERIOUS AND PERSISTENT LANGUAGE HANDICAP. THE SPRING TESTS INDICATED THAT THE SS CHILDREN GAINED ON THE AVERAGE LESS THAN THE ES CHILDREN IN READING AND ARITHMETIC. THE VARIABILITY OF SCORES IN BOTH THE SS AND ES GROUP WAS LARGE. THERE WAS EVIDENCE OF A POSITIVE RELATIONSHIP BETWEEN SOCIOECONOMIC LEVEL AND ACHIEVEMENT IN READING AND ARITHMETIC. IT IS CONCLUDED THAT THE PRESENCE OF THE LOW ACHIEVEMENT OF SS CHILDREN IN ANGLO-AMERICAN SCHOOLS INDICATES THEY SUFFER A SERIOUS

AND PERSISTENT LANGUAGE HANDICAP UP TO THE EIGHTH GRADE.

ACCN 000966

1130 AUTH **MANUEL, H. T.**
TITL PHYSICAL MEASUREMENTS OF MEXICAN CHILDREN IN AMERICAN SCHOOLS.
SRCE *CHILD DEVELOPMENT, 1935, 5(3), 237-252.*
INDX PHYSICAL DEVELOPMENT, MEXICAN AMERICAN, CHILDREN, EMPIRICAL, CROSS CULTURAL, TEXAS, SOUTHWEST
ABST A REPORT OF MEASURES OF HEIGHT, WEIGHT, WIDTH OF SHOULDERS, WIDTH OF HIPS, DEPTH OF CHEST, AND ARM GIRTH OF MEXICAN SCHOOL CHILDREN IN LAREDO AND EL PASO, TEXAS, IS PRESENTED. ON A MEASURE OF SKIN COLOR WITH 1,863 BOYS, AGES 5 TO 17, 18.7% WERE CLASSIFIED AS LIGHT, 40.3% AS MEDIUM, AND 41% AS DARK. OF 1,815 GIRLS OF THE SAME AGES, 25.3% WERE CLASSIFIED AS LIGHT, 36.7% AS MEDIUM, AND 38% AS DARK. BOTH MALES AND FEMALES OF DARKEST COMPLEXION SHOWED A TENDENCY TO BE A LITTLE SMALLER IN ALL PHYSICAL MEASUREMENTS THAN THOSE OF LIGHTER COLOR EXCEPT IN THE DEPTH OF CHEST MEASUREMENT. THE AVERAGE DIFFERENCE, HOWEVER, AT AGE LEVELS 7 TO 14 WAS LESS THAN AN INCH, A POUND, OR A CENTIMETER IN MEASUREMENT. THE HEIGHTS AND WEIGHTS OF MEXICAN CHILDREN FROM THE UNITED STATES CORRESPOND CLOSELY TO THOSE REPORTED FROM MEXICO. IN GENERAL, MEXICAN MALES FROM MEXICO WEIGH LESS THAN MEXICAN CHILDREN IN THE UNITED STATES, WHILE MEXICAN FEMALES FROM MEXICO ARE HEAVIER. COMPARED WITH ANGLO AMERICAN CHILDREN, MEXICAN MALES BETWEEN THE AGES OF 6 TO 14 AND FEMALES BETWEEN 6 TO 12 YEARS ARE APPROXIMATELY 2 INCHES SHORTER, AGE FOR AGE, AND APPROXIMATELY 4 TO 7 POUNDS LIGHTER. IT IS SUGGESTED THAT MEXICAN BOYS AND GIRLS MATURE MORE SLOWLY THAN THE ANGLO AMERICAN CHILDREN. 5 REFERENCES.

ACCN 000967

1131 AUTH **MANUEL, H. T.**
TITL SPANISH-SPEAKING CHILDREN OF THE SOUTHWEST: THEIR EDUCATION AND THE PUBLIC WELFARE.
SRCE *AUSTIN, TEXAS: UNIVERSITY OF TEXAS PRESS, 1965.*
INDX SOUTHWEST, REVIEW, MEXICAN AMERICAN, SES, POVERTY, EDUCATION, FARM LABORERS, MIGRANTS, DEMOGRAPHIC, CHILDREN, PREJUDICE, EQUAL OPPORTUNITY, CULTURAL PLURALISM, HISTORY, CULTURAL FACTORS, BILINGUALISM, ABILITY TESTING, ACHIEVEMENT TESTING, COMMUNITY INVOLVEMENT, SPANISH SURNAMED, EMPIRICAL, INTELLIGENCE TESTING, PERSONALITY, BILINGUAL-BICULTURAL EDUCATION, ATTITUDES, PARENTAL INVOLVEMENT
ABST THE EDUCATIONAL AND SOCIAL DIFFICULTIES EXPERIENCED BY SPANISH-SPEAKING CHILDREN ARE EXAMINED FROM AN HISTORICAL AND CULTURAL PERSPECTIVE. THE AUTHOR

TAKES INTO ACCOUNT THE CIRCUMSTANCES OF HISPANIC AND ANGLO MIGRATIONS INTO THE SOUTHWEST AND THEIR BACKGROUND OF INTERGROUP STRIFE. DEMOGRAPHIC CHARACTERISTICS OF THE SPANISH-SPEAKING POPULATION, PARTICULARLY THE SCHOOL AGE POPULATION, ARE ALSO DISCUSSED—WITH DETAILS PROVIDED BY 8 FIGURES AND 23 TABLES. IT IS CONCLUDED THAT SPANISH-SPEAKING STUDENTS ARE HANDICAPPED NOT ONLY BY DIVISIONS AND CULTURAL CONFLICTS BETWEEN ENGLISH- AND SPANISH-SPEAKING COMMUNITIES, BUT ALSO BY SPECIAL PROBLEMS OF LANGUAGE, POVERTY, AND MIGRATION WHICH RESULT IN DIFFICULT PERSONAL AND SOCIAL ADJUSTMENT. EMPHASIZING THE NECESSITY FOR COMMUNITY SUPPORT, THE AUTHOR ARGUES THAT THE PROBLEMS OF SPANISH-SPEAKING CHILDREN MUST BE RECOGNIZED NOT SIMPLY AS A PROBLEM IN EDUCATION, BUT AS A PROBLEM IN DEMOCRACY. 83 REFERENCES.

ACCN   002148

1132 AUTH   **MANUEL, H. T.**
TITL   TEACHING A SECOND LANGUAGE TO SPANISH SPEAKING CHILDREN OF THE SOUTHWEST.
SRCE   *IN J. C. STONE & D. P. DENEVI (EDS.), TEACHING MULTICULTURAL POPULATIONS: FIVE HERITAGES. NEW YORK: VAN NOSTRAND, 1971, PP. 262-271.*
INDX   BILINGUAL-BICULTURAL EDUCATION, LANGUAGE LEARNING, PUERTO RICAN-M, CHILDREN, ESSAY, INSTRUCTIONAL TECHNIQUES, CURRICULUM, TEACHERS, MEXICAN AMERICAN, READING
ABST   METHODS FOR TEACHING ENGLISH TO SPANISH-SPEAKING CHILDREN ARE PRESENTED. A SUGGESTED LANGUAGE PROGRAM INCLUDES THE FOLLOWING STEPS: (1) BEGIN TEACHING ENGLISH IN A PRE-FIRST GRADE PROGRAM FOR FIVE YEAR-OLDS WITH A GRADUAL TRANSITION FROM SPEAKING SPANISH TO SPEAKING ENGLISH AND AN EMPHASIS ON PREPARATION FOR READING ENGLISH; (2) BEGIN INSTRUCTION IN READING ENGLISH WHEN AN ADEQUATE STAGE OF READINESS IS REACHED; (3) BEGIN INSTRUCTION IN READING SPANISH WHEN THE CHILDREN HAVE MASTERED BASIC TECHNIQUES IN READING ENGLISH; (4) GIVE INSTRUCTION IN SPANISH AS A LANGUAGE THROUGH ALL THE ELEMENTARY GRADES TO ALL WHO QUALIFY; (5) FOR ENGLISH-SPEAKING CHILDREN ENROLLED IN THE SAME SCHOOL, GIVE INSTRUCTION IN ORAL SPANISH BEGINNING IN GRADE ONE, AND BEGIN READING IN SPANISH AFTER THEY HAVE MASTERED READING IN ENGLISH; AND (6) ENCOURAGE STUDENTS TO CONTINUE STUDY OF SPANISH BEYOND THE ELEMENTARY LEVEL. 1 REFERENCE.
ACCN   000968

1133 AUTH   **MANUEL, H. T., & HUGHES, L. S.**
TITL   THE INTELLIGENCE AND DRAWING ABILITY OF YOUNG MEXICAN CHILDREN.
SRCE   *JOURNAL OF APPLIED PSYCHOLOGY, 1932, 16(4), 382-387.*

INDX   GOODENOUGH DRAW-A-MAN TEST, INTELLIGENCE TESTING, MEXICAN AMERICAN, CHILDREN, CROSS CULTURAL, EMPIRICAL, TEXAS, SOUTHWEST
ABST   THE GOODENOUGH INTELLIGENCE TEST (GIT) WAS ADMINISTERED TO 440 MEXICAN AND 396 NON-MEXICAN CHILDREN TO COMPARE INTELLIGENCE AND DRAWING ABILITY. THE DRAWINGS WERE SELECTED BY A SAMPLING PROCESS FROM ABOUT TWELVE THOUSAND STUDENTS IN THE FIRST FOUR GRADES OF THE SAN ANTONIO PUBLIC SCHOOLS. INTELLIGENCE AND DRAWING ABILITY WERE CLOSELY RELATED INSOFAR AS MEASURED BY THE GIT. HOWEVER, THIS RELATION DECREASED WITH ADVANCE IN SCHOOL GRADE. PERHAPS THE FACTORS WHICH DIFFERENTIATE TALENT IN DRAWING ARE LESS OBVIOUS IN THE FIRST GRADE THAN THEY ARE IN LATER YEARS. THE AVERAGE ABILITY OF THE MEXICAN CHILDREN BOTH IN INTELLIGENCE AND IN DRAWING COMPARE FAVORABLY, GRADE FOR GRADE, WITH THAT OF THE OTHER CHILDREN. A COMPARISON BY AGES, HOWEVER, WAS LESS FAVORABLE. LOWER SCORES BOTH IN DRAWING AND IN INTELLIGENCE WERE SHOWN AT EACH AGE LEVEL (7-10) FOR THE MEXICAN CHILDREN. THE BELIEF THAT MEXICAN CHILDREN ARE GIFTED IN DRAWING AND HANDWORK IS NOT SUPPORTED BY A COMPARISON OF THE SCORES AT ANY AGE LEVEL. IT MAY BE THAT THE APPARENT TALENT OF MEXICAN CHILDREN IN DRAWING IS MORE A MATTER OF TRAINING AND INTEREST OR THAT THE TEST USED IN THIS STUDY IS NOT A SUITABLE ONE TO REVEAL THIS ABILITY. 3 REFERENCES.
ACCN   000969

1134 AUTH   **MANUEL, H. T., & WRIGHT, C. E.**
TITL   THE LANGUAGE DIFFICULTY OF MEXICAN CHILDREN.
SRCE   *JOURNAL OF GENETIC PSYCHOLOGY, 1929, 36(3), 458-466.*
INDX   ACHIEVEMENT TESTING, LINGUISTIC COMPETENCE, STANFORD ACHIEVEMENT TEST, TEST RELIABILITY, CROSS CULTURAL, MEXICAN AMERICAN, BILINGUALISM, EMPIRICAL, SCHOLASTIC ACHIEVEMENT, ADOLESCENTS, COLLEGE STUDENTS, TEXAS, SOUTHWEST, READING, BILINGUAL
ABST   THE LANGUAGE HANDICAP PROBLEM OF SPANISH-AMERICAN (SA) PUPILS WAS APPROACHED BY TESTING THE RELATIVE ABILITY OF STUDENTS IN BOTH ENGLISH AND SPANISH. FORMS A AND B OF THE PARAGRAPH MEANING TEST OF THE STANFORD ACHIEVEMENT READING EXAMINATION WERE TRANSLATED INTO SPANISH. TWO OF THE FOUR TESTS WERE GIVEN IN VARIOUS COMBINATIONS TO 669 HIGH SCHOOL STUDENTS AND 207 COLLEGE STUDENTS. OF THE 876 STUDENTS, 168 (19%) SPOKE SPANISH AS THEIR NATIVE LANGUAGE. THE FOLLOWING RESULTS WERE OBTAINED. (1) ENGLISH-SPEAKING STUDENTS SCORE HIGHER ON THE ENGLISH TEST THAN DO THE SA STUDENTS. (2) ENGLISH-SPEAKING STUDENTS ACHIEVE HIGHER SCORES ON THE ENGLISH TEST THAN THEY DO

ON THE SPANISH TEST. (3) THE SPANISH READING TEST REVEALS A WIDE RANGE OF ABILITIES BETWEEN THE ENGLISH-SPEAKING AND SA STUDENTS. (4) SA STUDENTS, AS A RULE, HAVE HIGHER RATINGS ON THE SPANISH TESTS THAN DO NATIVE SPEAKERS OF ENGLISH. (5) SLIGHTLY MORE THAN HALF OF THE SA STUDENTS ACHIEVE SCORES ON THE ENGLISH TEST HAVING A HIGHER NUMERICAL VALUE THAN THEIR SCORES ON THE SPANISH TEST. THESE RESULTS, HOWEVER, CANNOT BE EASILY INTERPRETED BECAUSE OF THE UNKNOWN RELATIVE DIFFICULTY OF THE ENGLISH AND SPANISH TESTS. IF THE ENGLISH AND SPANISH TESTS ARE OF EQUAL DIFFICULTY THEN THE FINDINGS CAN BE INTERPRETED AS SUGGESTIVE OF (1) A DIFFERENCE OF NATIVE ABILITY BETWEEN THE TWO GROUPS OR (2) A DUAL LANGUAGE HANDICAP ON THE PART OF THE SA STUDENTS. ON THE OTHER HAND, IF SA'S HAVE GREATER ABILITY TO READ IN SPANISH, THEN THE TRANSLATION OF THE TESTS HAS FAILED TO YIELD TESTS OF EQUAL DIFFICULTY IN BOTH LANGUAGES. 4 REFERENCES.

ACCN   000970

1135 AUTH   **MARCOS, L. R.**
TITL   LINGUISTIC DIMENSIONS IN THE BILINGUAL PATIENT.
SRCE   *THE AMERICAN JOURNAL OF PSYCHOANALYSIS, 1976, 36, 347-354.*
INDX   PSYCHOTHERAPY, BILINGUALISM, LINGUISTICS, COMPOUND-COORDINATE DISTINCTION, ESSAY, LINGUISTIC COMPETENCE
ABST   BILINGUAL INDIVIDUALS' MAJOR LINGUISTIC DIMENSIONS AS RELATED TO THE PROCESS OF DYNAMIC PSYCHOTHERAPY ARE DESCRIBED. ONE LINGUISTIC DIMENSION, THE DEGREE OF LINGUISTIC COMPETENCE OF BILINGUALS, IS USUALLY CLASSIFIED AS SUBORDINATE OR PROFICIENT. A FUNDAMENTAL CHARACTERISTIC OF SUBORDINATE BILINGUALS IS THE LANGUAGE BARRIER WHICH RESULTS FROM THE DIFFICULTY IN THE PROCESSING OF INFORMATION IN THE SECOND LANGUAGE. THE IMPLICATIONS FOR PSYCHOTHERAPY OF THE LANGUAGE BARRIER APPEAR TO BE: (1) PATIENTS TEND TO BE MORE OCCUPIED WITH HOW THEY SAY THINGS RATHER THAN WHAT THEY SAY; (2) PATIENTS' CONSTANT CONCERN ABOUT DICTION AND OVER USE OF CLICHES; (3) PATIENTS' INABILITY TO UNDERSTAND THE VOCAL OR PARALINGUISTIC CUES FROM THE THERAPIST; AND (4) THE BILINGUAL SITUATION POSES MORE DEMANDS FOR THE THERAPIST IN ATTEMPTING TO TREAT THE PATIENT. ANOTHER SIGNIFICANT ASPECT OF THE BILINGUAL PERSON IS THE CONTEXT BY WHICH THE SECOND LANGUAGE WAS ACQUIRED. LANGUAGE INCOMPATIBILITY, A FACTOR WHICH RESULTS FROM THE LACK OF TRANSLATION EQUIVALENTS FOR EVERYDAY TERMS AND DIFFERENCES IN PSYCHOSOCIAL MEANINGS OF WORDS, MUST BE TAKEN INTO CONSIDERATION. IT IS CONCLUDED THAT THE THERAPIST NEEDS TO ASSESS THE DEGREE OF LANGUAGE DOMINANCE AND THE DEGREE OF NONCONGRUENCY OF THE PA-

TIENT'S LANGUAGE SYSTEM IN THE TREATMENT PROCESS. 44 REFERENCES.

ACCN   000971

1136 AUTH   **MARCOS, L. R.**
TITL   NONVERBAL BEHAVIOR AND THOUGHT PROCESSING.
SRCE   *ARCHIVES OF GENERAL PSYCHIATRY, 1979, 36, 940-943.*
INDX   BILINGUAL, PSYCHOPATHOLOGY, SPANISH SURNAMED, STRESS, ADULTS, EMPIRICAL, PSYCHOTHERAPY, BILINGUALISM, LINGUISTIC COMPETENCE
ABST   THE RELATIONSHIP OF CENTRAL COGNITIVE PROCESSES TO HAND MOVEMENT BEHAVIORS WAS INVESTIGATED IN ORDER TO IDENTIFY ENCODING-RELATED MOTOR BEHAVIOR AMONG BILINGUAL PERSONS. THE METHOD EMPLOYED COMPARED THE HAND MOVEMENTS OF SUBORDINATE BILINGUAL SUBJECTS IN SITUATIONS OF DOMINANT AND NONDOMINANT LANGUAGE USE AND LOW- AND HIGH-IMAGERY VERBALIZATION. IN CONTRAST TO THE PARALLEL DOMINANT-LANGUAGE CONDITION, THE 16 ADULT SUBJECTS WHEN VERBALIZING IN THEIR NONDOMINANT LANGUAGE (ENGLISH OR SPANISH) PRODUCED MORE SPEECH-PRIMACY AND GROPING HAND MOVEMENTS. COMPARED TO THEIR VERBALIZATIONS ABOUT A HIGH-IMAGERY TOPIC, WHEN THE SUBJECTS ENCODED A LOW-IMAGERY TOPIC THEY DISPLAYED MORE POINTING MOVEMENTS. IT IS CONCLUDED THAT UNLESS CLINICIANS ARE AWARE OF HAND MOVEMENT DIFFERENCES IN BILINGUAL CLIENTS, THEY MAY, IN EVALUATING SUCH CLIENTS, INTERPRET AN INCREASE IN ENCODING-RELATED MOTOR ACTIVITY AS REFLECTING PSYCHOPATHOLOGY. APART FROM THIS PSYCHODIAGNOSTIC SIGNIFICANCE, HYPOTHETICAL IMPLICATIONS OF THESE FINDINGS FOR THE STUDY OF APHASIA AND INFORMATION PROCESSING MECHANISMS ARE DISCUSSED. 26 REFERENCES. (JOURNAL ABSTRACT MODIFIED)

ACCN   001826

1137 AUTH   **MARCOS, L. R., ALPERT, M., URCUYO, L., & KESSELMAN, M.**
TITL   THE EFFECT OF INTERVIEW LANGUAGE ON THE EVALUATION OF PSYCHOPATHOLOGY IN SPANISH-AMERICAN SCHIZOPHRENIC PATIENTS.
SRCE   *AMERICAN JOURNAL OF PSYCHIATRY, 1973, 130(5), 549-553.*
INDX   PSYCHOPATHOLOGY, SPANISH SURNAMED, CULTURAL FACTORS, BILINGUAL-BICULTURAL PERSONNEL, MENTAL HEALTH, ADULTS, EMPIRICAL, WAIS, EXAMINER EFFECTS, NEW YORK, EAST, BILINGUAL
ABST   THE BRIEF PSYCHIATRIC RATING SCALE (BPRS) WAS ADMINISTERED TO 10 NATIVE SPANISH-SPEAKING SCHIZOPHRENIC PATIENTS ADMITTED TO THE BELLEVUE PSYCHIATRIC HOSPITAL IN NEW YORK TO ASCERTAIN THE INTERRATER RELIABILITY BETWEEN ENGLISH- AND SPANISH-SPEAKING RATERS AND WHETHER THE LANGUAGE OF THE INTERVIEW WOULD

HAVE AN EFFECT ON THE AMOUNT OF PA-
THOLOGY DETECTED BY THE 4 RATERS. MORE
PSYCHOPATHOLOGY WAS DISCLOSED WHEN
THE SUBJECTS WERE INTERVIEWED IN THE EN-
GLISH LANGUAGE THAN WHEN THEY THEY
WERE INTERVIEWED IN SPANISH. EVIDENCE
SUGGESTS THAT THERE WERE IMPORTANT
CLINICAL CHANGES IN THE PATIENT ATTRIB-
UTABLE TO HIS PROBLEMS IN SPEAKING IN A
SECOND LANGUAGE. THE CLINICIAN-SUBJECT
FRAME OF REFERENCE MUST ALSO BE TAKEN
INTO ACCOUNT; FOR WHAT IS APPLICABLE TO
NATIVE ENGLISH-SPEAKING PATIENTS CANNOT
NECESSARILY BE DIRECTLY APPLIED TO THE
EVALUATION OF PERSONS FROM OTHER CUL-
TURES. 19 REFERENCES. (PASAR ABSTRACT
MODIFIED)

ACCN   000972

1138 AUTH   **MARCOS, L. R., & ALPERT, M.**
TITL   STRATEGIES AND RISKS IN PSYCHOTHERAPY
WITH BILINGUAL PATIENTS: THE PHENOME-
NON OF LANGUAGE INDEPENDENCE.
SRCE   *AMERICAN JOURNAL OF PSYCHIATRY, 1976,*
133(11), 1275-1278.
INDX   PSYCHOTHERAPY, PSYCHOTHERAPISTS, LIN-
GUISTICS, BILINGUALISM, ESSAY
ABST   THE PRESENCE OF TWO SEPARATE LAN-
GUAGES, EACH WITH ITS OWN LEXICAL, SYN-
TACTIC, SEMANTIC, AND IDEATIONAL COMPO-
NENTS, CAN COMPLICATE PSYCHOTHERAPY
WITH PROFICIENT BILINGUAL PATIENTS. IF ONLY
ONE LANGUAGE IS USED IN THERAPY, SOME
ASPECTS OF THE PATIENT'S EMOTIONAL EX-
PERIENCE MAY BE UNAVAILABLE TO TREAT-
MENT; IF BOTH LANGUAGES ARE USED, THE
PATIENT MAY USE LANGUAGE SWITCHING AS A
FORM OF RESISTANCE TO AFFECTIVELY
CHARGED MATERIAL. THE AUTHORS SUGGEST
THAT MONOLINGUAL THERAPISTS SHOULD
CAREFULLY ASSESS THE DEGREE OF LAN-
GUAGE INDEPENDENCE IN BILINGUALS IN OR-
DER TO MINIMIZE ITS IMPACT ON THERAPY.
THEY CONCLUDE THAT STUDY OF BILINGUAL
PATIENTS MAY PROVIDE IMPORTANT INSIGHTS
INTO THE NATURE OF THE THERAPEUTIC PRO-
CESS. 34 REFERENCES. (JOURNAL ABSTRACT)

ACCN   000973

1139 AUTH   **MARCUM, J. P., & BEAN, F. D.**
TITL   MINORITY GROUP STATUS AS A FACTOR IN THE
RELATIONSHIP BETWEEN MOBILITY AND FER-
TILITY: THE MEXICAN AMERICAN CASE.
SRCE   *SOCIAL FORCES, 1976, 55(1), 135-148.*
INDX   MEXICAN AMERICAN, SOCIAL MOBILITY, FER-
TILITY, FAMILY STRUCTURE, ACCULTURATION,
EMPIRICAL, ETHNIC IDENTITY, SES, ADULTS,
MARRIAGE, SURVEY, URBAN, CROSS GENERA-
TIONAL, TEXAS, SOUTHWEST
ABST   CONTRASTING HYPOTHESES ABOUT THE IN-
FLUENCE OF RACIAL AND ETHNIC GROUP
MEMBERSHIP ON THE RELATIONSHIP BE-
TWEEN MOBILITY AND FERTILITY ARE TESTED.
ONE HYPOTHESIS MAY BE TERMED THE MI-
NORITY GROUP STATUS APPROACH, AND THE
OTHER THE UNDERDEVELOPMENT AP-
PROACH. BOTH PERSPECTIVES OFFER BASES
FOR PREDICTING FERTILITY LEVELS THAT DE-

VIATE FROM THE LEVEL THAT IS ROUGHLY THE
AVERAGE OF THE FERTILITY LEVELS TYPICAL
OF THE SOCIAL STRATA BETWEEN WHICH MO-
BILITY HAS OCCURRED. THE FORMER IMPLIES
GREATER FERTILITY DEVIATIONS THE MORE IN-
TEGRATED THE MINORITY GROUP IS INTO THE
LARGER SOCIETY, WHEREAS THE LATTER SUG-
GESTS GREATER DEVIATIONS THE LESS INTE-
GRATED THE MINORITY GROUP IS INTO THE
LARGER SOCIETY. THESE HYPOTHESES WERE
TESTED USING DATA FROM A SAMPLE OF MEX-
ICAN AMERICAN COUPLES, SPLIT ACCORDING
TO GENERATIONAL DISTANCE FROM MEXICO.
THE RESULTS INDICATE MORE SUPPORT FOR
THE MINORITY GROUP STATUS THAN THE UN-
DERDEVELOPMENT HYPOTHESIS, AS RE-
VEALED BY LOWER THAN AVERAGE EXPECTED
FERTILITY ON THE PART OF COUPLES RE-
MOVED AT LEAST THREE GENERATIONS FROM
MEXICO. 29 REFERENCES. (JOURNAL AB-
STRACT MODIFIED)

ACCN   000974

1140 AUTH   **MARDEN, C. F., & MEYER, G.**
TITL   MEXICAN AMERICANS—LA RAZA (CHAPTER
11).
SRCE   *IN C. F. MARDEN, & G. MEYER (EDS.), MINORI-*
TIES IN AMERICAN SOCIETY. NEW YORK: VAN
NOSTRAND, 1973, PP. 304-331.
INDX   MEXICAN AMERICAN, REVIEW, HISTORY, POV-
ERTY, ECONOMIC FACTORS, MIGRATION, CEN-
SUS, CULTURE, ESSAY, SELF CONCEPT,
STEREOTYPES, FAMILY ROLES, EMPLOYMENT,
EDUCATION, EQUAL OPPORTUNITY, COMMU-
NITY INVOLVEMENT, POLICY, DISCRIMINATION,
RELIGION, SOCIAL MOBILITY, COMMUNITY, PO-
LITICAL POWER, JUDICIAL PROCESS, CHICANO
MOVEMENT, ACCULTURATION, FAMILY STRUC-
TURE, FATALISM, TIME ORIENTATION
ABST   THIS CHAPTER FOCUSES ON THE MIGRATION,
THE ESTABLISHMENT OF ANGLO DOMINANCE,
ANGLO AND MEXICAN AMERICAN RELATIONS,
AND THE RECENT STRIDES IN ACQUIRING PO-
LITICAL POWER AMONG THE MEXICAN AMERI-
CAN POPULATION. FOR THE MAJORITY OF
MEXICAN AMERICANS LA RAZA (THE RACE) IS
A CULTURAL CONCEPT REFLECTING THE
EVENTS OF FEUDALISM, OPPRESSION, AND
DISCRIMINATION THEY HAVE HISTORICALLY
EXPERIENCED. THE FATALISTIC ATTITUDE THAT
HAS BEEN ASSOCIATED WITH MEXICAN AMERI-
CANS IS LARGELY DUE TO THE INTERTWINING
OF CATHOLICISM AND CULTURE. THE CONSE-
QUENCES OF CATHOLICIZED FATALISM AMONG
MEXICAN AMERICANS WILL CONTINUE AS LONG
AS THE ANGLO SOCIETY PERSISTS IN ITS DE-
VALUATION OF AND LIMITATION OF OPPORTU-
NITY FOR PERSONS OF SPANISH DESCENT.
SINCE WORLD WAR II, THE MEXICAN AMERI-
CAN COMMUNITY HAS RALLIED BEHIND LA
RAZA AND MEXICAN AMERICANS HAVE BEGUN
TO DEVELOP ETHNIC PRIDE. AS A RESULT OF
THIS NEW SELF-IDENTITY, MEXICAN AMERI-
CANS ARE BEGINNING TO RECOGNIZE THEIR
POLITICAL POTENTIAL TO BRING ABOUT RELE-
VANT CHANGE TO INSURE THAT THEY WILL NO

LONGER BE THE FORGOTTEN PEOPLE. 32 REFERENCES.

ACCN   000975

1141 AUTH **MARES, R.**
TITL   LA PINTA: THE MYTH OF REHABILITATION.
SRCE   *ENCUENTRO FEMENIL, 1975, 1(2), 20-27.*
INDX   FEMALE, MEXICAN AMERICAN, CHICANO MOVEMENT, CORRECTIONS, CRIMINOLOGY, CALIFORNIA, SOUTHWEST, ESSAY, REVIEW, REHABILITATION, ADULTS, SOCIAL SERVICES, PROGRAM EVALUATION, VOCATIONAL COUNSELING, EMPLOYMENT, MOTHER-CHILD INTERACTION, POLICY, EDUCATION
ABST   FOCUSING ON THE LACK OF AN EFFECTIVE REHABILITATION PROGRAM AT THE CALIFORNIA INSTITUTION FOR WOMEN (CIW), A STATE PRISON FOR THE INCARCERATION OF FEMALE FELONS, THIS ARTICLE DESCRIBES CONDITIONS AND PRACTICES AFFECTING THE 650 INMATES, 11% OF WHOM ARE CHICANA. A 1971 STUDY CONDUCTED BY THE DEPARTMENT OF CORRECTIONS CONFIRMED THAT ONGOING VOCATIONAL AND EDUCATIONAL PROGRAMS HAD DONE LITTLE TO AID WOMEN ON PAROLE IN FINDING EMPLOYMENT IN THE FIELD IN WHICH THEY HAD RECEIVED TRAINING. OBVIOUS NEEDS OF THE WOMEN AT CIW INCLUDE VOCATIONAL PROGRAMS TO DEVELOP MARKETABLE SKILLS, PLACEMENT SERVICES TO ASSIST THE WOMEN IN FINDING EMPLOYMENT MATCHED TO THEIR SKILLS, AND SERVICES TO ASSIST IN FAMILY PROBLEMS ARISING FROM INCARCERATION. MARA, AN ORGANIZATION OF CHICANA INMATES, HAS BEEN ABLE TO PROVIDE MUCH-NEEDED RESOURCES AND COUNSELING, PARTICULARLY IN BRIDGING THE GAP BETWEEN "LA PINTA" (THE PRISON) AND THE CHICANO COMMUNITY. SPECIFIC COMPLAINTS REGARDING EMPLOYMENT AND TRAINING PROGRAMS, VOCATIONAL AND EDUCATIONAL CLASSES, AGENCY INVOLVEMENT AND ASSISTANCE, THE VISITATION SYSTEM, CHILD PLACEMENT, INDETERMINATE SENTENCING AND PAROLE, AND THE POLITICAL AND ETHNIC MAKEUP OF THE CIW GOVERNING BOARD ARE DISCUSSED. DESPITE THE TREND IN MODERN CRIMINOLOGY AWAY FROM PUNISHMENT AND TOWARD REHABILITATION, NO EFFECTIVE PROGRAM OF REHABILITATION FOR THE WOMEN AT CIW HAS YET BEEN DEVISED.
ACCN   002149

1142 AUTH **MARGOLIS, R. J.**
TITL   THE LOSERS.
SRCE   *IN J. C. STONE & D. P. DENEVI (EDS.), TEACHING MULTICULTURAL POPULATIONS: FIVE HERITAGES. NEW YORK: VAN NOSTRAND, 1971, PP. 148-162.*
INDX   EDUCATION, PUERTO RICAN-M, EMPIRICAL, MIGRATION, DISCRIMINATION, BILINGUALISM, ACHIEVEMENT TESTING, CULTURAL FACTORS, ENVIRONMENTAL FACTORS, EMPLOYMENT, TEACHERS, INSTRUCTIONAL TECHNIQUES, CONNECTICUT, NEW YORK, NEW JERSEY, ILLINOIS, PENNSYLVANIA, EAST, MIDWEST, URBAN, BILINGUAL-BICULTURAL EDUCATION, PARENTAL INVOLVEMENT, CULTURE

ABST   THE PREDICAMENT OF PUERTO RICAN CHILDREN IN PUBLIC SCHOOLS IN SEVEN CITIES (BRIDGEPORT, CHICAGO, PHILADELPHIA, NEWARK, HOBOKEN, PATTERSON, AND NEW YORK CITY) IS EXAMINED. THE PURPOSE OF THIS REPORT IS TO PUT THE PROBLEM (WHAT THESE CHILDREN ARE LEARNING AND NOT LEARNING, WHAT THE SCHOOLS ARE TEACHING AND NOT TEACHING) INTO SHARPER FOCUS USING CURRENT DATA FROM SCHOOLS NOT ONLY IN NEW YORK BUT IN OTHER AREAS WHERE THE PUERTO RICAN POPULATION IS GROWING. ALTHOUGH SPECIFIC CONCLUSIONS OR RECOMMENDATIONS ARE NOT GIVEN, THE FOLLOWING POINTS ARE STRONGLY EMPHASIZED: (1) PUERTO RICAN CHILDREN ARE "LOSERS," AS THEY LEARN LESS AND DROPOUT MORE THAN ANY OTHER ETHNIC GROUP IN THE CITIES STUDIED; (2) SCHOOLS AND TEACHERS HAVE NOT BEEN SUFFICIENTLY AWARE OF CULTURAL DIFFERENCES OR TRAINED TO TEACH CHILDREN FROM OTHER CULTURES; (3) SPANISH-SPEAKING AND PUERTO RICAN TEACHERS SHOULD BE HIRED TO TEACH PUERTO RICAN AND OTHER SPANISH-SPEAKING CHILDREN; (4) BILINGUAL PROGRAMS, IN PARTICULAR PROGRAMS WHICH TEACH PRIMARY GRADES IN SPANISH WITH ENGLISH TAUGHT IN THE CONTEXT OF OTHER SUBJECT MATTER, HAVE BEEN SUCCESSFUL; (5) PUERTO RICAN PARENTS CAN BE ENCOURAGED TO BECOME MORE INVOLVED IN SCHOOL ACTIVITIES BY USING BILINGUAL SCHOOL-COMMUNITY REPRESENTATIVES TO MEDIATE SCHOOL-PARENT PROBLEMS; AND (6) PUERTO RICAN ENROLLMENTS IN THE CITIES STUDIED ARE GOING UP AT ASTONISHING RATES, A SITUATION THE PUBLIC SCHOOLS SHOULD DEAL WITH BY IMPLEMENTING CHANGES IN SCHOOL POLICIES AND PROGRAMS. 7 REFERENCES.
ACCN   000977

1143 AUTH **MARIATEGUI, J., & SAMANEZ, F.**
TITL   SOCIOCULTURAL CHANGE AND MENTAL HEALTH IN THE PERU OF TODAY.
SRCE   *SOCIAL PSYCHIATRY, 1968, 3(1), 35-40.*
INDX   SOUTH AMERICA, ACCULTURATION, MIGRATION, CULTURAL CHANGE, MENTAL HEALTH, CULTURE, ECONOMIC FACTORS, CULTURAL FACTORS, HISTORY, ESSAY, DEMOGRAPHIC
ABST   A STUDY OF PERSONALITY AND ACCULTURATION PROBLEMS OF THE MESTIZO POPULATION OF PERU INCLUDES: (1) A COMPARISON OF RURAL AND URBAN POPULATION CHARACTERISTICS; (2) A DESCRIPTION OF THE IMPACT OF INTERNAL MIGRATION UPON MENTAL HEALTH; AND (3) AN EXPLORATION OF DYNAMIC ASPECTS IN THE ADAPTIVE MECHANISM OF UPROOTED INDIVIDUALS. THE IMPORTANCE OF ACCOMODATING THE PSYCHOSOCIAL CHARACTERISTICS OF THE NATIVE POPULATION WHEN PLANNING MENTAL HEALTH PROGRAMS IN UNDERDEVELOPED COUNTRIES IS STRESSED.
ACCN   000978

1144 AUTH **MARIN, R. C.**
TITL   A COMPREHENSIVE PROGRAM FOR MULTI-

PROBLEM FAMILIES: REPORT ON A FOUR-YEAR CONTROLLED EXPERIMENT.

SRCE *CARIBBEAN STUDIES, 1969, 9(2), 67-80.*

INDX FAMILY ROLES, FAMILY STRUCTURE, SURVEY, PUERTO RICAN-I, TAT, SES, PSYCHOPATHOLOGY, CULTURAL FACTORS, ECONOMIC FACTORS, ATTITUDES, DELINQUENCY, MARRIAGE, SEXUAL BEHAVIOR, CHILDREARING PRACTICES, OCCUPATIONAL ASPIRATIONS, SOCIAL MOBILITY, EMPIRICAL

ABST IN AN EFFORT TO EXPLORE THE DYNAMICS OF FAMILY CRISIS, JUVENILE DELINQUENCY, AND MOTIVES FOR BEHAVIOR AMONG MULTI-PROBLEM PUERTO RICAN FAMILIES, 240 ACTIVE WELFARE RECIPIENTS WERE STUDIED. THE FAMILIES WERE DIVIDED INTO TWO MAJOR GROUPS. THE EXPERIMENTAL GROUP OF 120 FAMILIES WAS AIDED BY VARIOUS FAMILY CENTERED SOCIAL WORK TREATMENT TECHNIQUES. THE CONTROL GROUP OF FAMILIES CONTINUED AS BEFORE RECEIVING THE REGULAR SERVICES THEY HAD BEEN GIVEN BY THE PUBLIC WELFARE AGENCY. TO ASSESS THE EFFECTS OF THE FAMILY CENTERED SOCIAL WORK PROGRAM, NUMEROUS QUESTIONNAIRES WERE ADMINISTERED BY MEANS OF INTERVIEWS TO VARIOUS MEMBERS OF THE FAMILIES AND THE THEMATIC APPERCEPTION TEST WAS ADMINISTERED TO THE 120 HEADS OF THE HOUSEHOLDS IN THE EXPERIMENTAL GROUP. ANALYSES OF DATA FOR THE 120 FAMILIES IN THE EXPERIMENTAL GROUP SHOWED THAT AT THE TERMINATION OF THE PROGRAM 11.7% OF THE FAMILIES SHOWED DETERIORATION, 31.7% SHOWED NO CHANGE, 30.8% INDICATED A SLIGHT POSITIVE CHANGE, AND 25.8% SHOWED EVIDENCE OF SUBSTANTIAL POSITIVE CHANGE. PROBLEMS IN ANALYZING FAMILY FUNCTIONING ARE DISCUSSED, AND FURTHER RESEARCH ON THE PUERTO RICAN FAMILY IS RECOMMENDED. 7 REFERENCES.

ACCN 000979

1145 AUTH **MARMOR, J.**

TITL THE PSYCHODYNAMICS OF PREJUDICE.

SRCE *IN E. R. PADILLA & A. M. PADILLA (EDS.), TRANSCULTURAL PSYCHIATRY: AN HISPANIC PERSPECTIVE (MONOGRAPH NO. 4). LOS ANGELES: UNIVERSITY OF CALIFORNIA, SPANISH SPEAKING MENTAL HEALTH RESEARCH CENTER, 1977, PP. 5-11.*

INDX PREJUDICE, AUTHORITARIANISM, ESSAY, STEREOTYPES, SPANISH SURNAMED, DEVIANCE, PSYCHOPATHOLOGY, EQUAL OPPORTUNITY

ABST THE PHENOMENON OF PREJUDICE IS NOT A LIMITED CONCEPT APPLICABLE ONLY TO DIFFERENCES IN RACIAL ORIGIN BUT ALSO MANIFESTS ITSELF REGARDING DIFFERENCES IN SEX, RELIGION, ETHNICITY, CLASS, POLITICS, AND AGE LEVELS. THE ACTUAL MEANING OF PREJUDICE IS PREJUDGMENT AND IMPLIES AN ATTITUDE BASED ON INSUFFICIENT KNOWLEDGE. PREJUDICE APPEARS TO HAVE TWO BASIC FEATURES: (1) GENERALIZATION FROM THE PARTICULAR; AND (2) A LACK OF RATIONALITY OR LOGIC. THESE CHARACTERISTICS OFTEN LEAD TO STEREOTYPING AND MU-

TUALLY CONTRADICTORY ATTITUDES THAT STEM FROM EMOTIONAL SOURCES. PREJUDICE IS ACQUIRED BY INDIVIDUALS IN TWO WAYS: (1) PASSIVE ADOPTION OF ENVIRONMENTAL ATTITUDES; AND (2) CERTAIN PERSONALITY PATTERNS THAT TEND TO BE PREJUDICE PRONE. THE DIFFERENCE BETWEEN PREJUDICE IN A GROUP AND GROUP IDENTITY IS THAT THE FORMER IS BASED ON ETHNOCENTRICISM WHILE THE LATTER IS AN INEVITABLE CONSTRUCTIVE ELEMENT OF HUMAN LIFE. ASSIMILATION AND TOLERANCE IS NOT THE ANSWER TO ELIMINATING PREJUDICE. RESOLVING THE NEGATIVE IMPACT OF PREJUDICE CAN ONLY BE ACCOMPLISHED BY LEARNING TO RESPECT INDIVIDUALS REGARDLESS OF THEIR RACE, CREED, OR COLOR AND PROVIDING EQUAL OPPORTUNITIES TO ALL MEMBERS IN OUR SOCIETY.

ACCN 000980

1146 AUTH **MARMORALE, A. M., & BROWN, F.**

TITL BENDER-GESTALT PERFORMANCE OF PUERTO RICAN, WHITE, AND NEGRO CHILDREN.

SRCE *JOURNAL OF CLINICAL PSYCHOLOGY, 1977, 33(1), 224-228.*

INDX PUERTO RICAN-M, BENDER VISUAL-MOTOR GESTALT TEST, SES, EMPIRICAL, SEX COMPARISON, LEARNING DISABILITIES, CROSS CULTURAL, CHILDREN, NEW YORK, EAST

ABST THE BENDER GESTALT PERFORMANCE OF 74 LOWER-CLASS PUERTO RICAN, 44 MIDDLE-CLASS ANGLO, AND 47 LOWER-CLASS NEGRO CHILDREN ENROLLED IN A NEW YORK CITY PUBLIC SCHOOL WAS INVESTIGATED OVER A TWO YEAR PERIOD. THE TEST, ADMINISTERED IN SPANISH AND ENGLISH, WAS GIVEN TO THE CHILDREN DURING THE FIRST THREE MONTHS OF FIRST GRADE AND AGAIN DURING THE LAST THREE MONTHS OF THIRD GRADE. RESULTS WERE SCORED BY THE KOPPITZ DEVELOPMENTAL BENDER SCORING SYSTEM AND ANALYZED BY T-TESTS. THE DEVELOPMENTAL LAG FOUND IN THE PUERTO RICAN AND NEGRO CHILDREN SUPPORTS PREVIOUS FINDINGS THAT WERE GENERALIZED TO INCLUDE PUERTO RICAN CHILDREN. THE BENDER WAS FOUND TO BE A VALID MEASURE OF DEVELOPMENTAL DIFFERENCES FOR NON-WHITE GROUPS. BY THE END OF THE THIRD GRADE THE PUERTO RICAN GROUP EQUALED THE SCORES OF THE WHITE GROUP, WHILE THE NEGRO GROUP DID NOT. DATA SUGGEST THAT THE KOPPITZ NORMS MAY BE TOO HIGH IN THE MIDDLE RANGE DEVELOPMENT YEARS REPRESENTED BY THIRD AND FOURTH GRADERS, AND NOT ACCURATE WHEN DIFFERENCES BETWEEN SCORES ARE SMALL. THE PRIMARY IMPLICATION OF THIS STUDY IS THAT VISUAL-MOTOR SKILL EVALUATION MUST BE DONE IN FIRST GRADE OR EARLIER SO THAT TRAINING IN THESE AREAS CAN BE GIVEN—IF NECESSARY, BEFORE FORMAL READING AND WRITING TASKS ARE BEGUN. 14 REFERENCES. (AUTHOR SUMMARY MODIFIED)

ACCN 000981

1147 AUTH **MARMORALE, A. M., & BROWN, F.**

TITL COMPARISON OF BENDER-GESTALT AND WISC CORRELATIONS FOR PUERTO RICAN, WHITE, AND NEGRO CHILDREN.

SRCE *JOURNAL OF CLINICAL PSYCHOLOGY, 1975, 31(3), 465-468.*

INDX PUERTO RICAN-M, PERSONALITY ASSESSMENT, WISC, CROSS CULTURAL, CULTURAL FACTORS, BENDER VISUAL-MOTOR GESTALT TEST, CHILDREN, INTELLIGENCE TESTING, PERSONALITY, EMPIRICAL, NEW YORK, EAST

ABST CORRELATIONS WERE OBTAINED BETWEEN BENDER GESTALT SCORES AND WISC IQS FOR 3 ETHNIC GROUPS—123 PUERTO RICAN, 82 WHITE, AND 61 BLACK CHILDREN IN THE 1ST GRADE. THE BENDER GESTALT TEST DID NOT SHOW ANY SIGNIFICANT RELATIONSHIP WITH THE WISC SCORES OF THE PUERTO RICAN CHILDREN. SIGNIFICANT CORRELATIONS BETWEEN THE BENDER GESTALT AND ALL THE WISC SCORES WERE FOUND FOR THE BLACK GROUP. FOR THE WHITE CHILDREN, THE RELATIONSHIP BETWEEN THE WISC AND BENDER GESTALT WAS SIGNIFICANT, BUT ONLY FOR THE PERFORMANCE AND FULL SCALE SCORES. THE DIFFERENCES IN IQS AMONG THE THREE ETHNIC GROUPS WERE ALL SIGNIFICANT, WITH THE WHITE SCORES ABOVE THOSE OF THE OTHER TWO GROUPS AND THE BLACK SCORES ABOVE THOSE OF THE PUERTO RICAN CHILDREN. THE ABSENCE OF A SIGNIFICANT CORRELATION BETWEEN THE BENDER AND THE WISC VERBAL IQ IN THESE CHILDREN IS ATTRIBUTED TO THE RELATIVE SUPERIORTITY OF THEIR VERBAL SCORES. 6 REFERENCES. (PASAR ABSTRACT MODIFIED)

ACCN 000982

1148 AUTH **MARMORALE, A. M., & BROWN, F.**

TITL MENTAL HEALTH INTERVENTION IN THE PRIMARY GRADES.

SRCE *COMMUNITY MENTAL HEALTH JOURNAL MONOGRAPH SERIES, 1974, (WHOLE NO. 7).*

INDX CHILDREN, MENTAL HEALTH, INTELLIGENCE TESTING, PUERTO RICAN-M, PSYCHOTHERAPY, HEALTH DELIVERY SYSTEMS, HEALTH, GOODENOUGH DRAW-A-MAN TEST, WISC, BENDER VISUAL-MOTOR GESTALT TEST, PEABODY PICTURE-VOCABULARY TEST, EMPIRICAL, CROSS CULTURAL, NEW YORK, EAST

ABST THE EFFECTIVENESS OF A COMPREHENSIVE MENTAL HEALTH PROGRAM IN THE ELEMENTARY GRADES (1ST-4TH) OF A PUBLIC SCHOOL IN EAST HARLEM, NEW YORK, WAS INVESTIGATED. SUBJECTS WERE 176 ANGLO, BLACK, AND PUERTO RICAN CHILDREN (111 BOYS, 65 GIRLS) FROM WELFARE AND LOW-MIDDLE INCOME FAMILIES. AN EXPERIMENTAL GROUP CONSISTED OF ALL CHILDREN IN THE SCHOOL'S FIRST GRADE CLASS, WHILE THE CONTROL GROUP WAS COMPRISED OF ALL THE CHILDREN IN THE FOLLOWING YEAR'S FIRST GRADE CLASS. SUBJECTS IN BOTH GROUPS WERE GIVEN A COMPREHENSIVE BATTERY OF TESTS TO OBTAIN BASELINE DATA AT THE BEGINNING OF THEIR FIRST GRADE YEAR. RETESTING WAS DONE AT THE END OF THEIR THIRD GRADE YEAR. DURING THE TWO AND A HALF YEARS BETWEEN TESTING PERIODS, THE EXPERIMENTAL GROUP HAD ACCESS TO EXTENSIVE MENTAL HEALTH SERVICES BUT THE CONTROL GROUP DID NOT. SOME OF THE STUDY'S FINDINGS WERE UNEXPECTED, IN PARTICULAR THAT THE EXPERIMENTAL GROUP SHOWED NO OVERALL SIGNIFICANT DIFFERENCES IN ACADEMIC ACHIEVEMENT OR PSYCHOLOGICAL GROWTH FROM THE CONTROL GROUP. THIS SUGGESTS THAT IN A REASONABLY ADEQUATE SCHOOL, THE GROWTH AND DEVELOPMENTAL FACTORS INHERENT IN THE SCHOOL ARE SUFFICIENT FOR THE PROGRESS OF MOST CHILDREN—ESPECIALLY FOR MINORITY CHILDREN WHO "CATCH UP" AFTER 2 TO 3 YEARS OF SCHOOLING. SCHOOL EXPERIENCE, HOWEVER, DOES NOT APPEAR TO BE SUFFICIENT FOR CHILDREN WITH SERIOUS PERSONALITY AND LEARNING PROBLEMS. SUCH CHILDREN NEED SPECIAL MENTAL HEALTH INTERVENTION IF THEY ARE TO GROW COGNITIVELY AND AFFECTIVELY; THEIR NEEDS CAN BE HANDLED IN AN AVERAGE SCHOOL BY A PERMANENT STAFF OF 1 OR 2 MENTAL HEALTH PROFESSIONALS. 25 REFERENCES.

ACCN 000983

1149 AUTH **MARTIN, P. P. (ED.)**

TITL LA FRONTERA PERSPECTIVE: PROVIDING MENTAL HEALTH SERVICES TO MEXICAN AMERICANS (MONOGRAPH NO. 1).

SRCE *TUCSON, ARIZ.: LA FRONTERA CENTER, INC., 1979.*

INDX MEXICAN AMERICAN, ARIZONA, SOUTHWEST, MENTAL HEALTH, RESOURCE UTILIZATION, DRUG ABUSE, ALCOHOLISM, HEALTH DELIVERY SYSTEMS, PSYCHOTHERAPY, SOCIAL SERVICES, BILINGUAL-BICULTURAL PERSONNEL, ATTITUDES, PSYCHOTHERAPISTS, ROLE EXPECTATIONS, POLICY, FAMILY ROLES, SEX ROLES, CULTURAL FACTORS, BOOK, MACHISMO

ABST THE AUTHORS OF THIS VOLUME'S SEVEN PAPERS ARE OR HAVE BEEN STAFF MEMBERS OF "LA FRONTERA"—AN OUTPATIENT MENTAL HEALTH FACILITY IN TUCSON. THE CENTER'S CATCHMENT AREA POPULATION IS PREDOMINANTLY MEXICAN AMERICAN, AND IT HAS THE CITY'S HIGHEST RATES OF VENEREAL DISEASE, POLICE ARRESTS, AND WELFARE RECIPIENTS. THE FIRST SECTION OF THE BOOK FOCUSES ON THE PROCESS BY WHICH MEXICAN AMERICANS DEFINE A SIGNIFICANT OTHER AS "MENTALLY ILL" AND, CONCOMITANTLY, HOW THEY PERCEIVE AND UTILIZE MENTAL HEALTH SERVICES. RECOMMENDATIONS FOR CULTURALLY APPROPRIATE THERAPY ARE ALSO OFFERED. THE BOOK'S SECOND SECTION ADDRESSES THE HISTORICAL AND CULTURAL FACTORS INVOLVED IN MEXICAN AMERICANS' ALCOHOL AND DRUG ABUSE, AND THEN THE IMPLICATIONS FOR PREVENTION AND TREATMENT STRATEGIES ARE DISCUSSED. THE FINAL SECTION EXAMINES MACHISMO AS WELL AS SEVERAL DYSFUNCTIONAL ASPECTS OF MEXICAN AMERICAN FAMILY LIFE IN ORDER TO IDENTIFY EFFECTIVE INTERVENTION AND FAMILY COUNSELING STRATEGIES. IN THE EDITOR'S CONCLUDING COMMENTS, IT IS NOTED THAT THE

BOOK MAY BE OF PARTICULAR VALUE TO SERVICE PROVIDERS AND THOSE WHO ARE IN THE PROCESS OF DEVELOPING MENTAL HEALTH SERVICES FOR MEXICAN AMERICANS. 25 REFERENCES.

ACCN   001793

1150   AUTH   **MARTINEZ, C.**

TITL   COMMUNITY MENTAL HEALTH AND THE CHICANO MOVEMENT.

SRCE   *AMERICAN JOURNAL OF ORTHOPSYCHIATRY, 1973, 43(4), 595-601.*

INDX   POLITICAL POWER, CHICANO MOVEMENT, COMMUNITY INVOLVEMENT, SELF CONCEPT, MENTAL HEALTH, PSYCHOPATHOLOGY, CULTURAL FACTORS, ESSAY, STEREOTYPES, HEALTH DELIVERY SYSTEMS, THERAPEUTIC COMMUNITY, HOMOSEXUALITY, REVIEW, SEX COMPARISON, CROSS CULTURAL, CHILDREN, ADOLESCENTS, ADULTS

ABST   THE CHICANO MOVEMENT IS DEFINED AS A GROUP OF OPPRESSED PEOPLE WHO, BY SHARING SIMILAR POLITICAL AND IDEOLOGICAL BELIEFS, ACT AS A COHESIVE UNIT TOWARD SOME COMMON GOAL. THIS MOVEMENT IN EMPHASIZING INCREASED SELF-AWARENESS AND POSITIVE ETHNIC IDENTIFICATION HAS MENTAL HEALTH IMPLICATIONS FOR THE INVOLVED INDIVIDUALS. THE RELATIONSHIP BETWEEN GOALS OF THE CHICANO MOVEMENT AND IMPROVED MENTAL HEALTH FOR MEXICAN AMERICANS ARE DISCUSSED. THE EFFECTS OF MEXICAN AMERICAN STEREOTYPES ARE EXAMINED WITH RESPECT TO MENTAL HEALTH. BOTH THE PSYCHIATRIC COMMUNITY AND THE CHICANO MOVEMENT SUPPORT A MENTAL HEALTH SYSTEM WHICH FOCUSES ON SPECIFIC CONCERNS FOR THE MEXICAN AMERICAN POPULATION AND INCORPORATES A CRISIS INTERVENTION MODEL THAT STRESSES RESPONSIVENESS AND AVAILABILITY OF MENTAL HEALTH WORKERS FOR INDIVIDUALS IN A CRISIS SITUATION. HOMOSEXUALITY AMONG MEXICAN AMERICAN MALES IS ALSO DISCUSSED. 8 REFERENCES.

ACCN   000985

1151   AUTH   **MARTINEZ, C.**

TITL   GROUP PROCESS AND THE CHICANO: CLINICAL ISSUES.

SRCE   *INTERNATIONAL JOURNAL OF GROUP PSYCHOTHERAPY, 1977, 27(2), 225-231.*

INDX   CROSS CULTURAL, CULTURAL FACTORS, ESSAY, GROUP DYNAMICS, MEXICAN AMERICAN, PSYCHOTHERAPY, ROLE EXPECTATIONS, ATTITUDES, INTERPERSONAL RELATIONS

ABST   IN THIS COMPARISON OF CHICANO AND ANGLO RESPONSES TO GROUP THERAPY, IT IS ARGUED THAT NEGATIVE STEREOTYPING HAS AFFECTED THE CHICANO SELF-IMAGE AND THAT CERTAIN CULTURAL TRADITIONS (SUCH AS A RELUCTANCE TO OPEN UP TO OTHERS AND A FORMALITY IN INTERPERSONAL RELATIONS) IMPEDE PSYCHOTHERAPEUTIC INTERVENTION. SPECIFICALLY, EXPERIENCE WITH CHICANO PATIENTS INVOLVED IN A DAY PROGRAM REVEALS THAT CHICANO PATIENTS IN GROUPS DO DIFFER FROM OTHERS, PRIMARILY

IN THEIR RETICENCE TO DEAL WITH FEELINGS TOWARD THE THERAPIST AND IN VARIOUS MANIFESTATIONS OF THE PRESENCE OF A SECOND LANGUAGE AND A UNIQUE ETHNIC BACKGROUND. IN OTHER AREAS, HOWEVER, CHICANO PATIENTS DO NOT DIFFER FROM OTHERS AS LONG AS LANGUAGE, ECONOMIC, AND CULTURAL FACTORS ARE TAKEN INTO ACCOUNT. 7 REFERENCES.

ACCN   002150

1152   AUTH   **MARTINEZ, C.**

TITL   PSYCHIATRIC CONSULTATION IN A RURAL MEXICAN-AMERICAN CLINIC.

SRCE   *PSYCHIATRIC ANNALS, 1977, 7(12), 74-80.*

INDX   TEXAS, COMMUNITY INVOLVEMENT, RURAL, MALE, THERAPEUTIC COMMUNITY, COMMUNITY, CULTURAL FACTORS, DRUG ABUSE, ALCOHOLISM, ESSAY, HEALTH DELIVERY SYSTEMS, SOUTHWEST, MENTAL HEALTH, PROGRAM EVALUATION, SOCIAL SERVICES, MEXICAN AMERICAN

ABST   THE CRYSTAL CITY MENTAL HEALTH AND OUTREACH CLINIC, A PILOT RURAL MENTAL HEALTH PROGRAM IN A TOWN HIGHLY POLITICIZED (BEING THE HOME OF LA RAZA UNIDA) IS EXAMINED. THE CLINIC WAS ESTABLISHED WITH THE COLLABORATION OF CHICANO RESIDENTS OF CRYSTAL CITY AND MEMBERS OF THE PSYCHIATRIC FACULTY OF THE UNIVERSITY OF TEXAS HEALTH SERVICES CENTER, SAN ANTONIO. THE FACULTY'S INVOLVEMENT HAS BEEN IN THE AREAS OF PROGRAM PLANNING, STAFF TRAINING, LIAISON WITH SOCIAL SERVICE AGENCIES, AND DIRECT SERVICES. DEMONSTRATION OF COMMUNITY ACCEPTANCE OF THE PROGRAM WAS MONITORED VIA ESCALATING NON-ALCOHOL AND DRUG-RELATED MALE USAGE—CONSIDERED TO REPRESENT A STEP BEYOND "MACHISMO," IN WHICH MALES MUST BE STRONG AND INDEPENDENT OF THE CONTROL OF SOCIAL AGENCIES. COMMUNITY ACCEPTANCE IS ALSO TRACED TO THE PROGRAM'S FIRST DIRECTOR (AN INDIGENOUS, EDUCATED COMMUNITY LEADER WHO HAD BECOME A RESPECTED MEMBER OF LA RAZA UNIDA) AND TO OTHER STAFF MEMBERS WHO REMAIN SOCIALLY AND POLITICALLY PROMINANT IN THE COMMUNITY. OTHER REASONS FOR COMMUNITY ACCEPTANCE ARE: (1) A TRADITION OF PROVIDING CONCRETE HELP TO PROSPECTIVE PATIENTS IN THE FORM OF CASEWORK ASSISTANCE, I.E., INFORMATION ABOUT FOOD STAMPS, GLASSES, TRANSPORTATION, AND WELFARE BENEFITS; (2) A COMMUTER PSYCHIATRIC STAFF, THUS AUGMENTING PATIENTS' SENSE OF URGENCY AND RESPECT TOWARD THE THERAPEUTIC PROCESS; (3) CENTRALIZATION OF MENTAL HEALTH ISSUES WITH ONE WORKER, WHO SERVES AS A CONDUIT FOR ALL PERSONAL INFORMATION ABOUT CLIENTS;. AND (4) COMMUNITY SIZE. THE SMALL SIZE ALLOWS THE STAFF TO MAINTAIN EXCELLENT FOLLOW-UP WITH PATIENTS AND WITH OTHER INSTITUTIONS, SUCH AS SCHOOL AND POLICE. THE PROGRAM CONTINUES TO THRIVE WITH LITTLE

OF THE INITIAL DEPENDENCE ON PSYCHIATRIC STAFF FROM SAN ANTONIO.

ACCN   002151

1153 AUTH   **MARTINEZ, C., JR.**
TITL   HISPANICS IN PSYCHIATRY.
SRCE   *IN E. L. OLMEDO & S. LOPEZ (EDS.), HISPANIC MENTAL HEALTH PROFESSIONALS (MONO-GRAPH NO. 5). LOS ANGELES: UNIVERSITY OF CALIFORNIA, SPANISH SPEAKING MENTAL HEALTH RESEARCH CENTER, 1977, PP. 7-11.*
INDX   MENTAL HEALTH PROFESSION, REPRESENTA-TION, MEXICAN AMERICAN, SPANISH SUR-NAMED, BILINGUAL-BICULTURAL PERSONNEL, EMPIRICAL, MEDICAL STUDENTS, CURRICU-LUM, PROFESSIONAL TRAINING, HIGHER EDU-CATION, ESSAY, FINANCING
ABST   THE NEED FOR MORE HISPANIC PSYCHIA-TRISTS, THE PRESENT STATUS OF HISPANICS IN PSYCHIATRY AND PSYCHIATRIC TRAINING, AND RECOMMENDATIONS FOR IMPROVING THE PRESENT SITUATION ARE DISCUSSED. IT IS SUGGESTED THAT MANY CHICANO STUDENTS ARE HESITANT IN APPLYING TO MEDICAL SCHOOL BECAUSE OF THE LENGTHY AND RIG-OROUS TRAINING THAT THE PROFESSION RE-QUIRES. HOWEVER, THE UNDERREPRESENTA-TION OF HISPANICS IN THE FIELD OF PSYCHIATRY HAS RESULTED IN MANY SPANISH SPEAKING PEOPLE RECEIVING INADEQUATE CARE AND A RELUCTANCE TO SEEK PROFES-SIONAL SERVICES BECAUSE OF LANGUAGE AND CULTURAL FACTORS. FOUR RECOMMEN-DATIONS ARE PRESENTED TO HELP INCREASE THE NUMBER OF HISPANIC PSYCHIATRISTS: (1) GREATER EMPHASIS ON RECRUITMENT AND ENCOURAGING HIGH SCHOOL STUDENTS TO ENTER HEALTH PROFESSIONS; (2) CURRICULA SHOULD BE INNOVATIVE, MOTIVATING, AND PROVIDE A BALANCE BETWEEN PSYCHOAN-ALYTIC THEORY AND OTHER PERSONALITY THEORIES; AND (3) GREATER FEDERAL FINAN-CIAL SUPPORT IN RECRUITMENT AND TRAIN-ING. IT IS CONCLUDED THAT INCREASING HIS-PANIC REPRESENTATION IN PSYCHIATRY WILL IMPROVE THE OVERALL MENTAL HEALTH SER-VICES TO HISPANICS. 8 REFERENCES.
ACCN   000986

1154 AUTH   **MARTINEZ, C., & MARTIN, H. W.**
TITL   FOLK DISEASES AMONG URBAN MEXICAN AMERICANS.
SRCE   *JOURNAL OF THE AMERICAN MEDICAL ASSO-CIATION, 1966, 196(2), 161-164.*
INDX   FOLK MEDICINE, CURANDERISMO, MEXICAN AMERICAN, EMPIRICAL, URBAN, SURVEY, ADULTS, FEMALE, ATTITUDES, PHYSICIANS, HEALTH, MENTAL HEALTH, TEXAS, SOUTHWEST
ABST   AN EXPLORATORY STUDY WAS CONDUCTED TO DETERMINE THE EXTENT OF KNOWLEDGE ABOUT DISEASE CONCEPTS (MAL OJO, EMPA-CHO, SUSTO, CAIDA DE MOLLERA, AND MAL PUESTO) AMONG 75 MEXICAN AMERICAN (MA) HOUSEWIVES AND TO OBTAIN A DETAILED AC-COUNT OF BELIEFS ABOUT ETIOLOGY, SYMP-TOMATOLOGY, AND MODES OF TREATMENT. THE AGE OF THE SUBJECTS RANGED FROM 18 TO 84 YEARS OF AGE WITH A MEDIAN OF

39 YEARS OF AGE AND A MEDIAN OF 6 YEARS OF EDUCATION. SUBJECTS WERE INTER-VIEWED IN THEIR HOMES. MORE THAN 97 PER-CENT OF THE SUBJECTS INTERVIEWED KNEW ABOUT EACH OF THE FIVE DISEASES, AND 85 PERCENT HAD SOME SPECIFIC KNOWLEDGE ABOUT SYMPTOMS AND ETIOLOGY OF THE DISEASES, EXCEPT FOR MAL PUESTO. EIGHTY-FIVE PERCENT OF THE SUBJECTS REPORTED THERAPEUTIC MEASURES FOR ALL THE DIS-EASES EXCEPT FOR MAL PUESTO. ALL BUT 5 PERCENT OF THE SUBJECTS REPORTED ONE OR MORE INSTANCES OF THESE ILLNESSES IN THEMSELVES, A FAMILY MEMBER, OR IN AC-QUAINTANCES. REPORTS OF OCCURRENCE OF THE DISEASES IN IMMEDIATE FAMILY MEMBERS WERE EMPLOYED AS AN INDEX OF BELIEF IN FOLK MALADIES; NO RELATIONSHIP AP-PEARED BETWEEN THIS INDEX AND SUCH CHARACTERISTICS AS AGE, EDUCATION, OR PLACE OF BIRTH. DISCUSSIONS OF THE TREAT-MENT FOR THE FIVE DISEASES AND THE UTILI-ZATION OF FOLK HEALERS AND PHYSICIANS ARE PRESENTED. THE FINDINGS PROVIDE AD-DITIONAL EVIDENCE THAT BELIEF IN FOLK ILL-NESSES AND THE USE OF FOLK HEALERS CON-TINUE TO BE WIDESPREAD AMONG URBANIZED MEXICAN AMERICANS. 6 REFERENCES.
ACCN   000987

1155 AUTH   **MARTINEZ, F. H.**
TITL   CHICANOS AND THE "NON-SYSTEM" FOR MEN-TAL HEALTH SERVICES.
SRCE   *IN A. M. PADILLA & E. R. PADILLA (EDS.), IM-PROVING MENTAL HEALTH AND HUMAN SER-VICES FOR HISPANIC COMMUNITIES: SE-LECTED PRESENTATIONS FROM REGIONAL CONFERENCES. WASHINGTON, D.C.: NA-TIONAL COALITION OF HISPANIC MENTAL HEALTH AND HUMAN SERVICE ORGANIZA-TIONS (COSSMHO), 1977, PP. 9-14.*
INDX   HEALTH DELIVERY SYSTEMS, MENTAL HEALTH, MEXICAN AMERICAN, PROFESSIONAL TRAIN-ING, CHICANO MOVEMENT, ESSAY, LEGISLA-TION, POLICY, POLITICAL POWER, REPRESENTATION
ABST   THE MENTAL HEALTH SERVICE DELIVERY SYS-TEM IS DESCRIBED AS A "NON-SYSTEM" IN WHICH ITS FOUR BASIC COMPONENTS ARE DIFFUSED, DIVERSE, AND DISCONNECTED. THESE FOUR STRUCTURES ARE: (1) THE GOV-ERNMENTAL STRUCTURES WHICH INVOLVE THE FEDERAL, STATE, AND LOCAL UNITS OF GOV-ERNMENT; (2) THE SERVICE DELIVERY SYSTEM WHICH IS COMPOSED OF CLINICS, COMMU-NITY MENTAL HEALTH CENTERS, HOSPITALS, SPECIALIZED SERVICE FACILITIES AND PRAC-TITIONERS AND FACILITIES IN THE PRIVATE SECTOR; (3) THE TRAINERS OF THE MENTAL HEALTH PROFESSIONALS, SUCH AS THE UNI-VERSITIES AND ALLIED TRAINING INSTITU-TIONS; AND (4) SPECIAL INTEREST GROUPS COMPOSED OF VARIOUS NATIONAL ADVO-CACY ASSOCIATIONS, PROFESSIONAL ASSO-CIATIONS, AND INSURANCE COMPANIES. SO FAR THE HISPANIC COMMUNITY HAS HAD LITTLE IMPUT IN THE MENTAL HEALTH SYSTEM. IT IS PROPOSED THAT THE NATIONAL COALITION OF

HISPANIC MENTAL HEALTH AND HUMAN SERVICES ORGANIZATIONS (COSSMHO) SHOULD ULTILIZE ITS NATIONAL AND STATE RESOURCES TO MONITOR AND INFLUENCE THE LEGISLATIVE PROCESS REGARDING HEALTH AND MENTAL HEALTH PROGRAMS AND PRIORITIES OF THEIR FUNDING. THERE NEEDS TO BE A CONCERTED EFFORT TO INTEREST YOUNG HISPANICS IN THE MENTAL HEALTH PROFESSIONS. THE MEMBER ORGANIZATIONS OF COSSMHO SHOULD ALSO PUT EFFORT IN APPLIED RESEARCH TO DEVELOP BETTER SERVICE MODELS. SINCE SPECIAL INTEREST GROUPS REPRESENT THE INTERESTS OF VARIOUS PROFESSIONS, SPECIFIC POPULATIONS AND NATIONAL ASSOCIATIONS AS WELL AS REFLECT PUBLIC ATTITUDES AND VOTES, THEN A LIAISON WITH AND PARTICIPATION IN SUCH ORGANIZATIONS WOULD BE ADVANTAGEOUS TO THE SPANISH-SPEAKING POPULATION. BY BECOMING INVOLVED IN THE BASIC STRUCTURES OF THE MENTAL HEALTH SYSYTEM, MEMBERS OF COSSMHO REDUCE THEIR DEPENDENCY ON FEDERAL GRANTS AND THEREBY INCREASE THE CERTAINTY OF THEIR EFFORTS IN DEVELOPING MEANINGFUL AND ADEQUATE MENTAL HEALTH SERVICES FOR HISPANICS.

ACCN   000988

1156 AUTH   **MARTINEZ, F. H.**
TITL   MENTAL HEALTH SERVICES FOR LA RAZA.
SRCE   *AGENDA, JULY 1974, 22-23.*
INDX   MENTAL HEALTH, PSYCHOTHERAPY, COMMUNITY INVOLVEMENT, HEALTH DELIVERY SYSTEMS, CULTURAL FACTORS, BILINGUAL-BICULTURAL PERSONNEL, ESSAY, MEXICAN AMERICAN, LEGISLATION, POLICY, REPRESENTATION
ABST   IN SPITE OF THE ELABORATE HEALTH CARE SYSTEM, THE MENTAL HEALTH NEEDS OF THE SPANISH-SPEAKING POPULATION HAVE BEEN GENERALLY NEGLECTED. THE COMMUNITY MENTAL HEALTH CENTERS ACT OF 1963—ESTABLISHING LOCAL COMMUNITY MENTAL HEALTH CENTERS TO PROVIDE SERVICES SUCH AS SHORT TERM HOSPITALIZATION, OUTPATIENT CARE, AND COMMUNITY EDUCATION AND CONSULTATION—HAVE FOR THE MOST PART BEEN UNABLE TO MEET THE NEEDS OF THE POOR, AND RACIAL AND ETHNIC MINORITIES. THE UNDERUTILIZATION OF THESE CENTERS IS A RESULT OF THE FOLLOWING CONDITIONS: (1) CENTERS TEND TO BE LOCATED A GREAT DISTANCE FROM THE BARRIOS; (2) LACK OF PRIVACY IN THE INTAKE PROCESS; (3) LACK OF BILINGUAL-BICULTURAL STAFF; (4) LACK OF SENSITIVITY TO CULTURAL DIFFERENCES; AND (5) LACK OF RELIANCE ON THE FAMILY STRUCTURE AND THE USE OF FOLK HEALERS. NEW HEALTH CARE PROGRAMS NEED TO CONSIDER AND INCORPORATE WITHIN THEIR FRAMEWORK THE FOLLOWING MATTERS IF THEY ARE TO SUCCESSFULLY MEET THE HEALTH AND MENTAL NEEDS OF THE SPANISH POPULATION: (1) CREATE AN OFFICE AT THE NATIONAL LEVEL THAT SERVES AS AN INFORMED AND EFFECTIVE FOCAL POINT FOR THE HEALTH

CONCERNS OF THE SPANISH-SPEAKING POPULATION; (2) DEVELOP MENTAL HEALTH DELIVERY SERVICES APPROPRIATE TO THE PROBLEM OF THE MINORITY POPULATION; (3) INCREASE THE NUMBER OF SPANISH-SPEAKING HEALTH PROFESSIONALS; AND (4) EVALUATE METHODS USED IN ORDER TO ADVOCATE BETTER SERVICES FOR THE SPANISH-SPEAKING. IT IS CONCLUDED THAT ADDRESSING SPECIFIC ISSUES SHOULD INVOLVE A COMBINED EFFORT OF THE VARIOUS RAZA ORGANIZATIONS.

ACCN   000989

1157 AUTH   **MARTINEZ, J.**
TITL   MINORITIES AND ALCOHOL/DRUG ABUSE.
SRCE   *AMERICAN JOURNAL OF DRUG AND ALCOHOL ABUSE, 1976, 3(1), 185-187.*
INDX   ALCOHOLISM, DRUG ABUSE, PUERTO RICAN-M, CROSS CULTURAL, COMMUNITY INVOLVEMENT, POLITICAL POWER, THERAPEUTIC COMMUNITY, PSYCHOTHERAPY, ESSAY, CULTURAL FACTORS, POLICY, NEW YORK, EAST
ABST   A BRIEF DISCUSSION IS PRESENTED BY THE EXECUTIVE DIRECTOR OF "PROJECT R.E.T.U.R.N." CONCERNING SOME OF THE PROBLEMS IN THE TREATMENT OF HISPANICS WITHIN THE ESTABLISHED THERAPEUTIC COMMUNITY. THE URGENCY AND NECESSITY OF RESOLVING THE ISSUE OF PROVIDING MEANINGFUL SERVICES TO THE MINORITY COMMUNITY IS REFLECTED IN THE FACT THAT A DISPROPORTIONATE NUMBER OF BLACKS AND PUERTO RICANS IN NEW YORK ARE REGISTERED NARCOTIC ADDICTS AND DRUG ABUSERS. AS LONG AS THE MIDDLE OR UPPER CLASS PROFESSIONALS DETERMINE THE DEFINITION OF MENTAL HEALTH, OF METHODS USED IN TREATMENT, AND THE CONDITIONS OF TREATMENT, THERE WILL EXIST A TENDENCY TO IGNORE THE UNIQUE NATURE OF THE HISPANIC SITUATION, AND THE THERAPEUTIC COMMUNITY WILL FAIL TO UNDERSTAND HISPANIC CULTURAL IDENTIFICATION. THE CONTINUED LACK OF GROUP COUNSELING WITH SPANISH-SPEAKING PERSONNEL, LACK OF BILINGUAL EDUCATION, AND LACK OF BILINGUAL PREVENTATIVE MATERIALS WHICH COULD INFORM THE COMMUNITY ALL REFLECT NEGLECT IN THE PROVISION OF REHABILITATIVE SERVICES FOR MINORITIES. UNLIKE OTHER PROGRAMS, PROJECT R.E.T.U.R.N. REPRESENTS AN ATTEMPT TO TREAT INDIVIDUALS HAVING ALCOHOL OR DRUG PROBLEMS WITHIN THEIR OWN CULTURAL CONTEXT.

ACCN   000991

1158 AUTH   **MARTINEZ, J. L. (ED.)**
TITL   CHICANO PSYCHOLOGY.
SRCE   *NEW YORK: ACADEMIC PRESS, 1977.*
INDX   MENTAL HEALTH, BILINGUALISM, INTELLIGENCE TESTING, CULTURAL PLURALISM, SEX ROLES, FEMALE, BOOK, MEXICAN AMERICAN, EMPIRICAL, REVIEW, HEALTH DELIVERY SYSTEMS, PSYCHOTHERAPISTS, EDUCATION, RESEARCH METHODOLOGY, PSYCHOTHERAPY, CHILDREN, ADULTS, BILINGUAL-BICULTURAL EDUCATION

ABST THE FIRST COMPREHENSIVE COLLECTION OF THE WORK OF CHICANO PSYCHOLOGISTS AND OTHERS DOING RESEARCH ABOUT CHICANOS SUMMARIZES PAST RESEARCH AND PROVIDES GUIDELINES FOR FUTURE EMPIRICAL INVESTIGATIONS RELEVANT TO CHICANOS. TWENTY-ONE AUTHORS ARE REPRESENTED IN FIVE BROAD TOPIC AREAS: (1) SOCIAL PSYCHOLOGY; (2) PSYCHOLOGICAL TESTING; (3) BILINGUALISM; (4) MENTAL HEALTH AND PSYCHOTHERAPY; AND (5) FOUNDATIONS FOR A CHICANO PSYCHOLOGY. THROUGHOUT THE BOOK THESE MAJOR CONCEPTS ARE EMPHASIZED: (1) HUMAN BEHAVIOR CAN BE UNDERSTOOD ONLY IF IT IS VIEWED WITHIN THE CULTURAL CONTEXT IN WHICH IT OCCURS; (2) OF THE THE MAJOR CONCERNS OF CHICANO PSYCHOLOGY—THE NEED FOR SOCIAL JUSTICE—CAN BE BROUGHT ABOUT BY THE CLARIFICATION, REINTERPRETATION AND CORRECTION OF PREVIOUS PSYCHOLOGICAL DATA ON INTELLIGENCE AND ACHIEVEMENT TESTING; AND (3) THERE IS A GREAT NEED FOR THE INCLUSION AND ANALYSIS OF SOCIOCULTURAL VARIABLES IN THOSE AREAS OF PSYCHOLOGICAL STUDY WHERE THEIR INFLUENCE IS MOST RELEVANT—LANGUAGE, COGNITIVE PROCESSING, INTERPERSONAL RELATIONS, AND PERSONALITY. THE WORKS PRESENTED, COMPREHENSIVE ENOUGH TO BE USED AS A REFERENCE SOURCE, WILL INTEREST THOSE WORKING IN CROSS-CULTURAL PSYCHOLOGY, RACE RELATIONS, PSYCHOLOGICAL ANTHROPOLOGY, CHICANO STUDIES, AND BILINGUAL EDUCATION.

ACCN 000992

1159 AUTH **MARTINEZ, J. L., JR., MARTINEZ, S. R., OLMEDO, E. L., & GOLDMAN, R. D.**
TITL THE SEMANTIC DIFFERENTIAL TECHNIQUE: A COMPARISON OF CHICANO HIGH SCHOOL STUDENTS.
SRCE *JOURNAL OF CROSS-CULTURAL PSYCHOLOGY, 1976, 7(3), 325-334.*
INDX CROSS CULTURAL, ATTITUDES, FAMILY ROLES, FAMILY STRUCTURE, SEX ROLES, CULTURAL FACTORS, ETHNIC IDENTITY, EMPIRICAL, CULTURE, SEX COMPARISON, ADOLESCENTS, PERFORMANCE EXPECTATIONS, ACCULTURATION, SEMANTICS, CALIFORNIA, SOUTHWEST
ABST OSGOOD'S SEMANTIC DIFFERENTIAL TECHNIQUE WAS USED TO INVESTIGATE RESPONSES OF 288 CHICANO AND ANGLO 11TH AND 12TH GRADE STUDENTS ON FIVE CONCEPTS VIEWED AS BASIC TO THE TRADITIONAL MEXICAN FAMILY STRUCTURE: (1) SELF (2) MALE, (3) FEMALE, (4) FATHER, (5) MOTHER. IT WAS FOUND THAT THE CHICANOS AND ANGLOS DIFFERED SIGNIFICANTLY ON THE FIVE CONCEPTS, SUGGESTING THAT THESE CONCEPTS HAVE DIFFERENT AFFECTIVE MEANINGS FOR THE TWO CULTURAL GROUPS. THE RESULTS SHOWED THAT THE DIFFERENCES SEEMED TO BE CENTERED AROUND THE POTENCY DIMENSION. IN ADDITION, THERE WERE SEX DIFFERENCES CENTERED AROUND THE POTENCY DIMENSION, AS WELL AS AN ETHNIC BY SEX INTERACTION. 8 REFERENCES. (JOURNAL ABSTRACT MODIFIED)

ACCN 000993

1160 AUTH **MARTINEZ, L. K.**
TITL ADULT EDUCATION: A KEY TO AIDING THE MEXICAN AMERICAN.
SRCE *EDUCATION, 1973, 94(2), 120-121.*
INDX ADULT EDUCATION, EDUCATION, MEXICAN AMERICAN, ADULTS, ESSAY, MODELING, POLICY
ABST THE MEXICAN AMERICANS AS A GROUP HAVE CONTINUED TO REMAIN AT THE LOWER SOCIOECONOMIC LEVEL, AND CHILDREN OF THIS CULTURAL GROUP CONTINUE TO HAVE THE HIGHEST DROPOUT RATE OF ANY ONE GROUP. THE AUTHOR FEELS THAT THIS IS DUE LARGELY TO EDUCATORS' FOCUS ON THE CHILD ALONE. IN ORDER TO REACH THE STUDENT, A PROGRAM IS NEEDED WHICH WILL INVOLVE THE PARENTS IN THE LEARNING PROCESS. BY PARTICIPATING IN AN ADULT EDUCATION PROGRAM, THE PARENT IS GIVEN THE OPPORTUNITY TO ACQUIRE SKILLS WHICH WILL AID IN HIS UNDERSTANDING AND ENCOURAGEMENT OF THE EDUCATION OF HIS CHILD. 4 REFERENCES. (JOURNAL ABSTRACT)

ACCN 000994

1161 AUTH **MARTINEZ, R. A. (ED.)**
TITL HISPANIC CULTURE AND HEALTH CARE: FACT, FICTION, FOLKLORE.
SRCE *ST. LOUIS: C. V. MOSBY COMPANY, 1978.*
INDX ATTITUDES, CULTURAL FACTORS, CURANDERISMO, DISEASE, FAMILY ROLES, FOLK MEDICINE, HEALTH, HEALTH DELIVERY SYSTEMS, MENTAL HEALTH, MEXICAN AMERICAN, NURSING, REVIEW, INSTITUTIONALIZATION, PSYCHOTHERAPY, RESOURCE UTILIZATION, BOOK
ABST THIS COLLECTION OF 19 SELECTED READINGS ABOUT HISPANIC HEALTH CARE BELIEFS AND PRACTICES DIRECTED TOWARD NURSES AND ALLIED HEALTH PERSONNEL IS DIVIDED INTO FOUR UNITS. THE FIRST DISCUSSES SIGNIFICANT ADAPTIVE MECHANISMS AND PARTICULAR LIFE STYLES THAT MAY CONTRIBUTE TO HISPANIC HEALTH CARE BELIEFS. AN OVERVIEW OF CULTURAL ATTITUDES IS PROVIDED, WITH PRIMARY FOCUS ON THE ROLE OF THE MEXICAN AMERICAN FAMILY. UNIT TWO EXPLORES THE SIGNIFICANCE OF SOCIETAL INFLUENCE ON THE HEALTH ATTITUDES AND BELIEFS OF HISPANICS. CULTURAL COMPONENTS SUCH AS RELIGION, LANGUAGE, FAMILY STRUCTURE, AND TRADITIONAL COMMUNITY LIFE STYLE, OFTEN CONSIDERED AS INHIBITING THE ACCEPTANCE OF MODERN TREATMENT REGIMENS, ARE EXAMINED. THE ANALYSIS OF FOLK MEDICINE AND DISEASE AS SOCIAL PHENOMENA IS THE UNIFYING THEME IN UNIT THREE. FOLK DISEASES, HEALTH RITUALS AND PRACTICES, AND THEIR INFLUENCE ON THE BIOPSYCHOSOCIAL REALMS OF THE HISPANIC ARE DISCUSSED. IMPLICATIONS FOR THE MUTUALLY SATISFACTORY COEXISTENCE OF FOLK AND SCIENTIFIC SYSTEMS ARE ALSO CONSIDERED. UNIT FOUR IS CONCERNED WITH COMMON BARRIERS THAT MEXICAN AMERICANS MUST OVERCOME IN SEEKING, ACQUIRING,

AND UTILIZING AVAILABLE INSTITUTIONAL AND COMMUNITY-BASED HEALTH SERVICES. SPECIFIC CASE STUDIES REFLECT SOME HISPANIC REACTIONS TO HOSPITALIZATION, INTERVENTION BY PUBLIC HEALTH NURSES, AND TREATMENT OF MENTAL ILLNESS. THE APPENDIX CONSISTS OF A TABLE OF COMMONLY USED "FOLK" HERBS AND THEIR INDICATED USE IN THE TREATMENT OF PARTICULAR ILLNESSES.

ACCN   001726

1162 AUTH   **MARTINEZ, S. R., MARTINEZ, J. L., JR., & OLMEDO, E. L.**
TITL   COMPARATIVE STUDY OF CHICANO AND ANGLO VALUES USING THE SEMANTIC DIFFERENTIAL TECHNIQUE.
SRCE   *ATISBOS: JOURNAL OF CHICANO RESEARCH, 1975, SUMMER, 93-98.*
INDX   MEXICAN AMERICAN, ACCULTURATION, FAMILY STRUCTURE, EMPIRICAL, RESEARCH METHODOLOGY, CROSS CULTURAL, SEX COMPARISON, CALIFORNIA, SOUTHWEST, SEMANTICS, VALUES
ABST   A COMPARATIVE STUDY WAS CONDUCTED AMONG 28 STUDENTS ATTENDING A STATE COLLEGE IN SAN BERNARDINO, CALIFORNIA, WHO WERE ADMINISTERED OSGOOD'S SEMANTIC DIFFERENTIAL TO INVESTIGATE RESPONSES OF CHICANOS AND ANGLOS ON FIVE CONCEPTS VIEWED AS BASIC TO THE MEXICAN FAMILY STRUCTURE. IT WAS FOUND THAT THE CHICANOS AND ANGLOS DIFFERED SIGNIFICANTLY ON FIVE PAIRS OF CONCEPTS: (1) SELF-MOTHER, (2) SELF-MALE, (3) SELF-FEMALE, (4) FATHER-FEMALE, AND (5) MALE-FEMALE. THE RESULTS INDICATE THAT THESE CONCEPTS HAVE DIFFERENT MEANINGS FOR THE TWO CULTURAL GROUPS. 9 REFERENCES. (JOURNAL ABSTRACT MODIFIED)
ACCN   000995

1163 AUTH   **MARTINEZ, T. M.**
TITL   ADVERTISING AND RACISM: THE CASE OF THE MEXICAN AMERICAN.
SRCE   *EL GRITO, 1969, 2(3), 3-13.*
INDX   PREJUDICE, STEREOTYPES, MASS MEDIA, MEXICAN AMERICAN, ESSAY
ABST   AN EXAMINATION OF THE ADVERTISING IN AMERICAN SOCIETY REVEALS RACIST IMPLICATIONS OF MASS MEDIA, ESPECIALLY REGARDING MEXICANS AND MEXICAN AMERICANS. EXAGGERATED MEXICAN RACIAL AND CULTURAL CHARACTERISTICS, TOGETHER WITH SOME OUTRIGHT MISCONCEPTIONS CONCERNING THEIR WAY OF LIFE, SYMBOLICALLY SUGGEST TO THE AUDIENCE THAT SUCH PEOPLE ARE COMICAL, LAZY, AND THIEVING. THE CONSEQUENCE IS THAT THE ETHNIC GROUP IS PERCEIVED AS "NATURALLY INFERIOR." NOT ONLY ARE ADVERTISERS EXHIBITING RACIST THINKING AT THE EXPENSE OF EVERYONE OF MEXICAN DESCENT, BUT THEY ARE ALSO CREATING, IN MANY CASES, UNFAVORABLE RACIAL AND CULTURAL STEREOTYPES. ALTHOUGH THE COMPLEXITY OF THE SITUATION DOES NOT WARRANT A SIMPLE EXPLANATION, THE EVIDENCE FOR PREJUDICE ON THE PART OF BOTH THE CORPORATIONS

AND ADVERTISING AGENCIES IS GLARING. 8 REFERENCES.
ACCN   000996

1164 AUTH   **MARTINEZ, V. S.**
TITL   ILLEGAL IMMIGRATION AND THE LABOR FORCE: AN HISTORICAL AND LEGAL VIEW.
SRCE   *AMERICAN BEHAVIORAL SCIENTIST, 1976, 19(3), 335-350.*
INDX   IMMIGRATION, UNDOCUMENTED WORKERS, ECONOMIC FACTORS, HISTORY, MEXICAN AMERICAN, ESSAY, DISCRIMINATION, LABOR FORCE
ABST   A DISCUSSION OF THE PROBLEMS FACING MEXICAN UNDOCUMENTED WORKERS AS WELL AS MEXICAN AMERICANS MISTAKEN FOR ALIENS IS PRESENTED ON BEHALF OF THE MEXICAN AMERICAN LEGAL DEFENSE AND EDUCATION FUND (MALDEF). SOME GOVERNMENT AND MEDIA SOURCES PLACE MUCH BLAME ON "ILLEGAL ALIENS" FOR REDUCING THE NUMBER OF JOBS, DRAINING WELFARE MONIES AND SERVICES, AND CONTRIBUTING TO HIGH CRIME RATES. MEXICAN IMMIGRANT EMPLOYMENT TRENDS AND U.S. IMMIGRATION POLICIES ARE TRACED HISTORICALLY; THE VAST DEPORTATION AND "REPATRIATION" PRACTICES WHICH CAUSED EVEN LEGAL IMMIGRANTS TO BE SENT TO MEXICO ARE DESCRIBED. CURRENTLY, ALIENS ARE LACKING ADEQUATE LEGAL REPRESENTATION AND ARE UNDERGOING HARASSMENT AND ILLEGAL SEARCH AND SEIZURE BY THE IMMIGRATION AND NATURALIZATION SERVICE (INS) OFFICIALS. CRITERIA SUCH AS SKIN COLOR, DEMEANOR, TYPES OF CLOTHES, AND MANNERISMS ARE OFTEN USED TO JUSTIFY SUSPICION OF ILLEGAL STATUS; THIS IS A POSSIBLE VIOLATION OF CONSTITUTIONAL RIGHTS. A TALK WITH MEXICO'S PRESIDENT ECHEVERRIA REVEALED HIS CONCERN WITH THE TREATMENT OF MEXICAN ALIENS BY U.S. AUTHORITIES. RECOMMENDATIONS MADE BY MALDEF, INCLUDING THOSE PRESENTED TO PRESIDENT FORD, INCLUDE: (1) GOVERNMENT RESEARCH INTO THE IMMIGRATION PROBLEM, LAWS, ENFORCEMENT OF THOSE LAWS, AND PRACTICES AND PROCEDURES OF INS; AND (2) GOVERNMENT PROTECTION OF THE CONSTITUTIONAL RIGHTS OF AMERICANS OF MEXICAN DESCENT, EMPHASIZING SPECIFIC INS GUIDELINES FOR STOPPING CITIZENS WHO LOOK "MEXICAN." OVERALL, THE ILLEGAL IMMIGRATION ISSUE PRESENTS QUESTIONS OF INTERNATIONAL LAW AND RELATIONS, INTERNATIONAL AGRICULTURAL ECONOMICS, DIPLOMACY AND CONSTITUTIONAL RIGHTS OF MEXICAN AMERICANS. 23 REFERENCES.
ACCN   000997

1165 AUTH   **MARTINEZ-DOMINGUEZ, G.**
TITL   LA FAMILIA MEXICANA. (THE MEXICAN FAMILY.)
SRCE   *REVISTA MEXICANA DE SOCIOLOGIA, 1949, 11(3), 337-353. (SPANISH)*
INDX   FAMILY ROLES, FAMILY STRUCTURE, MEXICAN, EMPIRICAL, CENSUS, MEXICO, DEMOGRAPHIC
ABST   THE 1930 AND 1940 CENSUS DATA OF MEXICO ARE REANALYZED TO PROVIDE NEW DEMO-

GRAPHIC INFORMATION ABOUT THE AVERAGE MEXICAN FAMILY. ARITHMETIC MEANS, MODES, PERCENTILES, AND GRAPHS ARE USED TO DESCRIBE THE DATA. FAMILY CHARACTERISTICS INCLUDE NUMBER OF PERSONS PER FAMILY, SEX OF THE HEAD OF HOUSEHOLD, AND APPROXIMATE RURAL-URBAN DIFFERENCES. DERIVING A MORE ACCURATE CHARACTERIZATION OF THE AVERAGE MEXICAN FAMILY, THE FINDINGS SHOW: (1) THAT MOST OF THE POPULATION LIVES IN FAMILIES; (2) THE AVERAGE FAMILY HAS SIX MEMBERS; (3) THE NUMBER OF FAMILIES UNIFORMLY DECREASES AS THE NUMBER OF MEMBERS INCREASES; (4) RURAL FAMILIES TEND TO BE LARGER THAN URBAN FAMILIES; (5) THE HEAD OF THE HOUSEHOLD IS USUALLY MALE, AND MALE-HEADED HOUSEHOLDS HAVE MORE MEMBERS THAN FAMILIES WITH FEMALE-HEADED HOUSEHOLDS; (6) FAMILIES WITH A FEMALE HEAD OF HOUSEHOLD ARE MARKED BY SOCIAL PROBLEMS AND HIGHER POVERTY; AND (7) THE DEGREE OF VARIANCE, DISPERSION, AND SYMMETRY WAS GENERALLY GREATER IN 1940 THAN IN 1930.

ACCN 000990

1166 AUTH **MARTINEZ-URRUTIA, A., & SPIELBERGER, C. D.**

TITL THE RELATIONSHIP BETWEEN STATE-TRAIT ANXIETY AND INTELLIGENCE IN PUERTO RICAN PSYCHIATRIC PATIENTS.

SRCE *REVISTA INTERAMERICANA DE PSICOLOGIA, 1973, 7(3-4), 199-214.*

INDX ANXIETY, INTELLIGENCE, MENTAL HEALTH, PUERTO RICAN-I, WAIS, INTELLIGENCE TESTING, PERSONALITY, PSYCHOTHERAPY, URBAN, EMPIRICAL, PSYCHOPATHOLOGY, ESCALA DE INTELIGENCIA WECHSLER, MALE

ABST FORTY MALE PUERTO RICAN PSYCHIATRIC PATIENTS—15 WERE NEWLY ADMITTED INPATIENTS AND 25 WERE OUTPATIENTS—AT THE SAN JUAN VETERANS ADMINISTRATION HOSPITAL IN PUERTO RICO WERE ADMINISTERED THE SPANISH VERSION OF THE WAIS, THE ESCALA DE INTELIGENCIA WECHSLER PARA ADULTOS (EIWA), AND THE SPANISH EDITION OF SPIELBERGER'S STATE-TRAIT ANXIETY INVENTORY (STAI). THE STAI A-STATE SCALE WAS ADMINISTERED IMMEDIATELY BEFORE THE EIWA (A-STATE-1), AND AGAIN, IMMEDIATELY AFTER THE EIWA (A-STATE-2). A SHORT FORM OF THE STAI A-STATE SCALE WAS ALSO GIVEN IMMEDIATELY AFTER EACH OF THE ELEVEN EIWA SUBTESTS. SIGNIFICANT NEGATIVE CORRELATIONS OF THE STAI A-TRAIT SCALE AND THE A-STATE-2 SCALE WERE OBTAINED WITH THE EIWA FULL SCALE, THE VERBAL AND PERFORMANCE SCALES, THE "WECHSLER TRIAD," AND THE TIMED AND UNTIMED EIWA SUBTESTS. IN ADDITION, SCORES ON EACH EIWA SUBTEST WERE INVERSELY CORRELATED WITH THE SHORT FORM A-STATE SCALES, EXCEPT FOR VOCABULARY AND ANALOGIES. PATIENTS WITH HIGH A-TRAIT SCORES SHOWED HIGHER LEVELS OF A-STATE INTENSITY WHILE PERFORMING ON THE EIWA THAN LOW A-TRAIT PATIENTS. MOREOVER, THE A-STATE LEVELS OF THE HA-TRAIT (HIGH ANXIETY) PATIENTS TENDED TO INCREASE DURING THEIR PERFORMANCE ON THE EIWA, WHILE LEVEL OF A-STATE FOR THE LA-TRAIT (LOW ANXIETY) PATIENTS REMAINED RELATIVELY CONSTANT FROM THE BEGINNING TO THE END OF THE EIWA. 30 REFERENCES. (AUTHOR ABSTRACT MODIFIED)

ACCN 000998

1167 AUTH **MASON, E. P.**

TITL COMPARISON OF PERSONALITY CHARACTERISTICS OF JUNIOR HIGH STUDENTS FROM AMERICAN INDIAN, MEXICAN, AND CAUCASIAN ETHNIC BACKGROUNDS.

SRCE *JOURNAL OF SOCIAL PSYCHOLOGY, 1967, 73(2), 145-155.*

INDX CPI, PERSONALITY, ADOLESCENTS, MEXICAN AMERICAN, CULTURAL FACTORS, SEX COMPARISON, PERSONALITY ASSESSMENT, EMPIRICAL, CROSS CULTURAL, WASHINGTON, WEST, INDIGENOUS POPULATIONS

ABST A COMPARATIVE ANALYSIS OF ETHNIC DIFFERENCES IN PERSONALITY CHARACTERISTICS IS PRESENTED. THE CALIFORNIA PSYCHOLOGICAL INVENTORY (CPI) WAS ADMINISTERED TO 49 CULTURALLY DISADVANTAGED JUNIOR HIGH STUDENTS PARTICIPATING IN A SUMMER EDUCATIONAL ENRICHMENT PROGRAM. THE PARTICIPANT GROUP INCLUDED 26 AMERICAN INDIANS (13 BOYS AND 13 GIRLS), 13 CAUCASIANS (6 BOYS AND 7 GIRLS), AND 10 MEXICAN AMERICANS (5 BOYS AND 5 GIRLS). DATA SHOWED THAT FEMALES, THOUGH EVIDENCING SPECIFIC ETHNIC DIFFERENCES, RESPONDED IN A CONSISTENTLY NEGATIVE PATTERN ACROSS THE 18 SUBTESTS. ETHNIC DIFFERENCES FOR MALES INDICATED THAT THE MEXICAN AND INDIAN GROUPS HAD LOWER SOCIAL PRESENCE THAN THE CAUCASIAN. THE MEXICAN MALE SCORED LOWER THAN THE CAUCASIAN OR INDIAN ON FLEXIBILITY, BUT HIGHER ON SOCIAL RESPONSIBILITY, TOLERANCE, AND INTELLECTUAL EFFICIENCY. THE GIRLS' CONSISTENTLY NEGATIVE RESPONSES CAN BE ATTRIBUTED TO EARLIER MATURING, AS THEY ACCEPTED THEIR ROLE IN LIFE WITH PASSIVITY AND WITH LITTLE EXPECTATION FOR CHANGE. IN CONTRAST TO THE MEXICAN FAMILIES, THE CONSIDERABLE FAMILY DISORGANIZATION FOUND IN BOTH THE CAUCASIAN AND INDIAN GROUPS SEEMED RELATED TO THEIR LOWER SCORES ON SOCIAL MATURITY AND MOTIVATION FOR INTELLECTUAL ACHIEVEMENT. THE RESULTS OF THIS STUDY ILLUSTRATE THAT CULTURAL DISADVANTAGE HAS DIFFERENTIAL EFFECTS BOTH IN RELATIONSHIP TO SEX OF THE RECIPIENT AND TO HIS ETHNIC GROUP. 10 REFERENCES.

ACCN 000999

1168 AUTH **MASON, E. P.**

TITL CROSS VALIDATION STUDY OF PERSONALITY CHARACTERISTICS OF JUNIOR HIGH STUDENTS FROM AMERICAN-INDIAN, MEXICAN, AND CAUCASIAN ETHNIC BACKGROUNDS.

SRCE *IN N. N. WAGNER & M. J. HAUG (EDS.), CHICANOS: SOCIAL AND PSYCHOLOGICAL PERSPEC-*

TIVES. SAINT LOUIS: C. V. MOSBY COMPANY, 1971, PP. 150-155.

INDX PERSONALITY, PERSONALITY ASSESSMENT, CROSS CULTURAL, EMPIRICAL, CPI, ADOLESCENTS, MEXICAN AMERICAN, BEHAVIOR MODIFICATION, ACHIEVEMENT MOTIVATION, SEX COMPARISON, INDIGENOUS POPULATIONS, WASHINGTON, WEST

ABST A REPLICATION OF A STUDY DONE IN 1967, WHICH COMPARED SEX AND ETHNICITY DIFFERENCES IN PERSONALITY CHARACTERISTICS OF AMERICAN INDIAN, MEXICAN AMERICAN AND ANGLO ADOLESCENTS, IS PRESENTED. JUNIOR HIGH GRADUATES IN A SPECIAL SUMMER PROGRAM, PROJECT CATCH-UP, DESIGNED TO RAISE THE ASPIRATION LEVEL AND ACADEMIC PERFORMANCE OF MINORITY STUDENTS ARE TESTED USING CALIFORNIA PSYCHOLOGICAL INVENTORY (CPI). STUDENTS WERE RANDOMLY ASSIGNED TO THE CONTROL OR PARTICIPANT GROUP. 47 (22 AMERICAN INDIANS, 9 MEXICAN AMERICAN AND 16 ANGLOS) COMPLETED THE CPI IN THE PARTICIPANT GROUP. ANALYSIS OF VARIANCE BY ETHNICITY, SEX AND TEST SHOWED AN OVERALL SIGNIFICANT ETHNIC DIFFERENCE, ORDERED WITH CAUCASION HIGHEST AND INDIAN LOWEST. THIS ORDERING DID NOT OCCUR IN THE 1967 STUDY AND RESULTED FROM THE MORE NEGATIVE RESPONSE OF THE MEXICAN MALE AND MORE POSITIVE RESPONSE OF THE MEXICAN FEMALE IN THIS SECOND STUDY. THE EVIDENCE OF A GENERALIZED MORE NEGATIVE RESPONSE BY FEMALES REGARDLESS OF ETHNIC BACKGROUND WAS VALIDATED. OF GREATEST SIGNIFICANCE WAS THE CONSISTENT, ALL PERVASIVE NEGATION OF BOTH MALE AND FEMALE AMERICAN INDIANS. 6 REFERENCES.

ACCN 001000

1169 AUTH **MASON, E. P.**
TITL PROGRESS REPORT: PROJECT CATCH-UP. AN EDUCATIONAL PROGRAM FOR JUNIOR HIGH STUDENTS FROM AMERICAN INDIAN, MEXICAN, AND CAUCASIAN ETHNIC BACKGROUNDS.
SRCE *PSYCHOLOGY IN THE SCHOOLS, 1968, 5(3), 272-276.*
INDX EDUCATION, DISCRIMINATION, MEXICAN AMERICAN, SCHOLASTIC ACHIEVEMENT, SELF CONCEPT, EDUCATIONAL COUNSELING, INSTRUCTIONAL TECHNIQUES, EDUCATIONAL MATERIALS, ADOLESCENTS, PROGRAM EVALUATION, EMPIRICAL, CPI, PSYCHOSOCIAL ADJUSTMENT, WASHINGTON, WEST, INDIGENOUS POPULATIONS
ABST PRELIMINARY RESULTS OF PROJECT CATCH-UP SUMMER 1966, ARE REPORTED. MEXICAN AMERICANS (MA) WERE RATED AS "MORE RESPONSIVE" ON PARTICIPANT IMPROVEMENT MEASURES OF RESPONSIBILITY, COOPERATION, AND INDEPENDENCE. TEST RESULTS OF THE CALIFORNIA PSYCHOLOGICAL INVENTORY SHOWED THAT MA FEMALES RESPONDED IN A CONSISTENTLY NEGATIVE PATTERN ACROSS THE 18 SUBTESTS. ETHNIC GROUP DIFFERENCES FOR MALES INDICATED

THAT MA AND INDIAN GROUPS HAD LOWER SOCIAL PRESENCE SCORES THAN THE CAUCASIAN MALES. FLEXIBILITY SCORES FOR MA MALES WERE LOWER THAN FOR THE CAUCASIAN AND INDIAN MALES, BUT MA MALES SCORED HIGHER IN SOCIAL RESPONSIBILITY, TOLERANCE, AND INTELLECTUAL EFFICIENCY THAN DID THE CAUCASIAN AND INDIAN GROUPS. THE ORAL READING SCORES IMPROVED FROM A MEAN OF 7.55 GRADE LEVEL TO A MEAN OF 8.19 GRADE LEVEL. SIGNIFICANT IMPROVEMENTS IN READING SPEED AND ARITHMETIC COMPUTATIONAL SKILLS WERE ALSO NOTED. THE PRE- AND POST-ADMINISTRATION OF THE READ GENERAL SCIENCE TEST SHOWED A STATISTICALLY SIGNIFICANT INCREMENT IN TEST SCORES. THE VOCATIONAL COUNSELING PROGRAM WAS ESPECIALLY SUCCESSFUL FOR THE GIRLS AND LEAST EFFECTIVE FOR THE BOYS. IN A FOLLOW-UP EVALUATION, NO SIGNIFICANT IMPROVEMENT OCCURRED WHEN SCHOOL PERFORMANCE IN 1966-1967 WAS COMPARED TO SCHOOL PERFORMANCE IN 1965-1966. 6 REFERENCES.

ACCN 001001

1170 AUTH **MASON, E. P.**
TITL PROJECT CATCH-UP: AN EDUCATIONAL PROGRAM FOR SOCIALLY DISADVANTAGED THIRTEEN AND FOURTEEN YEAR OLDS.
SRCE *PSYCHOLOGY IN THE SCHOOLS, 1969, 6(3), 253-257.*
INDX EDUCATION, DISCRIMINATION, MEXICAN AMERICAN, SCHOLASTIC ACHIEVEMENT, SELF CONCEPT, EDUCATIONAL COUNSELING, INSTRUCTIONAL TECHNIQUES, EDUCATIONAL MATERIALS, ADOLESCENTS, PROGRAM EVALUATION, EMPIRICAL, WASHINGTON, WEST, CPI, CASE STUDY, INDIGENOUS POPULATIONS
ABST A SUMMARY OF THE 1967 PROJECT CATCH-UP PROGRAM AND THE FOLLOW-UP EVALUATION OF 1966 AND 1967 PARTICIPANT GROUPS ARE PRESENTED. DURING THE SUMMERS OF 1966 AND 1967 ONE HUNDRED 13 AND 14 YEAR-OLD STUDENTS FROM AMERICAN INDIAN, MEXICAN, AND CAUCASIAN BACKGROUNDS WERE ENROLLED IN A 6-WEEK RESIDENCE PROGRAM OF ACADEMIC REMEDIATION AND ACCELERATION AND GENERAL CULTURAL ENRICHMENT. THE 1967 GROUP BEHAVED DIFFERENTLY FROM THE MORE COOPERATIVE 1966 GROUP PARTICIPANTS. THE RESULTS OF THE CALIFORNIA PSYCHOLOGICAL INVENTORY FOR THE 1967 GROUP REVEALED NEGATIVE FEELINGS OF SELF-WORTH, SOCIAL INEPTNESS, REBELLIOUSNESS, AND EXTREME INTOLERANCE. IN CONTRAST TO THE 1966 GROUP WHO REPORTED THAT THEY LIKED THE FIELD TRIPS AND COUNSELORS, THE 1967 GROUP REPORTED THAT THEY LIKED THE CLASSES BEST. A FOLLOW-UP EVALUATION, BY A COUNSELOR, OF EACH STUDENT MADE IT POSSIBLE TO DEVELOP APPROPRIATE PREVENTATIVE MEASURES TO INSURE SUCCESS IN SCHOOL. INDIVIDUAL CASE STUDIES ARE PROVIDED THAT DESCRIBE SOME OF THE POSITIVE AND NEGATIVE ASPECTS OF THE PROGRAM. 7 REFERENCES.

ACCN 001002

1171 AUTH **MASON, E. P.**
TITL SEX DIFFERENCES IN PERSONALITY CHARACTERISTICS OF DEPRIVED ADOLESCENTS.
SRCE *PERCEPTUAL AND MOTOR SKILLS, 1968, 27(3), 934.*
INDX CPI, PERSONALITY, PERSONALITY ASSESSMENT, MEXICAN AMERICAN, ADOLESCENTS, SEX COMPARISON, POVERTY, SES, EMPIRICAL, INDIGENOUS POPULATIONS, CROSS CULTURAL, PSYCHOSOCIAL ADJUSTMENT, WASHINGTON, WEST
ABST SEX DIFFERENCES WERE INVESTIGATED IN PERSONALITY CHARACTERISTICS OF DEPRIVED JUNIOR HIGH SCHOOL STUDENTS FROM AMERICAN INDIAN, MEXICAN, AND CAUSCASIAN ETHNIC BACKGROUNDS WHO PARTICIPATED IN A 6-WEEK SUMMER ENRICHMENT PROGRAM. THE STAFF RATINGS OF PARTICIPANT IMPROVEMENT IN INDEPENDENCE, RESPONSIBILITY, AND COOPERATION CONSISTENTLY RANKED THE BOYS ABOVE THE GIRLS. THE CALIFORNIA PSYCHOLOGICAL INVENTORY WAS ADMINISTERED TO PARTICIPANT GROUPS DURING EACH OF TWO CONSECUTIVE SUMMERS. IN BOTH SAMPLES, THE FEMALES, REGARDLESS OF ETHNIC GROUP, WERE MORE NEGATIVE, POORLY MOTIVATED, AND NONCONFORMING THAN THE MALES. FOLLOW-UP EVALUATION OF THE OVERALL EFFECTIVENESS OF THE PROGRAM INDICATES THAT ONE MEXICAN GIRL DROPPED OUT OF SCHOOL, WHILE 11 STUDENTS DROPPED OUT OF COMPARABLE CONTROL GROUPS. HOWEVER, TWO INDIAN GIRLS WERE OUT OF SCHOOL BECAUSE OF ILLEGITIMATE PREGNANCIES AND ONE INDIAN GIRL, PLANNING TO BE MARRIED, DROPPED OUT. RESULTS INDICATE THAT THE DEPRIVED ADOLESCENT GIRL MAY BE MORE DEFEATED THAN HER MALE COUNTERPART, AND THIS IS ESPECIALLY TRUE FOR THE AMERICAN INDIAN GIRL. 5 REFERENCES.
ACCN 001003

1172 AUTH **MASON, E. P., & LOCASSO, R. M.**
TITL EVALUATION OF THE POTENTIAL FOR CHANGE IN JUNIOR-HIGH-AGE YOUTH FROM AMERICAN INDIAN, MEXICAN, AND ANGLO ETHNIC BACKGROUNDS.
SRCE *PSYCHOLOGY IN THE SCHOOLS, 1972, 9(4), 423-427.*
INDX INTERPERSONAL RELATIONS, ADOLESCENTS, CURRICULUM, EDUCATION, ATTITUDES, SELF CONCEPT, SCHOLASTIC ACHIEVEMENT, MEXICAN AMERICAN, CROSS CULTURAL, CULTURAL FACTORS, EMPIRICAL, WEST, CALIFORNIA ACHIEVEMENT TESTS, CALIFORNIA TEST OF MENTAL MATURITY, PERSONALITY ASSESSMENT
ABST AN EVALUATION OF PROJECT CATCH-UP FOR THE YEARS 1968 AND 1969 IS PRESENTED. THE PRIMARY INTENT OF THE PROJECT WAS TO DECREASE THE EXPECTED HIGH DROPOUT RATE AND TO ALTER BEHAVIOR PATTERNS SO AS TO IMPROVE SCHOOL ACHIEVEMENT AMONG NATIVE AMERICANS, MEXICAN AMERICANS AND ANGLOS IN THE NORTHWEST. NINETY-EIGHT STUDENTS WERE SELECTED TO PARTICIPATE IN THE PROGRAM ON THE BASIS OF TEACHERS' JUDGMENT OF POSSESSING GREATER POTENTIAL FOR ACHIEVEMENT. DURING A 6-WEEK SUMMER PERIOD THESE STUDENTS WERE EXPOSED TO ACADEMIC REMEDIATION AND ACCELERATION AS WELL AS GENERAL CULTURAL ENRICHMENT. PRE- AND POST-TEST SCORES FROM THE CALIFORNIA TEST OF MENTAL MATURITY (CTMM), CALIFORNIA ACHIEVEMENT TEST (CAT, READING AND ARITHMETIC), AND THE CALIFORNIA PERSONALITY INVENTORY (CPI) WERE ANALYZED. THE RESULTS INDICATE THAT WITH THE EXCEPTION OF ARITHMETIC SCORES AND FEMALE RESPONSES TO THE CTMM, ALL OTHER MEASURES IMPROVED SIGNIFICANTLY. HOWEVER, THE ACTUAL IMPROVEMENT WAS AT A SLOWER RATE THAN EXPECTED FOR THE AVERAGE PUBLIC SCHOOL STUDENT. THE DATA ALSO REVEAL THAT, OVER TIME, ANGLOS CONTINUE TO SCORE THE HIGHEST, NATIVE AMERICANS SCORE THE LOWEST, AND MEXICAN AMERICANS SHOW THE LEAST IMPROVEMENT. THE FINDINGS SUGGEST THAT ALTHOUGH ATTITUDES AS MEASURED BY THE CPI DO CHANGE, THE ETHNIC DIFFERENCES REMAIN RELATIVELY CONSTANT OVER TIME. 8 REFERENCES.
ACCN 000965

1173 AUTH **MASSAD, C. E., YAMAMOTO, K., & DAVIS, O. L., JR.**
TITL STIMULUS MODES AND LANGUAGE MEDIA: A STUDY OF BILINGUALS.
SRCE *PSYCHOLOGY IN THE SCHOOLS, 1970, 7(1), 38-42.*
INDX BILINGUALISM, LINGUISTICS, COGNITIVE STYLE, LINGUISTIC COMPETENCE, RESEARCH METHODOLOGY, COLLEGE STUDENTS, EMPIRICAL
ABST ELEVEN ENGLISH-SPANISH BILINGUAL COLLEGE STUDENTS PARTICIPATED IN AN EXPERIMENT WHICH ASCERTAINED THE EFFECT OF THE PRINTED WORD AND PICTURE IN EVOKING SENSE-IMPRESSION RESPONSES. ALTHOUGH A HIGHER PROPORTION OF SENSE-IMPRESSION RESPONSES WAS ELICITED BY WORDS THAN BY PICTURES IN BOTH LANGUAGES, AND A HIGHER PROPORTION OF SENSORY RESPONSES WAS RECORDED IN SPANISH THAN IN BOTH MODES, THE OBSERVED DIFFERENCES DID NOT ATTAIN STATISTICAL SIGNIFICANCE. IT IS CONCLUDED THAT NEITHER THE STIMULUS MODES NOR THE LANGUAGE MEDIA AFFECTED THE PERFORMANCE ON THE ASSOCIATION TASK WHEN JUDGED BY THE PROPORTION OF SENSE-IMPRESSION RESPONSES. 16 REFERENCES.
ACCN 001004

1174 AUTH **MATHEWSON, G. C., & PEREYRA-SUAREZ, D. M.**
TITL SPANISH LANGUAGE INTERFERENCE WITH ACOUSTIC-PHONETIC SKILLS AND READING.
SRCE *JOURNAL OF READING BEHAVIOR, 1975, 7(2), 187-196.*
INDX PHONOLOGY, BILINGUALISM, READING, SEMANTICS, SES, EDUCATION, ENVIRONMENTAL FACTORS, MEXICAN AMERICAN, CHILDREN,

EMPIRICAL, CALIFORNIA, SOUTHWEST, CROSS CULTURAL

ABST THE EFFECTS OF SPANISH LANGUAGE INTERFERENCE WITH AUDITORY CONCEPTUALIZATION AND READING WERE STUDIED IN 80 SECOND GRADERS FROM RIVERSIDE, CALIFORNIA (34 MEXICAN AMERICAN AND 46 OF OTHER ETHNIC BACKGROUNDS). IT WAS PREDICTED THAT (1) MEXICAN AMERICAN SUBJECTS RECEIVE LOWER AUDITORY CONCEPTUALIZATION SCORES ON A SPANISH INTERFERENCE TEST THAN ON A NONINTERFERENCE TEST, (2) DEGREE OF INTERFERENCE IS POSITIVELY RELATED TO READING ABILITY AMONG MEXICAN AMERICAN CHILDREN, AND (3) AUDITORY CONCEPTUALIZATION IS POSITIVELY RELATED TO READING LEVEL, REGARDLESS OF ETHNIC GROUP. THE LINDAMOOD AUDITORY CONCEPTUALIZATION TEST, THE WIDE RANGE ACHIEVEMENT TEST, AND THE COOPERATIVE PRIMARY TEST BATTERY WERE USED TO TEST THE HYPOTHESES. THE FINDINGS SUPPORTED PREDICTIONS (1) AND (3), BUT NOT (2). IT IS CONCLUDED THAT THOUGH AUDITORY CONCEPTUALIZATION IS STRONGLY RELATED TO READING, SPANISH LANGUAGE INTERFERENCE WITH AUDITORY CONCEPTUALIZATION DOES NOT EXTEND TO READING SKILLS. IN ADDITION, CAUTION CONCERNING THE INTERPRETATION OF AUDITORY CONCEPTUALIZATION SCORES IS URGED IN LIGHT OF THEIR STRONG RELATIONSHIP WITH SES. 12 REFERENCES. (JOURNAL ABSTRACT MODIFIED)

ACCN 001005

1175 AUTH **MATLIN, N., & ALBIZU-MIRANDA, C.**
TITL THE LATENT FUNCTION OF PSYCHOLOGICAL TESTS IN THE COUNSELING PROCESS.
SRCE *REVISTA INTERAMERICANA DE PSICOLOGIA, 1968, 101-112.*
INDX ESSAY, PUERTO RICAN-I, MENTAL HEALTH, CULTURAL FACTORS, ROLE EXPECTATIONS, STEREOTYPES, VOCATIONAL COUNSELING, PSYCHOTHERAPY, PSYCHOTHERAPISTS, CULTURAL CHANGE, AUTHORITARIANISM, SELF CONCEPT, EDUCATIONAL COUNSELING
ABST PSYCHOLOGICAL TESTING INFLUENCES THE COUNSELOR-CLIENT RELATIONSHIP IN SUBTLE BUT SIGNIFICANT WAYS. TESTING ACTS TO REAFFIRM THE STATUS OF THE COUNSELOR AS AN EXPERT, BOTH TO HIMSELF AND TO HIS CLIENT. IT ALSO ENABLES THE COUNSELOR TO CONFIDENTLY PROVIDE ANSWERS THAT ARE BASED UPON THE OPINIONS OF THOSE MORE EXPERT THAN HIMSELF. THE CLIENT, IN TURN, BENEFITS BY THE PERCEPTION THAT THE COUNSELOR SEEMS TO BE DOING SOMETHING, SEEMS TO KNOW WHAT HE IS DOING, AND IS GOING ABOUT IT IN A SCIENTIFIC WAY. TEST RESULTS THUS FACILITATE THE CLIENT'S DECISION-MAKING BY PREDISPOSING HIM TO ACCEPT THE COUNSELOR'S SUGGESTIONS. THESE CONSIDERATIONS CAN BE APPLIED, THOUGH WITH LESS STRINGENCY, TO DEVELOPING COUNTRIES SUCH AS PUERTO RICO. ON THE ONE HAND, BECAUSE CONSULTATION WITH FRIENDS AND FAMILY IS MORE ACCEPTABLE IN SUCH COUNTRIES, THE COUNSELOR

IS UNDER LESS PRESSURE TO JUSTIFY HIS ROLE. ON THE OTHER HAND, MANY PROFESSIONALS ARE UNACCOSTUMED TO THEIR NEW POSITION IN SOCIETY AND MAY FEEL GREATER SELF-DOUBT. IN PARTICULAR, PUERTO RICAN SOCIETY CONTINUES TO BE CLASS-ORIENTED, CAUSING THE COUNSELOR-CLIENT RELATIONSHIP TO BE AFFECTED BY TRADITIONAL AUTHORITARIAN ROLES. TO COUNTERACT THIS, IT IS HOPED THAT IN PUERTO RICO NEW FORMS OF COUNSELING RELATIONSHIPS WILL EMERGE.

ACCN 002152

1176 AUTH **MATLUCK, J. A., & MACE B. J.**
TITL LANGUAGE CHARACTERISTICS OF MEXICAN-AMERICAN CHILDREN: IMPLICATIONS FOR ASSESSMENT.
SRCE *JOURNAL OF SCHOOL PSYCHOLOGY, 1973, 11(4), 365-386.*
INDX LINGUISTIC COMPETENCE, GRAMMAR, PHONOLOGY, LEARNING, BILINGUALISM, INTELLIGENCE TESTING, ACHIEVEMENT TESTING, SES, CHILDREARING PRACTICES, MEXICAN AMERICAN, CHILDREN, REVIEW, LINGUISTICS, LANGUAGE ASSESSMENT, SYNTAX
ABST A DETAILED DESCRIPTION IS PRESENTED OF THE LANGUAGE FEATURES CHARACTERIZING THE SPEECH OF MEXICAN AMERICAN CHILDREN WITH RESPECT TO THEIR DEVIATIONS FROM ACCEPTABLE STANDARDS IN BOTH SPANISH AND ENGLISH. ACCEPTABILITY REFERS TO HOW WELL THE CHILD FUNCTIONS IN EACH OF THE LANGUAGE SETTINGS IN WHICH THE CHILD LIVES. THE MOST CRITICAL PROBLEM IS THE LOSS OF LEXICAL AND GRAMMATICAL SIGNALS THROUGH UNDERDEVELOPED PERCEPTION OF ENGLISH PHONOLOGY. HOW THIS FAULTY PERCEPTION VITALLY AFFECTS NOT ONLY THE CHILD'S LEXICAL AND GRAMMATICAL FAILINGS BUT ALSO THE ABILITY TO LEARN AS FAST OR AS EFFICIENTLY AS THE MONOLINGUAL ENGLISH-SPEAKING CHILD IN EVERY AREA OF LEARNING IS DEMONSTRATED. SUGGESTIONS ARE MADE IN LANGUAGE ASSESSMENT WHICH MAY MORE ACCURATELY EVALUATE ACTUAL LANGUAGE ABILITIES AND THEREBY PROVIDE IMPROVED EDUCATIONAL PROGRAMS FOR THESE CHILDREN. FACTORS RELATED TO THE SOCIOECONOMIC STATUS OF THE FAMILY, CHILD-REARING PRACTICES AND TEST ORIENTATIONS MUST ALSO BE RECOGNIZED AS INFLUENCING THE SCORES THESE CHILDREN RECEIVE, AND THERFORE MUST BE CONSIDERED IN THE INTERPRETATION OF TEST STATISTICS AND ALSO IN PLANNING AND DESIGNING SCHOOL PROGRAMS. 38 REFERENCES. (AUTHOR ABSTRACT MODIFIED)

ACCN 001006

1177 AUTH **MATTHEWS, M. S.**
TITL FOSTERING UPWARD MOBILITY OF MEXICAN AMERICAN ADULTS THROUGH A CRITICAL INCIDENT (DOCTORAL DISSERTATION, OREGON STATE UNIVERSITY, 1971).
SRCE *DISSERTATION ABSTRACTS INTERNATIONAL,*

1971, 32(2), 722A. (UNIVERSITY MICROFILMS NO. 71-19,908.)

INDX   ADULT EDUCATION, SOCIAL MOBILITY, OCCUPATIONAL ASPIRATIONS, SCHOLASTIC ASPIRATIONS, EMPIRICAL, SES, EDUCATION, INSTRUCTIONAL TECHNIQUES, MALE, MEXICAN AMERICAN, FARM LABORERS, OREGON, WEST, MIGRANTS

ABST   THIS STUDY EXAMINED WHETHER THE MEXICAN AMERICAN MALE ADULT BELIEVES HIS FAMILY AND ETHNIC GROUP CAN BENEFIT FROM EDUCATION FOR ADULTS IN WHICH ENGLISH IS TAUGHT, AND WHETHER THE MEXICAN AMERICAN TAKING ADULT CLASSES THINKS HE WILL ACHIEVE UPWARD MOBILITY IN AN ADVANCING TECHNICAL SOCIETY THROUGH OCCUPATIONALLY ORIENTED ADULT EDUCATION. THE SUBJECTS WERE 18 MEXICAN AMERICAN MIGRANT WORKERS IN OREGON, NINE OF WHOM WERE CONTROLS. THE DESIGN OF THE STUDY INCLUDED A CRITICAL INCIDENT—BASED UPON THE CULTURAL STRENGTHS OF THIS MINORITY GROUP—WHICH WOULD CAUSE SUCH ADULT CLASS MEMBERS TO MAKE DECISIONS CONCERNING THE COMPONENTS OF THEIR NEED FOR UPWARD MOBILITY. THE EXPERIMENTAL GROUP ACKNOWLEDGED GREATER RAPPORT WITH EDUCATION COUNSELORS AND EXPRESSED GREATER NEED TO LEARN ANGLO RULES. THEY ALSO EXPRESSED A MUCH GREATER SELF-ASSURANCE THAN THE CONTROLS WHO WERE NOT EXPOSED TO THE CULTURALLY RELEVANT CRITICAL INCIDENT. THE TARGET POPULATION INDICATED A STRONG DESIRE TO LEARN ENGLISH AND TO HAVE CONTINUING ADULT EDUCATION, WITH THE PLEA FOR BILINGUAL AND BICULTURAL COMPONENTS. 118 REFERENCES.

ACCN   001007

1178 AUTH   **MATTLEMAN, M. S., & EMANS, R. L.**
TITL   THE LANGUAGE OF THE INNER-CITY CHILD: A COMPARISON OF PUERTO RICAN AND NEGRO THIRD GRADE GIRLS.
SRCE   *JOURNAL OF NEGRO EDUCATION, 1969, 38(2), 173-176.*
INDX   LINGUISTIC COMPETENCE, SYNTAX, GRAMMAR, SES, CROSS CULTURAL, PUERTO RICAN-M, EMPIRICAL, CHILDREN, FEMALE, URBAN
ABST   THE ORAL LANGUAGE OF FIVE NEGRO AND SIX PUERTO RICAN THIRD GRADE FEMALES WAS COMPARED ON FACILITY, SYNTACTIC STRUCTURE, AND FLUENCY, BY MEANS OF THE LANGUAGE FACILITY TEST. THE MEDIAN SCORE FOR THE PUERTO RICAN CHILDREN WAS 14.51 WHILE THE MEDIAN SCORE FOR THE NEGRO GROUP WAS 20.0 FROM A POSSIBLE 27.0 POINTS. ANALYSES INDICATE THAT THE TWO GROUPS DIFFER SIGNIFICANTLY IN LANGUAGE FACILITY. IN THE SYNTACTIC STRUCTURE, THE PUERTO RICAN CHILDREN USED TWICE AS MANY FRAGMENTS IN THEIR UTTERANCES AS DID NEGRO CHILDREN. WHILE NEGROES USED THE NON-VERB PATTERN IN 10 PERCENT OF THEIR SPEECH, PUERTO RICANS USED THIS CONSTRUCTION IN 19 PERCENT OF THEIR RESPONSES. THE NOUN-VERB-NOUN PATTERN WAS FOUND TO BE PREDOMINANT IN BOTH

GROUP RESPONSES. FLUENCY, AS MEASURED FROM A RAW WORD COUNT OF THE PROTOCOLS, SHOWED THE MEDIAN TOTAL NUMBER OF WORDS USED BY THE PUERTO RICAN GROUP AS 81 AND THE MEDIAN FOR THE NEGRO GROUP AS 289 WORDS. VARIATIONS IN THE LANGUAGE OF BOTH GROUPS SHOWED THE NEGROES USING MORE LINKING VERB CONSTRUCTIONS WHICH ACCOUNTED FOR THEIR PROFICIENCY IN LANGUAGE FACILITY. 12 REFERENCES.

ACCN   001008

1179 AUTH   **MAURER, R., & BAXTER, J. C.**
TITL   IMAGES OF THE NEIGHBORHOOD AND CITY AMONG BLACK-, ANGLO-, AND MEXICAN-AMERICAN CHILDREN.
SRCE   *ENVIROMENT AND BEHAVIOR, 1972, 4(4), 351-388.*
INDX   MEXICAN AMERICAN, CHILDREN, CROSS CULTURAL, IMAGERY, POVERTY, SES, ENVIRONMENTAL FACTORS, EMPIRICAL, ADOLESCENTS, PROJECTIVE TESTING, TEXAS, SOUTHWEST
ABST   TWENTY-FIVE MEXICAN AMERICAN, 36 BLACK AND 30 ANGLO MALE AND FEMALE CHILDREN (7 TO 14 YEARS-OLD) FROM POVERTY LEVEL FAMILIES IN HOUSTON, TEXAS, WERE INTERVIEWED. SUBJECT AND INTERVIEWER WERE MATCHED BY ETHNICITY. SUBJECTS WERE ASKED TO DRAW MAPS OF THEIR NEIGHBORHOOD AND CITY IN AN ATTEMPT TO ASSESS THEIR IMAGERY OF THEIR PHYSICAL ENVIRONMENT. STRONG ETHNIC DIFFERENCES APPEARED IN IMAGES AND DESCRIPTIONS OF THE HOME, THE NEIGHBORHOOD, THE CITY, AND PREFERRED PLAY SETTINGS. FEW OR NO AGE OR SEX DIFFERENCES WERE FOUND. CONTRASTS BETWEEN THESE RESULTS AND THOSE FROM OTHER STUDIES INVOLVING CHILDREN AND ADULTS ARE NOTED. A VARIETY OF HYPOTHESES ARE POSED TO EXPLAIN THE ETHNIC DIFFERENCES. IT IS CONCLUDED THAT BOTH MAP DRAWINGS AND INTERVIEWS ARE HIGHLY PRODUCTIVE MEANS OF ELICITING CHILDREN'S VIEWS OF THEIR PHYSICAL WORLD. 12 REFERENCES. (PASAR ABSTRACT MODIFIED)

ACCN   001009

1180 AUTH   **MAYESKE, G. W.**
TITL   ON THE EXPLANATION OF RACIAL-ETHNIC GROUP DIFFERENCES IN ACHIEVEMENT TEST SCORES.
SRCE   *UNPUBLISHED MANUSCRIPT, UNDATED. (AVAILABLE FROM DR. G. W. MAYESKE, DEPARTMENT OF HEALTH, EDUCATION AND WELFARE, OFFICE OF EDUCATION, WASHINGTON, D.C.)*
INDX   CULTURAL FACTORS, ACHIEVEMENT TESTING, MEXICAN AMERICAN, PUERTO RICAN-M, SES, SCHOLASTIC ACHIEVEMENT, ENVIRONMENTAL FACTORS, EMPIRICAL, INDIGENOUS POPULATIONS, FAMILY STRUCTURE, PARENTAL INVOLVEMENT, SURVEY, CROSS CULTURAL
ABST   AN ANALYSIS OF RACIAL-ETHNIC GROUP DIFFERENCES IN ACHIEVEMENT TEST SCORES BASED ON ONE OF FIVE DIFFERENT GRADE LEVELS FROM WHICH THE EDUCATIONAL OP-

PORTUNITIES SURVEY DATA WERE DERIVED IS PRESENTED. ANALYSIS OF THE DATA SHOWS THAT FOR 123,386 SIXTH-GRADE STUDENTS, 24% OF THE TOTAL DIFFERENCE IN ACADEMIC ACHIEVEMENT IS THE MAXIMUM NATIONAL VALUE THAT CAN BE ASSOCIATED WITH THE STUDENT'S MEMBERSHIP IN ONE OF SIX RACIAL-ETHNIC GROUPS (INDIAN, MEXICAN, PUERTO RICAN, NEGRO, ORIENTAL, OR CAUCASIAN). THIS RELATIONSHIP HOLDS TRUE EVEN BEFORE THE ALLOCATION OF THESE GROUPS TO DIFFERENT SOCIAL CONDITIONS HAS BEEN TAKEN INTO ACCOUNT. THE 24% IS REDUCED TO 1.2% WHEN A NUMBER OF CONFOUNDING SOCIAL CONDITIONS ARE CONSIDERED: (1) SOCIAL AND ECONOMIC WELL-BEING OF THE FAMILY; (2) PRESENCE OR ABSENCE OF KEY FAMILY MEMBERS; (3) ASPIRATIONS OF STUDENTS AND PARENTS FOR SCHOOLING; (4) BELIEFS ABOUT HOW ONE MIGHT BENEFIT FROM AN EDUCATION; (5) ACTIVITIES THAT ONE ENGAGES IN TO SUPPORT THESE ASPIRATIONS; (6) ONE'S REGION OF RESIDENCE; AND (7) ACHIEVEMENT AND MOTIVATIONAL LEVELS OF ONE'S FELLOW STUDENTS. NO INFERENCE ABOUT THE "INDEPENDENT EFFECT" OF MEMBERSHIP IN A PARTICULAR RACIAL-ETHNIC GROUP ON ACADEMIC ACHIEVEMENT CAN BE MADE. OTHER FINDINGS ARE THAT MOTIVATIONAL AND ATTITUDINAL ASPECTS OF FAMILY LIFE PLAY A GREATER INDEPENDENT ROLE IN ACADEMIC ACHIEVEMENT THAN DO RACIAL-ETHNIC GROUP MEMBERSHIP, SOCIAL CLASS MEMBERSHIP, OR THE TYPE OF SCHOOL ATTENDED. 9 REFERENCES.

ACCN   001010

1181 AUTH   **MAYESKE, G. W., WISCLER, C. E., BEATON, A. E., WEINFELD, F. D., COHEN, W. M., OKADA, T., PROSHEK, J. M., & TABLER, K. A.**

TITL   A STUDY OF OUR NATION'S SCHOOLS: A WORKING PAPER.

SRCE   *WASHINGTON, D.C.: U.S. DEPARTMENT OF HEALTH, EDUCATION, AND WELFARE, OFFICE OF EDUCATION, UNDATED.*

INDX   SURVEY, RESEARCH METHODOLOGY, EDUCATION, SPANISH SURNAMED, SCHOLASTIC ACHIEVEMENT, CHILDREN, CROSS CULTURAL, ADOLESCENTS, ACHIEVEMENT MOTIVATION, EMPIRICAL, SES, EDUCATIONAL ASSESSMENT, PROGRAM EVALUATION, ENVIRONMENTAL FACTORS

ABST   DATA FROM A NATIONWIDE SURVEY CONDUCTED IN 1965 BY DHEW WHICH SAMPLED 650,000 STUDENTS IN GRADES 1, 3, 6, 9 AND 12 FROM 4,000 SCHOOLS IS PRESENTED. A 5% STRATIFIED CLUSTER SAMPLE WITH AN EMPHASIS ON MINORITIES WAS USED TO COLLECT DATA ON (1) STUDENT'S SOCIAL BACKGROUND, (2) SCHOOL'S CHARACTERISTICS, AND (3) SCHOOL OUTCOMES WITH THE MAIN PURPOSE BEING TO IDENTIFY WHAT SCHOOL CHARACTERISTICS MOST AFFECT STUDENT OUTCOMES WHEN STUDENT SOCIAL BACKGROUND IS ACCOUNTED FOR. IN THIS STUDY, A SEQUEL TO "EQUALITY OF EDUCATIONAL OPPORTUNITY" ALSO PUBLISHED BY DHEW, THE UNIT OF ANALYSIS IS THE SCHOOL. STA-

TISTICAL TECHNIQUES EMPLOYED ARE REGRESSION ANALYSIS AND PARTITION OF MULTIPLE CORRELATION. FINDINGS ARE SUMMARIZED IN OVER 100 TABLES AND DIAGRAMS. AMONG THE PRINCIPAL FINDINGS ARE THE FOLLOWING: (1) VERY LITTLE SCHOOL INFLUENCE CAN BE SEPARATED FROM STUDENT SOCIAL BACKGROUND, AND CONVERSELY, VERY LITTLE OF STUDENT SOCIAL BACKGROUND CAN BE SEPARATED FROM SCHOOL INFLUENCE. (2) UNTIL 12TH GRADE, THE STUDENT'S SOCIAL BACKGROUND PLAYS A LARGER PART IN SCHOOL OUTCOME THAN DOES SCHOOL INFLUENCE. AT THE 12TH GRADE, THE DISTINGUISHABLE INFLUENCE OF THE SCHOOL IS GREATER ON THE CHILD'S MOTIVATIONAL AND ATTITUDINAL OUTCOMES, THOUGH THE OPPOSITE IS TRUE FOR ACHIEVEMENT AT THIS GRADE LEVEL. (3) SCHOOL VARIABLES MOST INFLUENTIAL IN SCHOOL OUTCOME ARE THOSE RELATED TO PERSONNEL CHARACTERISTICS AS DISTINGUISHED FROM PHYSICAL FACILITIES, PUPIL PROGRAMS OR POLICIES. CHIEF AMONG TEACHER'S CHARACTERISTICS RELATED TO SCHOOL OUTCOME ARE THOSE REFLECTING TRAINING IN RACIALLY IMBALANCED EDUCATIONAL SETTINGS, RESULTING IN LESS ADEQUATE TEACHER PREPARATION. (4) SCHOOLS, AS THEY ARE CURRENTLY CONSTITUTED, PRODUCE MORE LEARNING IN CHILDREN FROM HIGHER SES LEVELS, TWO PARENT HOMES AND IN ANGLOS OR ORIENTAL AMERICANS RATHER THAN MEXICAN AMERICAN, PUERTO RICAN OR OTHER MINORITY FAMILIES. ALTHOUGH MANY FINDINGS HAVE PREVIOUSLY BEEN PRESENTED ELSEWHERE, THIS STUDY DOCUMENTS THE EXTENT AND MAGNITUDE OF THESE RELATIONSHIPS WITH A NATIONAL SAMPLE FOR THE FIRST TIME. ITS FINDINGS AND RECOMMENDATIONS, THEREFORE, SHOULD MORE FREELY MEASURE AND INFLUENCE THE PROBLEMS CONFRONTING THE AMERICAN EDUCATIONAL SYSTEM. 23 REFERENCES.

ACCN   001011

1182 AUTH   **MCANDREW, C., & EDGERTON, R. B.**

TITL   DRUNKEN COMPORTMENT: A SOCIAL EXPLANATION.

SRCE   *CHICAGO: ALDINE PUBLISHING CO., 1969.*

INDX   ADULTS, CROSS CULTURAL, CULTURAL FACTORS, THEORETICAL, MEXICAN, RURAL, INDIGENOUS POPULATIONS, REVIEW, SOUTH AMERICA, ALCOHOLISM

ABST   WHILE CONCEDING THAT ALCOHOL IS A SENSORIMOTOR INHIBITOR, THE AUTHORS (BOTH CULTURAL ANTHROPOLIGISTS) CHALLENGE THE CONVENTIONAL NOTION THAT IT IS ALSO A SUPER-EGO DISINHIBITOR WHICH CAUSES THE DRINKER TO "LOSE CONTROL OF HIMSELF AND TO DO THINGS HE WOULD NOT OTHERWISE DO." THEY SUGGEST, INSTEAD, THAT INTOXICATION BEHAVIORS ARE LEARNED, AND THAT THE WAY PEOPLE COMPORT THEMSELVES WHEN DRUNK IS DETERMINED BY WHAT THEIR SOCIETY HOLDS THESE BEHAVIORS TO BE. IN SUPPORT OF THIS, THE AUTHORS SEARCHED THE ETHNOGRAPHIC LITERATURE

TO DESCRIBE THE DRUNKEN COMPORTMENT IN FIVE SOCIETIES: (1) THE YURUNA INDIANS OF THE PERUVIAN ANDES; (2) THE CAMBA OF EASTERN BOLIVIA; (3) THE IFALUK OF MICRONESIA; (4) THE ARITAMAN MESTIZOS OF NORTHERN COLUMBIA; AND (5) THE MIXTECOS OF OAXACA, MEXICO. IN EACH OF THESE SOCIETIES THE DISINHIBITING EFFECTS OF ALCOHOL ARE NOWHERE IN EVIDENCE, EVEN DURING PERIODS OF EXTREME INTOXICATION. FOLLOWING THIS BROAD SURVEY OF THESE SOCIETIES, THE AUTHORS DEVOTE TWO CHAPTERS TO AN HISTORICAL AND ETHNOGRAPHIC ANALYSIS OF THE STEREOTYPICAL PROPOSITION IN THE U.S. THAT "INDIANS CAN'T HOLD THEIR LIQUOR." IT IS CONCLUDED THAT SINCE SOCIETIES GET EXACTLY THE SORTS OF DRUNKEN COMPORTMENT THAT THEY ALLOW (AND HENCE DESERVE), A RE-EXAMINATION OF THE WHOLE PROBLEM OF THE EFFECTS OF ALCOHOL UPON BEHAVIOR IS WARRANTED. 211 REFERENCES.

ACCN   001756

1183 AUTH   **MCCLINTOCK, C. G.**
TITL   THE DEVELOPMENT OF SOCIAL MOTIVES IN ANGLO-AMERICAN AND MEXICAN-AMERICAN CHILDREN.
SRCE   *JOURNAL OF PERSONALITY AND SOCIAL PSYCHOLOGY, 1974, 29(3), 348-354.*
INDX   ACHIEVEMENT MOTIVATION, COOPERATION, COMPETITION, INTERPERSONAL RELATIONS, CROSS CULTURAL, MEXICAN AMERICAN, EMPIRICAL
ABST   THE CHOICE BEHAVIORS OF 108 MEXICAN AMERICAN AND 108 ANGLO AMERICAN SECOND, FOURTH, AND SIXTH GRADE CHILDREN IN A MAXIMIZING DIFFERENCE GAME ARE COMPARED. ALL SUBJECTS RECEIVED INFORMATION ABOUT OWN AND OTHER'S CHOICES AFTER EACH TRIAL, AS WELL AS OWN AND OTHER'S CUMULATIVE POINT SCORES ACROSS 100 PLAYS OF THE GAME. THE RESULTS INDICATE THAT: (1) FOR BOTH CULTURAL GROUPS, COMPETITIVE CHOICE BEHAVIOR BECAME MORE DOMINANT WITH INCREMENTS IN GRADE LEVEL; (2) THE ANGLO AMERICAN CHILDREN SAMPLED WERE MORE COMPETITIVE AT EACH GRADE LEVEL THAN MEXICAN AMERICAN CHILDREN SAMPLED; AND (3) FOR ALL CULTURAL AND GRADE GROUPS, COMPETITIVE CHOICES INCREASED OVER TRIAL BLOCKS. THE INCREASE IN COMPETITIVE RESPONDING AS A FUNCTION OF GRADE IS INTERPRETED IN TERMS OF A DEVELOPMENTAL THEORY OF ACHIEVEMENT MOTIVATION SET FORTH BY VEROFF (1969). SOME EDUCATIONAL IMPLICATIONS OF DIFFERENCES BETWEEN ANGLO AND MEXICAN AMERICAN CHILDREN ARE NOTED, AS WELL AS SOME CAUTIONARY STATEMENTS CONCERNING THE INTERPRETATION OF CROSS-CULTURAL DATA. 11 REFERENCES.
ACCN   001012

1184 AUTH   **MCCLINTOCK, E.**
TITL   A MULTI-FACET STUDY OF MEXICAN AMERICAN MOTHERS AND CHILDREN IN A PRESCHOOL PROGRAM (PROGRESS REPORT FOR THE OF-

FICE OF CHILD DEVELOPMENT GRANT NO. 90-C-620).
SRCE   *SANTA BARBARA, CALIFORNIA: SANTA BARBARA FAMILY CARE CENTER, MARCH 1976.*
INDX   BILINGUALISM, BILINGUAL-BICULTURAL EDUCATION, MEXICAN AMERICAN, EARLY CHILDHOOD EDUCATION, CHILDREN, SOCIALIZATION, MOTHER-CHILD INTERACTION, CHILDREARING PRACTICES, EMPIRICAL, SELF CONCEPT, INSTRUCTIONAL TECHNIQUES, SES, PARENTAL INVOLVEMENT, LANGUAGE ACQUISITION, CALIFORNIA, SOUTHWEST
ABST   CENTRO FAMILIAR, A UNIQUE BILINGUAL-BICULTURAL FAMILY EDUCATION PROGRAM IN SANTA BARBARA, CALIFORNIA, WAS STUDIED IN ORDER TO: (1) EVALUATE THE IMPACT OF THE PROGRAM ON THE BILINGUAL LANGUAGE DEVELOPMENT OF THE CHILDREN; (2) STUDY THE PROCESSES THAT CONTRIBUTE TO INVOLVEMENT OF LOW INCOME MEXICAN AMERICAN MOTHERS IN THE PROGRAM; (3) INVESTIGATE THE IMPACT OF THE PROJECT ON THE SOCIALIZATION STYLES OF PARTICIPATING MOTHERS; AND (4) ASSESS THE LONGITUDINAL EFFECTS OF THE CENTER ON THE MOTHERS' AND CHILDREN'S RELATIONSHIPS TO THE ELEMENTARY SCHOOL SYSTEM. THE PROGRAM, IN OPERATION FOR 5 YEARS, ITS OBJECTIVES, AND ITS METHODS OF IMPLEMENTATION AND EVALUATION ARE DESCRIBED IN DETAIL. EACH OF FOUR RESEARCH PROJECTS DESIGNED TO EVALUATE THE FOUR CONCEPTS LISTED ABOVE IS OUTLINED BY METHOD, INSTRUMENTS, SUBJECTS AND DATA ANALYSIS. THE STUDY DEMONSTRATES HOW SEVERAL DIFFERENT RESEARCH METHODOLOGIES CAN BE USED TO EVALUATE A MULTIFACETED PROGRAM FOR MEXICAN AMERICAN MOTHERS AND THEIR CHILDREN. 32 REFERENCES.
ACCN   001013

1185 AUTH   **MCCLINTOCK, E., BAYARD, M. P., BRANDES, P., CASTRO, S. K., & PEPITONE, T.**
TITL   A MULTIFACET STUDY OF MEXICAN AMERICAN MOTHERS AND CHILDREN IN A PRESCHOOL PROGRAM (SECOND YEAR PROGRESS REPORT FOR THE OFFICE OF CHILD DEVELOPMENT, OCD NO. 90-C-620).
SRCE   *SANTA BARBARA, CALIF.: SANTA BARBARA FAMILY CARE CENTER, MARCH 1977.*
INDX   BILINGUALISM, BILINGUAL-BICULTURAL EDUCATION, MEXICAN AMERICAN, EARLY CHILDHOOD EDUCATION, CHILDREN, SOCIALIZATION, MOTHER-CHILD INTERACTION, CHILDREARING PRACTICES, EMPIRICAL, SELF CONCEPT, SES, INSTRUCTIONAL TECHNIQUES, INTERPERSONAL RELATIONS, LANGUAGE ACQUISITION, PARENTAL INVOLVEMENT, CALIFORNIA, SOUTHWEST, CROSS GENERATIONAL
ABST   THE SECOND PROGRESS REPORT OF THE RESEARCH BEING CONDUCTED AT CENTRO FAMILIAR, A BILINGUAL-BICULTURAL FAMILY EDUCATION PROGRAM IN SANTA BARBARA, CALIFORNIA, IS PRESENTED. DATA WERE COLLECTED AT BOTH THE PROGRAM SITE AND FROM FAMILIES AND SCHOOLS IN THE COMMUNITY VIA OBSERVATIONS, VIDEOTAPES AND

INTERVIEWS IN AN EFFORT TO ASSESS THE LONG TERM IMPACT OF THE CENTER ON SCHOOL PARTICIPATION OF MOTHERS AND CHILDREN. THE MAJOR ACCOMPLISHMENTS REPORTED ARE: (1) REVISION OF THE CARROW'S TEST OF AUDITORY COMPREHENSION OF LANGUAGE TO ASSESS PROGRAM IMPACTS ON THE BILINGUAL DEVELOPMENT OF CHILDREN; (2) IMPLEMENTATION OF AN OBSERVATIONAL METHODOLOGY SENSITIVE TO THE DYNAMIC NATURE OF THE PROGRAM AND TO THE BICULTURALITY OF ITS PARTICIPANTS; (3) DEVELOPMENT OF A COMPUTER-AIDED TECHNIQUE TO ANALYZE NARRATIVE OBSERVATIONS COLLECTED AT THE CENTER; AND (4) FOLLOW-UP OF FORMER CENTER PARTICIPANTS. PRELIMINARY FINDINGS INDICATE THAT ONE OF THE MOST BENEFICIAL FUNCTIONS OF THE PROGRAM IS THE PROVISION OF OPPORTUNITIES FOR ROLE EXIT AND EXPANSION BY PARTICIPATING MOTHERS. PROGRAM PARTICIPATION AND GENERATIONAL STATUS OF THE MEXICAN AMERICAN PARTICIPANTS ARE FOUND TO AFFECT THEIR SOCIALIZATION STYLES. EMPIRICAL DATA AND ANALYSES ARE PRESENTED FOR PARTS OF THE STUDY. MORE DETAILED ANALYSES ARE TO BE PRESENTED IN FUTURE REPORTS. (AUTHOR SUMMARY MODIFIED)

ACCN   001014

1186 AUTH   **MCCLINTOCK, E., & BARON, J.**

TITL   EARLY INTERVENTION AND BILINGUAL LANGUAGE COMPREHENSION.

SRCE   *HISPANIC JOURNAL OF BEHAVIORAL SCIENCES, 1979, 1(3), 229-245.*

INDX   BILINGUAL, LANGUAGE COMPREHENSION, EMPIRICAL, CALIFORNIA, SOUTHWEST, MEXICAN AMERICAN, CHILDREN, BILINGUAL-BICULTURAL EDUCATION, BILINGUALISM, LINGUISTIC COMPETENCE

ABST   TO EXAMINE THE IMPACT OF A BILINGUAL INTERVENTION PROGRAM ON THE LANGUAGE COMPREHENSION OF MEXICAN AMERICAN PRESCHOOLERS, 28 BOYS AND 28 GIRLS IN A SOUTHERN CALIFORNIA CITY WERE TESTED TWICE IN BOTH ENGLISH AND SPANISH USING A REVISION OF CARROW'S TEST OF AUDITORY COMPREHENSION OF LANGUAGE (TACL). THE INTERVAL BETWEEN PRE- AND POSTTESTS RANGED FROM 2.5 TO 5 MONTHS. EACH CHILD'S NATIVE AND SECOND LANGUAGE WAS DETERMINED FROM MATERNAL REPORTS. SIGNIFICANT EFFECTS OF ATTENDANCE ON POSTTEST SCORES IN BOTH LANGUAGES WERE OBTAINED FROM MULTIPLE REGRESSION ANALYSES, HOLDING CONSTANT RELEVANT CONTROL VARIABLES. SOCIOECONOMIC AND ENVIRONMENTAL FACTORS WERE UNRELATED TO NATIVE LANGUAGE COMPREHENSION, BUT WERE SIGNIFICANTLY ASSOCIATED WITH SECOND LANGUAGE PROFICIENCY. THE RESULTS SUGGEST THAT EARLY BILINGUAL EDUCATION PROMOTES BILINGUAL LANGUAGE COMPREHENSION. SEVERAL LIMITATIONS OF THIS STUDY ARE DISCUSSED, AS IS THE NEED FOR RESEARCH CLARIFYING THE EFFECTS OF VARIOUS LINGUISTIC MILIEUS ON CHILDREN'S LANGUAGE COMPREHENSION. 14 REFERENCES. (JOURNAL ABSTRACT)

ACCN   001775

1187 AUTH   **MCCLURE, E.**

TITL   TEACHER-PUPIL QUESTIONS AND RESPONSES AND THE MEXICAN-AMERICAN CHILD.

SRCE   *PAPER PRESENTED AT THE ANNUAL MEETING OF THE AMERICAN ANTHROPOLOGICAL ASSOCIATION, SAN FRANCISCO, 1975.*

INDX   CULTURAL FACTORS, CLASSROOM BEHAVIOR, MIDWEST, INSTRUCTIONAL TECHNIQUES, INTERPERSONAL RELATIONS, GROUP DYNAMICS, EMPIRICAL, MEXICAN AMERICAN, CHILDREN, RURAL, CROSS CULTURAL

ABST   THE PASSIVITY OF MEXICAN AMERICAN STUDENTS COMPARED TO ANGLO STUDENTS WAS EXAMINED BY OBSERVING TEACHER-PUPIL VERBAL INTERACTION IN CLASSROOM SITUATIONS. SUBJECTS WERE FOUR TEACHERS (2 ANGLO, 1 BILINGUAL ANGLO AND 1 MEXICAN AMERICAN BILINGUAL), AND 70 KINDERGARTEN AND 1ST GRADE ANGLO AND MEXICAN AMERICAN STUDENTS IN A RURAL MIDWESTERN COMMUNITY INVOLVED IN A 3-YEAR PROJECT ON THE ACQUISITION OF COMMUNICATIVE COMPETENCE. THE MEXICAN AMERICAN STUDENTS WERE ENROLLED IN BOTH A BILINGUAL AND REGULAR CLASSROOM. DATA WERE OBTAINED FROM TAPE RECORDINGS, GENERAL OBSERVATIONS, AND TABULATIONS PERTAINING TO THE FREQUENCY AND TYPE OF QUESTIONS AND RESPONSES MADE BY THE TEACHERS AND THE PUPILS IN THE CLASSROOMS. THE FINDINGS INDICATE THE FOLLOWING: (1) MEXICAN AMERICAN CHILDREN ASK AS MANY QUESTIONS AS ANGLO CHILDREN; (2) MEXICAN AMERICAN KINDERGARTEN STUDENTS RESPOND LESS THAN ANGLOS TO TEACHER'S QUESTIONS; AND (3) MEXICAN AMERICAN 1ST GRADERS MATCH ANGLOS IN THEIR RESPONSE RATE. IT IS SUGGESTED THAT PERHAPS ADULT-INITIATED QUESTIONING ROUTINE DIFFERS IN THE ANGLO AND MEXICAN AMERICAN HOME. THE CHILDREN IN THIS STUDY APPEARED TO BE INTERESTED IN PARTICIPATING IN THE CLASSROOM AND PERHAPS THIS ENTHUSIASM CHANGES TO APATHY FOR MEXICAN AMERICAN STUDENTS AS THEY PROGRESS IN SCHOOL. 7 REFERENCES.

ACCN   001015

1188 AUTH   **MCCOY, G.**

TITL   CASE ANALYSIS: CONSULTATION AND COUNSELING.

SRCE   *ELEMENTARY SCHOOL GUIDANCE AND COUNSELING, 1971, 5(3), 221-225.*

INDX   CASE STUDY, EDUCATIONAL COUNSELING, PSYCHOTHERAPY, INSTRUCTIONAL TECHNIQUES, DISCRIMINATION, MEXICAN AMERICAN, TEXAS, SOUTHWEST

ABST   AN ANALYSIS IS PRESENTED OF A CASE DRAWN FROM THE COUNSELING PRACTICE OF A COUNSELOR FOR THREE ELEMENTARY SCHOOLS IN A MIDDLE CLASS, PREDOMINANTLY WHITE SECTION OF A CITY WITH AN APPROXIMATELY 5 PERCENT BLACK POPULATION AND THE BALANCE EQUALLY DIVIDED BE-

TWEEN MEXICAN AMERICANS AND ANGLO AMERICANS. A RECENT COURT ORDER RESULTED IN AN INFLUX OF MEXICAN AMERICAN CHILDREN FROM A LOWER SOCIOECONOMIC LEVEL INTO ONE OF THE THREE SCHOOLS. THE COUNSELOR IN THIS CASE STUDY WAS BLACK, THE HOMEROOM TEACHER, WHITE, AND THE STUDENT, MEXICAN AMERICAN. THERE WERE COMPLAINTS FROM SEVERAL TEACHERS ABOUT ATTITUDE AND BEHAVIOR PROBLEMS WITH THE STUDENT, AND THE HOMEROOM TEACHER REQUESTED ASSISTANCE FROM THE COUNSELOR. PRIOR GROUP GUIDANCE TECHNIQUES USED BY THE COUNSELOR FOR SEVERAL CLASSES, INCLUDING THIS TEACHER'S, RESULTED IN ANALYSIS OF SOME OF THE PROBLEMS INVOLVED IN THE SITUATION WITH THIS STUDENT AND THE RELATIONSHIP BETWEEN TEACHER AND STUDENT. THE BEGINNING OF A TEAM APPROACH TO THE SITUATION, INVOLVING THE STUDENT'S MOTHER AS WELL AS TEACHERS, PRINCIPAL, AND COUNSELOR, DEVELOPED ACCIDENTLY FOLLOWING A FIGHT BETWEEN THE STUDENT AND ANOTHER BOY. THE RESULTS OF "FEELINGS" CLASSES CONDUCTED BY THE COUNSELOR AND ATTENDED BY THE STUDENT APPARENTLY PLAYED A ROLE IN ESTABLISHING BETTER RELATIONSHIPS. THE STUDENT'S BEHAVIOR AND SCHOOL WORK IMPROVED, AND RELATIONSHIPS OF TRUST AND MUTUAL RESPECT WERE ESTABLISHED BETWEEN THE COUNSELOR AND HER COLLEAGUES.

ACCN   001016

1189 AUTH   **MCCRACKEN, J. H.**
TITL   SEX TYPING OF READING BY BOYS ATTENDING ALL MALE CLASSES.
SRCE   *DEVELOPMENTAL PSYCHOLOGY, 1973, 8(1), 148.*
INDX   SEX COMPARISON, STEREOTYPES, SEX ROLES, READING, TEACHERS, CHILDREN, EDUCATION, EDUCATIONAL MATERIALS, MEXICAN AMERICAN, PEER GROUP, CROSS CULTURAL, MALE
ABST   THE EFFECT OF THE SEXUAL COMPOSITION OF CLASSES ON THE SEX ROLE ASSOCIATION FOR READING WAS EXAMINED WITH 88 MIDDLE CLASS ANGLO AND MEXICAN AMERICAN BOYS, GRADES 1-3, ATTENDING FEMALE TAUGHT CLASSES. SUBJECTS SORTED 35 ITEMS INTO TWO GROUPS ASSOCIATED WITH MALE OR FEMALE USAGE, WITH SOME ITEMS SEX-TYPED, SOME MISCELLANEOUS, AND SOME DIRECTLY RELATED TO READING. THE RESULTS REVEALED THAT BOYS IN ALL MALE CLASSES ASSOCIATED READING-RELATED ITEMS WITH MALES MORE THAN BOYS IN COEDUCATIONAL CLASSES. THE STRONGEST AND MOST CONSISTENT EFFECTS ACROSS GRADES WERE FOR ITEMS USED IN ALL THREE GRADES (I.E., READER, PHONICS WORKBOOK, LIBRARY CARD). ITEMS USED PRIMARILY IN FIRST GRADE SHOWED A STRONGER GROUP EFFECT AT THIS GRADE THAN AT THE OTHER GRADES. FINALLY, ADULT READING ITEMS SHOWED WEAK AND INCONSISTENT GROUP DIFFERENCES IN ALL GRADES. 3 REFERENCES. (AUTHOR SUMMARY MODIFIED)
ACCN   001017

1190 AUTH   **MCCREARY, C., & PADILLA, E.**
TITL   MMPI DIFFERENCES AMONG BLACK, MEXICAN-AMERICAN, AND WHITE MALE OFFENDERS.
SRCE   *JOURNAL OF CLINICAL PSYCHOLOGY, 1977, 33(1), 171-177.*
INDX   MMPI, PERSONALITY, PERSONALITY ASSESSMENT, CROSS CULTURAL, MALE, MEXICAN AMERICAN, SES, CRIMINOLOGY, CULTURAL FACTORS, EMPIRICAL, PSYCHOPATHOLOGY
ABST   MMPI SCORES OF 40 BLACK, 36 MEXICAN-AMERICAN, AND 267 WHITE MALE OFFENDERS WERE COMPARED IN ORDER TO INVESTIGATE WHETHER CULTURAL AND/OR SOCIOECONOMIC FACTORS AFFECT THIS PERSONALITY INVENTORY. DATA WERE ANALYZED BY T-TEST COMPARISONS PERFORMED ON UNMATCHED AND MATCHED (EDUCATION AND OCCUPATION) GROUPS THAT UTILIZED ALL PROFILES OR VALID ONES ONLY AND EXAMINED BOTH TRAIT (INDIVIDUAL SCALES) AND TYPE (GOLDBERG INDICES) DIFFERENCES. BLACK/WHITE DIFFERENCES ON THE MA (MANIC), K (VALIDITY), AND HY (HYPOCHONDRIASIS) SCALES APPEARED TO REFLECT CULTURAL FACTORS, WHILE DIFFERENCES ON MF (MASCULINITY-FEMININITY) AND ALCOHOLISM SEEMED TO BE ACCOUNTED FOR BY SOCIOECONOMIC DIFFERENCES AMONG THE GROUPS. CULTURAL FACTORS SEEMED TO BE RELATED TO DIFFERENCES BETWEEN MEXICAN AMERICANS AND WHITES ON THE L (LIE), K, AND OVERCONTROLLED HOSTILITY SCALES, WHILE SOCIOECONOMIC FACTORS APPEARED TO EXPLAIN DIFFERENCES ON THE HS (HYSTERIA) SCALE. TYPE DIFFERENCES WERE NOT APPARENT EXCEPT THAT MEXICAN AMERICANS WERE CLASSIFIED MORE OFTEN AS PSYCHIATRIC, WHILE WHITES AND BLACKS SCORED WELL INTO THE SOCIOPATHIC RANGE. 16 REFERENCES. (AUTHOR ABSTRACT MODIFIED)
ACCN   001018

1191 AUTH   **MCCURRY, M. F. (ED.)**
TITL   VIVA LA DIFERENCIA...A CHICANO CULTURAL AWARENESS CONFERENCE WITH EMPHASIS ON HEALTH.
SRCE   *ALBUQUERQUE: REGIONAL MEDICAL PROGRAMS SERVICE AND THE NEW MEXICO REGIONAL MEDICAL PROGRAM, 1972.*
INDX   MEXICAN AMERICAN, CULTURE, ACCULTURATION, STEREOTYPES, PREJUDICE, ATTITUDES, PHYSICIANS, CROSS CULTURAL, CURANDERISMO, DISEASE, HEALTH, HISTORY, MENTAL HEALTH, TIME ORIENTATION, INTERPERSONAL SPACING, DEATH, ESSAY, CULTURAL FACTORS, PROCEEDINGS, SOUTHWEST
ABST   IN AN EFFORT TO ACHIEVE GREATER CROSS-CULTURAL UNDERSTANDING AND TO DISCUSS THE SPECIAL HEALTH NEEDS OF CHICANOS, THE CHICANO CULTURAL AWARENESS CONFERENCE WAS HELD IN NORTHERN NEW MEXICO IN 1972. THE CONFERENCE PAPERS FOCUSED ON THE FOLLOWING TOPICS: (1) CHICANO CULTURE AND HISTORY; (2) COMPARISONS OF ANGLO AND CHICANO CULTURES; (3) THE MYTH OF AZTLAN AS A CATALYST FOR CHANGE; (4) CHICANO ATTITUDES TOWARDS ANGLO MEDICINE; AND (5) CURAN-

DERISMO. PANEL DISCUSSIONS EXPLORED CULTURAL DIFFERENCES AMONG CHICANOS IN THE SOUTHWEST, LANGUAGE USAGE AS IT AFFECTS CULTURAL ATTITUDES, STEREOTYPES, AND THE USE OF CULTURAL AWARENESS AS A MEANS TO STIMULATE SOCIAL ACTION.

ACCN   000984

1192 AUTH   **MCDONAGH, E. C.**
TITL   ATTITUDES TOWARD ETHNIC FARM WORKERS IN COACHELLA VALLEY.
SRCE   *SOCIOLOGY AND SOCIAL RESEARCH, 1955, 40(1), 10-18.*
INDX   JOB PERFORMANCE, PERFORMANCE EXPECTATIONS, CROSS CULTURAL, FARM LABORERS, SOUTHWEST, MIGRANTS, EMPLOYMENT, LABOR FORCE, RURAL, EMPIRICAL, MEXICAN, MEXICAN AMERICAN, ADOLESCENTS, STEREOTYPES, ATTITUDES, PREJUDICE, ADULTS, CALIFORNIA, SOUTHWEST, ECONOMIC FACTORS
ABST   A SAMPLE OF 124 HIGH SCHOOL STUDENTS AND A SECOND OF 100 RANCHERS IN THE COACHELLA VALLEY, CALIFORNIA, WERE ADMINISTERED A QUESTIONNAIRE TO ASCERTAIN THEIR STEREOTYPED ATTITUDES TOWARD AMERICAN FILIPINOS, BLACKS, MEXICAN NATIONALS, AND MEXICAN "WETBACKS." BOTH SAMPLES WERE ASKED TO CLASSIFY THESE FOUR GROUPS IN TERMS OF FIVE STEREOTYPES: (1) AMBITION; (2) HONESTY; (3) HARDWORKING; (4) LAW-ABIDING; AND (5) MORALS. IN ADDITION, THE RANCHERS WERE GIVEN A QUESTIONNAIRE CONCERNING THE ADVANTAGES AND DISADVANTAGES IN THE EMPLOYMENT OF MEXICAN NATIONAL LABORERS COMPARED WITH ANY OTHER FARM LABOR SUPPLY. FINDINGS ON THE FIRST QUESTIONNAIRE WERE THAT THE STUDENTS AND RANCHERS ASSIGNED A RANGE OF STEREOTYPES TO THE FOUR GROUPS. BLACKS WERE VIEWED WITH MORE CRITICISM BY RANCHERS THAN BY THE STUDENTS, ESPECIALLY WITH REFERENCE TO THE STEREOTYPES OF HONESTY AND MORALITY. BOTH GROUPS OF RESPONDENTS INTERPRETED THE "WETBACK" AND MEXICAN NATIONAL AS THE HARDEST WORKING. MOREOVER, THE RANCHERS ASSIGNED TO THE MEXICAN "WETBACK" OR NATIONAL THE HIGHEST POSITIVE RANKING OF ALL ETHNIC GROUPS ON ALL FIVE STEREOTYPES. CONCERNING THE SECOND QUESTIONNAIRE, THE RANCHERS CITED PROBLEMS OF HOUSING, "RED TAPE," LANGUAGE BARRIERS, AND TRANSPORTATION AS THE CHIEF DISADVANTAGES ASSOCIATED WITH EMPLOYMENT OF MEXICAN NATIONALS. HOWEVER, THE RANCHERS CONSIDERED THE MEXICAN NATIONALS TO BE MORE EFFICIENT THAN DOMESTIC LABOR; AND OVERALL, IT APPEARS THAT RANCHERS HAVE COME TO RELY ON THE MEXICAN NATIONALS AS A DEPENDABLE SOURCE OF LABOR IN AN AREA OF FLUCTUATING LABOR SUPPLY AND PERISHABLE CROPS. 9 REFERENCES.
ACCN   001019

1193 AUTH   **MCDONALD, T. F., & MOODY, E.**

TITL   A BASIC COMMUNICATION PROJECT FOR MIGRANT CHILDREN.
SRCE   *READING TEACHER, 1970, 24(1), 29-32.*
INDX   LINGUISTIC COMPETENCE, LANGUAGE COMPREHENSION, READING, CURRICULUM, PHONOLOGY, INSTRUCTIONAL TECHNIQUES, PROGRAM EVALUATION, MEXICAN AMERICAN, RURAL, CHILDREN, POVERTY, SES, MIGRANTS, ARIZONA, SOUTHWEST, EMPIRICAL
ABST   THE TOLLESON ELEMENTARY SCHOOL DISTRICT IN ARIZONA USES A BASIC COMMUNICATION (ABC) CURRICULUM TO HELP MEXICAN AMERICAN CHILDREN OF MIGRANT FAMILIES WITH HANDICAPS INHERENT IN BILINGUAL SITUATIONS. THE CHILDREN ARE LIMITED IN THEIR ABILITY TO SPEAK EITHER SPANISH OR ENGLISH FLUENTLY. WITHIN THE CURRICULUM, CHILDREN ARE ENCOURAGED TO EXPRESS, IN ENGLISH, THEIR REACTIONS TO FIELD TRIPS AND TO AUDIO AND VISUAL PRESENTATIONS. EXPERIENCE STORIES, PUPPETRY, AND ROLE-PLAYING ARE MEDIA FOR ORAL EXPRESSION. THE ABC APPROACH USES NO PRESCRIBED TEXTS AND NO EMPHASIS IS PUT ON MASTERY OF SUBJECT MATTER AS AN END IN ITSELF. TEACHERS ASSUME THE ROLE OF FACILITATORS IN LEARNING INSTEAD OF SIMPLY DIRECTING STUDENT ACTIVITIES. EVALUATION OF THE PROGRAM AFTER ITS FIRST YEAR OF OPERATION INDICATES SIGNIFICANT ACHIEVEMENT IN ORAL LANGUAGE AND A POSITIVE BEHAVIORAL CHANGE. THE CURRICULUM IS PART OF A TOTAL PROGRAM THAT INCLUDES HEALTH CARE AND SUPPLEMENTAL NUTRITION. 3 REFERENCES.
ACCN   001020

1194 AUTH   **MCGEHEARTY, L., & WOMBLE, M.**
TITL   CASE ANALYSIS: CONSULTATION AND COUNSELING.
SRCE   *ELEMENTARY SCHOOL GUIDANCE AND COUNSELING, 1970, 5(2), 141-144; 147.*
INDX   CASE STUDY, EDUCATIONAL COUNSELING, PSYCHOTHERAPY, BILINGUAL, MALE, PSYCHOSOCIAL ADJUSTMENT, MEXICAN AMERICAN, CHILDREN, TEXAS, SOUTHWEST
ABST   THE TREATMENT OF A MEXICAN AMERICAN FIFTH GRADER WHO WAS UNRESPONSIVE IN SCHOOL BY A WHITE, MIDDLE CLASS COUNSELOR IS DESCRIBED. THE COUNSELOR SAW THIS AS A SITUATION WHERE A CHILD FROM A CULTURALLY DIFFERENT BACKGROUND DELIBERATELY PLAYED DUMB TO AVOID PRESSURE FROM THE TEACHER. THE PRIORITY THE COUNSELOR SET ON HELPING HIM LEARN THROUGH A GROUP SETTING APPEARED APPROPRIATE. HELPING HIM DEVELOP COPING MECHANISMS OF HIS OWN SEEMED A MORE REASONABLE APPROACH IN THIS SITUATION THAN WORKING WITH HIS PARENTS OR WITH HIS TEACHER AT ANY GREAT LENGTH. 1 REFERENCE.
ACCN   001021

1195 AUTH   **MCGINN, N. F.**
TITL   MARRIAGE AND FAMILY IN MIDDLE CLASS MEXICO.

SRCE   *JOURNAL OF MARRIAGE AND THE FAMILY, 1966, 28, 305-313.*

INDX   SES, FAMILY STRUCTURE, FAMILY ROLES, SEX ROLES, SEXUAL BEHAVIOR, MEXICAN, MEXICO, ESSAY, MARRIAGE, ROLE EXPECTATIONS, CULTURAL CHANGE, CHILDREARING PRACTICES, VALUES

ABST   A GENERAL DESCRIPTION OF NORMATIVE MARRIAGE AND FAMILY ROLES AS FOUND IN PRESENT-DAY MIDDLE CLASS MEXICO IS PRESENTED. AN ATTEMPT IS MADE TO SHOW HOW CULTURALLY DEFINED IDEALS OF MALE AND FEMALE ROLES IN COURTSHIP INFLUENCE MARITAL RELATIONSHIPS. IT IS CONTENDED THAT THE DISCONTINUITY OF ROLE EXPECTATIONS BY WOMEN IS REFLECTED IN CHILD-REARING PRACTICES. THESE PRACTICES LEAD TO A MALE-FEMALE ROLE DICHOTOMY WHICH IN TURN PERPETUATES THE CYCLE. CHANGES IN THESE TRADITIONAL PATTERNS HAVE BEEN SLOW AND THE EFFECTS OF INDUSTRIALIZATION ON THE RATE AND DIRECTION OF CHANGE IN MARRIAGE RELATIONSHIPS IS DIFFICULT TO ASCERTAIN AT THIS POINT. IT DOES APPEAR POSSIBLE, HOWEVER, THAT MEXICO'S MIDDLE-CLASS COULD DEVELOP VALUES OF EGALITARIAN MARRIAGE. 14 REFERENCES. (JOURNAL ABSTRACT MODIFIED)

ACCN   001022

1196 AUTH   **MCHUGH, J. P., KAHN, M. W., & HEIMAN, E.**
TITL   RELATIONSHIPS BETWEEN MENTAL HEALTH TREATMENT AND MEDICAL UTILIZATION OF LOW INCOME MEXICAN AMERICAN PATIENTS: SOME PRELIMINARY FINDINGS.
SRCE   *MEDICAL CARE, 1977, 15(5), 439-444.*
INDX   PHYSICIANS, MENTAL HEALTH, MENTAL HEALTH PROFESSION, PSYCHOTHERAPY, HEALTH DELIVERY SYSTEMS, HEALTH, MEXICAN AMERICAN, EMPIRICAL, POVERTY, SES, CULTURAL FACTORS, SOUTHWEST
ABST   THE HYPOTHESIS THAT MEDICAL VISITS DECREASE AS A FUNCTION OF MENTAL HEALTH TREATMENT WAS TESTED AMONG 119 LOWER SOCIOECONOMIC MEXICAN PATIENTS. THE NUMBER OF MEDICAL AND PSYCHOTHERAPY VISITS FOR ALL PATIENTS REFERRED FOR MENTAL HEALTH TREATMENT BEFORE, DURING AND AFTER, WERE OBTAINED AND ANALYZED TO DETERMINE RATE OF MEDICAL VISITS AS A FUNCTION OF PSYCHIATRIC SERVICES. RESULTS INDICATE CLEAR REJECTION OF THE HYPOTHESIS. MEDICAL VISITS SIGNIFICANTLY INCREASED RATHER THAN DECREASED. FACTORS WHICH MAY ACCOUNT FOR THESE FINDINGS BEING THE OPPOSITE OF PREVIOUS STUDIES ARE DISCUSSED AND INCLUDE PREVIOUS POOR MEDICAL SERVICE AVAILABILITY AND SOCIOECONOMIC DIFFERENCES IN POPULATIONS. 7 REFERENCES. (JOURNAL ABSTRACT MODIFIED)
ACCN   001023

1197 AUTH   **MCKAY, R. V.**
TITL   AMERICANS OF SPANISH ORIGIN IN THE LABOR FORCE: AN UPDATE.
SRCE   *AGENDA, JANUARY/FEBRUARY 1977, PP. 29-32.*
INDX   LABOR FORCE, DEMOGRAPHIC, ECONOMIC FACTORS, SPANISH SURNAMED, EMPLOYMENT, CROSS CULTURAL, EMPIRICAL, SEX COMPARISON, MALE
ABST   THE RECENT DEVELOPMENTS IN THE LABOR FORCE STATUS OF WORKERS OF SPANISH ORIGIN ARE ANALYZED AND COMPARED WITH THE EMPLOYMENT OF BLACKS AND WHITES. SPANISH ORIGIN WORKERS HAVE GENERALLY EXPERIENCED HIGHER THAN AVERAGE UNEMPLOYMENT AND HAVE BEEN OVER-REPRESENTED IN OCCUPATIONS THAT HAVE HIGH JOBLESS RATES. THE CURRENT ECONOMIC SITUATION, HOWEVER, HAS RESULTED IN INCREASING THE SEVERITY OF THEIR EMPLOYMENT STATUS. FOR EXAMPLE, THE UNEMPLOYMENT RATE FOR SPANISH ORIGIN WORKERS ROSE FROM 7.5% IN 1972 TO 12.2% IN 1975. ALTHOUGH SPANISH MALES EXPERIENCED THE GREATEST INCREASE OF UNEMPLOYMENT, JOBLESSNESS FOR SPANISH ADULT FEMALES AND TEENAGERS ALSO INCREASED. ADDITIONAL STATISTICS ARE PROVIDED WHICH EXAMINE THE CHARACTERISTICS OF THE SPANISH ORIGIN POPULATION, THEIR PARTICIPATION IN THE LABOR FORCE, AND THE DURATION OF THEIR UNEMPLOYMENT. 5 REFERENCES.
ACCN   001024

1198 AUTH   **MCKNIGHT, G. L.**
TITL   COMMUNICATION: THE KEY TO SOCIAL CHANGE.
SRCE   *IN M. M. MANGOLD (ED.), LA CAUSA CHICANA: THE MOVEMENT FOR JUSTICE. NEW YORK: FAMILY SERVICE ASSOCIATION OF AMERICA, 1971, PP. 192-210.*
INDX   HISTORY, CHICANO MOVEMENT, ETHNIC IDENTITY, COMMUNITY, LEADERSHIP, POLITICS, MASS MEDIA, ESSAY, COMMUNITY INVOLVEMENT, SOCIAL SERVICES
ABST   COMMUNICATION IS THE GREATEST ALLY OF INTER-GROUP RELATIONS, COMMUNITY ORGANIZATION, AND SOCIAL CHANGE. ALTHOUGH CHICANO COMMUNITIES ARE BEGINNING TO VOICE THEIR NEEDS, THERE ARE STILL MISSING LINKS IN THE LINES OF COMMUNICATION. AMONG THESE PROBLEM AREAS ARE: (1) THE CONTINUED SUPPRESSION OF MEXICAN AMERICAN HISTORY; (2) PARENTAL DENIAL OF CULTURAL IDENTITY IN ORDER TO ASSIMILATE AND MOVE UP ECONOMICALLY; AND (3) THE STEREOTYPING OF CHICANO CULTURAL PATTERNS AND FAMILY ROLES. THESE AND OTHER PROBLEMS CAN BE OVERCOME BY POLITICAL ACTION AND LEADERSHIP IN CHICANO COMMUNITIES, BASED UPON PRIDE OF ETHNIC IDENTITY AND ECONOMIC DEVELOPMENT. A PROFESSIONAL GROUP OF CHICANO SOCIAL WORKERS, LOS TRABAJADORES DE LA RAZA (TR), IS AN EXAMPLE OF CHICANO LEADERSHIP WHICH CAN COMMUNICATE THE NEEDS OF THE COMMUNITY AND MAKE COMMUNITY ORGANIZATION MORE EFFECTIVE. 12 REFERENCES.
ACCN   001025

1199 AUTH   **MCLEMORE, S. D.**
TITL   ETHNIC ATTITUDES TOWARD HOSPITALIZA-

TION: AN ILLUSTRATIVE COMPARISON OF AN-GLOS AND MEXICAN AMERICANS.

SRCE   *THE SOUTHWESTERN SOCIAL SCIENCE QUAR-TERLY, 1963, 43(4), 341-346.*

INDX   SES, HEALTH DELIVERY SYSTEMS, HEALTH, AT-TITUDES, CROSS CULTURAL, MEXICAN AMERI-CAN, EMPIRICAL, ADULTS, TEXAS, SOUTHWEST

ABST   THE RELATIONSHIP OF EDUCATIONAL LEVEL TO ATTITUDES TOWARD HOSPITALIZATION AMONG 30 ANGLO AMERICAN (AA) AND 28 MEXICAN AMERICAN (MA) PATIENTS IS EXAM-INED. THE FIRST HYPOTHESIS STATES THAT MA PATIENTS HOLD MORE UNFAVORABLE ATTI-TUDES TOWARD HOSPITALIZATION THAN AA PATIENTS. THE SECOND HYPOTHESIS MAIN-TAINS THAT THE OBSERVED ATTITUDINAL DIF-FERENCES CAN BE ACCOUNTED FOR BY DIF-FERENT LEVELS OF EDUCATION. A 20-ITEM HOSPITALIZATION ATTITUDE SCALE WAS AD-MINISTERED TO THE SUBJECTS IN THE EN-GLISH AND SPANISH FORMS. RESULTS OF THE FIRST HYPOTHESIS WERE INCONCLUSIVE. CONFLICTING ANALYSES DID NOT PERMIT A DECISION ON THE QUESTION OF WHETHER OR NOT MA'S HOLD MORE UNFAVORABLE ATTI-TUDES TOWARD HOSPITALIZATION THAN DO AA'S. WITH RESPECT TO THE SECOND HY-POTHESIS, HOWEVER, THERE WAS A DIRECT RELATION IN BOTH ETHNIC GROUPS BETWEEN LEVEL OF EDUCATION AND ATTITUDES TO-WARD HOSPITALIZATION, AND THERE WAS ONLY SLIGHT EVIDENCE OF AN ETHNIC DIFFERENCE PER SE IN ATTITUDES TOWARD HOSPITALIZA-TION. FINDINGS SUGGEST THAT IF THERE IS A CORRELATION BETWEEN MA AND AA ETHNI-CITY AND ATTITUDES TOWARD HOSPITALIZA-TION, AS REPORTED IN THE LITERATURE, IT MAY BE A REFLECTION OF AN UNDERLYING CONNECTION BETWEEN THOSE ATTITUDES AND DIFFERENCES IN AVERAGE EDUCATIONAL LEV-ELS OF MEMBERS OF TWO GROUPS. 8 REFER-ENCES.

ACCN   001026

1200 AUTH   **MCNAMARA, P.**

TITL   MEXICAN-AMERICANS IN LOS ANGELES COUNTY: A STUDY IN ACCULTURATION.

SRCE   *SAN FRANCISCO: R AND E RESEARCH ASSOCI-ATES, 1975. (REPRINTED FROM AN UNPUB-LISHED THESIS, ST. LOUIS UNIVERSITY, 1957.)*

INDX   ACCULTURATION, SOCIAL MOBILITY, HISTORY, OCCUPATIONAL ASPIRATIONS, CULTURE, FAMILY STRUCTURE, ROLE EXPECTATIONS, SCHOLAS-TIC ACHIEVEMENT, ECONOMIC FACTORS, SES, EMPIRICAL, MEXICAN AMERICAN, INTERPER-SONAL RELATIONS, MIGRATION, IMMIGRATION, CHILDREARING PRACTICES, FICTIVE KINSHIP, CULTURAL FACTORS, CULTURAL CHANGE, DE-MOGRAPHIC, RELIGION, FAMILY ROLES, COM-MUNITY, SOCIALIZATION, CALIFORNIA, SOUTH-WEST, CROSS GENERATIONAL

ABST   AN ANTHROPOLOGICAL APPROACH EXAMIN-ING THE EXTENT OF ACCULTURATION OCCUR-RING AMONG CONTEMPORARY MEXICAN AMERICAN FAMILIES IN LOS ANGELES COUNTY IS PRESENTED. THE FIRST SECTION IS DE-VOTED TO FOLLOWING THE PATHS OF IMMI-GRATION IN THIS AREA FROM THE AMERICAN

CONQUEST UNTIL THE END OF WORLD WAR II. THE CONDITIONS OF FAMILY DISORGANIZA-TION ARE BRIEFLY DESCRIBED BETWEEN GEN-ERATIONS. A THOROUGH DISCUSSION OF THE MAJOR CONCEPTS OF CULTURE, CULTURE OR-GANIZATION, AND ACCULTURATION ARE EX-AMINED WITHIN A THEORETICAL FRAMEWORK OF THE CHANGING FAMILY. CENSUS DATA ARE USED TO PROVIDE BACKGROUND INFORMA-TION REGARDING CONTEMPORARY CONDI-TIONS; PASTORS AND MEXICAN FAMILIES WERE INTERVIEWED CONCERNING VARIOUS FACETS OF CULTURAL CHANGE. THE MEXICAN IMMI-GRANT FAMILY IS SEEN AS HAVING MOVED FROM DISORGANIZATION TO A NEW "CULTURE REORGANIZATION;"YOUNGER FAMILIES ARE COMPARATIVELY MORE ASSIMILATED; AND CERTAIN ASPECTS OF EARLIER CULTURE PAT-TERNS HAVE BEEN RETAINED INCLUDING CA-THOLICISM, TEENAGE DATING CUSTOMS, AND FAMILY RECREATION. THE FINAL SECTION IN-TEGRATES THE FINDINGS PRESENTED EAR-LIER, PROVIDES AN ASSESSMENT OF THESE FINDINGS IN RELATION TO ACCULTURATION, AND DISCUSSES PROBLEMS AND SUGGES-TIONS FOR FURTHER RESEARCH. 74 REFER-ENCES.

ACCN   001027

1201 AUTH   **MCNEILL, R., & PATINO, L. E.**

TITL   ASPECTS OF THE LEGISLATIVE PROCESS RELE-VANT TO BETTER SERVICES DELIVERY AT THE FEDERAL AND STATE LEVEL.

SRCE   *IN A. M. PADILLA & E. R. PADILLA (EDS.), IM-PROVING MENTAL HEALTH AND HUMAN SER-VICES FOR HISPANIC COMMUNITIES: SE-LECTED PRESENTATIONS FROM REGIONAL CONFERENCES. WASHINGTON, D.C.: NA-TIONAL COALITION OF HISPANIC MENTAL HEALTH AND HUMAN SERVICES ORGANIZA-TIONS (COSSMHO), 1977, PP. 61-67.*

INDX   LEGISLATION, POLITICS, PROCEEDINGS, MEN-TAL HEALTH, FINANCING, POLICY, JUDICIAL PROCESS. SPANISH SURNAMED, POLITICAL POWER. HEALTH DELIVERY SYSTEMS

ABST   THE FOLLOWING ARE EXCERPTS OF WORK-SHOP PRESENTATIONS PERTAINING TO THE LEGISLATIVE PROCESSES AT THE FEDERAL AND STATE LEVEL REGARDING THE DEGREE AND EXTENT OF THE IMPROVEMENT OF MEN-TAL HEALTH HUMAN SERVICES. AT THE FED-ERAL LEVEL THE DEVELOPMENT, ENACTMENT, AND IMPLEMENTATION OF LEGISLATION COM-PRISES TWO MAJOR PROCESSES: (1) THE AU-THORIZATIONS PROCESS, TO ENACT LEGISLA-TION AUTHORIZING A PARTICULAR PROGRAM; AND (2) THE APPROPRIATIONS PROCESS, TO PROVIDE FUNDING FOR THE APPROVED PRO-GRAM. AN EXAMPLE OF THE STEPS TAKEN TO ENACT NEW LEGISLATION REGARDING OB-TAINING ADDITIONAL FUNDS FOR MENTAL RE-TARDATION PROGRAMS IS PRESENTED. AT THE STATE LEVEL IMPROVING THE DELIVERY OF MENTAL HEALTH AND HUMAN SERVICES TO THE SPANISH-SPEAKING IS DISCUSSED WITH RESPECT TO PROTECTING AND PROMOTING BILINGUALISM, SUCH AS THE 1973 BILINGUAL

SERVICES ACT AND THE BILINGUAL CON-
TRACTS ACT. COURT ACTION SUCH AS THE
WYATT VS. STICKNEY DECISION CONCERNING
PROTECTING THE RIGHTS OF MINORITIES CAN
ALSO BE AN EFFECTIVE MEANS FOR IMPROV-
ING MENTAL HEALTH TREATMENT FOR THE
SPANISH-SPEAKING. IT IS CONCLUDED THAT
JUST AS THE FLOW OF INFORMATION IS IM-
PORTANT FOR IMPLEMENTING PROGRAMS TO
PROVIDE EFFECTIVE SERVICES FOR THE SPAN-
ISH-SPEAKING COMMUNITY AT THE FEDERAL
LEVEL, THIS IS ALSO TRUE AT THE STATE
LEVEL.

ACCN   001028

1202 AUTH   **MEADOW, A., STOKER, D. H., & ZURCHER, L.
A.**
TITL   SEX ROLE AND SCHIZOPHRENIA: A CROSS-
CULTURAL STUDY.
SRCE   *THE BRITISH JOURNAL OF SOCIAL PSYCHIATRY,
1967, 1(4), 250-259.*
INDX   SCHIZOPHRENIA, CROSS CULTURAL, MEXICAN
AMERICAN, MEXICAN, MMPI, SEX COMPARI-
SON, SEX ROLES, POVERTY, EMPIRICAL, SES,
ADULTS, ADOLESCENTS, FAMILY ROLES, DE-
MOGRAPHIC, CULTURAL CHANGE, CULTURAL
FACTORS, ARIZONA, SOUTHWEST, FEMALE
ABST   A CROSS CULTURAL COMPARISON EXAMINING
THE RELATIONSHIP BETWEEN THE SOCIAL STA-
TUS OF SEX AND THE PREVALENCE OF
SCHIZOPHRENIA IS PRESENTED. THREE
SAMPLES WERE USED IN THIS STUDY: (1) 211
SCHIZOPHRENIC PATIENTS FROM ARIZONA
STATE HOSPITAL; (2) 968 SCHIZOPHRENIC PA-
TIENTS FROM MANICOMIO GENERAL HOSPI-
TAL IN MEXICO CITY; AND (3) 311 ANGLO
AMERICAN AND MEXICAN AMERICAN 10TH
GRADE STUDENTS ATTENDING TUCSON HIGH
SCHOOL IN ARIZONA WHO SCORED LOWER
THAN 70 ON THE F SCALE OF THE MMPI. THE
SUBJECTS' SEX-ETHNIC RATIOS WERE COM-
PARED TO SEX-ETHNIC RATIO POPULATION
FIGURES FOR ARIZONA AND MEXICO. THE
FINDINGS INDICATE THAT MEXICAN AMERICAN
FEMALES ARE LESS APT TO DEVELOP SCHIZO-
PHRENIA THAN MEXICAN AMERICAN MALES.
THE CONTRIBUTING FACTOR FOR THIS SEX
DIFFERENCE IS ATTRIBUTED TO THE TRADI-
TIONAL SEX ROLE ASSIGNED TO THE FEMALE.
17 REFERENCES.
ACCN   001029

1203 AUTH   **MEADOW, A., & BRONSON, L.**
TITL   RELIGIOUS AFFILIATION AND PSYCHOPATHOL-
OGY IN A MEXICAN AMERICAN POPULATION.
SRCE   *JOURNAL OF ABNORMAL PSYCHOLOGY, 1969,
74(2), 177-180.*
INDX   RELIGION, PSYCHOPATHOLOGY, ACCULTURA-
TION, EDUCATION, SES, COPING MECHA-
NISMS, GROUP DYNAMICS, ATTRIBUTION OF
RESPONSIBILITY, MEXICAN AMERICAN, EMPIR-
ICAL
ABST   AN INVESTIGATION OF THE RELATIONSHIP BE-
TWEEN RELIGIOUS AFFILIATION AND PSYCHO-
PATHOLOGY IN A MEXICAN AMERICAN (MA)
COMMUNITY IS PRESENTED. FIFTY-FOUR MA
PROTESTANT AND 54 MA CATHOLIC SUBJECTS
WERE MATCHED ON AGE, COUNTRY OF NATIV-

ITY, EDUCATION, AND SOCIOECONOMIC STA-
TUS. EVALUATIONS OF PSYCHOPATHOLOGY
WERE DERIVED FROM THE L-R (HABIT AND
TENSION) SECTIONS OF THE CORNELL MEDI-
CAL INDEX (CMI) AND FROM BEHAVIORAL OB-
SERVATIONS. THE PRINCIPAL FINDING WAS
THAT CATHOLICS PRODUCED A GREATER
NUMBER OF PATHOLOGICAL RESPONSES THAN
THE NON-CATHOLICS. THE MEAN M-R (INADE-
QUACY AND TENSION) CMI SCORE FOR THE
CATHOLICS WAS 9.4, FOR THE PROTESTANTS
4.6. THIS DIFFERENCE BETWEEN THE GROUPS
WAS HIGHLY SIGNIFICANT. SUBJECTS WITH 0
TO 5 YEARS OF EDUCATION HAD SIGNIFI-
CANTLY MORE PATHOLOGY THAN THOSE WITH
6 TO 11 YEARS OF EDUCATION, AND THOSE
WITH 12 YEARS OR MORE OF EDUCATION HAD
MORE SYMPTOMATOLOGY THAN THOSE WITH
6 TO 11 YEARS OF EDUCATION. DISCUSSION
OF THE CMI RESULTS IS PRESENTED. A LOWER
PATHOLOGY REPORTED BY PROTESTANTS IS
ATTRIBUTED TO SMALL SOCIAL GROUPS OF
THE PROTESTANT MA CHURCH, WHICH PRO-
VIDES GREATER SOCIAL SUPPORT THAN LARGE
CATHOLIC CONGREGATIONS. PROTESTANT
DOCTRINE PRODUCES A LESS PATHOLOGICAL
CHARACTER STRUCTURE THAN CATHOLIC RE-
LIGIOUS CONTENT. THE PROTESTANT MA
CHURCH APPEARS TO FILL MANY OF THE
GAPS IN WEAKENED MA TRADITIONAL CUL-
TURE. 7 REFERENCES.
ACCN   001030

1204 AUTH   **MEADOW, A., & STOKER, D.**
TITL   SYMPTOMATIC BEHAVIOR OF HOSPITALIZED
PATIENTS.
SRCE   *ARCHIVES OF GENERAL PSYCHIATRY, 1965,
12(3), 267-277.*
INDX   SYMPTOMATOLOGY, PSYCHOPATHOLOGY,
MEXICAN AMERICAN, ADULTS, CROSS CUL-
TURAL, EMPIRICAL, CULTURAL FACTORS, SES,
ALCOHOLISM, SCHIZOPHRENIA, AGGRES-
SION, PSYCHOSIS, NEUROSIS, ARIZONA,
SOUTHWEST, MENTAL HEALTH, ATTITUDES,
MACHISMO
ABST   THE QUANTITATIVE DIFFERENCES IN THE
SYMPTOMATIC BEHAVIOR OF 240 PATIENTS'
CASE HISTORY FILES, 120 MEXICAN AMERICAN
(MA) AND 120 ANGLO AMERICAN (AA) SUB-
JECTS, ARE DESCRIBED. A LIST OF 58 SYMP-
TOMATIC BEHAVIORS AND CHARACTERISTICS
TYPICAL OF MENTAL HOSPITAL PATIENTS WAS
CONSTRUCTED AND EACH CASE RECORD WAS
CAREFULLY EXAMINED FOR THE PRESENCE OF
THE VARIABLES (E.G., BELIEF IN WITCHES, PA-
TIENT VISITS CURERS) IN THE BEHAVIOR AND
HISTORY OF THE PATIENT. IN ADDITION, THE
SYMPTOM CHECKLIST WAS FILLED OUT BY A
MEMBER OF THE PATIENT'S FAMILY FOR FUR-
THER VALIDATION. FINDINGS INDICATED THAT
MA FEMALES (60) WERE THE MOST AFFEC-
TIVELY DISTURBED AND SHOWED CATATONIC
SYMPTOMATOLOGY. MA MALES (60) REVEALED
THE IMPORTANCE OF THE "MACHO" PATTERN
IN THEIR SYMPTOMATOLOGY. THEY WERE THE
MOST ALCOHOLIC AND ASSAULTIVE, AND
SHOWED AN UNDERLYING TENDENCY TO-
WARD CATATONIC SYMPTOMATOLOGY. AA FE-

MALES (60) AND MALES (60) WERE BOTH MORE PARANOID THAN THE MA SAMPLES. BEHAVIORS REPORTED BY ANGLO HOSPITAL PERSONNEL IN PATIENTS' CASE FILES MODERATELY CORRELATED WITH BEHAVIORS INDEPENDENTLY DESCRIBED BY FAMILY MEMBERS FOR BOTH PATIENT GROUPS. THIS CORRELATION SUGGESTS THAT A COMMON CORE OF AGREEMENT EXISTS BETWEEN MEMBERS OF THE TWO CULTURES IN THE PERCEPTION OF PATHOLOGICAL BEHAVIOR. 23 REFERENCES.

ACCN   001031

1205 AUTH   **MECH, E. V.**
TITL   ACHIEVEMENT MOTIVATION PATTERNS AMONG LOW-INCOME ANGLO-AMERICAN, MEXICAN-AMERICAN, AND NEGRO YOUTH.
SRCE   *PROCEEDINGS OF THE 80TH ANNUAL CONVENTION OF THE AMERICAN PSYCHOLOGICAL ASSOCIATION, 1972, 7(1), 279-280.*
INDX   ACHIEVEMENT MOTIVATION, POVERTY, SES, CROSS CULTURAL, TAT, ACHIEVEMENT TESTING, EMPIRICAL, ADOLESCENTS, SCHOLASTIC ASPIRATIONS, SCHOLASTIC ACHIEVEMENT, MALE, ARIZONA, SOUTHWEST, PERSONALITY ASSESSMENT
ABST   THE RELATIONSHIP BETWEEN ETHNIC-RACIAL FACTORS AND PATTERNS OF ACHIEVEMENT-MOTIVATION IN 605 ADOLESCENT MALES RAISED IN LOW-INCOME FAMILIES WAS STUDIED. INDICES UTILIZED WERE: LEVEL OF ASPIRATION, TAT, EPPS, SOCIAL ACHIEVEMENT TESTS, AND GPA'S. BLACK SUBJECTS RANKED HIGH ON COGNITIVE MEASURES OF ACHIEVEMENT-MOTIVATION BUT SCORED LOW ON MEASURES OF ACHIEVEMENT-PERFORMANCE. MEXICAN AMERICAN SUBJECTS DID LESS WELL ON INTERVIEW MEASURES OF ACHIEVEMENT-MOTIVATION BUT SURPASSED BLACK AND CAUCASIAN SUBJECTS IN GPA. BLACK SUBJECTS SHOWED A GREATER DISCREPANCY BETWEEN ACHIEVEMENT-COGNITION AND ACHIEVEMENT-BEHAVIOR THAN DID MEXICAN AMERICAN AND CAUCASIAN SUBJECTS. 5 REFERENCES. (PASAR ABSTRACT)
ACCN   001032

1206 AUTH   **MEEKER, F. B., & KLEINKE, C. L.**
TITL   KNOWLEDGE OF NAMES FOR IN- AND OUT-GROUP MEMBERS OF DIFFERENT SEX AND ETHNIC GROUPS.
SRCE   *PSYCHOLOGICAL REPORTS, 1972, 31(2), 832-834.*
INDX   INTERPERSONAL RELATIONS, STEREOTYPES, SEX COMPARISON, GROUP DYNAMICS, ETHNIC IDENTITY, EMPIRICAL, MEXICAN AMERICAN, COLLEGE STUDENTS, CALIFORNIA, SOUTHWEST
ABST   TWO STUDIES WERE CONDUCTED TO TEST THE NOTION THAT MEMBERS OF OUTGROUPS WOULD REPORT MORE NAMES FOR OUTGROUPS AND FOR INGROUPS THAN MEMBERS OF INGROUPS. IN THE FIRST STUDY, 20 BLACK AND 24 CHICANO STUDENTS LISTED MORE NAMES FOR THEMSELVES AND FOR WHITES THAN DID 106 WHITE STUDENTS. IN THE SECOND STUDY 36 FEMALE STUDENTS LISTED MORE NAMES FOR THEMSELVES AND FOR MALES THAN DID 31 MALE STUDENTS. ANALY-

SIS OF THE MOST COMMON NAMES LISTED SHOWED THAT IN- AND OUTGROUPS SHARE USE OF MANY NAMES BUT ALSO HAVE SOME NAMES WHICH ARE EXCLUSIVE TO THEIR OWN GROUP. IT IS SUGGESTED THAT THE NUMBER OF NAMES LISTED BY PERSONS MIGHT BE AFFECTED BY INTELLIGENCE OR OTHER PERSONALITY VARIABLES. 2 REFERENCES.

ACCN   001033

1207 AUTH   **MEEKER, M., & MEEKER, R.**
TITL   STRATEGIES FOR ASSESSING INTELLECTUAL PATTERNS IN BLACK, ANGLO, AND MEXICAN-AMERICAN BOYS—OR ANY OTHER CHILDREN—AND IMPLICATIONS FOR EDUCATION.
SRCE   *JOURNAL OF SCHOOL PSYCHOLOGY, 1973, 11(4), 341-350.*
INDX   INTELLIGENCE TESTING, MEXICAN AMERICAN, CROSS CULTURAL, CULTURAL FACTORS, WISC, STANFORD-BINET INTELLIGENCE TEST, REVIEW, TEST VALIDITY
ABST   METHODS OF ASSESSING INTELLECTUAL PROCESSES IN BLACK, ANGLO, MEXICAN AMERICAN OR OTHER CHILDREN ARE DISCUSSED ALONG WITH EDUCATIONAL IMPLICATIONS. IQ TEST RESULTS ARE ANALYZED USING A SPECIFIC AND PRESCRIPTIVE TECHNIQUE IN WHICH: (1) THE IQ TEST RESPONSES ON BINETS ARE SEPARATED FROM THE SCORE AND INTERPRETED AS INDICATORS OF INDIVIDUAL OR GROUP PROFILES OF ABILITIES; (2) THESE RESPONSES ARE MADE TO SERVE DIAGNOSTICALLY FOR AN INDIVIDUALIZED PROGRAM OF TRAINING INTELLECTUAL ABILITIES IN CHILDREN; AND (3) THIS INFORMATION IS SEEN AS COMING FROM THE PSYCHOLOGIST TO THE TEACHER OUT OF THE TRADITIONAL TESTING BATTERY, WITH LITTLE MORE EFFORT ON THE PART OF THE PSYCHOLOGIST. IT IS CONCLUDED THAT SPECIFIC, TREATMENT RELATED, INDIVIDUAL ASSESSMENT CAN BE AN IMMEDIATE REMEDY FOR INTELLIGENCE TESTING ABUSES. SEVERAL WAYS OF MAKING THE IQ TEST DATA RELEVANT TO TEACHING ARE OFFERED. 17 REFERENCES. (NCMHI ABSTRACT)

ACCN   001034

1208 AUTH   **MEGARGEE, E. I.**
TITL   DELINQUENCY IN THREE CULTURES: PROJECT FOLLOW-UP SUMMARY.
SRCE   *AUSTIN: HOGG FOUNDATION FOR MENTAL HEALTH, 1968.*
INDX   CRIMINOLOGY, DELINQUENCY, CROSS CULTURAL, MEXICAN, MEXICAN AMERICAN, ADOLESCENTS, SES, POVERTY, PHYSICAL DEVELOPMENT, PERSONALITY, EMPIRICAL, TEXAS, SOUTHWEST, VALUES
ABST   IN A CROSS-CULTURAL STUDY OF JUVENILE DELINQUENCY, 50 ADJUDICATED MALE DELINQUENTS, AGED 12 TO 17, AND 50 MATCHED LOWER-CLASS NONDELINQUENTS WERE SELECTED FROM EACH OF THREE ETHNIC GROUPS: MEXICAN NATIONALS LIVING IN MONTERREY, NUEVO LEON, MEXICO; MEXICAN AMERICANS (LATINS) RESIDING IN SAN ANTO-

NIO, TEXAS; AND NORTH AMERICANS (AN-GLOS) RESIDING IN SAN ANTONIO. ALL 300 SUBJECTS WERE EVALUATED ON SOCIOLOGI-CAL, PSYCHOLOGICAL, AND PHYSIOLOGICAL MEASURES, AND THE DELINQUENTS AND NON-DELINQUENTS IN EACH SAMPLE WERE COM-PARED. IT WAS HYPOTHESIZED: THAT FAMILIES OF DELINQUENTS WOULD BE CHARACTERIZED BY LESS COHESIVENESS; THAT DELINQUENTS' PARENTS WOULD EXHIBIT LESS WARMTH AND THAT THEY WOULD BE MORE LIKELY TO HAVE ANTISOCIAL ATTITUDES; THAT THE DISCIPLINE EXERCISED BY THESE PARENTS WOULD BE MORE PUNITIVE AND ERRATIC; AND THAT THEY WOULD BE LESS ACHIEVEMENT ORIENTED. THE DELINQUENTS WERE EXPECTED TO BE MORE DISRESPECTFUL OF AUTHORITY FIG-URES AND TO HAVE ANTISOCIAL VALUES, TO BE LESS ACHIEVEMENT ORIENTED, AND TO HAVE FEWER OF THE SKILLS NECESSARY FOR ACHIEVEMENT. MOST OF THE HYPOTHESES WERE CONFIRMED. THUS, QUALITIES DIFFER-ENTIATING THE DELINQUENTS WERE NOT MERE ARTIFACTS OF LOWER-CLASS STATUS. HOW-EVER, THERE WERE SOME NOTEWORTHY DIF-FERENCES BETWEEN THE ETHNIC SAMPLES: MEXICAN AND LATIN DELINQUENTS WERE CONSISTENTLY NEGATIVE IN THEIR ATTITUDE TOWARD THEIR FATHERS AND WERE AMBIVA-LENT TOWARD THEIR MOTHERS; ANGLO DE-LINQUENTS HAD MORE SIBLINGS THAN DID THE NONDELINQUENTS; AND IN THE MEXICAN SAMPLE, DELINQUENTS DEVELOPED LATER. THE RESULTS SUGGEST THAT MANY CHARAC-TERISTICS OF JUVENILE DELINQUENTS HAVE CROSS-CULTURAL VALIDITY.

ACCN   001035

1209 AUTH   **MEJIA, D. P.**

TITL   CROSS-ETHNIC FATHER ROLES: PERCEPTIONS OF MIDDLE CLASS ANGLO-AMERICAN AND MEXICAN-AMERICAN PARENTS (DOCTORAL DISSERTATION, UNIVERSITY OF CALIFORNIA, IRVINE, 1975).

SRCE   *DISSERTATION ABSTRACTS INTERNATIONAL, 1975, 36(10), 5355B. (UNIVERSITY MICROFILMS NO. 76-7255.)*

INDX   CHILDREARING PRACTICES, SOCIALIZATION, FAMILY ROLES, FATHER-CHILD INTERACTION, CROSS CULTURAL, SES, EMPIRICAL, CASE STUDY, PERCEPTION, LOCUS OF CONTROL, CALIFORNIA, SOUTHWEST, RELIGION

ABST   THIS STUDY INVESTIGATED PERCEPTIONS OF THE FATHER ROLE AMONG A CROSS-ETHNIC SAMPLE OF FOUR ANGLO AMERICAN AND FOUR MEXICAN AMERICAN MIDDLE CLASS IN-TACT CATHOLIC FAMILIES WITH AN ELDEST PRE-SCHOOL DAUGHTER AND RESIDING IN SOUTHERN ·CALIFORNIA. INFORMATION RE-GARDING THE FATHER'S ROLE WAS OBTAINED FROM UNSTRUCTURED OBSERVATIONS AND STRUCTURED QUESTIONNAIRES THAT WERE ADMINISTERED TO BOTH PARENTS IN THE HOME. THE INSTRUMENT SCHEDULE CON-TAINED MEASUREMENTS OF RISK-TAKING, LO-CUS OF CONTROL, PERMISSIVE-RESTRICTIVE CHILD-REARING PRACTICES, PARENTAL AU-THORITY, VALUE SYSTEMS, AND FATHER ROLE

PERCEPTIONS. WITH RESPECT TO ETHNICITY AND FATHER ROLE, THE FOLLOWING WAS CONCLUDED. FIRST, THE CROSS-ETHNIC SAMPLES DESCRIBED THE FATHER ROLE MORE SIMILAR THAN DISSIMILAR DESPITE SUBCUL-TURAL DIFFERENCES SUCH AS VARIATIONS IN THE GENERATIONAL FAMILIES' SOCIOECO-NOMIC STATUS AND FAMILY SIZE. SECOND, RAMIFICATIONS OF ROLE DEVELOPMENT AS HIERARCHIES OF CULTURAL MODALITIES WENT UNOBSERVED BECAUSE THE CROSS-ETHNIC GROUPS' SELF-DESCRIPTIONS WERE SO ALIKE. THIRD, MOTHERS AND FATHERS DID NOT DE-PICT THE FATHER OR HIS ROLE AS VESTIGIAL. FOURTH, WHEN COMPARED TO PREVIOUS RE-SEARCH, THE FAMILIES APPEARED TO BE UNDERGOING FURTHER DEMOCRATIZATION. 130 REFERENCES. (AUTHOR ABSTRACT MODI-FIED)

ACCN   001036

1210 AUTH   **MELGARES, R.**

TITL   OVERCOMING BARRIERS ASSOCIATED WITH INCREASING THE NUMBER OF MEXICAN-AMERICAN DENTISTS.

SRCE   *IN R. W. SUNNICHT & C. F. COLLINS (EDS.), WORKSHOP ON MINORITY DENTAL STUDENT RECRUITMENT, RETENTION AND EDUCATION. KANSAS CITY, MO.: SCHOOL OF DENTISTRY, UNIVERSITY OF MISSOURI-KANSAS CITY, 1975, PP. 67-73.*

INDX   PROFESSIONAL TRAINING, HEALTH, MEXICAN AMERICAN, HEALTH DELIVERY SYSTEMS, SCHOLASTIC ACHIEVEMENT, REPRESENTA-TION, PHYSICIANS, ESSAY, EQUAL OPPORTU-NITY, BILINGUAL-BICULTURAL PERSONNEL

ABST   THE PAUCITY OF MEXICAN AMERICAN (MA) DENTISTS IN THE U.S. IS DUE TO A NUMBER OF EDUCATIONAL BARRIERS FACING THE MA POPULATION—E.G., POVERTY, DISCRIMINA-TION, LANGUAGE, AND SCHOOL PRACTICES WHICH DISCOURAGE MA CHILDREN FROM ACADEMIC ADVANCEMENT. TO RECTIFY THIS, MA HIGH SCHOOL STUDENTS SHOULD BE EN-COURAGED TO PURSUE PROFESSIONAL CA-REERS, COLLEGE PROGRAMS SHOULD PRO-VIDE SPECIAL ASSISTANCE TO MA STUDENTS, AND IN GENERAL THE EDUCATIONAL SYSTEM SHOULD ELIMINATE DISCRIMINATORY PRAC-TICES AND ATTITUDES. WITH REGARD TO DEN-TISTRY—SPECIFICALLY, THE LACK OF BOTH MA DENTISTS AND DENTAL SERVICES IN MA COM-MUNITIES—IT IS RECOMMENDED THAT A RE-CRUITMENT AND TRAINING PROGRAM FOR MA'S BE INSTITUTED, INCLUDING: (1) ADE-QUATE STIPENDS AND SCHOLARSHIPS; (2) IN-SERVICE TRAINING OF NON-MA PERSONNEL TO PROMOTE AN UNDERSTANDING OF MA CULTURE; (3) FIELD PLACEMENT OF PROFES-SIONAL STUDENTS IN MA AREAS WHICH LACK DENTAL SERVICES; AND (4) INTERNSHIPS WITHIN HEALTH AGENCIES FOR MA HIGH SCHOOL AND COLLEGE STUDENTS.

ACCN   001037

1211 AUTH   **MELTON, J. V.**

TITL   CONCEPTIONS OF DRINKING PATTERNS AMONG

FARM WORKERS: A CROSS-CULTURAL COMPARISON.

SRCE   *UNPUBLISHED MASTER'S THESIS, CALIFORNIA STATE COLLEGE, BAKERSFIELD, 1976.*

INDX   ALCOHOLISM, ATTITUDES, FARM LABORERS, PSYCHOTHERAPISTS, MEXICAN AMERICAN, SURVEY, REVIEW, CROSS CULTURAL, PROFESSIONAL TRAINING, SES, EMPIRICAL, CALIFORNIA, SOUTHWEST

ABST   THIS STUDY INVESTIGATED DIFFERENCES IN ATTITUDES TOWARD ALCOHOL-RELATED BEHAVIORS AND PROBLEMS BETWEEN 137 FARM WORKERS OF MEXICAN CULTURE AND 81 COUNSELORS/THERAPISTS IN NORTHERN KERN COUNTY, CALIFORNIA. THE CHOICES OF THE FOUR MOST FREQUENT OF EIGHT BEHAVIORS ASSOCIATED WITH ALCOHOL CONSUMPTION AMONG FARM WORKERS WERE: (1) SPENDING MONEY MEANT FOR FAMILY USE; (2) FORGETTING PROBLEMS; (3) RETURNING HOME LATE AT NIGHT; AND (4) PERCEIVING THINGS AS BECOMING EASIER. COUNSELORS/THERAPISTS REPORTED SIMILAR ITEMS AS MAJOR BEHAVIORAL ASPECTS ACCOMPANYING DRINKING: (1) FORGETTING PROBLEMS; (2) SPENDING MONEY MEANT FOR FAMILY USE; (3) FEEL LIKE GETTING TOGETHER WITH FRIENDS; AND (4) RETURNING HOME LATE AT NIGHT. WITH RESPECT TO SERIOUS PROBLEMS RELATED TO DRINKING, FARM WORKERS LISTED THE FOLLOWING FOUR ITEMS: (1) BEING A HAZARD ON THE ROAD; (2) HARMFUL TO HEALTH; (3) LOSING WORK; AND (4) DRINKING ALCOHOL IS FATAL. THERAPISTS, ON THE OTHER HAND, INDICATED THE FOLLOWING PROBLEMS ASSOCIATED WITH DRINKING: (1) LOSING WORK; (2) BEING A HAZARD ON THE ROAD; (3) EMOTIONALLY UPSETTING TO FAMILIES; AND (4) ALCOHOL BECOMING A NECESSITY. CHI SQUARE TESTS OF INDEPENDENCE WERE CALCULATED FOR EACH ITEM OF THE BEHAVIORS AND PROBLEMS TO DETERMINE DIFFERENCES BETWEEN THE FARM WORKERS, BY SEX AND COUNTRY OF BIRTH, AND THE COUNSELORS. ONLY TWO OF THE EIGHT BEHAVIORS WERE FOUND TO BE SIGNIFICANTLY DIFFERENT. HOWEVER, SEVEN OF THE EIGHT ITEMS ON THE PROBLEM LIST WERE FOUND TO BE SIGNIFICANTLY DIFFERENT, SUGGESTING THE NEED FOR CROSS-CULTURAL EDUCATION OF ALCOHOL COUNSELORS/THERAPISTS WHO WORK WITH PROBLEM DRINKERS AMONG FARM WORKERS OF MEXICAN CULTURE. 21 REFERENCES. (AUTHOR ABSTRACT MODIFIED)

ACCN   001038

1212 AUTH   **MELUS, A.**

TITL   UNA COMUNIDAD HISPANA OPINA SOBRE EL ALCOHOLISMO. (AN HISPANIC COMMUNITY GIVES ITS OPINIONS ABOUT ALCOHOLISM.)

SRCE   *AGENDA, JANUARY/FEBRUARY 1977, PP. 23-24. (SPANISH)*

INDX   SURVEY, ALCOHOLISM, DEMOGRAPHIC, ATTITUDES, SPANISH SURNAMED, EMPIRICAL, URBAN, SEX ROLES, WASHINGTON D.C., EAST

ABST   THE SPANISH-SPEAKING COMMUNITY MAY BE ESPECIALLY VULNERABLE TO ALCOHOL PROBLEMS BECAUSE OF LOWER ECONOMIC AND EDUCATIONAL LEVELS, AS WELL AS ATTITUDES TOWARDS ALCOHOL ABUSE. IN ORDER TO STUDY ATTITUDES OF HISPANICS TOWARDS ALCOHOLISM, A QUESTIONNAIRE WAS GIVEN TO A SPANISH SURNAMED SAMPLE OF WASHINGTON, D.C. RESIDENTS, COMPRISED MAINLY OF PERSONS FROM CENTRAL AND SOUTH AMERICA, PUERTO RICO, AND MEXICO. THE QUESTIONNAIRE SOUGHT THE FOLLOWING: (1) HISPANIC ATTITUDES TOWARDS ALCOHOLISM AND THOSE WHO DRINK; (2) HOW, WHY, AND WHERE HISPANICS DRINK; AND (3) THE RELATIONSHIP BETWEEN DRINKING AND PERSONAL/FAMILY PROBLEMS. AFTER INTERVIEWING 200 PERSONS, THE FINDINGS SHOW THAT MOST HISPANICS BELIEVE ALCOHOL IS A SEVERE PROBLEM IN THEIR COMMUNITY AS WELL AS A CHIEF CAUSE OF FAMILY PROBLEMS. FEWER PEOPLE ADMITTED TO FREQUENT DRINKING THAN THOSE WHO SAID THEY DRINK ONCE OR TWICE A DAY, THE MAIN BEVERAGE BEING BEER. THE MAJORITY BELIEVE THAT MEN DRINK MORE AND THAT IT IS SHAMEFUL TO SEE AN INTOXICATED WOMAN. HOWEVER, A LARGE MAJORITY DO NOT SEE DRINKING AS BEING MASCULINE. A LITTLE OVER HALF VIEW ALCOHOLISM AS A DISEASE, WHILE THE REST SEE IT AS A VICE; AND MOST BELIEVE THERE IS A CURE. BECAUSE DRINKING IS A SOCIAL ACTIVITY IN HISPANIC CULTURE, PEOPLE SEE BEGINNING SIGNS OF ALCOHOLISM AS DRINKING ALONE AND IN THE MORNING. NO RELATION IS SEEN BETWEEN ALCOHOLISM AND CLASS. RECOMMENDATIONS ARE MADE FOR MORE EDUCATIONAL AND INFORMATIVE MATERIALS, BILINGUAL-BICULTURAL PROGRAMS DIRECTED AT ALCOHOLISM, AND PREVENTIVE MEASURES TO COMBAT ALCOHOLISM.

ACCN   001039

1213 AUTH   **MENDES, H. A.**

TITL   SINGLE FATHERHOOD.

SRCE   *SOCIAL WORK, 1976, 21(4), 308-312.*

INDX   FATHER-CHILD INTERACTION, FAMILY STRUCTURE, INTERPERSONAL ATTRACTION, PARENTAL INVOLVEMENT, MEXICAN AMERICAN, CROSS CULTURAL, SURVEY, CALIFORNIA, MALE, PSYCHOSOCIAL ADJUSTMENT, EMPIRICAL

ABST   RESULTS OF A COMPARATIVE STUDY OF THE PARENTAL EXPERIENCES OF 32 SINGLE FATHERS ARE SUMMARIZED. THE SUBJECTS ARE SINGLE PARENTS WHO WERE REFERRED BY TEACHERS, DOCTORS, SOCIAL WORKERS AND SELF-HELP GROUPS. DATA WERE COLLECTED BETWEEN JUNE 1974 AND MARCH 1975 IN SOUTHERN CALIFORNIA AND WERE OBTAINED THROUGH SEMISTRUCTURED INTERVIEWS HELD IN THE FATHERS' HOMES OR OFFICES PERTAINING TO (1) THE PROCESSES AND MOTIVATIONS THAT LED THEM TO BECOME SINGLE FATHERS AND (2) THE ONGOING ADJUSTMENTS EXPERIENCED AS SINGLE PARENTS. THE SUBJECTS, DIVERSE IN ETHNICITY, MARITAL STATUS AND SES, ARE DESCRIBED BY THESE CATEGORIES. THE MOST SALIENT PATTERNS OF THE FATHERS' PARENTAL EXPERIENCES AND THE ISSUE WHICH SERVED TO DIF-

FERENTIATE BETWEEN THE TWO SUBGROUPS OF THE SAMPLE WAS THE ISSUE OF CHOICE— WHETHER THE FATHER HAD ACTIVELY INITIATED BECOMING A SINGLE PARENT (SEEKER) OR HAD ONLY ACCEDED TO CIRCUMSTANCES OR SOMEONE ELSE'S WISHES (ASSENTER). INTERVIEW RESPONSES INDICATE THAT THIS ISSUE IS AN IMPORTANT FACTOR IN (1) THE FATHER-CHILD RELATIONSHIP, AND (2) THE ONGOING ADJUSTMENTS THAT THE SINGLE FATHER MAKES IN THAT NEW ROLE. THE IMPLICATIONS OF THIS ISSUE FOR THOSE WORKING WITH SINGLE FATHERS ARE DISCUSSED. 4 REFERENCES.

ACCN   001040

1214 AUTH   **MENDOZA-FRIEDMAN, M.**
TITL   SPANISH BILINGUAL STUDENTS AND INTELLIGENCE TESTING.
SRCE   *CHANGING EDUCATION, 1973, SPRING, 25-28.*
INDX   MEXICAN AMERICAN, BILINGUAL, INTELLIGENCE TESTING, ADOLESCENTS, ESSAY, BILINGUAL-BICULTURAL EDUCATION, EDUCATION, CHILDREN, BILINGUAL.-BICULTURAL PERSONNEL, PROGRAM EVALUATION, CULTURAL FACTORS, SPECIAL EDUCATION, REVIEW, CALIFORNIA, SOUTHWEST
ABST   THE USE OF STANDARDIZED INTELLIGENCE TESTING IN OUR EDUCATIONAL SYSTEM HAS HAD DETRIMENTAL CONSEQUENCES FOR SPANISH-SPEAKING CHILDREN. THESE TESTS HAVE CREATED THE MYTH THAT CHICANO CHILDREN ARE OF INFERIOR INTELLIGENCE AND RESULTED IN THEIR PLACEMENT IN CLASSES DESIGNED FOR MENTALLY RETARDED. THE PROPONENTS OF THE SO-CALLED MEASURES OF IQ HAVE FAILED TO CONSIDER THE DIFFERENCES BETWEEN THE ANGLO AND CHICANO CHILD, SUCH AS LANGUAGE AND THE EFFECTS OF POVERTY, AND HOW THESE FACTORS INFLUENCE TEST SCORES. ALTHOUGH BILINGUAL EDUCATION CAN REMEDY THE EXISTING INEQUALITIES WITHIN EDUCATIONAL SYSTEM, CAUTION MUST BE TAKEN CONCERNING THE DEVELOPMENT AND THE ASSESSMENT OF THE EFFECTIVENESS OF BILINGUAL PROGRAMS. FOR EXAMPLE, THE C-R FORM (CRITERION REFERENCE) TO ASSESS BILINGUAL PROGRAMS PROPOSED BY THE BAY AREA BILINGUAL EDUCATIONAL LEAGUE MAY RESULT IN POORLY FINANCED AND UNDERSTAFFED SCHOOLS. THE SUCCESS OF BILINGUAL EDUCATION DEPENDS LARGELY ON TRAINING BILINGUAL SPECIALISTS WHO WOULD BE QUALIFIED TO DEVELOP PROGRAMS AND PROCEDURES THAT WOULD REFLECT VALID ASSESSMENTS OF THE ACCOMPLISHMENTS OF BILINGUAL PROGRAMS.
ACCN   001042

1215 AUTH   **MERCADO, S. J., GUERRERO, R. D., & GARDENER, R. W.**
TITL   COGNITIVE CONTROL IN CHILDREN OF MEXICO AND THE UNITED STATES.
SRCE   *JOURNAL OF SOCIAL PSYCHOLOGY, 1963, 59(2), 199-208.*
INDX   CROSS CULTURAL, SEX COMPARISON, COGNI-

TIVE STYLE, CHILDREN, MEXICAN, PERSONALITY, EMPIRICAL
ABST   AN INTERCULTURAL INVESTIGATION OF CONCEPTUAL DIFFERENTIATION AND PREFERRED LEVELS OF ABSTRACTION IS REPORTED. THE OBJECT SORTING TEST WAS ADMINISTERED TO 29 MIDDLE-CLASS THIRD AND FOURTH GRADE MEXICAN CHILDREN AND TO 25 ANGLO AMERICAN CHILDREN OF THE SAME AGES AND/OR COMPARABLE SOCIOECONOMIC STATUS. THE SUBJECTS WERE REQUIRED TO DEFINE EACH GROUP CONTAINING TWO OR MORE OBJECTS, AND EACH DEFINITION WAS SCORED IN TERMS OF LEVEL OF ABSTRACTION. THE FINDINGS SHOW A GREATER DEGREE OF CONCEPTUAL DIFFERENTIAL FOR THE ANGLO CHILDREN. THAT IS, THEY FORMED A GREATER TOTAL NUMBER OF GROUPS. THE INTERPRETATION OF DIFFERENCES BETWEEN THE GROUPING BEHAVIOR OF THE TWO SAMPLES DEPENDS ON INTERPRETATION OF THE PHENOMENA OF LEAVING CERTAIN OBJECTS BY THEMSELVES. THE MEXICAN CHILDREN LEFT FEWER OBJECTS BY THEMSELVES, BUT THEY MAY HAVE BEEN SIMPLY SHOWING GREATER COMPLIANCE WITH THE INSTRUCTIONS WHICH IMPLIED THAT THE OBJECTS SHOULD BE GROUPED TOGETHER. THE ANGLO CHILDREN GAVE A SMALLER PERCENTAGE OF CONCRETE DEFINITIONS AND A MUCH LARGER PERCENTAGE OF ABSTRACT, CONCEPTUAL DEFINITIONS. THE GROUPS DID NOT DIFFER, HOWEVER, IN THE PERCENT OF FUNCTIONAL DEFINITIONS. THE MEXICAN BOYS PERFORMED AT SIGNIFICANTLY HIGHER MEAN LEVELS OF ABSTRACTION THAN DID THE MEXICAN GIRLS, BY GIVING A GREATER PERCENTAGE OF ABSTRACT, CONCEPTUAL DEFINITIONS, AND A SMALLER PERCENTAGE OF CONCRETE DEFINITIONS. NO SIGNIFICANT DIFFERENCES WERE FOUND BETWEEN ANGLO BOYS AND GIRLS. 7 REFERENCES.
ACCN   001043

1216 AUTH   **MERCER, J. R.**
TITL   IDENTIFYING THE GIFTED CHICANO CHILD.
SRCE   *IN J. L. MARTINEZ, JR. (ED.), CHICANO PSYCHOLOGY. NEW YORK: ACADEMIC PRESS, 1977, PP. 155-173.*
INDX   EDUCATIONAL ASSESSMENT, CHILDREN, ABILITY TESTING, CULTURAL FACTORS, EDUCATION, INTELLIGENCE TESTING, LEARNING, PERFORMANCE EXPECTATIONS, MEXICAN AMERICAN, INTELLIGENCE TESTING, ESSAY, REVIEW, CULTURE-FAIR TESTS, SCHOLASTIC ACHIEVEMENT, WISC
ABST   RELATIVELY FEW CHICANO CHILDREN ARE IDENTIFIED AS GIFTED BY THE PUBLIC SCHOOLS—A FACT WHICH SEVERELY LIMITS THE ACCESS OF SOME CHICANO CHILDREN TO EQUAL EDUCATIONAL OPPORTUNITIES. FOLLOWING A REVIEW OF THE PHILOSOPHICAL AND HISTORICAL BACKGROUND OF ASSESSMENT PRACTICES, BASED ON ANGLO-CONFORMITY MODELS, THIS PAPER PRESENTS AN ALTERNATIVE SYSTEM OF PLURALISTIC ASSESSMENT THAT MIGHT BE HELPFUL IN IDENTIFYING THE GIFTED CHICANO CHILD—THE

SYSTEM OF MULTICULTURAL PLURALISTIC ASSESSMENT (SOMPA). SOMPA IS DESIGNED TO ASSESS THE CURRENT LEVEL OF FUNCTIONING AND POTENTIAL OF ANGLO, CHICANO, AND BLACK CHILDREN ON THE BASIS OF THREE CONCEPTUAL MODELS: A MEDICAL MODEL, A SOCIAL SYSTEM MODEL, AND A PLURALISTIC MODEL. IDEALLY, AS IT SHOULD BE ADMINISTERED, THE SCHOOL PSYCHOLOGIST WOULD LOOK AT THE CHILD FIRST THROUGH A MEDICAL MODEL, SCREENING HIM OR HER FOR POSSIBLE PHYSICAL ANOMALIES WHICH MIGHT INTERFERE WITH OPTIMUM FUNCTIONING. THEN, USING A SOCIAL SYSTEM MODEL, THE PSYCHOLOGIST WOULD EXAMINE THE CHILD'S ROLE BEHAVIOR IN FAMILY, PEER GROUPS, COMMUNITY, AND EARNER/CONSUMER ROLES. FINALLY, VIA A PLURALISTIC MODEL, THE CHILD'S PERFORMANCE RELATIVE TO OTHERS FROM THE SAME SOCIOCULTURAL BACKGROUND ON THE WISC-R MEASURE OF SCHOOL FUNCTION WOULD BE EXAMINED, AND INFERENCES ABOUT THE CHILD'S ESTIMATED LEARNING POTENTIAL WOULD BE MADE. IT IS HOPED THAT THROUGH THIS PROCESS IT WILL BE POSSIBLE IN THE FUTURE TO IDENTIFY THE GIFTED CHICANO CHILD. 36 REFERENCES.

ACCN   002155

1217 AUTH   **MERCER, J. R.**
TITL   IMPRINTS OF CULTURE ON THE PERSONALITIES OF CHILDREN.
SRCE   *IN M. P. DOUGLASS (ED.), CLAREMONT READING CONFERENCE: THIRTY-FIRST YEARBOOK. CLAREMONT, CALIF.: CLAREMONT GRADUATE SCHOOL AND UNIVERSITY CENTER, 1967, PP. 55-62.*
INDX   SOCIALIZATION, PERSONALITY, COGNITIVE DEVELOPMENT, CULTURE, MEXICAN AMERICAN, CHILDREN, SES, CROSS CULTURAL, ACCULTURATION, RAVEN PROGRESSIVE MATRICES, PEABODY PICTURE-VOCABULARY TEST, SOCIAL STRUCTURE, ANXIETY, SURVEY, SELF CONCEPT, EMPLOYMENT, SPECIAL EDUCATION, ACHIEVEMENT TESTING, CALIFORNIA, SOUTHWEST, MENTAL RETARDATION, COMMUNITY
ABST   AN ANALYSIS OF THE INTERRELATIONSHIP BETWEEN SOCIALIZATION PRACTICES AND PERSONALITY VARIABLES OF ANGLO AMERICAN (AA), MEXICAN AMERICAN (MA), AND NEGRO (N) CHILDREN IN A COMMUNITY IS PRESENTED. INFORMATION WAS OBTAINED FROM INTERVIEWS WITH PARENTS, PEER RATINGS, TEACHER RATINGS, AND SCHOLASTIC RATINGS. SOCIOECONOMIC DIFFERENCES AMONG THE GROUPS INDICATE THAT MA FAMILIES ARE MORE DISADVANTAGED ECONOMICALLY, AND THEY HAVE LESS EDUCATIONAL PREPARATION. THE COMMUNITY STUDIED IS MARKED BY STRUCTURAL SEPARATION WHERE EACH SUBGROUP RESIDES IN THREE SEPARATE AREAS. PATTERNS OF INFORMAL INTIMATE ASSOCIATION SHOW EACH GROUP INTERACTING MAINLY WITH RELATIVES OR MEMBERS OF THE SAME SUBCULTURE. DIFFERENCES IN CULTURAL INTEGRATION OF THE GROUP APPEAR

IN THE MA FAMILIES. MA PARENTS ARE LESS LIKELY TO BE AWARE OF THE REALITY FACTORS GOVERNING THE RELATIONSHIPS BETWEEN EDUCATIONAL AND OCCUPATIONAL ACHIEVEMENT IN AMERICAN SOCIETY. OF THE PERSONS NOMINATED AS MENTALLY RETARDED, 52 PERCENT WERE AA, 33 PERCENT MA, AND 12 PERCENT N. COMPARED TO THE PROPORTION OF EACH OF THESE GROUPS IN THE COMMUNITY (84% AA, 9%, 6% N) THERE IS A REPRESENTATION OF ALMOST FOUR TIMES AS MANY MA'S AND TWICE AS MANY N'S CLASSIFIED AS MENTALLY RETARDED BY COMMUNITY AGENCIES. IN TERMS OF SCHOOL ACHIEVEMENT, THE MA AND N GROUPS WERE BEHIND THE EXPECTED GRADE LEVEL FOR THEIR CHRONOLOGICAL AGE. THE CHILDREN OF ALL GROUPS HAD A POSITIVE SELF-CONCEPT, ALTHOUGH THE MA CHILDREN SHOWED HIGHER SCHOOL ANXIETY THAN THE OTHER GROUPS IN TERMS OF EMOTIONAL ADJUSTMENT. 7 REFERENCES.

ACCN   001044

1218 AUTH   **MERCER, J. R.**
TITL   IQ: THE LETHAL LABEL.
SRCE   *PSYCHOLOGY TODAY, 1972, 6(4), PP. 44; 46-47; 95-96.*
INDX   INTELLIGENCE TESTING, MENTAL RETARDATION, MEXICAN AMERICAN, CROSS CULTURAL, STANFORD-BINET INTELLIGENCE TEST, WISC, TEST VALIDITY, SES, CULTURAL PLURALISM, REVIEW, SURVEY, RESEARCH METHODOLOGY, SPECIAL EDUCATION, SOUTHWEST, POLICY, CULTURE-FAIR TESTS, CALIFORNIA
ABST   THE INACCURACY OF THE IQ TEST AS THE PRIMARY CRITERION FOR CLASSIFICATION OF MENTAL RETARDATION AMONG MINORITY GROUP MEMBERS IS INVESTIGATED. THREE TESTS (THE STANFORD-BINET, THE KULHMAN-BINET, AND THE WECHSLER INTELLIGENCE SCALE FOR CHILDREN) AND AN ADAPTIVE BEHAVIOR SKILL MEASURE (E.G., TO SHOP AND TRAVEL ALONE; TO HOLD A JOB OR ACTIVITIES NOT APPROPRIATE FOR A 6-YEAR-OLD) WITH 28 AGE-GRADED SCALES WERE COMBINED TO ASSESS THE IQ OF SEPARATE SAMPLES EACH COMPOSED OF ANGLO, BLACK, AND CHICANO SUBJECTS. FINDINGS INDICATE ETHNIC GROUPS OF LOW SOCIOECONOMIC STATUS ARE THE MOST LIKELY TO BE PENALIZED BY THE IQ (SCORE BELOW 70) BUT NOT BY THE ADAPTIVE BEHAVIOR SKILL MEASURE. TO DEFINE PERSONS AS RETARDED BECAUSE THEY FAIL AN IQ TEST AT THE 70 LEVEL IS TO STIGMATIZE THOSE WHO ARE OTHERWISE COMPETENT TO FUNCTION NORMALLY. IQ TESTS THAT ARE NOW IN USE ARE CULTURE-SPECIFIC AND THEREFORE BIASED. SINCE IQ TESTS ARE ANGLOCENTRIC, THEY ONLY MEASURE THE EXTENT TO WHICH AN INDIVIDUAL'S BACKGROUND APPROXIMATES THE AVERAGE CULTURAL PATTERN OF AMERICAN SOCIETY. THE CHILDREN WHOSE FAMILIES WERE LEAST LIKE THE AVERAGE ANGLO FAMILY (E.G., A 5-ITEM SCALE RELATED ASPIRATIONS, NUMBER OF CHILDREN IN THE FAMILY, ETC.) HAD AN AVERAGE IQ OF 82.7, AND THOSE CHILDREN

WHOSE FAMILIES MATCHED THE ANGLO FAMILY HAD AN AVERAGE IQ OF 99.5. WHEN SOCIAL BACKGROUND WAS CONTROLLED THERE WERE NO DIFFERENCES IN INTELLIGENCE BETWEEN ANGLOS AND BLACKS, OR BETWEEN ANGLOS AND CHICANOS. A DIAGNOSTIC PROGRAM IS SUGGESTED WITH A PLURALISTIC ASSESSMENT THAT WOULD BASE ITS LABELS OF RETARDATION ON A SOCIOCULTURAL INDEX, AN ADAPTIVE BEHAVIOR SCALE, AND AN ETHNIC IQ NORM. 12 REFERENCES.

ACCN 001045

1219 AUTH **MERCER, J. R.**
TITL LABELING THE MENTALLY RETARDED: CLINICAL AND SOCIAL SYSTEM PERSPECTIVES ON MENTAL RETARDATION.
SRCE *BERKELEY: UNIVERSITY OF CALIFORNIA PRESS, 1973.*
INDX ABILITY TESTING, MENTAL RETARDATION, CASE STUDY, ADULTS, EDUCATION, CULTURE-FAIR TESTS, FAMILY ROLES, INTELLIGENCE, BILINGUALISM, SURVEY, SEX COMPARISON, STANFORD-BINET INTELLIGENCE TEST, WISC, WAIS, SES, WECHSLER MENTAL ABILITY SCALE, CALIFORNIA, SOUTHWEST, BOOK, POLICY, DISCRIMINATION, PREJUDICE, ATTITUDES, IMPAIRMENT, EMPIRICAL, CULTURAL PLURALISM
ABST THIS VOLUME CHALLENGES THE ASSUMPTIONS UNDERLYING TRADITIONAL DIAGNOSES OF 'NORMALITY' AND CONTENDS THAT THE PRESENT SYSTEM OFTEN UNFAIRLY PLACES MANY COMPETENT PEOPLE (PARTICULARLY THE POOR AND ETHNIC MINORITIES) IN THE ROLE OF RETARDATES. BASED ON AN 8-YEAR STUDY ANALYZING THE LABELING PROCESS IN EIGHT COMMUNITY AGENCIES IN A CALIFORNIA CITY (ESPECIALLY THE PUBLIC SCHOOL SYSTEM), IT WAS FOUND THAT ASSESSMENTS OF INDIVIDUALS' MENTAL ABILITY WAS FOUNDED SOLEY ON IQ TEST SCORES. CONCOMITANTLY, THERE WAS A GROSSLY DISPROPORTIONATE NUMBER OF BLACKS AND MEXICAN AMERICANS LABELED AS MENTALLY DEFICIENT. MOREOVER, FOLLOW-THROUGH PROCEDURES ALSO WORKED TO THE DISADVANTAGE OF THESE GROUPS. IN ONE SETTING, FOR EXAMPLE, OF THE 134 ELEMENTARY SCHOOL CHILDREN WHO HAD IQ TEST SCORES OF 79 OR BELOW, ONLY 64% WERE RECOMMENDED FOR PLACEMENT IN SPECIAL EDUCATION CLASSES—AND THESE TENDED TO BE MEXICAN AMERICANS FROM THE LOWEST SOCIOECONOMIC LEVELS. IN ORDER TO COUNTERACT THE EFFECTS OF SUCH MISLABELING, THE FOLLOWING RECOMMENDATIONS ARE OFFERED: (1) LOWER THE CUT-OFF POINT USED BY SCHOOLS IN DETERMINING RETARDATION; (2) USE THE TWO-DIMENSIONAL DEFINITION OF RETARDATION PROPOSED BY THE AMERICAN ASSOCIATION OF MENTAL DEFINCIENCY; AND (3) USE A PLURALISTIC APPROACH WHICH MEASURES BOTH IQ AND ADAPTIVE BEHAVIOR WITHIN THE TESTED PERSON'S SOCIOCULTURAL GROUP. AS AN ILLUSTRATION, AN EXPERIMENTAL APPLICATION OF PLURALISTIC, SOCIOCULTURALLY-SENSITIVE PROCEDURES IN A CALIFORNIA SCHOOL SET-

TING IS DESCRIBED. IT IS CONCLUDED THAT WITH THE LARGER FUND OF INFORMATION PROVIDED BY SUCH PROCEDURES, A MORE ACCURATE ASSESSMENT WILL BE POSSIBLE OF WHO IS NORMAL AND WHO IS NOT. 126 REFERENCES.

ACCN 001822

1220 AUTH **MERCER, J. R.**
TITL PLURALISTIC DIAGNOSIS IN THE EVALUATION OF BLACK AND CHICANO CHILDREN: A PROCEDURE FOR TAKING SOCIOCULTURAL VARIABLES INTO ACCOUNT IN CLINICAL ASSESSMENT.
SRCE *IN C. HERNANDEZ, M. J. HAUG & N. N. WAGNER (EDS.), CHICANOS: SOCIAL AND PSYCHOLOGICAL PERSPECTIVES. SAINT LOUIS: C. V. MOSBY COMPANY, 1976, PP. 183-195.*
INDX MENTAL RETARDATION, INTELLIGENCE TESTING, MEXICAN AMERICAN, CROSS CULTURAL, EMPIRICAL, SURVEY, SES, CULTURAL FACTORS, WISC, CHILDREN, SPECIAL EDUCATION, INTELLIGENCE, CALIFORNIA, SOUTHWEST
ABST THE PRESENT INADEQUACIES OF INTELLIGENCE ASSESSMENT HAVE LED TO A GREATER PROPORTION OF NON-ANGLO CHILDREN BEING LABELED MENTALLY RETARDED. THE PLURALISTIC DIAGNOTIC MODEL CONSISTING OF PROCEDURES THAT TAKE INTO ACCOUNT SOCIOCULTURAL FACTORS INFLUENCING INTELLIGENCE TEST SCORES IS DESCRIBED. THE DEVELOPMENT OF THE PLURALISTIC MODEL EVOLVED FROM A STUDY CONDUCTED IN RIVERSIDE, CALIFORNIA, THAT FOCUSED ON THE LABELING PROCESS AND CHARACTERISTICS OF SCHOOL CHILDREN WHO HAD BEEN LABELED MENTALLY RETARDED. THREE GENERAL FINDINGS OF THE RIVERSIDE DATA ARE DISCUSSED: (1) CUTOFF LEVEL FOR SUBNORMALITY SHOULD BE SET AT 3%; (2) BOTH IQ AND ADAPTIVE BEHAVIOR SHOULD BE EVALUATED IN MAKING DIAGNOSES; AND (3) SOCIOCULTURAL FACTORS SHOULD BE SYSTEMATICALLY TAKEN INTO ACCOUNT IN INTERPRETING CLINICAL SCORES. PLURALISTIC ASSESSMENT IS BASED ON FOUR TYPES OF INFORMATION: (1) A SOCIOCULTURAL MODALITY INDEX; (2) A MEASURE OF ADAPTIVE BEHAVIOR WITHIN A SOCIOCULTURAL NORMATIVE FRAMEWORK; (3) THE MEASURE OF ACADEMIC READINESS—IQ TEST; AND (4) THE IQ TEST INTERPRETED WITHIN STANDARD NORMS TO DETERMINE PLACEMENT IN A REGULAR OR SPECIAL ACADEMIC SCHOOL PROGRAM. IT IS SUGGESTED THAT A MORE SENSITIVE SYSTEM FOR IDENTIFYING CHILDREN NEEDING SPECIFIC TYPES OF ASSISTANCE BE INSTITUTED—THEREBY PROVIDING CHILDREN SPECIAL EDUCATION PROGRAMS THAT ALLOW THEM TO MAXIMIZE THEIR OWN POTENTIAL. 17 REFERENCES.

ACCN 001046

1221 AUTH **MERZ, W. R.**
TITL A FACTOR ANALYSIS OF THE GOODENOUGH-HARRIS DRAWING TEST ACROSS FOUR ETHNIC GROUPS (DOCTORAL DISSERTATION, UNIVERSITY OF NEW MEXICO, 1970).

SRCE *DISSERTATION ABSTRACTS, 1970, 31(4), 1647A. (UNIVERSITY MICROFILMS NO. 70-19,714.)*

INDX GOODENOUGH DRAW-A-MAN TEST, EMPIRICAL, INTELLIGENCE TESTING, CROSS CULTURAL, CHILDREN, SEX COMPARISON, INDIGENOUS POPULATIONS, RESEARCH METHODOLOGY, CALIFORNIA ACHIEVEMENT TESTS, SOUTHWEST, ARIZONA, TEXAS, NEW MEXICO, OKLAHOMA, MIDWEST

ABST A STUDY WAS CONDUCTED TO EXAMINE THE FACTOR STRUCTURE OF THE GOODENOUGH-HARRIS DRAWING TEST (DAP) ITEM RESPONSES ACROSS FOUR ETHNIC GROUPS. THE MAN SCALE OF THE TEST WAS USED; 1338 ANGLO, BLACK, MEXICAN AMERICAN, AND YUCCA INDIAN FIRST GRADE BOYS AND GIRLS WERE INCLUDED. THE CHILDREN WERE 6, 7, AND 8 YEARS-OLD. CALIFORNIA ACHIEVEMENT TEST (CAT) PERFORMANCE WAS INCLUDED IN THE INVESTIGATION. AGE AND SEX VARIABLES WERE CORRELATED WITH GOODENOUGH-HARRIS ITEM RESPONSES AND CAT SUBSCORES. CORRELATION MATRICES WERE REDUCED BY PRINCIPAL COMPONENTS ANALYSIS WITH ORTHOGONAL ROTATION TO SIMPLE STRUCTURE. SIMILAR FACTOR STRUCTURES WERE OBTAINED ACROSS THE FOUR ETHNIC GROUPS. FOUR TYPES OF FACTORS WERE OBTAINED FOR EACH GROUP: ONE RELATING TO CAT SUBSCORES, SEVERAL RELATING TO DAP ITEM RESPONSES, SOME RELATING TO AGE, AND SOME RELATING TO SEX. CAT SUBTESTS AND DAP ITEMS DID NOT ASSOCIATE; SEX AND AGE DID NOT ASSOCIATE WITH EACH OTHER NOR WITH CAT SUBTESTS AND DAP ITEMS. SOME OF THE COMMON FACTORS IDENTIFIED WERE ACHIEVEMENT, EYE DETAIL, HAIR, FACIAL FEATURES, LIMBS, PERSPECTIVE, PROPORTION, COORDINATION, AGE, AND SEX. 85 REFERENCES. (AUTHOR ABSTRACT)

ACCN 001047

1222 AUTH **MESTAS, L.**

TITL THE BILINGUAL/BICULTURAL EMOTIONALLY DISTURBED CHILD.

SRCE *SAN FERNANDO, CALIFORNIA: MONTAL EDUCATIONAL ASSOCIATES, 1972.*

INDX ITPA, SPECIAL EDUCATION, LEARNING DISABILITIES, PSYCHOPATHOLOGY, WISC, REVIEW, INSTRUCTIONAL TECHNIQUES, CURRICULUM, CHILDREN, CROSS CULTURAL, LEGISLATION, DEMOGRAPHIC, MEXICAN AMERICAN, PROGRAM EVALUATION, POLICY, SPECIAL EDUCATION, BILINGUAL-BICULTURAL EDUCATION, IMPAIRMENT

ABST THE DEVELOPMENT OF SPECIAL PROGRAMS IN PRIVATE AND PUBLIC SCHOOLS TO MEET THE NEEDS OF EMOTIONALLY DISTURBED CHILDREN WAS STUDIED. FINDINGS INDICATE THAT FEW SCHOOLS HAVE CONFRONTED THE ISSUE OF THE BILINGUAL/BICULTURAL (B/B) EMOTIONALLY DISTURBED CHILD UNLESS FEDERAL MONEY WAS AVAILABLE TO ASSIST THE SCHOOLS. THE NOTION THAT CURRICULUM GUIDES FOR EMOTIONALLY DISTURBED CHILDREN WHICH CONTAIN DETAILED INSTRUCTIONAL PLANNING, DIAGNOSTIC PLANNING, AND TESTING THAT CAN BE ADAPTED-

FOR THE (B/B) LOW-INCOME CHILD IS DISPUTED. IN A REVIEW OF EDUCATIONAL CURRICULUM GUIDELINES USED IN PUBLIC SCHOOLS, THE RESULTS SHOW MANY SCHOOLS MERELY UTILIZING THE STANDARD SPECIAL EDUCATION GUIDELINES WITH THE WORDS "BILINGUAL/BICULTURAL EMOTIONALLY DISTURBED" ADDED. THE WECHSLER INTELLIGENCE SCALE FOR CHILDREN, THE ILLINOIS TEST OF PSYCHOLINGUISTIC ABILITIES, THE FROSTY TEST OF VISUAL PERCEPTION, AND THE WEPMAN AUDITORY DISCRIMINATION TEST ARE TESTS NOT DEVELOPED FOR THE B/B CHILD AND ARE POTENTIALLY DAMAGING FOR THE B/B CHILD. RECOMMENDATIONS DESIGNED TO IMPROVE THE NEEDS OF EMOTIONALLY DISTURBED B/B STUDENTS ARE LISTED. 16 REFERENCES.

ACCN 001048

1223 AUTH **METROPOLITAN LATIN COMMITTEE.**

TITL REPORT ON THE GREATER WASHINGTON HEALTH CONFERENCE FOR THE SPANISH SPEAKING PEOPLE, DECEMBER 11, 1971.

SRCE *WASHINGTON, D.C.: METROPOLITAN LATIN COMMITTEE, 1971. (AVAILABLE FROM RON DIBENEDETTO, METROPOLITAN LATIN COMMITTEE, 3118 SIXTEENTH ST., N.W., WASHINGTON, D.C., 20010.)*

INDX ALCOHOLISM, COMMUNITY, NUTRITION, HEALTH, COMMUNITY INVOLVEMENT, DRUG ABUSE, SPANISH SURNAMED, SOCIAL SERVICES, PROCEEDINGS, HEALTH, MENTAL HEALTH, EAST, PROGRAM EVALUATION, HEALTH DELIVERY SYSTEMS, WASHINGTON D.C.

ABST THE FIRST GREATER WASHINGTON HEALTH CONFERENCE, HELD IN THE DISTRICT OF COLUMBIA (D.C.), WAS ORGANIZED BECAUSE OF AN HISPANIC COMMITTEE'S FINDINGS THAT HEALTH AND SOCIAL SERVICES AVAILABLE TO THE PEOPLE OF THE SPANISH-SPEAKING (SS) COMMUNITY IN D.C. WERE INADEQUATE OR TOTALLY LACKING. CONFERENCE OBJECTIVES WERE TO INVESTIGATE RESOURCES, TO FIND WAYS OF IMPROVING HEALTH SERVICES OF THE SS POPULATION OF D.C., TO INVOLVE SS CONSUMERS IN FORMULATING PLANS FOR NEW PROGRAMS AND WAYS OF IMPROVING EXISTING PROGRAMS, AND TO IDENTIFY NEEDED RESOURCES TO DEVELOP USEFUL HEALTH PROGRAMS FROM THE SS CONSUMER'S PERSPECTIVE. THE WORKSHOP COVERED: (1) NARCOTICS AND ALCOHOLISM, (2) GENERAL MEDICAL, SURGICAL AND DENTAL CARE, (3) MATERNAL AND CHILD CARE, (4) MENTAL HEALTH, (5) NUTRITION AND HEALTH EDUCATION, (6) TREATMENT AND PREVENTION OF COMMUNICABLE DISEASES, AND (7) COMMUNITY ORGANIZATION. OVERALL RECOMMENDATIONS ARE FOR MORE SS PERSONNEL, ADDITIONAL FUNDING OF SERVICE FACILITIES, THE ELICITING OF THE SS COMMUNITY'S SUPPORT AND PARTICIPATION, INCREASED EDUCATION AND CULTURAL SENSITIVITY, PROGRAM PLANNING AND PUBLICITY. IT IS BELIEVED THAT THE SS COMMUNITY SHOULD ASSESS ITS OWN PRESSING HEALTH NEEDS AND ADDRESS RECOMMENDATIONS TO THE MAYOR AND

OTHER REPRESENTATIVES FOR THEIR EN-DORSEMENT.

ACCN   001049

1224 AUTH   **MEYER, G. G.**
TITL   THE PROFESSIONAL IN THE CHICANO COM-MUNITY.
SRCE   *PSYCHIATRIC ANNALS, 1977, 7(12), 9-19.*
INDX   BILINGUAL-BICULTURAL PERSONNEL, COM-MUNITY INVOLVEMENT, CULTURAL FACTORS, MENTAL HEALTH, MENTAL HEALTH PROFES-SION, PARAPROFESSIONALS, PSYCHOTHERA-PISTS, PSYCHOTHERAPY OUTCOME, SOUTH-WEST, MEXICAN AMERICAN, PSYCHOTHERAPY
ABST   FROM HIS EXPERIENCE AS DIRECTOR OF A SAN ANTONIO MENTAL HEALTH CENTER THE AUTHOR MAKES THE FOLLOWING OBSERVA-TIONS AND SUGGESTIONS FOR THE ANGLO PROFESSIONAL WORKING IN THE CHICANO COMMUNITY. THE CLINICIAN PRACTICING IN A PREDOMINATELY MEXICAN AMERICAN LO-CALITY IS LIKELY TO CONFRONT PROBLEMS ARISING FROM THE INTERFACE BETWEEN VARIOUS CONTRACTING AGENCIES AND COM-MUNITY, DISTRICT, STATE, AND FEDERAL AGEN-CIES. IF THE PATIENT'S WELFARE IS TO BE FOREMOST, THE PRACTITIONER WILL DIS-COVER THAT CLINICAL EXPERTISE IS USEFUL IN THE POLITICAL ARENA AS WELL, AND THAT AN AWARENESS OF COMMUNITY DYNAMICS IS CRUCIAL FOR DELIVERY OF SERVICES TO THAT COMMUNITY. MOREOVER, SKILLS IN GROUP AS WELL AS IN FAMILY AND INDIVIDUAL DYNAMIC PROCESSES WILL BE HELPFUL. CLINICAL KNOWLEDGE OF SUCH INGRAINED CULTURAL FACTORS AS FEAR OF INSTITUTIONS—SO CHARACTERISTIC OF THE CHICANO—AND HIS RELUCTANCE TO SEPARATE HIMSELF FROM THE FAMILY ARE TWO FACTORS THAT CAN BE UTILIZED TO HELP THE MEXICAN AMERICAN MENTAL HEALTH PATIENT WITHIN THE CON-TEXT OF HIS OWN NEIGHBORHOOD. IF THE CLINICIAN IS SUCCESSFUL IN THIS AREA, MANY PSYCHOTIC PATIENTS WHO WOULD CUSTOM-ARILY REQUIRE HOSPITALIZATION WILL BE ABLE TO BE TREATED SUCCESSFULLY IN THE COM-MUNITY. IN GENERAL, THE CLINICIAN WHO BRINGS TO THE CHICANO COMMUNITY AN AC-TIVE INTEREST IN THAT CHANGING COMMU-NITY HELPS HIMSELF, HIS CO-WORKERS, AND HIS PATIENTS. 5 REFERENCES.
ACCN   002156

1225 AUTH   **MEYER, G. G., QUESADA, G. M., MARTIN, H. W., & MONTOYA, G. R.**
TITL   CURANDEROS AND PSYCHIATRISTS AS PROFESSIONAL HEALERS.
SRCE   *PAPER PRESENTED AT THE FIFTH WORLD CON-GRESS OF PSYCHIATRY, MEXICO CITY, 1971.*
INDX   CURANDERISMO, FOLK MEDICINE, MENTAL HEALTH PROFESSION, PSYCHOTHERAPY, CUL-TURAL FACTORS, ESSAY, POLICY, HEALTH DE-LIVERY SYSTEMS
ABST   ASSUMING THE EXISTENCE OF A PROFESSION-ALIZATION CONTINUUM, THIS ARTICLE ANA-LYZES HOW BOTH CURANDEROS AND PSY-CHIATRISTS FIT VARIOUS SELECTED SOCIOLOGICAL CHARACTERISTICS OF A

PROFESSION. ALTHOUGH BOTH PROFESSION-ALS DELIVER SERVICES AND HAVE TEACHABLE TECHNIQUES, CURANDEROS ARE SEEN AS HAVING MORE ASCRIBED AUTHORITY, RELA-TIVELY FEW ETHICAL PROBLEMS, AND FEWER RULES FOR THE CONTROL AND REGULATION OF THEIR PRACTICE. ALSO, PATIENTS COME TO THE CURANDERO EXPECTING TO BE TOLD WHAT THE PROBLEM IS, WHILE THE PSYCHIA-TRIST EXPECTS THE PATIENT TO HELP DE-VELOP A CURE. FACTORS WHICH HINDER DE-VELOPING COLLABORATION BETWEEN CURANDEROS AND PSYCHIATRISTS ARE THE DECREASE IN ABSOLUTE NUMBERS OF THE FORMER, INCREASING EDUCATION, URBANI-ZATION AND SOPHISTICATION OF THE MEXI-CAN AMERICAN POPULATION, AND GENERAL MISTRUST DUE TO SUPPRESSION OF CURAN-DERISMO. IT IS SUGGESTED THAT CURANDE-ROS BECOME ASSOCIATES OF PSYCHIATRISTS IN ORDER FOR AN AWARENESS OF FOLK BE-LIEFS AND RECOGNITION OF THE SUPPORTIVE AND INTEGRATIVE FUNCTION FOR THE PATIENT TO BE OBTAINED. 37 REFERENCES.
ACCN   001050

1226 AUTH   **MEYER, N. G.**
TITL   AGE, SEX, COLOR VARIATIONS IN THE DIAG-NOSTIC DISTRIBUTION OF ADMISSIONS TO IN-PATIENT SERVICES OF STATE AND COUNTY MENTAL HEALTH HOSPITALS, UNITED STATES, 1972 (DHEW PUBLICATION NO. ADM 75-158).
SRCE   *WASHINGTON, D.C.: NATIONAL INSTITUTE OF MENTAL HEALTH, DEPARTMENT OF HEALTH, EDUCATION AND WELFARE, 1974.*
INDX   SPANISH SURNAMED, ADULTS, CROSS CUL-TURAL, EMPIRICAL, DEMOGRAPHIC, ALCO-HOLISM, DRUG ABUSE, DRUG ADDICTION, SCHIZOPHRENIA, PSYCHOPATHOLOGY, SEX COMPARISON, PERSONALITY ASSESSMENT, ADOLESCENTS, CHILDREN, SYMPTOMA-TOLOGY, DEPRESSION, NEUROSIS, PSYCHOSIS
ABST   THE DIAGNOSTIC DISTRIBUTION OF THE 403,-924 ADMISSIONS TO THE INPATIENT SERVICES OF STATE AND COUNTY MENTAL HOSPITALS FOR 1972 IS PRESENTED. SPANISH AMERICANS CONSTITUTED 12,269 OF THE REPORTED TO-TAL. OVER HALF OF THE SPANISH AMERICANS WERE DIAGNOSED AS HAVING DRUG DISOR-DERS, ALCOHOLIC DISORDERS, OR SCHIZO-PHRENIA. THE AGE ADJUSTED ADMISSIONS RATE FOR DRUG DISORDERS (PER 100,000 POPULATION) FOR SPANISH AMERICAN (22.1) AND NONWHITE (19.4) WAS OVER TWICE THAT FOR "OTHER WHITES" (7.5). AMONG THE SPAN-ISH AMERICAN ADMISSIONS, 17 PERCENT WERE DIAGNOSED WITH DRUG DISORDERS, AS OP-POSED TO 6 PERCENT OF THE NONWHITE AND 4.2 PERCENT OF THE "OTHER WHITE." THE AGE ADJUSTED ADMISSION RATE FOR ALCOHOL DISORDERS AMONG SPANISH AMERICANS WAS ABOUT HALF THAT OF THE "OTHER WHITE" AND ABOUT A THIRD THAT OF THE NONWHITE RATE. THE AGE ADJUSTED NONWHITE RATE OF ALCOHOL ADMISSIONS, 77.2, EXCEEDED BY FAR THAT AMONG SPANISH AMERICANS (22.4) AND OTHER WHITES (48.9). THE AGE AD-JUSTED ADMISSION RATE FOR SCHIZOPHRE-

NIA AMONG NONWHITES (126.2) WAS OVER THREE TIMES THE CORRESPONDING RATE FOR SPANISH AMERICANS (41.1) AND MORE THAN TWO AND ONE-HALF TIMES THE "OTHER WHITE" RATE (49.1). 1 REFERENCE. (AUTHOR SUMMARY MODIFIED)

ACCN   001051

1227 AUTH   **MILLER, A. R., & STEWARD, R. A.**
TITL   PERCEPTION OF FEMALE PHYSIQUES.
SRCE   *PERCEPTUAL AND MOTOR SKILLS, 1968, 27(3), 721-722.*
INDX   MALE, STEREOTYPES, SEX ROLES, MEXICAN AMERICAN, ADOLESCENTS, FEMALE, ATTITUDES, EMPIRICAL, CALIFORNIA, SOUTHWEST
ABST   A STUDY OF STEREOTYPES OF FEMALE PHYSIQUES IS PRESENTED. THE SUBJECTS WERE 14 MEXICAN AMERICAN MALES WHOSE AGES RANGED FROM 13 TO 19 YEARS. SIX 3-INCH BY 4-INCH REPRODUCTIONS OF SOMATOTYPES, TWO ENDOMORPHIC, TWO ECTOMORPHIC, AND TWO MESOMORPHIC, WERE SELECTED. THE CONCEPTS USED TO JUDGE THE PICTURES WERE LAZY, MOTHER, INTELLIGENT, HOUSEWIFE, ALCOHOLIC, LIKED BEST, AND PROSTITUTE. KENDALLS' COEFFICIENT OF CONCORDANCE WAS USED TO TEST THE AGREEMENT AMONG SUBJECTS' RANKINGS. DATA INDICATE THAT OF SEVEN CONCEPTS TESTED, SIX ARE STATISTICALLY SIGNIFICANT, DEMONSTRATING THAT THE SAME CRITERIA ARE USED IN RANKING THE PICTURES BY THE MAJORITY OF 14 SUBJECTS. SINCE THE SAMPLE IS HOMOGENEOUS AND SMALL, THE AUTHORS STATE THAT FURTHER WORK IS NEEDED TO VERIFY THESE FINDINGS. 7 REFERENCES.

ACCN   001052

1228 AUTH   **MILLER, D. E., HIMELSON, A. N., & GEIS, G.**
TITL   COMMUNITY'S RESPONSE TO SUBSTANCE ABUSE: THE EAST LOS ANGELES HALFWAY HOUSE FOR FELON ADDICTS.
SRCE   *INTERNATIONAL JOURNAL OF THE ADDICTIONS, 1967, 2(2), 305-311.*
INDX   DRUG ADDICTION, REHABILITATION, THERAPEUTIC COMMUNITY, CORRECTIONS, CROSS CULTURAL, DRUG ABUSE, MALE, CRIMINOLOGY, EMPIRICAL, MEXICAN AMERICAN, SOUTHWEST, CALIFORNIA
ABST   MALE PAROLEES WHO HAD A HISTORY OF NARCOTIC USAGE WERE DIVIDED INTO TWO GROUPS, A CONTROL GROUP AND AN EXPERIMENTAL GROUP, WHICH WERE HOUSED IN THE EAST LOS ANGELES HALFWAY HOUSE. THE MAJORITY OF THE SUBJECTS WERE MEXICAN AMERICAN—116 WERE IN THE EXPERIMENTAL GROUP, 109 IN THE CONTROL GROUP. FOLLOWUP STUDIES WERE DONE. A SIMILAR INCIDENCE OF FURTHER CRIMINAL ACTIVITY WAS REPORTED IN BOTH GROUPS. NO ASSOCIATION WAS FOUND UPON EXAMINATION OF THE SOCIOCULTURAL VARIABLES. OF THE 63 RELEASED FROM THE HALFWAY HOUSE, 44% SHOWED NO EVIDENCE OF DRUG USE OF MAJOR DIFFICULTY AFTER A 1-YEAR PERIOD. THESE FINDINGS SHOULD, HOWEVER, BE INTERPRETED WITH RESERVATIONS. THE APPARENT LACK OF SUCCESS OF THE HALFWAY HOUSE PROJECT CREATES DOUBTS ABOUT THE EFFECTIVENESS OF THE THERAPEUTIC COMMUNITY CONCEPT IN TREATING FELON ADDICTS. THE MAJOR FAILURE WAS THE INABILITY TO ACHIEVE THE PROPER ATMOSPHERE. 9 REFERENCES.

ACCN   001053

1229 AUTH   **MILLER, M. V.**
TITL   CHICANO COMMUNITY CONTROL IN SOUTH TEXAS: PROBLEMS AND PROSPECTS.
SRCE   *JOURNAL OF ETHNIC STUDIES, 1975, 3(3), 70-89.*
INDX   ATTITUDES, CROSS CULTURAL, CULTURAL FACTORS, FARM LABORERS, LEADERSHIP, MEXICAN, MEXICAN AMERICAN, POLITICAL POWER, POVERTY, PREJUDICE, RURAL, SOCIAL MOBILITY, SPANISH SURNAMED, STEREOTYPES, POLITICS
ABST   POLITICAL PROBLEMS AND PROSPECTS FOR CHICANOS IN SOUTH TEXAS ARE ASSESSED. THE FOCUS IS ON THE PROBLEM OF CHICANO COMMUNITY CONTROL IN TRADITIONALLY ANGLO-DOMINATED AREAS WHERE IMPEDIMENTS CAN BE TRACED TO: (1) THE "PATRON" SYSTEM, WHICH BREEDS ECONOMIC DEPENDENCY AS WELL AS VULNERABILITY TO REPRISALS IN TERMS OF LESS FAVORABLE WORKING CONDITIONS, DEMOTIONS, WAGE REDUCTIONS, OR FIRINGS; AND (2) DISCRIMINATORY ELECTION PRACTICES WHICH WORK AGAINST LOW-CLASS PARTICIPATION IN LOCAL GOVERNMENT. OTHER FACTORS MILITATING AGAINST THE EFFECTIVE FORMATION OF CHICANO POLITICAL ORGANIZATIONS AT THE LOCAL LEVEL ARE EXAMINED, BASED ON RELEVANT SOCIAL SCIENCE LITERATURE AND RESEARCH IN CRYSTAL CITY AND OTHER SOUTH TEXAS CITIES. TYPES OF COMMUNITIES IN SOUTH TEXAS IN WHICH CHICANO POLITICAL ACTIVITY MAY SUCCEED ARE EVALUATED. 20 REFERENCES. (NCMHI ABSTRACT MODIFIED)

ACCN   002157

1230 AUTH   **MILLER, M. V.**
TITL   MEXICAN AMERICANS, CHICANOS, AND OTHERS: ETHNIC SELF-IDENTIFICATION AND SELECTED SOCIAL ATTRIBUTES OF RURAL TEXAS YOUTH.
SRCE   *RURAL SOCIOLOGY, 1976, 41(2), 234-247.*
INDX   ADOLESCENTS, BILINGUAL, EMPIRICAL, ENVIRONMENTAL FACTORS, ETHNIC IDENTITY, FARM LABORERS, LABOR FORCE, MEXICAN AMERICAN, POLITICS, SES, SELF CONCEPT, RURAL, TEXAS, SOUTHWEST
ABST   FOLLOWING THE THESIS THAT VARIATIONS IN ETHNIC IDENTIFICATION REFLECT SOCIAL DIFFERENTIATION WITHIN THE MEXICAN AMERICAN POPULATION, THIS PAPER SEEKS TO DELINEATE PRIMARY TERMS FOR ETHNIC SELF-IDENTIFICATION AMONG YOUTHS RESIDING IN A RELATIVELY HOMOGENEOUS AREA OF SOUTH TEXAS. DATA WERE COLLECTED FROM A QUESTIONNAIRE GIVEN TO 379 MEXICAN AMERICAN HIGH SCHOOL SOPHOMORES RESIDING IN THE BORDER REGION OF SOUTH TEXAS, AN AREA WITH A HIGH PERCENTAGE

OF MEXICAN AMERICANS AND—ATYPICAL OF MOST SUCH TOWNS—WITH A LONG TRADITION OF MEXICAN AMERICAN POLITICAL CONTROL. ANALYSIS REVEALED THAT ETHNIC SELF-IDENTIFICATION TENDS TO BE VARIED EVEN AMONG MEXICAN AMERICAN YOUTHS WITHIN A LIMITED GEOGRAPHICAL AREA. MOST PREDOMINANT WAS THE REFERENT "MEXICAN AMERICAN," WHICH WAS CHOSEN BY 50% OF THE RESPONDENTS. THE SECOND MOST FAVORED TERM WAS "CHICANO," CHOSEN BY 25% OF THE ADOLESCENTS. A SIGNIFICANT MINORITY, HOWEVER, PREFERRED LABELS DEVOID OF REFERENCE TO ETHNICITY. LABELING VARIATION WAS FOUND TO BE RELATED TO SUCH SPECIFIC VARIABLES AS RESIDENCE, SEX, SOCIOECONOMIC STATUS, MIGRANT FARM WORK EXPERIENCE, AND LANGUAGE USE PREDOMINANCE. A NECESSARY COURSE FOR FUTURE RESEARCH WOULD ENTAIL INVESTIGATIONS OF THE EXACT MEANINGS AND USES OF THESE LABELS. 26 REFERENCES.

ACCN   002158

1231 AUTH   **MILLER, M. V.**
TITL   VARIATIONS IN MEXICAN AMERICAN FAMILY LIFE: A REVIEW AND SYNTHESIS (REPORT NO. TAES-NC-128).
SRCE   *WASHINGTON D.C.: COOPERATIVE STATE RESEARCH SERVICE, DEPARTMENT OF AGRICULTURE, 1975. (ERIC DOCUMENT REPRODUCTION SERVICE NO. ED 111 536)*
INDX   MEXICAN AMERICAN, FAMILY ROLES, FAMILY STRUCTURE, REVIEW, URBAN, MARRIAGE, FICTIVE KINSHIP, SEX ROLES, CULTURAL CHANGE, CULTURAL FACTORS, SOCIAL MOBILITY, SOUTHWEST, MIDWEST
ABST   A REVIEW OF THE PUBLISHED EMPIRICAL LITERATURE ON FAMILIES IN THE SEVERAL AREAS OF CONCENTRATED MEXICAN AMERICAN SETTLEMENT (PRIMARILY CALIFORNIA, ARIZONA, COLORADO, NEW MEXICO, TEXAS, AND VARIOUS CITIES IN THE MIDWEST) IS PRESENTED TO PROVIDE A FRAME OF REFERENCE ON THE SOCIOLOGY OF MEXICAN AMERICAN FAMILIES. VARIATIONS IN FAMILY BEHAVIOR APPEAR TO BE LINKED TO SUCH FACTORS AS SOCIOECONOMIC STATUS, NATIVITY, AGE AND GENERATION, SPECIFIC PLACE OF RESIDENCE, AND LANGUAGE USE PATTERNS. STUDIES DEALING WITH THE FOLLOWING TOPICS ARE CITED: (1) THE EXTENDED FAMILY; (2) FAMILY ROLES; (3) DATING AND COURTSHIP; (4) RITUAL KINSHIP RELATIONS; AND (5) INTERMARRIAGE. THE PAPER CONCLUDES WITH SOME GENERAL COMMENTS ON FAMILY DISORGANIZATION AND FAMILY PERSISTENCE. 60 REFERENCES. (RIE ABSTRACT MODIFIED)
ACCN   001054

1232 AUTH   **MILLER, M. V., & PRESTON, J. D.**
TITL   VERTICAL TIES AND THE REDISTRIBUTION OF POWER IN CRYSTAL CITY.
SRCE   *SOCIAL SCIENCE QUARTERLY, 1973, 53(4), 772-773.*
INDX   COMMUNITY INVOLVEMENT, CROSS CULTURAL, CULTURAL FACTORS, EMPIRICAL, ECONOMIC FACTORS, ESSAY, FARM LABORERS, CASE STUDY, MEXICAN AMERICAN, POLITICAL POWER, SPANISH SURNAMED, TEXAS, SOUTHWEST, POLITICS, CHICANO MOVEMENT, MIGRANTS, RURAL, COMMUNITY
ABST   THIS CASE STUDY DESCRIBES THE WAY IN WHICH A FORMERLY POWERLESS MINORITY GROUP WRESTED POWER FROM THE DOMINANT GROUP IN A SMALL TEXAS COMMUNITY. CRYSTAL CITY, POPULATION 9,000, HAS AN ESTIMATED SPANISH SURNAMED POPULATION OF 80%. HISTORICALLY, THESE MEXICAN AMERICANS OWNED PRACTICALLY NO FARM LAND, HAD LOW LEVELS OF MEDIAN INCOME AND EDUCATION, AND WORKED MOSTLY AS MIGRANT FARM LABORERS. RESEARCH DATA TRACING THEIR GRADUAL ACHIEVEMENT OF POLITICAL DOMINANCE WERE GENERATED FROM LIMITED PARTICIPANT-OBSERVATION, INTERVIEWS WITH COMMUNITY RESIDENTS, AND A CONTENT ANALYSIS OF NEWSPAPERS AND OTHER AVAILABLE DOCUMENTS. VERTICAL INPUTS WHICH WERE SEEN TO INTRODUCE NEW RESOURCES AND SANCTIONS INTO THE COMMUNITY AND THUS ALTER THE POWER STRUCTURE WERE: (1) THE CITY COUNCIL ELECTION OF 1962; (2) THE SCHOOL BOYCOTT OF 1969; AND (3) THE CITY COUNCIL AND SCHOOL BOARD ELECTIONS OF 1970. SINCE THESE EVENTS CAN BE TAKEN AS A "WATERSHED" FOR MANY CHICANO COMMUNITIES, THE QUESTION IS POSED: "WHY DID THE MOVEMENT START HERE AND NOT IN OTHER SIMILAR SOUTHWESTERN COMMUNITIES?" A PARTIAL ANSWER IS PROVIDED BY A SUMMARY OF VERTICAL INPUTS WHICH ENHANCED AND REINFORCED MEXICAN AMERICAN POLITICAL ACTIVITY IN THE COMMUNITY. 15 REFERENCES.
ACCN   002159

1233 AUTH   **MILLER, N., & MARUYAMA, G.**
TITL   ORDINAL POSITION AND PEER POPULARITY.
SRCE   *JOURNAL OF PERSONALITY AND SOCIAL PSYCHOLOGY, 1976, 33(2), 123-131.*
INDX   FAMILY STRUCTURE, INTERPERSONAL RELATIONS, INTERPERSONAL ATTRACTION, CHILDREN, MEXICAN AMERICAN, PERSONALITY, ANXIETY, SELF CONCEPT, EMPIRICAL, CROSS CULTURAL, SEX COMPARISON, SES, ACHIEVEMENT TESTING, WISC, RAVEN PROGRESSIVE MATRICES, PEABODY PICTURE-VOCABULARY TEST, CALIFORNIA, SOUTHWEST
ABST   THE INTERACTION OF SIBLINGS WITHIN THE HOME MAY REQUIRE LATER-BORN CHILDREN (THOSE WITH LESS POWER THAN THEIR OLDER SIBLINGS) TO DEVELOP MORE EFFECTIVE INTERPERSONAL SKILLS. IF SO, THEIR POPULARITY SHOULD BE APPRECIABLY AFFECTED—I.E., THEY SHOULD BE BETTER LIKED. TO TEST THIS LINE OF REASONING, THE RELATIONSHIP BETWEEN ORDINAL POSITION OF A CHILD AND HIS POPULARITY AMONG PEERS WAS EXAMINED BY RELATING SCHOOL SETTING MEASURES OF POPULARITY IN FRIENDSHIP, PLAY, AND SCHOOLWORK SITUATIONS TO ORDINAL POSITION FOR A SAMPLE OF 1,750 GRADE SCHOOL CHILDREN FROM RIVERSIDE, CALIFORNIA. FOR FRIENDSHIP AND PLAY MEASURES, LATER-BORN CHILDREN WERE FOUND

TO BE MORE POPULAR THAN THEIR EARLY-BORN PEERS. THIS FINDING HELD ACROSS RACIAL/ETHNIC BACKGROUND (BLACK, MEXICAN AMERICAN, AND WHITE), AGE (KINDERGARTEN THROUGH SIXTH GRADE), AND SEX. IN ADDITION, TEACHERS' RATINGS OF CHILDREN SHOWED THAT LATER-BORNS DO POSSESS GREATER SOCIAL SKILLS THAN THEIR EARLY-BORN PEERS. FINALLY, THIS STUDY FAILED TO CONFIRM PREVIOUS FINDINGS RELATING ORDINAL POSITION TO (A) MEASURES OF ACHIEVEMENT AND INTELLIGENCE AND (B) PERSONALITY DIMENSIONS SUCH AS ANXIETY, SELF-CONCEPT, AND DEPENDENCE. 23 REFERENCES. (JOURNAL ABSTRACT)

ACCN 001055

1234 AUTH **MILLER, S. O.**

TITL CURRENT STATUS OF HISPANIC SOCIAL WORKERS.

SRCE *IN E. L. OLMEDO & S. LOPEZ (EDS.), HISPANIC MENTAL HEALTH PROFESSIONALS (MONOGRAPH NO. 5). LOS ANGELES: UNIVERSITY OF CALIFORNIA, SPANISH SPEAKING MENTAL HEALTH RESEARCH CENTER, 1977, PP. 13-21.*

INDX MENTAL HEALTH PROFESSION, PUERTO RICAN-M, MEXICAN AMERICAN, REVIEW, EMPIRICAL, PROFESSIONAL TRAINING, REPRESENTATION, BILINGUAL-BICULTURAL PERSONNEL, HIGHER EDUCATION, CURRICULUM, EQUAL OPPORTUNITY

ABST THE PROFESSION OF SOCIAL WORK IS PRIMARILY CONCERNED WITH PROVIDING ASSISTANCE TO INDIVIDUALS OF POVERTY STATUS. CHARACTERISTIC OF THE POOR IS THAT THEY USUALLY ARE MEMBERS OF ETHNIC MINORITIES. THIS IS ESPECIALLY TRUE OF HISPANICS, OF WHICH PRESENT STATISTICS INDICATE THAT 32% OF PUERTO RICAN FAMILIES AND 35% OF MEXICAN AMERICAN FAMILIES ARE BELOW THE POVERTY LEVEL. AT THE SAME TIME, HISPANICS WHO CAN MORE ADEQUATELY PROVIDE THE CLINICAL AND SOCIAL SERVICE NEEDS OF THIS POPULATION ARE UNDERREPRESENTED IN THE SOCIAL WORK PROFESSION. TO ALLEVIATE THIS SITUATION THE COUNCIL ON SOCIAL WORK EDUCATION (CSWE) WAS CREATED. THIS ORGANIZATION IN ITS ATTEMPTS TO INCREASE THE NUMBER OF HISPANIC SOCIAL WORKERS HAS SPONSORED NUMEROUS WORKSHOPS, DEVELOPED PROGRAMS AND POLICY RELEVANT TO THE NEEDS OF HISPANICS, AND IMPLEMENTED A FELLOWSHIP PROGRAM FOR THE TRAINING OF ETHNIC MINORTY RESEARCHERS. IT IS CONCLUDED, HOWEVER, THAT PLANS TO INCREASE THE NUMBER AND QUALITY OF HISPANIC SOCIAL WORKERS IS DEPENDENT UPON BASIC DATA THAT PERTAIN TO THE CHARACTERISTICS OF SOCIAL WORKERS, TRENDS IN SOCIAL BEHAVIOR OF MINORITIES AND THEIR COMMUNITIES, AND TRENDS OCCURRING IN SOCIAL POLICIES AND LEGISLATION. 12 REFERENCES.

ACCN 001056

1235 AUTH **MILLER, W.**

TITL THE RUMBLE THIS TIME.

SRCE *PSYCHOLOGY TODAY, 1977, 10(12), 52-54; 56; 58-59; 88.*

INDX ADOLESCENTS, AGGRESSION, CROSS CULTURAL, DELINQUENCY, EMPIRICAL, GANGS, EAST, SOUTHWEST, SURVEY, MIDWEST, CALIFORNIA, NEW YORK, ILLINOIS, PENNSYLVANIA, MICHIGAN, SPANISH SURNAMED, URBAN

ABST THE IMPRESSION THAT YOUTH GANGS HAVE RECENTLY RETURNED, HAVE A DEFINED TURF, AND RESTRICT VIOLENCE TO OTHER GANGS ONLY, ARE FICTIONALIZED ACCOUNTS SUPPORTED BY THE MEDIA. A SURVEY OF 150 REPRESENTATIVES FROM 60 AGENCIES, OVER ONE-HALF MINORITY MEMBERS, CONCENTRATED IN NEW YORK, LOS ANGELES, CHICAGO, PHILADELPHIA, DETROIT, AND SAN FRANCISCO REFUTE THESE IDEAS. THESE POLICE AND OTHER PUBLIC AND PRIVATE AGENCIES REPORT THAT GHETTO GUERRILLA FORAYS HAVE REPLACED LARGE SCALE RUMBLES AND THAT OBTAINING MONEY HAS TAKEN PRIORITY OVER DEFENDING ONE'S NEIGHBORHOOD. INCREASED FIREPOWER AS A FUNCTION OF GREATER ACCESSIBILITY OF SOPHISTICATED FIREARMS IS NOTED. TERRORISM IN SCHOOLS, INTIMIDATION OF OFFICIALS, AND AN INCREASED NUMBER OF VIOLENT ACTS AGAINST NON-GANG MEMBERS ARE ALSO NOTED. PRE-TEEN GANG MEMBERS OR FEMALE AUTONOMOUS GANGS WERE NOT FOUND FREQUENTLY. "WHITE FLIGHT" AND A 17% INCREASE IN THE 10 TO 20 YEAR-OLD'ETHNIC AND BLACK POPULATIONS PREDICT A RISE IN GANG ACTIVITY WITHIN THE NEXT FEW YEARS. AS OBTAINING MONEY HAS REPLACED THE SEEKING OF GANG REPUTATIONS, ROBBERIES AND BURGLARIES MAY INCREASE IN MIDDLE CLASS NEIGHBORHOODS WHERE GANGS HAVE PREVIOUSLY NOT BEEN A PROBLEM. THEREFORE, GANG-RELATED VIOLENCE IS NOT SEEN AS RESTRICTED TO THE INNER CITY AND, AS SUCH, IS A CITY-WIDE PROBLEM TO BE SOLVED. 4 REFERENCES.

ACCN 002576

1236 AUTH **MILLS, C. W., SENIOR, C., & GOLDSEN, R. K.**

TITL THE PUERTO RICAN JOURNEY: NEW YORK'S NEWEST MIGRANTS.

SRCE *NEW YORK: RUSSELL & RUSSELL, 1967.*

INDX PUERTO RICAN-I, HISTORY, CULTURE, BILINGUALISM, ECONOMIC FACTORS, SOCIAL SERVICES, INTERPERSONAL RELATIONS, STRESS, PSYCHOSOCIAL ADJUSTMENT, EMPLOYMENT, FAMILY ROLES, FAMILY STRUCTURE, ACCULTURATION, EMPIRICAL, SURVEY, DEMOGRAPHIC, EDUCATION, OCCUPATIONAL ASPIRATIONS, URBAN, RELIGION, SEX ROLES, DISCRIMINATION, CULTURAL FACTORS, LEGISLATION, POLICY, SES, POVERTY, PUERTO RICAN-M, IMMIGRATION, NEW YORK, EAST

ABST THIS 230 PAGE REPORT ON THE PUERTO RICAN MIGRATION TO NEW YORK CITY (SPECIFICALLY, TO SPANISH HARLEM, THE BRONX, AND BROOKLYN) EXAMINES THE FOLLOWING ISSUES: (1) WHO THE MIGRANTS ARE AND WHY THEY CAME; (2) HOW THEY COMPARE WITH THEIR COMPATRIOTS WHO REMAIN AT HOME; (3) WHAT THEIR MIGRATION MEANS IN TERMS OF OCCUPATION AND INCOME; (4) WHAT KIND

OF SOCIAL WORLD THEY INHABIT IN NEW YORK; AND (5) HOW THAT WORLD COMPARES WITH THE EXPERIENCES OF PREVIOUS IMMIGRANT GROUPS. THE STUDY WAS BEGUN IN 1947, INCLUDES DEMOGRAPHIC DATA FROM 1930 AND 1940, AND IS LARGELY BASED UPON A SURVEY QUESTIONNAIRE ADMINISTERED TO 1,113 PUERTO RICANS AGE 18 AND OVER. THE REPORT EMPHASIZES THAT PUERTO RICANS ARE A DISTINCTIVE IMMIGRANT GROUP BECAUSE THEY ARE RACIALLY MIXED, ARE OF LATIN AMERICAN CULTURE, AND CONSTITUTE THE FIRST SIZEABLE GROUP FROM OUTSIDE THE CONTINENT TO ENTER THE U.S. SINCE THE IMMIGRATION LAWS OF THE 1920S. THEREFORE, THEIR STORY NECESSITATES A RECONSIDERATION OF THE PROBLEMS OF MIGRATION. THE STUDY'S QUESTIONNAIRE IS INCLUDED IN AN APPENDIX, THE SAMPLING PROCEDURE IS DESCRIBED IN DETAIL, AND 96 TABLES ARE PRESENTED. 67 REFERENCES. (AUTHOR SUMMARY MODIFIED)

ACCN   001057

1237 AUTH   **MINGIONE, A. D.**
TITL   NEED ACHIEVEMENT IN NEGRO, WHITE, AND PUERTO RICAN CHILDREN.
SRCE   *JOURNAL OF CONSULTING AND CLINICAL PSYCHOLOGY, 1968, 32(1), 94-95.*
INDX   ACHIEVEMENT MOTIVATION, CROSS CULTURAL, ADOLESCENTS, PUERTO RICAN-M, EMPIRICAL, CONNECTICUT, EAST, URBAN, CHILDREN
ABST   A COMPARISON OF THE NEED FOR ACHIEVEMENT (N-ACH) OF NEGRO, WHITE, AND PUERTO RICAN FIFTH AND SEVENTH GRADERS FROM LOW-SOCIOECONOMIC AREAS OF A CONNECTICUT CITY IS PRESENTED. THE N-ACH TEST CONSISTS OF SIX TOPIC SENTENCES WHERE SUBJECTS WRITE A STORY IN RESPONSE TO EACH ITEM. STATISTICAL TESTS OF N-ACH SCORES REVEAL NO SIGNIFICANT DIFFERENCES AMONG THE GROUPS. THESE RESULTS CONTRADICT A PREVIOUS STUDY BY THE SAME AUTHOR WHERE WHITE CHILDREN HAD HIGHER N-ACH SCORES THAN NEGRO CHILDREN. COMPARED TO THE EARLIER STUDY, THERE WERE MORE WORDS PER STORY, GREATER VARIETY OF STORY THEMES, AND MORE STORIES CONCERNING FEMALES WRITTEN BY BOTH BOYS AND GIRLS. SCHOOL GRADES AND GROUP INTELLIGENCE TEST SCORES DID NOT CORRELATE WITH N-ACH SCORES. 10 REFERENCES.

ACCN   001058

1238 AUTH   **MINTZ, S. W., & WOLF, R. E.**
TITL   AN ANALYSIS OF RITUAL CO-PARENTHOOD (COMPADRAZGO).
SRCE   *SOUTHWESTERN JOURNAL OF ANTHROPOLOGY, 1950, 6(4), 341-368.*
INDX   ESSAY, CULTURE, ENVIRONMENTAL FACTORS, FICTIVE KINSHIP, EXTENDED FAMILY, FAMILY ROLES, FAMILY STRUCTURE, CROSS CULTURAL, CENTRAL AMERICA, MEXICAN, PUERTO RICAN-I, SOUTHWEST, ARIZONA, MEXICAN AMERICAN, CULTURAL CHANGE, ECONOMIC FACTORS, REVIEW, SOUTH AMERICA

ABST   THE HISTORY AND FUNCTION OF THE RITUAL KINSHIP MECHANISM OF COMPADRAZGO ARE PRESENTED. THE RELATIONSHIP BETWEEN LAND TENURE AND RITUAL KIN TIES ARE TRACED THROUGH EUROPEAN FEUDALISM AND PEASANT RIGHTS TO PRESENT DAY EUROPE AND INDUSTRIAL DEVELOPMENT. FIVE MODERN LATIN AMERICAN COMMUNITIES WERE ANALYZED TO SHOW THE FUNCTIONAL CORRELATES OF THE COMPADRE MECHANISM WITHIN THEIR POPULATIONS. WITHIN THESE COMMUNITIES IT WAS FOUND THAT: (1) WHERE THE RESIDENTS ARE A SELF-CONTAINED CLASS OR TRIBALLY HOMOGENEOUS, COMPADRAZGO IS PREDOMINANTLY HORIZONTAL; (2) WHERE THE COMMUNITY CONTAINS SEVERAL INTERACTING CLASSES, COMPADRAZGO IS VERTICAL; AND (3) WHERE RAPID SOCIAL CHANGE IS OCCURRING, COMPADRE MECHANISMS MAY MULTIPLY TO MEET THE ACCELERATED RATE OF CHANGE. 59 REFERENCES. (AUTHOR SUMMARY MODIFIED)

ACCN   001059

1239 AUTH   **MIRANDA DE JESUS, F., & CORDOVA, A. A.**
TITL   CARACTERISTICAS PSICO-SOCIALES DEL ESTUDIANTE DE PRIMER ANO DE LA UNIVERSIDAD DE PUERTO RICO, RIO PIEDRAS 1960-1961. (PSYCHOSOCIAL CHARACTERISTICS OF FIRST-YEAR STUDENTS AT THE UNIVERSITY OF PUERTO RICO, RIO PIEDRAS.)
SRCE   *REVISTA MEXICANA DE PSICOLOGIA, 1964, 1(4), 368-380. (SPANISH)*
INDX   INTELLIGENCE TESTING, PSYCHOSOCIAL ADJUSTMENT, LINGUISTIC COMPETENCE, PUERTO RICAN-I, EMPIRICAL, RAVEN PROGRESSIVE MATRICES, COLLEGE STUDENTS, PERSONALITY, VALUES
ABST   A SERIES OF TESTS TO DETERMINE INTELLIGENCE, PERSONALITY ADJUSTMENT AND VALUES, MASTERY OF VOCABULARY, AND READING SKILL (IN ENGLISH AND IN SPANISH) WERE ADMINISTERED TO A GROUP OF 130 FIRST-YEAR STUDENTS SELECTED AT RANDOM FROM THE UNIVERSITY OF PUERTO RICO (UPR) SCHOOLS OF GENERAL STUDIES, EDUCATION, AND COMMERCE. THE 53 MALE AND 77 FEMALE SUBJECTS, WITH A MEAN AGE OF 19.7 YEARS, WERE REPRESENTATIVE OF THE TOTAL FIRST-YEAR ENROLLMENT IN THE THREE COLLEGES AS TO SEX DISTRIBUTION, EDUCATIONAL BACKGROUND, NATIVE GEOGRAPHIC AREA, AND TENTATIVE SELECTION OF POST-FIRST-YEAR UNIVERSITY GOALS. ANALYSIS OF THE RESULTS INDICATES THAT SIGNIFICANT PSYCHOSOCIAL TRAITS EXIST FOR THIS GROUP, PARTICULARLY IN THE AREAS OF INTELLIGENCE AND OVERALL PERSONALITY ADJUSTMENT. WHEN MEASURED BY THE RAVEN GUIDE TO STANDARD PROGRESSIVE MATRICES, THE TEST GROUP SHOWED AN INTELLECTUAL CAPACITY SUPERIOR TO THAT OF THE GENERAL STUDENT POPULATION TESTED FOR ADMITTANCE TO UPR. COMPARED TO A SECONDARY SCHOOL POPULATION, THE FIRST-YEAR UNIVERSITY STUDENT SEEMS TO BE BETTER ADJUSTED IN HIS SOCIAL, EMOTIONAL, AND HOME ENVIRONMENT. THE TESTS FOR READING AND

VOCABULARY SKILLS IN SPANISH AND IN ENGLISH SHOWED THAT THE SUBJECTS HAVE EQUAL DOMINION OVER BOTH LANGUAGES. A MORE EXHAUSTIVE INVESTIGATION INTO THE PSYCHOSOCIAL CHARACTERISTICS OF UNIVERSITY STUDENTS IN PUERTO RICO IS SUGGESTED. 33 REFERENCES.

ACCN   001060

1240 AUTH   **MIRANDA, M. R. (ED.)**
     TITL   PSYCHOTHERAPY WITH THE SPANISH-SPEAKING: ISSUES IN RESEARCH AND IN SERVICE DELIVERY (MONOGRAPH NO. 3).
     SRCE   *LOS ANGELES: UNIVERSITY OF CALIFORNIA, SPANISH SPEAKING MENTAL HEALTH RESEARCH CENTER, 1976.*
     INDX   MENTAL HEALTH, HEALTH DELIVERY SYSTEMS, RESOURCE UTILIZATION, ACCULTURATION, PSYCHOTHERAPY, BEHAVIOR THERAPY, MENTAL HEALTH PROFESSION, MEXICAN AMERICAN, PSYCHOTHERAPISTS, SES, PSYCHOTHERAPY OUTCOME, CULTURAL FACTORS, EMPIRICAL, BOOK
     ABST   SEVEN ARTICLES BY LATINO MENTAL HEALTH RESEARCHERS AND CLINICIANS ATTEST TO THE INCREASING INTEREST IN PSYCHOTHERAPEUTIC PROCESSES AND THEIR EFFECT ON THE SPANISH-SPEAKING (SS). THE AUTHORS STRONGLY SUGGEST THAT TREATMENT APPROACHES FOR THE SS CLIENT SHOULD BE BASED ON MORE APPROPRIATE SERVICES AND THAT BASIC REVISIONS IN TRADITIONAL FORMS OF PSYCHOTHERAPY ARE NEEDED IF MENTAL HEALTH SERVICES IN THE LATINO COMMUNITY ARE TO BE MAXIMALLY EFFECTIVE. THE WIDELY PREVALENT NOTION THAT PSYCHOTHERAPY IS NOT THE TREATMENT OF CHOICE FOR LOW INCOME SS CLIENTS IS QUESTIONED. NEW INFORMATION ON PSYCHOTHERAPEUTIC APPROACHES, TECHNIQUES, AND GOALS APPROPRIATE TO THE SPANISH-SPEAKING ARE EMPHASIZED. ALL OF THE ARTICLES ATTEMPT TO STUDY THE MULTIPLICITY OF VARIABLES INVOLVED IN THE DEVELOPMENT OF EFFECTIVE MENTAL HEALTH SERVICES FOR LATINOS.

ACCN   001061

1241 AUTH   **MIRANDA, M. R., ANDUJO, E., CABALLERO, I. L., GUERRERO, C. C., & RAMOS, R. A.**
     TITL   MEXICAN AMERICAN DROPOUTS IN PSYCHOTHERAPY AS RELATED TO LEVELS OF ACCULTURATION.
     SRCE   *IN M. R. MIRANDA (ED.), PSYCHOTHERAPY WITH THE SPANISH SPEAKING: ISSUES IN RESEARCH AND SERVICE DELIVERY (MONOGRAPH NO. 3). LOS ANGELES: UNIVERSITY OF CALIFORNIA, SPANISH SPEAKING MENTAL HEALTH RESEARCH CENTER, 1976, PP. 35-50.*
     INDX   RESOURCE UTILIZATION, PSYCHOTHERAPY, PSYCHOTHERAPISTS, PSYCHOTHERAPY OUTCOME, MEXICAN AMERICAN, ADULTS, FEMALE, EMPIRICAL, BILINGUAL-BICULTURAL PERSONNEL, LOCUS OF CONTROL, HEALTH DELIVERY SYSTEMS, EDUCATION, SES, ACCULTURATION, CALIFORNIA, SOUTHWEST, TIME ORIENTATION
     ABST   PREVIOUS STUDIES ABOUT MEXICAN AMERICANS IN THERAPY SUGGEST A STRONG RELA-

TIONSHIP BETWEEN THE CLIENT'S IDENTIFICATION WITH MIDDLE CLASS VALUES AND THE LENGTH OF THERAPY. THIS STUDY TESTED THE FOLLOWING HYPOTHESIS: MEXICAN AMERICAN (MA) CLIENTS DEMONSTRATING BOTH A PSYCHOLOGICAL AND BEHAVIORAL IDENTIFICATION WITH THE DOMINANT CULTURE WILL BE MORE LIKELY TO SEEK OUT AND REMAIN IN THERAPY THAN THOSE WHO DEMONSTRATE LESS ACCULTURATION. SUBJECTS WERE 60 RANDOMLY SELECTED FEMALE OUTPATIENTS WHO HAD SOUGHT MENTAL HEALTH SERVICES AT EAST LOS ANGELES CLINICS; 30 CONTINUOUS SUBJECTS ATTENDED 5 OR MORE THERAPY SESSIONS, AND 30 DISCONTINUOUS SUBJECTS ATTENDED NO MORE THAN 2 SESSIONS FOLLOWING THE INTAKE INTERVIEW. EACH SUBJECT'S LEVEL OF PSYCHOLOGICAL AND BEHAVIORAL ACCULTURATION WAS DETERMINED BY AN INVENTORY OF TESTS MEASURING (1) INTERPERSONAL BEHAVIOR, (2) FEELING OF PERSONAL CONTROL, (3) FUTURE TIME PERSPECTIVE, (4) FORMAL EDUCATION, (5) ACCULTURATION, AND (6) OCCUPATION. BILINGUAL-BICULTURAL INTERVIEWERS ALSO COLLECTED PERSONAL DATA, PERCEPTIONS OF THERAPY, AND REASONS FOR ENTERING THERAPY. T-TEST AND CHI-SQUARE COMPUTATIONS SUPPORTED THE STUDY'S HYPOTHESIS: THOSE MA FEMALES ELECTING TO REMAIN IN PSYCHOTHERAPY FOR AT LEAST 5 SESSIONS DEMONSTRATED HIGHER LEVELS OF BOTH PSYCHOLOGICAL AND BEHAVIORAL ACCULTURATION THAN THOSE WHO PREMATURELY TERMINATED THERAPY. RESULTS IMPLY THAT MORE ATTENTION BE DIRECTED TO REASSESSING THE DELIVERY OF SERVICES TO CLIENTS NOT IDENTIFYING OR FAMILIAR WITH THE VALUES OF THE DOMINANT CULTURE. 17 REFERENCES.

ACCN   001062

1242 AUTH   **MIRANDA, M. R., & KITANO, H. H. L.**
     TITL   MENTAL HEALTH SERVICES IN THIRD WORLD COMMUNITIES.
     SRCE   *INTERNATIONAL JOURNAL OF MENTAL HEALTH, 1976, 5(2), 39-49.*
     INDX   ESSAY, MEXICAN AMERICAN, CROSS CULTURAL, MENTAL HEALTH, HEALTH DELIVERY SYSTEMS, RESOURCE UTILIZATION, PSYCHOTHERAPY, PROFESSIONAL TRAINING, ADMINISTRATORS
     ABST   THIRD WORLD (E.G., ASIAN AMERICAN, MEXICAN AMERICAN) COMMUNITY MENTAL HEALTH PROBLEMS ARE GENERALLY MISUNDERSTOOD BY MOST PROVIDERS OF MENTAL HEALTH SERVICES IN THIS COUNTRY. DIFFERENCES BETWEEN THE CULTURAL VALUES AND EXPERIENCES OF THE MINORITIES AND PROFESSIONALS TRAINED IN TRADITIONAL TECHNIQUES ARE GREAT. AN ANALYSIS OF THE PROBLEMS RELATED TO SERVICE DELIVERY TO MINORITIES FOCUSES ON (1) FRAGMENTATION OF SERVICES, (2) INACCESSIBILITY OF SERVICES, (3) DISCONTINUITY OF SERVICES, AND (4) UNACCOUNTABILITY OF SERVICES. THE INTERACTION OF THESE VARIABLES EXPLAINS THE LOW UTILIZATION OF MENTAL HEALTH

SERVICES BY THIRD WORLD COMMUNITIES. A WIDER VIEW OF MENTAL HEALTH INCLUDING PEOPLE'S FEELINGS OF WORTH WITHIN CULTURAL AND SOCIETAL SYSTEMS IS NEEDED. THE MAJOR RESPONSIBILITY FOR CHANGE LIES WITH THE SERVICE PROVIDERS, ESPECIALLY THE ADMINISTRATORS OF DELIVERY SYSTEMS. IT IS THEIR RIGIDITY, MODELS, CONCEPTS, AND ATTITUDES THAT CREATE BARRIERS FOR THIRD WORLD PEOPLE. (AUTHOR SUMMARY MODIFIED)

ACCN   001063

1243 AUTH   **MIRANDA, M., & KITANO, H. H. L.**
TITL   BARRIERS TO MENTAL HEALTH SERVICES: A JAPANESE-AMERICAN AND MEXICAN-AMERICAN DILEMMA.
SRCE   *IN C. HERNANDEZ, M. J. HAUG & N. N. WAGNER (EDS.), CHICANOS: SOCIAL AND PSYCHOLOGICAL PERSPECTIVES. SAINT LOUIS: C. V. MOSBY COMPANY, 1976, PP. 242-252.*
INDX   RESOURCE UTILIZATION, MEXICAN AMERICAN, CROSS CULTURAL, HEALTH DELIVERY SYSTEMS, CULTURAL FACTORS, REVIEW, ECONOMIC FACTORS, MENTAL HEALTH
ABST   SOME SIMILARITIES AND DIFFERENCES OF JAPANESE AMERICANS (JA) AND MEXICAN AMERICANS (MA) REGARDING MENTAL HEALTH NEEDS AND USE OF MENTAL HEALTH FACILITIES ARE DISCUSSED. SEVERAL HYPOTHESES CONCERNING THE UNDERREPRESENTATION OF THESE PARTICULAR ETHNIC GROUPS AMONG SERVICE USERS ARE PRESENTED: LACK OF INFORMATION, ETHNIC STYLES, FRAGMENTATION, INACCESSIBILITY, DISCONTINUITY, AND UNACCOUNTABILITY. ALTHOUGH NO SYSTEMATIC TESTING OF THESE VARIABLES AND THEIR IMPACT ON RESOURCE UTILIZATION BY EITHER THE JA OR MA HAS BEEN CONDUCTED, THE UNDERUTILIZATION BY BOTH OF THESE GROUPS IS BELIEVED TO BE DUE TO THE RIGIDITY, ATTITUDES, CONCEPTS, AND MODELS OF THE SERVICE PROVIDERS. BY FOCUSING ON TWO DIFFERENT ETHNIC GROUPS, THE AUTHORS BELIEVE THE TEMPTATION TO HYPOTHESIZE CULTURE AS THE CAUSE OF UNDERUTILIZATION IS REDUCED, AND THEREBY ATTENTION IS DIRECTED TO PROBLEMS IN SERVICE DELIVERY. 23 REFERENCES.

ACCN   001064

1244 AUTH   **MISHRA, S. P., & HURT, M. JR.**
TITL   THE USE OF METROPOLITAN READINESS TESTS WITH MEXICAN-AMERICAN CHILDREN.
SRCE   *CALIFORNIA JOURNAL OF EDUCATION RESEARCH, 1970, 21(4), 182-187.*
INDX   METROPOLITAN READINESS TEST, MEXICAN AMERICAN, CHILDREN, TEST VALIDITY, TEST RELIABILITY, ACHIEVEMENT TESTING, SCHOLASTIC ACHIEVEMENT, CULTURAL FACTORS, EMPIRICAL, ARIZONA, SOUTHWEST
ABST   A STUDY OF THE RELIABILITY OF METROPOLITAN READINESS TESTS WHEN USED ON CHILDREN OF MEXICAN DESCENT IS REPORTED. THE PRESTUDY HYPOTHESIS WAS THAT SUCH TESTS HAVE POOR RELIABILITY AND PREDICTIVE VALIDITY FOR THIS POPULATION. SEVENTY-THREE DISADVANTAGED CHILDREN WITH PRIMARILY NON-ENGLISH-SPEAKING BACKGROUNDS WERE USED AS SUBJECTS. METROPOLITAN READINESS TESTS (MRT) WERE ADMINISTERED TO THESE MEXICAN AMERICAN CHILDREN WHO WERE THEN BEGINNING FIRST GRADE. THE SAME CHILDREN WERE ALSO TESTED IN THIRD GRADE WITH CRITERION MEASURES FOR ESTABLISHING VALIDITY. SPLIT-HALF RELIABILITY COEFFICIENTS, CORRECTED WITH THE SPEARMAN AND BROWN FORMULA, REVEALED THAT TWO MRT SUBTESTS (THOSE MOST DEPENDENT ON LANGUAGE ABILITY) HAD SIGNIFICANTLY LOWER RELIABILITY. PREDICTIVE VALIDITY ALSO WAS FOUND TO BE LOWER FOR THESE CHILDREN. 5 REFERENCES.

ACCN   001065

1245 AUTH   **MISKIMINS, R. W., & BAKER, B. R.**
TITL   SELF CONCEPT AND THE DISADVANTAGED (MONOGRAPH SUPPLEMENT NO. 41).
SRCE   *BRANDON, VT.: CLINICAL PSYCHOLOGY PUBLISHING COMPANY, 1973.*
INDX   SELF CONCEPT, SES, POVERTY, ADULTS, EMPIRICAL, URBAN, CROSS CULTURAL, DEVIANCE, PERSONALITY ASSESSMENT, SEX COMPARISON, MEXICAN AMERICAN, VOCATIONAL COUNSELING, JOB PERFORMANCE, PSYCHOPATHOLOGY, COLORADO, SOUTHWEST
ABST   THE RELATIONSHIP OF BEING ECONOMICALLY DISADVANTAGED TO SELF-CONCEPT WAS EMPIRICALLY ASSESSED IN A SAMPLE OF 660 DISADVANTAGED URBAN ADULTS (APPROXIMATELY HALF MEXICAN AMERICAN) LIVING IN DENVER, COLORADO. FOUR TYPES OF DATA (ALL TYPES COLLECTED ON ONLY ABOUT 25% OF THE SAMPLE) ARE PRESENTED: (1) OVERALL MULTIDIMENSIONAL SELF-CONCEPT DESCRIPTION OF THE DISADVANTAGED; (2) DETAILED SELF-CONCEPT DESCRIPTION; (3) CONSIDERATION OF COUNSELING AND WORK INFORMATION AS RELATED TO SELF-CONCEPT DESCRIPTION; AND (4) CHANGES IN SELF-CONCEPT WITH WORK EXPERIENCES. MEASURES OF SELF-ESTEEM, CULTURAL REJECTION, SELF-DEROGATION, RELATIONSHIP PROBLEMS, SUSPICIOUSNESS AND LEVEL OF MALADJUSTMENT WERE COLLECTED WITH THE MISKIMINS SELF-GOAL-OTHER DISCREPANCY SCALE. RESULTS SUGGEST TWO IMPORTANT CONCLUSIONS: (1) SUCCESSFUL JOB EXPERIENCES HAVE POSITIVE EFFECTS UPON THE SELF-CONCEPT OF THE POOR, ESPECIALLY REGARDING MALADJUSTMENT, SELF-ESTEEM, RELATIONSHIPS AND SUSPICIOUSNESS; BUT AS IMPORTANT, (2) FAILURE IN WORK EXPERIENCES HAS NEGATIVE EFFECTS (INCREASES MALADJUSTMENT, CULTURAL REJECTION, SELF-DEROGATION WHILE SELF-ESTEEM DECREASES). COMPARISONS BETWEEN THE FAILURE GROUP AND THOSE DISADVANTAGED WHO WERE NEVER PLACED ON JOBS SUGGEST THAT IT IS BETTER NOT TO TRY WORKING AT ALL THAN TO WORK AND FAIL—FAILURE ONLY MAGNIFIES SELF-CONCEPT PROBLEMS. 34 REFERENCES. (AUTHOR SUMMARY MODIFIED)

ACCN   001066

1246 AUTH   **MITCHELL, A. J.**

TITL THE EFFECT OF BILINGUALISM IN THE MEASUREMENT OF INTELLIGENCE.

SRCE *ELEMENTARY SCHOOL JOURNAL, 1937, 38(1), 29-37.*

INDX BILINGUALISM, INTELLIGENCE TESTING, MEXICAN AMERICAN, CHILDREN, EMPIRICAL, TEST VALIDITY, ARIZONA, SOUTHWEST

ABST AN ATTEMPT TO DETERMINE WHETHER BILINGUALISM HAS AN APPRECIABLE EFFECT ON CHILDREN'S ABILITY TO THINK WITH EQUAL ACCURACY AND FACILITY IN EITHER LANGUAGE IS PRESENTED. BOTH FORMS (SPANISH AND ENGLISH) OF THE OTIS GROUP INTELLIGENCE SCALE WERE ADMINISTERED TO 236 1ST-3RD GRADE MEXICAN AMERICAN CHILDREN. THE LANGUAGE FACTOR WAS COUNTERBALANCED ACROSS SUBJECTS. THE MEAN DIFFERENCE IN THE OBTAINED IQ'S WAS IN FAVOR OF THE SPANISH TRANSLATION. THIS INDICATES THAT BILINGUAL CHILDREN WORK UNDER A SERIOUS HANDICAP IN AMERICAN SCHOOLS. IT IS SUGGESTED THAT AN EXHAUSTIVE STUDY OF THE EFFECTS OF BILINGUALISM ON INTELLIGENCE WILL PROVIDE BETTER MEANS FOR DETERMINING THE IQ'S OF FOREIGN LANGUAGE CHILDREN, FOR AT PRESENT THERE ARE MANY FACTORS WHICH IMPAIR THE VALUE OF IQ TEST RESULTS. 5 REFERENCES.

ACCN 001067

1247 AUTH **MITCHELL, M.**

TITL THE COOPERATIVE MOVEMENT IN PUERTO RICO.

SRCE *JOURNAL OF EDUCATION, 1967, 150(2), 39-42.*

INDX PUERTO RICAN-I, CULTURAL CHANGE, ADULTS, ACCULTURATION, EMPIRICAL

ABST A NONRANDOM SAMPLE OF SEVERAL PUERTO RICAN RESIDENTS' OPINIONS ABOUT THE COOPERATIVE MOVEMENT IN THEIR COUNTRY IS PRESENTED. THE SAMPLE CONSISTED OF 19 ADULTS FROM SEVERAL SUBCULTURES, SES LEVELS AND OCCUPATIONS. USING THE ANTHROPOLOGICAL CONCEPTS OF INNOVATION, ACCULTURATION, AND FOCUS IN HIS INTERVIEW QUESTIONS, THE AUTHOR VISITED SCHOOLS, FACTORIES AMD HACIENDAS TO COLLECT DATA. ANALYSIS INDICATES THAT COOPERATIVES HAVE NOT DEVELOPED AS RAPIDILY AS EXPECTED IN THE LAST TEN YEARS. THERE WERE NO OUTSTANDING INNOVATIONS READILY DISCOVERED FROM THE SMALL SAMPLE. SOME ACCULTURATION WAS TAKING PLACE IN MERCHANDIZING WITH SOME CO-OP STORES ADOPTING AMERICAN METHODS. OVERALL, THE COOPERATIVE MOVEMENT IN PUERTO RICO WAS NOT A FOCUS FOR CHANGE IN THE COUNTRY, ALTHOUGH THE POTENTIAL FOR THIS REMAINS GREAT. 5 REFERENCES.

ACCN 001068

1248 AUTH **MITTELBACH, F. G., & MOORE, J. W.**

TITL ETHNIC ENDOGAMY—THE CASE OF THE MEXICAN AMERICANS.

SRCE *AMERICAN JOURNAL OF SOCIOLOGY, 1968, 74(1), 50-62.*

INDX SES, ACCULTURATION, INTERMARRIAGE, MEXICAN AMERICAN, SEXUAL BEHAVIOR, EMPIRICAL, SEX ROLES, DEMOGRAPHIC, MARRIAGE, CROSS GENERATIONAL, CALIFORNIA, SOUTHWEST

ABST A THREE-GENERATIONAL ANALYSIS OF MARRIAGES INVOLVING MEXICAN AMERICANS SHOWS HIGHER RATES OF EXOGAMY THAN DO EARLIER STUDIES. EXOGAMY IS HIGHER FOR WOMEN AND INCREASES WITH REMOVAL FROM IMMIGRANT STATUS. THERE IS A STRONG PATTERN OF GENERATIONAL ENDOGAMY AND A STRONG SUGGESTION THAT SOCIAL DISTANCE BETWEEN GENERATIONS MAY BE AS IMPORTANT AS SOCIAL DISTANCE BETWEEN THE ETHNIC GROUP AND THE DOMINANT SOCIETY. EXOGAMY IS MORE PREVALENT AMONG HIGHER STATUS INDIVIDUALS AND OCCUPATION APPEARS TO BE A BETTER PREDICTOR OF EXOGAMY THAN GENERATION. FINDINGS HAVE IMPLICATIONS FOR UNDERSTANDING THE ASSIMILATION OF MEXICAN AMERICANS. 29 REFERENCES. (JOURNAL ABSTRACT MODIFIED)

ACCN 001069

1249 AUTH **MITTELBACH, F. G., MOORE, J. W., & MCDANIEL, R.**

TITL INTERMARRIAGE OF MEXICAN AMERICANS (MEXICAN AMERICAN STUDY PROJECT, ADVANCE REPORT NO. 6).

SRCE *LOS ANGELES: UNIVERSITY OF CALIFORNIA, GRADUATE SCHOOL OF BUSINESS ADMINISTRATION, 1966. (ERIC DOCUMENT REPRODUCTION SERVICE NO. ED 015 799)*

INDX MARITAL STABILITY, ACCULTURATION, INTERMARRIAGE, MARRIAGE, MEXICAN AMERICAN, SEXUAL BEHAVIOR, EMPIRICAL, SEX ROLES, DEMOGRAPHIC, CROSS GENERATIONAL, CALIFORNIA, SOUTHWEST

ABST BASED ON THE ASSUMPTION THAT MARRIAGE PATTERNS ARE GENERALLY A RELIABLE GUIDE TO THE SPEED WITH WHICH ANY ETHNIC GROUPS IS ASSIMILATING INTO THE LARGER AMERICAN SOCIETY, THIS STUDY ANALYZES INTERMARRIAGE PATTERNS OF 7,492 LOS ANGELES COUNTY MARRIAGE LICENSES BEARING SPANISH SURNAMES (SS) ISSUED DURING 1963. DATA FROM AREAS OTHER THAN LOS ANGELES AND FROM YEARS PRIOR TO 1963 ARE ALSO PRESENTED TO DEMONSTRATE TRENDS AND BROADEN THE APPLICABILITY OF THE FINDINGS. DESCRIPTIVE ANALYSES ARE USED TO EXPLORE THE RELATIONSHIPS BETWEEN THE BRIDE AND GROOM'S GENERATION, AGE, AREA OF RESIDENCE, PREVIOUS MARRIAGE AND TYPE OF CEREMONY, AND SOCIAL CLASS WITH THEIR PATTERNS OF INTERMARRIAGE AND ETHNICITY OF OUT GROUP SPOUSE. OVERALL IT IS FOUND THAT MEXICAN AMERICANS ARE MARRYING OUT OF THEIR ETHNIC COMMUNITY TO AN EXTENT FAR GREATER THAN DETERMINED FROM EARLIER STUDIES. INTERPRETATIONS OF THESE FINDINGS INCLUDE A DISCUSSION OF ETHNIC VS. SOCIAL CLASS CULTURE. ANTI-TRADITIONALISM AND ASSIMILATION AS MOTIVATIONS FOR INTERMARRIAGE BY MEXICAN AMERICANS ARE ALSO DISCUSSED. 27 REFERENCES.

ACCN 001070

1250 AUTH **MIZIO, E.**

TITL IMPACT OF EXTERNAL SYSTEMS ON THE PUERTO RICAN FAMILY.

SRCE *SOCIAL CASEWORK, 1974, 55(2), 76-83.*

INDX PUERTO RICAN-I, ESSAY, FAMILY STRUCTURE, EXTENDED FAMILY, CULTURAL CHANGE, SEX ROLES, HEALTH DELIVERY SYSTEMS, FICTIVE KINSHIP, FAMILY ROLES, EDUCATION, DISCRIMINATION

ABST STRUCTURAL DIFFERENCES OF EXTENDED FAMILIES IN RELATION TO SOCIOLEGAL SYSTEMS ARE DISCUSSED. THE PUERTO RICAN FAMILY IS, IN CONTRAST TO THE AMERICAN, AN EXTENDED FAMILY; INTIMATE RELATIONSHIPS WITH THE KINSHIP SYSTEM ARE OF HIGH VALUE AND A SOURCE OF PRIDE AND SECURITY. RELATIONSHIPS ARE INTENSE AND FREQUENT, EVEN IF THE PERSONS ARE NOT LIVING IN THE SAME HOUSEHOLD. IN THIS PATRIARCHAL FAMILY, ROLES ARE CLEARLY DEFINED AND STRICTLY MONITORED. THE ELDERLY ARE RESPECTED AND THE YOUNG ARE DEARLY LOVED. THE PUERTO RICAN FAMILY, HOWEVER, ENCOMPASSES NOT ONLY THOSE RELATED BY BLOOD AND MARRIAGE, BUT ALSO THOSE TIED TO IT THROUGH CUSTOM. 29 REFERENCES (PASAR ABSTRACT MODIFIED)

ACCN 001071

1251 AUTH **MOCHIZUKI, M.**

TITL DISCHARGES AND UNITS OF SERVICE BY ETHNIC ORIGIN: FISCAL YEAR 1973-1974.

SRCE *E & R ROWS AND COLUMNS, COUNTY OF LOS ANGELES, DEPARTMENT OF HEALTH SERVICES, MENTAL HEALTH SERVICES, 1975, 3(11), 1-15.*

INDX CROSS CULTURAL, HEALTH DELIVERY SYSTEMS, RESOURCE UTILIZATION, MEXICAN AMERICAN, SPANISH SURNAMED, EMPIRICAL, DEMOGRAPHIC, REPRESENTATION, CALIFORNIA, SOUTHWEST

ABST THE ETHNIC DISTRIBUTION OF INDIVIDUALS DISCHARGED FROM LOS ANGELES COUNTY SHORT-DOYLE SERVICES DURING THE FISCAL YEAR 1973-74 AND THE AMOUNT OF SERVICE ATTRIBUTED TO EACH OF THE IDENTIFIED ETHNIC GROUPS WERE EXAMINED, WITH A COMPARISON OF THE AMOUNT OF SERVICES PROVIDED TO EACH ETHNIC GROUP WITH THEIR DISTRIBUTION IN THE TOTAL LOS ANGELES COUNTY POPULATION. BESIDES SHORT-DOYLE RECORDS, DATA SOURCES INCLUDED 1970 CENSUS ETHNIC ORIGIN DATA AND AN APRIL 1974 ESTIMATE OF ETHNIC COMPOSITION DEVELOPED BY THE GREATER LOS ANGELES COMMUNITY ACTION AGENCY (GLACAA). DATA PRESENTED IN THE REPORT INDICATE THAT SPANISH SURNAME (SS), ASIAN, NATIVE AMERICAN AND OTHER NON-WHITE MINORITIES HAVE BEEN AND CONTINUE TO BE UNDERREPRESENTED IN SHORT-DOYLE SERVICES COMPARED TO THEIR REPRESENTATION IN THE TOTAL COUNTY POPULATION. THE EXTENT OF SS UNDERREPRESENTATION AMONG DISCHARGE AND UNITS OF SERVICE DATA IS NOTABLE. ALTHOUGH THESE DISPARITIES BETWEEN SERVICE STATISTICS AND DISTRIBUTION IN TOTAL COUNTY POPULATION ARE NOT DISCUSSED

WITHIN THE STUDY, POSSIBLE CAUSES ARE BRIEFLY MENTIONED. 4 REFERENCES.

ACCN 001072

1252 AUTH **MOERK, E.**

TITL THE ACCULTURATION OF THE MEXICAN-AMERICAN MINORITY TO THE ANGLO-AMERICAN SOCIETY IN THE UNITED STATES.

SRCE *JOURNAL OF HUMAN RELATIONS, 1972, 20(3), 317-325.*

INDX ACCULTURATION, MEXICAN AMERICAN, SES, BILINGUALISM, SCHOLASTIC ASPIRATIONS, OCCUPATIONAL ASPIRATIONS, ACHIEVEMENT MOTIVATION, REVIEW, CROSS CULTURAL, CHILDREN, ADOLESCENTS, EMPIRICAL, SOUTHWEST, VALUES

ABST THE ACCULTURATION OF THE MEXICAN AMERICAN (MA) INTO ANGLO-AMERICAN (AA) SOCIETY WAS INVESTIGATED IN A SAMPLE OF 446 ANGLO, BLACK, AND MEXICAN AMERICAN ELEMENTARY AND HIGH SCHOOL STUDENTS, AGES 11 TO 17. SUBJECTS WERE ADMINISTERED A QUESTIONNAIRE DESIGNED TO DETERMINE EDUCATIONAL ASPIRATIONS, OCCUPATIONAL ASPIRATIONS, INCOME EXPECTATIONS, IDEAL FAMILY SIZE, AND THE TYPE OF MATERIAL POSSESSIONS DESIRED. DATA INDICATE THAT THERE WERE NO SIGNIFICANT DIFFERENCES IN EDUCATIONAL ASPIRATIONS BETWEEN MA'S AND AA'S. MA'S EXPERIENCED THE SAME PRESSURE TO ATTEND COLLEGE AND TO ACHIEVE ACADEMICALLY AS DID OTHER GROUPS. IN ADDITION, NO SIGNIFICANT DIFFERENCES IN OCCUPATIONAL ASPIRATIONS BETWEEN AA'S AND MA'S WERE FOUND. A TREND TOWARD HAVING A SMALL NUMBER OF CHILDREN WAS NOTED. A CHANGE IN VALUES AND ASPIRATIONS IN THE MA GROUP WAS CLEARLY EVIDENT. IT IS SUGGESTED THAT THE "CHICANO" OR LA RAZA MOVEMENT APPEARS TO BE A PROBABLE CAUSAL LINK IN ATTITUDINAL CHANGE. THE DEVELOPMENT OF STRONG ETHNIC ORGANIZATIONS WHICH REPRESENT THESE NEW VALUES AND PROVIDE MODELS TO IDENTIFY WITH COULD BE OF IMPORTANCE TO THE YOUNGER MA POPULATION. 21 REFERENCES.

ACCN 001073

1253 AUTH **MOERK, E. L.**

TITL ACCULTURATION OF THE OFFSPRING OF ETHNIC MINORITIES OF THE ANGLO-AMERICAN SOCIETY IN THE UNITED STATES.

SRCE *IN J. L. M. DAWSON & W. J. LONNER (EDS.), READINGS IN CROSS CULTURAL PSYCHOLOGY: PROCEEDINGS OF THE INAUGURAL MEETING OF THE INTERNATIONAL ASSOCIATION FOR CROSS CULTURAL PSYCHOLOGY HELD IN HONG KONG, AUGUST, 1972. HONG KONG: HONG KONG UNIVERSITY PRESS, 1974, PP. 304-317.*

INDX ACCULTURATION, ATTITUDES, SOCIAL MOBILITY, OCCUPATIONAL ASPIRATIONS, SES, RESEARCH METHODOLOGY, URBAN, ADOLESCENTS, ADULTS, CROSS CULTURAL, EMPIRICAL, MEXICAN AMERICAN, CALIFORNIA, SOUTHWEST

ABST THE DYNAMICS OF MODEL TRANSMISSION

AND ACCULTURATION WERE EXPLORED THROUGH THE MEASUREMENT OF CHANGES IN FUTURE PLANS AND ASPIRATIONS OF 443 ANGLO, BLACK, MEXICAN AMERICAN, AND ORIENTAL ADOLESCENTS AND YOUNG ADULTS OVER A FOUR YEAR PERIOD. SUBJECTS WERE ADMINISTERED A QUESTIONNAIRE ON THEIR EDUCATIONAL, OCCUPATIONAL, AND INCOME ASPIRATIONS IN 1967 AND AGAIN IN 1971. INITIAL COMPARISON FOUND THAT THE ORIENTALS RANKED HIGHEST THROUGHOUT, THE ANGLOS OCCUPIED SECOND PLACE, AND MEXICAN AMERICANS RANKED LAST. BY 1971, HOWEVER, THE DIFFERENCES BETWEEN THE ETHNIC GROUPS HAD DIMINISHED CONSIDERABLY. THE ASPIRATIONS OF ANGLOS HAD DECLINED SOMEWHAT, WHILE THOSE OF THE MEXICAN AMERICANS AND ESPECIALLY THE BLACKS INCREASED CONSIDERABLY. SPECIFICALLY, BY 1971 BLACKS' ASPIRATIONS SURPASSED THOSE OF ANGLOS; AND THOUGH MEXICAN AMERICANS HAD VERY LOW ASPIRATIONS IN 1967, BY 1971 THEY CAME TO OCCUPY THE SAME POSITION IN RELATION TO ANGLOS THAT BLACKS OCCUPIED IN 1967. IT IS SUGGESTED THAT BY CLOSELY APPROACHING THE MAJORITY GROUP IN FINANCIAL AND EDUCATIONAL ASPIRATIONS, MEXICAN AMERICANS ARE MAKING THE FIRST MOVE TOWARD ASPIRATIONAL ASSIMILATION. IF SUCH ASPIRATIONS ARE PREDICTORS OF ECONOMIC SUCCESS, THEN THESE MINORITY GROUPS SHOULD ATTAIN ECONOMIC SUCCESS IN THE COURSE OF ONE GENERATION. MORE SYSTEMATIC APPROACHES MAY BE NEEDED, HOWEVER, TO ACQUAINT MINORITY GROUP MEMBERS WITH THE MEANS OF ACHIEVING THEIR ASPIRATIONS. 15 REFERENCES.

ACCN   002160

1254 AUTH   **MOERK, E. L.**
TITL   AGE AND EPOGENIC INFLUENCES ON ASPIRATIONS OF MINORITY AND MAJORITY GROUP CHILDREN.
SRCE   *JOURNAL OF COUNSELING PSYCHOLOGY, 1974, 21(4), 294-298.*
INDX   ADOLESCENTS, SCHOLASTIC ASPIRATIONS, EMPIRICAL, OCCUPATIONAL ASPIRATIONS, CHICANO MOVEMENT, MEXICAN AMERICAN, CROSS CULTURAL, ACHIEVEMENT MOTIVATION, SEX COMPARISON, SES, ENVIRONMENTAL FACTORS, CALIFORNIA, SOUTHWEST
ABST   THE ASPIRATIONS OF 48 ANGLO, 55 BLACK, AND 56 MEXICAN AMERICAN LOWER AND LOWER-MIDDLE SOCIOECONOMIC STATUS ADOLESCENTS WERE INVESTIGATED. THE STUDY COMBINED A CROSS-SECTIONAL APPROACH, A REPEATED MEASUREMENT DESIGN WITH MATCHED GROUPS, AND A LONGITUDINAL APPROACH. THE EXPECTATIONS OF MEXICAN AMERICANS WERE THE LOWEST AT THE TIME OF THE FIRST MEASUREMENT IN 1967, AND THOSE OF THE ANGLOS WERE THE HIGHEST. IN 1970, THE TIME OF THE SECOND MEASUREMENT, THE EXPECTATIONS OF THE MINORITY GROUPS HAD INCREASED AND THOSE OF THE ANGLO SUBJECTS HAD DECREASED OWING TO EPOGENIC INFLUENCES. IN THE

LONGITUDINAL STUDY THE ASPIRATIONS OF THE ANGLOS WERE STABLE, WHILE THE ASPIRATIONS OF THE MINORITY GROUP MEMBERS DECLINED. THE COUNTERACTING EFFECTS OF THE INCREASING AGE OF SUBJECTS AND OF THE EPOGENIC INFLUENCES ARE DISCUSSED. 8 REFERENCES. (JOURNAL ABSTRACT)
ACCN   001074

1255 AUTH   **MOERK, E., & BECKER, P.**
TITL   ATTITUDES OF HIGH SCHOOL STUDENTS TOWARD FUTURE MARRIAGE AND COLLEGE EDUCATION.
SRCE   *FAMILY COORDINATOR, 1971, 20(1), 67-73.*
INDX   CROSS CULTURAL, MEXICAN AMERICAN, ADOLESCENTS, ATTITUDES, SCHOLASTIC ACHIEVEMENT, SEXUAL BEHAVIOR, MARRIAGE, SEX COMPARISON, SES, BIRTH CONTROL, CALIFORNIA, SOUTHWEST, SCHOLASTIC ASPIRATIONS, VALUES
ABST   HIGH SCHOOL STUDENTS (119 MALE, 168 FEMALE) WERE ASKED TO JUDGE WHAT THE OPTIMAL AGES FOR MARRIAGE AND CHILBEARING WOULD BE FOR A YOUNG COUPLE, AND WHAT THEY SAW AS THE MOST CONVENIENT NUMBER OF CHILDREN IN THE FAMILY. THEIR COLLEGE PLANS AND THE IMPORTANCE THEY ATTRIBUTED TO HIGHER EDUCATION WERE ALSO DETERMINED. THE SUBJECTS WERE FROM LOWER CLASS NEIGHBORHOODS AND 40% WERE MEXICAN AMERICAN, 10% BLACK, 10% ORIENTAL AND 40% WHITE. THE RESULTS OF THE QUESTIONNAIRE STUDY WERE COMPARED WITH PREVIOUS INVESTIGATIONS, AND THE EFFECTS OF CULTURAL CHANGES, SOCIOECONOMIC CLASS, AGE AND SEX WERE ANALYZED AND PRESENTED. CONFLICTS BETWEEN FUTURE PLANS AND ACTUAL LIFE CHANCES OF THESE STUDENTS AND THE CONSEQUENCES OF THIS CONFLICT FOR THE INDIVIDUAL WERE CONSIDERED. SUGGESTED SOCIAL REFORMS WHICH ARE NEEDED TO KEEP UP WITH THE TRENDS IN VALUES AND EXPECTATIONS OF LOWER CLASS YOUTH ARE: (1) EDUCATIONAL INVESTMENT WITH REGARD TO SMALLER FAMILY SIZE; (2) MORE INTENSIVE VOCATIONAL COUNSELING TOGETHER WITH A DRASTIC REDIRECTION OF THE EDUCATIONAL GOALS AND INSTITUTIONS; (3) MORE SCHOLARSHIPS FOR STUDENTS FROM LOWER SOCIAL CLASS; AND (4) A JUNIOR HIGH SCHOOL CURRICULUM THAT HELPS FORM A WELL-ADAPTED VALUE SYSTEM WITH GOOD LIVING TECHNIQUES. 5 REFERENCES. (JOURNAL ABSTRACT MODIFIED)
ACCN   001075

1256 AUTH   **MOLL, L. C., RUEDA, R. S., REZA, R., HERRERA, J., & VASQUEZ, L. P.**
TITL   MENTAL HEALTH SERVICES IN EAST LOS ANGELES: AN URBAN COMMUNITY CASE STUDY.
SRCE   *IN M. R. MIRANDA (ED.), PSYCHOTHERAPY WITH THE SPANISH SPEAKING: ISSUES IN RESEARCH AND SERVICE DELIVERY (MONOGRAPH NO. 3). LOS ANGELES: UNIVERSITY OF CALIFORNIA, SPANISH SPEAKING MENTAL HEALTH RESEARCH CENTER, 1976, PP. 21-34.*
INDX   DEMOGRAPHIC, RESOURCE UTILIZATION,

HEALTH DELIVERY SYSTEMS, PSYCHOTHER-APY, ATTITUDES, PSYCHOTHERAPISTS, BILINGUAL-BICULTURAL PERSONNEL, POVERTY, PSYCHOPATHOLOGY, SES, EMPIRICAL, MEXICAN AMERICAN, ADULTS, URBAN, CALIFORNIA, SOUTHWEST

ABST   RESULTS OF A SURVEY CONDUCTED WITH BOTH THE CONSUMERS AND PROVIDERS OF A MENTAL HEALTH AGENCY IN EAST LOS ANGELES ARE PRESENTED. THE RESEARCH FOCUSES ON THESE AREAS: (1) A DEMOGRAPHIC PROFILE OF THE CONSUMER SAMPLE OF THE E.L.A. MENTAL HEALTH SERVICE; (2) THE CONSUMERS' AND PROVIDERS' PERCEPTIONS OF IMPORTANT FACTORS IN OBTAINING SERVICES; (3) AWARENESS OF ALTERNATIVE MENTAL HEALTH SYSTEMS AND PERCEPTIONS OF AVAILABLE SERVICES; (4) PERCEPTIONS OF THE SIGNIFICANCE OF LANGUAGE AND ETHNICITY IN SERVICE DELIVERY; (5) PERCEPTIONS OF UNMET MENTAL HEALTH NEEDS AND COMMUNITY PROBLEMS; AND (6) PERCEPTIONS OF CAUSES OF EMOTIONAL PROBLEMS. DIFFERENCES BETWEEN THIS STUDY'S FINDINGS AND PREVIOUS RESEARCH ARE DISCUSSED. AN INNOVATIVE STYLE OF INTERVIEWING USED IN COLLECTING DATA IS CREDITED WITH ELICITING MORE MEANINGFUL RESPONSES FROM CHICANO RESPONDENTS. 9 REFERENCES.

ACCN   001076

1257 AUTH   **MOLLER, D. A. T.**
TITL   FAMILY INTERACTION IN THE DEVELOPMENT OF GENDER IDENTITY IN MEXICAN-AMERICAN AND ANGLO ADOLESCENTS (DOCTORAL DISSERTATION, WASHINGTON STATE UNIVERSITY, 1976).
SRCE   *DISSERTATION ABSTRACTS INTERNATIONAL, 1975, 36(8), 5583A. (UNIVERSITY MICROFILMS NO. 76-4369.)*
INDX   FAMILY ROLES, CHILDREARING PRACTICES, SOCIALIZATION, GENDER IDENTITY, MEXICAN AMERICAN, CROSS CULTURAL, EMPIRICAL, SEX COMPARISON, WASHINGTON, WEST, ADOLESCENTS, RURAL
ABST   THE INFLUENCE OF CULTURAL AND FAMILY INTERACTIONAL VARIABLES ON THE DEVELOPMENT OF GENDER IDENTITY IN 158 MEXICAN AMERICAN AND 372 ANGLO ADOLESCENTS IS REPORTED. DATA ON SEX, ETHNICITY, PARENT SUPPORT, PARENT COMMUNICATION AND CONJUGAL POWER WERE OBTAINED FROM PERSONAL DATA BY INTERVIEW OR QUESTIONNAIRE AND FROM SCORES ON THE FOLLOWING SCALES: (1) PARENT-CHILD INTERACTION RATING SCALE; (2) FAMILY COMMUNICATION AND CLOSENESS SCALE; AND (3) CONJUGAL POWER SCALE. GENDER IDENTITY WAS MEASURED BY A MODIFIED VERSION OF THE TWENTY STATEMENTS TEST. THE FINDINGS REVEAL THAT GENDER IDENTITY IS MORE FREQUENT FOR MEXICAN AMERICANS THAN FOR ANGLOS. THE FAMILY INTERACTION VARIABLES OF CONJUGAL POWER AND COMMUNICATION/CLOSENESS WITH SAME-SEX OR CROSS-SEX PARENT HAD NO SIGNIFICANT EFFECT ON ADOLESCENT GENDER IDENTITY WITHOUT THE

CONTRIBUTING INFLUENCE OF ETHNICITY. SELF-SOCIALIZATION THEORY AND PATH ANALYSIS ARE USED TO DESCRIBE THE GENDER IDENTIFICATION PROCESS. THE NEED FOR FURTHER BREAKDOWN OF THIS CULTURAL VARIABLE—I.E., ITS FAMILIAL, SOCIAL AND ECONOMIC ASPECTS—IN EXPLAINING ETHNIC DIFFERENCES IN GENDER IDENTITY IS DISCUSSED. 90 REFERENCES.

ACCN   001077

1258 AUTH   **MONCARZ, R.**
TITL   EFFECTS OF PROFESSIONAL RESTRICTIONS ON CUBAN REFUGEES IN SELECTED HEALTH PROFESSIONS IN THE UNITED STATES 1959-1969.
SRCE   *INTERNATIONAL MIGRATION REVIEW, 1970, 4(2), 22-30.*
INDX   ACCULTURATION, CUBAN, OCCUPATIONAL ASPIRATIONS, DISCRIMINATION, EDUCATION, EMPIRICAL, PHYSICIANS, EQUAL OPPORTUNITY, LABOR FORCE, MIGRANTS, NURSING, PROFESSIONAL TRAINING, SURVEY, HEALTH, EMPLOYMENT
ABST   THIS STUDY ANALYZES THE EXTENT OF UTILIZATION OR UNDERUTILIZATION OF CUBAN-EDUCATED AND TRAINED PHYSICIANS, VETERINARIANS, OPTOMETRISTS, DENTISTS, PHARMACISTS, AND NURSES IN THE U.S. FROM 1959 TO 1969. THE TWO OBJECTIVES OF THE STUDY WERE TO (1) IDENTIFY INDIVIDUALS BY OCCUPATION OR PERSONAL CHARACTERISTICS WHO ADJUSTED WELL TO THE U.S., AND (2) IDENTIFY BARRIERS ENCOUNTERED BY CUBAN REFUGEES ATTEMPTING TO MAINTAIN THEIR PROFESSIONAL STATUS IN THE U.S. ONE HUNDRED QUESTIONNAIRES WERE SENT TO RANDOMLY SELECTED MEMBERS FROM EACH OCCUPATION. A SECOND QUESTIONNAIRE WAS SENT TO NON-RESPONDENTS, FOLLOWED BY DIRECT CONTACT WHENEVER POSSIBLE. FINALLY, PERSONAL INTERVIEWS WERE CONDUCTED WITH MEMBERS OF DIFFERENT HEALTH PROFESSIONS IN NEW YORK, CHICAGO, LOS ANGELES, AND MIAMI TO GAIN FURTHER INSIGHT INTO THE ADAPTATION PROCESS. THE CRUCIAL VARIABLES AFFECTING PROFESSIONAL ADAPTATION WERE: LEGAL STATUS; LANGUAGE; SEX; AGE; AVAILABILITY AND LENGTH OF RETRAINING PROGRAMS; ATTENDANCE IN SCHOOLS OR UNIVERSITIES; STATE AND LOCAL REQUIREMENTS TO PRACTICE A GIVEN PROFESSION; THE NEED FOR A LICENSE OR HIGHER DEGREE IN THE U.S.; AND EXTENT OF ABILITY TO CONTINUE IN THE FORMER PROFESSION. CLOSELY RELATED TO THE ADAPTATION PROCESS IS THE RECOGNITION EFFECT—I.E., FIRMS AND EMPLOYERS ACQUIRING CONFIDENCE IN THE ABILITY OF CUBANS AFTER THEY EMPLOY ONE. THE RECOGNITION EFFECT IS OF TREMENDOUS IMPORTANCE FOR ALL THE OCCUPATIONAL CATEGORIES UNDER STUDY BECAUSE OF THE LACK OF KNOWLEDGE ABOUT CUBANS MANIFESTED BY THE DIFFERENT NATIONAL ASSOCIATIONS, STATE BOARDS OF PROFESSIONAL PRACTICE, AND EMPLOYERS. 6 REFERENCES.

ACCN   002162

1259 AUTH **MONCARZ, R.**

TITL A MODEL OF PROFESSIONAL ADAPTATION OF REFUGEES: THE CUBAN CASE IN THE U.S. 1959-1970.

SRCE *INTERNATIONAL MIGRATION REVIEW, 1973, 11, 171-183.*

INDX EMPLOYMENT, IMMIGRATION, CUBAN, PHYSICIANS, NURSING, EDUCATION, PROFESSIONAL TRAINING, EMPIRICAL, ACCULTURATION

ABST TO ANALYZE THE EXTENT OF THE ADAPTIVE PROCESS OF REFUGEES TO A NEW ENVIRONMENT, THE EFFECT OF VARIOUS TRANSITION FACTORS WAS MEASURED AMONG 14 SELECTED OCCUPATIONAL GROUPS OF CUBANS. QUESTIONNAIRES WERE DISTRIBUTED TO 1,400 ARCHITECTS, CIVIL ENGINEERS, ELECTRICAL ENGINEERS, PHYSICIANS, OPTOMETRISTS, VETERINARIANS, PHARMACISTS, LAWYERS, TEACHERS, NURSES, PILOTS, TELEPHONE WORKERS, BEAUTICIANS, AND ACCOUNTANTS. LINEAR REGRESSION ANALYSIS OF DATA OBTAINED FROM 572 RESPONDENTS STRONGLY INDICATED THAT OCCUPATIONAL ADAPTATION IS A FUNCTION OF LEGAL STATUS, SELF-EMPLOYMENT, AVAILABILITY AND LENGTH OF RETRAINING PROGRAMS, ATTENDANCE AT SCHOOLS OR UNIVERSITIES, STATE AND LOCAL REQUIREMENTS TO PRACTICE A GIVEN PROFESSION, LICENSE OF HIGHER DEGREE IN THE UNITED STATES, EXTENT OF ABILITY TO CONTINUE IN FORMER PROFESSION, AND THE COMMON PRODUCTIVITY VARIABLES OF AGE AND SEX. ALSO CLOSELY RELATED WITH THE ADAPTATION PROCESS WERE THE AGE EFFECT (INVERSE RELATIONSHIP BETWEEN AGE AND ABILITY TO LEARN A LANGUAGE), AND THE RECOGNITION EFFECT (FIRMS AND EMPLOYERS ACQUIRING CONFIDENCE IN THE ABILITIES OF CUBANS AFTER THEY EMPLOY ONE). 3 REFERENCES.

ACCN 002161

1260 AUTH **MONDALE, W. F., GONZALEZ, H. B., & ROYBAL, E. R.**

TITL EDUCATION FOR THE SPANISH SPEAKING: THE ROLE OF THE FEDERAL GOVERNMENT.

SRCE *THE NATIONAL ELEMENTARY PRINCIPAL, 1970, 50(2), 116-122.*

INDX EDUCATION, EQUAL OPPORTUNITY, SPANISH SURNAMED, LEGISLATION, ESSAY, POLICY, BILINGUAL-BICULTURAL EDUCATION

ABST THREE VIEWS ON THE PROGRESS AND DEFICIENCIES OF THE NATIONAL BILINGUAL EDUCATION PROGRAM UNDER TITLE VII OF THE ELEMENTARY AND SECONDARY EDUCATION ACT, PASSED IN 1968, ARE PRESENTED. EACH POINTS OUT THAT FUNDING FOR BILINGUAL PROGRAMS HAS BEEN LIMITED AND SLOW TO COME EVEN WITH THIS NATIONAL LEGISLATION. EXISTING PROGRAMS IN TEXAS, FLORIDA AND CALIFORNIA CAN PROVIDE GUIDELINES FOR FUTURE PROGRAMS IN OTHER STATES. THE ROLE OF THE FEDERAL GOVERNMENT IN PROMOTING BILINGUAL EDUCATION FOR ALL WHO REQUIRE IT IS SEEN AS (1) PROVIDING FUNDS FOR THE DEVELOPMENT AND CONTINUED OPERATION OF ALL ASPECTS OF BILINGUAL EDUCATION—FROM THE TEACHING OF BILINGUAL TEACHERS TO THE DEVELOPMENT OF INSTRUCTIONAL MATERIALS, AND (2) COLLECTING AND DISSEMINATING RESEARCH AND EVALUATION DATA ON EXISTING PROGRAMS, METHODS AND MATERIALS. IT IS EMPHASIZED THAT THE WASTE, ABUSE AND HARM PAST EDUCATIONAL PROGRAMS HAVE CAUSED CAN BE REVERSED IF THE FEDERAL GOVERNMENT PROVIDES FORWARD-LOOKING, PROGRESSIVE LEADERSHIP IN BILINGUAL EDUCATION.

ACCN 001078

1261 AUTH **MONK, M., & WARSHAUER, E.**

TITL COMPLETED AND ATTEMPTED SUICIDE IN THREE ETHNIC GROUPS.

SRCE *AMERICAN JOURNAL OF EPIDEMIOLOGY, 1974, 100(4), 333-345.*

INDX CROSS CULTURAL, DEMOGRAPHIC, EMPIRICAL, ENVIRONMENTAL FACTORS, PUERTO RICAN-M, EAST, SUICIDE, SEX COMPARISON, NEW YORK

ABST TO EXAMINE ETHNIC DIFFERENTIALS IN SUICIDAL BEHAVIOR AND FACTORS ASSOCIATED WITH SUCH BEHAVIOR, COMPLETED AND ATTEMPTED SUICIDE RATES WERE DETERMINED FOR ADULT PUERTO RICANS, OTHER WHITES (HEREAFTER, WHITES) AND BLACKS LIVING IN EAST HARLEM. PUERTO RICAN MEN HAD THE HIGHEST RATES OF COMPLETED SUICIDE OF ALL GROUPS, AND PUERTO RICANS OF BOTH SEXES ATTEMPTED SUICIDE TWO TO THREE TIMES MORE OFTEN THAN EITHER BLACKS OR WHITES. WHITE WOMEN HAD RATES FOR COMPLETED SUICIDE AS HIGH AS THOSE FOR WHITE MEN AND THREE TIMES AS HIGH AS FOR BLACK WOMEN. OTHERWISE, WHITES HAD RATES OF COMPLETED AND ATTEMPTED SUICIDE ONLY SLIGHTLY HIGHER THAN BLACKS. IT IS SUGGESTED THAT PART OF THE DIFFERENCE BETWEEN WHITE AND BLACK SUICIDE RATES REPORTED ELSEWHERE MAY REFLECT DIFFERENTIAL REPORTING OR CLASSIFICATION OF DEATHS FOR THE TWO GROUPS. IN THIS STUDY, THE USE OF INFORMATION FROM MEDICAL EXAMINER RECORDS RESULTED IN HIGHER RATES THAN USUALLY REPORTED AND A VERY SMALL DIFFERENCE BETWEEN WHITE AND BLACK MEN. THE HIGH RATES FOR WHITE WOMEN RESULTED PARTLY FROM THE INCLUSION OF DEATHS FROM BARBITURATE INGESTION THAT HAD ORIGINALLY BEEN CLASSIFIED AS "UNDETERMINED." THE HIGH ATTEMPTED RATES FOR PUERTO RICANS REMAIN UNEXPLAINED, ALTHOUGH MIGRATION AND ECONOMIC CONDITIONS MAY PLAY A PART. 24 REFERENCES. (JOURNAL ABSTRACT MODIFIED)

ACCN 002385

1262 AUTH **MONTALVO, B.**

TITL HOME-SCHOOL CONFLICT AND THE PUERTO RICAN CHILD.

SRCE *SOCIAL CASEWORK, 1974, 55(2), 100-110.*

INDX PUERTO RICAN-M, CHILDREN, EDUCATION, CASE STUDY, CULTURAL FACTORS, FAMILY STRUCTURE, PARENTAL INVOLVEMENT

ABST THE DIFFICULTIES ENCOUNTERED BY BOTH SCHOOLS AND PARENTS IN THE EDUCATION

OF PUERTO RICAN CHILDREN IN THE U. S. ARE DISCUSSED. ALTHOUGH, ON A SUPERFICIAL LEVEL, SCHOOLS SEEM TO BE MORE RESPONSIVE TO THE NEEDS OF PUERTO RICAN STUDENTS, THEIR FAMILIES AND CULTURE, MANY INSTANCES OF MISUNDERSTANDING AND DISCRIMINATION STILL OCCUR, RESULTING IN A CONTINUED HIGH DROPOUT AND LOW EMPLOYMENT RATE FOR YOUNG PUERTO RICANS. SEVERAL CITIES WITH SUBSTANTIAL PUERTO RICAN ENROLLMENTS HAVE INTIATED SPECIAL SCHOOL PROGRAMS WITH TITLE VII FUNDS. DESPITE THESE SPECIAL PROJECTS AND GOOD INTENTIONS, THE EDUCATION OF PUERTO RICAN CHILDREN IS DETRIMENTALLY AFFECTED BY THE CONTINUED LACK OF KNOWLEDGE AND APPRECIATION OF PUERTO RICAN FAMILY AND CULTURAL PATTERNS BY SCHOOL PERSONNEL. THE MOST OUTSTANDING PROBLEMS CONTINUE TO BE THOSE MOST CLOSELY RELATED TO CULTURAL DIFFERENCES. SIX CASE STUDIES ILLUSTRATE THAT MANY YOUNGSTERS ARE STILL PLACED IN CONFLICT SITUATIONS REGARDING THEIR LANGUAGE, APPEARANCE, RELATIONSHIP STYLE AND ASPIRATIONS. THE REPARATORY APPROACHES DEVELOPED BY SCHOOLS TO DEAL WITH THESE CONFLICT SITUATIONS ARE UNSYSTEMATIC AND FRAGMENTARY, LEAVING UNTOUCHED THE OVERALL NEED FOR CHANGE IN THE RELATIONSHIPS OF SCHOOL, FAMILY, PEER GROUP, AND CHILD. THE PROBLEMS RESULTING FROM THIS INTERACTION WILL CONTINUE AS LONG AS THESE RELATIONSHIPS ARE MISUNDERSTOOD. IT IS FELT THAT MORE INFORMATION ABOUT THESE HOME-SCHOOL CONFLICTS IS NEEDED BEFORE THE REACHING-OUT TEACHER, CONSCIENTIOUS COUNSELOR, OR EVEN THE CHANGED TEACHER-TRAINING INSTITUTION OR COMPENSATORY BILINGUAL PROGRAM CAN BE EFFECTIVE. 2 REFERENCES.

ACCN   001079

1263 AUTH   **MONTENEGRO, M.**

TITL   CHICANOS AND MEXICAN-AMERICANS: ETHNIC SELF-IDENTIFICATION AND ATTITUDINAL DIFFERENCES.

SRCE   *SAN FRANCISCO: R AND E RESEARCH ASSOCIATES, 1976.*

INDX   ETHNIC IDENTITY, MEXICAN AMERICAN, DISCRIMINATION, ATTITUDES, OCCUPATIONAL ASPIRATIONS, SCHOLASTIC ASPIRATIONS, SOCIAL MOBILITY, EMPIRICAL, ADOLESCENTS, RELIGION, SEX ROLES, CALIFORNIA, SOUTHWEST, CULTURAL CHANGE

ABST   THE HYPOTHESIS THAT YOUNG PEOPLE OF LATIN EXTRACTION WILL TEND TO IDENTIFY THEMSELVES AS EITHER CHICANO OR MEXICAN AMERICAN AND THAT SUCH SELF-IDENTIFICATION WILL IMPLY ATTITUDINAL DIFFERENCES ON SOME SPECIFIC ACTIVITIES (I.E., MATERIAL SUCCESS, SERVICE IN THE ARMED FORCES, RELIGIOUS ATTACHMENT, EDUCATIONAL AND OCCUPATIONAL ASPIRATIONS, SEX ROLES AND DISCRIMINATION) WAS TESTED ON 109 11TH-12TH GRADE STUDENTS ATTENDING A HIGH SCHOOL IN EAST LOS ANGELES.

RESULTS INDICATE THAT THOSE WHO IDENTIFY THEMSELVES AS MEXICAN AMERICAN (1) ARE RELIGIOUS PEOPLE WHO ATTEND CHURCH REGULARLY, (2) WISH FOR HIGHER EDUCATION WHICH THEY MAY NOT OBTAIN, (3) SEE HARD WORK AS THE ROAD TO SUCCESS, (4) PLAN TO SERVE IN THE ARMED FORCES EVEN THOUGH THEY ARE NOT "PROWAR," (5) CONTINUE TO VIEW MEN AND WOMEN AS HAVING DISTINCT ROLES WITHIN THE FAMILY, AND (6) GENERALLY DO NOT BELIEVE THEY ARE VICTIMS OF DISCRIMINATION. CHICANOS, ON THE OTHER HAND, ARE (1) MOVING AWAY FROM CATHOLICISM TOWARD SECULARIZATION, (2) SEEKING HIGHER EDUCATION BUT OBTAINING IT ONLY A LITTLE MORE FREQUENTLY THAN MEXICAN AMERICANS, (3) REJECTING HARD WORK AND COMPETITION AS THE PRIMARY WORK VALUE, (4) NOT PLANNING SERVICE IN THE ARMED FORCES, (5) VIEWING BOTH MEN AND WOMEN AS SHARING ROLES AND FUNCTIONS WITHIN THE FAMILY, AND (6) VIEWING THEMSELVES AS VICTIMS OF DISCRIMINATION. CHANGES AND DIFFERENCES WITHIN THE ETHNIC GROUPS ARE DISCUSSED IN RELATION TO THESE FINDINGS. 66 REFERENCES. (AUTHOR SUMMARY MODIFIED)

ACCN   001080

1264 AUTH   **MONTIEL, M.**

TITL   THE CHICANO FAMILY: A REVIEW OF RESEARCH.

SRCE   *SOCIAL WORK, 1973, 18(2), 22-31.*

INDX   MEXICAN AMERICAN, FAMILY STRUCTURE, FAMILY ROLES, REVIEW, EXTENDED FAMILY, ACCULTURATION, SEX ROLES, RESEARCH METHODOLOGY, STEREOTYPES, MACHISMO

ABST   SOCIAL SCIENCE LITERATURE ON THE CHICANO HAS OFTEN POSED FALLACIOUS PREMISES TO EXPLAIN HIS LOW STATUS IN TERMS OF RECENT IMMIGRATION, MARGINALITY, TRADITIONAL CULTURE OR CULTURAL DEPRIVATION. NEW ALTERNATIVE MODELS ARE DISCUSSED TO PROVIDE A HOLISTIC RATHER THAN A PATHOLOGICAL OR CORRECTIVE MODE OF INTERVENTION. A REVIEW OF THE EXISTING LITERATURE REVEALS THE FOLLOWING GENERALIZATIONS, ALL OF WHICH HAVE NO REALITY BASIS: (1) THE CHICANO FAMILY, UNLESS ACCULTURATED OR MODERNIZED, IS CALLED A "TRADITIONAL EXTENDED FAMILY" DESPITE CONTRARY EMPIRICAL EVIDENCE; (2) OTHER INDICATORS OF FAMILY STRUCTURE (E.G., COMPADRAZGO AND MACHISMO) ARE STILL SEEN AS PREVAILING DESPITE CHANGES FROM TRADITIONAL NORMS; AND (3) THE MACHISMO CULT IS SEEN AS DETERMINING THE INDIVIDUAL'S ROLE WITHIN THE FAMILY AS WELL AS EXPLAINING THE PATHOLOGY WITHIN IT. FURTHER, REMEDIES AND INTERVENTION STRATEGIES FOR HELPING CHICANOS ARE SEEN AS TRYING TO CHANGE THE INDIVIDUALS' ATTITUDES AND LANGUAGE TO ASSIMILATE THEM MORE INTO THE MIDDLE CLASS ANGLO CULTURE. OVERALL, THE CHICANO IS REPRESENTED IN SOCIAL SCIENCE LITERATURE AS BEING LOW INCOME, CULTURALLY INFERIOR, AND RESPONSIBLE FOR HIS POVERTY;

INTERVENTION TECHNIQUES ARE AIMED AT DENYING THE INDIVIDUAL HIS CULTURE AND TAKING ON MAJORITY CULTURE CHARACTERISTICS. SUGGESTIONS ARE MADE FOR INTERVENTION PROGRAMS WHICH HAVE A GREATER SCOPE AND AN IMPLICIT UNDERSTANDING OF CHICANOS IN MANY CONTEXTS. 57 REFERENCES.

ACCN 001081

1265 AUTH **MONTIEL, M.**
TITL THE SOCIAL SCIENCE MYTH OF THE MEXICAN AMERICAN FAMILY.
SRCE *EL GRITO, 1970, 3(4), 56-63.*
INDX MEXICAN AMERICAN, FAMILY STRUCTURE, FAMILY ROLES, MEXICAN, ESSAY, SEX ROLES, STEREOTYPES, MACHISMO
ABST THE MYTH OF THE MEXICAN FAMILY HAS BEEN CREATED BECAUSE OF CERTAIN QUESTIONABLE ASSUMPTIONS THAT HAVE DOMINATED MEXICAN AND MEXICAN AMERICAN FAMILY STUDIES. SOCIAL SCIENTISTS HAVE REGARDED MACHISMO AS THE UNDERLYING CAUSE OF MEXICAN AND MEXICAN AMERICAN PROBLEMS. AS A RESULT, THESE POPULATIONS HAVE BEEN LABELED AS REFLECTING VARIOUS DEGREES OF SICKNESS. TERMS LIKE MACHISMO ARE ABSTRACT, VALUE-LADEN CONCEPTS THAT LACK THE EMPIRICAL REFERENTS NECESSARY FOR CONSTRUCTION OF SOUND EXPLANATIONS. ACCORDINGLY, AS LONG AS RESEARCH ON THE MEXICAN AND MEXICAN AMERICAN FAMILY IS GUIDED BY ANYTHING OTHER THAN SOUND OPERATIONAL DEFINITIONS ITS FINDINGS, CONCLUSIONS, AND INTERPRETATIONS MUST BE SEEN ONLY AS PHILOSOPHICAL AND IDEOLOGICAL SPECULATIONS, NOT AS EMPIRICAL TRUTHS. 14 REFERENCES. (AUTHOR SUMMARY MODIFIED)

ACCN 001082

1266 AUTH **MONTIEL, M. (ED)**
TITL HISPANIC FAMILIES: CRITICAL ISSUES FOR POLICY AND PROGRAMS IN HUMAN SERVICES.
SRCE *WASHINGTON, D.C.: NATIONAL COALITION OF HISPANIC MENTAL HEALTH AND HUMAN SERVICES ORGANIZATIONS (COSSMHO), 1978.*
INDX ESSAY, EMPIRICAL, PUERTO RICAN-I, CUBAN, MEXICAN AMERICAN, GERONTOLOGY, BOOK, FAMILY ROLES, FAMILY STRUCTURE, HEALTH DELIVERY SYSTEMS, POVERTY, ECONOMIC FACTORS, ADOLESCENTS, HEALTH, MENTAL HEALTH, POLICY, CULTURAL FACTORS, SPANISH SURNAMED, FOLK MEDICINE, SOCIAL SERVICES, ADULTS, CULTURAL PLURALISM, VALUES
ABST THIS COLLECTION OF EIGHT PAPERS EXAMINES THE HISTORICAL PROCESSES, CULTURAL VALUES, AND SOCIOECONOMIC CONDITIONS IMPACTING ON HISPANIC FAMILIES, AND IT EXPLORES THE IMPLICATIONS FOR IMPROVED SOCIAL POLICY AND PROGRAMS THAT WILL BENEFIT THESE FAMILIES. THE TOPICS COVERED IN THESE PAPERS INCLUDE: (1) A GENERAL REVIEW PROVIDING BACKGROUND INFORMATION ON THE HISPANIC FAMILY; (2) A HUMANISTIC MODEL FOR THE DELIVERY OF

SERVICES TO HISPANICS; (3) AN OVERVIEW OF THE HISTORICAL ECONOMIC DISPARITIES BETWEEN HISPANICS AND ANGLOS; (4) INTERGENERATIONAL SOURCES OF ROLE CONFLICT IN CUBAN AMERICAN MOTHERS; (5) THE VULNERABILITY OF POOR FAMILIES IN SAN JUAN, PUERTO RICO; (6) RECOMMENDATIONS FOR AMELIORATING THE PROBLEMS SUFFERED BY HISPANIC YOUTHS IN THE U.S.; (7) THE INSENSITIVITY OF HEALTH CARE SERVICES TO THE CULTURAL AND OTHER SPECIAL NEEDS OF HISPANIC ELDERLY; AND (8) AN ASSESSMENT OF THE RESPONSIVENESS OF THE OLDER AMERICANS ACT TO THE NEEDS OF MINORITY ELDERLY. THE BASIC MESSAGE EMPHASIZED THROUGHOUT THE BOOK IS THAT HISPANICS AS A GROUP ARE POOR, UNDEREDUCATED, AND UNDERSERVED; AND THE FUTURE FOR HISPANICS DOES NOT LOOK PROMISING UNLESS DRAMATIC ACTION IS TAKEN BY ACADEMICIANS, PLANNERS, POLICY MAKERS, AND PUBLIC OFFICIALS. 81 REFERENCES.

ACCN 001782

1267 AUTH **MONTIJO, J.**
TITL THE PUERTO RICAN CLIENT.
SRCE *PROFESSIONAL PSYCHOLOGY, 1975, 6(4), 475-477.*
INDX PUERTO RICAN-M, PSYCHOTHERAPISTS, ATTITUDES, PSYCHOTHERAPY, ROLE EXPECTATIONS, CONFORMITY, MENTAL HEALTH, SEX ROLES, FAMILY ROLES, CULTURAL FACTORS, ESSAY, POLICY, VALUES
ABST THE PROBLEMS OF PROVIDING RELEVANT PSYCHOTHERAPY TO PUERTO RICANS BY NONHISPANIC THERAPISTS ARE DISCUSSED. THE NONHISPANIC THERAPIST NEEDS TO BE AWARE THAT THE MAJORITY OF PUERTO RICAN PATIENTS COME FROM LOWER SOCIOECONOMIC FAMILIES AND THAT EITHER THEY OR THEIR PARENTS WERE BORN IN PUERTO RICO. THEREFORE, THEY ARE LIKELY TO SPEAK SPANISH AT HOME AND ADHERE TO THE ISLAND'S CUSTOMS AND VALUES. THE MIGRATION TO THE MAINLAND HAS, FOR MANY, PRODUCED FEELINGS OF POWERLESSNESS, FATALISM, MISTRUST, LOSS OF EXTERNAL CONTROL OVER THEIR LIVES, AND SUBMISSION TO THOSE OCCUPYING POSITIONS OF AUTHORITY. IN ADDITION, IT IS IMPORTANT FOR THE NONHISPANIC THERAPIST TO RECOGNIZE THE CULTURAL DIFFERENCES AND VALUES ASSOCIATED WITH THE FAMILY AND SEX ROLES OF PUERTO RICANS. THE THERAPEUTIC IMPLICATIONS AND SUGGESTIONS FOR DEVELOPING TRUST IN THESE CLIENTS ARE BRIEFLY DISCUSSED.

ACCN 001083

1268 AUTH **MONTOYA, J. M.**
TITL BILINGUAL-BICULTURAL EDUCATION: MAKING EQUAL EDUCATIONAL OPPORTUNITIES AVAILABLE TO NATIONAL ORIGIN MINORITY STUDENTS.
SRCE *THE GEORGETOWN LAW JOURNAL, 1973, 61(4), 991-1007.*
INDX EDUCATION, BILINGUAL-BICULTURAL EDUCATION, EQUAL OPPORTUNITY, LEGISLATION, RE-

VIEW, SPANISH SURNAMED, POLICY, FINANC-
ING, CROSS CULTURAL

ABST   A RECENT DEVELOPMENT IN THE MOVEMENT
TO ENSURE EQUAL EDUCATIONAL OPPORTU-
NITY HAS BEEN INCREASED CONCERN WITH
THE EDUCATIONAL TREATMENT OF NATIONAL
ORIGIN MINORITY STUDENTS IN AMERICA. THE
LINGUISTIC HANDICAPS OF NATIONAL ORIGIN
MINORITY STUDENTS, THEIR CONSEQUENT IN-
ABILITY TO TAKE FULL ADVANTAGE OF AN EN-
GLISH-SPEAKING EDUCATIONAL SYSTEM, AND
THE NEED FOR BILINGUAL-BICULTURAL EDU-
CATIONAL PROGRAMS ARE DISCUSSED. IN AD-
DITION, THE CONCEPT OF BILINGUAL-BICUL-
TURAL EDUCATION AND THE LEGAL RIGHT OF
NATIONAL ORIGIN MINORITY STUDENTS TO RE-
CEIVE SUCH AN EDUCATION ARE EXAMINED.
104 REFERENCES. (JOURNAL ABSTRACT MODI-
FIED)

ACCN   001084

1269 AUTH   **MONTOYA, R.**
TITL   TESTIMONY TO THE CALIFORNIA DEMOCRATIC
PLATFORM COMMISSION ON HEALTH AND
WELFARE COMMITTEE.
SRCE   *PAPER PRESENTED TO THE CALIFORNIA DEMO-
CRATIC PLATFORM COMMISSION ON HEALTH
AND WELFARE COMMITTEE, FEBRUARY 14, 1976.*
INDX   MEXICAN AMERICAN, HEALTH, PHYSICIANS,
MENTAL HEALTH PROFESSION, REPRESENTA-
TION, DISCRIMINATION, COLLEGE STUDENTS,
EQUAL OPPORTUNITY, POLICY, HIGHER EDU-
CATION, FINANCING, POLITICS, ESSAY
ABST   THE LACK OF MINORITY HEALTH PERSONNEL
IS CONSIDERED TO BE ONE OF THE MAJOR
CAUSES OF POOR HEALTH CARE AND POOR
HEALTH STATUS AMONG PEOPLE REPRESENT-
ING MINORITY COMMUNITIES. AS A RESULT OF
FEDERALLY SUPPORTED MINORITY RECRUIT-
MENT AND RETENTION PROGRAMS, THERE
HAS BEEN AN INCREASE IN THE NUMBER OF
MINORITY ENROLLMENTS IN HEALTH PROFES-
SIONAL SCHOOLS. HOWEVER, THIS INCREASE
HAS NOT REACHED THE POINT OF BEING REP-
RESENTATIVE OF THE MINORITY POPULATION.
THE CHARGE OF "REVERSE DISCRIMINATION"
WHICH THREATENS THE INCREASING MI-
NORITY APPLICANTS IS BASED ON THE FALLA-
CIOUS ARGUMENT THAT QUALIFIED NONMI-
NORITY APPLICANTS ARE REJECTED FOR
UNQUALIFIED MINORITY APPLICANTS. BUT THIS
IS NOT THE CASE; MORE NONMINORITY APPLI-
CANTS CONTINUE TO BE ACCEPTED INTO
HEALTH PROFESSIONAL SCHOOLS. CRITERIA
USED TO DETERMINE WHO IS QUALIFIED ARE
CULTURALLY BIASED, AND MINORITY STU-
DENTS WHO HAD LOWER QUALIFICATIONS
HAVE DONE FAIRLY WELL IN SCHOOL. TWO
FEDERAL PROGRAMS, THE NATIONAL HEALTH
SERVICES CORPS AND THE PUBLIC HEALTH
SERVICE SCHOLARSHIP PROGRAM, ARE VIEWED
AS HAVING POSITIVE IMPACT ON HEALTH CARE
WITHIN THE MINORITY COMMUNITY AND RE-
CRUITMENT OF MINORITY PERSONNEL IN
AREAS OF HEALTH. IT IS RECOMMENDED THAT
THE DEMOCRATIC PARTY ADOPT BOTH OF
THESE PROGRAMS IN THEIR PLATFORM. ADDI-
TIONAL EVIDENCE CONCERNING MINORITY

ENROLLMENT IN RELATED HEALTH FIELDS AND
QUESTIONS REGARDING THE VALIDITY OF AD-
MISSIONS REQUIREMENTS ARE INCLUDED IN
THIS TESTIMONY TO THE HEALTH AND WEL-
FARE COMMITTEE OF THE DEMOCRATIC PLAT-
FORM. 14 REFERENCES.

ACCN   001085

1270 AUTH   **MOORE, J. W.**
TITL   COLONIALISM: THE CASE OF THE MEXICAN
AMERICANS.
SRCE   *SOCIAL PROBLEMS, 1970, 17(4), 463-472.*
INDX   DISCRIMINATION, PREJUDICE, MEXICAN
AMERICAN, CULTURE, ECONOMIC FACTORS,
POLITICAL POWER, HISTORY, MIGRATION, IM-
MIGRATION, CULTURAL CHANGE, STEREO-
TYPES, SOUTHWEST, ESSAY
ABST   "COLONIALISM" HAS BEEN INCREASINGLY USED
BY MINORITY IDEOLOGUES TO ACCOUNT FOR
THEIR SITUATION IN THE UNITED STATES.
ADAPTING THE CONCEPT FOR SOCIAL SCI-
ENCES INVOLVES SERIOUS CONCEPTUAL
ANALYSIS. THIS IS AN ATTEMPT TO SPECIFY
THE CONCEPT IN THE CASE OF MEXICAN
AMERICANS, WITH POLITICAL PARTICIPATION
ON THE ELITE AND ON THE MASS LEVEL ILLUS-
TRATING THE VARIETIES OF INTERNAL COLO-
NIALISM TO WHICH THIS POPULATION HAS
BEEN SUBJECTED. THREE "CULTURE AREAS"
ARE DELINEATED: NEW MEXICO, WITH "CLAS-
SIC COLONIALISM"; TEXAS, WITH "CONFLICT
COLONIALISM"; AND CALIFORNIA, WITH "ECO-
NOMIC COLONIALISM." ECOLOGY OF SETTLE-
MENT, HISTORICAL DISCONTINUITIES, AND
PROPORTIONS OF VOLUNTARY-IMMIGRANT AS
COMPARED WITH CHARTER MEMBER DE-
SCENDANTS IN THE MINORITY ARE AMONG
THE FACTORS DISTINGUISHING THE THREE
TYPES. THE CHICANO MILITANT IDEOLOGY IN-
CORPORATES SYMBOLS WHICH ATTEMPT TO
TRANSCEND THESE REGIONAL DIFFERENCES.
14 REFERENCES.

ACCN   001087

1271 AUTH   **MOORE, J. W.**
TITL   MEXICAN AMERICANS AND CITIES: A STUDY IN
MIGRATION AND THE USE OF FORMAL RE-
SOURCES.
SRCE   *INTERNATIONAL MIGRATION REVIEW, 1971, 5(3),
292-308.*
INDX   ACCULTURATION, COPING MECHANISMS, CUL-
TURAL FACTORS, SES, FICTIVE KINSHIP, ECO-
NOMIC FACTORS, FAMILY STRUCTURE, PEER
GROUP, SOCIAL SERVICES, MALE, POLITICS,
MEXICAN, TEXAS, CALIFORNIA, SOUTHWEST,
HEALTH, HEALTH DELIVERY SYSTEMS, RE-
SOURCE UTILIZATION
ABST   CIRCUMSTANCES UNDER WHICH LOS ANGE-
LES MEXICAN AMERICAN MEN TURN TO FOR-
MAL OR INFORMAL, MEXICAN OR NON-MEXI-
CAN RESOURCES ARE EXPLORED. DATA WERE
DERIVED FROM A LARGE PROBABILITY SAMPLE
OF HOUSEHOLD HEADS AND SPOUSES (N UN-
SPECIFIED) OF DIVERSIFIED SES, INTERVIEWED
IN 1965-66. THE REPORT FOCUSES ON THE RE-
SPONSES TO FOUR SETS OF PROBLEM-RE-
SOURCE QUESTIONS: (1) PERSONAL PROB-
LEMS; (2) POLITICS; (3) MONEY MATTERS; AND

(4) RESOURCE UTILIZATION, I.E., WHERE TO GO IN THE CITY GOVERNMENT TO GET ASSISTANCE. THOUGH RESPONSES VARIED WIDELY, FORMAL SOURCES WERE MOST LIKELY TO BE UTILIZED FOR ADVICE OR HELP WITH, IN THIS ORDER: (1) THE CITY; (2) MONEY PROBLEMS; (3) POLITICAL MATTERS; AND (4) PERSONAL PROBLEMS. FORMALIZATION OF RESOURCES WAS ASSOCIATED WITH LENGTH OF RESIDENCE IN THE CITY, BUT BIRTHPLACE REVEALED A DIFFERENT PATTERN. THE DATA DO NOT SUPPORT THE THEORETICAL NOTION THAT URBANIZATION IS ASSOCIATED WITH ABANDONMENT OF PRIMARY-GROUP RESOURCES FOR THIS POPULATION. IN FACT, NATIVE ANGELENOS, WITH GREATER ACCESS TO "CHEAPER" SUPPORT SYSTEMS, STILL RESORT TO THEM. THE FINDINGS HAVE IMPLICATIONS FOR THEORIES OF URBANISM AS WELL AS FOR THE UNDERSTANDING OF MEXICAN AMERICANS. 21 REFERENCES.

ACCN   002163

1272 AUTH   **MOORE, J. W.**
TITL   MEXICAN AMERICANS.
SRCE   *GERONTOLOGIST, 1971, 2(1), 30-35.*
INDX   GERONTOLOGY, ESSAY, MEXICAN AMERICAN, CULTURE, FAMILY STRUCTURE
ABST   THE DISTINCTIVE AGE PATTERNS OF MEXICAN AMERICANS ARE DISCUSSED. IT IS CONCLUDED THAT MOST OF THE GROWING LITERATURE ON MEXICAN AMERICANS HAS INTERESTING IMPLICATIONS FOR A STUDY OF THE ELDERLY IN THE POPULATION. FAMILY STRUCTURE, COMMUNITY PATTERNS, GEOGRAPHIC, SOCIAL AND OCCUPATIONAL MOBILITY, AND THE DISTINCTIVE CHARACTERISTICS OF GENERATIONS AND OF INTERGENERATIONAL RELATIONS HAVE PARTICULARLY STRONG IMPLICATIONS FOR THE UNDERSTANDING OF NOT ONLY TODAY'S MEXICAN AMERICAN ELDERLY BUT ALSO THE PROCESS OF AGING PER SE AMONG MEXICAN AMERICANS. A FULL DELINEATION OF THE AGE-RELATED PATTERNS OF RESIDENCE, EDUCATION, INCOME, FAMILY STATUS, AND OTHER CHARACTERISTICS DERIVABLE FROM 1950, 1960, AND 1970 CENSUS DATA SHOULD BE A FIRST-ORDER PRIORITY IN RESEARCH. THE ACTUAL SOCIAL STRUCTURE OF AGE AS PERCEIVED BY THE ETHNIC GROUP SHOULD BE DELINEATED. 12 REFERENCES.
ACCN   001088

1273 AUTH   **MOORE, J. W.**
TITL   SITUATIONAL FACTORS AFFECTING MINORITY AGING.
SRCE   *GERONTOLOGIST, 1971, 11(PART 2), 88-93.*
INDX   GERONTOLOGY, ESSAY, SOCIAL STRUCTURE, DISCRIMINATION, STEREOTYPES, THEORETICAL, PREJUDICE, COPING MECHANISMS
ABST   RESEARCH ON MINORITY GROUPS AND MINORITY AGING CAN CONTRIBUTE GREATLY TO THE UNDERSTANDING OF AGING IN GENERAL. SEVERAL CHARACTERISTICS OF THE MINORITY SITUATION HAVE PARTICULAR RELEVANCE TO THE SITUATION IN WHICH THE ELDERLY FIND THEMSELVES. (1) EACH MINORITY HAS A SPE-

CIAL HISTORY AND COLLECTIVE EXPERIENCE SIMILAR TO THE "GENERATION GAP" EXPERIENCED BY THE ELDERLY. (2) THIS SPECIAL HISTORY HAS BEEN ACCOMPANIED BY SUBORDINATION, DISCRIMINATION, AND THE DEVELOPMENT OF NEGATIVE STEREOTYPES— A PATTERN REPEATED IN THE YOUNGER SOCIETY'S TREATMENT OF THE AGED. (3) EVERY MINORITY HAS DEVELOPED ITS OWN SUBCULTURE, INCLUDING VARIANT VALUES TOWARD WORK AND PERSONAL IDENTITY. (4) WITHIN THE MINORITY COMMUNITY, SUBSTRUCTURES HAVE BEEN DEVELOPED TO SUPPORT THE INDIVIDUAL IN COPING WITH ECONOMIC UNCERTAINTY AND A HOSTILE SOCIETY. THE DEVELOPMENT OF SUCH A SUPPORTIVE SOCIAL STRUCTURE IS CRUCIAL IN MEETING THE NEEDS OF THE ELDERLY. (5) ALTHOUGH DISCRIMINATORY PRACTICES AND ATTITUDES ARE CHANGING, EXPLOITATION AND PREJUDICE CONTINUE, OFTEN TAKING NEW FORMS. IN CONCLUSION, SPECIFIC ISSUES IN GERONTOLOGY (SUCH AS ISOLATION, COMMUNAL AND KIN-GROUP SUPPORT, NEW ROLES FOR OLD PEOPLE, AND SOCIETAL PLANNING FOR THE NEEDS OF THE ELDERLY) MAY BE EFFECTIVELY APPROACHED THROUGH MINORITY GROUP STUDIES. 7 REFERENCES.

ACCN   002164

1274 AUTH   **MOORE, J. W.**
TITL   SOCIAL CLASS, ASSIMILATION AND ACCULTURATION.
SRCE   *IN J. HELM (ED.), SPANISH-SPEAKING PEOPLE IN THE UNITED STATES, PROCEEDINGS OF THE 1968 ANNUAL SPRING MEETING OF THE AMERICAN ETHNOLOGICAL SOCIETY. SEATTLE: UNIVERSITY OF WASHINGTON PRESS, 1968, PP. 19-33.*
INDX   ACCULTURATION, SOCIAL MOBILITY, SES, CULTURE, ETHNIC IDENTITY, DEMOGRAPHIC, ENVIRONMENTAL FACTORS, TEXAS, CALIFORNIA, SOUTHWEST
ABST   A THEORETICAL APPROACH TO THE ANALYSIS OF SOCIAL CLASS STRATIFICATION AND ETHNIC AND RACIAL MINORITIES IS PRESENTED USING DATA GATHERED FROM MEXICAN AMERICAN ADULTS IN SAN ANTONIO AND LOS ANGELES. THE DATA SUGGEST: (1) THAT BOTH ASSIMILATION AND ACCULTURATION ARE OCCURRING AMONG THE MEXICAN AMERICANS STUDIED; (2) THAT BOTH ASSIMILATION AND ACCULTURATION OCCUR WITHIN A SOCIAL CLASS CONTEXT, BUT IN DIFFERENT WAYS FOR THOSE WHO REMAIN IN THE HIGH DENSITY MINORITY AREAS SUCH AS IN SAN ANTONIO AND THOSE WHO LIVE IN MORE MIXED NEIGHBORHOODS SUCH AS IN LOS ANGELES; AND (3) THAT MEXICAN AMERICAN "COLONIES" WILL PERSIST FOR GENERATIONS AS LONG AS ETHNIC EXCLUSIVENESS CONTINUES AND MIGRANTS MOVE INTO CITIES. IT IS POSITED THAT A REALISTIC APPROACH TO THE STUDY OF SOCIAL CLASS AND MINORITIES LIES IN SOME MIDDLE GROUND BETWEEN THE ASSIMILATIONIST AND THE PLURALIST MODELS. 8 REFERENCES.
ACCN   001089

1275 AUTH **MOORE, J. W.**

TITL SOCIAL CONSTRAINTS ON SOCIOLOGICAL KNOWLEDGE: ACADEMICS AND RESEARCH CONCERNING MINORITIES.

SRCE *SOCIAL PROBLEMS, 1973, 21(1), 65-77.*

INDX ESSAY, SOCIAL SCIENCES, SPANISH SURNAMED, RESEARCH METHODOLOGY, REPRESENTATION

ABST THE CURRENT STATUS OF ACADEMIC RESEARCH CONCERNING MINORITIES, FOCUSING ON THE CONSTRAINTS WHICH HINDER CREATIVITY IN THE FIELD OF SOCIOLOGY, IS DISCUSSED. MINORITY CRITICISMS OF SOCIOLOGICAL RESEARCH ON MINORITIES HAVE GENERATED PROFESSIONAL ACKNOWLEDGEMENT OF THE FOLLOWING UNRESOLVED DILEMMAS: (1) OMNISCIENCE, OR THE INCAPACITY OF RESEARCHERS TO EMPATHIZE WITH SUBJECTS BECAUSE THEY BELIEVE IN THE AUTONOMY OF THEIR KNOWLEDGE; AND (2) NEUTRALITY, WHEREBY ACADEMIC TRAINING IN THE USE OF SCIENTIFIC NORMS ENCOURAGES PATRONIZING ATTITUDES TOWARDS MINORITIES. THIS HAS CREATED OVERT METHODOLOGICAL STRUGGLES IN MINORITY STUDIES BETWEEN GROUPS OF CONVENTIONAL SOCIOLOGISTS WHO UPHOLD TRADITIONAL YET CULTURALLY BIASED METHODS, AND CRITICAL SOCIOLOGISTS WHO ATTEMPT TO DEVELOP ALTERNATIVE, EGALITARIAN METHODS. THE POLITICAL RAMIFICATIONS OF THE RELATIONSHIP BETWEEN ACADEMIC RESEARCHERS, UNIVERSITY ADMINISTRATORS, FUNDING SOURCES, AND MINORITIES IS EXAMINED. THE POLITICAL EFFECTS OF ACADEMIC RESEARCH ON MINORITY COMMUNITIES ARE OUTLINED AS FOLLOWS: (1) VALUABLE RESEARCH DATA ARE OFTEN NEVER PUT TO USE; (2) MINORITY EXCLUSION FROM PROJECTS RESULTS IN PROGRAMS THAT ARE NOT RELEVANT OR DO NOT BENEFIT MINORITY GROUPS; (3) INSTITUTIONAL RACISM INFLUENCES CONCEPTUAL FRAMEWORKS (I.E., 'BLAMING THE VICTIM'), THUS SUSTAINING AND GENERATING STEREOTYPES OF MINORITIES; AND (4) OMISSION OF SIGNIFICANT VARIABLES THAT RESULT IN THE MISINTERPRETATION OF RESEARCH FINDINGS. 21 REFERENCES.

ACCN 001090

1276 AUTH **MOORE, J., & MARTINEZ, A.**

TITL THE GRASS ROOTS CHALLENGE TO EDUCATIONAL PROFESSIONALISM IN EAST LOS ANGELES.

SRCE *IN A. CASTANEDA, M. RAMIREZ, III, C. E. CORTES & M. BARRERA (EDS.), MEXICAN AMERICANS AND EDUCATIONAL CHANGE. NEW YORK: ARNO PRESS, 1974, PP. 140-188.*

INDX PARAPROFESSIONALS, TEACHERS, PROFESSIONAL TRAINING, POLITICS, POLITICAL POWER, LEADERSHIP, SCHOLASTIC ACHIEVEMENT, MEXICAN AMERICAN, HISTORY, URBAN, SOCIAL SERVICES, CULTURAL FACTORS, DISCRIMINATION, PREJUDICE, SCHOLASTIC ACHIEVEMENT, PRIMARY PREVENTION, CHICANO MOVEMENT, ESSAY, CALIFORNIA, SOUTHWEST, COMMUNITY INVOLVEMENT, COMMUNITY

ABST AN HISTORICAL OVERVIEW OF THE CHALLENGE TO PROFESSIONAL AUTHORITY IN THE LOS ANGELES SCHOOL SYSTEM BY THE MEXICAN AMERICAN (MA) COMMUNITY CONCERNING THE SEMI-INSTITUTIONALIZATION OF THESE EFFORTS AND THE LEVEL OF BARRIO INVOLVEMENT IS PRESENTED. BEGINNING AS AN ELITE STRUGGLE WITHIN THE SYSTEM BY MA PROFESSIONALS, COMMUNITY CRITICISM OF THE SCHOOLS DEVELOPED INTO A GRASSROOTS ORIENTED MOVEMENT TO AFFECT CHANGE, EXEMPLIFIED BY THE EAST LOS ANGELES SCHOOL WALKOUTS AND THE ESTABLISHMENT OF THE EDUCATIONAL ISSUES COORDINATING COMMITTEE (EICC) IN 1968. AS AN OUTGROWTH OF THE EICC, THIS MOBILIZATION BECAME INSTITUTIONALIZED WITH THE CREATION OF THE MEXICAN AMERICAN EDUCATION COMMISSION WHICH ACTED AS THE "LEGITIMATE SPOKESMAN" FOR THE COMMUNITY. THE FINAL PHASES OF THIS OVERVIEW INCLUDE GRASSROOTS PARENTS ORGANIZING WITH REORIENTED TEACHERS AS WELL AS THE FORMATION OF YOUTH SERVING AGENCIES STAFFED BY COMMUNITY MEMBERS TO PROVIDE ALTERNATIVE EDUCATIONAL PROGRAMS FOR BARRIO YOUTH. IT IS RECOMMENDED THAT THERE IS A NEED FOR ALL PROFESSIONALS, SUCH AS SCHOOL OFFICIALS, TO INVOLVE BARRIO RESIDENTS IN THE DECISION-MAKING PROCESSES OF DEFINING AND RESOLVING PROBLEMS—ESPECIALLY WHEN THESE PROBLEMS DIRECTLY AFFECT BARRIO PEOPLE. 10 REFERENCES.

ACCN 001091

1277 AUTH **MORALES, A.**

TITL CHICANO-POLICE RIOTS.

SRCE *IN C. HERNANDEZ, M. J. HAUG & N. N. WAGNER (EDS.), CHICANOS: SOCIAL AND PSYCHOLOGICAL PERSPECTIVES. SAINT LOUIS: C. V. MOSBY COMPANY, 1976, PP. 64-83.*

INDX POLICE-COMMUNITY RELATIONS, CASE STUDY, HISTORY, DISCRIMINATION, MEXICAN AMERICAN, COMMUNITY INVOLVEMENT, AGGRESSION, CALIFORNIA, SOUTHWEST

ABST THE EAST LOS ANGELES (ELA) RIOTS OF 1970 ARE ANALYZED IN TERMS OF THE TYPES OF CONFRONTATIONS EXPERIENCED BETWEEN CHICANOS AND POLICE. TWO TYPES OF RIOTS HAVE BEEN DEFINED—"COMMUNAL" WHICH INVOLVES ONE ETHNIC-RACIAL GROUP FIGHTING A DIFFERENT ONE FOR A CONTESTED AREA, AND "COMMODITY" WHICH INVOLVES AN OUTBURST AGAINST PROPERTY AND RETAIL ESTABLISHMENTS, INCLUDING LOOTING. THE ELA RIOTS ARE SEEN AS "COMMUNAL" DUE TO CHICANO CONFRONTATION WITH INTRUDING ANGLO POLICEMEN, A BATTLE OVER A SPECIFIED AREA (I.E., A PARK), AND THEIR OCCURRENCE IN THE MEXICAN AMERICAN COMMUNITY. LOCAL GOVERNMENT ATTEMPTS AT "CONTROLLING THE SYMPTOM" BY ERECTING SPECIAL ENFORCEMENT BUREAUS IS SEEN AS CREATING ADDITIONAL PROBLEMS: (1) SOCIETY TENDS TO BELIEVE THAT CONTROL IS THE ANSWER TO URBAN UNREST; (2) THE URBAN AREAS MAY FULFILL THE EXPECTATIONS

DUE TO PSYCHOLOGICAL PROVOCATION; AND (3) IT CREATES A SANCTION FOR POLICE TO ACT OUT AGAINST MINORITIES. PERSONAL ACCOUNTS OF THE ELA RIOTS ARE GIVEN AND THE CIRCUMSTANCE-CONDITION FOUND IN THE 1960'S RIOTS ARE DESCRIBED. 45 REFERENCES.

ACCN   001092

1278 AUTH   **MORALES, A.**
TITL   THE COLLECTIVE PRECONSCIOUS AND RACISM.
SRCE   *IN M. M. MANGOLD (ED.), LA CHICANA: THE MOVEMENT FOR JUSTICE. NEW YORK: FAMILY SERVICE ASSOCIATION OF AMERICA, 1971, PP. 17-19.*
INDX   PREJUDICE, DISCRIMINATION, HISTORY, MASS MEDIA, MENTAL HEALTH PROFESSION, CASE STUDY
ABST   WHITE RACISM IN AMERICA, WITH A SPECIAL EMPHASIS ON ITS MANIFESTATIONS IN RELATION TO THE MEXICAN AMERICAN, IS DISCUSSED. THE CONCEPT OF THE COLLECTIVE PRECONSCIOUS IS DEVELOPED FROM WORKS OF A NUMBER OF WRITERS. IT IS A BEGINNING CONCEPT FOR AN UNDERSTANDING OF SOME OF THE COLLECTIVE, SOCIAL-PSYCHOLOGICAL DYNAMICS THAT MIGHT BE FOUND IN WHITE RACISM—A PHENOMENON THAT IS PASSED ON FROM GENERATION TO GENERATION. EXAMPLES OF THE MEDIA'S PORTRAYAL OF MEXICAN AMERICANS ARE PRESENTED TO DEMONSTRATE HOW THE MEDIA MAY UNINTENTIONALLY BE CONTRIBUTING TO WHITE RACISM. THAT IS, BY IMPLANTING A SUPERIOR RACIST MESSAGE IN THE MIND OF THE WHITE CHILD AND AN INFERIOR MESSAGE IN THE MIND OF THE MINORITY GROUP CHILD. THREE APPROACHES TO COMBATING RACISM ARE: (1) ETHNIC MINORITY STUDENTS AND FACULTY CAN MAKE A CONTRIBUTION TO SOCIAL WORK BY HELPING IT BECOME MORE CONSCIOUS OF RACISM IN AND OUT OF THE PROFESSION; (2) SOCIAL WORK CAN APPROACH THE TASK OF INFLUENCING, BY MEANS OF SOCIAL ACTION, THOSE FORCES THAT BECOME PART OF THE COLLECTIVE PRECONSCIOUS; AND (3) UNDERTAKE RESEARCH TO UNDERSTAND THE IMPACT OF WHITE RACISM ON MINORITY GROUP CHILDREN. 35 REFERENCES.
ACCN   001093

1279 AUTH   **MORALES, A.**
TITL   DISTINGUISHING PSYCHODYNAMIC FACTORS FROM CULTURAL FACTORS IN THE TREATMENT OF THE SPANISH-SPEAKING PATIENT.
SRCE   *IN N. N. WAGNER & M. J. HAUG (EDS.), CHICANOS: SOCIAL AND PSYCHOLOGICAL PERSPECTIVES. SAINT LOUIS: C. V. MOSBY COMPANY, 1971, PP. 279-280.*
INDX   MEXICAN AMERICAN, FEMALE, CASE STUDY, PSYCHOPATHOLOGY, ENVIRONMENTAL FACTORS, CULTURAL FACTORS, PERSONALITY ASSESSMENT, PSYCHOTHERAPY, ROLE EXPECTATIONS
ABST   PSYCHODYNAMIC AND CULTURAL FACTORS AFFECTING PSYCHOTHERAPY ARE DISTINGUISHED IN A CASE STUDY OF A MEXICAN

AMERICAN FEMALE. A THERAPIST IS DESCRIBED WHO EXPERIENCES DOUBTS ABOUT HIS ABILITY TO COMMUNICATE EFFECTIVELY IN SPANISH, PLACING TOO MUCH EMPHASIS ON CULTURAL FACTORS, AND THEREBY MINIMIZING HIS BASIC THERAPEUTIC SKILLS. WHILE CULTURAL FACTORS CAN BE AN IMPORTANT DETERMINANT IN THE THERAPEUTIC PROCESS, IT IS EMPHASIZED THAT OVERINTERPRETING CULTURAL FACTORS MAY IMPEDE THERAPY.

ACCN   001094

1280 AUTH   **MORALES, A.**
TITL   THE IMPACT OF CLASS DISCRIMINATION AND WHITE RACISM ON THE MENTAL HEALTH OF MEXICAN AMERICANS.
SRCE   *IN N. N. WAGNER & M. J. HAUG (EDS.), CHICANOS: SOCIAL AND PSYCHOLOGICAL PERSPECTIVES. SAINT LOUIS: C. V. MOSBY COMPANY, 1971, PP. 257-262.*
INDX   DISCRIMINATION, PREJUDICE, HEALTH DELIVERY SYSTEMS, RESOURCE UTILIZATION, REVIEW, HISTORY, MENTAL HEALTH, MENTAL HEALTH PROFESSION, ATTITUDES, POLICY, MEXICAN AMERICAN
ABST   AN INVESTIGATION OF THE IMPACT OF CLASS DISCRIMINATION AND WHITE RACISM ON THE MENTAL HEALTH OF MEXICAN AMERICANS IS PRESENTED. THE VARIOUS SOCIOECONOMIC CONDITIONS THAT BESET THE MA COMMUNITY ARE FOUND IN THE DISCRIMINATION AND RACISM THAT AMERICA PRACTICES TOWARD THE POOR. AN INSTITUTIONALIZED DELIVERY SYSTEM OF MENTAL HEALTH CARE EMPHASIZES QUALITY, INDIVIDUALIZED PSYCHIATRIC TREATMENT FOR THE AFFLUENT, AND AN ALMOST COMPLETE DENIAL OF QUALITY MENTAL HEALTH CARE FOR THE POOR. A HISTORICAL ANALYSIS OF THE ORIGINS OF DISCRIMINATION OF THE POOR IN THE CONTEXT OF A SOCIAL DARWINIST PHILOSOPHY IS PRESENTED. RACISM WAS THE UNDERLYING DYNAMIC OF THE MANIFEST DESTINY PREVALENT IN THE HISTORY OF THE U.S. AND MEXICO. STEREOTYPES WERE CREATED BY THE DOMINANT GROUP AS A LEVER OF NEGATIVELY IDENTIFYING AND MAINTAINING THE MINORITY GROUP IN A SUBORDINATE AND INFERIOR POSITION. THEY WERE DESCRIBED AS A "CHILD RACE" WITHOUT THE GENERATIONS OF CIVILIZATION AND CULTURE. IN THE AREA OF MENTAL HEALTH CARE, A HIGH INCIDENCE OF SCHIZOPHRENIA IS FOUND IN THE MA COMMUNITY. UNLIKE OTHER NATIONS THAT EXERCISE PROGRESSIVE APPROACHES IN THE TREATMENT OF SCHIZOPHRENIA, THE U.S. ASSIGNS THE DIFFICULT PSYCHOTIC PATIENTS TO PARAPROFESSIONALS AND AIDES, AND THE NEUROTIC PATIENTS ARE SEEN BY PSYCHIATRISTS AND PSYCHOLOGISTS. IT IS CONCLUDED THAT THE ROLE OF MENTAL HEALTH WORKERS SHOULD NOT ONLY BE TO PROVIDE TREATMENT TO PEOPLE IN NEED—NOT MERELY TO HELP THEM "ADJUST" TO SOCIETY'S DEVIANT

SYSTEMS—BUT TO ENDEAVOR TO CHANGE THOSE CONDITIONS WHICH UNDERLIE THE CAUSES OF THE PROBLEM BY INITIATING SOCIAL ACTION. 30 REFERENCES.

ACCN   001095

1281 AUTH   **MORALES, A.**
TITL   INSTITUTIONAL RACISM IN MENTAL HEALTH AND CRIMINAL JUSTICE.
SRCE   *SOCIAL CASEWORK, 1978, 59, 387-395.*
INDX   BILINGUAL-BICULTURAL PERSONNEL, COMMUNITY INVOLVEMENT, CRIMINOLOGY, CULTURAL PLURALISM, ESSAY, MENTAL HEALTH PROFESSION, POLICE-COMMUNITY RELATIONS, POLICY, REPRESENTATION, DEMOGRAPHIC, DISCRIMINATION, CALIFORNIA, SOUTHWEST
ABST   THE DYNAMICS OF INSTITUTIONAL RACISM IN THE MENTAL HEALTH AND CRIMINAL JUSTICE SYSTEM IN CALIFORNIA ARE ANALYZED IN THIS ESSAY. CONSIDERING THE PREVALENCE OF MENTAL DISORDER AND SUICIDE IN JAILS, PRESENT MENTAL HEALTH SERVICES ARE INADEQUATE—AND THIS IS ACUTELY SO FOR SPANISH-SPEAKING INMATES. RACISM IN POLICE DEPLOYMENT RESULTS IN GREATER ECONOMIC AND FAMILY DISRUPTION, AND THUS BECOMES A SPIRALING COMMUNITY MENTAL HEALTH PROBLEM. MINORITY EXCLUSION FROM MENTAL HEALTH POLICY-MAKING BOARDS RESULTS IN MORE RELEVANT MENTAL HEALTH PROGRAMS FOR WHITE THAN MINORITY POPULATIONS. MANY OF THE BARRIERS TO QUALITY MENTAL HEALTH SERVICES REFLECT STEREOTYPIC MYTHS AND INSTITUTIONAL RACISM AND ARE DISPROVEN BY AGENCIES WHICH PROVIDE PROFESSIONAL BILINGUAL-BICULTURAL STAFF IN THE COMMUNITY. MINORITY COMMUNITIES NEED MENTAL HEALTH PRACTITIONERS WHO INTERVENE ON BROADER SOCIAL PROBLEMS AS WELL AS WELL-TRAINED CLINICIANS WHO CARE FOR INDIVIDUAL CLINICAL NEEDS. WHETHER THE CHALLENGE AHEAD IS ADEQUATELY MET IN THE FUTURE DEPENDS ON PROFESSIONAL SCHOOLS, THE PROFESSIONS THEY REPRESENT, AND KNOWLEDGEABLE MINORITY PEOPLE IN AND OUT OF THE COMMUNITY. 19 REFERENCES.

ACCN   002390

1282 AUTH   **MORALES, A.**
TITL   MENTAL HEALTH AND PUBLIC HEALTH ISSUES: THE CASE OF THE MEXICAN AMERICANS IN LOS ANGELES.
SRCE   *EL GRITO, 1970, 3(2), 3-11.*
INDX   MEXICAN AMERICAN, MENTAL HEALTH, HEALTH DELIVERY SYSTEMS, RESOURCE UTILIZATION, DRUG ADDICTION, REHABILITATION, REVIEW, CALIFORNIA, SOUTHWEST
ABST   ASSUMPTIONS AND NOTIONS CONCERNING THE MEXICAN AMERICAN (MA) POPULATION AND MENTAL HEALTH ARE REVIEWED. FINDINGS INDICATE THAT MA'S DO HAVE MENTAL HEALTH PROBLEMS. PATIENTS SEEN AT THE EAST LOS ANGELES MENTAL HEALTH SERVICE (ELAMHS) HAVE MORE SEVERE PSYCHIATRIC DIAGNOSES. THEY DESIRE MENTAL HEALTH SERVICES AND HAVE THE HIGHEST SOURCE OF SELF AND FAMILY REFERRALS IN LOS ANGELES COUNTY WHEN COMPARED TO OTHER GROUPS. THERE IS A PAUCITY OF PSYCHIATRIC FACILITIES IN EAST LOS ANGELES AND A SEVERE SHORTAGE OF MENTAL HEALTH PROFESSIONALS, PARTICULARLY SPANISH-SPEAKING. THERE IS A RISK IN UTILIZING PARAPROFESSIONALS AS SUBSTITUTES FOR MENTAL HEALTH PROFESSIONALS. THIS COULD LEAD TO A DOUBLE STANDARD OF DELIVERY OF PSYCHIATRIC SERVICES TO THE POOR. REMEDIAL MEASURES—TO RECRUIT MENTAL HEALTH AIDES FROM THE COMMUNITY AND TO EXPAND PROFESSIONAL SCHOOLS FOR MA BILINGUAL STUDENTS—ARE MENTIONED. MA'S ARE GROSSLY OVERREPRESENTED IN PRISONS AND JAILS FOR OFFENSES RELATED TO NARCOTICS AND ALCOHOL, AND THERE ARE NO DETOXIFICATION PROGRAMS OR DRUG REHABILITATION PROGRAMS FOR THEM. A MODEST SATELLITE ALCOHOLIC REHABILITATION SERVICE HAS BEEN PROPOSED FOR EAST LOS ANGELES. AS WITH THE ELAMHS, IT IS EXPECTED THAT THE DEMAND FOR TREATMENT WILL FAR EXCEED THAT WHICH IS BEING OFFERED. 15 REFERENCES.

ACCN   001096

1283 AUTH   **MORALES, A.**
TITL   MENTAL HEALTH PROGRAM IMPLICATIONS OF DRINKING, DRUGS, AND VIOLENCE IN THE BARRIO.
SRCE   *PAPER PRESENTED AT THE SPANISH SPEAKING MENTAL HEALTH RESEARCH CENTER COLLOQUIUM SERIES, UNIVERSITY OF CALIFORNIA, LOS ANGELES, 1977.*
INDX   POLICE-COMMUNITY RELATIONS, ALCOHOLISM, MEXICAN AMERICAN, GANGS, SUICIDE, REVIEW, EMPIRICAL, ADOLESCENTS, INHALANT ABUSE, DRUG ABUSE, URBAN, ADULTS, DEMOGRAPHIC, DISCRIMINATION, COMMUNITY, HEALTH DELIVERY SYSTEMS, BILINGUAL-BICULTURAL PERSONNEL, CALIFORNIA, SOUTHWEST
ABST   THE TRADITIONAL MENTAL HEALTH PROGRAM MODEL DOES NOT ADEQUATELY MEET THE NEEDS OF ALL MEXICAN AMERICANS IN LOS ANGELES COUNTY. PROGRAMS THAT APPEAR TO BE SUCCESSFUL AND EFFECTIVE ARE STAFFED WITH BILINGUAL-BICULTURAL PERSONNEL AND CONTRARY TO STUDIES INDICATING UNDERUTILIZATION BY MEXICAN AMERICANS, THESE CLINICS TEND TO DEMONSTRATE OVERUTILIZATION OF FACILITIES. THREE PROBLEMS RELATED TO MENTAL HEALTH ARE DISCUSSED: DRINKING, GANGS, AND SUBSTANCE ABUSE. IN DEALING WITH ALCOHOLISM IT IS SUGGESTED THAT COMMUNITY ORGANIZATION AND COMPREHENSIVE PLANNING ARE NEEDED TO SOLVE MENTAL HEALTH PROBLEMS GENERATED BY LAW ENFORCEMENT DEPLOYMENT PRACTICES RELATED TO DRINKING OFFENSES. VIOLENCE IN THE BARRIO SHOULD NOT ONLY BE A POLICE MATTER BUT A COMMUNITY MENTAL HEALTH CONCERN. THERE ARE AT LEAST 8 INTERVENTIVE APPROACHES DESIGNED TO SOLVE THE GANG PROBLEM: (1) THE SOCIAL RECREATIONAL AP-

PROACH, (2) COMPETITIVE SPORTS, (3) LAW ENFORCEMENT APPROACH, (4) INSTITUTIONALIZATION, (5) STREET WORKERS, (6) COMMUNITY ORGANIZATIONAL APPROACH, (7) CLINICAL, AND (8) THE PSYCHO-SOCIAL AWARENESS APPROACH. THE LAST APPROACH DOES NOT DESTROY THE GANGS BUT REDIRECTS THEIR ACTIVITIES TOWARD HELPING THE ENVIRONMENT AND THUS REFLECTS A POSITIVE NONTRADITIONAL APPROACH. THE INCREASE OF SUBSTANCE ABUSE IN A RECENT STUDY CONDUCTED AMONG CHILDREN AND ADOLESCENTS IN HOUSING PROJECTS LOCATED IN EAST LOS ANGELES SUGGEST THAT IMMEDIATE ACTION BE TAKEN TO IMPLEMENT A VARIETY OF SOCIAL, RECREATIONAL, AND MENTAL HEALTH SERVICES IN BARRIOS. IT IS CONCLUDED THAT SCHOOLS OF PSYCHOLOGY, PSYCHIATRY, AND SOCIAL WORK NEED TO INCORPORATE CURRICULUM THAT IS RELEVANT TO MINORITY MENTAL HEALTH NEEDS. THE ULTIMATE CHALLENGE IS TO PROVIDE MEXICAN AMERICANS MENTAL HEALTH PERSONNEL AND SERVICES THAT ARE NONTRADITIONAL. 24 REFERENCES.

ACCN   001097

1284 AUTH   **MORALES, A.**
TITL   THE NEED FOR NONTRADITIONAL MENTAL HEALTH PROGRAMS IN THE BARRIO.
SRCE   *IN J. M. CASAS & S. E. KEEFE (EDS.), FAMILY AND MENTAL HEALTH IN THE MEXICAN AMERICAN COMMUNITY (MONOGRAPH NO. 7). LOS ANGELES: UNIVERSITY OF CALIFORNIA, SPANISH SPEAKING MENTAL HEALTH RESEARCH CENTER, 1978, PP. 125-142.*
INDX   CALIFORNIA, SOUTHWEST, URBAN, PSYCHOTHERAPISTS, POLICY, POLICE-COMMUNITY RELATIONS, GANGS, DRUG ABUSE, ADOLESCENTS, PROFESSIONAL TRAINING, MENTAL HEALTH, REVIEW, ESSAY, COMMUNITY, MEXICAN AMERICAN, PRIMARY PREVENTION
ABST   ALTHOUGH IN RECENT YEARS THERE HAVE BEEN SOME IMPROVEMENTS IN THE DELIVERY OF MENTAL HEALTH SERVICES TO MEXICAN AMERICANS (MA), THERE REMAINS AN URGENT NEED TO UNDERSTAND AND ACKNOWLEDGE THAT MA'S MENTAL HEALTH NEEDS EXTEND FAR BEYOND THE TRADITIONAL, CASEBY-CASE MODEL OF CLINICAL INTERVENTION. COMMUNITY ORGANIZATION AND COMPREHENSIVE MENTAL HEALTH PLANNING ARE NEEDED TO SOLVE MANY PROBLEMS IN THE BARRIO WHICH IMPACT ON MENTAL HEALTH— IN PARTICULAR, (1) ABUSIVE POLICE PRACTICES RELATED TO DRINKING OFFENSES AND RIOTS, AND (2) GANG BEHAVIOR AND SUBSTANCE ABUSE AMONG MA CHILDREN AND ADOLESCENTS. MOREOVER, MENTAL HEALTH PRACTITIONERS MUST GET INVOLVED IN AREAS PREVIOUSLY DELEGATED SOLEY TO THE POLICE. THEY MUST BE TRAINED AS CONSULTANTS, MEDIATORS, AND OMBUDSMEN BETWEEN THE COMMUNITY, THE POLICE, AND THE POLITICAL POWER STRUCTURE. THUS, WHAT IS CALLED FOR IS NONTRADITIONAL INTERVENTION APPROACHES WHICH BUILD UPON COMMUNITY COHESIVENESS AND PRIDE—E.G.,

THE COMMUNITY-ORGANIZATION APPROACH AND THE PSYCHOSOCIAL-AWARENESS APPROACH IN WORKING WITH GANGS. SUCH APPROACHES REQUIRE CHANGES IN CURRICULA IN SCHOOLS OF PSYCHIATRY, PSYCHOLOGY, AND SOCIAL WORK, AND THEY ALSO REQUIRE A NEW, PIONEERING BREED OF MENTAL HEALTH PRACTITIONERS THAT IS NOT BOUND BY RIGID, TRADITIONAL MODELS OF CLINICAL PRACTICE. 24 REFERENCES.

ACCN   001832

1285 AUTH   **MORALES, J. E., & DUBOIS, H.**
TITL   UN EXPERIMENTO EN LA ENSENANZA DE LA CONDUCTA HUMANA. (AN EXPERIMENT IN THE TEACHING OF HUMAN BEHAVIOR.)
SRCE   *IN J. A. ROSSELLO (ED.), MANUAL DE PSIQUIATRIA SOCIAL. SPAIN: INDUSTRIAS GRAFICAS "DIARIO-DIA," 1968, PP. 493-498. (SPANISH)*
INDX   ESSAY, PUERTO RICAN-I, HIGHER EDUCATION, CURRICULUM, INSTRUCTIONAL TECHNIQUES, MEDICAL STUDENTS, MENTAL HEALTH PROFESSION, PROFESSIONAL TRAINING, PSYCHOTHERAPISTS, SOCIAL SCIENCES
ABST   BASED UPON THEIR EXPERIENCE IN TEACHING THE STUDY OF HUMAN CONDUCT TO PSYCHIATRY STUDENTS IN PUERTO RICO, THE AUTHORS DISCUSS THE IMPORTANCE OF ACQUIRING KNOWLEDGE OF HUMAN CONDUCT IN DAILY LIFE BEFORE APPROACHING THE STUDY OF THE PSYCHOPATHOLOGY WHICH IS SEEN IN THE ARTIFICIAL ENVIRONMENT OF PSYCHIATRIC INSTITUTIONS. BEGINNING IN 1967, STUDENTS IN THE FIRST YEAR OF A PSYCHIATRY PROGRAM WERE INSTRUCTED IN THE SCIENCE OF HUMAN BEHAVIOR AS STUDIED IN THE FIELDS OF ANTHROPOLOGY, SOCIOLOGY, AND SOCIAL PSYCHOLOGY. SEMINARS INCLUDED DISCUSSIONS OF THE RELATIONSHIP BETWEEN DOCTOR AND PATIENT, THE ROLE OF THE FAMILY IN THE FORMATION OF NORMS AND ATTITUDES, THE EFFECTS OF SOCIAL STATUS IN INTERPERSONAL RELATIONS, AND THE RELATIONSHIP BETWEEN SCIENCE AND MAGIC. THE STUDENTS OBSERVED THEMSELVES IN ACTION, USING MUTUAL TEACHING TECHNIQUES UNDER THE SUPERVISION OF INSTRUCTORS. IT IS CONCLUDED THAT WITH A THOROUGH KNOWLEDGE OF THESE SCIENCES WHICH ARE CLOSELY RELATED TO PSYCHIATRY, THE STUDENTS WILL NOT ONLY GAIN GREATER INSIGHT INTO THE DETECTION AND EXPLANATION OF PSYCHOPATHOLOGY, BUT ALSO BE ABLE TO COMMUNICATE THEIR IDEAS MORE EFFECTIVELY.

ACCN   002286

1286 AUTH   **MORENO, P. R.**
TITL   VERTICAL DIFFUSION EFFECTS IN BLACK AND MEXICAN-AMERICAN FAMILIES PARTICIPATING IN THE FLORIDA PARENT EDUCATION MODEL (DOCTORAL DISSERTATION, UNIVERSITY OF FLORIDA, 1974).
SRCE   *DISSERTATION ABSTRACTS INTERNATIONAL, 1974, 36(3), 1358A. (UNIVERSITY MICROFILMS NO. 75-19,366.)*
INDX   PARENTAL INVOLVEMENT, ADULT EDUCATION, CROSS CULTURAL, MEXICAN AMERICAN, EM-

ABST PIRICAL, INSTRUCTIONAL TECHNIQUES, FLORIDA, SOUTH, CHILDREN, EDUCATION

ABST VERTICAL DIFFUSION EFFECTS ON THE YOUNGER SIBLINGS OF FAMILIES INVOLVED IN A PROGRAM DESIGNED TO INCREASE PARENTS' EFFECTIVENESS AS TEACHERS OF THEIR SCHOOL-AGE CHILDREN WERE INVESTIGATED IN TWO SEPARATE STUDIES. THE METHODS AND PROCEDURES OF STUDY I AND STUDY II WERE IDENTICAL. THE 93 CHILDREN IN STUDY I WERE ECONOMICALLY DISADVANTAGED BLACKS AND MEXICAN AMERICANS WHO: (1) ENTERED KINDERGARTEN IN THE FALL OF 1972; (2) WERE ADMINISTERED THE PRESCHOOL INVENTORY UPON ENTERING KINDERGARTEN; (3) HAD HAD PREVIOUS HEAD START EXPERIENCE; AND (4) HAD ELDER SIBLINGS AND PARENTS WHO HAD PARTICIPATED IN A PARENT EDUCATION PROJECT FROM ZERO TO TWO YEARS. THE 77 CHILDREN IN STUDY II ENTERED KINDERGARTEN IN THE FALL OF 1973, BUT OTHERWISE MET THE CRITERIA OUTLINED ABOVE FOR THE CHILDREN IN STUDY I. THE FINDINGS INDICATED THAT THE SPREAD OF TREATMENT EFFECTS TO YOUNGER SIBLINGS DID OCCUR, BUT ONLY AFTER TWO YEARS OF PARENT EDUCATION. WORKING DIRECTLY WITH PARENTS APPEARS TO PRODUCE VERTICAL DIFFUSION EFFECTS, BUT ONLY AFTER AN EXTENDED PERIOD. PARENT EDUCATION PROGRAMS, WHETHER HOME-BASED OR CENTER-BASED WITH A HOME VISITING COMPONENT, APPEAR TO OFFER AN EFFECTIVE AND ECONOMICAL WAY OF REACHING MORE CHILDREN AT LESS COST PER CHILD BECAUSE OF THE SPREAD OF TREATMENT EFFECTS TO YOUNGER CHILDREN. LIMITATIONS OF THE POST HOC DESIGN ARE DISCUSSED. 78 REFERENCES. (AUTHOR ABSTRACT MODIFIED)

ACCN 001098

1287 AUTH **MORGAN, R. R.**
TITL AN EXPLORATORY STUDY OF THREE PROCEDURES TO ENCOURAGE SCHOOL ATTENDANCE.
SRCE *PSYCHOLOGY IN THE SCHOOLS, 1975, 12(2), 209-215.*
INDX CHILDREN, GROUP DYNAMICS, INTERPERSONAL RELATIONS, PEER GROUP, CLASSROOM BEHAVIOR, BEHAVIOR MODIFICATION, MEXICAN AMERICAN, EMPIRICAL, ARIZONA, SOUTHWEST
ABST THE UTILITY OF MATERIAL PLUS SOCIAL REINFORCEMENT TECHNIQUES FOR IMPROVING SCHOOL ATTENDANCE WAS INVESTIGATED. EIGHTY-NINE LOWER SOCIOECONOMIC MEXICAN AMERICAN STUDENTS, WHO HAD EXCESSIVE UNEXCUSED ABSENSES, WERE RANDOMLY DIVIDED INTO THREE TREATMENT GROUPS—MATERIAL PLUS PEER SOCIAL REINFORCEMENT, MATERIAL REINFORCEMENT, AND TEACHER SOCIAL REINFORCEMENT—AND ONE CONTROL GROUP IN EACH SCHOOL. GROUPS WERE STRATIFIED ACCORDING TO GRADE LEVEL. SCHOOL ABSENTEEISM BEFORE CONDITIONING TRIALS WAS COMPARED DURING CONDITIONING TRIALS AND DURING EXTINCTION TRIALS FOR THE FOUR GROUPS.

THE RESULTS OF THIS STUDY OFFER SUPPORT FOR THE USE OF A COMBINATION OF MATERIAL PLUS PEER SOCIAL REINFORCEMENT, MATERIAL REINFORCEMENT ALONE, AND TEACHER SOCIAL REINFORCEMENT ALONE AS A MEANS OF IMPROVING SCHOOL ATTENDANCE. 8 REFERENCES. (AUTHOR SUMMARY MODIFIED)

ACCN 001099

1288 AUTH **MOSES, E. G., ZIRKEL, P. A., & GREENE, J. F.**
TITL MEASURING THE SELF-CONCEPT OF MINORITY GROUP PUPILS.
SRCE *JOURNAL OF NEGRO EDUCATION, 1973, 42(1), 93-98.*
INDX SELF CONCEPT, PERSONALITY, PUERTO RICANM, SES, ENVIRONMENTAL FACTORS, CROSS CULTURAL, TEACHERS, URBAN, TEST VALIDITY, TEST RELIABILITY, RESEARCH METHODOLOGY, CULTURAL FACTORS, CHILDREN, EMPIRICAL, CONNECTICUT, EAST
ABST AN INVESTIGATION OF MEASURING SELF-CONCEPT USING SELF-REPORT AND OBSERVER REPORT INSTRUMENTS WAS CONDUCTED AMONG 120 5TH AND 6TH GRADE DISADVANTAGED WHITE, BLACK, AND PUERTO RICAN STUDENTS RESIDING IN A LARGE CONNECTICUT CITY. THE STUDENTS WERE SELECTED FROM 3 SCHOOLS, EACH HAVING A DIFFERENT ETHNIC MAJORITY. THE COOPERSMITH SELF-ESTEEM INVENTORY (CSEI) CONTAINING 42 ITEMS MEASURING SELF-CONCEPT, SOCIAL SELF, AND SCHOOL SELF, WAS ADMINISTERED TO THE STUDENTS. THE MCDANIEL'S INFERRED SELF-CONCEPT SCALE (MISCS) CONSISTING OF 30 ITEMS CONCERNING THE CHILD'S BEHAVIOR WAS RATED BY THE CHILD'S TEACHER. THE FINDINGS REVEALED THE FOLLOWING: (1) PUERTO RICAN CHILDREN SCORED LOWER ON THE CSEI THAN BLACKS OR ANGLOS; (2) BLACK AND ANGLO CHILDREN APPEARED TO BE SIMILARLY AFFECTED BY SCHOOL ETHNIC COMPOSITION, WHEREAS THIS WAS NOT THE CASE FOR PUERTO RICAN CHILDREN; AND (3) MISCS RATINGS DID NOT INDICATE DIFFERENCES RELATED TO ETHNICITY OR THE SCHOOL'S ETHNIC COMPOSITION. THE DEGREE OF CORRELATION BETWEEN THE SELF- AND OBSERVER REPORTS SUGGEST THAT THEY ARE NOT NECESSARILY MEASURING THE SAME CONSTRUCT OF SELF-CONCEPT. THE EFFECTS OF BILINGUALISM AND BICULTURALISM MAY BE RESPONSIBLE FOR THE RELATIVELY LOW SELF-REPORT SCORES AND LOW INTER-INSTRUMENT CORRELATION COEFFICIENTS FOR THE PUERTO RICAN CHILDREN. 13 REFERENCES.

ACCN 001100

1289 AUTH **MOTE, T., NATALICIO, L. F., & RIVAS F.**
TITL COMPARABILITY OF THE SPANISH AND ENGLISH EDITIONS OF THE SPIELBERGER STATE-TRAIT ANXIETY INVENTORY.
SRCE *JOURNAL OF CROSS CULTURAL PSYCHOLOGY, 1971, 2(2), 205.*
INDX ANXIETY, TEST VALIDITY, TEST RELIABILITY, COLLEGE STUDENTS, RESEARCH METHODOLOGY, SPANISH SURNAMED, PERSONALITY ASSESSMENT, TEXAS, SOUTHWEST

ABST COMPARABILITY DATA RELATIVE TO THE EN-
GLISH EDITION OF THE SPIELBERGER STATE-
TRAIT ANXIETY INVENTORY (STAI) WERE OB-
TAINED FROM THE EXPERIMENTAL SPANISH
VERSION INVENTORY. THE SUBJECTS WERE 82
UNIVERSITY STUDENTS IN THIRD YEAR SPAN-
ISH CLASSES AT SAN ANTONIO, TEXAS. SEV-
ENTY OF THE SUBJECTS WERE NATIVE SPAN-
ISH SPEAKERS. SUBJECTS WERE RANDOMLY
ASSIGNED TO ONE OF THE FOUR FOLLOWING
SEQUENCES OF THE STAI: (1) ENGLISH-STATE,
SPANISH-STATE, ENGLISH-TRAIT, SPANISH-TRAIT;
(2) SPANISH-STATE, ENGLISH-STATE, SPANISH-
TRAIT, ENGLISH-TRAIT; (3) ENGLISH-TRAIT,
SPANISH-TRAIT, ENGLISH-STATE, SPANISH-
STATE; (4) SPANISH-TRAIT, ENGLISH-TRAIT,
SPANISH-STATE, ENGLISH-STATE. THE RESULTS
SHOW PRODUCT MOMENT CORRELATIONS BE-
TWEEN THE ENGLISH AND SPANISH EDITIONS
TO BE .941 AND .936 FOR THE STAI A-STATE
AND A-TRAIT SCALES, RESPECTIVELY. THE
CORRELATION COEFFICIENTS BETWEEN THE
ENGLISH AND SPANISH A-STATE SCALES FOR
SEQUENCES 1, 2, 3, AND 4 ARE .920, .967, .958,
AND .931, RESPECTIVELY, AND THE COMPA-
RABLE CORRELATION COEFFICIENTS FOR A-
TRAIT ARE .950, .922, .990, AND .903, RESPEC-
TIVELY. 6 REFERENCES.

ACCN 001101

1290 AUTH **MOXLEY, R. L.**
TITL SOCIAL SOLIDARITY, ETHNIC RIGIDITY AND
DIFFERENTIATION IN LATIN AMERICAN COM-
MUNITIES: A STRUCTURAL APPROACH.
SRCE *RURAL SOCIOLOGY, 1973, 38(4), 437-461.*
INDX DISCRIMINATION, COMMUNITY, ETHNIC IDEN-
TITY, SOCIAL MOBILITY, RURAL, EMPIRICAL,
SOUTH AMERICA, REVIEW, THEORETICAL
ABST THIRTY-NINE LATIN AMERICAN COMMUNITY
STUDIES WERE REVIEWED IN ORDER TO DE-
VELOP CROSS-NATIONAL STRUCTURAL MEA-
SURES OF THE CONCEPTS OF COMMUNITY SO-
CIAL SOLIDARITY AND ETHNIC RIGIDITY. THE
INTERRELATIONSHIPS AMONG THESE TWO SO-
CIAL PHENOMENA AND A THIRD STRUCTURAL
VARIABLE (COMMUNITY DIFFERENTIATION)
WERE EXAMINED UTILIZING GUTTMAN SCAL-
ING TECHNIQUES. THE TAUTOLOGICAL RELA-
TIONSHIP OF OPPOSING THEORETICAL AND
SOCIAL RIGIDITIES WAS ALSO INVESTIGATED.
IN CONCLUSION, THE RELATIONSHIP OF COM-
MUNITY SOLIDARITY, ETHNIC RIGIDITY, AND
MEASURES OF DEVELOPMENT ARE EXAMINED
IN LIGHT OF THEIR IMPLICATIONS FOR COM-
MUNITY THEORY, THE STUDY OF ETHNIC
GROUPS, AND COMMUNITY DEVELOPMENT. 45
REFERENCES. (JOURNAL ABSTRACT MODI-
FIED)
ACCN 001102

1291 AUTH **MULLER, D., & LEONETTI, R.**
TITL SELF-CONCEPTS OF PRIMARY LEVEL CHICANO
AND ANGLO STUDENTS.
SRCE *CALIFORNIA JOURNAL OF EDUCATIONAL RE-
SEARCH, 1974, 25(2), 57-60.*
INDX SPANISH SURNAMED, SELF CONCEPT, CHIL-
DREN, MEXICAN AMERICAN, CROSS CUL-

TURAL, SES, EMPIRICAL, NEW MEXICO, SOUTH-
WEST
ABST THE SELF-CONCEPTS OF 10 MEXICAN/SPANISH
AMERICAN AND 10 ANGLO KINDERGARTEN
THROUGH FOURTH GRADE CHILDREN FROM
LAS CRUCES, NEW MEXICO, PUBLIC SCHOOLS
CLASSROOMS WAS MEASURED BY THE PRI-
MARY SELF-CONCEPT SCALE (LEONETTI, 1973).
THE DATA WERE TESTED FOR HOMOGENEITY
OF VARIANCE AND THEN SUBJECTED TO AN
ANALYSIS OF VARIANCE. THE INSIGNIFICANT
MAIN EFFECT OF ETHNICITY SUGGESTS THAT
NO OVERALL OR CONSISTENT DIFFERENCES
EXIST BETWEEN ANGLO AND CHICANO CHIL-
DREN WITH REGARD TO SELF-CONCEPT. THE
SIGNIFICANT INTERACTION, HOWEVER, INDI-
CATES THAT THE EFFECT OF ETHNICITY ON
SELF-CONCEPT MAY BE DEPENDENT ON GRADE
LEVEL. MEAN DIFFERENCES BETWEEN CHIL-
DREN AT EACH GRADE LEVEL WERE TESTED
USING THE NEWMAN-KEULS PROCEDURE. THIS
ANALYSIS REVEALED THAT THE ONLY SIGNIFI-
CANT DIFFERENCE (P<.05) BETWEEN THE TWO
GROUPS WAS AT THE KINDERGARTEN LEVEL,
WITH ANGLO SUBJECTS HAVING HIGHER SELF-
CONCEPTS. 7 REFERENCES (AUTHOR SUM-
MARY MODIFIED)
ACCN 001103

1292 AUTH **MUNNS, J. G., GEIS, G., & BULLINGTON, B.**
TITL EX-ADDICT STREETWORKERS IN A MEXICAN-
AMERICAN COMMUNITY.
SRCE *CRIME AND DELINQUENCY, 1970, 16(4), 409-
416.*
INDX DRUG ADDICTION, DRUG ABUSE, REHABILITA-
TION, PARAPROFESSIONALS, EMPIRICAL, MEX-
ICAN AMERICAN, CALIFORNIA, FEMALE, MALE,
PREJUDICE, SOUTHWEST
ABST THE BOYLE HEIGHTS PROJECT, AN ATTEMPT
TO REDUCE NARCOTIC ADDICTION IN A MEXI-
CAN AMERICAN AREA BY EMPLOYING 30 FOR-
MER ADDICTS AS FIELD WORKERS, PRODUCED
THE FOLLOWING RESULTS IN ITS FIRST YEAR:
A HIGHER RATE OF RETURN TO ADDICTION
AMONG THE FIELD WORKERS THAN PREDIC-
TION TABLES MIGHT HAVE ANTICIPATED, WITH
NONE OF THE WOMEN WORKERS ABLE TO RE-
MAIN DRUG FREE; A CONTROVERSIAL EM-
PLOYMENT PROGRAM THAT BLATANTLY MA-
NIPULATED EMPLOYERS IN THE SERVICE OF
CLIENTS; A WELL-FUNCTIONING DETOXIFICA-
TION CENTER; AND AN EMERGING ROLE AS AN
AGENCY BRIDGING THE GAP BETWEEN THE
ADDICT AND THE FORCES OF SOCIETY BE-
FORE WHOM HE FEELS—AND OFTEN IS—
HELPLESS. 16 REFERENCES. (JOURNAL AB-
STRACT)
ACCN 001104

1293 AUTH **MUNOZ, C., JR.**
TITL THE POLITICS OF EDUCATIONAL CHANGE IN
EAST LOS ANGELES.
SRCE *IN A. CASTANEDA, M. RAMIREZ, III, C. E. CORTES,
& M. BARRERA (EDS.), MEXICAN AMERICANS
AND EDUCATIONAL CHANGE. NEW YORK: ARNO
PRESS, 1974, PP. 83-104.*
INDX LEGISLATION, POLITICS, POLITICAL POWER,
COMMUNITY INVOLVEMENT, CULTURAL

ABST A CASE STUDY ANALYSIS OF CHICANO PROTEST AGAINST THE LOS ANGELES CITY SCHOOL DISTRICT FROM THE 1968 SCHOOL WALKOUTS TO 1974 IS PRESENTED. PROTEST AS A POLITICAL RESOURCE IN EDUCATION IS CONSIDERED A VIABLE TOOL INSOFAR AS SCHOOLS HAVE CONTRIBUTED TOWARD DEFINING THE POWERLESS STATUS OF THE CHICANO. AS A RESULT OF THE HIGH SCHOOL WALKOUTS IN EAST LOS ANGELES (ELA), SCHOOLS BECAME SYMBOLIC OF CHICANO OPPRESSION AND POWERLESSNESS. THESE WALKOUTS, FOLLOWED BY MILITANT EFFORTS OF VARIOUS ORGANIZATIONS (E.G., MECHA, MAPA, BROWN BERETS), FURTHER ENHANCED THE CHICANO POWER MOVEMENT. THE FORMATION OF THE EDUCATIONAL ISSUES COORDINATING COMMITTEE (EICC), COMPRISED OF A CROSS-SECTION OF REPRESENTATIVES FROM CHICANO PROFESSIONAL AND GRASSROOTS COMMUNITY ORGANIZATIONS, IS VIEWED AS A UNIQUE POLITICAL EXPERIENCE FOR THE ELA BARRIOS WHICH PLACED SPECIFIC DEMANDS ON THE BOARD OF EDUCATION. ANALYSIS OF POST-1968 CHICANO REFORM INDICATES THAT THE ELA DROP-OUT RATE WAS REDUCED, THERE HAS BEEN AN INCREASE IN CHICANO REPRESENTATION IN ADMINISTRATION AND FACULTY, AND BILINGUAL-BICULTURAL PROGRAMS WERE INTRODUCED INTO TARGET SCHOOLS. HOWEVER, THE GENERAL GOAL OF COMMUNITY CONTROL WAS OBSCURED. IT IS BELIEVED THAT PROTEST ACTIVITY FAILED TO ACHIEVE THIS GOAL FOR TWO REASONS: (1) LACK OF ORGANIZATION AND STRATEGY WHICH FAILED TO TAKE INTO ACCOUNT THE NATURE OF THE SYSTEM; AND (2) THE BOARD OF EDUCATION SUCCESSFULLY CO-OPTED AND MANIPULATED BOTH LEADERSHIP AND EVENTS OF THE PROTEST ACTIVITY. OVERALL, THE FAILURE OF PAST PROTEST ACTIVITY PROVIDES A USEFUL LESSON TO CHICANOS COMMITTED TO THE DEVELOPMENT OF VIABLE ALTERNATIVES TO THE PRESENT EDUCATION STRUCTURE. 7 REFERENCES.

ACCN 001105

1294 AUTH **MUNOZ, L.**

TITL TRAINING CLASSROOM PERSONNEL IN DEALING WITH BILINGUAL/BICULTURAL HANDICAPPED CHILDREN.

SRCE *UNPUBLISHED MANUSCRIPT, 1972. (AVAILABLE FROM AUTHOR, TERRA SOUTHERN MEDICAL PLAZA, 1050 SOUTHER AVENUE, SUITE A-1, TEMPE, ARIZONA 85283.)*

INDX PROFESSIONAL TRAINING, TEACHERS, BILINGUAL-BICULTURAL PERSONNEL, BILINGUAL-BICULTURAL EDUCATION, PARAPROFESSIONALS, LEARNING DISABILITIES, PROGRAM EVALUATION, MEXICAN AMERICAN, CHILDREN, PHYSICAL DEVELOPMENT, REVIEW, ESSAY, BILINGUAL, CULTURAL FACTORS, BEHAVIOR MODIFICATION, CLASSROOM BEHAVIOR

ABST THE TRAINING PROCESS FOR DEVELOPING

BEHAVIOR MANAGEMENT SKILLS IN CLASSROOM PERSONNEL WHO DEAL WITH BILINGUAL-BICULTURAL CHILDREN IS DESCRIBED. SPECIFIC TRAINING PROCEDURES AND TECHNIQUES OFFERED ARE: (1) TEACHING TRAINEES TO OBSERVE BEHAVIOR; (2) DEVELOPING GOAL STATEMENTS; (3) MODELING BY TRAINING STAFF; (4) PROVIDING CORRECTIVE FEEDBACK; AND (5) DISCUSSING BEHAVIOR. IN PART II OF THE PAPER, A BRIEF LITERATURE REVIEW ADDRESSES ANGLO AND SPANISH AMERICAN VALUE ORIENTATION DIFFERENCES AS THESE PERTAIN TO THE SETTING OF APPROPRIATE GOALS. 35 REFERENCES.

ACCN 001106

1295 AUTH **MUNOZ, R. A., & ARBONA, G.**

TITL THE PUERTO RICAN MASTER SURVEY OF HEALTH AND WELFARE.

SRCE *IN I. I. KESSLER & M. L. LEVIN (EDS.), THE COMMUNITY AS AN EPIDEMIOLOGIC LABORATORY. BALTIMORE: JOHNS HOPKINS UNIVERSITY PRESS, 1970, PP. 279-295.*

INDX HEALTH, DEMOGRAPHIC, HEALTH DELIVERY SYSTEMS, PUERTO RICAN-I, URBAN, RURAL, SURVEY, PRIMARY PREVENTION, PROGRAM EVALUATION, POVERTY, SES, SOCIAL SERVICES, FERTILITY, RESEARCH METHODOLOGY, PSYCHOSOCIAL ADJUSTMENT, IMPAIRMENT, ATTITUDES, MIGRATION, EMPIRICAL, BIBLIOGRAPHY

ABST PUERTO RICO HAVING SUCCEEDED IN CONTROLLING INFECTIOUS DISEASE IS TURNING ITS ATTENTION TO AREAS OF CHRONIC DISEASE, MEDICAL CARE, AND HEALTH EDUCATION. THE DEVELOPMENT OF AN ONGOING MASTER SAMPLE SURVEY IS DISCUSSED AS WELL AS SOME OF ITS FINDINGS. USING A MULTI-STAGE STRATIFIED AREA PROBABILITY SAMPLE, 761 HOUSEHOLDS WERE INTERVIEWED BY TRAINED PERSONNEL REGARDING SOCIODEMOGRAPHIC INFORMATION, HEALTH HISTORY, DEGREE OF HAPPINESS, ATTITUDES TOWARD THE MENTALLY RETARDED, KNOWLEDGE OF DENGUE, AND LEVELS OF IMMUNIZATION. FINDINGS REVEAL THE FOLLOWING: (1) AGE, SEX, INCOME, AND PUBLIC ASSISTANCE ARE RELATED TO NUMBER OF ACUTE CONDITIONS REPORTED; (2) CHRONIC CONDITIONS INCREASE WITH AGE AND OCCUR MORE AMONG URBAN, POOR, AND THOSE OF MODERATE INCOME HAVING HEALTH INSURANCE; (3) NEGATIVE ATTITUDES TOWARD MENTALLY RETARDED ARE SOMEWHAT MORE FREQUENT AMONG OLDER PERSONS, FEMALES, RURAL DWELLERS, AND LESS EDUCATED; (4) COMPARED TO THE UNITED STATES, PUERTO RICANS REPORT BEING LESS HAPPY; (5) HAPPINESS IS RELATED TO HEALTH STATES; (6) OCCURRENCE OF DENGUE IN THE FAMILY DID NOT INCREASE KNOWLEDGE OF DENGUE; (7) AMONG THE YOUNG, THE MORE EDUCATED, AND URBANITES THERE IS GREATER KNOWLEDGE OF DENGUE; AND (8) ONLY A SMALL NUMBER OF CHILDREN UNDER 19 YEARS OF AGE REPORT HAVING BEEN IMMUNIZED. A BIBLIOGRAPHY OF THE SURVEY AND PROBLEM

AREAS AND THEIR RELATED VARIABLES ARE PROVIDED. 8 REFERENCES.

ACCN   001107

1296 AUTH   **MUNSINGER, H.**
TITL   CHILDREN'S RESEMBLANCE TO THEIR BIO-LOGICAL AND ADOPTING PARENTS IN TWO ETHNIC GROUPS.
SRCE   *BEHAVIOR GENETICS, 1975, 5(3), 239-254.*
INDX   CHILDREN, SES, INTELLIGENCE, FAMILY STRUCTURE, REPRESENTATION, EMPIRICAL, MEXICAN AMERICAN, CROSS CULTURAL, CALIFORNIA, SOUTHWEST
ABST   THE HYPOTHESIS THAT ADOPTED CHILDREN'S INDIVIDUAL IQ'S RESEMBLE THEIR BIOLOGICAL PARENTS' INDIVIDUAL SOCIAL-EDUCATION INDEX (SEI) RATHER THAN THOSE OF THEIR ADOPTED PARENTS' WAS TESTED. BACKGROUND DATA ON AGE, EDUCATION, AND OCCUPATION WERE COMPILED FROM 20 MEXICAN AMERICAN AND 21 WHITE BIOLOGICAL AND ADOPTING FAMILIES IN SAN DIEGO FOR WHOM THE IQ SCORE OF THE ADOPTED CHILD WAS AVAILABLE. PRODUCT-MOMENT CORRELATIONS WERE OBTAINED BETWEEN BIOLOGICAL AND ADOPTING MIDPARENT SEI, AND BETWEEN BOTH MIDPARENTS' SET AND THE ADOPTED CHILD'S IQ SCORES. BOTH THE WHITE AND THE MEXICAN AMERICAN SAMPLES SHOW THE SAME PATTERN OF RESULTS: NO SIGNIFICANT ASSORTIVE PLACEMENT OF THE CHILDREN IN ADOPTING HOMES; NO SIGNIFICANT RELATION BETWEEN THE SEI OF THE ADOPTING PARENTS AND THEIR ADOPTED CHILDREN'S INTELLIGENCE, BUT A STRONG CORRELATION BETWEEN BIOLOGICAL PARENTS' SEI AND THEIR CHILDREN'S IQ. THE HIGHER THAN EXPECTED OBSERVED CORRELATION BETWEEN BIOLOGICAL PARENTS AND THEIR OFFSPRING IS MOST LIKELY DUE TO SAMPLING ERROR, BASED ON THE RELATIVELY SMALL NUMBER OF FAMILIES IN THE STUDY. THE RESULT OF AN ANALYSIS OF VARIANCE OF THE SEI SHOWED THAT THERE IS A SIGNIFICANT DIFFERENCE IN SOCIAL STATUS BETWEEN THE BIOLOGICAL AND ADOPTING FAMILIES FROM BOTH ETHNIC GROUPS. IMPLICATIONS FOR ALTERNATE METHODS OF ASSESSING THE INFLUENCE THAT ADOPTION INTO A "SOCIALLY SUPERIOR" HOME ENVIRONMENT MIGHT EXERT ON THE AVERAGE GROUP INTELLIGENCE OF ADOPTED CHILDREN ARE DISCUSSED. 16 REFERENCES. (JOURNAL ABSTRACT MODIFIED)
ACCN   001108

1297 AUTH   **MURILLO, N.**
TITL   THE MEXICAN AMERICAN FAMILY.
SRCE   *IN N. N. WAGNER & M. J. HAUG (EDS.), CHICANOS: SOCIAL AND PSYCHOLOGICAL PERSPECTIVES. SAINT LOUIS: C.V. MOSBY COMPANY, 1971, PP. 97-108.*
INDX   ACCULTURATION, FAMILY ROLES, FAMILY STRUCTURE, CULTURE, CULTURAL FACTORS, ENVIRONMENTAL FACTORS, PERSONALITY, MEXICAN AMERICAN, ESSAY, CONFLICT RESOLUTION, SEX ROLES, VALUES
ABST   A DISCUSSION OF THE INTERCULTURAL CON-FLICTS AND DYNAMICS AS THEY APPLY TO THE MEXICAN AMERICAN (MA) FAMILY IS PROVIDED. SINCE THERE ARE A LARGE NUMBER OF MA FAMILIES, ALL DIFFERING SIGNIFICANTLY IN REGIONAL, HISTORICAL, POLITICAL, SOCIOECONOMIC, ACCULTURATION, AND ASSIMILATION FACTORS, ONE CANNOT PRESENT A STEREOTYPE MA FAMILY PATTERN. HOWEVER, BY MEANS OF COMPARISON, SOME CHARACTERISTICS IN THE WAY OF THOUGHT AND BEHAVIOR ARE MORE LIKELY TO APPEAR IN THE MA FAMILY THAN IN THE ANGLO FAMILY. SOME OF THESE DIFFERENCES ARE: (1) THE LATIN CULTURE SEEMS TO PROVIDE MORE EMOTIONAL SECURITY AND SENSE OF BELONGING TO ITS MEMBERS THAN DOES THE ANGLO CULTURE; (2) MA'S VALUE MATERIAL GOODS LESS THAN DO ANGLOS; (3) MA'S ARE PRESENT ORIENTED AND ANGLOS ARE FUTURE ORIENTED; (4) MA'S ENCOURAGE MORE DIPLOMACY AND TACTFULNESS THAN ANGLOS WHO ARE MORE BLUNT AND CONFRONTAL; (5) THE MA IS MORE SENSUAL THAN THE ANGLO; (6) THE FAMILY IS THE MOST IMPORTANT SOCIAL UNIT FOR THE MA; AND (7) THE ROLES FOR EACH OF THE FAMILY MEMBERS ARE MORE SHARPLY DEFINED FOR THE MA THAN FOR THE ANGLO. BECAUSE OF THE DIFFERENCE BETWEEN THE TWO CULTURES, A NUMBER OF CONFLICTS ARISE FOR THE MA INCLUDING PROBLEMS OF COMMUNICATION, IDENTIFICATION, SEX ROLE EXPECTATION, AND VALUES. THE MA HAS SEVERAL CHOICES IN COPING WITH THE DILEMMA, BUT THE ONE WHICH OFFERS HIM THE GREATEST POTENTIAL FOR ACHIEVING A SATISFYING LIFE IN THIS COUNTRY IS TO REALIZE HIS CREATIVE POTENTIAL FOR DEVELOPING HIS OWN UNIQUE IDENTITY. 7 REFERENCES.
ACCN   001109

1298 AUTH   **MURILLO, N.**
TITL   THE WORKS OF GEORGE I. SANCHEZ.
SRCE   *IN J. L. MARTINEZ, JR. (ED.), CHICANO PSYCHOLOGY. NEW YORK: ACADEMIC PRESS, 1977, PP. 1-10.*
INDX   BILINGUALISM, INTELLIGENCE TESTING, EDUCATION, MEXICAN AMERICAN, PREJUDICE, CHICANO MOVEMENT, CULTURAL PLURALISM, DISCRIMINATION, REVIEW, BILINGUAL-BICULTURAL EDUCATION, HISTORY, CHILDREN
ABST   A BIOGRAPHY IS PRESENTED OF G. I. SANCHEZ, EDUCATOR, WRITER, AND SOCIAL REFORMER, WHO DEVOTED HIS CAREER TO MAKING CONSTRUCTIVE CHANGES IN THE EDUCATIONAL SYSTEM AND TO EQUALIZING EDUCATIONAL OPPORTUNITIES IN NEW MEXICO AND NATIONWIDE. IN HIS EARLIEST PUBLISHED WORKS SANCHEZ CRITICIZED THE USE OF I.Q. TESTS BECAUSE THEY CREATED ARTIFICIAL INTELLIGENCE DIFFERENCES BETWEEN SPANISH-SPEAKING AND ENGLISH-SPEAKING CHILDREN. HE POSITED THAT OTHER INTERVENING FACTORS OUTSIDE OF HEREDITY EXPLAIN DIFFERENCES AND OFFERED EVIDENCE WHICH SHOWED THAT THE I.Q. SCORES OF SPANISH-SPEAKING CHILDREN IMPROVED ON REPEATED TESTS. SANCHEZ EMPHASIZED THE

IMPORTANCE OF A BASAL VOCABULARY IN ENGLISH FOR BILINGUAL CHILDREN BEFORE PROGRESS COULD BE MADE IN SCHOOL, WHICH LED HIM TO PROMOTE BILINGUAL-BICULTURAL PROGRAMS. THE NEED FOR THESE PROGRAMS GAVE HIM THE OPPORTUNITY TO CRITICIZE GOVERNMENTS FOR THE UNEQUAL DISTRIBUTION OF FUNDS. IN HIS LATER YEARS, SANCHEZ EXPOSED INSTITUTIONAL RACISM AS REFLECTED IN ETHNICALLY SEGREGATED SCHOOLS, AND TO A LARGER EXTENT, SOCIETY'S OVERALL PREJUDICE. THE APPLICATION OF SANCHEZ' LEADERSHIP TO CHICANO PSYCHOLOGISTS AND TO READVANCEMENT OF AWARENESS OF BILINGUAL AND BICULTURAL SPECIALIZATION IS DISCUSSED. 14 REFERENCES.

ACCN   001110

1299 AUTH   **MURILLO-ROHDE, I. M.**
TITL   FAMILY LIFE AMONG MAINLAND PUERTO RICANS IN NEW YORK CITY SLUMS.
SRCE   *PERSPECTIVES IN PSYCHIATRIC CARE, 1976, 14(4), 174-179.*
INDX   PUERTO RICAN-M, ENVIRONMENTAL FACTORS, PSYCHOSOCIAL ADJUSTMENT, MENTAL HEALTH, FAMILY STRUCTURE, INTERPERSONAL RELATIONS, FAMILY ROLES, FICTIVE KINSHIP, EXTENDED FAMILY, ESPIRITISMO, ACCULTURATION, ESSAY, REVIEW, BIRTH CONTROL, PREJUDICE, RELIGION, NEW YORK, EAST
ABST   THE CONDITIONS FACING MIGRANT AND SETTLED PUERTO RICAN FAMILIES IN NEW YORK CITY ARE EVIDENCED BY UNDESIRABLE HOUSING CONDITIONS, HIGH ECONOMIC INSECURITY DUE TO UNEMPLOYMENT, HIGH FERTILITY OF WOMEN, DISCRIMINATION, AND A LOW DEGREE OF ACCULTURATION. THE EXTENDED FAMILY WITH ITS STRONG SENSE OF KINSHIP STANDS IN SHARP CONTRAST TO THE AMERICAN FAMILY. MENTAL ILLNESS IN FAMILIES IS BROUGHT TO THE ATTENTION OF AN 'ESPIRITISTA' RATHER THAN CONVENTIONAL PSYCHIATRIC FACILITIES, AND PHYSICAL AND EMOTIONAL SUPPORT IS INCREASINGLY PROVIDED BY RELIGIOUS PENTECOSTAL MOVEMENTS. 12 REFERENCES.
ACCN   001111

1300 AUTH   **MURILLO-ROHDE, I. M.**
TITL   HISPANIC PSYCHIATRIC NURSING PERSONNEL IN THE UNITED STATES.
SRCE   *IN E. L. OLMEDO & S. LOPEZ (EDS.), HISPANIC MENTAL HEALTH PROFESSIONALS (MONOGRAPH NO. 5). LOS ANGELES: UNIVERSITY OF CALIFORNIA, SPANISH SPEAKING MENTAL HEALTH RESEARCH CENTER, 1977, PP. 23-29.*
INDX   MENTAL HEALTH PROFESSION, HIGHER EDUCATION, PUERTO RICAN-M, MEXICAN AMERICAN, SPANISH SURNAMED, REPRESENTATION, BILINGUAL-BICULTURAL PERSONNEL, EQUAL OPPORTUNITY, PROFESSIONAL TRAINING, POLITICAL POWER, EDUCATION, POLITICS
ABST   HISPANIC REPRESENTATION AMONG MENTAL HEALTH PROFESSIONALS AND, IN PARTICULAR, PSYCHIATRIC MENTAL HEALTH NURSES, IS VERY LOW. HOWEVER, RECENT SURVEYS BY

THE AMERICAN NURSES ASSOCIATION AND THE NATIONAL LEAGUE FOR NURSING INDICATE THAT A SMALL INCREASE IN ENROLLMENT AND COMPLETION OF ASSOCIATE, BACCALAUREATE AND GRADUATE NURSING PROGRAMS BY HISPANIC STUDENTS HAS OCCURRED FROM 1972 TO 1975. ALTHOUGH THESE FINDINGS COULD MEAN THAT EFFORTS TO RAISE HISPANIC REPRESENTATION IN NURSING AND SPECIFICALLY PSYCHIATRIC NURSING ARE BEGINNING TO SUCCEED, THE LACK OF ACCURATE RESOURCES ABOUT HISPANIC NURSES ILLUSTRATES THE NEED FOR MORE AND BETTER DATA AS WELL AS CONTINUED FUNDING FOR HISPANIC NURSING STUDENTS. RECOMMENDATIONS FOR IMPROVING THIS UNDERREPRESENTATION OF HISPANICS IN PSYCHIATRIC NURSING INCLUDE: (1) CONDUCTING A NATIONAL SURVEY TO ASCERTAIN AN ACCURATE COUNT OF HISPANIC PSYCHIATRIC NURSES IN THE U.S., AND (2) FORMING A COALITION OF MENTAL HEALTH PROFESSIONALS TO REQUEST FEDERAL FUNDING FOR BACCALAUREATE LEVEL NURSING EDUCATION AND PSYCHIATRIC MENTAL HEALTH NURSING. 6 REFERENCES.
ACCN   001112

1301 AUTH   **MURILLO-ROHDE, I. M.**
TITL   THE RELATIONSHIP BETWEEN PUERTO RICAN MOTHER-SON INTERPERSONAL COMPATIBILITY IN THE AREA OF CONTROL BEHAVIOR AND ADJUSTMENT IN SCHOOL (DOCTORAL DISSERTATION, NEW YORK UNIVERSITY, 1971).
SRCE   *DISSERTATION ABSTRACTS INTERNATIONAL, 1971, 32(7), 4030B. (UNIVERSITY MICROFILMS NO. 71-28549.)*
INDX   MOTHER-CHILD INTERACTION, PUERTO RICAN-M, EMPIRICAL, PSYCHOSOCIAL ADJUSTMENT, EDUCATION, CHILDREN, FAMILY STRUCTURE, CLASSROOM BEHAVIOR, DYADIC INTERACTION, NEW YORK, EAST, MALE
ABST   IT IS HYPOTHESIZED THAT A POSITIVE RELATIONSHIP EXISTS BETWEEN MOTHER-SON INTERPERSONAL COMPATIBILITY IN THE AREA OF EXPRESSED AND WANTED CONTROL BEHAVIOR AND THE BOY'S ADJUSTMENT IN SCHOOL. EIGHTY DYADS OF LOW INCOME PUERTO RICAN BOYS AND THEIR MOTHERS WERE SELECTED. THE FUNDAMENTAL INTERPERSONAL RELATIONS ORIENTATION BEHAVIOR SCALE (FIRO-B) WAS ADMINISTERED TO THE MOTHERS AND THE FIRO-BC TO THE SONS, USING EIGHTEEN ITEMS DEALING WITH EXPRESSED AND WANTED CONTROL BEHAVIOR. SCORES WERE USED TO COMPUTE RECIPROCAL INTERPERSONAL COMPATIBILITY BETWEEN MOTHER-SON DYADS. THE TEST RESULTS REVEAL THAT A CLOSE MOTHER-SON RELATIONSHIP IS POSITIVELY RELATED TO THE BOY'S SOCIAL AND BEHAVIORAL ADJUSTMENT IN SCHOOL; THIS IS ESPECIALLY SIGNIFICANT FOR BOYS IN FOURTH AND FIFTH GRADES AND IN HOMES WHERE THE FATHER IS ABSENT. RECOMMENDATIONS ARE MADE TO EVALUATE THE VARIABLES WITH OTHER ETHNIC GROUPS AND SOCIAL LEVELS, AND WITH GIRLS AS WELL AS BOYS. 53 REFERENCES. (AUTHOR ABSTRACT MODIFIED)

ACCN   001113

1302 AUTH   **MURPHY, S.**
TITL   LATINO THERAPY IN LOS ANGELES.
SRCE   *INNOVATIONS, 1975, 2(1), 12-15.*
INDX   BILINGUAL-BICULTURAL PERSONNEL, PSY-
CHOTHERAPY, PSYCHOTHERAPISTS, ESSAY,
SPANISH SURNAMED, ETHNIC IDENTITY, CALI-
FORNIA, SOUTHWEST, SELF CONCEPT, CUL-
TURAL FACTORS, CASE STUDY, PROGRAM
EVALUATION
ABST   THE COMMONLY HELD ASSUMPTION THAT LA-
TINOS ARE NOT AMENABLE TO PSYCHOTHER-
APY IS CHALLENGED BY A DESCRIPTION OF A
THERAPEUTIC PROGRAM FOR LATINOS IN
SOUTHERN CALIFORNIA. THE FOCUS IS ON
THE IMPROVEMENT OF SELF-IMAGE THROUGH
AN INCREASED UNDERSTANDING OF PSYCHO-
LOGICAL PROCESSES AND ACCEPTANCE AND
PRIDE IN THE PATIENTS' LATIN AMERICAN HER-
ITAGE. GAMES, FILMS, AND SMALL GROUP DIS-
CUSSIONS CONDUCTED IN SPANISH PROVIDE
A VEHICLE FOR SOCIALIZATION. THE SUCCESS
OF THE PROGRAM INDICATES THAT LATINOS
WILL ACCEPT AND BENEFIT FROM THERAPY
WHEN THEIR CULTURAL IDENTITY IS MAIN-
TAINED AND RECOGNIZED. 1 REFERENCE.
ACCN   001114

1303 AUTH   **MURRAY, M. E., WAITES, L., VELDMAN, D. J., &
HEATLY, M. D.**
TITL   ETHNIC GROUP DIFFERENCES BETWEEN WISC
AND WAIS SCORES IN DELINQUENT BOYS.
SRCE   *JOURNAL OF EXPERIMENTAL EDUCATION, 1973,
42(2), 68-72.*
INDX   CROSS CULTURAL, WISC, WAIS, DELINQUENCY,
INTELLIGENCE TESTING, MEXICAN AMERICAN,
CHILDREN, ADOLESCENTS, LINGUISTIC COM-
PETENCE, CROSS CULTURAL, EMPIRICAL, IN-
TELLIGENCE, MALE, TEXAS, SOUTHWEST
ABST   IN ORDER TO PROVIDE FURTHER INFORMA-
TION REGARDING PATTERNS OF INTELLEC-
TUAL FUNCTIONING IN DELINQUENT BOYS,
1007 ANGLO, 808 BLACK AND 683 CHICANO
STUDENTS AT THE GATESVILLE STATE SCHOOL
FOR BOYS IN TEXAS WERE ADMINISTERED THE
WISC AND WAIS. VARIABLES EXAMINED IN-
CLUDED AGE, ETHNICITY AND VERBAL PER-
FORMANCE AND FULL SCALE I.Q. SCORES. A
THREE-FACTOR ANALYSIS OF VARIANCE WAS
COMPUTED ON THE SCORES, INCLUDING ETH-
NIC GROUP, TEST-AGE LEVEL (WISC, WAIS),
AND SUBSCALE (VERBAL, PERFORMANCE). RE-
SULTS SHOW THAT THE MEAN I.Q. SCORES OF
THE SUBJECTS WERE SPREAD OVER A 15-
POINT RANGE WITH ANGLOS HIGHEST AND
BLACKS LOWEST. WISC SCORES WERE LOWER
THAN WAIS SCORES FOR ALL GROUPS, AL-
THOUGH THE DIFFERENCE WAS SIGNIFI-
CANTLY EXAGGERATED IN THE BLACKS. PER-
FORMANCE SUBSCALES ELICITED HIGHER
MEAN SCORES THAN VERBAL SUBSCALES,
WITH THEIR DIFFERENCE BEING TWICE AS
LARGE ON THE WISC AS ON THE WAIS. BLACKS
WERE FOUND TO PERFORM AT ABOUT THE
SAME LOW LEVEL ON BOTH SUBSCALES, WHILE
CHICANOS DID POORLY ON VERBAL I.Q., BUT
SCORED IN THE NORMAL RANGE ON PER-

FORMANCE SUBSCALE. RESULTS ARE DIS-
CUSSED IN THE LIGHT OF THE RECENT I.Q.
CONTROVERSY AS TO SOCIO-CULTURAL ENVI-
RONMENT, GENETIC PREDISPOSITION AND
EDUCATIONAL QUALITY. HOWEVER, AN EXAMI-
NATION OF I.Q. SCORE TRENDS IS SEEN AS IM-
PORTANT IN PROVIDING A REFERENCE POINT
ON WHICH TO BASE CLINICAL JUDGMENTS
AND DISCUSSIONS REGARDING INDIVIDUAL
INTELLECTUAL PERFORMANCES. 22 REFER-
ENCES. (AUTHOR ABSTRACT MODIFIED)
ACCN   001115

1304 AUTH   **MUSSEN P., & MALDONADO BEYTAGH, L. A.**
TITL   INDUSTRIALIZATION, CHILD-REARING PRAC-
TICES, AND CHILDREN'S PERSONALITY.
SRCE   *ANNUAL PROGRESS IN CHILD PSYCHIATRY AND
CHILD DEVELOPMENT, 1970, 3, 195-217. (RE-
PRINTED FROM JOURNAL OF GENETIC PSY-
CHOLOGY, 1969, 115, 195-216.)*
INDX   ACCULTURATION, CHILDREARING PRACTICES,
SOCIALIZATION, PUERTO RICAN-I, SES, OCCU-
PATIONAL ASPIRATIONS, ROLE EXPECTATIONS,
TAT, EMPIRICAL, PERSONALITY, CULTURAL
CHANGE, MIGRATION, PSYCHOSOCIAL AD-
JUSTMENT, FAMILY ROLES, MALE, FATHER-CHILD
INTERACTION, MOTHER-CHILD INTERACTION,
RURAL, URBAN
ABST   CONSEQUENCES OF THE FAMILY'S SHIFT FROM
AN AGRICULTURAL TO AN INDUSTRIAL WAY OF
LIFE ON CHILD-REARING PRACTICES AND ON
CHILDREN'S PERSONALITY WERE INVESTI-
GATED IN 63 PUERTO RICAN BOYS, AGED 9-12,
AND MANY OF THEIR PARENTS. THE SAMPLE,
BASED ON THE FATHER'S OCCUPATION AND
EDUCATION, WAS DIVIDED INTO (1) AGRICUL-
TURAL, (2) INDUSTRIAL-UNEDUCATED, AND (3)
INDUSTRIAL-EDUCATED. DATA CONSISTED OF:
(1) INTERVIEWS WITH MOTHERS AND FATHERS
ABOUT CHILD-REARING PRACTICES, PAREN-
TAL EXPECTATIONS OF THE CHILD, AND DISCI-
PLINE; (2) INTERVIEWS WITH THE BOYS ABOUT
THEIR GOALS AND VIEWS OF PARENTS; AND (3)
A TAT-LIKE PROJECTIVE TEST TAKEN BY THE
BOYS. DESCRIPTIVE ANALYSIS OF THE DATA
GAVE NO SUPPORT TO THE HYPOTHESIS THAT
INDUSTRIALIZATION LEADS TO PSYCHOLOGI-
CAL DISORGANIZATION OR MALADJUSTMENT.
ON THE CONTRARY, THE INDUSTRIALIZED PAR-
ENTS AND THEIR CHILDREN PRESENTED A PIC-
TURE OF PSYCHOLOGICAL HEALTH, STABILITY
AND OPTIMISM. WHILE AGRICULTURAL FATH-
ERS RETAINED THE TRADITIONAL COLD, ALOOF,
AUTHORITARIAN RELATIONSHIPS WITH THEIR
FAMILIES AND MADE STRONG DEMANDS FOR
OBEDIENCE AND CONFORMITY, THIS PATER-
NAL PATTERN IS BREAKING DOWN AMONG THE
INDUSTRIALIZED MEN, EVEN THE UNEDU-
CATED ONES. AGRICULTURAL MOTHERS, WHEN
COMPARED WITH INDUSTRIAL MOTHERS,
STRESSED TRADITIONAL VALUES AND WERE
LESS PERMISSIVE. EXPLANATIONS FOR THE AP-
PARENT SMOOTH TRANSITION FOR THESE
FAMILIES AND THEIR CHILDREN FROM AGRI-
CULTURE TO INDUSTRIALIZATION ARE PRE-
SENTED. 28 REFERENCES. (AUTHOR SUMMARY
MODIFIED)
ACCN   001116

1305 AUTH **MYERS, V.**
TITL DRUG USE AMONG MINORITY YOUTH.
SRCE *ADDICTIVE DISEASES: AN INTERNATIONAL JOURNAL, 1977, 3(2), 187-196.*
INDX ATTITUDES, ADULTS, ADOLESCENTS, DRUG ABUSE, MALE, MEXICAN AMERICAN, SPANISH SURNAMED, URBAN, RURAL, FEMALE, CROSS CULTURAL, EMPIRICAL
ABST INTERVIEWS WITH A NATIONWIDE SAMPLE OF YOUNG AND LOW-INCOME BLACK, CHICANO, AND CARIBBEAN MEN AND WOMEN, AS WELL AS THEIR NON-MINORITY COUNTERPARTS, REVEAL THAT THE MAJORITY DISAPPROVE OF ILLICIT DRUG USE. A DISPROPORTIONATE, STRATIFIED RANDOM SAMPLE OF 1,357 RESPONDENTS WAS DRAWN FROM A POPULATION OF ABOUT 20,000 ENROLLEES AT 19 JOB CORPS CENTERS IN 17 STATES. OF THESE RESPONDENTS, 53% WERE BLACK, 20% CHICANO, 8% CARIBBEAN, AND 19% WHITE; 70% WERE MEN; AND ALL WERE 16 TO 21 YEARS-OLD WHEN INTERVIEWED. THE SAMPLE REPRESENTED ALL AMERICAN STATES AND MANY OF ITS TERRITORIES. INTERVIEWERS WERE 3 BLACK MEN, 3 BLACK WOMEN, 2 CHICANOS, AND ONE CHICANA, ALL HAVING COMPLETED JOB CORPS TENURE AND ALL EXPERIENCED DRUG USERS. ALTHOUGH ONE-HALF OF THE YOUTH REPORTED HAVING HAD EXPERIENCE WITH ILLICIT DRUGS, MOST HAD RENOUNCED THEIR INVOLVEMENT AND NO LONGER USED THEM. OF THE RACIAL OR ETHNIC GROUPS INTERVIEWED, WHITE YOUTH WERE THE MOST LIKELY TO HAVE INGESTED ILLICIT DRUGS. THESE DATA, COUPLED WITH OTHER FINDINGS DRAWN FROM A MORE LENGTHY REPORT, LEAD TO THE CONCLUSION THAT DYSFUNCTIONAL PATTERNS OF DRUG INGESTION AMONG MANY LOW-INCOME MINORITIES ARE NOT PRONOUNCED. 5 REFERENCES. (AUTHOR ABSTRACT MODIFIED)
ACCN 002165

1306 AUTH **MYERS, V.**
TITL DRUG-RELATED COGNITIONS AMONG MINORITY YOUTH.
SRCE *JOURNAL OF DRUG EDUCATION, 1977, 7(1), 53-62.*
INDX DRUG ABUSE, ATTITUDES, MEXICAN AMERICAN, CROSS CULTURAL, SEX COMPARISON, URBAN, RURAL, EMPIRICAL, SURVEY, HEALTH EDUCATION, SPANISH SURNAMED
ABST DRUG RELATED SENTIMENTS, COGNITIONS, AND BEHAVIOR AMONG JOB CORP ENROLLEES WERE STUDIED TO AID JOB CORP OFFICIALS IN PLANNING AND DEVELOPING NEW DRUG EDUCATION AND HEALTH RELATED PROGRAMS. THE DATA WERE COLLECTED FROM A NATIONWIDE POPULATION OF YOUNG, MINORITY MEN AND WOMEN FROM LOWER SOCIOECONOMIC BACK GROUNDS, AS WELL AS FROM THEIR NON-MINORITY COUNTERPARTS. THE FINDINGS REVEAL: (1) THE MAJORITY OF SUBJECTS KNOW LITTLE ABOUT DRUGS OR ARE ILL INFORMED; (2) OF MALE–SUBJECTS, ANGLOS AND CARIBBEANS ARE MOST INFORMED AND OF FEMALE SUBJECTS, ANGLOS ARE MOST INFORMED; (3) AMONG CARIBBEAN

SUBJECTS, MALES ARE SIGNIFICANTLY MORE INFORMED THAN FEMALES; (4) AMONG OTHER MINORITIES, MEN AND WOMEN ARE RELATIVELY EQUAL IN DRUG KNOWLEDGE; AND (5) SUBJECTS WITH MORE EDUCATION AND THOSE FROM URBAN AREAS ARE GENERALLY BETTER INFORMED ABOUT DRUGS. THE NEED FOR DRUG ABUSE EDUCATION MATERIALS IN FORMS UNDERSTOOD WITHIN SUBCULTURES AND MORE ACCESSIBLE TO THEM IS DISCUSSED. 2 REFERENCES.
ACCN 001118

1307 AUTH **NADITCH, M. P., & MORRISSEY, R. F.**
TITL ROLE STRESS, PERSONALITY AND PSYCHOPATHOLOGY IN A GROUP OF IMMIGRANT ADOLESCENTS.
SRCE *JOURNAL OF ABNORMAL PSYCHOLOGY, 1976, 85(1), 113-118.*
INDX STRESS, PERSONALITY, PSYCHOPATHOLOGY, IMMIGRATION, ROLE EXPECTATIONS, ADOLESCENTS, CUBAN, ANXIETY, PERSONALITY ASSESSMENT, EMPIRICAL, FLORIDA, SOUTH
ABST THIS STUDY APPLIED A ROLE STRESS-PERSONALITY FRAMEWORK TO THE ANALYSIS OF PSYCHOPATHOLOGICAL SYMPTOMS IN A NON-CLINICAL SAMPLE OF 155 CUBAN REFUGEES IN MIAMI, FLORIDA. MEASURES INCLUDED THE EYSENCK PERSONALITY INVENTORY, CANTRIL'S SELF-ANCHORING STRIVING SCALE, AND ZUCKERMAN AND LUBIN'S DEPRESSION AND ANXIETY ADJECTIVE CHECKLIST. AMBIGUITY REGARDING EVALUATIONS OF PERFORMANCE IN THE DATING ROLE WAS MORE CONSISTENTLY RELATED TO SYMPTOMS OF PSYCHOPATHOLOGY THAN WERE EITHER ROLE CONFLICT OR AMBIGUITY REGARDING ROLE EXPECTATIONS. EXTROVERSION-INTROVERSION AND RELATIVE DISCONTENT WERE ALSO ASSOCIATED WITH PSYCHOPATHOLOGICAL SYMPTOMS, WITH SOME SEX DIFFERENCES. RESULTS SUGGEST THAT HIGH RATES OF MENTAL ILLNESS AMONG IMMIGRANT GROUPS MAY BE PARTIALLY A FUNCTION OF EVALUATION AMBIGUITY AND THE RESULTANT PROBLEMS OF IDENTITY FORMATION AMID CONFLICTING CULTURAL PATTERNS. 23 REFERENCES. (PASAR ABSTRACT MODIFIED)
ACCN 001120

1308 AUTH **NALL, F. C., & SPEILBERG J.**
TITL SOCIAL AND CULTURAL FACTORS IN THE RESPONSES OF MEXICAN-AMERICANS TO MEDICAL TREATMENT.
SRCE *JOURNAL OF HEALTH AND SOCIAL BEHAVIOR, 1967, 8(4), 299-308.*
INDX CONFLICT RESOLUTION, INTERPERSONAL RELATIONS, RESOURCE UTILIZATION, FOLK MEDICINE, HEALTH, ANOMIE, FAMILY STRUCTURE, FAMILY ROLES, MEXICAN AMERICAN, CULTURAL FACTORS, EMPIRICAL, CURANDERISMO, DISEASE, TEXAS, SOUTHWEST
ABST AN EXPLORATION OF THE CULTURAL AND SOCIETAL FACTORS RELATED TO THE ACCEPTANCE OR REJECTION OF A MODERN MEDICAL TREATMENT OF TUBERCULOSIS (TB) BY 53 LOW-SOCIOECONOMIC MEXICAN AMERICANS IS PRESENTED. THE RELATIONSHIP BETWEEN

FOLK MEDICAL BELIEFS AND PRACTICES, AND THE ACCEPTANCE OF A MODERN MEDICAL REGIME FOR THE TREATMENT OF A MAJOR ILLNESS WAS ANALYZED IN TERMS OF THE FOLLOWING CULTURAL TRAITS BELIEVED TO INHIBIT ACCEPTANCE OR REJECTION OF MODERN MEDICAL PRACTICES: (1) A SET OF TRADITIONAL FOLK BELIEFS AND PRACTICES; (2) THE USE OF FOLK MEDICAL CURERS (CURANDEROS); AND (3) A SET OF RITUALISTIC ACTS TRADITIONALLY CONSIDERED TO HAVE PROPITIATORY EFFECTS ON HEALTH. IN ORDER TO DETERMINE WHETHER SOCIAL INTEGRATION OF SUBJECTS BEARS ANY DISCERNIBLE RELATION TO THEIR ACCEPTANCE OR REJECTION OF MODERN MEDICAL TREATMENT, THE FOLLOWING FOUR DIMENSIONS WERE CONSIDERED: (1) INTEGRATION INTO THE FAMILY GROUP; (2) INTEGRATION INTO THE ETHNIC LOCALITY GROUP; (3) LANGUAGE OUTSIDE OF HOME; AND (4) SUBJECTIVE EXPRESSIONS OF SROLES' 5-ITEM ANOMIE SCALE OF INTEGRATION-ALIENATION. A CHI SQUARE ANALYSIS INDICATED THAT COMMITMENT TO FOLK BELIEFS, THE PRACTICE OF PROPITIATORY RELIGIOUS ACTS, AND THE USE OF CURANDEROS ARE NOT RELATED TO THE ACCEPTANCE OR REJECTION OF MODERN MEDICAL TREATMENT FOR TB. ONE SIGNIFICANT FINDING REVEALS THAT A WIDE VARIETY OF SOCIAL INTEGRATION INDICES ARE RELATED TO THE SUBJECTS' ACCEPTANCE OR REJECTION OF THE TREATMENT. THE FINDINGS IMPLY THAT THE MILIEU OF THE MEXICAN AMERICAN SUBCOMMUNITY IS UNFAVORABLE TO THE INTEGRATIVE, ADAPTIVE TECHNIQUES EMBODIED IN THE MEDICAL REGIME FOR TB TREATMENT. DETAILED DISCUSSION OF THE FINDINGS IS PROVIDED. 5 REFERENCES.

ACCN   001121

1309 AUTH   **NARDI, T. J., & DI SCIPIO, W. J.**
TITL   THE GANSER SYNDROME IN AN ADOLESCENT HISPANIC-BLACK FEMALE.
SRCE   *AMERICAN JOURNAL OF PSYCHIATRY, 1977, 134(4), 453-454.*
INDX   ADOLESCENTS, CASE STUDY, COPING MECHANISMS, FEMALE, PSYCHOPATHOLOGY, SPANISH SURNAMED, NEW YORK, EAST, DISEASE, SYMPTOMATOLOGY
ABST   A CASE STUDY OF THE GANSER SYNDROME IN A 15 YEAR-OLD HISPANIC BLACK FEMALE IS PRESENTED, AND THE SYNDROME IS DISCUSSED. THE GANSER SYNDROME IS CHARACTERIZED BY THE PATIENT GIVING SILLY ANSWERS TO QUESTIONS AND IS OFTEN OF SHORT DURATION. A NEUROLOGICAL EVALUATION, PERFORMED 1 WEEK AFTER THE FIRST COGNITIVE SCREENING, REPORTED THAT THE PATIENT IN THIS STUDY HAD A GOOD ATTENTION SPAN AND WAS ORIENTED AND COOPERATIVE. NO EVIDENCE OF IDENTIFIABLE BRAIN LESIONS WAS NOTED. THE CASE SUGGESTS ONE OF TWO POSSIBILITIES: (1) CLOSER EXAMINATION OF CHILDREN WHO GIVE FLIPPANT RESPONSES MAY LEAD TO FURTHER EVIDENCE OF THE GANSER SYNDROME IN THIS POPULATION; OR (2) THE VALIDITY OF THE GANSER

STATE AS A CLEARLY DEFINED BUT RARE PSYCHIATRIC ILLNESS IS QUESTIONABLE BECAUSE MANY OF THE SIGNS AND SYMPTOMS MAY APPEAR IN CHILDREN AS WELL AS IN ADULTS WITH LIMITED COPING MECHANISMS. THESE INDIVIDUALS, WHO DEMONSTRATE SOME FORM OF SOCIALLY UNACCEPTABLE BEHAVIOR, MAY BE RESPONDING TO STRESS ASSOCIATED WITH INSTITUTIONAL CONSTRAINTS IMPOSED UPON THEM IN THE INTEREST OF THERAPEUTIC INTERVENTION. 8 REFERENCES. (NCHHI ABSTRACT)

ACCN   002166

1310 AUTH   **NATALICIO, D. S., & NATALICIO L. F.**
TITL   A COMPARATIVE STUDY OF ENGLISH PLURALIZATION BY NATIVE AND NON-NATIVE ENGLISH SPEAKERS.
SRCE   *CHILD DEVELOPMENT, 1971, 42(4), 1302-1306.*
INDX   BILINGUALISM, SYNTAX, MEXICAN AMERICAN, CHILDREN, ADOLESCENTS, EMPIRICAL, LANGUAGE LEARNING, LINGUISTICS, MALE, TEXAS, SOUTHWEST
ABST   FOUR GROUPS OF 36 MALES IN THE FIRST, SECOND, THIRD AND TENTH GRADES, EQUALLY DIVIDED AT EACH GRADE LEVEL ACCORDING TO NATIVE LANGUAGE, WERE PRESENTED A RANDOMIZED LIST OF NONSENSE SYLLABLES DESIGNED TO ELICIT PLURAL FORMATIONS. EACH OF 24 FINAL CONSONANT PHONEMES WERE PAIRED WITH ONE OF THREE INITIAL CONSONANT-VOWEL COMBINATIONS, RESULTING IN A 24-TRIGRAM TEST INSTRUMENT. ALTHOUGH THE DATA REVEALED A DIFFERENCE BETWEEN NATIVE ENGLISH SPEAKERS (NES) AND NATIVE SPANISH SPEAKERS (NSS) IN OVERALL PROPORTION OF CORRECT RESPONSES, THE ORDER IN WHICH THE SEGMENTS WERE BROUGHT UNDER CONTROL SEEMED TO BE THE SAME (E.G., THOSE FINAL SEGMENTS PLURALIZED CORRECTLY IN THE SECOND GRADE BY NSS SUBJECTS WERE THE SAME AS THOSE WHICH THE NES SUBJECTS PLURALIZED BY THE END OF THE FIRST GRADE). THE DATA FAILED TO PROVIDE ANY INDICATION OF "INTERFERENCE" FROM SPANISH TO ENGLISH WITHIN THE CONSTRAINTS OF THE PLURALIZATION TASK. THE NSS SUBJECTS DID NOT APPEAR TO EMPLOY SPANISH PLURALIZATION STRATEGIES FOR FORMING ENGLISH PLURALS. IT IS SUGGESTED THAT THE NOTION OF INTERFERENCE IN SECOND-LANGUAGE TEACHING MAY WELL BE A SELF-FULFILLING PROPHECY IN THE TEACHING OF ENGLISH TO NON-NATIVE ENGLISH SPEAKERS IN THE ELEMENTARY GRADES. 7 REFERENCES.

ACCN   001122

1311 AUTH   **NATALICIO, L. F., & NATALICIO, D. S.**
TITL   THE EDUCATIONAL PROBLEMS OF ATYPICAL STUDENT GROUPS: THE NATIVE SPEAKER OF SPANISH.
SRCE   *URBAN EDUCATION, 1969, 4(3), 262-272.*
INDX   MEXICAN AMERICAN, LANGUAGE LEARNING, BILINGUALISM, EDUCATION, INSTRUCTIONAL TECHNIQUES, TEACHERS, PHONOLOGY, CURRICULUM, ESSAY, POVERTY, SES, TEXAS, SOUTHWEST, POLICY

ABST LINGUISTIC BARRIERS ARE PROBLEMS WHICH THE SPANISH-SPEAKING CHILD FACES IN THE EDUCATIONAL SYSTEM, AND LATER IN THE LABOR MARKET AND SOCIETY IN GENERAL. RESPONSIBILITY FOR AMELIORATING THE SITUATION IS SEEN AS RESIDING IN THE KIND OF TRAINING TEACHERS RECEIVE AS WELL AS THE EDUCATIONAL SYSTEM'S BASIC IDEOLOGIES. PRESENTED ARE STATISTICS FROM SURVEYS CONDUCTED IN TEXAS WHICH RELATE TO EMPLOYMENT OF VARIOUS ETHNIC GROUPS. BECAUSE OF THE DISPROPORTIONATE FIGURES AMONG THE SPANISH-SPEAKING, SUGGESTIONS ARE MADE FOR THE TRAINING OF TEACHERS IN A SECOND LANGUAGE AND KNOWLEDGE OF APPLIED LINGUISTICS AND ORAL TRADITION. ADMINISTRATIVE REASSESSMENT IS ALSO SEEN AS NECESSARY FOR PROGRAMS DEALING WITH EDUCATION PROBLEMS UNIQUE TO GROUPS DIFFERING IN CHARACTERISTICS FROM THE GENERAL NORM. A FINAL PROPOSAL IS MADE FOR POSITIVE LANGUAGE PROGRAMS. 12 REFERENCES.

ACCN 001123

1312 AUTH **NATIONAL COUNCIL OF LA RAZA.**
TITL LACK OF ACCESS TO POWER DOCUMENTED.
SRCE *AGENDA, NOVEMBER/DECEMBER 1976, PP. 1; 5.*
INDX REPRESENTATION, SPANISH SURNAMED, MEXICAN AMERICAN, POLITICAL POWER, POLITICS, REVIEW, SOUTHWEST, ESSAY, ECONOMIC FACTORS, LEADERSHIP
ABST HISPANICS ARE SIGNIFICANTLY UNDERREPRESENTED AT ALL LEVELS OF POWER AND DECISION MAKING IN THE UNITED STATES. IN A STATEMENT ENTITLED, "ACCESSIBILITY OF THE HISPANIC AMERICAN POPULATION TO THE DECISION AND POLICY MAKING PROCESS IN THE PRIVATE AND PUBLIC INSTITUTIONS OF THE U.S." (1975), RAUL YZAGUIRRE DOCUMENTS THIS LACK OF ACCESS TO POWER. STATISTICS REVEAL THAT ONLY A SMALL PERCENTAGE OF FEDERAL EMPLOYEES ARE HISPANIC, AND OF THESE A MAJORITY ARE AT THE LOWEST PAYING POSITIONS. THROUGHOUT THE SOUTHWEST, WHERE CHICANOS COMPRISE A SIGNIFICANT PROPORTION OF THE POPULATION, THEY HAVE LITTLE POLITICAL, JUDICIAL OR EDUCATIONAL REPRESENTATION. DUE TO THE LACK OF POWER AND INFLUENCE IN THESE AREAS, HISPANICS DO NOT RECEIVE A FAIR SHARE OF FUNDING AND FINANCIAL SUPPORT FROM FEDERAL OR PRIVATE FOUNDATIONS. THEREFORE, LACK OF ACCESS TO POWER MOST SEVERELY AFFECTS THE ECONOMIC SITUATION OF THE HISPANIC COMMUNITY. AS HISPANICS ARE SOON TO BECOME THE NATION'S LARGEST MINORITY, THE ACQUISITION OF POWER TO GAIN FULL PARTICIPATION IN U.S. SOCIETY IS THE MOST URGENT GOAL OF THIS GROUP.

ACCN 001124

1313 AUTH **NATIONAL INSTITUTE OF EDUCATION.**
TITL DESEGREGATION AND EDUCATION CONCERNS OF THE HISPANIC COMMUNITY: CONFERENCE REPORT, JUNE 26-28, 1977.
SRCE *WASHINGTON, D.C.: AUTHOR, OCTOBER 1977.*
INDX PROCEEDINGS, EDUCATION, MEXICAN AMERICAN, PROGRAM EVALUATION, CHILDREN, POLICY, EQUAL OPPORTUNITY, BILINGUAL-BICULTURAL EDUCATION, BILINGUAL, DISCRIMINATION, FINANCING, INTEGRATION, SPANISH SURNAMED
ABST THIS CONFERENCE WAS PLANNED BY HISPANIC SPOKESPERSONS CHOSEN BY THE NATIONAL INSTITUTE OF EDUCATION (NIE) TO GENERATE AN EXCHANGE OF IDEAS AMONG EDUCATIONAL RESEARCHERS ON DESEGREGATION AND HISPANIC EDUCATIONAL CONCERNS. THE SEVEN SESSIONS FOCUSED ON: (1) IDENTIFICATION AND CLARIFICATION OF RESEARCH ISSUES; (2) HEW POLICY TOWARDS DESEGREGATION; (3) LEGAL AND EDUCATIONAL IMPLICATIONS OF DESEGREGATION; (4) THE PROBLEMS AND NEEDS OF HISPANIC STUDENTS IN THE DESEGREGATION PROCESS; (5) CASE STUDIES PRESENTED BY PARENTS AND EDUCATORS FROM SELECTED AREAS; (6) THE PROS AND CONS OF DESEGREGATION FOR HISPANICS; AND (7) THE POTENTIAL ROLE OF NIE AND OTHER AGENCIES IN SPONSORING RESEARCH IN THESE AREAS. APPENDICES CONTAIN THE NIE PAPER ON LEGAL ISSUES RELATED TO SCHOOL DESEGREGATION, BIOGRAPHICAL SKETCHES OF THE 31 PARTICIPANTS, AND A LIST OF ATTENDEES.

ACCN 002167

1314 AUTH **NATIONAL INSTITUTE OF MENTAL HEALTH.**
TITL MENTAL HEALTH PLANNING CONFERENCE FOR THE SPANISH SPEAKING (DHEW PUBLICATION NO. HSM 73-9064).
SRCE *ROCKVILLE, MARYLAND: NATIONAL INSTITUTE OF MENTAL HEALTH, 1972.*
INDX HEALTH DELIVERY SYSTEMS, PSYCHOTHERAPY, BILINGUALISM, MENTAL HEALTH PROFESSION, PSYCHOTHERAPISTS, ALCOHOLISM, DRUG ABUSE, PROCEEDINGS, SPANISH SURNAMED
ABST THE PROCEEDINGS OF THE MENTAL HEALTH PLANNING CONFERENCE FOR THE SPANISH-SPEAKING (SS) ARE REPORTED. A PRESENTATION ENTITLED "MENTAL HEALTH AND THE SPANISH SPEAKING" EXAMINED THE PRESENT RELATIONSHIP BETWEEN GOVERNMENT AGENCIES AND THE SS. IN ADDITION, A DISCUSSION ON CURRENT PROBLEMS FOUND IN MENTAL HEALTH DELIVERY SYSTEMS EMPHASIZED THE IMPORTANCE OF COMPILING A BODY OF KNOWLEDGE OF THE SS FOR FUTURE PROGRAM PLANNING. A LIST OF 11 DEMANDS WAS PRESENTED BY THE SS PARTICIPANTS TO GENERATE NEW PROPOSALS, IDEAS, AND FUTURE PLANNING STRATEGIES. REPORTS ON GROUP WORKSHOPS CONCERNING SUCH TOPICS AS MENTAL HEALTH SERVICES, MANPOWER AND TRAINING PROGRAMS, SPECIAL MENTAL HEALTH PROGRAMS, ALCOHOLISM AND DRUG ABUSE PROGRAMS, AND RESEARCH DIRECTIONS ARE PROVIDED. EACH WORKSHOP INCLUDED THE SS CONFEREES AND REPRESENTATIVES FROM THE NATIONAL INSTITUTE OF MENTAL HEALTH (NIMH). RESPONSES FROM NIMH DIVISION MEMBERS DISCUSSED THE FEASIBILITY OF EACH GROUP'S REPORT. A SUMMARY OF THE RECOMMENDA-

TIONS PROPOSED BY EACH OF THE GROUP WORKSHOPS IS LISTED.

ACCN 001125

1315 AUTH **NATIONAL INSTITUTE OF MENTAL HEALTH.**
TITL PROCEEDINGS OF THE INSTITUTE ON NARCOTIC ADDICTION AMONG MEXICAN AMERICANS IN THE SOUTHWEST, APRIL 21-23, 1971 (DHEW PUBLICATION NO. (HSM) 73-9085).
SRCE *WASHINGTON, D.C.: U.S. GOVERNMENT PRINTING OFFICE, 1973.*
INDX DRUG ADDICTION, DRUG ABUSE, REHABILITATION, CULTURAL FACTORS, CULTURE, HISTORY, OCCUPATIONAL ASPIRATIONS, DEMOGRAPHIC, SES, METHADONE MAINTENANCE, ECONOMIC FACTORS, MEXICAN AMERICAN, PROCEEDINGS
ABST NIMH ESTABLISHED THIS CONFERENCE FOR THE EXCHANGE OF EMPIRICAL DATA AND PERSONAL EXPERIENCE IN ORDER TO DEVELOP GUIDELINES FOR THE TREATMENT OF MEXICAN AMERICAN ADDICTS, WHOSE PROBLEMS DIFFER FROM THOSE OF OTHER GROUPS IN OTHER PARTS OF THE COUNTRY. HELD IN SAN ANTONIO, TEXAS, APPROXIMATELY 150 PERSONS ATTENDED, REPRESENTING DRUG ADDICTION PROGRAMS IN 9 STATES. THE KEYNOTE PRESENTATIONS COVER HISTORICAL, PSYCHOHISTORICAL, AND SOCIOECONOMIC PERSPECTIVES OF THE MEXICAN AMERICAN OF TEXAS AND THE SOUTHWEST, SOCIAL AND COMMUNITY ACTION AMONG NARCOTIC ADDICTS, AND VOCATIONAL OPPORTUNITIES FOR THE EX-ADDICT. THE PANEL PRESENTATIONS DISCUSS ANALYSIS AND CAUSATION. WORKSHOP GROUPS FORMULATED RECOMMENDATIONS WHICH NOT ONLY CALL FOR SPECIFIC ACTIONS BUT APPEAL TO GENERAL IDEOLOGICAL PRINCIPLES. THESE INCLUDE: (1) A SYSTEMS APPROACH IN DEALING WITH THE CHICANO ADDICT; (2) INTER-DISCIPLINARY AND TEAM APPROACHES; (3) CHANGE IN EXPECTATIONS AND CRITERIA FOR SUCCESS; (4) FOLLOW-THROUGH SERVICES; AND (5) MORE INFORMATION ON AND MONITORING OF METHADONE AS PART OF A TREATMENT PROGRAM.
ACCN 001126

1316 AUTH **NATIONAL LEAGUE FOR NURSING.**
TITL EDUCATIONAL PREPARATION FOR NURSING—1972.
SRCE *NURSING OUTLOOK, 1973, 21, 586-593.*
INDX REPRESENTATION, PROFESSIONAL TRAINING, SPANISH SURNAMED, SURVEY, EMPIRICAL, NURSING
ABST SELECTED RESULTS ARE PRESENTED OF A 1970-71 SURVEY OF STATE-APPROVED SCHOOLS OF NURSING IN THE 56 U. S. JURISDICTIONS. THE PROGRAMS SURVEYED INCLUDE THOSE WHICH PREPARE FOR BEGINNING PRACTICE IN NURSING AND GRADUATE PROGRAMS WHICH LEAD TO MASTERS AND DOCTORAL DEGREES. THE DATA SHOW A MARKED INCREASE IN THE NUMBER OF A. D. PROGRAMS, A DECREASE IN DIPLOMA PROGRAMS, A SMALL INCREASE IN BACCALAUREATE PROGRAMS, AND AN INCREASE IN

PRACTICAL/VOCATIONAL PROGRAMS. THERE WAS INCREASED ENROLLMENT AND GRADUATION AT THE MASTERS LEVEL WITH THE DECREASE AT THE DOCTORAL. MINORITY DATA WERE EXPANDED, FOR THE FIRST TIME, TO INCLUDE SPANISH AMERICAN STUDENTS, AMERICAN INDIANS, AND ORIENTALS. THE FINDINGS SHOW THAT THE PERCENT OF SPANISH AMERICAN ADMISSIONS AND GRADUATIONS ARE SIGNIFICANTLY GREATER IN PRACTICAL NURSING PROGRAMS THAN IN REGISTERED NURSING PROGRAMS. THE SURVEY ALSO SHOWS THAT THE NUMBER OF MINORITY ADMISSIONS, ENROLLMENTS, AND GRADUATIONS HAVE CONTINUED TO INCREASE AND THAT THE PROPORTIONS OF MINORITY STUDENTS IN THE FOUR BASIC TYPES OF PROGRAMS HAVE ALSO RISEN. THE NLN BELIEVES THAT RECENT EFFORTS TO RECRUIT MINORITY STUDENTS HAVE BEGUN TO MATERIALIZE. 2 REFERENCES.
ACCN 001127

1317 AUTH **NATIONAL LEAGUE FOR NURSING.**
TITL EDUCATIONAL PREPARATION FOR NURSING—1975.
SRCE *NURSING OUTLOOK, 1976, 24, 568-573.*
INDX REPRESENTATION, HEALTH, PROFESSIONAL TRAINING, SURVEY, EMPIRICAL, SPANISH SURNAMED, NURSING, FEMALE
ABST SURVEY DATA ON THE ENROLLMENT AND DISTRIBUTION OF HISPANIC STUDENTS IN U.S. NURSING SCHOOLS ARE INCLUDED IN A STATISTICAL REPORT OF NURSING EDUCATION TRENDS. DATA ARE BASED UPON THE 1975 NATIONAL LEAGUE FOR NURSING'S ANNUAL SURVEY OF STATE APPROVED SCHOOLS OF NURSING, AND INCLUDE ADMISSIONS AND GRADUATIONS FOR THE PRECEEDING ACADEMIC YEAR, ADMISSIONS FOR THE CURRENT FALL TERM, AND ENROLLMENT AS OF OCTOBER, 1975. A CONTINUED REDUCED RATE OF GROWTH OF BASIC NURSING EDUCATION PROGRAMS IS NOTED IN THE 1975 SURVEY OF SCHOOLS OFFERING BACCALAUREATE, ASSOCIATE, DIPLOMA, R.N., AND PRACTICAL NURSING DEGREES. INFORMATION ON MINORITY (BLACK, SPANISH BACKGROUND, AMERICAN INDIAN, AND ORIENTALS) AND MALE ENROLLMENT COMMENCED IN 1972 AND IS COLLECTED EVERY 3 YEARS, AND THE NUMBER AND PERCENTAGE OF HISPANIC STUDENTS ADMITTED, ENROLLED, AND GRADUATED FROM NURSING PROGRAMS IS REPORTED FOR 1972 AND 1975. LARGER PROPORTIONS OF R.N. PROGRAMS REPORT ADMITTING AND GRADUATING MINORITY STUDENTS THAN DO PRACTICAL NURSING SCHOOLS. THIS IS ATTRIBUTABLE TO THE DIVERSE POPULATION FOUND IN GEOGRAPHIC AREAS FROM WHICH R.N.'S ARE DRAWN. THE LOCATION OF SPANISH NURSING STUDENTS REFLECTS THE U.S. GEOGRAPHIC DISTRIBUTION OF THE HISPANIC COMMUNITY. ALTHOUGH DIFFERENCES IN SCHOOLS' SURVEY RESPONSES IN 1972 AND 1975 MADE COMPARISONS DIFFICULT, CHANGES BETWEEN THESE YEARS APPEAR TO HAVE BEEN MODEST.

ACCN   001128

1318 AUTH   **NATIONAL MIGRANT INFORMATION CLEAR-INGHOUSE: JUAREZ-LINCOLN CENTER.**

TITL   A STATISTICAL PROFILE: 4344 MIGRANT FAMILIES IN SOUTH TEXAS/MARCH 1974.

SRCE   *EL PASO, TEXAS: NATIONAL MIGRANT INFORMATION CLEARINGHOUSE, JUAREZ-LINCOLN CENTER, 1974.*

INDX   FARM LABORERS, RURAL, MIGRATION, EMPLOYMENT, ECONOMIC FACTORS, DEMOGRAPHIC, FAMILY STRUCTURE, SURVEY, EMPIRICAL, MIGRANTS, TEXAS, SOUTHWEST

ABST   AS A SPECIAL REQUEST FROM THE MIGRANT DIVISION ON THE U. S. DEPARTMENT OF LABOR, THIS SURVEY WAS CONDUCTED TO DETERMINE WHETHER OR NOT THE ANTICIPATED GASOLINE SHORTAGES, PRECIPITATED BY THE ONSET OF THE "ENERGY CRISIS," WOULD AFFECT THE PLANS OF SOUTH TEXAS MIGRANT FARMWORKERS TO TRAVEL UP NORTH. WITH THE HELP OF SEVERAL ORGANIZATIONS, THE SURVEY WAS UNDERTAKEN IN TWO WEEKS COVERING 4344 MIGRANT FAMILIES IN SIX COUNTIES OF SOUTH TEXAS, INCLUDING THE CITIES OF LAREDO AND SAN ANTONIO. THE TOPICS FOR QUESTIONING INCLUDED: MIGRATION RATE, EMPLOYMENT, FUEL AND HOUSING ARRANGEMENTS, RECEIVER STATES, DEPARTURE MONTHS, MODES OF TRANSPORTATION, REASONS FOR NOT MIGRATING AND FAMILY SIZE. RESPECTIVELY, THE RESULTS SHOW THAT: (1) THE MAJORITY OF MIGRANT FAMILIES PLANNED TO MIGRATE (70.5%); (2) NEARLY 83% OF THE FAMILIES STATED THEY DI HAVE JOB COMMITTMENTS ALTHOUGH 80% HAD NOT MADE FULL ARRANGEMENTS; (3) 77% OF THE FAMILIES INDICATED THAT HOUSING ARRANGEMENTS HAD BEEN MADE FOR THEM; (4) MIGRANTS TRAVEL TO 36 STATES OUTSIDE OF TEXAS TO SECURE EMPLOYMENT, WITH THE LARGEST PERCENTAGE TRAVELING TO THE MIDWESTERN STATES; (5) MOST MIGRANTS (70%) LEAVE TEXAS DURING THE MONTHS OF MAY AND JUNE; (6) CARS OR TRUCKS ARE THE CHIEF MODE OF TRANSPORTATION; (7) WITH 25% OF THE FAMILIES NOT MIGRATING, 93% STATED SO FOR REASONS OF THE FUEL SHORTAGE; AND (8) THE SIZE OF MIGRANT FAMILIES RANGES FROM 4 TO 8 PERSONS.

ACCN   001129

1319 AUTH   **NATIONAL RESEARCH COUNCIL, COMMISSION ON HUMAN RESOURCES.**

TITL   MINORITY GROUPS AMONG UNITED STATES DOCTORATE-LEVEL SCIENTISTS, ENGINEERS, AND SCHOLARS, 1973 (VOL. 7).

SRCE   *WASHINGTON, D.C.: NATIONAL ACADEMY OF SCIENCES, 1974.*

INDX   HIGHER EDUCATION, CROSS CULTURAL, MENTAL HEALTH PROFESSION, SURVEY, PROFESSIONAL TRAINING, LABOR FORCE, REPRESENTATION, SPANISH SURNAMED

ABST   TWO SOURCES OF DATA WERE USED TO DETERMINE THE NUMBERS OF MINORITY GROUP MEMBERS (BLACK, ORIENTAL, LATIN, NATIVE AMERICAN) IN THE DOCTORATE-LEVEL POPULATION OF THE U.S. THE FIRST SOURCE CONTAINS THE NUMBER OF PEOPLE EARNING THIRD-LEVEL DEGREES (PHD., SCD., EDD., ETC., BUT EXCLUDING SUCH PROFESSIONAL DEGREES AS MD., DDS., DVM.) FROM U.S. UNIVERSITIES IN THE ACADEMIC YEAR 1972-73. THE SECOND SOURCE, WHICH IS RESTRICTED TO DOCTORATE-LEVEL ENGINEERS AND SCIENTISTS, INCLUDING SOCIAL SCIENTISTS, CONSISTS OF A LARGE STRATIFIED SAMPLE OF THE 1973 LABOR FORCE AT THIS LEVEL. THE DATA REVEAL: (1) APPROXIMATELY 975 BLACKS, 2430 ORIENTALS, 350 LATINS, AND 150 AMERICAN INDIANS ATTAINED DOCTORAL DEGREES, HOWEVER ONLY 37% OF THESE MINORITIES WERE U.S. CITIZENS; (2) BLACKS AND AMERICAN INDIANS WERE HEAVILY CONCENTRATED IN EDUCATION, ORIENTALS IN THE NATURAL SCIENCES, AND LATINS IN THE HUMANITIES; (3) AMONG DOCTORATE-LEVEL SCIENTISTS AND ENGINEERS, THERE WERE APPROXIMATELY 1,-860 BLACKS, 11,000 ORIENTALS, 1,400 LATINS, AND 100 AMERICAN INDIANS (OF THESE, 28% WERE U.S. CITIZENS); AND (4) ALTHOUGH THERE IS AN INCREASE OF MINORITIES IN THE SCIENTIFIC AND ENGINEERING POPULATION, THIS WAS DUE TO THE "BRAIN DRAIN" FROM FOREIGN COUNTRIES RATHER THAN FROM NATIVE U.S. CITIZENS. 11 REFERENCES. (AUTHOR SUMMARY MODIFIED)

ACCN   001130

1320 AUTH   **NAUN, R. J.**

TITL   COMPARISON OF GROUP COUNSELING APPROACHES WITH PUERTO RICAN BOYS IN AN INNER CITY HIGH SCHOOL (DOCTORAL DISSERTATION, FORDHAM UNIVERSITY, 1971).

SRCE   *DISSERTATION ABSTRACTS INTERNATIONAL, 1971, 32(2), 742A-743A. (UNIVERSITY MICROFILMS NO. 71-20,200.)*

INDX   EDUCATIONAL COUNSELING, PUERTO RICAN-M, PSYCHOTHERAPY, PSYCHOTHERAPY OUTCOME, ADOLESCENTS, EMPIRICAL, PROGRAM EVALUATION, MALE

ABST   EFFECTS OF TWO DIFFERENT METHODS OF COUNSELING ON 31 NINTH AND TENTH GRADE PUERTO RICAN BOYS LIVING IN A FEDERALLY DESIGNATED POVERTY AREA WERE INVESTIGATED. ONE GROUP RECEIVED INTERVENTIONIST COUNSELING, ONE RECEIVED ROGERIAN NONINTERVENTIONIST COUNSELING, AND ONE RECEIVED NO COUNSELING. THERE WAS A SIGNIFICANT DIFFERENCE IN COUNSELOR VERBAL RESPONSE RATE BETWEEN APPROACHES. THERE WERE NO SIGNIFICANT CHANGES IN LEVEL OF OCCUPATIONAL ASPIRATION FOR ANY GROUP. THERE WERE NO SIGNIFICANT DIFFERENCES IN ASPIRATION, SCHOOL BEHAVIOR, GRADE AVERAGE, TARDINESS OR TEACHER RATINGS. IN NEITHER EXPERIMENTAL APPROACH DID THE SUBJECTS PERCEIVE THE COUNSELOR IN TERMS THAT WOULD BE CONSIDERED MORE HELPFUL OR MORE CONDUCIVE TO COUNSELING. THE SUBJECTS GETTING NONINTERVENTIONIST TREATMENT RECEIVED SIGNIFICANTLY FEWER REFERRALS TO THE DEAN.

ACCN   001131

1321 AUTH   **NAVAR, I. N.**
     TITL   LA COMMUNIDAD HABLA: RACISM FROM THE
            EXPERIENCED REALITY—AN INVESTIGATION
            INTO THE RELEVANT VARIABLES AND THEIR
            MENTAL HEALTH CONSEQUENCES.
     SRCE   *UNPUBLISHED MANUSCRIPT, 1975. (AVAILABLE
            FROM DR. ISABELLE NAVAR, PSYCHOLOGY DE-
            PARTMENT, CALIFORNIA STATE COLLEGE,
            DOMINGUEZ HILLS, CALIFORNIA.)*
     INDX   PREJUDICE, DISCRIMINATION, COMMUNITY,
            MEXICAN AMERICAN, CULTURE, MARRIAGE,
            SELF CONCEPT, PSYCHOSOCIAL ADJUSTMENT,
            ACCULTURATION, ADOLESCENTS, ADULTS, UR-
            BAN, ENVIRONMENTAL FACTORS
     ABST   THE PURPOSE OF THIS EXPLORATORY-DE-
            SCRIPTIVE STUDY WAS TO ESTABLISH NEW
            CATEGORIES AND VARIABLES RELEVANT TO
            THE STUDY OF MENTAL HEALTH AND RACISM
            AS EXPERIENCED BY THE MEXICAN AMERICAN
            COMMUNITY. UNLESS THESE CONCEPTS ARE
            PROPERLY IDENTIFIED, MENTAL HEALTH SER-
            VICES ATTEMPTING TO RELATE TO THE CHI-
            CANO COMMUNITY WILL NOT BE EFFECTIVE
            NOR THERAPEUTIC. THE GOAL WAS AP-
            PROACHED THROUGH A RESEARCH DESIGN
            EMPLOYING AUDIO AND VIDEOTAPE INTER-
            VIEWS OF A WIDE RANGE OF MEXICAN AMERI-
            CANS INVOLVED IN DIFFERENT TYPES OF IN-
            TERACTION. THE VARIOUS EXPERIENCES
            INCLUDED ADOLESCENTS IN A GROUP, A WED-
            DING CELEBRATION, A FAMILY, A CHICANA
            GROUP, AND A DEMONSTRATION AND TALK BY
            TWO CURANDEROS. IN LOOKING AT THE SIG-
            NIFICANCE AND MEANING OF THESE EXPERI-
            ENCES, THE RELEVANT VARIABLES EXTRACTED
            WERE THE TYPES OF INTERACTION BETWEEN
            MEMBERS OF CERTAIN GROUPS AND THEIR
            PARTICULAR CONCERNS, SIGNS OF POSITIVE
            MENTAL HEALTH WELL-DEFINED VALUES, CON-
            VERGING OLD AND NEW TRADITIONS ALONG
            WITH THE PRESERVATION OF CUSTOMS. THE
            OVERALL NEED TO STUDY MINORITY CUL-
            TURES FROM THE VIEWPOINT OF MINORITY IN-
            DIVIDUALS IS EMPHASIZED IN ORDER TO IN-
            FLUENCE THE AMERICAN SYSTEM TOWARDS A
            MORE EQUITABLE SOCIETY.
     ACCN   001133

1322 AUTH   **NAVAR, I. N.**
     TITL   SOMOS ESTUDIANTES.
     SRCE   *UNPUBLISHED MANUSCRIPT, 1975. (AVAILABLE
            FROM DR. ISABELLE NAVAR, PSYCHOLOGY DE-
            PARTMENT, CALIFORNIA STATE COLLEGE,
            DOMINGUEZ HILLS, CALIFORNIA.)*
     INDX   BIBLIOGRAPHY, MEXICAN AMERICAN, ACCUL-
            TURATION, POVERTY, POLITICAL POWER, BIRTH
            CONTROL, HISTORY, ART, BILINGUALISM, CHI-
            CANO MOVEMENT, CHILDREN, CURANDER-
            ISMO, FARM LABORERS, LEARNING
     ABST   THIS MAGAZINE, DEVELOPED THROUGH THE
            EFFORTS OF A MEXICAN AMERICAN (MA) COL-
            LEGE PROFESSOR AND HER PSYCHOLOGY
            CLASS AT A CALIFORNIA STATE UNIVERSITY,
            CONTAINS THE WORK OF HER MA STUDENTS.
            SUBJECT THEMES COVER TWO AREAS: (1)
            EDUCATION AND (2) PERSONAL EXPERIENCE.

POETIC THEMES INCLUDE LIFE IN THE BARRIO,
CHICANO CONSCIOUSNESS, FARMWORKERS
AND FREE ASSOCIATION EXCERCISES. EDU-
CATIONAL TOPICS INCLUDE REJECTION OF BI-
LINGUALISM IN SCHOOLS, CONTRACEPTIVE
METHODS, MEXICAN AMERICAN HISTORY, AC-
CULTURATION, HOW TO WRITE TERM PAPERS,
LEARNING IN CHILDREN, CURANDEROS, AND
MEXICAN AMERICAN ART. 37 REFERENCES.
     ACCN   001132

1323 AUTH   **NAVARRO, A.**
     TITL   EDUCATIONAL CHANGE THROUGH POLITICAL
            ACTION.
     SRCE   *IN A. CASTANEDA, M. RAMIREZ, III, C. E. CORTES,
            & M. BARRERA (EDS.), MEXICAN AMERICANS
            AND EDUCATIONAL CHANGE. NEW YORK: ARNO
            PRESS, 1974, PP. 105-139.*
     INDX   HISTORY, POVERTY, PREJUDICE, EDUCATION,
            DISCRIMINATION, MEXICAN AMERICAN, REP-
            RESENTATION, POLITICS, POLITICAL POWER,
            LEADERSHIP, COMMUNITY INVOLVEMENT, SO-
            CIAL SERVICES, PARAPROFESSIONALS, COL-
            LEGE STUDENTS, ADMINISTRATORS, CHICANO
            MOVEMENT, CALIFORNIA, SOUTHWEST
     ABST   THE ORGANIZING EFFORTS OF A SOUTHERN
            CALIFORNIA CHICANO BARRIO TO AFFECT
            EDUCATIONAL CHANGE WITHIN THE CUCA-
            MONGA SCHOOL DISTRICT THROUGH THE
            POLITICIZATION AND MOBILIZATION OF COM-
            MUNITY MEMBERS IS PRESENTED. THE
            STRATEGIES OF THE MEXICAN AMERICAN PO-
            LITICAL ASSOCIATION (MAPA) AS THE MAIN
            ORGANIZING BODY ARE EXAMINED: (1) STIMU-
            LATION OF COMMUNITY INVOLVEMENT AND
            CULTURAL AWARENESS; (2) ACQUISITION OF
            BARRIO CONTROL OF THE DISTRICT'S BOARD
            OF TRUSTEES THROUGH VOTER REGISTRA-
            TION AND THE ELECTORAL PROCESS; AND (3)
            IMPLEMENTATION OF PROPOSALS CALLING
            FOR BILINGUAL/BICULTURAL EDUCATIONAL
            PROGRAMS AND MORE CHICANO TEACHERS,
            STAFF, AND NEW FACILITIES. INCLUDED IS A
            DISCUSSION OF THE RELATIONSHIP BETWEEN
            MAPA AND THE ANGLO COMMUNITY AND
            OTHER "MOVEMENT" ORIENTED GROUPS, SUCH
            AS MECHA AND THE BROWN BERETS. IN ADDI-
            TION, THE DEVELOPMENT OF EL PARTIDO DE
            LA RAZA UNIDA (PRU) IN THE CUCAMONGA
            AREA AS A NEW ENTITY TO ACHIEVE ECO-
            NOMIC AND SOCIAL CHANGE IS DISCUSSED.
            CULTURAL NATIONALISM IS STRESSED AS THE
            MAIN ORGANIZING TOOL OF THE PRU, WHILE
            ITS PRIMARY FUNCTION IS TO SERVE AS A
            MASS MOVEMENT AND PRESSURE GROUP.
     ACCN   001134

1324 AUTH   **NAYLOR, G. H.**
     TITL   LEARNING STYLES AT SIX YEARS IN TWO ETH-
            NIC GROUPS IN A DISADVANTAGED AREA
            (DOCTORAL DISSERTATION, UNIVERSITY OF
            SOUTHERN CALIFORNIA, 1971).
     SRCE   *DISSERTATION ABSTRACTS INTERNATIONAL,
            1971, 32(2), 794A. (UNIVERSITY MICROFILMS
            NO. 71-21,481.)*
     INDX   LEARNING, COGNITIVE STYLE, MEXICAN

AMERICAN, POVERTY, SES, CROSS CULTURAL, CHILDREN, EMPIRICAL, INSTRUCTIONAL TECHNIQUES, COGNITIVE DEVELOPMENT, FIELD DEPENDENCE-INDEPENDENCE, CALIFORNIA, SOUTHWEST, SEX COMPARISON

ABST THIS INVESTIGATION OF LEARNING STYLE AMONG 6 YEAR-OLD CHILDREN OF A DISADVANTAGED AREA FOCUSED ON THE RELATIONSHIP BETWEEN FOUR SELECTED LEARNING STYLES AND ETHNICITY. SUBJECTS WERE 40 MEXICAN AMERICAN AND 40 ANGLO AMERICAN CHILDREN IN FIRST GRADE WHO HAD A YEAR OF PUBLIC SCHOOL KINDERGARTEN. IT WAS EXPECTED THAT THE MEXICAN AMERICAN GROUPS WOULD DEMAND MORE INFORMATION IN DECISION MAKING, WOULD BE MORE FIELD DEPENDENT, LESS IMPULSIVE, AND LESS ORIGINAL THAN THE ANGLO AMERICAN GROUPS. NO SIGNIFICANT DIFFERENCES BETWEEN SAMPLE GROUPS WERE FOUND ON THE BASIS OF LEARNING STYLE TEST PERFORMANCE, WITH THE EXCEPTION OF THE IMPULSIVITY MEASURES WHERE THE ANGLO AMERICAN GROUP MADE MORE ERRORS THAN DID THE MEXICAN AMERICAN GROUP. THE INTERACTION OF SEX AND ETHNICITY FAILED TO RESULT IN SIGNIFICANT DIFFERENCES BETWEEN SAMPLE GROUPS FOR ANY OF THE LEARNING STYLE MEASURES.

ACCN 001135

1325 AUTH NEDLER, S., & SEBERA, P.
TITL INTERVENTION STRATEGIES FOR SPANISH-SPEAKING PRESCHOOL CHILDREN.
SRCE CHILD DEVELOPMENT, 1971, 42(1), 259-267.
INDX EARLY CHILDHOOD EDUCATION, LINGUISTIC COMPETENCE, POVERTY, BILINGUALISM, CHILDREN, PROGRAM EVALUATION, EMPIRICAL, PEABODY PICTURE-VOCABULARY TEST, MEXICAN AMERICAN, PARENTAL INVOLVEMENT, TEXAS, SOUTHWEST
ABST THREE EARLY INTERVENTION STRATEGIES TO INCREASE THE LANGUAGE AND COMMUNICATION SKILLS OF DISADVANTAGED 3 YEAR-OLD MEXICAN AMERICAN CHILDREN WERE COMPARED. TREATMENT GROUP I INCLUDED 16 CHILDREN IN A PLANNED BILINGUAL EARLY CHILDHOOD EDUCATIONAL PROGRAM. GROUP II INCLUDED 16 CHILDREN WHO WERE INDIRECTLY INVOLVED IN A PARENTAL INVOLVEMENT PROGRAM. GROUP III WAS COMPOSED OF 14 CHILDREN IN A TRADITIONAL DAY-CARE CENTER. BEFORE AND AFTER A 9-MONTH INTERVENTION PERIOD, ALL SUBJECTS WERE TESTED WITH THE LEITER INTERNATIONAL PERFORMANCE SCALE AND THE PEABODY PICTURE-VOCABULARY TEST IN ENGLISH AND SPANISH. ON ALL MEASURES, GROUP I MADE SIGNIFICANTLY GREATER GAINS THAN THE OTHER TWO GROUPS, INDICATING THE GREATER EFFECTIVENESS OF THE PLANNED BILINGUAL EARLY CHILDHOOD EDUCATION PROGRAM. LESSON ACTIVITIES FOR GROUP I WERE DESIGNED TO PROVIDE EXPERIENCES PROMOTING THE USE OF LANGUAGE TO ABSTRACT INFORMATION. BEGINNING WITH THE DEVELOPMENT OF COGNITIVELY DIRECTED PERCEPTIONS, THE SKILLS NEEDED FOR MAK-

ING OBSERVATIONS MEANINGFUL IN ANALYZING THE SURROUNDING "WORLD" ARE PROGRAMMED INTO LESSONS THROUGH CAREFUL, DELINEATED QUESTIONS. EXPANSION OF THIS ABILITY TO HANDLE THE CODING PROCESS FORMS THE BASE FOR THE DEVELOPMENT OF ABSTRACT THINKING SKILLS. 5 REFERENCES.
ACCN 001136

1326 AUTH NELSON, L., & KAGAN, S.
TITL COMPETITION: THE STAR SPANGLED SCRAMBLE.
SRCE PSYCHOLOGY TODAY, 1972, 6(4), PP. 53-54; 56; 90-91; 98.
INDX COOPERATION, COMPETITION, INTERPERSONAL RELATIONS, MEXICAN AMERICAN, MEXICAN, CROSS CULTURAL, CHILDREARING PRACTICES, EMPIRICAL, CHILDREN, CALIFORNIA
ABST THE COOPERATIVE-COMPETITIVE BEHAVIOR OF ANGLO AMERICAN (AA), MEXICAN AMERICAN (MA) AND MEXICAN (M) SCHOOL CHILDREN AGES 4, 5, 7, 9, AND 10 WAS EXAMINED BY FIVE VARIATIONS OF THE COOPERATION-BOARD GAME. ON A TASK TO MEASURE INHIBITION OF COMPETITIVENESS IN SOCIAL INTERACTION AMONG M AND AA SUBJECTS, M CHILDREN WERE FOUND TO AVOID CONFLICT MORE THAN AA'S. IT APPEARS THAT AA'S ENGAGED IN CONFLICT THAT WAS NOT ONLY IRRATIONALLY COMPETITIVE BUT ALMOST SADISTICALLY RIVALROUS. AA CHILDREN WERE MORE WILLING TO REDUCE THEIR OWN REWARDS IN ORDER TO REDUCE THE REWARDS OF THEIR PEERS. M CHILDREN, ON THE OTHER HAND, WERE MORE LIKELY TO ENGAGE IN COOPERATIVE BEHAVIOR WHERE EQUAL REWARDS WERE EARNED BY BOTH PLAYERS OF THE GAME. MA CHILDREN SEEMED TO BE CAUGHT BETWEEN THE STYLES OF BEHAVIOR OF AA AND M CHILDREN. THESE FINDINGS REVEAL DIFFERENCES IN COOPERATION-COMPETITION BETWEEN AA AND M RURAL CHILDREN WHICH APPEAR TO RESULT MORE FROM DIFFERENCES IN COMPETITIVENESS THAN FROM DIFFERENCES IN MOTIVATION OR ABILITY TO COOPERATE. DIFFERENT CHILD-REARING PATTERNS ARE SUGGESTED AS BEING RESPONSIBLE FOR THE DIFFERENCES IN COOPERATION-COMPETITION BEHAVIOR OF AA AND M. RESEARCH ON CHILD-REARING INDICATES THAT RURAL M MOTHERS TEND TO REINFORCE THEIR CHILDREN NONCONTINGENTLY, REWARDING THEM WHETHER THEY SUCCEED OR FAIL, WHEREAS AA MOTHERS TEND TO REINFORCE THEIR CHILDREN AS A RIGID FUNCTION OF THE CHILD'S ACHIEVEMENT. 10 REFERENCES.
ACCN 001137

1327 AUTH NEWMAN, L. E., & STEINBERG, J. L.
TITL CONSULTATION WITH POLICE ON HUMAN RELATIONS TRAINING.
SRCE AMERICAN JOURNAL OF PSYCHIATRY, 1970, 126(10), 1421-1429.
INDX POLICE-COMMUNITY RELATIONS, PROFESSIONAL TRAINING, COMMUNITY, MEXICAN AMERICAN, CASE STUDY, PARAPROFESSION-

ALS, PRIMARY PREVENTION, PROGRAM EVALUATION, CALIFORNIA, SOUTHWEST

ABST THIS STUDY INVESTIGATED THE LOS ANGELES POLICE ACADEMY'S HUMAN RELATIONS TRAINING PROGRAM WHICH WAS FOUNDED AFTER THE 1965 WATTS DISORDERS. THE PROGRAM IS DISCUSSED WITH RELATION TO THE VARIOUS METHODS OF PRESENTING THE MATERIAL TO THE POLICE TRAINEES AND CADETS. THE AREAS COVERED IN THE PROGRAM INCLUDE: (1) UNDERSTANDING AND RELATING TO ETHNIC MINORITY COMMUNITIES, ESPECIALLY THE MEXICAN AMERICAN AND NEGRO COMMUNITIES; (2) HANDLING SERVICE CALLS, E.G., PSYCHIATRIC EMERGENCIES, FAMILY DISPUTES, AND YOUTH CONTACTS; (3) UNDERSTANDING AND DEALING WITH PERSONAL STRESS ASSOCIATED WITH THE DAILY DEMANDS OF POLICE WORK; AND (4) THE MEANING OF POLICE PROFESSIONALISM. BY PRESENTING THE MATERIAL IN SMALL DISCUSSION GROUPS LED BY POLICE OFFICERS, THE PROGRAM WAS ABLE TO COMMUNICATE THE FAR-REACHING PROBLEMS CONFRONTING POLICE OFFICERS IN THEIR NONPUNITIVE RELATIONS WITH THE CITIZENS OF METROPOLITAN LOS ANGELES. A BRIEF MENTION OF OTHER SIMILAR PROGRAMS IN CITIES THROUGHOUT THE UNITED STATES IS ALSO GIVEN. 13 REFERENCES.

ACCN 001138

1328 AUTH **NEWMAN, R. G., CATES, M., TYTUN, A., & WERBELL, B.**

TITL NARCOTIC ADDICTION IN NEW YORK CITY: TRENDS FROM 1968 TO MID-1973.

SRCE *AMERICAN JOURNAL OF ALCOHOL AND DRUG ABUSE, 1974, 1(1), 53-66.*

INDX DRUG ABUSE, DRUG ADDICTION, URBAN, PUERTO RICAN-M, RESOURCE UTILIZATION, DEMOGRAPHIC, EMPIRICAL, CROSS CULTURAL, SEX COMPARISON, CRIMINOLOGY, NEW YORK, EAST, REHABILITATION

ABST BASED ON THE NEW YORK CITY NARCOTICS REGISTER, THIS PRESENTATION ANALYZES CHANGING TRENDS FROM 1968 THROUGH THE MIDDLE OF 1973. THE REGISTER INCLUDES MORE THAN 700,000 REPORTS SUBMITTED BY VARIOUS AGENCIES ON OVER 250,-000 KNOWN OR SUSPECTED DRUG ABUSERS. CASE RECORD ITEMS ANALYZED INCLUDE CONTACT DATE, ETHNIC GROUP, SEX, PRIMARY DRUG(S) OF ABUSE, AGE FIRST USED, MEDICAL COMPLICATIONS, AND REPORTING SOURCE. FOCUS IS ON (1) INDICATORS OF INCIDENCE AND PREVALENCE, (2) DISTRIBUTION BY AGE, SEX, AND ETHNICITY OF NEWLY REPORTED INDIVIDUALS, AND (3) RELATIVE VOLUME OF REPORTS RECEIVED FROM ADDICTION TREATMENT PROGRAMS AND LAW ENFORCEMENT AGENCIES. THE FINDINGS SHOW: (1) BOTH THE PREVALENCE AND INCIDENCE OF ADDICTION IN NEW YORK CITY HAVE BEEN DECLINING SINCE THE FIRST HALF OF 1972; (2) YOUNGER ADDICTS REPRESENT A SMALLER PROPORTION OF NEW CASES THAN IN THE PAST; (3) WOMEN COMPRISE A STEADILY INCREASING PROPORTION OF FIRST-REPORTED

INDIVIDUALS; (4) THERE HAS BEEN NO MARKED CHANGE IN ETHNIC DISTRIBUTION OF INDIVIDUALS FIRST REPORTED, WITH PUERTO RICANS COMPRISING THE LEAST (20%); (5) IN THE LAST HALF OF 1972, FOR THE FIRST TIME, ADDICTS WERE MORE LIKELY TO ENTER ADDICTION TREATMENT PROGRAMS THAN THEY WERE TO COME INTO CONTACT WITH LAW ENFORCEMENT AGENCIES; AND (6) EXPANSION OF ADDICTION TREATMENT FACILITIES AND THE OUTREACH EFFORTS TO ATTRACT NEW PATIENTS HAVE REACHED PREDOMINANTLY THE "OLDER" ADDICT POPULATION; "NEWER" ADDICTS REMAIN FAR MORE LIKELY TO BE REPORTED FROM LAW ENFORCEMENT THAN FROM ADDICTION TREATMENT AGENCIES. 4 REFERENCES.

ACCN 001139

1329 AUTH **NEWTON, F.**

TITL MEXICAN AMERICAN ELDERLY: PROBLEMS IN RESEARCH AND SERVICE DELIVERY.

SRCE *PAPER PRESENTED AT THE ANNUAL MEETING OF THE AMERICAN PUBLIC HEALTH ASSOCIATION, NEW YORK, NOVEMBER 1979. (AVAILABLE FROM AUTHOR, DEPARTMENT OF PSYCHOLOGY, UNIVERSITY OF CALIFORNIA, LOS ANGELES, CA 90024.)*

INDX MEXICAN AMERICAN, GERONTOLOGY, REVIEW, HEALTH DELIVERY SYSTEMS, POLICY, SOCIAL SERVICES·

ABST AN EXTENSIVE REVIEW OF THE LITERATURE ON MEXICAN AMERICAN ELDERLY REVEALS (1) MORE ARGUMENT THAN CONSENSUS IN THE INTERPRETATION OF THE AVAILABLE DATA, AND (2) A TENDENCY FOR RESEARCHERS TO TREAT THIS POPULATION AS IF IT WERE HOMOGENEOUS. REGARDING THE CURRENT CONTROVERSIES IN THE LITERATURE, ATTENTION IS GIVEN TO THREE MAIN ISSUES. FIRST, THERE IS CONFLICTING EVIDENCE ABOUT THE AMOUNT OF FAMILY SUPPORT RECEIVED BY MEXICAN AMERICAN ELDERLY. SECOND, THERE IS NO AGREEMENT ABOUT MALE-FEMALE DIFFERENCES IN THE HEALTH PROBLEMS OF THESE ELDERS. THIRD, THERE REMAINS A CONTROVERSY OVER WHETHER THESE ELDERS PREFER SUPPORT FROM RELATIVES OR GOVERNMENT SERVICES. IT IS CONCLUDED THAT THESE CONTROVERSIES ARE DUE TO THE LACK OF PRECISION IN STUDIES OF MEXICAN AMERICAN ELDERLY—PARTICULARLY, THE FAILURE OF RESEARCHERS TO CONSIDER THE HETEROGENEITY WITHIN THIS POPUALTION. TO RECTIFY THIS PROBLEM, IT IS RECOMMENDED THAT THE FOLLOWING INTRA-GROUP DIFFERENCES BE CAREFULLY EXAMINED IN FUTURE RESEARCH: AGE-COHORTS; ACCULTURATION LEVEL; SEX; RURAL-URBAN RESIDENCY; AND REGIONAL DIFFERENCES. IN ADDITION, RECOMMENDATIONS ARE OFFERED CONCERNING OUT-REACH EFFORTS AND CULTURAL FACTORS WHICH SERVICE PROVIDERS SHOULD TAKE INTO CONSIDERATION IN MEETING THE SPECIAL NEEDS OF THESE ELDERS. 36 REFERENCES. (AUTHOR ABSTRACT MODIFIED)

ACCN 001830

1330 AUTH **NEWTON, F.**

TITL THE MEXICAN AMERICAN EMIC SYSTEM OF MENTAL ILLNESS: AN EXPLORATORY STUDY.

SRCE *IN J. M. CASAS & S. E. KEEFE (EDS.), FAMILY AND MENTAL HEALTH IN THE MEXICAN AMERICAN COMMUNITY (MONOGRAPH NO. 7). LOS ANGELES: SPANISH SPEAKING MENTAL HEALTH RESEARCH CENTER, 1978, PP. 69-90.*

INDX MEXICAN AMERICAN, RESOURCE UTILIZATION, MENTAL HEALTH, PSYCHOPATHOLOGY, ATTITUDES, PSYCHOTHERAPY, COPING MECHANISMS, CALIFORNIA, SOUTHWEST, EMPIRICAL

ABST DIFFERENT CULTURAL PERSPECTIVES AND DEFINITIONS OF MENTAL DISORDERS PARTIALLY ACCOUNT FOR UNDERUTILIZATION OF MENTAL HEALTH SERVICES BY MEXICAN AMERICANS (MA). IN ORDER TO ESTABLISH WHAT THOSE PERCEPTIONS AND DEFINITIONS ARE, RESEARCH WAS CONDUCTED AMONG 24 MA'S, FROM AN ON-GOING PROJECT, IN THE FORM OF A SERIES OF HOME INTERVIEWS, TO OBTAIN INFORMATION ABOUT LIFE HISTORY, PERSONAL SUPPORT NETWORK, DEGREE OF PARTICIPATION IN AND IDENTIFICATION WITH MEXICAN AND ANGLO CULTURES, PERCEPTIONS AND DEFINITIONS OF MENTAL DISORDERS, AND ATTITUDES ABOUT AND UTILIZATION OF POTENTIAL SOURCES OF TREATMENT. THE FINDINGS SHOW NO SUPPORT FOR THE POSITION THAT MA'S ARE IGNORANT OF THE SIGNS AND SYMPTOMS OF MENTAL ILLNESS. IN FACT, ALL RESPONDENTS GENERATED LISTS OF DETAILED SYMPTOMS AND SIGNS OF ABNORMAL FUNCTIONING. SOME OF THE PARTICULAR ASPECTS OF MA'S PERCEPTIONS INCLUDE: THE DISTINCTION BETWEEN MENTAL AND EMOTIONAL; A UNITARY MODEL OF MENTAL DISORDERS RANGING FROM "MINOR" TO "INSANE"; THE CONCEPT OF STRONG AND WEAK CHARACTER; THE IMPORTANCE OF PRIDE IN SELF-IMAGE; AND THE LIKELIHOOD THAT PATIENTS REFERRED FOR THERAPY TEND TO PERCEIVE THEIR OWN CONDITION AS VERY SERIOUS AND BEYOND THEIR OWN MEANS OF CONTROL. THERE WAS SUBSTANTIAL COMPARABILITY BETWEEN THE RESPONDENTS' DESCRIPTIONS OF ETIOLOGY, SYMPTOMS, AND TYPES OF PROBLEMS, AND THE CLASSIFICATIONS OF THE AMERICAN PSYCHIATRIC ASSOCIATION. THERE WAS ALSO A MARKED ABSENCE OF REFERENCES TO SUPERNATURAL CAUSALITY OR FOLK-CONCEPTS. AMERICAN PSYCHOTHERAPISTS WERE VIEWED AS NEEDING TO BE MORE KNOWLEDGEABLE ABOUT AND SENSITIVE TO THE MA CULTURE AND LIFESTYLE. 15 REFERENCES.

ACCN 001140

1331 AUTH **NEY, J. W.·**

TITL BILINGUAL EDUCATION IN SUNDAY SCHOOL COUNTRY.

SRCE *ELEMENTARY ENGLISH, 1974, 51(2), 209-214.*

INDX BILINGUALISM, BILINGUAL-BICULTURAL EDUCATION, LINGUISTIC COMPETENCE, POLICY, SOUTHWEST, CULTURAL PLURALISM, PROGRAM EVALUATION, TEACHERS, CHILDREN, MEXICAN AMERICAN

ABST BILINGUAL EDUCATION IN THE SOUTHWEST CANNOT BE EXPECTED TO SOLVE ALL THE PROBLEMS OF THE BILINGUAL STUDENT. IT IS A MISTAKE TO TRY TO FORCE THE CULTURE OF MEXICO ON STUDENTS OF SPANISH ANCESTRY RESIDING IN THE SOUTHWEST. THE SYSTEMATIC DEROGATION OF SOUTHWEST SPANISH IN FAVOR OF "STANDARD SPANISH" FORCES THE STUDENT INTO A TRILINGUAL OR CUATROLINGUAL SITUATION. BILINGUAL PROGRAMS ARE USUALLY PROVIDED ONLY ON THE PRIMARY LEVELS AND ARE OFTEN VIEWED ONLY AS THE QUICKEST WAY FOR NON-ENGLISH SPEAKERS TO LEARN ENGLISH. AS A RESULT OF ALL THESE FACTORS, THE FAILURE RATE OF THE BILINGUAL STUDENT HAS BEEN EXCESSIVELY HIGH. UNLESS SOCIETY AS A WHOLE IS WILLING TO PROVIDE PROGRAMS TO ASSIST THE BILINGUAL-BICULTURAL STUDENT, THERE IS LITTLE THAT THE AVERAGE TEACHER CAN DO. NEVERTHELESS, TEACHERS CAN MAKE THE ATTEMPT TO BREAK AWAY FROM THEIR OWN CULTURAL ETHNOCENTRISM AND BECOME MORE SENSITIVE TO THE NEEDS OF THE STUDENTS. 7 REFERENCES.

ACCN 001141

1332 AUTH **NICOLETTI, J. A., & PATTERSON, T. W.**

TITL ATTITUDES TOWARD BUSING AS A MEANS OF DESEGREGATION.

SRCE *PSYCHOLOGICAL REPORTS, 1974, 35(1, PT 2), 371-376.*

INDX DISCRIMINATION, EDUCATION, COMMUNITY, ATTITUDES, CHILDREN, PREJUDICE, MEXICAN AMERICAN, CROSS CULTURAL, CULTURAL FACTORS, GROUP DYNAMICS, COLORADO, SOUTHWEST

ABST ATTITUDES TOWARD ENFORCED SCHOOL BUSING WERE STUDIED AMONG 24 BLACKS, 167 CAUCASIONS, AND 34 CHICANOS IN DENVER, COLORADO. SIGNIFICANT ASSOCIATIONS WERE FOUND BETWEEN TYPE OF ATTITUDE EXPRESSED AND RACE, CHILDREN ENROLLED IN SCHOOL, MEMBERSHIP IN PTA, EXPECTATION TOWARD THE QUALITY OF EDUCATION TO BE OBTAINED BY BUSING, AND HOME OWNERSHIP. THE NUMBER OF CONTACTS WITH THE SCHOOL BY THE ADULT RESPONDENTS WERE NOT RELATED TO ATTITUDES TOWARD BUSING. SUPPORTERS OF BUSING EMPHASIZED THE PROVISION OF EQUAL EDUCATIONAL OPPORTUNITIES FOR ALL CHILDREN AND IMPROVED COMMUNICATION AMONG ETHNIC GROUPS, WHILE THOSE OPPOSED TO BUSING EMPHASIZED THE DISRUPTION OF THE NEIGHBORHOOD SCHOOL CONCEPT AS THE BASIS FOR THEIR ATTITUDES. IT IS SUGGESTED THAT LACK OF PRIOR PLANNING IN PROGRAM IMPLEMENTATION IS THE CAUSE OF MANY OF THE BUSING PROBLEMS IN DENVER. IT IS RECOMMENDED THAT ASIDE FROM THE PHYSICAL PROBLEMS OF BUSING, A THOROUGH PLAN SHOULD INCLUDE PSYCHOLOGICAL PREPARATION OF CHILDREN AND PARENTS. DIFFERENCES IN ETHNICITY, CULTURE, VALUES, SES, AND PRIOR EXPECTATIONS NEED TO BE EXAMINED. SEVERAL DETAILED RECOMMENDATIONS ARE PRESENTED. 10 REFERENCES. (AUTHOR SUMMARY MODIFIED)

ACCN   001142

1333 AUTH   **NIES, C. M.**
TITL   SOCIAL PSYCHOLOGICAL VARIABLES RE-
            LATED TO FAMILY PLANNING AMONG MEXICAN
            AMERICAN FEMALES (DOCTORAL DISSERTA-
            TION, UNIVERSITY OF TEXAS AT AUSTIN, 1974).
SRCE   *DISSERTATION ABSTRACTS INTERNATIONAL,
            1974, 35(5), 2441B. (UNIVERSITY MICROFILMS
            NO. 74-24,914.)*
INDX   FAMILY STRUCTURE, ATTITUDES, MEXICAN
            AMERICAN, FEMALE, BIRTH CONTROL, SEX
            ROLES, SES, MARRIAGE, CPI, MMPI, TAT, EMPIR-
            ICAL, RESEARCH METHODOLOGY, TEXAS,
            SOUTHWEST, FAMILY PLANNING
ABST   AN EXPLORATORY STUDY WAS CONDUCTED
            TO INVESTIGATE FACTORS RELATED TO BIRTH
            PLANNING DECISIONS, AND TO DEVELOP A
            PSYCHOMETRIC INSTRUMENT WHICH A FAMILY
            PLANNING CLINIC OR HOSPITAL STAFF COULD
            USE TO PREDICT EACH CLIENT'S PROBABILITY
            OF "SUCCESS" WITH CONTRACEPTION. A
            SAMPLE OF 262 MEXICAN AMERICAN WOMEN
            WAS CHOSEN BECAUSE THEY CONSTITUTE A
            MAJOR ETHNIC MINORITY GROUP ABOUT
            WHOM THERE IS MEAGER BIRTH PLANNING IN-
            FORMATION. SUBJECTS WERE RANDOMLY SE-
            LECTED FROM AMONG MATERNITY PATIENTS
            AT A COUNTY HOSPITAL IN SAN ANTONIO,
            TEXAS, IN 1972. BETWEEN 2 AND 3 MONTHS
            AFTER DELIVERY, EACH WOMAN'S BIRTH-
            PLANNING STATUS WAS INVESTIGATED. INDE-
            PENDENT VARIABLES INCLUDED: SOCIAL AND
            DEMOGRAPHIC BACKGROUND; ATTITUDES
            TOWARD CHILDREN, BIRTH CONTROL AND
            FAMILY SIZE; INTENDED AND PAST CONTRA-
            CEPTIVE BEHAVIOR; HUSBAND'S ATTITUDE TO-
            WARD BIRTH CONTROL; AND PERSONALITY
            AND MODERNITY. DATA WERE GATHERED
            THROUGH VARIOUS GENERAL PERSONALITY
            INVENTORIES AND PROJECTIVE TECHNIQUES.
            TWO EQUATIONS WERE DEVELOPED TO PRE-
            DICT FUTURE USE OF CLINIC CONTRACEP-
            TIVES FOR SINGLE AND MARRIED WOMEN. THE
            WIFE'S PERCEPTION OF HER HUSBAND'S FEEL-
            INGS WAS THE STRONGEST SINGLE PREDIC-
            TOR OF LATER CONTRACEPTIVE USE, SUG-
            GESTING THE IMPORTANCE OF THE HUSBAND'S
            INVOLVEMENT IN DETERMINING BIRTH PLAN-
            NING BEHAVIOR. THE SINGLE WOMEN HAD A
            MUCH LOWER "SUCCESS" RATE THAN MAR-
            RIED WOMEN. INTENTIONS TO USE SPECIFIC
            BIRTH PLANNING METHODS WERE RELATED
            TO THEIR USE LATER. MORE MODERN WOMEN
            TENDED TO ADOPT BIRTH PLANNING METH-
            ODS MORE FREQUENTLY. VARIABLES SUCH AS
            EFFICACY AND IMPULSIVENESS FAILED TO
            MAINTAIN A SIGNIFICANT CORRELATION. SUG-
            GESTIONS ARE MADE TO INCLUDE THE HUS-
            BAND IN BIRTH PLANNING PROGRAMS. TO
            CREATE MORE EFFECTIVE PROGRAMS FOR
            SINGLE WOMEN, DATA ARE NEEDED ON HOW
            FREQUENTLY SECOND PREGNANCIES OUT-OF-
            WEDLOCK OCCUR. 71 REFERENCES. (AUTHOR
            ABSTRACT MODIFIED)
ACCN   001143

1334 AUTH   **NIETO-GOMEZ, A.**
TITL   CHICANAS IN THE LABOR FORCE.
SRCE   *ENCUENTRO FEMENIL, 1975, 1(2), 28-33.*
INDX   SOCIAL SERVICES, SOUTHWEST, SEX COM-
            PARISON, REPRESENTATION, CALIFORNIA, DE-
            MOGRAPHIC, ECONOMIC FACTORS, EMPLOY-
            MENT, FEMALE, LABOR FORCE, OCCUPATIONAL
            ASPIRATIONS, SES, STEREOTYPES, VOCA-
            TIONAL COUNSELING, MEXICAN AMERICAN,
            PREJUDICE
ABST   THE CHICANA, THOUGH A PARTICIPANT IN THE
            WORK FORCE AT EQUAL RATES TO THE TOTAL
            WORK FORCE IN CALIFORNIA AND LOS ANGE-
            LES, HAS A 2% HIGHER RATE OF UNEMPLOY-
            MENT AND IS AT THE BOTTOM OF THE LADDER
            ECONOMICALLY. THIS IMBALANCE IS EVIDENT
            WHEN COMPARING SALARIES OF CHICANAS
            WITH CHICANOS, WHICH REVEALS THAT
            THOUGH EDUCATIONAL LEVELS ARE SIMILAR
            THE MEDIAN INCOME OF THE CHICANO IS AL-
            MOST 3 TIMES AS MUCH AS THE CHICANA'S.
            THE SAME IS TRUE OF REPRESENTATION IN
            HIGHER PAYING JOBS—THE CHICANA IS PRI-
            MARILY A POORLY PAID WORKER WITH LITTLE
            OR NO JOB OPPORTUNITIES. THE EXPERIENCE
            OF THE CHICANA SERVICE ACTION CENTER OF
            LOS ANGELES VERIFIES THESE FINDINGS. 53%
            OF THE CHICANAS WERE FOUND IN LOW STA-
            TUS, LOW PAYING JOBS (E.G., DOMESTIC
            WORKERS, LAUNDRY, CLEANING, FOOD SER-
            VICE, AND FACTORY WORK), AND 42% OF THE
            MEXICAN AMERICAN FAMILIES HEADED BY
            WOMEN WERE AT THE POVERTY LEVEL OR UN-
            DER. AT THE CENTER, 50% OF THE CHICANAS
            LOOKING FOR WORK ARE UNSKILLED AND UN-
            TRAINED WOMEN UNDER 30, OR OLDER HEADS
            OF HOUSEHOLDS WHOSE LACK OF JOB EX-
            PERIENCE AND TRAINING REDUCES THEIR
            COMPETITIVE APPEAL TO PROSPECTIVE EM-
            PLOYERS. THREE MAJOR FACTORS AFFECT
            THIS SITUATION: COMMUNICATION BARRIERS,
            LACK OF INTERVIEWING SKILLS, AND LACK OF
            COMPETITIVE ENTRY LEVEL SKILLS. BETTER
            PAYING JOB OPPORTUNITIES OR JOB PLACE-
            MENT TRAINING ARE RARE BECAUSE THERE
            ARE NO BILINGUAL TRAINING PROGRAMS AND
            BECAUSE SO MANY COMPETE FOR SO FEW
            JOBS. RACIST SEXUAL STEREOTYPES ALSO
            WORK AS BARRIERS, REINFORCING THE IM-
            AGE OF THE CHICANA AS A NURTURING, PAS-
            SIVE, AND SUBMISSIVE WOMAN, GOOD ONLY
            FOR MENIAL EMPLOYMENT. TO DATE, THOUGH
            STATISTICS ABOUT ANGLO AND BLACK WOMEN
            ABOUND, INSUFFICIENT DATA EXIST ABOUT
            THE EMPLOYMENT SITUATION OF THE CHI-
            CANA. IT IS IMPORTANT THAT FURTHER DEMO-
            GRAPHIC STUDIES BE DONE TO SEPARATE HER
            OUT FROM THOSE WOMEN LISTED MERELY AS
            "SPANISH SPEAKING." THE CHICANA SERVICE
            ACTION CENTER IS CALLING ATTENTION TO
            THIS SITUATION SO THAT EDUCATORS, WOMAN-
            MANPOWER EXPERTS, AND EMPLOYERS CAN
            MORE ADEQUATELY HELP AND SERVE THIS
            POPULATION. 6 REFERENCES.
ACCN   002169

1335 AUTH   **NOEL, R. C., & ALLEN, M. J.**
TITL   SEX AND ETHNIC BIAS IN THE EVALUATION OF
            STUDENT EDITORIALS.

SRCE   *JOURNAL OF PSYCHOLOGY, 1976, 94, 53-58.*

INDX   ATTITUDES, CROSS CULTURAL, CULTURAL FACTORS, EMPIRICAL, MEXICAN AMERICAN, PERCEPTION, PREJUDICE, ROLE EXPECTATIONS, SEX ROLES, CALIFORNIA, SOUTHWEST, STEREOTYPES, ADULTS

ABST   THE GOLDBERG PARADIGM WAS USED TO ASSESS RACISM AND SEXISM AMONG A SAMPLE OF CALIFORNIA, NONCOLLEGE, CAUCASIAN ADULTS. RADICAL AND NEUTRAL STUDENT EDITORIALS, ATTRIBUTED TO AUTHORS VARYING IN SEX AND ETHNICITY (CAUCASIAN AND MEXICAN AMERICAN), WERE RATED BY 93 MALE AND 91 FEMALE S'S FOR QUALITY AND LEVEL OF AGREEMENT. THE RESULTS INDICATED THAT THE S'S WERE SIGNIFICANTLY LESS LIKELY TO AGREE WITH CONCLUSIONS REACHED BY THE MEXICAN AMERICAN AUTHORS AND RATED THE EDITORIALS WRITTEN BY FEMALES AND MEXICAN AMERICAN AUTHORS AS LOWER IN QUALITY. SECONDLY, THE "RADICAL" ISSUE THAT WAS PARTICULARLY RELEVANT TO MEXICAN AMERICAN INTERESTS (LOWER COLLEGE ADMISSION STANDARDS) LED TO LOWER RATINGS OF THE MEXICAN AMERICAN AUTHORS THAN DID THE NEUTRAL ARTICLE. WHILE THESE RESULTS WERE NOT CONCLUSIVE, THEY DID SUGGEST THAT THE PERCEIVED "PERSONAL GAIN" OF THE AUTHOR DOES INFLUENCE THE S'S RATINGS OF THE EDITORIALS. 8 REFERENCES. (AUTHOR ABSTRACT)

ACCN   002170

1336 AUTH   **NORMAN, R. D., & MARTINEZ, R.**

TITL   SOCIAL CLASS AND ETHNICITY EFFECTS ON CLINICAL JUDGMENTS.

SRCE   *PSYCHOLOGICAL REPORTS, 1978, 43, 91-98.*

INDX   COLLEGE STUDENTS, EMPIRICAL, NEW MEXICO, SOUTHWEST, MEXICAN AMERICAN, SES, CROSS CULTURAL, PREJUDICE, PSYCHOTHERAPY

ABST   THIS STUDY AT THE UNIVERSITY OF NEW MEXICO SOUGHT TO RESOLVE CONFLICTS BETWEEN EARLIER STUDIES OFFERING CONTRADICTORY RECOMMENDATIONS ON THE NEED FOR PROFESSIONAL HELP OF MIDDLE- VS. LOWER-CLASS PERSONS GIVEN NORMAL, NEUROTIC, AND PSYCHOTIC BEHAVIOR DESCRIPTIONS. NINETY-TWO COLLEGE STUDENTS (70 ANGLOS, 22 CHICANOS) RATED 24 FICTITIOUS BIOGRAPHICAL VIGNETTES IN TERMS OF THE STIMULUS PERSON'S (1) NEED FOR PROFESSIONAL HELP, (2) CANDIDACY FOR PSYCHOTHERAPY, (3) VOLUNTARY HOSPITAL COMMITMENT, (4) INVOLUNTARY COMMITMENT, AND (5) NEED FOR MEDICATION. A PRO-MIDDLE-CLASS BIAS WAS FOUND, CONSISTENT WITH ROUTH AND KING'S (1972) STUDY BUT INCONSISTENT WITH SCHOFIELD AND OAKES'S (1975) STUDY. ALSO CONTRARY TO THE LATTER, TREATMENT RECOMMENDATIONS AGREED WITH RATINGS. ETHNICITY BIAS APPEARED, AS ANGLOS RECOMMENDED CHICANOS MORE OFTEN FOR INVOLUNTARY HOSPITALIZATION. INCONSISTENCIES BETWEEN THE TWO EARLIER STUDIES ARE DISCUSSED IN TERMS OF METHODOLOGICAL VARIATIONS. 15 REFERENCES (JOURNAL ABSTRACT MODIFIED)

ACCN   001728

1337 AUTH   **NORMAN, R. D., & MEAD, D. F.**

TITL   SPANISH-AMERICAN BILINGUALISM AND THE AMMONS FULL-RANGE PICTURE-VOCABULARY TEST.

SRCE   *JOURNAL OF SOCIAL PSYCHOLOGY, 1960, 51, 319-330.*

INDX   BILINGUALISM, SPANISH SURNAMED, NEW MEXICO, SOUTHWEST, MILITARY, EMPIRICAL, INTELLIGENCE TESTING, TEST RELIABILITY, MALE, ADOLESCENTS, BILINGUAL, TEST VALIDITY

ABST   THE HOFFMAN BILINGUAL SCHEDULE (AN OBJECTIVE MEASURE OF BILINGUALISM) AND THE AMMONS FULL-RANGE PICTURE-VOCABULARY TEST (FRPV) WERE ADMINISTERED TO 150 SPANISH AMERICAN (SA) MALE, BILINGUAL SUBJECTS—50 EACH FROM THE AGE GROUPS OF 17, 18, AND 19 YEARS. THE PURPOSE OF THE INVESTIGATION WAS TO DISCOVER THE ASSOCIATION BETWEEN BILINGUALISM AND PERFORMANCE ON THE FRPV, AS WELL AS TO ESTABLISH TENTATIVE NORMS ON THE FRPV FOR THESE THREE SA AGE GROUPS. THE MAJOR FINDINGS OF THE STUDY WERE: (1) BILINGUALISM REMAINED CONSTANT IN THE THREE AGE GROUPS, ALTHOUGH IT WAS GREATER FOR THEM THAN FOR A NEW YORK CITY SAMPLE; (2) THERE WAS A LOW BUT SIGNIFICANT NEGATIVE ASSOCIATION (R OF -.26) BETWEEN AMOUNT OF SCHOOLING AND BILINGUAL BACKGROUND; (3) THERE WAS A STRONGER NEGATIVE ASSOCIATION (R OF -.49) BETWEEN BILINGUALISM AND FRPV, WITH THIS R DROPPING TO -.44 WHEN SCHOOLING WAS PARTIALED OUT; (4) A STRONGER POSITIVE ASSOCIATION (R OF .62) EXISTED BETWEEN SCHOOLING AND FRPV; (5) URBAN-RURAL DIFFERENCES WERE SIGNIFICANT IN BOTH MEASURES USED, WITH URBANITIES SCORING HIGHER ON FRPV AND LOWER IN BILINGUALISM; AND (6) THE SA'S SCORED CONSIDERABLY LOWER ON THE FRPV THAN DID ANGLOS IN PREVIOUS STUDIES. A DISCUSSION OF THE FINDINGS IS PRESENTED. 27 REFERENCES. (AUTHOR SUMMARY MODIFIED)

ACCN   001145

1338 AUTH   **NORMAND, W. C., IGLESIAS, J., & PAYN, S.**

TITL   BRIEF GROUP THERAPY TO FACILITATE UTILIZATION OF MENTAL HEALTH SERVICES BY SPANISH-SPEAKING PATIENTS.

SRCE   *AMERICAN JOURNAL OF ORTHOPSYCHIATRY, 1974, 44(1), 37-42.*

INDX   EMPIRICAL, HEALTH DELIVERY SYSTEMS, BILINGUAL-BICULTURAL PERSONNEL, ADULTS, PSYCHOTHERAPY, CUBAN, PUERTO RICAN-M, GROUP DYNAMICS, PSYCHOTHERAPY OUTCOME, RESOURCE UTILIZATION, NEW YORK, EAST

ABST   BARRIERS OF CULTURE AND LANGUAGE HAVE TENDED TO KEEP THE POOR SPANISH-SPEAKING FROM USING COMMUNITY MENTAL HEALTH CENTER TREATMENT FACILITIES. THIS PAPER DESCRIBES A PROGRAM OF BRIEF GROUP THERAPY AIMED AT HELPING POOR PATIENTS

ACCEPT REFERRAL TO THE LONGER TERM TREATMENT FACILITIES. FIFTY-FIVE PUERTO RICAN AND CUBAN PATIENTS WITH VARIOUS NON-SEVERE DISTURBANCES WERE ASKED TO ATTEND 8 GROUP SESSIONS WHICH WERE CONDUCTED TOTALLY IN SPANISH BY A BILINGUAL SOCIAL WORK ASSISTANT WITH PSYCHIATRIC CONSULTATION. AMID A WARM, ACCEPTING, AND SUPPORTIVE SETTING, PATIENTS WERE ENCOURAGED TO OPENLY DISCUSS MATTERS CONCERNING THEMSELVES AND OTHERS IN THE GROUP; NO FORMAL PSYCHOTHERAPY WAS USED. INFORMATION ABOUT COMMUNITY RESOURCES WAS IMPARTED WHENEVER SITUATIONAL PROBLEMS OCCURRED. A VERY HIGH PROPORTION OF PATIENTS ATTENDED SIX TO EIGHT SESSIONS. WHEN REFERRED FOR FURTHER THERAPY, APPROXIMATELY 75% FOLLOWED THROUGH ON THE REFERRAL. FINALLY, 70% OF THE PATIENTS IMPROVED DURING THE BRIEF THERAPY AS WAS EVIDENCED BY IMPROVEMENT IN THE INITIAL PROBLEM AND/OR WITH RELATIONSHIPS WITH OTHER PEOPLE. DESPITE THE PROBLEMS OF INFORMING POOR PEOPLE ABOUT COMMUNITY RESOURCES, THIS TYPE OF PREPARATION IS SEEN AS DESIRABLE AND PRACTICALLY EFFECTIVE IN BRINGING PEOPLE INTO MENTAL HEALTH FACILITIES. 10 REFERENCES. (JOURNAL ABSTRACT MODIFIED)

ACCN 001146

1339 AUTH **NOVACK, A. H., BROMET, E., NEILL, T. K., ABRAMOVITZ, R. H., & STORCH, S.**

TITL CHILDREN'S MENTAL HEALTH SERVICES IN AN INNER CITY NEIGHBORHOOD. 1. A 3-YEAR EPIDEMIOLOGICAL STUDY.

SRCE *AMERICAN JOURNAL OF PUBLIC HEALTH, 1975, 65(2), 133-138.*

INDX CHILDREN, EMPIRICAL, CROSS CULTURAL, RESOURCE UTILIZATION, SES, FAMILY STRUCTURE, HEALTH DELIVERY SYSTEMS, ADOLESCENTS, MENTAL HEALTH, SEX COMPARISON, ECONOMIC FACTORS, CONNECTICUT, EAST

ABST THE UTILIZATION OF MENTAL HEALTH SERVICES FOR CHILDREN WAS EXAMINED IN A LOW-INCOME NEIGHBORHOOD HEALTH CENTER LOCATED IN NEW HAVEN, CONNECTICUT. THE STUDY GROUP WAS COMPRISED OF PATIENTS UNDER 20 YEARS OF AGE WHO RECEIVED SERVICES OVER A THREE-YEAR PERIOD (1969-1971). TWO COMPARISON GROUPS WERE DEVELOPED FROM 320 CHILDREN REGISTERED AT THE GENERAL HEALTH CENTER AT THE TIME OF THE STUDY AND THE LARGER POPULATION OF CHILDREN LIVING IN THE SERVICED AREA. THE DATA, OBTAINED FROM HEALTH CENTER REGISTRATION CARDS AND 1970 CENSUS DATA, WERE ANALYZED BY AGE, SEX, ETHNIC GROUP OF CHILD, SEX OF HEAD OF HOUSEHOLD, INCOME, AND FAMILY SIZE. THE FINDINGS REVEALED THAT MALES RECEIVING MENTAL HEALTH SERVICES OUTNUMBERING FEMALES BY 2 TO 1. THIS TREND WAS INDEPENDENT OF ETHNIC GROUP, MOST SALIENT IN THE 5-14 YEAR-OLDS, AND IS SEEN AS A RESULT OF SOCIAL AND CULTURAL FACTORS. THE DISPROPORTIONATELY HIGH USE OF SER-

VICES BY ANGLOS COMPARED TO THE DEMOGRAPHIC POPULATION MAY BE EXPLAINED BY THE INCREASED NUMBER OF DISORGANIZED ANGLO FAMILIES. FEMALE AND MALE ADOLESCENT REFERRALS ARE MORE FREQUENTLY FROM HIGHER INCOME FAMILIES, WHILE YOUNGER MALES ARE PREDOMINANTLY LOW-INCOME. THE LOW UTILIZATION RATE BY SPANISH-SPEAKING CHILDREN IS ATTRIBUTED TO THE LACK OF BILINGUAL STAFF OR TO THE GREATER PROPORTION OF TWO PARENT-FAMILIES. THE NEED FOR SERVICES IS SEEN AS MORE OF A CONSEQUENCE OF ECONOMIC THAN ETHNIC FACTORS. 20 REFERENCES.

ACCN 001147

1340 AUTH **NUNEZ LOPEZ, J. A.**

TITL TRATAMIENTO DEL PACIENTE PSICOTICO: NUEVAS ALTERNATIVAS TERAPEUTICAS. (TREATMENT OF THE PSYCHOTIC PATIENT: NEW THERAPEUTIC ALTERNATIVES.)

SRCE *IN J. A. ROSSELLO (ED.), MANUAL DE PSIQUIATRIA SOCIAL. SPAIN: INDUSTRIAS GRAFICAS "DIARIO-DIA," 1968, PP. 435-464. (SPANISH)*

INDX PUERTO RICAN-I, ESSAY, MENTAL HEALTH, REHABILITATION, PERSONNEL, HEALTH DELIVERY SYSTEMS

ABST NEW MENTAL HEALTH TREATMENT METHODS IN PUERTO RICO ARE DISCUSSED AS AN ALTERNATIVE TO THE NEGATIVE EFFECTS AND SOCIAL STIGMA ATTACHED TO PROLONGED CONFINEMENT IN MENTAL INSTITUTIONS. IN RECENT YEARS IN PUERTO RICO, MENTAL PATIENTS HAVE BEEN TREATED PRIMARILY BY SUCH MEANS AS AMBULATORY TREATMENT, EMERGENCY ROOM TREATMENT, SHORT-TERM HOSPITALIZATION OF 1 TO 2 WEEKS, AND DAY CLINICS. ALL OF THESE METHODS SERVE TO KEEP THE PATIENT INTEGRATED INTO SOCIETY AS MUCH AS POSSIBLE DURING THERAPY AND ALSO REDUCE THE PUBLIC'S FEARS ABOUT MENTAL ILLNESS. THE USE OF EMERGENCY ROOMS HELPS GIVE BOTH THE PATIENT AND THE FAMILY A SENSE OF SECURITY AS THEY KNOW THAT HELP CAN BE OBTAINED WITHIN MINUTES OF A CRISIS. MOREOVER, IT LEADS THE PUBLIC TO ASSOCIATE MENTAL ILLNESS WITH PHYSICAL DISORDERS FOR WHICH EMERGENCY TREATMENT MAY BE NECESSARY. SIMILARLY, AMBULATORY TREATMENT, DAY CLINICS, AND SHORT-TERM HOSPITALIZATION SERVE TO ELIMINATE READJUSTMENT PROBLEMS WHICH PATIENTS MIGHT EXPERIENCE AFTER PROLONGED INSTITUTIONALIZATION. ALSO DISCUSSED IS THE CIRCUMSTANCE THAT TREATMENT DEPENDS NOT ONLY UPON THE STATE OF THE PATIENT BUT ALSO UPON THE RECEPTIVENESS AND DEGREE OF COOPERATION OF FAMILY MEMBERS. THE POINT IS THAT IT IS NECESSARY FOR MENTAL HEALTH STAFF (I.E., PSYCHOTHERAPISTS, NURSES, SOCIAL WORKERS, RECREATIONAL AND OCCUPATIONAL THERAPISTS, AND ADMINISTRATIVE PERSONNEL) TO HAVE APPROPRIATE INTERACTION WITH THE PATIENT AS WELL AS WITH FAMILY MEMBERS AND THE SOCIETY AT LARGE. FINALLY, BECAUSE THE GOAL OF THERAPY IS TO NOT ISOLATE THE PATIENT FROM SOCIETY,

IT IS RECOMMENDED THAT DRUGS BE USED AS SPARINGLY AS POSSIBLE. 7 REFERENCES.

ACCN 002287

1341 AUTH **NUNO, F. E.**
TITL DESCRIPTION AND EVALUATION OF A COMMUNITY MENTAL HEALTH AGENCY: THE EAST LOS ANGELES MENTAL HEALTH SERVICE.
SRCE *UNPUBLISHED MANUSCRIPT, UNIVERSITY OF CALIFORNIA, LOS ANGELES, JULY 20, 1976. (AVAILABLE FROM AMADO M. PADILLA, DEPARTMENT OF PSYCHOLOGY, UNIVERSITY OF CALIFORNIA, LOS ANGELES, CALIF. 90024.)*
INDX COMMUNITY, MENTAL HEALTH, MEXICAN AMERICAN, HEALTH DELIVERY SYSTEMS, ESSAY, URBAN, BILINGUAL-BICULTURAL PERSONNEL, PROGRAM EVALUATION, RESOURCE UTILIZATION, CALIFORNIA, SOUTHWEST
ABST A DESCRIPTION IS PRESENTED OF THE EAST LOS ANGELES MENTAL HEALTH SERVICE (ELAMHS), A COMMUNITY BASED AND ORIENTED CLINIC WHOSE FUNCTION IS TO PROVIDE MENTAL HEALTH SERVICES TO THE PREDOMINANTLY SPANISH-SPEAKING/SURNAMED (SSS) POPULATION IN EAST LOS ANGELES. ELAMHS IS FOUNDED ON THE COMMUNITY MENTAL HEALTH (CMH) MODEL—A MODEL WHICH FOCUSES ON SOCIAL FACTORS IN THE DEVELOPMENT AND TREATMENT OF MENTAL ILLNESS WITH BROAD SPECIFICATION OF TARGET POPULATIONS. MORE PRECISELY, ELAMHS' FORMAT, PERSONNEL MAKE-UP, AND PHILOSOPHY ARE GEARED TOWARDS SHORT-TERM THERAPY BY PROFESSIONAL AND PARAPROFESSIONAL STAFF, AND ITS GOAL IS PREVENTIVE PSYCHIATRY. THE CLIENT POPULATION (MAINLY LOW-INCOME YOUNGER MEN) AND THE LOCAL COMMUNITY HAVE BECOME MORE ACCEPTING OF PSYCHIATRY OVER THE YEARS. NEVERTHELESS, CMH FACILITIES ARE STILL UNDERUTILIZED BY THE SSS POPULATION, POSSIBLY DUE TO INADEQUACY OF SERVICES, LANGUAGE BARRIERS, GEOGRAPHIC ISOLATION, AND CULTURAL AND CLASS DIFFERENCES. RECOMMENDATIONS FOR ELAMHS, FORMULATED FROM THE CMH MODEL, INCLUDE: (1) AN INCREASE IN PARAPROFESSIONAL HELP; (2) CULTURAL SENSITIVITY; (3) PROGRAMS WHICH TAKE ADVANTAGE OF SSS STRONG FAMILIAL TIES; AND (4) THE USE OF A SYSTEMS APPROACH. 5 REFERENCES.
ACCN 001148

1342 AUTH **NUTTALL, R. L., NUTTALL, E. V., & SWEET, P. R.**
TITL CORRELATES OF FAMILY SIZE AND EXPECTED FAMILY SIZE AMONG PUERTO RICAN YOUTH.
SRCE *CATALOG OF SELECTED DOCUMENTS IN PSYCHOLOGY, 1972, 2(SUMMER), 111-112.*
INDX PUERTO RICAN-I, ADOLESCENTS, FAMILY STRUCTURE, EMPIRICAL, SES, RELIGION, PERSONALITY, DEMOGRAPHIC, FAMILY ROLES, SEX COMPARISON, ATTITUDES, FERTILITY, FAMILY PLANNING
ABST THIS THREE-PHASE STUDY CONDUCTED IN PUERTO RICO EXAMINED THE INFLUENCE OF FAMILY SIZE UPON THE PERSONALITIES AND FAMILY-SIZE EXPECTATIONS OF 5,000 ADOLESCENT PUERTO RICAN STUDENTS. THE FIRST PHASE DEALT WITH THE STUDENTS' NATURAL FAMILY AND THEIR PARENTS' SOCIOCULTURAL BACKGROUND AS IT RELATED TO THE NUMBER OF CHILDREN THEY HAD. THE SECOND PHASE DEALT WITH PARENT-CHILD RELATIONS AND THE CHILDREN'S PERSONALITIES, GOALS, AND ASPIRATIONS AS INFLUENCED BY NATURAL FAMILY SIZE. PHASE THREE DEALT WITH THE STUDENTS' PERSONALITIES AND THEIR FAMILY-SIZE EXPECTATIONS. DATA ANALYSIS REVEALED A VARIETY OF SIGNIFICANT FINDINGS. (1) SOCIOECONOMIC STATUS (SES) PROVED TO BE AN IMPORTANT VARIABLE FOR FAMILY SIZE, WITH THE HIGHER SES FAMILIES HAVING FEWER CHILDREN. (2) ONE-CHILD FAMILIES WERE DUE TO BIOLOGICALLY BASED SUB-FECUNDITY AND NOT TO SOCIOCULTURAL FACTORS. (3) PROTESTANT FAMILIES AVERAGED MORE CHILDREN PER FAMILY THAN CATHOLICS, AND RURAL FAMILIES MORE THAN URBAN. (4) PARENTAL REJECTION AND HOSTILE PSYCHOLOGICAL CONTROL WERE GREATER IN LARGER FAMILIES, AND THEREFORE IT APPEARS THAT THE BEST FAMILY SIZE FOR CHILDREN IS THE TWO-CHILD FAMILY. (5) FOR GIRLS, LARGER FAMILY SIZE WAS ASSOCIATED WITH POOR GRADES IN SCHOOL; MOREOVER, THESE GIRLS TENDED TO BE MORE AUTHORITARIAN AND INDIVIDUALISTIC. IN GENERAL, FAMILY SIZE HAD A GREATER IMPACT ON GIRLS THAN BOYS. (6) AMONG THOSE STUDENTS WHO DID HAVE FAMILY-SIZE EXPECTATIONS, THREE PERSONALITY TYPES WERE FOUND: (A) NONCONFORMING IN PERSONALITY, PLANNING TO HAVE ONE OR NO CHILDREN; (B) CONFORMING IN PERSONALITY, PLANNING TO HAVE TWO TO FIVE CHILDREN; AND (C) UNCONVENTIONAL, PLANNING TO HAVE EIGHT OR MORE CHILDREN.
ACCN 001149

1343 AUTH **NUTTALL, R. L., SMITH, D. H., & NUTTALL, E. V.**
TITL FAMILY BACKGROUND, PARENT-CHILD RELATIONSHIPS, AND ACADEMIC ACHIEVEMENT AMONG PUERTO RICAN JUNIOR AND SENIOR HIGH SCHOOL STUDENTS.
SRCE *PROCEEDINGS OF THE 78TH ANNUAL CONVENTION OF THE AMERICAN PSYCHOLOGICAL ASSOCIATION, 1970, 5, 307-308.*
INDX SES, CHILDREARING PRACTICES, SOCIALIZATION, ADOLESCENTS, RESEARCH METHODOLOGY, EDUCATION, POVERTY, FAMILY STRUCTURE, SCHOLASTIC ACHIEVEMENT, SCHOLASTIC ASPIRATIONS, EMPIRICAL, PUERTO RICAN-I
ABST THE CHILD'S REPORT OF PARENTAL BEHAVIOR (CRPBI) AND A SERIES OF OTHER INSTRUMENTS, INCLUDING A FAMILY BACKGROUND QUESTIONNAIRE, WERE GROUP ADMINISTERED IN THE SPRING OF 1968 TO 5,300 STUDENTS ATTENDING PUBLIC AND PRIVATE JUNIOR AND SENIOR HIGH SCHOOLS IN THE BAYAMON NORTE SCHOOL DISTRICT IN PUERTO RICO. THE OBJECTIVES WERE TO ASSESS (1) THE RELIABILITY AND VALIDITY OF A SPANISH ADAPTATION OF THE CRPBI IN A SPANISH-SPEAKING PUERTO RICAN SAMPLE, (2) THE EXTENT TO WHICH CRPBI SCORES WERE ASSO-

CIATED WITH FAMILY BACKGROUND VARI-
ABLES, AND (3) THE EXTENT TO WHICH THE
CRPBI CONTRIBUTED TO THE PREDICTION OF
ACADEMIC ACHIEVEMENT. THE TRANSLATED
ADAPTATION OF THE CRPBI YIELDED MEAN-
INGFUL AND VALID RESULTS. 21 PARENTAL
BACKGROUND VARIABLES (E.G., MOTHER'S
AND FATHER'S EDUCATION, FATHER'S OCCU-
PATIONAL PRESTIGE LEVEL) CORRELATED WITH
SIX CRPBI FACTOR SCORES, 3 FOR EACH PAR-
ENT (I.E., ACCEPTANCE, HOSTILE PSYCHO-
LOGICAL CONTROL, AND AUTONOMY). PAREN-
TAL EDUCATION AND FATHER'S OCCUPATIONAL
PRESTIGE WERE MOST POWERFULLY RELATED
TO THE CRPBI FACTORS. THE CRPBI FACTORS
AND BACKGROUND VARIABLES BOTH INDE-
PENDENTLY AFFECTED GRADE POINT AVER-
AGES AND COLLEGE PLANS (FROM 16% TO
24% OF PREDICTABLE VARIANCE). WEAK RE-
LATIONSHIPS (ABOUT 6% OF COMMON VARI-
ANCE), HOWEVER, WERE OBTAINED BETWEEN
THE CRPBI FACTORS AND OTHER BACK-
GROUND VARIABLES. THE SMALL PERCENT-
AGES OF ACCOUNTED FOR VARIANCE INDI-
CATE THAT THE CRPBI FACTORS ARE
DETERMINED BY MANY THINGS OTHER THAN
FAMILY BACKGROUND, AND THAT GRADES
AND COLLEGE PLANS ARE AFFECTED BY
THINGS OTHER THAN FAMILY BACKGROUND
AND PARENT-CHILD RELATIONSHIPS. 5
REFERENCES.

ACCN   001150

1344 AUTH   NUTTALL, R. L., & POGGIO, J. P.
TITL   A CROSS-CULTURAL, AMERICAN AND PUERTO
RICAN STUDY OF PERSONALITY STRUCTURE.
SRCE   CATALOG OF SELECTED DOCUMENTS IN PSY-
CHOLOGY, 1975, 5, 193.
INDX   CROSS CULTURAL, PERSONALITY, PERSONAL-
ITY ASSESSMENT, PUERTO RICAN-M, ADOLES-
CENTS, PSYCHOSOCIAL ADJUSTMENT, MEN-
TAL HEALTH, EMPIRICAL, CULTURAL FACTORS
ABST   THE PURPOSE OF THE INVESTIGATION WAS TO
COMPARE THE PERSONALITY STRUCTURE OF
AMERICAN AND PUERTO RICAN STUDENTS, AS
REFLECTED IN THE SECOND-ORDER FACTOR
STRUCTURE OF RESPONSES TO THE CATTELL
HIGH SCHOOL PERSONALITY QUESTION-
NAIRE, AND OF RESPONSES TO A SPANISH
VERSION OF THE QUESTIONNAIRE BY PUERTO
RICAN STUDENTS COLLECTED BY THE INVES-
TIGATORS. A TOTAL OF 4,782 PUERTO RICAN
JUNIOR AND SENIOR HIGH SCHOOL STU-
DENTS IN ONE SCHOOL DISTRICT IN PUERTO
RICO WERE TESTED. A PRINCIPLE COMPO-
NENTS SOLUTION YIELDED SEVEN SECOND-
ORDER FACTORS IN THE PUERTO RICAN DATA.
BOTH VERIMAX AND PROMAX ROTATIONS WERE
THEN EMPLOYED TO IDENTIFY FURTHER THE
SIGNIFICANT FACTORS. AS IN THE AMERICAN
DATA, ANXIETY AND SUPEREGO EMERGED AS
SECOND-ORDER FACTORS. EXVIA-INVIA WAS
ALSO FOUND, BUT IN THE FIRST PROMAX RO-
TATION, EXVIA-INVIA SPLIT INTO TWO FAC-
TORS. A NEW FACTOR APPEARED IN THE
PUERTO RICAN DATA, LINKING TENDERMIND-
EDNESS WITH RELAXATION, AS OPPOSED TO
TOUGHMINDEDNESS AND TENSENESS. (JOUR-
NAL ABSTRACT MODIFIED)

ACCN   001151

1345 AUTH   OAKLAND, T.
TITL   ASSESSING MINORITY GROUP CHILDREN:
CHALLENGES FOR SCHOOL PSYCHOLOGISTS.
SRCE   JOURNAL OF SCHOOL PSYCHOLOGY, 1973,
11(4), 294-303.
INDX   MENTAL HEALTH PROFESSION, TEACHERS,
CHILDREN, ADMINISTRATORS, ESSAY, PSY-
CHOSOCIAL ADJUSTMENT, EDUCATIONAL AS-
SESSMENT, CROSS CULTURAL, TEST RELIABIL-
ITY, CULTURAL FACTORS, CULTURAL
PLURALISM, EQUAL OPPORTUNITY, EDUCA-
TIONAL COUNSELING, CULTURE-FAIR TESTS
ABST   THE ROLE OF THE SCHOOL PSYCHOLOGIST IN
ASSESSING MINORITY CHILDREN IS DIS-
CUSSED, WITH EMPHASIS ON THE IMPACT OF
TESTING INSTRUMENTS ON MINORITY POPU-
LATIONS. RESPONSES TO AND CRITICISMS OF
ASSESSMENT PRACTICES BY EDUCATORS,
SCHOOL SYSTEMS, PROFESSIONAL ORGANI-
ZATIONS, AND FEDERAL AND STATE GOVERN-
MENTS ARE REVIEWED. WHILE NO ATTEMPT IS
MADE TO RESOLVE THE COMPLEX ISSUES IN-
VOLVED IN ASSESSING MINORITY CHILDREN, IT
IS MAINTAINED THAT VARIOUS FACTORS AS-
SOCIATED WITH MINORITY GROUPS AND
LOWER SES CAUSE CHILDREN TO SUFFER IN-
TELLECTUAL DEFICITS. THE DEVELOPMENT OF
CULTURE FAIR TESTING INSTRUMENTS, THE
RECOGNITION OF CULTURAL DIFFERENCES BY
SCHOOL SYSTEMS, AND THE ADAPTATION OF
EDUCATIONAL ENVIRONMENTS TO THESE DIF-
FERENCES ARE ESSENTIAL FOR THE IM-
PROVED EDUCATION OF MINORITY CHILDREN.
37 REFERENCES.

ACCN   001152

1346 AUTH   OAKLAND, T., & EMMER, E.
TITL   EFFECTS OF KNOWLEDGE OF CRITERION
GROUPS ON ACTUAL AND EXPECTED TEST
PERFORMANCE OF NEGRO AND MEXICAN
AMERICAN EIGHTH GRADERS.
SRCE   JOURNAL OF CONSULTING & CLINICAL PSY-
CHOLOGY, 1973, 40(1), 155-159.
INDX   MEXICAN AMERICAN, CHILDREN, CROSS CUL-
TURAL, EMPIRICAL, PERFORMANCE EXPECTA-
TIONS, EDUCATIONAL ASSESSMENT
ABST   PREVIOUS RESEARCH HAS INDICATED THAT
KNOWLEDGE OF THE CRITERION GROUP DIF-
FERENTIALLY AFFECTS TEST PERFORMANCE
OF MINORITY GROUP MEMBERS. TO TEST THIS,
102 BLACK AND 74 MEXICAN AMERICAN EIGHTH
GRADE STUDENTS FROM 2 DIFFERENT
SCHOOLS IN AUSTIN, TEXAS, WERE ADMINIS-
TERED A 75-ITEM QUICK WORD TEST. STU-
DENTS WERE ASKED TO SELF-RATE THEIR EX-
PECTED SUCCESS ON THE TEST AS COMPARED
TO ONLY ONE OF THE FOLLOWING REFERENCE
GROUPS: (1) AGE-MATES FROM THROUGHOUT
AUSTIN; (2) CHILDREN THROUGHOUT THE
UNITED STATES; (3) OWN AGE ETHNIC GROUP;
AND (4) STUDENTS THEIR AGE (CONTROL
GROUP). THERE WAS NO EVIDENCE THAT COM-
PARISON WITH ONE OF FOUR NORM GROUPS
AFFECTED PERFORMANCE THROUGH EITHER
AN APTITUDE X TREATMENT INTERACTION OR
THROUGH AN OVERALL TREATMENT EFFECT.

DATA ON EXPECTED PERFORMANCE INDICATED A SIGNIFICANT APTITUDE-TREATMENT EFFECT WITH BLACK STUDENTS ONLY. THESE RESULTS SUGGEST THAT KNOWLEDGE OF A CRITERION GROUP MAY NOT CONSISTENTLY ALTER THE TEST PERFORMANCE OF PERSONS FROM MINORITY GROUPS. 11 REFERENCES. (JOURNAL ABSTRACT MODIFIED).

ACCN   001153

1347 AUTH   **OBITZ, F. W., OZIEL, L. J., & UNMACHT, J. J.**
TITL   GENERAL AND SPECIFIC PERCEIVED LOCUS OF CONTROL IN DELINQUENT DRUG USERS.
SRCE   *INTERNATIONAL JOURNAL OF THE ADDICTIONS, 1973, 8(4), 723-727.*
INDX   SELF CONCEPT, DELINQUENCY, DRUG ABUSE, PERSONALITY, PERSONALITY ASSESSMENT, ADOLESCENTS, MEXICAN AMERICAN, LOCUS OF CONTROL, CROSS CULTURAL, ALCOHOLISM, ROTTER INTERNAL-EXTERNAL SCALE
ABST   THE PURPOSE OF THIS STUDY WAS TO ASCERTAIN WHETHER DRUG USERS ARE BELIEVERS IN INTERNAL OR EXTERNAL CONTROL WITH REGARD TO THEIR GENERAL PATTERNS OF ACTION AND TO THEIR DRUG-TAKING BEHAVIOR IN PARTICULAR. 44 MALE AND 36 FEMALE 12-18 YEAR-OLD DRUG USERS WERE ADMINISTERED THE ROTTER INTERNAL-EXTERNAL CONTROL SCALE (I-E) AND A SCALE DESIGNED TO MEASURE PERCEIVED LOCUS OF CONTROL OF DRUG-TAKING BEHAVIOR. SUBJECTS INCLUDED 40 WHITES, 14 MEXICAN AMERICANS, 4 AMERICAN INDIANS, AND 2 BLACKS. THEY SCORED AS EXTERNALS ON THE I-E SCALE BUT AS NEITHER INTERNAL NOR EXTERNAL ON THE MEASURE OF LOCUS OF CONTROL OF DRUG-TAKING BEHAVIOR. SCORES ON THE 2 SCALES WERE NOT SIGNIFICANTLY RELATED. COMPARED WITH PREVIOUS RESULTS, SUBJECTS WERE SIGNIFICANTLY MORE EXTERNAL THAN 18-26 YEAR-OLD PRISONERS, BLACK COLLEGE STUDENTS, AND A GROUP OF URBAN 18 YEAR-OLDS. 7 REFERENCES. (PASAR ABSTRACT MODIFIED)

ACCN   001154

1348 AUTH   **OBLEDO, M. G.**
TITL   MEXICAN AMERICANS AND THE MEDIA.
SRCE   *IN M. M. MANGOLD (ED.), LA CAUSA CHICANA: THE MOVEMENT FOR JUSTICE. NEW YORK: FAMILY SERVICE ASSOCIATION OF AMERICA, 1971, PP. 6-16.*
INDX   MEXICAN AMERICAN, MASS MEDIA, STEREOTYPES, ESSAY, DISCRIMINATION, ATTITUDES, PREJUDICE, CHICANO MOVEMENT
ABST   THE AMERICAN MASS MEDIA HAVE FAILED TO ACCURATELY PORTRAY THE MEXICAN AMERICAN PEOPLE AND HAVE OFFERED INSTEAD A STEADY DIET OF NEGATIVE STEREOTYPES. THESE CARICATURES REPRESENT THE ANTITHESIS OF THE POSITIVE CHICANO IDENTITY AND HAVE (1) CONTRIBUTED SUBSTANTIALLY TO THE SOCIAL AND ECONOMIC REPRESSION OF MEXICAN AMERICANS, (2) SUBTLY AND PERSUASIVELY INFLUENCED SOCIAL ATTITUDES, AND (3) REINFORCED FEELINGS OF RACIAL SUPERIORITY AND INFERIORITY. IT IS SUGGESTED THAT CHICANOS MONITOR RADIO

AND TELEVISION STATIONS IN THEIR COMMUNITIES AND INSIST UPON COMPLIANCE WITH THE FEDERAL COMMUNICATIONS COMMISION'S FAIRNESS DOCTRINE AS IT APPLIES TO ATTACKS MADE UPON THE HONESTY, CHARACTER OR PERSONAL QUALITIES OF MEXICAN AMERICANS AS AN IDENTIFIABLE GROUP. 38 REFERENCES.

ACCN   001155

1349 AUTH   **OGLETREE, E. J., & GARCIA, D. (EDS.)**
TITL   EDUCATION OF THE SPANISH-SPEAKING URBAN CHILD: A BOOK OF READINGS.
SRCE   *SPRINGFIELD, ILL.: CHARLES C. THOMAS, 1975.*
INDX   EDUCATION, CULTURAL PLURALISM, BILINGUAL-BICULTURAL EDUCATION, MEXICAN AMERICAN, SPANISH SURNAMED, PUERTO RICAN-M, CUBAN, CHILDREN, TEACHERS, ADMINISTRATORS, CULTURAL FACTORS, ABILITY TESTING, URBAN, BILINGUALISM, CURRICULUM, INTEGRATION, INTELLIGENCE TESTING, SCHOLASTIC ACHIEVEMENT, PREJUDICE, BOOK
ABST   A COLLECTION OF 41 PAPERS IS PRESENTED IN THIS 475-PAGE VOLUME, REPRESENTING THE STUDIES AND OBSERVATIONS OF 35 EDUCATORS AND SOCIAL SCIENTISTS REGARDING THE EDUCATIONAL PROBLEMS CONFRONTING URBAN SPANISH-SPEAKING CHILDREN. THE UNIFYING THESIS OF THE BOOK IS THAT THE U.S. SCHOOL SYSTEM—BY MEANS OF NEW CURRICULA AND TEACHER TRAINING PROGRAMS—MUST ELIMINATE FACTORS WHICH DISCOURAGE THE SUCCESS OF THESE CHILDREN. TO CLARIFY THE MAJOR PROBLEM AREAS IN THIS FIELD OF STUDY, THE TEXT IS DIVIDED INTO NINE THEMATIC SECTIONS: (1) A PROFILE OF THE CULTURAL BACKGROUND AND IMMIGRATION EXPERIENCES OF MEXICAN AMERICAN, PUERTO RICAN, CUBAN, AND OTHER HISPANIC CHILDREN; (2) THE EFFECTS OF RACE AND COLOR ON SEGREGATION AND INTEGRATION; (3) A PROFILE OF THESE CHILDREN'S SELF-CONCEPT AND PERFORMANCE EXPECTATIONS; (4) THE SCHOOL SYSTEM'S ORIENTATION TOWARD SPANISH-SPEAKING CHILDREN; (5) THE EFFECTS OF LANGUAGE ON SCHOOL ACHIEVEMENT; (6) ACHIEVEMENT AND INTELLIGENCE TESTING; (7) THE MEANING AND NECESSITY OF BILINGUAL-BICULTURAL EDUCATION; (8) NEW TEACHER TRAINING, EMPHASIZING IN-SERVICE TRAINING PROGRAMS WHICH ADDRESS THE HISTORY, CULTURE, AND PERSONALITY OF THESE CHILDREN; AND (9) GENERAL EDUCATIONAL AND SOCIAL ISSUES, SUCH AS THE CULTURAL BIASES EVIDENT IN TEXTBOOKS AND THE MANY SOCIOECONOMIC AND EDUCATIONAL INEQUALITIES IN U.S. SOCIETY. THE EDITORS' CONCLUDING COMMENT IS THAT THE PROBLEMS OF SPANISH-SPEAKING CHILDREN REQUIRE INSTITUTIONAL CHANGES RATHER THAN THE EDUCATIONAL SYSTEM'S CURRENT ATTITUDE OF "CHANGE THE CHILD." 202 REFERENCES.

ACCN   001753

1350 AUTH   **OLGUIN, L.**
TITL   SOLUTIONS IN COMMUNICATION.

SRCE   *ELEMENTARY ENGLISH, 1971, 48(3), 352-356.*

INDX   BILINGUALISM, MEXICAN AMERICAN, CHILDREN, ESSAY, LINGUISTICS, TEACHERS, LANGUAGE LEARNING, PHONOLOGY, CALIFORNIA, SOUTHWEST, PROFESSIONAL TRAINING

ABST   "SOLUTIONS IN COMMUNICATION" WAS DEVELOPED THROUGH THE CALIFORNIA STATE DEPARTMENT OF EDUCATION TO ALLEVIATE PROBLEMS ENCOUNTERED IN SCHOOLS BY SPANISH-SPEAKING CHILDREN. IT SHOWS TEACHERS SOME OF THE IDENTIFIABLE, PREDICTABLE, AND TESTABLE LANGUAGE BLOCKS THAT EXIST BETWEEN THE SPANISH AND ENGLISH LANGUAGES SUCH AS THE "SCHWA" SOUND (NON-EXISTENT IN SPANISH), VARIANT WORD ENDINGS, WORDS BEGINNING WITH "S," VARIANT AIR LEVELS OF SPEECH, AND THE "SH" COMBINATION. IT IS SUGGESTED THAT TEACHERS BECOME AWARE OF THE MAJOR AREAS OF BLOCKAGE FOR SPANISH-SPEAKING STUDENTS AND DEVISE EXERCISES WHICH INSTILL THE ENGLISH SOUNDS.

ACCN   001156

1351 AUTH   **OLGUIN, L.**

TITL   "SHUCK LOVES CHIRLEY": A NON-TECHNICAL TEACHING AID FOR TEACHERS OF BILINGUAL CHILDREN.

SRCE   *HUNTINGTON BEACH, CALIF.: GOLDEN WEST PUBLISHING HOUSE, 1968.*

INDX   INSTRUCTIONAL TECHNIQUES, BILINGUALISM, TEACHERS, CHILDREN, READING, MEXICAN AMERICAN, LINGUISTIC COMPETENCE

ABST   THIS HANDBOOK SERVES AS A TEACHING AID FOR TEACHERS WHO DEAL WITH THE LEARNING DIFFICULTIES OF THE BILINGUAL CHILD WHOSE LANGUAGE SKILLS SERVE HIM IN SPANISH-SPEAKING BUT NOT IN ENGLISH-SPEAKING ENVIRONS. VARIOUS BLOCKS TO THE ACQUISITION OF ENGLISH (E.G., MOUTH MUSCLES, TONE, WORD ORDER, ALPHABET SOUNDS, BREATH CONTROL) ARE DISCUSSED. SEVERAL DIAGNOSTIC TESTS FOR SOUND PROBLEMS AND FLUENCY, ALONG WITH DEMONSTRATION LESSONS, ARE INCLUDED. IT IS BELIEVED THAT IF THE BILINGUAL CHILD CAN BE TAUGHT TO HEAR AND SPEAK THE AMERICAN DIALECT EFFECTIVELY, READING AND SELF-IMAGE PROBLEMS WILL NOT ARISE. 4 REFERENCES.

ACCN   001157

1352 AUTH   **OLIVEIRA, A. L.**

TITL   A COMPARISON OF THE VERBAL TEACHING BEHAVIORS OF JUNIOR HIGH SCHOOL MEXICAN AMERICAN AND ANGLO AMERICAN TEACHERS OF SOCIAL STUDIES AND MATHEMATICS WITH CLASSES OF PREDOMINANTLY SPANISH-SPEAKING CHILDREN (DOCTORAL DISSERTATION, UNIVERSITY OF TEXAS AT AUSTIN, 1970).

SRCE   *DISSERTATION ABSTRACTS INTERNATIONAL, 1971, 31(7), 3396A. (UNIVERSITY MICROFILMS NO. 71-00168.)*

INDX   CLASSROOM BEHAVIOR, EDUCATIONAL ASSESSMENT, INTERPERSONAL RELATIONS, LANGUAGE COMPREHENSION, MATHEMATICS, TEACHERS, MEXICAN AMERICAN, EMPIRICAL, CROSS CULTURAL, INSTRUCTIONAL TECHNIQUES, TEXAS, SOUTHWEST

ABST   AN ATTEMPT TO DETERMINE IF ANY DIFFERENCES EXIST IN THE VERBAL TEACHING BEHAVIORS OF MEXICAN AMERICAN AND ANGLO AMERICAN TEACHERS OF EIGHTH GRADE MATHEMATICS AND SOCIAL STUDIES WITH CLASSES OF PREDOMINANTLY SPANISH-SPEAKING CHILDREN IS REPORTED. FORTY SECONDARY TEACHERS WERE SUBJECTS. THERE WERE 10 TEACHERS IN EACH OF 4 GROUPS: MEXICAN AMERICAN TEACHERS OF MATHEMATICS, MEXICAN AMERICAN TEACHERS OF SOCIAL STUDIES, AND CORRESPONDING SETS OF ANGLO AMERICAN TEACHERS. THROUGH OBSERVATION IT WAS DETERMINED THAT PUPIL RESPONSE STATEMENTS AND DIVERGENT QUESTIONS BY TEACHERS WERE MORE FREQUENT IN CLASSES WITH MEXICAN AMERICAN TEACHERS, WHILE INFORMING STATEMENTS WERE MORE FREQUENT IN CLASSES WITH ANGLO AMERICAN TEACHERS. A NUMBER OF DIFFERENCES BETWEEN MATHEMATICS TEACHERS AND SOCIAL STUDIES TEACHERS, INDEPENDENT OF LINGUISTIC OR ETHNIC BACKGROUND, WERE DISCOVERED.

ACCN   001158

1353 AUTH   **OLIVER, J. D.**

TITL   LOS OJOS: A STUDY IN BILINGUAL BEHAVIOR.

SRCE   *SAN FRANCISCO: R AND E RESEARCH ASSOCIATES, 1975.*

INDX   BILINGUALISM, CULTURE, ACCULTURATION, LANGUAGE COMPREHENSION, LANGUAGE ACQUISITION, LINGUISTICS, CULTURAL PLURALISM, EMPIRICAL, MEXICAN AMERICAN, STEREOTYPES, INTERPERSONAL RELATIONS, SEX COMPARISON, LANGUAGE ASSESSMENT, ADULTS, COMMUNITY, NEW MEXICO, ATTITUDES, PHONOLOGY, SOCIAL STRUCTURE, SES, MALE, SOUTHWEST, RURAL

ABST   A PARTICIPANT OBSERVATION STUDY IN LOS OJOS, NEW MEXICO, FROM APRIL 1970 TO MAY 1971, WAS CONDUCTED TO DESCRIBE THE SOCIAL CORRELATES AND DETERMINANTS OF LANGUAGE USE AND OTHER COMMUNICATIVE DEVICES IN A RURAL BILINGUAL COMMUNITY. LOS OJOS IS ONE OF THREE MAJOR POPULATION CENTERS (POPULATION 230) IN THE RIO CHAMA VALLEY OF NORTHERN NEW MEXICO. LOCAL HISTORICAL, SOCIAL, CULTURAL, ECONOMIC, AND POLITICAL STRUCTURES ARE REVIEWED. THE HISPANOS OF LOS OJOS USE A SOUTHWESTERN DIALECT OF AMERICAN ENGLISH AND A LOCAL DIALECT OF NEW MEXICAN SPANISH. INFORMAL OBSERVATION OF COMMUNICATIVE EVENTS OCCURRED IN HOMES OF UPPER AND LOWER CLASS PERSONS, OFFICES, STORES, THE BAR, SCHOOLS, AND CHURCHES. INVESTIGATORS USED SPANISH AND ENGLISH TO FORMALLY INTERVIEW TEN FRIENDS OF THE INVESTIGATOR (5 UPPER CLASS, 5 LOWER CLASS, 5 MALE, 5 FEMALE). RECORDINGS WERE MADE OF TOPICS DISCUSSED, PERSONS INVOLVED, LANGUAGE AND REGISTER USED, ADDRESS TERMS, KINEMICS

(COMMUNICATIVE BODY MOTIONS), AND PROXEMICS (MANAGEMENT OF PERSONAL SPACE). THE LINGUISTIC CHARACTERISTICS OF THE THREE REGISTERS OF THE TWO LANGUAGES (SIX DIATYPES) ARE DESCRIBED. AN ANALYSIS OF TWO-PERSON ENCOUNTERS CORRELATES LANGUAGE, PROXEMICS, AND KINEMICS AS ENTIRE COMMUNICATIVE OUTPUTS. THIRTEEN "PERSON FACTORS" THAT AFFECT COMMUNICATIVE OUTPUT ARE CONSIDERED—INCLUDING ETHNICITY, LANGUAGE COMPETENCE, SEX, CLASS, AGE, SOCIAL POSITION, AND INVOLVEMENT IN ENCOUNTER. OBSERVATIONS REVEALED THAT, IN GENERAL, SPANISH IS USED DOMINANTLY BY OLDER PERSONS, BY LOWER-CLASS PERSONS, AND BY MALES REGARDLESS OF AGE AND SOCIAL CLASS. SPANISH IS CONSIDERED THE IN-GROUP LANGUAGE, WHILE ENGLISH IS CONSIDERED A COLD LANGUAGE APPROPRIATE FOR PUNITIVE BEHAVIOR AND IMPERSONAL OR BUREAUCRATIC ENCOUNTERS. LOS OJOS COMMUNICATION BEHAVIOR IS CONSIDERED A COORDINATED PACKAGE WHICH IS AN EXPRESSION OF SOCIAL STRUCTURE. 247 REFERENCES.

ACCN   001159

1354 AUTH   **OLMEDO, E. L.**
     TITL   ACCULTURATION: A PSYCHOMETRIC PERSPECTIVE.
     SRCE   *AMERICAN PSYCHOLOGIST, 1979, 34(11), 1061-1070.*
     INDX   ACCULTURATION, CROSS CULTURAL, SPANISH SURNAMED, RESEARCH METHODOLOGY, REVIEW, THEORETICAL
     ABST   THE EMERGING PSYCHOMETRIC PERSPECTIVE IN THE STUDY OF ACCULTURATION IS PLACED WITHIN THE BROADER SCOPE OF BEHAVIORAL SCIENCE RESEARCH BY EXAMINING A NUMBER OF CONCEPTUAL AND OPERATIONAL ISSUES. A REVIEW OF RECENT RESEARCH INDICATES THAT THE MEASUREMENT OF INDIVIDUAL ACCULTURATION IS NOT ONLY A LEGITIMATE AREA OF INVESTIGATION, BUT CAN ALSO MEET CONVENTIONAL CRITERIA OF RELIABILITY AND VALIDITY. FURTHERMORE, PARTICULARLY WITHIN THE FRAMEWORK OF A FULL MEASUREMENT MODEL, PSYCHOMETRIC METHODS HAVE THE POTENTIAL TO CONTRIBUTE TO A BETTER UNDERSTANDING OF COMPLEX ISSUES SUCH AS THE IDENTIFICATION AND CROSS-CULTURAL EQUIVALENCE OF CULTURAL VARIABLES AS ANTECEDENTS OF BEHAVIOR. FINALLY, RECENT DEVELOPMENTS IN THE QUANTIFICATION OF ACCULTURATION ALONG MULTIPLE DIMENSIONS SUGGEST THAT THIS APPROACH IS MORE PROMISING THAN ARBITRARY CULTURAL GROUP OR GENERATIONAL TYPOLOGIES. 50 REFERENCES. (JOURNAL ABSTRACT MODIFIED)
     ACCN   001831

1355 AUTH   **OLMEDO, E. L.**
     TITL   HIGHER EDUCATION AND MENTAL HEALTH: AN HISPANIC PERSPECTIVE.
     SRCE   *PAPER PRESENTED AT THE W.I.C.H.E. PLANNING MEETING, SAN FRANCISCO, APRIL 29, 1977.*

INDX   HIGHER EDUCATION, HEALTH DELIVERY SYSTEMS, BILINGUAL-BICULTURAL PERSONNEL, MENTAL HEALTH, MENTAL HEALTH PROFESSION, CURRICULUM, PROFESSIONAL TRAINING, SPANISH SURNAMED, REPRESENTATION, ESSAY
ABST   THREE INTERRELATED ISSUES PERTINENT TO THE FUTURE OF MINORITY MENTAL HEALTH IN GENERAL AND HISPANIC MENTAL HEALTH IN PARTICULAR ARE DISCUSSED: (1) THE NEED FOR MINORITY MENTAL HEALTH SERVICE PROVIDERS AND RESEARCHERS; (2) THE NEED FOR A DATA BASE PERTAINING TO MINORITY MENTAL HEALTH; AND (3) THE NEED FOR IMPLEMENTING A COMPREHENSIVE MENTAL HEALTH CURRICULUM TRAINING PROGRAM THAT IS CULTURALLY SENSITIVE. HISPANICS ARE UNDERREPRESENTED AT ALL LEVELS OF PROFESSIONAL TRAINING AND EMPLOYMENT IN THE MENTAL HEALTH FIELDS. THE CURRENT LIMITED AND SEVERELY STEREOTYPIC KNOWLEDGE REFLECTS THE DATA BASE OF HISPANIC MENTAL HEALTH RESEARCH. THE FINAL ISSUE CONCERNS THE NECESSITY OF IMPLEMENTING PSYCHOLOGY PROGRAMS THAT CAN BE RESPONSIVE TO CULTURAL NEEDS WITHIN AND BETWEEN DIFFERENT ETHNIC GROUPS. TO RECTIFY THESE PROBLEMS, IT IS CONCLUDED THAT THE FOCUS OF THE PRESENT MEETING SHOULD BE THAT OF GENERATING EFFECTIVE ACTION AND NOT OF PRODUCING ADDITIONAL RECOMMENDATIONS. 8 REFERENCES.
ACCN   001160

1356 AUTH   **OLMEDO, E. L.**
     TITL   PATTERNS OF HISPANIC REPRESENTATION AMONG DOCTORAL LEVEL SCIENTISTS AND GRADUATE STUDENTS IN THE UNITED STATES.
     SRCE   *IN E. L. OLMEDO & S. LOPEZ (EDS.), HISPANIC MENTAL HEALTH PROFESSIONALS (MONOGRAPH NO. 5). LOS ANGELES: UNIVERSITY OF CALIFORNIA, SPANISH SPEAKING MENTAL HEALTH RESEARCH CENTER, 1977, PP. 59-76.*
     INDX   REPRESENTATION, PROFESSIONAL TRAINING, HIGHER EDUCATION, DEMOGRAPHIC, ECONOMIC FACTORS, EQUAL OPPORTUNITY, SPANISH SURNAMED, CROSS CULTURAL, MENTAL HEALTH PROFESSION, SOCIAL SCIENCES, EMPIRICAL, REVIEW, EMPLOYMENT
     ABST   AN EXAMINATION OF THE CURRENT STATUS AND DISCERNIBLE TRENDS OF HISPANIC REPRESENTATION IN THE U.S. PROFESSIONAL LABOR FORCE AT THE PH.D. LEVEL IS PRESENTED. THE STATUS OF HISPANIC REPRESENTATION IS DOCUMENTED IN THE FOLLOWING AREAS: (1) DOCTORAL LEVEL SCIENTISTS FOR 1973; (2) PH.D. RECIPIENTS FOR 1973-1975; (3) 1973 GRADUATE STUDENT ENROLLMENTS; AND (4) STUDENT SUPPORT PATTERNS FOR DOCTORATE RECIPIENTS DURING 1973-1974. IT IS CONCLUDED THAT DESPITE "AFFIRMATIVE ACTION EFFORTS" OF THE PAST, HISPANICS CONTINUE TO BE SEVERELY UNDERREPRESENTED IN THE U.S. PH.D.-LEVEL LABOR FORCE. PROFOUND AND EFFECTIVE

CHANGES MUST OCCUR AT ALL LEVELS OF EDUCATION TO IMPROVE THIS SITUATION, AND CURRENT LEVELS OF FINANCIAL ASSISTANCE SHOULD BE INCREASED. 9 REFERENCES. (AUTHOR SUMMARY MODIFIED)

ACCN 001161

1357 AUTH **OLMEDO, E. L.**
TITL PSYCHOLOGICAL TESTING AND THE CHICANO: A REASSESSMENT.
SRCE *IN J. L. MARTINEZ (ED), CHICANO PSYCHOLOGY. NEW YORK: ACADEMIC PRESS, 1977, PP. 175-195.*
INDX TEST RELIABILITY, INTELLIGENCE TESTING, PERSONALITY ASSESSMENT, REVIEW, ACCULTURATION, BILINGUALISM, CULTURE-FAIR TESTS, CULTURAL FACTORS, RESEARCH METHODOLOGY, MEXICAN AMERICAN
ABST DESPITE POSITIVE CHANGES IN PSYCHOLOGICAL TESTING, CHICANOS CONTINUE TO SUFFER ABUSES IN THIS AREA. THIS PAPER REASSESSES THE STATUS OF PSYCHOLOGICAL TESTING AND THE CHICANO, INCLUDING DISCUSSIONS ON THE NATURE AND USE OF PSYCHOLOGICAL TESTS, ASSUMPTIONS UNDERLYING PSYCHOLOGICAL TESTING, TEST BIAS, AND MODELS OF CULTURE FAIR TESTING. BILINGUALISM DOES NOT APPEAR TO IMPAIR COGNITIVE FUNCTIONING, WHILE OBSERVED DEFICITS ARE A RESULT OF FAILURE TO CONTROL THIS VARIABLE. IN ADDITION, SPANISH TRANSLATIONS OF STANDARD INSTRUMENTS HAVE BEEN FOUND UNPRODUCTIVE. THE PROBLEM OF CULTURAL BIAS IN CRITERIA, ESPECIALLY IN EDUCATIONAL SETTINGS, MUST BE RECOGNIZED AND SHOULD BE ONE OF THE PRIMARY FOCI OF FUTURE RESEARCH. 67 REFERENCES.
ACCN 001162

1358 AUTH **OLMEDO, E. L., MARTINEZ, J. L., JR., & MARTINEZ, S. R.**
TITL A MEASURE OF ACCULTURATION FOR CHICANO ADOLESCENTS.
SRCE *PSYCHOLOGICAL REPORTS, 1978, 42, 159-170.*
INDX ACCULTURATION, RESEARCH METHODOLOGY, FAMILY ROLES, SEX ROLES, BILINGUAL, SES, EMPIRICAL, MEXICAN AMERICAN, ADOLESCENTS, CALIFORNIA, SOUTHWEST, COLLEGE STUDENTS, TEST RELIABILITY, TEST VALIDITY
ABST A PAPER-AND-PENCIL MEASURE OF ACCULTURATION FOR CHICANO ADOLESCENTS WAS DEVELOPED USING MULTIPLE REGRESSION TECHNIQUES AND 924 CHICANO AND ANGLO HIGH SCHOOL STUDENTS IN THREE SOUTHERN CALIFORNIA COMMUNITIES. A LINEAR COMBINATION OF SOCIOCULTURAL AND SEMANTIC DIFFERENTIAL VARIABLES PROVIDED FOR OPTIMAL DISCRIMINATION BETWEEN CHICANOS AND ANGLOS. A DOUBLE CROSS-VALIDATION PROCEDURE INDICATED THAT THE 20-VARIABLE REGRESSION EQUATION WAS REASONABLY STABLE FROM THE FIRST SAMPLE TO THE NEXT, YIELDING VALIDITY COEFFICIENTS FROM .66 TO .80. AN ANCILLARY STUDY OF 129 CHICANO AND ANGLO JUNIOR COLLEGE STUDENTS SHOWED THAT TEST-RETEST RELIABILITY RANGED FROM .66 TO .89. A FACTORANA-

LYSIS OF THE ITEMS INCLUDED IN THE REGRESSION EQUATION RESULTED IN THREE FACTORS; TWO WERE SLIGHTLY INTERCORRELATED AND LOADED PRIMARILY WITH SOCIOCULTURAL VARIABLES PERTAINING TO LANGUAGE SPOKEN AT HOME, NATIONALITY, AND SOCIOECONOMIC STATUS OF THE HEAD OF HOUSEHOLD; THE THIRD FACTOR WAS ESSENTIALLY ORTHOGONAL TO THE OTHER TWO AND SHOWED HIGH LOADINGS FOR SEMANTIC DIFFERENTIAL SCALES FOR THE CONCEPTS "MOTHER," "FATHER," AND "MALE" ON THE POTENCY DIMENSION. THEORETICAL AND APPLIED IMPLICATIONS ARE DISCUSSED WITH RESPECT TO EDUCATIONAL AND PSYCHOLOGICAL ASSESSMENT. 21 REFERENCES. (AUTHOR ABSTRACT MODIFIED)

ACCN 001163

1359 AUTH **OLMEDO, E. L., & LOPEZ, S. (EDS.)**
TITL HISPANIC MENTAL HEALTH PROFESSIONALS (MONOGRAPH NO. 5).
SRCE *LOS ANGELES: UNIVERSITY OF CALIFORNIA, SPANISH SPEAKING MENTAL HEALTH RESEARCH CENTER, 1977.*
INDX MENTAL HEALTH PROFESSION, EQUAL OPPORTUNITY, SPANISH SURNAMED, MEXICAN AMERICAN, BILINGUAL-BICULTURAL PERSONNEL, REPRESENTATION, HIGHER EDUCATION, MENTAL HEALTH, BIBLIOGRAPHY, MEDICAL STUDENTS, PUERTO RICAN-M, EDUCATION, POLITICAL POWER, PROFESSIONAL TRAINING, REVIEW, EMPLOYMENT, DISCRIMINATION, NURSING, BOOK
ABST THE CURRENT STATUS OF HISPANIC REPRESENTATION IN THE MENTAL HEALTH FIELDS IS DOCUMENTED IN THIS COLLECTION OF REPORTS. DUE TO THE BARRIERS WITHIN MEDICAL SCHOOLS AND THE PSYCHIATRIC PROFESSION ITSELF, CHICANOS COMPRISE AN EXTREMELY SMALL PERCENTAGE OF PSYCHIATRISTS. THE PROPORTION OF PSYCHOLOGISTS WHO ARE HISPANIC IS 10 TO 16 TIMES SMALLER THAN THE PROPORTION OF AMERICANS WHO ARE OF HISPANIC DESCENT. FURTHERMORE, IN CLINICAL PSYCHOLOGY THERE IS AN INDICATION THAT HISPANIC REPRESENTATION IS DECREASING. ALTHOUGH THE PERCENTAGE OF HISPANICS IN SOCIAL WORK HAS YET TO REACH THE DEGREE OF HISPANIC REPRESENTATION IN THE U.S., HISPANICS ARE SUBSTANTIALLY REPRESENTED AT THE MSW AND DSW LEVELS AND THERE IS AN INCREASING NUMBER OF HISPANICS AMONG THE FACULTY RANKS. LASTLY, ALTHOUGH PSYCHIATRIC NURSING HAS NO DATA REGARDING REPRESENTATION, THE FIGURES FOR NURSING IN GENERAL ARE DISMAL. RECOMMENDATIONS ARE PROVIDED TO IMPROVE THE SEVERE UNDERREPRESENTATION OF HISPANICS. IN ADDITION, A SUMMARY WRITTEN IN SPANISH AND A COMPREHENSIVE ANNOTATED BIBLIOGRAPHY OF LITERATURE RELATED TO HISPANIC HUMAN RESOURCES ARE PROVIDED.
ACCN 001165

1360 AUTH **OLMEDO, E. L., & MARTINEZ, S. R.**
TITL A GENERAL MULTIDIMENSIONAL MODEL FOR

THE MEASUREMENT OF CULTURAL DIFFERENCES.

SRCE   *PAPER PRESENTED AT THE 85TH ANNUAL CONVENTION OF THE AMERICAN PSYCHOLOGICAL ASSOCIATION, SAN FRANCISCO, AUGUST 26-30, 1977. (AVAILABLE FROM DR. E. L. OLMEDO, AMERICAN PSYCHOLOGICAL ASSOCIATION, 1200 17TH ST., N.W., WASHINGTON D.C., 20036.)*

INDX   RESEARCH METHODOLOGY, ACCULTURATION, PERSONALITY ASSESSMENT, CULTURAL FACTORS, TEST VALIDITY, CROSS CULTURAL, EMPIRICAL, MEXICAN AMERICAN, BILINGUALISM, SES, FAMILY ROLES

ABST   A MULTIDIMENSIONAL MEASUREMENT MODEL (MCD) BASED ON FACTOR ANALYTIC THEORY AND TECHNIQUES IS PROPOSED. THE MODEL WAS TESTED WITH DATA PREVIOUSLY OBTAINED FROM 974 ANGLO AND MEXICAN AMERICAN SOUTHERN CALIFORNIA HIGH SCHOOL STUDENTS WHO WERE ADMINISTERED AN ACCULTURATION INVENTORY. THE ITEMS ON THE INVENTORY TAPPED SOCIOCULTURAL CHARACTERISTICS SUCH AS LANGUAGE, NATIONALITY, OCCUPATIONAL STATUS, AND RATINGS OF THE CONCEPTS "MOTHER," "FATHER," AND "MALE" ON THE POTENCY DIMENSION OF THE SEMANTIC DIFFERENTIAL. THE MODEL ASSUMES THAT A CULTURAL SPACE MAY BE DEFINED BY MEANS OF A RELATIVELY FEW ORTHOGONAL DIMENSIONS WHICH ARE LINEAR COMBINATIONS OF A MUCH LARGER NUMBER OF CULTURAL VARIABLES. ONCE A SUITABLE, CROSS-CULTURALLY EQUIVALENT FACTORIAL STRUCTURE IS ESTABLISHED, CULTURAL DIFFERENTIALS ARE OPERATIONALLY DEFINED AS DISTANCES WITHIN THE CULTURAL SPACE BETWEEN LOCI HAVING COORDINATES EQUAL TO FACTOR SCORES OR TRANSFORMS THEREOF. THE LOCI MAY REPRESENT INDIVIDUALS AS WELL AS GROUP CENTROIDS. ADDITIONALLY, MCD PROVIDES FOR QUANTITATIVE OPERATIONAL DEFINITIONS OF COMMONLY ENCOUNTERED CONSTRUCTS SUCH AS ACCULTURATION AND BICULTURALISM. 21 REFERENCES. (AUTHOR ABSTRACT MODIFIED)

ACCN   001166

1361 AUTH   **OLMEDO, E. L., & PADILLA, A. M.**

TITL   EMPIRICAL AND CONSTRUCT VALIDATION OF A MEASURE OF ACCULTURATION FOR MEXICAN AMERICANS.

SRCE   *JOURNAL OF SOCIAL PSYCHOLOGY, 1978, 105, 179-187.*

INDX   ACCULTURATION, ETHNIC IDENTITY, MEXICAN AMERICAN, CROSS CULTURAL, ADULTS, CALIFORNIA, SOUTHWEST, EMPIRICAL, CROSS GENERATIONAL

ABST   AN ACCULTURATION INVENTORY CONSISTING OF SOCIOCULTURAL AND SEMANTIC DIFFERENTIAL ITEMS WAS ADMINISTERED IN THREE SOUTHERN CALIFORNIA COMMUNITIES TO 68 ADULT MEN AND WOMEN—26 ANGLO AMERICANS, 16 FIRST GENERATION MEXICAN AMERICANS, AND 26 THIRD GENERATION MEXICAN AMERICANS. THE RESULTS INDICATED THAT ACCULTURATION SCORES DERIVED FROM THE INVENTORY CORRELATED HIGHLY WITH ETH-

NIC GROUP MEMBERSHIP (.83 R .85, P.01). FURTHERMORE, HYPOTHESES PERTAINING TO DIRECTIONAL DIFFERENCES IN ACCULTURATION SCORES AMONG GROUP MEANS WERE CONFIRMED. ANGLO AMERICANS SCORED SIGNIFICANTLY HIGHER (P.01) THAN THIRD GENERATION MEXICAN AMERICANS, WHO, IN TURN, SCORED SIGNIFICANTLY HIGHER (P<.05) THAN FIRST GENERATION MEXICAN AMERICANS. ADVANTAGES AND LIMITATIONS OF THE INVENTORY ARE DISCUSSED, AS WELL AS THEORETICAL IMPLICATIONS CONCERNING THE CONSTRUCT OF ACCULTURATION AND ITS RELATIONSHIP TO SOCIOCULTURAL CHARACTERISTICS. 15 REFERENCES. (JOURNAL ABSTRACT)

ACCN   001795

1362 AUTH   **ONODA, L., & MENDEZ, A.**

TITL   AFFIRMATIVE ACTION SURVEY OF COLLEGE COUNSELING CENTERS.

SRCE   *JOURNAL OF COLLEGE STUDENT PERSONNEL, 1977, 18(2), 102-104.*

INDX   EDUCATIONAL COUNSELING, REPRESENTATION, SURVEY, SPANISH SURNAMED, HIGHER EDUCATION, CROSS CULTURAL, EQUAL OPPORTUNITY, SEX COMPARISON, CALIFORNIA, SOUTHWEST

ABST   TO DETERMINE IF COLLEGE COUNSELING CENTERS ARE COMPLYING WITH AFFIRMATIVE ACTION GUIDELINES, A SURVEY WAS CONDUCTED TO MEASURE THEIR ETHNIC COMPOSITION. THE PERCENTAGE OF MINORITY STAFF IN 74 COUNSELING CENTERS IN CALIFORNIA WAS COMPARED TO THE EQUIVALENT MINORITY STUDENT ENROLLMENT IN TWO AND FOUR YEAR COLLEGES AND THE UNIVERSITY OF CALIFORNIA SYSTEM. ALSO COMPARED WAS THE PERCENTAGE OF COUNSELING STAFF BY SEX. EXCEPT FOR ASIAN AMERICANS AND WOMEN, THE RESULTS SHOW A GREATER PERCENTAGE OF MINORITY COUNSELING STAFF COMPARED TO THE EQUIVALENT ENROLLMENT OF MINORITY STUDENTS. THE PERCENTAGE OF SPANISH SURNAMED INDIVIDUALS ATTENDING BOTH TWO AND FOUR YEAR COLLEGES FELL BELOW THE RESPECTIVE POPULATION CENSUS PERCENTAGE; IF THE NUMBER OF STUDENTS INCREASED, THE PERCENTAGE OF SPANISH SURNAMED COUNSELING STAFF WOULD NOT CONFORM TO AFFIRMATIVE ACTION GUIDELINES. AN EXAMINATION OF THE PROBLEMS ASSOCIATED WITH THE ROLE OF MINORITY COUNSELORS AND THE RECRUITMENT OF MORE MINORITY STAFF ARE RECOMMENDED. 3 REFERENCES.

ACCN   001167

1363 AUTH   **ORIVE, R., & GERARD, H. B.**

TITL   SOCIAL CONTACT OF MINORITY PARENTS AND THEIR CHILDREN'S ACCEPTANCE BY CLASSMATES.

SRCE   *SOCIOMETRY, 1975, 38(4), 518-524.*

INDX   SES, CHILDREN, CROSS CULTURAL, CULTURE, DISCRIMINATION, EXTENDED FAMILY, FAMILY ROLES, FAMILY STRUCTURE, PEER GROUP, MEXICAN AMERICAN, SOCIALIZATION, EMPIRICAL, ACCULTURATION, SEX COMPARISON, IN-

TERPERSONAL ATTRACTION, CALIFORNIA, SOUTHWEST, INTEGRATION

ABST THE RELATIONSHIP BETWEEN SOCIOMETRIC CHOICES RECEIVED BY MEXICAN AMERICAN AND BLACK CHILDREN FROM ANGLO PEERS WAS EXAMINED, AND THE AMOUNT OF THE MINORITY PARENT'S CONTACT WITH HIS OWN IN-GROUP AS WELL AS OTHER ETHNIC GROUP MEMBERS WAS ASSESSED. A SAMPLE OF 549 ELEMENTARY SCHOOL CHILDREN AND THEIR PARENTS WAS CHOSEN FROM A DISTRICT WHICH HAD RECENTLY BEEN DESEGREGATED. RESULTS INDICATE THAT ONLY FATHER CONTACTS WERE SIGNIFICANTLY RELATED TO THE MINORITY CHILD'S ACCEPTANCE. CHILD SEX DIFFERENCES AND TYPE OF FATHER CONTACT INTERACTED IN DETERMINING ANGLO PEER ACCEPTANCE. FATHER'S INVOLVEMENT IN ORGANIZATIONS WAS SIGNIFICANTLY RELATED TO A BOY'S ACCEPTANCE, WHEREAS LESS CONTACT FOR FATHER WITH RELATIVES WAS RELATED TO A GIRL'S ACCEPTANCE. THIS OCCURRED REGARDLESS OF FAMILY SOCIOECONOMIC STATUS. 12 REFERENCES. (AUTHOR ABSTRACT MODIFIED)

ACCN 001169

1364 AUTH **ORR, R. G.**
TITL THE RELATIONSHIP OF SOCIAL CHARACTER AND DOGMATISM AMONG SPANISH AMERICAN YOUNG ADULTS IN THREE SELECTED INSTITUTIONS IN NEW MEXICO (DOCTORAL DISSERTATION, UNIVERSITY OF NEW MEXICO, 1967).
SRCE *DISSERTATION ABSTRACTS, 1967, 28(4), 1259A. (UNIVERSITY MICROFILMS NO. 67-11,763.)*
INDX ADULTS, ADULT EDUCATION, EMPIRICAL, SPANISH SURNAMED, ATTITUDES, PERSONALITY ASSESSMENT, CONFORMITY, EDUCATIONAL COUNSELING, EMPLOYMENT, VOCATIONAL COUNSELING, INTELLIGENCE, NEW MEXICO, SOUTHWEST
ABST THE EMERGING POST-SECONDARY SYSTEM OF VOCATIONAL TRAINING REPRESENTS A FURTHER DIFFERENTIATION OF THE FUNCTION OF EDUCATION IN THE SOCIALIZATION AND ROLE ALLOCATION PROCESS. THIS STUDY INVESTIGATED THE EFFECTS OF THE SYSTEM ON 193 YOUNG SPANISH SURNAMED ADULTS ENROLLED IN JOB TRAINING COURSES AT THREE DIFFERENT INSTITUTIONS IN NEW MEXICO DURING 1966. THE STUDY (1) COMPARED GROUPS OF SPANISH AMERICANS, AGES 18-24, IDENTIFIED DEMOGRAPHICALLY AND BY JOB TRAINING COURSE BY MEASURES OF THEIR SOCIAL CHARACTER AND DOGMATISM, (2) INVESTIGATED THE RELATIONSHIPS BETWEEN SOCIAL CHARACTER AND DOGMATISM, BETWEEN SOCIAL CHARACTER AND INTELLIGENCE, AND BETWEEN DOGMATISM AND INTELLIGENCE IN THESE YOUNG ADULTS, AND (3) EXAMINED THE EFFECTS OF A TWO MONTH BASIC EDUCATION ORIENTATION COURSE ON THE SOCIAL CHARACTER AND DOGMATISM OF THE SAMPLE GROUPS. SOME MAJOR FINDINGS INDICATE: (1) THERE ARE SOME PRONOUNCED DIFFERENCES IN SOCIAL CHARACTER, BUT NOT IN DOGMATISM, AMONG THE STUDENTS ATTENDING DIFFERENT VOCA-

TIONAL PROGRAMS; (2) STUDENTS FROM POORER, LESS POPULATED AREAS SHOW A SLIGHT TENDENCY TOWARD INNER-DIRECTEDNESS IN SOCIAL CHARACTER AND A DEFINITE TENDENCY TOWARD CLOSED-MINDEDNESS IN DOGMATISM; (3) SOCIAL CHARACTER, DOGMATISM, AND INTELLIGENCE DO NOT SHOW A GENERAL RELATIONSHIP WITH EACH OTHER; AND (4) SOCIAL CHARACTER AND DOGMATISM ARE RELATIVELY DIFFICULT TO CHANGE BY A SHORT TERM BASIC EDUCATION ORIENTATION COURSE. RECOMMENDATIONS BASED ON THE STUDY RESULTS ARE INCLUDED. 62 REFERENCES.

ACCN 001170

1365 AUTH **ORTEGA, F.**
TITL SPECIAL EDUCATION PLACEMENT AND MEXICAN AMERICANS.
SRCE *EL GRITO, 1971, 4(4), 29-35.*
INDX CHILDREN, MEXICAN AMERICAN, EMPIRICAL, ACHIEVEMENT TESTING, INTELLIGENCE TESTING, CROSS CULTURAL, MENTAL RETARDATION, CULTURAL FACTORS, IMPAIRMENT, SPECIAL EDUCATION, REPRESENTATION, PROGRAM EVALUATION, CALIFORNIA, SOUTHWEST
ABST USING DATA FROM A CALIFORNIA STATE DEPARTMENT OF EDUCATION REPORT ON SPECIAL EDUCATION, THIS STUDY VERIFIES THAT THERE IS A DISPROPORTIONATE PLACEMENT OF MEXICAN AMERICAN (MA) CHILDREN IN CLASSES FOR THE EDUCABLE MENTALLY RETARDED (EMR). HYPOTHESES BASED ON THE ASSUMPTION THAT THE PLACEMENT OF MA CHILDREN IN SPECIAL CLASSES WILL FOLLOW A NORMAL CURVE DISTRIBUTION WHEN COMPARED TO TOTAL SCHOOL AND GENERAL POPULATIONS WERE REJECTED AFTER CHI-SQUARE ANALYSIS. FINDINGS INDICATE THAT OUT OF ALL PUPILS IN CALIFORNIA SCHOOLS, 1.16% HAVE BEEN DIAGNOSED AS EMR, WHILE AMONG MA, 2.14% HAVE BEEN SO DIAGNOSED AND PLACED IN EMR CLASSES, AND ONLY .71% OF "OTHER WHITE" PUPILS HAVE BEEN SO DIAGNOSED. SEVERAL CONCLUSIONS ARE DRAWN: (1) THE DISPROPORTIONATE REPRESENTATION OF SPANISH-SPEAKING STUDENTS IN EMR CLASSES IS A STATEWIDE PROBLEM; (2) THE CONCEPT OF INTELLIGENCE IN CALIFORNIA IS CONTRADICTORY TO THE NORMAL CURVE DISTRIBUTION WHICH IS THE BASIC PREMISE UPON WHICH SPECIAL CLASSES ARE BASED; AND (3) THE PROCEDURE USED TO IDENTIFY STUDENTS AS MENTALLY RETARDED, AS USED IN CALIFORNIA, IS AMBIGUOUS. CALIFORNIA EDUCATORS' UNWILLINGNESS TO ACCEPT LANGUAGE AND CULTURAL DIFFERENCES AND TO MODIFY CURRICULA ACCORDINGLY IS POSITED AS THE MAJOR PROBLEM.

ACCN 001171

1366 AUTH **ORTEGO, P. D.**
TITL THE CHICANO RENAISSANCE.
SRCE *IN M. M. MANGOLD (ED.), LA CAUSA CHICANA: THE MOVEMENT FOR JUSTICE. NEW YORK: FAMILY SERVICE ASSOCIATION OF AMERICA, 1971, PP. 42-61.*

INDX   MEXICAN AMERICAN, HISTORY, ESSAY, ART, STEREOTYPES, MIGRATION, CHICANO MOVEMENT, CULTURE, ETHNIC IDENTITY

ABST   THE REBIRTH OF CHICANO LITERATURE, ART, POETRY, AND THEATER IS DISCUSSED IN TERMS OF EACH BEING A MEDIUM BY WHICH THE CHICANO MOVEMENT CAN BE EXTENDED INTO AMERICAN SOCIETY. BRIEF HISTORICAL REVIEWS AND CONTEMPORARY DEVELOPMENTS WITHIN EACH AREA ARE PRESENTED. THE CHICANO RENAISSANCE HAS COME ABOUT NOT IN RELATION TO THE TRADITIONAL PAST BUT RATHER IN RESPONSE TO A GROWING AWARENESS BY MEXICAN AMERICANS OF THEIR INDIAN IDENTITY. THIS AWARENESS OF THEIR ARTISTIC AND LITERARY HERITAGE HAS PARALLELED A SIMILAR INCREASE IN THE SOCIAL AND POLITICAL CONSCIOUSNESS OF MEXICAN AMERICANS OVER THE LAST TWO OR THREE DECADES. OVERALL, THE ARTICLE PROVIDES A CONCISE DESCRIPTION OF THE CHICANO MOVEMENT IN THE ARTS. 32 REFERENCES.

ACCN   001172

1367 AUTH   **ORTEGO, P. D.**

TITL   FABLES OF IDENTITY: STEREOTYPE AND CARICATURE OF CHICANOS IN STEINBECK'S "TORTILLA FLAT."

SRCE   *THE JOURNAL OF ETHNIC STUDIES, 1973, 1(1), 39-43.*

INDX   ETHNIC IDENTITY, STEREOTYPES, MEXICAN AMERICAN, PREJUDICE, ESSAY, ART

ABST   A CRITICAL REVIEW OF JOHN STEINBECK'S NOVEL, "TORTILLA FLAT," PUBLISHED IN 1935, IS PRESENTED. DISCUSSION FOCUSES ON THE FOLLOWING POINTS OF CRITICISM: (1) THE IMAGE PRESENTED IN THE NOVEL PERPETUATES A SOCIAL AND ETHNIC STEREOTYPE DAMAGING TO ALL CHICANOS; (2) STEREOTYPE AND CARICATURE SERIOUSLY FLAW THE ARTISTRY AND/OR VERACITY OF NOVELS USING THESE STYLES; AND (3) THE "ETHNIC" NOVEL IS MOST SUCCESSFUL AND TRUE-TO-LIFE WHEN RENDERED ARTISTICALLY BY AN "ETHNIC" WRITER. BECAUSE STEINBECK'S NOVEL DRAWS HEAVILY ON MYSTICAL IDENTITIES, STEREOTYPES, AND EXAGGERATED CARICATURES, IT MISREPRESENTS CHICANOS TO ANY READER WHO UNWITTINGLY ACCEPTS THE FIDELITY OF THIS REPRESENTATION. THIS IS CERTAINLY DETRIMENTAL TO CHICANOS AND, WHEN SEEN IN THIS LIGHT, THE NOVEL IS ONE OF STEINBECK'S LEAST SUCCESSFUL.

ACCN   001173

1368 AUTH   **OSIPOW, S. H.**

TITL   VOCATIONAL BEHAVIOR AND CAREER DEVELOPMENT, 1975: A REVIEW.

SRCE   *JOURNAL OF VOCATIONAL BEHAVIOR, 1976, 9, 129-145.*

INDX   ACHIEVEMENT MOTIVATION, ATTITUDES, CROSS CULTURAL, CULTURAL FACTORS, EMPLOYMENT, EQUAL OPPORTUNITY, FEMALE, LABOR FORCE, JOB PERFORMANCE, MEXICAN AMERICAN, OCCUPATIONAL ASPIRATIONS, RESEARCH METHODOLOGY, REVIEW, ROLE EXPECTATIONS, SEX ROLES, VOCATIONAL COUNSELING, TEST VALIDITY, STEREOTYPES

ABST   A REVIEW OF LITERATURE AND RESEARCH IN THE FIELDS OF VOCATIONAL BEHAVIOR AND CAREER DEVELOPMENT FOR 1975 IS PRESENTED. NOTABLE BOOKS PUBLISHED ON THE TOPIC IN 1975 ARE LISTED WHICH COVER THE THEORY OF INTEREST DEVELOPMENT, THE PSYCHOLOGY OF LEISURE, AND CAREER ANALYSIS AND OUTLOOKS FOR WOMEN, INCLUDING THE WORKING WOMAN'S INTERESTS, BARRIERS, AND THE EFFECTS OF MARRIAGE. STUDIES ON SEX STEREOTYPING IN CAREER DEVELOPMENT ARE REVIEWED, AND CAREER ORIENTATION IN WOMEN IS DISCUSSED. RESEARCH INTO ASPECTS OF WOMEN'S CAREERS ARE PRESENTED WITH THE CONCLUSION THAT SEX ROLE STEREOTYPING STILL CONTINUES ALTHOUGH IT APPEARS TO BE MODERATING. RECENT DEVELOPMENTS IN INTEREST MEASUREMENT AND THE THEORY OF CAREER DEVELOPMENT AND CURRENT RESEARCH DEALING WITH IT ARE DISCUSSED. VALIDITY RESEARCH ON THE VARIOUS HOLLAND MEASUREMENT INSTRUMENTS HAS CONTINUED TO SHOW THE TESTS' APPROPRIATENESS. RESEARCH INTO THE LIFE-SPAN ASPECTS OF CAREERS AND CAREER INTERVENTIONS AND CAREER WORKSHOPS IS PRESENTED, AS WELL AS SOME STUDIES OF JOB SATISFACTION AND WORK MOTIVATION. STUDIES OF OCCUPATIONAL ENVIRONMENTS ARE SUMMARIZED, AND RESEARCH ON RACIAL DIFFERENCES IS PRESENTED. OCCUPATIONAL PRESTIGE STABILITY, INCLUDING A STUDY OF MEXICAN AMERICANS, IS REVIEWED. IT IS CONCLUDED THAT 1975 WAS A PROLIFIC YEAR FOR RESEARCH ON CAREER DEVELOPMENT FOR WOMEN AND MINORITIES AND IN THE FIELD OF MEASUREMENT. 69 REFERENCES. (NCMHI ABSTRACT)

ACCN   002171

1369 AUTH   **OUR SUNDAY VISITOR, INC.**

TITL   A GALLUP STUDY OF RELIGIOUS AND SOCIAL ATTITUDES OF HISPANIC-AMERICANS.

SRCE   *PRINCETON, N.J.: THE GALLUP ORGANIZATION, INC., 1978.*

INDX   RELIGION, SURVEY, EAST, MIDWEST, SOUTH, WEST, SOUTHWEST, SEX COMPARISON, ADULTS, ATTITUDES, CULTURAL FACTORS, COMMUNITY INVOLVEMENT, DEMOGRAPHIC, SES, MALE, FEMALE, ECONOMIC FACTORS, MEXICAN AMERICAN, PUERTO RICAN-M, CUBAN, EMPIRICAL, RESOURCE UTILIZATION, BOOK

ABST   THE RESULTS OF A NATIONWIDE (13 STATES) TELEPHONE SURVEY OF 1,003 HISPANICS CONCERNING THE ROMAN CATHOLIC CHURCH ARE PRESENTED. THE STUDY FOCUSED ON ADULT HISPANICS' ATTITUDES REGARDING: (1) THE BASIC IMPORTANCE OF RELIGION; (2) THE ROLE OF THE CATHOLIC CHURCH WITH RESPECT TO PERSONAL, FAMILY, AND COMMUNITY PROBLEMS; (3) RELIGIOUS PRACTICES, CHURCH ATTENDANCE, AND INVOLVEMENT IN CHURCH ACTIVITIES; (4) THE PERCEIVED DEGREE OF HISPANIC REPRESENTATION IN THE CLERGY; (5) NAME AWARENESS AND READER-

SHIP OF CATHOLIC PUBLICATIONS; (6) PROT-
ESTANTS AND EVANGELICALS; AND (7) HAVING
ONE'S CHILDREN ENTER THE CLERGY. IN GEN-
ERAL, IT WAS FOUND THAT ALTHOUGH RELI-
GION IS IMPORTANT TO 90% OF HISPANICS
AND OVER HALF DESCRIBE THEMSELVES AS
"GOOD" CATHOLICS, A LARGE PERCENTAGE
DO NOT OUTWARDLY PRACTICE THEIR RELI-
GION. AMONG THOSE WHO DO, RELIGION IS
MOST IMPORTANT TO WOMEN, THE ELDERLY,
AND THOSE IN LOWER SES LEVELS. THE MA-
JORITY SEE THE CHURCH AS A PLACE OF WOR-
SHIP, BUT NOT AS A SOURCE OF HELP FOR
FAMILY OR COMMUNITY PROBLEMS. MORE-
OVER, 90% DO NOT DO ANY KIND OF WORK
FOR THE CHURCH. OVERALL, HISPANICS WANT
MORE RECOGNITION FROM THE CATHOLIC
CHURCH, MORE HISPANIC REPRESENTATION
IN THE CLERGY, AND MORE EVIDENCE OF HIS-
PANIC CULTURE AND TRADITIONS IN CHURCH
SERVICES. WITH REGARD TO THE VOLUME IT-
SELF, THE TEXT IS DIVIDED INTO A BRIEF OV-
ERVIEW OF RESULTS AND A 95-PAGE SUM-
MARY OF THE FINDINGS. THE CAREFULLY
DETAILED APPENDICES INCLUDE: (1) THE
COMPOSITION OF THE SAMPLE; (2) THE DE-
SIGN OF THE SAMPLE; (3) SAMPLE TOLER-
ANCES; (4) THE SURVEY QUESTIONNAIRE IN
SPANISH AND ENGLISH; AND (5) 133 TABLES
PROVIDING THE STATISTICAL BREAKDOWN BY
SEX, AGE, AND REGION FOR EACH OF THE
QUESTIONNAIRE ITEMS.

ACCN   001784

1370 AUTH   **O'DONNELL, H.**
TITL   CULTURAL BIAS: A MANY-HEADED MONSTER.
SRCE   *ELEMENTARY ENGLISH, 1974, 51(2), 181-184;
214.*
INDX   CULTURAL FACTORS, PREJUDICE, TEST VA-
LIDITY, TEACHERS, ATTITUDES, MEXICAN
AMERICAN, EDUCATION, REVIEW, ESSAY, CUL-
TURAL PLURALISM
ABST   CULTURAL BIAS IN THE CLASSROOM EVI-
DENCED BY ETHNIC STEREOTYPES IN CHIL-
DREN'S BOOKS, THROUGH THE USE OF STAN-
DARDIZED TESTS BASED ON ANGLO MIDDLE
CLASS NORMS, AND THROUGH BIASED
TEACHER ATTITUDES IS EXPLORED IN THIS AR-
TICLE. MOST OF THESE BIASES STEM FROM AN
ANGLICIZED NORM WHICH IS NOT TOLERANT
OR SENSITIVE TO NONMIDDLE CLASS BEHAV-
IOR. THE EFFECT ON VARIOUS ETHNIC MI-
NORITY GROUPS IS DESCRIBED THROUGH
SEVERAL SURVEYS AND STUDIES. CULTURAL
BIAS IN TEACHER ATTITUDES IS CONSIDERED
DETRIMENTAL TO SPANISH-SPEAKING CHIL-
DREN WHO ARE EVALUATED NEGATIVELY BE-
CAUSE THE TEACHER DOES NOT UNDERSTAND
THE LANGUAGE NOR THE CULTURAL BEHAV-
IOR. ALSO, BY STEREOTYPING MEXICAN
AMERICANS, MANY CHILDREN ARE BEING
FORCED TO REJECT THE DOMINANT CULTURE
AS WELL AS THEMSELVES. THE NEED IS SEEN
FOR TEACHERS TO DEVELOP CROSS-CUL-
TURAL UNDERSTANDING, THEREBY BECOM-
ING SENSITIVE TO THEIR OWN AND OTHERS'
VALUES. 9 REFERENCES.
ACCN   001174

1371 AUTH   **O'FLANNERY, E.**
TITL   SOCIAL AND CULTURAL ASSIMILATION.
SRCE   *THE AMERICAN CATHOLIC SOCIOLOGICAL RE-
VIEW, 1961, 22(1), 195-206.*
INDX   ACCULTURATION, PUERTO RICAN-M, MIGRA-
TION, CULTURE, COMMUNITY, RELIGION, ADO-
LESCENTS, FEMALE, CASE STUDY, NEW YORK,
SOUTHWEST
ABST   A FORMULATION OF AN IMMIGRANT ADAPTA-
TION PROCESS WHICH ATTEMPTS TO DIFFER-
ENTIATE BETWEEN SOCIAL AND CULTURAL AS-
SIMILATION   IS   PRESENTED   VIA   BOTH
ANALYTICAL AND EMPIRICAL DATA FROM
PUERTO RICAN MIGRANTS IN NEW YORK CITY.
GENERAL REVIEW OF THE LITERATURE ON
PUERTO RICAN MIGRANTS AND OBSERVA-
TIONS AND INTERVIEWS OF MEMBERS OF A
PARTICULAR CATHOLIC PARISH (INCLUDING 12
FEMALE ADOLESCENTS) SUPPORTS THE AU-
THOR'S CONTENTION THAT SOCIAL AND CUL-
TURAL ASSIMILATION ARE, TO A DEGREE, IN-
DEPENDENT PROCESSES. 24 REFERENCES.
ACCN   001175

1372 AUTH   **O'NELL, C. W.**
TITL   AN INVESTIGATION OF REPORTED FRIGHT AS A
FACTOR IN THE ETIOLOGY OF SUSTO, MAGI-
CAL FRIGHT.
SRCE   *ETHOS, 1975, 3(1), 41-63.*
INDX   CURANDERISMO, FOLK MEDICINE, STRESS,
SYMPTOMATOLOGY,   CULTURAL   FACTORS,
MEXICAN, EMPIRICAL, PSYCHOPATHOLOGY
ABST   SUSTO OR MAGICAL FRIGHT HAS BEEN WIDELY
REPORTED IN HISPANIC AMERICAN CULTURES.
THE FUNCTIONAL IMPORTANCE AND ADAPTA-
TIONAL PROPERTIES OF INDIGENOUS EXPLA-
NATIONS IN FOLK ILLNESS ETIOLOGY MERIT
SERIOUS ATTENTION BY WESTERN MEDICAL
AND SOCIAL SCIENTISTS. USING DATA FROM
24 ACTIVE CASES OF SUSTO OCCURRING OVER
A 12 MONTH PERIOD IN A ZAPATEC COMMU-
NITY IN OAXACA, MEXICO, THIS STUDY DEM-
ONSTRATES THAT THE TWO EXPLANATORY
SYSTEMS, ONE SCIENTIFIC AND THE OTHER IN-
DIGENOUS, CAN SUCCESSFULLY BE USED TO-
GETHER TO MORE COMPLETELY UNDERSTAND
THE ETIOLOGY OF SUSTO. FINDINGS INDICATE:
(1) THAT THERE ARE COGNITIVE ASSOCIA-
TIONS, BUT NOT NECESSARILY FULLY CON-
SCIOUS ONES, BETWEEN ROLE STRESS AND
FRIGHT IN THE SUSTO SYNDROME; (2) THAT
MORE INCIDENTS OF SUSTO ARE REPORTED
WHICH ARE CHARACTERIZED BY NONHUMAN
RATHER THAN HUMAN FRIGHT ELEMENTS; AND
(3) THAT MORE INCIDENTS OF SUSTO ARE RE-
PORTED CHARACTERIZED BY A DELAYED DE-
VELOPMENT OF SYMPTOMS THAN RAPID
SYMPTOM DEVELOPMENT. 21 REFERENCES.
ACCN   001176

1373 AUTH   **O'NELL, C. W.**
TITL   SEVERITY OF FRIGHT AND SEVERITY OF SYMP-
TOMS IN THE SUSTO SYNDROME.
SRCE   *INTERNATIONAL MENTAL HEALTH RESEARCH
NEWSLETTER, 1972, 14(2), 2; 4-5.*
INDX   ADULTS, ATTITUDES, CHILDREN, CULTURAL
FACTORS, DISEASE, EMPIRICAL, FOLK MEDI-

CINE, HEALTH, MENTAL HEALTH, STRESS, MEXICO, MEXICAN

ABST SUSTO IS A FOLK ILLNESS FOUND IN ASSOCIATION WITH MANY HISPANIC-AMERICAN CULTURES. THE BELIEF IS THAT THE SUFFERER HAS LOST HIS SOUL TO A MALEVOLENT SPIRIT AS THE RESULT OF A FRIGHTENING EXPERIENCE. CASE HISTORY DATA FROM PEOPLE WHO HAD SUFFERED SUSTO WERE COLLECTED IN A ZAPOTEC VALLEY COMMUNITY IN OAXACA, MEXICO, IN 1970-71 TO TEST THE FOLLOWING INDIGENOUS EXPLANATION OF SUSTO: THAT THE SEVERITY OF REPORTED SUSTO SYMPTOMS VARIES WITH THE SEVERITY OF THE FRIGHT CAUSALLY ATTRIBUTED TO THE CONDITION. THE SAMPLE CONSISTED OF 12 MALES AND 12 FEMALES RANGING FROM 7 TO 70 YEARS OF AGE. SEVERITY OF FRIGHT SCORES VARIED FROM 1 TO 4. ALL REPORTS OF FRIGHT LEADING TO SUSTO WERE GIVEN A BASE SCORE OF 1. IF THE REPORTED FRIGHT WAS CHARACTERIZED BY ONE OF THREE CONDITIONS (BODILY HARM, EXTRAORDINARY CONDITIONS, PATIENT'S STATEMENT OF HIGH INTENSITY), ONE WAS ADDED TO THE BASE SCORE. THE SEVERITY OF SYMPTOMS WAS MEASURED IN TERMS OF (1) THE NUMBER OF REPORTED SYMPTOMS, (2) LENGTH OF TIME FOR CURE, (3) DURATION OF THE SUSTO EPISODE, AND (4) INDICATORS OF TREATMENT DIFFICULTY. THE RESULTS OF THE LAMBDA B TEST—A NONPARAMETRIC REGRESSION ANALYSIS OF THE INFLUENCE OF X (SEVERITY OF FRIGHT) UPON Y (SEVERITY OF SYMPTOMS)—WERE NEGATIVE, INDICATING THAT THE SEVERITY OF FRIGHT DOES NOT SERVE AS A PREDICTOR OF SEVERITY OF SYMPTOMS. THIS FINDING CONTRADICTS THE INDIGENOUS EXPLANATION OF THE RELATIONSHIP BETWEEN FRIGHT AND SYMPTOMS OF SUSTO.

ACCN 002172

1374 AUTH **O'NELL, C. W., & SELBY, H. A.**

TITL SEX DIFFERENCE IN THE INCIDENCE OF SUSTO IN TWO ZAPOTEC PUEBLOS. AN ANALYSIS OF THE RELATIONSHIPS BETWEEN SEX ROLE EXPECTATIONS AND A FOLK ILLNESS.

SRCE *ETHNOLOGY, 1968, 7(1), 95-105.*

INDX SEX ROLES, STRESS, EMPIRICAL, MEXICAN, FOLK MEDICINE, DREAMS, ROLE EXPECTATIONS, FICTIVE KINSHIP, FAMILY STRUCTURE, FAMILY ROLES, FEMALE, INDIGENOUS POPULATIONS, MENTAL HEALTH, PSYCHOPATHOLOGY

ABST THE HYPOTHESIS THAT THE SEX WHICH EXPERIENCES THE GREATER INTRACULTURAL STRESS IN THE PROCESS OF MEETING SEX ROLE EXPECTATIONS WILL EVIDENCE GREATER SUSCEPTIBILITY TO SUSTO IS EXAMINED. SUBJECTS FROM TWO ZAPOTEC VILLAGES WERE ASKED ABOUT THEIR PERSONAL EXPERIENCES WITH SUSTO. FINDINGS REVEAL THAT OF THE 70 SUBJECTS (HALF OF WHOM WERE FEMALE), WOMEN STAND THE GREATER LIKELIHOOD OF EXPERIENCING ROLE STRESS DUE TO THEIR MORE NARROWLY DEFINED SEX ROLES AND TO THE LACK OF ESCAPE OUTLETS FROM STRESS WITHIN THE CULTURE. IT IS

CONCLUDED THAT SUSTO REPRESENTS AN IMPORTANT SOCIOCULTURALLY SANCTIONED MECHANISM OF ESCAPE AND REHABILITATION FOR PERSONS SUFFERING FROM INTRACULTURALLY INDUCED STRESS RESULTING FROM FAILURE IN SEX ROLE PERFORMANCE. 15 REFERENCES.

ACCN 001177

1375 AUTH **PADILLA, A. M.**

TITL BILINGUAL SCHOOLS: GATEWAYS TO INTEGRATION OR ROADS TO SEPARATION.

SRCE *BILINGUAL REVIEW, 1977, 4(1), 52-68. (REPRINTED AS "OCCASIONAL PAPER NO. 1." LOS ANGELES: UNIVERSITY OF CALIFORNIA, SPANISH SPEAKING MENTAL HEALTH RESEARCH CENTER, 1976.)*

INDX BILINGUAL-BICULTURAL EDUCATION, CHILDREN, CURRICULUM, DISCRIMINATION, EARLY CHILDHOOD EDUCATION, EDUCATION, EQUAL OPPORTUNITY, MEXICAN AMERICAN, ESSAY, BILINGUALISM, REVIEW, CULTURAL FACTORS, CULTURAL PLURALISM

ABST ALTHOUGH BILINGUAL-BICULTURAL SCHOOLING HAS BEEN CRITICIZED FOR NURTURING ETHNIC SEPARATENESS IN THIS COUNTRY, IT CAN PROVIDE ONE OF THE BEST ALTERNATIVE MEANS FOR DIMINISHING SUCH SEPARATION. THIS CONCLUSION IS POSITED AFTER: (1) A REVIEW OF THE HISTORY OF BILINGUAL EDUCATION IN THE U.S. INCLUDING THE BILINGUAL EDUCATION ACT (1965); (2) A DISCUSSION OF THE RATIONALE FOR BILINGUAL SCHOOLING INCLUDING THESE PHILOSOPHIES—CULTURAL ASSIMILATION, CULTURAL PLURALISM, AND CULTURAL SEPARATION; AND (3) A PRESENTATION OF BILINGUAL EDUCATION TYPOLOGIES DEVELOPED FROM THE ABOVE PHILOSOPHIES. ALSO PRESENTED ARE GUIDELINES AND RECOMMENDATIONS FOR MAKING BILINGUAL-BICULTURAL EDUCATION INTO A MEANINGFUL ALTERNATIVE BY WHICH ALL STUDENTS CAN LEARN ABOUT AND EXPERIENCE THE BENEFITS OF A PLURALISTIC SOCIETY. 20 REFERENCES.

ACCN 001178

1376 AUTH **PADILLA, A. M.**

TITL CHILD BILINGUALISM: INSIGHTS TO ISSUES.

SRCE *IN J. L. MARTINEZ, JR. (ED.), CHICANO PSYCHOLOGY. NEW YORK: ACADEMIC PRESS, 1977, PP. 111-126.*

INDX BILINGUALISM, CHILDREN, LANGUAGE ACQUISITION, LANGUAGE LEARNING, REVIEW, LANGUAGE COMPREHENSION, LINGUISTIC COMPETENCE, GRAMMAR, COGNITIVE DEVELOPMENT, INTELLIGENCE TESTING, BILINGUAL-BICULTURAL EDUCATION, ESSAY, LINGUISTICS

ABST CHILD BILINGUALISM HAS NOT RECEIVED ADEQUATE ATTENTION DUE TO (1) WIDESPREAD CONFUSION OVER WHAT CONSTITUTES BILINGUALISM, AND (2) MISCONCEPTIONS ABOUT CHILD BILINGUALISM IN PARTICULAR. THIS REVIEW ANALYZES SOME OF THE SALIENT ISSUES SURROUNDING THE SUBJECT. BILINGUALISM EXISTS AS A CONTINUUM OF ENCODING AND DECODING SKILLS IN

TWO LANGUAGES. LINGUISTIC INTERACTION, OR THE MIXING OF TWO LANGUAGES, IS NOT REFLECTIVE OF A LACK OF FLUENCY BUT IS RATHER A PHENOMENON OBSERVED IN ALL BILINGUAL COMMUNITIES AND AMONG SPEAKERS OF ALL LANGUAGES. RECENT LITERATURE SUGGESTS THAT CHILD BILINGUALISM HAS A POSITIVE AND FACILITORY EFFECT ON COGNITIVE DEVELOPMENT. IT IS ARGUED THAT INSTRUCTION IN TWO LANGUAGES SHOULD BEGIN EARLY FOR BOTH NEUROLOGICAL AND SOCIAL MODELING REASONS. THE ONE PERSON-ONE LANGUAGE STRATEGY IS PROPOSED AS THE BEST POSSIBLE METHOD OF INSTRUCTION. 30 REFERENCES.

ACCN   002173

1377 AUTH **PADILLA, A. M.**
TITL   COMPETENT COMMUNITIES: A CRITICAL ANALYSIS OF THEORIES AND PUBLIC POLICY.
SRCE   *ADDRESS PRESENTED AT THE SIXTH ANNUAL CLINICAL-COMMUNITY WORKSHOP, INSTITUTIONAL RACISM: IMPEDIMENT TO COMMUNITY COMPETENCE, BALTIMORE, NOVEMBER 1976.*
INDX   MENTAL HEALTH PROFESSION, ACCULTURATION, PUERTO RICAN-M, BILINGUALISM, HISTORY, PREJUDICE, DISCRIMINATION, DEVIANCE, POVERTY, PSYCHOPATHOLOGY, COMMUNITY, CRIMINOLOGY, CULTURAL PLURALISM, POLITICAL POWER, ESSAY, MEXICAN AMERICAN
ABST   AN OVERVIEW OF MINORITY GROUPS IN THE UNITED STATES, SOCIAL SCIENCE PARADIGMS, AND THE ROLE OF SOCIAL SCIENCE RESEARCH IN PUBLIC POLICY ARE DISCUSSED AROUND THE ISSUE OF MINORITY COMMUNITIES' COMPETENCE IN THE ORGANIZATION AND CONDUCT OF THEIR AFFAIRS. IT IS BELIEVED THAT THE VARIOUS PEOPLE "OF COLOR" HAVE SURVIVED ADVERSE SOCIAL CONDITIONS BY REMAINING RESILIENT TO ENCOUNTERS WITH THE MAJORITY CULTURE, ALTHOUGH MANY SOCIAL PROBLEMS STILL EXIST. IN THE STUDY OF SOCIAL PROBLEMS OF MINORITY GROUPS, SOCIAL SCIENTISTS ARE SEEN AS ADHERING TO PARTICULAR "PARADIGMS" WHICH OFTEN LEAVE MINORITY COMMUNITIES DIVESTED OF PRIDE AND DIGNITY AND RESTRICT MORE OPEN EXAMINATIONS. FOUR SOCIAL PROBLEM PARADIGMS (SOCIAL PATHOLOGY, SOCIAL DEVIANCE, SOCIAL DISORGANIZATION, AND CULTURAL DEFICIT) ARE DESCRIBED. BECAUSE THE PREPONDERANCE OF RESEARCH, AND THUS SOCIAL POLICY, HAS FOCUSED ON THE WEAKNESSES OF MINORITY PEOPLE, SOCIAL AND EDUCATIONAL PROGRAMS ARE VIEWED AS CONFLICTING WITH THE VALUES AND TRADITIONS OF THESE PEOPLE AS WELL AS ATTEMPTING TO TRANSFORM THEM IN A CARICATURE OF THE MAJORITY GROUP. HOWEVER, MINORITY COMMUNITIES ARE SEEN AS MAINTAINING THEIR COMPETENCE IN THE FACE OF INSTITUTIONAL RACISM AND BIAS IN SOCIAL SCIENCE RESEARCH PARADIGMS AND PUBLIC POLICIES. RECOMMENDATIONS FOR RESEARCH INTO INSTITUTIONAL RACISM AND THE DEVEL-

OPMENT OF A "CULTURAL STRENGTH" MODEL ARE MADE. 26 REFERENCES.

ACCN   001179

1378 AUTH **PADILLA, A. M.**
TITL   LATINOS IN THE UNITED STATES: SOME RESEARCH PRIORITIES.
SRCE   *BOLETIN DE LA SOCIEDAD INTERAMERICANA DE PSICOLOGIA, 1975, NO. 42, 2-6.*
INDX   REVIEW, ESSAY, INTELLIGENCE TESTING, PSYCHOTHERAPY, RESOURCE UTILIZATION, PERSONALITY ASSESSMENT, ACHIEVEMENT TESTING, BILINGUALISM, COGNITIVE DEVELOPMENT, BILINGUAL-BICULTURAL EDUCATION, REPRESENTATION, MENTAL HEALTH PROFESSION, PROFESSIONAL TRAINING
ABST   A BRIEF OVERVIEW OF RESEARCH PRIORITIES REGARDING LATINO PSYCHOLOGY IN THE UNITED STATES IS PRESENTED WITH THE INTENT OF ASSESSING ACCURATELY THE STATE OF KNOWLEDGE CONCERNING MENTAL HEALTH PROBLEMS OF LATINOS, IDENTIFYING PROBLEMS REQUIRING ADDITIONAL RESEARCH ON SOCIAL CHANGE PROGRAMS AND RECOMMENDING AMELIORATIVE PROGRAMS BASED ON EXPERIMENTAL DATA. A REVIEW OF LATINO MENTAL HEALTH STUDIES AND JOURNALS IS INCLUDED WITH EMPHASIS ON UNDERUTILIZATION OF SERVICES, DIAGNOSTIC ASSESSMENT, IQ TESTS, AND BILINGUAL-BICULTURAL EDUCATION OF CHILDREN. RECOMMENDATIONS ARE MADE FOR MORE EXPERIMENTAL INVESTIGATION OF THE COGNITIVE PROCESSING OF BILINGUALS, BETTER EDUCATIONAL PROGRAMS TO MEET CULTURAL DIFFERENCES THROUGH CLASSROOM RESEARCH, AND INCREASED TRAINING OF LATINOS IN THE MENTAL HEALTH PROFESSIONS WHO CAN MAKE SUBSTANTIAL CONTRIBUTIONS BECAUSE OF THEIR SENSE OF THE SOCIOPSYCHOLOGICAL ISSUES OF THEIR COMMUNITY. 18 REFERENCES.

ACCN   001180

1379 AUTH **PADILLA, A. M.**
TITL   MEASURING ETHNICITY AMONG MEXICAN AMERICANS: SOME QUESTIONS FOR CHICANOS IN MENTAL HEALTH.
SRCE   *IN A. M. PADILLA & E. R. PADILLA (EDS.), IMPROVING MENTAL HEALTH AND HUMAN SERVICES FOR HISPANIC COMMUNITIES. WASHINGTON, D.C.: NATIONAL COALITION OF HISPANIC MENTAL HEALTH AND HUMAN SERVICES ORGANIZATIONS (COSSMHO), 1977, PP. 23-34.*
INDX   ETHNIC IDENTITY, ACCULTURATION, CULTURAL FACTORS, MEXICAN AMERICAN, PSYCHOTHERAPY, TEST VALIDITY
ABST   IN ORDER FOR MENTAL HEALTH SPECIALISTS TO DEVELOP THERAPEUTIC TECHNIQUES THAT ARE BICULTURAL IN NATURE AND ACKNOWLEDGE THE MARKED DIVERSITY OF CULTURAL AWARENESS AND ETHNIC IDENTIFICATION THAT EXISTS AMONG CHICANOS, A NEW SCALE IS PROPOSED. THE INTENTION OF THE CULTURAL AWARENESS AND LOYALTY SCALE (CALS) IS TO LOCATE INDIVIDUALS ON A CONTINUUM RANGING FROM HIGH MEXICAN CULTURAL

IDENTITY, AWARENESS AND LOYALTY, TO THE ADOPTION OF HIGH ANGLO AMERICAN IDENTITY ACROSS SIX DIMENSIONS: LANGUAGE FAMILIARITY AND USAGE, CULTURAL HERITAGE, ETHNIC INTERACTION, ETHNIC PRIDE AND IDENTITY, ETHNIC PRIDE AND PERCEIVED DISCRIMINATION, AND GENERAL PROXIMITY TO MEXICO. BY MEANS OF THE CALS, CATEGORIES ARE EXPECTED TO BE DEVELOPED WHICH ALLOW THE SOCIAL SCIENTIST TO ANALYZE THE RANGE OF CULTURAL HETEROGENEITY WITHIN ETHNIC IDENTITY, AND THEREBY ADD GREATER PRECISION TO SOCIAL SCIENCE RESEARCH INVOLVING MEXICAN AMERICANS. IDENTIFICATION WITH MEXICAN VALUES AND NORMS IS CORRELATED WITH EFFECTIVE INTEGRATION OF THE INDIVIDUAL INTO FAMILIAL AND KIN NETWORKS, WHILE LOW IDENTIFICATION IS BELIEVED TO PREDISPOSE THE INDIVIDUAL TO NEED AND USE MENTAL HEALTH SERVICES. FIVE CASE HISTORIES ARE PRESENTED TO ILLUSTRATE HOW MENTAL HEALTH PROFESSIONALS WOULD APPROACH THEM. OVERALL, MENTAL HEALTH WORKERS ARE CALLED UPON TO CONSIDER THE IMPORTANCE OF ETHNIC IDENTIFICATION AND THE DYNAMICS OF DIVERSITY IN THEIR INTERVENTION AND PREVENTION PROGRAMS. 7 REFERENCES.

ACCN   001181

1380 AUTH   **PADILLA, A. M.**
TITL   PSYCHOLOGY AND THE MEXICAN AMERICAN: AN AWARENESS OF CULTURAL AND SOCIAL FACTORS.
SRCE   *IN M. M. MANGOLD (ED.), LA CAUSA CHICANA: THE MOVEMENT FOR JUSTICE. NEW YORK: FAMILY SERVICE ASSOCIATION OF AMERICA, 1972, PP. 65-77. (REPRINTED IN C. A. HERNANDEZ, M. J. HAUG & N. N. WAGNER (EDS.), CHICANOS: SOCIAL AND PSYCHOLOGICAL PERSPECTIVES. ST. LOUIS: C. V. MOSBY CO., 1976, PP. 152-159.)*
INDX   CULTURAL FACTORS, HEALTH DELIVERY SYSTEMS, STEREOTYPES, CHILDREARING PRACTICES, INTELLIGENCE TESTING, BILINGUALISM, NUTRITION, SES, POVERTY, SELF CONCEPT, MENTAL HEALTH, FOLK MEDICINE, PSYCHOTHERAPY
ABST   OBJECTIVES WHICH ARE POSITED INCLUDE: (1) TO SHOW HOW SOME PSYCHOLOGISTS, BECAUSE OF THEIR RIGIDITY IN ADHERING TO THE LABORATORY MODEL AND THEIR ETHNOCENTRISM, HAVE CREATED A SITUATION WHICH IS INTOLERABLE TO TODAY'S MEXICAN AMERICAN (MA); (2) TO SHOW HOW SUCH APPROACHES HAVE RESULTED IN INADEQUATE AND IRRELEVANT PSYCHOLOGICAL SERVICES; AND (3) TO OFFER RECOMMENDATIONS FOR CHANGE. THE APPROACH IS THROUGH AN EXAMINATION OF THE PSYCHOLOGICAL LITERATURE CENTERING ON ISSUES OF FAMILY-CHILD RELATIONSHIPS, BILINGUALISM AND TESTS OF INTELLIGENCE, AND MENTAL ILLNESS AND MENTAL HEALTH PRACTICES AMONG MA'S. PSYCHOLOGISTS HAVE ALLOWED STEREOTYPED CONCEPTIONS OF MA FAMILY-CHILD RELATIONSHIPS TO PERSIST BECAUSE OF THEIR

ACCEPTANCE OF THESE SAME STEREOTYPES AND THEIR FAILURE TO ENGAGE IN MEANINGFUL RESEARCH OF THE MA FAMILY. PSYCHOLOGISTS HAVE ALSO PROGRAMED THE MA INTO A "SELF-FULFILLING PROPHECY" OF FAILURE THROUGH THE USE OF INAPPROPRIATE PSYCHOLOGICAL MEASURING INSTRUMENTS. IN ADDITION, MA'S HAVE BEEN FORCED TO SEEK MENTAL HEALTH CARE IN SETTINGS WHICH HAVE DISCRIMINATED AGAINST THEM AND/OR HAVE BEEN OFFERED SERVICES WHICH ARE IRRELEVANT, BOTH CULTURALLY AND EMOTIONALLY. RECOMMENDATIONS FOR CHANGE CALL FOR INTERDISCIPLINARY AND SENSITIVE INVESTIGATIONS TOWARD THE MA CULTURE. THERE MUST BE MORE CONCERN FOR INDIVIDUAL DIFFERENCES BOTH WITHIN A GROUP AS WELL AS BETWEEN CULTURALLY DIFFERENT PEOPLE. THERE SHOULD BE LESS ARROGANCE ON THE PART OF THE PSYCHOLOGIST BY ENCOURAGING COMMUNITY PARTICIPATION. THERE MUST BE AN INCREASE IN CHICANO PSYCHOLOGISTS AND, FINALLY, MENTAL HEALTH SERVICES SHOULD INCLUDE BILINGUAL AND BICULTURAL SERVICES. 29 REFERENCES.

ACCN   001183

1381 AUTH   **PADILLA, A. M.**
TITL   RESEARCHING THE SPANISH SPEAKING COMMUNITY: ISSUES IN THE HUMAN SERVICE ENTERPRISE.
SRCE   *SSMHRC RESEARCH BULLETIN. LOS ANGELES: UNIVERSITY OF CALIFORNIA, SPANISH SPEAKING MENTAL HEALTH RESEARCH CENTER, 1979, 4(1), 1-4; 8.*
INDX   ESSAY, RESEARCH METHODOLOGY, ADMINISTRATORS, HEALTH DELIVERY SYSTEMS, SOCIAL SERVICES, POLITICAL POWER, PROGRAM EVALUATION, POLICY
ABST   THE RESPONSIBILITY AND ROLE OF RESEARCHERS AND PRACTITIONERS IN THE HEALTH AND HUMAN SERVICE NEEDS OF THE SPANISH-SPEAKING (SS) COMMUNITY ARE DISCUSSED. RESEARCHERS AND PRACTITIONERS ARE SEEN AS NEEDING TO SHARE THE COMMON GOAL OF RATIONAL PROGRAM DEVELOPMENT FOR THE GOOD OF THE HISPANIC POPULATION—THE RESEARCHER OBJECTIVELY INVESTIGATING THE PROBLEM AND THE PRACTITIONER ATTEMPTING TO ALLEVIATE HUMAN SUFFERING. POSITED REALITIES OF RESEARCH ARE THAT: (1) IT TAKES PLACE IN A POLITICAL CONTEXT; (2) IT IS TIME CONSUMING; (3) IT IS NOT AGREED UPON BY POLITICAL DECISION MAKERS; (4) PRACTITIONERS AND HUMAN SERVICE AGENCIES HAVE DIFFERENT GOALS THAN RESEARCHERS; AND (5) IMPROVED HUMAN SERVICES IN SS COMMUNITIES CAN ONLY COME ABOUT THROUGH THE JOINT AND CONCERTED EFFORTS OF RESEARCHERS, PRACTITIONERS, AND COMMUNITY MEMBERS. PARAMETERS NEEDED FOR RESEARCH (DEMOGRAPHIC AND SOCIOCULTURAL DIMENSIONS, GENERAL HEALTH STATUS AND ROLE FUNCTIONING, AND ATTITUDES AND RESPONSE TO ILLNESS AND HEALTH SERVICES) ARE DESCRIBED. RECOMMENDATIONS

ARE THAT INCREASED MONEY BE MADE AVAILABLE, THAT RESEARCH BE BUILT INTO THE HUMAN SERVICE AGENCY AND DECISION-MAKING PROCESS, AND THAT EMPHASIS BE GIVEN TO THE TRAINING OF HEALTH AND HUMAN SERVICE RESEARCHERS. 9 REFERENCES.

ACCN   001184

1382   AUTH   **PADILLA, A. M.**
      TITL   A SET OF CATEGORIES FOR COMBINING PSYCHOLOGY AND HISTORY IN THE STUDY OF CULTURE.
      SRCE   *IN J. W. WILKIE, M. C. MEYER & E. MONZON DE WILKIE (EDS.), CONTEMPORARY MEXICO: PAPERS OF THE IV INTERNATIONAL CONGRESS OF MEXICAN HISTORY. BERKELEY: UNIVERSITY OF CALIFORNIA PRESS, 1976, PP. 581-597.*
      INDX   HISTORY, CULTURE, ESSAY, REVIEW, ACCULTURATION, BILINGUALISM, RESEARCH METHODOLOGY, THEORETICAL, MEXICAN AMERICAN
      ABST   A CONCEPTUAL FRAMEWORK THAT COMBINES PSYCHOLOGY AND HISTORY IN THE STUDY OF THE CHICANO CULTURE IS DESCRIBED AND DISCUSSED. THE FRAMEWORK IS DEVELOPED AROUND CONCEPTS BASIC TO PSYCHOLOGY AND HISTORY: (1) LEVEL OF ANALYSES—OBJECTIVE AND PSYCHOLOGICAL; (2) TIME PERSPECTIVE—HISTORICAL AND CONTEMPORANEOUS; AND (3) EVENT LINKAGE—DETERMINISTIC AND ACCIDENTAL. EIGHT ARRANGEMENTS OF THESE CONCEPTUAL CATEGORIES ARE PROPOSED; ALSO A BRIEF DEMONSTRATION OF HOW EACH COULD BE USED TO ANALYZE SEVERAL EVENTS IN MEXICAN AMERICAN HISTORY OR CHARACTERISTICS OF MEXICAN AMERICAN CULTURE IS PRESENTED. IT IS HOPED THAT THIS CONCEPTUAL FRAMEWORK WILL PROVIDE A FIRST STEP TOWARD AN ANALYSIS OF THE CHICANO BASED ON AN APPRECIATION OF THE PSYCHOLOGICAL AND HISTORICAL PROCESSES SPECIFIC TO A CULTURE WITH ROOTS IN BOTH MEXICO AND THE UNITED STATES. 29 REFERENCES.
      ACCN   001185

1383   AUTH   **PADILLA, A. M.**
      TITL   SPECIAL REPORT TO THE PLANNING BRANCH OF THE NATIONAL INSTITUTE OF MENTAL HEALTH ON THE MENTAL HEALTH NEEDS OF THE SPANISH-SPEAKING IN THE UNITED STATES.
      SRCE   *UNPUBLISHED MANUCRIPT, 1971. (AVAILABLE FROM AMADO PADILLA, SPANISH SPEAKING MENTAL HEALTH RESEARCH CENTER, UNIVERSITY OF CALIFORNIA, LOS ANGELES, 90024.)*
      INDX   SPANISH SURNAMED, MENTAL HEALTH, HEALTH DELIVERY SYSTEMS, PROFESSIONAL TRAINING, ESSAY, EMPIRICAL, FINANCING, POLICY, REPRESENTATION
      ABST   THE EXTENT TO WHICH THE NATIONAL INSTITUTE OF MENTAL HEALTH (NIMH) EXTENDS SUPPORT TO THE SPANISH-SPEAKING (SS) IN THE AREAS OF SERVICE, TRAINING, AND RESEARCH IS ASSESSED. ONE OF THE LARGEST OBSTACLES FOR THE EFFECTIVE PLANNING OF MENTAL HEALTH SERVICES FOR THE SS IS THE ABSENCE OF AN ADEQUATE EPIDEMIOLOGICAL SURVEY ON THE INCIDENCE AND PREVA-

LENCE OF MENTAL DISORDERS OF THE SS. ALTHOUGH 47 COMMUNITY MENTAL HEALTH CENTERS WHICH SERVE THE SS WERE IDENTIFIED, THE EXTENT OF THE SERVICES OFFERED AND THE UTILIZATION OF SUCH SERVICES BY THE SS ARE QUESTIONABLE. SIXTEEN TRAINING PROGRAMS SUPPORTED BY NIMH FOR THE SS ARE IDENTIFIED. THE OVERALL SUPPORT FOR THESE TRAINING CENTERS ACCOUNTS FOR ONLY 1 PERCENT OF THE TOTAL NIMH TRAINING BUDGET. MORE INNOVATIVE RECRUITING AND TRAINING PROGRAMS ARE SUGGESTED FOR RECTIFYING THE UNDERREPRESENTATION OF SS IN THE MENTAL HEALTH DISCIPLINES. AN ANALYSIS OF 43 NIMH RESEARCH GRANTS DURING THE FISCAL YEARS 1965-1971 REVEALS THAT NOT ONE PROJECT WAS ACTION ORIENTED AND DIRECTED AT SPECIFIC PROBLEMS. MANY OF THE RECOMMENDATIONS CONCERNING THE IMPROVEMENT AND EXTENSION OF MENTAL HEALTH SERVICES FOR THE SS WILL DEPEND ON THE EXPANSION OF THE MINORITY STUDIES CENTER FOR NEW MONIES FOR SERVICE, TRAINING, AND RESEARCH PROGRAMS. ELEVEN TABLES DOCUMENTING FINDINGS ARE PROVIDED.

ACCN   001186

1384   AUTH   **PADILLA, A. M., CARLOS, M. L., & KEEFE, S. E.**
      TITL   MENTAL HEALTH SERVICE UTILIZATION BY MEXICAN AMERICANS (FIRST YEAR PROGRESS REPORT GRANT NO. MH26099-01).
      SRCE   *SANTA BARBARA: UNIVERSITY OF CALIFORNIA, SOCIAL PROCESSES RESEARCH INSTITUTE, 1976.*
      INDX   SURVEY, RESOURCE UTILIZATION, DEMOGRAPHIC, MENTAL HEALTH, FAMILY STRUCTURE, EXTENDED FAMILY, FICTIVE KINSHIP, FOLK MEDICINE, CURANDERISMO, PARAPROFESSIONALS, EMPIRICAL, CALIFORNIA, SOUTHWEST
      ABST   IT IS HYPOTHESIZED THAT MEXICAN AMERICANS UNDERUTILIZE MENTAL HEALTH FACILITIES FOR THE FOLLOWING REASONS: (1) DISCOURAGING MENTAL HEALTH FACILITY POLICIES, (2) USAGE OF FOLK MEDICINE, AND (3) DEPENDENCE ON THE EXTENDED FAMILY FOR EMOTIONAL SUPPORT. A SURVEY OF 666 MEXICAN AMERICANS IN 3 SOUTHERN CALIFORNIA TOWNS WAS CONDUCTED TO TEST THESE EXPLANATIONS. BILINGUAL INTERVIEWERS WERE EMPLOYED. DETAILED DESCRIPTIVE STATISTICS DESCRIBE THE SAMPLE IN THE FOLLOWING AREAS: AGE, HOUSEHOLD COMPOSITION, LANGUAGE SPOKEN, GENERATION AND ETHNIC IDENTITY OF THE RESPONDENT, YEARS OF RESIDENCE, AND SOCIOECONOMIC INDICATORS. THE RESULTS INDICATE THAT MEXICAN AMERICANS GENERALLY HAVE FAVORABLE ATTITUDES ABOUT MENTAL HEALTH CARE AND WOULD BE WILLING TO SEEK CARE AT THE LOCAL FACILITIES. SECONDLY, THERE IS LIMITED USE OF CURANDEROS OR FOLK MEDICINE. AND LASTLY, THIS ETHNIC GROUP GENERALLY RELIES UPON EXTENDED FAMILY MEMBERS, AS OPPOSED TO MENTAL HEALTH CLINICS. IT IS ALSO NOTED THAT THE MORE

ACCULTURATED AND SOCIALLY MOBILE MEXI-CAN AMERICANS ARE MOST LIKELY TO RECEIVE ADEQUATE CARE, WHEREAS THOSE WHO LACK FLUENCY IN ENGLISH, ARE POOR AND PROBABLY SUBJECT TO GREATER EMOTIONAL STRESS, ARE FORCED TO GO WITHOUT PROPER MENTAL HEALTH CARE. THE NEEDS OF THIS LATTER GROUP MUST BE RECOGNIZED IN PLANNING SUCCESSFUL MENTAL HEALTH SERVICES FOR THE MEXICAN AMERICAN COMMUNITY. 10 REFERENCES.

ACCN   001187

1385 AUTH   **PADILLA, A. M., CARLOS, M. L., & KEEFE, S. E.**
TITL   MENTAL HEALTH SERVICE UTILIZATION BY MEXICAN AMERICANS.
SRCE   *IN M. R. MIRANDA (ED.), PSYCHOTHERAPY WITH THE SPANISH SPEAKING: ISSUES IN RESEARCH AND SERVICE DELIVERY (MONOGRAPH NO. 3). LOS ANGELES: UNIVERSITY OF CALIFORNIA, SPANISH SPEAKING MENTAL HEALTH RESEARCH CENTER, 1976, PP. 9-20.*
INDX   SURVEY, RESOURCE UTILIZATION, DEMOGRAPHIC, FICTIVE KINSHIP, FAMILY STRUCTURE, RELIGION, IMMIGRATION, ACCULTURATION, SES, EDUCATION, COMMUNITY, COPING MECHANISMS, PHYSICIANS, CURANDERISMO, MENTAL HEALTH PROFESSION, DEVIANCE, PSYCHOPATHOLOGY, ATTITUDES, PSYCHOTHERAPY, EMPIRICAL, CALIFORNIA, SOUTHWEST
ABST   THE HYPOTHESES THAT CULTURAL AND LINGUISTIC BARRIERS, CLASS DISCREPANCIES BETWEEN THE THERAPIST AND CLIENT, AND THE USE OF CURANDEROS OR FOLK MEDICINE BEST EXPLAIN THE UNDERUTILIZATION OF MENTAL HEALTH FACILITIES BY MEXICAN AMERICANS WERE INVESTIGATED. BILINGUAL INTERVIEWERS COLLECTED DATA FROM 666 MEXICAN AMERICAN ADULTS (77% RESPONSE RATE) IN THREE SOUTHERN CALIFORNIA TOWNS. THE RESULTS INDICATE THAT THE RESPONDENTS (1) GENERALLY HAVE POSITIVE ATTITUDES ABOUT MENTAL HEALTH SERVICES, AND (2) DO NOT RELY EXTENSIVELY UPON CURANDEROS. THE MOST SIGNIFICANT REASON FOR THE LOW USE OF MENTAL HEALTH SERVICES IS THE PREFERENCE FOR ALTERNATIVE RESOURCES IN TIMES OF EMOTIONAL STRIFE. THE MEXICAN AMERICAN RESPONDENTS INDICATED THAT DURING THE YEAR BEFORE THE INTERVIEW, THEY SOUGHT EMOTIONAL SUPPORT FROM PRIMARILY EXTENDED FAMILY MEMBERS (36% OF RESPONDENTS), THEN FRIENDS (26%), PHYSICIANS (24%), AND PRIESTS OR MINISTERS (16%). MENTAL HEALTH CLINICS WERE VISITED BY ONLY 2% OF THE RESPONDENTS OVER A TWO YEAR PERIOD. THUS, THE MENTAL HEALTH CLINIC TENDS TO BE THE LAST RESORT FOR MEXICAN AMERICANS WITH EMOTIONAL PROBLEMS AFTER OTHER ALTERNATIVES HAVE PROVEN UNSUCCESSFUL. 7 REFERENCES.

ACCN   001188

1386 AUTH   **PADILLA, A. M., RUIZ, R. A., & ALVAREZ, R.**
TITL   COMMUNITY MENTAL HEALTH SERVICES FOR THE SPANISH-SPEAKING/SURNAMED POPULATION.

SRCE   *AMERICAN PSYCHOLOGIST, 1975, 30(9), 892-905.*
INDX   MENTAL HEALTH, SPANISH SURNAMED, ESSAY, CULTURAL FACTORS, HEALTH DELIVERY SYSTEMS, RESOURCE UTILIZATION, MEXICAN AMERICAN, PUERTO RICAN-M, POLICY, PSYCHOTHERAPY, PSYCHOTHERAPISTS, BILINGUAL-BICULTURAL PERSONNEL, COMMUNITY INVOLVEMENT, PARAPROFESSIONALS, PROFESSIONAL TRAINING
ABST   THE SPANISH-SPEAKING/SURNAMED (SSS) POPULATION RECEIVES PROPORTIONATELY LESS MENTAL HEALTH CARE THAN ANY OTHER U.S. ETHNIC GROUP. YET, BECAUSE THEY ARE ONLY PARTIALLY ACCULTURATED AND MARGINALLY INTEGRATED AND CONSEQUENTLY SUBJECT TO A GREAT DEAL OF STRESS, THEY ACTUALLY NEED AS MUCH OR MORE MENTAL HEALTH CARE. CULTURALLY INAPPROPRIATE AND INFLEXIBLE ORGANIZATIONAL FACTORS AND INSTITUTIONAL POLICIES ARE LARGELY RESPONSIBLE FOR SSS UNDERUTILIZATION OF MENTAL HEALTH FACILITIES. AND SSS SELF-REFERRALS ARE FURTHER MINIMIZED BY THE LANGUAGE BARRIER AND THEIR GEOGRAPHIC ISOLATION FROM MENTAL HEALTH CENTERS. TO RECTIFY THIS PROBLEM, THREE MODELS OFFERING IMPROVED CARE TO THE SSS POPULATION ARE PRESENTED: (1) A PROFESSIONAL ADAPTATION MODEL IN WHICH SPECIALIZED, NONSTANDARD TRAINING ALLOWS STAFF TO ADAPT TO THE SPECIFIC NEEDS OF THE SSS POPULATION; (2) A FAMILY ADAPTATION MODEL IN WHICH THE THERAPIST ASSUMES TRAITS WHICH ARE CHARACTERISTIC OF SSS FAMILY MEMBERS (E.G., A MALE THERAPIST ASSUMES A FATHERLY, DOMINANT ROLE); AND (3) A BARRIO SERVICE CENTER MODEL IN WHICH A COMMUNITY-BASED STAFF INTERVENES ON BEHALF OF THE SSS TO GET JOBS, BANK LOANS, AND OTHER BASIC ECONOMIC SERVICES. EIGHT OTHER RECOMMENDATIONS TO IMPROVE MENTAL HEALTH CARE DELIVERY TO THE SSS ARE ALSO PRESENTED. 39 REFERENCES.

ACCN   001190

1387 AUTH   **PADILLA, A. M., SAUNDERS, F., LINDHOLM, K., LIEBMAN, E., MEDINA, S., PEREGOY-FAULT, S., RIVAS, H., & DAVIS-WELSH, J.**
TITL   THE STUDY OF BILINGUAL LANGUAGE ACQUISITION.
SRCE   *UNPUBLISHED MANUSCRIPT, 1974. (AVAILABLE FROM THE NATIONAL SCIENCE FOUNDATION, GRANT NO. GY11534.)*
INDX   BILINGUALISM, LANGUAGE ACQUISITION, CHILDREN, MEXICAN AMERICAN, EMPIRICAL, LANGUAGE LEARNING, LINGUISTICS, CALIFORNIA, SOUTHWEST
ABST   THE LINGUISTIC DEVELOPMENT OF ENGLISH AND SPANISH AMONG 19 BILINGUAL MEXICAN AMERICAN CHILDREN FROM 2 TO 7 YEARS OF AGE IS THE FOCUS OF THIS CROSS-SECTIONALLY DESIGNED STUDY. A LANGUAGE SAMPLE, ONE IN ENGLISH AND IN SPANISH, WAS OBTAINED FROM THE CHILDREN BASED ON THEIR TAPED INTERACTION WITH THE EXPERIMENTERS. DATA ANALYSIS DEALT WITH PRIMARY

AND SECONDARY CATEGORIZATIONS OF UT-TERANCES, MIXED UTTERANCES, PARTS OF SPEECH, AND OVER-REGULARIZATIONS. THE FINDINGS REVEAL THAT MOST CHILDREN FROM MONOLINGUAL SPANISH-SPEAKING HOMES BEGIN LEARNING ENGLISH BETWEEN THE AGES OF 3 AND 5 YEARS, AND CANNOT BE DISTIN-GUISHED FROM CHILDREN SPEAKING TWO LANGUAGES ALL THEIR LIVES. HOWEVER, SPANISH IS THEIR PREFERRED LANGUAGE. CHILDREN FROM BILINGUAL HOMES HAVE BOTH LANGUAGES MAINTAINED AND LEARNED SIMULTANEOUSLY, WITH ENGLISH BEING THE DOMINANT LANGUAGE. BILINGUAL CHILDREN DEVELOP FROM A STAGE OF PRE-LINGUISTIC TO LINGUISTIC DIFFERENTIATION, WITH IN-CREASED PROFICIENCY AND AWARENESS OF BILINGUALISM. SUGGESTIONS ARE MADE FOR FURTHER RESEARCH USING A LONGITUDINAL DESIGN, REANALYZING SEMANTIC DEVELOP-MENT IN BILINGUAL CHILDREN, AND OBSERV-ING BILINGUAL CHILDREN IN VERBAL INTER-ACTION WITH PEERS, SIBLINGS, AND SIGNIFICANT OTHERS IN THEIR LANGUAGE COMMUNITY. 19 REFERENCES.

ACCN   001191

1388 AUTH   **PADILLA, A. M., WAGNER-GOUGH, J., AMARO-PLOTKIN, H., & AMODEO, L. B.**

TITL   PRESCHOOL BILINGUAL/BICULTURAL EDUCA-TION FOR SPANISH-SPEAKING/SURNAMED CHILDREN: A RESEARCH REVIEW AND STRATEGY PAPER.

SRCE   *IN BILINGUAL-BICULTURAL EARLY CHILDHOOD DEVELOPMENT RESEARCH WORKSHOP PRO-CEEDINGS. U.S. DEPARTMENT OF HEALTH, EDUCATION, AND WELFARE, OFFICE OF HU-MAN DEVELOPMENT AND OFFICE OF CHILD DEVELOPMENT, FEBRUARY 1976.*

INDX   BILINGUAL-BICULTURAL EDUCATION, MEXI-CAN AMERICAN, CHILDREN, LANGUAGE AC-QUISITION, LANGUAGE LEARNING, EARLY CHILDHOOD EDUCATION, REVIEW, PROGRAM EVALUATION, POLICY

ABST   THIS STATE-OF-THE-ART REVIEW AND RE-SEARCH STRATEGY PAPER IDENTIFIES ISSUES AND MAKES RECOMMENDATIONS TO THE OF-FICE OF CHILD DEVELOPMENT (OCD) REGARD-ING THE IMPROVEMENT OF BILINGUAL-BICUL-TURAL EDUCATION FOR THE 3 TO 5 YEAR-OLD SPANISH-SPEAKING/SURNAMED (SSS) CHILD. PRESENTED ARE AN HISTORICAL OVERVIEW OF THE DEVELOPMENT OF BILINGUAL-BICUL-TURAL EDUCATION, ALONG WITH PARENTAL AND COMMUNITY ATTITUDES, SOCIALIZATION PRACTICES AMONG SSS PARENTS, CURRENT RESEARCH IN LANGUAGE ACQUISITION AND BILINGUALISM, AND MAJOR ISSUES FOR PRE-SCHOOL BILINGUAL-BICULTURAL EDUCATION SPECIALISTS. A TOTAL OF 43 RECOMMENDA-TIONS URGE THE OCD TO DEMONSTRATE ITS COMMITMENT TO PRESCHOOL BILINGUAL-BI-CULTURAL EDUCATION BY ADEQUATELY FUND-ING PROGRAMMATIC DEVELOPMENT AND RE-SEARCH ACTIVITIES. 103 REFERENCES.

ACCN   001192

1389 AUTH   **PADILLA, A. M., & ARANDA, P.**

TITL   LATINO MENTAL HEALTH: BIBLIOGRAPHY AND ABSTRACTS (DHEW PUBLICATION NO. (HSM) 73-9144).

SRCE   *WASHINGTON, D.C.: U.S. GOVERNMENT PRINT-ING OFFICE, 1974.*

INDX   MENTAL HEALTH, SPANISH SURNAMED, BIBLI-OGRAPHY, MEXICAN AMERICAN, PUERTO RI-CAN-M, EDUCATION, HEALTH, BILINGUALISM, CHILDREN, ADULTS, ADOLESCENTS, HEALTH DELIVERY SYSTEMS, PUERTO RICAN-I

ABST   A BIBLIOGRAPHY WITH ABSTRACTS OF 497 REFERENCES ON THE PSYCHOLOGICAL AND MENTAL HEALTH LITERATURE OF THE LATINO COMMUNITY OF THE UNITED STATES IS PRO-VIDED. THE LATINO COMMUNITY IS CONSID-ERED TO BE ALL GROUPS IDENTIFYING THEM-SELVES AS SPANISH-SPEAKING, SPANISH SURNAMED OR OF SPANISH ORIGIN. DUE TO THE LIMITED LITERATURE, HOWEVER, THE BIB-LIOGRAPHY IS PRIMARILY COMPRISED OF RE-SEARCH ON MEXICAN AMERICANS AND, TO A LESSER EXTENT, PUERTO RICANS. REFER-ENCES WERE OBTAINED FROM A VARIETY OF SOURCES, OF WHICH THE MAJORITY WERE FROM ANTHROPOLOGICAL, PSYCHOLOGICAL, PSYCHIATRIC, SOCIOLOGICAL AND SOCIAL WORK JOURNALS. THIS WORK IS INTENDED TO INCREASE THE ACCESSIBILITY TO MENTAL HEALTH PRACTITIONERS, RESEARCHERS, AND STUDENTS OF ALL THE LITERATURE WHICH BEARS ON THE MENTAL HEALTH, DIRECTLY OR INDIRECTLY, OF THE LATINO PEOPLE. (AUTHOR SUMMARY MODIFIED)

ACCN   001193

1390 AUTH   **PADILLA, A. M., & GARZA, B. M.**

TITL   IQ TESTS: A CASE OF CULTURAL MYOPIA.

SRCE   *NATIONAL ELEMENTARY PRINCIPAL, 1975, 54(4), 53-58. (REPRINTED IN P. L. HOUTS (ED.), THE MYTH OF MEASURABILITY. NEW YORK: HART PUBLISHING CO., 1977, PP. 124-136.*

INDX   INTELLIGENCE, INTELLIGENCE TESTING, SPAN-ISH SURNAMED, ESSAY, EDUCATIONAL AS-SESSMENT, CULTURE-FAIR TESTS, TEST VA-LIDITY, CULTURAL FACTORS, CHILDREN, BILINGUALISM, WISC, STANFORD-BINET INTEL-LIGENCE TEST, PROGRAM EVALUATION, EDU-CATION

ABST   SINCE IQ TESTING OF SPANISH-SURNAMED CHILDREN FREQUENTLY RESULTS IN MISLA-BELING AND MISTAKEN DIAGNOSES, THESE TESTS ARE IN PART RESPONSIBLE FOR THE LARGE NUMBER OF THESE CHILDREN IN CLASSES FOR SLOW LEARNERS AND THE HIGH RATE OF HIGH SCHOOL DROPOUTS. THIS DIS-CUSSION EXAMINES THE ALTERNATIVES OF CULTURE-FREE TESTS, TRANSLATED TESTS, NO TESTING AT ALL, AND CULTURE SENSITIVE TESTS. CULTURE-FREE TESTS ARE REJECTED BECAUSE NO TEST CAN BE DIVORCED FROM THE CULTURAL CONTEXT IN WHICH THE EX-AMINEE IS EXPECTED TO PERFORM. TRANS-LATED TESTS ARE ALSO INADEQUATE BE-CAUSE THEY FAIL TO DEAL WITH THE SUBTLETIES AND COLLOQUIALISMS OF LAN-GUAGE AND HAVE NEVER BEEN STANDARD-IZED ON SPANISH-SPEAKING CHILDREN IN THE U.S. THE THIRD ALTERNATIVE—NO TESTING AT

ALL—LEAVES SCHOOL PERSONNEL WITH THE PROBLEM OF ASSESSING ACADEMIC PROGRESS. THE AUTHOR THEREFORE RECOMMENDS THE FOURTH ALTERNATIVE OF CULTURALLY SENSITIVE TESTING—A PROGRAM WHICH INCLUDES: (A) THE ASSESSMENT OF NON-COGNITIVE CHARACTERISTICS; (B) GREATER COOPERATION BETWEEN PSYCHOMETRICIAN, SCHOOL PERSONNEL, AND PARENTS IN PLANNING THE EDUCATIONAL PROGRAM; AND (C) THE EMPLOYMENT OF BILINGUAL-BICULTURAL PSYCHOMETRICIANS. IN VIEW OF THE UNLIKELIHOOD THAT MANY SCHOOL DISTRICTS WOULD BE WILLING TO ADOPT SUCH PROGRAMS, THE AUTHOR ADVOCATES A MORATORIUM ON IQ TESTING OF SPANISH-SURNAMED AND OTHER MINORITY GROUP CHILDREN UNTIL CULTURALLY SENSITIVE TESTING CAN BE IMPLEMENTED. 10 REFERENCES.

ACCN   001194

1391 AUTH   **PADILLA, A. M., & LEIBMAN, E.**
TITL   LANGUAGE ACQUISITION IN THE BILINGUAL CHILD.
SRCE   *THE BILINGUAL REVIEW/LA REVISTA BILINGUE, 1975, 2, 34-55.*
INDX   BILINGUALISM, CHILDREN, LANGUAGE ACQUISITION, MEXICAN AMERICAN, EMPIRICAL, CASE STUDY, LINGUISTIC COMPETENCE, CALIFORNIA, SOUTHWEST
ABST   TO GAIN AN INSIGHT INTO THE PROCESS INVOLVED IN BILINGUALISM, THREE MEXICAN AMERICAN CHILDREN WHO WERE SIMULTANEOUSLY ACQUIRING SPANISH AND ENGLISH WERE OBSERVED FOR 3 TO 6 MONTHS. THE SUBJECTS WERE FIRST-BORN, ONLY CHILDREN (TWO BOYS AND ONE GIRL, AGES 1 AND 2) LIVING IN SANTA BARBARA, CALIFORNIA. THEY WERE VISITED ON THE AVERAGE OF ONCE A WEEK FOR ONE HOUR, AND THE SESSIONS WERE TAPE RECORDED AND LATER TRANSCRIBED. THE MEAN LENGTH OF UTTERANCE WAS USED AS THE INDEX OF LANGUAGE ACQUISITION SINCE IT INCREASES WITH AGE AND WITH THE DEVELOPMENT OF COMPLEX GRAMMATICAL STRUCTURES. THE DATA WERE COMPARED TO MONOLINGUAL AND BILINGUAL ACQUISITION STUDIES. DATA ANALYSIS REVEALED THAT THESE THREE SUBJECTS ACQUIRED THE TWO LANGUAGES AT A RATE COMPARABLE TO THAT OF ENGLISH- AND SPANISH-SPEAKING MONOLINGUAL CHILDREN, AND THEY DEMONSTRATED THE USE OF INDEPENDENT SETS OF RULES FOR EACH LANGUAGE. IN LIGHT OF THESE FINDINGS, IT SEEMS FALLACIOUS TO SUGGEST THAT GRAMMATICAL STRUCTURES APPEAR IN ONE LANGUAGE EARLIER THAN IN A SECOND BECAUSE THE LANGUAGES DIFFER IN LINGUISTIC COMPLEXITY. IT IS THEREFORE RECOMMENDED THAT TO OBTAIN A BETTER UNDERSTANNDING OF LINGUISTIC DIFFERENTIATION, MORE DESCRIPTIVE STUDIES OF MIXED (ENGLISH AND SPANISH) UTTERANCES SHOULD BE UNDERTAKEN. 30 REFERENCES.

ACCN   001195

1392 AUTH   **PADILLA, A. M., & LINDHOLM, K. J.**
TITL   ACQUISITION OF BILINGUALISM: A DESCRIPTIVE ANALYSIS OF THE LINGUISTIC STRUCTURES OF SPANISH/ENGLISH SPEAKING CHILDREN.
SRCE   *IN G. D. KELLER, R. V. TESCHNER, & S. VIERA (EDS,), BILINGUALISM IN THE BICENTENNIAL AND BEYOND. NEW YORK: BILINGUAL PRESS, 1976, PP. 97-142.*
INDX   BILINGUAL, BILINGUAL-BICULTURAL EDUCATION, BILINGUALISM, CHILDREN, COGNITIVE DEVELOPMENT, EDUCATION, EMPIRICAL, LANGUAGE ACQUISITION, LANGUAGE LEARNING, LINGUISTICS, MEXICAN AMERICAN
ABST   THIS STUDY ASKS: (1) DO CHILDREN LEARNING TWO LANGUAGES DEVELOP PARALLEL GRAMMATICAL STRUCTURES OR ARE SOME STRUCTURES ACQUIRED IN ONE LANGUAGE AND LATER TRANSFERRED TO THE SECOND?; AND (2) DOES INTERFERENCE FROM ONE LANGUAGE TO ANOTHER HAVE HARMFUL EFFECTS ON HOW CHILDREN LEARN A LANGUAGE? SUBJECTS WERE 19 BILINGUAL SECOND GENERATION MEXICAN AMERICAN CHILDREN, AGES 2 TO 6 (11 MALES, 8 FEMALES). FOUR PAIRS OF FEMALE EXPERIMENTERS OBTAINED, VIA RECORDED AND WRITTEN HOME INTERVIEWS, REPRESENTATIVE SAMPLES OF EACH CHILD'S SPONTANEOUS UTTERANCES BOTH IN SPANISH AND IN ENGLISH. THREE GRAMMATICAL STRUCTURES WERE ANALYZED: INTERROGATIVES, ADVERBS, AND ADJECTIVES. ANALYSIS OF THE INTERROGATIVES REVEALED THAT CHILDREN SEEM TO LEARN THE STRUCTURES SEPARATELY. FURTHER, ADVERB AND ADJECTIVE STRUCTURES WERE FOUND TO BE ACQUIRED AT APPROXIMATELY THE SAME AGES IN SPANISH AND ENGLISH—SUGGESTING THAT THESE CHILDREN LEARNED THEIR LANGUAGES SEPARATELY AND DID NOT TRANSFER THE STRUCTURES OF ONE LANGUAGE TO THE OTHER. THE ONLY CASE WHERE INTERFERENCE FROM ONE LANGUAGE TO THE OTHER CAN BE SUGGESTED IS IN THE USE OF DOUBLE NEGATIVES IN THE ENGLISH SPEECH OF THE BILINGUAL CHILDREN. HOWEVER, SINCE ENGLISH MONOLINGUAL CHILDREN ALSO PASS THROUGH A STAGE WHERE DOUBLE NEGATION OCCURS, IT IS CONCLUDED THAT LITTLE, IF ANY, INTERFERENCE WAS APPARENT IN THE SPEECH OF THE 19 BILINGUAL CHILDREN. 18 REFERENCES.

ACCN   001196

1393 AUTH   **PADILLA, A. M., & LINDHOLM, K. J.**
TITL   DEVELOPMENT OF INTERROGATIVE, NEGATIVE AND POSSESSIVE FORMS IN THE SPEECH OF YOUNG SPANISH/ENGLISH BILINGUALS.
SRCE   *THE BILINGUAL REVIEW/LA REVISTA BILINGUE, 1976, 3(2), 122-152.*
INDX   BILINGUALISM, CHILDREN, LANGUAGE ACQUISITION, GRAMMAR, EMPIRICAL, LINGUISTICS, MEXICAN AMERICAN
ABST   SPONTANEOUS LANGUAGE SAMPLES WERE OBTAINED FROM 19 SPANISH/ENGLISH BILINGUAL CHILDREN RANGING FROM 2 YEARS OF AGE TO 6 YEARS, 4 MONTHS OF AGE. THE SPEECH OF THE CHILDREN WAS ANALYZED

FOR THE DEVELOPMENT OF INTERROGATIVE, NEGATIVE, AND POSSESSIVE FORMS IN EACH LANGUAGE. A DEVELOPMENTAL STAGE ANALYSIS WAS USED TO COMPARE AND CONTRAST THE RATE OF DEVELOPMENT OF EACH OF THE GRAMMATICAL STRUCTURES. IT WAS FOUND THAT THE CHILDREN ATTAINED THE ADULT MODEL FOR INTERROGATIVES AT DIFFERENT TIMES (I.E., TWO STAGES IN SPANISH VERSUS THREE STAGES IN ENGLISH). THIS DIFFERENCE WAS NOT OBSERVED IN THE ACQUISITION OF EITHER THE NEGATIVE (THREE STAGES) OR THE POSSESSIVE (TWO STAGES) FORMS. THE RESULTS ARE DISCUSSED IN TERMS OF THE OFTEN-CLAIMED DELETERIOUS EFFECTS OF CHILD BILINGUALISM. 16 REFERENCES. (JOURNAL ABSTRACT)

ACCN   001197

1394 AUTH   **PADILLA, A. M., & PADILLA, E. R. (EDS.)**
TITL   IMPROVING MENTAL HEALTH AND HUMAN SERVICES FOR HISPANIC COMMUNITIES: SELECTED PRESENTATIONS FROM REGIONAL CONFERENCES.
SRCE   *WASHINGTON, D.C.: NATIONAL COALITION OF HISPANIC MENTAL HEALTH AND HUMAN SERVICES ORGANIZATIONS (COSSMHO), 1977.*
INDX   MENTAL HEALTH, HEALTH DELIVERY SYSTEMS, MEXICAN AMERICAN, ETHNIC IDENTITY, ALCOHOLISM, PUERTO RICAN-M, ACCULTURATION, MENTAL HEALTH PROFESSION, PRIMARY PREVENTION, POVERTY, SES, LEGISLATION, DRUG ABUSE, DRUG ADDICTION, GERONTOLOGY, DELINQUENCY, PROFESSIONAL TRAINING, PROCEEDINGS, BOOK
ABST   THE NATIONAL COALITION OF HISPANIC MENTAL HEALTH AND HUMAN SERVICES ORGANIZATIONS (COSSMHO) HAS SPONSORED SEVERAL CONFERENCES OVER THE PAST THREE YEARS (1974-1976) RELATED TO THE PLANNING AND DELIVERY OF MENTAL HEALTH SERVICES TO HISPANIC COMMUNITIES. IN ORDER TO DISSEMINATE THE INFORMATION AND IDEAS GATHERED AT TWO OF THESE REGIONAL FORUMS, SEVERAL PAPERS AND REPORTS PRESENTED AT THE CONFERENCES IN LOS ANGELES AND SAN ANTONIO IN 1975 HAVE BEEN GATHERED IN THIS BOOK. SUBJECT AREAS INCLUDED ARE: (1) ALCOHOLISM AMONG CHICANOS; (2) PREVENTIVE MENTAL HEALTH STRATEGIES FOR THE LOW INCOME SPANISH-SPEAKING; (3) A MENTAL HEALTH RESEARCH PROGRAM FOR THE SPANISH-SPEAKING; (4) ASPECTS OF THE LEGISLATIVE PROCESS RELEVANT TO BETTER SERVICES DELIVERY; (5) MAKING PSYCHIATRY MEANINGFUL: IMPLICATIONS FOR CHICANOS; AND (6) WORKSHOP SUMMARIES ON BARRIO MENTAL HEALTH, DRUG ABUSE, DELINQUENCY PREVENTION AND SPANISH-SPEAKING ELDERLY. BECAUSE THESE CONFERENCES HAVE BROUGHT TOGETHER NOT ONLY COSSMHO'S MEMBER ORGANIZATIONS BUT ALSO REPRESENTATIVES FROM GOVERNMENT AGENCIES, RESEARCHERS, EDUCATORS, STUDENTS, SERVICE PROVIDERS AND CONSUMERS, THE OUTCOMES ARE RECOGNIZED AS THE FRAMEWORK FOR DETERMINING NATIONAL POLICY CONCERNING THE

MENTAL HEALTH NEEDS AND INTERESTS OF THE HISPANIC PEOPLE THROUGHOUT THE UNITED STATES.

ACCN   001198

1395 AUTH   **PADILLA, A. M., & ROMERO, A.**
TITL   VERBAL FACILITATION OF CLASS-INCLUSION REASONING: CHILDREN TESTED IN THEIR DOMINANT OR SUBORDINATE LANGUAGE.
SRCE   *PERCEPTUAL AND MOTOR SKILLS, 1976, 42, 727-733.*
INDX   BILINGUALISM, CHILDREN, COGNITIVE DEVELOPMENT, EMPIRICAL, MEXICAN AMERICAN, CALIFORNIA, SOUTHWEST
ABST   TWO EXPLANATIONS FOR VERBAL FACILITATION OF CLASS-INCLUSION REASONING (I.E., THE CONSTRUCTION OF HIERARCHICAL CLASSIFICATION) WERE INVESTIGATED IN A STUDY OF 44 MALE AND 44 FEMALE LOS ANGELES SCHOOL DISTRICT, MEXICAN AMERICAN CHILDREN CATEGORIZED AS ENGLISH OR SPANISH-LANGUAGE DOMINANT. ONE THEORY ATTRIBUTES VERBAL FACILITATION TO DIFFERENCES IN THE INTERPRETATION OF LINGUISTIC CUES (WINER), WHILE THE OTHER ATTRIBUTES VERBAL FACILITATION TO DISTRACTING PERCEPTUAL CUES (WOHLWILL). IT WAS HYPOTHESIZED THAT IF THE INTERPRETATION OF DISTRACTING PERCEPTUAL CUES WAS ACCURATE, THEN CHILDREN PERFORMING IN EITHER THEIR DOMINANT OR SUBORDINATE LANGUAGE WOULD FIND THE PICTORIAL FORMAT MORE DIFFICULT THAN THE VERBAL FORMAT. IF THE LINGUISTIC ENCODING HYPOTHESIS WERE CORRECT, HOWEVER, ONLY CHILDREN PERFORMING IN THEIR DOMINANT LANGUAGE SHOULD PERFORM BETTER ON THE VERBAL FORMAT. THE STUDY DESIGN WAS A FOUR-WAY FACTORIAL, WITH THE FOUR FACTORS BEING GRADE (THIRD AND FIFTH), LANGUAGE DOMINANCE (ENGLISH AND SPANISH), TEST LANGUAGE (ENGLISH AND SPANISH), AND TEST FORMAT (VERBAL AND PICTORIAL). HALF THE CHILDREN WERE TESTED IN THEIR DOMINANT LANGUAGE, THE OTHER HALF IN THEIR SUBORDINATE LANGUAGE. RESULTS DEMONSTRATE THAT CLASS-INCLUSION PROBLEMS PRESENTED IN A PURELY VERBAL FORMAT ARE LESS DIFFICULT THAN PICTORIAL ITEMS, REGARDLESS OF TEST LANGUAGE. THUS, FINDINGS SUPPORT THE HYPOTHESIS THAT VERBAL FACILITATION IS DUE TO ABSENCE OF DISTRACTING PERCEPTUAL CUES. 5 REFERENCES.

ACCN   001199

1396 AUTH   **PADILLA, A. M., & RUIZ, R. A.**
TITL   LATINO MENTAL HEALTH: A REVIEW OF LITERATURE (DHEW PUBLICATION NO. (HSM) 73-9143).
SRCE   *WASHINGTON, D.C.: U.S. GOVERNMENT PRINTING OFFICE, 1973.*
INDX   SPANISH SURNAMED, MENTAL HEALTH, REVIEW, DEMOGRAPHIC, POVERTY, HEALTH DELIVERY SYSTEMS, FAMILY STRUCTURE, SEX ROLES, INTELLIGENCE TESTING, PERSONALITY ASSESSMENT, EDUCATION, SCHOLASTIC ACHIEVEMENT, PREJUDICE, DISCRIMINATION, COOPERATION, COMPETITION, BILINGUALISM,

PUERTO RICAN-M, MEXICAN AMERICAN, EMPIRICAL, PUERTO RICAN-I, RESOURCE UTILIZATION, PSYCHOTHERAPY

ABST A REVIEW OF THE MENTAL HEALTH LITERATURE THROUGH 1972 PERTAINING TO THE SPANISH-SPEAKING/SPANISH SURNAMED (SSSS) POPULATION IS PRESENTED. THE PURPOSE OF THIS REVIEW IS THREEFOLD: (1) TO ACCURATELY ASSESS THE KNOWLEDGE BASE CONCERNING MENTAL HEALTH PROBLEMS OF THE SSSS; (2) TO IDENTIFY PROBLEMS REQUIRING ADDITIONAL RESEARCH OR SOCIAL CHANGE PROGRAMS; AND (3) TO RECOMMEND AMELIORATIVE PROGRAMS BASED ON EXPERIMENTAL DATA RATHER THAN SUBJECTIVE IMPRESSION OR SPECULATION. AREAS OF INTEREST INCLUDED IN THIS REVIEW ARE THE DELIVERY OF MENTAL HEALTH SERVICES TO SSSS COMMUNITIES, THE IDENTIFICATION OF COPING BEHAVIORS CHARACTERISTIC OF THIS ETHNIC GROUP, PERSONALITY AND TEST ASSESSMENT, THE SCHOOL PERFORMANCE OF HISPANIC CHILDREN, THE EFFECTS OF PREJUDICE AND DISCRIMINATION, COOPERATIVE AND COMPETITIVE BEHAVIORS AMONG CHILDREN, AND THE SOCIAL AND PSYCHOLOGICAL IMPLICATIONS OF BILINGUALISM. IT IS CONCLUDED THAT NOT ONLY IS THERE A SEVERE PAUCITY OF MENTAL HEALTH RESEARCH ON THE SSSS, BUT WHAT RESEARCH LITERATURE IS AVAILABLE IS OFTEN OF QUESTIONABLE VALIDITY (E.G., POOR RESEARCH METHODOLOGY). FURTHERMORE, THERE IS ALMOST NO RESEARCH ON OTHER HISPANIC GROUPS BESIDES MEXICAN AMERICANS AND PUERTO RICANS. PROGRAMMATIC, LONGITUDINAL AND WELL CONTROLLED RESEARCH ARE RECOMMENDED. (AUTHOR SUMMARY MODIFIED)

ACCN 001200

1397 AUTH **PADILLA, A. M., & RUIZ, R. A.**
TITL PERSONALITY ASSESSMENT AND TEST INTERPRETATION OF MEXICAN AMERICANS: A CRITIQUE.
SRCE *JOURNAL OF PERSONALITY ASSESSMENT, 1975, 38, 103-109. (REPRINTED IN R. ALVAREZ (ED.), DELIVERY OF SERVICES FOR LATINO COMMUNITY MENTAL HEALTH (MONOGRAPH NO. 2). LOS ANGELES: UNIVERSITY OF CALIFORNIA, SPANISH SPEAKING MENTAL HEALTH RESEARCH CENTER, 1975, PP. 39-48.)*
INDX PERSONALITY ASSESSMENT, RESEARCH METHODOLOGY, PROJECTIVE TESTING, RORSCHACH TEST, TAT, CPI, MMPI, ESSAY, REVIEW, TEST VALIDITY, EXAMINER EFFECTS
ABST THE LITERATURE ON PERSONALITY TEST ASSESSMENT OF MEXICAN AMERICANS IS REVIEWED. ALTHOUGH THERE IS A PAUCITY OF AVAILABLE RESEARCH, THERE ARE SOME INDICATIONS THAT MEXICAN AMERICANS DIFFER IN RESPONSE PATTERNING ON PROJECTIVE DEVICES. ON OBJECTIVE INSTRUMENTS, PROBLEMS INVOLVING FLUENCY IN ENGLISH OBSCURE THE FINDINGS. SEVERAL RECOMMENDATIONS ARE OFFERED FOR INCREASING THE EFFICIENCY OF THESE INSTRUMENTS FOR USE WITH MEXICAN AMERICAN CLIENTS. THE NEED FOR NORMATIVE STUDIES OF PERSON-

ALITY ASSESSMENT INSTRUMENTS FOR MEXICAN AMERICAN SUBJECTS IS EMPHASIZED, AND THE INFLUENCE OF EXAMINER CHARACTERISTICS ON TEST PERFORMANCES OF MEXICAN AMERICANS MUST BE ASSESSED. 19 REFERENCES. (NCMHI ABSTRACT)

ACCN 001201

1398 AUTH **PADILLA, A. M., & RUIZ, R. A.**
TITL PREJUDICE AND DISCRIMINATION.
SRCE *IN C. A. HERNANDEZ, M. J. HAUG & N. N. WAGNER (EDS.), CHICANOS: SOCIAL AND PSYCHOLOGICAL PERSPECTIVES. ST. LOUIS: C. V. MOSBY CO., 1976, PP. 110-119.*
INDX PREJUDICE, DISCRIMINATION, REVIEW, STEREOTYPES, MEXICAN AMERICAN, EDUCATION, HISTORY, PUERTO RICAN-M, SELF CONCEPT, SCHOLASTIC ACHIEVEMENT, ETHNIC IDENTITY
ABST A REVIEW OF THE RESEARCH ON PREJUDICE AND DISCRIMINATION TOWARDS THE SPANISH-SPEAKING/SPANISH SURNAMED (SSSS) POPULATION IS PRESENTED. PREJUDICE ATTRIBUTED TO ANGLO FEELINGS OF SUPERIORITY WHICH CAUSE THEM TO BE INTOLERANT OF INDIVIDUALS WHO DO NOT SHARE ANGLO WAYS, THUS MAKING SSSS SEEM "INFERIOR." THIS ASCRIBED ROLE CAUSES ETHNIC INSULATION AND FEELINGS OF LOW SELF-ESTEEM TO OCCUR IN SSSS PERSONS AS WELL AS OVERALL ECONOMIC, JUDICIAL, AND EDUCATIONAL DISCRIMINATION. RECOMMENDATIONS ARE MADE FOR THE ENFORCEMENT OF NONDISCRIMINATORY LEGISLATION, CULTURALLY SENSITIVE EDUCATION, AND MORE RESEARCH ON THE EFFECTS OF DISCRIMINATION ON SSSS PERSONALITY DEVELOPMENT. SEVERAL STUDIES ARE CITED DEALING WITH THE DEVELOPMENT OF RACIAL DISCRIMINATION AND RACIAL PREFERENCE AMONG CHILDREN, CULTURAL STEREOTYPES AMONG PROFESSIONALS, AND LOW SELF-IMAGE AMONG SSSS INDIVIDUALS. 27 REFERENCES.

ACCN 001203

1399 AUTH **PADILLA, E.**
TITL UP FROM PUERTO RICO.
SRCE *NEW YORK: COLUMBIA UNIVERSITY PRESS, 1958.*
INDX PUERTO RICAN-M, URBAN, MIGRATION, RESEARCH METHODOLOGY, SOCIAL SERVICES, ETHNIC IDENTITY, SES, POVERTY, ACCULTURATION, CULTURAL CHANGE, HOUSING, HISTORY, FAMILY ROLES, FAMILY STRUCTURE, STRESS, PSYCHOSOCIAL ADJUSTMENT, BILINGUALISM, SCHOLASTIC ACHIEVEMENT, INTERPERSONAL RELATIONS, PEER GROUP, SOCIALIZATION, HEALTH, MENTAL HEALTH, NEW YORK, EAST, EMPIRICAL, BOOK
ABST THE SOCIAL ADAPTATION OF PUERTO RICANS TO THE AMERICAN SLUM LIFE IS EXAMINED IN THIS ANTHROPOLOGICAL STUDY OF A NEW YORK CITY SLUM NAMED EASTVILLE. PARTICIPANT OBSERVATIONS, INFORMAL INTERVIEWS AND OPEN-ENDED QUESTIONNAIRES WERE USED TO COLLECT DATA ON THE COMMUNITY RESIDENTS, BOTH PUERTO RICAN AND NON-PUERTO RICAN. AN "IRRECONCILABLE DUAL-

ITY" CHARACTERIZES THIS ETHNIC GROUP IN EASTVILLE. BECAUSE OF SIMILAR CIRCUMSTANCES THERE ARE BONDS OF SOLIDARITY AND LOYALTY AMONG THE GROUP; HOWEVER, THERE IS A TENDENCY TO SEPARATE AND FRAGMENT THEMSELVES DUE TO DISLIKE, REJECTION AND INTOLERANCE. GREAT INTRA-ETHNIC VARIABILITY CONTRIBUTES TO THIS SOCIAL DISSENSION AMONG PUERTO RICANS. OTHER AREAS OF THE EASTVILLE PUERTO RICAN COMMUNITY EXAMINED IN THIS BOOK ARE: (1) THE DEVELOPMENT OF THE CHILD FROM INFANCY ON; (2) THE SOCIAL FUNCTION OF VARIOUS GROUPS AND ORGANIZATIONS; (3) THE RELATIONSHIP WITH AMERICAN INSTITUTIONS (E.G., SOCIAL AGENCIES, EMPLOYERS, POLITICS, AND THE CHURCH); AND (4) ATTITUDES TOWARD HEALTH, DISEASE AND MEDICINE. TO CONCLUDE, THE ADVANTAGES AND DISADVANTAGES OF THE PUERTO RICAN WAY OF LIFE ON THE MAINLAND AND ISLAND ARE CONTRASTED.

ACCN   001204

1400 AUTH   **PADILLA, E. R.**
TITL   CONSULTATION TO THE OBSTETRICAL SERVICE: THE SPANISH-SPEAKING PATIENT.
SRCE   *PAPER PRESENTED AT THE 84TH ANNUAL CONVENTION OF THE AMERICAN PSYCHOLOGICAL ASSOCIATION, WASHINGTON, D.C., SEPTEMBER 1976.*
INDX   HEALTH DELIVERY SYSTEMS, FEMALE, MOTHER-CHILD INTERACTION, PROFESSIONAL TRAINING, BILINGUAL-BICULTURAL PERSONNEL, SPANISH SURNAMED, NURSING, INSTRUCTIONAL TECHNIQUES, HEALTH EDUCATION
ABST   THE JUDGMENTS OF AN OBSTETRICS-NEONATAL STAFF WERE ASSESSED REGARDING THEIR PERCEIVED EFFECTIVENESS IN PROVIDING SERVICES TO ENGLISH- AND SPANISH-SPEAKING PATIENTS. NURSES AND CLINICAL SPECIALISTS UTILIZED A 53-ITEM CHECKLIST RATING THEIR EFFECTIVENESS IN TEACHING PATIENTS ABOUT AREAS SUCH AS BREAST/BOTTLE FEEDING, WARD OPERATING PROCEDURES, AND NORMAL DISCOMFORTS AND BODY CHANGES. THE MEAN TEACHING EFFECTIVENESS RATINGS WERE CONSISTENTLY MUCH LOWER FOR SPANISH-SPEAKING THAN ENGLISH-SPEAKING PATIENTS. (NO STATISTICAL TESTS WERE USED.) ALTHOUGH OTHER DATA ARE IN THE PROCESS OF BEING COLLECTED AND/OR ANALYZED, THE DATA THUS FAR ANALYZED HAVE CONVINCED THE HOSPITAL STAFF OF THE NECESSITY TO BEGIN DEVELOPING AN EDUCATIONAL VIDEOTAPE PROGRAM TO IMPROVE THE STAFF'S TEACHING EFFECTIVENESS. THIS FUTURE PROGRAM WILL CONTAIN VIDEOTAPED TEACHING GUIDES REGARDING INFANT AND MATERNAL CARE TO BE BROADCASTED IN SPANISH AND ENGLISH TO THE PATIENTS' ROOMS. IT IS ARGUED THAT SUCH AN EDUCATIONAL PROGRAM WOULD BE AN IMPORTANT ADDITION TO PRIMARY AND PREVENTATIVE HEALTH CARE OF OBSTETRICS-NEONATAL PATIENTS.
ACCN   001205

1401 AUTH   **PADILLA, E. R.**
TITL   HISPANICS IN CLINICAL PSYCHOLOGY: 1970-1976.
SRCE   *IN E. L. OLMEDO & S. LOPEZ (EDS.), HISPANIC MENTAL HEALTH PROFESSIONALS (MONOGRAPH NO. 5). LOS ANGELES: UNIVERSITY OF CALIFORNIA, SPANISH SPEAKING MENTAL HEALTH RESEARCH CENTER, 1977, PP. 43-57.*
INDX   MENTAL HEALTH PROFESSION, REPRESENTATION, PROFESSIONAL TRAINING, HIGHER EDUCATION, EMPIRICAL, SURVEY, PERSONNEL, SOCIAL SCIENCES
ABST   THIS 1976 SURVEY EXAMINES MINORITY REPRESENTATION IN DOCTORAL PROGRAMS OF CLINICAL PSYCHOLOGY. THE RESULTS ARE COMPARED WITH TWO PREVIOUS SURVEYS TO EXAMINE THE TREND OVER A SIX YEAR PERIOD WITHIN STUDENT AND FACULTY RANKS. DATA ARE PROVIDED FOR THE MAJOR ETHNIC GROUPS INCLUDING CHICANOS, CUBANS AND PUERTO RICANS. QUESTIONNAIRES WERE MAILED TO 128 DIRECTORS OF CLINICAL TRAINING OF WHICH 77% REPLIED. THE RESULTS INDICATE THAT THERE HAS BEEN AN INCREASE IN THE NUMBER OF HISPANIC FACULTY (4 IN 1970 TO 10 IN 1976), ALTHOUGH THESE FIGURES COMPRISE CONSIDERABLY LESS THAN 1% OF THE TOTAL CLINICAL PSYCHOLOGY FACULTY. HISPANIC STUDENTS, ON THE OTHER HAND, HAVE INCREASED MUCH MORE IN ABSOLUTE NUMBERS, FROM 25 IN 1970 TO 130 IN 1976. HOWEVER, THE PERCENTAGE OF FIRST YEAR HISPANIC AND OTHER MINORITY STUDENTS HAS DECREASED FROM 1972. THESE RESULTS SUGGEST THAT MINORITY REPRESENTATION MAY STABILIZE AT THE FOLLOWING APPROXIMATE RATES: 7% FOR BLACKS AND 1%-1.5% FOR HISPANICS. IN LIGHT OF THIS UNDERREPRESENTATION, RECOMMENDATIONS ARE PROVIDED TO INCREASE THE PERCENTAGE OF HISPANICS AND OTHER MINORITY GROUP MEMBERS IN DOCTORAL PROGRAMS OF CLINICAL PSYCHOLOGY. 5 REFERENCES.
ACCN   001206

1402 AUTH   **PADILLA, E. R.**
TITL   THE RELATIONSHIP BETWEEN PSYCHOLOGY AND CHICANOS: FAILURES AND POSSIBILITIES.
SRCE   *IN C. A. HERNANDEZ, M. J. HAUG & N. N. WAGNER (EDS.), CHICANOS: SOCIAL AND PSYCHOLOGICAL PERSPECTIVES. SAINT LOUIS: C. V. MOSBY COMPANY, 1976, PP. 282-290.*
INDX   MEXICAN AMERICAN, ESSAY, CULTURAL FACTORS, MENTAL HEALTH, MENTAL HEALTH PROFESSION, PROFESSIONAL TRAINING, ECONOMIC FACTORS, RESOURCE UTILIZATION, REPRESENTATION, SOCIAL SCIENCES
ABST   AN EXAMINATION OF THE RELATIONSHIP BETWEEN PSYCHOLOGY AND THE CHICANO IS PRESENTED, ALONG WITH A CRITICAL REVIEW OF THE PSYCHOLOGY TRAINING PROGRAMS WHICH DEAL WITH A NARROW STRATUM OF SOCIETY AND EXCLUDE MOST MINORITY INDIVIDUALS. THE LACK OF A STRONG CHICANO ORGANIZATION AT THE PROFESSIONAL AND GRADUATE LEVEL LIMITS THE POTENTIAL IMPACT FOR CHANGE WITHIN THE AMERICAN

PSYCHOLOGICAL ASSOCIATION. THE TRAINING PROGRAMS OFTEN EMPHASIZE THE CREATION OF RESEARCHERS AND TEACHERS RATHER THAN PROFESSIONAL PRACTITIONERS. THEREFORE, FINANCING AND STAFFING MORE MENTAL HEALTH CENTERS WITH MORE PROFESSIONALS IN POVERTY AREAS ARE PROBLEMMATICAL. UNLESS PSYCHOLOGY AND MENTAL HEALTH PROFESSIONS CREATE THEIR OWN INSTITUTIONAL STRUCTURE FOR DEVELOPING METHODS FOR THE DELIVERY OF SERVICES AND ACTIVELY SEEK ALTERNATIVES TO THE DISEASE MODEL FOR MENTAL DISORDER, THE PROFESSIONAL MANPOWER SHORTAGE WILL CONTINUE TO GROW. ONLY WHEN THE DISEASE MODEL IS DISCONTINUED WILL THE RELATIONSHIP BETWEEN PSYCHOLOGY AS A PROFESSION AND CHICANOS IMPROVE. IT IS SUGGESTED THAT PSYCHOLOGISTS CONSIDER THE IDEAS OF ALBEE AND OTHERS TO MAKE PSYCHOLOGY SOCIALLY RELEVANT. 45 REFERENCES.

ACCN   001207

1403 AUTH   **PADILLA, E. R., BOXLEY, R., & WAGNER, N. N.**
TITL   THE DESEGREGATION OF CLINICAL PSYCHOLOGY TRAINING.
SRCE   *PROFESSIONAL PSYCHOLOGY, 1973, 4, 259-264.*
INDX   REPRESENTATION, PROFESSIONAL TRAINING, MENTAL HEALTH PROFESSION, EQUAL OPPORTUNITY, MEXICAN AMERICAN, SURVEY, EMPIRICAL, SOCIAL SCIENCES
ABST   DATA ARE PRESENTED ON MINORITY REPRESENTATION OF DOCTORAL PROGRAMS OF CLINICAL PSYCHOLOGY. IMPROVEMENT IN MINORITY REPRESENTATION OF BOTH FACULTY MEMBERS AND STUDENTS IS MEASURED THROUGH THE COMPARISON OF THIS SURVEY WITH A SIMILAR 1970 SURVEY. QUESTIONNAIRES WERE MAILED TO 114 DIRECTORS OF CLINICAL TRAINING OF WHICH OVER 80% REPLIED. BLACK, CHICANO, FILIPINO, AND PUERTO RICAN FACULTY MEMBERS WERE THE GROUPS MOST UNDERREPRESENTED, WITH THE PERCENTAGES OF 2.40%, .08%, 0%, AND .08%, RESPECTIVELY. EACH OF THESE FIGURES WERE STATISTICALLY SIGNIFICANT IN COMPARISON WITH EACH ETHNIC GROUP'S RESPECTIVE PERCENTAGES WITHIN THE UNITED STATES POPULATION. MINORITY STUDENTS ALSO CONTINUE TO BE SEVERELY UNDERREPRESENTED, DESPITE SIGNIFICANT INCREASES DURING THE LAST TWO YEARS. BLACKS (5.04%), CHICANOS (.82%), FILIPINOS (.02%), AND PUERTO RICANS (.76%) ARE AGAIN THE GROUPS MOST UNDERREPRESENTED. IN 1972, HOWEVER, THERE WAS A SIGNIFICANTLY GREATER PERCENTAGE OF BLACKS, CHICANOS, JAPANESE, AND PUERTO RICANS ADMITTED THAN THE PERCENTAGE OF ADVANCED MINORITY STUDENTS. ALTHOUGH THE 1972 ADMISSION RATE HAD INCREASED, EVEN GREATER RATES OF MINORITY ADMISSIONS ARE NECESSARY FOR MORE EQUAL REPRESENTATION. DATA ARE ALSO REPORTED REGARDING SPECIAL ADMISSION PROCEDURES, FINANCIAL SUPPORT, AND RELEVANT COURSES AND CLINICAL PLACEMENTS FOR MINORITIES.

IN SHORT, THERE (1) HAS BEEN NO SIGNIFICANT CHANGE IN THE NUMBER OF MINORITY FACULTY, AND (2) THE CHANGES OF MINORITY REPRESENTATION AMONG GRADUATE STUDENTS HAVE BEEN FAVORABLE, ALTHOUGH STILL GREATER EFFORTS ARE NEEDED. 4 REFERENCES.

ACCN   001208

1404 AUTH   **PADILLA, E. R., PADILLA, A. M., RAMIREZ, R., MORALES, A., & OLMEDO, E. L.**
TITL   INHALANT, MARIJUANA AND ALCOHOL ABUSE AMONG BARRIO CHILDREN AND ADOLESCENTS.
SRCE   *INTERNATIONAL JOURNAL OF THE ADDICTIONS, 1979, 14, 943-964. (REPRINTED AS "OCCASIONAL PAPER NO. 4." LOS ANGELES: UNIVERSITY OF CALIFORNIA, SPANISH SPEAKING MENTAL HEALTH RESEARCH CENTER, 1977.)*
INDX   ALCOHOLISM, DRUG ABUSE, CHILDREN, ADOLESCENTS, MEXICAN AMERICAN, INHALANT ABUSE, EMPIRICAL, CALIFORNIA, SOUTHWEST, URBAN
ABST   PREVALENCE OF INHALANT, MARIJUANA AND ALCOHOL ABUSE WAS STUDIED IN A SAMPLE OF 457 MALE AND FEMALE MEXICAN AMERICAN CHILDREN AND ADOLESCENTS BETWEEN THE AGE OF 9 AND 17 YEARS. SUBJECTS INTERVIEWED RESIDED IN FOUR HOUSING PROJECTS LOCATED IN EAST LOS ANGELES. ALL INTERVIEWS WERE CONDUCTED BY ADOLESCENTS WHO RESIDED IN THE SAME HOUSING PROJECTS. RESULTS INDICATED THAT COMPARED TO A NATIONAL SAMPLE, MEXICAN AMERICAN ADOLESCENTS WERE AT LEAST 14 TIMES MORE LIKELY TO BE CURRENTLY ABUSING INHALANTS. THE PREVALENCE RATE OF MARIJUANA WAS DOUBLE THE NATIONAL RATE, BUT THE PREVALENCE OF ALCOHOL WAS EQUAL TO THAT FOUND NATIONALLY. REASONS FOR ELEVATED SUBSTANCE ABUSE RATES ARE DISCUSSED. 21 REFERENCES. (AUTHOR ABSTRACT)

ACCN   001209

1405 AUTH   **PADILLA, E. R., & PADILLA, A. M. (EDS.)**
TITL   TRANSCULTURAL PSYCHIATRY: AN HISPANIC PERSPECTIVE (MONOGRAPH NO. 4).
SRCE   *LOS ANGELES: UNIVERSITY OF CALIFORNIA, SPANISH SPEAKING MENTAL HEALTH RESEARCH CENTER, 1977.*
INDX   MENTAL HEALTH PROFESSION, PREJUDICE, ESSAY, BOOK, REVIEW, HEALTH DELIVERY SYSTEMS, MENTAL HEALTH, ADMINISTRATORS, COMMUNITY, MEXICAN AMERICAN, PUERTO RICAN-M, PARAPROFESSIONALS, CORRECTIONS, CHILD ABUSE, CHILDREN, PSYCHOTHERAPY, EMPIRICAL, PUERTO RICAN-I, PROCEEDINGS, HEALTH
ABST   THIS MONOGRAPH DEVELOPED OUT OF A JOINT MEETING OF THE SECTION OF PSYCHIATRY, NEUROLOGY, AND NEUROSURGERY OF THE PUERTO RICAN MEDICAL ASSOCIATION AND THE CARIBBEAN AND AMERICAN PSYCHIATRIC ASSOCIATION HELD IN SAN JUAN, PUERTO RICO, IN 1976. THE PURPOSE WAS TO

EVALUATE PARTICULAR SERVICES RENDERED TO THE FOREIGN-BORN AND CULTURALLY DIFFERENT POPULATIONS IN THE UNITED STATES AND TO DETERMINE WHETHER THEY ARE RECEIVING THEIR SHARE OF HEALTH CARE. BECAUSE CONTRIBUTORS REPRESENT VARIOUS COUNTRIES AND DISTINCT REGIONS WITHIN COUNTRIES, AS WELL AS MANY DISCIPLINES, THERE IS CONSIDERABLE EMPIRICAL, CLINICAL AND COMMUNITY-BASED MATERIAL ON AN ASSORTMENT OF MULTIETHNIC VIEWS ABOUT MENTAL HEALTH SERVICES TO THE HISPANIC POPULATION OF AMERICA. TOPICS WITHIN THE COLLECTION OF 18 ARTICLES INCLUDE PSYCHODYNAMICS OF PREJUDICE, EVALUATION OF MENTAL HEALTH CENTERS AND PSYCHIATRIC SERVICES FOR HISPANICS, PHARMACOTHERAPY, CHILD ABUSE, THE CRIMINAL JUSTICE SYSTEM, AND SPIRITISM. THE OBJECTIVE IS TO SENSITIZE POLICY MAKERS AND PROFESSIONALS TO THE MENTAL HEALTH SERVICE NEEDS OF THE HISPANIC POPULATION.

ACCN   001210

1406 AUTH   **PADILLA, E. R., & RONA, E.**
TITL   LA PSICOLOGIA COMO INSTRUMENTO DEL ESTADO. (PSYCHOLOGY AS AN INSTRUMENT OF THE STATE.)
SRCE   *IN D. R. MACIEL (ED.), LA OTRA CARA DE MEXICO: EL PUEBLO CHICANO. MEXICO: EDICIONES EL CABALLITO, 1977, PP. 192-223. (SPANISH)*
INDX   ESSAY, ABILITY TESTING, CULTURE-FAIR TESTS, DISCRIMINATION, INTELLIGENCE TESTING, HISTORY, EDUCATION, EQUAL OPPORTUNITY, MEXICAN AMERICAN, TEST VALIDITY, PERFORMANCE EXPECTATIONS, CHILDREN, EDUCATIONAL ASSESSMENT, CULTURAL PLURALISM
ABST   THE EFFECTS OF INTELLIGENCE AND ABILITY TESTS UPON EDUCATIONAL AND OCCUPATIONAL ADVANCEMENT ARE DISCUSSED IN RELATION TO THE POOR SOCIAL POSITION OF MEXICAN AMERICANS IN THE U.S. THE HISTORY OF INTELLIGENCE TESTS IN THE U.S., BEGINNING IN 1905, REVEALS THAT SUCH EXAMS HAVE TRADITIONALLY BEEN FORMULATED BY AND DIRECTED TOWARDS MEMBERS OF THE DOMINANT LANGUAGE AND CULTURE. IN FACT THE MAJORITY OF EXAMS, FUNDED BY CORPORATE ORGANIZATIONS, HAVE TENDED TO PROTECT THE INTERESTS OF THESE SPONSORING COMPANIES. AS A RESULT, LINGUISTIC AND CULTURAL MINORITIES (E.G., BLACKS, INDIANS, AND MEXICAN AMERICANS) HAVE NOT PERFORMED WELL ON THESE TESTS; AND AS THESE CHILDREN HAVE BEEN INFORMED ABOUT THEIR LOW APTITUDES, THEY HAVE ENDED UP ASSUMING A SELF-CONCEPT AND ROLE IN ACCORDANCE WITH THESE LOW EXPECTATIONS. SUCH PROBLEMS HAVE PERSISTED IN SPITE OF STUDIES REFUTING BIOLOGICAL EXPLANATIONS OF INTELLIGENCE. IN CONCLUSION, IT IS RECOMMENDED EITHER THAT CULTURE-FAIR TESTS BE CREATED (E.G., COMPARING MINORITY STUDENTS ONLY WITH ETHNIC PEERS) OR ELSE THAT A MORATORIUM

BE DECLARED ON THE USE OF INTELLIGENCE TESTS WITH SUCH STUDENTS. 52 REFERENCES.
ACCN   002175

1407 AUTH   **PAINE, H. J.**
TITL   ATTITUDES AND PATTERNS OF ALCOHOL USE AMONG MEXICAN AMERICANS.
SRCE   *JOURNAL OF STUDIES ON ALCOHOL, 1977, 38(3), 544-553.*
INDX   ALCOHOLISM, ATTITUDES, COMMUNITY, CROSS GENERATIONAL, CULTURAL FACTORS, EMPIRICAL, EXTENDED FAMILY, FAMILY ROLES, FAMILY STRUCTURE, FICTIVE KINSHIP, HEALTH DELIVERY SYSTEMS, MENTAL HEALTH, MEXICAN AMERICAN, SOCIAL SERVICES, SPANISH SURNAMED, URBAN, SOUTHWEST, TEXAS, SURVEY
ABST   THE DRINKING PATTERNS AND ATTITUDES OF MEXICAN AMERICANS ARE DESCRIBED IN THE CONTEXT OF DEVELOPING ALCOHOLISM TREATMENT PROGRAMS WHICH CONSIDER THE UNIQUE ASPECTS OF MEXICAN AMERICAN CULTURE. THE SURVEY INSTRUMENT, ADMINISTERED IN BOTH SPANISH AND ENGLISH, WAS DESIGNED TO RECORD THE BELIEFS, ATTITUDES, AND DRINKING HABITS OF A MEXICAN AMERICAN COMMUNITY IN HOUSTON, TEXAS. THE COMMUNITY IS A WORKING-CLASS AREA OF 67 BLOCKS AND 6,912 PEOPLE IN 1910 HOUSING UNITS. THE POPULATION IS 75% MEXICAN AMERICAN. THE RESULTS OF THE SURVEY ARE PRESENTED IN 5 SECTIONS: COMMUNITY PROFILE; DRINKING PATTERNS; PERCEPTIONS REGARDING ALCOHOL USE AS PROBLEMATIC; ATTITUDES REGARDING ALCOHOL USE; AND PREFERENCES IN UTILIZING RESOURCES. WITHIN THIS GROUP, ALCOHOL USE IS BOTH CULTURALLY INTEGRATED AND SOCIALLY PROBLEMATIC. SUGGESTIONS ARE MADE FOR INCORPORATING BICULTURAL DIMENSIONS IN SERVICE DELIVERY. 6 REFERENCES. (NCAI ABSTRACT)
ACCN   002176

1408 AUTH   **PALLONE, N. J., & HURLEY, R. B., & RICKARD, F. S.**
TITL   FURTHER DATA ON KEY INFLUENCERS OF OCCUPATIONAL EXPECTATIONS AMONG MINORITY YOUTH.
SRCE   *JOURNAL OF COUNSELING PSYCHOLOGY, 1973, 20(5), 484-486.*
INDX   ADOLESCENTS, EMPLOYMENT, FEMALE, SES, CROSS CULTURAL, PUERTO RICAN-M, EMPIRICAL, URBAN, OCCUPATIONAL ASPIRATIONS, VOCATIONAL COUNSELING, EAST
ABST   KEY INFLUENCES ON EXPECTED ADULT OCCUPATION SELECTION WERE EXAMINED IN A SAMPLE OF 73 PUERTO RICAN, 211 BLACK AND 200 ANGLO HIGH SCHOOL FEMALES FROM WORKING CLASS FAMILIES IN A MAJOR CITY. NINE KEY FIGURES INCLUDE IMMEDIATE FAMILY, PEERS, TEACHERS, COUNSELORS AND PEOPLE WITHIN THE SAME OCCUPATION. RANK-ORDER COEFFICIENTS REVEALED THE LEAST SIMILARITY IN CITATION OF KEY FIGURES BETWEEN ANGLO AND PUERTO RICAN SUBJECTS AND VIRTUALLY NO DIFFERENCE BETWEEN BLACK AND PUERTO RICAN OR BLACK AND ANGLO

SUBJECTS. ALL SUBJECTS RANKED THEIR MOTHERS AS FIRST, WITH FATHERS OR NEIGHBORS LAST AS KEY FIGURES. SCHOOL COUNSELORS RANKED WITH CONSIDERABLY GREATER FREQUENCY AMONG BLACK AND PUERTO RICANS, BUT NOT FOR ANGLOS FROM THE SAME SOCIAL CLASS. 4 REFERENCES. (AUTHOR ABSTRACT MODIFIED)

ACCN   001211

1409 AUTH   **PALMER, M. B.**
TITL   EFFECTS OF CATEGORIZATION, DEGREE OF BILINGUALISM, AND LANGUAGE UPON RECALL OF SELECTED MONOLINGUALS AND BILINGUALS.
SRCE   *JOURNAL OF EDUCATIONAL PSYCHOLOGY, 1972, 63(2), 160-164.*
INDX   BILINGUALISM, EMPIRICAL, MEMORY, SES, BILINGUAL-BICULTURAL EDUCATION, LANGUAGE COMPREHENSION, BILINGUAL, SOUTHWEST
ABST   A FREE-RECALL PROCEDURE, UTILIZING CATEGORIZED AND NONCATEGORIZED WORD LISTS IN ENGLISH, SPANISH, AND A MIXED CONDITION, WAS USED WITH THREE GROUPS OF SPANISH-ENGLISH BILINGUALS AND A MONOLINGUAL ENGLISH GROUP. THE AMOUNT OF RECALL ACROSS ALL LISTS WAS GREATER FOR A CATEGORIZED THAN FOR A NONCATEGORIZED CONDITION. THE PREFERRED LANGUAGE OF RECALL AND CLUSTERING WAS ENGLISH, REGARDLESS OF THE GROUP'S DEGREE OF BILINGUALISM. THE POORER PERFORMANCE IN SPANISH WAS INTERPRETED AS A STATE OF PERCEPTUAL UNREADINESS, WHICH WAS SHOWN TO CREATE "INTERFERENCE" FOR THE SUBJECTS WHEN THEY WERE PRESENTED WITH A TASK REQUIRING SIMULTANEOUS SWITCHING BETWEEN ENGLISH AND SPANISH. IT IS SHOWN THAT THE RELATIVE DEGREE OF BILINGUALISM DOES NOT SIGNIFICANTLY AFFECT RECALL. IN ADDITION, THE AMOUNT OF RECALL AND THE EXTENT OF CATEGORY CLUSTERING CAN BE USED AS A REFLECTION OF LINGUISTIC INDEPENDENCE. THESE RESULTS SUGGEST THAT CHILDREN BE PLACED IN A BILINGUAL PROGRAM TO ENABLE THEM TO USE THEIR "STRONGER" LANGUAGE TO FACILITATE THE LEARNING OF THEIR "WEAKER" LANGUAGE—IN THIS INSTANCE, BEGINNING WITH THE SPANISH LANGUAGE AND LEADING TO THE MASTERY OF THE ENGLISH LANGUAGE. 15 REFERENCES.
ACCN   001212

1410 AUTH   **PALMER, M., & GAFFNEY, P. D.**
TITL   EFFECTS OF ADMINISTRATION OF THE WISC IN SPANISH AND ENGLISH AND RELATIONSHIP OF SOCIAL CLASS TO PERFORMANCE.
SRCE   *PSYCHOLOGY IN THE SCHOOLS, 1972, 9(1), 61-64.*
INDX   ESCALA DE INTELIGENCIA WECHSLER, WISC, BILINGUALISM, MEXICAN AMERICAN, CHILDREN, SES, EMPIRICAL, ENVIRONMENTAL FACTORS, ARIZONA, SOUTHWEST
ABST   THE EFFECTS OF BILINGUALISM AND THE FAMILY'S SOCIAL POSITION UPON THE PERFORMANCE OF MEXICAN AMERICAN CHIL-

DREN ON THE WISC WERE ASSESSED. ONE HUNDRED FIFTY CHILDREN WERE GIVEN THE WISC IN ENGLISH, AND 30 FROM THE INITIAL 150 WERE RANDOMLY CHOSEN FOR TESTING WITH THE SPANISH VERSION A YEAR LATER. THE DATA SHOWED NO SIGNIFICANT DIFFERENCE BETWEEN THE ENGLISH AND SPANISH TESTINGS ON ANY OF THE SUBTEST SCALED SCORES. THERE WAS, HOWEVER, A DEFINITE OBSERVABLE TREND IN THE RELATIONSHIP BETWEEN SOCIOECONOMIC STATUS LEVEL AND THE SUBTEST SCALED SCORES. THESE RESULTS SUGGEST THAT THESE CHILDREN ARE NOT BEING PENALIZED BECAUSE THEY HAVE TO FUNCTION IN AN ENGLISH-SPEAKING SCHOOL. HOWEVER, A REVIEW OF THE MEAN SCALED SCORES SUGGESTS THAT THERE IS LITTLE ABILITY IN EITHER LANGUAGE. THE LACK OF ABILITY IN EITHER LANGUAGE, TOGETHER WITH THE SOCIOECONOMIC STATUS LEVEL, SUGGEST THAT LANGUAGE ITSELF MAY NOT BE THE IMPORTANT FACTOR BUT RATHER AN IMPOVERISHED BACKGROUND. IT IS OBVIOUS, THEN, THAT A RISE IN SOCIOECONOMIC STATUS COULD MEAN A RISE IN PERFORMANCE. THE IMPLICATION FOR SCHOOL DISTRICTS WITH A LARGE PERCENTAGE OF BILINGUALS IS THAT THEY MIGHT WANT TO EXERCISE CAUTION IN INSTITUTING A BILINGUAL PROGRAM SINCE THERE IS NOW EVIDENCE TO SUGGEST THAT NOTHING WOULD BE GAINED IN TERMS OF TEST PERFORMANCE. 9 REFERENCES.
ACCN   001213

1411 AUTH   **PALMIERI, R. G., & SUAREZ, Y.**
TITL   THE FUTURE OUTLOOK OF PUERTO RICAN VIETNAM-ERA HOSPITALIZED PSYCHIATRIC PATIENTS.
SRCE   *JOURNAL OF CLINICAL PSYCHOLOGY, 1972, 28(3), 394-399.*
INDX   PUERTO RICAN-I, PSYCHOTHERAPY, PSYCHOSOCIAL ADJUSTMENT, FAMILY ROLES, RELIGION, DEATH, SOCIALIZATION, EMPIRICAL, CULTURAL FACTORS, MALE
ABST   THE EXPECTATIONS AND PERCEPTIONS OF LIFE OUTSIDE THE HOSPITAL FOR 85 PUERTO RICAN HOSPITALIZED VIETNAM-ERA PSYCHIATRIC PATIENTS WERE EXPLORED. THE SPANISH VERSION OF THE FUTURE OUTLOOK INVENTORY (FOI), ADMINISTERED WITHIN A 2-WEEK PERIOD PRIOR TO DISCHARGE FROM A VA HOSPITAL, FOCUSED ON NINE AREAS OF CONCERN INCLUDING FUTURE OUTLOOK, FAMILY AND FRIEND RELATIONSHIPS, POSSIBILITY OF RELAPSE, MATURE ADJUSTMENT, AND COMMUNITY AND RELIGIOUS AFFILIATIONS. HIGH RATINGS WERE GIVEN FOR SUPPORT AND UNDERSTANDING FROM THEIR FAMILIES, CONCERN OVER THE ADULT ROLE, AND ACTIVITY IN A RELIGIOUS ORGANIZATION. UNCERTAINTY AND AMBIVALENCE WERE ALSO NOTED WITH REGARD TO THE PATIENTS' GENERAL VIEW OF THE FUTURE, POSSIBILITY OF RELAPSE, COMMUNITY UNDERSTANDING, AND EXPECTANCIES OF FRIENDSHIP AND UNDERSTANDING FROM OTHERS. LOW RATINGS WERE FOUND FOR MORBID THOUGHTS ABOUT

HEALTH AND DEATH AND ESTABLISHING FORMALIZED SOCIAL CONTACTS. PATIENT VARIABILITY WAS OBSERVED ON ALL FACTORS OF FOI WHEN DATA WERE BROKEN DOWN ACCORDING TO MARITAL STATUS, PLACE OF RESIDENCE, EDUCATION, LENGTH OF ILLNESS, EMPLOYMENT STATUS, AFFILIATIONS AND IQ. 7 REFERENCES. (PASAR ABSTRACT MODIFIED)

ACCN   001214

1412 AUTH   **PALOMARES, U. H.**
TITL   NUESTROS SENTIMIENTOS SON IGUALES, LA DIFERENCIA ES EN LA EXPERIENCIA. (OUR SENTIMENTS ARE THE SAME, THE DIFFERENCE IS IN THE EXPERIENCE.)
SRCE   *PERSONNEL AND GUIDANCE JOURNAL, 1971, 50(2), 137-144.*
INDX   PROFESSIONAL TRAINING, CULTURAL PLURALISM, ESSAY, PREJUDICE, SPANISH SURNAMED, PSYCHOTHERAPISTS, DYADIC INTERACTION
ABST   AN ATTEMPT IS MADE TO FACILITATE THE COMMUNICATION PROCESS BETWEEN ETHNICALLY DIVERGENT PERSONS IN A COUNSELING PARADIGM. SOME BASIC HUMAN ENCOUNTER SITUATIONS WHICH GENERATE RACIAL OR CULTURALLY ANTAGONISTIC RESPONSES ARE STUDIED AND IDENTIFIED. RACISM, OR THE USE OF COLOR AND ETHNIC CHARACTERISTICS AS AN ASPECT OF DIFFERENTIAL TREATMENT, EXISTS IN EVERYBODY IN VARYING DEGREES. THE EVIDENCE TO DATE INDICATES A DIRECT RELATIONSHIP BETWEEN SKIN COLOR AND THE DISTANCE A PERSON TENDS TO STAND FROM OTHER PEOPLE. THERE ALSO APPEARS TO BE A RELATIONSHIP BETWEEN SKIN COLOR AND THE FREQUENCY OF PHYSICAL CONTACT BETWEEN PEOPLE. MANY INDIVIDUALS HAVE ADOPTED VALUE SYSTEMS THAT ARE RELATED TO ONE'S PERCEPTIONS OF COLOR, BEAUTY, INTELLIGENCE, AND NONVERBAL COMMUNICATION. DESPITE A PROFESSED BELIEF IN EQUAL AND FAIR TREATMENT OF ALL PERSONS, A COUNSELOR MAY RELAY A DIFFERENT MESSAGE THROUGH HIS INDIRECT VERBAL AND NONVERBAL BEHAVIOR. IN TRAINING, A COUNSELOR SHOULD UNDERGO AN INTENSIVE SCRUTINY OF HIS VERBAL BEHAVIOR AS WELL AS PARTICIPATE IN INTERETHNIC ENCOUNTER GROUPS. A FOUR-STEP PROCESS FOR OVERCOMING PROBLEMS IN INTERRACIAL AND INTERCULTURAL COMMUNICATIONS IS PROVIDED. IT IS SUGGESTED THAT COUNSELORS AND EDUCATORS ACCEPT PLURALISTIC ACCULTURATION AS AN ALTERNATIVE TO THE TRADITIONAL THEORY AND PRACTICE OF ASSIMILATION. THIS APPROACH GUARDS AGAINST THE DEPERSONALIZATION INHERENT IN ENFORCED CULTURAL ASSIMILATION AND ENABLES COUNSELORS TO UNDERSTAND THE RICH DIVERSITY OF CULTURES AND OF HUMAN NATURE.
ACCN   001215

1413 AUTH   **PALOMARES, U. H.**
TITL   PUERTO RICAN YOUTH SPEAKS OUT.
SRCE   *PERSONNEL AND GUIDANCE JOURNAL, 1971, 50(2), 91-95.*
INDX   PUERTO RICAN-M, ENVIRONMENTAL FACTORS,

STEREOTYPES, POVERTY, ACCULTURATION, ADOLESCENTS, EDUCATIONAL COUNSELING, DISCRIMINATION, NEW YORK, EAST, CULTURAL FACTORS, ATTITUDES
ABST   ELEVEN PERCEPTIVE PUERTO RICAN YOUTHS FROM NEW YORK CITY PARTICIPATED IN A DISCUSSION CONCERNING THEIR OPINIONS ABOUT COUNSELORS. THEY RESPONDED TO THE FOLLOWING QUESTIONS: (1) ARE THERE PROBLEMS THAT ARE SPECIAL TO THE PUERTO RICAN?; (2) WHAT ARE SOME POSITIVE CHARACTERISTICS OF THE PUERTO RICAN THAT EDUCATORS DO NOT KNOW ABOUT?; (3) WHY DOES A COUNSELOR OR TEACHER NOT RECOGNIZE THESE CHARACTERISTICS?; AND (4) WHAT CAN THEY DO TO OVERCOME THIS PROBLEM? A NUMBER OF POSSIBLE SOLUTIONS TO STUDENT-COUNSELOR INTERACTIONS WERE OFFERED. SOME STUDENTS BELIEVE THAT IF THE RATIO OF STUDENTS TO COUNSELORS IS HIGH, THEN ANY COUNSELING SERVICE WILL BE MINIMAL. THERE WAS SOME DISCUSSION OF THE EFFECT OF RACISM AND POVERTY ON THE COUNSELING PROCESS. ATTENTION WAS GIVEN TO THE EFFECT OF CULTURAL STEREOTYPING IN THE EDUCATIONAL AND COUNSELING SETTING. THE ACCULTURATION PROCESS WAS CRITICALLY QUESTIONED BY THE PUERTO RICAN YOUTHS. IT IS RECOMMENDED THAT COUNSELORS SHOULD HAVE SOME BASIC KNOWLEDGE OF PUERTO RICAN LANGUAGE, CULTURE, CUSTOMS, AND FAMILY STRUCTURE.
ACCN   001216

1414 AUTH   **PANDO, J. R.**
TITL   APPRAISAL OF VARIOUS CLINICAL SCALES OF THE SPANISH VERSION OF THE MINI-MULT WITH SPANISH AMERICANS (DOCTORAL DISSERTATION, ADELPHI UNIVERSITY, 1974).
SRCE   *DISSERTATION ABSTRACTS INTERNATIONAL, 1974, 34, 5688B. (UNIVERSITY MICROFILMS NO. 74-11,677.)*
INDX   PERSONALITY ASSESSMENT, TEST VALIDITY, MMPI, SPANISH SURNAMED, PUERTO RICAN-I, MALE, ANXIETY, DEPRESSION, SCHIZOPHRENIA, EMPIRICAL, ADULTS, FLORIDA, SOUTH, PSYCHOPATHOLOGY, CUBAN, VETERANS
ABST   THE DIAGNOSTIC ASSESSMENT OF SPANISH-SPEAKING INDIVIDUALS WAS INVESTIGATED AMONG 115 SUBJECTS WHO WERE SPANISH AMERICAN PSYCHIATRIC PATIENTS RANGING FROM 17 TO 57 YEARS OLD IN THE MIAMI AND PUERTO RICO VETERANS ADMINISTRATION HOSPITALS. THEY WERE DIVIDED INTO FOUR GROUPS ON THE BASIS OF DIAGNOSIS: ANXIETY REACTION (N=25), DEPRESSIVE (N=25), PARANOID SCHIZOPHRENIA (N=30), AND UNDIFFERENTIATED SCHIZOPHRENIA (N=35). THE SUBJECTS WERE ADMINISTERED THE SPANISH VERSION OF THE MINI-MULT AND RATED ON THE INPATIENT MULTIDIMENSIONAL PSYCHIATRIC SCALES (IMPS) AND THE PSYCHOTIC INPATIENT PROFILE (PIP). MMPI PROFILES WERE DONE BY USING THE MEAN T SCORE ELEVATIONS ON EACH OF THE MINI-MULT SCALES. THE RESULTS INDICATE THAT THE PATHOLOGICAL LIMIT OF (T>70) IS OF NO VALUE IN DIF-

FERENTIATING PSYCHOPATHOLOGY. SECOND, MEAN PROFILE ELEVATIONS, ALTHOUGH IN SOME CASES SIGNIFICANTLY INDICATIVE OF A CERTAIN PSYCHOPATHOLOGY, WERE NOT CONCLUSIVE AS TO EMPOWER THE MINI-MULT WITH A HIGH DEGREE OF DIAGNOSTICALLY SIGNIFICANT PREDICTABILITY. THIRD, THE KIND OF PSYCHOPATHOLOGY AS SHOWN BY THE SUBJECTS' PERFORMANCE ON THE MINI-MULT SHOWED LITTLE CORRESPONDENCE WITH THEIR BEHAVIOR AS ASSESSED BY THE IMPS AND THE PIP. IT IS CONCLUDED THAT THE USE OF THE SPANISH VERSION OF THE MINI-MULT WITH SPANISH-SPEAKING PSYCHIATRIC PATIENTS USING NORTH AMERICAN STANDARDS FOR INTERPRETATION IS NOT WARRANTED AS AN ACCURATE PREDICTOR OF TYPE OF PSYCHOPATHOLOGY. 58 REFERENCES. (AUTHOR SUMMARY MODIFIED)

ACCN   001217

1415 AUTH   **PAREDES, A.**
TITL   FOLK MEDICINE AND THE INTERCULTURAL JEST.
SRCE   *IN J. HELM (ED.), SPANISH-SPEAKING PEOPLE IN THE UNITED STATES: PROCEEDINGS OF THE 1968 ANNUAL SPRING MEETING OF THE AMERICAN ETHNOLOGICAL SOCIETY. SEATTLE: UNIVERSITY OF WASHINGTON PRESS, 1968, PP. 104-119.*
INDX   FOLK MEDICINE, CURANDERISMO, MEXICAN AMERICAN, CULTURE, ATTITUDES, CONFLICT RESOLUTION, ADULTS, CASE STUDY, TEXAS, SOUTHWEST, RURAL, EMPIRICAL
ABST   A DISCUSSION OF SIX MOTIFS OF JEST OR "TALLAS," TOLD IN SPANISH, FROM THE LOWER END OF THE TEXAS-MEXICAN BORDER IS PRESENTED IN AN ATTEMPT TO COLLECT FOLKLORE WHICH MAKES COVERT OR DIRECT EXPRESSION OF ATTITUDES TOWARD ANGLO AMERICANS AND THEIR CULTURE. A TALLA SESSION WAS RECREATED AT A SMALL CITY RESIDENCE IN WHICH STORIES WERE RECORDED FROM MEXICAN AMERICAN MALES FOR FOUR-HOUR PERIODS. THE CONTENT WAS CONTROLLED THROUGH THE SUGGESTIONS OF A STUDY "PLANT." ALL SIX TALLAS HAD A GENERAL SITUATION IN COMMON: THERE WAS A SICK PERSON AND A GROUP OF PEOPLE WHO SOUGHT A CURE FOR HIM, EITHER FROM A DOCTOR OR A CURANDERO. THE TEXT OF EACH MOTIF IS INCLUDED WITH AN IN-DEPTH DISCUSSION OF THE CULTURAL ASPECTS. AS PARODIES OF THE CURANDERO TYPE OF BELIEF TALE, THE TALLAS EXPRESS THE MEXICAN AMERICAN'S REJECTION OF HIS TRADITIONAL CULTURE TO SOME EXTENT. HOWEVER, PARODY IS COMBINED WITH A GREAT DEAL OF RESENTMENT AGAINST THE ANGLO CULTURE, WHICH IS EXPRESSED IN A STEREOTYPIC VIEW OF AMERICAN PHYSICIANS AND HOSPITAL ATTENDANTS. IN GENERAL, THE JESTS HELP PEOPLE RESOLVE CONFLICTS BROUGHT ABOUT BY ACCULTURATION INVOLVING NOT ONLY A CHANGE FROM RURAL TO URBAN VALUES BUT FROM A BASICALLY MEXICAN CULTURE TO THE GENERALIZED, ENGLISH-SPEAKING CULTURE OF THE MAJORITY. 7 REFERENCES.

ACCN   001219

1416 AUTH   **PAREDES, A.**
TITL   TEXAS' THIRD MAN: THE TEXAS MEXICAN.
SRCE   *RACE, 1963, 4, 49-58.*
INDX   DISCRIMINATION, PREJUDICE, HEALTH, EDUCATION, HISTORY, COMMUNITY INVOLVEMENT, LEADERSHIP, ESSAY, SES, POVERTY, SCHOLASTIC ACHIEVEMENT, MEXICAN AMERICAN, RESOURCE UTILIZATION, HEALTH DELIVERY SYSTEMS, TEXAS, SOUTHWEST
ABST   THIS ESSAY EXAMINES THE NOTION THAT THE TEXAS-MEXICAN ENJOYS ALMOST FULL CITIZENSHIP IN AREAS RELATED TO HUMAN DIGNITY AND PERSONAL RIGHTS, BUT APPEARS TO BE OFTENTIMES WORSE OFF THAN BLACKS IN AREAS OF HEALTH, EMPLOYMENT, AND EDUCATION. UNLIKE THE BLACK, THE TEXAS-MEXICAN HAS ACHIEVED THE BENEFITS OF INTEGRATION (I.E., THE OFFICIAL ACCEPTANCE INTO BARS, HOTELS, RESTAURANTS AND SWIMMING POOLS). HOWEVER, IN TEXAS, MEXICANS HAVE THE HIGHEST INCIDENCE OF DISEASES (E.G., INFANTILE DIARRHEA, AND DEATH RATE FROM TUBERCULOSIS) THAT REFLECT POVERTY AND A LACK OF EDUCATION. COVERT DISCRIMINATION IS RESPONSIBLE FOR THIS SEEMINGLY PARADOXICAL SITUATION. THE PREJUDICE AGAINST THE MEXICAN IS BASED ON CULTURAL FACTORS IN WHICH HISTORICAL, POLITICAL, AND ECONOMIC FACTORS HAVE PLAYED A LARGE ROLE. IN PARTICULAR, ALTHOUGH THE MEXICAN GOVERNMENT HAS BEEN EFFECTIVE IN DECREASING THE OVERT DISCRIMINATION AGAINST MEXICAN NATIONALS AND TEXAS-MEXICANS IN AGRICULTURAL LABOR, THERE HAS BEEN LITTLE EFFECT ON THE DEPRESSED WAGES. WITHOUT ECONOMIC GAINS THE TEXAS-MEXICAN CONTINUES TO HAVE LOW LEVELS OF HEALTH AND EDUCATION, RESULTING IN LOW SOCIAL STATUS. IT IS CONCLUDED THAT TEXAS-MEXICANS MUST BECOME A POLITICAL FORCE BEFORE ANY SOCIAL CHANGES IN THEIR FAVOR WILL OCCUR.

ACCN   001221

1417 AUTH   **PARKER, W. S.**
TITL   BLACK-WHITE DIFFERENCES IN LEADER BEHAVIOR RELATED TO SUBORDINATES' REACTIONS.
SRCE   *JOURNAL OF APPLIED PSYCHOLOGY, 1976, 61(2), 140-147.*
INDX   INTERPERSONAL RELATIONS, MEXICAN AMERICAN, CROSS CULTURAL, CONFORMITY, GROUP DYNAMICS, CULTURAL FACTORS, COMPETITION, ACHIEVEMENT MOTIVATION, JOB PERFORMANCE, EMPIRICAL, LEADERSHIP, MIDWEST
ABST   DIFFERENCES WERE INVESTIGATED IN 4 MANAGERIAL LEADERSHIP MEASURES (MANAGERIAL SUPPORT, GOAL EMPHASIS, WORK FACILITATION, AND INTERACTION FACILITATION) AMONG 72 BLACK, 36 ANGLO, AND 15 CHICANO SUBORDINATES OF 16 BLACK AND 17 ANGLO SUPERVISORS IN 3 INDUSTRIAL PLANTS. RESULTS INDICATE THAT THE BEHAVIOR OF SUPERVISORS TOWARD THEIR SUBORDINATES IS

A COMPLEX FUNCTION OF (1) THE SUPERVISOR'S OWN RACE AND ROLE IN COMBINATION WITH (2) THE RACE OF SUBORDINATES, AND (3) THE MAJORITY OR MINORITY POSITIONS OF RACIAL GROUPS WITHIN THE GROUP SUPERVISED. THE STUDY SUPPORTS THE CONCLUSIONS THAT: (1) BLACK SUPERVISORS ARE SEEN BY SUBORDINATES AS MORE EFFECTIVE THAN ANGLO SUPERVISORS; (2) THERE IS NO EVIDENCE THAT SUBORDINATES VIEW SUPERVISORS OF THEIR OWN RACE MORE FAVORABLY THAN SUPERVISORS OF A DIFFERENT RACE; (3) ANGLO SUBORDINATES OF ANGLO SUPERVISORS IN PREDOMINANTLY BLACK GROUPS SEE THEIR SUPERVISORS MORE FAVORABLY THAN THOSE IN PREDOMINANTLY ANGLO GROUPS; AND (4) CHICANO SUBORDINATES SEE BLACK SUPERVISORS MORE FAVORABLY ONLY ON TASK-RELATED LEADERSHIP DIMENSION, NOT IN INTERPERSONAL LEADERSHIP AREAS. 7 REFERENCES. (PASAR ABSTRACT MODIFIED)

ACCN   001222

1418 AUTH   **PASAMANICK, B.**
TITL   THE INTELLIGENCE OF AMERICAN CHILDREN OF MEXICAN PARENTAGE: A DISCUSSION OF UNCONTROLLED VARIABLES.
SRCE   *JOURNAL OF ABNORMAL AND SOCIAL PSYCHOLOGY, 1951, 46(4), 598-602.*
INDX   INTELLIGENCE, MEXICAN AMERICAN, CHILDREN, EMPIRICAL, SES, NUTRITION, CULTURAL FACTORS, TEST RELIABILITY, TEST VALIDITY, REVIEW
ABST   A CRITICAL ANALYSIS OF THE EFFECT OF UNCONTROLLED VARIABLES UPON THE MEASURED INTELLIGENCE OF MEXICAN AMERICAN CHILDREN IS PRESENTED. A SPECIFIC ARTICLE WHICH PURPORTS TO CONTROL A NUMBER OF FACTORS THAT ARE FREQUENTLY IGNORED BY OTHERS PROVIDES THE BASIS FOR SUCH AN ANALYSIS. THE AUTHORS OF THAT ARTICLE INDICATE THAT THEY LEFT UNCONTROLLED THE FACTORS OF RURAL-URBAN PARENTAL BACKGROUND, THE CHILD'S VOCABULARY LIMITATION, AND THE MOTIVATION DURING TESTING. THEY FURTHER STATED THAT THESE FACTORS MIGHT ACCOUNT FOR THEIR FINDING OF INTELLECTUAL INFERIORITY FOR A PARTICULAR ETHNIC GROUP. HOWEVER, THE READER IS LEFT WITH THE IMPRESSION THAT THE THREE VARIABLES REPORTEDLY LEFT UNCONTROLLED ARE NOT OF SUFFICIENT IMPORTANCE TO BE RESPONSIBLE FOR THE MAGNITUDE OF THE DIFFERENCES IN IQ SCORES. A CRITICAL OBSERVATION REVEALS THAT THE AUTHORS EITHER IGNORED OR MISTAKENLY BELIEVED THAT THEY HAD CONTROLLED SUCH IMPORTANT VARIABLES AS: (1) THE SUBJECT'S NUTRITIONAL DIET; (2) THE FAMILY'S SOCIO-ECONOMIC LEVEL; (3) THE SUBJECT'S TOTAL CULTURAL COMPLEX; AND (4) THE EDUCATIONAL TRAINING FOR BOTH GROUPS OF SUBJECTS. IT IS CONCLUDED THAT THERE IS A NEED FOR A DIFFERENT TYPE OF STUDY IN THE SPHERE OF ETHNIC GROUP DIFFERENCES, SINCE SATISFACTORY CONTROL OF THE ABOVE MENTIONED FACTORS IS INADEQUATE AT THIS

TIME. WHAT ARE NEEDED ARE LONGITUDINAL STUDIES POSSIBLY BEGINNING EVEN PRIOR TO CONCEPTION AND FOLLOWING THE INDIVIDUAL TO MATURITY. 15 REFERENCES.

ACCN   001223

1419 AUTH   **PASCHAL, F. D., & SULLIVAN, L. R.**
TITL   RACIAL DIFFERENCES IN THE MENTAL AND PHYSICAL DEVELOPMENT OF MEXICAN CHILDREN.
SRCE   *COMPARATIVE PSYCHOLOGY MONOGRAPHS, 1925, 3(1), 1-76.*
INDX   COGNITIVE DEVELOPMENT, PHYSICAL DEVELOPMENT, TEST VALIDITY, TEST RELIABILITY, MEXICAN AMERICAN, CHILDREN, SES, DISCRIMINATION, PREJUDICE, EXAMINER EFFECTS, INTELLIGENCE, ARIZONA, SOUTHWEST
ABST   COMBINED PSYCHOLOGICAL AND ANTHROPOLOGICAL TECHNIQUES WERE USED TO INVESTIGATE RACIAL DIFFERENCES IN THE MENTAL AND PHYSICAL DEVELOPMENT OF MEXICAN CHILDREN. TO ASSESS MENTAL CAPACITY, THE SUBJECTS, 9 AND 12 YEAR-OLD MEXICAN MALES AND FEMALES, WERE ADMINISTERED SIX PERFORMANCE SCALES. ANTHROPOMETRIC OBSERVATIONS AND MEASUREMENTS WERE USED TO DETERMINE THE RACIAL COMPOSITION OF THE GROUP AND TO DEFINE ITS PHYSICAL STATUS. LENGTHY DISCUSSION IS GIVEN TO: (1) INDIAN BLOODS AND SOCIAL AND MENTAL STATUS; (2) CORRELATIONS OF MENTAL SCORES WITH PHYSICAL TRAITS; (3) PLACE OF BIRTH AND MENTAL SCORE WITH PHYSICAL TRAITS; AND (4) SOCIAL STATUS AND PHYSICAL, RACIAL AND MENTAL STATUS. ANALYSES OF THE INTERCORRELATIONS OF RACIAL, SOCIAL, AND MENTAL FACTORS INDICATE: (1) THERE IS AN AGREEMENT WITH EARLIER INVESTIGATORS WHO HAVE FOUND A DEFINITE RELATIONSHIP BETWEEN THE PROPORTION OF INDIAN BLOOD AND MENTAL STATUS; (2) MEXICANS LIVING IN TUCSON WHO ARE PARTIALLY OF INDIAN ORIGIN HAVE A LOWER MENTAL SCORE, A LOWER SOCIAL OR ECONOMIC STATUS, A LOWER SCHOOL STANDING IN GRADE, THAN DO THOSE TUCSON MEXICANS WHO ARE WHOLLY OF WHITE ORIGIN; (3) APPROXIMATELY 85 PERCENT OF THE GERM PLASM OF MEXICANS IN TUCSON IS WHITE GERM PLASM; (4) CHILDREN FROM THE BETTER SOCIAL OR ECONOMIC CLASSES EXCEED THOSE FROM THE POORER HOMES IN STATURE, IN SCHOOL GRADE, AND IN MENTAL SCORE; AND (5) THE CORRELATIONS BETWEEN MENTAL SCORE AND INDIVIDUAL RACE CHARACTERISTICS INDICATE SKIN COLOR AS THE HIGHEST CORRELATION WITH MENTAL SCORE. A DISCUSSION OF THE FINDINGS IS PROVIDED. 25 REFERENCES.

ACCN   001224

1420 AUTH   **PATELLA, V., & KUVLESKY, W. P.**
TITL   SITUATIONAL VARIATION IN LANGUAGE PATTERNS OF MEXICAN AMERICAN BOYS AND GIRLS.
SRCE   *SOCIAL SCIENCE QUARTERLY, 1973, 53(4), 855-864.*

INDX MEXICAN AMERICAN, ADOLESCENTS, BILIN-
GUALISM, SEX COMPARISON, EMPIRICAL, CUL-
TURAL FACTORS, MASS MEDIA, RURAL, SCHO-
LASTIC ACHIEVEMENT, TEXAS, SOUTHWEST,
ENVIRONMENTAL FACTORS, LINGUISTIC COM-
PETENCE, SEX ROLES, MALE, FEMALE

ABST INTERVIEWS ASSESSING LANGUAGE PREFER-
ENCE VARIATION BY SITUATION AND SEX WERE
GIVEN TO 596 HIGH SCHOOL SOPHOMORES
AND 73 DROPOUT PEERS IN 4 RURAL TEXAS
COUNTIES CLOSE TO THE MEXICAN BORDER.
THE CHARACTERISTICS OF THE INTERVIEWEES
WHO HAD IDENTIFIED THEMSELVES AS MEXI-
CAN AMERICAN WERE: LARGE FAMILIES, LOW
OCCUPATIONAL LEVEL OF FATHERS, BOTH
PARENTS PRESENT, LOW EDUCATIONAL LEVEL
OF PARENTS, AND NON-WORKING MOTHERS.
PATTERNS OF SPANISH OR ENGLISH IN VARI-
OUS SITUATIONS WERE STUDIED. THE RE-
SULTS FOR BOTH GROUPS WERE AS FOLLOWS:
(1) FREQUENCY OF SPANISH DECREASES AND
ENGLISH INCREASES AS ONE GOES FROM
FAMILY, TO NEIGHBORHOOD, TO SCHOOL OR
WORK; (2) SPANISH IS ALMOST ALWAYS USED
WITH PARENTS; (3) SPANISH AND ENGLISH ME-
DIA ARE BOTH UTILIZED; AND (4) EXCEPT FOR
PRINTED MEDIA, GIRLS USE SPANISH LESS
FREQUENTLY THAN BOYS. ONE OF THE MAJOR
DIFFERENCES BETWEEN STUDENTS AND
DROPOUTS IS THAT THE LATTER GROUP USES
MORE SPANISH THAN ENGLISH. ALSO, DROP-
OUTS' USE OF SPANISH BROADCASTS IS FIVE
TIMES THAT OF STUDENTS'. FREQUENCY OF
USE IS SUGGESTED TO BE RELATED TO
FLUENCY. LANGUAGE VARIATION ACROSS
SITUATIONS IS DISCUSSED IN TERMS OF AS-
SIMILATION PATTERNS. SEX DIFFERENCES ARE
SUGGESTED TO BE A FUNCTION OF SEX ROLE
TRAINING. 17 REFERENCES. (SOCIOLOGY AB-
STRACT MODIFIED)

ACCN 001225

1421 AUTH **PATON, S. M., & KANDEL, D. B.**
TITL PSYCHOLOGICAL FACTORS AND ADOLESCENT
ILLICIT DRUG USE: ETHNICITY AND SEX DIF-
FERENCES.
SRCE *ADOLESCENCE, 1978, 13(50), 188-200.*
INDX ADOLESCENTS, MALE, FEMALE, CULTURAL
FACTORS, DRUG ABUSE, DEPRESSION, SELF
CONCEPT, ETHNIC IDENTITY, URBAN, RURAL,
NEW YORK, EAST, EMPIRICAL, PUERTO RICAN-
M, DEPRESSION, ANOMIE, SEX COMPARISON
ABST THIS STUDY SOUGHT TO CLARIFY THE RELA-
TIONSHIP BETWEEN FOUR PSYCHOLOGICAL
FACTORS (DEPRESSIVE MOOD, NORMLESS-
NESS, SENSE OF ISOLATION FROM THE WORLD,
AND SELF-ESTEEM) AND DRUG USE IN A RAN-
DOM SAMPLE OF NEW YORK STATE PUBLIC
HIGH SCHOOL STUDENTS. THE ANALYSIS WAS
BASED ON A LARGE, MULTIPHASIC RANDOM
SAMPLE OF ADOLESCENTS (N = 8,206) DRAWN
FROM 18 PUBLIC SECONDARY SCHOOLS—SIX
LOCATED IN NEW YORK CITY, SIX IN SUBURBAN
AREAS, AND SIX IN SMALL TOWNS OR RURAL
AREAS IN UPPER NEW YORK STATE. STRUC-
TURED, SELF-ADMINISTERED QUESTION-
NAIRES, DESIGNED TO EVALUATE THE ADO-
LESCENTS' DRUG USE AND PSYCHOLOGICAL

STATES, WERE GIVEN IN A CLASSROOM SET-
TING. OF THE FOUR PSYCHOLOGICAL FAC-
TORS EXAMINED, ONLY TWO—DEPRESSIVE
MOOD AND NORMLESSNESS—SHOWED A
POSITIVE RELATIONSHIP WITH THE USE OF IL-
LICIT DRUGS, ESPECIALLY DRUGS OTHER THAN
MARIJUANA. THE ASSOCIATION OF DEPRES-
SIVE MOOD AND NORMLESSNESS WITH ILLE-
GAL MULTIPLE DRUG USE VARIED BY ETHNI-
CITY AND SEX—BEING CONSISTENTLY
STRONGER AMONG GIRLS AND AMONG
WHITES. IN ADDITION, DEPRESSIVE MOOD WAS
NEGATIVELY RELATED TO MULTIPLE DRUG USE
FOR BLACK AND PUERTO RICAN BOYS. THESE
FINDINGS SUGGEST THAT PSYCHOLOGICAL
FACTORS PLAY A DIFFERENT ROLE IN ADOLES-
CENT DRUG INVOLVEMENT WITHIN VARIOUS
SOCIAL AND CULTURAL GROUPS. 33 REFER-
ENCES.

ACCN 002177

1422 AUTH **PAULSTON, C. B.**
TITL IMPLICATIONS OF LANGUAGE LEARNING
THEORY FOR LANGUAGE PLANNING: CON-
CERNS IN BILINGUAL EDUCATION (BILING SE-
RIES NO. 1).
SRCE *ARLINGTON, VA.: CENTER FOR APPLIED LIN-
GUISTICS, 1974.*
INDX LANGUAGE LEARNING, BILINGUAL-BICUL-
TURAL EDUCATION, INSTRUCTIONAL TECH-
NIQUES, LINGUISTICS, BILINGUALISM, EDUCA-
TION, CHILDREN, ESSAY, LANGUAGE
ACQUISITION, LINGUISTIC COMPETENCE
ABST THE CONTRIBUTIONS OF LANGUAGE LEARN-
ING THEORY TO LANGUAGE PLANNING AT THE
NATIONAL LEVEL ARE EXAMINED FROM THE
POINT OF VIEW OF THE LANGUAGE TEACHING
SPECIALIST. THE PAPER IS COMPRISED OF
THREE PARTS. FIRST, A CONCEPTUAL FRAME-
WORK OF LANGUAGE PLANNING IS PRE-
SENTED, IDENTIFYING AREAS IN WHICH THE
LANGUAGE SPECIALIST MIGHT CONTRIBUTE.
THIS ENTAILS A DISTINCTION BETWEEN "LAN-
GUAGE CULTIVATION" (I.E., PROBLEMS OF LAN-
GUAGE LEARNING) AND "LANGUAGE POLICY"
(I.E., PROBLEMS INVOLVING SOCIAL AND CUL-
TURAL FACTORS), AND THE DEVELOPMENT OF
CRITERIA IN THE AREAS OF LANGUAGE DETER-
MINATION, DEVELOPMENT, AND IMPLEMENTA-
TION WHICH ENABLE THE ASSIGNMENT OF
PLANNING EVENTS TO EITHER THE LANGUAGE
CULTIVATION OR POLICY APPROACHES. SEC-
OND, IN A DISCUSSION OF LANGUAGE LEARN-
ING THEORY THE APPROACH, METHOD, AND
TECHNIQUE OF FOREIGN LANGUAGE AND
SECOND LANGUAGE LEARNING ARE DISTIN-
GUISHED. TWO LANGUAGE LEARNING THEO-
RIES ARE CONSIDERED—I.E., LANGUAGE
LEARNING AS A RESULT OF HABIT FORMATION
(SKINNER); AND LANGUAGE AS AN INNATE,
SPECIES-SPECIFIC, BIOLOGICALLY DETER-
MINED BEHAVIOR (LENNEBERG; CHOMSKY).
THIRD, THE RELATIVE MERITS OF THREE LAN-
GUAGE TEACHING APPROACHES (THE AUDIO
LINGUAL, THE COGNITIVE CODE, AND THE DI-
RECT METHOD) ARE EVALUATED IN AN EXAMI-
NATION OF CASE STUDIES ON BILINGUAL EDU-
CATION. THIS COMPARISON OF CASE STUDIES

IN BILINGUAL PRIMARY EDUCATION IN MEXICO, CANADA, KENYA, SOUTH AFRICA, AND THE PHILIPPINES REVEALS THAT DIFFERENCES IN THESE THREE TEACHING METHODS ARE OF MINOR IMPORTANCE BECAUSE: (1) STUDENTS DO NOT SEEM TO SUFFER IN ACADEMIC SUBJECT ACHIEVEMENT WHEN TAUGHT IN A SECOND LANGUAGE; (2) PROFICIENCY IN A SECOND LANGUAGE DOES NOT BRING ABOUT ILL EFFECTS ON NATIVE LANGUAGE; AND (3) FOLLOWING SOCIAL CLASS, THE MOST IMPORTANT FACTOR IN SCHOOL ACHIEVEMENT IS QUALITY OF THE INSTRUCTIONAL PROGRAM. IT IS THEREFORE CONCLUDED THAT IMPLICATIONS ABOUT LANGUAGE PLANNING DRAWN FROM LANGUAGE PLANNING THEORY ARE LIMITED. RECOMMENDED, INSTEAD, IS THE ADOPTION OF A SOCIOLINGUISTIC AND ANTHROPOLOGICAL FRAMEWORK FOR EXAMINING SOLUTIONS TO SOCIOLINGUISTIC PROBLEMS. 106 REFERENCES.

ACCN   001226

1423 AUTH   **PAYNE, B. F., & DUNN, C. J.**
TITL   AN ANALYSIS OF THE CHANGE IN SELF CONCEPT BY RACIAL DESCENT.
SRCE   *JOURNAL OF NEGRO EDUCATION, 1972, 41(2), 156-163.*
INDX   SELF CONCEPT, ATTITUDES, CHILDREN, EDUCATIONAL COUNSELING, PEER GROUP, GROUP DYNAMICS, CULTURAL FACTORS, CROSS CULTURAL, MEXICAN AMERICAN, EMPIRICAL, TEXAS, SOUTHWEST
ABST   THE EFFECT OF GROUP GUIDANCE ON THE SELF-CONCEPT OF CULTURALLY DIFFERENT LOWER SOCIOECONOMIC STUDENTS WAS STUDIED IN A PROGRAM FUNDED UNDER THE ELEMENTARY AND SECONDARY EDUCATION ACT, TITLE I. THIRTY 4TH AND 5TH GRADE PUPILS IN TEXAS (10 MEXICAN AMERICANS, 9 ANGLOS, AND 11 BLACKS) WERE ADMINISTERED THE BROWN IDS SELF-CONCEPT REFERENT TEST BEFORE AND AFTER 18 WEEKLY GROUP GUIDANCE SESSIONS. THE CHILD RATED HIMSELF ON 14 BIPOLAR DIMENSIONS (E.G., HAPPYSAD) AS HE PERCEIVES HIMSELF AND AS HIS TEACHER, MOTHER AND PEERS WOULD PERCEIVE HIM. TEST ITEMS WERE SUBDIVIDED FURTHER AND SCORES WERE OBTAINED FOR "SELF AS SUBJECT" AND "SELF AS OBJECT." THEIR PERFORMANCES WERE COMPARED TO A CONTROL GROUP OF 6 MEXICAN AMERICANS, 6 ANGLOS, AND 3 BLACKS. MEAN DIFFERENCES AMONG ETHNIC GROUPS WERE COMPARED FOR THE CONTROL GROUP AND REVEALED THAT ANGLOS BEGAN AND ENDED WITH THE HIGHER SELF AS SUBJECT REFERENT SCORE, BLACKS AND ANGLOS IMPROVED THEIR SELF AS OBJECT SCORES, BUT MEXICAN AMERICANS REGRESSED IN THEIR PERCEPTION OF SELF AS OBJECT. MEXICAN AMERICANS SHOWED THE GREATEST AMOUNT OF CHANGE IN MEAN DIFFERENCES ON THE SUBTEST SELF AS SUBJECT, WHILE BLACKS AND ANGLOS MADE THE GREATEST AMOUNT OF IMPROVEMENT ON SELF AS OBJECT SCORES. THE RESULTS INDICATE THAT GROUP GUIDANCE IS EFFECTIVE IN FORMAL ENCOUR-

AGEMENT OF PEER INTERACTION, OPPORTUNITY FOR VERBALIZATION, AND PERSONAL ACCEPTANCE THROUGH POSITIVE SOCIAL EXPERIENCES. 8 REFERENCES. (PASAR ABSTRACT MODIFIED)

ACCN   001227

1424 AUTH   **PEARSON, A. W.**
TITL   TRATAMIENTO DE ALCOHOLISMO DE MEXICANOS QUE VIVEN EN LOS ESTADOS UNIDOS. (THE TREATMENT OF ALCOHOLISM IN MEXICANS IN THE UNITED STATES.)
SRCE   *REVISTA MEXICANA DE PSICOLOGIA, 1964, 1(4), 358-362. (SPANISH)*
INDX   MEXICAN AMERICAN, ALCOHOLISM, REHABILITATION, CALIFORNIA, SOUTHWEST, PROGRAM EVALUATION
ABST   THE DEVELOPMENT OF THE LOS ANGELES ALCOHOLIC REHABILITATION CLINIC IS REPORTED AND THE CHARACTERISTICS OF THE MEXICAN AMERICANS (MA) WHO CONSTITUTE 20 PERCENT OF THOSE SEEKING TREATMENT FOR ALCOHOLISM ARE ANALYZED. THE CLINIC IS ADMINISTERED ON A PART-TIME BASIS BY A DIRECTOR, FIVE PRACTICING PHYSICIANS AND A PSYCHIATRIST, AND ON A FULL-TIME BASIS BY A PUBLIC HEALTH EDUCATOR, A PUBLIC HEALTH NURSE, A CLINICAL NURSE AND AN ADMINISTRATIVE SECRETARY WITH THREE STAFF MEMBERS. A SHELTER CLINIC SPECIFICALLY FOR PATIENT EVALUATION IS UNDER THE SAME DIRECTOR BUT WITH A SEPARATE ADMINISTRATIVE STAFF. ONE SPANISH-SPEAKING EMPLOYEE CONDUCTS TRAINING SESSIONS FOR NON-SPANISH-SPEAKING SOCIAL WORKERS WHO ARE INVOLVED WITH MEXICAN AMERICANS. THE CHARACTERISTICS OF THE MA ALCOHOLIC WHO SEEKS TREATMENT WERE ANALYZED ON THE BASIS OF ASSIMILATION AND NONASSIMILATION, USING THE FOLLOWING CRITERIA: (1) LANGUAGE SPOKEN IN THE HOME; (2) RELIGION; (3) THE WOMAN'S ROLE WITHIN THE HOME AND IN SOCIETY; (4) FAMILY OBEDIENCE AND OBLIGATIONS (TO MEMBERS OF THE IMMEDIATE AND EXTENDED FAMILY); AND (5) VALUE GIVEN TO OCCUPATIONAL SUCCESS. OF THE MA GROUP UNDER TREATMENT, 48 WERE CONSIDERED NONASSIMILATED AND 15 AS ASSIMILATED. ALL OF THE NONASSIMILATED MEXICAN AMERICANS HAVE SHOWN IMPROVEMENT THROUGH TREATMENT, WHEREAS ONLY 30 PERCENT OF THE ASSIMILATED GROUP HAS IMPROVED. REASONS FOR THE SUCCESS WITH THE NONASSIMILATED MA COULD BE DUE TO: (1) ACCEPTANCE AND COOPERATION OF THE ENTIRE FAMILY; (2) RESPECT OF AND COOPERATION WITH AUTHORITATIVE FIGURES SUCH AS THE DOCTORS, NURSES AND SOCIAL WORKERS; (3) TREATMENT BY A SPANISH-SPEAKING STAFF; AND (4) THE ACCEPTANCE OF ALCOHOLISM AS AN ILLNESS. A DISCUSSION OF THE RANGES OF ALCOHOLISM AND THE ALCOHOLIC IS PROVIDED.

ACCN   001228

1425 AUTH   **PECK, E. C.**
TITL   THE RELATIONSHIP OF DISEASE AND OTHER STRESS TO SECOND LANGUAGE.

SRCE *INTERNATIONAL JOURNAL OF SOCIAL PSY-CHIATRY, 1974, 20(1-2), 128-133.*

INDX BILINGUAL, BILINGUALISM, HEALTH, STRESS, LANGUAGE ACQUISITION, CASE STUDY, PSYCHOTHERAPY, MENTAL HEALTH, PHYSICIANS, MENTAL HEALTH PROFESSION, CALIFORNIA, MEXICAN AMERICAN, ATTITUDES, LINGUISTIC COMPETENCE, PREJUDICE, SOUTHWEST, PSYCHOTHERAPISTS

ABST INSIGHTS INTO THE PHENOMENON OF BILINGUALISM ARE APPLICABLE TO THE GENERAL PRACTICE OF PSYCHIATRY. A CASE FROM THE AUTHOR'S CLINICAL EXPERIENCE ILLUSTRATES THE EFFECT OF STRESS ON SELF-EXPRESSION IN A SECOND LANGUAGE. DURING A PERIOD OF ILLNESS, COMPETENCE IN THE SECOND LANGUAGE SUDDENLY DIMINISHED, CAUSING FEELINGS OF SHAME, ANGER, AND LOSS OF SELF-WORTH. IT IS RECOMMENDED THAT CLINICAL ASSESSMENT OF THE BILINGUAL PATIENT INCLUDE INQUIRY AS TO (1) THE AGE AND PLACE AT WHICH THE SECOND LANGUAGE WAS LEARNED, (2) ATTITUDES TOWARD HIS FIRST AND SECOND LANGUAGE IN HIS PRESENT ENVIRONMENT, AND (3) THE EFFECT OF ANY PRESENT STRESS ON HIS SELF-EXPRESSION IN EITHER LANGUAGE. THEORETICAL ISSUES OF THE EFFECT OF AGE UPON LEARNING A SECOND LANGUAGE AND THE PARTICULAR DIFFICULTY PRESENTED BY IDIOMATIC STRUCTURES ARE SUGGESTED FOR FURTHER CONSIDERATION. 14 REFERENCES.

ACCN 002178

1426 AUTH **PECK, H. B., KAPLAN, S. R., & ROMAN, M.**

TITL PREVENTION, TREATMENT, AND SOCIAL ACTION: A STRATEGY OF INTERVENTION IN A DISADVANTAGED URBAN AREA.

SRCE *AMERICAN JOURNAL OF ORTHOPSYCHIATRY, 1966, 36(1), 57-69.*

INDX PRIMARY PREVENTION, COMMUNITY, MENTAL HEALTH, PARAPROFESSIONALS, PSYCHOTHERAPY, HEALTH DELIVERY SYSTEMS, ESSAY, POLICY

ABST AN EFFECTIVE COMMUNITY MENTAL HEALTH PROGRAM FOR URBAN DISADVANTAGED AREAS REQUIRES TECHNIQUES DERIVED FROM SOCIAL ACTION AS WELL AS THE MORE TRADITIONAL SERVICES. THE USE OF SMALL GROUP APPROACHES AND STAFFING OF NEIGHBORHOOD STOREFRONT CENTERS WITH NON-PROFESSIONALS ARE EXAMPLES OF INNOVATIVE PROGRAMS DESIGNED TO BRING ABOUT SUBSTANTIAL CHANGES IN THE COMMUNITY'S MENTAL HEALTH STATUS. 8 REFERENCES. (JOURNAL ABSTRACT)

ACCN 001229

1427 AUTH **PECK, R. F., MANASTER, G. J., BORICH, G., ANGELINI, A. L., DIAZ-GUERRERO, R., & KUBO, S.**

TITL A TEST OF THE UNIVERSALITY OF AN "ACCULTURATION GRADIENT" IN THREE CULTURE-TRIADS.

SRCE *IN K. F. RIEGEL & J. A. MEACHAM (EDS.), THE DEVELOPING INDIVIDUAL IN A CHANGING WORLD, VOL 1: HISTORICAL AND CULTURAL ISSUES. CHICAGO: ALDINE PUBLISHERS, 1976, PP. 355-363.*

INDX ACCULTURATION, ACHIEVEMENT MOTIVATION, CHILDREN, EMPIRICAL, ADOLESCENTS, ATTITUDES, CROSS CULTURAL, MEXICAN, MEXICAN AMERICAN, MIGRATION, OCCUPATIONAL ASPIRATIONS, SOCIAL MOBILITY, SOUTH AMERICA, CULTURAL FACTORS, TEXAS, SOUTHWEST, IMMIGRATION, SES, VALUES

ABST A LINEAR ACCULTURATION MODEL SUGGESTS THAT IMMIGRANTS BRING THE VALUES OF THEIR "CORE CULTURE" OF ORIGIN TO THEIR NEW LOCALE. BUT OVER TIME THE VALUES OF THE OLD SOCIETY ARE GRADUALLY REPLACED BY THOSE OF THE NEW "CORE CULTURE." THIS "ACCULTURATION GRADIENT" MODEL WAS TESTED WITH DATA ON SCHOOL CHILDREN FROM THREE DIFFERENT "CULTURE TRIADS" (TAKEN FROM THE EIGHT-NATION CROSS-NATIONAL STUDY OF COPING STYLES AND MECHANISMS, 1965-1973, FROM THE U.S. OFFICE OF EDUCATION): (1) NATIVE JAPANESE (TOKYO)-JAPANESE-BRAZILIAN (SAO PAOLO)-BRAZILIAN (SAO PAOLO); (2) NATIVE MEXICAN (MEXICO CITY)-MEXICAN AMERICAN (AUSTIN, TEXAS)-ANGLO AMERICAN (AUSTIN); AND (3) SOUTHERN BLACKS (AUSTIN)-NORTHERN BLACKS (GARY, IND. AND CHICAGO)-ANGLO AMERICANS (CHICAGO): THE TOTAL SAMPLE CONSISTED OF 2,640 GIRLS AND BOYS, AGED 10 OR 14 YEARS, WHOSE FAMILIES WERE CLASSIFIED AS UPPER LOWER OR SKILLED WORKING CLASS. THIS PRESENT, PRELIMINARY REPORT IS AN ANALYSIS OF THE CHILDREN'S OCCUPATIONAL ASPIRATIONS AND CAREER VALUES AS MEASURED BY THE OCCUPATIONAL INTEREST INVENTORY AND THE OCCUPATIONAL VALUES INVENTORY WITH THE CAVEAT THAT THE "MIGRANT" SAMPLES PROBABLY DID NOT ORIGIATE IN THE SAME CULTURE GROUPS FROM WHICH THE "CORE CULTURE" OF ORIGIN SAMPLES WERE DRAWN. THE AUTHORS REPORT THAT THE "MIGRANT" SAMPLES FROM EACH TRIAD SHOWED PATTERNS OF VALUES AND EXPECTATIONS THAT ARE UNIQUE—A FUNCTION MORE OF THE REALITIES OF ECONOMIC CONDITIONS AND OPPORTUNITY IN THE "NEW" SOCIETY RATHER THAN A GRADUAL REJECTION OF "OLD" VALUES IN FAVOR OF THE "NEW." 2 REFERENCES.

ACCN 002179

1428 AUTH **PECK, R. F., & DIAZ-GUERRERO, R.**

TITL TWO CORE-CULTURE PATTERNS AND THE DIFFUSION OF VALUES ACROSS THEIR BORDER.

SRCE *INTERNATIONAL JOURNAL OF PSYCHOLOGY, 1967, 4(2), 272-282.*

INDX CULTURAL FACTORS, MEXICAN, CROSS CULTURAL, PEER GROUP, COLLEGE STUDENTS, ATTITUDES, MEXICAN AMERICAN, EMPIRICAL, ENVIRONMENTAL FACTORS, CULTURAL CHANGE, HIGHER EDUCATION, TEXAS, SOUTHWEST, VALUES

ABST A QUESTIONNAIRE OF 20 STATEMENTS WHICH ASSESSED THE VARIOUS MEANINGS OF "RESPECT" WAS ADMINISTERED TO 1,814 STUDENTS ATTENDING COLLEGE IN THE UNITED STATES AND MEXICO. TWO "CORE-CULTURE PATTERNS," ONE TYPIFYING STUDENTS IN

MEXICO CITY AND THE OTHER TYPIFYING STUDENTS IN TEXAS, WERE REVEALED. THE AMERICAN PATTERN IS CHARACTERIZED BY A RELATIVELY DETACHED, SELF-ASSURED EQUALITARIANISM, WHILE THE MEXICAN PATTERN IS ONE OF CLOSE-KNIT, HIGHLY EMOTIONALIZED, RECIPROCAL DEPENDENCE AND DUTIFULNESS WITHIN A FIRMLY AUTHORITARIAN FRAMEWORK. WHEN SAMPLES FROM THE BORDER ZONE (MONTERREY IN MEXICO AND EDINBURG IN TEXAS) WERE INCLUDED, THE RESPONSE-SIMILARITY ANALYSIS SUGGESTED CONSIDERABLE DIFFUSION OF VALUES IN THE BORDER AREA. THE LARGEST EFFECT APPEARS TO BE AN ASSIMILATIVE SEMIACCULTURATION OF MEXICAN AMERICANS IN EDINBURG TO THE "AMERICAN PATTERN." THERE IS ALSO EVIDENCE WHICH SUGGESTS SOME ACCULTURATION OF BORDER ANGLO AMERICANS TO MEXICAN VALUES. "THE BORDER EFFECT" PHENOMENON SOMETIMES OCCURS WHEREIN PEOPLE ON ONE OR BOTH SIDES OF THE BORDER ARE MORE DIFFERENT FROM EITHER "CORE-CULTURAL PATTERN" THAN MEMBERS OF THE CORE CULTURES ARE FROM EACH OTHER. 4 REFERENCES.

ACCN 001230

1429 AUTH **PECK, R. F., & GALLANI, C.**
TITL INTELLIGENCE, ETHNICITY AND SOCIAL ROLES IN ADOLESCENT SOCIETY.
SRCE *SOCIOMETRY, 1962, 25(1), 64-72.*
INDX ROLE EXPECTATIONS, ADOLESCENTS, CALIFORNIA TEST OF MENTAL MATURITY, CROSS CULTURAL, EMPIRICAL, SPANISH SURNAMED, INTELLIGENCE TESTING, CULTURAL FACTORS, LEADERSHIP, PEER GROUP, INTELLIGENCE, TEXAS, SOUTHWEST, INTERPERSONAL ATTRACTION
ABST THE RELATIONSHIP OF INTELLIGENCE TO SOCIAL VISIBILITY, THE DIFFERENTIATION OF SOCIAL ROLE GROUPS ACCORDING TO THEIR INTELLIGENCE, AND THE POSSIBILITY OF ETHNIC INFLUENCES ON SOCIAL VISIBILITY WERE INVESTIGATED. SPECIFIC HYPOTHESES WERE: (1) ADOLESCENTS WITH ABOVE AVERAGE INTELLIGENCE ARE MORE LIKELY TO BE SOCIALLY VISIBLE TO THEIR AGE-MATES THAN ADOLESCENTS OF BELOW AVERAGE INTELLIGENCE; (2) ADOLESCENTS TEND TO ESTIMATE EACH OTHER'S INTELLIGENCE WITH REASONABLE ACCURACY AND ASSIGN SOCIAL ROLES IN KEEPING WITH ACTUAL CAPACITIES; AND (3) ADOLESCENTS FROM ANGLO AMERICAN BACKGROUNDS ARE NOMINATED MORE FREQUENTLY FOR ANY ROLE, BY THE TOTAL GROUP OF THEIR AGE-MATES, THAN ARE THEIR CLASSMATES FROM LATIN AMERICAN BACKGROUNDS IN SCHOOLS OF MIXED ETHNIC COMPOSITION. A SAMPLE OF 1,217 SEVENTH GRADE STUDENTS WERE ADMINISTERED THE CALIFORNIA TEST OF MENTAL MATURITY (CTMM), MCGUIRRE'S ROLE NOMINATIONS INSTRUMENT, AND A NUMBER OF OTHER SOCIOLOGICAL AND PSYCHOLOGICAL TESTS. THE DATA CONFIRMED ALL THREE HYPOTHESES. WHATEVER "GENERAL" INTELLIGENCE MAY BE REFLECTED IN APTITUDE TEST SCORES, THIS

INTELLIGENCE ALSO INFLUENCES THE EFFECTIVENESS OF ADOLESCENTS' SOCIAL BEHAVIOR. ADOLESCENTS ALSO RESPECT SOCIAL BEHAVIOR THAT IS CHARACTERIZED BY INTELLIGENT ACTION, AND THEY TEND TO CHOOSE AS THEIR LEADERS THOSE WHO HAVE MORE THAN AVERAGE MENTAL ABILITY. IT APPEARS THAT ETHNIC FACTORS DECIDEDLY BIAS THE JUDGMENTS OF ADOLESCENTS IN THESE MIXED COMMUNITIES. ADOLESCENTS OF BOTH ETHNIC GROUPS UNITE IN ASSIGNING BRIGHTER-THAN-AVERAGE ANGLO YOUTHS TO LEADING OR ADMIRED ROLES. IT IS CONCLUDED THAT "LATIN INVISIBILITY" IS NOT JUST THE RESULT OF DISCRIMINATION FROM NON-LATIN YOUTHS BUT THE CREATION OF LATIN BOYS AND GIRLS THEMSELVES. THE IMPLICATION IS THAT THE ASSIMILATION OF LATIN AMERICAN YOUTH INTO ACTIVE PARTICIPATION IN THE SOCIAL AND CIVIC LIFE OF THE UNITED STATES MAY BE MUCH SLOWER AND LESS CERTAIN THAN WITH MOST OTHER IMMIGRANT GROUPS. 9 REFERENCES.

ACCN 001231

1430 AUTH **PEDHAZUR, L., & WHEELER, L.**
TITL LOCUS OF PERCEIVED CONTROL AND NEED ACHIEVEMENT.
SRCE *PERCEPTUAL AND MOTOR SKILLS, 1971, 33(3), 1281-1282.*
INDX PUERTO RICAN-M, EMPIRICAL, CHILDREN, CROSS CULTURAL, PERSONALITY ASSESSMENT, NEW YORK, EAST, LOCUS OF CONTROL, ACHIEVEMENT MOTIVATION
ABST FORTY-FIVE BLACK AND EIGHT PUERTO RICAN CHILDREN INDICATED MORE PERCEIVED EXTERNAL CONTROL THAN DID A COMPARISON GROUP OF 23 JEWISH SUBJECTS IN GRADES FIVE AND SIX; THIS WAS RELATED TO LOW NEED ACHIEVEMENT. OF THE ORIGINAL 53 BLACK AND PUERTO RICAN SUBJECTS, ONLY 44 OUT OF THE TOTAL MINORITY GROUP WERE INCLUDED IN THE ANALYSIS. WITHIN THE CONTEXT OF A READING ASSIGNMENT OF SEVERAL STORIES, MINORITY CHILDREN READ A PARAGRAPH ILLUSTRATING EITHER EXTERNAL OR INTERNAL CONTROL. WHEN THE MINORITY CHILDREN READ A STORY MAKING PERCEIVED INTERNAL CONTROL MORE SALIENT, MEASUREMENTS INDICATED AN INCREASE IN BOTH NEED ACHIEVEMENT AND INTERNAL CONTROL. 3 REFERENCES. (JOURNAL ABSTRACT MODIFIED)

ACCN 001232

1431 AUTH **PEELE, R.**
TITL PSYCHIATRY AND THE CRIMINAL JUSTICE SYSTEM: THE INVISIBLE BARRIER. A SUMMARY OF A PANEL DISCUSSION.
SRCE *IN E. R. PADILLA & A. M. PADILLA (EDS.), TRANSCULTURAL PSYCHIATRY: AN HISPANIC PERSPECTIVE (MONOGRAPH NO. 4). LOS ANGELES: UNIVERSITY OF CALIFORNIA, SPANISH SPEAKING MENTAL HEALTH RESEARCH CENTER, 1977, PP. 101-103.*
INDX CORRECTIONS, JUDICIAL PROCESS, REHABILITATION, ESSAY, MENTAL HEALTH PROFESSION, PROFESSIONAL TRAINING

ABST   A PANEL DISCUSSION OF THE INTERFACE BE-
TWEEN PSYCHIATRY AND THE CRIMINAL JUS-
TICE SYSTEM REVEALS THAT THEY HAVE (1)
DIFFERENT GOALS, (2) DIFFERENT ASSUMP-
TIONS, (3) DIFFERENT DEFINITIONS OF KEY
WORDS, AND (4) DIFFERENT WAYS OF AP-
PROACHING A PROBLEM. THE GOAL OF THE
MENTAL HEALTH SYSTEM IS THE CARE AND
TREATMENT OF THE MENTALLY ILL. A DETER-
MINISTIC MODEL OF THE MIND IS ADOPTED,
THEREBY PROVIDING PREDICTABILITY FOR
THERAPEUTIC INTERVENTIONS. AND TRUTH,
MEASURED IN GRADATIONS, IS APPROACHED
EMPIRICALLY. IN CONTRAST, THE JUDICIAL
SYSTEM ACHIEVES ITS GOAL OF JUSTICE BY
UTILIZING A RATIONAL MODEL OF BEHAVIOR
WHICH ASSUMES THAT INDIVIDUALS HAVE FREE
WILL (CONTRAPOSED TO THE DETERMINISTIC
MODEL); AND IN THIS RATIONALISTIC AP-
PROACH, TRUTH IS DEFINED IN ABSOLUTE
TERMS. BECAUSE OF SUCH FUNDAMENTAL
DIFFERENCES, CONFLICTS ARISE BETWEEN
THOSE IN THE PSYCHIATRIC AND LEGAL
PROFESSIONS. TO MITIGATE SUCH CON-
FLICTS, SEVERAL RECOMMENDATIONS ARE
OFFERED: (1) GREATER EXPOSURE OF LAW-
YERS AND PSYCHIATRISTS TO ONE ANOTHER
DURING TRAINING; (2) MINIMAL INVOLVEMENT
BY PSYCHIATRISTS IN THE DETERMINATION OF
GUILT AT CRIMINAL TRIALS; AND (3) FORMA-
TION OF AN AMALGAM OF LAW, PSYCHIATRY,
AND SOCIAL WORK TO PRESIDE AS JUDGES. A
PUERTO RICAN PROGRAM (TASC-TREATMENT
AS AN ALTERNATIVE TO STREET CRIME, IN
WHICH DRUG ADDICTS HAVE BEEN DIVERTED
FROM THE CRIMINAL JUSTICE SYSTEM TO THE
MENTAL HEALTH SYSTEM) IS PRESENTED AS A
MODEL TO BE EXPLORED FOR FURTHER USE.

ACCN   001233

1432 AUTH   **PENA, A. A.**
TITL   CREATING POSITIVE ATTITUDES TOWARDS BI-
LINGUAL-BICULTURAL EDUCATION.
SRCE   *IN A. CASTANEDA, M. RAMIREZ, III, C. E. CORTES,
& M. BARRERA (EDS.), MEXICAN AMERICANS
AND EDUCATIONAL CHANGE. NEW YORK: ARNO
PRESS, 1974, PP. 363-372.*
INDX   MEXICAN AMERICAN, BILINGUAL-BICULTURAL
EDUCATION, EDUCATION, ATTITUDES, COM-
MUNITY INVOLVEMENT, CULTURE, CULTURAL
PLURALISM, LANGUAGE LEARNING, BILIN-
GUALISM, CULTURE, INSTRUCTIONAL TECH-
NIQUES
ABST   CHANGES IN ATTITUDES TOWARDS BILIN-
GUAL/BICULTURAL EDUCATION (B/BE) ARE
NECESSARY FOR THE IMPLEMENTATION OF B/
BE AS A VIABLE APPROACH TO EQUAL EDU-
CATIONAL OPPORTUNITY AND CROSS CUL-
TURAL LEARNING. MONOCULTURAL ATTI-
TUDES WITHIN THE SCHOOLS FORCE
STUDENTS OF DIFFERENT ETHNIC BACK-
GROUNDS TO REJECT BOTH THEIR OWN CUL-
TURE AND LANGUAGE. INSISTENCE ON MON-
OLINGUAL ATTITUDES HAVE DEPRIVED NON-
ENGLISH SPEAKING STUDENTS THE OPPOR-
TUNITY TO LEARN SIMILAR CONCEPTS AT THE
SAME RATE AS THEIR ENGLISH SPEAKING
PEERS. THE IMPLEMENTATION OF B/BE AT-

TACKS THESE TWO FACTORS BY: (1) REDUC-
ING CULTURAL INSENSITIVITY THROUGH THE
PRACTICE OF APPRECIATING DIVERSE CUL-
TURES AND STIMULATING ETHNIC PRIDE; AND
(2) ALTERING THE MEDIUM OF INSTRUCTION
TO TEACH EDUCATIONAL CONCEPTS IN THE
LANGUAGE OF THE NON-ENGLISH SPEAKING
STUDENT WHILE PROVIDING INSTRUCTION IN
THE ENGLISH LANGUAGE. MISCONCEPTIONS
ABOUT B/BE STEM FROM THREE FACTORS: (1)
LACK OF ADEQUATE RESEARCH ON THE PART
OF ADMINISTRATORS AND FACULTY TO PLAN
AND IMPLEMENT SUCCESSFUL B/BE PRO-
GRAMS; (2) ABSENCE OF COMMUNITY LEVEL
PARTICIPATION IN B/BE PROGRAM DEVELOP-
MENT; AND (3) THE INSISTENCE OF EDUCA-
TORS IN UTILIZING INADEQUATE AND OUT-
DATED TEACHING METHODS. TO CREATE
POSITIVE ATTITUDES TOWARDS B/BE AND AS-
SURE SUCCESS: (1) SCHOOL ADMINISTRA-
TORS MUST LEND FULL SUPPORT TO B/BE
PROGRAMS IN THEIR DISTRICTS; (2) THE AF-
FECTED COMMUNITIES MUST BE THOR-
OUGHLY INFORMED OF THE NECESSITY FOR
AND THE FUNCTION OF B/BE, AND AT THE
SAME TIME BE INVOLVED IN THE PLANNING
AND IMPLEMENTATION OF THESE PROGRAMS;
AND (3) TEACHING STAFF MUST BE TOTALLY
SENSITIVE TO THE NEEDS AND LEARNING
STYLES OF MINORITY GROUP CHILDREN. CO-
OPERATION IS THE KEY TO THE SUCCESS OF
BILINGUAL/BICULTURAL EDUCATION.

ACCN   001234

1433 AUTH   **PENALOSA, F.**
TITL   CLASS CONSCIOUSNESS AND SOCIAL MOBIL-
ITY IN A MEXICAN AMERICAN COMMUNITY
(DOCTORAL DISSERTATION, UNIVERSITY OF
SOURTHERN CALIFORNIA, 1963).
SRCE   *DISSERTATION ABSTRACTS, 1964, 24(9), 3872.
(UNIVERSITY MICROFILMS NO. 64-02598.)*
INDX   SOCIAL MOBILITY, OCCUPATIONAL ASPIRA-
TIONS, SES, MEXICAN AMERICAN, EMPIRICAL,
COMMUNITY, ECONOMIC FACTORS, CALIFOR-
NIA, SOUTHWEST, CROSS GENERATIONAL,
ETHNIC IDENTITY
ABST   THE HYPOTHESES THAT VARIABLES INDICA-
TIVE OF HIGH ECONOMIC STATUS AND ORIEN-
TATION TO AMERICAN CULTURE WOULD BE
POSITIVELY ASSOCIATED WITH THE ABILITY TO
PERCEIVE CLAN DIVISIONS IN THE MEXICAN
AMERICAN COMMUNITY, WITH HIGH SELF-
PLACEMENT, AND WITH HIGH SOCIAL CLASS
STATUS WERE TESTED. A 6% RANDOM SAMPLE
OF ALL ADULTS OF MEXICAN DESCENT RESID-
ING IN POMONA, CALIFORNIA (N=147) WAS
OBTAINED FOR INTERVIEWS. OF THE 108 RE-
SPONDENTS WHO PERCEIVED A SOCIAL CLASS
SYSTEM IN THE MEXICAN AMERICAN COMMU-
NITY, 23.1% PERCEIVED ONE CLASS, 41.7%
TWO CLASSES, 31.5% THREE CLASSES, AND
3.7% FOUR CLASSES. RESPONDENTS GENER-
ALLY DESCRIBED A POOR, SEMILITERATE
GROUP OF UNACCULTURATED AND UN-
SKILLED WORKERS AND THEIR FAMILIES AS
THE BOTTOM STRATUM AND A "MIDDLE CLASS"
AS THE UPPER STRATUM. RESPONDENTS DE-
SCRIBED A MORE COMPLEX CLASS SYSTEM

FOR THE ANGLO THAN FOR THE MEXICAN COMMUNITY. OF THE 101 RESPONDENTS WHO CATEGORIZED THEMSELVES AS TO SOCIAL CLASS, 3.0% SAID THEY WERE UPPER CLASS, 58.4% MIDDLE, 22.8% WORKING, AND 15.8% LOWER. THE HIGHER A RESPONDENT RATED HIMSELF, THE LARGER WAS THE NUMBER OF SOCIAL CLASSES HE PERCEIVED. IN TERMS OF INTERGENERATIONAL OCCUPATIONAL MOBILITY, 40.1% OF ALL RESPONDENTS HAD BEEN UPWARDLY MOBILE, 31.3% NONMOBILE, AND 27.2% DOWNWARDLY MOBILE. UPWARDLY MOBILE PERSONS DID NOT TAKE ON A "SPANISH" IDENTIFICATION, AS OFTEN SUGGESTED IN THE LITERATURE, TO ANY SIGNIFICANT DEGREE. THE SECOND GENERATION HAS BEEN THE MOST UPWARDLY MOBILE, THE IMMIGRANT GENERATION THE LEAST. LASTLY, THE INTERCORRELATIONS OF KEY ECONOMIC AND CULTURAL VARIABLES WERE STUDIED FOR THE PURPOSE OF CONSTRUCTING STATUS AND SOCIOCULTURAL TYPOLOGIES FOR THE MEXICAN AMERICAN COMMUNITY. 95 REFERENCES. (JOURNAL ABSTRACT MODIFIED)

ACCN   001235

1434 AUTH   **PENALOSA, F.**
TITL   EDUCATION-INCOME DISCREPANCIES BETWEEN SECOND AND LATER-GENERATION MEXICAN-AMERICANS IN THE SOUTHWEST.
SRCE   *SOCIOLOGY AND SOCIAL RESEARCH, 1969, 53(4), 448-454.*
INDX   SES, ECONOMIC FACTORS, SCHOLASTIC ACHIEVEMENT, MEXICAN AMERICAN, EMPIRICAL, SOCIAL MOBILITY, CROSS GENERATIONAL, SOUTHWEST, ACCULTURATION, CALIFORNIA, ADULTS
ABST   RECENT CENSUS DATA CONTRADICT THE COMMON ASSUMPTION THAT FOR MEXICAN AMERICANS INCREASED EDUCATION LEADS TO BETTER JOB OPPORTUNITIES AND SUBSEQUENTLY HIGHER INCOME. THESE DATA SHOW THAT WHILE 3RD OR LATER GENERATION MEXICAN AMERICANS HAVE A HIGHER LEVEL OF SCHOOLING THAN 2ND GENERATION, THEIR INCOME LEVEL IS LOWER. THIS INCLUDES MEXICAN AMERICANS IN URBAN, RURAL-NONFARM, AND RURAL FARM AREAS IN FIVE SOUTHWESTERN STATES. A STUDY WAS CONDUCTED IN POMONA, CALIFORNIA, TO CLARIFY THE RELATIONSHIP BETWEEN EDUCATION AND INCOME AND TO EXAMINE THE CHARACTERISTICS OF THIRD OR LATER GENERATION GROUPS. A RANDOM SAMPLE OF 6% OF ALL MEXICAN AMERICAN ADULTS (N = 147) IN THE CITY WAS GIVEN A FORMAL, STRUCTURED INTERVIEW. THE RESULTS WERE CONSISTENT WITH THE MORE GENERAL, SOUTHWESTERNURBAN CENSUS DATA RELECTING LOWER INCOME AND HIGHER EDUCATION FOR THE THIRD GENERATION GROUP. IT WAS ALSO FOUND THAT THIRD OR LATER GENERATION RESPONDENTS WERE EITHER GRANDCHILDREN OR GREAT GRANDCHILDREN OF RECENT IMMIGRANTS, DESCENDENTS FROM 17TH CENTURY SPANISH COLONIALS, OR HAD ONE PARENT FROM EACH GROUP. IT IS SUGGESTED THAT A HIGH PROPORTION OF RELATIVELY UNACCULTURATED SPANISH COLONIAL DESCENDENTS HAVE BEEN UNABLE TO TRANSLATE HIGHER EDUCATION LEVELS INTO BETTER OCCUPATIONS. IN THE POMONA STUDY, SPANISH COLONIAL DESCENDENTS WERE FOUND TO BE IN THE GREATER PROPORTION OF THE THIRD OR LATER GENERATIONAL GROUP AND TO HAVE CONSISTENTLY LOWER OCCUPATIONAL AND INCOME LEVELS. YEARS OF SCHOOLING IS SEEN AS AN INACCURATE INDEX OF ACCULTURATION FOR THESE DESCENDENTS AND A LOW LEVEL OF ACCULTURATION IS SEEN AS A FACTOR IN LOWER OCCUPATIONAL STATUS. 6 REFERENCES.

ACCN   001236

1435 AUTH   **PENALOSA, F.**
TITL   MEXICAN FAMILY ROLES.
SRCE   *JOURNAL OF MARRIAGE AND THE FAMILY, 1968, 30(4), 680-689.*
INDX   FAMILY ROLES, MEXICAN, SEX ROLES, ROLE EXPECTATIONS, SOCIALIZATION, SOCIAL MOBILITY, ECONOMIC FACTORS, CULTURAL CHANGE, REVIEW, MALE, FEMALE, FAMILY STRUCTURE, MACHISMO
ABST   A SYNTHESIS OF THE WRITINGS OF MEXICAN SOCIAL SCIENTISTS SUGGESTS THAT MEXICAN FAMILY ROLES ARE PRIMARILY DETERMINED BY THE SUBMISSION OF FEMALE TO MALE AND OF THE YOUNGER TO THE OLDER. THE HUSBANDWIFE RELATIONSHIP EMPHASIZES HIS MANLINESS OR MACHISMO AND HIS ROLE AS AN AUTHORITARIAN PATRIARCH. THE FATHER-SON RELATIONSHIP TENDS TO BE DISTANT, RESPECTFUL, AND FREQUENTLY SEVERE. THE MOTHER HELPS PREPARE THE SON FOR DOMINANCE AND INDEPENDENCE. THE FATHERDAUGHTER RELATIONSHIP IS DISTANT THOUGH RELATIVELY CONFLICT FREE. THE MOTHERDAUGHTER RELATIONSHIP IS VERY CLOSE, THE DAUGHTER ACHIEVING AN EARLY IDENTIFICATION WITH THE FEMALE ROLE. YOUNGER CHILDREN RESPECT OLDER SIBLINGS AND GIRLS SHOW RESPECT FOR THEIR BROTHERS. SISTER-SISTER RELATIONS REMAIN CLOSE THROUGHOUT LIFE. FAMILY PATTERNS ARE BEING MODIFIED IN THE DIRECTION OF THE GREATER MOBILITY THAT IS INCREASINGLY CHARACTERIZING MEXICAN SOCIETY AS IT BECOMES MORE AND MORE INDUSTRIALIZED. AT THE SAME TIME, THE RAPID URBANIZATION PROCESS SEEMS TO BE WEAKENING THE AUTHORITARIAN-PATRIARCHAL FAMILY TRADITION. THE PATRIARCHAL SOCIETY IS BASED ON THE ABSOLUTE ECONOMIC DEPENDENCE OF THE FAMILY ON THE FATHER. WITH AN EXPANDING AND MODERNIZING ECONOMY, THERE ARE INCREASING OPPORTUNITIES FOR WOMEN TO GAIN ADVANCED EDUCATION AND EMPLOYMENT OUTSIDE THE HOME AND FOR YOUNG MEN TO ACHIEVE SOCIAL POSITIONS HIGHER THAN THOSE OF THEIR FATHERS. IT IS EXPECTED THEREFORE THAT, IN THE MORE MODERNIZED, INDUSTRIALIZED, AND URBANIZED UNITED STATES, THE MEXICAN FAMILY IS UNDERGOING ATTENUATIONS OF THE TRADITIONAL PATRIARCHAL, AUTHORITARIAN FAMILY. 24 REFERENCES.

ACCN   001237

1436 AUTH   **PENALOSA, F.**
     TITL   RECENT CHANGES AMONG THE CHICANOS.
     SRCE   *SOCIOLOGY AND SOCIAL RESEARCH, 1970, 55(1), 47-52.*
     INDX   MEXICAN AMERICAN, ESSAY, ETHNIC IDENTITY, ACCULTURATION, CHICANO MOVEMENT, CULTURAL CHANGE
     ABST   THE TERM "CHICANO" IS RAPIDLY REPLACING THE TERM "MEXICAN AMERICAN" AS THE SELF-CHOSEN TERM FOR THE GROUP, ESPECIALLY AMONG ITS MORE MILITANT AND BETTER INFORMED MEMBERS. A STRONGER SENSE OF COMMUNITY IS DEVELOPING AMONG THE CHICANOS, AT THE SAME TIME THAT PRIDE IN THE BARRIO SUBCULTURE IS INCREASING AND A RENEWED INTEREST IS MANIFESTED IN MEXICO'S SCIENTIFIC AND HUMANISTIC ACHIEVEMENTS. SOCIAL AND POLITICAL ACTION IS TAKING MORE MILITANT FORMS. SOME OF THE MOST SIGNIFICANT RECENT GAINS HAVE BEEN IN HIGHER EDUCATION, WITH THE INCREASE IN MEXICAN AMERICAN ENROLLMENT AND THE INSTITUTION OF CHICANO STUDIES PROGRAMS. 10 REFERENCES.
     ACCN   001238

1437 AUTH   **PENALOSA, F., & MCDONAGH, E. C.**
     TITL   EDUCATION, ECONOMIC STATUS AND THE SOCIAL-CLASS AWARENESS OF MEXICAN-AMERICANS.
     SRCE   *PHYLON, 1968, 29, 119-126.*
     INDX   MEXICAN AMERICAN, SES, ACCULTURATION, OCCUPATIONAL ASPIRATIONS, SCHOLASTIC ASPIRATIONS, DISCRIMINATION, SCHOLASTIC ACHIEVEMENT, BILINGUAL, BILINGUALISM
     ABST   TWO HYPOTHESES WERE TESTED: (1) THAT MEXICAN AMERICANS OF HIGHER SOCIAL CLASS STATUS WOULD HAVE A GREATER DEGREE OF CLASS AWARENESS THAN LOWER CLASS MEXICAN AMERICANS; AND (2) THAT MEASURES OF ACCULTURATION WOULD BE BETTER ASSOCIATED WITH SOCIAL CLASS AWARENESS THAN ECONOMIC STATUS WERE TESTED. A 6% RANDOM SAMPLE OF ALL ADULTS OF MEXICAN DESCENT RESIDING IN POMONA, CALIFORNIA, WAS OBTAINED (N=147). INTERVIEWS WERE CONDUCTED TO ACQUIRE PERSONAL DATA (E.G., AGE AND EDUCATIONAL LEVEL), THE RESPONDENTS' PERCEPTIONS OF THE SOCIAL CLASS STRUCTURE OF MEXICAN AMERICANS, AND THE RESPONDENTS' IDENTIFICATION OF THEIR OWN SOCIAL CLASS. THE FINDINGS INDICATE THAT: (1) MEXICAN AMERICANS IN A HIGHER SOCIAL CLASS WERE MORE AWARE OF THEIR OWN SOCIAL CLASS POSITION THAN MEXICAN AMERICANS IN LOWER CLASSES; (2) HIGHER CLASS MEXICAN AMERICANS PERCEIVED MORE CLASS DIVISIONS IN THEIR ETHNIC COMMUNITY THAN THOSE OF THE LOWER CLASSES; (3) THE MORE ACCULTURATED MEXICAN AMERICANS IN TERMS OF LANGUAGE, EDUCATION, AGE AND GENERATION, WERE ALSO MORE AWARE OF THEIR SOCIAL CLASS POSITION AND OF THE CLASS DIVISIONS WITHIN THE MEXICAN AMERICAN COMMUNITY; AND (4) ACCULTURATION INDICES WERE MORE STRONGLY RELATED TO THE MEXICAN AMERICANS' PERCEPTIONS OF THE MEXICAN AMERICAN CLASS STRUCTURE AND OF THEIR PERSONAL CLASS POSITION THAN WERE ECONOMIC INDICES (E.G., OCCUPATION, INCOME, RESIDENTIAL AREA). THESE RESULTS ARE SUPPORTIVE OF THE NEED FOR MEXICAN AMERICANS TO HAVE QUALITY EDUCATION IF SOCIAL MOBILITY AND ACCULTURATION ARE TO BE ENHANCED. 18 REFERENCES.
     ACCN   001239

1438 AUTH   **PENALOSA, F., & MCDONAGH, E. C.**
     TITL   SOCIAL MOBILITY IN A MEXICAN AMERICAN COMMUNITY.
     SRCE   *IN N. N. WAGNER & M. J. HAUG (EDS.), CHICANOS: SOCIAL AND PSYCHOLOGICAL PERSPECTIVES. SAINT LOUIS: C. V. MOSBY COMPANY, 1971, PP. 85-92.*
     INDX   SOCIAL MOBILITY, MEXICAN AMERICAN, COMMUNITY, ACCULTURATION, ADULTS, CROSS GENERATIONAL, ETHNIC IDENTITY, EMPIRICAL, SURVEY, SOUTHWEST, CALIFORNIA
     ABST   THE HYPOTHESIS THAT UPWARD SOCIAL MOBILITY INCREASES IN A MEXICAN AMERICAN (MA) POPULATION BY GENERATION AND THAT MORE ACCULTURATED INDIVIDUALS HAVE BEEN THE MOST MOBILE IS INVESTIGATED. A STRUCTURED INTERVIEW SCHEDULE WAS ADMINISTERED TO 6 PERCENT OF THE MEXICAN DESCENDED SPANISH SURNAMED ADULTS LIVING IN EACH OF FIVE AREAS OF POMONA, CALIFORNIA. DATA INDICATE THAT 40.1 PERCENT OF MA ADULTS ARE UPWARDLY MOBILE, 31.3 PERCENT NONMOBILE, AND 27.2 PERCENT DOWNWARDLY MOBILE. THE SECOND GENERATION OF MEXICAN AMERICANS EXPERIENCE A HIGHER PERCENTAGE OF UPWARDLY MOBILE RESPONDENTS (51.2%) AND A LOWER PERCENTAGE OF DOWNWARDLY MOBILE RESPONDENTS (22.1%) THAN EARLIER OR LATER GENERATIONS. THE SECOND GENERATION SIMILARLY ENJOYS THE HIGHEST AVERAGE INCOME, THE HIGHEST OCCUPATIONAL STATUS, AND IS OVERREPRESENTED IN THE HIGHEST STATUS RESIDENTIAL AREAS. UPWARDLY MOBILE MA RESPONDENTS ARE BETTER EDUCATED, MORE OFTEN PREFER ENGLISH, ARE MORE LIKELY TO BE CATHOLIC, AND HAVE A GREATER DEGREE OF CLASS AWARENESS. UPWARDLY MOBILE MEXICAN AMERICANS RETAIN THEIR MEXICAN ETHNIC IDENTIFICATION AND NO SIGNIFICANT RELATIONSHIP IS FOUND BETWEEN VERTICAL AND HORIZONTAL MOBILITY IN THIS MA POPULATION. IT IS SUGGESTED THAT THE SHEDDING OF LOWER CLASS CULTURE RATHER THAN ETHNICITY IS MOST RELATED WITH UPWARD MOBILITY. 27 REFERENCES.
     ACCN   001240

1439 AUTH   **PEREZ, M. S.**
     TITL   COUNSELING SERVICES AT UNIVERSITY OF CALIFORNIA-SANTA CRUZ: ATTITUDES AND PERSPECTIVES OF CHICANO STUDENTS.
     SRCE   *UNPUBLISHED MANUCRIPT, UNIVERSITY OF CALIFORNIA, SANTA CRUZ, 1975.*

INDX RESOURCE UTILIZATION, HIGHER EDUCATION, COLLEGE STUDENTS, MEXICAN AMERICAN, PSYCHOTHERAPY, EDUCATIONAL COUNSELING, SES, STRESS, ATTITUDES, ACCULTURATION, PSYCHOTHERAPISTS, EMPIRICAL, CULTURAL PLURALISM, CALIFORNIA, SOUTHWEST, POLICY

ABST REASONS FOR UNDERUTILIZATION OF PSYCHIATRIC/MENTAL HEALTH SERVICES BY CHICANO STUDENTS AT THE UNIVERSITY OF CALIFORNIA AT SANTA CRUZ WERE EXPLORED BY MEANS OF A TWO-PART QUESTIONNAIRE. THE FIRST PART OF THE QUESTIONNAIRE WAS ADMINISTERED TO 100 CHICANO STUDENTS, ALMOST ALL FROM LOW SOCIOECONOMIC BACKGROUNDS AND HAVING CLOSE CULTURAL TIES WITH MEXICO. THE QUESTIONNAIRE'S SECOND PART WAS ALSO ADMINISTERED TO THESE 100 STUDENTS AS WELL AS TO 76 NON-MINORITY STUDENTS. FINDINGS WERE THAT THE CHICANO STUDENTS: (1) HAD LITTLE OR NO DIRECT EXPERIENCE WITH MENTAL HEALTH SERVICES PRIOR TO THEIR ENROLLMENT IN COLLEGE; (2) WERE MOST AWARE OF AND ALSO LISTED "MINORITY COUNSELORS" AS THEIR MOST PREFERRED RESOURCE; (3) MORE OFTEN CITED SOURCES OF STRESS DIRECTLY RELATED TO PRESSURES BROUGHT TO BEAR UPON THEM BY THE UNIVERSITY SYSTEM; AND (4) HAD LESS POSITIVE ATTITUDES TOWARD PSYCHOTHERAPY IN GENERAL THAN DID NON-MINORITY STUDENTS. BASED UPON THESE FINDINGS, THE FOLLOWING RECOMMENDATIONS WERE PROPOSED TO IMPROVE THE UNIVERSITY'S COUNSELING SERVICES TO CHICANOS: (1) A MALE CHICANO COUNSELOR MUST BE ADDED AS A FULL-TIME POSITION TO THE COUNSELING STAFF; (2) AN OUTREACH PROGRAM MUST BE PLANNED, FINANCED, AND IMPLEMENTED TO IMPROVE PRESENT SERVICE DELIVERY; (3) ALTERNATIVE METHODS OF PSYCHOTHERAPY WHICH ARE MORE CULTURALLY RELEVANT MUST BE EXPLORED; AND (4) AN IN-SERVICE PROGRAM SHOULD BE PROVIDED BY WHICH THE COUNSELING STAFF CAN GAIN A BETTER UNDERSTANDING OF THE CULTURAL BACKGROUNDS OF CHICANO STUDENTS. 13 REFERENCES.

ACCN 001242

1440 AUTH **PEREZ, R., PADILLA, A. M., RAMIREZ, A., RAMIREZ, R., & RODRIGUEZ, M.**

TITL CORRELATES AND CHANGES OVER TIME IN DRUG AND ALCOHOL USE WITHIN A BARRIO POPULATION (OCCASIONAL PAPER NO. 9).

SRCE *LOS ANGELES: UNIVERSITY OF CALIFORNIA, SPANISH SPEAKING MENTAL HEALTH RESEARCH CENTER, 1979.*

INDX DRUG ABUSE, ADOLESCENTS, SELF CONCEPT, CALIFORNIA, SOUTHWEST, URBAN, PEER GROUP, ATTITUDES, INHALANT ABUSE, ALCOHOLISM, SEX COMPARISON, SURVEY, MEXICAN AMERICAN, EMPIRICAL

ABST THE EXTENT AND DETERMINANTS OF THE USE OF ALCOHOL, MARIJUANA, INHALANTS, AND PCP (I.E., ANGEL DUST) WERE EXPLORED IN A GROUP OF 339 MEXICAN AMERICAN YOUTHS LIVING IN EAST LOS ANGELES HOUSING PROJ-

ECTS. RESULTS OF THE STUDY WERE COMPARED WITH THOSE FROM A SIMILAR STUDY CONDUCTED TWO YEARS PREVIOUSLY. THIS COMPARISON REVEALED THAT THE USE OF INHALANTS HAD DECLINED MARKEDLY DURING THE TWO YEARS. HOWEVER, USE OF ALCOHOL AND MARIJUANA HAD INCREASED ACROSS ALL AGE AND SEX COHORTS. PREVALENCE OF PCP USE, EXPLORED FOR THE FIRST TIME IN THIS STUDY, PROVED TO BE EXTREMELY HIGH. THE USE OF ALL DRUGS WAS GENERALLY PREDICTED BY AGE, SEX, AND NUMBER OF PEERS REPORTING USE. SELF-CONCEPT FACTORS, ESPECIALLY ONE'S SELF-EVALUATION WITH RESPECT TO OTHERS, WERE ALSO SIGNIFICANT PREDICTORS TO USE OF MARIJUANA, INHALANTS, AND PCP. HOWEVER, ALCOHOL USE WAS NOT RELATED TO ANY SELF-CONCEPT FACTORS. LANGUAGE (SPANISH-ENGLISH) USED BOTH IN THE HOME AND WITH PEERS WAS RELATED TO USE OF ALL SUBSTANCES STUDIED. LIMITATIONS IN THE GENERALIZATION OF THIS STUDY'S FINDINGS DUE TO SAMPLING PROBLEMS ARE DISCUSSED. 32 REFERENCES. (AUTHOR ABSTRACT)

ACCN 001834

1441 AUTH **PEREZ, R., PADILLA, A. M., & RAMIREZ, A.**

TITL EXPECTATIONS TOWARD SCHOOL BUSING IN MEXICAN AMERICAN BARRIO YOUTH (OCCASIONAL PAPER NO. 10).

SRCE *LOS ANGELES: UNIVERSITY OF CALIFORNIA, SPANISH SPEAKING MENTAL HEALTH RESEARCH CENTER, 1979.*

INDX MEXICAN AMERICAN, ADOLESCENTS, CALIFORNIA, SOUTHWEST, URBAN, INTEGRATION, ATTITUDES, EMPIRICAL, INTERPERSONAL ATTRACTION, CULTURAL FACTORS, SELF CONCEPT

ABST EXPECTATIONS HELD TOWARD VARIOUS DIMENSIONS OF ENFORCED DESEGREGATION THROUGH BUSING WERE EXPLORED IN A GROUP OF 150 NINE TO SEVENTEEN YEAR-OLD MEXICAN AMERICAN STUDENTS IN EAST LOS ANGELES. THESE EXPECTATIONS WERE MEASURED ABOUT 30 DAYS PRIOR TO THE ONSET OF A CITYWIDE BUSING PLAN. STUDENTS HELD NEGATIVE OPINIONS TOWARD BUSING AND PREFERRED NOT BE PERSONALLY INVOLVED IN THE PROGRAM. THE EXPECTED EFFECTS OF BUSING ON INTERPERSONAL RELATIONS WERE CONSIDERABLY MORE SALIENT TO THE STUDENTS THAN WERE THE EXPECTED BUSING-RELATED EDUCATIONAL BENEFITS. STUDENTS GENERALLY EXPECTED GOOD INTERPERSONAL RELATIONS WITH THEIR ANGLO CLASSMATES, ALTHOUGH THEY ALSO ADMITTED THE POSSIBILITY OF SOME INTERPERSONAL CONFLICTS IN THE NEWLY DESEGREGATED SITUATION. THOSE STUDENTS WHO FIRMLY EXPECTED PERSONAL INVOLVEMENT IN BUSING TENDED TO HOLD MORE POSITIVE EXPECTATIONS ABOUT THE PROGRAM. VARIOUS SOCIODEMOGRAPHIC AND CULTURAL VARIABLES AND SEVERAL FACTOR-ANALYZED DIMENSIONS OF SELF-CONCEPT ARE ALSO EXPLORED FOR THEIR RELEVANCE TO EXPECTA-

TIONS ABOUT BUSING. 24 REFERENCES. (AUTHOR ABSTRACT)

ACCN   001833

1442 AUTH   **PERRY, J. B., JR., & SNYDER, E. E.**
TITL   OPINIONS OF FARM EMPLOYERS TOWARDS WELFARE ASSISTANCE FOR MEXICAN AMERICAN IMMIGRANT WORKERS.
SRCE   *SOCIOLOGY AND SOCIAL RESEARCH, 1971, 55, 161-169.*
INDX   LABOR FORCE, FARM LABORERS, MEXICAN AMERICAN, SES, POVERTY, SOCIAL SERVICES, EMPIRICAL, OHIO, MIDWEST, MIGRANTS, SURVEY, ATTITUDES
ABST   THE OPINIONS HELD BY EMPLOYERS OF MEXICAN AMERICAN AGRICULTURAL MIGRANTS ABOUT WELFARE ASSISTANCE FOR THEIR EMPLOYEES WERE STUDIED. QUESTIONNAIRES WERE MAILED TO FARM OPERATORS IN OHIO WITH LICENSED MIGRANT CAMPS. A 46% RESPONSE RATE WAS OBTAINED. CHI-SQUARE TESTS WERE CONDUCTED TO TEST THE RELATIONSHIP BETWEEN THE FARMERS' OPINIONS AND STATUS DISTANCE, AMOUNT OF CONTACT WITH MEXICAN AMERICANS, AND SOCIAL DEMOGRAPHIC DATA. THE FINDINGS INDICATE THAT (1) 79% OF THE SAMPLE FAILED TO NOTICE THAT WELFARE AID WAS FOLLOWED BY AN ABSENCE FROM WORK, AND (2) 49% BELIEVED THAT WELFARE ASSISTANCE INTERFERED TOO MUCH WITH FARM ACTIVITY WHILE 51% WERE EITHER NEUTRAL OR EXPRESSED FAVORABLE OPINIONS ABOUT THE WELFARE AGENCIES. ALTHOUGH EMPLOYERS OF MEXICAN AMERICAN MIGRANTS WERE NOT OVERWHELMINGLY NEGATIVE TOWARD WELFARE AID, THE FOLLOWING VARIABLES WERE ASSOCIATED WITH THE NEGATIVISM THAT EXISTED: RELIGION, STATUS DISTANCE AND EDUCATIONAL BACKGROUND. TENTATIVE EXPLANATIONS ARE OFFERED FOR THESE FINDINGS. 18 REFERENCES.

ACCN   001243

1443 AUTH   **PERRY, R. R., PHILLIPS, B. U., & MAHAN, J. M.**
TITL   A FOLLOW-UP EVALUATION OF A SUMMER HEALTH CAREER PROGRAM FOR MINORITY STUDENTS.
SRCE   *JOURNAL OF MEDICAL EDUCATION, 1975, 51(3), 175-180.*
INDX   EMPIRICAL, HEALTH, PROGRAM EVALUATION, OCCUPATIONAL ASPIRATIONS, MEXICAN AMERICAN, CROSS CULTURAL, TEXAS, SOUTHWEST, ADOLESCENTS
ABST   IN AN EFFORT TO ATTRACT MINORITY STUDENTS TO HEALTH CAREERS, A SPECIAL SUMMER EDUCATION HEALTH CAREER EXPERIENCE WAS DEVELOPED. A MATCHED COMPARISON GROUP DESIGN WAS UTILIZED TO DETERMINE THE VALUE OF THIS PROGRAM. DATA WERE COLLECTED ON BOTH THE 17 YEAR-OLD PARTICIPANTS AND A MATCHED COMPARISON GROUP THREE MONTHS BEFORE AND SIX MONTHS AFTER THE PROGRAM. DIFFERENCES ON MOST OF THE MEASURES WERE NOT SIGNIFICANT; HOWEVER, THERE WAS A SIGNIFICANT DIFFERENCE ON STABILITY OF FIRST CAREER CHOICE, INDICATING

THAT A SPECIAL SUMMER PROGRAM CAN AND DOES HAVE AN EFFECT ON THE PARTICIPANTS. THE STUDY MAKES IT CLEAR THAT PROGRAM EFFECTS CANNOT BE ASSUMED UNLESS A FOLLOW-UP EVALUATION IS UNDERTAKEN. THEREFORE, TO EVALUATE THE PROGRAM EFFECTS, IT IS SUGGESTED THAT THE FOLLOW-UP PERIOD BE EXTENDED AND ADDITIONAL QUESTIONS BE INCLUDED IN THE QUESTIONNAIRE. A RECOMMENDATION IS ALSO MADE FOR A COOPERATIVE EFFORT BETWEEN THE PLANNER AND THE EVALUATOR OF THESE PROGRAMS. 11 REFERENCES. (JOURNAL ABSTRACT MODIFIED)

ACCN   001244

1444 AUTH   **PETERSEN, B., & RAMIREZ, M., III.**
TITL   REAL IDEAL SELF DISPARITY IN NEGRO AND MEXICAN AMERICAN CHILDREN.
SRCE   *PSYCHOLOGY, 1971, 8(3), 22-28.*
INDX   MEXICAN AMERICAN, CROSS CULTURAL, CHILDREN, SELF CONCEPT, ETHNIC IDENTITY, CONFLICT RESOLUTION, EMPIRICAL, ADOLESCENTS
ABST   AN ATTEMPT TO OBTAIN A QUANTITATIVE MEASURE OF DEGREE OF SELF-REJECTION AMONG MINORITY GROUP CHILDREN IS REPORTED. SUBJECTS WERE 23 BLACK, 15 MEXICAN AMERICAN, AND 67 ANGLO STUDENTS IN THE 5TH THROUGH 8TH GRADES. IT WAS PREDICTED THAT NEGRO AND MEXICAN AMERICAN CHILDREN WOULD OBTAIN A GREATER DISCREPANCY BETWEEN THEIR REAL AND IDEAL SELVES THAN WOULD ANGLO CHILDREN. THE RESULTS SUPPORTED THE HYPOTHESIS. BOTH GROUPS OF MINORITY SUBJECTS OBTAINED SIGNIFICANTLY HIGHER SCORES THAN THE ANGLO SUBJECTS. THE REAL/IDEAL SCALE PROVED TO BE A PRODUCTIVE RESEARCH INSTRUMENT SINCE, THROUGH ITEM ANALYSIS, THE ASPECTS OF SELF-CONCEPT WHICH MEXICAN AMERICAN AND NEGRO CHILDREN SHARE AS MINORITY GROUP MEMBERS WERE REVEALED. IT ALSO PROVIDED EVIDENCE OF ASPECTS OF THE SELF-CONCEPT WHICH ARE UNIQUE TO EACH ETHNIC GROUP.

ACCN   001245

1445 AUTH   **PETERSON, P. Q.**
TITL   MIGRANT HEALTH—FUTURE OUTLOOK.
SRCE   *PAPER PRESENTED AT THE WESTERN REGIONAL MIGRANT HEALTH CONFERENCE, LOS ANGELES, JUNE 1967.*
INDX   HEALTH, FARM LABORERS, RURAL, POVERTY, HEALTH DELIVERY SYSTEMS, BILINGUAL-BICULTURAL PERSONNEL, SOCIAL SERVICES, DISCRIMINATION, PREJUDICE, POLITICAL POWER, POLITICS, LEGISLATION, ESSAY, MIGRANTS, PROGRAM EVALUATION, HEALTH EDUCATION
ABST   A DESCRIPTION AND EVALUATION OF THE MIGRANT HEALTH PROGRAM (MHP) IS PRESENTED. THE MHP, FEDERALLY MANDATED UNDER THE MIGRANT HEALTH ACT, WAS DESIGNED TO EXTEND HEALTH CARE TO PERSONS WHO MOVE ONE OR MORE TIMES EACH YEAR BEYOND NORMAL COMMUTING DISTANCE OF THEIR HOMES, AND WHO MUST ESTABLISH A

TEMPORARY RESIDENCE AWAY FROM HOME TO WORK IN AGRICULTURE. BEING GRANT-ASSISTED BY THE PUBLIC HEALTH SERVICE AND COMMUNITY-BASED, THE PROGRAM PURPORTS TO ENCOURAGE AND HELP THE COMMUNITY RECOGNIZE AND ASSUME ITS RESPONSIBILITY TO INCLUDE MIGRANTS IN ITS PLANNING AND PROVISION OF HEALTH SERVICES. STATE AGENCIES ARE ALSO ENCOURAGED TO BECOME INVOLVED IN THE MHP. THE ACHIEVEMENTS OF THE PROGRAM INCLUDE IMPROVED OUTREACH AND MULTIDISCIPLINARY APPROACHES IN ENCOURAGING MIGRANTS TO ADOPT IMPROVED HEALTH PRACTICES, INCREASED SUPPORT FROM THE PUBLIC SECTOR, GREATER USE OF PARAPROFESSIONAL HELP, AND LOCAL-STATE-FEDERAL PARTNERSHIP. INHERENT DIFFICULTIES ARE DISCUSSED THROUGH CASE EXAMPLES. MAJOR IMPROVEMENTS ARE PROJECTED THROUGH INCREASED PROGRAM IMPLEMENTATION AND ADDITIONAL FEDERAL LEGISLATION. 6 REFERENCES.

ACCN   001246

1446 AUTH   **PHILIPS, B. V., MAHAN, J. M., & PERRY, R. R.**
TITL   A FORMATIVE AND SUMMATIVE EVALUATION MODEL FOR SPECIAL EDUCATIONAL PROGRAMS.
SRCE   *JOURNAL OF MEDICAL EDUCATION, 1976, 51(10), 836-843.*
INDX   CULTURAL FACTORS, EDUCATION, EDUCATIONAL COUNSELING, EMPIRICAL, HEALTH EDUCATION, HIGHER EDUCATION, LEARNING, MEDICAL STUDENTS, MEXICAN AMERICAN, PROGRAM EVALUATION, SCHOLASTIC ASPIRATIONS, SPANISH SURNAMED, SOUTHWEST, EQUAL OPPORTUNITY, TEXAS
ABST   A DESIGN FOR EVALUATING EDUCATIONAL PROGRAMS IMPLEMENTED BY MEDICAL AND ALLIED HEALTH SCIENCE SCHOOLS FOR RECRUITING MINORITY STUDENTS TO THE HEALTH PROFESSIONS IS EXAMINED. THE AREA HEALTH EDUCATION CENTER AT THE UNIVERSITY OF TEXAS MEDICAL BRANCH SPONSORED A SUMMER PROGRAM FOR PREDOMINATELY MEXICAN AMERICAN, BILINGUAL, HIGH SCHOOL AND COLLEGE AGE STUDENTS TO INTRODUCE THEM TO CAREERS IN THE HEALTH PROFESSIONS, HELP THEM DEVELOP STUDY SKILLS, INTERPERSONAL AND COMMUNICATION SKILLS, PROVIDE INFORMATION ABOUT EDUCATION REQUIREMENTS FOR ENTRY INTO HEALTH FIELDS, AND TO HELP SOLIDIFY THEIR CAREER DECISIONS. THE EVALUATION DESIGN, CONTAINING BOTH FORMATIVE AND SUMMATIVE PHASES, IS TRACED THROUGH: (1) CAREER AREA PRETESTING; (2) ROTATION CAREER EXPERIENCE EVALUATION; (3) DAILY INTEGRATION FEEDBACK REPORTS; AND (4) FOLLOW-UP STUDIES COMPARING RESPONSES OF PARTICIPANTS WITH A MATCHED SAMPLE OF NONPARTICIPANTS CONCERNING CAREER INTERESTS, CHANGES, AND CURRENT AND FUTURE EDUCATIONAL PLANS. THE CONSIDERABLE SUCCESS OF THIS EVALUATION MODEL IS DISCUSSED IN LIGHT OF THE ACCOMPLISHMENT OF THE PROGRAM'S OBJECTIVES, AS WELL AS THE EFFICIENCY OF THE MODEL ITSELF IN PROVIDING USEFUL, SYSTEMATIC INPUT THROUGHOUT THE PROGRAM. IT IS CONCLUDED THAT GOOD EVALUATION OF SUCH A PROGRAM IS NOT BASED ON A SINGLE DATA COLLECTION POINT BUT BEGINS PRIOR TO THE PROGRAM, CONTINUES THROUGHOUT ITS DURATION, AND ENDS AFTER ITS COMPLETION. 10 REFERENCES.

ACCN   002180

1447 AUTH   **PHILLIPS, B. N.**
TITL   SCHOOL RELATED ASPIRATIONS OF CHILDREN WITH DIFFERENT CULTURAL BACKGROUNDS.
SRCE   *JOURNAL OF NEGRO EDUCATION, 1972, 41(1), 48-52.*
INDX   CROSS CULTURAL, SCHOLASTIC ACHIEVEMENT, SCHOLASTIC ASPIRATIONS, MEXICAN AMERICAN, CHILDREN
ABST   TO ASSESS CHILDREN'S REACTIONS TO SOCIAL AND ACADEMIC ACHIEVEMENT OPPORTUNITIES, 76 MIDDLE CLASS WHITE, 73 MEXICAN AMERICAN, AND 87 BLACK 4TH GRADE STUDENTS FROM 4 DIFFERENT ELEMENTARY SCHOOLS WERE ADMINISTERED 30 ITEMS FROM THE CHILDREN'S SCHOOL QUESTIONNAIRE PERTAINING TO SCHOOL RELATED ACHIEVEMENT ASPIRATIONS. THE RESULTS INDICATE THE FOLLOWING: (1) BLACKS USUALLY HAVE THE HIGHEST HOPES AND DESIRES FOR SCHOOL ACHIEVEMENT; (2) DIFFERENCES BETWEEN MIDDLE AND UPPER-LOWER CLASS WHITES ARE SIMILAR TO THOSE BETWEEN BLACKS AND MEXICAN AMERICANS IN THAT MEXICAN AMERICANS HAVE LOWER SOCIAL ASPIRATIONS THAN BLACKS, WHILE MIDDLE CLASS WHITES HAVE LOWER SOCIAL ASPIRATIONS THAN LOWER CLASS WHITES; AND (3) MEXICAN AMERICANS HAVE LOWER ACADEMIC ASPIRATIONS THAN BLACKS, BUT MIDDLE CLASS WHITES HAVE HIGHER ACADEMIC ASPIRATIONS THAN LOWER CLASS WHITES. THE DISCREPANCY BETWEEN SUCCESS AND ASPIRATIONS IS GREATEST FOR BLACKS, AND IT IS SUGGESTED THAT THIS CONTRIBUTES TO THE HIGHEST SCHOOL ANXIETY FOR THAT GROUP FOLLOWED BY MEXICAN AMERICANS, LOWER CLASS WHITES, AND FINALLY, MIDDLE CLASS WHITES. THIS CONCLUSION IS SUPPORTED BY PREVIOUS STUDIES. 9 REFERENCES. (PASAR ABSTRACT MODIFIED)

ACCN   001247

1448 AUTH   **PHILLIPUS, M. J.**
TITL   SUCCESSFUL AND UNSUCCESSFUL APPROACHES TO MENTAL HEALTH SERVICES FOR AN URBAN HISPANO-AMERICAN POPULATION.
SRCE   *JOURNAL OF PUBLIC HEALTH, 1971, 61(4), 820-830.*
INDX   MENTAL HEALTH, HEALTH DELIVERY SYSTEMS, PSYCHOTHERAPY, COMMUNITY, ESSAY, CULTURAL FACTORS, BILINGUAL-BICULTURAL PERSONNEL, PSYCHOSOCIAL ADJUSTMENT, CALIFORNIA, SOUTHWEST, PROGRAM EVALUATION
ABST   THE EXPERIENCES OF A MENTAL HEALTH TEAM IN DETERMINING SUCCESSFUL AND UNSUC-

CESSFUL APPROACHES TO MENTAL HEALTH SERVICES IN AN URBAN HISPANO POPULATION DURING A 2-YEAR PERIOD ARE PRESENTED. AN OUTLINE OF SUCCESSFUL METHODS THAT MIGHT BE UTILIZED IS PROVIDED. SUCCESSFUL APPROACHES AND RECOMMENDATIONS FOUND ARE AS FOLLOWS. (1) ACCESSIBILITY; A TEAM COMPOSED OF MEMBERS FROM DIFFERENT DISCIPLINES SHOULD BE PLACED DIRECTLY WITHIN THE NEIGHBORHOOD WHICH IS TO BE SERVED. (2) MENTAL HEALTH PATIENTS REGISTERED BY MENTAL HEALTH PERSONNEL; A BILINGUAL RECEPTIONIST IS INDISPENSABLE AND IS ONE OF THE MOST IMPORTANT TEAM MEMBERS. (3) CRISIS ORIENTATION OF TEAM PERSONNEL; A NEW PATIENT SHOULD BE SEEN AS SOON AS POSSIBLE AND NO WAITING LISTS SHOULD BE ESTABLISHED. (4) NECESSITY OF HAVING SPANISH-SPEAKING PERSONNEL; THE MORE SPANISH-SPEAKING STAFF IN MENTAL HEALTH THE GREATER THE EFFECTIVENESS ON THE HISPANO POPULATION. (5) USE OF DROP-IN ROOM; SERVICES SHOULD BE ACCESSIBLE AND IMMEDIATE IN RESPONSE TO ANTICIPATED RECURRING CRISES. (6) COMMUNITY INVOLVEMENT; A BOARD CONSISTING OF REPRESENTATIVES INDIGENOUS TO THE COMMUNITY SHOULD SERVE TO REFLECT THE NEEDS OF THE GENERAL COMMUNITY. (7) RELATIONSHIPS WITH MEDICAL SERVICES IN THE HEALTH CENTERS; IT IS IMPORTANT NOT TO SEPARATE THE TWO SERVICES BUT TO MAKE THEM EASILY ACCESSIBLE TO THE COMMUNITY. 5 REFERENCES.

ACCN   001248

1449 AUTH   PIERCE, R. C., CLARK, M. M., & KIEFER, C. W.
TITL   A "BOOTSTRAP" SCALING TECHNIQUE.
SRCE   HUMAN ORGANIZATION, 1972, 31(4), 403-410.
INDX   RESEARCH METHODOLOGY, ACCULTURATION, CROSS CULTURAL, MEXICAN AMERICAN, EMPIRICAL, CULTURE, TEST VALIDITY, TEST RELIABILITY, CALIFORNIA, SOUTHWEST
ABST   THE DEVELOPMENT OF A PICTORIAL, LANGUAGE-FREE METHOD FOR ASSESSING SOME OF THE COGNITIVE ASPECTS OF ACCULTURATION AMONG MEXICAN AMERICANS AND JAPANESE AMERICANS IS PRESENTED. SPECIFICALLY, THE KNOWLEDGE OF THESE ETHNIC GROUP MEMBERS OF THEIR OWN POPULAR CULTURE AND THAT OF THE ANGLO AMERICAN CULTURE WAS MEASURED. TWENTY-SEVEN MEXICAN AMERICANS AND 22 JAPANESE AMERICANS, OF WHICH FIRST, SECOND AND THIRD GENERATIONS WERE REPRESENTED, WERE ADMINISTERED A PICTURE-IDENTIFICATION TEST, WHICH INCLUDED POPULAR FIGURES, HISTORICAL PERSONAGES, WELL-KNOWN GEOGRAPHICAL SITES, AND FAMILIAR ARTIFACTS. THE CONSTRUCTION OF FOUR SCALES MEASURING AN ACQUAINTANCE WITH MEXICAN CULTURE, JAPANESE CULTURE AND AMERICAN CULTURE (ONE SCALE FOR MEXICAN AMERICANS AND ANOTHER FOR JAPANESE AMERICANS) WAS ACCOMPLISHED USING A CORRELATIONAL APPROACH TO GUARANTEE INTERNAL CONSISTENCY. A

METHOD TO OBTAIN A SINGLE SCORE REFLECTING ONE RELATIVE BALANCE BETWEEN THE TRADITIONAL CULTURE AND THE ADOPTED CULTURE WAS CONSTRUCTED AND STANDARIZED (ACCULTURATIVE BALANCE SCALE). THIS MEASURE MEETS THE CRITERIA OF BEING RELATED TO GENERATION BUT INDEPENDENT OF EDUCATION AND AGE WITHIN GENERATIONS. 4 REFERENCES.

ACCN   001249

1450 AUTH   PIERCE, R. C., CLARK, M., & KAUFMAN, S.
TITL   EXPLORATIONS OF ACCULTURATION AND ETHNIC IDENTITY: A TYPOLOGICAL ANALYSIS.
SRCE   UNPUBLISHED MANUSCRIPT, UNDATED. (AVAILABLE FROM DR. M. CLARK, UNIVERSITY OF CALIFORNIA, SAN FRANCISCO, CALIF.)
INDX   ACCULTURATION, ETHNIC IDENTITY, CROSS CULTURAL, MEXICAN AMERICAN, CULTURE, RESEARCH METHODOLOGY, EMPIRICAL
ABST   INTERVIEW DATA FROM A THREE GENERATIONAL SAMPLE OF JAPANESE AMERICANS AND MEXICAN AMERICANS WERE EXAMINED WITH THE AIM OF IDENTIFYING DIMENSIONS OF ACCULTURATION THAT COULD BE STUDIED QUANTITATIVELY. THREE MAJOR DIMENSIONS WERE DERIVED BY SCALING AND CLUSTER ANALYSIS—ACCULTURATIVE BALANCE, "TRADITIONAL ORIENTATION," AND "ANGLO FACE." SIX TYPES DISCOVERED IN A TYPOLOGICAL ANALYSIS ARE DESCRIBED. IT IS CONCLUDED THAT AT LEAST TWO COMPONENTS OF ACCULTURATION ARE ADEQUATELY ANALYZED AND THAT WITH MORE ITEMS AND BETTER MEASURES FURTHER DIMENSIONS MAY APPEAR. THE ANALYSIS INDICATES THAT THE MANNER OF ADAPTATION TO A NEW CULTURE IS DETERMINED BY PERSONAL FACTORS AS WELL AS BY AGE AND GENERATION. REFINEMENT OF THE DIMENSIONS UNCOVERED IS RECOMMENDED FOR FUTURE RESEARCH IN THIS AREA. 6 REFERENCES. (AUTHOR ABSTRACT MODIFIED)

ACCN   001250

1451 AUTH   PIERCE-JONES, J., REID, J. B., & KING, F. J.
TITL   ADOLESCENT RACIAL AND ETHNIC GROUP DIFFERENCES IN SOCIAL ATTITUDES AND ADJUSTMENT.
SRCE   PSYCHOLOGICAL REPORTS, 1959, 5(3), 549-552.
INDX   ADOLESCENTS, CULTURAL FACTORS, PERSONALITY, ANXIETY, CALIFORNIA ACHIEVEMENT TESTS, EDUCATION, ATTITUDES, PSYCHOSOCIAL ADJUSTMENT, CROSS CULTURAL, SPANISH SURNAMED, EMPIRICAL, TEXAS, SOUTHWEST
ABST   THE HYPOTHESIS THAT WHITE (ANGLO AND LATIN AMERICAN) AND NEGRO ADOLESCENTS OF SIMILAR MENTAL ABILITY LEVELS DIFFER IN SELECTED ORIENTATIONS TOWARD SOCIETY AND ITS INSTITUTIONS AND IN PERSONAL-SOCIAL ADJUSTMENT WAS TESTED. SUBJECTS WERE 252 TEXAS SEVENTH GRADE PUPILS (84 ANGLOS, 84 LATIN AMERICANS, 84 NEGROES). THE SELF-REPORT INSTRUMENTS USED WERE THE CHILDREN'S ANXIETY SCALE (CAS) AND SEVERAL COOPERATIVE YOUTH STUDY (CYS) SCALES DESIGNED TO MEASURE: NEGATIVISM

TOWARD SOCIETY; CRITICISM OF EDUCATION; FAMILY TENSIONS; FEELINGS OF SOCIAL INADEQUACY; AND PERSONAL ADJUSTMENT STATUS. DATA INDICATE THAT THE ONLY MEASURE WHICH DISTINGUISHES RELIABLY BETWEEN WHITE AND NEGROES IS THE CYS SCALE, "NEGATIVE ORIENTATION TO SOCIETY," ON WHICH NEGROES SCORE HIGHEST AND ANGLOS LOWEST. THIS DIFFERENCE IS INTERPRETED IN TERMS OF INTERGROUP RELATIONS AND SOCIALIZATION THEORY RATHER THAN BY MEANS OF ANY BIRACIAL CONCEPTS. OTHER SIGNIFICANT DIFFERENCES OBTAINED APPEAR TO BE INTERPRETABLE WITHIN A FRAMEWORK EMPHASIZING THE RELATIONS OF THE LATIN AMERICANS TO A MORE SOCIALLY VISIBLE, ACCESSIBLE, OR PSYCHOLOGICALLY UNIFIED CULTURAL GROUP. 6 REFERENCES.

ACCN   001251

1452 AUTH   **PINE, G. J.**
TITL   COUNSELING MINORITY GROUPS: A REVIEW OF THE LITERATURE.
SRCE   *COUNSELING AND VALUES, 1972, 17(1), 35-44.*
INDX   EDUCATIONAL COUNSELING, CROSS CULTURAL, CULTURAL FACTORS, MEXICAN AMERICAN, REVIEW, PSYCHOTHERAPY, PSYCHOTHERAPISTS, PSYCHOTHERAPY OUTCOME, ATTITUDES, ROLE EXPECTATIONS
ABST   THE ISSUES IN COUNSELING MINORITY GROUP MEMBERS, PRIMARILY BLACKS AND TO A LESSER DEGREE HISPANICS, ARE REVIEWED. IT HAS BEEN DEMONSTRATED THAT LOW SES CLIENTELE RECEIVE LOWER QUALITY SERVICES THAN HIGHER SES MEMBERS. THE MARKED CLASS AND ETHNIC DIFFERENCES BETWEEN THE THERAPIST AND LOW SES MINORITY CLIENT MAY LEAD TO POORER COUNSELING SERVICES. THE LITERATURE SUGGESTS THAT COUNSELORS SHOULD BECOME MORE SENSITIVE AND AWARE OF THEIR OWN VALUES (INCLUDING PREJUDICES) AS WELL AS THE VALUES OF THEIR CLIENTELE. INCREASED SELF-AWARENESS MAY LEAD TO INCREASED GENUINENESS, A NECESSARY CHARACTERISTIC IN COUNSELING MINORITY CLIENTS. THE ARGUMENTS FOR AND AGAINST THE THERAPIST BEING OF THE SAME SEX AND/OR ETHNICITY OF THE CLIENT ARE ALSO PRESENTED. FURTHERMORE, DIFFERENT VIEWS OF WHAT MINORITY CLIENTS EXPECT FROM COUNSELING ARE DISCUSSED. 96 REFERENCES.
ACCN   001252

1453 AUTH   **PINKNEY, A.**
TITL   PREJUDICE TOWARD MEXICAN AND NEGRO AMERICANS: A COMPARISON.
SRCE   *PHYLON, 1963, 24(4), 353-359. (REPRINTED IN J. H. BURMA, MEXICAN-AMERICANS IN THE UNITED STATES: A READER. CAMBRIDGE, MASSACHUSETTS: SCHENKMAN PUBLISHING CO., 1970, PP. 73-80.)*
INDX   ATTITUDES, MEXICAN AMERICAN, CROSS CULTURAL, PREJUDICE, EMPIRICAL, SOUTHWEST, ADULTS
ABST   A RANDOM SAMPLE OF 319 ANGLO AMERICAN (AA) ADULTS WERE INTERVIEWED WITH REF-

ERENCE TO THEIR ATTITUDES TOWARD TWO LOCAL ETHNIC MINORITY GROUPS—MEXICAN AMERICAN (MA) AND NEGRO AMERICAN (NA). FINDINGS INDICATE THAT ON THE WHOLE, AA'S APPROVED OF GREATER INTEGRATION OF MA'S THAN NA'S INTO THE COMMUNITY. THE ORDER IN WHICH AA'S ARE WILLING TO APPROVE OF THE POLICY ITEMS IS THE SAME: GREATEST DISAPPROVAL OF INTEGRATED HOUSING AND GREATEST APPROVAL OF INTEGRATION IN EMPLOYMENT IN DEPARTMENT STORES. THE DIFFERENCES IN RESPONSES ARE SIGNIFICANTLY MORE IN FAVOR OF INTEGRATION WITH THE MA THAN WITH THE NA. MANY OF THE AA'S FEEL THAT MA'S AND NA'S SHOULD BE DEPRIVED OF THE RIGHTS THEY THEMSELVES ENJOY. IN EACH CASE AA'S ARE WILLING TO ACCORD GREATER RIGHTS TO MA'S THAN TO NA'S. A MAJORITY OF THE RESPONDENTS FEEL THAT BOTH GROUPS SHOULD HAVE THE RIGHT TO EQUAL EMPLOYMENT, WHILE FEW FEEL THAT THEY SHOULD HAVE THE RIGHT TO EQUALITY IN HOUSING. THERE APPEARS TO BE A GREATER WILLINGNESS TO GRANT RIGHTS AS A MATTER OF LOCAL POLICY THAN TO ACCEPT THEM. THE DIFFERENCES IN ATTITUDES MAY BE ATTRIBUTED, IN PART, TO THE GENERAL FEELING AMONG AA'S THAT RACE IS A FUNCTION OF SKIN COLOR AND THAT THE CLOSER A MINORITY APPROACHES THE DOMINANT GROUP TRAIT, THE MORE ACCEPTABLE ARE ITS MEMBERS. 6 REFERENCES.
ACCN   001253

1454 AUTH   **PIORE, M. J.**
TITL   THE "NEW IMMIGRATION" AND THE PRESUMPTIONS OF SOCIAL POLICY.
SRCE   *IN J. L. STERN & B. D. DENNIS (EDS.), INDUSTRIAL RELATIONS RESEARCH ASSOCIATION SERIES: PROCEEDINGS OF THE TWENTY-SEVENTH ANNUAL WINTER MEETING (VOL. 9). MADISON, WISC.: INDUSTRIAL RELATIONS RESEARCH ASSOC., 1975, PP. 350-358.*
INDX   IMMIGRATION, SOCIAL SCIENCES, SOUTH AMERICA, ECONOMIC FACTORS, UNDOCUMENTED WORKERS, EMPLOYMENT, ESSAY, LABOR FORCE, MASSACHUSETTS, EAST, PUERTO RICAN-M
ABST   A NEW WAVE OF IMMIGRATION TO THE UNITED STATES FROM LATIN AMERICAN AND THE CARIBBEAN IS EXAMINED. THIS IMMIGRATION WHICH IS PRIMARILY ILLEGAL IS NO LONGER HEAVILY CONCENTRATED ALONG THE MEXICAN BORDER BUT RATHER APPEARS TO BE IN INDUSTRIALIZED URBAN AREAS THROUGHOUT THE COUNTRY. USING BOSTON AS A CASE IN POINT, IT IS ARGUED THAT THIS NEW IMMIGRATION IS A RESULT OF THE SHIFT IN THE COMPOSITION OF THE NATIVE BLACK LABOR FORCE FROM "FIRST" GENERATION BOSTONIANS WHO WERE RAISED IN THE SOUTH TO A SECOND GENERATION RAISED IN BOSTON. THE SECOND GENERATION IS UNWILLING TO ACCEPT THE POSITIONS WHICH THEIR PARENTS FILLED, LEAVING A SHORTAGE AT THE LOWER LEVELS OF THE LABOR MARKET. SINCE THE LABOR RESERVES IN THE RURAL SOUTH HAVE BEEN VIRTUALLY EXHAUSTED, THE LA-

BOR POSITIONS CANNOT BE REPLACED BY LOCAL RECRUITS. CONSEQUENTLY, INDUSTRIES ARE INCREASINGLY BECOMING DEPENDENT UPON FOREIGN WORKERS. ILLEGAL POPULATIONS RISK BECOMING PART OF AN "UNDERGROUND LABOR MARKET." IF SO, THEN WORKERS WILL SUFFER THE CONSEQUENCES OF INDUSTRY VIOLATION OF LABOR STATUTES. (AUTHOR SUMMARY MODIFIED)

ACCN   001254

1455 AUTH   **PLANT, W. T., & SOUTHERN, M. L.**
TITL   THE INTELLECTUAL AND ACHIEVEMENT EFFECTS OF PRESCHOOL COGNITIVE STIMULATION OF POVERTY MEXICAN-AMERICAN CHILDREN.
SRCE   *GENETIC PSYCHOLOGY MONOGRAPHS, 1972, 86, 141-173.*
INDX   ACHIEVEMENT TESTING, INTELLIGENCE TESTING, EARLY CHILDHOOD EDUCATION, COGNITIVE DEVELOPMENT, POVERTY, MEXICAN AMERICAN, CHILDREN, EMPIRICAL, SES, PEABODY PICTURE-VOCABULARY TEST, STANFORD-BINET INTELLIGENCE TEST, WISC, METROPOLITAN READINESS TEST, METROPOLITAN ACHIEVEMENT TEST, CALIFORNIA, SOUTHWEST
ABST   IN A FIVE-YEAR, LONGITUDINAL INVESTIGATION IN CENTRAL CALIFORNIA OF THE EFFECTS OF A COGNITIVELY ORIENTED PRESCHOOL FOR DISADVANTAGED MEXICAN AMERICAN (MA) CHILDREN, SEVEN GROUPS OF MA CHILDREN FROM LOW SOCIOECONOMIC FAMILY BACKGROUNDS WERE STUDIED. TWO GROUPS (108 TOTAL SUBJECTS) WERE EXPOSED TO TWO 10-WEEK SUMMER SESSIONS OF COGNITIVELY ORIENTED PRESCHOOL PRIOR TO ENTRY INTO KINDERGARTEN. SESSIONS WERE LED BY MA HIGH SCHOOL STUDENTS, AND ALL ACTIVITIES WERE DESIGNED TO HELP STUDENTS GAIN RELEVANT SCHOOL-RELATED ABILITIES AND EXPERIENCE. THE OTHER FIVE GROUPS (237 TOTAL SUBJECTS) OF MA CHILDREN SERVED AS COMPARISON GROUPS; THEY DID NOT RECEIVE THE COGNITIVELY ORIENTED TRAINING. FOR PURPOSES OF COMPARISON, PSYCHOMETRICS WERE CONDUCTED TO ASSESS INTELLECTUAL SKILLS, ORAL LANGUAGE FUNCTION, AND SCHOOL ACHIEVEMENT. THE BATTERY OF INSTRUMENTS INCLUDED: (1) THE STANFORD-BINET; (2) THE PEABODY PICTURE VOCABULARY TEST; (3) THE PICTORIAL TEST OF INTELLIGENCE; (4) THE WECHSLER PRESCHOOL AND PRIMARY SCALE OF INTELLIGENCE; (5) THE AUDITORY-VOCAL AND VOCAL-ENCODING SUBTESTS OF THE ILLINOIS TEST OF PSYCHOLINGUISTIC ABILITY; (6) THE METROPOLITAN READINESS TEST; AND (7) TWO FORMS OF THE METROPOLITAN ACHIEVEMENT TEST. THE RESULTS FROM THESE TESTS SUPPORTED FOUR HYPOTHESES OF THE STUDY— IN SUM, THE CHILDREN RECEIVING THE COGNITIVELY ORIENTED TRAINING DID SHOW EARLY GAINS OVER THE COMPARISON GROUPS. NEVERTHELESS, IT WAS ALSO FOUND THAT THESE EARLY GAINS DID NOT PERSIST THROUGH 1ST AND 2ND GRADES. THE POS-

SIBLE REASONS FOR THIS APPARENT LOSS BY THE TRAINING SUBJECTS OF THEIR EARLY ADVANTAGE ARE THEREFORE DISCUSSED. 22 REFERENCES.

ACCN   001255

1456 AUTH   **PLATA, M.**
TITL   STABILITY AND CHANGE IN THE PRESTIGE RANKING OF OCCUPATIONS OVER 49 YEARS.
SRCE   *JOURNAL OF VOCATIONAL BEHAVIOR, 1975, 6(1), 95-99.*
INDX   OCCUPATIONAL ASPIRATIONS, ATTITUDES, SEX COMPARISON, COLLEGE STUDENTS, MEXICAN AMERICAN, CROSS CULTURAL, REVIEW, EMPLOYMENT, TEXAS, SOUTHWEST, ADULTS, EMPIRICAL
ABST   A SURVEY ON THE RANKINGS OF THE SOCIAL STATUS OF OCCUPATIONS, REPLICATING DEEG (1968) AND BRAUN AND BAYER (1973), AND A COMPARISON OF THE RESULTS WITH THOSE OF 1925, 1947, 1968, 1973 STUDIES, ARE PRESENTED USING 129 MEXICAN AMERICANS (MA) AND 117 ANGLO (AA) POST-HIGH SCHOOL AGE SUBJECTS FROM TEXAS. IT WAS HYPOTHESIZED THAT THE MA VIEW WOULD DIFFER FROM THE AA VIEW AND FROM THE VIEWS OF SUBJECTS IN THE PREVIOUS STUDIES. THE RESULTS INDICATE VERY LITTLE CHANGE IN THE OVERALL PRESTIGE RANKING OF OCCUPATIONS, IRRESPECTIVE OF POPULATION SAMPLE-TYPE. BLACKS (FROM 1973 STUDY) AND MA'S RANKED ELECTRICIANS AND PLUMBERS HIGHER THAN BOTH AA'S IN THE PRESENT STUDY AND THE SUBJECTS IN THE 1925, 1947 AND 1968 STUDIES. THIS RANKING IS POSSIBLY DUE TO A PERCEPTION OF THEIR PARENTS IN THESE POSITIONS. SINCE THE STUDIES DID NOT SURVEY THE REASONS BEHIND EACH RANKING. SPECULATION AS TO THE DIFFERENCES WILL ALWAYS EXIST. IMPLICATIONS FOR VOCATIONAL TRAINING PROGRAMS AND COUNSELING ARE SUGGESTED. 4 REFERENCES.

ACCN   001256

1457 AUTH   **PLEMONS, G.**
TITL   A COMPARISON OF MMPI SCORES OF ANGLO- AND MEXICAN-AMERICAN PSYCHIATRIC PATIENTS.
SRCE   *JOURNAL OF CONSULTING AND CLINICAL PSYCHOLOGY, 1977, 45(1), 149-150.*
INDX   MMPI, PERSONALITY, PERSONALITY ASSESSMENT, MEXICAN AMERICAN, ADULTS, PSYCHOPATHOLOGY, NEUROSIS, TEST VALIDITY, EMPIRICAL, CALIFORNIA, SOUTHWEST, BILINGUAL
ABST   THE ENGLISH LANGUAGE MINNESOTA MULTIPHASIC PERSONALITY INVENTORIES (MMPIS) WERE ADMINISTERED TO 40 BILINGUAL MEXICAN AMERICAN AND 109 ANGLO AMERICAN PSYCHIATRIC PATIENTS IN A COMMUNITY MENTAL HEALTH CENTER TO DETERMINE WHETHER THERE WERE ANY SIGNIFICANT DIFFERENCES. THERE WERE CONTROLS FOR THE MAJOR VARIABLES OF AGE, SEX, ETHNICITY, SOCIOECONOMIC STATUS, AND PRESENTING PROB-

LEM. MULTIVARIATE ANALYSES OF VARIANCE AND COVARIANCE WERE CONDUCTED WITH AND WITHOUT THE STANDARD K-CORRECTED T SCORES. WITH K-CORRECTIONS, MEXICAN AMERICAN SUBJECTS SCORED HIGHER ON THE L-SCALES AND K-SCALES BUT NO SIGNIFICANT DIFFERENCES WERE FOUND ON THE CLINICAL SCALES OF THE MMPI. HOWEVER, WITH K-CORRECTIONS, MEXICAN AMERICANS SCORED SIGNIFICANTLY LOWER ON THE PD, PT, AND MA SCALES. ANGLO AMERICAN MALES SCORED HIGHER THAN MEXICAN AMERICAN MALES ON THE MF SCALE. THE SUPPRESSOR EFFECTS OF THE L AND K ELEVATIONS ARE DISCUSSED IN VIEW OF DIFFERENCES FOUND BETWEEN THE TWO CULTURE GROUPS ON THE MMPI. IT IS SUGGESTED THAT THE STANDARD WEIGHTS OF THE K-CORRECTION MAY NOT BE SUITABLE FOR MEXICAN AMERICAN PSYCHIATRIC PATIENTS. FURTHER RESEARCH ON THIS AND ON THE DEPRESSIVE EFFECT OF THE L-SCALE IS RECOMMENDED. 2 REFERENCES. (JOURNAL ABSTRACT MODIFIED)

ACCN   001257

1458 AUTH   **POLITZER, R. L., & RAMIREZ, A. G.**
TITL   JUDGING PERSONALITY FROM SPEECH: A PILOT STUDY OF THE ATTITUDES TOWARD ETHNIC GROUPS.
SRCE   *CALIFORNIA JOURNAL OF EDUCATIONAL RESEARCH, 1975, 26(1), 16-26.*
INDX   PERSONALITY ASSESSMENT, ATTITUDES, PERSONALITY, LINGUISTICS, PHONOLOGY, CHILDREN, ADOLESCENTS, STEREOTYPES, GROUP DYNAMICS, ETHNIC IDENTITY, FEMALE, SES, CULTURAL FACTORS, MEXICAN AMERICAN, CALIFORNIA, SOUTHWEST
ABST   THE ATTITUDES OF MEXICAN AMERICAN AND ANGLO AMERICAN STUDENTS TOWARD DIFFERENT TYPES OF SPEECH REPRESENTATIVE OF DIFFERENT SOCIAL AND ETHNIC GROUP WERE INVESTIGATED. THE OBJECT WAS TO DETERMINE TO WHAT EXTENT THEIR ATTITUDES DIFFERED FROM EACH OTHER AND WHETHER THESE DIFFERENT ATTITUDES OCCURRED AT DIFFERENT AGE LEVELS. 149 SUBJECTS WERE CHOSEN RANDOMLY FROM THE THIRD, SIXTH, NINTH, AND TWELFTH GRADES IN TWO DIFFERENT SCHOOLS IN NORTHERN CALIFORNIA. THE TECHNIQUE FOR MEASURING STUDENTS' REACTIONS TOWARD A SOCIAL OR ETHNIC GROUP WAS PRIMARILY BASED ON THE MATCHED GUISE METHOD, WHEREBY SUBJECTS WERE ASKED TO EVALUATE VOICES BY RATING THEM ACCORDING TO A SEMANTIC DIFFERENTIAL SCALE OF BIPOLAR ADJECTIVES. ANALYSIS OF THE SUBJECTS' JUDGMENTS CONCERNING THE SAME SPEECH VARIETY INDICATES THAT THE MAIN DIFFERENCE LAY IN THEIR REACTION TO THE SPANISH GUISE, WHICH WAS PERCEIVED MORE FAVORABLE BY THE MEXICAN AMERICANS, BY THE FEMALES, AND BY THE STUDENTS IN THE UPPER GRADES. ANOTHER NOTEWORTHY ALTHOUGH PREDICTABLE RESULT WAS THE RELATIVE DOWNGRADING BY BOTH MEXICAN AMERICANS AND ANGLOS OF ENGLISH SPO-

KEN WITH A SPANISH ACCENT. 5 REFERENCES. (NCMHI ABSTRACT)

ACCN   001258

1459 AUTH   **POLLACK, E. W., & MENACKER, J.**
TITL   SPANISH-SPEAKING STUDENTS AND GUIDANCE (GUIDANCE MONOGRAPH SERIES NO. VI).
SRCE   *BOSTON: HOUGHTON MIFFLIN CO., 1971.*
INDX   EDUCATION, CULTURAL PLURALISM, MEXICAN AMERICAN, PUERTO RICAN-M, EDUCATIONAL COUNSELING, SES, POVERTY, ACCULTURATION, STEREOTYPES, DEMOGRAPHIC, CULTURAL FACTORS, BILINGUAL-BICULTURAL EDUCATION, INTELLIGENCE TESTING, PARENTAL INVOLVEMENT, ESSAY, BOOK
ABST   THE MONOGRAPH APPROACHES THE GUIDANCE OF SPANISH-SPEAKING STUDENTS FROM A CULTURALLY PLURALISTIC POINT OF VIEW. THE CULTURAL VALUES THAT PUERTO RICAN AND MEXICAN AMERICAN STUDENTS MIGHT HAVE ARE OUTLINED WHILE EMPHASIZING THAT THERE ARE MANY INDIVIDUAL DIFFERENCES. THE ISSUE OF POVERTY AND ITS RELATIONSHIP TO CULTURAL DIFFERENCES IS ALSO ADDRESSED. THE GENERAL RECOMMENDATION IS THAT SCHOOL COUNSELORS MUST REFRAIN FROM STEREOTYPING THE STUDENT; INSTEAD, THEY SHOULD OBJECTIVELY ASSESS THE STUDENT'S STRENGTHS AND WEAKNESSES AND WORK WITH THESE. FIVE GUIDELINES ARE PROVIDED FOR THE COUNSELOR WORKING WITH SPANISH-SPEAKING STUDENTS: (1) GROUP TECHNIQUES ARE SUPERIOR TO INDIVIDUAL GUIDANCE AND COUNSELING; (2) NON-TRADITIONAL AND MORE PERSONAL METHODS OF SEEKING COMMUNITY INVOLVEMENT SHOULD BE USED; (3) GUIDANCE SHOULD HELP THE STUDENTS TO FEEL COMFORTABLE IN BOTH THEIR INDIGENOUS CULTURE AND THE DOMINANT AMERICAN CULTURE; (4) A CONCRETE APPROACH TO GUIDANCE IS MORE EFFECTIVE THAN SYMBOLIC VERBAL TREATMENTS; AND (5) GUIDANCE PRACTICES SHOULD BE FLEXIBLE ENOUGH TO ACCOMMODATE THE CLIENTS' CULTURAL BACKGROUND. 69 REFERENCES.

ACCN   001259

1460 AUTH   **POLLOCK, D., & VALDEZ, H.**
TITL   DEVELOPMENTAL ASPECTS OF SEXUALITY AND AGGRESSION.
SRCE   *JOURNAL OF GENETIC PSYCHOLOGY, 1973, 123(2), 179-184.*
INDX   SEX COMPARISON, SEX ROLES, AGGRESSION, CHILDREN, ADOLESCENTS, MEXICAN AMERICAN, CROSS CULTURAL, EMPIRICAL, COGNITIVE DEVELOPMENT, SOCIALIZATION
ABST   IN AN ATTEMPT TO MEASURE DEVELOPMENTAL ASPECTS OF AGGRESSION AND SEXUALITY, 70 ANGLO AMERICAN AND 70 MEXICAN AMERICAN CHILDREN, RANGING IN AGE FROM 9 TO 15, OF BOTH SEXES, WERE TESTED ON A 60-ITEM SENTENCE-COMPLETION TEST (SET). RESULTS SHOWED ANGLO AMERICANS SCORING HIGHER THAN MEXICAN AMERICANS ON BOTH PERSONALITY TRAITS, WITH AGGRESSION SCORES BEING HIGHER THAN SEXUALITY SCORES FOR BOTH GROUPS. A

SIGNIFICANT FINDING WAS OF GREATER LA-
BILITY IN SCORES OF THE MEXICAN AMERICAN
GROUPS, WHILE THE ANGLO AMERICAN GROUP
WAS AT A PLATEAU. NO SEX DIFFERENCE WAS
FOUND. THERE WAS NO INCREASE IN SEXUAL-
ITY OR AGGRESSION WITH AGE TO SUPPORT A
LATENCY STAGE. RATHER, THESE TRAITS AP-
PEAR TO HAVE BEEN LEARNED MUCH EARLIER
IN LIFE. 23 REFERENCES. (JOURNAL SUM-
MARY)

ACCN 001260

1461 AUTH **PORTES, A.**
TITL DILEMMAS OF A GOLDEN EXILE: INTEGRATION
OF CUBAN REFUGEE FAMILIES IN MILWAUKEE.
SRCE *AMERICAN SOCIOLOGICAL REVIEW, 1969, 34,*
505-518.
INDX CUBAN, IMMIGRATION, HISTORY, ACCULTURA-
TION, EMPIRICAL, SES, ECONOMIC FACTORS,
WISCONSIN, MIDWEST, PSYCHOSOCIAL AD-
JUSTMENT
ABST THE CUBAN REVOLUTION REMOVED THE OLD
UPPER AND MIDDLE STRATA FROM THEIR
DOMINANT POSITIONS. MANY OF THESE
PEOPLE CAME TO THE U.S. WITH THE INTEN-
TION OF OVERTHROWING CASTRO AND RE-
TURNING TO CUBA. AFTER 1962, HOWEVER,
THEY HAD TO START RESETTLING IN U.S. COM-
MUNITIES. THIS PAPER EXAMINES THEIR INTE-
GRATION AS A FUNDAMENTAL SHIFT FROM
STRONG PSYCHOLOGICAL ATTACHMENTS TO
THE PAST TO VALUES AND IDENTITIES CON-
GRUENT WITH THE NEW ENVIRONMENT. AMONG
48 REFUGEE FAMILIES IN MILWAUKEE, IT WAS
FOUND THAT INTEGRATION IS STRONGLY IN-
FLUENCED BY RELATIVE LEVEL OF PRESENT
SOCIOECONOMIC REWARDS. RESULTS ARE IN-
TERPRETED AS CONSEQUENCES OF THE RA-
TIONAL-INDIVIDUALISTIC ETHIC CHARACTER-
IZING FAMILIES FROM THESE FORMERLY
DOMINANT SECTORS OF CUBA. 21 REFER-
ENCES. (JOURNAL ABSTRACT)

ACCN 001261

1462 AUTH **POSTON, D. L., & ALVIREZ D.**
TITL ON THE COST OF BEING A MEXICAN AMERI-
CAN WORKER.
SRCE *SOCIAL SCIENCE QUARTERLY, 1973, 53(4), 697-*
709.
INDX MEXICAN AMERICAN, MALE, SES, DISCRIMINA-
TION, ECONOMIC FACTORS, SCHOLASTIC
ACHIEVEMENT, EQUAL OPPORTUNITY, LABOR
FORCE, EMPIRICAL, CROSS CULTURAL,
SOUTHWEST, URBAN, EMPLOYMENT
ABST INCOME DIFFERENCE BETWEEN ANGLOS AND
MEXICAN AMERICANS IS WELL DOCUMENTED.
MEXICAN AMERICAN INCOME HAS RANGED
FROM 49% TO 81% OF THAT WHICH ANGLOS
EARN. EDUCATIONAL AND OCCUPATIONAL
DIFFERENCES ACCOUNT FOR PART OF THIS
DISCREPANCY BUT BEYOND THESE COMPOSI-
TIONAL FACTORS, DISCRIMINATION CONTRIB-
UTES TO THE COST OF BEING A MEXICAN
AMERICAN WORKER. 1960 CENSUS DATA ARE
ANALYZED FOR MEXICAN AMERICAN AND AN-
GLO MEN BETWEEN THE AGES OF 20 AND 40,
LIVING IN FIVE SOUTHWESTERN STATES AND
EMPLOYED FULL TIME IN PREDOMINATELY UR-

BAN OCCUPATIONS. THESE CONTROLS MORE
CLEARLY DEFINE THE POPULATION AND GUARD
AGAINST INFLATED DIFFERENCES IN INCOME
DUE TO EXTRANEOUS FACTORS. THE AVER-
AGE INCOMES FOR BOTH GROUPS AT VARIOUS
LEVELS OF EDUCATIONAL ATTAINMENT AND
OCCUPATIONAL CATEGORIES REVEAL THAT
ANGLOS HAVE CONSISTENTLY HIGHER IN-
COMES THAN MEXICAN AMERICANS. THE EF-
FECTS OF DISCRIMINATION WITHIN OCCUPA-
TIONAL CATEGORIES AND WITH A DIFFERENT
SAMPLE ARE DISCUSSED. 17 REFERENCES.

ACCN 001262

1463 AUTH **PREBLE, E.**
TITL THE PUERTO RICAN-AMERICAN TEENAGER IN
NEW YORK CITY.
SRCE *IN E. B. BRODY (ED.), MINORITY GROUP ADO-*
LESCENTS IN THE UNITED STATES. BALTIMORE:
THE WILLIAMS AND WILKINS COMPANY, 1968,
PP. 48-72.
INDX PUERTO RICAN-M, ADOLESCENTS, POVERTY,
MIGRATION, HISTORY, CULTURE, EDUCATION,
FAMILY STRUCTURE, SEX ROLES, INTERMAR-
RIAGE, ESSAY, URBAN, EMPIRICAL, ETHNIC
IDENTITY, NEW YORK, EAST
ABST INFORMATION DESCRIBING PUERTO RICAN
ADOLESCENTS WAS OBTAINED FROM CON-
TACTS OBTAINED THROUGH SERVICE PRO-
GRAMS AND VOLUNTARY PERSONAL AND SO-
CIAL RELATIONSHIPS IN 4 DIFFERENT
COMMUNITIES OF NEW YORK CITY OVER A 10
YEAR PERIOD. SOCIO-DEMOGRAPHIC DATA ARE
PROVIDED, AS WELL AS NUMEROUS CASE
STUDIES OF WHICH SOME REFLECT A TECH-
NIQUE KNOWN AS PSYCHO-DIAGNOSTIC LIFE
HISTORY INTERVIEWING. TOPICS DISCUSSED
ARE HISTORY AND CULTURE OF PUERTO RICO,
MIGRATION TO THE MAINLAND, RELATIONS OF
PUERTO RICANS TO NON-PUERTO RICANS, RA-
CIAL IDENTITY, EDUCATION AND EMPLOYMENT,
THE PUERTO RICAN FAMILY, AND THE ADOLES-
CENT IN THE COMMUNITY. 26 REFERENCES.

ACCN 001263

1464 AUTH **PRESS, I.**
TITL THE URBAN CURANDERO.
SRCE *AMERICAN ANTHROPOLOGIST, 1971, 73(3), 741-*
756.
INDX CURANDERISMO, FOLK MEDICINE, MEXICAN
AMERICAN, PHYSICIANS, ADULTS, CHILDREN,
SOUTH AMERICA, CASE STUDY, URBAN,
STEREOTYPES
ABST ACCOUNTS OF THE CURANDERO IN LATIN
AMERICA INDICATE RELIANCE UPON A LARGELY
PEASANT-DERIVED STEREOTYPE. THE UTILITY
OF SUCH STEREOTYPES FOR UNDERSTANDING
CURANDERISMO IN AN URBAN CONTEXT IS
QUESTIONED. FIVE CASE STUDIES OF CURAN-
DEROS IN BOGOTA, COLOMBIA, ARE PRE-
SENTED AND THEIR APPROACH TO CURAN-
DERISMO AND THEIR CLIENTS' RESPONSE TO
THEM IS DESCRIBED. CURANDEROS DO NOT
FOLLOW A SINGLE MODEL AND RESEARCHERS
OUGHT TO BE AWARE OF THE MANY INDI-
VIDUAL DIFFERENCES. THE CONCEPT OF AN
"URBAN CURING COMPLEX—A HOLISTIC AP-
PROACH TO CURATIVE FACILITIES IN THE CITY—

SHOULD REPLACE PRESENT OVER-RELIANCE UPON THE PEASANT MODEL OF CURER STYLE AND HEALING. 25 REFERENCES. (AUTHOR ABSTRACT MODIFIED)

ACCN 001264

1465 AUTH **PRESS, I.**
TITL URBAN ILLNESS: PHYSICIANS, CURERS AND DUAL USE IN BOGOTA.
SRCE *JOURNAL OF HEALTH AND SOCIAL BEHAVIOR, 1969, 10(3), 209-218.*
INDX PHYSICIANS, CURANDERISMO, FOLK MEDICINE, SOUTH AMERICA, SPANISH SURNAMED, HEALTH, COMMUNITY, RESOURCE UTILIZATION, SES, ACCULTURATION, ADULTS, URBAN, EMPIRICAL
ABST A PILOT STUDY OF URBAN CURERS, COMPRISED BOTH OF PHYSICIANS AND CURANDEROS, WAS CONDUCTED BY A SOCIAL ANTHROPOLOGIST AND A PHYSICIAN TO ANALYZE THE DUAL USE OF PHYSICIANS AND CURERS IN BOGOTA, COLOMBIA. FORTY-FOUR OUTPATIENTS AT A SEMI-CHARITY HOSPITAL AND FORTY-EIGHT CURER PATIENTS BEING TREATED BY A CURANDERO WERE INTERVIEWED. THE TECHNIQUES USED BY THE PHYSICIAN AND THE CURER ARE DESCRIBED. SOCIOECONOMIC STATUS (SES) AND LOW-ACCULTURATION TO THE URBAN MILIEU ARE CORRELATED TO THE USE OF CURERS; THE HIGHER THE SES AND LEVEL OF ACCULTURATION THE LESS LIKELY A PERSON WILL UTILIZE THE SERVICES OF A CURANDERO. THE FINDINGS INDICATE THAT THREE PATTERNS OF USE OF CURERS HAS EMERGED: (1) COMPETITION BETWEEN THE PHYSICIAN AND CURER; (2) COMPARTMENTALIZATION IN WHICH THE PATIENT WILL CHOOSE BETWEEN THE TWO FOR A PARTICULAR PROBLEM; AND (3) EXPLOITATION WHERE SOCIAL STATUS, SUBGROUP OR CULTURAL IDENTITY DETERMINES THE CHOICE. NEVERTHELESS, DUAL USE AMONG THE MIDDLE CLASS OR ELITE DOES EXIST. 15 REFERENCES.

ACCN 001265

1466 AUTH **PRESTON, J. D., & FRY, P. A.**
TITL MARIJUANA USE AMONG HOUSTON HIGH SCHOOL STUDENTS.
SRCE *SOCIAL SCIENCE QUARTERLY, 1971, 51(1), 170-178.*
INDX ADOLESCENTS, DRUG ABUSE, SOUTHWEST, TEXAS, EMPIRICAL, CROSS CULTURAL, SEX COMPARISON, SES, PEER GROUP, ATTITUDES, URBAN, MEXICAN AMERICAN
ABST THE RELATIONSHIP BETWEEN SOCIOCULTURAL VARIABLES AND MARIJUANA USE AMONG ADOLESCENTS WAS INVESTIGATED AT FIVE HIGH SCHOOLS IN THE METROPOLITAN HOUSTON AREA. TWO PREDOMINATELY BLACK, LOWER SOCIOECONOMIC CLASS SCHOOLS, TWO PREDOMINATELY ANGLO UPPER AND LOWER MIDDLE-CLASS SCHOOLS, AND ONE MIDDLE-CLASS ETHNICALLY HETEROGENEOUS SCHOOL WITH A LARGE NUMBER OF MEXICAN AMERICANS WERE SELECTED. AMONG THE 535 STUDENTS INTERVIEWED, MARIJUANA USE VARIED BY SEX (MALES WERE MORE LIKELY TO BE USERS THAN FEMALES) AND BY ETHNICITY (ANGLOS WERE MORE LIKELY TO BE USERS THAN MEXICAN AMERICANS, AND BLACKS HAD THE LOWEST INCIDENCE OF USE). PARENTAL USE OF PRESCRIPTION AND NON-PRESCRIPTION DRUGS WAS FOUND TO BE SIGNIFICANTLY RELATED TO MARIJUANA USE; FAMILY STABILITY WAS NOT. MOST STRIKING WAS THE EXTENT TO WHICH NORMS DEFINING DRUG USE VARIED AMONG SCHOOLS SINCE, CONTROLLING FOR SCHOOL, ORIGINAL RELATIONSHIPS BETWEEN MARIJUANA USE AND OTHER VARIABLES SUCH AS GRADE AND SEX WERE MODIFIED. IT IS INDICATED THAT ADOLESCENTS USE MARIJUANA BECAUSE THEIR PEER GROUPS REWARD AND SUPPORT SUCH BEHAVIOR. 11 REFERENCES.

ACCN 002181

1467 AUTH **PRICE, D. O.**
TITL RURAL TO URBAN MIGRATION OF MEXICAN AMERICANS, NEGROES AND ANGLOS.
SRCE *INTERNATIONAL MIGRATION REVIEW, 1971, 5(3), 281-290.*
INDX URBAN, RURAL, MIGRATION, MEXICAN AMERICAN, CROSS CULTURAL, ECONOMIC FACTORS, EMPLOYMENT, HOUSING, ATTITUDES, EMPIRICAL, SOUTH, SOUTHWEST, ILLINOIS, INDIANA, MISSISSIPPI, TEXAS, MIDWEST, LABOR FORCE, ADULTS, KENTUCKY
ABST MEXICAN AMERICAN, NEGRO, AND ANGLO MIGRANTS FROM THREE SOUTHERN RURAL AREAS WERE INTERVIEWED AND COMPARED WITH NON-MIGRANTS WHO CONTINUED TO RESIDE IN THE SAME AREA. ANALYSIS OF 2,700 SCREENING QUESTIONNAIRES INDICATED THAT THOSE WHO MIGRATED WERE BETTER EDUCATED, YOUNGER, AND, IN THE CASE OF MINORITIES, HAD HIGHER INCOMES BEFORE MIGRATION. CONSIDERABLE ETHNIC DIFFERENCES EXISTED IN THE PERCENTAGE OF MIGRANTS WHO HAD JOB LEADS IN THE CITIES AND IN THE LENGTH OF TIME NEEDED TO OBTAIN STEADY EMPLOYMENT. ECONOMIC FACTORS WERE THE PRIME MOTIVATING FORCE AMONG ALL GROUPS, WHO GENERALLY EXPRESSED THAT THEY FELT THEY WERE HAPPIER AND BETTER OFF FINANCIALLY IN THE CITY. MEXICAN AMERICANS SEEMED TO BE THE HAPPIEST AND LEAST FRUSTRATED, WHILE NEGROES, ALTHOUGH EXPERIENCING THE GREATEST ECONOMIC IMPROVEMENT, WERE THE MOST DISAPPOINTED IN URBAN LIFE. ANGLOS MAINTAINED THE CLOSEST TIES TO THEIR HOME AREAS AND EXPRESSED THE GREATEST DESIRE TO RETURN HOME IF THE ECONOMIC OPPORTUNITY PRESENTED ITSELF.

ACCN 002182

1468 AUTH **PRICE, D. O.**
TITL A STUDY OF ECONOMIC CONSEQUENCES OF RURAL-URBAN MIGRATION (VOL. 3).
SRCE *AUSTIN: TRACOR, INC., 1969. (ERIC DOCUMENT REPRODUCTION SERVICE NO. ED 054325)*
INDX ECONOMIC FACTORS, RURAL, URBAN, MIGRATION, MEXICAN AMERICAN, FAMILY STRUCTURE, CROSS CULTURAL, PSYCHOSOCIAL ADJUSTMENT, FAMILY ROLES, EMPIRICAL, SOCIAL

MOBILITY, CULTURAL FACTORS, ATTITUDES, MIGRATION, SOUTH

ABST   THIS IS THE THIRD AND LAST VOLUME OF A STUDY THAT ANALYZED RURAL MIGRATION PATTERNS OF MEXICAN AMERICANS, NEGROES, AND ANGLO AMERICANS WHO MOVED FROM THE SOUTHERN STATES TO URBAN AREAS. SIX OF THE 14 CHAPTERS ARE INCLUDED IN THIS REPORT. THE STUDY EXAMINES DIFFERENCES IN FAMILY CHARACTERISTICS BETWEEN MIGRANTS AND NONMIGRANTS, MIGRANTS' PERCEPTIONS ABOUT ANTICIPATED CONDITIONS IN THE CITY AND ACTUAL CONDITIONS, AND ADJUSTMENT OF URBAN MIGRANTS TO THEIR NEW SURROUNDINGS. THE REPORT ALSO REVIEWS THE ADVICE OF URBAN MIGRANTS ON STEPS TO BE TAKEN BEFORE MOVING, THE CONDITIONS NECESSARY FOR MIGRANTS TO RETURN TO THEIR FORMER RESIDENCES, AND THE EFFECT OF OUT-MIGRATION ON RURAL AREAS. 106 REFERENCES. (RIE ABSTRACT)

ACCN   001266

1469 AUTH   **PRICE-WILLIAMS, D. R., & RAMIREZ, M., III.**

TITL   ETHNIC DIFFERENCES IN DELAY OF GRATIFICATION.

SRCE   *THE JOURNAL OF SOCIAL PSYCHOLOGY, 1974, 93(JUNE), 23-30.*

INDX   ETHNIC IDENTITY, CULTURAL FACTORS, MEXICAN AMERICAN, CHILDREN, SES, EMPIRICAL, ATTITUDES, PERSONALITY, TIME ORIENTATION, CROSS CULTURAL, SEX COMPARISON, EXAMINER EFFECTS, SOUTHWEST, COGNITIVE DEVELOPMENT

ABST   QUESTIONS RELATED TO THE PROBLEM OF ACCEPTING A SMALL REWARD IMMEDIATELY OR WAITING FOR A BIGGER REWARD WERE GIVEN TO 180 FOURTH-GRADE CHILDREN COMPOSED OF THREE ETHNIC GROUPS SAMPLED FROM A RELATIVELY POOR SOCIO-ECONOMIC REGION OF A SOUTH-WESTERN AREA IN THE UNITED STATES. IN ADDITION, QUESTIONS RELATED TO THE FACTOR OF TRUST IN THE PROMISES OF INVESTIGATORS TO DELIVER THE BIGGER REWARD WERE UNDERTAKEN. THE SAMPLE CONSISTED OF 60 ANGLOS, BLACKS, AND MEXICAN AMERICANS, RESPECTIVELY; EACH ETHNIC GROUP WAS DIVIDED IN TURN INTO AN EQUAL NUMBER OF BOYS AND GIRLS. RESULTS SHOW THAT AT THE FOURTH-GRADE LEVEL BLACK AND MEXICAN AMERICAN CHILDREN WERE MORE PRONE THAN ANGLO CHILDREN TO ACCEPT THE IMMEDIATE GRATIFICATION RATHER THAN CHOOSE THE LATER AND BIGGER REWARD. NO SEX DIFFERENCES WITHIN EACH ETHNIC GROUP WERE FOUND, WITH THE EXCEPTION OF THE MEXICAN AMERICAN GROUP FOR ONE OUT OF THE THREE CONDITIONS TESTED. THE FACTOR OF MISTRUST IN THE PROMISES OF THE INVESTIGATORS WAS NOTICEABLE IN THE BLACK CHILDREN, DESPITE THE FACT THAT THEY WERE TESTED BY BLACK INVESTIGATORS. 14 REFERENCES. (JOURNAL ABSTRACT)

ACCN   001267

1470 AUTH   **PROJECT MASP: MINORITY AGING & SOCIAL POLICY.**

TITL   FAMILY SUPPORTS FACTSHEET.

SRCE   *ETHEL PERCY ANDRUS GERONTOLOGY CENTER, UNIVERSITY OF SOUTHERN CALIFORNIA, SEPTEMBER 1979.*

INDX   GERONTOLOGY, MEXICAN AMERICAN, CALIFORNIA, SOUTHWEST, URBAN, SURVEY, EMPIRICAL, CROSS CULTURAL, HEALTH, HEALTH DELIVERY SYSTEMS, FAMILY ROLES, RESOURCE UTILIZATION, ATTITUDES, FINANCING, FAMILY STRUCTURE

ABST   A LOS ANGELES COUNTY SURVEY OF ANGLOS, MEXICAN AMERICANS (MA), AND BLACKS (AGES 45 TO 72) EXAMINED INTER-GROUP DIFFERENCES IN (1) OVERALL HEALTH, (2) HEALTH INSURANCE COVERAGE, (3) ACCESS TO HEALTH CARE, AND (4) WILLINGNESS TO RELY ON FAMILY IN TIMES OF NEED. REGARDING HEALTH STATUS, MOST ELDERLY RESPONDENTS—ESPECIALLY BLACKS AND MA'S—REPORTED THAT HEALTH PROBLEMS SERIOUSLY IMPAIRED THEIR ABILITY TO PERFORM DAILY TASKS. CONCERNING HEALTH CARE, MINORITY RESPONDENTS REPORTED HAVING LESS ACCESS TO PROVIDERS AND FACILITIES THAN DID ANGLO RESPONDENTS. MOREOVER, OLDER LOW-INCOME BLACKS AND MA'S WERE MORE LIKELY THAN ANGLOS TO HAVE NO HEALTH INSURANCE. BUT DESPITE SUCH FINDINGS, THE MINORITY RESPONDENTS—ESPECIALLY THE MA'S—WERE LESS LIKELY TO BE INSTITUTIONALIZED. THE CRUCIAL VARIABLE ACCOUNTING FOR THIS WAS FAMILY SUPPORT. SPECIFICALLY, OLDER MA'S WERE THE MOST LIKELY TO EXPECT SUPPORT FROM RELATIVES (TWO-THIRDS COMPARED TO ONE-THIRD OF THE ANGLOS AND ONE-SIXTH OF THE BLACKS). THE OLDER MA'S WERE ALSO THE MOST LIKELY TO BE LIVING WITH AN ADULT CHILD (24% COMPARED TO 5% AND 6% OF THE ANGLOS AND BLACKS, RESPECTIVELY). THUS, THE OLDER MA'S WERE THE MOST POSITIVE ABOUT RECEIVING INFORMAL SUPPORT FROM THEIR FAMILIES. IT IS CONCLUDED THAT A HEALTH CARE APPROACH TO ELDERLY MA'S WILL BE SUCCESSFUL IN PREVENTING UNNECESSARY INSTITUTIONALIZATION IF IT FITS MA'S EXPECTATIONS AND CUSTOMS ABOUT INFORMAL SUPPORT—E.G., AN APPROACH WHICH PROMOTES FAMILY ASSISTANCE AND FACILITATES INDEPENDENT LIVING. 8 REFERENCES.

ACCN   001783

1471 AUTH   **QUESADA, G. M.**

TITL   CORRELATES OF MENTAL HEALTH KNOWLEDGE FROM THREE URBAN SAMPLES IN SOUTH TEXAS.

SRCE   *PAPER PRESENTED AT THE SOUTHWESTERN SOCIOLOGICAL ASSOCIATION MEETING, DALLAS, MARCH 1973.*

INDX   MEXICAN AMERICAN, MENTAL HEALTH, HEALTH DELIVERY SYSTEMS, SES, POVERTY, ANOMIE, SURVEY, EMPIRICAL, DEMOGRAPHIC, PROGRAM EVALUATION

ABST   DATA MEASURING MENTAL HEALTH KNOWLEDGE AND PREDICTING LEVELS OF KNOWLEDGE WHICH CORRELATE WITH SPECIFIC SO-

CIO-DEMOGRAPHIC CHARACTERISTICS WAS OBTAINED FROM A 3-YEAR STUDY EVALUATING THE FIELD MENTAL HEALTH PROGRAM OF SAN ANTONIO. INTERVIEWS CONDUCTED AMONG 173 MEXICAN AMERICANS IN SAN ANTONIO, 56 MEXICAN AMERICANS IN AUSTIN, AND 48 BLACKS IN SAN ANTONIO REVEALED THESE FINDINGS: (1) ALTHOUGH BLACKS POSSESSED THE HIGHEST KNOWLEDGE, THEY REPORTED THE LOWEST INCOME BUT A HIGHER EDUCATIONAL LEVEL THAN MEXICAN AMERICANS; (2) MASS MEDIA EXPOSURE, USE OF THE WELFARE SYSTEM, OR EXPERIENCE AS A MIGRANT WORKER WERE NOT CORRELATED WITH MENTAL HEALTH KNOWLEDGE; AND (3) FOR ALL 3 SAMPLES THE GREATER THE ALIENATION AND MEDICAL NEGATIVISM, THE GREATER MENTAL HEALTH KNOWLEDGE. 12 REFERENCES.

ACCN   001268

1472 AUTH   **QUESADA, G. M.**
TITL   THE EPIDEMIOLOGY OF ACCEPTANCE OF MENTAL HEALTH SERVICES: DATA COMPARISONS BETWEEN THE 1972 AND 1973 SURVEYS FOR THREE URBAN SAMPLES IN SOUTH TEXAS (TECH. REP. NO. 3).
SRCE   *LUBBOCK, TEXAS: TEXAS TECH UNIVERSITY, DEPARTMENTS OF HEALTH COMMUNICATIONS AND SOCIOLOGY, 1974.*
INDX   PROGRAM EVALUATION, SURVEY, MENTAL HEALTH, ATTITUDES, MEXICAN AMERICAN, CROSS CULTURAL, TEXAS, SOUTHWEST, RESOURCE UTILIZATION, DEMOGRAPHIC
ABST   DATA WERE COLLECTED DURING THE YEARS 1972 AND 1973 FROM A RANDOM SAMPLE OF HOUSEHOLDS WITHIN THE SAN ANTONIO AND AUSTIN MODEL CITIES AREAS IN TEXAS. FOR EACH YEAR, A SURVEY WAS CONDUCTED AMONG MEXICAN AMERICANS IN AUSTIN (MAA) AND SAN ANTONIO (MASA), AND BLACKS IN SAN ANTONIO (BSA). THE PRIMARY OBJECTIVE OF THIS TREND STUDY WAS TO EVALUATE THE FIELD MENTAL HEALTH PROGRAM OF SAN ANTONIO. THE REPORT LISTS THE ITEMS USED IN THE QUESTIONNAIRE AS WELL AS THE FREQUENCY DISTRIBUTIONS OF THE RESPONSES OF EACH ITEM FOR THE MAA, MASA, AND BSA SAMPLES OBTAINED DURING THE SURVEY YEARS. QUESTIONS ON THE INSTRUMENT SCHEDULE ARE COMPRISED OF SOCIOCULTURAL DEMOGRAPHIC VARIABLES, ATTITUDES TOWARDS MENTAL HEALTH, FAMILIARITY OF MENTAL HEALTH AGENCIES, AND UTILIZATION OF MENTAL HEALTH FACILITIES.
ACCN   001269

1473 AUTH   **QUESADA, G. M.**
TITL   MEXICAN-AMERICANS: MEXICANS OR AMERICANS?
SRCE   *PRESENTED AT THE SOUTHWEST COUNCIL OF LATIN AMERICAN STUDIES, LUBBOCK, TEXAS, FEBRUARY 1973.*
INDX   STEREOTYPES, MEXICAN AMERICAN, SELF CONCEPT, ETHNIC IDENTITY, CROSS CULTURAL, HIGHER EDUCATION, ADULTS, EMPIRICAL
ABST   IN A STUDY INVESTIGATING ETHNIC IDENTIFICATION, 16 MEXICAN AMERICAN AND 8 ANGLO AMERICAN ADULTS RATED 25 SEMANTIC DIFFERENTIAL ITEMS REFLECTING THE CONCEPTS OF "MEXICAN AMERICAN" AND "ANGLO AMERICAN" AT THE BEGINNING AND AT THE END OF AN ETHNICALLY CONSCIOUS NIGHT COLLEGE COURSE. SCALE ITEMS FACTORED ON TWO DIMENSIONS: MORAL ATTRIBUTES AND PHYSICAL SUCCESS OF THE ETHNIC GROUP. THE RESULTS INDICATE A SIMILARITY BETWEEN MEXICAN AMERICAN AND ANGLO AMERICAN STUDENTS' RATING OF THE TWO CONCEPTS OVER TIME. AT TIME 1, EACH GROUP RATED THE MORAL CHARACTERISTICS AND PHYSICAL SUCCESS OF "MEXICAN AMERICAN" NEGATIVELY AND "ANGLO AMERICAN" POSITIVELY. THE SCORES AT TIME 2 REVEALED THAT EACH GROUP RATED THE MORAL ATTRIBUTES OF BOTH "MEXICAN AMERICAN" AND "ANGLO AMERICAN" POSITIVELY, HOWEVER, THE PHYSICAL SUCCESS SCORES FOR THE TWO CONCEPTS RECEIVED NEGATIVE RATINGS FROM BOTH ETHNIC GROUPS. IT IS CONCLUDED THAT THE MEXICAN AMERICAN ENTERING AN ANGLO SCHOOL LEARNS TO ADOPT THE VALUES OF THE ANGLO AMERICAN CULTURE. 11 REFERENCES.
ACCN   001270

1474 AUTH   **QUESADA, G. M., & AGUILAR, M.**
TITL   THE COMMUNICATION OF ANGLO MENTAL HEALTH TO A CHICANO COMMUNITY.
SRCE   *PAPER PRESENTED AT THE 19TH ANNUAL CONFERENCE OF THE INTERNATIONAL COMMUNICATION ASSOCIATION, PHOENIX, 1971.*
INDX   MENTAL HEALTH, MEXICAN AMERICAN, COMMUNITY, HEALTH DELIVERY SYSTEMS, PSYCHOTHERAPISTS, STEREOTYPES, FINANCING, ESSAY, PROGRAM EVALUATION, TEXAS, SOUTHWEST
ABST   BERLO'S SOURCE-MESSAGE-CHANNEL-RECEIVER MODEL IS USED TO HELP DESCRIBE THE DEVELOPMENT OF AN INNOVATIVE APPROACH IN MENTAL HEALTH SERVICE DELIVERY IN THE WESTSIDE OF SAN ANTONIO, TEXAS. THE STAFF OF THIS FIELD MENTAL HEALTH PROGRAM IS COMPOSED OF A DIRECTOR, A FIELD SUPERVISOR, A YOUTH COORDINATOR, A UNIT CLERK, AND NINE FIELDWORKERS. THE FIELDWORKERS MAINTAIN THE ASSUMPTION THAT TO SOLVE HUNGER AND UNEMPLOYMENT IS OF MORE IMMEDIATE IMPORTANCE THAN DETERMINATION OF AN INDIVIDUAL'S SPECIFIC MENTAL DISORDER. THIS PROGRAM IS OPERATED BY THE MEXICAN AMERICAN COMMUNITY, AND ITS GOAL IS TO DECREASE THE INTERCULTURAL GAP AND TO INCREASE THE FEEDBACK AND CROSS-CULTURAL COMMUNICATION BETWEEN LOWER CLASS CLIENTELE AND MENTAL HEALTH PROFESSIONALS. 9 REFERENCES.
ACCN   001271

1475 AUTH   **QUESADA, G. M., & HELLER, P. L.**
TITL   SOCIOCULTURAL BARRIERS TO MEDICAL CARE AMONG MEXICAN AMERICANS IN TEXAS: A SUMMARY REPORT OF RESEARCH CONDUCTED BY THE SOUTHWEST MEDICAL SOCIOLOGY AD HOC COMMITTEE.

SRCE   *MEDICAL CARE, 1977, 15(5), 93-101.*

INDX   HEALTH, MEXICAN AMERICAN, HEALTH DELIVERY SYSTEMS, RESOURCE UTILIZATION, FOLK MEDICINE, CURANDERISMO, DEATH, SEX COMPARISON, POVERTY, BILINGUAL-BICULTURAL PERSONNEL, POLITICAL POWER, FAMILY STRUCTURE, REVIEW, INTERPERSONAL RELATIONS, POLICY, TEXAS, SOUTHWEST

ABST   THE SOUTHWEST MEDICAL SOCIOLOGY AD HOC COMMITTEE MEMBERS STUDIED A NUMBER OF FACTORS CONCERNING MEXICAN AMERICAN MEDICAL CARE IN TEXAS SUCH AS: (1) MORTALITY, MORBIDITY, AND OTHER HEALTH STATUS INDICATORS; (2) HEALTH MANPOWER AND EDUCATIONAL NEEDS; (3) POLITICAL FACTORS IMPEDING ECONOMICAL HEALTH CARE; (4) ALIENATION, FAMILISM, AND THEIR RELATIONSHIP TO UTILIZATION OF THE HEALTH SERVICES; (5) LANGUAGE AND COMMUNICATION BARRIERS; AND (6) FOLK MEDICINE. FINDINGS INCLUDE DOCUMENTATION THAT STRUCTURAL ALIENATION OF MEXICAN AMERICANS FROM MAINSTREAM ANGLO AMERICAN MIDDLE-CLASS SOCIETY IS CARRIED OVER INTO THEIR RELATION WITH AND UTILIZATION OF THE HEALTH CARE DELIVERY SYSTEM; THAT THEIR EMPHASIS ON FAMILISM WORKS ALTERNATIVELY TO ENCOURAGE AND DISCOURAGE THEIR SEEKING ACCESS TO HEALTH CARE; THAT LANGUAGE DIFFERENCES SERVE TO PERPETUATE CERTAIN CULTURAL DIFFERENCES THAT ARE INIMICAL TO HEALTH CARE DELIVERY; AND THAT CURANDERISMO CAN BE SEEN AS COMPLEMENTING OTHER TYPES OF HEALTH CARE. THE REPORT CONCLUDES WITH A NUMBER OF RECOMMENDATIONS FOR ACCOMPLISHING CULTURAL INTEGRATION THAT WILL LEAD TO BETTER HEALTH CARE FOR THIS SEGMENT OF THE POPULATION. 11 REFERENCES. (JOURNAL ABSTRACT MODIFIED)

ACCN   001273

1476 AUTH   **QUIROGA, I. R.**

TITL   THE USE OF A LINEAR DISCRIMINANT FUNCTION OF THE MINNESOTA MULTIPHASIC PERSONALITY INVENTORY SCORES IN THE CLASSIFICATION OF PSYCHOTIC AND NONPSYCHOTIC MEXICAN-AMERICAN PSYCHIATRIC PATIENTS (DOCTORAL DISSERTATION, UNIVERSITY OF OKLAHOMA, 1972).

SRCE   *DISSERTATION ABSTRACTS INTERNATIONAL, 1972, 33, 448B. (UNIVERSITY MICROFILMS NO. 72-19,752).*

INDX   MMPI, PERSONALITY ASSESSMENT, PERSONALITY, PSYCHOPATHOLOGY, PSYCHOSIS, NEUROSIS, SCHIZOPHRENIA, MEXICAN AMERICAN, CROSS CULTURAL, SEX COMPARISON, SES, SCHOLASTIC ACHIEVEMENT, EMPIRICAL, TEXAS, SOUTHWEST, MENTAL HEALTH

ABST   THE PRIMARY PURPOSE OF THIS STUDY WAS TO DEVELOP A RELATIVELY FAST, MMPI BASED, ACTUARIAL PROCEDURE FOR THE CLASSIFICATION OF PSYCHOTIC AND NON-PSYCHOTIC MEXICAN AMERICAN PSYCHIATRIC PATIENTS. THE PROCEDURE CHOSEN WAS FISHER'S (1936) LINEAR DISCRIMINANT FUNCTION (LDF). SUBJECTS WERE ALL PSYCHIATRIC PATIENTS WHO HAD BEEN REFERRED FOR DIAGNOSTIC TESTING TO THE DIVISION OF PSYCHOLOGY AT THE UNIVERSITY OF TEXAS MEDICAL BRANCH. IN ASPECT I OF THIS STUDY AN ATTEMPT WAS MADE TO PROVIDE AN EMPIRICAL JUSTIFICATION FOR THE DEVELOPMENT OF THE MMPI-BASED LDF FOR MEXICAN AMERICAN PATIENTS. THE RESULTS INDICATED THAT WHETHER IT BE TWO GROUPS OF PSYCHOTICS, TWO GROUPS OF NON-PSYCHOTICS, OR TWO COMBINED GROUPS OF DIAGNOSTICALLY HETEROGENEOUS PSYCHIATRIC PATIENTS, THERE ARE SIGNIFICANT DIFFERENCES ON MMPI PERFORMANCE ASSOCIATED WITH DIFFERENCES IN CULTURAL GROUP MEMBERSHIP BETWEEN MEXICAN AMERICAN AND ANGLO AMERICAN PSYCHIATRIC PATIENTS. THESE FINDINGS JUSTIFIED ASPECT II OF THE STUDY IN WHICH AN LDF FOR CLASSIFYING PSYCHOTIC AND NON-PSYCHOTIC MEXICAN AMERICAN PSYCHIATRIC PATIENTS WAS DEVELOPED AND CROSS VALIDATED. ALTHOUGH THIS PROCEDURE WAS SIGNIFICANT AT THE .01 LEVEL, IT IS PREMATURE TO LABEL IT A SOUND PSYCHOMETRIC TOOL TO BE USED CLINICALLY IN ASSESSING PSYCHIATRIC PATIENTS. 114 REFERENCES. (AUTHOR SUMMARY MODIFIED)

ACCN   001274

1477 AUTH   **RABKIN, J. G., & STRUENING, E. L.**

TITL   ETHNICITY, SOCIAL CLASS AND MENTAL ILLNESS (WORKING PAPER NO. 17).

SRCE   *NEW YORK: INSTITUTE ON PLURALISM AND GROUP IDENTITY, MAY 1976.*

INDX   PSYCHOPATHOLOGY, CROSS CULTURAL, PUERTO RICAN-M, CHILDREN, ADULTS, SES, SCHIZOPHRENIA, MIGRATION, REVIEW, EMPIRICAL, RESEARCH METHODOLOGY, CULTURAL FACTORS, ESPIRITISMO, NEW YORK, EAST, MENTAL HEALTH

ABST   AN INVESTIGATION EXAMINING THE EXTENT TO WHICH ETHNICITY AND SOCIAL CLASS ACCOUNT FOR VARIATION IN RATES OF MENTAL HOSPITALIZATION FOR WOMEN AND MEN BETWEEN THE AGES OF 21 TO 64 YEARS WAS CONDUCTED IN TWO GEOGRAPHICAL SECTORS OF NEW YORK CITY. INFORMATION WAS OBTAINED FROM CENSUS DATA AND FROM RECORDS OF THE NEW YORK STATE DEPARTMENT OF MENTAL HYGIENE. RESULTS INDICATE ETHNICITY (JEWS, BLACKS, PUERTO RICANS, ITALIANS, AND IRISH) IS STRONGLY ASSOCIATED WITH MENTAL HOSPITAL ADMISSION RATES; INCREASED PRESENCE OF WHITE, MIDDLE-INCOME ETHNIC GROUPS IS NEGATIVELY RELATED TO HOSPITALIZATION RATES; AND THE INCREASED PRESENCE OF LOW-INCOME BLACKS AND PUERTO RICANS IS POSITIVELY RELATED TO HIGH HOSPITALIZATION RATES. IN ADDITION, THE FIVE ETHNIC GROUPS IN THIS STUDY ACCOUNT FOR MORE THAN 50 PERCENT OF THE PSYCHIATRIC HOSPITALIZATION RATE VARIATION. IT IS RECOMMENDED THAT THERE IS A DEFINITE NEED FOR ONGOING RESEARCH TO EXAMINE ETHNIC AS WELL AS SOCIAL CLASS FACTORS IN THE MAINTENANCE OR BREAKDOWN OF SUPPORT SYS-

TEMS IN COMMUNITIES. 70 REFERENCES. (AUTHOR ABSTRACT MODIFIED)

ACCN 001275

1478 AUTH **RACHLIN, S., MILTON, J., & PAM, A.**
TITL COUNTERSYMBIOTIC SUICIDE.
SRCE *ARCHIVES OF GENERAL PSYCHIATRY, 1977, 34(8), 965-967.*
INDX ADOLESCENTS, ADULTS, MALE, CASE STUDY, COPING MECHANISMS, DEVIANCE, DYADIC INTERACTION, ESSAY, MENTAL HEALTH, MOTHER-CHILD INTERACTION, PSYCHOSIS, PUERTO RICAN-M, NEW YORK, EAST, SUICIDE
ABST THREE CASES OF SUICIDE BY SEVERELY DISTURBED 17 TO 21 YEAR-OLD PUERTO RICAN MALE SCHIZOPHRENICS, WHO DEMONSTRATED PATHOLOGICALLY SYMBIOTIC RELATIONSHIPS WITH THEIR MOTHERS, ARE REPORTED. THE INCIDENTS OCCURRED WHILE EACH PATIENT WAS ON ROUTE TO, OR AT, THE MATERNAL HOME ON AN AUTHORIZED LEAVE FROM A SPECIAL WARD FOR SEVERELY DISTURBED SCHIZOPHRENICS AT THE BRONX PSYCHIATRIC CENTER, NEW YORK. NONE HAD A HISTORY OF OVERT SUICIDE ATTEMPTS PRIOR TO THEIR ACTUAL DEATH BY JUMPING. IT IS POSITED THAT IN EACH CASE THE SUICIDE REPRESENTED AN UNDERLYING DESIRE TO KILL THE MOTHER—A DESIRE THAT WAS NOT PERMISSIBLE. ALTERNATIVELY, THE PATIENTS' EGO BOUNDARIES WERE NOT SUFFICIENTLY CLEAR TO PERMIT DIFFERENTIATION OF SELF AND MOTHER. BECAUSE THE PATIENTS SAW ANY ATTEMPT, SHORT OF SUICIDE, TO LOOSEN THE SYMBIOTIC BOND AS BEING FUTILE, THE TERMINOLOGY "COUNTERSYMBIOTIC SUICIDE" IS GIVEN TO THE EVENT. 11 REFERENCES. (JOURNAL ABSTRACT MODIFIED)

ACCN 002183

1479 AUTH **RAGAN, P. K., & SIMONIN, M. (EDS.).**
TITL SOCIAL AND CULTURAL CONTEXTS OF AGING: AGING AMONG BLACKS AND MEXICAN AMERICANS IN THE UNITED STATES—A SELECTED BIBLIOGRAPHY.
SRCE *LOS ANGELES: ANDRUS GERONTOLOGY CENTER, UNIVERSITY OF SOUTHERN CALIFORNIA, 1977.*
INDX ADULTS, BIBLIOGRAPHY, CROSS CULTURAL, GERONTOLOGY, MEXICAN AMERICAN
ABST A SELECTED BIBLIOGRAPHY OF 311 REFERENCES ON SOCIOCULTURAL ASPECTS OF BLACK AND MEXICAN AMERICAN AGING WERE COMPILED DURING THE COURSE OF A FIVE YEAR RESEARCH PROJECT AT THE ANDRUS GERONTOLOGY CENTER, UNIVERSITY OF SOUTHERN CALIFORNIA. THERE ARE 184 REFERENCES TO PUBLICATIONS, PAPERS, DISSERTATIONS, AND GOVERNMENT DOCUMENTS ON BLACK AGING, 72 ON MEXICAN AMERICAN AGING, AND 46 ON BLACK AND MEXICAN AMERICAN AGING. IN ADDITION, 9 OTHER BIBLIOGRAPHIES ON BLACK AND MEXICAN AMERICAN AGING ARE CITED. 311 REFERENCES.

ACCN 002184

1480 AUTH **RALPH, J. R.**

TITL VOODOO, SPIRITUALISM AND PSYCHIATRY: A SUMMARY OF A PANEL DISCUSSION.
SRCE *IN E. R. PADILLA & A. M. PADILLA (EDS.), TRANSCULTURAL PSYCHIATRY: AN HISPANIC PERSPECTIVE (MONOGRAPH NO. 4). LOS ANGELES: UNIVERSITY OF CALIFORNIA, SPANISH SPEAKING MENTAL HEALTH RESEARCH CENTER, 1977, PP. 97-99.*
INDX FOLK MEDICINE, CURANDERISMO, ESPIRITISMO, PSYCHOTHERAPY, PSYCHOTHERAPISTS, CULTURAL FACTORS, ESSAY, PUERTO RICAN-I, CASE STUDY
ABST A SUMMARY OF A SERIES OF PRESENTATIONS ON FOLK HEALING IS PRESENTED, WITH A MAJOR FOCUS ON THE AREA OF ESPIRITISMO. BASED ON A VISIT TO AN ESPIRISTA TEMPLE IN SAN JUAN, PUERTO RICO, THE DOCTRINE AND PRACTICE OF ESPIRITISMO ARE DISCUSSED. IN MANY PUERTO RICAN COMMUNITIES THESE FOLK HEALERS ARE SOUGHT IN CASES OF EMOTIONAL DISTURBANCES. A SECOND AREA OF INTEREST IS THE PRACTICE OF WITCHCRAFT IN THE WEST INDIES KNOWN AS OBEAH. A BRIEF HISTORY OF THE DEVELOPMENT OF OBEAH AND A CASE PRESENTATION OF A FEMALE PSYCHIATRIC PATIENT BELIEVED TO HAVE BEEN CURSED ARE DISCUSSED. LASTLY, THE PRACTICE OF VOODOO IS BRIEFLY MENTIONED. FOLLOWING THIS REVIEW OF THE PANEL DISCUSSION, THE CONCLUSION EMPHASIZES THE IMPORTANCE FOR MENTAL HEALTH PROFESSIONALS TO BE FAMILIAR WITH AND "ACCORD RESPECT" TO CULTURALLY DIFFERENT BELIEF SYSTEMS.

ACCN 001276

1481 AUTH **RAMIREZ, A.**
TITL CHICANO POWER AND INTER-RACIAL GROUP RELATIONS.
SRCE *PRESENTED AT THE FIRST SYMPOSIUM ON CHICANO PSYCHOLOGY, UNIVERSITY OF CALIFORNIA, IRVINE, MAY 15-16, 1976.*
INDX CHICANO MOVEMENT, INTERPERSONAL RELATIONS, POLITICAL POWER, CULTURAL PLURALISM, EQUAL OPPORTUNITY, CONFLICT RESOLUTION, CULTURAL CHANGE, ETHNIC IDENTITY, REVIEW
ABST IF CONTACT BETWEEN CHICANOS AND ANGLOS IS TO RESULT IN POSITIVE RELATIONS, THE TWO GROUPS MUST MEET ON EQUAL TERMS. A REVIEW OF THE INTERDEPENDENCY BETWEEN SOCIAL POWER—THE ABILITY OF ONE GROUP OR PERSON TO INFLUENCE ANOTHER—AND INTERGROUP RELATIONS IS PRESENTED. IT IS CLEAR FROM THE RESEARCH CITED THAT ANGLOS HAVE GREATER SOCIAL POWER; TO IMPROVE INTERETHNIC RELATONS, THE SOCIAL POWER OF CHICANOS MUST BE INCREASED. PSYCHOLOGISTS CAN PLAY A VITAL ROLE IN THIS PROCESS THROUGH RESEARCH AND THE DEVELOPMENT OF PROGRAMS. FUTURE DIRECTIONS FOR RESEARCH IN THIS AREA ARE DISCUSSED.

ACCN 001277

1482 AUTH **RAMIREZ, H. M.**
TITL RESEARCH FOR A CHANGE—FOR A CHANGE.

SRCE IN A. CASTANEDA, M. RAMIREZ, III, C. E. CORTES & M. BARRERA (EDS.), MEXICAN AMERICANS AND EDUCATIONAL CHANGE. NEW YORK: ARNO PRESS, 1974, PP. 189-204.

INDX RESEARCH METHODOLOGY, EDUCATION, SCHOLASTIC ACHIEVEMENT, EQUAL OPPORTUNITY, CURRICULUM, ACCULTURATION, BILINGUALISM, ETHNIC IDENTITY, LEADERSHIP, POLITICAL POWER, MEXICAN AMERICAN, ADMINISTRATORS, BILINGUAL-BICULTURAL EDUCATION, LEGISLATION, PROGRAM EVALUATION, SES, POVERTY, CHICANO MOVEMENT, SOUTHWEST, CULTURAL PLURALISM

ABST THE MEXICAN AMERICAN EDUCATION STUDY (MAES) EXAMINES SCHOOLS, THEIR CONDITIONS, PRACTICES, AND POLICIES TO DETERMINE THE PRESENT EDUCATIONAL SYSTEM'S EFFECTIVENESS IN PROVIDING EQUAL EDUCATION TO MINORITY STUDENTS. IT WAS DEVELOPED TO COMPILE NEW DATA ASSESSING THE STATUS OF MEXICAN AMERICAN (MA) EDUCATION IN THE SOUTHWEST AND TO UTILIZE THE DATA AS A FOUNDATION TO STIMULATE EDUCATIONAL CHANGE AT THE FEDERAL, STATE, AND LOCAL LEVELS. AT THE FEDERAL AND STATE LEVELS, THE STUDY IS AN EFFECTIVE TOOL FOR: (1) MAKING RECOMMENDATIONS TO CONGRESS FOR PROGRESSIVE LEGISLATION; (2) DEVELOPING AWARENESS AND SENSITIVITY TO MA EDUCATION AMONG POLICY MAKERS AND FUNDING SOURCES; (3) FEDERAL PROGRAM ASSESSMENT; AND (4) THE CREATION OF METHODS TO DETERMINE THE EFFECTIVENESS OF EDUCATIONAL PROGRAMS FOR MINORITIES. AT THE LOCAL LEVEL, IT PROVIDES A BASIS FOR CHANGE IN THE CLASSROOM, COUNSELING, AND SCHOOL ADMINISTRATION. TO DETERMINE IF THE MA EDUCATIONAL EXPERIENCE DIFFERS QUANTITATIVELY AND QUALITATIVELY FROM THE ANGLO EXPERIENCE, THE FLANDERS VERBAL INTERACTION ANALYSIS WAS APPLIED TO 600 CLASSROOMS IN THE SOUTHWEST. THE FINDINGS REVEALED: (1) MA STUDENTS, TEACHERS, AND ADMINISTRATORS ARE SEVERELY SEGREGATED; (2) MINORITY STUDENTS DO NOT OBTAIN EQUAL BENEFITS OF PUBLIC EDUCATION; (3) SCHOOL SYSTEMS DO NOT RECOGNIZE MA LANGUAGE AND TRADITION AS VIABLE; AND (4) DISPARITIES EXIST IN SCHOOL FINANCES, FACILITIES, AND EXPENDITURES PER PUPIL FOR MA STUDENTS. THE MAES FOCUS ON THE SCHOOL, RATHER THAN ON THE STUDENT, RESULTED IN THE ACCURATE AND OBJECTIVE MEASUREMENT OF THE DENIAL OF EQUAL EDUCATIONAL OPPORTUNITIES TO MA STUDENTS. ANOTHER FEATURE OF THE MAES WAS THAT IT SHIFTED THE RESPONSIBILITY OF ACQUIRING AN EQUAL EDUCATION FROM THE STUDENT AND THE FAMILY TO THE PROFESSIONAL EDUCATOR.

ACCN 001278

1483 AUTH **RAMIREZ, M., III.**

TITL BILINGUAL EDUCATION AS A TOOL FOR INSTITUTIONAL CHANGE.

SRCE IN A. CASTANEDA, M. RAMIREZ, III, C. E. CORTES, & M. BARRERA (EDS.), MEXICAN AMERICANS AND EDUCATIONAL CHANGE. NEW YORK: ARNO PRESS, 1974, PP. 387-407.

INDX BILINGUAL-BICULTURAL EDUCATION, BILINGUALISM, EDUCATION, MEXICAN AMERICAN, CULTURE, CULTURAL PLURALISM, ACCULTURATION, POLITICAL POWER, ETHNIC IDENTITY, CULTURAL FACTORS, FAMILY STRUCTURE, PARENTAL INVOLVEMENT, COOPERATION, COGNITIVE STYLE, BILINGUAL-BICULTURAL PERSONNEL, STEREOTYPES, CURRICULUM, INSTRUCTIONAL TECHNIQUES, CALIFORNIA, SOUTHWEST, CLASSROOM BEHAVIOR, POLICY

ABST AN EXAMINATION OF THE MAJOR FACTORS AFFECTING THE SUCCESS OF BILINGUAL EDUCATION PROGRAMS REVEALS: (1) FAILURE OF PROGRAMS TO REPLACE THE CULTURAL EXCLUSIONIST OR CULTURE-IS-DAMAGING MODEL WITH THAT OF CULTURAL DEMOCRACY; (2) LACK OF CONCERN WITH TEACHING STRATEGIES; (3) IGNORANCE OF THE HETEROGENOUS MAKE-UP OF CHICANOS THROUGHOUT THE SOUTHWEST; AND (4) THAT PROGRAM COMPONENTS ARE NOT BASED ON RESEARCH DATA RELEVANT TO THE PSYCHODYNAMICS OF CHICANO CHILDREN AND THEIR PARENTS. BASED ON THESE FINDINGS, THE BILINGUAL-BICULTURAL FOLLOW THROUGH MODEL AT THE UNIVERSITY OF CALIFORNIA, RIVERSIDE, FOCUSED ON 3 AREAS IN DEVELOPING A GUIDANCE TOOL FOR IMPLEMENTING INSTITUTIONAL CHANGE. THESE AREAS INCLUDED: (1) ACTIVE PARENT INVOLVEMENT UTILIZING PARENTS AS TEACHER TRAINERS AND INSTRUCTORS; (2) CULTURE MATCHING CURRICULA AND TEACHING STYLES EXAMINING THE EXTENT TO WHICH SPANISH IS USED IN THE CLASSROOM, ACKNOWLEDGEMENT OF THE CHILD'S FAMILY, LIFE STYLE, AND COMMUNITY IN CURRICULUM AND RECOGNITION OF THE MEXICAN CULTURAL HERITAGE; AND (3) SELECTION OF CRITERIA FOR EVALUATING THE EFFECTIVENESS OF BILINGUAL EDUCATION WHICH EMPHASIZES THE ETHNIC PRIDE EXHIBITED BY STUDENTS AND THEIR ABILITY TO RELATE WITH OTHER GROUPS. THE SUCCESS OF BILINGUAL EDUCATION PROGRAMS IS DEPENDENT UPON THE ACCEPTANCE OF CULTURAL DEMOCRACY BY THE EDUCATIONAL SYSTEM. SIGNIFICANT INSTITUTIONAL CHANGE, THEREFORE, WILL ONLY OCCUR WHEN CHICANOS HAVE THE RIGHT TO MAINTAIN THEIR CULTURAL IDENTITY THROUGHOUT THE EDUCATIONAL PROCESS. 11 REFERENCES.

ACCN 001279

1484 AUTH **RAMIREZ, M., III.**

TITL COGNITIVE STYLES AND CULTURAL DEMOCRACY IN EDUCATION.

SRCE SOCIAL SCIENCE QUARTERLY, 1973, 53(4), 895-904. (REPRINTED IN C. HERNANDEZ, M. J. HAUG & N. N. WAGNER (EDS.), CHICANOS: SOCIAL AND PSYCHOLOGICAL PERSPECTIVES. SAINT LOUIS: C. V. MOSBY COMPANY, 1976, PP. 196-203.)

INDX EDUCATION, CULTURE, CULTURAL PLURALISM, COGNITIVE STYLE, SOCIALIZATION, MEXICAN

AMERICAN, CHILDREN, REVIEW, FIELD DEPENDENCE-INDEPENDENCE, CURRICULUM

ABST THE RESEARCH SUPPORTING THE NOTION THAT CHICANOS HAVE DISTINCT LEARNING STYLES WHICH ARE PRESENTLY NOT BEING RECOGNIZED BY EDUCATIONAL INSTITUTIONS IS REVIEWED. STUDIES HAVE SHOWN THAT DUE TO UNIQUE SOCIALIZATION PRACTICES, MEXICAN AMERICAN CHILDREN ARE MORE FIELD DEPENDENT OR FIELD SENSITIVE (I.E., MORE INFLUENCED BY OR MORE SENSITIVE TO THE HUMAN ELEMENT IN THE ENVIRONMENT) THAN ANGLOS. THE FAILURE OF EDUCATIONAL INSTITUTIONS TO MEET THE NEEDS OF MOST MEXICAN AMERICANS IS BELIEVED TO BE DUE TO THE ORIENTATION OF SCHOOLS TOWARD SERVING THE PERSON WHO IS RELATIVELY MORE FIELD INDEPENDENT. THE PHILOSOPHY OF CULTURAL DEMOCRACY, THAT IS, THE RIGHT OF EACH INDIVIDUAL TO BE EDUCATED IN HIS OWN LEARNING STYLE, IS STRONGLY RECOMMENDED TO IMPROVE EDUCATION FOR CHICANOS. IT IS HOPED THAT INSTRUCTIONAL TECHNIQUES, CURRICULA, AND ASSESSMENT INSTRUMENTS WILL BE DEVELOPED TO REFLECT BOTH FIELD SENSITIVE AND FIELD INDEPENDENT COGNITIVE STYLES SO THAT CHILDREN OF ANY CULTURAL BACKGROUND CAN BE ABLE TO FUNCTION IN THEIR TYPE OF LEARNING ENVIRONMENT AND CONSEQUENTLY INCREASE THEIR LEVEL OF ACHIEVEMENT. 21 REFERENCES.

ACCN 001280

1485 AUTH **RAMIREZ, M., III.**
TITL COMMUNITY PSYCHOLOGY FOR HISPANOS.
SRCE IN I. ISCOE, B. L. BLOOM, & C. D. SPIELBERGER (EDS.), COMMUNITY PSYCHOLOGY IN TRANSITION: PROCEEDINGS OF THE NATIONAL CONFERENCE ON TRAINING IN COMMUNITY PSYCHOLOGY. NEW YORK: JOHN WILEY & SONS, 1977, PP. 271-274.
INDX CULTURAL FACTORS, CULTURAL PLURALISM, ESSAY, SPANISH SURNAMED, SOCIAL SCIENCES
ABST SINCE TRADITIONAL PSYCHOLOGY REFLECTS THE ANGLO-WESTERN EUROPEAN WORLD VIEW, PSYCHOLOGY'S CONCEPTS, THEORIES, AND INSTRUMENTS ARE ORIENTED TOWARD AN ANGLO CONFORMITY MODEL. HISPANOS ARE VIEWED AS HAVING A CULTURE INFERIOR TO THE MAINSTREAM AMERICAN MIDDLE CLASS, AND THUS AS FUNCTIONING WITHIN A PATHOLOGY-GENERATING MILIEU. THE COMMUNITY PSYCHOLOGY MOVEMENT, HOWEVER, IS SENSITIVE TO CULTURAL DIFFERENCES AND ENCOURAGES CULTURAL DEMOCRACY. FROM THIS PERSPECTIVE, BICULTURALISM IS AN ASSET, AND THE HISPANO COMMUNITY IS SEEN AS A POTENTIALLY RICH RESOURCE IN THE DEVELOPMENT OF THE "COMPETENT COMMUNITY." IT IS NECESSARY FOR PSYCHOLOGY TO BE KNOWLEDGEABLE OF AND RESPONSIVE TO THE MESTIZO WORLD VIEW. CLOSE FAMILIAL AND ETHNIC IDENTIFICATION, PERSONALIZATION OF RELATIONSHIPS, HUMANISM, COOPERATION, AND HARMONY WITH THE ENVIRONMENT ARE VIEWED AS POSITIVE ASPECTS OF

THIS WORLD VIEW. MOREOVER, COMMUNITY PSYCHOLOGY CAN FACILITATE THE GOALS OF CULTURAL DEMOCRACY AND HELP ENFRANCHIZE HISPANOS IN THEIR COMMUNITIES. FUTURE CONFERENCES, RESEARCH AND TRAINING EFFORTS, AND ONGOING DEDICATION ARE NECESSARY FOR THESE GOALS TO BECOME AN ACTIVE REALITY. 1 REFERENCE.

ACCN 002391

1486 AUTH **RAMIREZ, M., III.**
TITL CULTURAL DEMOCRACY: A NEW PHILOSOPHY FOR EDUCATING THE MEXICAN AMERICAN CHILD.
SRCE THE NATIONAL ELEMENTARY PRINCIPAL, 1970, 50(2), 45-46.
INDX CULTURAL PLURALISM, BILINGUAL-BICULTURAL EDUCATION, MEXICAN AMERICAN, CHILDREN, ETHNIC IDENTITY, EDUCATION, CURRICULUM, ESSAY
ABST THE "MELTING POT" PHILOSOPHY OF EDUCATION HAS HAD NEGATIVE CONSEQUENCES FOR CHICANO CHILDREN. IN THE SCHOOLS' ATTEMPT TO MAKE THE CHICANO CHILD IN THE IMAGE OF ANGLO MIDDLE CLASS CHILDREN, AN IDENTITY CRISIS IN THE CHILD BECOMES EXACERBATED. SHOULD HE REJECT HIS CULTURE TO SUCCEED IN THE EDUCATIONAL SYSTEM OR SHOULD HE REJECT THE EDUCATION AND MAINTAIN HIS CULTURE? THE CIVIL RIGHTS MOVEMENT AND THE BILINGUAL EDUCATION ACT NOW PROVIDE THE EDUCATIONAL SYSTEM AN OPPORTUNITY TO RID ITSELF OF THE "MELTING POT" PHILOSOPHY AND ACCEPT CULTURAL DEMOCRACY—A PHILOSOPHY THAT FOSTERS THE CHILD'S ACCEPTANCE OF HIS ETHNIC IDENTITY. TRULY EFFECTIVE BILINGUAL-BICULTURAL PROGRAMS MUST HAVE (1) ACTIVE PARENT INVOLVEMENT, (2) MEXICAN AND CHICANO HERITAGE CURRICULUM, AND (3) CURRICULUM AND TEACHING STYLES TAILORED TO THE UNIQUE LEARNING AND INCENTIVE-MOTIVATIONAL STYLES OF CHICANO CHILDREN. IN CONCLUSION, CULTURAL DEMOCRACY STATES THAT THE EDUCATIONAL SYSTEM MUST CHANGE TO FIT THE CHILD AS OPPOSED TO THE CHILD CHANGING TO FIT THE INSTITUTION. 4 REFERENCES.

ACCN 001281

1487 AUTH **RAMIREZ, M., III.**
TITL CURRENT EDUCATIONAL RESEARCH: THE BASIS FOR A NEW PHILOSOPHY FOR EDUCATING MEXICAN-AMERICANS.
SRCE UNPUBLISHED MANUSCRIPT, UNIVERSITY OF CALIFORNIA, RIVERSIDE, 1972.
INDX EDUCATION, MEXICAN AMERICAN, CHILDREN, ESSAY, CULTURAL FACTORS, CULTURAL PLURALISM, EDUCATION, COGNITIVE STYLE, BILINGUAL-BICULTURAL EDUCATION
ABST A PHILOSOPHY OF EDUCATION TERMED "CULTURAL DEMOCRACY" IS DISCUSSED AS IT RELATES TO THE EDUCATION OF MEXICAN AMERICANS. THIS PHILOSOPHY STATES THAT A PERSON CAN BE BICULTURAL AND AT THE SAME TIME BE A RESPONSIBLE MEMBER OF A LARGER SOCIETY. EDUCATIONAL SYSTEMS HAVE ADHERED TO AN EXCLUSIONIST MELT-

ING POT PHILOSOPHY, WHICH RESEARCH IN-
DICATES HAS HAD NEGATIVE CONSEQUENCES
FOR MEXICAN AMERICAN STUDENTS IN TERMS
OF EDUCATIONAL ATTAINMENT AND CUL-
TURAL VALUE CONFLICTS. RECENT STUDIES
HAVE DEMONSTRATED THAT LEARNING STYLES
(E.G., COGNITIVE, INCENTIVE-MOTIVATIONAL,
AND HUMAN RELATIONAL) CAN BE CULTUR-
ALLY DISTINCT. TO IMPROVE EDUCATION FOR
MEXICAN AMERICANS, IT IS VITAL THAT LEARN-
ING ENVIRONMENTS WHICH ARE CONSISTENT
WITH THE CULTURAL LEARNING STYLES OF
MEXICAN AMERICANS BE DEVELOPED. A RE-
SEARCH AND DEVELOPMENT PROJECT THAT IS
DEVISING STRATEGIES TO FOLLOW THE CUL-
TURAL DEMOCRATIC MODEL IS DESCRIBED IN
DETAIL. LASTLY, IT IS RECOMMENDED THAT
UNIVERSITIES AND COLLEGES BEGIN TO IM-
PLEMENT THE PHILOSOPHY OF CULTURAL DE-
MOCRACY. 15 REFERENCES.

ACCN 001282

1488 AUTH **RAMIREZ, M., III.**
TITL IDENTIFICATION WITH MEXICAN FAMILY VAL-
UES AND AUTHORITARIANISM IN MEXICAN-
AMERICANS.
SRCE *JOURNAL OF SOCIAL PSYCHOLOGY, 1967, 73(1),
3-11.*
INDX ETHNIC IDENTITY, ATTITUDES, AUTHORITARI-
ANISM, MEXICAN AMERICAN, FAMILY ROLES,
ACCULTURATION, EMPIRICAL, COLLEGE STU-
DENTS, CONFLICT RESOLUTION, STRESS, CUL-
TURAL FACTORS, VALUES
ABST AN ASSESSMENT OF THE DEGREE TO WHICH
MEXICAN AMERICANS IDENTIFY WITH MEXI-
CAN FAMILY VALUES AND AN INVESTIGATION
OF WHETHER A POSITIVE RELATIONSHIP EX-
ISTS BETWEEN AUTOCRATIC FAMILY IDEOLOGY
AND AUTHORITARIAN IDEOLOGY IN MEXICAN
AMERICANS IS PRESENTED. THE SUBJECTS, 70
MEXICAN AMERICAN AND 70 ANGLO AMERI-
CAN MIDDLE-CLASS, CATHOLIC COLLEGE
STUDENTS, WERE ADMINISTERED CONCUR-
RENTLY A MEXICAN FAMILY ATTITUDE SCALE
AND THE CALIFORNIA F SCALE. RESULTS INDI-
CATE THAT MEXICAN AMERICANS SCORED
HIGHER ON BOTH SCALES THAN DID THE AN-
GLO AMERICANS. A SIGNIFICANT POSITIVE RE-
LATIONSHIP BETWEEN HIGH AGREEMENT WITH
THE ITEMS OF THE ATTITUDE SCALE AND HIGH
SCORES ON THE F SCALE WAS FOUND FOR
MEXICAN AMERICANS. THE RESULTS CONFIRM
THE OBSERVATIONS OF ADORNO ET AL., AND
LEVINSON AND HUFFMAN. COMPARISON OF
THE FAMILY ATTITUDE PATTERN OF THE MEXI-
CAN AMERICAN WITH THAT OF MEXICANS AND
PUERTO RICANS DISCLOSES THAT THE MEXI-
CAN AMERICAN VALUE SYSTEMS REVEAL SIGNS
OF AMERICANIZATION IN THE FORM OF A DE-
CREASE IN THE AUTHORITY OF THE MALE.
MEXICAN AMERICANS AGREED ON THE MEXI-
CAN FAMILY VALUES OF CONFORMITY, STRICT
CHILDREARING, AND AUTHORITARIAN SUB-
MISSION. A DETAILED DISCUSSION OF THE
FINDINGS IS PRESENTED. 11 REFERENCES.

ACCN 001283

1489 AUTH **RAMIREZ, M., III.**

TITL IDENTIFICATION WITH MEXICAN-AMERICAN
VALUES AND PSYCHOLOGICAL ADJUSTMENT
IN MEXICAN-AMERICAN ADOLESCENTS.
SRCE *THE INTERNATIONAL JOURNAL OF SOCIAL
PSYCHIATRY, 1969, 15(2), 151-156.*
INDX ETHNIC IDENTITY, ATTITUDES, PSYCHOSOCIAL
ADJUSTMENT, MEXICAN AMERICAN, ADOLES-
CENTS, CONFLICT RESOLUTION, EMPIRICAL,
ACCULTURATION, INTERPERSONAL RELA-
TIONS, SEX COMPARISON, CULTURAL FAC-
TORS, CALIFORNIA, SOUTHWEST, VALUES
ABST AN INVESTIGATION OF VALUE CONFLICTS AND
PSYCHOLOGICAL ADJUSTMENT AMONG THIRD
GENERATION MEXICAN AMERICAN (MA) HIGH
SCHOOL STUDENTS IS PRESENTED. AN EQUAL
NUMBER OF LOWER-MIDDLE SOCIOECO-
NOMIC CLASS MALES AND FEMALES BETWEEN
THE AGES OF 13 TO 18 WERE ADMINISTERED A
29-ITEM ATTITUDE SCALE OF MEXICAN AMERI-
CAN VALUES. THE ITEMS WERE RESPONDED
TO ON A 7-POINT SCALE RANGING FROM
"AGREE VERY MUCH" TO "DISAGREE VERY
MUCH." THE 10 SUBJECTS WHO SCORED THE
HIGHEST ON THE ATTITUDE SCALE WERE LA-
BELED 1-G'S (GREATEST AGREEMENT WITH MA
VALUES) AND THE 10 WHO SCORED THE LOW-
EST WERE CLASSIFIED AS R'S (REJECTION OF
MA VALUES). SUBJECTS IN BOTH THE R AND 1-
G GROUPS WERE ALSO ADMINISTERED THE
200-ITEM BELL ADJUSTMENT INVENTORY. DATA
REVEAL THAT THE SCORES OBTAINED BY BOTH
R MALES AND FEMALES ON THE HOME AD-
JUSTMENT SCALE ARE WITHIN THE UNSATIS-
FACTORY AND POOR RANGE, RESPECTIVELY.
THE MEAN SCORE OF THE R FEMALES ON THE
HEALTH ADJUSTMENT SCALE IS ALSO INDICA-
TIVE OF MALADJUSTMENT. THE SCORE OF 1-G
FEMALES IN THE SUBMISSIVENESS SCALE IS
INTERPRETED AS EXTREME SUBMISSIVENESS
IN INTERPERSONAL RELATIONS. BICULTURAL
INDIVIDUALS EXPERIENCE A VARIETY OF AD-
JUSTMENT PROBLEMS WHICH APPEAR TO BE
RELATED TO THE ATTITUDES THEY ADOPT AND
VALUE CONFLICTS EXPERIENCED IN THE PRO-
CESS OF CULTURAL TRANSFER. THE SEVERE
INTERPERSONAL CONFLICTS WITH PARENTS
AND OTHER MEMBERS OF THE FAMILY RE-
PORTED BY R SUBJECTS MAY BE RELATED TO
THEIR HEALTH PROBLEMS AND STRESS. IT IS
SUGGESTED THAT WHENEVER A PERSON IS
CAUGHT BETWEEN TWO OPPOSING SETS OF
VALUES AND DECIDES TO REJECT ONE OF THE
SETS, HE/SHE BECOMES OVERWHELMED BY
FEELINGS OF GUILT AND SELF-DEROGATION.
THIS OCCURS BECAUSE THE VALUES RE-
JECTED ARE ASSOCIATED WITH A PERSON IM-
PORTANT TO THE SUBJECT, USUALLY A PAR-
ENT. 11 REFERENCES.

ACCN 001284

1490 AUTH **RAMIREZ, M., III.**
TITL RECOGNIZING AND UNDERSTANDING DIVER-
SITY: THE CHICANO PSYCHOLOGY MOVEMENT.
SRCE *IN J. L. MARTINEZ, JR. (ED.), CHICANO PSY-
CHOLOGY. NEW YORK: ACADEMIC PRESS, 1977,
PP. 343-353.*
INDX CULTURAL PLURALISM, MEXICAN AMERICAN,
CHICANO MOVEMENT, PERSONALITY, PSYCHO-

SOCIAL ADJUSTMENT, CALIFORNIA, SOUTH-WEST, THEORETICAL, ETHNIC IDENTITY, REVIEW

ABST   A SURVEY OF THE LITERATURE YIELDS MANY EXAMPLES OF MINORITY GROUP MEMBERS BEING VIEWED AS "MARGINAL," SUBJECT TO LOSS OF SELF-IDENTITY, CAUGHT BETWEEN TWO DISSIMILAR AND DEMANDING CULTURAL SYSTEMS, AND CONSEQUENTLY EXPERIENCING CONFLICT AND ARRESTED DEVELOPMENT. IN CONTRAST TO THESE NEGATIVE THEORIES OF BICULTURALISM, CHICANO PSYCHOLOGY IS EVOLVING THE VIEW THAT PARTICIPATION IN MORE THAN ONE SOCIOCULTURAL SYSTEM IS A POSITIVE PHENOMENON WHICH ENCOURAGES FLEXIBILITY AND DIVERSITY OF FUNCTIONING. TO BETTER UNDERSTAND THIS, RESEARCH IS BEING CONDUCTED WITH CHICANO COLLEGE STUDENTS THROUGHOUT CALIFORNIA. AN INITIAL SERIES OF LIFE HISTORY INTERVIEWS PROVIDED THE BASIS FOR A QUESTIONNAIRE, "THE CHICANO BICULTURALISM/MULTICULTURALISM INVENTORY." THOSE IDENTIFIED BY THIS QUESTIONNAIRE AS BEING MOST BICULTURAL WILL BE SELECTED FOR INTENSIVE INTERVIEWING AND TESTING ON A VARIETY OF PERSONALITY TRAITS. PRELIMINARY DATA THUS FAR HAVE RESULTED IN A TENTATIVE MODEL—THE FLEXIBILITY/SYNTHESIS MODEL—IN WHICH THE BICULTURAL PERSON'S VALUES, ATTITUDES, COPING STYLES, PERCEPTUAL MODES, AND WORLD VIEWS SPECIFIC TO EACH CULTURE ARE DEVELOPED, INTEGRATED, AND FINALLY SYNTHESIZED INTO HIS OR HER MODE OF BEING. THE PRODUCT IS A MORE SOCIALLY FLEXIBLE AND WELL DEVELOPED INDIVIDUAL. THE DIFFERENCE BETWEEN THIS NEW MODEL AND PREVIOUS MODELS OF BICULTURALISM IS THAT DIVERSITY IS VIEWED AS CONTRIBUTING POSITIVELY TO SELF-ACTUALIZATION THROUGH THE BLENDING OF RICH AND DIVERSE CULTURES. IT IS HOPED THAT CHICANO PSYCHOLOGISTS WILL FURTHER EXPLORE SUCH METHODS AS THIS SO AS TO COUNTERACT THE TENDENCY IN TRADITIONAL SOCIAL SCIENCE TO VIEW DIVERSITY AS MERELY A SIGN OF INFERIORITY.

ACCN   001285

1491 AUTH **RAMIREZ, M., III.**
TITL   THE RELATIONSHIP OF ACCULTURATION TO EDUCATIONAL ACHIEVEMENT AND PSYCHOLOGICAL ADJUSTMENT IN CHICANO CHILDREN AND ADOLESCENTS: A REVIEW OF THE LITERATURE.
SRCE   *EL GRITO, 1971, 4(4), 21-28.*
INDX   ACCULTURATION, SCHOLASTIC ACHIEVEMENT, PSYCHOSOCIAL ADJUSTMENT, MEXICAN AMERICAN, CHILDREN, ADOLESCENTS, REVIEW, ETHNIC IDENTITY, SELF CONCEPT, VALUES
ABST   THE LITERATURE IS REVIEWED IN ORDER TO DETERMINE WHETHER IDENTIFICATION WITH ONE'S ETHNIC GROUP IS AN ASSET OR A LIABILITY FOR THE CHICANO. STUDIES RELATING ACCULTURATION TO EDUCATION INDICATE THAT THE REINFORCEMENT A CHILD RECEIVES FROM THE SCHOOL FOR IDENTIFICATION WITH THE

MEXICAN AMERICAN VALUE SYSTEM IS CRITICAL IN UNDERSTANDING THE RELATIONSHIP BETWEEN ACCULTURATION AND ACADEMIC ACHIEVEMENT. IN SCHOOLS WHERE THE CHILD IS SUPPORTED FOR HIS "CHICANISMO," ACHIEVEMENT IS NOT DIFFERENT FROM NON-CHICANO COMPARISON GROUPS. IT IS ALSO NOTED THAT SOCIOECONOMIC VARIABLES ARE CENTRAL TO THE ISSUE: ONE STUDY INDICATED THAT MIDDLE-CLASS SPANISH SURNAMED STUDENTS' ACCULTURATION TO FAMILY VALUES WAS NEGATIVELY RELATED TO PERFORMANCE IN SCHOOL. RESULTS OF STUDIES RELATING ACCULTURATION TO PERSONALITY SHOW THAT ACCULTURATION WHICH REDUCES THE CHICANO'S IDENTITY WITH HIS ETHNIC GROUP RESULTS IN NEGATIVE CONSEQUENCES FOR PSYCHOLOGICAL ADJUSTMENT. LONGITUDINAL RESEARCH FOCUSING ON HOW THE SOCIAL MILIEU AND SOCIOECONOMIC CLASS INTERACT WITH ACCULTURATION TO AFFECT PERSONALITY AND EDUCATIONAL ACHIEVEMENT IS RECOMMENDED. 10 REFERENCES.

ACCN   001286

1492 AUTH **RAMIREZ, M., III.**
TITL   SOCIAL RESPONSIBILITIES AND FAILURE IN PSYCHOLOGY: THE CASE OF THE MEXICAN-AMERICAN.
SRCE   *IN G. J. WILLIAMS & S. GORDON (EDS.), CLINICAL CHILD PSYCHOLOGY: CURRENT PRACTICES AND FUTURE PRESPECTIVES. NEW YORK: BEHAVIORAL PUBLICATIONS, 1974, PP. 326-332.*
INDX   MEXICAN AMERICAN, ESCALA DE INTELIGENCIA WECHSLER, WISC, MENTAL RETARDATION, INTELLIGENCE TESTING, CALIFORNIA TEST OF MENTAL MATURITY, CHILDREN, BILINGUAL-BICULTURAL EDUCATION, CULTURAL FACTORS, REVIEW, HIGHER EDUCATION, REPRESENTATION, MENTAL HEALTH PROFESSION
ABST   THE RESULTS OF A SURVEY CONDUCTED BY THE ASSOCIATION OF PSYCHOLOGISTS FOR LA RAZA ILLUSTRATE THE UNDERREPRESENTATION OF THE MEXICAN AMERICAN (MA) IN PSYCHOLOGY. ONLY 13 MA'S WITH DOCTORATE DEGREES IN PSYCHOLOGY WERE FOUND. CERTAIN ISSUES OF THE CIVIL RIGHTS MOVEMENT WHICH REQUIRE A PSYCHOLOGIST'S EXPERTISE ARE AFFECTED BY THE SHORTAGE OF TRAINED PSYCHOLOGISTS. FOR EXAMPLE, CHICANO PSYCHOLOGISTS ARE NEEDED TO DEVELOP NEW INSTRUMENTS WHICH NOT ONLY REFLECT THE COMMUNICATION STYLE OF THE MA CHILD, BUT HIS COGNITIVE AND INCENTIVE-MOTIVATIONAL STYLES AS WELL. IN PARTICULAR, SINCE MA'S MAY BE MISDIAGNOSED AS PATHOLOGICAL BY MANY PERSONALITY ASSESSMENT INSTRUMENTS WHICH CONTAIN CULTURALLY-LOADED ITEMS SUCH AS ARE FOUND IN THE CHILD MANIFEST ANXIETY SCALE AND THE MINNESOTA MULTIPHASIC PERSONALITY INVENTORY, A REEXAMINATION OF THESE INSTRUMENTS AND THEIR INTERPRETATIONS IS NECESSARY. RESEARCH IS ALSO NEEDED TO PROBE THE THEORIES OF PSYCHOLOGICAL DEVELOPMENT WHICH HAVE LED SOCIAL SCIENTISTS AND EDUCATORS TO THE CONCLU-

SION THAT THE MA CULTURE INTERFERES WITH THE INTELLECTUAL AND SOCIAL DEVELOPMENT OF THE CHICANO CHILD. FINALLY, THE QUALITY OF MENTAL HEALTH SERVICES TO MA'S IS QUESTIONABLE SINCE FEW MENTAL HEALTH PERSONNEL ARE BILINGUAL AND FAMILIAR WITH THE VALUE SYSTEM OF THE MA. ACTIVE RECRUITMENT OF CHICANOS INTO THE FIELD OF PSYCHOLOGY IS RECOMMENDED SO THAT THESE PROBLEMS CAN BE SOLVED OR ALLEVIATED. 8 REFERENCES.

ACCN 001287

1493 AUTH **RAMIREZ, M., III.**
TITL TOWARDS CULTURAL DEMOCRACY IN MENTAL HEALTH: THE CASE OF THE MEXICAN-AMERICAN.
SRCE *INTERAMERICAN JOURNAL OF PSYCHOLOGY, 1972, 6, 45-50.*
INDX MENTAL HEALTH, REHABILITATION, MEXICAN AMERICAN, CULTURAL PLURALISM, PSYCHOTHERAPY, BILINGUAL-BICULTURAL PERSONNEL, PARAPROFESSIONALS, HEALTH DELIVERY SYSTEMS, ATTITUDES, CULTURAL FACTORS, INTERPERSONAL RELATIONS, ESSAY
ABST THE MENTAL HEALTH NEEDS OF MEXICAN AMERICANS ARE DISCUSSED IN RELATION TO PROBLEMS OF CULTURAL PLURALITY, BICULTURALITY, AND BILINGUALISM. CHARACTERISTICS OF CHICANO CULTURE DEEMED IMPORTANT IN PSYCHOTHERAPEUTIC PROCESS INCLUDE: (1) A STRONG IDENTIFICATION WITH FAMILY AND ETHNIC GROUP; (2) RESPECT FOR PARENTS, MARRIAGE PARTNER, AND AUTHORITY; (3) IDENTIFICATION WITH THE IDEOLOGY OF THE MEXICAN CATHOLIC CHURCH; (4) A HIGH DEGREE OF PERSONALIZATION OF INTERPERSONAL RELATIONSHIPS; AND (5) SENSITIVITY TO HUMAN ENVIRONMENT. THE NEED FOR TRAINING OF CHICANO PROFESSIONALS IS EMPHASIZED. THE REEVALUATION OF TRADITIONAL THEORIES AND ASSESSMENT INSTRUMENTS IS URGED TO MAKE PSYCHOTHERAPY FOR MEXICAN AMERICANS CONSONANT WITH THEIR COMMUNICATION, MOTIVATION, AND LEARNING STYLES. 4 REFERENCES. (PASAR ABSTRACT)

ACCN 001289

1494 AUTH **RAMIREZ, M., III, CASTANEDA, A., & HEROLD, P. L.**
TITL THE RELATIONSHIP OF ACCULTURATION TO COGNITIVE STYLE AMONG MEXICAN AMERICANS.
SRCE *JOURNAL OF CROSS-CULTURAL PSYCHOLOGY, 1974, 5(4), 424-432.*
INDX ACCULTURATION, COGNITIVE STYLE, MEXICAN AMERICAN, EMPIRICAL, CHILDREN, MOTHER-CHILD INTERACTION, CALIFORNIA, SOUTHWEST, FIELD DEPENDENCE-INDEPENDENCE, ADULTS, SURVEY, FEMALE, VALUES
ABST TO ASSESS FIELD DEPENDENCY IN COGNITIVE STYLE, THE PORTABLE ROD AND FRAME TEST AND A FIGURE DRAWING TEST WERE ADMINISTERED TO 541 MEXICAN AMERICAN CHILDREN AND THEIR MOTHERS IN THREE COMMUNITIES IN SOUTHERN CALIFORNIA. APPROXIMATELY EQUAL NUMBERS OF BOTH SEXES, FROM MIDDLE AND LOWER SES GROUPS, WERE SELECTED FROM EACH GRADE LEVEL IN EACH COMMUNITY. ONLY THOSE CHILDREN WHOSE PARENTS HAD RESIDED IN THE U.S. FOR AT LEAST 4 YEARS AND WERE OF MEXICAN DESCENT WERE INCLUDED IN THE SAMPLE. QUESTIONNAIRES ON SOCIALIZATION PRACTICES AND MEXICAN AMERICAN FAMILY VALUES WERE ADMINISTERED TO THE MOTHERS. SUBJECTS FROM THE "TRADITIONAL" COMMUNITY, IN WHICH MEMBERS WERE MOST IDENTIFIED WITH THE SOCIOCULTURAL SYSTEM OF MEXICAN CULTURE, SCORED IN A FIELD-DEPENDENT DIRECTION. SUBJECTS FROM THE "ATRADITIONAL" COMMUNITY, WHOSE MEMBERS WERE MOST INFLUENCED BY MAINSTREAM AMERICAN MIDDLE-CLASS VALUES, WERE MOST FIELD-INDEPENDENT IN COGNITIVE STYLE. CHILDREN AND MOTHERS OF THE COMMUNITY INFLUENCED BY BOTH CULTURES, THE "DUALISTIC" COMMUNITY, OBTAINED SCORES BETWEEN THOSE OF THE OTHER TWO GROUPS. MOTHERS FROM THE TRADITIONAL COMMUNITY WERE MOST FREQUENTLY IN AGREEMENT WITH ITEMS REFLECTING INDICATORS OF THE FIELD-DEPENDENT "SOCIALIZATION" CLUSTER, AND ALSO WITH ITEMS REFLECTING THE SOCIOCULTURAL SYSTEM OF MEXICAN AMERICAN CULTURE. THE RESULTS INDICATE THAT THE REARING ENVIRONMENT IS IMPORTANT FOR THE DEVELOPMENT OF TYPE OF COGNITIVE STYLE AND THAT THE MEXICAN AMERICAN GROUP IS A HETEROGENEOUS ONE. THE IMPLICATIONS OF THESE FINDINGS ON THE DEVELOPMENT OF EDUCATIONAL PROGRAMS ARE DISCUSSED. 7 REFERENCES. (JOURNAL ABSTRACT MODIFIED)

ACCN 001290

1495 AUTH **RAMIREZ, M., III, HEROLD, P. L., & CASTANEDA, A.**
TITL DEVELOPING COGNITIVE FLEXIBILITY.
SRCE *IN P. HARPER (ED.), NEW APPROACHES TO BILINGUAL, BICULTURAL EDUCATION (REV. ED.). AUSTIN, TEXAS: THE DISSEMINATION AND ASSESSMENT CENTER FOR BILINGUAL EDUCATION, 1978, PP. 85-91.*
INDX BILINGUAL-BICULTURAL EDUCATION, COGNITIVE DEVELOPMENT, MEXICAN AMERICAN, CHILDREN, CURRICULUM, COGNITIVE STYLE, INSTRUCTIONAL TECHNIQUES, PROFESSIONAL TRAINING, TEACHERS, FIELD DEPENDENCE-INDEPENDENCE, EDUCATION, CULTURAL PLURALISM
ABST SIXTH IN A SERIES OF SEVEN MANUALS AND SELF-ASSESSMENT UNITS DESIGNED AS TEACHER TRAINING MATERIALS FOR USE IN BILINGUAL-BICULTURAL PROJECTS, THIS MANUAL COVERS A WIDE RANGE OF EDUCATIONAL ISSUES WITH PARTICULAR REFERENCE TO DEVELOPING COGNITIVE FLEXIBILITY IN BICOGNITIVE STYLE. COGNITIVE FLEXIBILITY IS DEFINED IN TERMS OF FIELD SENSITIVITY OR INDEPENDENCE, IMPERSONAL OR SOCIAL ABSTRACTIONS, AND INDUCTIVE OR DEDUCTIVE REASONING. THE IMPORTANCE OF THIS CONCEPT FOR MEXICAN AMERICAN CHILDREN IN

HUMAN RELATIONS, COMMUNICATION, AND THINKING ADAPTATIONS IS DISCUSSED. INSTRUCTION IN THE ASSESSMENT AND CONTINUAL EVALUATION OF INDIVIDUAL COGNITIVE STYLES IS STRESSED, AND CLASSROOM STRUCTURE AND CURRICULUM ISSUES ARE EXAMINED IN DETAIL. SUGGESTIONS FOR TRAINING OF TEACHERS TO DEVELOP BICOGNITIVE STYLES INCLUDE WORKSHOPS WITH VIDEOTAPED FEEDBACK AND SHARED LESSON PLANS. THE IMPORTANCE OF PROMOTING COGNITIVE FLEXIBILITY IN CHILDREN IN DEVELOPING CULTURALLY DEMOCRATIC EDUCATIONAL ENVIRONMENTS IS STRESSED IN TERMS OF FULL SCHOLASTIC OPPORTUNITY, PRESERVATION OF CULTURAL VALUES, DIVERSITY IN INTELLECTUAL AND SOCIAL ENVIRONMENTS, AND EXPOSURE TO ALTERNATIVE LIFE STYLES.

ACCN   001291

1496 AUTH   **RAMIREZ, M., III, HEROLD, P. L., & CASTANEDA, A.**

TITL   FIELD SENSITIVITY AND FIELD INDEPENDENCE IN CHILDREN.

SRCE   *IN P. HARPER (ED.), NEW APPROACHES TO BILINGUAL, BICULTURAL EDUCATION (REV. ED.). AUSTIN, TEXAS: THE DISSEMINATION AND ASSESSMENT CENTER FOR BILINGUAL EDUCATION, 1978, PP. 51-60.*

INDX   BILINGUAL-BICULTURAL EDUCATION, COGNITIVE STYLE, TEACHERS, CLASSROOM BEHAVIOR, CHILDREN, FIELD DEPENDENCE-INDEPENDENCE, CURRICULUM, BILINGUALISM, EDUCATION, EDUCATIONAL ASSESSMENT

ABST   FOURTH IN A SERIES OF SEVEN MANUALS AND SELF-ASSESSMENT UNITS DESIGNED AS TEACHER TRAINING MATERIALS FOR USE IN BILINGUAL-BICULTURAL PROJECTS, THIS MANUAL FAMILIARIZES TEACHERS WITH WAYS OF MEASURING A CHILD'S DOMINANT COGNITIVE STYLE (WHETHER FIELD SENSITIVE, FIELD INDEPENDENT OR "BICOGNITIVE") AS WELL AS THE CHILD'S DEVELOPING NONDOMINANT COGNITIVE STYLE. THE PORTABLE ROD AND FRAME TEST (PRFT) AND THE CHILD EMBEDDED FIGURES TEST (CEFT) ARE DESCRIBED IN DETAIL AS INSTRUMENTS DESIGNED TO MEASURE COGNITIVE STYLES. HOWEVER, DUE TO THEIR FIELD INDEPENDENT BIAS, THEY DO NOT AID IN DETERMINING THE EXTENT TO WHICH A CHILD IS ATTAINING MENTAL FLEXIBILITY OR COMPETENCIES IN BOTH COGNITIVE STYLES. THE OBSERVABLE BEHAVIOR RATING SYSTEM (OBRS) AND THE CHILD RATING FORMS (CRF) ARE SEEN AS APPROPRIATE FOR DETERMINING THESE. A GOAL OF CULTURALLY DEMOCRATIC EDUCATION IS HELPING CHILDREN BECOME BICOGNITIVE—TO FUNCTION COMFORTABLY AND COMPETENTLY IN BOTH COGNITIVE STYLES. SINCE BICOGNITIVE CHILDREN ARE OFTEN BILINGUAL-BICULTURAL AND HAVE ACHIEVED LINGUISTIC AND CULTURAL FLEXIBILITY, MEXICAN AMERICAN CHILDREN ARE SEEN AS BELONGING TO THIS CATEGORY. FINALLY, IN PROMOTING BICOGNITIVE DEVELOPMENT IN CHILDREN, THE FOLLOWING SEQUENCE IS RECOMMENDED FOR TEACHERS: (1) A GLOBAL RATING IS USED TO DETERMINE

THE DOMINANT COGNITIVE STYLE; (2) ASSIGNMENT TO A GROUP WITH CORRESPONDING INSTRUCTION; (3) GRADUAL INTRODUCTION TO THE FUNCTIONING IN THE UNFAMILIAR COGNITIVE STYLE; AND (4) OBSERVATION TO DETERMINE THE EXTENT TO WHICH HE DISPLAYS BEHAVIORS OF THE UNFAMILIAR COGNITIVE STYLE, THEREBY BECOMING BICOGNITIVE. 2 REFERENCES.

ACCN   001292

1497 AUTH   **RAMIREZ, M., III, HEROLD, P. L., & CASTANEDA, A.**

TITL   INTRODUCTION TO COGNITIVE STYLES.

SRCE   *IN P. HARPER (ED.), NEW APPROACHES TO BILINGUAL, BICULTURAL EDUCATION (REV. ED.). AUSTIN, TEXAS: THE DISSEMINATION AND ASSESSMENT CENTER FOR BILINGUAL EDUCATION, 1978, PP. 37-48.*

INDX   BILINGUAL-BICULTURAL EDUCATION, COGNITIVE STYLE, CULTURAL PLURALISM, MEXICAN AMERICAN, CHILDREN, ESSAY, ATTITUDES, FIELD DEPENDENCE-INDEPENDENCE, CULTURAL FACTORS, SOCIALIZATION, ETHNIC IDENTITY, EDUCATION

ABST   THIRD IN A SERIES OF SEVEN MANUALS AND SELF-ASSESSMENT UNITS DESIGNED AS TEACHER TRAINING MATERIALS FOR USE IN BILINGUAL-BICULTURAL PROJECTS, THIS MANUAL CONSIDERS THE INFLUENCE OF SOCIALIZATION PRACTICES ON CHILDREN'S COGNITIVE STYLES AND, IN PARTICULAR, CHILDREN'S PREFERRED LEARNING STYLES. DEFINED AND CONSIDERED IN ITS BROADEST PSYCHOLOGICAL SENSE, COGNITIVE STYLE IS SEEN AS RELATING TO DIFFERENCES BETWEEN PERSONS IN HUMAN RELATIONAL, COMMUNICATION, INCENTIVE-MOTIVATIONAL AND LEARNING STYLES. A REVIEW OF SEVERAL STUDIES, DEMONSTRATING DIFFERENCES IN COGNITIVE STYLES BETWEEN AMERICAN MIDDLE CLASS AND TRADITIONAL MEXICAN AMERICAN CULTURAL AND SOCIALIZATION VALUES, SUGGESTS THAT FIELD INDEPENDENCE IS COMMON AMONG CHILDREN WHOSE FAMILIES EMPHASIZE DEVELOPMENT OF A SEPARATE IDENTITY (AS IN ANGLO FAMILIES), WHILE FIELD SENSITIVITY IS COMMON AMONG CHILDREN WHOSE FAMILIES STRESS CLOSENESS BETWEEN MEMBERS AND THE CHILD'S IDENTIFICATION WITH THE FAMILY (AS IN MEXICAN AMERICAN FAMILIES). BECAUSE CULTURE CLEARLY INFLUENCES A PERSON'S WAY OF PERCEIVING AND THINKING ABOUT THE ENVIRONMENT, PLANNING CULTURALLY DEMOCRATIC EDUCATIONAL ENVIRONMENTS MUST FOLLOW FROM AN APPRECIATION OF DIVERSITY. AN APPENDIX CONTAINING RESEARCH FINDINGS RELEVANT TO COMPARISONS BETWEEN FIELD SENSITIVE AND FIELD INDEPENDENT PERSONS IS INCLUDED. 21 REFERENCES.

ACCN   001293

1498 AUTH   **RAMIREZ, M., III, HEROLD, P. L., & CASTANEDA, A.**

TITL   MEXICAN AMERICAN VALUES AND CULTUR-

ALLY DEMOCRATIC EDUCATIONAL ENVIRON-MENTS.

SRCE   *IN P. HARPER (ED.), NEW APPROACHES TO BI-LINGUAL, BICULTURAL EDUCATION (REV. ED.). AUSTIN, TEXAS: THE DISSEMINATION AND AS-SESSMENT CENTER FOR BILINGUAL EDUCA-TION, 1978, PP. 17-33.*

INDX   BILINGUAL-BICULTURAL EDUCATION, MEXI-CAN AMERICAN, ATTITUDES, CULTURAL PLU-RALISM, EDUCATIONAL ASSESSMENT, ENVI-RONMENTAL FACTORS, ESSAY, PROFESSIONAL TRAINING, TEACHERS, SOCIALIZATION, CON-FLICT RESOLUTION, ETHNIC IDENTITY, CUL-TURAL FACTORS, EDUCATION, CULTURE, VAL-UES

ABST   SECOND IN A SERIES OF SEVEN MANUALS AND SELF-ASSESSMENT UNITS DESIGNED AS TEACHER TRAINING MATERIALS FOR USE IN BI-LINGUAL-BICULTURAL PROJECTS, THIS MANUAL PRESENTS THE PHILOSOPHY OF CULTURAL DEMOCRACY WHICH EMPHASIZES A CHILD'S RIGHT TO PREPARE HIMSELF TO FUNCTION COMPETENTLY IN FAMILIAL, OCCUPATIONAL AND SOCIAL SETTINGS WHICH MAY OR MAY NOT RESEMBLE THOSE FAMILIAR TO EITHER HIS PARENTS OR TEACHERS. CONFLICTS ARIS-ING WHEN SCHOOLS UNDERMINE CULTURAL LOYALTIES ARE SEEN AS CAUSING THE MEXI-CAN AMERICAN (MA) STUDENT TO BECOME DISCOURAGED, TO SEE EVERYTHING THE SCHOOL HAS TO OFFER AS IRRELEVANT, OR TO INTERPRET HIS INABILITY TO RESOLVE THE HOME/SCHOOL CONFLICT AS A MEASURE OF HIS OWN INADEQUACY. IGNORANCE ABOUT CULTURAL VALUES IS BELIEVED TO LEAD TO NEGATIVE JUDGMENTS AND SUBTLE COER-CIVE POLICIES CONCERNING BEHAVIORS WHICH FOLLOW FROM THOSE VALUES. WHETHER RESIDING IN TRADITIONAL, DUALIS-TIC, OR ATRADITIONAL COMMUNITIES, MA'S ARE VIEWED AS SHARING VALUES FROM THE FOLLOWING CLUSTERS: (1) IDENTIFICATION WITH FAMILY, COMMUNITY AND ETHNIC GROUP; (2) PERSONALIZATION OF INTERPERSONAL RE-LATIONSHIPS; (3) STATUS AND ROLE DEFINI-TION IN FAMILY AND COMMUNITY; AND (4) MEXICAN CATHOLIC IDEOLOGY. IN ORDER TO MAINTAIN AN IDENTITY BASED ON THESE SO-CIALIZATION EXPERIENCES, BICULTURALISM IS A NECESSARY VALUE FOR TEACHERS. VARI-OUS TECHNIQUES AND STRATEGIES TO HELP TEACHERS WITH MA-VALUED CHILDREN ARE INCLUDED. 5 REFERENCES.

ACCN   001294

1499 AUTH   **RAMIREZ, M., III, MACAULAY, R. K. S., GONZA-LEZ, A., COX, B., & PEREZ, M.**

TITL   SPANISH-ENGLISH BILINGUAL EDUCATION IN THE UNITED STATES: CURRENT ISSUES, RE-SOURCES AND RECOMMENDED FUNDING PRIORITIES FOR RESEARCH (NIE-C-74-0151).

SRCE   *UNPUBLISHED MANUSCRIPT, UNDATED. (AVAIL-ABLE FROM PRIMARY AUTHOR, SYSTEMS AND EVALUATIONS IN EDUCATION, P.O. BOX 2148, EAST SANTA CRUZ, CA 95063.)*

INDX   BILINGUAL-BICULTURAL EDUCATION, MEXI-CAN AMERICAN, RESEARCH METHODOLOGY, PROGRAM EVALUATION, BILINGUALISM, LIN-

GUISTICS, INTELLIGENCE, COGNITIVE STYLE, CULTURAL FACTORS, EDUCATIONAL ASSESS-MENT, MEXICAN AMERICAN, POLICY, ESSAY, CULTURAL PLURALISM

ABST   THIS REPORT IDENTIFIES CURRENT ISSUES, RESOURCES, AND FUNDING PRIORITIES IN U.S. SPANISH/ENGLISH BILINGUALISM AND BICUL-TURAL EDUCATION. LINGUISTIC ASPECTS ARE EXAMINED IN TERMS OF PAST SURVEYS, LAN-GUAGE DOMINANCE, VARIETY, USAGE AND TEACHING, ATTITUDES TOWARDS LANGUAGE IN THE CLASSROOM, AND COMMUNITY AND TEACHER TRAINING. INTELLECTUAL DEVEL-OPMENT IS DISCUSSED IN TERMS OF IQ, BILIN-GUALISM, AND RESPECT FOR CULTURAL DI-VERSITY. ISSUES REGARDING EDUCATIONAL ASSESSMENT FOCUS ON THE ASSIMILATION VERSUS CULTURAL DEMOCRACY CONTRO-VERSY, THE NATURE OF THE ASSESSMENT, PERSONNEL, INSTRUMENTS, AND MODELS EM-PLOYED IN THE ASSESSMENT. BILINGUAL EDU-CATION IS CONSIDERED ESSENTIAL FOR TRUE EQUALITY, TO MAINTAIN CULTURAL DIVERSITY, AND TO MAKE A WORTHWHILE CONTRIBUTION TO THE NATION'S RESOURCES. IT IS FURTHER BELIEVED THAT THE SPANISH-SPEAKING CHILD CAN SLOWLY INTEGRATE INTO AMERICAN CUL-TURE WITHOUT SACRIFICING HIS OWN IDEN-TITY OR HIS MOTHER-TONGUE. MAJOR REC-OMMENDATIONS INCLUDE ORGANIZATIONAL PRIORITIES (E.G., FUNDING OF BILINGUAL RE-SEARCH AND INFORMATION CENTERS) AND RESEARCH PRIORITIES WHICH STUDY ATTI-TUDES TOWARDS BILINGUAL-BICULTURAL EDUCATION, THE NEED FOR DEVELOPING CONCEPTUAL MODELS, AND THE LEARNING ABILITIES OF CHILDREN. BIBLIOGRAPHIES ARE INCLUDED AFTER EACH MAJOR SECTION. AND A FINAL SECTION ON RESOURCES AND CUR-RICULUM MATERIALS IS ALSO INCLUDED. 196 REFERENCES.

ACCN   001295

1500 AUTH   **RAMIREZ, M., III, TAYLOR, C., JR., & PETER-SEN, B.**

TITL   MEXICAN AMERICAN CULTURAL MEMBERSHIP AND ADJUSTMENT TO SCHOOL.

SRCE   *DEVELOPMENTAL PSYCHOLOGY, 1971, 4(2), 141-148.*

INDX   MEXICAN AMERICAN, ATTITUDES, ADOLES-CENTS, CROSS CULTURAL, SES, EDUCATION, PSYCHOSOCIAL ADJUSTMENT, SCHOLASTIC ACHIEVEMENT, CULTURAL FACTORS, MALE, FE-MALE, CALIFORNIA, SOUTHWEST, PROJECTIVE TESTING

ABST   TO TEST THE HYPOTHESIS THAT THERE ARE DIFFERENCES IN MOTIVES, ATTITUDES, AND BEHAVIORS TOWARD EDUCATION AMONG AN-GLO AMERICAN (AA) AND MEXICAN AMERICAN (MA) STUDENTS, MA AND AA JUNIOR AND SEN-IOR HIGH SCHOOL STUDENTS OF THE LOWER SOCIOECONOMIC CLASS WERE ADMINIS-TERED AN ATTITUDES-TOWARD-EDUCATION SCALE AND A PROJECTIVE TEST. THE RESULTS SHOW THAT THE MA'S EXPRESS VIEWS TO-WARD EDUCATION WHICH ARE LESS POSITIVE THAN THOSE OF AA'S. ON THE PROJECTIVE TEST, MA'S SCORED HIGHER ON NEED POWER

AND NEED REJECTION AND LOWER ON NEED ACHIEVEMENT THAN DID AA'S. MA MALES SCORED HIGHER THAN AA MALES ON NEED SUCCORANCE AND NEED AGRESSION TOWARD FEMALES. MA FEMALES SCORED HIGHER ON NEED AUTONOMY THAN DID AA FEMALES. THE MA'S ADJUSTMENT TO SCHOOL IS HINDERED BY HIS AVOIDANCE REACTION TO SCHOOL AND SCHOOL PERSONNEL, AS EVIDENCED BY HIS HIGH SCORE ON NEED REJECTION. IT IS CONCLUDED THAT THESE FINDINGS RESULT FROM THE DIFFERING VALUE ORIENTATIONS OF AA AND MA GROUPS. RECOMMENDATIONS FOR IMPROVING THE ACADEMIC SUCCESS OF MA STUDENTS ARE OFFERED. 11 REFERENCES.

ACCN   001296

1501 AUTH   **RAMIREZ, M., III, & CASTANEDA, A.**

TITL   CULTURAL DEMOCRACY, BICOGNITIVE DEVELOPMENT, AND EDUCATION.

SRCE   *NEW YORK: ACADEMIC PRESS, 1974.*

INDX   MEXICAN AMERICAN, CHILDREN, COGNITIVE STYLE, COGNITIVE DEVELOPMENT, EDUCATION, CULTURAL PLURALISM, POLICY, INSTRUCTIONAL TECHNIQUES, REVIEW, CULTURE, CROSS CULTURAL, EDUCATIONAL ASSESSMENT, FIELD DEPENDENCE-INDEPENDENCE, TEACHERS, CHILDREARING PRACTICES, CULTURAL FACTORS, BILINGUAL-BICULTURAL PERSONNEL, BOOK

ABST   WITH A FOCUS ON THE MEXICAN AMERICAN CHILD, THE THEME OF THIS VOLUME IS "CULTURAL DEMOCRACY" IN EDUCATION—A CONCEPT ASSERTING THAT A BICULTURAL CHILD WHO IS MANDATED TO LEARN THE VALUES OF THE DOMINANT CULTURE ALSO HAS A RIGHT TO REMAIN IDENTIFIED WITH THE VALUES AND CUSTOMS OF HIS/HER OWN ETHNIC GROUP. THE TOPICS ADDRESSED IN THE EIGHT CHAPTERS INCLUDE: (1) THE AMERICAN IDEOLOGY OF ASSIMILATION; (2) BICULTURALISM IN AMERICAN PUBLIC EDUCATION; (3) FOUR KEY VALUE CLUSTERS IN MEXICAN AMERICAN CULTURE WHICH INFLUENCE THE EDUCATIONAL PROCESS; (4) COGNITIVE STYLE DIFFERENCES BETWEEN MEXICAN AMERICAN AND ANGLO CHILDREN; (5) SOCIALIZATION PRACTICES PERTAINING TO COGNITIVE STYLES; AND (6) CULTURALLY DEMOCRATIC EDUCATIONAL ENVIRONMENTS. SPECIAL EMPHASIS IS GIVEN TO RESEARCH INDICATING THAT MEXICAN AMERICAN VS. ANGLO DIFFERENCES IN COGNITIVE, MOTIVATIONAL, AND HUMAN-RELATIONAL STYLES MAY BE DUE TO CEREBRAL HEMISPHERE SPECIALIZATIONS—WITH MEXICAN AMERICAN CHILDREN BEING PRIMARILY FIELD-SENSITIVE, WHILE ANGLO CHILDREN ARE FIELD-INDEPENDENT. THUS, TO PROMOTE RESEARCH AND NEW EDUCATIONAL PROGRAMS WHICH ADDRESS THIS DICHOTOMY, THE APPENDICES INCLUDE: (1) A REVIEW OF INSTRUMENTS FOR ASSESSING COGNITIVE AND MOTIVATIONAL STYLES IN CHILDREN; (2) INSTRUMENTS FOR IDENTIFYING FIELD-SENSITIVE AND FIELD-INDEPENDENT CHILDREN; AND (3) RECOMMENDATIONS FOR IMPLEMENTING CULTURALLY

DEMOCRATIC TEACHING STRATEGIES. 142 REFERENCES.

ACCN   001745

1502 AUTH   **RAMIREZ, M., III, & GONZALEZ, A.**

TITL   MEXICAN AMERICANS AND INTELLIGENCE TESTING.

SRCE   *IN M. M. MANGOLD (ED.), LA CAUSA CHICANA: THE MOVEMENT FOR JUSTICE. NEW YORK: FAMILY SERVICE ASSOCIATION OF AMERICA, 1971, PP. 137-147.*

INDX   INTELLIGENCE TESTING, MEXICAN AMERICAN, CULTURAL PLURALISM, EDUCATION, REVIEW, COGNITIVE STYLE, EDUCATIONAL ASSESSMENT, CHILDREN, CULTURAL FACTORS

ABST   THE WEAKNESSES ATTRIBUTED TO THE STANDARD ASSESSMENT OF INTELLIGENCE IN REGARDS TO MEXICAN AMERICANS ARE REVIEWED. INTELLIGENCE TESTS HAVE BEEN USED IN EDUCATIONAL SYSTEMS TO HELP CHANGE MEXICAN AMERICANS AND OTHER ETHNIC GROUP MEMBERS TO CONFORM TO THE IMAGE OF THE MAINSTREAM AMERICAN MIDDLE CLASS. LITTLE CONSIDERATION HAS BEEN GIVEN TO THE CULTURALLY DISTINCT LANGUAGE AND LEARNING STYLES OF MEXICAN AMERICAN CHILDREN. FURTHERMORE, THE CONTENT OF THE ASSESSMENT TOOLS AND THE TESTING PHEONOMENON ARE OFTEN FOREIGN TO THIS GROUP. RESEARCH INDICATES THAT WHEN SOME OF THESE FACTORS ARE TAKEN INTO ACCOUNT (E.G., LANGUAGE), MEXICAN AMERICANS' INTELLIGENCE SCORES IMPROVE CONSIDERABLY. THE MOST IMPORTANT ROLE THAT ASSESSMENT CAN PLAY IN EDUCATION IS TO ASSESS THE CHILD'S CULTURALLY UNIQUE COGNITIVE STYLE. AS SUCH, ASSESSMENT CAN THEN BE USED TO DETERMINE HOW THE INSTITUTION CAN CHANGE TO BE MORE COMPATIBLE WITH THE CHILD. THIS ORIENTATION, TERMED "CULTURAL DEMOCRACY," MUST BE APPLIED TO TEACHING METHODOLOGY AND CURRICULUM DEVELOPMENT. 21 REFERENCES.

ACCN   001297

1503 AUTH   **RAMIREZ, M., III, & PRICE-WILLIAMS, D.**

TITL   COGNITIVE STYLES IN CHILDREN: TWO MEXICAN COMMUNITIES.

SRCE   *INTERAMERICAN JOURNAL OF PSYCHOLOGY, 1974, 8(1-2), 93-101.*

INDX   COGNITIVE STYLE, CHILDREN, FIELD DEPENDENCE-INDEPENDENCE, MOTHER-CHILD INTERACTION, MEXICAN, SOCIALIZATION, CULTURAL FACTORS, BILINGUAL, EMPIRICAL, SEX COMPARISON, ADULTS, VALUES

ABST   ONE HUNDRED THIRTY-SIX CHILDREN OF TWO MEXICAN COMMUNITIES (ONE MORE IDENTIFIED WITH TRADITIONAL MEXICAN VALUES) WERE TESTED WITH THE PORTABLE ROD AND FRAME TEST (PRFT). THEIR MOTHERS WERE INTERVIEWED AND ADMINISTERED A SOCIALIZATION QUESTIONNAIRE. IT WAS HYPOTHESIZED THAT CHILDREN FROM THE MORE TRADITIONAL MEXICAN-VALUED COMMUNITY WOULD BE MORE FIELD DEPENDENT AND THAT THEIR

MOTHERS WOULD MORE FREQUENTLY AGREE WITH QUESTIONNAIRE ITEMS WHICH REFLECTED ATTITUDES AND BEHAVIORS OF THE FIELD DEPENDENT "SOCIALIZATION" CLUSTER. PRFT SCORES SHOWED THAT CHILDREN IN THE MORE TRADITIONAL COMMUNITY SCORED IN A SIGNIFICANTLY MORE FIELD DEPENDENT DIRECTION THAN THE OTHER COMMUNITY. MOREOVER, FEMALES AND YOUNGER CHILDREN SCORED IN A MORE FIELD DEPENDENT DIRECTION THAN MALES AND OLDER CHILDREN. RESULTS FROM THE QUESTIONNAIRE INDICATED THAT MOTHERS IN THE MORE TRADITIONAL COMMUNITY AGREED MORE WITH THE ITEMS THAN THE OTHER MOTHERS, BUT THE DIFFERENCE WAS NOT SIGNIFICANT. SOCIALIZATION RESULTS ALSO SHOWED A NEED FOR MODIFICATION OF THE FIELD DEPENDENT "SOCIALIZATION" CLUSTER FOR STUDY OF COGNITIVE STYLE DEVELOPMENT IN THE MEXICAN CULTURE—PARTICULARLY IN THOSE COMMUNITIES WHICH MORE STRONGLY IDENTIFY WITH THE TRADITIONAL MEXICAN SYSTEM OF VALUES. 9 REFERENCES. (JOURNAL ABSTRACT MODIFIED)

ACCN 001298

1504 AUTH **RAMIREZ, M., III, & PRICE-WILLIAMS, D.**
TITL COGNITIVE STYLES OF CHILDREN OF THREE ETHNIC GROUPS IN THE UNITED STATES.
SRCE *JOURNAL OF CROSS-CULTURAL PSYCHOLOGY, 1974, 5(2), 212-219.*
INDX CHILDREN, BILINGUAL, EMPIRICAL, MEXICAN AMERICAN, COGNITIVE STYLE, CROSS CULTURAL, SOCIALIZATION, FIELD DEPENDENCE-INDEPENDENCE, FAMILY STRUCTURE, SCHOLASTIC ACHIEVEMENT, CULTURAL FACTORS
ABST TO ASSESS CULTURAL DIFFERENCES OF COGNITIVE STYLE, 60 ANGLO, 60 BLACK AND 60 MEXICAN AMERICAN FOURTH GRADE CHILDREN WERE ADMINISTERED THE PORTABLE ROD AND FRAME TEST. THE RESULTS SHOWED THAT BLACK AND MEXICAN AMERICAN CHILDREN, AND FEMALES IN ALL THREE GROUPS, SCORED IN A SIGNIFICANTLY MORE FIELD DEPENDENT DIRECTION THAN ANGLO MALES. THE RESULTS CONFIRMED PREVIOUS FINDINGS THAT MEMBERS OF GROUPS WHICH EMPHASIZE RESPECT FOR FAMILY AND RELIGIOUS AUTHORITY AND GROUP IDENTITY AND WHICH ARE CHARACTERIZED BY SHARED-FUNCTION FAMILY AND FRIENDSHIP GROUPS TEND TO BE FIELD DEPENDENT IN COGNITIVE STYLE. MEMBERS OF GROUPS WHICH ENCOURAGE QUESTIONING OF CONVENTION AND AN INDIVIDUAL IDENTITY AND ARE CHARACTERIZED BY FORMALLY ORGANIZED FAMILY AND FRIENDSHIP GROUPS, ON THE OTHER HAND, TEND TO BE MORE FIELD INDEPENDENT. THE IMPLICATIONS OF THIS STUDY ARE THAT EDUCATIONAL SETTINGS WHICH HAVE BEEN SHOWN TO BE BIASED IN THE DIRECTION OF FIELD INDEPENDENCE MAY NOT BE CONSONANT WITH THE FIELD DEPENDENT COGNITIVE STYLES OF MEXICAN AMERICANS, BLACKS AND SOME ANGLO FEMALES. FURTHERMORE, THIS LACK OF CONSONANCE MAY CONTRIBUTE TO THE FAILURE WHICH MEMBERS OF

THESE GROUPS EXPERIENCE IN SCHOOL. 11 REFERENCES. (JOURNAL ABSTRACT MODIFIED)

ACCN 001299

1505 AUTH **RAMIREZ, M., III, & PRICE-WILLIAMS, D. R.**
TITL ACHIEVEMENT MOTIVATION IN CHILDREN OF THREE ETHNIC GROUPS IN THE UNITED STATES.
SRCE *JOURNAL OF CROSS-CULTURAL PSYCHOLOGY, 1976, 7(1), 49-60.*
INDX CHILDREN, CROSS CULTURAL, CULTURAL FACTORS, ACHIEVEMENT MOTIVATION, SCHOLASTIC ACHIEVEMENT, FAMILY STRUCTURE, SEX COMPARISON, MEXICAN AMERICAN, EMPIRICAL, TEXAS, SOUTHWEST
ABST TO STUDY THE RELATIONSHIP BETWEEN ETHNICITY AND ACHIEVEMENT MOTIVATION, CHILDREN OF THREE ETHNIC GROUPS IN THE UNITED STATES—ANGLOS, BLACKS, AND MEXICAN AMERICANS—WERE ASKED TO TELL A STORY OF EACH OF SEVEN LINE DRAWINGS DEPICTING PERSONS IN A SETTING RELATED TO EDUCATION. STORIES WERE SCORED FOR N ACHIEVEMENT AND FAMILY ACHIEVEMENT (ORIENTED TOWARD ACHIEVEMENT GOALS FROM WHICH THE FAMILY WOULD BENEFIT OR THAT WOULD GAIN RECOGNITION FROM FAMILY MEMBERS). RESULTS SHOW THAT MEXICAN AMERICAN AND BLACK CHILDREN SCORED HIGHER ON FAMILY ACHIEVEMENT THAN DID ANGLO CHILDREN, WHILE ANGLOS SCORED HIGHER ON N ACHIEVEMENT. ON THOSE CARDS DEPICTING PARENTAL FIGURES, HOWEVER, MEXICAN AMERICAN AND BLACK CHILDREN TENDED TO SCORE HIGHER ON N ACHIEVEMENT THAN ANGLO CHILDREN. FEMALES IN ALL THREE ETHNIC GROUPS SCORED LOWER ON N ACHIEVEMENT BUT HIGHER ON FAMILY ACHIEVEMENT THAN MALES. IT IS CONCLUDED THAT CONTEXTUAL CONDITIONS ARE MOST IMPORTANT IN EXPRESSION OF ACHIEVEMENT MOTIVATION AND THAT THE PARTICULAR FORM IN WHICH ACHIEVEMENT IS EXPRESSED IS DETERMINED BY THE DEFINITION THAT CULTURE GIVES TO IT. 15 REFERENCES. (NCMHI ABSTRACT)

ACCN 001300

1506 AUTH **RAMIREZ, P. C.**
TITL MIGRANT HEALTH CARE: A MIXTURE OF HOPE AND DESPAIR.
SRCE *AGENDA, MARCH/APRIL 1977, PP. 19-22.*
INDX HEALTH, FARM LABORERS, MIGRATION, POVERTY, EDUCATION, LEGISLATION, HEALTH DELIVERY SYSTEMS, DISEASE, ESSAY, MEXICAN AMERICAN, RURAL, PUERTO RICAN-M, POLICY, MIGRANTS
ABST APPROXIMATELY 3 MILLION MIGRANT FARM WORKERS AND THEIR FAMILIES (MEXICAN AMERICAN, PUERTO RICAN, BLACK, AND WHITE) IN THE U.S. SUFFER UNIQUE HEALTH PROBLEMS AND ALSO FACE SEVERE BARRIERS TO QUALITY HEALTH CARE. PROBLEMS INCLUDE: (1) POOR ACCESS TO HEALTH CARE IN RURAL COMMUNITIES; (2) INADEQUATE MEDICAL INSURANCE COVERAGE AND INELIGIBILITY FOR MEDICAID AND WORKMAN'S COMPENSATION; (3) POOR HOUSING WHICH HAS SUBSTAND-

ARD PLUMBING AND INADEQUATE WATER SUPPLIES; (4) NUTRITIONAL DEFICIENCIES; AND (5) POOR EDUCATIONAL OPPORTUNITIES FOR MIGRANT CHILDREN. THIS POOR HEALTH STANDARD FOR MIGRANTS IS REFLECTED IN VITAL STATISTICS. THE MIGRANT LIFE EXPECTANCY IS 49 YEARS, COMPARED TO THE NATIONAL AVERAGE OF 70, AND THE INFANT MORTALITY RATE IS 25% HIGHER THAN THE NATIONAL AVERAGE. THE MIGRANT HEALTH PROGRAM (MANDATED BY PL 94-439 ENACTED JULY 29, 1975) AUTHORIZES THE HEW SECRETARY TO MAKE GRANTS TO PUBLIC AND NON-PROFIT PRIVATE ORGANIZATIONS TO PLAN, DEVELOP, AND OPERATE MIGRANT HEALTH CENTERS AND PROJECTS WHICH PROVIDE EMERGENCY AND PRIMARY HEALTH CARE. IN 1977, 125 HEW FUNDED CENTERS WERE IN OPERATION. RECOMMENDATIONS TO ENSURE AN IMPROVEMENT OF MIGRANT HEALTH STATUS INCLUDE: (1) INCREASE FEDERAL FUNDING TO MIGRANT HEALTH CENTERS; (2) IMPROVE INSPECTION OF MIGRANT CAMPS TO ENSURE COMPLIANCE WITH HOUSING AND SANITATION STANDARDS; (3) IMPROVE EDUCATION IN AREAS OF BASIC NUTRITION, PRENATAL CARE, PREVENTIVE HEALTH MEASURES, DENTAL HYGIENE, AND WAYS OF GAINING ACCESS TO MEDICAL CARE; (4) PREVENT DUPLICATION OF SERVICES; (5) ASSURE CONTINUITY OF CARE THROUGH ESTABLISHMENT OF A COMPUTERIZED NETWORK FOR THE TRANSFER OF MEDICAL RECORDS; (6) MEET TRANSPORTATION NEEDS; AND (7) TRAIN MIGRANTS AS HEALTH AIDS TO PROVIDE EDUCATION AND PRELIMINARY SCREENING SERVICES IN MIGRANT CAMPS. 1 REFERENCE.

ACCN   001301

1507 AUTH   **RAMIREZ, S., & PARRES, R.**
TITL   SOME DYNAMIC PATTERNS IN ORGANIZATION OF THE MEXICAN FAMILY.
SRCE   *INTERNATIONAL JOURNAL OF SOCIAL PSYCHIATRY, 1957, 3(1), 18-21.*
INDX   MEXICAN, FAMILY ROLES, FAMILY STRUCTURE, INTERPERSONAL RELATIONS, EMPIRICAL, SELF CONCEPT, CULTURAL FACTORS, MARITAL STABILITY, MEXICO, FERTILITY, PERSONALITY, MALE, SES
ABST   A SAMPLE OF 635 FAMILIES (500 OBTAINED FROM THE RECORDS OF THE HOSPITAL INFANTIL IN MEXICO CITY AND 135 FROM THE CENTERS FOR MENTAL HYGIENE) WERE ANALYZED TO EXAMINE THE ORGANIZATION OF THE MEXICAN FAMILY. THREE BASIC DYNAMIC TENDENCIES MENTIONED ARE: (1) THE INTENSE MOTHER-CHILD RELATIONSHIP DURING THE FIRST YEAR OF LIFE, WHICH PROBABLY EXPLAINS THE MAJORITY OF THE POSITIVE VALUES IN THE MEXICAN CULTURE; (2) THE DILUTION OF THE FATHER-CHILD RELATIONSHIP; AND (3) THE TRAUMATIC RUPTURE OF THE MOTHER-CHILD RELATIONSHIP AT THE BIRTH OF THE NEXT SIBLING. GENERAL DATA INDICATE THAT THE MEXICAN FAMILY IS FORMED IN 65 PERCENT OF THE CASES BY A BIOSOCIAL UNIT—THE FATHER, THE MOTHER, AND THE OFFSPRING. IN 32 PERCENT OF THE CASES THE FATHER IS ABSENT BECAUSE OF DEATH

OR ABANDONMENT. THE ABANDONMENT BY THE FATHER COINCIDES IN 70 PERCENT OF THE CASES WITH THE WIFE'S PREGNANCY. IN THE FAMILIES SAMPLED, THE NUMBER OF PREGNANCIES WAS 5.8 CHILDREN PER MOTHER, WITH 0.98 PERCENT OF ABORTIONS PER MOTHER. THE PERCENTAGE OF LIVE CHILDREN WAS ALMOST FIVE PER FAMILY. IT IS FREQUENTLY THE CASE THAT THESE CHILDREN ARE OF DIFFERENT FATHERS, AND ALL THE MORE SO AS THE SOCIOCULTURAL LEVEL GOES DOWN. DISCUSSIONS OF THE EFFECTS OF ABANDONMENT BY THE FATHER ARE PROVIDED. 1 REFERENCE.

ACCN   001302

1508 AUTH   **RAMIREZ-MURGADO, J. O.**
TITL   CONSULTATION AND EDUCATION IN A CHICANO COMMUNITY.
SRCE   *SOCIAL CASEWORK, 1975, 56(9), 558-561.*
INDX   MENTAL HEALTH, HEALTH DELIVERY SYSTEMS, ATTITUDES, PSYCHOPATHOLOGY, PROGRAM EVALUATION, COMMUNITY INVOLVEMENT, FOLK MEDICINE, COMMUNITY, ESSAY, MEXICAN AMERICAN, CULTURAL FACTORS
ABST   IF MENTAL HEALTH CENTERS ARE TO BE EFFECTIVE WITHIN THE CHICANO COMMUNITY, ETHNIC CONCEPTS OF MENTAL HEALTH MUST BE RECOGNIZED AND INCORPORATED WITHIN THE HEALTH DELIVERY SYSTEM. DIFFERENT LABELS, SUCH AS "LOCO" AND "NERVIOSO," ATTACHED TO DIFFERENT LEVELS OF DYSFUNCTIONAL BEHAVIOR, AND TREATMENT FOR THESE MALADIES CANNOT BE OFFERED FROM AN ANGLO FRAME OF REFERENCE. IN DEVELOPING A CONSULTATIVE AND EDUCATIONAL MENTAL HEALTH PROGRAM TO SERVE THE COMMUNITY, THE FIRST STEP IS TO ASSESS WHAT IS PERCEIVED AS DYSFUNCTIONAL WITHIN THE CULTURE. THIS CAN BE ACCOMPLISHED THROUGH A SURVEY OF ATTITUDES TOWARD MENTAL ILLNESS AND INTERVIEWS WITH LOCALLY ACKNOWLEDGED HEALERS. COMMUNITY RESIDENTS WHO HAVE ACQUIRED A REPUTATION AS UNDERSTANDING INDIVIDUALS, AND MEMBERS OF THE CLERGY. 4 REFERENCES. (NCMHI ABSTRACT MODIFIED)
ACCN   001303

1509 AUTH   **RAMOS, R.**
TITL   A CASE IN POINT: AN ETHNOMETHODOLOGICAL STUDY OF A POOR MEXICAN AMERICAN FAMILY.
SRCE   *SOCIAL SCIENCE QUARTERLY, 1973, 53(4), 905-919.*
INDX   MEXICAN AMERICAN, CONFLICT RESOLUTION, PSYCHOSOCIAL ADJUSTMENT, ECONOMIC FACTORS, CASE STUDY, RESEARCH METHODOLOGY, COLORADO, SOUTHWEST, EMPIRICAL
ABST   ATTENTION IS DRAWN TO THE BACKGROUND KNOWLEDGE WHICH MEXICAN AMERICANS USE AS INTERPRETATIVE SCHEMES TO COPE WITH THE PROBLEMATIC FEATURES IN THEIR DAILY LIVES. THROUGH A CASE HISTORY GATHERED BY PARTICIPANT OBSERVATION AND INTERVIEW WITH ONE MEXICAN AMERICAN FAMILY THROUGH USE OF AN INTERACTION APPROACH, IT IS SHOWN THAT MEXICAN AMERI-

CANS USE THEIR BACKGROUND KNOWLEDGE OR COMMON SENSE UNDERSTANDING OF SOCIETAL STRUCTURE TO COPE WITH THE PROBLEMATIC SITUATIONS ENCOUNTERED IN EVERYDAY LIFE. THE CASE STUDY RELATES THAT MRS. MARTINEZ DID NOT ATTEND A COURT HEARING ON HER SON'S TRUANCY FROM SCHOOL BECAUSE THIS WOULD HAVE MEANT MISSING A DAY'S WORK WHICH SHE COULD NOT AFFORD. THE COURT HEARING WAS SCHEDULED DURING THE PEAK SEASON AT THE TURKEY PLANT WHERE MRS. MARTINEZ WORKED. PLANT FOREMEN INTIMIDATED EMPLOYEES BY THREATENING TO FIRE THEM IF THEY MISSED A DAY'S WORK. THE CASE ILLUSTRATES HOW MRS. MARTINEZ COPES WITH THE PRACTICAL CIRCUMSTANCES IN HER EVERYDAY LIFE NOT AS SEPARATE EVENTS, BUT AS EVENTS THAT ARE VERY MUCH RELATED TO EACH OTHER. HER UNDERSTANDING OF THE RELATIONSHIPS THAT EXIST BETWEEN THESE EVENTS CONSTITUTES THE BACKGROUND KNOWLEDGE SHE USES TO MANAGE THOSE EVENTS. IT IS RECOMMENDED THAT RESEARCHERS TAKE THIS BACKGROUND KNOWLEDGE INTO ACCOUNT IN ORDER TO AVOID DISTORTED INTERPRETATIONS OF MEXICAN AMERICANS' BEHAVIORS. 5 REFERENCES. (SOCIOLOGY ABSTRACT MODIFIED)

ACCN   001304

1510 AUTH   **RAMOS, S.**
TITL   PROFILE OF MAN AND CULTURE IN MEXICO (P. G. EARLE, TRANS.).
SRCE   *AUSTIN: UNIVERSITY OF TEXAS PRESS, 1962.*
INDX   MEXICO, CULTURE, HISTORY, MEXICAN, SELF CONCEPT, SEX ROLES, RELIGION, RURAL, URBAN, EDUCATION, PERSONALITY, ESSAY, BOOK
ABST   AN ANALYSIS OF THE MEXICAN PEOPLE IS MADE WITH RESPECT TO HISTORICAL EUROPEAN AND FRENCH INFLUENCE, EVOLUTION OF IDEOLOGIES, AND INDIGENOUS CULTURAL PATTERNS. MEXICANS ARE SEEN AS SUFFERING FROM UNDERLYING FEELINGS OF INFERIORITY WHICH CAUSE THEM TO WANT TO IMITATE AND ADOPT THE SEMBLANCES OF WESTERN CULTURE, THUS NEGATING THEIR INDIGENOUS CULTURE. MOREOVER, THEIR SENSE OF DEEP "NATIONALISM" IS SEEN AS DECEPTIVE AND COUNTERPRODUCTIVE DUE TO THEIR UNWILLINGNESS TO ACCEPT THEMSELVES. THREE MEXICAN CHARACTER TYPES ARE PSYCHOANALYZED: THE "PELADO" (A BUM; A GOOD-FOR-NOTHING), THE MEXICAN OF THE CITY, AND THE MIDDLE-CLASS MEXICAN. THE PELADO, THROUGH HIS COARSE LANGUAGE AND SEXUALLY-SUGGESTIVE MANNERISMS, DISPLAYS THE MOST SOCIAL INFERIORITY; THE CITY-DWELLER IS CHARACTERIZED AS BEING DISTRUSTFUL OF SOCIAL RELATIONSHIPS, ACADEMICS, AND SCIENCE BECAUSE OF HIS OWN SELF-NEGATIVITY; AND THE MIDDLE-CLASS MEXICAN, WHO POSSESSES INTELLECTUAL GIFTS AND RESOURCES, EXPRESSES HIS FEELINGS OF INFERIORITY THROUGH NATIONALISM AND SOCIAL POSITION. THE INDIAN, ALTHOUGH NOT UNDER STUDY, IS SEEN AS PASSIVE YET FREE FROM A POOR SELF-IMAGE.

ALTHOUGH HEAVILY AFFECTED BY THE MECHANIZATION OF THE UNITED STATES. MEXICO IS APPROACHING A BETTER BALANCE BOTH ECONOMICALLY AND IDEOLOGICALLY. CHANGES OCCURING IN THE ARTS. SOCIAL THOUGHT, AND THE NEW GENERATION ARE VIEWED AS HELPING MEXICO ACHIEVE ITS OWN UNIQUE IDENTITY.

ACCN   001305

1511 AUTH   **RAND, C.**
TITL   THE PUERTO RICANS.
SRCE   *NEW YORK: OXFORD UNIVERSITY PRESS, 1958.*
INDX   PUERTO RICAN-M, HISTORY, CULTURE, BILINGUALISM, URBAN, SOCIAL SERVICES, INTERPERSONAL RELATIONS, MIGRATION, STRESS. MENTAL HEALTH, PSYCHOSOCIAL ADJUSTMENT, EMPLOYMENT, LABOR FORCE, PHYSICIANS, NUTRITION, FAMILY ROLES. FAMILY STRUCTURE, DRUG ABUSE, DRUG ADDICTION. CRIMINOLOGY, GANGS, HOUSING, SES. POVERTY, PUERTO RICAN-I, NEW YORK, EAST. EMPIRICAL, BOOK, BOOK
ABST   THIS DESCRIPTIVE ACCOUNT OF NEW YORK'S PUERTO RICANS, THEIR LIFE STYLE, AND MIGRATION FROM THE ISLAND IS BASED UPON PARTICIPANT OBSERVATION RESEARCH, INTERVIEWS. AND SOME STATISTICAL DATA. TOPICS INCLUDE (1) THEIR DRESS, DIET, AND LANGUAGE, (2) AN ACCOUNT OF LIFE IN THE ISLAND, AND (3) THE ECONOMIC AND HISTORICAL BASIS FOR THEIR MIGRATION TO THE MAINLAND. THE PRESENT SOCIAL STATUS OF PUERTO RICANS IN NEW YORK CITY IS ANALYZED IN TERMS OF HOUSING, WELFARE, EDUCATION, AND EMPLOYMENT; AND THIS IS RELATED TO ISSUES OF ASSIMILATION AMONG PUERTO RICANS.

ACCN   001306

1512 AUTH   **RAPIER, J. L.**
TITL   EFFECTS OF VERBAL MEDIATION UPON THE LEARNING OF MEXICAN-AMERICAN CHILDREN.
SRCE   *CALIFORNIA JOURNAL OF EDUCATIONAL RESEARCH, 1967, 18(1), 40-48.*
INDX   LEARNING, MEXICAN AMERICAN, CHILDREN. CROSS CULTURAL, COGNITIVE DEVELOPMENT, LEARNING DISABILITIES, CALIFORNIA, SOUTHWEST, EMPIRICAL, POLICY, MENTAL RETARDATION, LINGUISTIC COMPETENCE, INTELLIGENCE, BILINGUAL
ABST   AN INVESTIGATION INTO THE ROLE OF VERBAL MEDIATION IN THE LEARNING OF MEXICAN AMERICAN CHILDREN IS PRESENTED. TWO EXPERIMENTS WERE CONDUCTED WITH THIRD AND FOURTH GRADE MEXICAN AMERICAN (MA) AND ANGLO AMERICAN (AA) CHILDREN SERVING AS SUBJECTS. THE FIRST EXPERIMENT STUDIED THE ROLE OF VERBAL MEDIATION IN THE FACILITATION OF CONCEPT DISCOVERY. THE SECOND EXPERIMENT STUDIED THE EFFECTS OF SUPPLYING THE NECESSARY MEDIATING LINKS ON PAIRED-ASSOCIATE LEARNING. SIX FINDINGS ARE PRESENTED. (1) OLDER CHILDREN MAKE MORE FREQUENT USE OF MEDIATING CUES TO FACILITATE THEIR LEARNING THAN YOUNGER CHILDREN. (2) ON THE TRAINING DISCRIMINATION THE DIFFERENCE

BETWEEN THE TWO NATIONALITY GROUPS FELL SHORT OF SIGNIFICANCE. (3) DULL MA'S DID NOT PERFORM AS WELL AS THE OTHER GROUPS ON REVERSAL SHIFT. (4) REVERSAL SHIFT WAS EASIER THAN NONREVERSAL SHIFT FOR THE TOTAL SAMPLING. (5) MEDIATED LEARNING OCCURRED IN BOTH NATIONALITY GROUPS. (6) THE DULL MA'S SHOWED MUCH BETTER ABILITY TO MAKE USE OF MEDIATED LINKS IN LEARNING NEW CONNECTIONS THAN DID DULL AA'S. THE FINDINGS SUGGEST THAT THE MA'S LEARNING DISABILITY MAY NOT BE DUE TO AN INABILITY TO SPONTANEOUSLY VERBALLY MEDIATE, BUT TO THE LACK OF A RESERVOIR OF VERBAL ASSOCIATIONS WHICH CAN BE EVOKED IN ANY NEW LEARNING SITUATION. AS A RESULT, MA'S MUST CONTINUALLY LEARN NEW CONNECTIONS AND THEIR LEARNING CONSEQUENTLY RESEMBLES THAT OF A RETARDED CHILD. PLANNED LANGUAGE EXPERIENCES ARE RECOMMENDED FOR CHILDREN FROM VERBALLY DEPRIVED ENVIRONMENTS IN ORDER TO HELP THEM PASS THROUGH VARIOUS STAGES OF VERBAL DEVELOPMENT. 4 REFERENCES.

ACCN   001307

1513 AUTH   **RAZA ASSOCIATION OF SPANISH SURNAMED AMERICANS.**

TITL   LA LUZ REPORT: SOCIO/ECONOMIC CHARACTERISTICS OF THE SPANISH SPEAKING POPULATION.

SRCE   *LA LUZ, MARCH-APRIL 1975, P. 34.*

INDX   RURAL, URBAN, SES, POVERTY, ECONOMIC FACTORS, SPANISH SURNAMED, DEMOGRAPHIC, REVIEW, EDUCATION, EMPLOYMENT

ABST   A SUMMARY IS PROVIDED OF 1972 TO 1974 DATA PERTAINING TO THE SOCIOECONOMIC STATUS OF THE U.S. SPANISH-SPEAKING (SS) POPULATION. REGARDING 1973 INCOME LEVELS, 21.9% OF THE SS POPULATION WAS CLASSIFIED IN THE LOW INCOME BRACKET, COMPARED TO 11.1% OF THE TOTAL U.S. POPULATION. FURTHERMORE, THE MEDIAN INCOME FOR SPANISH-SPEAKING INDIVIDUALS 25 YEARS AND OLDER WAS $5,369 WHILE $6,289 WAS THE MEDIAN INCOME FOR THOSE IN THIS AGE CATEGORY IN THE U.S. UNEMPLOYMENT FIGURES FOR THE THIRD QUARTER OF 1974 SHOW THAT 325,000 OR 8% OF THE SS POPULATION WERE UNEMPLOYED, WHICH COMPARES TO A 5% UNEMPLOYMENT FIGURE FOR ANGLO WORKERS AND A 10.5% FIGURE FOR BLACKS. OF THESE THREE ETHNIC CATEGORIES, THE SPANISH-SPEAKING SUFFERED THE GREATEST RATE OF INCREASE IN UNEMPLOYMENT FROM THE THIRD QUARTER OF 1973, 29%. WITH RESPECT TO EDUCATION, 1974 FIGURES INDICATE THAT THE DROP-OUT RATE FOR THE SS WAS 55%, FOR BLACKS 40% AND FOR ANGLOS 20%. SPANISH-SPEAKING INDIVIDUALS COMPLETED AN AVERAGE OF 7.1 YEARS OF SCHOOLING IN COMPARISON TO 12.1 YEARS COMPLETED BY ANGLOS. LASTLY, SPANISH-SPEAKING OWNED BUSINESSES CLAIMED APPROXIMATELY .2% OF THE TOTAL U.S. BUSINESS RECEIPTS ACCORDING TO A 1972 REPORT. MORE SPECIFIC DATA ARE PRO-

VIDED IN THE BUSINESS AREA AS WELL AS THE OTHER AREAS MENTIONED.

ACCN   001308

1514 AUTH   **REAL, D., & REAL, J.**

TITL   RAISING A NEW GENERATION OF ADDICTS.

SRCE   *HUMAN BEHAVIOR, 1973, 2(1), 8-15; 76.*

INDX   DRUG ABUSE, DRUG ADDICTION, REHABILITATION, HEALTH DELIVERY SYSTEMS, METHADONE MAINTENANCE, PRIMARY PREVENTION, SPANISH SURNAMED, ESSAY, MEXICAN AMERICAN, COMMUNITY, PERSONNEL, BILINGUAL-BICULTURAL PERSONNEL, CALIFORNIA, SOUTHWEST, ADMINISTRATORS, PROGRAM EVALUATION, CULTURAL FACTORS

ABST   IT IS OFTEN ASSUMED THAT DRUG PREVENTION AND TREATMENT AGENCIES ARE DEVELOPED AND IMPLEMENTED ON THE BASIS OF A COHERENT, COMPREHENSIVE GOVERNMENTAL POLICY TOWARDS SUBSTANCE ABUSE. HOWEVER, THE LOS ANGELES COUNTY'S DRUG PROGRAM DEMONSTRATES THAT INEFFECTIVE PROGRAMS ARE PARTIALLY DUE TO OVER EXTENDED BUREAUCRACY AND STAFF WHO TEND TO BE PREOCCUPIED WITH THE CONTINUED MAINTENANCE OF THEIR FEDERAL FUNDS. THE VARIOUS DRUG CLINICS IN LOS ANGELES ARE DISCUSSED IN TERMS OF THEIR DEVELOPMENT, THE POPULATION SERVED, AND THE DIFFICULTIES OF SECURING STATE AND COUNTY FUNDS. IN EXAMINING PROGRAMS IN THE BARRIO AND THE INDIVIDUALS WHO RUN THEM, IT IS SUGGESTED THAT THEIR SUCCESS CAN BE ATTRIBUTED TO THE CULTURAL RELEVANCE THEY PROVIDE FOR CHICANOS. OTHER PROGRAMS WITHOUT THIS CULTURAL RELEVANCE REPORT LESS SUCCESS WITH CHICANOS. HOSPITAL DRUG-RELATED CASES AND VERBATIM PERSONAL ACCOUNTS OF DRUG USAGE ARE PRESENTED, AND THE LIMITATIONS AND THE IRRELEVANCE OF SEVERAL LOS ANGELES COUNTY FACILITIES ARE DISCUSSED.

ACCN   001309

1515 AUTH   **RECIO, M.**

TITL   WASHINGTON, D.C.: ONE COMMUNITY'S ATTEMPTS TO IMPROVE POLICE-COMMUNITY RELATIONS.

SRCE   *AGENDA, JANUARY/FEBRUARY 1977, PP. 36-37.*

INDX   POLICE-COMMUNITY RELATIONS, URBAN, ESSAY, REPRESENTATION, SOCIAL SERVICES, CRIMINOLOGY, WASHINGTON D.C., EAST

ABST   THE NUMBER OF LATINOS IN THE WASHINGTON, D.C. AREA IS ESTIMATED TO BE CLOSE TO 70,000. A HIGH CRIME RATE, INCLUDING AN ALARMING INCIDENCE OF RAPE, PROMPTED SEVERAL LATINO LEADERS TO CALL FOR A CONFERENCE ADDRESSING THEIR SPECIFIC CONCERNS. THE CONFERENCE ON THE ADMINISTRATION OF JUSTICE AND THE LATINO COMMUNITY WAS HELD IN 1976 AND LOCAL AND NATIONAL OFFICIALS WERE REPRESENTED. ELEVEN ISSUES REGARDING POLICE AND COMMUNITY RELATIONS WERE RAISED. THESE INCLUDED SENSITIVITY OF POLICE TO CULTURAL AND IMMIGRATION CONCERNS, STEPS TO ALLEVIATE THE VICTIMIZATION OF WOMEN, AND A CALL FOR INCREASED SER-

VICES FOR LATINOS. A DETAILED DESCRIPTION OF PROPOSALS AND ACTIONS THAT WERE TAKEN WITH RESPECT TO ADDRESSING THESE ISSUES IS PRESENTED. ALTHOUGH GREATER RESPONSE IN THE FORM OF ACTION IS NEEDED, THE DIALOGUE THAT WAS INITIATED BETWEEN THE HISPANIC COMMUNITY AND THE POLICE IS SEEN AS BOTH FACILITATING FUTURE RELATIONS AND PROVIDING AN EXAMPLE TO OTHER HISPANIC COMMUNITIES.

ACCN   001310

1516 AUTH   **REDLINGER, L. J., & MICHEL, J. B.**
TITL   ECOLOGICAL VARIATIONS IN HEROIN ABUSE.
SRCE   *SOCIOLOGICAL QUARTERLY, 1970, 11(2), 219-229.*
INDX   SES, SCHOLASTIC ACHIEVEMENT, DRUG ADDICTION, EMPIRICAL, MEXICAN AMERICAN, CROSS CULTURAL, DEMOGRAPHIC, DRUG ABUSE, ADULTS, TEXAS, SOUTHWEST
ABST   A STUDY WAS MADE OF THE RELATIONSHIP BETWEEN THE ECOLOGICAL DISTRIBUTION OF HEROIN ADDICTION IN SAN ANTONIO, TEXAS, AND MEASURES OF SOCIOECONOMIC STATUS AND MINORITY GROUP STATUS. CENSUS TRACTS CONSTITUTED THE BASIC UNIT OF ANALYSIS; A SAMPLE OF 185 ADDICTS WAS OBTAINED (143 VOLUNTEER PATIENTS AND 42 PATIENTS UNDER FEDERAL SENTENCE). MEDIAN YEARS OF SCHOOLING COMPLETED, MEDIAN FAMILY INCOME, PERCENTAGE OF UNEMPLOYED MALES, AND PERCENTAGE OF OVERCROWDED DWELLINGS WERE USED AS INDICATORS OF SOCIOECONOMIC STATUS. FINDINGS LARGELY CORROBORATED PRIOR SOCIOLOGICAL RESEARCH ON HEROIN ABUSE. RATES WERE INVERSELY RELATED TO SOCIAL RANK, MEDIAN FAMILY INCOME, AND MEDIAN YEARS OF SCHOOL COMPLETED. ADDICTION HAD DIRECT RELATIONSHIPS WITH PERCENTAGE OF MALE UNEMPLOYMENT AND OVERCROWDED HOUSING. THE STRONGEST PREDICTOR OF HEROIN ADDICTION WAS THE PERCENTAGE OF MEXICAN AMERICANS IN THE TRACT POPULATION, BUT FOR THEM, EDUCATIONAL AND ETHNICITY VARIABLES INTERACT. RATES OF HEROIN ABUSE IN SAN ANTONIO WERE NOT ASSOCIATED WITH PERCENTAGES OF BLACKS—AN ANOMALY SINCE IN OTHER AREAS THERE IS A HIGH ASSOCIATION. DIFFERENTIAL ACCESSIBILITY OF DRUGS WAS THE MAJOR FACTOR IN GREATER NARCOTICS ABUSE BY MEXICAN AMERICANS THAN BY BLACKS. SUPPLIES OF ILLICIT DRUGS COME FROM MEXICO AND ARE ONLY SOLD TO MEXICAN AMERICANS, AND MEXICAN AMERICANS DO NOT TRUST BLACKS AND WILL NOT SELL TO THEM. 19 REFERENCES.
ACCN   001311

1517 AUTH   **REED, E. T.**
TITL   ETHNIC CLASSIFICATION OF MEXICAN AMERICANS.
SRCE   *SCIENCE, 1974, 185, 283.*
INDX   MEXICAN AMERICAN, DEMOGRAPHIC, RESEARCH METHODOLOGY, DISEASE, TEXAS, SOUTHWEST
ABST   THE ETHNIC CLASSIFICATION OF RACIAL HYBRIDS POSES PROBLEMS FOR EPIDEMIOLOGICAL AND DEMOGRAPHIC STUDIES. FOR EXAMPLE, IN THE CASE OF MENCK, CASAGRANDE, AND HENDERSON'S STUDY ON THE EFFECTS OF AIR POLLUTION ON RISK OF LUNG CANCER, THEIR SAMPLE CLASSIFIED MEXICAN AMERICANS AS CAUCASIAN. IN CALIFORNIA. HOWEVER. ABOUT ONE-THIRD OF THE ANCESTRY OF MEXICAN AMERICANS IS MEXICAN INDIAN. SINCE THE "R" GENE OF THE RH BLOOD GROUP SYSTEM IS ABSENT IN PURE MEXICAN INDIANS BUT COMMON IN CAUCASIANS, THE AMOUNT OF CAUCASIAN ANCESTRY OF MEXICAN AMERICANS CAN BE ASCERTAINED. THE ACTUAL GENETIC COMPOSITION OF HYBRID POPULATIONS MUST BE RECOGNIZED AS AN IMPORTANT PROBLEM IN THE STUDY OF DISEASE SINCE BIRACIAL HYBRIDS MAY HAVE DISTINCT DISEASE SUSCEPTIBILITIES. 6 REFERENCES.
ACCN   001312

1518 AUTH   **REEDER, L. G., & BERKANOVIC, E.**
TITL   SOCIOLOGICAL CONCOMITANTS OF HEALTH ORIENTATIONS: A PARTIAL REPLICATION OF SUCHMAN.
SRCE   *JOURNAL OF HEALTH AND SOCIAL BEHAVIOR, 1973, 14, 134-143.*
INDX   THEORETICAL, SOUTHWEST, CALIFORNIA, URBAN. DEMOGRAPHIC, REVIEW, SES, CULTURAL FACTORS. CROSS CULTURAL, ATTITUDES, HEALTH. ADULTS, MEXICAN AMERICAN, SEX COMPARISON, COMMUNITY INVOLVEMENT. EMPIRICAL. RESOURCE UTILIZATION
ABST   DATA WERE OBTAINED AS PART OF THE LOS ANGELES METROPOLITAN AREA SURVEY ON A REPRESENTATIVE SAMPLE OF 1,026 COUNTY RESIDENTS. INTERVIEW QUESTIONS INCLUDED MEDICAL ORIENTATION, HEALTH KNOWLEDGE. AND PREVENTATIVE BEHAVIOR ITEMS FROM SUCHMAN'S WASHINGTON HEIGHTS. N.Y., STUDIES ON THE RELATIONSHIP BETWEEN SOCIODEMOGRAPHIC AND SOCIOSTRUCTURAL VARIABLES AND MEDICAL ORIENTATION. THE DATA—ANALYZED FOR MEXICAN AMERICANS, BLACKS, ANGLOS AT ALL SOCIOECONOMIC LEVELS—INDICATE THAT THE RELATIONSHIPS DESCRIBED BY SUCHMAN ARE MORE COMPLEX THAN HIS FINDINGS SUGGESTED. IN PARTICULAR, THE EVIDENCE DIRECTLY CONTRADICTS HIS FINDINGS ABOUT THE RELATIONSHIP BETWEEN COSMOPOLITAN-PAROCHIALISM AND MEDICAL ORIENTATION. THESE DIFFERENCES MAY BE ATTRIBUTED TO SUCH FACTORS AS TIME, PLACE, AND ITEM CONTENT. FURTHERMORE, THE LAST DECADE HAS SEEN THE GROWTH OF CONSUMERISM IN THE HEALTH CARE FIELD AND THE MOVEMENT AMONG MINORITIES FOR LOCAL CONTROL OF HEALTH CARE FACILITIES AND SERVICES. IT IS CONCLUDED THAT RELIANCE ON EITHER SOCIODEMOGRAPHIC OR COMMUNITY ORIENTATION VARIABLES AS PREDICTORS OF MEDICAL ORIENTATION IS A WEAK PROCEDURE. AND THAT THE RELATIONSHIP BETWEEN MEDICAL ORIENTATIONS AND HEALTH

BEHAVIOR REMAINS TO BE ESTABLISHED. 16 REFERENCES.

ACCN   002187

1519 AUTH   **REEVE, S. B.**
TITL   A COMPARISON BY SOCIOECONOMIC CLASS OF THE POWER STRUCTURE OF MEXICAN AMERICAN AND ANGLO-AMERICAN FAMILIES IN THE LOWER RIO GRANDE VALLEY OF SOUTH TEXAS (DOCTORAL DISSERTATION, FLORIDA STATE UNIVERSITY, 1975).
SRCE   *DISSERTATION ABSTRACTS INTERNATIONAL, 1975, 36(8), 5585A. (UNIVERSITY MICROFILMS NO. 76-2693.)*
INDX   CROSS CULTURAL, MEXICAN AMERICAN, SES, FAMILY STRUCTURE, EMPIRICAL, ATTITUDES, CULTURAL FACTORS, SEX COMPARISON, FAMILY ROLES, COLLEGE STUDENTS, TEXAS, SOUTHWEST
ABST   HYPOTHESIZING THAT THE POWER STRUCTURE OF A GIVEN FAMILY CAN BE DETERMINED BY THE DECISION-MAKING PRACTICES OF HUSBANDS AND WIVES, THIS STUDY ADMINISTERED QUESTIONNAIRES ABOUT PARENTS' DECISION-MAKING PRACTICES TO A RANDOM SAMPLE OF 233 MEXICAN AMERICAN AND 71 ANGLO AMERICAN STUDENTS. THE QUESTIONNAIRE INCORPORATED THE BLOOD AND WOLFE INSTRUMENTS, WITH ADDITIONAL QUESTIONS TO DETERMINE ETHNIC BACKGROUND, SOCIOECONOMIC CLASS, AND SEX OF THE RESPONDENTS. THE FINDINGS SUGGEST THAT NO DIFFERENCES EXIST BETWEEN MEXICAN AMERICAN AND ANGLO AMERICAN FAMILIES IN POWER STRUCTURE. MOST COLLEGE STUDENTS BELIEVED THEIR PARENTS TO BE EGALITARIAN. MOREOVER, WHEN COMPARISONS WERE MADE BY THE SEX OF THE RESPONDENT, THERE WAS NO DIFFERENCE BETWEEN ANGLO MALES AND FEMALES. MEXICAN AMERICAN STUDENTS BELIEVED THEIR PARENTS WERE EGALITARIAN, BUT FEMALES REPORTED MORE WIFE DOMINANCE AND MALES REPORTED WIFE AND HUSBAND DOMINANCE. THIS DIFFERENCE MAY INDICATE THAT SOME STEREOTYPED CONCEPTS ABOUT POWER STRUCTURE PERSIST EVEN THOUGH NOT SUPPORTED BY ACTUAL PRACTICES. IT IS SUGGESTED THAT FUTURE STUDIES GATHER MORE SPECIFIC INFORMATION ABOUT THE FAMILY'S SIZE, NUMBER OF GENERATIONS REMOVED FROM MEXICAN NATIONALITY, AND THE NATURE OF SPECIFIC CONTACTS WITH ANGLO CULTURE. QUESTIONING HIGH SCHOOL AND JUNIOR HIGH SCHOOL STUDENTS ABOUT THEIR PARENTS' DECISION-MAKING PRACTICES AND CONDUCTING PERSONAL INTERVIEWS OF A RANDOM SAMPLE OF HUSBANDS AND WIVES ACROSS THE RIO GRANDE VALLEY WOULD ALSO BE VALUABLE. 30 REFERENCES. (DISSERTATION ABSTRACT MODIFIED)
ACCN   001313

1520 AUTH   **REGALADO, J.**
TITL   THE CHICANO URBAN HEALTH STUDY—A BRIEF.
SRCE   *IN COMMUNITY HEALTH BULLETIN (SPECIAL REPORT NO. 3). LOS ANGELES: EAST LOS ANGELES HEALTH SYSTEM, INC., UNDATED.*
INDX   URBAN, MEXICAN AMERICAN, SPANISH SURNAMED, HEALTH, DEATH, SURVEY, SES. HEALTH DELIVERY SYSTEMS, CALIFORNIA, SOUTHWEST
ABST   ALTHOUGH PERTINENT HEALTH INFORMATION IS OFTEN GENERATED FOR SPECIFIC WHITE, BLACK, AND OTHER POPULATIONS IN CALIFORNIA, CHICANOS HAVE BEEN LARGELY IGNORED. TO EXPLORE THIS SEEMING INSENSITIVITY TOWARD THE STATE'S LARGEST ETHNIC MINORITY, THE CHICANO URBAN HEALTH STUDY UNDERTOOK IN 1972 AN EXTENSIVE ANALYSIS OF HEALTH INFORMATION RETRIEVAL AND HEALTH CARE DELIVERY SYSTEMS FOR THE CHICANO POPULATION. FINDINGS WERE THAT IN EIGHT URBAN INNER-CITY AREAS IN CALIFORNIA IN WHICH CHICANOS/LATINOS REPRESENT THE OVERWHELMING PROPORTION OF THE POPULATION, HIGH RATES OF INFANT, NEONATAL, AND FETAL MORTALITY, INFECTIOUS REPORTABLE DISEASES, MENTAL ILLNESS AND RETARDATION, AND SOCIOECONOMIC DEPRIVATION COEXIST WITH LOW LEVELS OF REPRESENTATION IN PRIVATE AND PUBLIC SECTOR HEALTH CARE SERVICES AND FACILITIES AS COMPARED TO THE COUNTY POPULATION AT LARGE. WHAT IS MORE, DUE TO POOR REPRESENTATION IN HEALTH STATUS INDICATORS, FUNDAMENTAL PLANNING TO IMPROVE HEALTH CARE DELIVERY TO THE STATE'S LARGEST ETHNIC MINORITY POPULATION HAS BEEN NOTICEABLY ABSENT. IMPROVED REPRESENTATION IN HEALTH INFORMATION RETRIEVALS (THE MOST BASIC TOOLS OF HEALTH CARE PLANNING) IS STRONGLY RECOMMENDED. 2 REFERENCES.
ACCN   001314

1521 AUTH   **REILLEY, R. R., & KNIGHT, G. E.**
TITL   MMPI SCORES OF MEXICAN-AMERICAN COLLEGE STUDENTS.
SRCE   *JOURNAL OF COLLEGE STUDENT PERSONNEL, 1970, 11(6), 419-422.*
INDX   MMPI, MEXICAN AMERICAN, COLLEGE STUDENTS, PERSONALITY ASSESSMENT, CROSS CULTURAL, EMPIRICAL, SOUTHWEST, SEX COMPARISON, MALE, FEMALE
ABST   AN INVESTIGATION OF THE DIFFERENCES IN MINNESOTA MULTIPHASIC PERSONALITY INVENTORY (MMPI) SCORES OF SPANISH SURNAMED (SS) AND NON-SPANISH SURNAMED (NSS) FRESHMEN COLLEGE STUDENTS AT A SOUTHWESTERN AMERICAN UNIVERSITY IS PRESENTED. THE PERSONALITY INVENTORY WAS ADMINISTERED TO APPROXIMATELY 200 SUBJECTS; 136 WERE RANDOMLY SELECTED AND DIVIDED INTO TWO GROUPS OF 68 EACH. A TWO-BY-TWO FACTORIAL ANALYSIS OF VARIANCE WAS USED TO ANALYZE THE DATA. SEVEN SIGNIFICANT DIFFERENCES BETWEEN MEAN SCORES OF GROUPS WERE FOUND: L SCORES BETWEEN RACES; D SCORES BETWEEN SEXES; PA SCORES BETWEEN RACES; INTERACTION ON PT; INTERACTION ON SC; SI SCORES BETWEEN SEXES; AND INTERACTION ON SI. THE HIGHER L SCORE OF THE SS GROUP COULD REFLECT STRICT MORAL PRINCIPLES OR OVERTLY CONVENTIONAL ATTITUDES. THE NSS

GROUP'S HIGHER PA SCALE SCORE COULD INDICATE A TENDENCY TOWARD BEING MORE SUBJECTIVE, SENSITIVE, CONCERNED WITH SELF, AND LESS TRUSTING OF OTHERS. THE SS MALE AND THE NSS FEMALE SUBJECTS SCORED HIGHER THAN THEIR COUNTERPARTS ON: PT, INDICATING WORRY AND ANXIETY; SC, REFLECTING SOCIAL ALIENATION, SENSITIVITY, WORRY, AND THE TENDENCY TO AVOID REALITY BY USE OF FANTASY; AND SI, TENDING TOWARD INTROVERSION, MODESTY, AND SHYNESS. FEMALE SUBJECTS SCORED HIGHER THAN MALES ON D AND SI SCALES. BOTH OF THESE HIGH SCORES RELATE TO INTROVERSION, SHYNESS, AND MODESTY, WHILE THE D SCORE HAS THE ADDED IMPLICATION OF TENDENCY TO WORRY, LACK OF SELF-CONFIDENCE, AND REACTION TO STRESS WITH DEPRESSION. CAUTION IN THE INTERPRETATION OF PROFILES OF COLLEGE STUDENTS IS SUGGESTED. 12 REFERENCES.

ACCN   001315

1522 AUTH   **REISS, R. L.**
TITL   CONSIDERATIONS ON THE HEALTH STATUS ALONG MEXICO'S NORTHERN BORDER.
SRCE   *IN S. R. ROSS, (ED.), VIEWS ACROSS THE BORDER: THE UNITED STATES AND MEXICO. ALBUQUERQUE: UNIVERSITY OF NEW MEXICO PRESS, 1978, PP. 241-255.*
INDX   MEXICO, HEALTH, HEALTH DELIVERY SYSTEMS, DEMOGRAPHIC, REVIEW, ECONOMIC FACTORS, PERSONNEL, PROGRAM EVALUATION, PHYSICIANS, MEXICAN, DISEASE
ABST   FROM THE VIEW POINT OF PUBLIC HEALTH, TWO MAJOR AREAS OF CONCERN EXIST IN BORDER REGIONS: (1) THE PREVENTION OF THE SPREAD OF COMMUNICABLE DISEASE, AND (2) THE PREVENTION OF ENVIRONMENTAL AND SOCIAL CONDITIONS BROUGHT ABOUT BY DISEASE. USING DATA RELATING TO MEXICO, ITS SIX BORDER STATES AND 36 BORDER MUNICIPALITIES, A BROAD PICTURE OF PREVALENT HEALTH PROBLEMS, HEALTH RESOURCES AND SERVICES, AND RELEVANT CONDITIONING FACTORS ARE PRESENTED. TEN TABLES PRESENT DEMOGRAPHIC DATA AND INFORMATION ON HOSPITAL FACILITIES, HEALTH AND WELFARE AGENCIES, AND HEALTH RESOURCE PERSONNEL. IT IS CONCLUDED THAT THE HEALTH STATUS ALONG MEXICO'S NORTHERN BORDER IS BETTER THAN THAT OF THE NATION AS A WHOLE, AND THAT THIS IS DUE MORE TO A HIGHER STANDARD OF LIVING THAN TO SPECIFIC HEALTH PROGRAMS.
ACCN   002188

1523 AUTH   **REMMERS, H. H.**
TITL   CROSS-CULTURAL STUDIES OF TEENAGERS' PROBLEMS.
SRCE   *JOURNAL OF EDUCATIONAL PSYCHOLOGY, 1962, 53(6), 254-261.*
INDX   CROSS CULTURAL, ADOLESCENTS, PUERTO RICAN-I, TEST RELIABILITY, CULTURAL FACTORS, HEALTH, SURVEY, ANXIETY, EMPIRICAL
ABST   REPRESENTATIVE STRATIFIED SAMPLES OF MORE THAN 5,000 TEENAGERS IN SCHOOL IN THE UNITED STATES, PUERTO RICO, WEST GERMANY AND INDIA WERE COMPARED ON A SCIENCE RESEARCH ASSOCIATES YOUTH INVENTORY. THIS INVENTORY CONSISTS OF A PROBLEMS CHECK-LIST WHICH WAS ADAPTED TO EACH OF THE CULTURES SURVEYED. MEAN SCORES, RELIABILITY ESTIMATES, INTERCORRELATIONS OF SUBSCALE SCORES, AND FACTOR ANALYSES OF THESE MATRICES ALL LED TO THE CONCLUSION THAT (1) THE MEASURING INSTRUMENT IS HIGHLY RELIABLE, (2) TEENAGERS' SELF-PERCEIVED PROBLEMS CAN BE COMPARABLY MEASURED ACROSS WIDELY DIFFERENT CULTURES, (3) RANKINGS OF PROBLEM AREAS ACROSS CULTURES ARE HIGHLY SIMILAR, AND (4) HEALTH PROBLEMS ARE OF LEAST CONCERN AND POST-HIGH-SCHOOL PROBLEMS OF MOST CONCERN. THE AMOUNT AND INTENSITY OF WORRY VARIED GREATLY ACROSS CULTURES. 13 REFERENCES.
ACCN   001316

1524 AUTH   **RENDON, M.**
TITL   TRANSCULTURAL ASPECTS OF PUERTO RICAN MENTAL ILLNESS IN NEW YORK.
SRCE   *INTERNATIONAL JOURNAL OF SOCIAL PSYCHIATRY, 1974, 20(1-2), 18-24.*
INDX   ETHNIC IDENTITY, PUERTO RICAN-M, MENTAL HEALTH, SCHIZOPHRENIA, CULTURAL FACTORS, ADOLESCENTS, DEMOGRAPHIC, PSYCHOPATHOLOGY, PSYCHOSOCIAL ADJUSTMENT, SES, LINGUISTIC COMPETENCE, SEXUAL BEHAVIOR, FAMILY STRUCTURE, ENVIRONMENTAL FACTORS, SURVEY, ACCULTURATION, CROSS CULTURAL, EMPIRICAL
ABST   EPIDEMIOLOGICAL STUDIES INDICATE THAT MENTAL ILLNESS IS EXCEPTIONALLY HIGH AMONG PUERTO RICANS IN NEW YORK. STATISTICS OBTAINED FROM NEW YORK STATE AND CITY CENSUS AND SURVEY DATA PERTAINING TO THE DISTRIBUTION OF MENTAL HEALTH CATEGORIES AMONG PUERTO RICANS AND NON-PUERTO RICANS WITH RESPECT TO VARIOUS SOCIODEMOGRAPHIC FACTORS ARE PRESENTED. THE DATA SUGGEST THAT ADOLESCENTS ARE THE MOST AFFECTED, AFTER THE AGE GROUPS WITH SENILE DISEASES. THIS CONTRASTS WITH THE RELATIVELY LOW INCIDENCE OF MENTAL ILLNESS AMONG NON-PUERTO RICAN ADOLESCENTS. BESIDES POVERTY, CROWDING, ILLITERACY, LACK OF SKILL FOR QUALIFIED JOBS, AND OTHER SOURCES OF STRESS, TRANSCULTURATION SEEMS TO EXPLAIN SOME OF THESE FACTS. THE TRANSCULTURATION OF PUERTO RICANS TO NEW YORK IMPLIES LEARNING A DIFFERENT LANGUAGE AND ADJUSTING TO DIFFERENT ROLES AND VALUES. THE STRUCTURE OF THE FAMILY IN NEW YORK DIFFERS FROM THAT FOUND IN PUERTO RICO. IN DEALING WITH AGGRESSION AND SEXUALITY, THERE ARE OPPOSITE PATTERNS IN BOTH CULTURES. THIS HAS PARTICULAR SIGNIFICANCE FOR THE PUERTO RICAN ADOLESCENT IN HIS TASK OF IDENTITY FORMATION. DISSOCIATION IS THE PREDOMINANT DEFENSE IN DEALING WITH THOSE CONFLICTS, AND DISSOCIATIVE PHENOMENA MAY BE MISDIAGNOSED AS SCHIZOPHRENIA BECAUSE OF LACK OF UNDERSTANDING OF CUL-

TURAL DIFFERENCES. SOME CONSIDERATION IS GIVEN TO THE DIFFERENTIAL DIAGNOSIS. 11 REFERENCES. (AUTHOR SUMMARY MODIFIED)

ACCN 001317

1525 AUTH **RESCHLY, D. J.**

TITL WISC-R FACTOR STRUCTURES AMONG ANGLOS, BLACKS, CHICANO, AND NATIVE-AMERICAN PAPAGOS.

SRCE *JOURNAL OF CONSULTING AND CLINICAL PSYCHOLOGY, 1978, 46(3), 417-422.*

INDX WISC, CROSS CULTURAL, CHILDREN, SOUTHWEST, ARIZONA, INTELLIGENCE TESTING, CULTURAL FACTORS, EMPIRICAL, MEXICAN AMERICAN, URBAN, RURAL, SEX COMPARISON

ABST WECHSLER INTELLIGENCE SCALE FOR CHILDREN-REVISED (WISC-R) FACTOR STRUCTURES WERE COMPARED FOR SAMPLES OF ANGLO, BLACK, CHICANO, AND NATIVE-AMERICAN PAPAGO CHILDREN FROM PIMA COUNTY, ARIZONA. THE SAMPLES WERE RANDOMLY SELECTED FROM SCHOOL ENROLLMENT ROSTERS AND STRATIFIED BY ETHNICITY, GRADE LEVEL, SEX, AND URBAN-RURAL RESIDENCE (N = 950). APPLICATION OF TWO OBJECTIVE PROCEDURES FOR DETERMINING THE APPROPRIATE NUMBER OF FACTORS FOR EACH GROUP SUGGESTED A THREE-FACTOR SOLUTION FOR ANGLOS, A TWO- OR THREE-FACTOR SOLUTION FOR CHICANOS DEPENDING ON PROCEDURE USED, AND TWO-FACTOR SOLUTIONS FOR BLACKS AND NATIVE-AMERICAN PAPAGOS. THE TWO-FACTOR SOLUTIONS WERE HIGHLY SIMILAR FOR THE FOUR GROUPS. THE THREE-FACTOR SOLUTIONS WERE SIMILAR FOR ANGLOS AND CHICANOS BUT WERE SUBSTANTIALLY DIFFERENT FOR THE OTHER GROUPS. THE GROUPS WERE HIGHLY SIMILAR IN TERMS OF THE PROPORTION OF VARIANCE ACCOUNTED FOR BY A GENERAL FACTOR, AND THE VERBAL-PERFORMANCE SCALE DISTINCTION APPEARED EQUALLY APPROPRIATE FOR ALL GROUPS. 11 REFERENCES. (JOURNAL ABSTRACT)

ACCN 002189

1526 AUTH **RESCHLY, D. J., & JIPSON, F. J.**

TITL ETHNICITY, GEOGRAPHIC LOCALE, AGE, SEX, AND URBAN-RURAL RESIDENCE AS VARIABLES IN THE PREVALENCE OF MILD RETARDATION.

SRCE *AMERICAN JOURNAL OF MENTAL DEFICIENCY, 1976, 81(2), 154-161.*

INDX MENTAL RETARDATION, EMPIRICAL, ARIZONA, SOUTHWEST, CROSS CULTURAL, MEXICAN AMERICAN, WISC, CHILDREN, INTELLIGENCE TESTING, RURAL, URBAN, SEX COMPARISON

ABST THE WECHSLER INTELLIGENCE SCALE FOR CHILDREN-REVISED (WISC-R) WAS ADMINISTERED TO 950 OF A STRATIFIED RANDOM SAMPLE OF 1,040 CHILDREN IN PIMA COUNTY, ARIZONA. THE SAMPLE WAS STRATIFIED FOR ETHNICITY (ANGLO, BLACK, MEXICAN AMERICAN, AND PAPAGO INDIAN), URBAN-RURAL RESIDENCE, SEX, AND GRADE LEVEL. THE THREE WISC-R IQ SCORES AND CUTOFF POINTS OF 69 AND 75 WERE USED IN COMPARISONS OF PREVALENCE OF MILD MENTAL RETARDATION. PREVALENCE IN PIMA COUNTY EX-

CEEDED THE NATIONAL PREVALENCE ESTIMATES FOR VERBAL AND FULL-SCALE IQ. USING A CUTOFF SCORE OF 69, SIGNIFICANT DISPROPORTIONALITY WAS EVIDENT ACROSS ETHNIC GROUPS. THIS OVERREPRESENTATION BY ETHNICITY WAS ELIMINATED FOR MEXICAN AMERICANS AND GREATLY REDUCED FOR BLACKS AND PAPAGO INDIANS WHEN THE PERFORMANCE IQ WAS USED AS THE CRITERION. A CUTOFF SCORE OF 75, HOWEVER, YIELDED DRAMATIC ETHNIC DIFFERENCES REGARDLESS OF THE WISC-R IQ SCORE USED. SEX, URBAN-RURAL RESIDENCE, AND GRADE LEVEL WERE FOUND TO HAVE NO RELATION TO PREVALENCE. 31 REFERENCES. (JOURNAL ABSTRACT MODIFIED)

ACCN 002190

1527 AUTH **REVELES, R. A.**

TITL BICULTURALISM AND THE UNITED STATES CONGRESS: THE DYNAMICS OF POLITICAL CHANGE.

SRCE *IN A. CASTANEDA, M. RAMIREZ, III, C. E. CORTES, & M. BARRERA (EDS.), MEXICAN AMERICANS AND EDUCATIONAL CHANGE. NEW YORK: ARNO PRESS, 1974, PP. 205-225.*

INDX POLITICAL POWER, LEADERSHIP, EDUCATION, BILINGUAL-BICULTURAL EDUCATION, CHICANO MOVEMENT, ADMINISTRATORS, LEGISLATION

ABST THE POLITICS OF EDUCATIONAL CHANGE CAN BE EXEMPLIFIED BY THE EVENTS WHICH OCCURRED AT A CONFERENCE ON THE BILINGUAL EDUCATION ACT, HELD IN ALBUQUERQUE IN 1966. AT THIS CONFERENCE, SPONSORED BY THE EQUAL EMPLOYMENT OPPORTUNITY COMMISSION (EEOC), A COALITION OF CHICANO ORGANIZATIONS WALKED OUT OF THE CONFERENCE IN PROTEST OF MEXICAN AMERICAN UNDERREPRESENTATION IN THE STAFFING OF EEOC AS WELL AS EEOC'S INSENSITIVITY TO THE EDUCATIONAL NEEDS OF MEXICAN AMERICANS. THIS COALITION LATER PRESENTED A LIST OF DEMANDS TO PRESIDENT JOHNSON: (1) APPOINTMENT OF A MEXICAN AMERICAN AS COMMISSIONER IN EEOC; (2) CHANGES IN EEOC'S STAFF HIRING PRACTICES SO AS TO ELIMINATE ETHNIC IMBALANCE; AND (3) INCLUSION OF MEXICAN AMERICANS' PROBLEMS IN THE WHITE HOUSE CONFERENCE ON CIVIL RIGHTS. AT THE ALBUQUERQUE CONFERENCE THE COMMITTMENT BY GOVERNMENT OFFICIALS WAS SEEN AS STRONGLY SUPPORTING BILINGUAL EDUCATION, YET RESERVATIONS WERE MAINTAINED BY SOME AS TO THE "EXCLUSIVE" LEGISLATION REQUIRED FOR IT. OTHERS FELT THAT FEDERAL REVENUES WERE NOT SUFFICIENT TO IMPLEMENT A MEANINGFUL PROGRAM. POSITED IS THE NEED FOR THE MEXICAN AMERICAN COMMUNITY AND THE EDUCATION COMMUNITY TO FORM AN ALLIANCE FOR FEDERAL ADOPTION OF BILINGUAL EDUCATION. IN ADDITION, ACTIVISM IS CONSIDERED A NECESSITY FOR GAINING A WIDER BASE OF NATIONAL SUPPORT. 7 REFERENCES.

ACCN 001318

1528 AUTH **REYES DE AHUMADA, I., AHUMADA, R., & DIAZ-GUERRERO, R.**

TITL CONSIDERACIONES ACERCA DE LA ESTANDARIZACION DE PRUEBAS A LATINO AMERICA, CON ILUSTRACIONCES DE LA ADAPTACION DEL WISC A MEXICO. (CONSIDERATIONS REGARDING THE STANDARDIZATION OF TESTS TO LATIN AMERICA, WITH ILLUSTRATIONS OF THE ADAPTION OF THE WISC TO MEXICO).

SRCE *REVISTA MEXICANA DE PSICOLOGIA, 1966, 2(10), 813-823.*

INDX WISC, INTELLIGENCE TESTING, SES, ECONOMIC FACTORS, CHILDREN, ADOLESCENTS, RESEARCH METHODOLOGY, TEST VALIDITY, TEST RELIABILITY, MEXICAN

ABST THE BASIC PROBLEMS IN ADAPTING AND STANDARDIZING AN INTELLIGENCE TEST TO A CULTURE WHICH DIFFERS FROM THAT IN WHICH THE TEST ORIGINATED ARE DISCUSSED. THE SAMPLE EMPLOYED FOR OBTAINING THE DATA CONSISTED OF 444 STUDENTS IN THREE MEXICO CITY SCHOOLS, TAKEN IN EQUAL NUMBERS FROM THE FIRST AND FOURTH YEARS OF PRIMARY SCHOOL AND FIRST YEAR OF SECONDARY SCHOOL. THE OBSTACLES ENCOUNTERED IN STANDARDIZING THE UNITED STATES' VERSION OF THE WECHSLER INTELLIGENCE SCALE FOR CHILDREN (WISC) TO MEXICO ARE SEPARATED INTO TWO MAJOR CATEGORIES—GENERIC CRITERIA AND SPECIFIC STEPS. GENERIC CRITERIA REFERS TO THE RIGOROUS MAINTENANCE OF THE SAME SCIENTIFIC METHODOLOGY EMPLOYED IN CREATING THE ORIGINAL TEST, AND THE JUSTIFICATION FOR ALL MODIFICATIONS IN THE ORDER OF DIFFICULTY AND SOCIOCULTURAL AND SOCIOECONOMIC DIFFERENCES. THE SPECIFIC STEPS DISCUSSED AND ILLUSTRATED ARE: (1) OBTAINING A SAMPLE THAT IS BOTH EXTENSIVE AND REPRESENTATIVE OF THE POPULATION TO WHICH THE SCALE WILL BE STANDARDIZED; (2) TRANSLATION AND ADAPTATION OF THE TEST ITEMS TO MORE ADEQUATELY MODIFY THEM FOR THE MEXICAN VERSION; (3) ADMINISTERING THE COMPLETE SCALE TO THE SUBJECTS, USING ALL THE ITEMS OF EACH SUBTEST; (4) DETERMINING AND REARRANGING THE NEW ORDER OF DIFFICULTY THAT WILL HAVE TO BE APPLIED ON A GIVEN SUBTEST; AND (5) RELATING THE DIFFICULT PROBLEMS THAT MUST BE CONSIDERED WHEN MODIFYING THE WISC FOR USE IN A DIFFERENT SOCIOCULTURAL AND SOCIOECONOMIC CONTEXT. 16 REFERENCES.

ACCN 001319

1529 AUTH **REYES, D. J. (ED.)**

TITL TEACHING THE LATINO STUDENT.

SRCE *THRESHOLDS IN SECONDARY EDUCATION, 1976, 2(WHOLE ISSUE NO. 2).*

INDX SPANISH SURNAMED, ESSAY, EMPIRICAL, BILINGUALISM, MEXICAN AMERICAN, EDUCATION, INTELLIGENCE TESTING, CROSS CULTURAL, CULTURAL PLURALISM, COGNITIVE DEVELOPMENT, BILINGUAL-BICULTURAL EDUCATION, OCCUPATIONAL ASPIRATIONS

ABST CURRENTLY, BILINGUAL/BICULTURAL EDUCATIONAL PROGRAMS, DESIGNED TO EQUALIZE ACCESS TO EDUCATION, ARE NOT WIDESPREAD ENOUGH TO SIGNIFICANTLY ALTER THE EDUCATIONAL PROSPECTS OF LATINO YOUNGSTERS. THE EDUCATION OF THIS POPULATION REMAINS ALMOST EXCLUSIVELY IN THE HANDS OF NON-LATINO EDUCATORS. THIS ISSUE OF THRESHOLDS WAS ORGANIZED TO DISSEMINATE USEFUL INFORMATION RELEVANT TO LATINO EDUCATION TO EDUCATORS WHO ARE WORKING WITH THIS POPULATION. INCLUDED ARE THE FOLLOWING ARTICLES: (1) LATINO? OR SHOULD ONE SAY CHICANO?; (2) THE CHICANO STUDENT AND ANGLO AMERICAN FICTION; (3) NEW PERSPECTIVES IN TESOL: INTERDISCIPLINARY APPROACHES; (4) CULTURAL DEMOCRACY, COGNITIVE FLEXIBILITY AND EDUCATION OF MEXICAN AMERICANS; (5) ANGLO AMERICAN LAW IN THE MULTI-CULTURAL SCHOOL; (6) WHERE AND HOW: ACQUISITION AND EVALUATION OF SPANISH BILINGUAL MATERIALS FOR SECONDARY SCHOOLS; (7) TEACHING SPANISH TO CHICANOS; (8) BILINGUAL EDUCATION: WHAT? WHY? WHEN? HOW? WHERE?; (9) BEYOND THE IQ TESTS: PROBLEMS IN ALTERNATIVE TESTING PROCEDURES WITH CHICANO CHILDREN; AND, (10) A SURVEY OF CAREER ASPIRATIONS FOR SECONDARY SCHOOL STUDENTS. EMPHASIS ON THE SCHOOLS TO ALTER THEIR METHODS RATHER THAN ON INDIVIDUAL STUDENTS TO REJECT THEIR CULTURE IS A RECURRENT THEME THROUGHOUT THE ISSUE.

ACCN 001320

1530 AUTH **REYES, J. A., & ASSOCIATES, INC.**

TITL MODEL MENTAL HEALTH PROGRAM FOR HISPANIC PATIENTS AT ST. ELIZABETHS HOSPITAL.

SRCE *WASHINGTON, D.C.: AUTHOR, 1978.*

INDX ESSAY, POLICY, BILINGUAL-BICULTURAL PERSONNEL, COMMUNITY, CULTURAL FACTORS, EMPIRICAL, ENVIRONMENTAL FACTORS, FAMILY THERAPY, HEALTH DELIVERY SYSTEMS, MENTAL HEALTH, RESOURCE UTILIZATION, SPANISH SURNAMED, EAST, WASHINGTON D.C., URBAN

ABST THE FINDINGS OF A YEAR LONG PROJECT TO RESEARCH AND DESIGN A MODEL MENTAL HEALTH PROGRAM FOR HISPANIC PATIENTS AT ST. ELIZABETHS HOSPITAL (SEH) IN WASHINGTON, D.C. ARE REPORTED. THE PROJECT WAS COMPLETED IN THREE PHASES: (1) A BACKGROUND REVIEW WHICH INCLUDED AN ASSESSMENT OF THE LITERATURE DEALING WITH LATINO MENTAL HEALTH AND A SURVEY OF U.S. HISPANIC MENTAL HEALTH PROGRAMS; (2) COMPLETION OF COMMUNITY AND CLIENT PROFILES, INCLUDING A DEMOGRAPHIC PROFILE OF THE HISPANIC POPULATION IN WASHINGTON, D.C., A PROFILE OF RESIDENT SEH HISPANIC PATIENTS, AND A SURVEY OF MENTAL HEALTH RESOURCES WITHIN THE LOCAL HISPANIC COMMUNITY AND AT SEH; AND (3) SITE VISITS TO SIX SELECTED HISPANIC MENTAL HEALTH PROGRAMS FOR PURPOSES OF OBSERVATION AND DATA COLLECTION. UPON COMPLETION OF THESE TASKS, A CULTURALLY RELEVANT, MODEL MENTAL HEALTH PROGRAM WAS PROPOSED WHICH WOULD ADDRESS THE

PROBLEM OF HISPANIC UNDERUTILIZATION OF MENTAL HEALTH SERVICES. THIS MODEL PROGRAM INCLUDES: (1) BILINGUAL-BICULTURAL STAFF; (2) AN ENVIRONMENT REFLECTIVE OF HISPANIC CULTURE; (3) FAMILY INVOLVEMENT IN THERAPY AS MUCH AS POSSIBLE; (4) STRONG COMMUNITY OUTREACH EFFORTS; (5) DEVELOPMENT OF A POSITIVE IMAGE AMONG PROFESSIONALS AND WITHIN THE HISPANIC COMMUNITY; AND (6) A BASE OF STRONG HOSPITAL SUPPORT FOR THE CONCEPT OF A CULTURALLY SPECIFIC PROGRAM. SPECIFIC RECOMMENDATIONS FOR THE MODEL PROGRAM (INCLUDING GOALS, SERVICES, ADMINISTRATIVE REQUIREMENTS, THERAPEUTIC AND ENVIRONMENTAL CONSIDERATION, COMMUNITY OUTREACH, RECORD-KEEPING AND EVALUATION, AND BUDGETARY CONSIDERATIONS) ARE DISCUSSED IN THE REPORT. 54 REFERENCES.

ACCN   002191

1531 AUTH   **REYES, S.**
TITL   CHICANO STUDENTS IN GRADUATE SCHOOLS OF SOCIAL WORK AS REFLECTED IN THE STATISTICS ON SOCIAL WORK EDUCATION, 1969.
SRCE   *SOCIAL WORK EDUCATION, 1971, 19(2), 19-20.*
INDX   MEXICAN AMERICAN, COLLEGE STUDENTS, EDUCATION, REPRESENTATION, MENTAL HEALTH, PROFESSIONAL TRAINING, ESSAY, HIGHER EDUCATION, MENTAL HEALTH PROFESSION
ABST   THE 1969 EDITION OF "STATISTICS ON SOCIAL WORK EDUCATION" INDICATES THE HIGH PRIORITY THE COUNCIL OF SOCIAL WELFARE EDUCATION IS PLACING ON INCREASING THE NUMBERS OF ALL ETHNIC MINORITIES IN SOCIAL WORK EDUCATION. FOR THE FIRST TIME, STATISTICS ARE PROVIDED FOR CHICANOS AND OTHER ETHNIC GROUPS IN GRADUATE SCHOOLS OF SOCIAL WELFARE. ALSO, THE 1969 DATA COMPARED WITH A 1967 STUDY SHOW A SIGNIFICANT INCREASE IN CHICANO ENROLLMENT. HOWEVER, TAKING INTO CONSIDERATION OTHER FACTORS, CHICANOS APPEAR TO BE THE FORGOTTEN MINORITY IN SCHOOLS OF SOCIAL WORK. FOR EXAMPLE, FEWER SCHOOLS ATTRACTED CHICANOS IN 1969 THAN IN 1967; AND, OTHER THAN NATIVE AMERICANS, CHICANOS ARE LEAST REPRESENTED. STEPS TO INCREASE THE OPPORTUNITIES FOR CHICANOS IN SOCIAL WORK EDUCATION MUST BE TAKEN. 1 REFERENCE.
ACCN   001321

1532 AUTH   **REYNOLDS, D. K., & KALISH, R. A.**
TITL   ANTICIPATION OF FUTURITY AS A FUNCTION OF ETHNICITY AND AGE.
SRCE   *JOURNAL OF GERONTOLOGY, 1974, 29(2), 224-231.*
INDX   CROSS CULTURAL, EMPIRICAL, DEATH, CULTURAL FACTORS, FATALISM, GERONTOLOGY, ATTITUDES, MEXICAN AMERICAN, CALIFORNIA, SOUTHWEST, SURVEY
ABST   AS PART OF A LARGER STUDY OF DEATH ATTITUDES AND EXPECTATIONS, 434 RESIDENTS OF GREATER LOS ANGELES, APPROXIMATELY EQUALLY DIVIDED BY FOUR ETHNIC AND THREE AGE GROUPS, STATED HOW LONG THEY WISH TO LIVE AND HOW LONG THEY EXPECT TO LIVE. AS ANTICIPATED, THE OLDER PERSONS EXPECTED TO AND WANTED TO LIVE LONGER THAN THE YOUNGER AGE COHORTS. BLACK RESPONDENTS WERE SIGNIFICANTLY MORE LIKELY TO EXPECT TO LIVE AND WANT TO LIVE LONGER THAN JAPANESE AMERICANS, MEXICAN AMERICANS, AND WHITE AMERICANS; OTHER DIFFERENCES BETWEEN ETHNIC GROUPS WERE MINIMAL. RESULTS ARE DISCUSSED FROM TWO THEORETICAL POINTS OF VIEW. 14 REFERENCES. (JOURNAL ABSTRACT)
ACCN   001322

1533 AUTH   **REYNOLDS, D. K., & KALISH, R. A.**
TITL   DEATH RATES, ATTITUDES, AND THE ETHNIC PRESS.
SRCE   *ETHNICITY, 1976, 3, 305-316.*
INDX   MASS MEDIA, DEATH, CROSS CULTURAL, SUICIDE, ATTITUDES, DEMOGRAPHIC, EMPIRICAL, MEXICAN AMERICAN, CALIFORNIA, SOUTHWEST, CULTURAL FACTORS, URBAN, ADULTS, SURVEY
ABST   ATTITUDES TOWARD DEATH, IMAGES OF DEATH PRESENTED IN ETHNIC COMMUNITY NEWSPAPERS, AND STATISTICAL INCIDENCE OF DEATH WERE EACH EXAMINED IN A STUDY OF THE MEANING OF DEATH IN A CROSS-ETHNIC CONTEXT. IN LOS ANGELES, 434 BLACK, JAPANESE AMERICAN, MEXICAN AMERICAN, AND ANGLO RESIDENTS WERE INTERVIEWED CONCERNING THEIR EXPECTATIONS, EXPERIENCES AND PREFERENCES RELATED TO DEATH; SIMULTANEOUSLY, A CONTENT ANALYSIS OF ARTICLES INVOLVING DEATH IN THREE ETHNIC COMMUNITY NEWSPAPERS AND ONE GENERAL CIRCULATION DAILY WAS CONDUCTED. FINDINGS INDICATED THAT THE "LOS ANGELES SENTINEL," SERVING THE BLACK COMMUNITY, REPORTED THE LARGEST PROPORTION OF DEATHS BY HOMICIDE, WHILE THE BILINGUAL JAPANESE-ENGLISH "RAFU SHIMPO" PRIMARILY CONTAINED DESCRIPTIONS OF NATURAL DEATHS. THE "LOS ANGELES TIMES" AND THE SPANISH-LANGUAGE "LA OPINION" BOTH REPORTED MORE DEATHS BY ACCIDENT. ATTITUDES OF EACH ETHNIC GROUP RESEMBLED THE KINDS OF DEATHS PUBLICIZED BY THE NEWSPAPERS AND COINCIDED WITH OFFICIAL DEATH STATISTICS. ALTHOUGH OFFICIAL DEATH STATISTICS FOR EACH ETHNIC GROUP WERE REFLECTED IN THE EMPHASIS OF EACH PAPER, VIOLENT DEATHS WERE FOUND TO BE REPORTED FAR OUT OF PROPORTION TO THEIR ACTUAL OCCURRENCE. A DISCUSSION IS PRESENTED AS TO THE ROLE OF EDITORIAL POLICY IN REPORTING DEATHS, AND THE EXTENT TO WHICH THE NEWSPAPERS REFLECT OR SHAPE WHAT IS OCCURRING IN THE COMMUNITY. 2 REFERENCES.
ACCN   002192

1534 AUTH   **RICE, A. S., RUIZ, R. A., & PADILLA, A. M.**
TITL   PERSON PERCEPTION, SELF-IDENTITY, AND ETHNIC GROUP PREFERENCE IN ANGLO, BLACK, AND CHICANO PRESCHOOL AND THIRD-GRADE CHILDREN.

SRCE JOURNAL OF CROSS-CULTURAL PSYCHOLOGY, 1974, 5(1), 100-108.

INDX CHILDREN, SELF CONCEPT, ETHNIC IDENTITY, CROSS CULTURAL, GROUP DYNAMICS, EMPIRICAL, PREJUDICE, DISCRIMINATION, SES, MEXICAN AMERICAN

ABST AN INVESTIGATION OF THE ETHNIC AND RACIAL AWARENESS, SELF-IDENTIFICATION, AND ETHNIC GROUP PREFERENCE IN ANGLO, BLACK, AND CHICANO CHILDREN IS PRESENTED. SEVENTY-TWO PRESCHOOL AND 68 THIRD-GRADE CHILDREN WERE SHOWN COLOR PHOTOGRAPHS OF YOUNG MALE ADULTS FROM THE SAME THREE ETHNIC GROUP GROUPS. ALL CHILDREN WERE ABLE TO DISCRIMINATE BETWEEN THE PHOTOGRAPHS OF THE ANGLO AND BLACK MALES, BUT THE PRESCHOOL S'S WERE UNABLE TO MAKE THE FINE DISCRIMINATION BETWEEN THE ANGLO AND CHICANO PHOTOGRAPHS. IT MAY BE THAT THIS DISTINCTION IS TOO FINE FOR 5-6 YEAR-OLD CHILDREN TO ACCURATELY MAKE, OR THEY MAY BE UNFAMILIAR WITH THE TERM "CHICANO." ANOTHER MAJOR FINDING IS THAT ALL SUBJECTS INDICATED THE APPROPRIATE PHOTOGRAPH WHEN ASKED WHICH LOOKED MOST LIKE THEM. ADDITIONALLY, AMONG THE PRESCHOOL CHILDREN NEITHER THE BLACKS NOR THE CHICANOS EXPRESSED A SIGNIFICANT PREFERENCE FOR THEIR OWN ETHNIC GROUP, WHILE A SIGNIFICANT NUMBER OF THE ANGLO SUBJECTS SELECTED THE ANGLO PHOTOGRAPH AS THE ONE THEY LIKED THE MOST. AT THE THIRD GRADE LEVEL, ONLY THE CHICANO SUBJECTS DISPLAYED A STRONG PREFERENCE FOR THEIR OWN ETHNIC GROUP. THIS LAST FINDING IS DISCUSSED IN TERMS OF THE STRONG SENSE OF SELF-ESTEEM AND ETHNIC GROUP PRIDE AMONG THE OLDER CHICANO GROUP. 11 REFERENCES. (JOURNAL ABSTRACT MODIFIED)

ACCN 001323

1535 AUTH **RICHARDSON, S. A., & ROYCE J.**

TITL RACE AND PHYSICAL HANDICAP IN CHILDREN'S PREFERENCE FOR OTHER CHILDREN.

SRCE CHILD DEVELOPMENT, 1968, 39(2), 467-480.

INDX PUERTO RICAN-M, CHILDREN, PEER GROUP, SES, CULTURAL FACTORS, INTERPERSONAL ATTRACTION, SEX COMPARISON, NEW YORK, EAST

ABST THE RELATIVE SALIENCE OF SKIN COLOR AND PHYSICAL DISABILITY IN ESTABLISHING CHILDREN'S PREFERENCE FOR OTHER CHILDREN IS EXAMINED. A RANK-ORDER PREFERENCE OF DRAWINGS IN WHICH COLOR AND HANDICAP WERE SYSTEMATICALLY VARIED WAS OBTAINED FROM 298 MALES AND 389 FEMALES, AGES 10 TO 12 FROM LOWER INCOME NEGRO, WHITE, AND PUERTO RICAN FAMILIES. THE RESULTS SHOW THAT THE SUBJECTS' PREFERENCE RANKING OF THE MOST AND LEAST LIKED DRAWING OF CHILDREN WITH AND WITHOUT PHYSICAL HANDICAPS WAS NOT ALTERED BY THE ADDITIONAL VARIABLE OF SKIN COLOR. FOR ALL SUBJECTS, THE NONHANDICAPPED DRAWING WAS JUDGED "MOST LIKED" REGARDLESS OF COLOR, AND THE OBESE

DRAWING (FOR GIRLS) OR THE FOREARM AMPUTATION DRAWING (FOR BOYS) WAS THE "LEAST LIKED" REGARDLESS OF COLOR. THERE WAS SLIGHT EVIDENCE THAT SKIN COLOR INFLUENCES THE FEMALE SUBJECTS' CHOICES MORE THAN MALES BY THEIR PREFERENCE FOR THE WHITE PICTURE. OTHER STUDIES THAT PROVIDE GENERALLY CONSISTENT RESULTS ARE ALSO DISCUSSED. 14 REFERENCES.

ACCN 001324

1536 AUTH **RICHMOND, A. H., MANNING, R., MALDONADO, J., & ROSS, M.**

TITL DAY TREATMENT OF HISPANIC ADOLESCENTS INVOLVED WITH THE COURTS.

SRCE IN E. R. PADILLA & A. M. PADILLA (EDS.), TRANSCULTURAL PSYCHIATRY: AN HISPANIC PERSPECTIVE (MONOGRAPH NO. 4). LOS ANGELES: UNIVERSITY OF CALIFORNIA, SPANISH SPEAKING MENTAL HEALTH RESEARCH CENTER, 1977, PP. 85-87.

INDX PSYCHOTHERAPY, PRIMARY PREVENTION, CORRECTIONS, DELINQUENCY, ESSAY, PUERTO RICAN-M, ADOLESCENTS, MENTAL HEALTH ·

ABST A BRIEF RATIONALE FOR AND DESCRIPTION OF A DAY TREATMENT PROGRAM FOR HISPANIC ADOLESCENT DELINQUENTS IN THE SOUTH BRONX ARE PRESENTED. SOME OF THE PROBLEMS IN ASSISTING DELINQUENT ADOLESCENTS IN A HIGH DELINQUENCY AREA ARE DISCUSSED. THIS TREATMENT PROGRAM FOR YOUTHS BETWEEN THE AGES OF 11 AND 15 PROVIDES A SERIES OF TREATMENT MODALITIES WHICH EMPHASIZE ACTIVE INTERVENTION AND COMMUNITY INVOLVEMENT. AMONG THE PROGRAM GOALS ARE: (1) PROVISION OF A MILIEU OF GROWTH AND UNDERSTANDING; (2) PROVISION OF A VOLUNTARY PROGRAM WITHIN THE PSYCHIATRIC MODEL IN WHICH EMOTIONS CAN BE EXPRESSED; (3) PROVISION OF A STRUCTURED ACTIVITY PROGRAM. (4) MANAGEMENT OF LOW CLIENT-FRUSTRATION THRESHOLD; AND (5) ERADICATION OF VIOLENT BEHAVIOR SYMPTOMS AND PATTERNS. THE UTILIZATION OF GROUPS AND GROUP THERAPY ALLOWS FOR THE DEVELOPMENT OF MEANINGFUL PEER RELATIONSHIPS FOR THESE YOUTHS. BOTH CONTRACTING AND BEHAVIOR MODIFICATION ARE UTILIZED TO ENCOURAGE ACTIVITY PARTICIPATION AND CONTINUANCE IN THE PROGRAM. STAFFING IS MULTIDISCIPLINARY, AND SERVICES AND ACTIVITIES ARE PROVIDED THROUGH THE COOPERATION OF A WIDE RANGE OF COMMUNITY AGENCIES. (NCMHI ABSTRACT MODIFIED)

ACCN 001325

1537 AUTH **RICHMOND, M. L.**

TITL BEYOND RESOURCE THEORY: ANOTHER LOOK AT FACTORS ENABLING WOMEN TO AFFECT FAMILY INTERACTION.

SRCE JOURNAL OF MARRIAGE AND THE FAMILY, 1976, 38(2), 257-266.

INDX FEMALE, MARRIAGE, INTERPERSONAL RELATIONS, FAMILY STRUCTURE, SEX ROLES, SES, SURVEY, CUBAN, EMPIRICAL, FLORIDA, SOUTH, FAMILY ROLES

ABST THIS STUDY INVESTIGATED THE INTERACTION OF AN EGALITARIAN NORM AND THE WIFE'S CONTRIBUTION OF RESOURCES WITH HER ABILITY TO AFFECT THE DECISION MAKING AND THE DIVISION OF LABOR IN THE FAMILIES OF RECENT CUBAN IMMIGRANTS. BASED ON THE INTERVIEW RESPONSES OF THE WIVES OF 120 INTACT EXILE FAMILIES AND A SUBSAMPLE OF 30 HUSBANDS, IT IS CONCLUDED THAT THE WIFE'S CONTRIBUTION OF RESOURCES IS NOT AS IMPORTANT IN DETERMINING INTER-CHANGE IN THE FAMILY AS ARE THE JOINT EF-FECTS OF RESOURCES OF THE DYAD AND THE ADHERENCE OF THE COUPLE TO AN EGALI-TARIAN IDEOLOGY. IF THE HUSBAND'S RE-SOURCES ARE HIGH OR IF THE WIFE IS NOT IN A CULTURAL CONTEXT THAT SUPPORTS HER EXERCISE OF POWER, HER RESOURCES ARE ONLY MINIMALLY EFFECTIVE. THE GREATEST DEGREE OF EGALITARIAN INTERACTION OC-CURS WHEN THE HUSBAND'S RESOURCES ARE MODERATE, WHEN THE WIFE IS CONTRIBUTING ECONOMIC RESOURCES, AND THE COUPLE HAS HIGH EXPOSURE TO EGALITARIAN NORMS. THE STUDY HAS IMPLICATIONS FOR AMERICAN FAMILIES AND THE CURRENT WOMEN'S LIBER-ATION MOVEMENT AS IT POINTS OUT THE NEED TO FOCUS ON SOURCES OF NORMS AS INFLUENTIAL FACTORS IN CHANGING THE PO-SITION OF WOMEN IN THE U.S. 29 REFER-ENCES. (PASAR ABSTRACT MODIFIED)

ACCN 001326

1538 AUTH **RIEBER, M., & WOMACK, M.**
TITL THE INTELLIGENCE OF PRE-SCHOOL CHIL-DREN AS RELATED TO ETHNIC AND DEMO-GRAPHIC VARIABLES.
SRCE *EXCEPTIONAL CHILDREN, 1968, 34(8), 609-614.*
INDX INTELLIGENCE, EARLY CHILDHOOD EDUCA-TION, DEMOGRAPHIC, PEABODY PICTURE-VO-CABULARY TEST, CHILDREN, CROSS CUL-TURAL, SES, CULTURAL FACTORS, SPANISH SURNAMED, INTELLIGENCE TESTING, TEXAS, SOUTHWEST
ABST TO COMPARE INTELLIGENCE AND ETHNICITY, A GROUP OF 568 NEGRO, LATIN AMERICAN, AND ANGLO CHILDREN FROM FAMILIES WITH INCOMES IN THE LOWEST 20 PERCENT FOR THE COMMUNITY WERE ADMINISTERED THE PEABODY PICTURE-VOCABULARY TEST. AP-PROXIMATELY ONE-FOURTH WERE RETESTED AFTER 5 WEEKS IN A HEADSTART PRESCHOOL PROGRAM. THE AVERAGE IQ FOR ANGLOS WAS 85.0, FOR NEGROES 69.0, AND FOR LAT-INS 50.3. CHILDREN WHO SCORED IN THE LOWEST QUARTILE WERE COMPARED WITH THOSE IN THE HIGHEST ON A NUMBER OF ECONOMIC AND FAMILY VARIABLES. INCOME AND EDUCATIONAL LEVEL OF PARENTS, SIZE OF FAMILY, AND MATERNAL EMPLOYMENT WERE FOUND TO DIFFER FOR THE TWO GROUPS. THOSE CHILDREN WHO WERE RETESTED ALL MADE SIGNIFICANT GAINS. THESE RESULTS IN-DICATE THAT THE TYPE OF EXPERIENCES OF-FERED BY THE HEADSTART PROGRAM ARE GENERALLY MISSING IN THEIR HOME ENVI-RONMENT AND PERHAPS THEIR POOR SHOW-

ING ON THE PEABODY CAN PRIMARILY BE AT-TRIBUTED TO A BROAD FORM OF STIMULUS DEPRIVATION. THE LARGE DIFFERENCES IN AV-ERAGE IQ'S OF THE LATIN, ANGLO, AND NE-GRO CHILDREN ARE DIFFICULT TO ACCOUNT FOR BECAUSE COMPARISONS ACROSS RACIAL GROUPS INVOLVE DIFFERENCES IN CASTE AS WELL AS IN SOCIAL CLASS—AND CONTROL-LING FOR ONE DOES NOT ELIMINATE THE OTHER. 10 REFERENCES.

ACCN 001327

1539 AUTH **RIEGEL, K. F., RAMSEY R. M., & RIEGEL R. M.**
TITL A COMPARISON OF THE FIRST AND SECOND LANGUAGES OF AMERICAN AND SPANISH STU-DENTS.
SRCE *JOURNAL OF VERBAL LEARNING AND VERBAL BEHAVIOR, 1967, 6(4), 536-544.*
INDX BILINGUALISM, COLLEGE STUDENTS, SPANISH SURNAMED, CROSS CULTURAL, GRAMMAR, LANGUAGE COMPREHENSION, LINGUISTIC COMPETENCE, EMPIRICAL, MIDWEST, MICHI-GAN, SOUTH AMERICA, CENTRAL AMERICA, MEXICAN, CUBAN
ABST THE ASSUMPTION THAT SECOND-LANGUAGE LEARNING SHOULD RESULT NOT ONLY IN AN INCREASE IN VOCABULARY BUT ALSO IN AN APPROXIMATION TO THE CONCEPTUAL SE-MANTIC STRUCTURE OF THE TARGET LAN-GUAGE IS TESTED. TWENTY-FOUR AMERICAN AND 24 LATIN AMERICAN SUBJECTS GAVE RE-STRICTED ASSOCIATIONS BOTH IN ENGLISH AND IN SPANISH TO 35 STIMULI UNDER SEVEN DIFFERENT INSTRUCTIONS. SECOND-LAN-GUAGE LEARNERS LEFT MORE BLANKS IN THEIR RECORDS THAN NATIVE SPEAKERS. THIS WAS ESPECIALLY TRUE FOR AMERICAN SUB-JECTS STUDYING SPANISH. IN BOTH LAN-GUAGES, THE RESPONSE VARIABILITY WAS GREATER FOR THE NATIVE SPANISH SPEAKERS THAN FOR AMERICAN SUBJECTS. HOWEVER, AMERICAN SUBJECTS WERE SUPERIOR WHEN THE DEGREE OF CONCEPTUAL CLARITY WAS ANALYZED BY COUNTING THE RESPONSE REPETITIONS PER STIMULUS THAT OCCUR UN-DER DIFFERENT TASK INSTRUCTIONS. INTER-PRETATIONS ARE IN TERMS OF GROWTH OF VOCABULARY AND THE ACQUISITION OF THE CONCEPTUAL AND SEMANTIC SYSTEMS OF THE TARGET LANGUAGE. RESULTS SUGGEST THAT FORMAL LANGUAGE TRAINING IN COL-LEGE SETTINGS ENCOURAGES THE IDENTIFI-CATION OF THE CONCEPTUAL SEMANTIC STRUCTURE OF THE TARGET LANGUAGE, WHEREAS THE INFORMAL TRAINING IN EVERY-DAY COMMUNICATION LEADS TO A FAST IN-CREASE IN BOTH VOCABULARY AND VERBAL FLUENCY. 19 REFERENCES. (JOURNAL AB-STRACT MODIFIED)

ACCN 001328

1540 AUTH **RIVERA, J.**
TITL ON THE CONCEPT OF LA RAZA: A PRELIMI-NARY STATEMENT.
SRCE *PAPER PRESENTED AT THE SOUTHWESTERN SOCIOLOGICAL ASSOCIATION ANNUAL MEET-INGS, SAN ANTONIO, TEXAS, MARCH 1972.*

INDX HISTORY, CULTURE, CHICANO MOVEMENT, ES-
SAY, MEXICAN AMERICAN, ETHNIC IDENTITY

ABST SOME OF THE PHILOSOPHICAL AND IDEO-
LOGICAL IMPLICATIONS OF THE MEANINGS OF
LA RAZA FOR THE CHICANO MOVEMENT ARE
REVIEWED. THE HISTORICAL DEVELOPMENT
OF LA RAZA FROM THE SPANISH EMPHASIS ON
RACE TO JOSE VASCONCELOS' ACCOUNT OF
LA RAZA COSMICA IS DISCUSSED. THE CHI-
CANO MOVEMENT HAS SHARPENED ITS PHILO-
SOPHICAL AND IDEOLOGICAL CONTENT AND
IMPORT. THE EMPHASIS IS NOW ON CULTURAL
COMMITMENTS, THE IDEA OF COMMENSALITY,
AND PARTICIPATORY SHARING AMONG THOSE
DEDICATED TO THE MOVEMENT. THE PHILO-
SOPHICAL UNDERSTANDING OF LA RAZA MUST
BE COUPLED WITH SOCIAL ACTION. STATE-
MENTS BY CORKY GONZALEZ, JOSE ANGEL
GUTIERREZ, AND REIES TIJERINA REFLECT
BOTH THE IDEOLOGY OF LA RAZA AND THE
COMMITMENT TO LA CAUSA OR SOCIAL AC-
TION. 21 REFERENCES.

ACCN 001329

1541 AUTH **RIVERA, J.**
TITL RECRUITMENT OF PUERTO RICAN STUDENTS
INTO SCHOOLS OF SOCIAL WORK.
SRCE *SOCIAL WORK EDUCATION, 1971, 19(1), 43-44.*
INDX EDUCATION, ESSAY, MENTAL HEALTH, MENTAL
HEALTH PROFESSION, PUERTO RICAN-M, REP-
RESENTATION, HIGHER EDUCATION

ABST DESPITE THE GREAT NEED FOR PUERTO RICAN
SOCIAL WORKERS, THE PERCENTAGE OF
PUERTO RICAN GRADUATE STUDENTS IN SO-
CIAL WORK PROGRAMS IS CONSIDERABLY LESS
THAN THE PERCENTAGE OF PUERTO RICANS
IN THE COMMUNITY. A NUMBER OF EXCUSES
FOR THE LOW NUMBERS OF PUERTO RICAN
STUDENTS ARE DELINEATED BY THE SCHOOLS
OF SOCIAL WORK. A MAJOR REASON IS THE
LACK OF SCHOLARSHIP FUNDS. SPECIAL EF-
FORTS MUST BE MADE TO ACQUIRE FUNDS AS
THE PUERTO RICANS INTERESTED IN SOCIAL
WORK ARE UNABLE TO AFFORD THE EDUCA-
TIONAL EXPENSES. SOME RECOMMENDA-
TIONS ARE PROVIDED TO ASSIST SOCIAL WORK
SCHOOLS IN INCREASING THE NUMBER OF
PUERTO RICAN STUDENTS.

ACCN 001330

1542 AUTH **RIVERA, J. J.**
TITL GROWTH OF A PUERTO RICAN AWARENESS.
SRCE *SOCIAL CASEWORK, 1974, 55(2), 84-89.*
INDX PUERTO RICAN-M, PREJUDICE, ETHNIC IDEN-
TITY, POLITICAL POWER, SOCIAL SERVICES, IM-
MIGRATION, ESSAY, CULTURE, POVERTY, UR-
BAN, PUERTO RICAN-I, CULTURAL CHANGE

ABST THE EMERGING PUERTO RICAN STRUGGLE
FOR SELF-DETERMINATION AND A FAIR SHARE
OF INFLUENCE IS DIRECTED AT A VICIOUS
CIRCLE OF POVERTY AND LACK OF POWER.
ONE OF THE FIRST TASKS IS IDENTIFICATION
OF THE SOURCES OF OPPRESSION. SECOND,
THE MULTI-RACIAL PUERTO RICAN ETHNIC
IDENTITY MUST BE RECOGNIZED AND PRE-
SERVED. PUERTO RICO'S UNIQUE POLITICAL
STATUS AND GEOGRAPHIC PROXIMITY TO THE
U.S., COMBINED WITH THE FREQUENT MIGRA-
TION TO AND FROM THE ISLAND, HAVE RE-
SULTED IN A PUERTO RICAN DIASPORA. BUT
DESPITE MANY PROBLEMS, PUERTO RICANS
HAVE MADE CONSIDERABLE PROGRESS IN
EDUCATIONAL ACHIEVEMENT, THE ESTABLISH-
MENT OF THEIR OWN SOCIAL SERVICE AGEN-
CIES, AND THE DEVELOPMENT OF SMALL BUSI-
NESSES AND SKILLED MANPOWER. AND THE
RECENT INFLUX OF UNIVERSITY PROFESSORS
AND OTHER PROFESSIONALS HAS BROUGHT
ABOUT AN INCREASED AWARENESS OF PUERTO
RICAN IDENTITY AND CULTURE. ALTHOUGH
COALITION WITH OTHER OPPRESSED GROUPS
MAY AT TIMES BE APPROPRIATE, IT IS EMPHA-
SIZED THAT PUERTO RICANS ARE THE ONLY
EXPERTS ON PUERTO RICANS, AND THERE-
FORE THEY MUST DEVELOP THEIR OWN AP-
PROACHES AND STRATEGIES TOWARD AC-
COMPLISHING THEIR GOALS.

ACCN 002193

1543 AUTH **ROBERTS, A. H., & ERICKSON, R. V.**
TITL DELAY OF GRATIFICATION, PORTEUS MAZE
TEST PERFORMANCE, AND BEHAVIORAL AD-
JUSTMENT IN A DELINQUENT GROUP.
SRCE *JOURNAL OF ABNORMAL PSYCHOLOGY, 1968,
73(5), 449-453.*
INDX CROSS CULTURAL, DELINQUENCY, TIME ORI-
ENTATION, PSYCHOSOCIAL ADJUSTMENT,
ABILITY TESTING, ADOLESCENTS, CALIFORNIA
TEST OF MENTAL MATURITY, EMPIRICAL, NEW
MEXICO, SOUTHWEST

ABST THE RELATIONSHIPS AMONG A BEHAVIORAL
AND VERBAL MEASURE OF DELAY OF GRATIFI-
CATION, PORTEUS MAZE TEST MEASURES OF
PLANNING ABILITY AND FORESIGHT (TQ) AND
IMPULSE CONTROL (Q), AND SCHOOL ADJUS-
TEMNT RATINGS FOR DELINQUENT ADOLES-
CENT MALES WERE EXPLORED. THE SUBJECTS
CONSISTED OF 30 SPANISH AMERICANS, 10
ANGLO AMERICANS, 5 NAVAJO INDIANS, AND
5 NEGROES. BOTH MEASURES OF DELAY OF
GRATIFICATION WERE SIGNIFICANTLY RELATED
TO THE PORTEUS MEASURES AND THE AD-
JUSTMENT RATINGS. ABILITY OR WILLINGNESS
TO DELAY GRATIFICATION WAS RELATED TO
SHORT-TERM ADJUSTMENT IN A RESTRICTIVE
TRAINING SCHOOL SITUATION, AND DELAY OF
GRATIFICATION WAS ALSO FOUND TO BE RE-
LATED, IN PART, TO AGE AND ETHNIC GROUP
MEMBERSHIP, BUT NOT IQ. THE FINDINGS WERE
REPLICATED IN A SPANISH AMERICAN SUB-
GROUP OF THE TOTAL SAMPLE EXCEPT FOR
THE RELATIONSHIP BETWEEN TQ AND THE BE-
HAVIORAL MEASURE OF DELAY. WITH THE EX-
CEPTION OF TQ, A HIGH DEGREE OF COMMUN-
ALITY AMONG THE VARIOUS MEASURES WAS
DEMONSTRATED. THE FINDINGS SUPPORT THE
CONSTRUCT VALIDITY OF THE PORTEUS MAZE
TEST AND FURTHER SUGGEST THAT THE DE-
LAY OF GRATIFICATION CONSTRUCT IS A PAR-
TICULARLY POWERFUL ONE DESERVING FUR-
THER INVESTIGATION. 17 REFERENCES.
(JOURNAL ABSTRACT MODIFIED)

ACCN 001331

1544 AUTH **ROBERTS, A. H., & GREENE, J. E.**
TITL CROSS-CULTURAL STUDY OF RELATIONSHIPS

AMONG FOUR DIMENSIONS OF TIME PERSPECTIVE.

SRCE *PERCEPTUAL AND MOTOR SKILLS, 1971, 33, 163-173.*

INDX CROSS CULTURAL, SPANISH SURNAMED, EMPIRICAL, TIME ORIENTATION, CHILDREN, ADOLESCENTS, CULTURAL FACTORS, NEW MEXICO, SOUTHWEST

ABST THE PRESENT INVESTIGATION WAS DESIGNED (1) TO DESCRIBE THE INTERNAL STRUCTURE OF THE CONCEPT OF TIME PERSPECTIVE IN TERMS OF DIMENSIONS DERIVED FROM PERFORMANCE ON ONE TASK AND (2) TO DETERMINE WHETHER OR NOT THIS INTERNAL STRUCTURE WAS IN ANY WAY DIFFERENT FOR THREE ETHNIC GROUPS (32 SPANISH AMERICAN, 32 AMERICAN INDIAN, AND 32 ANGLO AMERICAN), TWO AGE GROUPS (10 AND 16 YEARS), AND TWO THEMATIC CONTENT AREAS (RELIGIOUS AND SOCIAL). MEASURES OF TEMPORAL EXTENSION, LOCATION, AND KINESIS WERE DERIVED FROM A STORY-TELLING TASK. DATA WERE ANALYZED BY A MULTI-DIMENSIONAL CHI-SQUARE ANALYSIS. THE THREE MEASURES WERE DIFFERENTIALLY SENSITIVE TO VARIABLES INTRODUCED. FOR EXAMPLE, ETHNIC DIFFERENCES WERE MOST CLEARLY SHOWN BY THE KINETIC MEASURE AND CONTENT DIFFERENCES BY EXTENSION. CLUES TO THE MEANING OF TIME IN VARIOUS CULTURES MUST BE EXAMINED AGAINST THE BACKGROUND OF CONTENT. THERE IS LIKELY TO BE NO GENERAL CULTURAL PREFERENCE FOR ONE TEMPORAL MODALITY ACROSS VARIOUS CONTENTS, AND STEREOTYPING OF A CULTURAL GROUP CLOUDS SIGNIFICANT VALUE AND ORIENTATIONAL DIFFERENCES. 20 REFERENCES. (JOURNAL SUMMARY MODIFIED)

ACCN 001332

1545 AUTH **ROBERTSON, D. J., & TREPPER, T. S.**
TITL THE EFFECTS OF I.T.A. ON THE READING ACHIEVEMENT OF MEXICAN-AMERICAN CHILDREN.
SRCE *READING WORLD, 1974, 14(2), 132-139.*
INDX READING, SCHOLASTIC ACHIEVEMENT, CHILDREN, INSTRUCTIONAL TECHNIQUES, TEACHERS, CURRICULUM, BILINGUAL, BILINGUAL-BICULTURAL EDUCATION, MEXICAN AMERICAN, EMPIRICAL
ABST TO DETERMINE WHETHER THE INITIAL TEACHING ALPHABET (I.T.A.) HAS A GREATER EFFECT ON THE READING SCORES OF BILINGUAL CHILDREN THAN DOES TRADITIONAL ORTHOGRAPHY, 52 MEXICAN AMERICAN BILINGUAL FOURTH GRADERS FROM LOW-INCOME FAMILIES IN EAST LOS ANGELES WERE STUDIED. THE SAMPLE WAS EQUALLY DIVIDED INTO TWO GROUPS, EACH HAVING BEEN RANDOMLY ASSIGNED TO EITHER KIND OF INSTRUCTION IN THE FIRST THREE ELEMENTARY YEARS. SUBJECTS WERE POST TESTED WITH A VARIETY OF TESTS MEASURING READING ACHIEVEMENT, INSTRUCTIONAL AND INDEPENDENT LEVEL, CONSONANT SOUNDS, ETC. USING A T-TEST FOR UNCORRELATED DATA, THE I.T.A. GROUP SCORED SIGNIFICANTLY HIGHER ON 8 OF 9 TESTS, AND ITS OVERALL GRADE LEVEL IN

READING WAS HIGHER ON BOTH STANDARDIZED ACHIEVEMENT AND DIAGNOSTIC TESTS. THREE FACTORS SEEN IN THE I.T.A. THAT FACILITATE READING ACQUISITION IN THE MEXICAN AMERICAN CHILD ARE: (1) IT OFFERS FEW STRUCTURAL IRREGULARITIES LEADING TO LINGUISTIC CONFUSION; (2) IT DOES NOT DEPEND ON A LARGE SIGHT VOCABULARY FOR READING FLUENCY; AND (3) IT EXPEDITES PRODUCTION SPONTANEITY OF WORDS AND PHRASES. SUGGESTIONS ARE MADE FOR TESTING THE I.T.A. AGAINST OTHER NEW PROGRAMS FOR MEXICAN AMERICAN CHILDREN AND IN OTHER TYPES OF BILINGUAL COMMUNITIES. 7 REFERENCES.

ACCN 001333

1546 AUTH **ROBINSON, T. N., JR.**
TITL A CRITICAL ASSESSMENT OF PSYCHOLOGICAL RESEARCH RELATING TO FACTORS OF GROWTH AND DEVELOPMENT IN MINORITY GROUPS WITH RECOMMENDATIONS FOR FUTURE RESEARCH (ORDER NO. 74-SP-0859).
SRCE *WASHINGTON, D.C.: NATIONAL SCIENCE FOUNDATION, AUGUST 1974.*
INDX RESEARCH METHODOLOGY, DISCRIMINATION, PREJUDICE, INTELLIGENCE TESTING, INTELLIGENCE, TEST VALIDITY, REPRESENTATION, POVERTY, SES, SELF CONCEPT, ETHNIC IDENTITY, LANGUAGE ACQUISITION, SCHOLASTIC ACHIEVEMENT, EXAMINER EFFECTS, LINGUISTICS, CHILDREN, ATTRIBUTION OF RESPONSIBILITY, WISC, WAIS, CATTELL CULTURE-FREE INTELLIGENCE TEST, ROTTER INTERNAL-EXTERNAL SCALE, REVIEW, ADULTS, CROSS CULTURAL, BIBLIOGRAPHY, MEXICAN AMERICAN, PUERTO RICAN-M
ABST AN EXAMINATION OF THE PROMINENT AREAS OF PSYCHOLOGICAL RESEARCH WITH REGARD TO MINORITY CHILDREN AND ADULTS IS PROVIDED. RESEARCH REPORTED IN THE PSYCHOLOGICAL ABSTRACTS DURING 1965-1974 IS CRITICALLY ASSESSED. IN ADDITION, RECOMMENDATIONS FOR FUTURE RESEARCH ARE PROVIDED FOR SPECIFIC AREAS. THE TOPICS REVIEWED ARE THE FOLLOWING: INTELLECTIVE ABILITY, LINGUISTIC EFFICIENCY, RACIAL/ETHNIC AWARENESS AND ATTITUDES, SELF-CONCEPT, AND LOCUS OF CONTROL. IN GENERAL, RESEARCH FINDINGS OF BLACKS, MEXICAN AMERICANS, AMERICAN INDIANS, ORIENTAL AMERICANS, PUERTO RICANS, ETC., PRESENT A DISMAL PICTURE OF THEIR PSYCHOLOGICAL WELL-BEING. WITH THE INCREASE OF MINORITY RESEARCH THERE APPEARS TO BE A STRONG TREND TOWARD A REVERSAL OF THE PAST NEGATIVE FINDINGS. LASTLY, THE APPENDICES (1) SUMMARIZE THE 1973-1974 DATA ON FEDERAL AND NON-FEDERAL SUPPORT OF MINORITY RESEARCH, (2) LIST PRIVATE INSTITUTIONS AND FOUNDATIONS SUPPORTIVE OF THIS RESEARCH, AND (3) LIST THE JOURNALS THAT HAVE PUBLISHED MINORITY GROUP RELATED RESEARCH. 97 REFERENCES.

ACCN 001334

1547 AUTH **ROCA, P.**

TITL   PROBLEMS OF ADAPTING INTELLIGENCE SCALES FROM ONE CULTURE TO ANOTHER.

SRCE   *REVISTA DE LA ASOCIACION DE MAESTROS, 1954, 13(2), 46-47; 66-67.*

INDX   INTELLIGENCE TESTING, CULTURAL FACTORS, CHILDREN, PUERTO RICAN-I, WISC, STANFORD ACHIEVEMENT TEST, GOODENOUGH DRAW-A-MAN TEST, CROSS CULTURAL, EMPIRICAL, CULTURE-FAIR TESTS, STANFORD-BINET INTELLIGENCE TEST

ABST   THE TRANSLATION AND ADAPTATION OF THREE INTELLIGENCE TESTS (THE WECHSLER INTELLIGENCE SCALE FOR CHILDREN (WISC), THE STANFORD-BINET (S-B) SCALE REVISED, FORM L, AND THE GOODENOUGH INTELLIGENCE TEST) INTO SPANISH FOR USE WITH PUERTO RICAN SCHOOL CHILDREN ARE PRESENTED. USE OF THE TRANSLATED VERSIONS OF THE WISC AND S-B INDICATES THAT NUMEROUS CHANGES IN VOCABULARY ITEMS AND PLACEMENT OF TRANSLATED ITEMS ARE NECESSARY FOR MAINTAINING DIFFICULTY LEVEL. DESPITE THESE CHANGES, DATA INDICATE THAT IN GENERAL THE PUERTO RICAN CHILD SCORES LOWER THAN THE AMERICAN CHILD. WITH THE WISC, THE AVERAGE IQ FOR PUERTO RICAN CHILDREN IS 87.94 AND WITH THE S-B, FORM L, IT IS 95.65. IN THE CASE OF THE GOODENOUGH TEST THE NORMS FOR THE DIFFERENT AGES WERE ALSO FOUND TO BE LOWER WITH THE EXCEPTION OF AGES 5 AND 6, WHICH WERE SELECTED FROM PRIVATE SCHOOLS. THERE IS NO DOUBT THAT NO MATTER HOW WELL AN INTELLIGENCE SCALE IS ADAPTED FROM ONE CULTURE TO ANOTHER, THERE ARE CULTURAL DIFFERENCES WHICH MAKE THE CHILDREN FROM THE SECOND CULTURE (E.G., PUERTO RICAN) SCORE LOWER THAN THOSE FROM THE FIRST. THE PROPER INTERPRETATION OF THESE FACTS IS TO CONSIDER WHATEVER AVERAGE IS OBTAINED AS EQUIVALENT TO AN IQ OF 100. 2 REFERENCES.

ACCN   001335

1548 AUTH **RODRIGUEZ DEL VALLE, J., & ROSADO, M.**
TITL   ESTUDIO LONGITUDINAL SOBRE LA SALUD MENTAL DE UN GRUPO DE FAMILIAS PUERTORRIQUENAS Y LOS FACTORES EMOCIONALES, SOCIALES Y ECONOMICOS QUE LE AFECTAN. (LONGITUDINAL STUDY OF THE MENTAL HEALTH OF A GROUP OF PUERTO RICAN FAMILIES AND THE EMOTIONAL, SOCIAL AND ECONOMIC FACTORS WHICH AFFECT THEM.)

SRCE   *REVISTA DE PSIQUIATRIA Y SALUD MENTAL DE PUERTO RICO, 1970, 2(2), 34-45. (SPANISH)*

INDX   PUERTO RICAN-I, EMPIRICAL, URBAN, RURAL, FAMILY STRUCTURE, MENTAL HEALTH, ENVIRONMENTAL FACTORS, INTERPERSONAL RELATIONS, EXTENDED FAMILY

ABST   FIFTY FAMILIES IN PUERTO RICO WERE INTERVIEWED TO DISCERN THE EFFECTS OF SOCIAL AND ECONOMIC FACTORS ON THE ISLAND UPON FAMILY "EMOTIONAL CLIMATE" (I.E., THE LEVEL OF HARMONY AND COMMUNICATION AMONG FAMILY MEMBERS). THE 50 FAMILIES WERE IN RURAL AND URBAN AREAS, NUCLEAR OR EXTENDED IN STRUCTURE, AND LARGE OR SMALL (I.E., LESS THAN FIVE MEMBERS). A LOOSELY STRUCTURED INTERVIEW WAS CONDUCTED WITH THE ENTIRE FAMILY IN ITS OWN HOME, AND QUESTIONS DEALT WITH ROLES AND RELATIONSHIPS WITHIN THE FAMILY. FAMILY EMOTIONAL CLIMATE WAS CLASSIFIED AS (1) "ADEQUATE." A HARMONIOUS ATMOSPHERE IN WHICH FAMILY MEMBERS COMMUNICATED FREELY AND OPENLY, (2) "MARGINAL," AN INTERMEDIATE CONDITION, AND (3) "INADEQUATE," CHARACTERIZED BY FEAR OF SELF-EXPRESSION AND RIGID OR DOMINEERING INTERRELATIONSHIPS. THE RESULTS INDICATE THAT RURAL FAMILIES ARE MORE MARGINAL THAN URBAN FAMILIES, LARGE FAMILIES ARE MORE INADEQUATE THAN SMALL FAMILIES, AND NUCLEAR FAMILIES ARE MORE INADEQUATE THAN EXTENDED FAMILIES. HOWEVER, BECAUSE INSUFFICIENT NUMBERS OF SMALL EXTENDED FAMILIES AND LARGE NUCLEAR FAMILIES WERE INTERVIEWED, IT IS SUGGESTED THAT FURTHER RESEARCH CONCENTRATE ON THESE GROUPS IN ORDER TO CONFIRM THE CONSISTENCY OF THESE FINDINGS. IT IS CONCLUDED, NEVERTHELESS, THAT SEEMINGLY INTANGIBLE PHENOMENA, SUCH AS "EMOTIONAL CLIMATE" OF A FAMILY, CAN BE MEASURED AND ANALYZED. 21 REFERENCES.

ACCN   002291

1549 AUTH **RODRIGUEZ, I. D.**
TITL   GROUP WORK WITH HOSPITALIZED PUERTO RICAN PATIENTS.

SRCE   *HOSPITAL AND COMMUNITY PSYCHIATRY, 1971, 22(7), 219-220.*

INDX   PSYCHOTHERAPY, PUERTO RICAN-M, ADULTS, ESSAY, GROUP DYNAMICS, MENTAL HEALTH, CASE STUDY, INSTITUTIONALIZATION

ABST   THE PROGRESS AND TERMINATION OF AN OPEN-ENDED GROUP WITH PUERTO RICAN PATIENTS OF A LARGE PSYCHIATRIC HOSPITAL IS DISCUSSED. BECAUSE THERE WERE A NUMBER OF PUERTO RICAN PATIENTS WITH LIMITED ENGLISH FLUENCY, A SPANISH-SPEAKING SOCIAL WORKER ORGANIZED A VOLUNTARY GROUP OF 21 MEN, OF WHICH 5 TO 9 MEMBERS ATTENDED WEEKLY. THE GROUP PROVIDED SUPPORT FOR EACH MEMBER, PARTICULARLY IN MAKING PLANS TO LEAVE THE HOSPITAL. SPECIFIC CASES ARE DISCUSSED IN DETAIL. IT IS CONCLUDED THAT THIS GROUP PROJECT IS A FURTHER STEP IN MEETING THE SPECIAL NEEDS OF PATIENTS WHOSE LIMITED ENGLISH-SPEAKING SKILLS ONLY COMPOUND THEIR EMOTIONAL AND REALITY PROBLEMS.

ACCN   001336

1550 AUTH **RODRIGUEZ, L., & KIMMEL, H. D.**
TITL   DISCREPANCIA ENTRE EL YO REAL Y EL YO IDEAL EN PUERTO RICO Y LOS ESTADOS UNIDOS. (THE DISCREPANCY BETWEEN THE REAL-SELF AND THE IDEAL-SELF IN PUERTO RICO AND THE UNITED STATES.)

SRCE   *REVISTA LATINOAMERICANA DE PSICOLOGIA, 1970, 2(3), 353-365. (SPANISH)*

INDX   COLLEGE STUDENTS, PUERTO RICAN-I, PERSONALITY ASSESSMENT, SELF CONCEPT, CON-

FLICT RESOLUTION, CROSS CULTURAL, EMPIR-ICAL

ABST IN THIS CROSS-CULTURAL PERSONALITY STUDY, THE FOLLOWING HYPOTHESIS WAS TESTED: THE DISCREPANCY BETWEEN PERSONALITY TEST PERFORMANCE UNDER INSTRUCTIONS TO DESCRIBE YOURSELF THE WAY YOU ACTU-ALLY ARE (REAL-SELF) AND PERFORMANCE UNDER INSTRUCTIONS TO DESCRIBE YOUR-SELF THE WAY YOU WOULD LIKE TO BE (IDEAL-SELF) DEPENDS UPON THE RELATIVE STABIL-ITY OF CULTURAL VALUES AND IDEALS. IN A CULTURE WITH RELATIVELY STABLE AND LONG-TERM VALUES, SUCH AS THE UNITED STATES, A LARGE DISCREPANCY BETWEEN REAL- AND IDEAL-SELF HAS BEEN REPORTED, THE IDEAL BEING MORE CLOSELY IN LINE WITH THE "CUL-TURALLY DESIRABLE." IN A CULTURE RECOG-NIZED TO BE IN A STATE OF CONSIDERABLE FLUX, SUCH AS PUERTO RICO, A SMALLER DIS-CREPANCY BETWEEN REAL- AND IDEAL-SELF IS EXPECTED SINCE THE CULTURAL IDEAL IS NOT CLEARLY IDENTIFIED. ONE HUNDRED EIGHTEEN FEMALE AND 105 MALE, PUERTO RI-CAN COLLEGE STUDENTS BETWEEN THE AGES OF 18 AND 21 YEARS WERE ADMINISTERED A SPANISH TRANSLATION OF THE PENSACOLA Z PERSONALITY SURVEY. THE RESULTS SHOW THAT WHILE THE PUERTO RICAN SAMPLE MATCHED THE ORIGINAL U.S. SAMPLE UNDER THE REAL-SELF INSTRUCTIONS, THEIR REAL-IDEAL DISCREPANCY IS SIGNIFICANTLY SMALLER AS PREDICTED. THE RESULTS SUP-PORT THE POTENTIAL USEFULNESS OF THE REAL-IDEAL DISCREPANCY METHODOLOGY IN THE STUDY OF CULTURAL INFLUENCES ON PERSONALITY. 21 REFERENCES. (JOURNAL AB-STRACT MODIFIED)

ACCN 001337

1551 AUTH **RODRIGUEZ, R.**
TITL GOING HOME AGAIN: THE NEW AMERICAN SCHOLARSHIP BOY.
SRCE *THE AMERICAN SCHOLAR, 1974-1975, 44(1), 15-28.*
INDX MEXICAN AMERICAN, ETHNIC IDENTITY, ESSAY, ACCULTURATION, SOCIALIZATION, HIGHER EDUCATION, SELF CONCEPT, STRESS, CASE STUDY, COLLEGE STUDENTS, EDUCATION, COPING MECHANISMS
ABST FOR CHICANOS, SUCCESS IN ACADEMIA HAS TYPICALLY BEEN POSITIVELY VALUED IN TERMS OF INCREASED OPPORTUNITY, SOCIAL MOBIL-ITY, AND HIGHER INCOME. HOWEVER, AS THIS AUTOBIOGRAPHY ILLUSTRATES, THE LOSS OF CULTURE THROUGH THE NECESSARY ADOP-TION OF ACADEMIC VALUES AND PERSPEC-TIVES IS NOT GENERALLY RECOGNIZED. THIS CULTURAL SCHISM IS PORTRAYED AS THE "SCHOLARSHIP BOY," ONE WHO MUST CHOOSE BETWEEN TWO MUTUALLY EXCLUSIVE WORLDS. THE PRESSURES TO BECOME PART OF THE ACADEMIC CULTURE IN ORDER TO SUCCEED HAVE A SIGNIFICANT EFFECT ON PERSONAL-ITY AND SELF-CONCEPT. RELATIONSHIPS WITH FAMILY AND RELATIVES CHANGE AS A FUNC-TION OF INCREASED CULTURAL DISTANCE AND A SENSE OF LOSS IS INEVITABLE. THE THIRD

WORLD STUDENT MOVEMENT COMPLICATES SCHOLASTIC LIFE IN MANY WAYS, ALTHOUGH IT DOES CONTRIBUTE TO A RENEWED INTER-EST IN ETHNIC BACKGROUND. YET, CHANGE IS INEVITABLE AND THIS SELF-PORTRAIT PRE-SENTS A PERSPECTIVE OF ONE PERSON'S STRUGGLE FOR PERSONAL, CULTURAL, AND ACADEMIC GROWTH.

ACCN 001338

1552 AUTH **ROGENESS, G. A., STOKES, J. P., BEDNAR, R. A., & GORMAN, B. L.**
TITL SCHOOL INTERVENTION PROGRAM TO IN-CREASE BEHAVIORS AND ATTITUDES THAT PROMOTE LEARNING.
SRCE *UNPUBLISHED MANUSCRIPT, UNDATED. (AVAIL-ABLE FROM DR. G.A. ROGNESS, DEPARTMENT OF PSYCHIATRY, UNIVERSITY OF TEXAS HEALTH SCIENCE CENTER, 7703 FLOYD CURL DRIVE, SAN ANTONIO, TEXAS, 78284.)*
INDX EDUCATION, TEACHERS, INSTRUCTIONAL TECHNIQUES, ADMINISTRATORS, GROUP DY-NAMICS, BEHAVIOR MODIFICATION, EMPIRI-CAL, PROGRAM EVALUATION, SCHOLASTIC ACHIEVEMENT, ANXIETY, CHILDREN, TEXAS, SOUTHWEST
ABST THE RESULTS OF A 2-YEAR INTERVENTION PROGRAM IN A LARGE MIDWESTERN CITY PUBLIC ELEMENTARY SCHOOL, OF WHICH LA-TINS COMPRISED 68% OF THE STUDENT BODY, ARE DISCUSSED. THE TWO OBJECTIVES OF THIS PROGRAM WERE: (1) TO DEVELOP A COUNSELING AND CONSULTATION PROGRAM THAT ASSISTED FACULTY IN DEFINING BEHAV-IORS AND ATTITUDES THAT EITHER PROMOTED OR INTERFERED WITH LEARNING; AND (2) TO DEVELOP AND IMPLEMENT BEHAVIORAL METHODS THAT WOULD INCREASE THE FRE-QUENCY OF DESIRABLE BEHAVIORS AND DE-CREASE UNDESIRABLE BEHAVIORS. THE RE-SULTS INDICATE THAT FOR THE FIRST YEAR THERE WERE NO SIGNIFICANT DIFFERENCES BETWEEN THE CONTROL AND TREATMENT GROUPS IN READING AND MATH SCORE CHANGES; HOWEVER, THE TREATMENT GROUP DID REFLECT POSITIVE CHANGES IN ANXIETY, BEHAVIOR PROBLEMS, AND IMPULSE CON-TROL. THE SECOND YEAR RESULTS SHOWED, IN GENERAL, NO POSITIVE CHANGE. POSSIBLE REASONS FOR THE FAILURE OF THE PROGRAM IN THE SECOND YEAR AND A REVIEW OF THE PROGRAM BY SCHOOL PERSONNEL ARE RE-PORTED. 11 REFERENCES.

ACCN 001339

1553 AUTH **ROGLER, L. H.**
TITL A BETTER LIFE: NOTES FROM PUERTO RICO.
SRCE *TRANS-ACTION, 1965, 2(3), 34-36.*
INDX ACHIEVEMENT MOTIVATION, COMMUNITY, CULTURE, ECONOMIC FACTORS, ENVIRON-MENTAL FACTORS, PUERTO RICAN-I, HOUS-ING, ESSAY, CASE STUDY, POVERTY, SOCIAL MOBILITY, FAMILY ROLES, FAMILY STRUCTURE, SEX ROLES, ATTITUDES, MARITAL STABILITY, VALUES
ABST A CASE STUDY IS PRESENTED OF A LOW IN-COME PUERTO RICAN FAMILY THAT HAS ASPI-RATIONS OF SOCIAL MOBILITY IN SPITE OF

THEIR SOCIOECONOMIC LIMITATIONS. LIKE MANY PUERTO RICANS, THE PARENTS OF THE VILA FAMILY HAVE LIMITED EDUCATIONAL BACKGROUNDS AND ARE FROM POOR RURAL AREAS OF PUERTO RICO. DURING THE EARLY PART OF THEIR MARRIAGE, LUIS VILA SPENT MUCH TIME AWAY FROM THE FAMILY WITH DRINKING COMPANIONS AND OTHER WOMEN. LUIS HAS CHANGED AND NOW MAINTAINS A STRONG WORK ETHIC AND A CONVICTION THAT HE BELONGS TO THE MIDDLE CLASS (THOUGH SOCIOECONOMIC INDICATORS PLACE HIM IN THE LOWER CLASS). AS IN THE PAST, MRS. VILA GREATLY VALUES A STRONG, STABLE FAMILY. THESE ATTITUDES CONTRIBUTE SIGNIFICANTLY TO THE VILA'S ABILITY TO ACHIEVE A HOME THAT IS CONDUCIVE TO THE SOCIAL AND ACADEMIC EDUCATION OF THEIR CHILDREN. SOON THEY WILL MOVE AWAY FROM A LARGE HOUSING PROJECT INTO A HOME IN A MIDDLE CLASS NEIGHBORHOOD—THEIR SOCIAL ASPIRATIONS ACHIEVED IN PART.

ACCN   001341

1554 AUTH   **ROGLER, L. H.**
    TITL   THE CHANGING ROLE OF A POLITICAL BOSS IN A PUERTO RICAN MIGRANT COMMUNITY.
    SRCE   *AMERICAN SOCIOLOGICAL REVIEW, 1974, 39(1), 57-67.*
    INDX   EMPIRICAL, PUERTO RICAN-M, COMMUNITY, HISTORY, POLITICS, ETHNIC IDENTITY, ACCULTURATION, POLITICAL POWER, URBAN, LEADERSHIP, GROUP DYNAMICS, COMMUNITY INVOLVEMENT, IMMIGRATION
    ABST   OBSERVATIONS IN A FIELD STUDY OF A PUERTO RICAN MIGRANT COMMUNITY AND HISTORICAL DATA COVERING ALMOST FOUR DECADES ARE USED TO DISCUSS THE EMERGENCE OF POLITICAL BOSSISM IN AN ETHNIC COMMUNITY AND THE SOCIAL FORCES SUSTAINING IT. ALSO DISCUSSED ARE THE ASCENT OF POLITICALLY INDEPENDENT ETHNIC ORGANIZATIONS IN THE FACE OF THE BOSS'S UNOFFICIAL POLITICAL SYSTEM, THE VIABILITY OF SUCH ORGANIZATIONS, AND THEIR RELATIONSHIP TO THE ROLE OF THE POLITICAL BOSS. IT IS FOUND THAT A DEVELOPING MODERN POLITICAL MACHINE CONVERTS A GRASSROOTS CENTRALIZED ETHNIC LEADERSHIP INTO THE ROLE OF THE POLITICAL BOSS. THE PUERTO RICANS' INCENTIVE TO FORM POLITICALLY INDEPENDENT ORGANIZATIONS ARISES FROM THE EVOLUTION OF THEIR ETHNIC IDENTITY, AS THE HOST SOCIETY COMES INCREASINGLY TO FAVOR SUCH SELECTED GROUPS AND AS THE BOSS SYSTEM CEASES TO BE ABLE TO CONTAIN OR CHANNEL INWARDLY THE THRUST OF ASSIMILATION. AS PUERTO RICAN ACTIVISM CHANGES TO FIT THE PREVAILING ETHOS OF URBAN LIFE, THE BOSS'S ROLE IS DISRUPTED BY NEW ORGANIZATIONAL PRESSURES. 23 REFERENCES. (AUTHOR ABSTRACT MODIFIED)

ACCN   001342

1555 AUTH   **ROGLER, L. H.**
    TITL   DOES SCHIZOPHRENIA DISORGANIZE THE

FAMILY: THE MODIFICATION OF AN HYPOTHESIS.
    SRCE   *IN D. ROSENTHAL & S. S. KETTY (EDS.), THE TRANSMISSION OF SCHIZOPHRENIA. OXFORD: PERGAMON PRESS, 1968, PP. 129-135.*
    INDX   PROCEEDINGS, SCHIZOPHRENIA, PUERTO RICAN-I, FAMILY STRUCTURE, INTERPERSONAL RELATIONS, SES, FAMILY ROLES, SEX ROLES, MENTAL HEALTH, EMPIRICAL
    ABST   AS PART OF A CONFERENCE PRESENTATION ON THE TRANSMISSION OF SCHIZOPHRENIA, A STUDY OF ITS DISORGANIZING EFFECT ON THE FAMILY IS DISCUSSED. THE HYPOTHESIS IS THAT SUCH A SEVERE MENTAL DISORDER WOULD HAVE A MARKED DISRUPTIVE EFFECT, BASED ON THE ASSUMPTION THAT PERSONAL AND SOCIAL DISORGANIZATION ARE INTERRELATED. EMPHASIS IS PLACED ON THE EFFECT OF SCHIZOPHRENIA ON THE LOWER-CLASS PUERTO RICAN FAMILY. THE DATA INDICATE THAT SCHIZOPHRENIA'S DESTRUCTIVE EFFECT ON THE FAMILY IS DEPENDENT UPON THE SEX ROLE OF THE AFFLICTED FAMILY MEMBER; THE HYPOTHESIS THEREFORE APPLIES TO THE FAMILIES IN WHICH THE HUSBAND IS AFFLICTED. 1 REFERENCE.

ACCN   001343

1556 AUTH   **ROGLER, L. H.**
    TITL   MIGRANT IN THE CITY: THE LIFE OF A PUERTO RICAN ACTION GROUP.
    SRCE   *NEW YORK: BASIC BOOKS, 1972.*
    INDX   EAST, PUERTO RICAN-M, LEADERSHIP, POLITICS, POLITICAL POWER, CASE STUDY, EMPIRICAL, URBAN, IMMIGRATION, ACCULTURATION, GROUP DYNAMICS, INTERPERSONAL RELATIONS, FEMALE, MALE, RESEARCH METHODOLOGY, CULTURAL FACTORS, BOOK
    ABST   TO ACCOUNT FOR THE REPEATED FAILURE OF PUERTO RICAN IMMIGRANTS TO FORM VIABLE COMMUNITY ACTION GROUPS, A 44-MONTH ETHNOGRAPHIC STUDY WAS CONDUCTED OF SUCH A GROUP IN AN EASTERN INDUSTRIAL CITY. BY MEANS OF FIELDNOTES TAKEN AT GROUP MEETINGS, STRUCTURED INTERVIEWS WITH ALL GROUP MEMBERS, AND LIFE HISTORIES OF TWO LEADERS IN THE PUERTO RICAN COMMUNITY, THE STUDY CAREFULLY EXPLAINS (1) HOW THE GROUP ORIGINATED, (2) HOW GROUP NORMS AND GOALS DEVELOPED, AND (3) HOW INTRA-GROUP RELATIONSHIPS PROGRESSED FROM AN EARLY PERIOD OF FREQUENT CONFLICTS TO A UNIFIED AND SUCCESSFUL POLITICAL STANCE AGAINST THE CITY GOVERNMENT. THE REPORT CONCLUDES THAT PUERTO RICAN COMMUNITY GROUPS OFTEN FAIL BECAUSE PUERTO RICANS HAVE NO EXPERIENCE WITH SUCH GROUPS IN THEIR HOMELAND; BUT ONCE THEY LEARN THE REQUISITES FOR GROUP ORGANIZATION AND ALSO DEVELOP A SENSE OF UNITY AGAINST THE NON-PUERTO RICAN ESTABLISHMENT, THEN THEY CAN FORM STABLE AND SUCCESSFUL COMMUNITY GROUPS. THE REPORT ALSO INCLUDES IMPORTANT INSIGHTS BY THE AUTHOR CONCERNING THE PROBLEMS A MINORITY RESEARCHER ENCOUNTERS IN WORKING WITHIN A MINORITY COMMUNITY.

ACCN   001340

1557 AUTH   **ROGLER, L. H. & HOLLINGSHEAD, A. B.**
TITL   LA CLASE SOCIAL Y EL LENGUAJE DESARTI-
CULADO EN LOS ENFERMOS MENTALES. (SO-
CIAL CLASS AND VERBAL INCOHERENCY
AMONG THE MENTALLY ILL.)
SRCE   *REVISTA DE CIENCIAS SOCIALES, 1961, 5(3),
515-528. (SPANISH)*
INDX   MENTAL HEALTH, PSYCHOSIS, SCHIZOPHRE-
NIA, ADULTS, PUERTO RICAN-I, EMPIRICAL,
LINGUISTIC COMPETENCE, SES
ABST   TO EXPLORE THE RELATIONSHIP BETWEEN
SOCIAL CLASS AND THE ABILITY OF MENTALLY
ILL PERSONS TO CONVERSE IN A COHERENT,
RATIONAL MANNER, 278 MENTAL PATIENTS IN
SAN JUAN, PUERTO RICO, WERE STUDIED. THE
FIRST PHASE OF DATA ANALYSIS COMPARED
SCHIZOPHRENIC AND NON-SCHIZOPHRENIC
PATIENTS. IT WAS FOUND THAT SCHIZOPHREN-
ICS WERE SIGNIFICANTLY LESS ABLE TO RE-
SPOND COHERENTLY IN AN INTERVIEW SITUA-
TION, THUS INDICATING THAT VERBAL
COHERENCE IS RELATED TO THE SEVERITY OF
THE MENTAL DISORDER. IN THE SECOND PHASE
OF ANALYSIS, THE SUBJECTS' SOCIAL CLASS
WAS DETERMINED BY A SCALE COMPRISING
OCCUPATIONAL STATUS, YEARS OF SCHOOL-
ING, WEEKLY INCOME, PLACE OF RESIDENCE,
AND HOUSEHOLD HEAD MARITAL STATUS.
THEREBY, SUBJECTS WERE GROUPED INTO A
VERY LOW SES (N = 208) OR A SLIGHTLY HIGHER,
ESSENTIALLY LOWER-MIDDLE CLASS SES
(N = 70) CATEGORY. THE LOW SES PATIENTS
WERE SIGNIFICANTLY LESS COHERENT IN THEIR
CONVERSATIONS THAN THE HIGHER SES PA-
TIENTS, AND THIS RELATIONSHIP HELD ACROSS
THE VARIABLES OF (1) AGE, (2) MARITAL STA-
TUS, (3) PSYCHIATRIC TREATMENT, (4) SOCIAL
CLASS OF THE INTERVIEWER, AND (5) SCHIZO-
PHRENICS VS. NON-SCHIZOPHRENICS. TO AC-
COUNT FOR THIS, IT IS REASONED THAT THE
PROBLEMS OF SEVERE POVERTY COMPOUND
THE MENTAL DISORDERS SUFFERED BY INDI-
VIDUALS. THUS, THOSE PERSONS IN THE LOW-
EST SOCIAL CLASS EXPERIENCE THE MOST SE-
VERE MENTAL DISORIENTATION. 12 REF-
ERENCES.
ACCN   002680

1558 AUTH   **ROGLER, L. H., & HOLLINGSHEAD, A. B.**
TITL   THE PUERTO RICAN SPIRITUALIST AS A PSY-
CHIATRIST.
SRCE   *AMERICAN JOURNAL OF SOCIOLOGY, 1961,
67(1), 17-21.*
INDX   PUERTO RICAN-I, FOLK MEDICINE, PSYCHO-
THERAPY, SCHIZOPHRENIA, NEUROSIS, ADULTS,
SES, EMPIRICAL, ESPIRITISMO
ABST   A PRELIMINARY STUDY OF SCHIZOPHRENIA IN
THE LOWER CLASS IN SAN JUAN, PUERTO
RICO, SUGGESTS THAT SPIRITUALISTS OFTEN
SERVE AS PSYCHIATRISTS AND THAT SPIRITU-
ALISM FUNCTIONS AS A THERAPEUTIC OUTLET
FOR MENTAL ILLNESS. SYSTEMATIC INTER-
VIEWS WERE OBTAINED FROM MENTALLY ILL
PERSONS (RANGING FROM MILD NEUROTICS
TO SEVERE PSYCHOTICS), FROM THEIR
SPOUSES, AND FROM A SERIES OF INDIVIDU-

ALS DIAGNOSED AS HAVING "NO MENTAL ILL-
NESS" BY QUALIFIED PSYCHIATRISTS. INTER-
VIEWS WITH SPIRITUALISTS AND SUBSEQUENT
PARTICIPATION IN THEIR SESSIONS IN ORDER
TO OBSERVE THE INTERACTIONS AND REAC-
TIONS OF THEIR PATIENTS PROVIDED ADDI-
TIONAL DATA. SPIRITUALISM ACTIVELY PRO-
VIDES SOCIAL MEANING TO ITS TROUBLED
PARTICIPANTS. IN THE LOWER CLASS, IT IS
COTERMINOUS WITH SOCIAL LIFE, WOVEN
INTO THE INTIMATE TRIALS, STRIFE AND PER-
SONAL TURMOIL THAT ENMESH THE MEMBERS
OF A SOCIALLY AND ECONOMICALLY DE-
PRIVED STRATUM. A MENTALLY AFFLICTED IN-
DIVIDUAL, ALIENATED FROM HIS SOCIAL GROUP
BY HIS DEVIANT BEHAVIOR, MAY FIND THAT A
GROUP OF SPIRITUALISTS ACCEPTS HIS BE-
HAVIOR. PARTICIPATION IN A SPIRITUALIST
GROUP SERVES TO STRUCTURE, DEFINE, AND
RENDER THE ABERRANT BEHAVIOR INSTITU-
TIONALLY MEANINGFUL. SPIRITUALISM SERVES
THE AFFLICTED WITHOUT THE STIGMA OF AT-
TENDING A PSYCHIATRIC CLINIC. 15 REFER-
ENCES.

ACCN   001344

1559 AUTH   **ROGLER, L. H., & HOLLINGSHEAD, A. B.**
TITL   TRAPPED: FAMILIES AND SCHIZOPHRENIA.
SRCE   *NEW YORK: JOHN WILEY AND SONS, INC., 1965.*
INDX   EMPIRICAL, FAMILY STRUCTURE, FAMILY ROLES,
SCHIZOPHRENIA, ROLE EXPECTATIONS,
ADULTS, PSYCHOSOCIAL ADJUSTMENT, PUERTO
RICAN-I, PSYCHOPATHOLOGY, BOOK
ABST   THREE QUESTIONS WERE INVESTIGATED IN A
THREE GENERATIONAL STUDY OF INTERRELA-
TIONS BETWEEN THE PERFORMANCE OF SO-
CIAL ROLES IN PUERTO RICAN FAMILIES AND
SCHIZOPHRENIA: (1) DO THE LIFE HISTORIES
OF PERSONS WHO DEVELOP SCHIZOPHRENIA
DIFFER FROM THOSE OF PERSONS WHO ARE
NOT SCHIZOPHRENIC?; (2) WHEN AND UNDER
WHAT CIRCUMSTANCES DO PERSONS WHO
BECOME SCHIZOPHRENIC EXHIBIT THE SYMP-
TOMS CHARACTERISTIC OF SCHIZOPHRENIA?;
AND (3) WHAT EFFECT DOES SCHIZOPHRENIA
IN A HUSBAND OR A WIFE HAVE ON THE
FAMILY? FORTY FAMILIES WERE SELECTED FOR
STUDY. IN THE CONTROL GROUP OF 20 FAMI-
LIES NEITHER THE HUSBAND NOR WIFE SUF-
FERED FROM SCHIZOPHRENIA. IN THE EXPERI-
MENTAL GROUP ONE OR BOTH OF THE
SPOUSES WAS AFFLICTED WITH SCHIZOPHRE-
NIA. ALL SUBJECTS WERE BETWEEN 20 AND 39
YEARS OF AGE, WERE IN THE LOWEST SOCIO-
ECONOMIC CLASS, AND HAD NEVER BEEN
TREATED FOR MENTAL ILLNESS. EXTENSIVE IN-
TERVIEWS WITH THE FAMILIES REVEALED THAT
THE HUSBANDS OR WIVES WHO WERE
SCHIZOPHRENIC DID NOT DIFFER IN CHILD-
HOOD, YOUTH, OR EARLY ADULT LIFE HISTO-
RIES FROM THE MENTALLY HEALTHY MEN AND
WOMEN. ANALYSES SHOWED THAT IN THE
YEAR PRECEDING THE ONSET OF SCHIZO-
PHRENIA, THE SICK MEN AND WOMEN RE-
PORTED MORE ECONOMIC, SOCIAL, AND

PHYSICAL PROBLEMS THAN THE WELL FAMI-
LIES. AS THE STRESSES CONTINUED TO IN-
CREASE, THE SUBJECTS BEGAN TO EXHIBIT
THE BEHAVIOR THAT SOCIETY DEFINES AS LO-
CURA (CRAZY). ONCE SCHIZOPHRENIA IS
CLEARLY APPARENT, THE EXTENDED FAMILY
STRUCTURE OFFERS AID TO THE AFFLICTED
FAMILY, RANGING FROM TOKEN TO TOTAL
SUPPORT. WHETHER THE HUSBAND OR
WIFE'S FAMILY OFFERS SUPPORT DEPENDS ON
WHICH OF THE TWO IS AFFLICTED. WOMEN
ARE SHOWN TO BE BETTER ABLE TO COPE
WITH THEIR SICK HUSBANDS WHILE THE FAMI-
LIES OF SICK WIVES OFTEN FALL INTO DISOR-
GANIZATION. 45 REFERENCES.

ACCN   001345

1560 AUTH **ROJAS, G. F.**
TITL   LA FAMILIA RURAL MEXICANA Y SU INDUSTRIA
DOMESTICA. (THE MEXICAN RURAL FAMILY
AND ITS DOMESTIC INDUSTRY).
SRCE   *ESTUDIOS SOCIOLOGICOS: PRIMER CON-
GRESO NACIONAL DE SOCIOLOGIA, 1950, 1,
69-76.*
INDX   RURAL, MEXICAN, FAMILY STRUCTURE, ECO-
NOMIC FACTORS, FAMILY ROLES
ABST   THE AUTHOR SUMMARIZES HIS 20 YEARS OF
RESEARCH BY DISCUSSING THE MODAL CHAR-
ACTERISTICS OF THE RURAL MEXICAN FAMILY—
ITS FRAMEWORK, EDUCATIONAL FUNCTION,
ECONOMY, DOMESTIC INDUSTRY, AND RECENT
SOCIAL CHANGE. COMPRISED NOT ONLY OF A
LARGE NUMBER OF IMMEDIATE FAMILY MEM-
BERS, THE RURAL FAMILY INCLUDES IN-LAWS
AND SERVANTS, AND ADHERES TO THE FOR-
MULA "MORE HANDS, MORE LABOR." THE EDU-
CATION CONDUCTED BY THE MOTHER IS TO-
TALLY PRACTICAL IN NATURE, RELATING ONLY
TO THE NEEDS OF AGRICULTURAL LIFE. AS
BOTH SEXES PARTICIPATE IN THE FARM LABOR
NECESSARY TO THE FAMILY'S SURVIVAL, THE
DIVISION OF LABOR HAS TRADITIONALLY BEEN
BY AGE RATHER THAN BY SEX. THE FAMILY'S
WOMEN ARE ALSO RESPONSIBLE FOR A SMALL
DOMESTIC INDUSTRY (E.G., SPINNING OR
WEAVING). ALTHOUGH THE DOMESTIC INDUS-
TRY HAS TRADITIONALLY MET ONLY THOSE
NEEDS REQUIRED FOR THE FAMILY'S OWN
CONSUMPTION, URBAN DEMAND FOR GOODS
PRODUCED BY THESE INDUSTRIES HAS ADDED
THE PROFIT MOTIVE TO THE FAMILY'S ECO-
NOMIC LIFE. THIS AND SUCH OTHER FACTORS
AS (1) THE MIGRATIONS OF THE YOUNG TO
THE CITIES AND ABROAD IN SEARCH OF BET-
TER PAYING JOBS, (2) THE MULTIPLICATION OF
RURAL SCHOOLS, AND (3) THE SUBSTITUTION
OF SPANISH FOR INDIGENOUS LANGUAGES
ARE BRINGING GRADUAL SOCIAL CHANGES.
ALTHOUGH THE NATURE OF THESE CHANGES
IS NOT DISCUSSED, THEY ARE VIEWED IN A
POSITIVE LIGHT AS A STEP IN THE INCORPO-
RATION OF THE RURAL FAMILY INTO THE MAIN-
STREAM OF MEXICAN LIFE.

ACCN   001346

1561 AUTH **ROLL, S., HINTON, R., & GLAZER, M.**
TITL   DREAMS OF DEATH: MEXICAN-AMERICANS VS.
ANGLO-AMERICANS.

SRCE   *INTERAMERICAN JOURNAL OF PSYCHOLOGY,
1974, 8(1-2), 111-115.*
INDX   DREAMS, DEATH, MEXICAN AMERICAN, CROSS
CULTURAL, CULTURAL FACTORS, SEX COM-
PARISON, COLLEGE STUDENTS, EMPIRICAL
ABST   IN ORDER TO TEST THE HYPOTHESIS THAT
MEXICAN AMERICANS HAVE MORE DEATH-RE-
LATED CONCERNS APPEARING IN THE RE-
PORTS OF THEIR DREAMS, 65 MEXICAN AMERI-
CAN AND 243 ANGLO AMERICAN UNIVERSITY
STUDENTS WERE GIVEN A DREAM SURVEY IN
WHICH 12 DEATH RELATED DREAMS WERE IN-
CLUDED IN A 48-ITEM QUESTIONNAIRE. MORE
MEXICAN AMERICANS THAN ANGLO AMERI-
CANS REPORTED HAVING 8 OF THE 12 DEATH
RELATED DREAMS AT LEVELS OF STATISTICAL
SIGNIFICANCE. THE CULTURAL RELEVANCE OF
DEATH FOR MEXICAN AMERICANS AND SEX
DIFFERENCES ARE DISCUSSED. 7 REFER-
ENCES. (JOURNAL ABSTRACT MODIFIED)

ACCN   001347

1562 AUTH **ROLL, S., RABOLD, K., & MCARDLE, L.**
TITL   DISCLAIMED ACTIVITY IN DREAMS OF CHICA-
NOS AND ANGLOS.
SRCE   *JOURNAL OF CROSS-CULTURAL PSYCHOLOGY,
1976, 7(3), 335-345.*
INDX   COLLEGE STUDENTS, EMPIRICAL, DREAMS,
CROSS CULTURAL, PERSONALITY, CULTURE,
MEXICAN AMERICAN, CULTURAL FACTORS,
COPING MECHANISMS
ABST   THE RELATIONSHIP BETWEEN CULTURE AND
DREAMING HAS BEEN USEFUL IN STUDYING
THE INTERACTION BETWEEN THE NATURE OF
THE CULTURE AND THE PSYCHOLOGICAL EX-
PERIENCES OF ITS MEMBERS. TO TEST THE HY-
POTHESIS THAT CHICANOS WOULD REPORT
THEIR DREAMS IN TERMS WHICH RELIED MORE
HEAVILY ON A PASSIVE APPROACH TO LIFE, 109
CHICANO COLLEGE STUDENTS (43 MALES AND
66 FEMALES) WERE ASKED TO SUBMIT WRIT-
TEN REPORTS OF THEIR DREAMS. THE SPE-
CIFIC TYPE OF PASSIVITY INVESTIGATED WAS
DISCLAIMED ACTIVITY, IN WHICH THE DREA-
MER NEGATES THE EXISTENCE OF A SELF-
CONSCIOUS AND KNOWING ACTION. THIS IS
DONE BY ATTRIBUTING THE RESPONSIBILITY
FOR THE ACTIVITY IN THE DREAMS TO SOME-
ONE ELSE, TO THE PARTS OF THE BODY, TO
PARTS OF THE MIND, TO FATE, AND TO OTHER
OBJECTS. THE PASSIVE APPROACH WOULD
ALSO MANIFEST ITSELF IN A GREAT AMOUNT
OF CROSSING OUT WHAT WAS REPORTED AS A
MEANS OF TAKING BACK WHAT WAS ALREADY
WRITTEN. THE CHICANOS DISPLAYED SIGNIFI-
CANTLY MORE DISCLAIMED ACTIVITY, AS WELL
AS USED MORE CROSSOUTS THAN DID THE
ANGLOS. THIS SUPPORTS THE GENERALIZA-
TION THAT CHICANOS TEND TO BE MORE PAS-
SIVE THAN ANGLOS IN THEIR COPING STYLES.
HOWEVER, THE TENDENCY FOR PASSIVITY TO
BE NEGATIVELY WEIGHTED IN AMERICAN CUL-
TURE AND THE LACK OF RECOGNITION OF THE
HETEROGENEITY OF THE CHICANO CULTURE,
TOGETHER CALL FOR CONSIDERABLE CAU-
TION IN INTERPRETING THESE FINDINGS. 14
REFERENCES. (JOURNAL ABSTRACT MODI-
FIED)

ACCN   001348

1563 AUTH   **ROLL, S., & BRENNEIS, C. B.**
TITL   CHICANO AND ANGLO DREAMS OF DEATH.
SRCE   *JOURNAL OF CROSS-CULTURAL PSYCHOLOGY, 1975, 6(3), 377-383.*
INDX   DREAMS, DEATH, MEXICAN AMERICAN, CROSS CULTURAL, COLLEGE STUDENTS, EMPIRICAL, CULTURAL FACTORS, SEX COMPARISON
ABST   RESEARCH ON DREAM CONTENT AND ORGANIZATION IS USEFUL IN UNDERSTANDING THE PERSON'S VIEW OF HIMSELF, OF HUMAN RELATIONSHIPS, AND OF THE WORLD. CROSS CULTURAL INVESTIGATIONS HELP TO CLARIFY THE RELATIONSHIP BETWEEN CULTURE AND DREAMS. TO REPLICATE AN EARLIER STUDY IN WHICH CHICANOS REPORTED HAVING MORE DREAMS OF DEATH THAN DID THEIR ANGLO COUNTERPARTS, DREAM REPORTS WERE OBTAINED FROM 80 CHICANO (40 MALES AND 40 FEMALES) AND 80 ANGLO (40 MALES AND 40 FEMALES) COLLEGE STUDENTS. THE DREAMS WERE SCORED FOR THE PRESENCE OF DEATH-RELATED DREAM CONTENT. CHI-SQUARE TESTS REVEALED A STATISTICALLY HIGHER NUMBER OF CHICANO FEMALES REPORTING DREAMS OF DEATH, BUT NO SIGNIFICANT DIFFERENCE WAS FOUND BETWEEN CHICANO AND ANGLO MALES. RESULTS ARE LINKED TO THE GREATER PHENOMENOLOGICAL EMPHASIS ON DEATH IN CHICANO CULTURE AND THE GREATER TENDENCY FOR CHICANO WOMEN TO CARRY THE INFLUENCES OF THE CULTURE. IT IS SUGGESTED THAT A HIGH DEGREE OF INVOLVEMENT WITH DEATH MAY NOT BE SPECIFIC TO MEXICAN CULTURE, BUT PART OF A PERVASIVE SYSTEM OF HISPANIC BELIEFS. 5 REFERENCES. (JOURNAL ABSTRACT MODIFIED)
ACCN   001349

1564 AUTH   **ROMANO-V., O. I.**
TITL   THE ANTHROPOLOGY AND SOCIOLOGY OF THE MEXICAN AMERICANS.
SRCE   *EL GRITO, 1968, 2(1), 13-26.*
INDX   REVIEW, MEXICAN AMERICAN, CULTURE, STEREOTYPES, SOCIAL SCIENCES, CULTURAL FACTORS
ABST   A REVIEW OF CONTEMPORARY SOCIAL SCIENCE LITERATURE PERTAINING TO THE MEXICAN AMERICAN (MA) IS PRESENTED. ALL SOCIAL SCIENTISTS HAVE RELIED UPON THE CONCEPT OF TRADITIONAL CULTURE IN ORDER TO DESCRIBE THE FOUNDATIONS OF MA CULTURE. SOCIAL SCIENCE STUDIES HAVE DEALT WITH MA'S AS AN HISTORIC PEOPLE. A LIST OF STEREOTYPES DERIVED FROM CONTEMPORARY SOCIAL SCIENTISTS WERE COMPARED TO THOSE HELD BY PEOPLE DURING THE AMERICAN FRONTIER, REVEALING THAT THERE HAS BEEN NO SIGNIFICANT CHANGE IN VIEWS TOWARD THE MA FOR THE PAST 100 YEARS. THE VIEWS ARE PERNICIOUS AND DEGRADING IN THAT THEY ELIMINATE THE HISTORICAL SIGNIFICANCE OF MA'S. HISTORICALLY, MA'S HAVE BEEN, AND CONTINUE TO BE, A PLURALISTIC PEOPLE. THEY CANNOT BE DESCRIBED ACCORDING TO A SIMPLISTIC FORMULA. IT IS RECOMMENDED THAT THE CONCEPT OF TRADITIONAL CULTURE AS PRESENTLY USED BY SOCIAL SCIENTISTS BE DISMISSED AND THE CONCEPT OF THE HISTORICAL CULTURE BE ADOPTED. 8 REFERENCES.
ACCN   001350

1565 AUTH   **ROMANO-V., O. I.**
TITL   CHARISMATIC MEDICINE, FOLK HEALING, AND FOLK SAINTHOOD.
SRCE   *AMERICAN ANTHROPOLOGIST, 1965, 67(5), 1151-1173.*
INDX   FOLK MEDICINE, ESSAY, MEXICAN AMERICAN, SES, CURANDERISMO, PERSONALITY, CASE STUDY, TEXAS, SOUTHWEST, THEORETICAL, SOCIAL STRUCTURE
ABST   AN ELABORATION UPON THE NATURE OF DIFFERENCES BETWEEN FOLK HEALERS IS ADVANCED IN THE HOPE THAT NEW THEORETICAL DIRECTIONS FOR STUDIES WILL FOCUS UPON THE FOLK-MEDICAL WORLD. THE PAPER BEGINS WITH AN OUTLINE OF AN EMPIRICAL MODE CONSISTING OF TRADITIONAL BEHAVIORAL DIRECTIONS WHICH GOVERN THE LIFE OF THE SOUTH TEXAS MEXICAN AMERICAN (I.E., COMMUNITY VS. THE ATOMISTIC SOCIAL ORDER). FOLLOWING THE OUTLINE IS THE PRESENTATION OF A HEALING HIERARCHY CONSISTING OF RELATIVE SOCIAL POSITIONS ASSOCIATED WITH DIFFERENTIAL HEALING ACHIEVEMENT. FINALLY, A SPECIFIC CASE OF DON PEDRITO JARAMILLO IS DISCUSSED IN TERMS OF HIS ASCENDANCY IN THE HEALING HIERARCHY FROM AN OBSCURE FIGURE TO A FAMOUS HEALER WITH A REPUTATION OF FOLK SAINTHOOD. THE ANALYSIS OF DON PEDRITO'S SOCIAL COMMITMENT SHOWS HIM OCCUPYING THE BEHAVIORAL SECTOR OF COMMUNALITY, COOPERATIVENESS, AND MUTUAL ASSISTANCE. IN ADDITION, DON PEDRITO SHOWED MANY OTHER TRAITS WHICH POINT TOWARD AN INDIVIDUAL MANIFESTATION OF AN INFLUENCE WHICH APPEARS TO BE FUNDAMENTALLY CHARISMATIC. THE CASE OF DON PEDRO JARAMILLO SUGGESTS A REEXAMINATION OF HISTORICAL CASES WHICH HAVE BEEN CALLED CHARISMATICALLY INNOVATIVE. IT IS FURTHER SUGGESTED THAT FOR FOLK MEDICINE IN GENERAL, FUTURE RESEARCH IS POSSIBLE IN TERMS OF DIFFERENTIAL HEALER ACHIEVEMENT AND SOCIAL THEORY. 19 REFERENCES.
ACCN   001351

1566 AUTH   **ROSEN, B. M., LAWRENCE, L., GOLDSMITH, H. F., WINDLE, C. D., & SHAMBAUGH, J. P.**
TITL   MENTAL HEALTH DEMOGRAPHIC SYSTEM PROFILE: PURPOSE, CONTENTS, AND SAMPLER OF USES (SERIES C, NO. 11).
SRCE   *ROCKVILLE, MD.: U.S. DEPARTMENT OF HEALTH, EDUCATION AND WELFARE; ALCOHOL, DRUG ABUSE AND MENTAL HEALTH ADMINISTRATION, UNDATED.*
INDX   CENSUS, DEMOGRAPHIC, COMMUNITY, MENTAL HEALTH, SURVEY, SPANISH SURNAMED, RESOURCE UTILIZATION, HEALTH DELIVERY SYSTEMS
ABST   A DESCRIPTION OF THE MENTAL HEALTH DEMOGRAPHIC PROFILE SYSTEM (MHDPS) IS PROVIDED, ILLUSTRATING WHAT IS INCLUDED

AND HOW DATA FROM THIS SYSTEM MAY BE OBTAINED. IN ADDITION, CERTAIN PRODUCTS AND USES OF THE SYSTEM ARE CITED AND AN ANNOTATED BIBLIOGRAPHY IS INCLUDED. THE MHDPS IS A DATA SOURCE PROVIDING INFORMATION ON THE DEMOGRAPHIC, SOCIAL, AND ECONOMIC CHARACTERISTICS OF EACH COMMUNITY MENTAL HEALTH CENTER CATCHMENT AREA IN THE U.S. DATA IN THIS SYSTEM ARE BASED ON SOCIAL AND ECONOMIC CONDITIONS AS REPORTED IN THE 1970 CENSUS.

ACCN   001352

1567 AUTH   **ROSEN, C. L., & ORTEGO, P. D.**

TITL   LANGUAGE AND READING PROBLEMS OF SPANISH SPEAKING CHILDREN IN THE SOUTHWEST.

SRCE   *JOURNAL OF READING BEHAVIOR, 1969, 1(1), 51-70.*

INDX   REVIEW, LANGUAGE ACQUISITION, CHILDREN, BILINGUALISM, READING, SPANISH SURNAMED, SOUTHWEST

ABST   FIVE MAJOR CATEGORIES OF LANGUAGE PROBLEMS OF SPANISH-SPEAKING CHILDREN ARE REVIEWED: (1) THE VAGUE DEFINITION OF BILINGUALISM, (2) INADEQUATE TIMING OF SECOND LANGUAGE INSTRUCTION, (3) IMPROPER LEARNING CONTEXT FOR SECOND LANGUAGE INSTRUCTION, (4) LANGUAGE EQUIVALENCE ON A BILINGUAL SCALE, AND (5) DEALING WITH INDIVIDUAL DIFFERENCES ATTRIBUTABLE TO INDIVIDUAL CHILD STATUS. THE DIFFICULTIES INVOLVED IN A NUMBER OF CURRENT APPROACHES USED TO TEACH READING TO SPANISH-SPEAKING CHILDREN ARE DISCUSSED, AND THE NECESSITY FOR DEVELOPING NEW AND MORE APPROPRIATE TECHNIQUES, I.E., LINGUISTICALLY ORIENTED READING MATERIALS, A LANGUAGE EXPERIENCE APPROACH, AND A BILINGUAL APPROACH BASED UPON THE UNIQUE NEEDS OF THE SPANISH-SPEAKING CHILD IS EMPHASIZED. IT IS CONCLUDED THAT WHILE NO APPROACH SHOULD BE CONSIDERED A PANACEA, A NUMBER OF TECHNIQUES APPEAR PROMISING. 70 REFERENCES.

ACCN   001353

1568 AUTH   **ROSENBERG, B., & BENSMAN, J.**

TITL   SEXUAL PATTERNS IN THREE ETHNIC SUBCULTURES OF AN AMERICAN UNDERCLASS.

SRCE   *ANNALS OF THE AMERICAN ACADEMY OF POLITICAL AND SOCIAL SCIENCES, 1968, 376, 61-75. (REPRINTED IN H. THORNBURG (ED.), CONTEMPORARY ADOLESCENCE: READINGS. BELMONT, CALIF: BROOKS/COLE, 1971, PP. 94-107.)*

INDX   SEX ROLES, CROSS CULTURAL, EMPIRICAL, ADOLESCENTS, SES, PUERTO RICAN-M, ATTITUDES, SEXUAL BEHAVIOR, NEW YORK, EAST, ILLINOIS, MIDWEST, WASHINGTON D.C., POVERTY, HOMOSEXUALITY, BIBLIOGRAPHY

ABST   THREE AMERICAN ETHNIC SUBCULTURES, ALL CONSISTING OF TRANSMIGRATED GROUPS LIVING IN POVERTY, WERE STUDIED AND THE SEXUAL PATTERNS OF THE YOUTH DESCRIBED. THE GROUPS CONSISTED OF WHITE APPALACHIANS LIVING IN CHICAGO, NEGROES IN WASHINGTON, D.C., AND PUERTO RICANS IN

NEW YORK. SHARPLY DIFFERENTIATED PATTERNS OF SEXUAL BEHAVIOR, INVOLVING CONQUEST, SEX EDUCATION, SEX MISINFORMATION, ATTITUDES TOWARD FEMALES, RESPONSIBILITY, AND AFFECT WERE DISCOVERED, AND THESE PATTERNS WERE REFLECTED IN THE LANGUAGE OF THE SUBCULTURES, PARTICULARLY IN THE ARGOT. THE UNDERCLASS SEXUAL MORES DIFFER FROM THOSE OF THE AMERICAN MIDDLE CLASS, BUT NOT MORE THAN THEY DIFFER FROM EACH OTHER AMONG THE THREE ETHNIC GROUPS. SEXUAL PRACTICES ARE RELATED TO GENERAL LIFE-STYLES, AND REFLECT GHETTOIZATION, SUBCULTURAL ISOLATION, AND SHORT-RANGE HEDONISM IN GROUPS ONLY RECENTLY TRANSPLANTED FROM THEIR RURAL AREAS OF ORIGIN. 48 REFERENCES. (JOURNAL ABSTRACT)

ACCN   001354

1569 AUTH   **ROSENBERG, B., & SILVERSTEIN, H.**

TITL   FIGHTING.

SRCE   *IN B. ROSENBERG (ED.), THE VARIETIES OF DELINQUENT EXPERIENCE. WALTHAM, MASS: BLAISDELL, 1969.*

INDX   AGGRESSION, CROSS CULTURAL, EMPIRICAL, PUERTO RICAN-M, ADOLESCENTS, DELINQUENCY

ABST   A STUDY REGARDING JUVENILE DELINQUENCY, AGGRESSION, STEALING, SEXUAL BEHAVIOR, AND LEVEL OF ASPIRATION AMONG 40 BLACK, 52 PUERTO RICAN AND 41 ANGLO ADOLESCENTS, 13-17 YEARS-OLD, WHERE MORE THAN 95% HAD COMMITTED AT LEAST ONE DELINQUENT ACT, WAS CONDUCTED IN WASHINGTON, D.C., CHICAGO, AND EAST HARLEM. THE RESPONDENTS GAVE PERSONAL ACCOUNTS OF THEIR VARIOUS DELINQUENT EXPERIENCES, INCLUDING THEIR PERCEPTIONS OF SCHOOL, WORK, WELFARE, AND THE POLICE. RESPONSES FROM THE DIFFERENT URBAN CENTERS WERE COMPARED AND CONTRASTED. SEXUAL BEHAVIOR WAS APPROACHED IN TERMS OF FIRST EXPERIENCE, USE OF CONTRACEPTIVES, MALE-FEMALE ROLES, AND MORALITY; FIGHTING AND VIOLENCE WERE A CODE OF HONOR, RACIAL STRIFE, AND GANG INITIATION; STEALING WAS TO A COLLECTIVE ACTIVITY, DRUG HABIT, AND DEPRIVATION. OVERALL, FINDINGS SHOW THAT ALTHOUGH IMPOVERISHED YOUTH ARE ALIKE IN SHARING ECONOMIC CIRCUMSTANCES, HOW THEY INTERPRET AND RESPOND TO THEIR CONDITION DIFFERS. CROSS-CULTURAL VARIATIONS AMONG THE POOR ARE MARKED IN DELINQUENCY AND OTHER SOCIAL ACTIVITIES. ALTHOUGH THE PREPONDERANCE OF THE SAMPLE (75%) RANKED LOW IN ASPIRATION, THERE WAS NO ESTABLISHED LINK BETWEEN HIGH ASPIRATION AND DELINQUENCY. FINALLY, MORAL ANOMIE IS AS SOCIETY-WIDE, DERIVING NOT FROM ECONOMIC PRIVATION BUT FROM THE MORAL CURRENTS OF CONTEMPORARY SOCIAL DEVELOPMENT. 51 REFERENCES.

ACCN   001355

1570 AUTH **ROSENBERG, T. J., & LAKE, R. W.**
TITL TOWARD A REVISED MODEL OF RESIDENTIAL SEGREGATION AND SUCCESSION: PUERTO RICANS IN NEW YORK, 1960-1970.
SRCE *AMERICAN JOURNAL OF SOCIOLOGY, 1976, 81(5), 1142-1150.*
INDX ACCULTURATION, HOUSING, CULTURE, PUERTO RICAN-M, COMMUNITY, ECONOMIC FACTORS, ENVIRONMENTAL FACTORS, ETHNIC IDENTITY, POVERTY, REVIEW, THEORETICAL
ABST GENERALLY ACCEPTED MODELS OF RESIDENTIAL SEGREGATION AND SUCCESSION WERE TESTED WITH THE PUERTO RICAN POPULATION IN NEW YORK. THESE MODELS DESCRIBE ETHNIC ASSIMILATION IN TERMS OF HOUSING AND OUTLINE A PATTERN OF DECREASING RESIDENTIAL SEGREGATION WHICH IS ASSOCIATED WITH INCREASING SIMILARITY TO NATIVE CAUCASIANS (E.G., IN SOCIOECONOMIC STATUS). SIMILAR MODELS FOR THE BLACK POPULATION POSIT CONTINUING RESIDENTIAL CONCENTRATION COMBINED WITH RAPID TURNOVER AND SUCCESSION. AN ANALYSIS OF 258 CENSUS TRACTS IN THE NEW YORK STANDARD METROPOLITAN STATISTICAL AREA FOR 1960 AND 1970 INDICATE THAT PUERTO RICAN SETTLEMENT PATTERNS ARE NOT CONFORMING TO EITHER TYPE OF PREVIOUSLY ACCEPTED MODEL. COMPETITION BETWEEN THE PUERTO RICAN MINORITY AND THE LARGER, MORE ECONOMICALLY ADVANTAGED BLACK MINORITY, A NEW SET OF PUBLIC HOUSING NITIES, AND THE RETURN MIGRATION OF SUCCESSFUL PUERTO RICANS ARE FACTORS THAT ARE NOT CONSIDERED IN PREVIOUSLY DEVELOPED MODELS. A NEW MODEL OF RESIDENTIAL SEGREGATION AND SUCCESSION MUST INCORPORATE THESE REALITIES OF CONTEMPORARY URBANIZATION. 12 REFERENCES. (JOURNAL ABSTRACT MODIFIED)
ACCN 001358

1571 AUTH **ROSENBLATT, A., & WIGGINS, L. M.**
TITL CHARACTERISTICS OF THE PARENTS SERVED.
SRCE *SOCIAL CASEWORK, 1967, 48(10), 639-647.*
INDX PARENTAL INVOLVEMENT, ADULTS, MEXICAN AMERICAN, EMPIRICAL, EDUCATION, SES, CHILDREARING PRACTICES, ADULT EDUCATION, COMMUNITY, CROSS CULTURAL, COMMUNITY INVOLVEMENT
ABST CHARACTERISTICS OF PARTICIPANTS IN THE EDUCATION AND NEIGHBORHOOD ACTION FOR BETTER LIVING PROJECT WERE COMPARED WITH FAMILIES SEEN BY FAMILY SERVICE AGENCIES AND THOSE SEEN IN A PARENT EDUCATION PROGRAM. PROJECT PARTICIPANTS WERE SIGNIFICANTLY DIFFERENT FROM REGULAR ATTENDERS IN THE OTHER GROUPS AND, IN FACT, DIFFERED LITTLE FROM THE NONATTENDERS AND REFUSERS IN THESE OTHER GROUPS. WITHIN THE PROJECT ITSELF, FEW DIFFERENCES WERE FOUND BETWEEN REGULAR ATTENDERS AND DROPOUTS. DATA SUGGEST THAT THE PERSONS REACHED WERE MORE DEPRIVED THAN THOSE IN THE COMPARISON GROUPS, THAT THE MORE ENTERPRISING RESIDENTS IN THE DISADVANTAGED COMMUNITIES REFUSED TO JOIN THE PROJ-

ECT, AND THAT THE PROJECT WAS SLIGHTLY LESS SUCCESSFUL IN RETAINING AS MEMBERS NEGROES, MEXICAN AMERICANS, AND PERSONS WITH LESS THAN A HIGH SCHOOL EDUCATION THAN IT WAS IN RETAINING WHITE CLIENTELE AND PERSONS WITH MORE EDUCATION. 6 REFERENCES.
ACCN 001359

1572 AUTH **ROSENQUIST, C. M., & MEGARGEE, E. I.**
TITL DELINQUENCY IN THREE CULTURES.
SRCE *AUSTIN, TEXAS: HOGG FOUNDATION FOR MENTAL HEALTH, 1969.*
INDX DELINQUENCY, CROSS CULTURAL, MEXICAN AMERICAN, EMPIRICAL, ADOLESCENTS, URBAN, PERSONALITY ASSESSMENT, WAIS, PROJECTIVE TESTING, BOOK
ABST RESULTS OF A CROSS-CULTURAL, CROSS-NATIONAL INVESTIGATION TO COMPARE DIFFERENCES BETWEEN DELINQUENTS AND NONDELINQUENTS IN ANGLO AMERICAN, MEXICAN AMERICAN AND MEXICAN NATIONAL ETHNIC GROUPS ARE REPORTED. DATA WERE OBTAINED FROM 300 SUBJECTS REGARDING SOCIOLOGICAL, PSYCHOLOGICAL, AND PHYSIOLOGICAL VARIABLES THAT ARE CONSIDERED TO BE MAJOR CHARACTERISTICS OF DELINQUENT BEHAVIOR. AN ATTEMPT WAS MADE TO DETERMINE IF FACTORS THAT DIFFERENTIATE DELINQUENTS FROM NONDELINQUENTS IN URBAN AREAS OF THE NORTHEASTERN UNITED STATES WOULD ALSO DIFFERENTIATE SAMPLE POPULATIONS FROM OTHER CULTURAL GROUPS. SEVERAL PATTERNS WERE TRACED IN THE BEHAVIOR OF SUBJECTS IN ALL THREE GROUPS, AND THE CONSISTENCY WITH OTHER REPORTS IS EXAMINED. GENERAL AGREEMENT IN THE CHARACTERISTICS OF DELINQUENT BEHAVIOR AMONG THE GROUPS WAS FOUND, ALTHOUGH SOME NOTEWORTHY DIFFERENCES WERE RELATED TO VARIATIONS IN FAMILY STRUCTURE, CHILD-REARING PRACTICES, AND ECONOMIC OPPORTUNITIES. THE IMPLICATIONS OF THE FINDINGS FOR THE MAJOR THEORIES OF DELINQUENCY ARE DISCUSSED IN DETAIL, AS WELL AS THEIR CONTRIBUTION TO PREVENTIVE AND REHABILITATION PROGRAMS. 228 REFERENCES.
ACCN 001360

1573 AUTH **ROSENTHAL, T. L., COXON, M., HURT, M., JR., ZIMMERMAN, B. J., & GRUBBS, C. F.**
TITL PEDAGOGICAL ATTITUDES OF CONVENTIONAL AND SPECIALLY-TRAINED TEACHERS.
SRCE *PSYCHOLOGY IN THE SCHOOLS, 1970, 7(1), 61-66.*
INDX ATTITUDES, TEACHERS, EMPIRICAL, MEXICAN AMERICAN, EDUCATIONAL ASSESSMENT, CHILDREN, INSTRUCTIONAL TECHNIQUES, ARIZONA, SOUTHWEST, PROGRAM EVALUATION
ABST THE PEDAGOGICAL ATTITUDES OF ELEMENTARY SCHOOL TEACHERS IN AN EXPERIMENTAL PROGRAM (EP) FOR DISADVANTAGED MEXICAN AMERICANS ARE REPORTED. THE ATTITUDES DEALT WITH THE APPLICATIONS OF CONTEMPORARY REINFORCEMENT AND SOCIAL LEARNING PRINCIPLES, AS WELL AS WITH THE NEEDS OF CULTURALLY DISADVANTAGED

CHILDREN. THE EP CONSISTED OF MAKING AVAILABLE RESOURCE PERSONNEL TO ASSIST TEACHERS IN THEIR DAY-TO-DAY ACTIVITIES FOR A PERIOD OF AT LEAST 1 YEAR. RESULTS REVEAL THAT EP TEACHERS SCORED SIGNIFICANTLY HIGHER THAN TEACHERS NOT INCLUDED IN THE EP IN: (1) ENCOURAGING FREE ACCESS TO, AND EXPLORATION OF, A WIDE RANGE OF MATERIAL AND EXPERIENCE DESPITE CONSIDERATIONS OF TIDINESS OF UNIFORMITY; (2) EMPHASIZING MOTIVATIONAL PRACTICE FACTORS IN SHAPING SCHOOL PERFORMANCE AND ULTIMATE, RATHER THAN IMMEDIATE, ACQUISITION; (3) DISCOURAGING THE REPETITION OF GRADES AND GRADE PLACEMENT BASED ON JUDGMENTS OF INNATE INTELLIGENCE OR "MATURATIONAL" READINESS; AND (4) DISCOURAGING USE OF CENSURE AND CRITICISM AS GUIDANCE DEVICES. IT IS ALSO SHOWN THAT WITHOUT TRAINING, ONGOING CONTACT WITH CULTURALLY DISADVANTAGED YOUNGSTERS LED TEACHERS TO INDUCE ATTITUDES IN GENERAL CONCORDANCE WITH EP PHILOSOPHY BUT OF LOWER INTENSITY THAN WAS ACCOMPLISHED THROUGH TEACHER RETRAINING. IT FURTHER APPEARED THAT, WITHOUT MAINTAINING SUCH ATTITUDES BY CONTINUED TRAINING, WHEN TEACHERS STOPPED WORKING WITH UNDERPRIVILEGED CHILDREN, TEACHER ATTITUDES BECAME STATISTICALLY INDISTINGUISHABLE FROM THOSE OF COLLEAGUES ACCUSTOMED TO WORKING WITH MIDDLE- AND UPPER-CLASS CHILDREN. A SECOND STUDY REVEALS THAT A SHORT 6-WEEK INTENSIVE TRAINING PROGRAM ALSO RESULTS IN TEACHER ATTITUDE CHANGE. 16 REFERENCES.

ACCN   001361

1574 AUTH   ROSENTHAL, T. L., HENDERSON, R. W., HOBSON, A., & HURT, M., JR.
TITL   SOCIAL STRATA AND PERCEPTION OF MAGICAL AND FOLK-MEDICAL CHILD-CARE PRACTICES.
SRCE   JOURNAL OF SOCIAL PSYCHOLOGY, 1969, 77(1), 3-13.
INDX   FOLK MEDICINE, SES, CROSS CULTURAL, MEXICAN AMERICAN, EMPIRICAL, ADULTS, ATTITUDES, CHILDREARING PRACTICES, FEMALE, ARIZONA, SOUTHWEST
ABST   A SAMPLE OF 139 FEMALE SUBJECTS—37 MEXICAN AMERICANS (MA), 52 LOWER INCOME ANGLOS (LOW-A) AND 50 UPPER INCOME ANGLOS (UP-A)—RATED 10 MAIN ASSERTIONS RELATED TO MAGICAL CHILD CARE HEALING CURES ON A 7-POINT SCALE DURING A HOME INTERVIEW. THE DATA REVEAL THAT THE MA GROUP ACCEPTS THE MAGICAL CURES SIGNIFICANTLY MORE THAN DO THE LOW-A GROUP, WHICH IN TURN DISPLAYS LESS REJECTION OF EACH BELIEF AND THEIR AGGREGATE THAN DOES THE UP-A GROUP. THUS NOT ONLY CULTURAL MILIEU BUT ALSO SOCIOECONOMIC LEVEL WITHIN ANGLO AMERICAN SOCIETY AFFECTS ACCEPTANCE OF THE HEALING PRACTICES. THE SIZABLE GROUP DIFFERENCES DERIVE MORE FROM INTENSE DISAGREEMENT OF ANGLO WOMEN THAN FROM

STRONG AGREEMENT WITH THE BELIEF COMPLEX BY THE MA GROUP. ALL GROUPS JUDGED THAT SUCH CURES WOULD BE USED LESS OFTEN, IF AT ALL, BY THE NEXT GENERATION OF MOTHERS. 12 REFERENCES.

ACCN   001362

1575 AUTH   ROSENTHAL, T. L., UNDERWOOD, B., & MARTIN, M.
TITL   ASSESSING CLASSROOM INCENTIVE PRACTICES.
SRCE   JOURNAL OF EDUCATIONAL PSYCHOLOGY, 1969, 60(5), 370-376.
INDX   EDUCATIONAL ASSESSMENT, EMPIRICAL, CHILDREN, MEXICAN AMERICAN, INSTRUCTIONAL TECHNIQUES, ARIZONA, SOUTHWEST, TEACHERS, CLASSROOM BEHAVIOR
ABST   THE MOTIVATIONAL EFFECTS OF AN EXPERIMENTAL PROGRAM OF PEDAGOGY, DESIGNED FOR CULTURALLY DISADVANTAGED CHILDREN, WERE EVALUATED RELATIVE TO A CONTROL GROUP OF CONVENTIONAL CLASSROOMS. THE SAMPLE COMPRISED 155 PRIMARY GRADE CLASSROOMS IN TUCSON, DISTRICT I. OBSERVATIONS WERE MADE ON THREE ASPECTS OF INTERACTIVE BEHAVIOR: (1) THE TARGET TO WHOM THE TEACHER DISPENSED INCENTIVES; (2) THE NATURE OF THE INCENTIVES DELIVERED; AND (3) THE ACTION OF THE CHILDREN WHICH ELICITED REINFORCEMENT FROM THE TEACHER. RESULTS REVEALED EXPERIMENTAL CLASSROOMS TO BE CHARACTERIZED BY SIGNIFICANTLY MORE TEACHER APPROVAL, LESS TEACHER DISAPPROVAL, AND BY MORE STUDENT SOLICITATION OF TEACHER ATTENTION THAN WAS FOUND IN CONVENTIONAL CLASSROOMS. THESE DIFFERENCES, GENERALLY OBTAINED IN VERBAL, GESTURAL, AND PHYSICAL-CONTACT RESPONSE MODES, AS WELL AS THEIR SUMS, WERE FURTHER MAINTAINED WHEN EXPERIMENTAL ROOMS WERE COMPARED WITH CONVENTIONAL ROOMS WITHIN HIGHER AND LOWER SOCIOECONOMIC STATUS LEVELS SEPARATELY. A BRIEF OBSERVATIONAL METHOD FOR ASSESSING SPECIFIC CLASSROOM INCENTIVE PRACTICES IS PROVIDED, AND IMPLICATIONS OF THE QUANTITATIVE RESULTS ARE DISCUSSED. 17 REFERENCES.
ACCN   001363

1576 AUTH   ROSENTHAL, T. L., & ZIMMERMAN, B. J.
TITL   MODELING BY EXEMPLIFICATION AND INSTRUCTION IN TRAINING CONSERVATION.
SRCE   DEVELOPMENTAL PSYCHOLOGY, 1972, 6(3), 392-401.
INDX   MODELING, EMPIRICAL, MEXICAN AMERICAN, CROSS CULTURAL, CHILDREN, COGNITIVE DEVELOPMENT, ARIZONA, SOUTHWEST
ABST   FOUR OBSERVATIONAL LEARNING EXPERIMENTS INVOLVING MULTIDIMENSIONAL PIAGETIAN CONSERVATION TASKS WERE CONDUCTED ON GROUPS OF CHILDREN IN TUCSON. SUBJECTS WERE MIDDLE-CLASS ANGLO AND ECONOMICALLY DISADVANTAGED CHICANO BOYS AND GIRLS IN FIRST GRADE OR NURSERY SCHOOL, AGES 4 TO 7. WITHOUT FURTHER TRAINING, IMITATIVE CONSERVATION WAS

544

GENERALIZED TO NEW STIMULI. VERBALLY PRAISING THE MODEL'S RESPONSES DID NOT AFFECT PERFORMANCE. A NONCONSERVING MODEL REDUCED INITIALLY CONSERVING CHILDREN'S SCORES. A NONMODELING INSTRUCTION PROCEDURE DID NOT ALTER CONSERVATION. PROVIDING A RULE TO EXPLAIN STIMULUS EQUIVALENCE IMPROVED RESPONSES WHEN BOTH JUDGED EQUIVALENCE AND EXPLANATION WERE REQUIRED, BUT NOT WHEN JUDGED EQUIVALENCE ALONE WAS REQUIRED. OBSERVING A MODEL CONSERVE WITHOUT GIVING EXPLANATIONS INCREASED CORRECT JUDGMENTS PLUS RULE RESPONSES IN IMITATION. THIS INDICATED INFERENTIAL THINKING ELICITED BY MODELING. THE EFFICIENCY OF MODELING TECHNIQUES FOR TRANSMITTING ABSTRACT INFORMATION AND FOR USE IN PRACTICAL PEDAGOGY IS DISCUSSED. 12 REFERENCES. (JOURNAL ABSTRACT MODIFIED)

ACCN   001364

1577 AUTH   **ROSS, H., & GLASER, E. M.**
TITL   MAKING IT OUT OF THE GHETTO.
SRCE   *PROFESSIONAL PSYCHOLOGY, 1973, 4(3), 347-356.*
INDX   SOCIAL MOBILITY, ACHIEVEMENT MOTIVATION, PARENTAL INVOLVEMENT, MALE, MEXICAN AMERICAN, GANGS, SOCIALIZATION, CROSS CULTURAL, CULTURAL FACTORS, GROUP DYNAMICS, CHILDREARING PRACTICES, URBAN, EMPIRICAL, CALIFORNIA, SOUTHWEST, SELF CONCEPT
ABST   A PILOT STUDY WAS CONDUCTED TO IDENTIFY FACTORS DIFFERENTIATING UPWARDLY AND NONUPWARDLY MOBILE MEN. SIXTY MEN—SUCCESSFUL OR UNSUCCESSFUL BLACKS AND MEXICAN AMERICANS—WERE INTERVIEWED USING A QUESTIONNAIRE STRUCTURED AROUND 14 LIFE FACTORS DISTILLED FROM THE LITERATURE. THEY ALSO TOOK THE SCIENCE RESEARCH ASSOCIATES NON-VERBAL FORM MENTAL ABILITY TEST AND PARTICIPATED IN GROUP SESSIONS. RESULTS REVEALED THAT 34 ITEMS (CENTERING AROUND SELF-CONCEPT AND THE QUALITY OF FAMILY SUPPORT) DIFFERENTIATED SUCCESSFUL AND NONSUCCESSFUL SUBJECTS IN BOTH ETHNIC GROUPS, WHILE MENTAL ABILITY WAS NOT SIGNIFICANTLY DIFFERENT. THE RESULTANT CLUSTERS OF DIFFERENCES WERE COMPARED TO THE CHARACTERISTICS OF MAINSTREAM LIFE AND STREET OR GANG LIFE AND TO DIFFERENCES IN PARENTAL INFLUENCE BETWEEN ETHNIC GROUPS. RECOMMENDATIONS FOR MODIFYING TRAINING AND EMPLOYMENT PROGRAMS INCLUDE: (1) EXPLAINING THE STEPS TO PROGRAM COMPLETION; (2) BREAKING PROGRAMS INTO SUBGOALS; (3) MINIMIZING FAILURE AND MAXIMIZING SUCCESS; (4) FOSTERING GROUP COHESIVENESS; (5) UTILIZING COUNSELORS TO PROVIDE PERSONAL RELATIONSHIPS, INTERPRET EXPECTATIONS, AND DISCUSS VALUES AND GOALS; (6) USING THE UNSUCCESSFUL SUBJECTS' EXPERTISE FOR PLANNING; AND (7) USING FORMER UN-

SUCCESSFUL SUBJECTS FOR RECRUITING. 15 REFERENCES. (PASAR ABSTRACT MODIFIED)

ACCN   001366

1578 AUTH   **ROSSELLO, J. A.**
TITL   APUNTES PARA UNA HISTORIA DE LA PSIQUIATRIA EN PUERTO RICO. (NOTES ON THE HISTORY OF PSYCHIATRY IN PUERTO RICO.)
SRCE   *IN J. A. ROSSELLO (ED.), TRATADO GENERAL DE PSIQUIATRIA. PUERTO RICO: UNIVERSIDAD DE PUERTO RICO, 1962, PP. 41-83. (SPANISH)*
INDX   ESSAY, PUERTO RICAN-I, HISTORY, INSTITUTIONALIZATION, MENTAL HEALTH, CULTURE, INDIGENOUS POPULATIONS
ABST   IN THIS SHORT COLLECTION OF ANECDOTES AND DOCUMENTS, THE HISTORY OF PSYCHIATRY IN PUERTO RICO IS DISCUSSED FROM THE EARLY MEDICINAL PRACTICES OF INDIAN TRIBES TO THE ESTABLISHMENT AND DEVELOPMENT OF THE CASA DE BENEFICENCIA IN SAN JUAN DURING THE 19TH CENTURY. GENERAL CHARACTERISTICS OF THE SOCIAL STRUCTURE OF THE ISLAND'S PRIMITIVE INDIAN TRIBES INCLUDED A VERY SYSTEMATIC AND THOROUGH METHOD OF "PUBLIC ASSISTANCE." THIS IS IN DIRECT CONTRAST TO THE EARLY YEARS OF THE CASA DE BENEFICENCIA (FIRST OPENED IN 1844), WHERE MENTAL PATIENTS AS WELL AS ORPHANS AND OTHER TYPES OF SOCIAL MARGINALS WERE CONFINED TOGETHER AND EXPOSED TO CRUEL TREATMENT, VICE, AND DEGENERATION. IN 1863, UNDER THE DIRECTION OF THE SPANISH SISTERS OF CHARITY, THIS ASYLUM UNDERWENT A GREAT DEAL OF CHANGE AND PATIENTS WERE AWARDED MORE FREEDOM AND PRIVILEGES. SECULARIZED IN 1871, THE ASYLUM WAS SUBSEQUENTLY DIVIDED INTO DEPARTMENTS ACCORDING TO THE AGE AND SEX OF THE PATIENTS. DOCUMENTS REGARDING THE ESTABLISHMENT AND FUNCTIONS OF THE ASYLUM ARE REPRODUCED, AS ARE PORTIONS OF ITS OFFICIAL REGULATIONS CONCERNING PURPOSE, BUDGET, DIVISION OF LABOR, NUTRITIONAL AND HYGIENE SYSTEMS, AND SECURITY. STATISTICS CONCERNING THE NUMBERS OF PATIENTS RESIDING IN THE CASA DE BENEFICENCIA ARE GIVEN. MATERIAL IN THIS CHAPTER MAY BE OF IMPORTANCE TO THOSE INTERESTED IN HISTORICAL PSYCHIATRY OR IN THE DEVELOPMENT OF MENTAL HEALTH INSTITUTIONS IN PUERTO RICO.

ACCN   002500

1579 AUTH   **ROSSELLO, J. A.**
TITL   LA INVESTIGACION CIENTIFICA EN EL PROGRAMA DE SALUD MENTAL. (SCIENTIFIC INVESTIGATION IN THE MENTAL HEALTH PROGRAM.)
SRCE   *IN J. A. ROSSELLO (ED.), MANUAL DE PSIQUIATRIA SOCIAL. SPAIN: INDUSTRIAS GRAFICAS "DIARIO-DIA," 1968, PP. 573-589. (SPANISH)*
INDX   PUERTO RICAN-I, RESOURCE UTILIZATION, DEMOGRAPHIC, PROGRAM EVALUATION, RESEARCH METHODOLOGY, EMPIRICAL
ABST   CONSIDERING STATISTICAL ANALYSIS TO BE OF THE UTMOST IMPORTANCE IN THE INVESTIGATION AND PLANNING OF PROGRAMS FOR

MENTAL HEALTH IN PUERTO RICO. THE AU-
THOR PRESENTS STATISTICAL DATA FROM THE
PSYCHIATRIC HOSPITAL IN RIO PIEDRAS,
PUERTO RICO. THE HOPE IS THAT THIS WILL
SERVE AS A MODEL UPON WHICH THE COL-
LECTION OF DATA FROM ALL HOSPITALS AND
CLINICS IN THE ISLAND MAY BE BASED. COM-
PARING THE FISCAL YEARS 1965-66 TO 1964-
65, DATA INCLUDE NEW ADMISSIONS, READ-
MISSIONS, RELEASES, DEATHS, LENGTH OF
STAYS, REASONS FOR CONFINEMENT, AGES
AND SEXES OF PATIENTS, GEOGRAPHIC RE-
GION OF PATIENTS, AND ADMISSIONS TO THE
INTENSIVE TREATMENT AND GERIATRIC UNITS.
SOME OF THE MORE SIGNIFICANT FINDINGS
INCLUDE (1) A 56% INCREASE IN THE NUMBER
OF PATIENTS ADMITTED WITH PERSONALITY
DISORDERS, (2) A 34% INCREASE IN PATIENTS
WITH PSYCHONEUROTIC DISORDERS, AND (3)
A 52% INCREASE IN THE ADMISSION OF CHIL-
DREN AGE 17 OR YOUNGER. HOWEVER, NO
DISCUSSION OF THE DATA IS GIVEN NOR ARE
ANY CONCLUSIONS DRAWN. 14 GRAPHS AND
TABLES ARE INCLUDED. MATERIAL PRESENTED
MAY BE OF INTEREST TO THOSE DESIRING
PUERTO RICAN MENTAL HEALTH STATISTICS
FOR THE MID-SIXTIES FOR PURPOSES OF COM-
PARISON WITH PRESENT CONDITIONS.

ACCN   002293

1580 AUTH   **ROSSELLO, J. A.**
TITL   LA PSIQUIATRIA Y LA LEY. (PSYCHIATRY AND
THE LAW.)
SRCE   *IN J. A. ROSSELLO (ED.), MANUAL DE PSIQUIA-
TRIA SOCIAL. SPAIN: INDUSTRIAS GRAFICAS,
"DIARIO-DIA," 1968, PP. 591-607. (SPANISH)*
INDX   PUERTO RICAN-I, LEGISLATION, MENTAL
HEALTH, ESSAY
ABST   PUERTO RICAN LEGISLATION PERTAINING TO
THE ADMISSION AND TREATMENT OF THE MEN-
TALLY ILL IN PSYCHIATRIC HOSPITALS IS VIEWED
IN A POSITIVE LIGHT BY THE AUTHOR. AL-
THOUGH NO COMMENT IS MADE ABOUT SPE-
CIFIC ARTICLES IN THE LAW, IT IS STATED IN
THE INTRODUCTION THAT PUERTO RICO'S
MENTAL HEALTH LAW IS CLEAR, PRECISE, AND
RESPECTFUL TO THE INDIVIDUAL, AND IT IS
ALSO BENEFICIAL TO BOTH PSYCHIATRIC RE-
SEARCH AND TREATMENT. IT IS EXPLAINED, AS
WELL, THAT AMENDMENTS IN RECENT DEC-
ADES HAVE MADE A GREAT STEP FORWARD IN
COMPARISON TO EARLY LEGISLATION. THE
SECTIONS OF THE LAW DEALT WITH IN THE DIS-
CUSSION CONCERN THE ADMISSION OF PA-
TIENTS TO MENTAL HOSPITALS, FORCED COM-
MITMENTS, UNAUTHORIZED EXIT OF PATIENTS,
APPREHENSION, COSTS OF HOSPITALIZATION,
PERSONAL COSTS TO PATIENTS, AND CRUELTY
TOWARDS THE INSANE. THOSE LAWS DEALING
WITH FORENSIC AND PENAL PSYCHIATRY ARE
NOT DISCUSSED BECAUSE REVISIONS TO THE
PENAL CODE IN THIS AREA ARE PENDING. THE
MATERIAL PRESENTED HERE MAY BE OF INTER-
EST TO THOSE STUDYING THE RELATIONSHIP
BETWEEN PSYCHIATRIC RESEARCH, TREAT-
MENT, AND NATIONAL LEGISLATION IN AN EN-
VIRONMENT   WHICH   IS   PARTICULARLY
FAVORABLE.

ACCN   002294

1581 AUTH   **ROSSELLO, J. A.**
TITL   PROCEDIMIENTO DE INGRESO AL HOSPITAL
DE PSIQUIATRIA Y LEYES DE HIGIENE MENTAL
DE PUERTO RICO. (ADMISSION PROCEDURES
TO PSYCHIATRIC HOSPITALS AND THE MENTAL
HYGIENE LAWS OF PUERTO RICO.)
SRCE   *IN J. A. ROSSELLO (ED.), TRATADO GENERAL
DE PSIQUIATRIA. PUERTO RICO: UNIVERSIDAD
DE PUERTO RICO, 1962, PP. 525-544. (SPANISH)*
INDX   PUERTO RICAN-I, LEGISLATION, MENTAL
HEALTH, POLICY, INSTITUTIONALIZATION, ES-
SAY, PSYCHOTHERAPY
ABST   THE LAWS OF THE PUERTO RICAN LEGISLA-
TIVE ASSEMBLY WHICH PERTAIN TO MENTAL
HEALTH ARE EXAMINED IN TERMS OF THEIR IM-
PACT UPON THE PROCESS OF ADMITTING AND
MAINTAINING PATIENTS IN PSYCHIATRIC HOS-
PITALS. THOSE PORTIONS OF THE MENTAL
HEALTH LAWS WHICH ARE DISCUSSED CON-
CERN ADMISSIONS, UNAUTHORIZED EXIT OF
PATIENTS AND THE ENSUING APPREHENSION
PROCEDURES, DECLARATIONS OF RECLU-
SION, PAYMENT FOR TREATMENT, AND CRU-
ELTY TOWARDS THE INSANE. REGARDING AD-
MISSIONS IN THE CASE OF ORAL SOLICITATION,
THE PATIENT RECEIVES ATTENTION IMMEDI-
ATELY. IF MENTAL AND PHYSICAL EXAMINA-
TIONS DEEM HOSPITALIZATION NECESSARY,
THE PATIENT'S CONFINEMENT IS KEPT TO THE
SHORTEST POSSIBLE TIME, WITH A MAXIMUM
OF FREEDOM GRANTED. OVERALL, THE GOAL
OF PUERTO RICAN MENTAL HEALTH IS TO RE-
TURN THE PATIENT TO AN ACTIVE ROLE IN SO-
CIETY; AND WHENEVER POSSIBLE, PATIENTS
RECEIVE OUT-PATIENT TREATMENT WHICH AL-
LOWS THEM TO REMAIN WITH THEIR FAMILIES.
IN 1959-60, OVER 40,000 PATIENTS THROUGH-
OUT PUERTO RICO RECEIVED SUCH OUT-PA-
TIENT TREATMENT.

ACCN   002468

1582 AUTH   **ROSSELLO, J. A. (ED.)**
TITL   TRATADO GENERAL DE PSIQUITRIA. (GENERAL
TOPICS IN PSYCHIATRY.)
SRCE   *PUERTO RICO: UNIVERSIDAD DE PUERTO RICO,
1962. (SPANISH)*
INDX   PUERTO RICAN-I, MENTAL HEALTH, MENTAL
HEALTH PROFESSION, PROFESSIONAL TRAIN-
ING, HIGHER EDUCATION, EDUCATIONAL MA-
TERIALS, HISTORY, NEUROSIS, PSYCHOSIS,
PSYCHOPHARMACOLOGY,   PSYCHOPATHOL-
OGY, ALCOHOLISM, DRUG ABUSE, CRIMINOL-
OGY, ADMINISTRATORS, PROGRAM EVALUA-
TION, ESSAY, REVIEW, JUDICIAL PROCESS, BOOK
ABST   THIS TEXT BOOK—COMPRISED OF 27 CHAP-
TERS—IS INTENDED TO PROVIDE TEACHING
GUIDELINES FOR BOTH THE MEDICAL AND SO-
CIAL ASPECTS OF PSYCHIATRY AT THE UNIVER-
SITY OF PUERTO RICO'S DEPARTMENT OF PSY-
CHIATRY   AND   PUERTO   RICO'S   STATE
PSYCHIATRIC HOSPITAL AND MENTAL HEALTH
PROGRAM. ITS AUTHORS INCLUDE PROFES-
SORS OF PSYCHIATRY, PRACTICING PSYCHIA-
TRISTS, SOCIAL PSYCHOLOGISTS, PEDIATRI-
CIANS, AND REGISTERED NURSES. MOST OF
THE CHAPTERS ARE OF A GENERAL NATURE,

DEALING WITH SUCH PROBLEMS AS NEURO-LOGICAL FUNCTIONS AND DISORDERS, MENTAL ILLNESS SYMPTOMATOLOGY, PSYCHO-PHYSIOLOGICAL REACTIONS, ALCOHOLISM, AND DRUG ADDICTION. THERE ARE, HOWEVER, OTHER CHAPTERS WHICH DEAL SPECIFICALLY WITH THE PRACTICE OF PSYCHIATRY AND THE STATE OF MENTAL DISORDERS IN PUERTO RICO. THESE CHAPTERS CONCERN FORENSIC AND PENAL PSYCHIATRY, CRIMINAL RESPONSIBILITY, CONFIDENTIALITY AND PRIVILEGED COMMUNICATION, PROGRAM ADMINISTRATION, SOCIAL WORK, THE TEACHING OF PSYCHIATRY, THE USE OF NARCOTICS, THE HISTORY OF PUERTO RICAN PSYCHIATRIC INSTITUTIONS, AND THE ISLAND'S LEGISLATION AND LAWS PERTAINING TO MENTAL HEALTH. APPENDED TO THE TEXT ARE AN EXTENSIVE INDEX AND A BILINGUAL GLOSSARY OF PSYCHIATRIC TERMINOLOGY.

ACCN   002499

1583 AUTH   **ROTHENBERG, A.**
TITL   PUERTO RICO AND AGGRESSION.
SRCE   *AMERICAN JOURNAL OF PSYCHIATRY, 1964, 120(10), 962-970.*
INDX   PUERTO RICAN-I, AGGRESSION, ESSAY, EMPIRICAL, CULTURAL FACTORS, STRESS, PSYCHOPATHOLOGY, CRIMINOLOGY
ABST   THE DIFFICULTY OF PUERTO RICANS TO SELF-REGULATE FEELINGS OF AGGRESSION AND ANGER IS EXAMINED. CULTURAL IDEALS WHICH TEND TO EMPHASIZE PERSONALITY QUALITIES SUCH AS DIGNIDAD (DIGNITY) AND HOSPITALIDAD (HOSPITALITY) TEND TO PRESERVE A SOCIAL APPEARANCE AT THE EXPENSE OF INNER PSYCHOLOGICAL NEEDS. THUS THE ADHERENCE TO THESE IDEALS RESULTS IN SUPPRESSION AND REPRESSION OF ASSERTIVENESS AND AGGRESSIVENESS. SINCE SOCIALLY DIRECT ASSERTIVENESS IS FROWNED UPON, MALADAPTIVE WAYS OF EXPRESSING AGGRESSION SUCH AS ANGRY OUTBURSTS, SUDDEN VIOLENCE OR SELF-DESTRUCTIVENESS LEAD TO SERIOUS SOCIAL PROBLEMS. FOR EXAMPLE, NON-NEGLIGENT MANSLAUGHTER IN PUERTO RICO IN 1961 WAS 7.1 PER 100,000 POPULATION AS COMPARED TO 4.7 PER 100,-000 POPULATION IN THE UNITED STATES. MOST MURDERS APPEAR TO BE NON-PREMEDITATED OR CRIMES OF PASSION (SO-CALLED CRIMENES PERSONALES). PREMEDITATED MURDER FOR MONETARY GAIN IS ALMOST UNHEARD OF ON THE ISLAND. CRIMES OF VIOLENCE DO NOT SEEM TO RESULT PRIMARILY FROM ANTICOLONIAL FEELINGS, ETHNIC PROBLEMS, OR PECUNIARY MOTIVATIONS BUT MORE FROM SUDDEN LOSS OF CONTROL IN PERSONAL RELATIONSHIPS. IT IS CONCLUDED THAT MUCH OF THE PRESENT PROBLEM IS GENERATED BY THE IMPACT OF CULTURE CHANGE AND A NEED TO ADAPT TO NEW VALUES AND ECONOMIC PROBLEMS. LARGE FAMILIES AND CONSEQUENT PROBLEMS IN CHILDREARING PRACTICES SERVE TO PERPETUATE PROBLEMS IN HANDLING AGGRESSION. 39 REFERENCES.

ACCN   001367

1584 AUTH   **ROZYNKO, V., & WENK, E.**
TITL   INTELLECTUAL PERFORMANCE OF THREE DELINQUENT GROUPS OF DIFFERENT ETHNIC ORIGIN.
SRCE   *JOURNAL OF CONSULTING PSYCHOLOGY, 1965, 29(3), 282.*
INDX   INTELLIGENCE, CALIFORNIA TEST OF MENTAL MATURITY, DELINQUENCY, CROSS CULTURAL, EMPIRICAL, MEXICAN AMERICAN, INTELLIGENCE TESTING
ABST   AN INVESTIGATION OF INTELLECTUAL TEST DIFFERENCES AMONG DELINQUENT WHITE, NEGRO, AND MEXICAN AMERICAN (MA) CALIFORNIA YOUTH AUTHORITY (CYA) INMATES IS PRESENTED. THE SUBJECTS WERE ADMINISTERED THE CALIFORNIA TEST OF MENTAL MATURITY (CTMM) AND THE GENERAL APTITUDE TEST BATTERY (GATB). THREE INDEPENDENT STUDIES WERE CONDUCTED, WITH ALL SUBJECTS RANDOMLY DISTRIBUTED. THE FIRST STUDY CONTAINED 78 SUBJECTS IN EACH OF THE THREE SUBGROUPS WHILE THE SECOND AND THIRD CONTAINED 50 IN EACH SUBGROUP. AN ANALYSIS OF VARIANCE SHOWED THAT ON THE CTMM FOR ALL THREE STUDIES, THE WHITE GROUP SCORED HIGHEST, THE NEGRO GROUP LOWEST. THE MA GROUP WAS EQUAL TO THE NEGRO GROUP IN THE LANGUAGE PORTION OF THE TEST AND TENDED TO OCCUPY AN INTERMEDIATE POSITION BETWEEN THE NEGRO AND WHITE GROUPS ON THE NONLANGUAGE PORTIONS OF THE TEST. THE NEGROES SCORED CONSISTENTLY LOW ON BOTH THE VERBAL AND NONVERBAL SECTIONS OF THE GATB, WHEREAS THE WHITES SCORED CONSISTENTLY HIGH. THE MA'S OCCUPIED AN INTERMEDIATE POSITION ON THE NONVERBAL TESTS BUT WERE AS LOW AS NEGROES ON THE VERBAL TESTS. THE MA GROUP PERFORMED MOST POORLY WHEN GOOD PERFORMANCE DEPENDED ON EITHER LANGUAGE ABILITY OR KNOWLEDGE OF MATERIAL TAUGHT IN SCHOOL; THEY PERFORMED BEST ON NON-ACADEMIC SUBJECTS. TEST DIFFERENCES BETWEEN THE WHITE AND MA GROUP PARALLELED THE DIFFERENCES IN EDUCATIONAL LEVELS.

ACCN   001368

1585 AUTH   **RUBEL, A. J.**
TITL   CONCEPTS OF DISEASE IN MEXICAN-AMERICAN CULTURE.
SRCE   *AMERICAN ANTHROPOLOGIST, 1960, 62(5), 795-814.*
INDX   HEALTH, FOLK MEDICINE, MEXICAN AMERICAN, CULTURE, FAMILY STRUCTURE, DISEASE, CASE STUDY, THEORETICAL, RURAL, CURANDERISMO, TEXAS, SOUTHWEST, ATTITUDES, CULTURAL CHANGE, SYMPTOMATOLOGY
ABST   THE MANNER IN WHICH TRADITIONAL CONCEPTS OF HEALTH AND DISEASE CONTRIBUTE TO THE MAINTENANCE OF THE MEXICAN AMERICAN (MA) SOCIAL SYSTEM IN TEXAS IS EXAMINED. FIVE ILLNESSES WHICH ARE CULTURALLY CONFINED TO THE MA ARE CAIDA DE LA MOLLERA (FALLEN FONTANEL), EMPACHO (INTESTINE BLOCK BY A BOLUS OF FOOD), MAL OJO (EVIL EYE), SUSTO (SHOCK), AND

MAL PUESTO (SORCERY). THE FIRST FOUR ILLNESSES ARE CATEGORIZED AS "MALES NATURALES" (SICKNESSES FROM NATURAL CAUSE WITHIN THE REALM OF GOD), WHILE MAL PUESTO IS CONSIDERED ARTIFICIAL OR OUTSIDE THE REALM OF GOD. A DESCRIPTION OF EACH OF THE FOUR ILLNESSES WHICH ARE CONCEPTUALLY BOUND TOGETHER BY MA'S IS PRESENTED WITH CASE STUDY ILLUSTRATIONS. A DISCUSSION OF THE MA FAMILIAL STRUCTURE WHICH EXAMINES THE ROLES OF HERMANOS, PRIMO HERMANOS, CONCUNOS, HIJAS, SOBRINAS, PADRINOS, AND COMPADRES IS PRESENTED. IT IS SHOWN THAT THE FOUR ILLNESSES HAVE REMAINED FIRMLY EMBEDDED IN THE MA SOCIOCULTURAL FRAMEWORK DESPITE THE INTRODUCTION OF AN ALTERNATE SYSTEM OF BELIEF AND COMPETING HEALING WAYS. IT IS ARGUED THAT THREE OF THE FOUR ILLNESSES FUNCTION TO SUSTAIN SOME OF THE DOMINANT VALUES OF MA CULTURE BY EMPHASIZING MAINTENANCE OF THE SOLIDARITY OF A SMALL, BILATERAL FAMILY UNIT AND BY PRESCRIBING THE APPROPRIATE ROLE BEHAVIORS OF MALES AND FEMALES AND OF OLDER AND YOUNGER INDIVIDUALS. THOSE WHOSE ORIENTATION IS TOWARD ADOPTION OF ANGLO AMERICAN SOCIOCULTURAL BEHAVIOR TEND TO DISPARAGE THESE CONCEPTS OF ILLNESS AS INGENUOUS BELIEFS. BUT THE MORE CREDULOUS INDIVIDUALS SEIZE UPON EVERY AVAILABLE OPPORTUNITY TO VOUCH FOR THE AUTHENTICITY OF THE ILLNESS. 7 REFERENCES.

ACCN   001369

1586 AUTH   **RUBEL, A. J.**
TITL   THE EPIDEMIOLOGY OF A FOLK ILLNESS: SUSTO IN HISPANIC AMERICA.
SRCE   *ETHNOLOGY, 1964, 3(3), 268-283.*
INDX   MEXICAN AMERICAN, PEER GROUP, INTERPERSONAL RELATIONS, ADOLESCENTS, MALE, RESEARCH METHODOLOGY, HEALTH, EMPIRICAL, CULTURAL FACTORS, CURANDERISMO, MENTAL HEALTH
ABST   A PRELIMINARY DISCUSSION OF SOME OF THE METHODOLOGICAL PROBLEMS IN STUDYING FOLK ILLNESSES IS FOLLOWED BY AN EXAMINATION OF ONE SUCH ILLNESS—"SUSTO" (FRIGHT), AN HISPANIC-AMERICAN FOLK ILLNESS. THE SUSTO SYNDROME IS FOUNDED UPON THE BELIEF THAT AN INDIVIDUAL IS COMPOSED OF BOTH A CORPOREAL BEING AND ONE OR MORE IMMATERIAL SOULS OR SPIRITS. SUSTO OCCURS IF THESE SOULS BECOME DETACHED FROM THE BODY, OFTEN AS THE CONSEQUENCE OF AN UNSETTLING, FRIGHTENING EXPERIENCE. THE CHARACTERISTICS OF THE SYNDROME ARE AS FOLLOWS: (1) DURING SLEEP THE PATIENT EVIDENCES RESTLESSNESS; AND (2) AWAKE, THE PATIENT IS CHARACTERIZED BY LISTLESSNESS, LOSS OF APPETITE, LACK OF INTEREST IN DRESS AND PERSONAL HYGIENE, LOSS OF STRENGTH, DEPRESSION, AND INTROVERSION. ELEVEN CASE STUDIES ILLUSTRATE THE CIRCUMSTANCES SURROUNDING THE ONSET OF SUSTO AND PROVIDE SOME OF THE SOCIAL AND PERSONALITY CHARACTERISTICS OF THE PATIENTS. A DISCUSSION IS ALSO PRESENTED OF THE CURING RITES ASSOCIATED WITH THE SUSTO SYNDROME. A TENTATIVE HYPOTHESIS PROPOSES THAT SUSTO AMONG HISPANIC AMERICANS MAY BE UNDERSTOOD TO BE THE PRODUCT OF A COMPLEX INTERACTION BETWEEN AN INDIVIDUAL'S STATE OF HEALTH AND THE ROLE EXPECTATIONS WHICH HIS SOCIETY PROVIDES, MEDIATED BY ASPECTS OF THE INDIVIDUAL'S PERSONALITY. 31 REFERENCES.

ACCN   001370

1587 AUTH   **RUBEL, A. J.**
TITL   THE MEXICAN AMERICAN PALOMILLA.
SRCE   *ANTHROPOLOGICAL LINGUISTICS, 1965, 7(4), 92-97.*
INDX   MEXICAN AMERICAN, ESSAY, PEER GROUP, INTERPERSONAL RELATIONS, ADOLESCENTS, MALE, CASE STUDY, FICTIVE KINSHIP, COMMUNITY, TEXAS, SOUTHWEST, SEX ROLES, SOCIAL STRUCTURE, DEVIANCE, CULTURE
ABST   THE BASIC ORGANIZATIONAL FEATURES OF THE MEXICAN AMERICAN (MA) PALOMILLA, A VOLUNTARY FRIENDSHIP ORGANIZATION, IN SOUTH TEXAS ARE DISCUSSED. GENERICALLY, PALOMILLA REFERS TO AN EGOCENTRIC ASSOCIATION OF YOUNG MA MALES WHO INTERACT WITH SOME FREQUENCY. PALOMILLAS ARE PARTICULARISTIC, PERSONAL, VOLUNTARY, AND NONINSTRUMENTAL; THEY LACK SUCH CORPORATE ATTRIBUTES AS GROUP NAME, IDENTIFICATION WITH A PARTICULAR TERRITORY, IN-GROUP SENTIMENTS, OR EVEN PERSISTENCE OVER TIME. THE ABSENCE OF INSTRUMENTAL LEADERS AND THE FAILURE OF THE PARTICIPANTS TO CONSISTENTLY ALLOCATE DIFFERENTIAL ROLES TO ONE ANOTHER ARE NOTED. IT IS IN THE PALOMILLA, RATHER THAN IN THE FAMILY, THAT A BOY BECOMES A MAN AND LEARNS TO EXPRESS HIMSELF AS SUCH. IT HAS BEEN SUGGESTED THAT PALOMILLAS PERMIT YOUNG MEN TO CONDUCT THEMSELVES IN A MANNER WHICH IS QUITE INCOMPATIBLE WITH THE KIND OF BEHAVIOR DEMANDED OF THEM WITHIN THE STRUCTURE AND VALUES OF THE MA FAMILY. THE SUPPORTIVE ROLE OF THE PALOMILLA IN TWO LIFE CRISES SITUATIONS, THE TRANSITION PERIOD BETWEEN BETROTHAL AND MARRIAGE, AND BEREAVEMENT IS SHOWN. EMPIRICAL DATA DEMONSTRATE THAT THESE AMORPHOUS FRIENDSHIP ASSOCIATIONS ARE IMPORTANT BOTH TO THE INDIVIDUAL PARTICIPANTS AND TO THE SOCIETY OF WHICH THEY ARE A PART. AN MA'S INVOLVEMENT IN PALOMILLA ACTIVITIES IS A PERIOD IN HIS DEVELOPMENT WITHIN THE STRUCTURE OF MA CULTURE AND SOCIALIZATION. 8 REFERENCES.

ACCN   001371

1588 AUTH   **RUBINSTEIN, D.**
TITL   BEYOND THE CULTURAL BARRIERS: OBSERVA-

TIONS ON EMOTIONAL DISORDERS AMONG CUBAN IMMIGRANTS.

SRCE *INTERNATIONAL JOURNAL OF MENTAL HEALTH, 1976, 5(2), 69-79.*

INDX CUBAN, IMMIGRATION, RELIGION, ATTITUDES, MENTAL HEALTH, FOLK MEDICINE, PSYCHOTHERAPY, ACCULTURATION, FAMILY STRUCTURE, CASE STUDY, ADOLESCENTS, ADULTS, PSYCHOPATHOLOGY, CULTURAL FACTORS, SYMPTOMATOLOGY, STRESS, DEPRESSION, ANOMIE

ABST TWO CASE STUDIES ARE PRESENTED AS ILLUSTRATIVE OF CERTAIN ASPECTS OF EMOTIONAL DISORDERS AMONG CUBAN IMMIGRANTS. SOCIAL AND CULTURAL FACTORS ARE EMPHASIZED WHICH TEND TO INFLUENCE THE DISORDER. THE STRESSES OF EMIGRATION AND THE LOSS OF TRADITIONAL WAYS OF DEALING WITH EMOTIONAL DIFFICULTIES ARE DISCUSSED, AND THE PREDOMINANCE OF MAGIC AND RELIGIOUS/MYSTIC PHENOMENA IN THE MANIFESTATION OF EMOTIONAL DISORDER IS NOTED. DESPITE THE FREQUENCY OF HALLUCINATIONS AND DELUSIONS, SUCH DISORDERS ARE MORE LIKELY TO BE DEPRESSIVE RATHER THAN SCHIZOPHRENIC AND THEY RESPOND WELL TO ANTIDEPRESSANTS. 4 REFERENCES. (PASAR ABSTRACT MODIFIED)

ACCN 001372

1589 AUTH **RUEBENS, E. P.**
TITL OUR URBAN GHETTOS IN BRITISH PERSPECTIVE.
SRCE *URBAN AFFAIRS QUARTERLY, 1971, 6(3), 319-340.*
INDX URBAN, COMMUNITY, PUERTO RICAN-I, ESSAY, CROSS CULTURAL, PREJUDICE
ABST SOME ESSENTIAL AND CRUCIAL FEATURES OF U.S. URBAN GHETTO PROBLEMS ARE TENDING TO BE SUBMERGED AND POSTPONED RATHER THAN FACED AND RESOLVED. AMONG THE MOST CRUCIAL FEATURES IS THE INTERRELATIONSHIP BETWEEN THE ECONOMIC AND THE SOCIAL ASPECTS OF THE GHETTO. IN GREAT BRITAIN A COMPARABLE PATTERN OF COLORED MINORITIES MOVING INTO AN INDUSTRIAL ECONOMY AND A WHITE SOCIETY IS FOUND. IT IS A FLOW OF IMMIGRANTS INTO BRITAIN MAINLY FROM THE NEW COMMONWEALTH AREAS OF ASIA, AFRICA, AND THE WEST INDIES. MOST HAVE COME SINCE 1954 AND SETTLED PRIMARILY IN THE GREAT URBAN CENTERS, PARTICULARLY IN CERTAIN DISTRICTS. ALTHOUGH MUCH SMALLER IN SCALE, THIS PATTERN IS SIMILAR IN MANY FEATURES TO THE MIGRATIONS OF SOUTHERN NEGROES AND SPANISH-CULTURE PUERTO RICANS TO THE NORTHERN CITIES IN THE UNITED STATES. LIKEWISE, THE IMPACT IN BRITAIN HAS COME OUT IN COLORED PROTESTS AND WHITE BACKLASHES, A FEW VIOLENT OUTBREAKS, AND EVEN THE BEGINNINGS OF BLACK POWER MOVEMENTS AND WHITE YOUTH RACIST GANGS. HOWEVER, SO FAR NOTHING HAS OCCURRED THERE ON THE ORDER OF THE GREAT URBAN RACE RIOTS IN THE UNITED STATES DURING THE LAST FEW YEARS. 16 REFERENCES.
ACCN 001373

1590 AUTH **RUEDA, R., & PEROZZI, J. A.**
TITL A COMPARISON OF TWO SPANISH TESTS OF RECEPTIVE LANGUAGE.
SRCE *JOURNAL OF SPEECH AND HEARING DISORDERS, 1977, 42(2), 210-215.*
INDX BILINGUAL, BILINGUALISM, CHILDREN, EMPIRICAL, LANGUAGE ACQUISITION, LANGUAGE ASSESSMENT, LINGUISTIC COMPETENCE, MEXICAN AMERICAN, SOUTHWEST, SYNTAX, TEST VALIDITY
ABST FOR SPANISH-SPEAKING CHILDREN, MINIMAL ENGLISH LANGUAGE SKILLS CAN BE COMPOUNDED BY LINGUISTIC DEFICITS IN SPANISH. IDENTIFICATION AND ASSESSMENT OF CHILDREN DEVELOPMENTALLY DELAYED IN SPANISH LANGUAGE ACQUISITION IS NECESSARY BUT SHOULD FOLLOW CAREFUL ASSESSMENT OF SPANISH DOMINANCE. IN THE PRESENT STUDY, THE JAMES LANGUAGE DOMINANCE TEST WAS ADMINISTERED TO 20 SPANISH-DOMINANT MEXICAN AMERICAN CHILDREN PRIOR TO THE ADMINISTRATION OF TWO DEVELOPMENTAL SPANISH TESTS OF RECEPTIVE LANGUAGE ABILITY: THE RECEPTIVE PORTION OF THE SCREENING TEST OF SPANISH GRAMMAR (STSG) AND THE SPANISH VERSION OF THE TEST OF AUDITORY COMPREHENSION OF LANGUAGE (TACL). THE CORRELATION OBTAINED BETWEEN THE TWO TESTS WAS NOT STATISTICALLY SIGNIFICANT. THE CORRELATION OBTAINED BETWEEN 24 SYNTACTICAL ITEMS COMMON TO BOTH TESTS WAS ALSO NOT STATISTICALLY SIGNIFICANT. IT IS HYPOTHESIZED THAT THESE NONSIGNIFICANT CORRELATIONS REFLECT THE FACT THAT THE TACL ITEMS ARE DIRECT ENGLISH TRANSLATIONS, A PROCEDURE OF DUBIOUS VALIDITY. THE TRANSLATION OF ENGLISH LANGUAGE TESTS INTO SPANISH IS SEEN AS AN INAPPROPRIATE MEANS OF MEASURING SPANISH-SPEAKING CHILDREN'S LINGUISTIC ABILITIES BECAUSE THE TRANSLATED TESTS REFLECT CULTURAL AND LINGUISTIC VALUES WHICH MAY NOT BE PRESENT AMONG THE SPANISH-SPEAKING POPULATION. FURTHER, CRITICAL ANALYSIS OF THE TACL ITEMS REVEAL BOTH TRANSLATION DIFFICULTIES AND AMBIGUOUS PICTORIAL REPRESENTATIONS OF STIMULI. 8 REFERENCES. (AUTHOR ABSTRACT MODIFIED)
ACCN 002533

1591 AUTH **RUEVENI, U.**
TITL USING SENSITIVITY TRAINING WITH JUNIOR HIGH SCHOOL STUDENTS.
SRCE *CHILDREN, 1971, 18(2), 69-72.*
INDX ADOLESCENTS, EMPIRICAL, PUERTO RICAN-M, AGGRESSION, GROUP DYNAMICS, TEACHERS, ATTITUDES, BEHAVIOR THERAPY, URBAN, PENNSYLVANIA, EAST
ABST A SUCCESSFUL PROGRAM OF SENSITIVITY TRAINING FOR 15 AGGRESSIVE JUNIOR HIGH SCHOOL STUDENTS WHOSE BEHAVIOR HAD BEEN CHARACTERIZED BY DESTRUCTIVENESS, TRUANCY, AND FIGHTING IS DESCRIBED. THE EXPERIMENT WAS CONDUCTED FOR 2 HOURS ONCE A WEEK OVER A PERIOD OF 5 MONTHS IN A SCHOOL IN A DENSELY POPULATED BLACK NEIGHBORHOOD OF PHILADELPHIA. SUB-

JECTS INCLUDED 10 BLACK AND 5 PUERTO RI-
CAN STUDENTS FROM 13 TO 15 YEARS OF AGE
(EIGHT BOYS AND SEVEN GIRLS) WHO WERE
VOLUNTEERS FROM A LIST OF NAMES SUBMIT-
TED BY THEIR TEACHER. OBJECTIVES OF THE
PROGRAM WERE TO HELP THE STUDENTS IN-
CREASE THEIR SOCIAL SENSITIVITY AND THEIR
BEHAVIORAL FLEXIBILITY. VARIOUS GROUP
THERAPY TECHNIQUES AND EXERCISES WERE
USED TO ENHANCE THE GROUP PROCESS, IN-
CLUDING STRENGTH BOMBARDMENT OF
POSITIVE FEELINGS AND FREE EXPRESSION OF
NEGATIVE FEELINGS. STUDENTS IN THE EX-
PERIMENT WERE ENTHUSIASTIC AND INCI-
DENCES OF TRUANCY AND AGGRESSION
AMONG THEM DECREASED. MOREOVER, MANY
TEACHERS INDICATED THAT THEIR OWN ATTI-
TUDES TOWARD STUDENTS IN THE GROUP
HAD BECOME MORE POSITIVE. SUCCESS OF
THE EXPERIMENT LED TO FORMATION OF AN-
OTHER TRAINING GROUP IN THE CURRENT
YEAR. 7 REFERENCES.

ACCN   001374

1592 AUTH   **RUIZ, A. S.**
    TITL   THE CHICANO AND TRANSACTIONAL ANALY-
    SIS.
    SRCE   *TRANSACTIONAL ANALYSIS, 1976, 6(1), 37-40.*
    INDX   MEXICAN AMERICAN, PSYCHOTHERAPY, ES-
    SAY, MENTAL HEALTH, CULTURAL PLURALISM,
    PROFESSIONAL TRAINING, POLICY
    ABST   LANGUAGE AND CULTURAL DIFFERENCES HAVE
    NOT TYPICALLY BEEN PART OF THE FORMAL
    EDUCATIONAL PROCESS FOR PSYCHOTHER-
    APY. WITHIN THE CONTEXT OF THE TRANSAC-
    TIONAL ANALYSIS MODEL, INFORMATION AND
    CONSIDERATIONS OF CHICANO CULTURE ARE
    PRESENTED AND CHICANO LANGUAGE AND
    CULTURAL IMPLICATIONS ARE DISCUSSED IN
    TERMS OF THE PSYCHOLOGICAL ASSESSMENT
    OF CHICANOS. EGO STATE ANALYSIS SHOULD
    BE DONE WITH AWARENESS OF UNIQUE LAN-
    GUAGE AND CULTURE AS WELL AS KNOWL-
    EDGE OF PAST INTERACTIONAL PATTERNS.
    SCRIPT ANALYSIS, GAME ANALYSIS, STROKES,
    AND DISCOUNTS CAN ALL BE RECAST BY IN-
    CORPORATING CHICANO CULTURAL AND LAN-
    GUAGE EXPRESSIONS AND BY RECOGNIZING
    THE CHICANO EXPERIENCE OF OPPRESSION
    AND RACISM. FINALLY, A RECOMMENDATION IS
    MADE TO REVIEW TRANSACTIONAL ANALYSIS
    VOCABULARY AND REMOVE SUCH INACCUR-
    ATE, INAPPROPRIATE TERMINOLOGY AS
    "MACHO" AND "BROWN STAMPS." 7 REFER-
    ENCES.

ACCN   001375

1593 AUTH   **RUIZ, A. S.**
    TITL   CHICANO GROUP CATALYSTS.
    SRCE   *PERSONNEL AND GUIDANCE JOURNAL, 1975,*
    53(6), 462-466.
    INDX   MEXICAN AMERICAN, PSYCHOTHERAPY, PSY-
    CHOTHERAPY OUTCOME, ETHNIC IDENTITY, BI-
    LINGUAL, GROUP DYNAMICS, ESSAY, EDUCA-
    TIONAL COUNSELING, COLLEGE STUDENTS,
    ADOLESCENTS, CULTURAL PLURALISM
    ABST   ETHNICITY IS A FACTOR WHICH HAS GENER-
    ALLY BEEN IGNORED BY THE GROWTH GROUP

THERAPY MOVEMENT. RECOGNIZING THE IM-
PORTANCE OF LANGUAGE AND CULTURE FOR
CHICANOS, SEVEN INTERACTION FACILITATION
TECHNIQUES WERE DEVELOPED BY MEANS OF
CHICANO GROUP CATALYSTS TO DEMON-
STRATE HOW ETHNICITY CAN BE INCORPO-
RATED INTO GROWTH GROUPS. TECHNIQUES
INCLUDED ARE: RESOLVING UNFINISHED BUSI-
NESS, RECLAIMING IGNORED PARTS OF THEM-
SELVES, VALIDATING GROUP ETHNICITY AND
COHESION, TAPPING POTENTIAL AND EN-
HANCING GROWTH, AND FACILITATING THE
SELF-ACTUALIZATION OF GROUP MEMBERS.
THE TECHNIQUES WERE USED WITH CHICANO
UNIVERSITY STUDENTS, CHICANO HIGH
SCHOOL STUDENTS, NEIGHBORHOOD YOUTH
CORPS STUDENTS, AND PROGRAM COORDI-
NATORS. WITH MINOR SUBSTITUTIONS OR
MODIFICATIONS, COUNSELORS CAN MAKE USE
OF SOME OF THE CATALYSTS WITH OTHER
CULTURAL GROUPS. PARTICIPANT EVALUA-
TIONS OF EFFECTIVENESS SUGGEST IN-
CREASED ACCEPTANCE OF ETHNICITY AND
CHICANO CULTURAL FACTORS. 5 REFER-
ENCES. (NCMHI ABSTRACT MODIFIED)

ACCN   001376

1594 AUTH   **RUIZ, E. J.**
    TITL   INFLUENCE OF BILINGUALISM ON COMMUNI-
    CATION IN GROUPS.
    SRCE   *INTERNATIONAL JOURNAL OF GROUP PSY-*
    CHOLOGY, 1975, 25(4), 391-395.
    INDX   BILINGUALISM, PSYCHOTHERAPY, REVIEW, ES-
    SAY, CULTURAL FACTORS, ACCULTURATION,
    BILINGUAL-BICULTURAL PERSONNEL, PER-
    SONALITY, SPANISH SURNAMED, INTERPER-
    SONAL RELATIONS
    ABST   COMMUNICATION IS AFFECTED BY THE INTER-
    PLAY OF CONSCIOUS AND UNCONSCIOUS
    IDEAS WITHIN THE INDIVIDUAL, AND IN THE BI-
    LINGUAL PERSON, THIS CONFLICT BETWEEN
    CONSCIOUS AND UNCONSCIOUS MATERIAL IS
    INTENSIFIED. SINCE UNCONSCIOUS MATERIAL
    OFTEN COMES OUT MORE EASILY IN THE
    MOTHER TONGUE, THE LANGUAGE IN WHICH
    PSYCHIATRIC INTERVIEWS ARE TAKEN CAN RE-
    SULT IN SIGNIFICANT DIFFERENCES IN MEA-
    SURES OF DEPRESSION, SCHIZOPHRENIA, AND
    SUCH CULTURAL TRAITS AS FATALISM. A SEC-
    OND FACET OF SUCH COMMUNICATION FAC-
    TORS PERTAINS TO THE SOCIAL FUNCTION OF
    LANGUAGE AMONG ACCULTURATING MI-
    NORITY GROUPS. FOR EXAMPLE, IN-GROUP/
    OUT-GROUP VARIATION IN COMMUNICATION
    IS EVIDENT IN THE FINDING THAT BILINGUAL,
    SOCIAL SERVICE PROFESSIONALS HAVE MORE
    INTELLECTUALIZED AND STRUCTURED DIS-
    CUSSIONS IN ENGLISH; WHILE IN SPANISH,
    THEY EXPRESS MORE SINCERE INTERPER-
    SONAL REACTIONS AND EMOTIONS. IT IS CON-
    CLUDED THAT FEELINGS AND THOUGHT PRO-
    CESSES ARE NURTURED IN THE NATIVE
    LANGUAGE, AND THUS THE NATIVE LAN-
    GUAGE IS MORE BASIC TO PERSONALITY DE-
    VELOPMENT. 4 REFERENCES.

ACCN   002195

1595 AUTH   **RUIZ, P.**

TITL CULTURE AND MENTAL HEALTH: A HISPANIC PERSPECTIVE.

SRCE *JOURNAL OF CONTEMPORARY PSYCHOTHERAPY, 1977, 9(1), 24-27.*

INDX ATTITUDES, CULTURAL FACTORS, EMPIRICAL, FOLK MEDICINE, ESPIRITISMO, PUERTO RICAN-M, PARAPROFESSIONALS, PSYCHOTHERAPISTS, SPANISH SURNAMED, STRESS, ACCULTURATION, URBAN, NEW YORK, EAST, POLICY

ABST "ESPIRITISMO" AMONG STRESSED, ACCULTURATING PUERTO RICAN MIGRANTS IN NEW YORK CITY IS DISCUSSED IN LIGHT OF ITS ALLIANCE WITH A MENTAL HEALTH CENTER IN THE SOUTH BRONX. IT IS NOTED THAT, UNLIKE TRADITIONAL PSYCHOTHERAPISTS WHO CLASSIFY AND TREAT "INNER" PSYCHIC CONFLICTS, FOLK HEALERS IDENTIFY "OUTER" PSYCHIC CONFLICTS AND ADVERSARIES. THEIR PROFICIENCY WITH "ATAQUE" AND OTHER SUCH CULTURAL PHENOMENA ARE EXPLAINED VIA ORGANIZED DIALOGUES BETWEEN LOCAL FOLK HEALERS AND PROFESSIONALS AT THE MENTAL HEALTH CENTER OF SOUTH BRONX. ONCE BARRIERS WERE LOWERED, EACH GROUP COULD APPRECIATE THE SKILLS OF THE OTHER, AND TREATMENT COULD BE COORDINATED FOR PATIENTS USING BOTH SYSTEMS SIMULTANEOUSLY. AN IN-SERVICE TRAINING PROGRAM WAS SUBSEQUENTLY DEVELOPED FOR PROFESSIONALS AND NON-PROFESSIONALS ALIKE TO ACQUAINT THEM WITH THE CULTURAL VALUES OF THE PATIENT POPULATION AND THEIR IMPLICATIONS FOR TREATMENT. IT IS SUGGESTED THAT FURTHER TRAINING AND RECOGNIZED STATUS FOR FOLK HEALERS MIGHT AUGMENT THE RANKS OF QUALIFIED MENTAL HEALTH MANPOWER ABLE TO SERVE THE MANY HISPANICS WHO REQUIRE MENTAL HEALTH SERVICES. 5 REFERENCES.

ACCN 002295

1596 AUTH **RUIZ, P.**

TITL FOLK HEALERS AS ASSOCIATE THERAPISTS.

SRCE *CURRENT PSYCHIATRIC THERAPIES, 1976, 16, 269-275.*

INDX FOLK MEDICINE, ESPIRITISMO, PUERTO RICAN-M, NEW YORK, EAST, PARAPROFESSIONALS, MENTAL HEALTH PROFESSION, HEALTH DELIVERY SYSTEMS, ESSAY

ABST TO GAIN A BETTER UNDERSTANDING OF AN HISPANIC COMMUNITY'S SOCIAL AND EMOTIONAL SUPPORT SYSTEMS AND TO ENLIST THESE SYSTEMS IN THE PREVENTION AND EARLY TREATMENT OF PSYCHOSOCIAL PATHOLOGY, A SOUTH BRONX COMMUNITY MENTAL HEALTH CENTER STAFF MADE AN EFFORT TO FAMILIARIZE THEMSELVES WITH PUERTO RICAN FOLK HEALING PRACTICES. THE PRACTICES OF ESPIRITISMO AND THE MEANING OF CERTAIN SYMPTOMS AND BEHAVIORS WITHIN THE CONTEXT OF THE HISPANIC CULTURE WERE EXPLORED. EFFORTS WERE MADE TO EFFECT A WORKABLE ALLIANCE BETWEEN THE PROFESSIONAL PSYCHIATRIC STAFF AND THE COMMUNITY'S FOLK HEALERS, AND TREATMENT OF MENTAL HEALTH PROBLEMS WAS COORDINATED USING BOTH SYSTEMS SIMULTA-

NEOUSLY. ALTHOUGH INITIALLY REGARDED AS A MATTER OF EXPEDIENCY, THE IDENTIFICATION AND ACKNOWLEDGMENT OF FOLK HEALERS ENABLED CENTER STAFF TO OVERCOME THEIR PREJUDICE AGAINST WHAT THEY HAD BEEN TRAINED TO VIEW AS MYSTICAL AND NONRATIONAL. ULTIMATELY, THE STAFF ACCEPTED THE VALUE OF SPIRITIST PRACTICES IN THE MENTAL HEALTH OF THE COMMUNITY. 7 REFERENCES.

ACCN 002297

1597 AUTH **RUIZ, P.**

TITL A SEVEN-YEAR EVALUATION OF A CAREER ESCALATION TRAINING PROGRAM FOR INDIGENOUS NONPROFESSIONALS.

SRCE *HOSPITAL AND COMMUNITY PSYCHIATRY, 1976, 27(4), 253-257.*

INDX PROGRAM EVALUATION, MENTAL HEALTH, PROFESSIONAL TRAINING, PARAPROFESSIONALS, NEW YORK, EAST, HIGHER EDUCATION, MENTAL HEALTH PROFESSION, PUERTO RICAN-M, EMPIRICAL, POLICY, SPANISH SURNAMED

ABST A COMMUNITY MENTAL HEALTH CENTER IN SOUTHEAST BRONX, N.Y., OFFERS A CAREER-ESCALATION PROGRAM IN WHICH INDIGENOUS NONPROFESSIONAL MENTAL HEALTH WORKERS CAN EARN A MASTER'S DEGREE IN THE BEHAVIORAL SCIENCES. AN EVALUATION OF THE FIRST SEVEN YEARS OF THE PROGRAM SHOWED THAT ONLY 56 OF THE 91 STAFF MEMBERS WHO WERE ELIGIBLE FOR THE PROGRAM ENTERED IT, AND 23 SUBSEQUENTLY DROPPED OUT. ONLY THREE TRAINEES EARNED A MASTER'S DEGREE, ALTHOUGH 24 WERE PURSUING OR HAD RECEIVED AN ASSOCIATE-IN-ARTS DEGREE. THE AUTHOR BRIEFLY DISCUSSES CHANGES THAT COULD MAKE THE PROGRAM MORE EFFECTIVE, BUT HE BELIEVES A COMMUNITY MENTAL HEALTH CENTER IS NOT THE BEST SETTING FOR A CAREER-ESCALATION PROGRAM. 4 REFERENCES. (NCMHI ABSTRACT MODIFIED)

ACCN 002292

1598 AUTH **RUIZ, P., LANGROD, J., LOWINSON, J., & MARCUS, N. J.**

TITL SOCIAL REHABILITATION OF ADDICTS: A TWO YEAR EVALUATION.

SRCE *INTERNATIONAL JOURNAL OF THE ADDICTIONS, 1977, 12(1), 173-181.*

INDX DRUG ADDICTION, DRUG ABUSE, NEW YORK, EAST, PUERTO RICAN-M, CROSS CULTURAL, METHADONE MAINTENANCE, PROGRAM EVALUATION, RESOURCE UTILIZATION, POLICY, PERSONNEL, SES, EMPIRICAL, REHABILITATION

ABST ONE HUNDRED-FIFTY PATIENTS AT A PREDOMINANTLY WHITE, MIDDLE CLASS METHADONE MAINTENANCE CLINIC WERE COMPARED WITH 232 AT A PREDOMINANTLY LOWER CLASS, PUERTO RICAN CLINIC IN ORDER TO ASSESS THE RELATIVE EFFICACY OF TREATMENT APPROACHES. ALTHOUGH A LOWER RATE OF REHABILITATION WAS EXPECTED FOR THE HISPANIC GROUP, THE DATA REVEALED THAT BOTH CLINICS SHOWED SIMILAR PROGRESS AS

MEASURED BY EMPLOYMENT, ABSENCE OF ARRESTS, AND RETENTION IN TREATMENT. SECONDARY DRUG ABUSE WAS FOUND TO BE MUCH HIGHER AT THE WHITE CLINIC (54%) THAN AT THE PUERTO RICAN CLINIC (36%). ALTHOUGH THE RATE OF TERMINATION WAS THE SAME AT BOTH CLINICS, THE REASONS FOR TERMINATION WERE MARKEDLY DIFFERENT. THE MORE STRUCTURED MIDDLE CLASS CLINIC HAD A HIGHER RATE OF VOLUNTARY DETOXIFICATION AND WAS FAR MORE LIKELY TO TERMINATE PATIENTS INVOLUNTARILY. AT THE HISPANIC CLINIC, NEARLY TWO-THIRDS OF THE TERMINATIONS WERE PATIENT DROPOUTS. IT IS SPECULATED THAT DIFFERENT ATTITUDES AT THE TWO CLINICS PROMOTE CONTRASTING ENVIRONMENTS THAT ARE SELECTIVELY DETRIMENTAL TO THE PATIENTS. 4 REFERENCES.

ACCN   002296

1599 AUTH   **RUIZ, P., & LANGROD, J.**
TITL   THE ANCIENT ART OF FOLK HEALING: AFRICAN INFLUENCE IN A NEW YORK CITY COMMUNITY MENTAL HEALTH CENTER.
SRCE   *IN P. SINGER (ED.), TRADITIONAL HEALING: NEW SCIENCE OR NEW COLONIALISM? NEW YORK: CONCH MAGAZINE LIMITED, 1977, PP. 80-95.*
INDX   FOLK MEDICINE, ESPIRITISMO, PUERTO RICAN-M, MENTAL HEALTH, HEALTH DELIVERY SYSTEMS, NEW YORK, COMMUNITY, EAST, EMPIRICAL, CULTURAL FACTORS, RELIGION, PARAPROFESSIONALS, PROFESSIONAL TRAINING, PHYSICIANS, PSYCHOTHERAPISTS, HEALTH, CULTURAL CHANGE, CUBAN, URBAN
ABST   AN INVESTIGATION OF THE INTERACTION BETWEEN MEDICAL HEALTH CARE AND TRADITIONAL HEALING PRACTICES PREVALENT AMONG THE PUERTO RICAN POPULATION SERVED BY A NEW YORK COMMUNITY MENTAL HEALTH CENTER REVEALS THE GROWING INFLUENCE OF THE AFRO-CUBAN CULT OF SANTERIA AMONG LOCAL PUERTO RICAN PRACTITIONERS OF ESPIRITISMO. ALTHOUGH SOCIAL PRESSURES TO ASSIMILATE ARE STRONG WITHIN THE PUERTO RICAN COMMUNITY, ESPIRITISMO APPEARS TO BE REACHING TOWARDS AFRICA, RATHER THAN AMERICA, FOR ITS SYMBOLS AND RITUALS. A DETAILED ACCOUNT OF ONE SEANCE, THREE CONSULTATIONS ACCORDING TO THE PRACTICE OF ESPIRITISMO, AND A DESCRIPTION OF A SANTERIA HEALING RITUAL ARE PRESENTED. FURTHERMORE, AN INTERVIEW WITH A PRACTICING ESPIRITISTA WHO IS ALSO A NONPROFESSIONAL HEALTH WORKER AT THE COMMUNITY MENTAL HEALTH CENTER GIVES EVIDENCE OF THE ECLECTIC NATURE OF THE FOLK HEALING SYSTEM. PRESENT PSYCHIATRIC TRAINING IS BASED ON THE SCIENTIFICALLY ORIENTED AND ETHNOCENTRIC CLASSIC MODEL WHICH DENIES THE EXISTENCE OF SUPERNATURAL FORCES. HOWEVER, BELIEF IN SUPERNATURAL FORCES IS POSSIBLY AN INTRINSIC ASPECT OF HISPANIC CULTURE WHICH CLASHES WITH MODERN PSYCHIATRY. THEREFORE, IF PSYCHIATRISTS ARE TO PROMOTE A MENTALLY HEALTHY SOCIETY, THEY MUST LEARN MORE

ABOUT THE CULTURAL VALUES OF THE HISPANIC PEOPLES. 5 REFERENCES.
ACCN   002196

1600 AUTH   **RUIZ, P., & LANGROD, J.**
TITL   PSYCHIATRY AND FOLK HEALING: A DICHOTOMY?
SRCE   *AMERICAN JOURNAL OF PSYCHIATRY, 1976, 133(1), 95-97.*
INDX   CULTURAL FACTORS, PSYCHOTHERAPY, PSYCHOTHERAPY OUTCOME, FOLK MEDICINE, PROFESSIONAL TRAINING, SPANISH SURNAMED, HEALTH DELIVERY SYSTEMS, POLICY, NEW YORK, EAST, PUERTO RICAN-M, STRESS, COPING MECHANISMS, URBAN, PROGRAM EVALUATION, CULTURAL PLURALISM, ESPIRITISMO
ABST   A COMMUNITY MENTAL HEALTH CENTER'S EXPERIENCE WITH FOLK HEALERS IN A HISPANIC URBAN GHETTO IS DESCRIBED. FINDINGS REVEAL THE EXISTENCE OF A CULTURALLY ACCEPTED BELIEF SYSTEM WHICH IS BASED ON A BODY OF EMPIRICAL KNOWLEDGE AND WHICH HELPS ITS MEMBERS TO COPE WITH STRESS. IT IS SUGGESTED THAT INCLUDING FOLK HEALERS AS TEAM MEMBERS IN THE DELIVERY OF MENTAL HEALTH SERVICES IS A VALUABLE CONTRIBUTION TO PSYCHIATRY. 9 REFERENCES. (NCMHI ABSTRACT)
ACCN   001377

1601 AUTH   **RUIZ, P., & LANGROD, J.**
TITL   THE ROLE OF FOLK HEALERS IN COMMUNITY MENTAL HEALTH SERVICES.
SRCE   *COMMUNITY MENTAL HEALTH JOURNAL, 1976, 12(4), 392-398.*
INDX   FOLK MEDICINE, MENTAL HEALTH, CULTURAL FACTORS, PUERTO RICAN-M, URBAN, RELIGION, ESPIRITISMO, PSYCHOTHERAPY, PSYCHOTHERAPISTS, PROGRAM EVALUATION, HEALTH DELIVERY SYSTEMS, ATTITUDES, NEW YORK, EAST, ESSAY, POLICY
ABST   DATA DRAWN FROM A 6-YEAR COLLABORATIVE UNDERTAKING BETWEEN THE LINCOLN COMMUNITY MENTAL HEALTH CENTER AND TWO LOCAL SPIRITIST CENTERS IN NEW YORK WERE USED TO ASSESS THE RELATIONSHIP BETWEEN SOCIOCULTURAL FACTORS AND PSYCHOPATHOLOGY IN HISPANIC GROUPS IN A DISADVANTAGED URBAN AREA. COMPARISONS WERE MADE BETWEEN CLASSICAL MENTAL HEALTH PRACTITIONERS AND INDIGENOUS FOLK HEALERS, WITH EMPHASIS ON TERMINOLOGY, MEANS OF COMMUNICATION, DIAGNOSTIC TECHNIQUES, AND UTILIZATION OF SOCIAL BEHAVIOR AND MORAL VALUES. ALTHOUGH SPIRITUALISTIC PRACTICES HAVE BEEN ASCRIBED ONLY TO PRIMITIVE CULTURES OR AREAS WHERE MEDICAL FACILITIES ARE NOT AVAILABLE, THE AUTHORS CONCLUDE THAT IT IS THE UNCERTAINTY CONCERNING THE ACHIEVEMENT OF SOCIALLY VALUED GOALS WHICH LEADS URBAN HISPANICS TO SEEK HELP FROM BOTH MENTAL HEALTH CLINICS AND SPIRITIST CENTERS. SINCE THE UNIQUE ASPECTS OF A CULTURE MUST BE IDENTIFIED

AND UTILIZED WITHIN ANY MENTAL HEALTH PROGRAM, A MUTUAL ALLIANCE BETWEEN PROFESSIONAL MENTAL HEALTH WORKERS AND FOLK HEALERS IS RECOMMENDED. 8 REFERENCES. (JOURNAL ABSTRACT MODIFIED)

ACCN 002197

1602 AUTH **RUIZ, R.**
TITL IMPROVING POLICE-PUERTO RICAN RELATIONS.
SRCE *IN A. PFEFFER (ED.), PROCEEDINGS OF THE JOHN JAY COLLEGE FACULTY SEMINARS. NEW YORK: JOHN JAY FACULTY SEMINARS, 2, 1971.*
INDX POLICE-COMMUNITY RELATIONS, ESSAY, PUERTO RICAN-M, CULTURAL FACTORS, PROCEEDINGS, IMMIGRATION, EAST, POLICY, ECONOMIC FACTORS
ABST DIFFICULTIES ENCOUNTERED BY PUERTO RICANS WHO COME TO THE UNITED STATES, PARTICULARLY IN THEIR RELATIONS WITH THE POLICE, ARE DISCUSSED. ALTHOUGH CRIME IS INCREASING IN PUERTO RICO, DUE LARGELY TO OUTSIDE INFLUENCES, THE PUERTO RICANS ARE BASICALLY A LAW-ABIDING PEOPLE WITH RESPECT FOR THE POLICE. THEY OFTEN BECOME INVOLVED WITH THE LAW WHEN THEY FIRST COME TO THE UNITED STATES BECAUSE THEY ARE IGNORANT OF THE LAWS HERE AND THEIR CUSTOMS ARE DIFFERENT. THE LANGUAGE BARRIER AND POOR ECONOMIC CONDITIONS ARE CONTRIBUTING FACTORS. COMMUNITY RELATIONS UNITS ESTABLISHED IN POLICE DEPARTMENTS SHOULD TRAIN THE POLICE TO UNDERSTAND THE PUERTO RICAN MORES AND CULTURE, AND SHOULD TRAIN PRIVATE CITIZENS TO UNDERSTAND AND COOPERATE WITH THE POLICE. THE POLICE SHOULD BE GIVEN MORE AUTHORITY AND THE POPULATION WILL HAVE MORE RESPECT FOR THEM. RECRUITING POLICEMEN WITH HISPANIC ORIGINS WOULD ALSO HELP.

ACCN 001378

1603 AUTH **RUIZ, R. A.**
TITL THE DELIVERY OF MENTAL AND SOCIAL CHANGE SERVICES FOR CHICANOS: ANALYSIS AND RECOMMENDATIONS.
SRCE *IN J. L. MARTINEZ (ED.), CHICANO PSYCHOLOGY. NEW YORK: ACADEMIC PRESS, 1977, PP. 233-248.*
INDX HEALTH DELIVERY SYSTEMS, MENTAL HEALTH, MEXICAN AMERICAN, STRESS, PERSONALITY, CULTURAL FACTORS, SOCIAL SERVICES, ACCULTURATION, ESSAY, CULTURAL PLURALISM
ABST THIS DISCUSSION SUMMARIZES INFORMATION ABOUT CHICANOS IN THE AREAS OF DEMOGRAPHIC CHARACTERISTICS, ETHNOHISTORY, CULTURAL DIVERSITY, ASSIMILATION AND ACCULTURATION, SOURCES OF STRESS, AND FACTORS REDUCING SELF-REFERRAL TO MENTAL HEALTH FACILITIES. THE OBJECTIVE IS TO HELP MENTAL HEALTH AND SOCIAL WELFARE PERSONNEL TO IDENTIFY SOURCES OF STRESS SO THAT THEY CAN FORMULATE APPROPRIATE REMEDIAL OR INTERVENTION STRATEGIES FOR CHICANO CLIENTS. TWO KINDS OF STRESS—INTRAPSYCHIC AND EXTRAPSYCHIC—ARE IDENTIFIED AS SIGNIFICANT, AS BOTH AFFECT

MENTAL ILLNESS AND SOCIAL MALADJUSTMENT. INTRAPSYCHIC STRESS IS PRIMARILY DETERMINED BY SUCH INTERNAL FACTORS AS THE INDIVIDUAL'S LIFESTYLE AND PERSONAL ADJUSTMENT; EXTRAPSYCHIC STRESS IS THAT WHICH ORIGINATES IN SOCIETY—E.G., SOCIETAL DISCRIMINATION. TO UNDERSTAND THESE STRESS FACTORS AS WELL AS OTHER PROBLEMS SUFFERED BY CHICANOS, WELL-FOUNDED, EMPIRICALLY BASED RESEARCH IS ESSENTIAL. SPECIFICALLY, THE RESEARCH AREAS OF HIGHEST PRIORITY ARE: (1) THE INTRAPSYCHIC-EXTRAPSYCHIC DIMENSIONS OF STRESS; (2) IDENTIFICATION OF CULTURAL DIVERSITY; (3) MEASURES OF THE VARYING DEGREES OF ASSIMILATION AND ACCULTURATION; (4) INTELLIGENCE TESTING; (5) THE EFFECTS OF BILINGUALISM; (6) COGNITIVE STYLE; AND (7) SEX ROLES WITHIN CHICANO CULTURE. TO PROMOTE SUCH MEANINGFUL RESEARCH, AN INTENSIVE DIALOGUE BETWEEN MENTAL HEALTH PRACTIONERS AND SCIENTISTS IS REQUIRED. FURTHERMORE, THE NEW TESTS, TREATMENT METHODS, AND INTERVENTION STRATEGIES WHICH HAVE BEEN DEVELOPED FOR CHICANOS MUST BE TESTED FOR VALIDITY AND EFFICIENCY. IN CONCLUSION, RECOMMENDATIONS ARE OFFERED WHICH CAN INCREASE CHICANO UTILIZATION OF MENTAL HEALTH SERVICES. 25 REFERENCES.

ACCN 001379

1604 AUTH **RUIZ, R. A.**
TITL FREQUENCY COUNT OF SELF-IDENTIFIED CUBAN, MEXICAN-AMERICAN, PUERTO RICAN, AND SPANISH PSYCHOLOGISTS, PSYCHIATRISTS, AND SOCIOLOGISTS IN THE UNITED STATES.
SRCE *UNPUBLISHED MANUSCRIPT, DEPT. OF PSYCHOLOGY, UNIVERSITY OF MISSOURI, KANSAS CITY, 1971.*
INDX CUBAN, MEXICAN AMERICAN, PUERTO RICAN-M, SPANISH SURNAMED, MENTAL HEALTH PROFESSION, SOCIAL SCIENCES, REPRESENTATION, REVIEW
ABST AN ANALYSIS OF SPANISH-SURNAME (SS) ETHNIC MINORITY GROUP MEMBERSHIP IN ASSOCIATIONS OF PSYCHOLOGY, PSYCHIATRY AND SOCIOLOGY IS PRESENTED. MEMBERSHIP LISTS OF THESE ASSOCIATIONS WERE EXAMINED IN ORDER TO IDENTIFY THOSE INDIVIDUALS WHOSE SURNAMES MIGHT BE SPANISH. FROM A TOTAL POOL OF ALMOST 60,000 MEMBERS, A SUBPOOL OF 501 WAS IDENTIFIED AS SS. FOLLOWING TWO ATTEMPTS TO OBTAIN ACCURATE SS ETHNIC BACKGROUND INFORMATION BY MAIL, A TOTAL OF 379 RESPONSES WERE ANALYZED (76 PERCENT RETURN). DATA INDICATE THAT 105 INDIVIDUALS IDENTIFIED THEMSELVES AS "SPANISH-SURNAME ETHNIC MINORITY GROUP AMERICAN RESIDENTS." THIS GROUP BREAKS DOWN INTO 58 PSYCHOLOGISTS, 20 PSYCHIATRISTS, AND 26 SOCIOLOGISTS WHO IDENTIFY THEMSELVES AS FOLLOWS: 30 CUBANS, 30 MEXICAN AMERICANS, 10 PUERTO RICANS, AND 35 SPANIARDS. A MAILING LIST WHICH IDENTIFIES CUBANS, MEXICAN AMERICAN, PUERTO RICANS AND

SPANIARDS BY PROFESSION IS PROVIDED. IT IS SUGGESTED THAT THESE PROFESSIONALS HAVE THE POTENTIAL TO SERVE AS RESOURCE PERSONNEL TO INCREASE THE NUMBER OF SS ETHNIC MINORITY GROUP MEMBERS IN THESE DISCIPLINES. RECOMMENDATIONS TO CREATE SUPPORT PROGRAMS FOR THE ACTIVE RECRUITMENT OF SS INDIVIDUALS INTO THE VARIOUS DISCIPLINES ARE DISCUSSED. 3 REFERENCES.

ACCN   001381

1605 AUTH **RUIZ, R. A.**
TITL   INCREASING EDUCATIONAL OPPORTUNITIES FOR MEXICAN AMERICANS IN PSYCHOLOGY.
SRCE   *WORKING PAPER PRESENTED AT THE UNIVERSITY OF CALIFORNIA, RIVERSIDE, MAY 17-18, 1973.*
INDX   ESSAY, MEXICAN AMERICAN, REPRESENTATION, PROFESSIONAL TRAINING, MENTAL HEALTH PROFESSION, SCHOLASTIC ACHIEVEMENT, HIGHER EDUCATION, POVERTY, EQUAL OPPORTUNITY, POLICY, DISCRIMINATION, EDUCATION
ABST   THE DEGREE OF UNDERREPRESENTATION OF CHICANOS IN PSYCHOLOGY AND EXPLANATIONS FOR THIS CONDITION ARE DISCUSSED. USING A CONSERVATIVE ESTIMATE OF THE CHICANO POPULATION (5.5 MILLION), DATA INDICATE THAT THERE IS A RATIO OF 1 CHICANO MEMBER OF THE AMERICAN PSYCHOLOGICAL ASSOCIATION (APA) FOR EVERY 400,000 CHICANOS, WHILE THERE IS 1 APA MEMBER FOR EVERY 6,500 NON-CHICANOS. IN 1972, CHICANOS COMPRISED LESS THAN 1.4% OF NATIONAL GRADUATE ENROLLMENT IN PSYCHOLOGY. SIMILAR PATTERNS EXIST IN OTHER PROFESSIONS REQUIRING GRADUATE STUDY. POVERTY, INADEQUATE NUTRITION, AND POOR MEDICAL CARE ARE FACTORS WHICH CAN IMPAIR ACADEMIC PERFORMANCE AMONG CHICANOS. SCHOOL SEGREGATION, DISCRIMINATION, AND THE LACK OF VIABLE BILINGUAL-BICULTURAL EDUCATIONAL PROGRAMS RESULT IN FEWER CHICANOS ATTAINING HIGHER EDUCATION AND ENTERING PROFESSIONAL SCHOOLS. RECOMMENDATIONS TO RESOLVE THOSE PROBLEMS INCLUDE: (1) INCREASED RECRUITMENT, ADMISSIONS, FINANCIAL AID, AND SUPPORTIVE SERVICES FOR CHICANOS IN HIGHER EDUCATION; (2) INCREASED PROFESSIONAL APPOINTMENTS FOR CHICANO PSYCHOLOGISTS; AND (3) SUPPORT FOR THE INCREASED USE OF CULTURE-FAIR TESTING INSTRUMENTS TO PREVENT THE EDUCATIONAL FAILURE OF CHICANO STUDENTS AT ALL LEVELS. 16 REFERENCES.
ACCN   001382

1606 AUTH **RUIZ, R. A.**
TITL   AN OVERVIEW OF RESEARCH NEEDS IN LATINO MENTAL HEALTH.
SRCE   *IN A. M. PADILLA (CHAIR), LATINO RESEARCH TRENDS. WORKSHOP PRESENTED AT THE ANNUAL MEETING OF THE NATIONAL COUNCIL OF COMMUNITY MENTAL HEALTH CENTERS AND THE NATIONAL INSTITUTE FOR COMMU-*

NITY MENTAL HEALTH, DENVER, COLORADO, FEBRUARY 22-25, 1976.
INDX   PROGRAM EVALUATION. MENTAL HEALTH, RESEARCH METHODOLOGY, SPANISH SURNAMED, MENTAL HEALTH, RESOURCE UTILIZATION, CULTURAL FACTORS, ESSAY, PROCEEDINGS
ABST   THE 9 MILLION LATINOS IN THE UNITED STATES SHARE COMMON PROBLEMS—POVERTY; PREJUDICE; URBAN LIFESTYLES; UNEMPLOYMENT; POOR EDUCATION; AND INADEQUATE COMMUNICATION SKILLS. THESE ARE STRESS INDICATORS WHICH WOULD POINT TO HIGH UTILIZATION OF MENTAL HEALTH FACILITIES. BUT SINCE THE OPPOSITE IS TRUE (I.E., COMMUNITY MENTAL HEALTH FACILITIES ARE UNDERUTILIZED BY LATINOS), SEVERAL BROAD SUBJECT AREAS REQUIRE FURTHER RESEARCH: (1) CULTURAL DIFFERENCES AMONG SUBGROUPS; (2) TYPES OF SERVICE, AS STANDARD THERAPEUTIC SERVICES ARE NOT ALWAYS APPROPRIATE FOR THE LATINO INDIVIDUAL; (3) TESTING, AS MORE VALID PSYCHODIAGNOSTIC MEASURES ARE NEEDED; (4) THE LATINO FAMILY'S ABILITY TO MITIGATE STRESS; (5) SEX ROLES, SUCH AS THE EFFECTS OF MACHISMO AND THE WOMEN'S LIBERATION MOVEMENT; (6) COGNITIVE STYLE DIFFERENCES BETWEEN LATINOS AND ANGLO AMERICANS; AND (7) THE VARIABLES OPERATING IN LATINO INDIVIDUALS WHO ACHIEVE OR FAIL TO ACHIEVE PERSONAL SUCCESS IN THE FACE OF DIFFICULT LIFE SITUATIONS. 4 REFERENCES.
ACCN   001383

1607 AUTH **RUIZ, R. A.**
TITL   RELATIVE FREQUENCY OF AMERICANS WITH SPANISH SURNAMES IN ASSOCIATIONS OF PSYCHOLOGY, PSYCHIATRY, AND SOCIOLOGY.
SRCE   *AMERICAN PSYCHOLOGIST, 1971, 26(11), 1022-1024.*
INDX   SPANISH SURNAMED, MENTAL HEALTH PROFESSION, SOCIAL SCIENCES, REPRESENTATION, REVIEW
ABST   AN ATTEMPT TO QUANTIFY THE RELATIVE FREQUENCY OF AMERICANS WITH SPANISH SURNAMES (SS) WHO ARE IN ASSOCIATIONS OF PSYCHOLOGY, PSYCHIATRY AND SOCIOLOGY AND WHO RESIDE IN THE U.S. OR ELSEWHERE IS SUMMARIZED. TWO INDEPENDENT JUDGES IDENTIFIED SS FROM DIRECTORIES AND REGISTRIES OF FIVE ORGANIZATIONS RELATED TO THE THREE DISCIPLINES MENTIONED ABOVE. THE POSSIBLE LIST WAS FURTHER REDUCED BY DELETING SS THAT FAILED TO APPEAR IN A STANDARD 12-VOLUME WORK ON SPANISH GENEALOGY AND HERALDRY. RESULTS SHOW A TOTAL OF 1,091 SS FROM THE THREE DISCIPLINES, WITH 501 RESIDING IN THE U.S. AND 590 ELSEWHERE. THE AMERICAN PSYCHIATRIC ASSOCIATION WITH A TOTAL MEMBERSHIP OF 15,799 SHOWS 544 (3.4%) SS. HOWEVER, ONLY 85 (0.5%) RESIDE IN THE U.S. THE GUIDE TO GRADUATE DEPARTMENTS AND SOCIOLOGISTS WITH A TOTAL MEMBERSHIP OF 3,250 SHOWS 89 (2.8%) SS, WITH THE EXCEPTION OF SEVEN SS, THE REMAINDER RESIDE IN THE U.S.

THE AMERICAN SOCIOLOGICAL ASSOCIATION HAS 152 (1.6%) SS OUT OF 9,566 MEMBERS. FINALLY, THE AMERICAN PSYCHOLOGICAL ASSOCIATION, WITH THE LARGEST MEMBERSHIP OF 28,488, LISTS 302 (1.1%) SS MEMBERS, AND ONLY 250 (0.88%) SS MEMBERS RESIDE IN THE U.S. EVEN THOUGH THE SS FIGURES APPEAR RELATIVELY SMALL, IT IS BELIEVED THAT THESE NUMBERS ARE SOMEWHAT INFLATED.

ACCN 001384

1608 AUTH **RUIZ, R. A., CASAS, J. M., & PADILLA, A. M.**
TITL CULTURALLY RELEVANT BEHAVIORISTIC COUNSELING (OCCASIONAL PAPER NO. 5).
SRCE *LOS ANGELES: UNIVERSITY OF CALIFORNIA, SPANISH SPEAKING MENTAL HEALTH RESEARCH CENTER, 1977.*
INDX EDUCATIONAL COUNSELING, PSYCHOTHERAPY, REVIEW, MEXICAN AMERICAN, ESSAY, CULTURAL PLURALISM, ETHNIC IDENTITY, BEHAVIOR THERAPY, RESOURCE UTILIZATION, COLLEGE STUDENTS, BILINGUAL-BICULTURAL PERSONNEL
ABST A BEHAVIORISTIC COUNSELING MODEL FOR BILINGUAL-BICULTURAL CHICANO COLLEGE STUDENT CLIENTELE IS OFFERED IN RESPONSE TO THE PROBLEM OF CHICANOS' UNDERUTILIZATION OF MENTAL HEALTH SERVICES. THE ESSENTIAL CHARACTERISTICS OF THIS MODEL INCLUDE A BEHAVIORISTIC ORIENTATION AND THERAPEUTIC INTERVENTION STRATEGIES WHICH ARE DIRECTIVE, RESTRICTIVE, AND CONTRACTUAL. THE HIGH FREQUENCY OF PROBLEMS REPORTED BY THIS POPULATION ARE REVIEWED, CITING NEGATIVE SELF-IMAGES, SKILL DEFICIENCIES IN LANGUAGE AND EDUCATION, LACK OF IDENTIFICATION WITH THE UNIVERSITY, AND CULTURE CONFLICT. COUNSELOR RESPONSES TO VARIOUS PROBLEMS ARE ALSO DISCUSSED. UNDERUTILIZATION OF MENTAL HEALTH SERVICES BY CHICANOS IS ATTRIBUTED TO INSTITUTIONAL POLICIES WHICH DISCOURAGE SELF-REFERRAL, LACK OF SPANISH SPEAKING PERSONNEL, AND CULTURE AND CLASS DIFFERENCES WHICH IMPEDE COMMUNICATION BETWEEN CLIENT AND COUNSELOR. CULTURALLY RELEVANT MODELS OF COUNSELING AND THE USE OF BILINGUAL-BICULTURAL PERSONNEL ARE ESSENTIAL FOR THE INCREASED UTILIZATION OF MENTAL HEALTH SERVICES BY CHICANOS. 35 REFERENCES.
ACCN 001385

1609 AUTH **RUIZ, R. A., PADILLA, A. M., & ALVAREZ, R.**
TITL ISSUES IN THE COUNSELING OF SPANISH-SPEAKING/SURNAMED CLIENTS: RECOMMENDATIONS FOR THERAPEUTIC SERVICES.
SRCE *IN G. R. WALZ & L. BENJAMIN (EDS.), TRANSCULTURAL COUNSELING: NEEDS, PROGRAMS, AND TECHNIQUES. NEW YORK: HUMAN SCIENCES PRESS, 1978, PP. 13-56.*
INDX MENTAL HEALTH, PSYCHOTHERAPY, PROGRAM EVALUATION, SPANISH SURNAMED, HEALTH DELIVERY SYSTEMS, COMMUNITY INVOLVEMENT, PROFESSIONAL TRAINING, ETHNIC IDENTITY, DEMOGRAPHIC, ESSAY, REVIEW, CULTURAL FACTORS, RESOURCE UTILIZATION, ACCULTURATION, POLICY, CULTURAL PLURALISM
ABST TO ENABLE COUNSELORS TO COMMUNICATE MORE EFFECTIVELY WITH SPANISH-SPEAKING/SURNAMED (SSS) CLIENTS, THE FOLLOWING THEMES ARE DISCUSSED: (1) ISSUES OF ETHNIC IDENTIFICATION AND MARGINAL ASSIMILATION; (2) DEMOGRAPHIC CHARACTERISTICS OF THE SSS GROUP; (3) UTILIZATION PATTERNS OF COUNSELING SERVICES; AND (4) FACTORS OPERATING TO REDUCE SELF-REFERRALS. THREE CASE HISTORIES ILLUSTRATE THE KINDS OF PROBLEMS AND COMPLAINTS SSS CLIENTS TYPICALLY BRING TO COUNSELING. THESE ISSUES TEND TO CREATE A PATTERN OF LIFE PROBLEMS THAT ARE DIFFERENT FROM AND EXCLUSIVE OF THOSE EXPERIENCED BY OTHER AMERICANS. IT IS RECOMMENDED THAT COUNSELING SERVICE FACILITIES PROVIDE BETTER ACCESS TO SERVICES, MORE PERSONALIZED SERVICE, AND ALSO ADOPT A MORE AGGRESSIVE MODE OF ADVERTISING THEIR SERVICES. COMMUNITY INVOLVEMENT IS ESSENTIAL IN THE OPERATION OF COUNSELING PROGRAMS. RELEVANT PROFESSIONAL TRAINING PROGRAMS MUST BE CREATED TO MEET THE NEEDS OF THE SSS POPULATION, AND TRADITIONAL COUNSELING METHODS MODIFIED. SUGGESTED COUNSELING INNOVATIONS INCLUDE: (1) DRAWING ON THE STRENGTH AND UNITY OF THE EXTENDED FAMILY SYSTEM; (2) RELAXATION OF INSTITUTIONAL RIGIDITY IN SCHEDULING, PRIORITIES, ETC.; (3) A PROGRAM TO ASSESS THE NEEDS OF THE SSS COMMUNITY; (4) INTERVENTION IN CLIENT EMPLOYABILITY; (5) EXTENSION OF COUNSELING SERVICES TO COVER BOTH PHYSICAL AND PSYCHOLOGICAL NEEDS; AND (6) THE ESTABLISHMENT OF A CULTURALLY RELEVANT CRISIS INTERVENTION SERVICE. 27 REFERENCES.
ACCN 002199

1610 AUTH **RUIZ, R. A., & PADILLA, A. M.**
TITL COUNSELING LATINOS.
SRCE *PERSONNEL AND GUIDANCE JOURNAL, 1977, 55(7), 401-408.*
INDX MENTAL HEALTH, STRESS, SPANISH SURNAMED, CULTURAL FACTORS, EDUCATIONAL COUNSELING, DEMOGRAPHIC, REVIEW, PSYCHOTHERAPY, RESOURCE UTILIZATION, CULTURE, ACCULTURATION, HEALTH DELIVERY SYSTEMS, CASE STUDY, DISCRIMINATION
ABST LITERATURE PERTAINING TO LATINOS AND PSYCHOTHERAPEUTIC COUNSELING IS REVIEWED IN AN ATTEMPT TO ASSIST COUNSELORS TO BETTER UNDERSTAND LATINO CLIENTELE AND THEREBY IMPROVE COUNSELING SERVICES. DEMOGRAPHIC DATA WHICH DESCRIBE THE LATINO POPULATION IN GENERAL AS URBAN DWELLERS, POOR, LOW PAID, AND UNDEREDUCATED ARE FIRST PRESENTED. A BRIEF HISTORICAL AND CULTURAL OVERVIEW OF THIS POPULATION POINTS OUT THE SIMILARITIES AND DIFFERENCES OF THE LATINO SUBGROUPS. FURTHER, THE SOURCES OF STRESS, THE UTILIZATION OF MENTAL HEALTH SERVICES, AND THE FACTORS WHICH INFLU-

ENCE UTILIZATION ARE DISCUSSED. TO CLARIFY IMPORTANT ISSUES IN COUNSELING LATINOS AND TO FACILITATE THE PRESENTATION OF SPECIFIC RECOMMENDATIONS, CASE HISTORIES OF TWO CHICANO CLIENTS ARE PRESENTED. A CONCLUDING SECTION PROVIDES GENERAL RECOMMENDATIONS FOR COUNSELORS AND THE SETTINGS IN WHICH THEY FUNCTION. 26 REFERENCES.

ACCN   001386

1611 AUTH   **RUMBAUT, R. D., & RUMBAUT, R. G.**
TITL   THE EXTENDED FAMILY IN EXILE: CUBAN EXPATRIATES IN THE UNITED STATES.
SRCE   *AMERICAN JOURNAL OF PSYCHIATRY, 1976, 133(4), 395-399.*
INDX   CUBAN, ACCULTURATION, IMMIGRATION, EXTENDED FAMILY, HISTORY, PSYCHOSOCIAL ADJUSTMENT, MENTAL HEALTH, PSYCHOPATHOLOGY, ESSAY, SOCIAL MOBILITY, SES
ABST   FOR THE NEARLY ONE MILLION CUBAN EXILES IN THE U.S., EXPATRIATION HAS MEANT ANGUISH, UPROOTEDNESS, CHALLENGE, AND ACCOMPLISHMENT. SEVERAL FACTORS ACCOUNT FOR THE COMPARATIVELY SUCCESSFUL ASPECTS OF THEIR STRUGGLE: RELATIVELY HIGH OCCUPATIONAL AND EDUCATIONAL LEVELS, FORMATION OF VIGOROUS COMMUNITIES THAT PERMIT A POSITIVE ETHNIC CONSCIOUSNESS AND THE CREATION OF STRONG SOCIAL TIES, AND EFFECTIVELY ORGANIZED RECEPTION BY THE U.S. IT IS NOTED THAT EXPATRIATION IS ALWAYS TRAUMATIC, BUT MASTERY OF THE STRUGGLES IT INVOLVES CAN LEAD TO PERSONAL GROWTH AND EXPANDED HORIZONS. IT IS CONCLUDED THAT THE CUBAN EXPERIENCE SHOWS THAT THE INFLUX OF LARGE NUMBERS OF REFUGEES CAN BE AN ENRICHING PROCESS FOR BOTH THE HOST COUNTRY AND THE INDIVIDUAL REFUGEE. 10 REFERENCES. (JOURNAL ABSTRACT)
ACCN   001387

1612 AUTH   **RUSHING, W. A.**
TITL   CLASS, CULTURE, AND "SOCIAL STRUCTURE AND ANOMIE."
SRCE   *AMERICAN JOURNAL OF SOCIOLOGY, 1971, 76(5), 857-872.*
INDX   SES, SOCIALIZATION, ANOMIE, EMPIRICAL, MEXICAN AMERICAN, CROSS CULTURAL, ADULTS, SOCIAL STRUCTURE, FARM LABORERS, OCCUPATIONAL ASPIRATIONS, WASHINGTON, WEST, BILINGUAL, SCHOLASTIC ASPIRATIONS, CULTURAL FACTORS
ABST   HYPOTHESES DERIVED FROM MERTON'S THEORY OF SOCIAL STRUCTURE AND ANOMIE, WHICH VIEWS DEVIANT BEHAVIOR AND DEVIANT ATTITUDES AS DUE TO THE MALINTEGRATION OF CULTURAL GOALS AND SOCIAL NORMS, WERE TESTED ON 240 AFFLUENT FARMERS AND 1,031 POOR FARM WORKERS IN WASHINGTON. FARM WORKERS CONSISTED OF ANGLO AMERICANS, BILINGUAL MEXICAN AMERICAN, AND NON-ENGLISH-SPEAKING MEXICAN AMERICANS. RESULTS INDICATE THAT DISJUNCTION BETWEEN EDUCATIONAL ASPIRATIONS FOR CHILDREN AND PERCEIVED OP-

PORTUNITY IS GREATER AMONG ANGLO AMERICAN FARM WORKERS THAN FARMERS. IN BOTH CLASSES, HOWEVER, DISJUNCTION IS RELATED TO NORMATIVE ALIENATION (NORMLESSNESS). THE RELATIONSHIP APPEARS TO DEPEND UPON CULTURAL BACKGROUND, SINCE THE RELATIONSHIP HOLDS FOR ANGLO AMERICANS AND, LESS CONSISTENTLY, BILINGUALS, BUT NOT AT ALL FOR NON-ENGLISH SPEAKERS. RESULTS THUS SUGGEST THAT THE RELATIONSHIP BETWEEN ASPIRATION PERCEIVED OPPORTUNITY DISJUNCTION AND NORMLESSNESS TRANSCENDS CLASS LEVELS BUT MAY BE SPECIFIC TO A CULTURE THAT EMPHASIZES AN OPEN-CLASS IDEOLOGY. HENCE IT IS THE CULTURAL INTERPRETATION GIVEN TO ASPIRATION PERCEIVED OPPORTUNITY DISJUNCTION RATHER THAN DISJUNCTION PER SE THAT MAY BE CRUCIAL IN NORMLESSNESS. 41 REFERENCES.

ACCN   001388

1613 AUTH   **RUSTIN, S. L.**
TITL   THE GRINGO AND COUNSELING PUERTO RICAN COLLEGE STUDENTS.
SRCE   *HANDBOOK OF INTERNATIONAL SOCIOMETRY, 1973, 8(1), 37-42.*
INDX   EDUCATIONAL COUNSELING, COLLEGE STUDENTS, CONFLICT RESOLUTION, CULTURAL FACTORS, SEX ROLES, ETHNIC IDENTITY, ACCULTURATION, RELIGION, DISCRIMINATION, SES, GROUP DYNAMICS, ESSAY, CROSS CULTURAL, PUERTO RICAN-M, INTERPERSONAL RELATIONS, NEW YORK, EAST
ABST   THE CHANGING ROLE OF A NON-PUERTO RICAN COUNSELOR IN RELATION TO A PUERTO RICAN STUDENT ORGANIZATION (PRO) AT QUEENSBOROUGH COMMUNITY COLLEGE, BAYSIDE, NEW YORK, WAS EXAMINED OVER A FIVE YEAR PERIOD. DURING THE FIRST YEAR OF OPERATION THE PRO PROVIDED A FORUM FOR SPEAKERS, AN OPPORTUNITY FOR INTERPERSONAL SUPPORT, AND AN ACADEMIC TUTORING PROGRAM. A NON-PUERTO RICAN COUNSELOR WAS SOUGHT BY GROUP MEMBERS DURING THE PRO'S THIRD YEAR TO INITIATE A SENSITIVITY GROUP. THE FOLLOWING YEAR A GROUP WAS FORMED CONCENTRATING ON THREE MAJOR STUDENT CONFLICTS: (1) CONFLICT BETWEEN TRADITIONAL PUERTO RICAN VALUES AND MIDDLE CLASS AMERICAN VALUES; (2) PERSONAL IDENTITY CONFUSION; AND (3) SEXUAL ROLE CONFLICTS. IN THE FIFTH YEAR A GROUP OF NEW STUDENTS STRESSED SELF-HELP WITHOUT NON-PUERTO RICAN INPUT. NEW STUDENTS DID NOT HAVE A BASIS FOR TRUSTING THE NON-PUERTO RICAN COUNSELOR AND FELT THAT SENSITIVITY TRAINING HAD DEFLECTED THE GROUP FROM POLITICAL OBJECTIVES. THE SENSITIVITY GROUP DISBANDED TO ALIGN WITH THE NEW POLITICALLY MOTIVATED MAJORITY. THE REJECTION OF THE NON-PUERTO RICAN COUNSELOR IS SAID TO REFLECT THE STUDENTS' NEED TO ESTABLISH THEMSELVES WITHOUT OUTSIDE HELP—HELP WHICH THEY CONSIDERED PATRONIZING AND A CONTINUATION OF

556

ROLES THAT HAD PREVIOUSLY DOMINATED THEIR LIVES.

ACCN 001390

1614 AUTH **RYAN, E. B., CARRANZA, M. A., & MOFFIE, R. W.**

TITL REACTIONS TOWARD VARYING DEGREES OF ACCENTEDNESS IN THE SPEECH OF SPANISH-ENGLISH BILINGUALS.

SRCE *LANGUAGE AND SPEECH, 1977, 20(PART 3), 267-273.*

INDX BILINGUALISM, COLLEGE STUDENTS, EMPIRICAL, STEREOTYPES, MIDWEST, PREJUDICE, RESEARCH METHODOLOGY

ABST THE RELATIONSHIP BETWEEN THE AMOUNT OF ACCENTEDNESS HEARD FROM SPANISH-ENGLISH BILINGUAL SPEAKERS AND THE CHARACTERISTICS ATTRIBUTED TO THOSE SPEAKERS WAS INVESTIGATED. APPROXIMATELY 100 MIDWESTERN COLLEGE STUDENTS—CHARACTERIZED AS MIDDLE CLASS AND NATIVE ENGLISH SPEAKERS—WERE ASKED TO EVALUATE BILINGUAL SPEAKERS ON THE BASIS OF TAPED READINGS OF AN ENGLISH TEXT. THE SPEAKERS WERE CHOSEN TO REPRESENT A WIDE RANGE OF ACCENTEDNESS. THE RESULTS SHOW THAT THE STUDENTS MADE RATHER FINE DISCRIMINATIONS AMONG VARYING DEGREES OF ACCENTEDNESS IN RATING SPEAKERS' PERSONAL ATTRIBUTES AND SPEECH. SUPPORT WAS THUS FOUND FOR THE PROPOSITION THAT SPANISH-ACCENTED ENGLISH IS NEGATIVELY STEREOTYPED AND THAT THE MORE ACCENTED THE SPEECH, THE STRONGER THE STEREOTYPE. A SECOND CONCERN OF THE STUDY WAS THE METHODOLOGY. AS OPPOSED TO THE COMPLICATED SCALING TECHNIQUES PREVIOUSLY EMPLOYED IN SUCH RESEARCH, THE PRESENT STUDY USED A COMPARATIVELY SIMPLE SEVEN-POINT RATING SCALE WHICH CAN BE GROUP-ADMINISTERED. THIS TECHNIQUE WAS EFFECTIVE AND CONVENIENT. IT IS CONCLUDED THAT RESEARCH CONCERNED WITH REACTIONS TO A RANGE OF ACCENTEDNESS CAN NOW PROGRESS RAPIDLY. 17 REFERENCES. (AUTHOR ABSTRACT MODIFIED)

ACCN 001391

1615 AUTH **RYAN, E. B., & CARRANZA, M. A.**

TITL EVALUATIVE REACTIONS OF ADOLESCENTS TOWARD SPEAKERS OF STANDARD ENGLISH AND MEXICAN AMERICAN ACCENTED ENGLISH.

SRCE *JOURNAL OF PERSONALITY AND SOCIAL PSYCHOLOGY, 1975, 31(5), 855-863.*

INDX CROSS CULTURAL, MEXICAN AMERICAN, ETHNIC IDENTITY, ADOLESCENTS, EMPIRICAL, DISCRIMINATION

ABST TWENTY-ONE BILINGUAL MEXICAN AMERICAN, 21 BLACK, AND 21 ANGLO ADOLESCENT FEMALE SUBJECTS FROM CHICAGO RATED PERSONALITIES OF MALE SPEAKERS OF STANDARD ENGLISH AND MEXICAN AMERICAN ACCENTED ENGLISH. IN ORDER TO DEMONSTRATE THAT THE FUNCTIONAL SEPARATION OF SPEECH STYLES WOULD BE REFLECTED IN THESE EVALUATIVE REACTIONS, TWO SPEECH

CONTEXTS (HOME AND SCHOOL) AND TWO SETS OF RATING SCALES (STATUS STRESSING AND SOLIDARITY STRESSING) WERE EMPLOYED. ALTHOUGH STANDARD ENGLISH SPEAKERS RECEIVED MORE FAVORABLE RATINGS IN EVERY CASE, THE DIFFERENCES WERE SIGNIFICANTLY GREATER IN THE SCHOOL CONTEXT THAN IN THE HOME CONTEXT AND FOR STATUS RATINGS THAN FOR SOLIDARITY RATINGS. CONTRARY TO EXPECTATIONS, MEXICAN AMERICANS DID NOT PREFER ACCENTED ENGLISH IN THE HOME CONTEXT OR ON SOLIDARITY SCALES. 32 REFERENCES. (JOURNAL ABSTRACT MODIFIED)

ACCN 001392

1616 AUTH **RYAN, E. B., & CARRANZA, M. A.**

TITL INGROUP AND OUTGROUP REACTIONS TO MEXICAN AMERICAN LANGUAGE VARIETIES.

SRCE *IN H. GILES (ED.), LANGUAGE, ETHNICITY, AND INTERGROUP RELATIONS. LONDON: ACADEMIC PRESS, 1976.*

INDX BILINGUALISM, STEREOTYPES, REVIEW, RESEARCH METHODOLOGY, CROSS CULTURAL, PREJUDICE, ACCULTURATION, ETHNIC IDENTITY, ATTITUDES

ABST VARIOUS STUDIES ARE SUMMARIZED CONCERNING INGROUP AND OUTGROUP ATTITUDES TOWARDS MEXICAN AMERICAN (MA) LANGUAGE VARIETIES. EVALUATIVE REACTIONS OF LISTENERS TOWARD TAPE RECORDED SPEAKERS REPRESENTATIVE OF PARTICULAR SPEECH STYLES ARE REVIEWED. RESULTS OF THESE STUDIES INDICATE SOME APPRECIATION FOR THE SPANISH LANGUAGE BY BOTH MA'S AND ANGLOS. STANDARD SPANISH WAS VIEWED MORE FAVORABLY THAN LOCAL SPANISH DIALECTS, AND DEFINITE NEGATIVE ATTITUDES EXISTED TOWARD MA ACCENTED ENGLISH. INDIVIDUALS WITH STRONGER ACCENTS ARE ASSUMED TO BE CLOSELY TIED TO MEXICO AND ITS TRADITIONS. IT IS CONCLUDED THAT ATTITUDES TOWARD LANGUAGE VARIETIES CAN BE USED AS A METHOD OF STUDYING FACTORS RELATED TO ETHNIC IDENTIFICATION AMONG MEXICAN AMERICANS. 40 REFERENCES.

ACCN 001393

1617 AUTH **SAAVEDRA, P.**

TITL THE FEDERAL GOVERNMENT—WASHINGTON'S BIGGEST INDUSTRY HIRES FEW HISPANICS.

SRCE *AGENDA, JANUARY/FEBRUARY 1977, PP. 10-13.*

INDX REPRESENTATION, EMPLOYMENT, EQUAL OPPORTUNITY, PROGRAM EVALUATION, HISTORY, DISCRIMINATION, EMPIRICAL, SPANISH SURNAMED, LABOR FORCE

ABST HISPANIC REPRESENTATION IN THE WORK FORCE OF THE FEDERAL GOVERNMENT IS VERY POOR AND THE NEEDS OF THE HISPANIC COMMUNITY REMAIN LARGELY UNANSWERED. THE U.S. CIVIL SERVICE COMMISSION'S 1969 REPORT ON MINORITY EMPLOYMENT IN THE FEDERAL GOVERNMENT DOCUMENTED THIS FACT, AND THEREFORE THE SPANISH-SPEAKING PROGRAM (SSP) WAS SET UP TO REMEDY THE SITUATION. TO ASSESS THE EFFORTS OF SSP, DATA FROM LATER COMMISSION RE-

PORTS FROM 1971 AND 1972 PLUS STATISTICS ON THE DISTRIBUTION OF HISPANICS ACROSS JOB LEVELS ARE PRESENTED. THESE DATA REVEAL THE FAILURE OF SSP TO INCREASE HISPANIC EMPLOYMENT MORE THAN .5 PERCENT. BOTH AN OPTIMISTIC AND CRITICAL VIEW OF SSP ARE DISCUSSED, BUT THE CONTINUING UNDERREPRESENTATION SUPPORTS A REASSESSMENT OF SSP AND ITS MANNER OF ACHIEVING ITS GOALS. IT IS RECOMMENDED THAT HISPANICS BE INCLUDED IN POLICY-MAKING POSITIONS AND THAT THE MAJOR OBSTACLES TO AN INCREASED NUMBER OF HISPANIC EMPLOYEES BE REEXAMINED. MOREOVER, AREAS OF THE FEDERAL GOVERNMENT THAT DEAL CLOSELY WITH THE LATINO COMMUNITY SHOULD BE CLOSELY MONITORED AND THEIR RECRUITMENT AND UPWARD MOBILITY EFFORTS FOR HISPANICS SHOULD BE CRITICALLY ASSESSED. 2 REFERENCES.

ACCN 001394

1618 AUTH **SAAVEDRA, P.**
TITL THE WELFARE SYSTEM: NEW PROMISES OF REFORM.
SRCE *THE NATION, MARCH/APRIL 1977, PP. 11-13.*
INDX SOCIAL SERVICES, POVERTY, ESSAY, ECONOMIC FACTORS, LEGISLATION, MIGRATION, EMPLOYMENT, MEXICAN AMERICAN, POLICY, POLITICS, SES
ABST IN LIGHT OF OUTSTANDING WELFARE PROBLEMS, THE CARTER ADMINISTRATION'S CAMPAIGN PROMISES AND INITIAL ACTIVITIES WITH REGARD TO WELFARE SYSTEM REFORM ARE EXAMINED. WELFARE SYSTEM PROBLEMS REPORTED INCLUDE: (1) SIZE (OVER 100 PROGRAMS GIVE AID ADMINISTERED BY HUNDREDS OF FEDERAL, STATE, AND LOCAL AGENCIES); (2) DUPLICATION OF SERVICES; (3) INEQUITY IN DISTRIBUTION; (4) LANGUAGE BARRIERS BETWEEN AGENCY STAFF AND RECIPIENTS; (5) REGIONAL VARIATION IN ELIGIBILITY REQUIREMENTS; (6) HIGH ADMINISTRATIVE COSTS; (7) LACK OF BUILT-IN WORK INCENTIVES; (8) SYSTEM ENCOURAGEMENT OF FAMILY DISPERSION; AND (9) OUTDATED POVERTY AND ELIGIBILITY MEASURES. A WELFARE REFORM CONSULTING GROUP FORMED WITHIN HEW IN MAY, 1977, WAS CHARGED WITH EVALUATING ALTERNATIVES TO THE PRESENT SYSTEM AND MAKING RECOMMENDATIONS TO THE PRESIDENT. WITHIN THE GROUP WERE REPRESENTATIVES FROM CONGRESSIONAL COMMITTEES, DEPARTMENTS OF HOUSING AND URBAN DEVELOPMENT, THE TREASURY, AGRICULTURE, LABOR, THE COUNCIL OF ECONOMIC ADVISORS, AND STATE AND LOCAL LEGISLATURES. HISPANIC REPRESENTATION INCLUDED HEW ASSISTANT SECRETARY FOR HUMAN DEVELOPMENT, ARABELLA MARTINEZ. PROPOSALS FOR REFORM INCLUDED: (1) TOTAL FEDERALIZATION OF THE WELFARE SYSTEM; (2) ESTABLISHMENT OF A NATIONAL INCOME FLOOR OR MINIMUM STANDARD OF BENEFITS; (3) WORKER REGISTRATION REQUIREMENTS FOR RECIPIENTS; (4) COORDINATION OF FEDERAL JOB POLICIES WITH INCOME TRANSFER PROGRAMS; AND (5) ELIMINATION OF ELIGIBIL-

ITY REQUIREMENTS BASED ON SUCH CATEGORIES AS FEMALE-HEADED HOUSEHOLDS. MAJOR CONCERNS WITHIN THE HISPANIC COMMUNITY WERE THE LACK OF ACCURATE DATA ON THE IMPACT OF WELFARE ON HISPANICS AND INADEQUATE BILINGUAL/BICULTURAL STAFFING IN WELFARE AGENCIES. THE INPUT OF MAJOR INTEREST GROUPS THROUGH PUBLIC FORUMS WAS ENCOURAGED BY THE WELFARE REFORM COUNSELING GROUP.

ACCN 001041

1619 AUTH **SABIN, J. E.**
TITL TRANSLATING DESPAIR.
SRCE *AMERICAN JOURNAL OF PSYCHIATRY, 1975, 132(2), 197-199.*
INDX BILINGUAL, BILINGUAL-BICULTURAL PERSONNEL, BILINGUALISM, CASE STUDY, EMPIRICAL, MENTAL HEALTH, MOTHER-CHILD INTERACTION, PSYCHOPATHOLOGY, PSYCHOTHERAPISTS, PSYCHOTHERAPY OUTCOME, SOUTH AMERICA, PUERTO RICAN-M, SPANISH SURNAMED, SUICIDE, EAST, ADULTS, POLICY
ABST THE AUTHOR REVIEWS TWO CASES OF SUICIDE BY SPANISH-SPEAKING PATIENTS—A 45 YEAR-OLD SOUTH AMERICAN WOMAN AND A 71 YEAR-OLD PUERTO RICAN MAN—WHO WERE BOTH EVALUATED AND TREATED BY ENGLISH-SPEAKING PSYCHIATRISTS USING A TRANSLATOR. BY TRACING KEY EVENTS LEADING TO THE SUICIDAL EPISODES, HE SUGGESTS THAT THE PATIENTS' EMOTIONAL SUFFERING MAY BE SELECTIVELY UNDERESTIMATED WHEN THE CLINICIAN WORKS BY MEANS OF TRANSLATION. SO EVEN THOUGH THE CLINICIAN IS BEING PROVIDED WITH DATA WHICH ALLOW HIM TO RECOGNIZE THE PSYCHOTIC FEATURES OF THE ILLNESS, HE MAY NOT HAVE THE INTERPERSONAL CLOSENESS NECESSARY FOR AN APPRECIATION OF THE PATIENT'S AFFECTIVE STATE. CONSEQUENTLY, THE RISK OF SUICIDE MAY BE UNDERESTIMATED OR OVERLOOKED. GIVEN SUCH A RISK, IT IS PROPOSED THAT MENTAL HEALTH CLINICIANS AND THEIR TRANSLATOR COLLEAGUES TAKE SPECIAL PRECAUTIONS. THEY SHOULD RECOGNIZE THAT WHILE TRANSLATION ALLOWS EFFECTIVE GATHERING OF DATA ON LIFE HSITORY, BEHAVIOR, AND PSYCHOTIC PHENOMENA, THE PROCESS MAY SELECTIVELY MISS RECOGNITION OF THE PATIENT'S DESPAIR. 4 REFERENCES.

ACCN 002200

1620 AUTH **SAEGERT, J., KAZARIAN, S., & YOUNG, R. K.**
TITL PART/WHOLE TRANSFER WITH BILINGUALS.
SRCE *AMERICAN JOURNAL OF PSYCHOLOGY, 1973, 86(3), 537-546.*
INDX CROSS CULTURAL, COLLEGE STUDENTS, MEXICAN AMERICAN, LINGUISTICS, LANGUAGE ASSESSMENT, LANGUAGE COMPREHENSION, LINGUISTIC COMPETENCE, EMPIRICAL, BILINGUALISM, ADOLESCENTS, TEXAS, SOUTHWEST, BILINGUAL
ABST LANGUAGE STORAGE FOR BILINGUALS IS HYPOTHESIZED TO BE EITHER AN INDEPENDENT SYSTEM FOR EACH LANGUAGE OR SOME SYSTEM OF SHARED INTERDEPENDENCE. IN STUDYING SUBJECTIVE WORD GROUPINGS,

RESEARCHERS HAVE USED THE PART/WHOLE TRANSFER PARADIGM AND HAVE FOUND AN INITIAL POSITIVE TRANSFER WHICH THEN SHIFTS TO A NEGATIVE TRANSFER. THIS TRANSFER OR INTERFERENCE PARADIGM IS USED TO TEST THE HYPOTHESES OF INDEPENDENT VERSUS INTERDEPENDENT STORAGE FOR BILINGUALS. SUBJECTS WERE 64 ENGLISH/ SPANISH BILINGUALS IN HIGH SCHOOLS IN AUSTIN, TEXAS, AND 64 ARABIC/ENGLISH COLLEGE BILINGUALS FROM BERUIT. THESE BILINGUAL SUBJECTS WERE FOUND TO EXHIBIT TYPICAL NEGATIVE TRANSFER EFFECTS IN PART/ WHOLE LEARNING WHEN BOTH PART AND WHOLE LISTS WERE IN THE SAME LANGUAGE. HOWEVER, IN A BILINGUAL VERSION OF THE EXPERIMENT, ONLY WHEN SUBJECTS WERE SWITCHED FROM A PART LIST IN THEIR DOMINANT LANGUAGE TO A WHOLE LIST IN THEIR NONDOMINANT LANGUAGE WAS NEGATIVE TRANSFER OBSERVED. THE HYPOTHESIS OF INTERLINGUAL INTERDEPENDENT STORAGE BEST EXPLAINS THESE RESULTS. HOWEVER, ALTERNATIVE EXPLANATIONS OF INTERLINGUAL INDEPENDENCE AND DIFFERENTIAL ATTENTION EFFECTS ARE ALSO DISCUSSED. 12 REFERENCES. (JOURNAL ABSTRACT MODIFIED)

ACCN   001396

1621 AUTH **SAFA, H. I.**
TITL   FROM SHANTY TOWN TO PUBLIC HOUSING: A COMPARISON OF FAMILY STRUCTURE IN TWO URBAN NEIGHBORHOODS IN PUERTO RICO.
SRCE   *CARIBBEAN STUDIES, 1964, 4(1), 3-12.*
INDX   POVERTY, HOUSING, COMMUNITY, PUERTO RICAN-I, FAMILY ROLES, URBAN, FAMILY STRUCTURE, INTERPERSONAL RELATIONS, SES
ABST   AN EFFORT IS MADE TO ASCERTAIN THE BASIC PATTERNS OF FAMILY AND COMMUNITY LIFE IN A SHANTY TOWN AND THE WAY IN WHICH THESE PATTERNS ARE ALTERED IN PUBLIC HOUSING. DATA WERE COLLECTED BY MEANS OF INTENSIVE PARTICIPANT OBSERVATION AND A FORMAL INTERVIEW SCHEDULE ADMINISTERED TO A SAMPLE OF 474 INDIVIDUALS IN 100 HOUSEHOLDS IN EACH NEIGHBORHOOD. AN ATTEMPT WAS MADE TO INTERVIEW MALE AND FEMALE ADULTS AS WELL AS ADOLESCENTS. THE ETHNOHISTORICAL APPROACH TO WEST INDIAN FAMILY STRUCTURE CANNOT EXPLAIN THE DIFFERENTIAL EMPHASIS ON MATRIFOCALITY IN A CULTURALLY HOMOGENEOUS POPULATION LIKE THE SHANTY TOWN AND PUBLIC HOUSING PROJECT. JOB INSTABILITY, LIMITED OPPORTUNITIES FOR UPWARD MOBILITY, THE STRICT DIVISION OF LABOR IN THE HOUSEHOLD, AND THE STRONG EMOTIONAL BOND BETWEEN A MOTHER, HER CHILDREN, AND HER FEMALE RELATIVES ALL CONTRIBUTE TO THE MARGINAL POSITION OF THE MAN IN BOTH THE SHANTY TOWN AND THE PROJECT HOUSEHOLD. IN PUBLIC HOUSING HIS STATUS IS WEAKENED FURTHER BY A PATERNALISTIC PROJECT MANAGEMENT WHICH TAKES OVER MANY OF HIS RESPONSIBILITIES WHILE THE WOMAN'S ROLE IN RUNNING THE HOUSEHOLD AND REARING THE CHILDREN IS LEFT LARGELY INTACT. WHILE SLAVERY AND WEST AFRICAN HERITAGES MAY HAVE CONTRIBUTED TO THE ORIGIN OF THE MATRIFOCAL FAMILY IN THE CARIBBEAN, WE MUST LOOK TO PRESENT-DAY STRUCTURAL FACTORS FOR ITS CONTINUATION. 6 REFERENCES.

ACCN   001397

1622 AUTH **SAFA, H. I.**
TITL   STIMULUS/RESPONSE: THE POOR ARE LIKE EVERYONE ELSE, OSCAR.
SRCE   *PSYCHOLOGY TODAY, 1970 (SEPTEMBER), PP. 26; 28; 30; 32.*
INDX   POVERTY, SES, PUERTO RICAN-I, CASE STUDY, SOCIAL MOBILITY, OCCUPATIONAL ASPIRATIONS, SCHOLASTIC ASPIRATIONS, ATTITUDES, ADULTS, FATALISM
ABST   A STUDY OF PUERTO RICO'S POOR REFUTES THAT PORTION OF THE OSCAR LEWIS STUDY WHICH FOUND THEM TO BE FATALISTIC, LAZY, IGNORANT PEOPLE WHO DON'T KNOW HOW TO SPEND THEIR MONEY. ON THE CONTRARY, THOSE PUERTO RICAN POOR INTERVIEWED IN THE CURRENT STUDY BELIEVE FIRMLY IN UPWARD MOBILITY BASED ON INDIVIDUAL INITIATIVE, THRIFT, EDUCATION, AND OTHER ATTITUDES COMMONLY ASSOCIATED WITH THE PROTESTANT ETHIC. UNFORTUNATELY, THE POOR IN PUERTO RICO ARE CONTENT WITH THE RELATIVELY SMALL GAINS MADE IN THE LAST DECADE: A SMALL HOUSE, A STABLE MINIMUM INCOME, AND EDUCATION FOR THEIR CHILDREN. THEIR MODEST GAINS HAVE PLAYED A STRATEGIC ROLE IN MAINTAINING THE EXISTING SOCIAL SYSTEM IN PUERTO RICO, CONVINCING THE POOR THAT UPWARD MOBILITY IS POSSIBLE AND THAT ANYONE WHO WANTS TO CAN GET AHEAD. THIS COMMITMENT TO THE STATUS QUO EXTENDS TO PUERTO RICO'S CONTINUED DEPENDENCE ON THE UNITED STATES AND ITS REJECTION OF COMMUNISM. THEIR HANDICAP IS THAT THEY DO NOT EVIDENCE A CURRENT CAPACITY TO RECOGNIZE THEIR POTENTIAL AND CHANGE THE SOCIOECONOMIC STRUCTURE THAT PLACES LIMITATIONS ON THEIR CONTINUED ADVANCEMENT.

ACCN   001398

1623 AUTH **SALAS, G., & SALAS, I.**
TITL   THE MEXICAN COMMUNITY OF DETROIT.
SRCE   *IN M. M. MANGOLD (ED.), LA CAUSA CHICANA: THE MOVEMENT FOR JUSTICE. NEW YORK: FAMILY SERVICE ASSOCIATION OF AMERICA, 1971, PP. 161-178.*
INDX   MIGRATION, MEXICAN AMERICAN, FARM LABORERS, LEADERSHIP, COMMUNITY, POLITICAL POWER, CASE STUDY, URBAN, RELIGION, REPRESENTATION, DISCRIMINATION, PREJUDICE, EMPLOYMENT, MICHIGAN, MIDWEST
ABST   DETROIT, MICHIGAN, IS GENERALLY REFERRED TO AS A BLACK-WHITE CITY, AND CENSUS FORMS WHICH ONLY LIST BLACK, WHITE OR OTHER CATEGORIES FOR ETHNIC IDENTIFICATION HAVE RESULTED IN A SEVERE UNDERESTIMATION OF THE SIZE OF THE MEXICAN AMERICAN COMMUNITY IN THIS AREA. A CASE STUDY OF A MEXICAN AMERICAN FAMILY MI-

GRATING FROM TEXAS IS PRESENTED AS TYPICAL OF OTHER CHICANOS WHO HAVE MOVED TO THIS REGION. ACCOMPANYING THE GROWTH OF THE CHICANO COMMUNITY HAS BEEN THE FORMATION OF CULTURAL, RELIGIOUS, AND LABOR ORGANIZATIONS WHICH PROVIDE A NETWORK OF SUPPORT FOR CHICANO RESIDENTS. WITH THE FORMATION OF THE LATIN AMERICANS FOR SOCIAL AND ECONOMIC DEVELOPMENT (LASED), CREATED SPECIFICALLY TO DEAL WITH PROBLEMS WITHIN THIS COMMUNITY, CHICANOS ACHIEVED A RECOGNIZED POLITICAL VOICE AND SUCCESSFULLY COMPETED FOR PROGRAM FUNDS. ALTHOUGH THE CHICANO COMMUNITY OF DETROIT HAS MADE SOME STRIDES, MANY SERIOUS PROBLEMS STILL EXIST. 5 REFERENCES.

ACCN   001399

1624 AUTH   **SALDATE, M., IV.**
TITL   FACTORS INFLUENCING ACADEMIC PERFORMANCE OF HIGH AND LOW ACHIEVING MEXICAN-AMERICAN CHILDREN (DOCTORAL DISSERTATION, UNIVERSITY OF ARIZONA, 1972).
SRCE   *DISSERTATION ABSTRACTS INTERNATIONAL, 1973, 33(9), 4987A. (UNIVERSITY MICROFILMS NO. 73-06724.)*
INDX   MEXICAN AMERICAN, CHILDREN, ACHIEVEMENT MOTIVATION, PERFORMANCE EXPECTATIONS, SCHOLASTIC ACHIEVEMENT, EMPIRICAL, FAMILY STRUCTURE, SCHOLASTIC ASPIRATIONS, CLASSROOM BEHAVIOR, SELF CONCEPT, TEACHERS, SES, BILINGUAL, ENVIRONMENTAL FACTORS, CULTURAL FACTORS, ARIZONA
ABST   AN INVESTIGATION OF FACTORS WHICH INFLUENCE THE ACADEMIC ACHIEVEMENT AND ATTITUDES OF MEXICAN AMERICAN CHILDREN INVOLVED 23 HIGH-ACHIEVING AND 23 LOW-ACHIEVING 6TH GRADE STUDENTS IN NOGALES, ARIZONA. THESE SUBJECTS HAD OBTAINED SIMILAR SCORES ON THE LORGE-THORNDIKE FORM A INTELLIGENCE TEST AND ON THE CALIFORNIA ACHIEVEMENT TEST. INFORMATION WAS OBTAINED FROM INTERVIEWS WITH THE MOTHERS OF THE SUBJECTS, TEACHERS' RATINGS OF THE CHILDREN'S BEHAVIORAL CHARACTERISTICS, AND ASSESSMENTS OF THE SUBJECTS' SELF-CONCEPT, ACADEMIC VALUES, AND SCHOLASTIC ASPIRATIONS. THE RESULTS REVEALED THAT HOME VARIABLES (SUCH AS PARENTAL EDUCATION AND INCOME, LANGUAGE USAGE, AND ENVIRONMENTAL REINFORCEMENT MODES) WERE NOT SIGNIFICANTLY RELATED TO THE SUBJECTS' HIGH OR LOW LEVELS OF ACHIEVEMENT. HOWEVER, PARENTAL OCCUPATIONS PROVED TO BE HIGHER AMONG THE HIGH ACHIEVERS, WHILE GUIDANCE FROM PARENTS WAS GREATER AMONG LOW ACHIEVERS. WHILE THERE WERE NO SIGNIFICANT DIFFERENCES IN THE SUBJECTS' ACADEMIC VALUES AND ASPIRATIONS, HIGH ACHIEVERS RECEIVED HIGHER RATINGS FROM TEACHERS AND SCORED SIGNIFICANTLY HIGHER ON THE SELF-ESTEEM INVENTORY. THESE FINDINGS SUGGEST THAT VARIABLES (SUCH AS LANGUAGE USAGE) SHOULD BE RE-EVALUATED AND THAT GREATERATTENTION SHOULD BE GIVEN TO SELF-CONCEPT AND TEACHER PERCEPTIONS BY THOSE INVOLVED IN EDUCATING OR COUNSELING MEXICAN AMERICANS. 78 REFERENCES. (AUTHOR ABSTRACT MODIFIED)
ACCN   001400

1625 AUTH   **SALINAS, G.**
TITL   MEXICAN-AMERICANS AND THE DESEGREGATION OF SCHOOLS IN THE SOUTHWEST.
SRCE   *HOUSTON LAW REVIEW, 1971, 8(5), 929-951.*
INDX   DISCRIMINATION, EDUCATION, INTEGRATION, JUDICIAL PROCESS, LEGISLATION, MEXICAN AMERICAN, ESSAY, HOUSING, HISTORY
ABST   THE COURT DECISION OF CISNEROS VS. CORPUS CHRISTI INDEPENDENT SCHOOL DISTRICT (1970) HELD THAT MEXICAN AMERICANS ARE AN "IDENTIFIABLE ETHNIC GROUP" FOR THE PURPOSE OF PUBLIC SCHOOL DESEGREGATION. THIS LANDMARK RULING CHALLENGES THE VIEW THAT MEXICAN AMERICANS ARE WHITE AND IS HENCE HAILED BY THE AUTHOR AS CAUSE FOR OPTIMISM: (1) IT INTRODUCES A NEW GROUP INTO THE DESEGREGATION PROCESS; (2) UNDERSCORES THE CONCEPT THAT FEDERAL COURTS SHOULD CONSIDER MEXICAN AMERICAN STUDENTS IN DETERMINING WHETHER A SCHOOL SYSTEM IS RACIALLY BALANCED; AND (3) MOST IMPORTANTLY, IT SHOULD SERVE TO RESTRAIN THOSE SCHOOL DISTRICTS WHO SEEK TO CIRCUMVENT COURT DESEGREGATION ORDERS BY ONLY INTEGRATING MEXICAN AMERICANS WITH NEGROES. AGAINST THE BACKDROP OF THE CISNEROS LEGISLATION, THIS ESSAY CHRONICLES VARIOUS CIVIL RIGHTS STRUGGLES BY CHICANO GROUPS IN THE SOUTHWEST FROM THE 1940'S TO THE PRESENT TO ACHIEVE EDUCATIONAL PARITY WITH ANGLO POPULATIONS. CAUSE FOR HOPE IN THIS EFFORT IS SEEN TO BE CONSISTENT WITH PRIOR JUDICIAL DEVELOPMENTS WHICH HAVE GRANTED MEXICAN AMERICANS PROTECTION FROM DISCRIMINATION IN HOUSING, EMPLOYMENT, PUBLIC ACCOMMODATIONS, VOTING, THE ADMINISTRATION OF JUSTICE, AND IN THE FIELD OF EDUCATIONAL OPPORTUNITY. 110 REFERENCES.
ACCN   001401

1626 AUTH   **SAMORA, J.**
TITL   CONCEPTIONS OF HEALTH AND DISEASE AMONG SPANISH-AMERICANS.
SRCE   *THE AMERICAN CATHOLIC SOCIOLOGICAL REVIEW, 1961, 22(1), 314-323.*
INDX   HEALTH, DISEASE, ATTITUDES, SPANISH SURNAMED, RELIGION, FOLK MEDICINE, CURANDERISMO, ESSAY, RURAL, POLICY, SOUTHWEST, CULTURE
ABST   CONCEPTIONS OF HEALTH AND DISEASE AS PERCEIVED BY SPANISH AMERICAN VILLAGERS ARE DISCUSSED IN TERMS OF THE IMPACT OF CULTURAL AND RELIGIOUS ORIENTATIONS. A GENERAL FRAMEWORK WITH AN EMPHASIS ON THE ROLE OF RELIGIOUS BELIEFS ON THESE CONCEPTIONS IS PRESENTED. VIEWS OF DISEASE PREVENTION, CAUSATION, DIAGNOSIS, TREATMENT, AND GENERAL HEALTH

ORIENTATION FOR SPANISH AMERICANS ARE CONSIDERED WITHIN THIS FRAMEWORK. IT IS SUGGESTED THAT A STRONG RELIGIOUS COMPONENT, SUCH AS SUPERNATURAL PUN-ISHMENTS AND DIVINE PREDESTINATION, IS PART OF A GENERAL LIFE ORIENTATION AND AMONG THIS POPULATION REPRESENTS A CENTRAL THEME IN HEALTH AND DISEASE CONCEPTIONS. THESE BELIEFS SHOULD BE TAKEN INTO ACCOUNT WHEN CONSIDERING ETIOLOGICAL FACTORS, PREVENTIVE MEA-SURES, DIAGNOSTIC PERCEPTIONS, AND THERAPEUTIC PROCEDURES AS THEY ARE CONCEPTUALIZED BY SPANISH AMERICAN VIL-LAGERS IN THE RURAL SOUTHWEST. 7 REFER-ENCES.

ACCN 001402

1627 AUTH **SAMORA, J.**
TITL LOS MOJADOS: THE WETBACK STORY.
SRCE *NOTRE DAME, IND.: UNIVERSITY OF NOTRE DAME PRESS, 1971.*
INDX MEXICAN, UNDOCUMENTED WORKERS, JUDI-CIAL PROCESS, STEREOTYPES, SOUTHWEST, MIDWEST, ECONOMIC FACTORS, MALE, EMPIR-ICAL, CASE STUDY, DEMOGRAPHIC, BOOK, POLICY, WEST, ATTITUDES, IMMIGRATION
ABST TO UNDERSTAND THE MOTIVES, STRATEGIES, AND PROBLEMS OF MEXICANS WHO ILLE-GALLY ENTER THE U.S. IN SEARCH OF WORK, 493 SUCH MEN WHO WERE AWAITING DEPOR-TATION WERE INTERVIEWED AT IMMIGRATION & NATURALIZATION SERVICE (INS) DETENTION CENTERS IN THE SOUTHWEST. SUPPLEMEN-TARY DATA ARE PROVIDED BY INS STATISTICS PLUS A NARRATIVE BY ONE RESEARCH WHO POSED AS A WETBACK "TO LEARN WHAT IT FEELS LIKE TO AVOID 'LA MIGRA' (THE BORDER PATROL)." INCLUDED IN THIS REPORT OF THE STUDY ARE: (1) THE HISTORY OF MEXICAN IM-MIGRATION; (2) METHODOLOGICAL DIFFICUL-TIES WITH THIS SUBJECT POPULATION; (3) THE PROCESS OF INS APPREHENSION AND DEPOR-TATION; (4) THE ARRANGEMENTS MADE FOR CROSSING THE BORDER ILLEGALLY; (5) THE IMMIGRANTS' PERCEPTIONS AND ASPIRA-TIONS REGARDING THE U.S.; (6) THE IMMI-GRANTS' WORK EXPERIENCES AND THEIR EF-FORTS TO AVOID THE INS; AND (7) GOVERNMENT POLICIES IN MEXICO AND THE U.S. CONCERNING ILLEGAL IMMIGRANTS. AT A GENERAL, MORE MEANINGFUL LEVEL, THIS STUDY REVEALED THAT ILLEGAL ENTRY IS LIKE A "GAME" RATHER THAN A SERIOUS LEGAL OF-FENSE. NEVERTHELESS, IT IS A DESPERATE GAME WHICH PROVES BENEFICIAL ONLY TO THE U.S., AS THE MEXICANS TAKE DANGER-OUS RISKS AND SUFFER COUNTLESS ABUSES FOR A NONEXISTENT UTOPIA. THUS, THE FINAL CHAPTER OFFERS SEVERAL RECOMMENDA-TIONS FOR ALLEVIATING THE PROBLEM—E.G., FOR THE U.S. TO FINE EMPLOYERS WHO HIRE UNDOCUMENTED WORKERS, AND FOR MEXICO TO IMPLEMENT A REALISTIC ECONOMIC DE-VELOPMENT PROGRAM. 63 REFERENCES.
ACCN 001842

1628 AUTH **SAMORA, J., SAUNDERS, L., & LARSON, R. F.**
TITL KNOWLEDGE ABOUT SPECIFIC DISEASES IN FOUR SELECTED SAMPLES.
SRCE *JOURNAL OF HEALTH AND HUMAN BEHAVIOR, 1962, 3(3), 176-185.*
INDX SEX COMPARISON, SES, INDIANA, COLORADO, PENNSYLVANIA, MIDWEST, SOUTHWEST, EAST, SES, MEXICAN AMERICAN, ADOLESCENTS, ADULTS, DISEASE, HEALTH, HEALTH EDUCA-TION, PHYSICIANS, SYMPTOMATOLOGY, CROSS CULTURAL
ABST IN AN EFFORT TO INCREASE EFFECTIVE COM-MUNICATION BETWEEN PHYSICIANS AND PA-TIENTS, THE LEVEL OF MEDICAL KNOWLEDGE ABOUT 10 COMMON DISEASES AMONG RE-SPONDENTS IN 3 DIFFERENT SETTINGS WAS INVESTIGATED. THE SAMPLE INCLUDED 118 IN-PATIENTS IN A DENVER, COLORADO HOSPITAL, 102 PATIENTS FROM A READING, PENNSYLVA-NIA HOSPITAL OUTPATIENT CLINIC AND RA-DIOLOGY LABORATORY, AND 150 SUBJECTS FROM A QUOTA SAMPLING IN SOUTH BEND, IN-DIANA. RESPONSES FROM THESE SAMPLES WERE COMPARED TO DATA PREVIOUSLY RE-PORTED FOR OUTPATIENTS IN A NEW YORK CLINIC. THE VARIABLES OF AGE AND SEX WERE NOT SIGNIFICANTLY ASSOCIATED WITH HEALTH KNOWLEDGE. ETHNICITY WAS ONLY CRUCIAL WHERE CULTURAL DIFFERENCES ARE SIGNIFICANT, SUCH AS BETWEEN ANGLOS AND MEXICAN AMERICANS IN THE SOUTHWEST. EDUCATION WAS THE VARIABLE MOST POSI-TIVELY ASSOCIATED WITH POSSESSION OF HEALTH KNOWLEDGE. FINDINGS REVEALED THAT THE LOW LEVEL OF HEALTH KNOWLEDGE AMONG RESPONDENTS MAY BE A POTENTIAL BARRIER TO EFFECTIVE PHYSICIAN-PATIENT COMMUNICATION. 7 REFERENCES.
ACCN 001403

1629 AUTH **SAMUDA, R. J.**
TITL PSYCHOLOGICAL TESTING OF AMERICAN MI-NORITIES ISSUES AND CONSEQUENCES.
SRCE *NEW YORK: HARPER & ROW PUBLISHERS, 1975.*
INDX ABILITY TESTING, INTELLIGENCE TESTING, CROSS CULTURAL, WISC, STEREOTYPES, STANFORD-BINET INTELLIGENCE TEST, CUL-TURE-FAIR TESTS, CULTURAL FACTORS, CUL-TURAL PLURALISM, TEST VALIDITY, TEST RELI-ABILITY, SES, REVIEW, BOOK, EDUCATION, PREJUDICE, READING, ENVIRONMENTAL FAC-TORS
ABST A SUMMARY AND CRITICAL ANALYSIS ARE PRESENTED OF THE PERSPECTIVES, TRENDS, AND PITFALLS IN THE USE OF STANDARDIZED, NORM-REFERENCED TESTS WITH AMERICAN MINORITIES. THE BOOK'S SIX CHAPTERS BE-GIN WITH A GENERAL CONSIDERATION OF TESTING ISSUES AND THE PROBLEMS OF MEA-SURING INTELLIGENCE. THEN, ATTENTION FO-CUSES ON THE MAIN CONTROVERSY OF HE-REDITY VS. ENVIRONMENT REGARDING THE DEVELOPMENT OF INTELLIGENCE. IN THIS, A SPECIAL CONCERN IS WITH ENVIRONMENTAL FACTORS (SUCH AS VERBAL DEPRIVATION, MA-TERNAL MALNUTRITION, BILINGUALISM) WHICH MAY NEGATIVELY INFLUENCE THE TEST PER-FORMANCE OF MINORITIES AND THEREBY HAVE DAMAGING SOCIAL, EDUCATIONAL, AND ECO-

NOMIC CONSEQUENCES THROUGHOUT THEIR LIVES. TO AVOID SUCH PROBLEMS AND BIASES, ALTERNATIVE TESTING STRATEGIES ARE ADVOCATED—FOR EXAMPLE, CULTURE-FREE/CULTURE-FAIR TESTS, MEASURES OF THE ENVIRONMENT, AND CRITERION-REFERENCED TESTS. THE AUTHOR CONCLUDES THAT THIS BOOK DEALS MORE WITH SOCIAL JUSTICE THAN WITH PSYCHOMETRICS, SINCE PSYCHOLOGICAL TESTING CAN IMPEDE THE PARITY WHICH AMERICAN MINORITIES DESERVE. FINALLY, THE APPENDIX SECTION OFFERS A REFERENCE GUIDE TO 137 PSYCHOLOGICAL TESTS (IN THE AREAS OF ACHIEVEMENT, APTITUDE, PERSONALITY/ATTITUDES, AND MISCELLANEOUS/SENSORY-MOTOR) FOR USE WITH MINORITY ADOLESCENTS AND ADULTS. 398 REFERENCES.

ACCN 001843

1630 AUTH **SANCHEZ, A.**
TITL DRUG ABUSE AND TREATMENT OF THE "TECATO, OR MEXICAN AMERICAN "JUNKIE.
SRCE *PAPER PRESENTED AT A SYMPOSIUM ON THE HEALTH OF THE MEXICAN AMERICAN POPULATION, UNIVERSITY OF ARIZONA, TUCSON, 1975.*
INDX DRUG ADDICTION, ESSAY, METHADONE MAINTENANCE, PSYCHOTHERAPY, MEXICAN AMERICAN, SES, REHABILITATION, DRUG ABUSE, CULTURAL FACTORS, BILINGUAL-BICULTURAL PERSONNEL, ARIZONA, SOUTHWEST
ABST THE CAUSES AND TREATMENT OF THE MEXICAN AMERICAN HEROIN ADDICT ARE DISCUSSED BY A DRUG ABUSE COUNSELOR IN TUCSON, ARIZONA. DRUG ABUSE IS FOR MANY MEXICAN AMERICANS A MEANS OF COPING WITH A SOCIETY THAT IMPOSES LIMITATIONS AND FRUSTRATIONS. LOW SES, LACK OF IDENTITY, NEGATIVE SELF-IMAGES CREATED BY RACISM, DISCRIMINATION, DISTRUST OF GOVERNMENTAL INSTITUTIONS, AND LACK OF EDUCATION ARE FACTORS WHICH CONTRIBUTE TO DRUG ABUSE. PROGRAMS DESIGNED TO REHABILITATE MEXICAN AMERICAN DRUG ADDICTS MUST ACKNOWLEDGE THE CULTURAL DIFFERENCES OF THIS POPULATION, WHILE INCREASING THE NUMBER OF BILINGUAL-BICULTURAL COUNSELING PERSONNEL. 1 REFERENCE.
ACCN 001404

1631 AUTH **SANCHEZ, A. J.**
TITL THE DEFINERS AND THE DEFINED: A MENTAL HEALTH ISSUE.
SRCE *EL GRITO, 1971, 4(4), 4-11.*
INDX MENTAL HEALTH, ESSAY, RESOURCE UTILIZATION, HEALTH DELIVERY SYSTEMS, MEXICAN AMERICAN, CALIFORNIA, SOUTHWEST
ABST THE CENTRAL ISSUE EXPLORED IS THAT THE NONUTILIZATION BY CHICANOS OF PUBLIC OUTPATIENT AND INPATIENT MENTAL HEALTH FACILITIES THROUGHOUT CALIFORNIA IS DUE TO THE FACT THAT THESE SERVICES ARE PLANNED BY INSTITUTIONS OUTSIDE OF THE BARRIO. LITERATURE CITED SHOWS THAT THE NONUTILIZATION OF MENTAL HEALTH FACILITIES DOES NOT OCCUR BECAUSE OF LOWER RATES OF PSYCHOLOGICAL DISTRESS, BUT

BECAUSE THE SERVICES ARE IRRELEVANT TO THE CHICANO. MENTAL ILLNESS CAN ONLY BE DEFINED IN RELATION TO THE SOCIAL PROBLEMS WHICH CAUSE STRESS. SINCE THE MENTAL HEALTH SERVICES OFFERED CHICANOS FAIL TO ALLEVIATE THE SOCIAL PROBLEMS WHICH INTENSIFY PSYCHOLOGICAL PROBLEMS, THEY ARE OF LITTLE USE. MENTAL ILLNESS MUST BE DEFINED WITHIN THE FRAMEWORK OF THE CHICANO PHILOSOPHY OF LIFE, AND THIS CAN ONLY BE ACHIEVED WHEN THE COMMUNITY IS ALLOWED TO DEFINE MENTAL ILLNESS AND PLAN MENTAL HEALTH SERVICES. 12 REFERENCES.

ACCN 001405

1632 AUTH **SANCHEZ, G. I.**
TITL BILINGUALISM AND MENTAL MEASURES.
SRCE *THE JOURNAL OF APPLIED PSYCHOLOGY, 1934, 18(6), 765-772.*
INDX ACHIEVEMENT TESTING, ESSAY, BILINGUAL-BICULTURAL EDUCATION, BILINGUALISM, CHILDREN, INTELLIGENCE TESTING, EDUCATION, EQUAL OPPORTUNITY, TEST VALIDITY, CULTURE-FAIR TESTS
ABST A CRITICAL ANALYSIS OF MENTAL MEASURES AS THEY RELATE TO BILINGUAL SUBJECTS REVEALS THE INJUSTICES COMMITTED WHEN TESTS ARE MISAPPLIED. THOSE WHO BLINDLY ACCEPT THE DOCTRINE OF INDIVIDUAL DIFFERENCE FAIL TO RECOGNIZE THE IMPORTANCE OF PERSONAL, SOCIAL AND CULTURAL DIFFERENCES OF PEOPLE. IN THIS REGARD, SIX ISSUES ARE DISCUSSED. (1) TESTS ARE NOT STANDARDIZED ON THE SPANISH-SPEAKING POPULATION OF THIS COUNTRY. (2) TEST ITEMS ARE NOT REPRESENTATIVE OF THE SPANISH-SPEAKING CULTURE. (3) THE ENTIRE NATURE OF INTELLIGENCE IS STILL A CONTROVERSIAL ISSUE. (4) TEST RESULTS FROM THE SPANISH-SPEAKING CONTINUE TO BE ACCEPTED UNCRITICALLY. (5) REVISED OR TRANSLATED TESTS ARE NOT NECESSARILY AN IMPROVEMENT ON TEST MEASURES. (6) ATTITUDES AND PREJUDICES OFTEN DETERMINE THE USE OF TEST RESULTS. IT IS SUGGESTED THAT A NOTE OF CAUTION IN THE USE OF MENTAL TESTS IS IN ORDER, AND THAT THEIR USE MUST BE SUPPLEMENTED BY INTELLIGENT AND PROFESSIONAL APPLICATION AND EVALUATION FOR THE BEST INTERESTS OF THE CHILD AND THE GROUP CONCERNED. 9 REFERENCES.
ACCN 001406

1633 AUTH **SANCHEZ, G. I.**
TITL EDUCATIONAL CHANGE IN HISTORICAL PERSPECTIVE.
SRCE *IN A. CASTANEDA, M. RAMIREZ, III, C. E. CORTES, & M. BARRERA (EDS.), MEXICAN AMERICANS AND EDUCATIONAL CHANGE. NEW YORK: ARNO PRESS, 1974, PP. 14-21.*
INDX EDUCATION, HISTORY, MEXICAN AMERICAN, LEGISLATION, ESSAY, BILINGUAL-BICULTURAL EDUCATION, EQUAL OPPORTUNITY, TEXAS, SOUTHWEST, PREJUDICE
ABST FOR MEXICAN AMERICANS THERE HAS BEEN VERY LITTLE EDUCATIONAL CHANGE. AL-

THOUGH THERE HAVE BEEN "FREE" MONIES FROM PUBLIC AND PRIVATE SOURCES TO IMPLEMENT PROGRESSIVE CHANGE, MANY PROGRAMS HAVE BEEN NO MORE THAN "SHOWCASES." SEGREGATION, DISCRIMINATION, AND THE LACK OF VIABLE BILINGUAL-BICULTURAL EDUCATIONAL PROGRAMS IN TEXAS ARE PRESENTED AS BARRIERS TO EDUCATIONAL CHANGE. FROM ELEMENTARY SCHOOL TO HIGHER EDUCATION THE MEXICAN HERITAGE IS IGNORED, WHILE THE SCHOOL SYSTEM CONTINUES TO ATTEMPT TO FIT THE MEXICAN AMERICAN CHILD INTO A STANDARD MOLD OF MIDDLE CLASS, PROTESTANT TRADITION. EDUCATION FOR THE MEXICAN AMERICAN REMAINS A DISMAL PICTURE, WHILE EDUCATIONAL CHANGE IS NONEXISTENT.

ACCN   001407

1634 AUTH   **SANCHEZ, G. I.**
     TITL   GROUP DIFFERENCES AND SPANISH-SPEAKING CHILDREN: A CRITICAL REVIEW.
     SRCE   *JOURNAL OF APPLIED PSYCHOLOGY, 1932, 16(5), 549-558.*
     INDX   REVIEW, CHILDREN, CULTURAL FACTORS, SPANISH SURNAMED, BILINGUALISM, INTELLIGENCE, INTELLIGENCE TESTING
     ABST   A CRITICAL LITERATURE REVIEW OF GROUP DIFFERENCES AS REVEALED BY INTELLIGENCE TESTS FOR SPANISH-SPEAKING (SS) CHILDREN IS PRESENTED. IT IS SHOWN THAT SS CHILDREN RECEIVE ATTENTION IN NUMEROUS INVESTIGATIONS WHERE THEY HAVE BEEN CLASSIFIED AS INFERIOR TO THE ENGLISH-SPEAKING AMERICAN CHILDREN ON THE BASIS OF TESTS RESULTS. THREE EXPLANATIONS FOR GROUP DIFFERENCES ARE OFFERED: (1) INNATE CAPACITY IS DIFFERENTIATED RACIALLY, AND INTELLIGENCE TESTS MEASURE SUCH DIFFERENTIATION; (2) ENVIRONMENT IS LARGELY RESPONSIBLE FOR "INTELLIGENCE" AS MEASURED BY TESTS, AND INTELLIGENCE TESTS ARE, IN PART, MEASURES OF ENVIRONMENTAL EFFECTS; AND (3) BILINGUALISM, OVER AND ABOVE ITS ENVIRONMENTAL ATTRIBUTES, IS A HANDICAP ACTING NOT ONLY UPON LANGUAGE EXPRESSION AND LANGUAGE UNDERSTANDING BUT UPON MORE INTRICATE PSYCHOLOGICAL PROCESSES. AT THE VERY LEAST, BILINGUALISM PRESENTS AN EXTRA OBSTACLE IN THE LEARNING PROCESS OF FOREIGN-LANGUAGE CHILDREN. THESE EXPLANATIONS HAVE LED INVESTIGATORS TO RECOGNIZE THAT THE SCIENTIFIC VALUE OF TEST RESULTS IS NOT ENTIRELY DETERMINED BY THE RELIABILITY OF THE MEASURE USED BUT IS CONDITIONED BY THE EXTENT TO WHICH THE COMPLEX FACTORS OF HEREDITY, ENVIRONMENT, AND LANGUAGE INDIVIDUALLY AND COLLECTIVELY IMPACT UPON IQ SCORES. DETAILED EXAMINATIONS OF EACH OF THE ABOVE EXPLANATIONS FOR GROUP DIFFERENCES ARE PRESENTED. 40 REFERENCES.
     ACCN   001408

1635 AUTH   **SANCHEZ, G. I.**
     TITL   HISTORY, CULTURE AND EDUCATION.
     SRCE   *IN J. SAMORA (ED.), LA RAZA: FORGOTTEN*

AMERICANS. SOUTH BEND, IND.: UNIVERSITY OF NOTRE DAME PRESS, 1966, PP. 1-26.
     INDX   HISTORY, CULTURAL FACTORS, MEXICAN AMERICAN, SPANISH SURNAMED, BILINGUALISM, BILINGUAL-BICULTURAL EDUCATION, CULTURE, EDUCATION, ESSAY, SOUTHWEST
     ABST   THE COMPLEX FACTORS WHICH HAVE CONTRIBUTED TO THE CONTINUING USAGE OF THE SPANISH LANGUAGE BY MEXICAN AMERICANS IN THE SOUTHWEST ARE EXAMINED. THE VALUE OF LANGUAGE IN EDUCATION, INTELLECTUAL DEVELOPMENT, AND PERSONALITY FORMATION HAS BEEN IGNORED IN THE TEACHING OF SPANISH SPEAKING CHILDREN. SPANISH HAS BEEN RETAINED BY THIS GROUP PARTIALLY BY DEFAULT—I.E., THE SCHOOLS SOUGHT TO MAKE MEXICAN AMERICAN CHILDREN MONOLINGUAL, ENGLISH-SPEAKING BUT FAILED IN THAT ENDEAVOR. THE FOLLOWING APPROACHES TO THE BILINGUAL EDUCATION OF MEXICAN AMERICANS ARE SUGGESTED: (1) THE HOME LANGUAGE SHOULD BE THE SPRINGBOARD FOR THE PROPER DEVELOPMENT OF THE SECOND LANGUAGE; (2) THE MOTHER TONGUE MUST BE USED PARTIALLY IN THE INSTRUCTION PROGRAM; (3) BILINGUAL TEACHERS SHOULD BE EMPLOYED TO INSTILL CULTURAL PRIDE; (4) THE ECONOMICALLY DISADVANTAGED BACKGROUND OF MEXICAN AMERICAN STUDENTS MUST BE ACKNOWLEDGED AND THE CURRICULUM ADOPTED TO MEET THE SPECIAL NEEDS OF THIS GROUP; AND (5) READING READINESS PROGRAMS SHOULD BE EXTENDED FOR THE FUTURE EDUCATIONAL SUCCESS OF MEXICAN AMERICAN STUDENTS. 28 REFERENCES.
     ACCN   001409

1636 AUTH   **SANCHEZ, G. I.**
     TITL   THE IMPLICATIONS OF A BASAL VOCABULARY TO THE MEASUREMENT OF THE ABILITIES OF BILINGUAL CHILDREN.
     SRCE   *JOURNAL OF SOCIAL PSYCHOLOGY, 1934, 5(3), 395-402.*
     INDX   SPANISH SURNAMED, BILINGUAL, CHILDREN, STANFORD-BINET INTELLIGENCE TEST, PERFORMANCE EXPECTATIONS, INTELLIGENCE TESTING, CULTURE-FAIR TESTS, EDUCATION, EMPIRICAL, TEST VALIDITY
     ABST   THE EMPHASIS ON A BASAL VOCABULARY AS A PREREQUISITE TO THE MEASUREMENT OF THE MENTAL ABILITIES OF BILINGUAL CHILDREN IS PRESENTED. SPECIFICALLY, A STANDARD BASAL VOCABULARY LIST OF 660 WORDS WAS DESIGNED AND CHECKED AGAINST THE STANFORD-BINET VOCABULARY, YEARS 3 TO 8 INCLUSIVELY. UNDER PRESENT CONDITIONS IN THE SCHOOLS ATTENDED BY THE SPANISH-SPEAKING CHILDREN, THIS BASAL VOCABULARY REPRESENTS THE DESIDERATUM—NOT ACTUAL ACHIEVEMENT. THEREFORE, THE FOLLOWING COMPARISONS MAY BE JUDGED AS ULTRACONSERVATIVE IN PORTRAYING ACTUAL LANGUAGE HANDICAPS. RESULTS OF THE COMPARISON SHOW THAT THERE ARE 8 "UNKNOWN" WORDS FOUND IN THE STANFORD-BINET TEST, WITH SOME OF THE WORDS AFFECTING AS MANY AS SIX SEPARATE TESTS. IN

ADDITION TO THE FACT THAT MANY OF THE WORDS ARE "UNKNOWN" TO THE CHILDREN, THERE ARE DIFFICULTIES WITH HOMONYMS AND WORD USAGE. THE EXAMINATION OF VOCABULARY DIFFICULTIES PRESENTED TO SPANISH-SPEAKING CHILDREN BY THE STANFORD-BINET SUGGESTS THAT SCHOOLS HAVE BEEN FAILING AT THEIR JOBS. THE IMPROVEMENT OF THE INSTRUCTION OF THESE CHILDREN IS ESSENTIAL TO PROPER MEASUREMENT. SCHOOLS SHOULD MAKE EXPERIENCES TO THE SPANISH-SPEAKING CHILDREN AS COMMON AS THEY ARE TO THE CHILDREN UPON WHOM THE NORMS OF THE TEST MEASURE ARE BASED. 15 REFERENCES.

ACCN   001410

1637 AUTH   **SANCHEZ, G. I.**
TITL   SCORES OF SPANISH-SPEAKING CHILDREN ON REPEATED TESTS.
SRCE   *JOURNAL OF GENETIC PSYCHOLOGY, 1932, 40(1), 223-231.*
INDX   SPANISH SURNAMED, CHILDREN, EMPIRICAL, STANFORD ACHIEVEMENT TEST, SCHOLASTIC ACHIEVEMENT, INTELLIGENCE TESTING, TEST RELIABILITY, NEW MEXICO, SOUTHWEST, INTELLIGENCE
ABST   THE EFFECTS OF ADMINISTERING A NUMBER OF INTELLIGENCE TESTS TO SPANISH-SPEAKING CHILDREN ARE EXAMINED. BOTH THE STANFORD ACHIEVEMENT TEST (SAT), FORMS A, B, V, V (PRIMARY AND ADVANCE), AND THE HAGGERTY INTELLIGENCE TEST (HIT) WERE GIVEN TO 45 SPANISH-SPEAKING CHILDREN, GRADES THREE TO EIGHT IN NEW MEXICO OVER A 1-YEAR PERIOD. RESULTS SHOW THAT: (1) AS A GENERAL RULE, THE MEAN QUOTIENTS IN THE VARIOUS ABILITIES TESTED WERE INCREASINGLY GREATER WITH SUCCESSIVE APPLICATIONS OF THE TEST; (2) THE INCREASES IN MENTAL ABILITY WERE LARGEST, FOLLOWED BY INCREASES IN READING ABILITY; (3) CHILDREN IN THE UPPER GRADES HAD HIGHER QUOTIENTS ON THE FIRST TESTING BUT MADE SMALLER GAINS ON THE RETESTS THAN DID CHILDREN IN THE LOWER GRADES; (4) THE BRIGHTEST CHILDREN HAD THE HIGHEST EDUCATIONAL QUOTIENTS ON THE FIRST TEST, BUT ON THE RETESTS THE DULLER CHILDREN MADE GREATER GAINS IN BOTH MENTAL AND EDUCATIONAL ABILITY; (5) READING CORRELATED MOST HIGHLY WITH OTHER ABILITIES; AND (6) QUOTIENTS HAD NEGATIVE CORRELATIONS WITH OTHER CHANGES. THE STUDY SHOWS THAT FOR BOTH MENTAL AND EDUCATIONAL ABILITIES OF SPANISH-SPEAKING CHILDREN, THE CHANGES BEYOND THE SECOND TEST VARY NOT ONLY FOR GRADE GROUPS BUT ALSO FOR DIFFERENT AGES, FOR DIFFERENT SCHOOL SUBJECTS, AND FOR BRIGHTER AND DULLER CHILDREN. THE OBTAINED VARIATION MAKES EVALUATION OF THE MERITS OF THE TESTS' APPLICATION VERY DIFFICULT. THE VARIOUS FACTORS WHICH ACCOUNT FOR THE VARIATION ARE DISCUSSED IN DETAIL. 31 REFERENCES.

ACCN   001411

1638 AUTH   **SANCHEZ, R.**
TITL   THE CHICANA LABOR FORCE.
SRCE   *IN R. SANCHEZ & R. M. CRUZ (EDS.), ESSAYS ON LA MUJER, (ANTHOLOGY NO. 1). LOS ANGELES: UNIVERSITY OF CALIFORNIA, CHICANO STUDIES CENTER, 1977, PP. 3-15.*
INDX   MEXICAN AMERICAN, FEMALE, LABOR FORCE, EMPLOYMENT, DEMOGRAPHIC, SES, ECONOMIC FACTORS, CAPITALISM, ESSAY, REVIEW, MARXIAN THEORY, CHICANO MOVEMENT
ABST   TO IDENTIFY AND ASSESS DETERMINANTS OF THE CHICANA SOCIOECONOMIC CONDITION, SUCH FACTORS AS EMPLOYMENT STATUS, OCCUPATIONAL CATEGORY, AGE BRACKET, EDUCATIONAL ATTAINMENT, FAMILY INCOME, AND HUSBAND'S OR FATHER'S OCCUPATION ARE DISCUSSED. A MAJOR PROBLEM IS THAT ECONOMIC CONDITIONS DIVIDE THE MEXICAN ORIGIN POPULATION ALONG CLASS LINES: 82.9% OF CHICANAS IN THE LABOR FORCE ARE EMPLOYED AS CLERICAL WORKERS OR OPERATIVES, OR IN THE SERVICE OCCUPATIONS, AND THEIR NEEDS AND INTERESTS ARE VASTLY DIFFERENT FROM THOSE FEW CHICANAS (4.5,) ATTAINING PROFESSIONAL STATUS. IT IS IMPERATIVE, THEREFORE, THAT HIGH SES CHICANAS RECOGNIZE THE LOW STATUS OF THE MAJORITY AND IDENTIFY WITH THEIR STRUGGLE RATHER THAN WITH MIDDLE CLASS FEMINIST ASPIRATIONS. 15 REFERENCES.

ACCN   002201

1639 AUTH   **SANCHEZ, R. B.**
TITL   DRAFT STATEMENT ON HISPANIC RECOMMENDATIONS.
SRCE   *PAPER PRESENTED AT THE ANNUAL LEGISLATIVE AND POLITICAL WORKSHOP OF EL CONGRESO, KANSAS CITY, MISSOURI, DECEMBER 1976.*
INDX   PROCEEDINGS, RESEARCH METHODOLOGY, FAMILY ROLES, FAMILY STRUCTURE, PROFESSIONAL TRAINING, REPRESENTATION, PARAPROFESSIONALS, MENTAL HEALTH, ALCOHOLISM, DRUG ABUSE, DRUG ADDICTION, PROGRAM EVALUATION, FARM LABORERS, HEALTH DELIVERY SYSTEMS, POLITICS, POLITICAL POWER, SES, POVERTY, LEGISLATION, SOCIAL SERVICES, GERONTOLOGY, CHILDREN, FEMALE
ABST   THIS DRAFT REPRESENTS A PRELIMINARY COMPILATION OF THE CONCERNS, ISSUES, AND RECOMMENDATIONS THAT WERE GENERATED IN WORKSHOPS AND CAUCUSES HELD DURING THE FIRST HISPANIC CONFERENCE ON HEALTH AND HUMAN SERVICES CONVENED BY THE NATIONAL COALITION OF HISPANIC MENTAL HEALTH AND HUMAN SERVICES ORGANIZATIONS (COSSMHO) IN LOS ANGELES ON SEPTEMBER 22-25, 1976. IT INCLUDES A BRIEF BACKGROUND STATEMENT ON THE CONFERENCE ITSELF, FOLLOWED BY A PRESENTATION OF MAJOR CONCERNS RELATED TO THE CONFERENCE'S WORKSHOPS AND CAUCUSES. PRESENTATIONS COVER TEN KEY SUBJECT AREAS: (1) THE HISPANIC FAMILY IN TRANSITION, INCLUDING ATTENTION TO THE PARTICULAR NEEDS OF YOUTH AND THE ELDERLY; (2) RESEARCH; (3) PERSPECTIVES ON

TRAINING; (4) PLANNING; (5) AFFIRMATIVE ACTION TO INCREASE HISPANIC PARTICIPATION IN HEALTH, MENTAL HEALTH, AND HUMAN SERVICE PROFESSIONS; (6) MENTAL HEALTH NEEDS AND DRUG AND ALCOHOL ABUSE; (7) MIGRANT HEALTH AND RELATED SERVICES; (8) REGIONALIZATION OF SERVICES AND ITS IMPACT ON LOCAL PLANNING AND DELIVERY SYSTEMS; (9) PROPOSED METHODS OF HEALTH CARE FINANCING; AND (10) MAJOR HEALTH AND HUMAN SERVICES LEGISLATION. THE OBJECTIVE OF THESE DELIBERATIONS WAS TO ASSIST HISPANOS ACTIVE IN THESE FIELDS, TOGETHER WITH THEIR NON-HISPANIC COUNTERPARTS, TO CONTRIBUTE THEIR KNOWLEDGE, EXPERIENCE, AND EXPERTISE TOWARD IMPROVING LEGISLATION, PUBLIC POLICY, AND PROFESSIONAL PRACTICES THAT SIGNIFICANTLY AFFECT THE PLANNING AND DELIVERY OF THESE SERVICES TO HISPANICS.

ACCN   001413

1640 AUTH   **SANCHEZ, R. B.**
TITL   HISPANIC CONCERNS ABOUT DRUG INFORMATION FOR PATIENTS: A STATEMENT ON BEHALF OF THE NATIONAL COALITION OF HISPANIC MENTAL HEALTH AND HUMAN SERVICE ORGANIZATIONS (COSSMHO).
SRCE   *PAPER PRESENTED AT THE JOINT DIA/AMA/FDA/PMA SYMPOSIUM ON DRUG INFORMATION FOR PATIENTS, WASHINGTON, D.C., NOVEMBER 1976.*
INDX   ADULT EDUCATION, PROFESSIONAL TRAINING, PHYSICIANS, HEALTH DELIVERY SYSTEMS, BILINGUAL-BICULTURAL PERSONNEL, SPANISH SURNAMED, HEALTH EDUCATION
ABST   A DISCUSSION OF THE IMPROVEMENT OF CONSUMER INFORMATION ON PRESCRIPTION DRUGS—WITH EMPHASIS ON THE NEEDS OF HISPANICS—RECOMMENDS THAT GREATER RESPONSIBILITY IS REQUIRED OF OVER-THE-COUNTER DRUG MANUFACTURERS, PHYSICIANS, AND PHARMACIES TO DECREASE INAPPROPRIATE DRUG USE. GENERALLY, THERE IS A NEED FOR INCREASED CONSUMER AWARENESS ABOUT THE EFFECTS OF DRUG INGREDIENTS. THIS NEED IS PARTICULARLY URGENT FOR HISPANICS DUE TO LANGUAGE AND CULTURAL BARRIERS WHICH IMPEDE THEIR UNDERSTANDING OF MEDICAL PROVIDERS AND DRUG MANUFACTURERS. THE PROBLEM CAN BE RECTIFIED BY PROVIDING BILINGUAL MATERIALS THAT INFORM CONSUMERS ABOUT THE DRUGS THEY ARE USING. IN THIS VEIN, A MODEL PROGRAM HAS RECENTLY BEEN ESTABLISHED AT THE LOS ANGELES COUNTY-USC MEDICAL CENTER. THE PROGRAM INCLUDES THREE BILINGUAL PHARMACISTS AS WELL AS DRUG LABELS IN ENGLISH AND SPANISH. IT IS RECOMMENDED THAT MORE SUCH PROGRAMS BE DEVELOPED. 4 REFERENCES.
ACCN   001414

1641 AUTH   **SANCHEZ, R. B.**
TITL   NATIONAL LEGISLATION AND LATINO MENTAL HEALTH: THE IMPACT OF HISTORY ON MENTAL HEALTH AND WAYS SPECIFIC LAWS CAN IMPROVE SERVICE DELIVERY TO HISPANOS.
SRCE   *PAPER PRESENTED AT THE ANNUAL MEETING OF THE NATIONAL COUNCIL OF COMMUNITY MENTAL HEALTH CENTERS, DENVER, COLORADO, FEBRUARY 22-25, 1976.*
INDX   LEGISLATION, MENTAL HEALTH, HISTORY, HEALTH DELIVERY SYSTEMS, SES, ESSAY, PROCEEDINGS, MEXICAN AMERICAN, SPANISH SURNAMED, POLITICS
ABST   THE SPANISH-SPEAKING COMMUNITY, BECAUSE OF ITS UNIQUE HISTORY, HAS SPECIFIC MENTAL HEALTH NEEDS, BUT THESE NEEDS ARE NOT BEING ADEQUATELY MET BY HEALTH DELIVERY SYSTEMS TODAY. THE COMMUNITY MENTAL HEALTH CENTER (CMHC) PROGRAM, FOR EXAMPLE, IS A HEALTH SYSTEM WHICH HAS BEEN PLANNED AND OPERATED WITH LITTLE INPUT FROM LATINOS. FURTHERMORE, ONLY RECENTLY HAS NATIONAL LEGISLATION (I.E., THE 1975 AMENDMENTS TO THE COMMUNITY MENTAL HEALTH CENTER ACT AND THE 1974 HEALTH PLANNING AND RESOURCES DEVELOPMENT ACT) SOUGHT TO MAKE THE CMHC PROGRAM MORE RESPONSIVE TO LATINO NEEDS BY EXPANDING THE NUMBER AND KINDS OF SERVICES PROVIDED AND REQUIRING BILINGUAL-BICULTURAL STAFF AND SERVICES. HISPANOS ARE ENCOURAGED TO STUDY THESE TWO ACTS AND KEEP INFORMED OF THEIR PROGRESS BY STAYING IN CONTACT WITH STATE AND LOCAL HEALTH DEPARTMENTS. ALSO DISCUSSED IS THE FINANCIAL ASSISTANCE FOR HEALTH CARE ACT, AS PROPOSED IN THE ADMINISTRATION'S 1977 BUDGET. THIS REVENUE SHARING BLOCK GRANT IN THE AREA OF HEALTH ELIMINATES STATE MATCHING-FUND REQUIREMENTS, AND IT HAS IMPORTANT IMPLICATIONS FOR THE LATINO COMMUNITY IN TERMS OF SERVICES COVERED, TARGET POPULATIONS, AND PROGRAM STANDARDS. THE CONCLUDING POINT IS THAT AN ACTIVE AND POSITIVE ROLE IN POLICY PLANNING AND IMPLEMENTATION MUST BE TAKEN BY THE LATINO COMMUNITY TO ENSURE GREATER EQUITY TO MINORITY COMMUNITIES IN THE DELIVERY OF SOCIAL SERVICES AT ALL LEVELS.
ACCN   001415

1642 AUTH   **SANCHEZ, R. B.**
TITL   REPORT ON CONFERENCE WORKSHOPS TO DEVELOP BACKGROUND INFORMATION ESSENTIAL TO PRODUCTION OF SPANISH LANGUAGE TV AND RADIO SPOTS RELATING TO MENTAL HEALTH (CONTRACT NO. 278-76-0080(SP)).
SRCE   *ROCKVILLE, MD.: DIVISION OF SCIENTIFIC AND PUBLIC INFORMATION, NATIONAL INSTITUTE OF MENTAL HEALTH, FEBRUARY 1977.*
INDX   PROCEEDINGS, SPANISH SURNAMED, CULTURAL PLURALISM, ESSAY, MASS MEDIA
ABST   WITH FUNDS FROM AN NIMH CONTRACT, THE NATIONAL COALITION OF HISPANIC MENTAL HEALTH AND HUMAN SERVICES ORGANIZATIONS (COSSMHO) HELD TWO SYMPOSIA ON THE POSSIBLE USE OF MASS MEDIA IN THE PREVENTION OF MENTAL ILLNESS—THE FIRST

IN LOS ANGELES, JANUARY, 1976; THE SECOND IN WASHINGTON, D.C., JANUARY, 1977. A TOTAL OF 38 PARTICIPANT/CONSULTANTS WERE PRESENT, REPRESENTING MENTAL HEALTH PROFESSIONALS, MEDIA EXPERTS, AND CONSUMERS FROM EACH OF THE HISPANIC SUBGROUPS AND FROM EVERY GEOGRAPHIC REGION OF THE U.S. THE PROJECT'S OBJECTIVES INCLUDED THE FOLLOWING TASKS: (1) IDENTIFY MAJOR CONCENTRATIONS OF HISPANIC POPULATION; (2) IDENTIFY LOCAL SPANISH LANGUAGE TELEVISION AND RADIO STATIONS SERVING HISPANIC COMMUNITIES; (3) DEVELOP CONCEPTS AND THEMES FOR PUBLIC TV AND RADIO PUBLIC SERVICE ANNOUNCEMENTS; (4) IDENTIFY THEATER GROUPS, ARTISTS, AND OTHER PERSONS CAPABLE OF WRITING SCRIPTS; AND (5) RECOMMEND AT LEAST THREE FILM PRODUCTION ORGANIZATIONS WITH EXPERTISE IN DEVELOPING TV AND RADIO MATERIAL FOR HISPANIC GROUPS. THERE WAS GENERAL CONSENSUS THAT IF PROBLEMS OF LOW SELF-ESTEEM AND LACK OF CULTURAL PRIDE COULD BE SQUARELY AND EFFECTIVELY ADDRESSED, THEN MANY OTHER PROBLEMS WOULD BE REDUCED. IN THE APPENDIX TO THIS REPORT, THE FOLLOWING ARE ATTACHED: (1) NAMES OF ALL PARTICIPANTS AT THE SYMPOSIA; (2) SPANISH LANGUAGE TV AND RADIO STATIONS ACROSS THE U.S.; (3) MEDIA CONFERENCE PARTICIPANTS' SUGGESTIONS AND SCRIPTS FOR PUBLIC SERVICE ANNOUNCEMENTS; (4) A LIST OF THEATER GROUPS, ARTISTS, AND OTHER PERSONS CAPABLE OF WRITING SCRIPTS AND DRAMATIC EPISODES; AND (5) ADDITIONAL INFORMATION ON RECOMMENDED PRODUCTION COMPANIES.

ACCN   001416

1643 AUTH   **SANCHEZ, R., & CRUZ, R. M. (EDS.)**
TITL   ESSAYS ON LA MUJER. (ANTHOLOGY NO. 1)
SRCE   *LOS ANGELES: UNIVERSITY OF CALIFORNIA, CHICANO STUDIES CENTER PUBLICATIONS, 1977.*
INDX   FEMALE, CHICANO MOVEMENT, LABOR FORCE, HISTORY, ESSAY, REVIEW, HEALTH, MEXICAN AMERICAN, SEX ROLES, MARXIAN THEORY, ECONOMIC FACTORS, EMPLOYMENT, CAPITALISM, BOOK
ABST   PART ONE OF THIS COLLECTION OF ARTICLES FOCUSES UPON THE SITUATION OF THE CHICANA WITHIN HER SPECIAL HISTORICAL, SOCIAL, AND ECONOMIC CONTEXT; AND IN PARTICULAR, IT EMPHASIZES THAT THE CHICANA'S SITUATION SHOULD BE VIEWED FROM AN ECONOMIC PERSPECTIVE. THE ESSAYS ADDRESS THE ROLE OF THE CHICANA WITHIN THE LABOR FORCE, WITHIN THE STUDENT MOVEMENT, AND WITHIN THE CHICANO FAMILY. A COMMENTARY ON AVAILABLE HEALTH SERVICES IS PROVIDED, AND A CRITICAL REVIEW IS PRESENTED OF THE NOVEL "HASTA NO VERTE JESUS MIO," BY ELENA PONIATOWSKA. THE ARTICLES IN PART TWO FOCUS UPON THE HISTORICAL ROOTS OF THE CHICANA. INCLUDED ARE A REVIEW OF THE LITERATURE ON CHICANA HISTORY, AND AN ARTICLE ON

THE AZTEC HISTORICAL FIGURE "MALITZIN TENEPAL" (ALSO KNOWN AS "LA MALINCHE"). THE CONCLUDING ESSAYS PROVIDE A STATISTICAL PROFILE OF THE INDUSTRIAL AND OCCUPATIONAL DISTRIBUTION OF CHICANA WORKERS, AND A MOVING DISCOURSE ON THE STRUGGLE OF THE CHICANA WORKING CLASS.

ACCN   002684

1644 AUTH   **SANCHEZ-HIDALGO, E.**
TITL   PSICOLOGIA Y CURRICULO. (PSYCHOLOGY AND CURRICULUM).
SRCE   *REVISTA MEXICANA DE PSICOLOGIA, 1966, 2(9), 785-793. (SPANISH)*
INDX   ESSAY, CURRICULUM, COGNITIVE DEVELOPMENT, INTELLIGENCE, LANGUAGE COMPREHENSION, PERCEPTION, ACHIEVEMENT MOTIVATION, CHILDREN, SES, LANGUAGE LEARNING, EDUCATION, POLICY, INSTRUCTIONAL TECHNIQUES, TEACHERS
ABST   FIVE RECENT CONTRIBUTIONS OF PSYCHOLOGY TO EDUCATION, PARTICULARLY WITH REGARD TO CURRICULUM DEVELOPMENT, ARE SUMMARIZED. (1) INTELLECTUAL DEVELOPMENT. HERE INTELLIGENCE TESTING, MENTAL DEFICIENCY AND MENTAL SUPERIORITY, AND JUVENILE DELINQUENCY ARE DISCUSSED IN RELATION TO CURRICULUM PLANNING. (2) SOCIOECONOMIC AND CULTURAL DEPRIVATION. RELATING CURRICULUM TO THE STUDENTS' DAILY LIFE IS SEEN AS A NECESSITY FOR ACHIEVING MOTIVATION AND EDUCATIONAL DEVELOPMENT. THIS IS ESPECIALLY TRUE IN THE CASE OF ECONOMICALLY AND SOCIALLY DEPRIVED CHILDREN WHOSE HOME ENVIRONMENT IS NOT EDUCATIONALLY STIMULATING. (3) LANGUAGE. LANGUAGE LEARNING IS CONSIDERED THE KEY TO HUMANIZATION AND THE LEARNING OF TWO OR MORE LANGUAGES IS HIGHLY RECOMMENDED. (4) PERCEPTION AND MEANING. EFFECTIVE TEACHING CREATES AN ENVIRONMENT THAT PERMITS THE EXPLORATION OF MEANINGFUL LEARNING. TO ATTAIN THIS ENVIRONMENT THE EDUCATOR MUST BE AWARE OF THE STUDENTS' ATTITUDES AND PERCEPTIONS TOWARD EDUCATION BEFORE A CURRICULUM PROGRAM OF "WHAT IS IMPORTANT" CAN BE DESIGNED. (5) MOTIVATION. THE EDUCATOR SHOULD BE PROVIDED WITH AS MUCH KNOWLEDGE AS POSSIBLE OF CONTEMPORARY PSYCHOLOGICAL INVESTIGATIONS THAT RELATE TO MOTIVATION. WITH THIS KNOWLEDGE, THE TEACHER CAN BETTER UNDERSTAND THE DYNAMICS THAT STIMULATE, DIRECT, AND SUSTAIN STUDENT CONDUCT. 6 REFERENCES.

ACCN   001412

1645 AUTH   **SANDERS, M., SCHOLZ, M. P., & KAGAN, S.**
TITL   THREE SOCIAL MOTIVES AND FIELD INDEPENDENCE-DEPENDENCE IN ANGLO AMERICAN AND MEXICAN AMERICAN CHILDREN.
SRCE   *JOURNAL OF CROSS CULTURAL PSYCHOLOGY, 1976, 7(4), 451-460.*
INDX   PERSONALITY, COGNITIVE STYLE, MEXICAN AMERICAN, CROSS CULTURAL, CHILDREN, EMPIRICAL, FIELD DEPENDENCE-INDEPENDENCE,

ACHIEVEMENT MOTIVATION, SEX COMPARISON, CALIFORNIA, SOUTHWEST

ABST   PREVIOUS RESEARCH HAS INDICATED THAT MEXICAN AMERICAN CHILDREN HAVE HIGHER NEED (N) AFFILIATION AND ARE MORE FIELD DEPENDENT THAN ANGLO AMERICAN CHILDREN, WHO ARE MORE FIELD INDEPENDENT AND TEND TO HAVE HIGHER N ACHIEVEMENT. THREE SOCIAL MOTIVES (N ACHIEVEMENT, N AFFILIATION, N POWER) AND FIELD DEPENDENCE-INDEPENDENCE WERE COMPARED AMONG 184 ANGLO AND MEXICAN AMERICAN FIFTH- AND SIXTH-GRADE CHILDREN. APPROXIMATELY HALF OF EACH GROUP WAS MALE AND HALF FEMALE. THE SAMPLE WAS DRAWN FROM THREE SCHOOLS IN A LOWER-INCOME AREA IN SOUTHERN CALIFORNIA. ALL CHILDREN SPOKE FLUENT ENGLISH. AS PREDICTED, ANGLO AMERICAN CHILDREN WERE SIGNIFICANTLY MORE FIELD INDEPENDENT, HIGHER ON N ACHIEVEMENT, AND TENDED TO BE HIGHER ON N POWER; MEXICAN AMERICAN CHILDREN TENDED TO BE HIGHER ON N AFFILIATION. CONTRARY TO PREDICTIONS, FIELD INDEPENDENCE-DEPENDENCE WAS NOT RELATED TO N AFFILIATION OR N POWER; ONLY THE PREDICTED POSITIVE RELATIONSHIP BETWEEN FIELD INDEPENDENCE AND N ACHIEVEMENT WAS CONFIRMED. RESULTS ARE INCONSISTENT WITH SOME PREVIOUS CONCLUSIONS THAT FIELD DEPENDENCE IS RELATED TO THE GREATER N AFFILIATION OF MEXICAN AMERICAN COMPARED TO ANGLO AMERICAN CHILDREN. 34 REFERENCES. (JOURNAL ABSTRACT MODIFIED)

ACCN   001417

1646 AUTH   **SANDIS, E. V.**
TITL   CHARACTERISTICS OF PUERTO RICAN MIGRANTS TO, AND FROM, THE UNITED STATES.
SRCE   *INTERNATIONAL MIGRATION REVIEW, 1970, 4(2), 22-43.*
INDX   MIGRATION, PUERTO RICAN-I, PUERTO RICAN-M, CENSUS, SURVEY, SES, SCHOLASTIC ACHIEVEMENT, SEX COMPARISON, EMPLOYMENT, LABOR FORCE, ECONOMIC FACTORS, SOCIAL MOBILITY, EMPIRICAL
ABST   TO ASSESS WHAT SEGMENT OF THE POPULATION PUERTO RICO IS LOSING OR GAINING DUE TO MIGRATION, A COMPARISON WAS CONDUCTED OF THE SOCIOECONOMIC AND MOTIVATIONAL CHARACTERISTICS OF PUERTO RICAN MIGRANTS TO AND FROM THE UNITED STATES. DATA SOURCES INCLUDED (1) THE 1960 CENSUS OF BOTH PUERTO RICO AND THE U.S., (2) A SURVEY BY THE PUERTO RICO DEPARTMENT OF LABOR, AND (3) A HOUSEHOLD SURVEY BY THE PUERTO RICO BUREAU OF ECONOMIC AND SOCIAL ANALYSIS. DATA ANALYSIS COMPARED THREE POPULATIONS: (1) PUERTO RICAN MIGRANTS TO THE U.S.; (2) PUERTO RICAN RESIDENTS; AND (3) MIGRANTS RETURNING FROM THE U.S. TO PUERTO RICO. RESULTS INDICATE THAT MIGRANTS TO THE U.S. TEND TO BE DRAWN FROM THE MIDDLE EDUCATIONAL AND OCCUPATIONAL STRATA IN PUERTO RICO. ECONOMICS APPEARS TO BE THE PRIMARY MOTIVATION FOR MIGRATION.

PERHAPS A SOCIAL MOBILITY PROCESS IS INVOLVED, IN WHICH THE MORE MOTIVATED MIGRATE TO THE MAINLAND TO IMPROVE THEIR SOCIOECONOMIC STATUS. FOR THE MIGRANT, ARRIVAL IN THE U.S. OFTEN RESULTS IN HIGHER INCOME BUT A DOWNWARD MOVEMENT IN OCCUPATIONAL STATUS. THE EFFECT FOR PUERTO RICO IS A LOSS OF ITS MORE HIGHLY TRAINED WORKERS. IT APPEARS THAT THOSE WHO EXPERIENCE THE MOST SUCCESS IN THE U.S. ARE THE ONES MOTIVATED TO RETURN TO PUERTO RICO, BUT MORE RESEARCH IS NECESSARY ON THE MOTIVATIONS OF RETURNING MIGRANTS AS WELL AS ON THE IMPACT OF THEIR RETURN ON SOCIETAL CHANGE IN PUERTO RICO. 18 REFERENCES.

ACCN   001418

1647 AUTH   **SANDLER, I., HOLMEN, M., & SCHOPPER, A.**
TITL   SELF VERSUS COUNSELOR PERCEPTIONS OF INTERPERSONAL CHARACTERISTICS OF FEMALE WELFARE RECIPIENTS: A CROSS-CULTURAL COMPARISON.
SRCE   *JOURNAL OF COMMUNITY PSYCHOLOGY, 1978, 6, 179-188.*
INDX   INTERPERSONAL RELATIONS, SES, CROSS CULTURAL, POVERTY, STEREOTYPES, PSYCHOSOCIAL ADJUSTMENT, MEXICAN AMERICAN, VOCATIONAL COUNSELING, CULTURAL FACTORS, EMPIRICAL, PERSONALITY, PERSONNEL
ABST   EXPLORING FOR CULTURAL FACTORS WHICH WOULD ACCOUNT FOR DIFFERENCES BETWEEN WELFARE RECIPIENTS' SELF-DESCRIBED PERSONALITY CHARACTERISTICS AND THE CHARACTERISTICS ATTRIBUTED TO THEM BY COUNSELORS IN A MANPOWER DEVELOPMENT PROGRAM (WIN), A COMPARISON WAS MADE BETWEEN SELF-RATINGS AND COUNSELOR RATINGS OF 108 ANGLO, 69 BLACK, AND 55 MEXICAN AMERICAN FEMALE ENROLLEES. EACH ENROLLEE COMPLETED A PERSONALITY TEST BATTERY, INCLUDING A SELF-RATING ON THE INTERPERSONAL CHECK LIST (ICL); THE FIVE PARTICIPATING COUNSELORS ALSO USED THE ICL TO RATE THEIR CLIENTS. RESULTS DEMONSTRATED THAT THE DIFFERENCE BETWEEN COUNSELOR AND ENROLLEE PERSONALITY DESCRIPTIONS WAS APPRECIABLY GREATER FOR MEXICAN AMERICANS THAN FOR ANGLOS AND BLACKS. THE COUNSELORS DESCRIBED THE MEXICAN AMERICAN WOMEN AS LESS COMPETITIVE, MORE APOLOGETIC, MORE DOCILE, AND LESS DOMINANT. THESE ATTRIBUTIONS ARE SIMILAR TO WHAT HAS BEEN CALLED THE MEXICAN AMERICAN STEREOTYPE. SINCE MEXICAN AMERICAN INTERPERSONAL STYLE EMPHASIZES COURTESY, TACT, AND DIPLOMACY—AS OPPOSED TO MORE OPEN, FRANK, AND DIRECT INTERACTION STYLES—IT IS POSSIBLE THAT THE COUNSELORS WERE MISINTERPRETING THEIR MEXICAN AMERICAN CLIENTS' BEHAVIORS. ONE CONSEQUENCE OF THIS IS THAT MEXICAN AMERICAN CLIENTS MAY BE SUBJECTED TO MORE DOMINANT OR DIRECTIVE FORMS OF COUNSELING THAN OTHER CLIENTS. IN GENERAL, THE IMPLICATON IS THAT MEXICAN AMERICAN CLIENTS MAY RECEIVE INAPPRO-

PRIATE COUNSELING. IT IS CONCLUDED THAT BECAUSE THE ABILITY TO UNDERSTAND OTHERS IS CRUCIAL FOR EFFECTIVE THERAPEUTIC RELATIONSHIPS, SUCH STEREOTYPES AND MISINTERPRETATIONS OF CULTURAL DIFFERENCES AS THOSE FOUND IN THIS STUDY MAY WEAKEN THE EFFECTIVENESS AND AVAILABILITY OF COUNSELING SERVICES. 33 REFERENCES.

ACCN   001419

1648 AUTH   **SANDOVAL, M. C.**
TITL   LA RELIGION AFROCUBANA.
SRCE   *MADRID: PLAYOR, S.A., 1975. (SPANISH)*
INDX   CUBAN, RELIGION, HISTORY, CULTURE, ACCULTURATION, ESPIRITISMO, MIGRATION, CULTURAL CHANGE, BIBLIOGRAPHY
ABST   A STUDY OF THE AFROCUBAN RELIGIOUS COMPLEX IN CUBA, COMMONLY KNOWN BY THE NAME OF SANTERIA, IS VIEWED IN THE LIGHT OF ITS AFRICAN ORIGINS—THE CULTS OF ORICHAS AND VODUNS IN THE LANDS OF YORUBA AND DAHOMEY. SANTERIA IS THE PRODUCT OF THE FUSION OF AFRICAN AND CATHOLIC BELIEFS AND PRACTICES. IN THIS CULTURAL PROCESS THE AFRICAN RELIGIOUS FORMS WERE PROJECTED MORE STRONGLY THAN THE CHRISTIAN FORMS AND BECAME THE BASIS FOR THE NEW RELIGIOUS SYSTEM. SANTERIA HAS INCORPORATED MANY AFRICAN CULTURAL FORMS INTO THE CUBAN CULTURE. IT WAS THROUGH THE RELIGION THAT THE MOST DIVERSE CULTURAL FORMS WERE ABLE TO LIVE IN A STRANGE AND SOMETIMES HOSTILE ENVIRONMENT. ONLY THROUGH THE CULT, ONE OF THE MOST IMPORTANT MEANS OF SOCIAL COMMUNICATION, COULD THE SLAVES TRANSMIT TO THEIR CHILDREN THEIR MORAL VALUES, ATTITUDES, AND BELIEFS. THIS STUDY IS THE FIRST ONE TO PRESENT A SYSTEMATIC COMPARISON OF THE YORUBA GODS FROM BOTH SIDES OF THE ATLANTIC. THE YORUBA GODS ARE STUDIED AS THEY ARE KNOWN IN CUBA AND AFRICA. SANTERIA AMONG THE CUBAN COMMUNITY IN MIAMI IS BRIEFLY DISCUSSED. INCLUDED ARE A GLOSSARY OF TERMS AND AN AFRICAN AND AFROAMERICAN BIBLIOGRAPHY.
ACCN   000339

1649 AUTH   **SANDOVAL, M. C.**
TITL   PATTERNS OF DRUG ABUSE AMONG THE SPANISH-SPEAKING-GAY-BAR CROWD.
SRCE   *UNPUBLISHED MANUSCRIPT, UNDATED. (AVAILABLE FROM DR. M. CROS SANDOVAL, DEPARTMENT OF PSYCHIATRY, UNIVERSITY OF MIAMI, 1120 NE 85TH ST., MIAMI, FLORIDA, 33158.)*
INDX   HOMOSEXUALITY, DRUG ABUSE, ALCOHOLISM, INTERPERSONAL RELATIONS, INTERPERSONAL ATTRACTION, SEXUAL BEHAVIOR, CASE STUDY, FLORIDA, SOUTH, EMPIRICAL, DEVIANCE
ABST   THE LIFE STYLE AND VALUE SYSTEM OF SPANISH-SPEAKING POLYDRUG USERS WHO ATTEND THE GAY BARS IN MIAMI, FLORIDA, ARE DESCRIBED. THE STUDY OF 32 VOLUNTEER SUBJECTS, BASED ON INFORMAL INTERVIEWS AND OBSERVATIONS, WAS UNDERTAKEN TO BETTER UNDERSTAND THIS GROUP'S NEEDS AND PROBLEMS SO AS TO ALLOW IDENTIFICATION OF SOURCES OF SUPPORT WHICH COULD BE TAPPED FOR REHABILITATIVE PURPOSES. THROUGH A DESCRIPTION OF THE GAY BAR "SCENE," THE CHARACTERISTICS OF THE SAMPLE, AND THE RANGE OF DRUG USE, IT IS POINTED OUT THAT THIS GAY "CROWD" HAS AN INORDINATE NEED FOR RECOGNITION, ADMIRATION AND ACCEPTANCE. IT IS CONCLUDED THAT ANY REHABILITATIVE PROGRAM MUST FOCUS ON A SPECIAL TYPE OF COUNSELING THAT IS SENSITIVE TO THE BEHAVIORAL PATTERNS WHICH EXPRESS AND SATISFY THEIR NEEDS. PEER COUNSELING AND PARENTAL THERAPY AS MODES OF TREATMENT ARE SUGGESTED. 6 REFERENCES.
ACCN   000340

1650 AUTH   **SANDOVAL, M. C.**
TITL   SANTERIA: AFROCUBAN CONCEPTS OF DISEASE AND ITS TREATMENT IN MIAMI.
SRCE   *JOURNAL OF OPERATIONAL PSYCHIATRY, 1977, 8(2), 52-63.*
INDX   RELIGION, CUBAN, FLORIDA, ACCULTURATION, STRESS, HEALTH, CULTURAL FACTORS, IMMIGRATION, SES, SOCIAL MOBILITY, ESSAY, REVIEW, ANXIETY, SOUTH, ESPIRITISMO
ABST   THE AFRO-CUBAN RELIGIOUS COMPLEX OF SANTERIA HAS BEEN INSTRUMENTAL IN THE ADJUSTMENT OF CUBAN IMMIGRANTS IN THE UNITED STATES. SANTERIA'S ABILITY NOT ONLY TO SURVIVE BUT TO EXPAND IN ITS NEW ENVIRONMENT IS DUE TO THE FOLLOWING: (1) SANTERIA IS A TASK-ORIENTED, PRESENT-ORIENTED SYSTEM WHICH IS FLOURISHING AMONG THE SOCIALLY MOBILE MIDDLE CLASS WHO WERE FORMERLY OF THE LOWER STRATA; (2) IT OFFERS SUPERNATURAL CONTACT, FILLING THE GAP LEFT BY THE CATHOLIC CHURCH'S LOSS OF POSITION, AND STIMULATED BY THE CURRENT AMERICAN INTEREST IN EXOTIC RELIGIONS; (3) SANTERIA OFFERS RELIEF FROM THE GUILT PRODUCED BY LOSS OF ONE'S HOMELAND AND THE TENSIONS PRODUCED BY THE PRESSURES OF ACCULTURATION; AND (4) SANTERIA IS A FLEXIBLE, NON-ETHICAL SYSTEM, AND ITSELF IS THE PRODUCT OF 300 YEARS OF ACCULTURATION. FUNDAMENTALLY, "SANTEROS" OFFER INTENSIVE SUPPORT TO PEOPLE RAISED IN A CULTURE IN WHICH AUTHORITY AND INTERDEPENDENCE ARE HIGHLY VALUED, AND FOR WHOM TREATMENT MODALITIES DEVELOPED IN AN INDIVIDUALISTIC SOCIETY MAY BE INAPPROPRIATE. AN UNDERSTANDING OF THIS BELIEF SYSTEM AND THE NEEDS IT FULFILLS IS INDISPENSABLE TO PROFESSIONALS AND PARAPROFESSIONALS SERVING THE CUBAN COMMUNITY. 20 REFERENCES.
ACCN   002203

1651 AUTH   **SANDOVAL, M. C., & TOZO, L.**
TITL   AN EMERGENT CUBAN COMMUNITY.
SRCE   *PSYCHIATRIC ANNALS, 1975, 5(8), 48-63.*
INDX   CUBAN, COMMUNITY, MENTAL HEALTH, HEALTH DELIVERY SYSTEMS, PARAPROFESSIONALS,

RESOURCE UTILIZATION, COMMUNITY IN-VOLVEMENT, FLORIDA, SOUTH, ESSAY

ABST AN HISTORICAL ACCOUNT IS PROVIDED OF THE DEVELOPMENT OF A MENTAL HEALTH CENTER FOR CUBANS RESIDING IN THE ALL-PATTAH COMMUNITY OF MIAMI, FLORIDA. IT IS EMPHASIZED THAT THE PROCESS OF STAFF-ING THE CENTER AND CREATING EFFECTIVE SERVICE DELIVERY STRATEGIES INVOLVED CONSIDERABLE INPUT FROM COMMUNITY MEMBERS. AS A RESULT, A STRONG SENSE OF "COMMUNITY" EMERGED FOR THIS CUBAN POPULATION. BASED ON THIS EXPERIENCE, IT IS CONCLUDED THAT IF COMMUNITY MENTAL HEALTH CENTERS ARE TO BE ECONOMICALLY FEASIBLE AND EFFECTIVE, THEN SEVERAL FACTORS MUST BE INTEGRATED: (1) THE LINK-AGE BETWEEN THE IDENTIFICATION OF NEEDS AND THE MATCHING OF RESOURCES; (2) THE SOCIAL ASSISSTANCE CONCERNED WITH SOLVING PROBLEMS; (3) THE MENTAL HEALTH SERVICES INVOLVED WITH EARLY DETECTION AND TREATMENT; AND (4) THE SOCIAL PLAN-NING AND COMMUNITY DEVELOPMENT STRATEGIES WHICH ATTEMPT TO REWEAVE THE WEB OF SOCIETY. 4 REFERENCES. (NCMHI ABSTRACT MODIFIED)

ACCN 001420

1652 AUTH **SANTA CRUZ, L. A., & HEPWORTH, D. H.**
TITL EFFECTS OF CULTURAL ORIENTATION ON CASEWORK.
SRCE *SOCIAL CASEWORK, 1975, 56(1), 52-57.*
INDX EMPIRICAL, MEXICAN AMERICAN, PSYCHOTH-ERAPY, CULTURAL FACTORS, CROSS CUL-TURAL, PSYCHOTHERAPY OUTCOME, HEALTH DELIVERY SYSTEMS
ABST THE DELIVERY OF SERVICES TO ETHNIC MI-NORITIES WAS STUDIED FROM THE PERSPEC-TIVE OF THE EFFECTS OF CULTURAL SIMI-LARITY OR DIFFERENCE ON THE CASEWORK RELATIONSHIP. SIX CASEWORKERS AND 48 CLIENTS COMPRISED SIX STUDY GROUPS HAV-ING A CULTURAL MIX OF MEXICAN AMERICANS AND WHITES. CLIENTS WERE GIVEN THE BAR-RETT-LENNARD RELATIONSHIP INVENTORY, WHICH OPERATIONALIZES CARL ROGER'S FA-CILITATIVE CONDITIONS OF EMPATHIC UNDER-STANDING, LEVEL OF REGARD, UNCONDITION-ALITY OF REGARD, AND CONGRUENCE. THE RESULTS OF THE BICULTURAL STUDY SHOW THAT THE SIMILARITIES AND DIFFERENCES BE-TWEEN WORKER AND CLIENT ACROSS THE VARIABLES OF CULTURAL ORIENTATION AND SEX PRODUCED NO MEASURABLE EFFECTS ON CLIENTS' PERCEPTIONS OF THE HELPING RELATIONSHIP DEFINED IN TERMS OF WORKER OFFERED EMPATHY, WARMTH, AND GENUINE-NESS. THE FINDINGS SUGGEST THAT INORDI-NATE EMPHASIS SHOULD NOT BE ACCORDED THE NEGATIVE EFFECTS OF CULTURAL DIFFER-ENCES BETWEEN HELPERS AND HELPEES. IT IS CONCLUDED THAT COMPETENCE IN COMMU-NICATION IS A MORE POWERFUL DETERMI-NANT OF THE QUALITY OF A WORKER-CLIENT RELATIONSHIP THAN ARE LIKENESSES IN ETH-NIC BACKGROUND OR SEX. 15 REFERENCES. (NCMHI ABSTRACT MODIFIED)

ACCN 001421

1653 AUTH **SANTILLAN, R., & TEIXIERA, S.**
TITL THE CONCEPT OF CHICANO POLITICAL SELF-DETERMINATION WITHIN A CAPITALIST SOCI-ETY: A CASE STUDY OF THE ATTEMPTED IN-CORPORATION OF EAST LOS ANGELES.
SRCE *PAPER PRESENTED AT THE NATIONAL ASSO-CIATION OF CHICANO SOCIAL SCIENCES CON-FERENCE, EL PASO, TEXAS, APRIL 23-25, 1976.*
INDX MEXICAN AMERICAN, POLITICS, ECONOMIC FACTORS, CAPITALISM, SES, DISCRIMINATION, DEMOGRAPHIC, POLITICAL POWER, COMMU-NITY, CHICANO MOVEMENT, ESSAY, CALIFOR-NIA
ABST IN THIS DIALECTICAL ANALYSIS OF THE STRUGGLE BY EAST LOS ANGELES TO BE-COME INCORPORATED INTO THE CITY OF LOS ANGELES, IT IS ARGUED THAT CHICANO PO-LITICAL VISIBILITY WITHIN THE SUPERSTRUC-TURE OF CAPITALISM DOES NOT DIRECTLY LEAD TO ECONOMIC PROGRESS. THE PRI-MARY OBSTACLE TO CHICANO POLITICAL SELF-DETERMINATION LIES IN THE CIRCUMSTANCE THAT ALTHOUGH CHICANOS FORM A MASSIVE PORTION OF THE WAGE-EARNING POPULA-TION, THEY DO NOT CONTROL THE MEANS OF PRODUCTION. OTHER OBSTACLES—SUCH AS GERRYMANDERING, TOKENISM, AND "RACE—ARE SECONDARY MANIFESTATIONS WHICH MERELY REINFORCE THE EXISTING ECONOMIC ORDER. EVEN IF EAST LOS ANGELES HAD WON ITS 1974 FIGHT FOR INCORPORATION, THE POVERTY, GANG VIOLENCE, AND INADEQUATE HEALTH CARE FACILITIES WOULD HAVE PER-SISTED—EVIDENT IN THE FACT THAT OTHER MEXICAN AMERICAN COMMUNITIES WHICH ARE INCORPORATED IN LOS ANGELES STILL FACE THE SAME SEVERE SOCIAL AND ECONOMIC PROBLEMS SUFFERED BY EAST LOS ANGELES. IT IS CONCLUDED THAT THE PREVAILING BE-LIEF THAT POLITICAL POWER CAN RESULT IN UPWARD SOCIAL AND ECONOMIC MOBILITY FOR THE CHICANO WORKING CLASS IS DE-MONSTRABLY FALSE. INDEED, WITHIN THE LAST FEW YEARS THE ELECTION AND APPOINTMENT OF CHICANOS TO POSITIONS OF "POWER" HAVE NOT RESULTED IN SOCIAL IMPROVE-MENTS IN THE BARRIO; INSTEAD, THIS HAS CO-INCIDED WITH THE DOWNWARD TREND OF THE SOCIOECONOMIC STATUS OF THE MEXICAN NATIONAL MINORITY WORKING CLASS. ANY PARADIGM OF CHICANO POLITICAL SELF-DE-TERMINATION—AND SELF-DETERMINATION FOR THE ENTIRE WORKING CLASS, REGARDLESS OF RACE—MUST BE FOUNDED UPON CLASS ANALYSIS; AND TRUE POLITICAL SELF-DETER-MINATION CAN ONLY BE ACHIEVED WHEN THE PRIVATE MEANS OF PRODUCTION BECOME SO-CIAL. 15 REFERENCES.

ACCN 001422

1654 AUTH **SANUA, V. D.**
TITL A NOTE OF THE SPANISH LANGUAGE FORM OF THE ORAL DIRECTIONS TEST OF INTELLI-GENCE.
SRCE *THE JOURNAL OF APPLIED PSYCHOLOGY, 1956, 40(5), 350-352.*

INDX   SES, ENVIRONMENTAL FACTORS, TEST VA-
        LIDITY, CULTURE-FAIR TESTS, EMPIRICAL,
        ADULTS, INTELLIGENCE TESTING, TEST RELIA-
        BILITY, LABOR FORCE, NEW YORK, EAST

ABST   JOB HIRING PROCEDURES WITH PUERTO RI-
        CANS IN NEW YORK CITY REVEAL SERIOUS IN-
        ADEQUACIES IN TOOLS FOR MEASURING THEIR
        INTELLIGENCE. AT THE LEVEL OF INDIVIDUAL
        JOB DECISIONS, INFORMATION ON AN APPLI-
        CANT'S JOB LEVEL CLASSIFICATION AND PO-
        TENTIAL FOR JOB TRAINING ARE DIFFICULT TO
        OBTAIN. THE EXPERIMENTAL SPANISH FORM
        OF THE WECHSLER SCALES ARE TOO TIME
        CONSUMING FOR INDUSTRIAL SCREENING OR
        FOR QUICK CLASSIFICATION IN GUIDANCE
        AGENCIES. MOREOVER, THE NEED FOR A
        SPANISH SPEAKING PSYCHOLOGIST FOR ITS
        ADMINISTRATION IS UNREALISTIC. WHAT IS
        NEEDED IS A SHORT ORAL GROUP TEST WHICH
        CAN BE ADMINISTERED TO SPANISH SPEAKING
        ADULTS BY A TRAINED NON-PROFESSIONAL.
        TO THAT END, THE ORAL DIRECTIONS TEST—
        DESIGNED SPECIFICALLY FOR USE IN SCREEN-
        ING JOB APPLICANTS AT A LARGE REFINERY IN
        VENEZUELA—IS RECOMMENDED. THE ENTIRE
        TEST, INCLUDING ALL DIRECTIONS IN SPANISH,
        IS ORALLY ADMINISTERED BY A 15-MINUTE
        MAGNETIC TAPE RECORDING. THE TEST AD-
        MINISTRATOR NEED ONLY KNOW GROUP TEST-
        ING MANAGEMENT. ITS TIMING IS AUTOMATI-
        CALLY STANDARDIZED BY THE RECORDED
        PRESENTATION OF ALL INSTRUCTION AND TEST
        ITEMS. TO TEST WHETHER SLIGHT DIFFER-
        ENCES IN LANGUAGE BETWEEN THE TWO
        COUNTRIES WOULD POSE PROBLEMS, IT WAS
        ADMINISTERED TO 3 GROUPS OF NIGHT
        SCHOOL STUDENTS IN PUERTO RICO: THE
        FIRST GROUP HAD REACHED ONLY A FIFTH
        GRADE LEVEL OF EDUCATION, THE SECOND
        WERE TRAINEES IN AVIATION MECHANICS, THE
        THIRD WERE HIGH SCHOOL GRADUATES WHO
        WERE UNIVERSITY BOUND. RESULTS WERE
        THAT THE TEST EFFECTIVELY COVERS A WIDE
        RANGE OF ABILITY AND TRANSFERS EASILY
        FROM A VENEZUELAN TO A PUERTO RICAN
        POPULATION. THE MANAGEMENT OF THE MA-
        TERIALS WAS EASY, AND THE STUDENTS EN-
        JOYED THE EXPERIENCE. IN VIEW OF THE
        ACUTE PROBLEM OF TESTING PUERTO RICANS
        IN NEW YORK CITY AND ELSEWHERE, THIS
        SPANISH FORM OF THE ORAL DIRECTIONS
        TEST SHOULD PROVE USEFUL WHERE AN IN-
        TELLIGENCE SCORE IS NEEDED FOR SCREEN-
        ING, GUIDANCE, OR PLACEMENT IN TRAINING.
        1 REFERENCE.

ACCN   001423

1655 AUTH   **SANUA, V. D.**
     TITL   SOCIO-CULTURAL ASPECTS.
     SRCE   *IN L. BELLAK AND L. LOEB (EDS.), THE SCHIZO-
             PHRENIC SYNDROME. NEW YORK: GRUNE &
             STRATTON, 1969, PP. 256-309.*
     INDX   SCHIZOPHRENIA, SES, REVIEW, PUERTO RI-
             CAN-M, MIGRATION, CULTURAL FACTORS,
             POVERTY, CROSS CULTURAL, DEMOGRAPHIC,
             IMMIGRATION, BIBLIOGRAPHY
     ABST   THE RELATIONSHIP OF SCHIZOPHRENIA TO
             POVERTY IS REPORTED BY A GREAT MANY IN-

VESTIGATORS, THOUGH THIS IS NOT A UNIVER-
SAL FINDING. A MAJOR EPIDEMIOLOGIC STUDY
FOUND THAT THE CLASS POSITION OF A GIVEN
SCHIZOPHRENIC IS A FUNCTION OF THE DIS-
EASE—I.E., THE POTENTIAL SCHIZOPHRENIC
IS MORE LIKELY TO END UP IN A LOWER-CLASS
POSITION. IN RELATION TO PROGNOSIS, ONE
STUDY FOUND THAT SCHIZOPHRENICS IN
LOWER CLASSES TENDED TO STAY LONGER IN
MENTAL HOSPITALS. ANOTHER STUDY FOUND
THAT THE LOWER-CLASS SCHIZOPHRENICS
RELEASED FROM THE HOSPITAL HAD A MUCH
BETTER MENTAL STATUS THAN THE UPPER-
CLASS RELEASED SCHIZOPHRENICS. DESPITE
THE PREVALENCE OF THIS DISEASE AMONG
THE LOWER CLASSES, IT DOES NOT NECES-
SARILY HOLD FOR THE EDUCATIONAL LEVEL:
THE RATE IS NOT HIGHER AMONG THOSE WITH
A LOW LEVEL OF EDUCATION. OVERSEAS EMI-
GRATION AND INTRACONTINENTAL EMIGRA-
TION WERE FOUND TO CORRELATE WITH AN
INCREASE IN MENTAL ILLNESS. MIGRATION
WITHIN THE SAME COUNTRY APPEARS TO BE
DELETERIOUS IN THE UNITED STATES BUT NOT
IN THE SCANDINAVIAN COUNTRIES. FROM
STUDIES OF VARIOUS ETHNIC AND NATIONAL-
ITY GROUPS, THE HIGHEST INCIDENCE IS
AMONG THE NEGROES AND PUERTO RICANS;
THE TOTAL JEWISH RATE WAS FOUND LOWER
(35.5%) THAN THE PROTESTANT (41.7%) OR
CATHOLIC (41.2%) RATES. STUDIES IN LATIN
AMERICA, THE CARIBBEAN ISLANDS, EURO-
PEAN COUNTRIES, ASIATIC COUNTRIES, AF-
RICA AND THE MIDDLE EAST ARE REVIEWED.
SOME BELIEVE THAT THE SOCIAL ENVIRON-
MENT INFLUENCES THE INCREASE OR DE-
CREASE OF SCHIZOPHRENIA AND OTHERS IN-
SIST THAT THE PREVALENCE OF THIS DISEASE
IS THE SAME IN ALL COUNTRIES, DIFFERENCES
IN STATISTICS BEING ATTRIBUTED TO THE
AVAILABLE HOSPITAL FACILITIES. RESEARCH
IN THIS AREA SHOULD BE CONDUCTED ON AN
INTERNATIONAL LEVEL. 450 REFERENCES.

ACCN   001424

1656 AUTH   **SARGENT, C.**
     TITL   BY-PASS ON THE ROAD.
     SRCE   *AMERICAN EDUCATION, 1975, 11(1), 29-33.*
     INDX   MIGRATION, EDUCATION, ADULT EDUCATION,
             SES, INSTRUCTIONAL TECHNIQUES, SOCIAL
             SERVICES, FLORIDA, SOUTH, MIGRANTS
     ABST   TO IMPROVE EDUCATIONAL OPPORTUNITIES
             AMONG MIGRANT CHILDREN, THE PROGRAM
             "LEARN AND EARN" WAS IMPLEMENTED IN
             FLORIDA. THE PROGRAM IS FUNDED BY THE
             U.S. OFFICE OF EDUCATION AND IS ADMINIS-
             TERED BY THE FLORIDA MIGRANTRY CHILD
             COMPENSATORY PROGRAM. "LEARN AND
             EARN" IS DESIGNED TO DEVELOP JOB ENTRY
             SKILLS TO STUDENTS AND THEREBY PROVIDE
             ALTERNATIVES TO "GOING UP THE ROAD."
             GOING UP THE ROAD" MEANS FOLLOWING
             THE CROP AND BEING BOUNCED AROUND
             FROM SCHOOL TO SCHOOL. STUDENTS PAR-
             TICIPATE IN THE PROGRAM ON A VOLUNTARY
             BASIS FOR UP TO THREE HOURS A DAY. THE
             REST OF THEIR SCHOOL TIME IS SPENT IN
             REGULAR CLASSROOMS. TO PROVIDE ACCESS

TO THE PROGRAM, MOBIL VANS WHICH SERVE AS LEARNING LABS ARE LOCATED AT VARIOUS SCHOOLS. THE "LEARN" ASPECT OF THE PROGRAM INCLUDES INSTRUCTIONAL TRAINING IN AREAS SUCH AS AUTOMOBILE TUNE-UP, HOSPITAL HOUSEKEEPING AND PATIENT CARE, TYPING, AND BUSINESS EDUCATION. THE "EARN" PART OF THE PROGRAM REFERS TO THE PARTICIPANTS WORKING IN THE NEARBY COMMUNITIES IN JOBS RELATED TO THE SKILLS THEY ARE ACQUIRING IN THE LEARNING LABS. AS PART OF THE PROGRAM, STUDENTS ARE PAID STIPENDS FOR THEIR JOB EXPERIENCE. THE RESPONSE OF THE PARENTS WHOSE CHILDREN ARE INVOLVED IN THE PROGRAM HAS BEEN EXTREMELY FAVORABLE. IN ADDITION, BY PROVIDING JOB ENTRY SKILLS, THE PROGRAM HAS HELPED TO IMPROVE THE SELF-CONCEPT OF THESE STUDENTS.

ACCN   001425

1657 AUTH   **SATTERFIELD, D. M. O.**
TITL   ACCULTURATION AND MARRIAGE ROLE PATTERNS: A COMPARATIVE STUDY OF MEXICAN-AMERICAN WOMEN (DOCTORAL DISSERTATION, UNIVERSITY OF ARIZONA, 1966).
SRCE   *DISSERTATION ABSTRACTS, 1966, 27(7), 2517B. (UNIVERSITY MICROFILMS NO. 66-15251.)*
INDX   ACCULTURATION, MARRIAGE, FAMILY ROLES, ROLE EXPECTATIONS, MEXICAN AMERICAN, FEMALE, EMPIRICAL, CROSS CULTURAL, SOUTHWEST
ABST   TO DETERMINE THE EFFECT OF ACCULTURATION ON MARRIAGE ROLES, INTERVIEWS WERE CONDUCTED WITH 42 ENGLISH-SPEAKING (HIGH ACCULTURATION) AND 42 SPANISH-SPEAKING (LOW ACCULTURATION) MEXICAN AMERICAN WIVES IN A SOUTHWESTERN U.S. CITY. THE SURVEY INSTRUMENT WAS THE KELLY-THARP MARRIAGE ROLE QUESTIONNAIRE. THE RESULTS FROM THESE TWO GROUPS OF WIVES WERE COMPARED WITH THOSE FROM ANGLO WIVES INTERVIEWED BY THARP IN 1961. THE DATA INDICATE THAT ROLE EXPECTATIONS AND ROLE ENACTMENTS VARY IN DIFFERENT WAYS AMONG ALL THREE GROUPS OF WIVES. IN ROLE EXPECTATIONS THE ENGLISH-SPEAKING MEXICAN AMERICAN WIVES LINKED THEIR DESIRE FOR A COMPANIONATE RELATIONSHIP WITH THE HUSBAND TO EXPECTATIONS OF LEADERSHIP BY THE HUSBAND. IN ROLE ENACTMENTS, SPOUSE INTIMACY WAS LINKED TO UNDERSTANDING AND TOGETHERNESS. AMONG THE SPANISH-SPEAKING WIVES, ROLE EXPECTATIONS DERIVED FROM TRADITIONAL MEXICAN HUSBAND AND WIFE ROLES—I.E., HUSBAND LEADERSHIP WAS EXPECTED, AND SPOUSE TOGETHERNESS EXPECTATIONS WERE MINOR. REGARDING ROLE ENACTMENTS, THESE WIVES PERCEIVED SOLIDARITY IN TERMS OF FAMILINESS, AND DECISION-MAKING RELATED TO TRADITIONAL DIVISIONS OF INFLUENCE. MAJOR DIFFERENCES IN SELF EXPECTATIONS, SEXUAL SATISFACTION, FAMILY ACTIVITY, AND COMMUNITY ACTIVITY ARE ALSO DISCUSSED. IT IS CONCLUDED THE ENGLISH- AND SPANISH-SPEAKING WIVES WERE QUITE DIFFERENT AND MUST BE CONSIDERED AS TWO SEPARATE POPULATIONS. FINALLY, BOTH MEXICAN AMERICAN GROUPS WERE DIFFERENT FROM THE ANGLO WIVES, INDICATING THAT MARRIAGE ROLE DIMENSIONS WHICH ADEQUATELY DESCRIBE MIDDLE CLASS ANGLO MARRIAGES ARE NOT SUFFICIENT TO DESCRIBE THOSE OF OTHER CULTURES, NOR OF SUBGROUPS IN ACCULTURATIVE TRANSITION. 51 REFERENCES. (AUTHOR ABSTRACT MODIFIED)

ACCN   001426

1658 AUTH   **SATTLER, J. M., & KUNCIK, T. M.**
TITL   ETHNICITY, SOCIOECONOMIC STATUS, AND PATTERN OF WISC SCORES AS VARIABLES THAT AFFECT PSYCHOLOGISTS' ESTIMATES OF "EFFECTIVE INTELLIGENCE."
SRCE   *JOURNAL OF CLINICAL PSYCHOLOGY, 1976, 32(2), 362-366.*
INDX   SES, WISC, ETHNIC IDENTITY, INTELLIGENCE TESTING, MEXICAN AMERICAN, CROSS CULTURAL, CHILDREN, EMPIRICAL
ABST   ETHNICITY, SOCIOECONOMIC STATUS, AND PATTERN OF WECHSLER INTELLIGENCE SCALE FOR CHILDREN (WISC) SCORES WERE INVESTIGATED AS BIASING FACTORS IN PSYCHOLOGISTS' ESTIMATES OF EFFECTIVE INTELLIGENCE. PSYCHOLOGISTS ESTIMATED TRUE IQ'S, OR EFFECTIVE INTELLIGENCE, FROM WISC PROFILES THAT VARIED FOR ETHNICITY (BLACK, MEXICAN AMERICAN, OR WHITE), SOCIAL CLASS (LOWER OR MIDDLE), PROFILE (THREE SCATTER PATTERNS), AND DIRECTION OF VERBAL/PERFORMANCE SCALE DISCREPANCY. PSYCHOLOGISTS GAVE HIGHER IQ ESTIMATES TO BLACK AND MEXICAN AMERICAN CHILDREN'S PROFILES THAN TO THE SAME PROFILES OF WHITE CHILDREN. SOCIAL CLASS WAS NOT A SIGNIFICANT FACTOR. PROFILES WITH MUCH SCATTER RECEIVED HIGHER IQ'S THAN PROFILES WITH LIMITED SCATTER. THE PATTERN OF SUBTEST SCORES ALSO AFFECTED ESTIMATES, WHILE THE DIRECTION OF THE VERBAL/PERFORMANCE DISCREPANCY WAS NOT SIGNIFICANT. FINALLY, THE WISC WAS JUDGED TO BE MORE VALID FOR WHITE THAN FOR BLACK AND MEXICAN AMERICAN CHILDREN. REASONS FOR THE DECREASE IN VALIDITY INCLUDE: CULTURAL BIAS OF THE TEST; CULTURAL AND/OR EDUCATIONAL DEPRIVATION; LACK OF APPROPRIATE STANDARDIZATION; AND BILINGUALISM FOR THE MEXICAN AMERICAN CHILDREN. 3 REFERENCES. (AUTHOR SUMMARY MODIFIED)

ACCN   001427

1659 AUTH   **SAUNDERS, L.**
TITL   CULTURAL DIFFERENCE AND MEDICAL CARE: THE CASE OF THE SPANISH-SPEAKING PEOPLE OF THE SOUTHWEST.
SRCE   *NEW YORK: RUSSELL SAGE FOUNDATION, 1954.*
INDX   HEALTH, HEALTH DELIVERY SYSTEMS, CASE STUDY, MEXICAN AMERICAN, URBAN, SES, POVERTY, CULTURAL FACTORS, FAMILY ROLES, INTERPERSONAL RELATIONS, ACCULTURATION, HEALTH, EMPIRICAL, CURANDERISMO, FOLK MEDICINE, DEMOGRAPHIC, RELIGION,

DISCRIMINATION, LEADERSHIP, EDUCATION, CULTURE, TIME ORIENTATION, ACHIEVEMENT MOTIVATION, OCCUPATIONAL ASPIRATIONS, SOUTHWEST, BOOK

ABST THE SPANISH-SPEAKING PEOPLE OF THE SOUTHWEST SHARE A DISTINCTIVE CULTURE WHICH INFLUENCES THEIR BEHAVIOR IN MANY SITUATIONS. ALTHOUGH THIS INFLUENCE VARIES ACROSS INDIVIDUALS AND SITUATIONS, THE CULTURAL BELIEFS, PRACTICES, AND PATTERNS OF RELATIONSHIPS ARE DIFFERENT FROM THOSE OF THE NATIVE ENGLISH-SPEAKING POPULATION OF THE U.S. THE MAIN PURPOSE OF THIS BOOK IS TO LOOK AT THOSE CULTURAL DIFFERENCES AND TO ANALYZE THE RELATIONSHIP BETWEEN THE VARIOUS PROFESSIONAL MEDICAL SERVICES AND THE SPANISH-SPEAKING POPULATION. IN GENERAL, MEDICINE IS SEEN AS PART OF A CULTURE, CONSISTING OF ALL THE COMPLEX ASPECTS OF A FUNCTIONING INSTITUTION. A HYPOTHETICAL HOUSEHOLD IS DESCRIBED TO ILLUSTRATE BOTH THE ROLE OF MEDICAL CARE WITHIN THE SPANISH-SPEAKING CULTURE AND IN RELATION TO MAJORITY SERVICES. DEMOGRAPHIC, ECONOMIC, HISTORICAL, EDUCATIONAL, POLITICAL, SES, ACCULTURATION, AND OTHER PSYCHOSOCIAL VARIABLES ARE PRESENTED TO FURTHER DESCRIBE THIS GROUP. ALTERNATIVE HEALING METHODS AND BELIEFS ARE DISCUSSED RELATING FOLK MEDICINE PRACTICES TO MAINSTREAM PROFESSIONAL SERVICES. FOLLOWING A DISCUSSION OF MAJOR CULTURAL DIFFERENCES, RECOMMENDATIONS ARE MADE FOR BRIDGING THE GAP BETWEEN ANGLO MEDICAL AND HEALTH PERSONNEL AND THE SPANISH-SPEAKING PEOPLE WITH WHOM THEY WORK.

ACCN 001428

1660 AUTH **SAUNDERS, L.**
TITL HEALING WAYS IN THE SPANISH SOUTHWEST.
SRCE *IN E. G. JACO (ED.), PATIENTS, PHYSICIANS AND ILLNESS. GLENCOE, ILL.: THE FREE PRESS, 1958, PP. 188-206.*
INDX HEALTH, FOLK MEDICINE, PHYSICIANS, SPANISH SURNAMED, ESSAY
ABST THE SOCIOCULTURAL ASPECTS OF MEDICAL CARE AND TREATMENT OF THE SPANISH SPEAKING (SS) IN THE SOUTHWEST ARE EXAMINED. THE SS'S MEDICAL KNOWLEDGE OF ILLNESS AND TREATMENT STEMS FROM FOUR SOURCES: (1) FOLK-MEDICAL LORE OF MEDIEVAL SPAIN AS REFINED IN SEVERAL CENTURIES OF ISOLATION FROM ITS SOURCE; (2) CULTURES OF ONE OR MORE AMERICAN INDIAN TRIBES; (3) ANGLO FOLK MEDICINE AS PRACTICED IN RURAL AND URBAN AREAS; AND (4) "SCIENTIFIC" MEDICAL SOURCES. IN A GIVEN INSTANCE OF ILLNESS, ELEMENTS FROM ANY OF THE ABOVE SOURCES MAY BE UTILIZED FOR TREATMENT. THREE OF THE FOUR SOURCES ARE CLASSIFIED AS FOLK MEDICINE. FOLK MEDICINE DIFFERS FROM SCIENTIFIC MEDICINE IN THAT IT IS THE COMMON POSSESSION OF THE GROUP AND THERE IS LITTLE DIVISION OF KNOWLEDGE WITH RESPECT TO MEDICINE AMONG THE GROUP MEMBERS; STILL, FOLK MEDICINE IS A WELL-ORGANIZED AND FAIRLY CONSISTENT THEORY OF MEDICINE. DETAILED DESCRIPTIONS OF MEXICAN FOLK MEDICINE AND SPANISH AMERICAN FOLK MEDICINE ARE PRESENTED ALONG WITH COMPARISONS OF FOLK MEDICINE AND SCIENTIFIC MEDICINE AND FOLK PRACTITIONERS. REASONS FOR ANGLO MEDICINE NOT BEING MORE EXTENSIVELY USED ARE THE GEOGRAPHICAL DISTANCE FACTORS, THE COST FACTOR, THE LACK OF KNOWLEDGE OF ANGLO MEDICAL WAYS, AND THE FEAR FACTOR. ANGLO MEDICINE IS RAPIDLY BECOMING MORE ACCEPTED DESPITE THE MANY OBSTACLES THAT OPERATE IN THE SOCIOCULTURAL ENVIRONMENT.

ACCN 001429

1661 AUTH **SAUNDERS, L., & SAMORA, J.**
TITL A MEDICAL CARE PROGRAM IN A COLORADO COUNTY.
SRCE *IN B. D. PAUL & W. B. MILLER (EDS.), HEALTH, CULTURE, AND COMMUNITY. NEW YORK: RUSSEL SAGE FOUNDATION, 1955, PP. 377-400.*
INDX HEALTH, HEALTH DELIVERY SYSTEMS, RURAL, COMMUNITY, SPANISH SURNAMED, COMMUNITY INVOLVEMENT, POLITICS, CULTURAL FACTORS, FINANCING, CASE STUDY, PROGRAM EVALUATION, COLORADO, SOUTHWEST
ABST THE SUCCESS OF A MEDICAL CARE PROGRAM WHICH WAS ORGANIZED AND BEGAN FUNCTIONING IN BRAZOS COUNTY, COLORADO, AN AREA INHABITED PRIMARILY BY RURAL SPANISH AMERICANS (SA), IS DESCRIBED. MEMBERSHIP DRIVES TWICE SUCCEEDED IN OBTAINING THE 540 MEMBERS NECESSARY TO SUSTAIN THE ASSOCIATION; HOWEVER, MEMBERSHIP DECLINED AS SOON AS THE ORGANIZING IMPETUS DIMINISHED. THE FAILURE OF THE ASSOCIATION, WHICH CEASED TO FUNCTION IN 1952, CAN BE EXPLAINED BY THE FACT THAT ITS INCEPTION, ORGANIZATION, PROMOTION, AND MANAGEMENT WERE THE EFFORTS OF PERSONS NOT CULTURALLY REPRESENTATIVE OF THE MAJORITY OF THE COUNTY'S POPULATION (SA), AND THAT THE PROGRAM ITSELF CONTAINED MANY ELEMENTS INCOMPATIBLE WITH TRADITIONAL PRACTICES AND BELIEFS. A NEW EFFORT TO PROVIDE MEDICAL CARE FOR THE PEOPLE OF BRAZOS COUNTY HAS BEEN UNDERTAKEN. IT EMBODIES SUBSTANTIAL MODIFICATIONS OF THE ORIGINAL PLAN BUT IT INCORPORATES FEATURES MORE IN HARMONY WITH LOCAL BELIEFS AND PRACTICES. THIS NEW PERSPECTIVE SHOULD RECEIVE MORE POPULAR ACCEPTANCE THAN THE FIRST PROGRAM. 6 REFERENCES.

ACCN 001430

1662 AUTH **SAVILLE-TROIKE, M.**
TITL BILINGUAL CHILDREN: A RESOURCE DOCUMENT (BILINGUAL EDUCATION SERIES NO. 2).
SRCE *ARLINGTON, VA.: CENTER FOR APPLIED LINGUISTICS, 1973.*
INDX BILINGUALISM, LANGUAGE LEARNING, BILINGUAL-BICULTURAL EDUCATION, BILINGUAL-BICULTURAL PERSONNEL, LINGUISTICS,

GRAMMAR, PHONOLOGY, SYNTAX, COGNITIVE DEVELOPMENT, MOTHER-CHILD INTERACTION, PHYSICAL DEVELOPMENT, SES, SEX COMPARISON, RESEARCH METHODOLOGY, SOCIALIZATION, MEXICAN AMERICAN, PUERTO RICAN-M, ESSAY, REVIEW, CULTURAL FACTORS, CHILDREN, EDUCATION, EDUCATIONAL ASSESSMENT, EARLY CHILDHOOD EDUCATION, CURRICULUM, LANGUAGE ACQUISITION, LINGUISTIC COMPETENCE

ABST THIS REPORT IS INTENDED TO PROVIDE AN UNDERSTANDING OF THE NATURE OF LANGUAGE, THE LANGUAGE ACQUISITION PROCESS, AND CULTURAL FACTORS AFFECTING THE EDUCATION OF THE BILINGUAL CHILD. DIRECTED TOWARD EARLY CHILDHOOD EDUCATION PERSONNEL, AN ATTEMPT IS MADE TO CORRECT COMMON MISCONCEPTIONS REGARDING MEXICAN AMERICAN, PUERTO RICAN, AND AMERICAN INDIAN CHILDREN. ATTENTION IS GIVEN TO THE SYSTEMATIC, SYMBOLIC, AND SOCIAL NATURE OF LANGUAGE, AND THE IMPLICATIONS OF LANGUAGE DIVERSITY. DIFFERENCES IN FIRST AND SECOND LANGUAGE ACQUISITION ARE EXPLAINED, WITH REFERENCE TO THE INTERFERENCE PHENOMENON AND OPTIMUM AGE FOR SECOND LANGUAGE LEARNING. SUGGESTIONS ARE MADE FOR EARLY CHILDHOOD EDUCATION PROGRAM DEVELOPMENT IN THE AREAS OF RESEARCH, SPECIFICATION OF COMPETENCIES, PERSONNEL TRAINING, AND CURRICULUM. APPENDICES PROVIDE A REVIEW OF RESEARCH ON THE MEXICAN AMERICAN PRESCHOOL CHILD, PLUS AN EXTENSIVE DISCUSSION ON THE EDUCATIONAL AND CULTURAL PROBLEMS AFFECTING MEXICAN AMERICAN, PUERTO RICAN, AND AMERICAN INDIAN CHILDREN. 490 REFERENCES.

ACCN 001431

1663 AUTH SAWYER, J., & SENN, D. J.
TITL INSTITUTIONAL RACISM AND THE AMERICAN PSYCHOLOGICAL ASSOCIATION.
SRCE JOURNAL OF SOCIAL ISSUES, 1973, 29(1), 67-79.
INDX EMPLOYMENT, EQUAL OPPORTUNITY, DISCRIMINATION, REPRESENTATION, PREJUDICE, SOCIAL SCIENCES
ABST INSTITUTIONAL RACISM DOES NOT REQUIRE INDIVIDUAL PREJUDICE OR INSTITUTIONAL INTENT, BUT IS A BY-PRODUCT OF BUSINESS AS USUAL. AS A CASE IN POINT, THIS REPORT BY PSYCHOLOGISTS FOR SOCIAL ACTION SHOWS HOW THE AMERICAN PSYCHOLOGICAL ASSOCIATION (APA) PRACTICED INSTITUTIONAL RACISM BY CONDONING EMPLOYMENT PRACTICES OF LANCASTER PRESS, APA'S MAJOR PRINTER. IN MAY 1969, THE PRESS EMPLOYED 1 BLACK (WASH-UP MAN) OUT OF 300 EMPLOYEES, THOUGH LANCASTER'S 63,000 POPULATION INCLUDED OVER 15% BLACKS AND PUERTO RICANS. BOTH THE PRESS AND THE APA CENTRAL OFFICE ATTRIBUTED THIS TO LOW EDUCATIONAL LEVEL. COLLECTIVE EFFORTS INFLUENCED THE PRESS TO HIRE 9 BLACKS OUT OF 18 NEW EMPLOYEES BETWEEN OCTOBER 1, 1969 AND SEPTEMBER 30,

1970. NEVERTHELESS, A MAY 1973 POSTSCRIPT DOCUMENTS APA'S CONTINUED HESITANCY TO INFLUENCE ITS SUPPLIERS TOWARD EQUAL EMPLOYMENT PRACTICES. 8 REFERENCES. (JOURNAL ABSTRACT MODIFIED)
ACCN 001432

1664 AUTH SCHALLERT, D. L., & CATERINO, L. C.
TITL CROSS LANGUAGE MEMORY RECONSTRUCTIVE PROCESSES IN SPANISH-ENGLISH BILINGUALS.
SRCE PAPER PRESENTED AT THE ANNUAL MEETING OF THE SOUTHWESTERN PSYCHOLOGICAL ASSOCIATION, HOUSTON, APRIL 1975.
INDX MEMORY, SEMANTICS, BILINGUALISM, COLLEGE STUDENTS, LANGUAGE COMPREHENSION, LINGUISTIC COMPETENCE, SPANISH SURNAMED, EMPIRICAL, BILINGUAL
ABST AN INVESTIGATION TESTING THE HYPOTHESIS THAT MEMORY FOR VERBAL MATERIALS IS DUE TO SEMANTIC RECONSTRUCTION, RATHER THAN BEING VERBATIM IN NATURE, WAS CONDUCTED AMONG 18 SPANISH-ENGLISH BILINGUAL AND 18 ENGLISH MONOLINGUAL COLLEGE STUDENTS. THE SUBJECTS HEARD FIVE PARAGRAPHS IN EACH OF TWO LANGUAGES. BILINGUAL SUBJECTS IDENTIFIED MOST OF THE EXACT ORIGINAL SENTENCES THAT AGREED SEMANTICALLY WITH THE INFORMATION ACTUALLY PRESENTED AND REJECTED SENTENCES THAT DEVIATED IN MEANING. THE LANGUAGE OF A SENTENCE IN THE RECOGNITION TEST DID NOT INFLUENCE THE JUDGMENTS OF THE BILINGUAL SUBJECTS. MONOLINGUAL SUBJECTS, HOWEVER, WERE LESS LIKELY TO REPORT RECOGNITION OF ANY OF THE SENTENCES, IMPLIED OR ORIGINAL. THE FINDINGS SUPPORT THE RECONSTRUCTIVE MEMORY HYPOTHESIS SINCE THE BILINGUAL SUBJECTS BASED RECOGNITION DECISIONS ON SEMANTIC REPRESENTATION, OVERLOOKING STRUCTURAL AND LANGUAGE CHANGES. 9 REFERENCES. (AUTHOR ABSTRACT MODIFIED)
ACCN 001433

1665 AUTH SCHEFLEN, A. E.
TITL LIVING SPACE IN AN URBAN GHETTO.
SRCE FAMILY PROCESS, 1971, 10(4), 429-450.
INDX EMPIRICAL, URBAN, COMMUNITY, PUERTO RICAN-M, INTERPERSONAL SPACING, SURVEY
ABST THE IDEA OF HUMAN TERRITORIALITY IS OUTLINED, AND SOME TERRITORIAL ARRANGEMENTS AND BEHAVIORS IN URBAN GHETTO HOUSEHOLDS ARE DISCUSSED. RESULTS OF STUDIES OF THE PRESTRUCTURAL LIVING AND THE TERRITORIAL BEHAVIOR OF URBAN PEOPLE IN A CENTRAL BRONX GHETTO INDICATE THAT THE ENVIRONMENT OF PEOPLE IS PRESTRUCTURED SOCIALLY AND TEMPORALLY. INTERVIEWS WERE CONDUCTED IN ABOUT 1,800 HOUSEHOLDS, SPACE LAYOUTS WERE PHOTOGRAPHICALLY SURVEYED IN 35, AND SPACE USAGE AND TERRITORIAL BEHAVIOR WERE VIDEOTAPED IN SIX. MOST OF THE DATA PERTAIN TO PUERTO RICANS AND AFRO-AMERICANS.
ACCN 001434

1666 AUTH **SCHEIDLINGER, S., STRUENING, E. L., & RABKIN, J. G.**

TITL EVALUATION OF A MENTAL HEALTH CONSULTATION SERVICE IN THE GHETTO AREA.

SRCE *AMERICAN JOURNAL OF PSYCHOTHERAPY, 1970, 24(3), 485-492.*

INDX PROGRAM EVALUATION, HEALTH DELIVERY SYSTEMS, MENTAL HEALTH, COMMUNITY, ATTITUDES, ADMINISTRATORS

ABST AN EVALUATION DESIGNED TO GAUGE THE ATTITUDES OF THE ADMINISTRATORS OF CONSULTEE AGENCIES TOWARD A MENTAL HEALTH CONSULTATION SERVICE IN AN INNER CITY AREA IS PRESENTED. TWENTY-ONE DIRECTORS OF THE COMMUNITY AGENCIES AFFILIATED WITH THE CONSULTATION SERVICE (CS) ANSWERED A SERIES OF QUESTIONS DESIGNED TO ELICIT THEIR ATTITUDES TOWARD THE CONSULTATION PROGRAM, TO ASCERTAIN WHETHER AND HOW THEY HAD FOUND IT HELPFUL, AND TO SOLICIT THEIR OPINION AS TO WHAT, IF ANYTHING, SHOULD BE DONE DIFFERENTLY IN THE FUTURE. WHILE THERE WERE DEFINITE DIFFERENCES REGARDING THE RESPONDENTS' PREFERENCES FOR INDIVIDUAL COMPONENTS OF THE CONSULTATION SERVICE, A LARGE MAJORITY CLAIMED TO HAVE BENEFITED FROM THIS PROGRAM AND ASKED THAT IT BE CONTINUED. MOST RESPONDENTS ALSO INDICATED A DEFINITE APPRECIATION OF THE DIRECTORS' GROUP MEETINGS AND OF THE TRAINING WORKSHOPS. THE WORKSHOPS RECEIVING MOST FAVORABLE COMMENT WERE ARTS AND CRAFTS AND SHORT-TERM COUNSELING. SUGGESTIONS FOR FUTURE DIRECTIONS OF THE CS INCLUDE: (1) MORE COMMUNITY AGENCIES SHOULD BE INVOLVED IN THE COLLABORATIVE SERVICE; (2) MORE SPANISH-SPEAKING MEMBERS SHOULD BE INCLUDED IN THE CS STAFF; AND (3) THE CS SHOULD NOT ONLY TEACH METHODOLOGY BUT ALSO PROVIDE RESOURCE INFORMATION REGARDING SUCH WIDESPREAD PROBLEMS AS WELFARE AND HOUSING. OTHER SUGGESTIONS INCLUDE HAVING WORKSHOPS ON PROBLEMS OF UNWED MOTHERS AND ADDICTION. ENCOUNTER GROUPS FOR STAFF MEMBERS ARE ALSO MENTIONED AS A FUTURE IMPROVEMENT. THE ULTIMATE TEST OF THE EFFECTIVENESS OF MENTAL HEALTH CONSULTATION, THE CHANGE IN THE QUALITY OF SERVICES OFFERED BY CONSULTEE AGENCIES AND THE REDUCED INCIDENCE OF SOCIAL AND PSYCHIATRIC DISABILITY, IS NOT MEASURABLE IN THE TERMS OF THIS STUDY. 4 REFERENCES.

ACCN 001435

1667 AUTH **SCHENSUL, S. L.**

TITL SKILLS NEEDED IN ACTION ANTHROPOLOGY: LESSONS FROM EL CENTRO DE LA CAUSA.

SRCE *HUMAN ORGANIZATION, 1974, 33(2), 203-209.*

INDX HEALTH DELIVERY SYSTEMS, MENTAL HEALTH, COMMUNITY, CULTURAL FACTORS, CASE STUDY, PROGRAM EVALUATION, URBAN, LEADERSHIP, MEXICAN AMERICAN, COMMUNITY INVOLVEMENT, ILLINOIS, MIDWEST

ABST A DISCUSSION IS PRESENTED OF SOCIAL ACTION RESEARCH AS APPLIED TO EL CENTRO DE LA CAUSA—A LATINO COMMUNITY-CONTROLLED SERVICE ORGANIZATION IN CHICAGO'S WEST SIDE. THE CONSULTATIVE RELATIONSHIP BETWEEN A TEAM OF APPLIED ANTHROPOLOGISTS AND THE DEVELOPMENT OF EL CENTRO IS REVIEWED, INCLUDING THE INFORMATION GATHERING EFFORTS OF THE RESEARCHERS FOR THE SUPPORT OF EL CENTRO'S PROGRAMS. ACTIVITIES AND SKILLS OF THE RESEARCH TEAM ARE PRESENTED, OUTLINING THEIR PARTICIPATION IN (1) THE COLLECTION OF USEFUL DATA FOR PROGRAM DEVELOPMENT, (2) FACILITATING COMMUNICATION WITH OUTSIDE GROUPS, (3) THE CREATION OF INFORMATION ARCHIVES, AND (4) ESTABLISHING FUNDING SOURCES FOR PROGRAM EXPANSION. IN ORDER FOR SOCIAL ACTION RESEARCH TO BECOME A SIGNIFICANT PART OF GRADUATE TRAINING, MORE INFORMATION IS NEEDED ON THE OPERATION, ACTIVITIES, METHODS, AND STRATEGIES OF APPLIED ANTHROPOLOGISTS IN A VARIETY OF SITUATIONS. 5 REFERENCES.

ACCN 001436

1668 AUTH **SCHEPERS, E. M.**

TITL VOICES, VISIONS AND STRANGE IDEAS: HALLUCINATIONS AND DELUSIONS IN A MEXICAN ORIGIN POPULATION (DOCTORAL DISSERTATION, NORTHWESTERN UNIVERSITY, 1974). .

SRCE *DISSERTATION ABSTRACTS INTERNATIONAL, 1974, 35, 3199A. (UNIVERSITY MICROFILMS NO. 74-28,736).*

INDX MEXICAN AMERICAN, ACCULTURATION, SCHIZOPHRENIA, NEUROSIS, CULTURAL FACTORS, FOLK MEDICINE, CURANDERISMO, EMPIRICAL, SYMPTOMATOLOGY, PSYCHOSOCIAL ADJUSTMENT, ILLINOIS, MIDWEST

ABST THE CULTURAL PATTERNING OF DELUSIONS AND HALLUCINATIONS WAS EXAMINED AMONG THE MEXICAN ORIGIN POPULATION IN CHICAGO. THE THEORETICAL AND PRACTICAL IMPLICATIONS OF THIS PATTERNING ARE PRESENTED. ATTITUDES TOWARD MENTAL ILLNESS WITHIN THIS POPULATION ARE PATTERNED, IN PART, BY A COMPLEX OF IDEAS DERIVED FROM MEXICAN FOLK CULTURE, SPIRIT MEDIUMSHIP, AND OTHER FACTORS, AND MODIFIED BY LOCAL CONDITIONS. THESE AND OTHER ASPECTS OF THE ADAPTIVE SYSTEMS OF MEXICAN ORIGIN POPULATIONS ARE REFLECTED IN THE DELUSIONAL AND HALLUCINATORY PATTERNS OF HOSPITALIZED AND NONHOSPITALIZED PATIENTS. NONPSYCHOTIC INDIVIDUALS FREELY EXPERIENCE VISIONS AND VOICES INTERPRETED AS THOSE OF SPIRITS OF THE DEAD—A PATTERN WHICH CAN BE ANALYZED IN TERMS OF ITS RELATIONSHIP BOTH TO THE BELIEF SYSTEM AND TO DISSOCIATION OF THE PERSONALITY. 195 REFERENCES. (NCMHI ABSTRACT)

ACCN 001437

1669 AUTH **SCHMIDT, D. E., GOLDMAN, R. D., & FEIMER, N. R.**

TITL PHYSICAL AND PSYCHOLOGICAL FACTORS ASSOCIATED WITH PERCEPTIONS OF CROWD-

ING: AN ANALYSIS OF SUBCULTURAL DIFFER-
ENCES.

SRCE   *JOURNAL OF APPLIED PSYCHOLOGY, 1976,
61(3), 279-289.*

INDX   URBAN, INTERPERSONAL SPACING, PSYCHO-
SOCIAL ADJUSTMENT, STRESS, EMPIRICAL,
ENVIRONMENTAL FACTORS, MEXICAN AMERI-
CAN, CROSS CULTURAL, CULTURAL FACTORS,
SURVEY, CALIFORNIA, SOUTHWEST

ABST   A FIELD STUDY WAS CONDUCTED TO DETER-
MINE IF A NUMBER OF PSYCHOLOGICAL AND
PHYSICAL FACTORS THAT HAD BEEN PREVI-
OUSLY ASSOCIATED WITH PERCEPTIONS OF
ENVIRONMENTAL CROWDING DIFFERED WITH
THE CULTURAL CHARACTERISTICS OF URBAN
RESIDENTS. SIX HUNDRED NINETY-SEVEN
SUBJECTS LIVING IN THE RIVERSIDE AND SAN
BERNARDINO, CALIFORNIA, AREA WERE SUR-
VEYED TO ASCERTAIN PERCEIVED CROWDING
IN THE RESIDENCE, NEIGHBORHOOD, AND
CITY. IT WAS FOUND BY MULTIPLE REGRES-
SION ANALYSIS THAT PSYCHOLOGICAL FAC-
TORS INDICATIVE OF THE IMPACT OF PHYSICAL
CONDITIONS ON THE INDIVIDUAL PROVIDED
THE BEST EXPLANATION FOR THE PERCEPTION
OF CROWDING FOR WHITE SUBJECTS. BLACK
AND CHICANO GROUPS, HOWEVER, TENDED
TO VIEW CROWDING AT EACH OF THE ANALY-
SIS LEVELS IN TERMS OF THE TOTAL URBAN
GESTALT, ASSOCIATING PHYSICAL MEASURES
BEYOND THEIR IMPLICATED IMPACT. 43 REF-
ERENCES. (NCMHI ABSTRACT)

ACCN   001438

1670 AUTH   **SCHMIDT, L., & GALLESSICH, J.**

TITL   ADJUSTMENT OF ANGLO-AMERICAN AND MEX-
ICAN-AMERICAN PUPILS IN SELF-CONTAINED
AND TEAM-TEACHING CLASSROOMS.

SRCE   *JOURNAL OF EDUCATIONAL PSYCHOLOGY, 1971,
62(4), 328-332.*

INDX   MEXICAN AMERICAN, CROSS CULTURAL, GROUP
DYNAMICS, EDUCATIONAL ASSESSMENT, IN-
STRUCTIONAL   TECHNIQUES,   CHILDREN,
TEACHERS, CULTURAL FACTORS, SEX COM-
PARISON, ANXIETY, EMPIRICAL, TEXAS, SOUTH-
WEST

ABST   PUPIL ADJUSTMENT IN SELF-CONTAINED AND
TEAM-TEACHING CLASSROOMS WAS COM-
PARED. THE SUBJECTS WERE 160 FIRST-GRADE
AND 382 SIXTH-GRADE PUPILS FROM EXPERI-
MENTAL TEAM-TEACHING SCHOOLS, ONE PRE-
DOMINATELY ANGLO AMERICAN (AA) AND ONE
PREDOMINATELY MEXICAN AMERICAN (MA),
AND SELF-CONTAINED CLASSROOM SCHOOLS
WITH COMPARABLE POPULATIONS. ANXIETY
WAS MEASURED WITH THE PICTURE ANXIETY
TEST (FIRST-GRADE SUBJECTS) AND THE PHIL-
LIPS ANXIETY TEST (SIXTH-GRADE SUBJECTS);
PUPIL EVALUATION OF TEACHERS WAS MEA-
SURED WITH THE PUPIL OBSERVATION SURVEY
REPORT. RESULTS INDICATED THAT THE ANXIETY
LEVEL REPORTED BY MA SUBJECTS OF BOTH
GRADE LEVELS AND IN BOTH TEACHING OR-
GANIZATIONS WAS SIGNIFICANTLY HIGHER
THAN THE ANXIETY REPORTED BY AA SUB-
JECTS. FIRST-GRADE MA SUBJECTS ALSO
VIEWED THEIR TEACHERS LESS FAVORABLY
THAN DID AA FIRST-GRADE SUBJECTS, BUT

THIS DIFFERENCE DID NOT APPEAR IN SIXTH-
GRADE SUBJECTS. IN SUMMARY, THE DATA IN-
DICATE THAT TEAM-TEACHING IS NOT DETRI-
MENTAL TO THE ELEMENTARY GRADE CHIL-
DREN OF THIS STUDY—REGARDLESS OF
ETHNICITY OR SEX—AND MAY IN FACT BE AD-
VANTAGEOUS FOR SOME CHILDREN. 14 REF-
ERENCES. (NCMHI ABSTRACT)

ACCN   001439

1671 AUTH   **SCHNEER, H. I., PERLSTEIN, A., & BROZOV-
SKY, M.**

TITL   HOSPITALIZED SUICIDAL ADOLESCENTS: TWO
GENERATIONS.

SRCE   *JOURNAL OF THE AMERICAN ACADEMY OF
CHILD PSYCHIATRY, 1975, 14(2), 268-280.*

INDX   SUICIDE, MENTAL HEALTH, ADOLESCENTS,
CROSS CULTURAL, SES, DRUG ABUSE, DRUG
ADDICTION, DELINQUENCY, DEVIANCE, EMPIR-
ICAL, PUERTO RICAN-M, SEX COMPARISON,
ENVIRONMENTAL FACTORS, SURVEY

ABST   A REVIEW OF THE KINGS COUNTY PSYCHIAT-
RIC HOSPITAL (NEW YORK) RECORDS FOR
366 LOW-SOCIOECONOMIC ADOLESCENTS
TREATED IN 1959 AND 356 IN 1969-70 REVEAL
THAT THE TOTAL NUMBER OF SUICIDAL ADO-
LESCENTS ALMOST DOUBLED AND THE PER-
CENTAGE OF SUICIDAL ADOLESCENTS DOU-
BLED FROM BEFORE THE DECADE OF THE 60'S
TO JUST AFTER IT. A CHANGE IN THE SEX RATIO
FOR ADOLESCENT SUICIDAL BEHAVIOR ALSO
APPEARED. THERE WAS A GREATER INCREASE
IN FREQUENCY OF SUICIDAL BEHAVIOR AMONG
THE BOYS THAN AMONG THE GIRLS. COMPAR-
ING THE TWO GENERATIONS OF ADOLES-
CENTS ON ETHNIC, SEXUAL, AND SOCIAL VARI-
ABLES REVEALS ADDITIONAL TRENDS: (1) THE
SUICIDAL RATE FOR BLACK GIRLS INCREASED
FOUR TO FIVE FOLD, WHILE THERE WAS ONLY
A MODERATE INCREASE FOR ANGLO AND
PUERTO RICAN GIRLS; AND (2) THE RATE FOR
SUICIDAL PUERTO RICAN MALES INCREASED
FOUR TO FIVE TIMES, WHILE FOR ANGLO MALES
IT MORE THAN DOUBLED, AND FOR BLACK
MALES LESS THAN DOUBLED. BEFORE THE
DECADE, ONE-FOURTH OF THE SUICIDAL ADO-
LESCENTS WERE DIAGNOSED PSYCHOTIC AND/
OR SCHIZOPHRENIC, WHILE IN 1969-70 ONE-
HALF WERE SO DIAGNOSED. REPORTS OF
HALLUCINATIONS ALMOST DOUBLED, RUN-
AWAYS WERE FOUR TIMES AS FREQUENT, AND
DRUG ABUSE AS A DIAGNOSTIC SYMPTOM OC-
CURRED TEN TIMES MORE FREQUENTLY IN
1969-70 THAN IN 1959. AT THE END OF THE
DECADE THE ADOLESCENTS TREATED WERE
MORE DRUG-ABUSING, EMOTIONALLY DIS-
TURBED, TRUANT, AGGRESSIVE, AND REPETI-
TIOUSLY SUICIDAL. SCHOOL ADJUSTMENT AND
ACADEMIC   PERFORMANCE   WERE   POOR
AMONG BOTH GENERATIONS. DISTURBED AND
ONE-PARENT (USUALLY FATHER ABSENT) FAMILY
PATTERNS WERE FREQUENT AMONG ALL THE
SAMPLE ADOLESCENTS, WITH NO STRIKING
DIFFERENCE AMONG SUICIDAL AND NONSUI-
CIDAL GROUPS. HOWEVER, EARLY DEATH OF
THE FATHER FOLLOWED BY OTHER EGO-
THREATENING EVENTS ARE POSSIBLY SIGNIFI-

CANT FACTORS IN DETERMINING SUICIDAL BE-HAVIOR IN ADOLESCENTS. 22 REFERENCES.

ACCN 001440

1672 AUTH **SCHRATZ, M. M.**
TITL A DEVELOPMENTAL INVESTIGATION OF SEX DIFFERENCES IN SPATIAL (VISUAL-ANALYTIC) AND MATHEMATICAL SKILLS IN THREE ETHNIC GROUPS.
SRCE *DEVELOPMENTAL PSYCHOLOGY, 1978, 14(3), 263-267.*
INDX ABILITY TESTING, ADOLESCENTS, CHILDREN, COGNITIVE STYLE, CROSS CULTURAL, EMPIRICAL, LEARNING, EXAMINER EFFECTS, MATHEMATICS, SPANISH SURNAMED, SEX COMPARISON, NEW YORK, EAST, URBAN, SES
ABST THIS STUDY INVESTIGATED SEX DIFFERENCES IN MATHEMATICAL AND SPATIAL SKILLS IN THREE ETHNIC GROUPS—BLACK, WHITE, AND HISPANIC—PRIOR TO AND DURING ADOLESCENCE. THERE WERE 20 SUBJECTS, WITH AN EQUAL NUMBER OF MALES AND FEMALES FORMING A PREADOLESCENT AND AN ADOLESCENT GROUP. SUBJECTS WERE TAKEN FROM 2 ELEMENTARY SCHOOLS AND 3 HIGH SCHOOLS IN AN ETHNICALLY MIXED, LOW SES NEIGHBORHOOD. TO CONTROL FOR POSSIBLE EXAMINER EFFECTS OF SEX AND ETHNIC MEMBERSHIP, BOTH MALE AND FEMALE EXAMINERS OF EACH ETHNIC GROUP WERE EMPLOYED. THE EXAMINERS ADMINISTERED FORMS OF THE EMBEDDED FIGURES TEST AND THE MODERN MATHEMATICS SUPPLEMENT TO THE IOWA TEST OF BASIC SKILLS. SIGNIFICANT INTERACTION EFFECTS WERE DISCOVERED BETWEEN ETHNIC GROUP MEMBERSHIP AND SEX FOR BOTH MATHEMATICAL AND SPATIAL SKILLS. IN HISPANIC ADOLESCENT GROUPS, SIGNIFICANT SEX DIFFERENCES WERE FOUND IN SCORES ON BOTH SKILLS IN FAVOR OF THE FEMALES. A SIMILAR BUT NOT SIGNIFICANT TREND WAS SEEN IN THE SCORES OF BLACK ADOLESCENT GROUPS. IN CONTRAST, WHITE ADOLESCENT MALES SCORED HIGHER THAN WHITE ADOLESCENT FEMALES, BUT NOT SIGNIFICANTLY SO. NO PRIOR STUDY HAS REPORTED THIS OBSERVED PATTERN OF SEX DIFFERENCES IN HISPANIC SUBJECTS. 10 REFERENCES. (JOURNAL ABSTRACT MODIFIED)
ACCN 002204

1673 AUTH **SCHROTH, M. L.**
TITL THE USE OF IQ AS A MEASURE OF LEARNING RATE WITH MINORITY CHILDREN.
SRCE *JOURNAL OF GENETIC PSYCHOLOGY, 1976, 128(MARCH), 101-128.*
INDX INTELLIGENCE TESTING, SES, MEXICAN AMERICAN, TEST VALIDITY, LEARNING, EMPIRICAL, CHILDREN, CALIFORNIA, SOUTHWEST
ABST THE PURPOSE OF THIS STUDY WAS TO INVESTIGATE THE USE OF IQ AS A MEASURE OF LEARNING RATE WITH CHILDREN OF SIMILAR ETHNIC ORIGIN BUT DIFFERENT SOCIOECONOMIC BACKGROUNDS. THE THEORETICAL BASIS FOR THIS EXPERIMENT WAS THE OPPOSING HYPOTHESES OF WEIR AND ZIGLER CONCERNING THE USE OF IQ OR MA AS THE BEST

MEASURE OF LEARNING RATE. SPECIFICALLY, A DIMENSION-ABSTRACTED ODDITY TASK WAS PRESENTED TO 180 MEXICAN AMERICAN CHILDREN WITH DIFFERENT IQ'S FROM LOWER AND MIDDLE SOCIOECONOMIC BACKGROUNDS. THEY WERE MATCHED ON MA. THE RESULTS SUPPORT WEIR'S HYPOTHESIS AS IQ WAS FOUND TO DETERMINE THE RATE OF LEARNING THE TASK. ALSO, MIDDLE-SES CHILDREN LEARNED THE TASK FASTER THAN THEIR MATCHED LOW-SES PEERS. 17 REFERENCES. (JOURNAL ABSTRACT)

ACCN 001441

1674 AUTH **SCHULMAN, S.**
TITL RURAL HEALTHWAYS IN NEW MEXICO.
SRCE *ANNALS OF THE NEW YORK ACADEMY OF SCIENCES, 1960, 84(17), 950-958.*
INDX MEXICAN AMERICAN, ESSAY, HEALTH DELIVERY SYSTEMS, HEALTH, FOLK MEDICINE, RURAL, NEW MEXICO, SOUTHWEST, DISEASE
ABST A CASE DESCRIPTION OF THE HEALTHWAYS OF RURAL SPANISH AMERICANS IN A NORTHERN NEW MEXICAN VILLAGE IS PRESENTED. THROUGH VIRTUAL ISOLATION THE VILLAGE DEVELOPED A DISTINGUISHABLE AND SPECIFIC SUBCULTURE ANALOGOUS TO THE LARGER HISPANIC-AMERICAN WORLD. THE HEALTH/DISEASE COMPLEX OF THE VILLAGE HAS ITS ROOTS IN MEDIEVAL SPAIN AND PRECOLONIAL AMERICA AND, CONSEQUENTLY, THE MEDICAL SYSTEM IS RELATIVELY STATIC AND TRADITIONAL. MAJOR FACTORS OF THE HEALTH/DISEASE COMPLEX ARE HYGIENIC ASPECTS OF HOME LIFE, DIETARY HABIT, PRECAUTIONARY HEALTH MEASURES, MENTAL ILLNESS, AND THE IDENTIFICATION AND TREATMENT OF DISEASE. THE CURATIVE PROCESS ENTAILS BOTH IDENTIFICATION AND TREATMENT OF THE DISEASE. ILLNESSES INCLUDE THE FOLLOWING TYPES: PHYSICAL, EMOTIONAL, AND MAGICO-RELIGIOUS. THE THERAPIES AND THERAPISTS DIFFER ACCORDING TO THE PARTICULAR DISEASE. DISCUSSION OF REMEDIOS (FOLK REMEDIES), SOBANDO AND TRAQUEANDO (MASSAGING AND BONE CRACKING) TECHNIQUES, AND MEDICOS CURANDEROS, PARTERAS, ARBOLARIOS AND BRUJOS (CURING PRACTITIONERS) IS PROVIDED; AND NOTED IS THE TREND TOWARD THE INCLUSION OF MODERN MEDICAL TREATMENT AS AN ACCEPTABLE ALTERNATIVE IN THERAPY. 26 REFERENCES.

ACCN 001442

1675 AUTH **SCHWARTZ, A. J.**
TITL A COMPARATIVE STUDY OF VALUE AND ACHIEVEMENT: MEXICAN AMERICANS AND ANGLO YOUTH.
SRCE *SOCIOLOGY OF EDUCATION, 1971, 44(4), 438-462.*
INDX CROSS CULTURAL, MEXICAN AMERICAN, ADOLESCENTS, ATTITUDES, SCHOLASTIC ACHIEVEMENT, EMPIRICAL, SES, URBAN, ACHIEVEMENT TESTING, CULTURAL FACTORS, TIME ORIENTATION, SEX COMPARISON, SOUTHWEST, CALIFORNIA, VALUES
ABST SEVERAL VALUE ORIENTATIONS AND THEIR RE-

LATIONS WITH SCHOOL ACHIEVEMENT AMONG BLUE-COLLAR AND WHITE-COLLAR NINTH- AND TWELFTH-GRADE MEXICAN AMERICAN (MA) PUPILS ARE CONTRASTED WITH SIMILAR DATA FOR AN ANGLO (AA) SAMPLE. A QUESTION-NAIRE MEASURING IDEALIZED SCHOOL GOALS, INSTRUMENTAL ORIENTATION, EXPRESSIVE ORIENTATION, FORMAL SCHOOL COMPLI-ANCE, FAITH IN HUMAN NATURE, FUTURE ORI-ENTATION, INDEPENDENCE FROM PEERS, IN-DEPENDENCE FROM FAMILY, AND CONCERN FOR FAMILY OVER PEERS, WAS ADMINISTERED TO THE SUBJECTS. THE FINDINGS SHOW THAT THOSE MA PUPILS WITH VALUE ORIENTATIONS MOST SIMILAR TO ANGLO PUPILS HAD THE HIGHEST SCHOLASTIC ACHIEVEMENT. WHILE IT IS RECOGNIZED THAT PUPILS' VALUES AND ACHIEVEMENT ARE SUBSTANTIALLY INTERDE-PENDENT, THE FINDINGS SUGGEST THAT AF-FECTIVE FACTORS IN THE CULTURAL BACK-GROUND OF THE MA PUPIL (LOW FUTURE ORIENTATION) HINDER THEIR GENERAL ACA-DEMIC ACHIEVEMENT. EARLIER STUDIES HAVE CONCLUDED THAT CHILDREN REARED IN THE TRADITIONAL MA CULTURE HAVE LOWER GOAL ORIENTATION, ARE MORE EXPRESSIVE, MORE PARTICULARISTIC, MORE FATALISTIC, AND HAVE GREATER ORIENTATION TOWARD AUTHORITY THAN THOSE REARED IN ANGLO CULTURE. FINDINGS SUPPORT THESE CONCLUSIONS FOR ALL VALUES EXCEPT GOAL ORIENTATION, AS MA AND AA PUPILS WERE SIMILAR IN GOAL ORIENTATION. OF THOSE VALUES THAT DISTIN-GUISH THE TWO CULTURES, PARTICULARISM AND FATALISM (LOW FAITH IN HUMAN NATURE AND LOW FUTURE ORIENTATION) ARE RE-LATED SIGNIFICANTLY AND NEGATIVELY TO ACHIEVEMENT FOR ALL PUPILS, WHILE ORIEN-TATION TOWARD FAMILY AUTHORITY (NOT SCHOOL AUTHORITY) IS RELATED NEGATIVELY TO ACHIEVEMENT FOR BOTH MA AND BLUE-COLLAR AA PUPILS. 27 REFERENCES.

ACCN   001443

1676 AUTH   **SCHWIRIAN, K. P., & RICO-VELASCO, J.**
TITL   THE RESIDENTIAL DISTRIBUTION OF STATUS GROUPS IN PUERTO RICO'S METROPOLITAN AREAS.
SRCE   *DEMOGRAPHY, 1971, 8(1), 81-90.*
INDX   URBAN, PUERTO RICAN-I, EMPIRICAL, ECO-NOMIC FACTORS, DISCRIMINATION, DEMO-GRAPHIC, SES, HOUSING
ABST   THE PURPOSE OF THIS PAPER IS TO INVESTI-GATE THE PATTERN OF RESIDENTIAL SEGRE-GATION OF STATUS GROUPS IN PUERTO RICO'S THREE METROPOLITAN AREAS. THE FINDINGS SHOWED THAT IN ALL THREE AREAS: (1) AS THE SOCIAL STATUS DISTANCE BETWEEN GROUPS INCREASES SO TOO DOES THE DE-GREE OF DISSIMILARITY OF THEIR RESIDEN-TIAL DISTRIBUTIONS; (2) THE STATUS GROUPS MOST RESIDENTIALLY SEGREGATED ARE THOSE AT THE TOP AND AT THE BOTTOM OF THE STA-TUS PYRAMID; AND (3) THE PATTERN OF RESI-DENTIAL CENTRALIZATION OF STATUS GROUPS FOR PONCE AND MAYAGUEZ ARE SUCH THAT THE HIGHEST STATUS GROUPS ARE THE MOST CENTRALIZED, WHILE THE LOWEST STATUS

GROUPS ARE THE MOST DECENTRALIZED, BUT IN SAN JUAN, IT IS THE HIGHEST STATUS GROUPS THAT ARE THE MOST DECENTRAL-IZED AND THE LOWEST STATUS GROUPS THAT ARE THE MOST CENTRALIZED. THE DATA ARE FROM THE 1960 CENSUS. INDICATORS OF STA-TUS EMPLOYED ARE EDUCATION, OCCUPA-TION, AND INCOME. DIFFERENCES IN FIND-INGS ABOUT CENTRALIZATION BETWEEN SAN JUAN AND THE OTHER CITIES ARE EXPLAINED IN TERMS OF DIFFERENTIAL ECONOMIC DE-VELOPMENT. 14 REFERENCES. (JOURNAL AB-STRACT)

ACCN   001444

1677 AUTH   **SCOTT, C. S.**
TITL   HEALTH AND HEALING PRACTICES AMONG FIVE ETHNIC GROUPS IN MIAMI, FLORIDA.
SRCE   *PUBLIC HEALTH REPORTS, 1974, 89(6), 524-532.*
INDX   CULTURE, HEALTH, CROSS CULTURAL, CUBAN, PUERTO RICAN-M, FOLK MEDICINE, HEALTH DELIVERY SYSTEMS, MENTAL HEALTH, RE-SOURCE UTILIZATION, CULTURAL FACTORS, EMPIRICAL
ABST   TO DEVELOP MODELS FOR IMPROVED HEALTH CARE DELIVERY, THE HEALTH AND ECOLOGY PROJECT INVESTIGATED THE UTILIZATION OF ORTHODOX AND TRADITIONAL HEALTH SYS-TEMS BY FIVE ETHNIC GROUPS IN INNER-CITY MIAMI. HEALTH BELIEFS AND PRACTICES OF BAHAMIANS, CUBANS, HAITIANS, PUERTO RI-CANS, AND SOUTHERN U.S. BLACKS WERE IN-VESTIGATED BY FEMALE INTERVIEWERS, ETH-NICALLY-MATCHED WITH SUBJECTS. THE RESEARCH PROTOCOL INCLUDED (1) A QUES-TIONNAIRE TO 100 HOUSEHOLD HEADS IN EACH ETHNIC GROUP AND (2) MONTH-LONG PARTICIPANT-OBSERVATION OF 30-40 FAMILIES SELECTED FROM THE SURVEY GROUP (IN-CLUDING IN-DEPTH INTERVIEWS OF MOTHERS AND A REVIEW OF A HEALTH CALENDAR RE-CORDED BY THE FAMILY CARE-PROVIDER). BA-HAMIAN HEALTH CALENDARS INDICATE CHRONICALLY POOR HEALTH AND A RELIANCE ON THE ORTHODOX HEALTH SYSTEM ONLY FOR EMERGENCIES OR IN CONJUNCTION WITH FOLK THERAPY. CUBANS EXPERIENCE LESS ILLNESS THAN DO OTHER GROUPS AND USE ALL MEDICAL RESOURCES, BOTH ORTHODOX AND TRADITIONAL, AVAILABLE TO THEM. HAI-TIANS, RECENT EMIGRANTS TO MIAMI, PREFER TO USE HERBS AND HOME REMEDIES FOR HEALTH CONCERNS. PUERTO RICANS SHOW LEAST USE OF THE ORTHODOX HEALTH SYS-TEM. SOUTHERN BLACKS SHOW A BROAD RANGE OF TRADITIONAL HEALING SYSTEMS INCLUDING HOME REMEDIES, FAITH HEALERS, SPIRITUALISTS, AND "ROOT DOCTORS. DE-SCRIPTIONS OF HEALTH CARE PATTERNS RE-VEAL THAT WHILE THE FIVE ETHNIC GROUPS HAVE UNIQUE UTILIZATION PATTERNS FOR IN-DIGENOUS AND ORTHODOX HEALTH SYS-TEMS, ALL USE BOTH SYSTEMS CONCUR-RENTLY. THE SCIENTIFIC HEALTH CARE SYSTEM IS FOUND TO BE NOT SUFFICIENTLY RELEVANT TO MULTI-ETHNIC POPULATIONS IN URBAN U.S. AREAS, LEADING INVESTIGATORS TO SUG-GEST PRACTICAL MEASURES WHICH HEALTH

PERSONNEL MIGHT ADOPT: (1) INCREASING AWARENESS OF ETHNIC HEALTH BELIEFS AND (2) ACCOMMODATING TRADITIONAL HEALTH BELIEFS IN PRESCRIBED MEDICAL REGIMENS. 16 REFERENCES.

ACCN 001445

1678 AUTH **SCOTT, J. D., & PHELAN, J. G.**
TITL EXPECTANCIES OF UNEMPLOYABLE MALES RE-GARDING SOURCE OF CONTROL OF REIN-FORCEMENT.
SRCE *PSYCHOLOGICAL REPORTS, 1969, 25(3), 911-913.*
INDX MALE, ECONOMIC FACTORS, ATTITUDES, AN-OMIE, CROSS CULTURAL, MEXICAN AMERICAN, SES, ROTTER INTERNAL-EXTERNAL SCALE, EM-PIRICAL, ADULTS, EMPLOYMENT, WAIS, CALI-FORNIA, SOUTHWEST
ABST THE DEGREE OF EXPRESSED ATTITUDES OF ALIENATION AS AN EFFECT OF SUBJECTS HAV-ING BEEN UNEMPLOYED OVER LONG PERIODS OF TIME AND PRESUMABLY UNEMPLOYABLE IS EXPLORED. WHITE, MEXICAN AMERICAN, AND BLACK MALE GROUPS OF 60 SUBJECTS EACH (MATCHED FOR AGE, SOCIOECONOMIC STA-TUS AND SCHOLASTIC APTITUDE, AND CLASSI-FIED AS HARD CORE UNEMPLOYABLES) WERE TESTED ON THE ROTTER INTERNAL-EXTERNAL SCALE. THE RESULTS SHOW NO SIGNIFICANT DIFFERENCES IN ALIENATION SCORES BE-TWEEN THE WHITE UNEMPLOYABLE GROUP AND WHITE COLLEGE STUDENTS FROM A PRE-VIOUS STUDY. THE BLACK SUBJECTS WERE SIGNIFICANTLY MORE EXTERNALLY CON-TROLLED WITH GREATER VARIABILITY OF SCORES. THE MEXICAN AMERICAN GROUP SHOWED AN EVEN GREATER VARIABILITY THAN THE OTHERS. BLACKS AND MEXICAN AMERI-CANS DID NOT DIFFER SIGNIFICANTLY IN EXPRESSION OF EXTERNAL CONTROL. LACK OF FEELING FOR ANY RELATION BETWEEN IN-DIVIDUAL EFFORT AND REWARD MAY AC-COUNT FOR THE DIFFICULTY IN EQUIPPING THESE GROUPS WITH KNOWLEDGE AND SKILL TO IMPROVE THEIR LOT. 9 REFERENCES.

ACCN 001446

1679 AUTH **SCOTT, J., & GAITZ, C. M.**
TITL ETHNIC AND AGE DIFFERENCES IN MENTAL HEALTH MEASUREMENTS.
SRCE *DISEASES OF THE NERVOUS SYSTEM, 1975, 36(7), 389-393.*
INDX MENTAL HEALTH, GERONTOLOGY, ANXIETY, CROSS CULTURAL, CULTURAL FACTORS, SES, MEXICAN AMERICAN, DEPRESSION, ADULTS, EMPIRICAL, SYMPTOMATOLOGY, TEXAS, SOUTHWEST, URBAN
ABST A SURVEY OF 1,441 ADULTS IN HOUSTON IN-VESTIGATED THE INFLUENCE OF CHRONO-LOGICAL AGE AND ETHNICITY ON MENTAL HEALTH MEASURES. THE SAMPLE IS UNIQUE IN THAT THERE WAS AN ALMOST EQUAL REPRE-SENTATION OF SIX AGE GROUPS (20-29, 30-39, 40-54, 55-64, 65-74, 75-94), AND THREE ETHNIC GROUPS (BLACKS, ANGLOS, MEXICAN AMERI-CANS). THE SAMPLE ALSO INCLUDED EQUAL REPRESENTATION OF BOTH SEXES AND TWO SOCIOECONOMIC LEVELS. THE TWENTY-TWO ITEM SCREENING SCALE OF PSYCHIATRIC SYMPTOMS AND THE AFFECT BALANCE SCALE WERE USED AS MEASURES OF MENTAL HEALTH. THE ANALYSIS REVEALED AGE-RELATED AND ETHNIC-RELATED PATTERNS; EACH PATTERN, HOWEVER, WAS INDEPENDENT OF THE OTHER. THE AGE-RELATED PATTERN WAS THE SAME WITHIN THE THREE ETHNIC GROUPS, AND THE ETHNIC PATTERN WAS INDEPENDENT OF AGE. ANGLOS REPORTED SIGNIFICANTLY MORE PSYCHIATRIC SYMPTOMS, ESPECIALLY THOSE OF ONE FACTOR GROUPING NAMED "ANXIETY," AND THEY REPORTED MORE RECENT EXPERI-ENCES WITH BOTH POSITIVE AND NEGATIVE AFFECT THAN DID MEXICAN AMERICANS AND BLACKS. THE ELDERLY PERSONS "WELL ENOUGH" TO PARTICIPATE IN A LONG INTER-VIEW EXPRESSED NO SIGNIFICANT INCREASE IN SYMPTOMATOLOGY COMPARED WITH YOUNGER GROUPS, EXCEPT ON THE FACTOR OF DEPRESSION. THE OLDER GROUPS, COM-PARED WITH MIDDLE-AGED AND YOUNGER GROUPS, REPORTED LESS POSITIVE AND NEGATIVE AFFECT EXPRESSION. RESULTS ARE DISCUSSED IN TERMS OF THE POSSIBLE LIM-ITS OF THE TEST ITSELF AND THE PSYCHO-LOGICAL DIFFERENCES BETWEEN GROUPS. 13 REFERENCES. (AUTHOR SUMMARY MODIFIED)

ACCN 001447

1680 AUTH **SCOTT, N. R., ORZEN, W., MUSILLO, C., & COLE, P. T.**
TITL METHADONE IN THE SOUTHWEST: A THREE YEAR FOLLOW-UP OF CHICANO HEROIN AD-DICTS.
SRCE *AMERICAN JOURNAL OF ORTHOPSYCHIATRY, 1973, 43(3), 355-361.*
INDX METHADONE MAINTENANCE, MEXICAN AMERI-CAN, DRUG ADDICTION, ALCOHOLISM, PRO-GRAM EVALUATION, REHABILITATION, BEHAV-IOR MODIFICATION, PSYCHOSOCIAL ADJUST-MENT, EMPIRICAL, ADULTS, SOUTHWEST, NEW MEXICO
ABST A THREE-YEAR OUTCOME STUDY OF THE ORIGINAL 61 CHICANO PARTICIPANTS IN THE ALBUQUERQUE METHADONE MAINTENANCE PROGRAM IS PRESENTED. THIS STUDY CON-TRASTS WITH PREMETHADONE MEDICAL KNOWLEDGE OF NARCOTICS ADDICTION THAT CHARACTERISTICALLY PROVIDES LIMITED KNOWLEDGE OF PATHOGENESIS AND DOCU-MENTATION OF THE EFFECTS OF PSYCHO-THERAPY. DATA FROM THE FOLLOW-UP STUDY REVEALED THE FOLLOWING: (1) OVERALL HEALTH IMPROVEMENT AMONG THE PARTICI-PANTS; (2) ALCOHOLISM WAS CONSIDERED THE MAJOR HEALTH COMPLICATION; AND (3) MODEST EVIDENCE OF SOCIAL REHABILITA-TION. CHARACTERISTICS OF THE ADDICT POPULATION, INCLUDING ENVIRONMENTAL FACTORS ASSOCIATED WITH ADDICTION AND THE RELATIVE ABUNDANCE OF FAMILY RE-SOURCES, ARE ALSO DISCUSSED. 3 REFER-ENCES. (JOURNAL ABSTRACT MODIFIED)

ACCN 001448

1681 AUTH **SEAGOE, M. V.**

TITL CHILDREN'S PLAY IN THREE AMERICAN SUB-CULTURES.

SRCE *JOURNAL OF SCHOOL PSYCHOLOGY, 1971, 9(2), 167-172.*

INDX CHILDREN, CROSS CULTURAL, SOCIALIZATION, EMPIRICAL, MEXICAN AMERICAN, SEX COMPARISON, CULTURAL FACTORS, EDUCATION, MENTAL RETARDATION, CALIFORNIA, SOUTHWEST

ABST A STUDY WAS DESIGNED TO ANALYZE CHILDREN'S PLAY AS AN INDEX OF DEGREE OF SOCIALIZATION IN THREE ETHNIC GROUPS, INDEPENDENT SCHOOLS, AND SCHOOL PROGRAMS FOR EXCEPTIONAL CHILDREN. COMPARED WITH CAUCASIANS, MEXICAN AMERICAN AND NEGRO BOYS WERE SLIGHTLY LOWER, MEXICAN AMERICAN GIRLS EQUIVALENT, AND NEGRO GIRLS MARKEDLY LOWER IN LATE CHILDHOOD. INDEPENDENT SCHOOL COMPARISONS SHOWED SMALL DIFFERENCES BETWEEN PUBLIC AND PROTESTANT SCHOOLS, BUT MUCH GREATER EMPHASIS ON STRUCTURED PLAY IN CATHOLIC SCHOOLS. THERE WAS LITTLE DIFFERENCE BETWEEN NORMAL AND GIFTED, EDUCABLE MENTALLY RETARDED, AND LEARNING DISORDER GROUPS, BUT THE TRAINABLE MENTALLY RETARDED WERE MARKEDLY LOWER. 2 REFERENCES.

ACCN 001449

1682 AUTH **SEDA BONILLA, E.**

TITL PATRONES DE ACOMODO DEL EMIGRANTE PUERTORRIQUENO EN LA ESTRUCTURA SOCIAL NORTEAMERICANA. (PATTERNS OF ACCOMMODATION OF THE IMMIGRANT PUERTO RICAN IN THE AMERICAN SOCIAL STRUCTURE.)

SRCE *REVISTA DE CIENCIAS SOCIALES, 1958, 2, 189-200.*

INDX SES, ETHNIC IDENTITY, ACCULTURATION, PUERTO RICAN-M, MIGRATION, URBAN, RURAL, EMPIRICAL, PSYCHOSOCIAL ADJUSTMENT, STRESS, SOCIAL STRUCTURE, PREJUDICE, CROSS GENERATIONAL, NEW YORK, EAST

ABST PUERTO RICAN IMMIGRANTS TO THE UNITED STATES ARE CONFRONTED WITH A SYSTEM OF SOCIAL-RACIAL STRATIFICATION AND STATUS ASCRIPTION QUITE DIFFERENT FROM THAT IN LATIN AMERICA. IN LATIN AMERICA THE OFFSPRING OF RACIALLY MIXED MARRIAGES ASSUME A SOCIAL-RACIAL STATUS INTERMEDIATE TO THAT OF THE PARENTS; BUT IN THE U.S. THERE IS NO INTERMEDIATE RACIAL STATUS, AND SO SUCH OFFSPRING MUST EITHER "PASS" AS WHITE OR ELSE BE CLASSIFIED AS NEGRO. TO EXAMINE THE VARIOUS WAYS IMMIGRANTS ADAPT TO THIS SITUATION, AN UNSPECIFIED NUMBER OF PUERTO RICAN IMMIGRANTS WERE INTERVIEWED IN THREE NEIGHBORHOODS OF NEW YORK CITY. RESULTS DEMONSTRATE THAT ADAPTIVE STRATEGIES VARY ACCORDING TO THE RACE OF THE IMMIGRANTS. (1) PUERTO RICAN BLACKS ASSIMILATE READILY INTO AMERICAN NEGRO SOCIETY. (2) PUERTO RICANS OF MIXED RACIAL ANCESTRY, HOWEVER, EXPERIENCE A DROP IN STATUS FROM THAT WHICH THEY HELD IN PUERTO RICO. IN RESPONSE, THEY SEEK TO BE CONSPICUOUS AS A FOREIGN LANGUAGE GROUP RATHER THAN AS NEGROES. (3) LOWER CLASS WHITE PUERTO RICAN IMMIGRANTS SEEK RAPID ASSIMILATION BY ABANDONING THEIR PUERTO RICAN HERITAGE, IDENTIFYING THEIR FOREBEARERS AS "SPANISH," OFTEN ANGLICIZING THEIR NAMES, SPEAKING ONLY ENGLISH IN PUBLIC, AND EVEN DENYING ANY KNOWLEDGE OF THE SPANISH LANGUAGE. (4) IN CONTRAST, MIDDLE CLASS WHITE PUERTO RICANS ORGANIZE THEMSELVES INTO COHESIVE GROUPS, IDENTIFY AS PUERTO RICAN, AND TAKE PRIDE IN THEIR CULTURAL HERITAGE WHILE ALSO ACHIEVING EDUCATIONAL AND OCCUPATIONAL MOBILITY. 10 REFERENCES.

ACCN 001450

1683 AUTH **SENA-RIVERA, J.**

TITL CASA AND FAMILIA: AN ALTERNATIVE MODEL OF THE TRADITIONAL CHICANO EXTENDED FAMILY—A REPORT ON EXPLORATORY INVESTIGATION.

SRCE *PRESENTED AT THE ANNUAL MEETING OF THE AMERICAN SOCIOLOGICAL ASSOCIATION, GALVESTON, TEXAS, AUGUST 1976.*

INDX MEXICAN AMERICAN, EXTENDED FAMILY, EMPIRICAL, CULTURE, FAMILY STRUCTURE, MEXICAN, SES, DEMOGRAPHIC, AUTHORITARIANISM, CROSS GENERATIONAL, FAMILY ROLES, URBAN

ABST THE ISOLATED NUCLEAR PARSONIAN FAMILY MODEL VERSUS THE KIN-INTEGRATED LITWAK AND SUSSMAN FAMILY MODEL IS DISCUSSED. REVIEW OF THE LITERATURE ON THE MEXICAN DESCENT POPULATION IN THE U.S. REVEALS AN ISOLATED-NUCLEAR FAMILY MODEL, WITH THE EXTENDED FAMILY SYSTEM AMONG CHICANOS PERCEIVED AS EITHER A DISPLAY OF PASSING REMNANTS OF THE "CLASSICAL" EXTENDED FAMILY OR EVIDENCE OF LOWER SOCIOECONOMIC CLASS OR CULTURE OF POVERTY, AND AS DYSFUNCTIONAL IN AN URBAN INDUSTRIAL SOCIETY. IT IS ASSERTED THAT THE TRI-GENERATIONAL HOUSEHOLD HAS NEVER BEEN THE NORM FOR MEXICO OR FOR MEXICANS IN THE U.S. INSTEAD, WHAT IS NORMATIVE IS A SUBJECTIVELY COMPACT SOCIAL ORGANIZATIONAL UNIT CLUSTERING (FAMILIA) OF ESSENTIALLY INDEPENDENT NUCLEAR OR CONJUGAL HOUSEHOLDS (CASAS). CITED IS A 1970-72 STUDY OF AN URBAN SOUTHERN CALIFORNIA TOWN AND ITS SOCIAL ENVIRONS WHICH CONFIRMS THE KIN-INTEGRATED FAMILY. THE TRUE TRADITIONAL MEXICAN AND CHICANO EXTENDED FAMILY DOES NOT DEMONSTRATE A FACT OF DEVELOPMENT IN AN INDUSTRIAL SOCIETY, BUT RATHER A CULTURAL CONSTANT OF SEVERAL HUNDRED YEARS DURATION TRANSCENDING PRE-COLUMBIAN, SPANISH-COLONIAL, AND NATIONALISTIC URBAN-INDUSTRIAL SOCIETIES. 108 REFERENCES. (AUTHOR ABSTRACT MODIFIED)

ACCN 001452

1684 AUTH **SENIOR, C.**

TITL PUERTO RICANS: STRANGERS—THEN NEIGHBORS.

SRCE *CHICAGO: QUADRANGLE BOOKS, 1965.*

INDX PUERTO RICAN-M, RELIGION, IMMIGRATION,

POLICY, ATTITUDES, COMMUNITY INVOLVE-MENT, DEMOGRAPHIC, CROSS GENERA-TIONAL, CULTURAL FACTORS, CULTURAL CHANGE, REVIEW, URBAN, HISTORY, MIGRA-TION, DISCRIMINATION, STEREOTYPES, POV-ERTY, EMPLOYMENT, HOUSING, EDUCATION

ABST A DETAILED PORTRAYAL OF PUERTO RICANS (THEIR HISTORY, MIGRATION AND IMMIGRANT STATUS, EMPLOYMENT, HOUSING, RELIGION, ORGANIZATIONAL SYSTEMS, AND COMMUNITY DEVELOPMENT) IS PRESENTED. DEMO-GRAPHIC STATISTICS COMPARING FIRST AND SECOND GENERATION DIFFERENCES ARE DIS-CUSSED REGARDING EMPLOYMENT, ECO-NOMIC STATUS, MIGRATION, AND GROWTH PATTERNS. IMMIGRATION POLICY AND ITS TRENDS ARE DESCRIBED IN A HISTORICAL CONTEXT. VARIOUS ASPECTS OF DISCRIMINA-TION AND STEREOTYPES BY THE DOMINANT CULTURE INCLUDING THE POLICIES, ATTI-TUDES AND RELATIONS BETWEEN THE UNITED STATES AND PUERTO RICO ARE EXAMINED. IT IS THE INTENT OF THIS COMPREHENSIVE OV-ERVIEW TO PROVIDE INFORMATION WHICH MORE ACCURATELY DESCRIBES THE PUERTO RICAN IN THE UNITED STATES, SO THAT BET-TER RELATIONS BETWEEN THIS MINORITY AND THE DOMINANT CULTURE WILL BE ESTAB-LISHED. 188 REFERENCES.

ACCN 001451

1685 AUTH **SENOUR, M. N.**
TITL PSYCHOLOGY OF THE CHICANA.
SRCE *IN J. L. MARTINEZ (ED.), CHICANO PSY-CHOLOGY. NEW YORK: ACADEMIC PRESS, 1977, PP. 329-342.*
INDX MEXICAN AMERICAN, FEMALE, SEX ROLES, RE-VIEW, RESEARCH METHODOLOGY, STEREO-TYPES, CULTURAL FACTORS, ACCULTURATION, CROSS CULTURAL, SEX COMPARISON
ABST THIS REVIEW DESCRIBES THE TRADITIONAL ROLE OF THE MEXICAN AMERICAN WOMEN AS PORTRAYED IN THE AVAILABLE, ALBEIT LIM-ITED, LITERATURE. A COMPARISON IS MADE WITH FINDINGS ON THE PSYCHOLOGY OF AN-GLO FEMALES, AND THE INFLUENCES OF BI-OLOGY AND THE ACCULTURATION PROCESS ARE EXAMINED. STUDIES INDICATE THAT CHI-CANAS, COMPARED TO MEXICAN AMERICAN MALES, EXHIBIT LOWER SELF-ESTEEM, MORE FIELD DEPENDENCE, MORE CONCERN FOR AND AWARENESS OF THEIR PHYSICAL SELVES, LESS WELL-DEFINED PSYCHIC SELVES, AND MORE DEPRESSION. THEY APPEAR TO BE MORE PROSOCIAL AND LESS COMPETITIVE THAN MALES AND HAVE A LOWER LEVEL OF SCHO-LASTIC ACHIEVEMENT. HOWEVER, THEY SEEM TO BE MORE RESPONSIVE TO POSITIVE ACA-DEMIC INTERVENTION, AND THEY EXHIBIT GREATER ENHANCEMENT OF SELF-IMAGE AS A RESULT OF BILINGUAL-BICULTURAL EDUCA-TIONAL PROGRAMS. RECENT STUDIES ON SEX ROLES AND ETHNICITY REVEAL THAT CHI-CANAS ARE MORE SEX-TYPED IN THEIR RE-SPONSES THAN ANGLO WOMEN. COMPARED TO ANGLOS AND BLACKS, CHICANOS OF BOTH SEXES DEMONSTRATE THE GREATEST TEN-DENCY TO ENDORSE FEMININE ITEMS OVER

MASCULINE ONES. IN CONCLUSION, IT IS CAU-TIONED THAT THIS PROFILE OF THE CHICANA CANNOT BE ACCEPTED AT FACE VALUE BE-CAUSE OF VARIOUS WEAKNESSES IN THE RE-SEARCH WHICH HAS BEEN CONDUCTED: (1) DATA ARE INSUFFICIENT; (2) FINDINGS ARE CONTRADICTORY; (3) ANGLOCENTRIC TEST BIAS; (4) USE OF FREUDIAN ANALYSIS; (5) AN ABSENCE OF EMPIRICAL DATA IN MUCH OF THE DESCRIPTION OF SEX ROLES; AND (6) THE LACK OF RESEARCH CONDUCTED BY CHI-CANA INVESTIGATORS. DUE TO SUCH PROB-LEMS AND, IN PARTICULAR, THE DYNAMICS OF RECENT CULTURE CHANGE, FURTHER RE-SEARCH ON THE EMERGING CHICANA IS NEEDED. 52 REFERENCES.

ACCN 001453

1686 AUTH **SENTER, D.**
TITL ACCULTURATION AMONG NEW MEXICAN VIL-LAGERS IN COMPARISON TO ADJUSTMENT PATTERNS OF OTHER SPANISH-SPEAKING AMERICANS.
SRCE *RURAL SOCIOLOGY, 1945, 10(1), 31-47.*
INDX ACCULTURATION, MEXICAN AMERICAN, PSY-CHOSOCIAL ADJUSTMENT, STRESS, HISTORY, SOCIAL STRUCTURE, SES, NEW MEXICO, SOUTHWEST, CALIFORNIA
ABST A COMPARISON OF ACCULTURATION AND AD-JUSTMENT PATTERNS AMONG THREE GROUPS OF SPANISH-SPEAKING AMERICANS IS PRE-SENTED. IT IS SHOWN THAT MINORITY GROUPS FACE THREE POSSIBILITIES OF ADJUSTMENT: (1) THEY MAY ATTEMPT TO MAINTAIN THEIR ORIGINAL CULTURE; (2) THEY MAY ATTEMPT QUICK ACCEPTANCE OF THE NEW CULTURE, THUS LEADING TO EVENTUAL ASSIMILATION, ALTHOUGH THE PATH WILL BE ROUGHENED BY PREJUDICE; OR (3) THEY MAY DEVELOP SOME-THING FOREIGN TO BOTH THEIR ANCESTRAL CULTURE AND THAT OF THE PRESENT MA-JORITY GROUP. ALL THREE OF THESE POSSI-BILITIES HAVE BEEN TRIED OUT BY DIFFERENT GROUPS OF SPANISH-SPEAKING PEOPLES WITHIN THE UNITED STATES. THE "MANITOS," OR SPANISH AMERICANS OF NEW MEXICO, DI-VIDE THEMSELVES BETWEEN THE FIRST AND SECOND POSSIBILITY. THE BORDER MEXICANS CONTENT THEMSELVES WITH THE FIRST POS-SIBILITY, WHILE THE "POCHOS" OF SOUTHERN CALIFORNIA ATTEMPT SOMETHING OF ALL THREE. THE DEVELOPMENT OF THE LAWLESS ZOOT SUIT PACHUCO GANGS AMONG THE YOUNG PEOPLE OF THE LOS ANGELES AREA IS PERHAPS THE MOST EXTREME EXAMPLE OF GROUP REFUSAL TO ACCEPT A MINORITY PO-SITION IN THIS COUNTRY. IF WE CONTRAST THE THREE PEOPLES, IT BECOMES APPARENT THAT EVEN THOUGH THE MANITOS ARE SUB-JECT TO SEVERE STRESS IN THE ACCULTURA-TION PROCESS, THE OTHER TWO GROUPS ARE AT EVEN GREATER IMMEDIATE OR EVENTUAL DISADVANTAGE. THIS GRADIENT OF STRESS IS A MAJOR DETERMINANT IN SELECTION OF AD-JUSTMENT MECHANISMS, EVEN THOUGH THE PROCESS OF SELECTION MAY BE UNCON-SCIOUS. 10 REFERENCES. (AUTHOR ABSTRACT MODIFIED)

ACCN   001454

1687 AUTH   **SENTER, D.**
TITL   WITCHES AND PSYCHIATRISTS.
SRCE   *PSYCHIATRY, 1947, 10(1), 49-56.*
INDX   FOLK MEDICINE, MENTAL HEALTH PROFESSION, HEALTH, ESSAY, PSYCHOTHERAPY, CURANDERISMO, MEXICAN AMERICAN, ATTITUDES, DISEASE, CROSS CULTURAL, HEALTH DELIVERY SYSTEMS, NEW MEXICO, SOUTHWEST

ABST   IN THIS EXAMINATION OF WITCHES AND PSYCHIATRISTS IN NEW MEXICO, IT IS NOTED THAT SEVENTEENTH CENTURY WITCHCRAFT HAS BEEN A BASIS FOR CONSTANT ANXIETY AMONG SPANISH AMERICAN (SA) VILLAGERS IN NEW MEXICO. CASE DESCRIPTIONS EXHIBIT THE NATURE OF WITCHCRAFT PRACTICES AND THE ROLE OF THE CURANDERO. THE THEORY OF DISEASE, ACCORDING TO BOTH SA'S AND PUEBLO INDIANS, IS BASED ON THE CONCEPT OF FOREIGN MATERIAL ENTERING THE BODY OF THE VICTIM. THE DISEASE IS CAUSED BY SOMETHING BEING POINTED AT THE VICTIM, AS A RESULT OF WHICH IT OR ANOTHER OBJECT ENTERS HIS BODY; OR HE EATS FOOD MADE DANGEROUS BY HAIR OR SPELLS; OR A DOLL REPRESENTING HIM IS PUNCHED WITH PINS. DISCUSSIONS OF THE VARIOUS PRESCRIPTIONS FOR TREATMENT ARE PRESENTED. THE PRESENT CLASH OF ANGLO AND SA CULTURE IS DISRUPTING THE FOUNDATIONS OF THE OLD NATIVE SYSTEM. SOME CURANDEROS HAVE MADE EFFORTS TO MODERNIZE SOME OF THEIR TREATMENTS AND HAVE COOPERATED IN PUBLIC HEALTH PROJECTS BY ADVISING THEIR CLIENTELE TO JOIN THE ORGANIZATION AND SUBMIT THEIR AILMENTS TO THE NEW THERAPY.
ACCN   001455

1688 AUTH   **SENTER, D., & HAWLEY, F.**
TITL   THE GRAMMAR SCHOOL AS THE BASIC ACCULTURATING INFLUENCE FOR NATIVE NEW MEXICANS.
SRCE   *SOCIAL FORCES, 1945-46, 24(4), 398-407.*
INDX   ACCULTURATION, EDUCATIONAL ASSESSMENT, ENVIRONMENTAL FACTORS, ESSAY, CHILDREN, SPANISH SURNAMED, CULTURE, EDUCATION, MEXICAN AMERICAN, CULTURAL FACTORS, NEW MEXICO, SOUTHWEST

ABST   AN ANALYSIS OF THE EDUCATIONAL AND SOCIAL PROBLEMS OF THE NEW MEXICAN IS PRESENTED. IMPOVERISHED AND SUFFERING FROM POOR HEALTH, NEW MEXICANS CANNOT MOVE OUT INTO SUCCESSFUL PARTICIPATION IN THE SOCIAL AND COMMERCIAL WORLD OF THE DOMINANT ANGLO CULTURE BECAUSE THEIR CULTURAL CHARACTERISTICS ARE TOO DIFFERENT. EXCEPT IN INDIVIDUAL INSTANCES, THE NEW MEXICAN PEOPLE DO NOT UNDERSTAND ANGLO CULTURE SUFFICIENTLY WELL TO ADAPT SUCCESSFULLY TO IT. AS ONE OF THE MOST PRACTICAL SOLUTIONS TO THE ACCULTURATION PROBLEM, THE GRAMMAR SCHOOL, WHICH COULD COORDINATE THE CUSTOMARY STUDIES WITH A PLAN FOR TEACHING SOCIAL ORIENTATION AND IMPROVED HEALTH WITHIN THE VILLAGES, IS PROPOSED AS OFFERING THE NECESSARY BACKGROUND FOR MOVEMENT TOWARD GENERAL REHABILITATION AND PROSPERITY. THIS PLAN SHOULD AID STUDENTS IN MAKING THE ACCULTURATION PROCESS QUICKER AND LESS OF A PSYCHOLOGICAL STRAIN THAN IT IS AT PRESENT. THE INSTRUCTOR SHOULD BE A SPANISH AMERICAN WHO, WHILE RETAINING RAPPORT WITH THE VILLAGERS, WOULD REPRESENT THE SUCCESSFUL ANGLICIZATION OF THE PRESENT AND FUTURE GENERATIONS. 16 REFERENCES.
ACCN   001456

1689 AUTH   **SERENO, R.**
TITL   BORICUA: A STUDY OF LANGUAGE, TRANSCULTURATION AND POLITICS.
SRCE   *PSYCHIATRY, 1949, 12(2), 167-184.*
INDX   CULTURE, ACCULTURATION, PUERTO RICAN-I, HISTORY, POLITICS, LINGUISTICS, ESSAY, CULTURAL CHANGE, CULTURAL FACTORS, PSYCHOSOCIAL ADJUSTMENT

ABST   THE PASSAGE OF INDIVIDUALS FROM ONE CULTURE TO ANOTHER IS HERE CALLED TRANSCULTURATION. TO THE EXTENT THAT CULTURE CAN BE IDENTIFIED WITH LANGUAGE, A CHANGE IN CULTURE IS A POLITICAL CHANGE AFFECTING LANGUAGE AND SPEECH HABITS. ASSUMING LANGUAGE TO BE THE MOST IMPORTANT INSTRUMENTALITY OF THE PROCESS OF PERSONAL INTEGRATION, AN EXAMINATION IS MADE OF THE VICISSITUDES OF THE LANGUAGE SPOKEN IN PUERTO RICO AND THE MANNER IN WHICH THE PASSAGE FROM SPANISH TO AMERICAN SOVEREIGNTY AFFECTS PERSONAL INTEGRATION AND PERSONAL SECURITY. THE STUDY INDICATES THAT BY ANALYZING THE RELATIONSHIP BETWEEN LANGUAGE, TRANSCULTURATION, AND POLITICS IT IS POSSIBLE TO SHOW BOTH THE FARREACHING, NONCALCULATED EFFECTS OF SHIFTS IN POWER AND THE NONCALCULATED RESULTS OF POLITICAL PLANNING. 36 REFERENCES.
ACCN   001457

1690 AUTH   **SERENO, R.**
TITL   CRYPTOMELANISM: A STUDY OF COLOR RELATIONS AND PERSONAL INSECURITY IN PUERTO RICO.
SRCE   *PSYCHIATRY, 1947, 10(3), 261-269.*
INDX   SELF CONCEPT, PUERTO RICAN-I, EMPIRICAL, ADULTS, DISCRIMINATION, SES, ATTITUDES, PREJUDICE, VETERANS

ABST   TO STUDY THE RELATIONSHIP BETWEEN RACIAL COLOR PROBLEMS AND PERSONAL INSECURITY IN PUERTO RICO, A GROUP OF 160 VETERANS WAS DIVIDED INTO GROUPS TO DISCUSS SOCIAL PROBLEMS. ALL THE SUBJECTS EXPERIENCED DISCRIMINATION WHILE IN THE ARMY AND HAD BEEN CONSTANTLY UPBRAIDED FOR THEIR LACK OF FLUENCY IN ENGLISH OR THEIR IGNORANCE OF AMERICAN WAYS. THE NON-NEGRO (NN) PUERTO RICANS WERE AWARE OF THE RACIAL DISCRIMINATION THAT PUERTO RICANS OF OBVIOUS NEGROID TRAITS WERE SUBJECTED TO. THE AMERICAN PATTERN OF DISCRIMINATION AND SEGREGA-

TION AROUSED DOUBTS AMONG THE NN PUERTO RICANS OF THEIR COLOR ANCESTRY AND PERSONAL SECURITY. AS A REACTION TO THIS SYSTEM NN PUERTO RICANS ORGANIZED A FRATERNITY WHICH, BOUND TOGETHER BY A COMMON FEELING OF PERSONAL INSECURITY, DISCRIMINATED AGAINST THEIR FELLOW NEGRO PUERTO RICANS. THE RESISTANCE TO RACIAL ANCESTRY SEEMS TO BE AN UPPER- AND MIDDLE-CLASS PHENOMENON. LOW-INCOME PEOPLE SHOW NO EVIDENCE OF EXTREME OR PATHOLOGICAL CONSEQUENCES OF CONCEALMENT OF COLOR. A MEMBER OF THE MIDDLE-CLASS IS NOT ONLY NEWLY RICH BUT NEWLY WHITE. THIS IS THE GROUP THAT DEMONSTRATES THE MOST HOSTILITY TO NEGRO PUERTO RICANS. THE IMPACT OF AMERICAN CULTURE FORCES THE PUERTO RICAN COLOR PROBLEM INTO A MORE RIGID AND INTOLERABLE STATE OF RACIAL DISCRIMINATION AMONG NN PUERTO RICANS AND NEGRO PUERTO RICANS. 11 REFERENCES.

ACCN   001458

1691 AUTH   **SERRANO, A. C., & GIBSON, G.**
TITL   MENTAL HEALTH SERVICES TO THE MEXICAN AMERICAN COMMUNITY IN SAN ANTONIO, TEXAS.
SRCE   *AMERICAN JOURNAL OF PUBLIC HEALTH, 1973, 63(12), 1055-1057.*
INDX   MENTAL HEALTH, HEALTH DELIVERY SYSTEMS, MEXICAN AMERICAN, CULTURAL FACTORS, PSYCHOTHERAPY, PARAPROFESSIONALS, CASE STUDY, COMMUNITY
ABST   IMPROVED MENTAL HEALTH SERVICES FOR MEXICAN AMERICANS AS THE RESULT OF CHANGES IN PHILOSOPHY AND PERSONNEL IN A BEXAR COUNTY, TEXAS, OUTPATIENT FACILITY ARE DESCRIBED. INCREASED EFFORTS WERE MADE TO DISCOVER HOW TO (1) BEST MEET THE GROWING DEMAND FOR MENTAL HEALTH SERVICES, (2) MAKE SERVICES MORE RELEVANT TO THE ENTIRE COMMUNITY, INCLUDING LOWER SOCIOECONOMIC AND MINORITY FAMILIES, AND (3) PROVIDE MORE COMPREHENSIVE SERVICES. WAITING LISTS FOR EVALUATION AND TREATMENT WERE ELIMINATED THROUGH A FAMILY-CENTERED ORIENTATION PROGRAM EMPHASIZING BRIEF THERAPIES, CRISIS INTERVENTION, GROUP AND FAMILY TECHNIQUES, AND BEHAVIOR THERAPIES. MENTAL HEALTH SERVICES ARE COORDINATED THROUGH HOSPITAL AND PUBLIC AGENCIES, RELIGIOUS ORGANIZATIONS, AND VOLUNTEER PROGRAMS. BARRIO RESIDENT FIELD WORKERS ARE USED TO PROVIDE MORE OPEN, FLEXIBLE, AND REALISTIC COMMUNICATION AND NEGOTIATION TO CLOSE THE GAP BETWEEN EXISTING ESTABLISHMENTS AND THE CHICANO COMMUNITY. IT IS PROPOSED THAT THE BEST ROLE FOR THE MENTAL HEALTH PROFESSIONAL IS THAT OF A CONSULTANT AND A FACILITATOR, WITH THE ROLE OF DIRECT THERAPIST BEING GRADUALLY DECREASED. 6 REFERENCES. (NCMHI ABSTRACT MODIFIED)
ACCN   001459

1692 AUTH   **SERRANO, J.**
TITL   CULTURE, MENTAL HEALTH AND MEXICAN AMERICANS.
SRCE   *UNPUBLISHED MANUSCRIPT, UNIVERSITY OF SOUTHERN CALIFORNIA, MAY 20, 1970.*
INDX   MENTAL HEALTH, HEALTH DELIVERY SYSTEMS, MEXICAN AMERICAN, CULTURE, STEREOTYPES, PARAPROFESSIONALS, REVIEW, CULTURAL FACTORS, POVERTY, PSYCHOTHERAPY, ATTITUDES, FATALISM
ABST   DISTORTIONS, GENERALIZATIONS, AND MISINTERPRETATIONS OF MEXICAN AMERICANS AND MEXICAN AMERICAN CULTURE ARE DISCUSSED AS OBSTACLES TO SUCCESSFUL PSYCHOTHERAPY OF MEXICAN AMERICAN PATIENTS. A REVIEW OF THE LITERATURE ON MEXICAN AMERICANS DESCRIBES ATTITUDES ASSOCIATED WITH MEXICAN AMERICANS AND THE CULTURE OF POVERTY, SUCH AS ORIENTATION TO THE PRESENT, PASSIVITY, AND CYNICISM. IT IS MAINTAINED THAT OVEREMPHASIS ON CULTURAL FACTORS AND DIFFERENCES MAY MINIMIZE PSYCHOTHERAPEUTIC TREATMENT AND DIAGNOSIS OF MEXICAN AMERICAN PATIENTS. 11 REFERENCES.
ACCN   001460

1693 AUTH   **SHANKMAN, A.**
TITL   THE IMAGE OF MEXICO AND THE MEXICAN AMERICAN IN THE BLACK PRESS, 1890-1935.
SRCE   *THE JOURNAL OF ETHNIC STUDIES, 1975, 3(2), 43-56.*
INDX   MEXICO, MEXICAN AMERICAN, IMMIGRATION, MASS MEDIA, ATTITUDES, STEREOTYPES, PREJUDICE, CROSS CULTURAL, LABOR FORCE
ABST   PERCEPTIONS OF MEXICO AND MEXICAN AMERICANS BY THE BLACK COMMUNITY FROM 1890 TO 1935 ARE PRESENTED. ALTHOUGH MEXICO WAS GENERALLY PERCEIVED AS FAVORABLE TOWARDS BLACKS, THESE PERCEPTIONS BEGAN TO CHANGE IN THE EARLY 20TH CENTURY. FROM 1910-1935, THE BLACK PRESS VIEWED MEXICANS AS A BACKWARD AND IGNORANT PEOPLE. MEXICAN IMMIGRANTS AND MEXICAN AMERICANS WERE PERCEIVED AS A THREAT IN TERMS OF LABOR COMPETITION, AND THE FACT THAT MEXICANS IN THE U.S. WERE RACIALLY CLASSIFIED AS "WHITE" AND EXEMPT FROM JIM CROW LEGISLATION ALSO CAUSED JEALOUSY. THIS PERIOD FINDS BLACKS AND MEXICANS AS RIVALS IN A CHEAP LABOR MARKET AND UNSUPPORTIVE OF EACH OTHER IN THE STRUGGLE TOWARDS EQUAL OPPORTUNITY. 80 REFERENCES.
ACCN   001461

1694 AUTH   **SHANNON, L.**
TITL   AGE CHANGE IN TIME PERCEPTION IN NATIVE AMERICANS, MEXICAN AMERICANS, AND ANGLO AMERICANS.
SRCE   *JOURNAL OF CROSS CULTURAL PSYCHOLOGY, 1976, 7(1), 117-122.*
INDX   MEXICAN AMERICAN, CROSS CULTURAL, TIME ORIENTATION, ADOLESCENTS, CHILDREN, COGNITIVE DEVELOPMENT, ACHIEVEMENT MOTIVATION, CULTURAL FACTORS, MALE
ABST   TO ASSESS THE EFFECTS OF ETHNICITY AND AGE ON TIME PERCEPTION, NATIVE AMERICAN,

MEXICAN AMERICAN, AND ANGLO AMERICAN SUBJECTS (60 BOYS AGE 10 TO 12 AND 60 BOYS AGE 14 TO 17) ESTIMATED EQUAL INTERVALS OF IDLE TIME AND TIME SPENT WORKING AT MEANINGFUL TASKS. YOUNGER ANGLO AMERICANS AND ALL OLDER GROUPS PERCEIVED IDLE TIME AS LONGER. YOUNGER MINORITY CULTURE GROUPS PERCEIVED NO DIFFERENCE IN THE TWO TIMES. THESE FINDINGS SUGGEST A PERCEPTION OF IDLE TIME AS WASTED AND THUS APPEARING LONG AS CONTRASTED WITH THE PERCEPTION OF TIME SPENT ACHIEVING. IT IS PROPOSED THAT CULTURAL DIFFERENCES EXIST IN THE STRENGTH OF THE TENDENCY TO VIEW ACHIEVEMENT AS OCCURRING IN SEQUENCES OF TIME. THE TEMPORAL PROBLEMS OF MINORITY CULTURES IN MAJORITY CULTURE SCHOOLS ARE RELATED TO THIS ASPECT ON TIME. 14 REFERENCES. (NCMHI ABSTRACT MODIFIED)

ACCN   001462

1695 AUTH   **SHANNON, L.**
TITL   DEVELOPMENT OF TIME PERSPECTIVE IN THREE CULTURAL GROUPS: A CULTURAL DIFFERENCE OR AN EXPECTANCY INTERPRETATION.
SRCE   *DEVELOPMENTAL PSYCHOLOGY, 1975, 11(1), 114-115.*
INDX   CROSS CULTURAL, TIME ORIENTATION, CULTURAL FACTORS, MALE, SES, INDIGENOUS POPULATIONS, MEXICAN AMERICAN, ADOLESCENTS, CHILDREN, COGNITIVE DEVELOPMENT
ABST   AN EXPERIMENT WAS CONDUCTED TO PROVIDE INSIGHT INTO THE DEVELOPMENT OF TEMPORAL PERSPECTIVES IN DISADVANTAGED SUBCULTURES IN COMPARISON TO THE MAJORITY CULTURE AND TO DETERMINE THE COGNITIVE STRUCTURES UNDERLYING THOSE PERSPECTIVES. THE SUBJECTS WERE 120 MALES, COMPRISED OF 20 ANGLO AMERICANS, INDIAN AMERICANS, AND MEXICAN AMERICANS FROM EACH OF TWO AGE GROUPS: AGES 10 TO 12 AND 14 TO 17 YEARS. THE MEASURE OF TIME PERSPECTIVE WAS THE "LINES TEST," IN WHICH SUBJECTS INDICATED THEIR PERSPECTIVE OF THE PAST, PRESENT, AND FUTURE BY MARKING OFF SEGMENTS OF A 100 MILLIMETER LINEAR REPRESENTATION OF THE LIFE SPACE. RESULTS REVEALED SIGNIFICANT MAIN EFFECTS FOR CULTURAL GROUP, AGE LEVEL, AND GROUP X AGE. ANGLO AMERICANS DEPICTED MORE EXTENDED FUTURES AND SHORTER PRESENTS THAN DID INDIAN AMERICANS AND MEXICAN AMERICANS. THUS, DESPITE CONSIDERABLE EXPOSURE TO MIDDLE-CLASS ATTITUDES TOWARD TIME, INDIAN AMERICAN AND MEXICAN AMERICAN ADOLESCENTS RETAIN AN AWARENESS THAT MEMBERS OF DISADVANTAGED SUBCULTURES ARE NOT LIKELY TO REALIZE SUBSTANTIAL REWARD IN THE FUTURE. THIS LATTER ATTITUDE CONFLICTS WITH THE MORE AFFLUENT MAJORITY CULTURE NORMS OF FUTURE ORIENTATION. 2 REFERENCES. (PASAR ABSTRACT)
ACCN   001463

1696 AUTH   **SHANNON, L. W.**
TITL   THE ECONOMIC ABSORPTION AND CULTURAL

INTEGRATION OF IMMIGRANT WORKERS: CHARACTERISTICS OF THE INDIVIDUAL VERSUS THE NATURE OF THE SYSTEM.
SRCE   *IN E. B. BRODY (ED.), BEHAVIOR IN NEW ENVIRONMENTS: ADAPTATION OF MIGRANT POPULATIONS. BEVERLY HILLS: SAGE PUBLICATIONS, 1970, PP. 167-185.*
INDX   ECONOMIC FACTORS, INTEGRATION, IMMIGRATION, COMMUNITY, SOCIAL MOBILITY, CROSS GENERATIONAL, RELIGION, CULTURAL FACTORS, OCCUPATIONAL ASPIRATIONS, SCHOLASTIC ASPIRATIONS, EMPIRICAL, CROSS CULTURAL, MEXICAN AMERICAN, ACCULTURATION
ABST   AN INVESTIGATION WAS MADE OF HOW PARTICIPATION IN OR IDENTIFICATION WITH PARAMETERS OF DIFFERENT SUBCULTURES INFLUENCES THE RATE OF ECONOMIC ABSORPTION AND CULTURAL INTEGRATION OF IMMIGRANTS. ANALYSIS OF DATA SHOWS THAT, ALTHOUGH INCOME AND OTHER CHARACTERISTICS OF THE IMMIGRANTS AND LONG-TIME RESIDENTS ARE RELATED TO WORLD VIEW, MORE VARIATION IS EXPLAINED BY RACE AND ETHNICITY THAN BY ANY OTHER VARIABLES. FURTHER ANALYSIS INDICATES THAT ANGLO PROTESTANT MALES ARE AT THE EXTREME ACTIVE END OF THE WORLD VIEW SCALE, WHILE MEXICAN AMERICAN CATHOLIC AND PROTESTANT FEMALES ARE AT THE PASSIVE END OF THE SCALE. WORLD VIEW IS FOUND TO CORRELATE SIGNIFICANTLY WITH THREE OF THE FOUR VARIABLES FOR ONE GROUP ONLY—THE MEXICAN AMERICAN CATHOLIC MALES. THE CORRELATIONS OF THE GREATEST MAGNITUDE ARE FOR ANGLO CATHOLIC AND NEGRO PROTESTANT FEMALES. THUS, WITH CONTROLS FOR RACE AND ETHNICITY, RELIGION, AND SEX, THE HYPOTHESIS THAT THE HIGHEST CORRELATIONS BETWEEN WORLD VIEW AND OTHER VARIABLES WOULD BE IN THE ANGLO GROUP AND THE LOWEST CORRELATIONS IN THE MEXICAN AMERICAN GROUP MUST BE REJECTED. THE GENERAL IDEA OF SUBCULTURES BEING REPRESENTED BY DIFFERENCES IN THE INTERRELATIONSHIP OF VARIABLES IS NOT REJECTED, ALTHOUGH THE SPECIFIC PATTERN OF DIFFERENCES HYPOTHESIZED FOR THE GROUPS OBSERVED WAS NOT PRESENT.
ACCN   001464

1697 AUTH   **SHANNON, L. W.**
TITL   FALSE ASSUMPTIONS ABOUT THE DETERMINANTS OF MEXICAN AMERICAN AND NEGRO ECONOMIC ABSORPTION.
SRCE   *THE SOCIOLOGICAL QUARTERLY, 1975, 16(1), 3-15.*
INDX   MEXICAN AMERICAN, CROSS CULTURAL, ECONOMIC FACTORS, SES, MIGRATION, SOCIAL MOBILITY, ADULTS, DEMOGRAPHIC, EMPLOYMENT, URBAN, EMPIRICAL, WISCONSIN, MIDWEST
ABST   ACCULTURATION CHANGES IN RURAL-REARED AND URBAN-REARED MINORITIES WERE EXAMINED IN A LONGITUDINAL STUDY OF 973 FAMILIES IN RACINE, WISCONSIN. INTERVIEWS WERE CONDUCTED WITH 280 MEXICAN AMERICAN, 280 NEGROES, AND 413 ANGLOS IN 1960.

THE FOLLOW-UP SAMPLE IN 1971 CONTAINED 75% OF THE ORIGINAL SAMPLE. ADDITIONAL DATA FROM 20% OF THE BALANCE OF THE ORIGINAL RESPONDENTS WERE OBTAINED FROM RELATIVES AND OTHER SOURCES. LITTLE SIGNIFICANT CHANGE (1960-1971) IN THE RELATIVE POSITION OF MEXICAN AMERICANS AND BLACKS WAS FOUND ON OCCUPATIONAL LEVEL, INCOME AND LEVEL OF LIVING, EVEN THOUGH CONTROLS FOR AGE, EDUCATION, URBAN WORK EXPERIENCE, TIME IN THE COMMUNITY, AND OTHER PERTINENT VARIABLES WERE INTRODUCED. ALTHOUGH NUMEROUS PROGRAMS WERE INTRODUCED DURING THE 1960'S WITH THE PURPOSE OF AIDING THE LESS FORTUNATE IN SOCIETY, THESE FINDINGS SUGGEST THAT THE COMMUNITY IS ORGANIZED TO FACILITATE THE ECONOMIC ABSORPTION OF ANGLO IMMIGRANTS. IN VIEW OF THESE FINDINGS, RACE/ETHNICITY REMAINS THE MOST POWERFUL DETERMINANT OF A FAMILY'S POSITION IN THE COMMUNITY. 12 REFERENCES. (AUTHOR ABSTRACT MODIFIED)

ACCN   001465

1698 AUTH   **SHANNON, L. W., & KRASS, E.**
TITL   THE URBAN ADJUSTMENT OF IMMIGRANTS: THE RELATIONSHIP OF EDUCATION TO OCCUPATION AND TOTAL FAMILY INCOME.
SRCE   *PACIFIC SOCIOLOGICAL REVIEW, 1963, 6(1), 37-42.*
INDX   URBAN, IMMIGRATION, SCHOLASTIC ACHIEVEMENT, OCCUPATIONAL ASPIRATIONS, SES, MEXICAN AMERICAN, FAMILY STRUCTURE
ABST   THIS 1960 SURVEY OF 284 ANGLO, 236 MEXICAN AMERICAN, AND 280 BLACK HOUSEHOLD HEADS IN A NORTHERN INDUSTRIAL COMMUNITY CHALLENGES THE CONCEPT THAT EDUCATION IS A GREAT ECONOMIC EQUALIZER. THE STUDY EXPLICITLY GUARDED AGAINST LINKING EDUCATION AND ECONOMIC SUCCESS BY CONTROLLING FOR RACE, ETHNICITY AND LENGTH OF RESIDENCY IN THE COMMUNITY. FOR RECENT IMMIGRANTS WITH LIMITED EDUCATION, FEW ETHNIC DIFFERENCES WERE FOUND. BUT, BEYOND 7 YEARS OF EDUCATION AND 9 YEARS OF RESIDENCY, ANGLOS CONSISTENTLY HAD HIGHER TOTAL FAMILY INCOME AND OCCUPATIONAL LEVELS THAN MEXICAN AMERICANS AND BLACKS, REGARDLESS OF ANY OTHER CONTROLS THAT WERE INTRODUCED. THE REPORT CONCLUDES THAT HIGHER LEVELS OF EDUCATION AND LONGER PERIODS OF TIME IN THE URBAN, INDUSTRIAL COMMUNITY ARE ASSOCIATED WITH HIGHER OCCUPATIONAL LEVELS AND HIGHER INCOMES FOR ANGLOS BUT NOT NECESSARILY FOR BLACKS OR MEXICAN AMERICANS. 10 REFERENCES.

ACCN   001466

1699 AUTH   **SHANNON, L. W., & MORGAN, P.**
TITL   THE PREDICTION OF ECONOMIC ABSORPTION AND CULTURAL INTEGRATION AMONG MEXICAN AMERICANS, NEGROES, AND ANGLOS IN A NORTHERN INDUSTRIAL COMMUNITY.
SRCE   *HUMAN ORGANIZATION, 1966, 25(2), 154-162.*

INDX   ECONOMIC FACTORS, CULTURAL FACTORS, INTEGRATION, MEXICAN AMERICAN, CROSS CULTURAL, COMMUNITY, SES, SCHOLASTIC ACHIEVEMENT, ACCULTURATION, EMPIRICAL, ADULTS, MIGRATION, OCCUPATIONAL ASPIRATIONS, EMPLOYMENT, SOCIAL MOBILITY, SCHOLASTIC ASPIRATIONS
ABST   THE ANTECEDENT SOCIOLOGICAL AND INTERVENING SOCIAL-PSYCHOLOGICAL FACTORS WHICH FACILITATE ECONOMIC ABSORPTION AND CULTURAL INTEGRATION ARE EXAMINED. THE SAMPLE CONSISTED OF 284 ANGLOS, 236 MEXICAN AMERICANS, AND 280 NEGROES. MEXICAN AMERICANS ARE THE MOST HANDICAPPED IN TERMS OF OCCUPATIONAL STATUS, FAMILY INCOME, AND EDUCATION, WHILE ANGLOS ARE THE LEAST, WITH NEGROES IN THE MIDDLE. WHEN THE COMBINED SAMPLES OF SUBJECTS ARE EXAMINED WITHOUT HOLDING ETHNICITY OR RACE CONSTANT, A RELATIVELY HIGH CORRELATION BETWEEN MEASURES OF ECONOMIC ABSORPTION AND CULTURAL INTEGRATION AND THEIR PREDICTIVE SET OF SCALE SCORES IS FOUND. IT IS DISCLOSED THAT ON EACH OF THE VARIABLES RELATED GENERALLY TO WORK EXPERIENCE, EDUCATION, OCCUPATIONAL STATUS, WORLD VIEW, PATTERN OF SOCIAL PARTICIPATION, AND LEVEL OF ASPIRATION, ANGLOS SCORE THE HIGHEST, WITH NEGROES USUALLY NEXT AND MEXICAN AMERICANS LOWEST. IN REFERRING TO CULTURAL INTEGRATION IN THE ETHNIC AND ANGLO MIDDLE-CLASS SUBCULTURES, THE IMPORTANCE OF THE SOCIAL CLASS ELEMENT MUST NOT BE OVERLOOKED. INTEGRATION INTO THE LARGE CULTURE AT THE LOWEST SOCIOECONOMIC LEVEL OR CORRESPONDING SOCIAL CLASS DOES NOT HAVE THE SAME MEANING OR CONSEQUENCE AS DOES INTEGRATION INTO THE LARGER CULTURE AT A HIGHER SOCIOECONOMIC LEVEL OR CORRESPONDING SOCIAL CLASS. IT IS FOR THIS REASON THAT ECONOMIC ABSORPTION AND CULTURAL INTEGRATION ARE SO CLOSELY LINKED. 20 REFERENCES.

ACCN   001467

1700 AUTH   **SHANNON, L. W., & SHANNON, M.**
TITL   MINORITY MIGRANTS IN THE URBAN COMMUNITY: MEXICAN AMERICAN AND NEGRO ADJUSTMENT TO INDUSTRIAL SOCIETY.
SRCE   *BEVERLY HILLS, CALIF.: SAGE PUBLICATIONS, 1973.*
INDX   MIGRATION, URBAN, PSYCHOSOCIAL ADJUSTMENT, EMPLOYMENT, ENVIRONMENTAL FACTORS, MEXICAN AMERICAN, CROSS CULTURAL, SES, ESSAY, IMMIGRATION, WISCONSIN, MIDWEST, BOOK
ABST   THE ADJUSTMENT PROBLEMS OF IMMIGRANT MEXICAN AMERICANS AND NEGROES IN THE NORTHERN INDUSTRIAL COMMUNITY OF RACINE, WISCONSIN, ARE DESCRIBED. THE EXTENT TO WHICH EACH GROUP HAS BEEN ABSORBED INTO THE INDUSTRIAL ECONOMY AND INTEGRATED INTO THE LARGER URBAN SOCIETY, CONTRASTED TO INTEGRATION INTO EITHER THE MEXICAN AMERICAN OR NEGRO

SUBCOMMUNITIES, IS FEATURED. FINDINGS SUGGEST THAT ECONOMIC ABSORPTION OF PERSONS WITH RURAL ANTECEDENTS PROCEEDS WITH TIME IN THE COMMUNITY, BUT THAT THE EFFECT OF TIME IN THE COMMUNITY ON THE ECONOMIC ABSORPTION OF MEXICAN AMERICANS AND NEGROES WHO ARE PREDOMINATELY RURAL IN ORIGIN IS LIMITED BY WHATEVER OCCUPATIONAL CEILINGS HAVE BEEN FORMALLY OR INFORMALLY ESTABLISHED IN THE URBAN SETTING. IT IS CONCLUDED THAT THE SOCIAL ORGANIZATION OF THE URBAN COMMUNITY LIMITS THE INFLUENCE OF BOTH TIME IN THE COMMUNITY AND LEVEL OF ASPIRATION OF THE IMMIGRANTS AS A PREDICTOR OF ECONOMIC ABSORPTION. (NCMHI ABSTRACT)

ACCN   001468

1701 AUTH   **SHAW, M. E., BRISCOE, M. E., & GARCIA-ES-TEVE, J.**
TITL   A CROSS CULTURAL STUDY OF ATTRIBUTION OF RESPONSIBILITY.
SRCE   *INTERNATIONAL JOURNAL OF PSYCHOLOGY, 1968, 3(1), 51-60.*
INDX   CROSS CULTURAL, ATTRIBUTION OF RESPONSIBILITY, CUBAN, PUERTO RICAN-I, CHILD-REARING PRACTICES, CHILDREN, ADOLESCENTS, EMPIRICAL, FLORIDA, SOUTHWEST
ABST   AN EXPERIMENT TO DETERMINE WHETHER THE ATTRIBUTION OF RESPONSIBILITY (AR) VARIABLES OPERATE IN CUBAN, PUERTO RICAN AND AMERICAN CULTURES IS PRESENTED. TWENTY SUBJECTS WERE SELECTED FROM EACH OF FOUR AGE GROUPS (7-8, 9-10, 11-13, AND 16-18) IN EACH OF THE THREE CULTURES. WITHIN EACH AGE GROUP, SUBJECTS WERE MATCHED ACROSS CULTURES WITH RESPECT TO SEX, IQ SCORES, AND SOCIAL CLASS. THE BASIC INSTRUMENT, THE AR QUESTIONNAIRE WHICH CONSISTS OF 40 SHORT STORIES WITH POSITIVE AND NEGATIVE OUTCOMES, WAS ADMINISTERED TO THE SUBJECTS. DATA INDICATE THAT, IN GENERAL, CUBANS SHOW SOMEWHAT GREATER SOPHISTICATION THAN DO EITHER PUERTO RICANS OR AMERICANS WITH HIGH INTENSITY, NEGATIVE OUTCOMES. WITH POSITIVE OUTCOMES, BOTH CUBANS AND PUERTO RICANS SHOW GREATER SOPHISTICATION THAN DO AMERICANS. HOWEVER, THE LATIN CULTURES DO NOT SHOW THE EXPECTED GREATER AR FOR POSITIVE OUTCOMES; CUBANS GENERALLY ATTRIBUTE LESS FOR POSITIVE OUTCOMES THAN DO PUERTO RICANS AND AMERICANS. IN ALL CULTURES, SOPHISTICATION APPEARS TO DEVELOP MORE RAPIDLY WITH RESPECT TO NEGATIVE EVENTS THAN POSITIVE EVENTS. THERE IS ALSO SOME INDICATION THAT SOPHISTICATION FOR POSITIVE EVENTS DEVELOPS MORE RAPIDLY IN LATIN CULTURES THAN IN THE UNITED STATES. THE LATIN CULTURE SEEMS TO GIVE MORE ATTENTION TO REWARD AND PRAISE AND LESS TO PUNISHMENT THAN AMERICAN CULTURES, AND THIS SENSITIZES INDIVIDUALS TO ATTRIBUTE RESPONSIBILITY FOR POSITIVE OUTCOMES. 12 REFERENCES.

ACCN   001470

1702 AUTH   **SHELDON, W. H.**
TITL   THE INTELLIGENCE OF MEXICAN CHILDREN.
SRCE   *SCHOOL AND SOCIETY, 1924, 19, 139-142.*
INDX   INTELLIGENCE, MEXICAN, CHILDREN, STANFORD-BINET INTELLIGENCE TEST, CROSS CULTURAL
ABST   A CROSS-CULTURAL COMPARISON OF INTELLIGENCE OF CHILDREN OF THE SAME AGE AND SCHOOL ENVIRONMENT DISCOVERED APPRECIABLE DIFFERENCES BETWEEN THE 100 WHITE AND 100 MEXICAN CHILDREN TESTED. SUBJECTS WERE ADMINISTERED A COLE-VINCENT GROUP TEST AND IMMEDIATELY THEREAFTER A STANFORD-BINET INDIVIDUAL TEST. A SUMMARY OF THE RESULTS INDICATES: (1) THE AVERAGE MEXICAN CHILD IS 14 MONTHS BELOW THE NORMAL MENTAL DEVELOPMENT OF THE WHITE CHILD; (2) THE MEXICANS AS A GROUP POSSESS ABOUT 85 PERCENT OF THE INTELLIGENCE OF A SIMILAR GROUP OF WHITE CHILDREN; (3) THROUGH A COMBINED EFFORT OF STUDIES, MEXICAN CHILDREN ARE FOUND TO BE LESS INTELLIGENT THAN AMERICAN, ENGLISH, HEBREW, AND CHINESE CHILDREN, BUT MORE INTELLIGENT THAN INDIAN, SLAVIC, ITALIAN, AND NEGRO CHILDREN; AND (4) AS CHRONOLOGICAL AGE INCREASES, THESE RESULTS SHOW THAT THE PROPORTIONATE DIFFERENCES IN MENTAL AGE BETWEEN MEXICAN AND WHITE CHILDREN BECOME GREATER. THE AVERAGE MENTAL AGE OF THE MEXICAN GROUP SEEMS TO HAVE REACHED ITS MAXIMUM AT AROUND 9 YEARS.

ACCN   001471

1703 AUTH   **SHLIFER, E., & BARRIOS, A.**
TITL   UNDERCOUNTING OF SPANISH AMERICAN CLIENTS IN OUR REPORTING SYSTEM.
SRCE   *EXCHANGE, 1974, 2(5), 10-12.*
INDX   DEMOGRAPHIC, EMPIRICAL, RESEARCH METHODOLOGY, SPANISH SURNAMED, RESOURCE UTILIZATION, CALIFORNIA
ABST   TO DETERMINE IF SPANISH AMERICANS IN SANTA CLARA, CALIFORNIA, WERE RECEIVING THEIR SHARE OF COUNTY MENTAL HEALTH SERVICES, JANUARY-APRIL ADMISSIONS RECORDS WERE EXAMINED AT 2 HOSPITALS AND 4 COMMUNITY MENTAL HEALTH CENTERS. EVIDENCE OF CLIENT ETHNICITY WAS BASED UPON SPANISH SURNAME OR SPANISH-SPEAKING IRRESPECTIVE OF SURNAME. IT WAS DISCOVERED THAT HEALTH SERVICE CLERICAL STAFF WERE FAILING TO RECOGNIZE SOME CLIENTS AS SPANISH AMERICAN: (1) 2% TO 7% OF THE CLIENT POPULATION WERE INCORRECTLY LISTED IN CATEGORIES OTHER THAN SPANISH AMERICAN; AND (2) RECORDS OF THE NUMBER OF SPANISH AMERICAN CLIENTS AT THE SIX FACILITIES HAD TO BE REVISED UPWARDS FROM 8% TO AS MUCH AS 71%. THE FINDINGS WERE USED TO CORRECT SUMMARY REPORTS ON THE NUMBER, PROPORTION, AND RATE OF SPANISH AMERICAN CLIENTS BEING SEEN IN COUNTY MENTAL HEALTH SERVICE FACILITIES.

ACCN   001472

1704 AUTH   **SHONTZ, O. J.**

TITL   LAND OF POCO TIEMPO: A STUDY IN MEXICAN FAMILY RELATIONSHIPS IN A CHANGING SOCIAL ENVIRONMENT.

SRCE   *FAMILY; 1927, 8, 74-79.*

INDX   MEXICAN, SOCIALIZATION, ACCULTURATION, CULTURAL CHANGE, ESSAY, MARRIAGE, FAMILY STRUCTURE

ABST   A REVIEW OF THE MEXICAN LEGAL CODES RELATING TO MARRIAGE AND FAMILY RELATIONSHIPS REVEALS A SYSTEM SAFEGUARDING THE CONVENTIONAL MARRIAGE AND FAMILY UNIT. UNLIKE AMERICAN LAW, THE RESPONSIBILITY FOR SUPPORT OF FAMILY MEMBERS EXTENDS BEYOND THE HUSBAND AND WIFE TO SECOND DEGREE RELATIVES, GIVING THE MEXICAN A FEELING OF SECURITY. WITH INCREASED IMMIGRATION TO THE U.S. TO SUPPLY AGRICULTURAL LABOR, THE MEXICAN IS CONFRONTED WITH CHANGING IDEAS AND STANDARDS OF FAMILY MORALITY. ATTEMPTS TO ADOPT AMERICAN CULTURAL NORMS EMPHASIZING THE INDIVIDUAL OVER FAMILY ARE OFTEN DISRUPTIVE TO INDIGENOUS FAMILY COHESIVENESS. THE IMPINGING AMERICAN COURTS OF LAW, TEACHERS, SOCIAL WORKERS, AND MISSIONARIES SERVE AS SOLVENTS TO MEXICAN IDEALS AND HABITS. IT IS RECOMMENDED THAT SOCIAL AGENCIES APPROACH THE MEXICAN FAMILY WITH RESPECT AND A FAMILIARITY WITH ITS UNDERLYING LEGAL BASIS AND SPIRITUAL TRADITION. 3 REFERENCES.

ACCN   001473

1705 AUTH   **SHOTWELL, A. M.**

TITL   ARTHUR PERFORMANCE RATINGS OF MEXICAN AND AMERICAN HIGH-GRADE MENTAL DEFECTIVES.

SRCE   *AMERICAN JOURNAL OF MENTAL DEFICIENCY, 1945, 49(4), 445-449.*

INDX   PERFORMANCE EXPECTATIONS, MEXICAN AMERICAN, CROSS CULTURAL, MENTAL RETARDATION, EMPIRICAL, STANFORD-BINET INTELLIGENCE TEST, INTELLIGENCE TESTING

ABST   A COMPARISON OF THE ARTHUR PERFORMANCE SCALE BETWEEN MEXICAN AND AMERICAN HIGH-GRADE MENTAL DEFECTIVES OF COMPARABLE AGE AND BINET IQ RATINGS IS PRESENTED. THE SUBJECTS TESTED CONSIST OF 80 MEXICAN AND 80 AMERICAN NONEPILEPTIC PATIENTS. THE RESULTS SHOW THAT THE MEXICAN PATIENTS MADE, ON THE AVERAGE, AN ARTHUR IQ WHICH IS 14 POINTS HIGHER THAN THAT MADE BY THE AMERICANS, ALTHOUGH ON THE BINET THE MEXICANS HAVE AN AVERAGE THREE POINTS LOWER THAN THE AMERICANS. BOTH GROUPS SHOW AN INCREASE IN ARTHUR OVER BINET IQ, BUT WHEREAS THE AMERICANS AVERAGED 5 POINTS HIGHER ON THE ARTHUR THE MEXICANS AVERAGED 22 POINTS HIGHER. THE AVERAGE ARTHUR IQ FOR THE MEXICANS IS 83 AND 69 FOR THE AMERICANS. ONE POSSIBLE EXPLANATION FOR THE FINDINGS IS THAT THE MEXICAN'S ACQUISITION OF A SECOND LANGUAGE MAY RESULT IN CONFUSION OF THOUGHT AND EXPRESSION WHICH IS REFLECTED IN LOWER BINET IQ THAN IS REPRE-SENTATIVE OF THE INDIVIDUAL'S TRUE MENTAL ABILITY. ANOTHER EXPLANATION FOR THE DISCREPANCY IN IQ SCORES FROM THE TESTS IS THAT MEXICANS OF LOWER INTELLIGENCE HAVE A SPECIAL APTNESS ALONG MANUAL LINES THAT IS NOT FOUND IN AMERICANS WHO ARE SIMILARLY RETARDED MENTALLY. IT IS CONCLUDED THAT MEXICANS ARE INADEQUATELY MEASURED AND UNDULY PENALIZED WHEN THEIR INTELLIGENCE IS MEASURED BY A VERBAL TEST ALONE—ESPECIALLY A TEST WHICH HAS BEEN STANDARDIZED ONLY ON AMERICAN WHITES. 9 REFERENCES.

ACCN   001474

1706 AUTH   **SHUTT, D. L., & HANNON, T. A.**

TITL   THE VALIDITY OF THE HNTLA FOR EVALUATION OF THE ABILITIES OF BILINGUAL CHILDREN.

SRCE   *EDUCATIONAL AND PSYCHOLOGICAL MEASUREMENT, 1974, 32(2), 429-432.*

INDX   BILINGUAL-BICULTURAL EDUCATION, BILINGUALISM, TEST VALIDITY, SPECIAL EDUCATION, COMMUNITY, MEXICAN AMERICAN, WISC, SCHOLASTIC ACHIEVEMENT, COGNITIVE DEVELOPMENT, CHILDREN, CROSS CULTURAL, INTELLIGENCE TESTING, ARIZONA

ABST   THE VALIDITY OF THE HISKEY NEBRASKA TEST OF LEARNING APTITUDE (HNTLA) FOR PLACEMENT OF BILINGUAL CHILDREN IN APPROPRIATE SPECIAL CLASSES WAS INVESTIGATED AND ASSESSED. RANDOM GROUPS OF 50 MEXICAN AMERICAN AND 50 NAVAJO STUDENTS ENROLLED IN SPECIAL EDUCATION CLASSES THROUGHOUT ARIZONA WERE ADMINISTERED THE INSTRUMENT BY SIX ADMINISTRATORS. LEARNING AGES BASED ON THE USE OF DEAF NORMS WERE COMPARED WITH MENTAL TEST AGES FROM THE PERFORMANCE SCALE RESULTS OF THE WECHSLER INTELLIGENCE SCALE FOR CHILDREN (WISC). THE WISC IQ'S WERE THEN RELATED TO THOSE FROM THE HNTLA. IN ADDITION, EACH SUBTEST OF THE HNTLA WAS CORRELATED WITH EACH SUBTEST OF THE WISC PERFORMANCE SCALE. IT IS CONCLUDED THAT THE HNTLA IS A VALID INSTRUMENT FOR USE IN THE PLACEMENT OF NAVAJO AND MEXICAN AMERICAN PUPILS IN SPECIAL EDUCATION CLASSES. 8 REFERENCES. (NCMHI ABSTRACT)

ACCN   001476

1707 AUTH   **SIEGEL, A. I.**

TITL   THE SOCIAL ADJUSTMENTS OF PUERTO RICANS IN PHILADELPHIA.

SRCE   *JOURNAL OF SOCIAL PSYCHOLOGY, 1957, 46(1), 99-110.*

INDX   PSYCHOSOCIAL ADJUSTMENT, PUERTO RICAN-M, EMPIRICAL, SOCIALIZATION, ATTITUDES, DISCRIMINATION, INTERPERSONAL RELATIONS

ABST   FOLLOWING AN INTERETHNIC CLASH BETWEEN WHITES AND PUERTO RICANS (PR) IN JULY OF 1953, THE SOCIAL ADJUSTMENT OF 209 PUERTO RICANS WAS ASSESSED BY MEANS OF INTERVIEWS. WITH RESPECT TO QUESTIONS PERTAINING TO FLUENCY IN ENGLISH, THE DATA SUGGEST THAT THE MIGRANT PR POPULATION IS WEAK IN ENGLISH LANGUAGE

ABILITY, BUT AWARE OF THEIR DEFICIENCY. ITEMS WHICH WERE INCLUDED TO DETERMINE PERCEIVED SOCIAL DISTANCE SHOW THAT PR'S VIEW OTHER PHILADELPHIANS TO BE MODERATELY DISTANT TOWARD THEM AND REPORT THAT MOST OF THEIR FRIENDS ARE PR'S. IT WAS ALSO SEEN THAT 44 PERCENT OF THE ANSWERS TO THE QUESTION, "DO YOU THINK THAT CONTINENTAL AMERICANS WOULD LIKE TO EXCLUDE PUERTO RICANS FROM THIS COUNTRY?," WERE AFFIRMATIVE. SPANISH LANGUAGE RADIO AND TV PROGRAMS, AS WELL AS NEWSPAPERS, WERE PREFERRED BY MOST OF THE SAMPLE INTERVIEWED. ADJUSTMENT TO POLICE AND LAWS REVEALS THAT 31 PERCENT OF THE RESPONDENTS FELT THAT THE POLICE TREATED THEM UNJUSTLY, BUT ONLY 4 PERCENT FELT THAT THE LAWS SHOULD BE CHANGED. AS FOR LEADERSHIP, MOST PR'S STATE THAT THEY PREFER TO GO TO ANOTHER PR FOR ADVICE. MOST OF THE RESPONDENTS STATE THAT THEIR MAJOR PROBLEMS IN PHILADELPHIA CENTER ON LACK OF EMPLOYMENT OR LOW WAGES. MANY OF THE SUBJECTS INDICATE A DISCREPANCY BETWEEN THEIR LEVEL OF VOCATIONAL ASPIRATION AND LEVEL OF ACHIEVEMENT. A VOCATIONAL PESSIMISM WAS ALSO OBSERVED BY MANY OF THE PR'S WHEN THEY INDICATED THAT ANY KIND OF "STEADY" WORK WAS SATISFACTORY. THIS SAME PESSIMISM WAS NOT SHOWN WHEN RESPONDENTS INDICATED THAT THEY DESIRED WHITE-COLLAR OR PROFESSIONAL JOBS FOR THEIR CHILDREN. 1 REFERENCE.

ACCN   001477

1708 AUTH   **SILVERSTEIN, A. B.**
TITL   FACTOR STRUCTURE OF THE WECHSLER INTELLIGENCE SCALE FOR CHILDREN FOR THREE ETHNIC GROUPS.
SRCE   *JOURNAL OF EDUCATIONAL PSYCHOLOGY, 1973, 65(3), 408-410.*
INDX   WISC, CHILDREN, CULTURAL FACTORS, TEST VALIDITY, CROSS CULTURAL, INTELLIGENCE TESTING
ABST   CORRELATIONS AMONG THE WECHSLER INTELLIGENCE SCALE FOR CHILDREN (WISC) SUBTESTS WERE FACTORED FOR GROUPS OF ANGLO, BLACK, AND CHICANO PUBLIC SCHOOLCHILDREN, AND TWO FACTORS (VERBAL COMPREHENSION AND PERCEPTUAL ORGANIZATION) WERE FOUND FOR EACH GROUP. THE RESULTS OF TWO METHODS OF ASSESSING FACTORIAL INVARIANCE SUGGEST THAT THE WISC MEASURES THE SAME ABILITIES IN CHILDREN OF ALL THREE GROUPS. 14 REFERENCES. (JOURNAL ABSTRACT)
ACCN   001478

1709 AUTH   **SIMMONS, O. G.**
TITL   THE MUTUAL IMAGES AND EXPECTATIONS OF ANGLO AMERICANS AND MEXICAN AMERICANS.
SRCE   *DAEDALUS, 1961, 90(2), 286-299.*
INDX   MEXICAN AMERICAN, CROSS CULTURAL, INTERPERSONAL RELATIONS, GROUP DYNAMICS, COMMUNITY, PEER GROUP, ATTITUDES, STEREOTYPES, TEXAS, SOUTHWEST

ABST   THE INTERGROUP RELATIONS BETWEEN AN ANGLO AMERICAN (AA) AND MEXICAN AMERICAN (MA) SAMPLE IN A SOUTH TEXAS COMMUNITY ARE STUDIED. THE ASSUMPTIONS AND EXPECTATIONS OF EACH GROUP ARE COMPARED. FINDINGS INDICATE THAT THERE ARE MAJOR INCONSISTENCIES IN THE ASSUMPTIONS THAT AA'S AND MA'S HOLD ABOUT ONE ANOTHER. AA'S ASSUME THAT MA'S ARE THEIR POTENTIAL PEERS, BUT AT THE SAME TIME ASSUME THAT THEY ARE THEIR INFERIORS. THE BELIEFS ATTRIBUTING UNDESIRABLE CHARACTERISTICS TO MA'S AND PRESUMABLY DEMONSTRATING MA'S INFERIORITY TEND TO PLACE THEM OUTSIDE THE ACCEPTED MORAL ORDER AND FRAMEWORK OF AA SOCIETY. THESE NEGATIVE IMAGES PROVIDE NOT ONLY A RATIONALIZED DEFINITION OF THE INTERGROUP RELATION THAT MAKES IT PALATABLE FOR AA'S BUT ALSO A SUBSTANTIAL SUPPORT FOR MAINTAINING THE RELATION AS IT IS. THE ASSUMPTIONS OF MA'S ABOUT AA'S ARE SIMILARLY INCONSISTENT, AND THEIR IMAGES OF AA'S ARE PREDOMINANTLY NEGATIVE AND PRIMARILY DEFENSIVE RATHER THAN JUSTIFICATORY. THE MUTUAL EXPECTATIONS OF THE TWO GROUPS CONTRAST SHARPLY IN THAT AA'S EXPECT MA'S TO BECOME LIKE THEMSELVES, IF THEY ARE TO BE ACCORDED EQUAL STATUS, WHEREAS MA'S WANT FULL ACCEPTANCE, REGARDLESS OF THE EXTENT TO WHICH THEY GIVE UP THEIR MORES AND ACQUIRE THOSE OF THE AA GROUP. 16 REFERENCES.
ACCN   001479

1710 AUTH   **SIMON, A. J., & JOINER, L. M.**
TITL   A MEXICAN VERSION OF THE PEABODY PICTURE VOCABULARY TEST.
SRCE   *JOURNAL OF EDUCATIONAL MEASUREMENT, 1976, 13(2), 137-143.*
INDX   PEABODY PICTURE-VOCABULARY TEST, MEXICAN, CHILDREN, INTELLIGENCE TESTING, EMPIRICAL, TEST VALIDITY, TEST RELIABILITY, MENTAL RETARDATION, MEXICAN AMERICAN
ABST   DUE TO THE RELATIVE SCARCITY OF PSYCHOMETRIC SCREENING DEVICES FOR MEXICAN AND MEXICAN AMERICAN CHILDREN, AN ATTEMPT WAS MADE TO IMPROVE A MEXICAN VERSION OF THE PEABODY PICTURE-VOCABULARY TEST (PPVT). FORMS A & B OF THE AMERICAN TEST WERE DIRECTLY TRANSLATED, AND BY MEANS OF A SET OF DECISION PROCEDURES TO SELECT THE BETTER ITEM FROM EACH PAIR OF ITEMS (N = 150), A REORDERING OF THE SELECTED ITEMS WAS CONDUCTED. THE RESULTING VERSION (PPVT-RT) WAS ADMINISTERED TO A SAMPLE OF 120 MEXICAN ELEMENTARY SCHOOL CHILDREN. WHEREAS SIMPLE TRANSLATION OF FORMS A AND B RESULTED IN AN ALTERNATE FORMS RELIABILITY OF .85 (AS CONTRASTED WITH .95 REPORTED FOR THE ORIGINAL TEST), REVISION OF THE SIMPLE TRANSLATIONS SIGNIFICANTLY INCREASED THE INTERNAL CONSISTENCY OF THE TEST. FURTHER STUDIES INTO THE PPVT-RT SHOULD ADDRESS THE PREDICTIVE VALIDITY OF THE TEST USING KNOWN MENTAL

RETARDATION OR GIFTEDNESS AS CLASSIFI-
CATION VARIABLES. 17 REFERENCES.

ACCN 002207

1711 AUTH **SIMON, H. J., & COVELL, J. W.**
TITL PERFORMANCE OF MEDICAL STUDENTS AD-
MITTED VIA REGULAR AND ADMISSION-VARI-
ANCE ROUTES.
SRCE *JOURNAL OF MEDICAL EDUCATION, 1975, 50(3),
237-241.*
INDX CALIFORNIA, HIGHER EDUCATION, COLLEGE
STUDENTS, CROSS CULTURAL, EDUCATIONAL
ASSESSMENT, EMPIRICAL, PROFESSIONAL
TRAINING, MEDICAL STUDENTS, MEXICAN
AMERICAN, SOUTHWEST
ABST TWENTY-THREE MEDICAL STUDENTS FROM
SOCIOECONOMICALLY DISADVANTAGED
BACKGROUNDS AND DRAWN CHIEFLY FROM
CHICANO AND BLACK RACIAL MINORITY
GROUPS WERE GRANTED ADMISSION VARI-
ANCES TO THE UNIVERSITY OF CALIFORNIA,
SAN DIEGO, SCHOOL OF MEDICINE IN 1970
AND 1971. THIS GROUP WAS COMPARED WITH
21 REGULARLY ADMITTED JUNIOR AND SEN-
IOR MEDICAL STUDENTS WITH RESPECT TO
SPECIFIC ADMISSIONS CRITERIA, SCORES ON
PART I OF THE NATIONAL BOARD OF MEDICAL
EXAMINERS (NBME) TEST, AND PERFORMANCE
IN AT LEAST TWO CLINICAL CLERKSHIPS. THE
TWO GROUPS DIFFERED MARKEDLY ON AD-
MISSION. THE USUAL SCREENING WOULD HAVE
PRECLUDED ADMISSION OF ALL BUT ONE OF
THE STUDENTS GRANTED VARIANCES. AT THE
END OF THE SECOND YEAR, AVERAGE NBME
SCORES AGAIN IDENTIFIED TWO DISTINCT
POPULATIONS, BUT THE AVERAGE SCORES OF
BOTH GROUPS WERE CLEARLY ABOVE THE
MINIMUM PASSING LEVEL. THE GROUPS STILL
DIFFERED ON ANALYSIS OF THEIR AGGREGATE
PERFORMANCES ON THE CLINICAL SERVICES,
BUT THE DIFFERENCE FOLLOWING COMPLE-
TION OF TWO OF THREE MAJOR CLINICAL
CLERKSHIPS HAD BECOME THE DISTINCTION
BETWEEN A "SLIGHTLY ABOVE AVERAGE" LEVEL
OF PERFORMANCE FOR THE REGULARLY AD-
MITTED STUDENTS AND AN "AVERAGE" LEVEL
FOR STUDENTS ADMITTED ON VARIANCES.
THE FACULTY ATTRIBUTES THESE FINDINGS TO
A FLEXIBLE CURRICULUM, INDIVIDUALIZED DI-
AGNOSIS OF ACADEMIC PROBLEMS, AND AN
EXTENSIVE, INTENSIVE SYSTEM OF TUTORIALS
IN PRECLINICAL SUBJECTS. 1 REFERENCE.
(AUTHOR ABSTRACT MODIFIED)

ACCN 002644

1712 AUTH **SIMPSON, M.**
TITL AUTHORITARIANISM AND EDUCATION: A COM-
PARATIVE APPROACH.
SRCE *SOCIOMETRY, 1972, 35(2), 223-234.*
INDX AUTHORITARIANISM, EDUCATION, CROSS CUL-
TURAL, TEACHERS, ATTITUDES, INSTRUC-
TIONAL TECHNIQUES, CULTURAL FACTORS,
ADULTS, MEXICAN, CENTRAL AMERICA
ABST THE RELATIONSHIP BETWEEN AUTHORITARI-
ANISM AND EDUCATION WAS EXAMINED, US-
ING CROSS-CULTURAL DATA OBTAINED BY
MICHIGAN STATE UNIVERSITY'S NATIONS STUDY
WHICH SURVEYED OVER 1,000 PERSONS IN

EACH OF FOUR COUNTRIES—COSTA RICA,
FINLAND, MEXICO, AND THE UNITED STATES.
ALTHOUGH PREVIOUS STUDIES HAVE INDI-
CATED A STRONG INVERSE RELATIONSHIP BE-
TWEEN AUTHORITARIANISM AND EDUCATION,
THE PRESENT RESEARCH FOUND THAT EDU-
CATION REDUCES AUTHORITARIANISM ONLY
(1) WHERE THE EDUCATIONAL SYSTEM EM-
PHASIZES DIALECTIC AND COGNITIVE AP-
PROACHES RATHER THAN ROTE LEARNING,
AND (2) WHERE THE MAJORITY OF THE SCHOOL
SYSTEM'S TEACHERS ARE NON-AUTHORI-
TARIAN. IN COSTA RICA, EDUCATION REDUCED
AUTHORITARIANISM ONLY AFTER 8TH GRADE.
IN MEXICO, EDUCATION PROVED TO HAVE
LITTLE EFFECT ON AUTHORITARIANISM UNTIL
AFTER THE 11TH YEAR OF SCHOOLING. IN
CONTRAST, THE EDUCATIONAL SYSTEMS OF
FINLAND AND THE U.S, AT ALL LEVELS RE-
DUCED AUTHORITARIANISM. FURTHER RE-
SEARCH IS SUGGESTED ON THE RELATIVE IM-
PACT OF DIFFERENT KINDS OF EDUCATIONAL
SYSTEMS AND TEACHERS UPON STUDENT
CHARACTER. 32 REFERENCES.

ACCN 001480

1713 AUTH **SIMPSON, M. L.**
TITL IDEAL FAMILY SIZE IN MONTERREY, MEXICO.
SRCE *HUMAN MOSAIC, 1968, 3(1), 105-123.*
INDX MEXICO, MEXICAN, FAMILY STRUCTURE, ATTI-
TUDES, FERTILITY, SES, SOUTH AMERICA, UR-
BAN, CULTURAL FACTORS, DEMOGRAPHIC,
ADULTS, MALE
ABST THIS STUDY COMPARED IDEAL AND ACTUAL
FAMILY SIZE IN EIGHT LATIN AMERICAN CITIES,
AND THEN ATTEMPTED TO IDENTIFY FACTORS
AFFECTING IDEAL AND ACTUAL FAMILY SIZE IN
ONE CITY—MONTERREY, MEXICO. IDEAL FAMILY
SIZE WAS FOUND TO BE LARGER THAN AC-
TUAL FAMILY SIZE IN EACH OF THE CITIES.
AMONG THE 448 MARRIED MEN SURVEYED IN
MONTERREY, IT WAS FOUND THAT THE MA-
JORITY OF THOSE HAVING THE LARGEST FAMI-
LIES EXPRESSED A SMALLER IDEAL FAMILY
SIZE. SECOND, THE SMALLER THE COMMU-
NITY OF ORIGIN, THE LARGER THE NUMBER OF
CHILDREN CONSIDERED IDEAL. THIRD, LONGER
RESIDENTS IN THE CITY TENDED TO PREFER
MEDIUM-SIZED FAMILIES. IN GENERAL, THOSE
WHO AGREED THAT CHILDREN WERE OB-
STACLES TO MOBILITY AND FAVORED FAMILY
LIMITATION ALSO FAVORED SMALLER FAMI-
LIES. FINALLY, EDUCATION, OCCUPATIONAL
LEVEL, AND AGE OF ARRIVAL IN MONTERREY
SHOWED NO EFFECT ON THE SIZE OF THE
FAMILY CONSIDERED IDEAL. IT IS SUGGESTED
THAT PERHAPS THE INTRODUCTION OF AN AP-
PROPRIATE THIRD VARIABLE OR COMBINATION
OF VARIABLES (E.G., COMMUNITY OF ORIGIN
AND AGE OF ARRIVAL) WOULD OFFER THE
STRONGEST EXPLANATION OF VARIABILITY. 16
REFERENCES.

ACCN 001481

1714 AUTH **SIMPSON, M. L., & WILLIAMSON, D.**
TITL THE COMPLETED FAMILY IN MONTERREY,
MEXICO: FERTILITY, MOBILITY AND MIGRATION.
SRCE *HUMAN MOSAIC, 1968, 3(1), 81-104.*

INDX   MEXICO, MEXICAN, FAMILY STRUCTURE, ATTITUDES, FERTILITY, MIGRATION, EMPIRICAL, CROSS GENERATIONAL, MALE, ADULTS, DEMOGRAPHIC

ABST   A SURVEY IN MONTERREY, MEXICO, OF 526 MARRIED MALES (AGE 40 OR OLDER) SOUGHT TO DETERMINE IF FERTILITY WAS IN FACT INCREASING IN THAT RAPIDLY URBANIZING CITY. DATA ANALYSIS EXAMINED THE RELATIONSHIP BETWEEN FERTILITY, MIGRATION, AND SOCIAL MOBILITY; AND FINDINGS REVEALED SIGNIFICANT RELATIONSHIPS BETWEEN FERTILITY, OCCUPATION LEVELS, EDUCATION, COMMUNITY OF ORIGIN, AND ATTITUDES ABOUT FAMILY SIZE. THE HIGHEST RATE OF FERTILITY WAS FOUND AMONG THE LOWEST OCCUPATIONAL STATUSES, THOSE WHO HAD LITTLE OR NO EDUCATION, THOSE WHO WERE RURAL IMMIGRANTS, AND THOSE WHO FAVORED NO LIMITATION ON FAMILY SIZE. THE IMMIGRANT'S AGE UPON ARRIVAL TO THE CITY WAS SIGNIFICANT, AS THOSE WHO ARRIVED AT A YOUNG AGE HAD A RELATIVELY LOW FERTILITY RATE. UPWARD SOCIAL MOBILITY ALSO LOWERED FERTILITY RATE, IRRESPECTIVE OF COMMUNITY OF ORIGIN. THE RESULTS PERTAIN TO THE PREVAILING SOCIOLOGICAL THEORY THAT TRANSITIONAL SOCIETIES PASS THROUGH A STAGE OF DECREASING FERTILITY. 16 REFERENCES.

ACCN   001482

1715 AUTH   **SIMPSON, R. L.**
TITL   STUDY OF THE COMPARABILITY OF THE WISC AND THE WAIS.
SRCE   *JOURNAL OF CONSULTING AND CLINICAL PSYCHOLOGY, 1970, 34(2), 156-158.*
INDX   WISC, WAIS, CROSS CULTURAL, MEXICAN AMERICAN, INTELLIGENCE TESTING, ADOLESCENTS, EMPIRICAL, SEX COMPARISON, CALIFORNIA, SOUTHWEST, URBAN
ABST   IN TEN JUNIOR AND SENIOR HIGH SCHOOLS IN LOS ANGELES, STUDENTS OF BELOW-AVERAGE INTELLIGENCE WERE TESTED TO ASSESS THE COMPARABILITY OF THE WESCHLER INTELLIGENCE SCALE FOR CHILDREN (WISC) AND THE WESCHLER ADULT INTELLIGENCE SCALE (WAIS). THE SAMPLE CONSISTED OF 40 ANGLO, 40 BLACK, AND 40 MEXICAN AMERICAN MALES AND FEMALES WHO WERE WITHIN THREE MONTHS OF THEIR SIXTEENTH BIRTHDAY AND WHO HAD SCORES BELOW 90 ON A RECENT GROUP OR INDIVIDUAL INTELLIGENCE TEST. ANALYSIS OF VARIANCE INDICATED SIGNIFICANTLY HIGHER IQ SCORES FOR THE WAIS THAN FOR THE WISC ON VERBAL, PERFORMANCE, AND FULL SCALES. RACIAL DIFFERENCES BETWEEN THE TWO TESTS WERE SIGNIFICANT BEYOND THE .05 LEVEL FOR ALL THREE SCALES. THE DISPARITY BETWEEN THE TWO TESTS WAS SIGNIFICANTLY GREATER FOR THE BLACKS THAN FOR THE MEXICAN AMERICANS AND ANGLOS. THERE WERE NO SIGNIFICANT SEX DIFFERENCES. IT IS CONCLUDED THAT STUDENTS WHO ARE BELOW THE AVERAGE RANGE IN INTELLIGENCE OBTAINED SIGNIFICANTLY HIGHER WAIS THAN WISC IQ'S. THE DISCREPANCY WAS GREATEST IN THE VER-

BALSCALE FOLLOWED BY THE FULL SCALE AND LEAST ON THE PERFORMANCE SCALE. IN SPITE OF THE SIMILARITIES IN ADMINISTRATION AND FORMAT, THE TWO INSTRUMENTS CANNOT BE CONSIDERED COMPARABLE WHEN USED WITH BELOW-AVERAGE INTELLIGENCE STUDENTS. 3 REFERENCES.

ACCN   001483

1716 AUTH   **SINGER, H. A.**
TITL   POLICE ACTION—COMMUNITY ACTION.
SRCE   *JOURNAL OF SOCIAL ISSUES, 1975, 31(1), 99-106.*
INDX   POLICE-COMMUNITY RELATIONS, COMMUNITY INVOLVEMENT, ATTITUDES, ADOLESCENTS, PUERTO RICAN-M, SOCIAL SERVICES, CROSS CULTURAL, CULTURAL FACTORS, EMPIRICAL, CONNECTICUT, EAST, PROGRAM EVALUATION
ABST   THE POLICE COMMUNITY AWARENESS LABORATORY (PCAL), A PROGRAM INVOLVING A BATTERY OF QUESTIONNAIRES AND SIX-WEEK 15-HOUR COMMUNITY SESSIONS, WAS CONDUCTED WITH 300 POLICE OFFICERS AND 150 ANGLO, BLACK AND PUERTO RICAN CIVILIANS FROM CONNECTICUT. THE PURPOSE OF PCAL WAS TO REDUCE CRIME AND ELICIT CITIZEN COOPERATION. THE QUESTIONNAIRE ADMINISTERED TO THE POLICE OFFICERS PRIOR TO THE SESSIONS MEASURED ATTITUDES TOWARDS YOUTH, MINORITY MEMBERS, PEERS, SELF, CIVIL RIGHTS AND VIOLENCE. AMONG THE ISSUES RAISED IN THE COMMUNITY SESSIONS WERE ABUSE OF POLICE POWER, HOSTILITY TOWARDS MINORITIES, MINORITY UNCOOPERATIVENESS WITH POLICE, MISUNDERSTANDING OF POLICE FUNCTION IN THE INNER-CITY, AND LACK OF COMMUNICATION. THESE SESSIONS WERE FOLLOWED BY JOINT EVALUATIONS. RESULTS OF THE PROGRAM SUGGEST: (1) PARTICIPATING CITIES EXPERIENCED A DROP IN THEIR CRIME RATE; (2) POLICE OFFICERS WERE ABLE TO VENTILATE ABOUT THEIR OWN "MINORITY" STATUS AS OFFICERS; (3) POLICE ATTITUDES TOWARDS PUERTO RICANS IMPROVED; (4) POLICE ATTITUDES TOWARDS YOUTH IMPROVED; (5) NEGATIVE ATTITUDES TOWARDS BLACKS DID NOT CHANGE SIGNIFICANTLY; AND (6) THE COURSE WAS RATED ABOVE AVERAGE, WITH THE INSTRUCTOR RECEIVING THE HIGHEST RATING. OVERALL, THE PCAL DID PROVE EFFECTIVE, ESPECIALLY AS THE OFFICER'S RATING OF HIMSELF AND HIS PEERS IMPROVED SIGNIFICANTLY. 4 REFERENCES.

ACCN   001484

1717 AUTH   **SMITH, G. M.**
TITL   PERSONALITY CORRELATES OF ACADEMIC PERFORMANCE IN THREE DISSIMILAR POPULATIONS.
SRCE   *PROCEEDINGS OF THE 77TH ANNUAL CONVENTION OF THE AMERICAN PSYCHOLOGICAL ASSOCIATION, 1969, 4(1), 303-304.*
INDX   PERSONALITY ASSESSMENT, SCHOLASTIC ACHIEVEMENT, CROSS CULTURAL, PUERTO RICAN-M
ABST   FORTY-TWO PERSONALITY VARIABLES, DERIVED FROM PEER RATINGS, WERE FACTOR

ANALYZED AND STUDIED IN RELATION TO GPA (USING UNIVARIATE AND MULTIVARIATE PROCEDURES) IN A SAMPLE OF 1,022 SPANISH-SPEAKING PUERTO RICAN HIGH SCHOOL STUDENTS AND TWO ENGLISH-SPEAKING SAMPLES (348 UNDERGRADUATES AND 798 STUDENT NURSES). FACTOR ANALYTIC STRUCTURE WAS STABLE ACROSS POPULATIONS. THE PREDICTIVE VALIDITY OF VARIABLES BELONGING TO THE FACTOR CALLED "STRENGTH OF CHARACTER" SURPASSED THAT OF MOST OTHER VARIABLES. THE RELATIONS BETWEEN PERSONALITY AND ACADEMIC PERFORMANCE WERE HIGHLY CONSISTENT ACROSS THE THREE DISSIMILAR POPULATIONS—ESPECIALLY FOR THE "STRENGTH OF CHARACTER" VARIABLES. 4 REFERENCES.

ACCN   001485

1718 AUTH   **SMITH, I. L., & RINGLER, L. H.**
TITL   PREFERRED SENSORY MODALITY, READING READINESS, AND READING ACHIEVEMENT IN FIRST-GRADE CHILDREN.
SRCE   *PERCEPTUAL AND MOTOR SKILLS, 1971, 32(3), 764-766.*
INDX   READING, SCHOLASTIC ACHIEVEMENT, CHILDREN, CROSS CULTURAL, PUERTO RICAN-M, SES, COGNITIVE STYLE, EMPIRICAL, NEW YORK,EAST
ABST   THE RELATIONSHIP AMONG READING READINESS, PREFERRED SENSORY MODALITY, AND READING ACHIEVEMENT WERE STUDIED USING FIRST-GRADE BOYS AND GIRLS FROM A LOW-SOCIOECONOMIC AREA OF NEW YORK CITY. THE CHILDREN WERE OF PUERTO RICAN, NEGRO, CHINESE, AND CAUCASIAN DESCENT, AND WERE CONSIDERED TO HAVE ADEQUATE ENGLISH-LANGUAGE BACKGROUND. THE NEW YORK STATE READING READINESS TEST WAS ADMINISTERED AT THE BEGINNING OF THE SCHOOL YEAR. TO DETERMINE PREFERRED MODALITY OF THE PUPILS FROM AMONG AUDITORY, VISUAL, AND KINESTHETIC MODALITIES, THE NEW YORK UNIVERSITY MODALITY TEST (1968) WAS USED. READING ACHIEVEMENT WAS MEASURED BY THE METROPOLITAN READING TEST-PRIMARY I, ADMINISTERED AT THE END OF THE FIRST-GRADE. DATA WERE ANALYZED THROUGH USE OF A STEPWISE MULTIPLE REGRESSION ANALYSIS, WHICH INDICATED THAT THE MAJOR VARIABLE RELATED TO PREDICTING FIRST-GRADE READING ACHIEVEMENT WAS READING READINESS. 3 REFERENCES. (AUTHOR SUMMARY MODIFIED)
ACCN   001486

1719 AUTH   **SMITH, L. W.**
TITL   SOCIOECONOMIC CHARACTERISTICS OF THE SPANISH ORIGIN HIRED FARM WORKING FORCE, 1973.
SRCE   *PRESENTED AT THE ANNUAL MEETING OF THE RURAL SOCIOLOGICAL SOCIETY, SAN FRANCISCO, CALIFORNIA, AUGUST 22, 1975.*
INDX   SES, FARM LABORERS, LABOR FORCE, SEX COMPARISON, MIGRATION, ENVIRONMENTAL FACTORS, SOCIAL MOBILITY, EDUCATION, CROSS CULTURAL, CULTURAL FACTORS, ECONOMIC FACTORS, EMPLOYMENT, SPANISH SURNAMED, CALIFORNIA, SOUTHWEST, SOUTHWEST, MIGRANTS
ABST   TO ASCERTAIN THE PARTICULAR CHARACTERISTICS, PROBLEMS, AND NEEDS OF SPANISH ORIGIN HIRED FARM WORKERS, A COMPARATIVE ANALYSIS WAS CONDUCTED OF SPANISH ORIGIN, WHITE, BLACK, AND OTHER ETHNIC MINORITY FARM WAGEWORKERS IN CALIFORNIA. DATA WERE OBTAINED FROM THE ANNUAL HIRED FARM WORKING FORCE SURVEY OF THE U.S. DEPARTMENT OF AGRICULTURE, CONDUCTED BY THE BUREAU OF THE CENSUS IN DECEMBER, 1973. SIGNIFICANT FINDINGS REVEALED THAT SPANISH ORIGIN FARM WORKERS WERE HIGHLY DEPENDENT UPON AGRICULTURAL WORK FOR A LIVELIHOOD AND HAD VERY FEW VIABLE ALTERNATIVES FOR EMPLOYMENT OUTSIDE OF FARM LABOR. GENERALLY, SPANISH ORIGIN FARM WORKERS HAVE VERY LOW LEVELS OF EDUCATION AND FEW SKILLS FOR NONFARM EMPLOYMENT, ESPECIALLY COMPARED TO WHITES; THUS, WHEREAS WHITE FARM WORKERS TEND TO MOVE ON TO BETTER PAYING NONAGRICULTURAL JOBS, SPANISH ORIGIN FARM LABORERS CONTINUE IN AGRICULTURAL WORK ALL OR MOST OF THEIR WORKING LIVES. THE ECONOMIC PROBLEMS AND LACK OF JOB MOBILITY OF SPANISH ORIGIN FARM WORKERS ARE FURTHER COMPLICATED BY THEIR MIGRATORY LABOR PATTERN AND THEIR LARGE HOUSEHOLD SIZES; THESE FACTORS PROHIBIT THEM FROM SAVING SUFFICIENT CAPITAL TO ESTABLISH THEIR OWN BUSINESSES. IT IS CONCLUDED THAT ECONOMIC IMPROVEMENT FOR THIS POPULATION DEPENDS UPON INCREASED ACCESS TO NONFARM EMPLOYMENT THROUGH EDUCATION AND JOB TRAINING. HOWEVER, MANPOWER PROGRAMS WHICH HAVE THIS AIM MUST TAKE INTO CONSIDERATION THE PARTICULAR SOCIOECONOMIC AND CULTURAL CHARACTERISTICS OF SPANISH ORIGIN FARM WORKERS—I.E., THEIR HIGH DEGREE OF MIGRANCY, STRONG AGRICULTURAL DEPENDENCE, SEVERE EDUCATIONAL DISABILITIES, ETHNIC SOLIDARITY, AND LANGUAGE PROBLEMS. 19 REFERENCES.
ACCN   001487

1720 AUTH   **SMITH, M. E.**
TITL   THE SPANISH-SPEAKING POPULATION OF FLORIDA.
SRCE   *IN J. HELM (ED.), SPANISH-SPEAKING PEOPLE IN THE UNITED STATES: PROCEEDINGS OF THE 1968 ANNUAL SPRING MEETING OF THE AMERICAN ETHNOLOGICAL SOCIETY. SEATTLE: UNIVERSITY OF WASHINGTON PRESS, 1968, PP. 120-133.*
INDX   PUERTO RICAN-M, CUBAN, MEXICAN AMERICAN, ESSAY, CULTURAL FACTORS, ACCULTURATION, RESEARCH METHODOLOGY, ECONOMIC FACTORS, CASE STUDY, SOCIAL MOBILITY, FAMILY STRUCTURE, RELIGION, FLORIDA, SOUTH, EMPIRICAL
ABST   AN ETHNOLOGICAL STUDY OF THE SPANISH-SPEAKING PEOPLES IN FOUR FLORIDA COMMUNITIES—INCLUDING PUERTO RICANS,

OLDER CUBANS AND NEW CUBAN REFUGEES, AND MEXICAN AMERICANS—IS PRESENTED. PERSONAL ACCOUNTS BY INFORMANTS OF EACH GROUP ARE INCLUDED. FOR PUERTO RICANS, THE DATA REVEAL THERE IS HIGH INTERNAL MOBILITY; THE "BROKERAGE" SYSTEM IS SEEN AS AN EFFECTIVE MEANS OF OBTAINING EMPLOYMENT; SOCIAL OR POLITICAL CLUBS PLAY AN IMPORTANT FUCTION; AND PREJUDICE IS DIRECTED MORE AGAINST THIS GROUP, USUALLY IN THE FORM OF DISDAIN. THE CUBANS, PREDOMINANTLY CASTRO REFUGEES, WITH MANY INTENDING TO RETURN TO CUBA, PRESENT A LESS TIGHTLY KNIT FAMILY UNIT ALTHOUGH STRICT SOCIAL ETIQUETTE IS MAINTAINED; RELIGIOUS ACTIVITIES ARE MORE IMPORTANT THAN AMONG PUERTO RICANS; CLASS DISTINCTIONS ARE EMPHASIZED; AND WHILE RELATIVELY RAPID ACCULTURATION AND ADJUSTMENT TO THE ECONOMIC SYSTEM IS TAKING PLACE AMONG THE YOUNGER NEW CUBANS, THEY APPEAR TO DEVALUATE OTHER AMERICAN FOLKWAYS MORE THAN THE PUERTO RICANS. A BRIEF HISTORY OF YBOR CITY, A CUBAN ENCLAVE ESTABLISHED IN TAMPA AROUND 1869, IS PRESENTED. THE LAST GROUP, THE MEXICANS (A GENERIC TERM USED BY FLORIDIANS TO REFER TO ANY SPANISH-SPEAKING MIGRANT WORKER FROM WEST OF THE MISSISSIPPI), IS SEEN AS MAINTAINING RELATIVE COHESIVENESS, STABLE MEMBERSHIP AND STABLE MIGRATORY CYCLES OVER THREE GENERATIONS; PHILOSOPHICAL ELEMENTS OF RELIGION ARE MINIMAL; AND MARRIAGE BETWEEN MIGRANT CREWS IS ENCOURAGED MORE THAN OUT OF THE MIGRANT GROUP. THE VALIDITY OF THE GENERIC "SPANISH-SPEAKING" CLASSIFICATION AND WHAT KIND OF ANTHROPOLOGY IS TO BE EMPLOYED IS ALSO DISCUSSED. POSITED IS A MORE STRINGENT APPLICATION OF ANTHROPOLOGICAL CONSTRUCTS SUCH AS "PRIMITIVE," "PEASANT," "ETHNOGRAPHIC PRESENT" AND "THE CITY." 4 REFERENCES.

ACCN   001488

1721 AUTH   **SMITH, P. A.**
TITL   NONPENAL REHABILITATION FOR THE CHRONIC ALCOHOLIC OFFENDER.
SRCE   *FEDERAL PROBATION, 1968, 32(3), 46-50.*
INDX   REHABILITATION, ALCOHOLISM, CORRECTIONS, MEXICAN AMERICAN, ADULTS, EMPIRICAL, CROSS CULTURAL, BEHAVIOR MODIFICATION
ABST   AN EXPERIMENTAL PROGRAM FOR VOLUNTARY TREATMENT WITH A NONPENAL REHABILITATIVE SETTING FOR THE ALCOHOLIC OFFENDER WITH A HISTORY OF MULTIPLE ARRESTS, SENT 191 MEN TO TWO LOS ANGELES COUNTY REHABILITATION CENTERS IN LIEU OF DETENTION AT A SHERIFF'S CLOSED FACILITY. THE CRITERION FOR SUCCESS WAS VOLUNTARY COMPLETION OF A 60-DAY MODIFIED SENTENCE AND PARTICIPATION IN THE REHABILITATION CENTER TREATMENT PROGRAMS. ALL WERE CHRONIC ALCOHOLIC OFFENDERS, WITH THE TYPICAL OFFENDER HAVING BETWEEN 60 AND 70 ARRESTS. THE MEN

INCLUDED A GREATER PERCENTAGE OF MINORITY GROUP MEMBERS THAN THE GENERAL POPULATION, AND THE SPANISH-SPEAKING MINORITY HAD THE BEST SUCCESS RATE. SUCCESS OR FAILURE IN THE STUDY WAS NOT RELATED TO EITHER EDUCATION OR INTELLIGENCE. YOUNGER MEN DID NOT DO WELL IN THE PROGRAM, BUT AFTER 40, AGE WAS NOT A SIGNIFICANT FACTOR IN CONTRIBUTING TO SUCCESS OR FAILURE. DESPITE THEIR CHRONICITY AND RESISTANCE TO OTHER FORMS OF TREATMENT, 64% OF MEN OVER AGE 40 SHOWED FAVORABLE SIGNS OF RESPONSE TO THE NONPENAL REHABILITATIVE SETTING. THE RESULTS HAVE IMPLICATIONS FOR TREATMENT OF THE ALCOHOLIC OFFENDER IN VIEW OF RECENT COURT DECISIONS WHICH REGARD SUCH PERSONS AS DISABLED OR DISORDERED INDIVIDUALS RATHER THAN LAWBREAKERS. 13 REFERENCES.
ACCN   001489

1722 AUTH   **SNARR, R. W., & BALL, J. C.**
TITL   INVOLVEMENT IN A DRUG SUBCULTURE AND ABSTINENCE FOLLOWING TREATMENT AMONG PUERTO RICAN NARCOTIC ADDICTS.
SRCE   *BRITISH JOURNAL OF ADDICTION, 1974, 69(3), 243-248.*
INDX   DRUG ABUSE, DRUG ADDICTION, PUERTO RICAN-I, SES, REHABILITATION, PEER GROUP, PSYCHOSOCIAL ADJUSTMENT, PERFORMANCE EXPECTATIONS, MALE
ABST   THE RESULTS OF A FOLLOW-UP STUDY OF 108 MALE NATIVE PUERTO RICAN OPIATE ADDICTS INDICATED THAT 38% OF THOSE WITH LITTLE INVOLVEMENT IN A DRUG SUBCULTURE WERE CURED, WHEREAS ONLY 10% OF THOSE WITH EXTENSIVE INVOLVEMENT WERE CURED. FURTHER ANALYSIS SHOWED THAT INVOLVEMENT IN A SUBCULTURE AMONG THOSE WHO BEGAN OPIATE USE BY THE AGE OF 20 OR BEFORE HAD LITTLE RELATIONSHIP TO BEING CURED, BUT INVOLVEMENT AMONG THOSE WHO BEGAN OPIATE USE AT AGE 21 OR OVER WAS HIGHLY RELATED TO BEING CURED. THESE FINDINGS INDICATE DIFFERENCES IN SOME BASIC SOCIAL DIMENSIONS AMONG A RELATIVELY HOMOGENEOUS SAMPLE OF ADDICTS AND SUGGEST FACTORS WHICH MIGHT BE USEFUL CONSIDERATIONS FOR SUCCESSFUL TREATMENT. 10 REFERENCES. (PASAR ABSTRACT)
ACCN   001490

1723 AUTH   **SNIBBE, H. M., FABRICATORE, J., AZEN, S. P., & SNIBBE, J. R.**
TITL   RACE DIFFERENCES IN POLICE PATROLMEN: A FAILURE TO REPLICATE THE CHICAGO STUDY.
SRCE   *AMERICAN JOURNAL OF COMMUNITY PSYCHOLOGY, 1976, 4(2), 155-160.*
INDX   STRESS, MEXICAN AMERICAN, CROSS CULTURAL, TEST RELIABILITY, PERSONALITY ASSESSMENT, JOB PERFORMANCE, CALIFORNIA, SOUTHWEST, URBAN, ADULTS, PERSONNEL, EMPIRICAL, MALE, POLICE-COMMUNITY RELATIONS, TEST VALIDITY
ABST   TWO PSYCHOLOGICAL QUESTIONNAIRES AND A PRESSURE TOLERANCE TEST WERE ADMIN-

ISTERED TO 425 WHITE, 32 BLACK, AND 34 MEXICAN AMERICAN LOS ANGELES COUNTY SHERIFF'S DEPARTMENT (LASD) PATROLMEN. THE TESTS CONSISTED OF: (1) THE PERSONAL HISTORY INDEX, WHICH ATTEMPTS TO PREDICT JOB SUCCESS ON THE BASIS OF REPORTED PAST PERFORMANCE AND EXPERIENCE; (2) THE CREE QUESTIONNAIRE, WHICH ASSESSES ASPECTS OF TEMPERAMENT AND PERSONALITY DISTINGUISHING CREATIVE FROM NON-CREATIVE INDIVIDUALS; AND (3) THE PRESS TEST, WHICH MEASURES ABILITY TO WORK UNDER STRESS. RESULTS WERE COMPARED TO THOSE OBTAINED FROM IDENTICAL INSTRUMENTS ADMINISTERED TO 358 WHITE AND 154 BLACK CHICAGO POLICE DEPARTMENT (CPD) PATROLMEN. SIGNIFICANT DIFFERENCES BETWEEN ETHNIC GROUPS WERE NOT FOUND IN THE LASD SAMPLE, WHICH CONTRADICTED THE RESULTS OF THE CPD STUDY. WHEN COMPARED TO THE CPD OFFICERS, LASD PATROLMEN TENDED TO SCORE SIGNIFICANTLY HIGHER ON MOST TEST SCALES. THE GOAL OF ESTABLISHING NATIONWIDE SELECTION CRITERIA FOR PATROLMEN WAS JUDGED UNREALISTIC, AND CAUTION IS ADVISED IN OVERGENERALIZING FROM SINGLE SAMPLE RESULTS. 7 REFERENCES. (AUTHOR ABSTRACT MODIFIED)

ACCN   002209

1724 AUTH   **SOLIS, F.**
TITL   SOCIOECONOMIC AND CULTURAL CONDITIONS OF MIGRANT WORKERS.
SRCE   *IN M. MANGOLD (ED.), LA CAUSA CHICANA: THE MOVEMENT FOR JUSTICE. NEW YORK: FAMILY SERVICE ASSOCIATION OF AMERICA, 1971, PP. 179-191.*
INDX   SES, CULTURAL FACTORS, MIGRATION, FARM LABORERS, MEXICAN AMERICAN, ESSAY, EMPLOYMENT, HISTORY, HEALTH DELIVERY SYSTEMS, SOCIAL SERVICES, RURAL, MIGRANTS
ABST   THE MAJOR SOCIOECONOMIC AND CULTURAL CHARACTERISTICS OF MEXICAN ORIGIN FARMWORKERS ARE DESCRIBED IN ORDER TO UNDERSTAND FARMWORKERS' EFFORTS TO UTILIZE SERVICES AND MOBILIZE THEIR COMMUNITY. HISTORICAL OVERVIEWS OF FARM LABOR IN THE U.S. AND UNIONIZATION EFFORTS OF AGRICULTURAL WORKERS ARE PROVIDED. THE MIGRATORY CONDITIONS OF FAMILIES DEPENDENT UPON FARM LABOR FOR SURVIVAL NECESSITATE SOCIAL SERVICES, ESPECIALLY PUBLIC ASSISTANCE AND PUBLIC HEALTH. IN THE PAST, THESE SERVICES HAVE TENDED TO BE MINIMAL AND FUNDING UNCERTAIN. IT IS THE TASK OF SOCIAL WORK, THROUGH ITS ADVOCACY PROGRAMS, TO RECOGNIZE THE STATUS OF FARM LABORERS AND PROVIDE THE NECESSARY MECHANISMS FOR SOCIAL CHANGE. 3 REFERENCES.

ACCN   001492

1725 AUTH   **SOLOMON, D., ALI, F. A., KFIR, D., HOULIHAN, K. A., & YAEGER, J.**
TITL   THE DEVELOPMENT OF DEMOCRATIC VALUES AND BEHAVIOR AMONG MEXICAN AMERICAN CHILDREN.

SRCE   *CHILD DEVELOPMENT, 1972, 43(2), 625-638.*
INDX   COOPERATION, VALUES, MEXICAN AMERICAN, CHILDREN, EMPIRICAL, ILLINOIS, MIDWEST
ABST   AN INVESTIGATION TO DETERMINE THE AGE AT WHICH DEMOCRATIC VALUES AND BEHAVIOR ARE ESTABLISHED AND REFLECTED WITHIN THE VALUE SYSTEM OF MEXICAN AMERICAN (MA) CHILDREN IS PRESENTED. VALUES ON EQUALITY OF REPRESENTATION, EQUALITY OF PARTICIPATION, EQUALITY OF RESOURCE DISTRIBUTION, ASSERTION, AND COMPROMISE WERE ASSESSED IN INTERVIEWS WITH 174 MA CHILDREN IN GRADES TWO, FOUR, FIVE, SIX, AND EIGHT. BEHAVIORAL REPRESENTATIONS OF THE SAME FIVE VALUES WERE MEASURED IN FOUR-PERSON, GROUP PROBLEM-SOLVING AND DART THROWING SESSIONS. DATA INDICATE THAT THE RESPONSES TO QUESTIONS REPRESENTING FOUR OF THE FIVE DEMOCRATIC VALUES SHOW DISTINCT INCREASES ACROSS GRADES. RESPONSES REFLECTING ASSERTION AND EQUALITY OF PARTICIPATION BEGAN TO INCREASE IN THE MIDDLE ELEMENTARY GRADES, WHILE COMPROMISE AND EQUALITY OF REPRESENTATION DID NOT INCREASE SUBSTANTIALLY UNTIL THE LATE ELEMENTARY GRADES. THE ONLY CLEAR GRADE EFFECT ON GROUP BEHAVIOR WAS OBTAINED FOR THE MEASURE OF RESOURCE DISTRIBUTION, WHICH BECAME MORE EQUALITARIAN WITH INCREASING GRADE. IT IS SUGGESTED THAT THE DIFFERENCES IN TRENDS FOR DEMOCRATIC VALUES AND BEHAVIOR ARE THE PRODUCTS OF TWO DISTINCT AND SEPARATE LEARNING PROCESSES. DEMOCRATIC FORMS OF BEHAVIOR MAY BE LEARNED RELATIVELY EARLY, AND THIS LEARNING MAY OCCUR LONG BEFORE THE VALUE-RELATED VERBAL JUSTIFICATIONS FOR THE SAME TYPES OF BEHAVIORS ARE ACQUIRED. 28 REFERENCES.

ACCN   001493

1726 AUTH   **SOMERS, B. J.**
TITL   PSYCHOLOGY EDUCATION AND MENTAL HEALTH SERVICES IN CUBA IN 1968.
SRCE   *AMERICAN PSYCHOLOGIST, 1969, 24, 940-943.*
INDX   CUBAN, MENTAL HEALTH PROFESSION, PROFESSIONAL TRAINING, HEALTH DELIVERY SYSTEMS, POLITICS, CULTURAL CHANGE, HIGHER EDUCATION, MENTAL HEALTH, CURRICULUM, ESSAY
ABST   OBSERVATIONS OF THE TEACHING AND PRACTICE OF PSYCHOLOGY AND THE STATUS OF MENTAL HEALTH SERVICES IN CUBA ARE REPORTED IN THE CONTEXT OF THE ONGOING CUBAN REVOLUTION. ALTHOUGH PSYCHOLOGY HAD FORMERLY BEEN VIEWED AS AN ESOTERIC FIELD OF STUDY, SINCE 1959 PSYCHOLOGISTS HAVE BEEN EMPLOYED AT THE UNIVERSITY ON A FULLTIME BASIS, RECEIVE HIGH PAY, AND STUDY PROBLEMS THAT ARE OF MAJOR CONCERN TO SOCIETY AS A WHOLE—SUCH AS TRUANCY AND RURAL-URBAN MIGRATION. PSYCHOLOGY IS TAUGHT IN AN ECLECTIC FASHION, WITH STUDENTS MATRICULATING IN A LIBERAL ARTS CURRICULUM, PARTICIPATING IN FIELD ACTIVITIES, AND SPENDING A FIFTH YEAR IN ONE CHOSEN SPE-

CIALTY. A DESCRIPTION OF MENTAL HEALTH SERVICES ON THE LOCAL AND NATIONAL LEVELS IS GIVEN, PARTICULARLY OF ONE LARGE CUSTODIAL HOSPITAL FOR CHRONIC PATIENTS. ALTHOUGH NATIONAL PRIORITIES DO NOT PLACE PRIMARY EMPHASIS ON TRADITIONAL PSYCHOLOGY AND MENTAL HEALTH SERVICES, THE REORGANIZATION OF THE UNIVERSITY AND THE UPGRADING OF MENTAL HEALTH FACILITIES HAS BEEN TO THE ADVANTAGE OF PSYCHOLOGY AS A WHOLE.

ACCN   002210

1727 AUTH   **SOMMER, G.**
TITL   A SHORT-TERM STUDY OF ELOPEMENT FROM A STATE HOSPITAL.
SRCE   *JOURNAL OF COMMUNITY PSYCHOLOGY, 1974, 2(1), 60-62.*
INDX   MENTAL HEALTH, CROSS CULTURAL, PUERTO RICAN-M, EMPIRICAL, INSTITUTIONALIZATION, SEX COMPARISON, PSYCHOPATHOLOGY, NEW YORK, EAST, MALE
ABST   THIS STUDY ATTEMPTED TO CHARCTERIZE THE TYPICAL PATIENT WHO ELOPES FROM BRONX (NEW YORK) STATE HOSPITAL AND ALSO EXAMINED THE NATURE OF HIS/HER UNCONSENTED LEAVE. A GROUP OF 70 PATIENTS WHO ELOPED DURING ONE MONTH WAS COMPARED TO A GROUP OF 105 PATIENTS DISCHARGED DURING THAT MONTH AND TO A GROUP OF 224 PATIENTS GRANTED HOME LEAVE DURING THE SAME MONTH. ALL PATIENTS IN THE 3 GROUPS SHARED A WILLINGNESS AND ABILITY TO LEAVE THE HOSPITAL. THOSE VARIABLES WHICH DISTINGUISHED SIGNIFICANTLY BETWEEN THOSE WHO ELOPED AND THOSE ON PASS OR DISCHARGED WERE AGE, ETHNIC GROUP, PREVIOUS ADMISSIONS, AND PREVIOUS ELOPEMENTS. ELOPERS WERE MORE LIKELY TO BE MALE, PUERTO RICAN, BETWEEN 20 AND 29 YEARS OF AGE, AND TO HAVE HAD A PREVIOUS ADMISSION AND A PREVIOUS LEAVE WITHOUT CONSENT. TWO IMPORTANT FINDINGS ARE CITED: (1) THE GREAT MAJORITY OF PATIENTS WHO LEFT WITHOUT CONSENT RETURNED, USUALLY WITHIN A SHORT TIME; AND (2) MOST LEAVES WITHOUT CONSENT OCCURRED OVER OR PARTIALLY OVER A WEEKEND. 1 REFERENCE. (PASAR ABSTRACT MODIFIED)
ACCN   001494

1728 AUTH   **SOMMERS, V. S.**
TITL   THE IMPACT OF DUAL-CULTURAL MEMBERSHIP ON IDENTITY.
SRCE   *PSYCHIATRY, 1964, 27(4), 332-344.*
INDX   CULTURAL PLURALISM, ETHNIC IDENTITY, CASE STUDY, PUERTO RICAN-M, SELF CONCEPT, PSYCHOTHERAPY, MEXICAN AMERICAN, MALE, ADULTS, CULTURAL FACTORS, PSYCHOSOCIAL ADJUSTMENT, PERSONALITY, ACCULTURATION
ABST   AN INVESTIGATION OF THE IMPACT OF DUAL CULTURAL MEMBERSHIP ON IDENTITY IS PRESENTED THROUGH FOUR REPRESENTATIVE CASE STUDIES. THE EXAMINATION FOCUSES ON THE INTIMATE INTERDEPENDENCE AND CROSS INFLUENCE OF PSYCHOLOGICAL AND SOCIOCULTURAL PROCESSES IN PERSONALITY FUNCTIONING, PARTICULARLY WITH REGARD TO IDENTITY DISORDERS AND THE MANNER IN WHICH A DEPRECIATED SELF-IMAGE CAN BECOME THE KEYSTONE OF AN ENTIRE DEFENSE SYSTEM. THE CASES WERE AS FOLLOWS: (1) RODRIGO THE "ALL AMERICAN BOY" IMPOSTER; (2) A STRUGGLE WITH INCOMPATIBLE IDENTITIES, A JEWISH INDIVIDUAL; (3) A FLIGHT FROM AN IDENTITY OF BLACK AND WHITE, A STUDY OF PABLO, A PUERTO RICAN NEGRO; AND (4) A PSYCHOCULTURAL NEUROSIS, A STUDY OF AN ORIENTAL PERSON. A BRIEF DISCUSSION OF THE COMMON FACTORS THAT AFFLICTED THESE MEN IS PRESENTED, TOGETHER WITH THE GENERAL TYPES OF EGO IDEALS THAT RANGE FROM REALITY-ADJUSTED CHOICES THROUGH EXTREMELY UNREALISTIC MODEL CHOICES. THERE ARE THREE SOURCES OF IDENTITY DISORDERS WHICH MUST BE CONSIDERED AND DEALT WITH IF PSYCHOTHERAPEUTIC EFFORTS ARE TO SUCCEED: (1) THE SENSE OF IDENTITY THAT A PERSON FORMS DEPENDS LARGELY UPON HOW PERSONAL NEEDS ARE SATISFIED IN HIS EARLY LIFE AND HOW HE IS THOUGHT OF BY HIS PARENTS AND OTHER SIGNIFICANT PEOPLE IN HIS FAMILY; (2) HOW THE PARENTAL OBJECTS ARE THOUGHT OF AND VALUED BY THE INFLUENTIAL MAJORITY GROUP; AND (3) THE INNER CONFUSION ENGENDERED BY CONFLICTING LOYALTIES. ONCE FREED FROM THIS "IDENTITY NEUROSIS," THESE MEN CAN NOW ENJOY A NEW-FOUND SENSE OF BELONGING WITH THEIR OWN FAMILY AND THEIR PARENTAL HERITAGE, AS WELL AS A BELONGING TO THE COUNTRY AND CULTURE OF THEIR BIRTH. 11 REFERENCES.
ACCN   001495

1729 AUTH   **SONGUIST, H.**
TITL   A MODEL FOR LOW-INCOME AND CHICANO PARENT EDUCATION (REPORT NO. OCD-CB-127 (2)).
SRCE   *WASHINGTON, D.C.: CHILDRENS BUREAU, DEPARTMENT OF HEALTH, EDUCATION AND WELFARE, 1975. (ERIC DOCUMENT REPRODUCTION SERVICE NO. ED 113 063)*
INDX   MODELING, SES, MEXICAN AMERICAN, ADULT EDUCATION, PARENTAL INVOLVEMENT, SOCIAL SERVICES, RESOURCE UTILIZATION, INSTRUCTIONAL TECHNIQUES, CHILDREN, MOTHER-CHILD INTERACTION, CHILDREARING PRACTICES, FEMALE
ABST   DESIGNED PRIMARILY FOR LOW-INCOME MEXICAN AMERICAN FAMILIES, THE PROGRAM'S GOALS WERE TO: (1) EXPAND THE MOTHER'S SKILL AND KNOWLEDGE OF CHILDREARING PRACTICES AND THEIR DAILY USE; (2) DEVELOP HER SELF-CONFIDENCE AND PERCEIVED ABILITY TO INFLUENCE HER CHILD'S DEVELOPMENT; (3) INCREASE HER SKILLS IN DEALING WITH HER INSTITUTIONAL ENVIRONMENT; (4) NURTURE HER INVOLVEMENT WITH AND RESPONSIBILITY FOR THE PROGRAM; AND (5) EXPAND HER HUMAN RELATIONS SKILLS AND PREVENTIVE MENTAL HEALTH PRACTICES IN DEALING WITH HER OWN AND HER FAMILY'S NEEDS AND EMOTIONS. TO BEST ACHIEVE

THESE GOALS, A 3-FACETED APPROACH WAS INITIATED WHICH CONSISTED OF A PROGRAM FOR MOTHERS, A CHILDREN'S PROGRAM, AND A SERVICE COMPONENT. FROM JANUARY 1972 TO JUNE 1974, 126 MOTHERS AND 250 CHILDREN PARTICIPATED IN THE PROGRAM. THE PROGRAM WAS EVALUATED TO IDENTIFY THE PARTICIPANTS' SOCIAL AND DEMOGRAPHIC CHARACTERISTICS, THEIR UTILIZATION OF EXISTING COMMUNITY RESOURCES, THEIR ATTITUDES TOWARD THE PROGRAM, AND THE PROGRAM'S IMPACT ON THE MOTHERS' CHILD-REARING REPERTOIRE AND SELF-CONCEPTS. SOME DATA WERE COLLECTED ON A COMPARISON GROUP, CONSISTING OF MOTHERS WHOSE CHILDREN PARTICIPATED IN THE 1972-73 AND 1973-74 HEADSTART PROGRAM. OVERALL, IT WAS FOUND THAT MOTHERS INCREASED THEIR PARTICIPATION AND SENSE OF RESPONSIBILITY AT THE CENTRO, HAD BETTER RESOURCES AND SKILLS TO SOLVE THEIR PROBLEMS, AND VALUED THEIR CHILD'S AND THEIR OWN LEARNING PROCESS. THIS REPORT DISCUSSES THE PROGRAM'S GOALS, PROGRESS, AND EVALUATION. 63 REFERENCES. (ERIC ABSTRACT)

ACCN   001496

1730 AUTH   **SOTOMAYOR, M.**
TITL   LANGUAGE, CULTURE, AND ETHNICITY IN DEVELOPING SELF-CONCEPT.
SRCE   *SOCIAL CASEWORK, 1977, 58(4), 195-203.*
INDX   ESSAY, SELF CONCEPT, LINGUISTICS, CULTURE, SOCIALIZATION, ACCULTURATION, ETHNIC IDENTITY, MEXICAN AMERICAN, COGNITIVE DEVELOPMENT, ENVIRONMENTAL FACTORS, COPING MECHANISMS, PSYCHOSOCIAL ADJUSTMENT
ABST   SOME PHILOSOPHICAL AND THEORETICAL UNDERPINNINGS OF LANGUAGE, CULTURE, AND ETHNICITY ARE TRACED TO DETERMINE THEIR IMPACT ON HUMAN BEHAVIOR. THE ROLE OF LANGUAGE AND CULTURE IN THE MENTAL PROCESSES WHICH DETERMINE PERCEPTIONS AND DEFINITIONS OF REALITY ARE EMPHASIZED. SPECIAL ATTENTION IS GIVEN TO THE CHICANO, FOR WHOM LANGUAGE, CULTURE, AND ETHNICITY PLAY A MAJOR ROLE IN THE DEVELOPMENT OF COGNITIVE SKILLS AND COPING PATTERNS. THE COLONIZED STATUS OF THIS GROUP, AFFECTED BY EXTERNAL ECONOMIC AND POLITICAL FACTORS (E.G., POVERTY, RACISM, POOR NUTRITION, LOW EDUCATIONAL ATTAINMENT), IS AN IMPORTANT VARIABLE IN UNDERSTANDING THE DEVELOPMENT AND SELECTION OF COPING PATTERNS, BEHAVIOR PATTERNS, AND SELF-CONCEPT. 29 REFERENCES.

ACCN   001497

1731 AUTH   **SOTOMAYOR, M.**
TITL   MEXICAN AMERICAN INTERACTION WITH SOCIAL SYSTEMS.
SRCE   *IN M. MANGOLD (ED.), LA CAUSA CHICANA: THE MOVEMENT FOR JUSTICE. NEW YORK: FAMILY SERVICE ASSOCIATION OF AMERICA, 1971, PP. 148-160.*
INDX   MEXICAN AMERICAN, ESSAY, DISCRIMINATION,

ENVIRONMENTAL FACTORS, CULTURAL FACTORS, STEREOTYPES, FAMILY STRUCTURE
ABST   WEAKNESSES FORMERLY ATTRIBUTED TO THE DYNAMICS OF MEXICAN AMERICAN (MA) FAMILIES ARE SHOWN TO RESULT FROM THE LIMITATIONS CREATED BY THE EXTERNAL SOCIAL SYSTEMS. HOW THESE LIMITATIONS AFFECT THE INTERNAL INTEGRATION OF THE FAMILY UNIT IS ALSO ILLUSTRATED. THE SOCIALIZATION PROCESS HAS BEEN DELEGATED TO OUTSIDE INSTITUTIONS OF SOCIETY. THESE INSTITUTIONS ARE DESCRIBED AS MAINTAINING RACIST POLICIES THAT SYSTEMATICALLY EXCLUDE MA'S FROM ACTIVE PARTICIPATION IN COMMUNITY ACTIVITIES. THUS MA FAMILIES ARE DENIED A POSITIVE STATUS AND IDENTITY. THEY ARE LEFT WITH A FEELING OF ALIENATION, MARGINALITY, AND ANOMIE. THESE CONDITIONS PLACE THE MA FAMILIES IN A POSITION WHERE THEY ARE UNABLE TO REORGANIZE AND MOBILIZE THEIR INTERNAL RESOURCES TO DEAL WITH THE DESTRUCTIVE EXTERNAL SYSTEMS. IT IS SUGGESTED THAT SOCIOCULTURAL STRENGTHS OF THE MA FAMILY BE IDENTIFIED, EVALUATED, AND SUPPORTED. SPECIFIC SUPPORTIVE ELEMENTS ARE THE EXTENDED FAMILY PATTERN, RESPECT FOR THE AGED, FAMILY ROLE PATTERNS, THE BARRIO, AND THE USE OF THE SPANISH LANGUAGE. FURTHERMORE, DESTRUCTIVE EXTERNAL FORCES SHOULD BE CHANGED THROUGH SOCIAL WORK INTERVENTION, OPEN FORUM DISCUSSIONS ON THE CONSEQUENCES OF RACISM, DECENTRALIZATION OF THE FUNCTIONS OF THE GOVERNMENT, AND BY THE SELF-HELP PROCESS CHARACTERISTIC OF THE CHICANO MOVEMENT. 10 REFERENCES.

ACCN   001498

1732 AUTH   **SOUFLEE, F.**
TITL   HEALTH PERCEPTIONS IN THE CHICANO COMMUNITY.
SRCE   *PAPER PRESENTED AT THE NATIONAL CONFERENCE ON SOCIAL WELFARE, SAN FRANCISCO, MAY 11-15, 1975. (AVAILABLE FROM THE AUTHOR, CHICANO TRAINING CENTER, HOUSTON, TEXAS.)*
INDX   SOCIAL SERVICES, MEXICAN AMERICAN, HEALTH DELIVERY SYSTEMS, BILINGUAL-BICULTURAL PERSONNEL, CURANDERISMO, FOLK MEDICINE, CULTURE, ESSAY, DISEASE, HEALTH
ABST   A BILINGUAL-BICULTURAL APPROACH TO MENTAL HEALTH AND SOCIAL SERVICES TO CHICANOS AS APPLIED TO HEALTH PERCEPTIONS IN THE CHICANO COMMUNITY IS PRESENTED. CHICANO COMMUNITIES MAINTAIN PRESCIENTIFIC HEALTH THEORIES AND PRACTICES, AND CULTURAL ISOLATION AND LACK OF ENVIRONMENTAL SUPPORT ACCOUNT FOR THE PREVALENCE OF FOLK HEALING METHODS. CURANDERISMO, AS A COMBINATION OF HEALING AND WORSHIP, IS DISCUSSED AS A PSEUDOSCIENTIFIC APPROACH TO ALL AILMENTS. CURANDERISMO MUST BE UNDERSTOOD AND APPRECIATED BY HEALTH AND WELFARE SERVICES FOR THE SUCCESSFUL DELIVERY OF HEALTH CARE TO THE CHICANO COMMUNITY. 17 REFERENCES.

ACCN   001499

1733 AUTH **SPALDING, N.**
TITL   LEARNING PROBLEMS OF MEXICAN AMERI-
        CANS.
SRCE   *READING IMPROVEMENT, 1970, 7(2), 33-36.*
INDX   MEXICAN AMERICAN, ESSAY, SCHOLASTIC
        ACHIEVEMENT, PSYCHOSOCIAL ADJUSTMENT,
        EDUCATION, HIGHER EDUCATION, COLLEGE
        STUDENTS, TIME ORIENTATION
ABST   PSYCHOSOCIAL FACTORS PERTINENT TO
        LEARNING PROBLEMS OF MEXICAN AMERI-
        CANS ARE DISCUSSED. MEXICAN AMERICANS
        FACE AN INTENSIFIED FAILURE-PRODUCING
        SYSTEM WHEN THEY ATTEMPT COLLEGE. THEY
        KNOW THEIR GRAMMAR AND ACCENT ARE
        NONSTANDARD AND THEY ARE INHIBITED
        ABOUT PARTICIPATING IN CLASSROOM DIS-
        CUSSIONS FOR FEAR OF RIDICULE. SOME
        HAVE A TENDENCY TO ATTEND CLASSES IR-
        REGULARLY, TO BE TARDY, AND TO HAND IN
        ASSIGNMENTS LATE. A MULTITUDE OF REA-
        SONS LIE BEHIND THESE LAST THREE BEHAV-
        IORS, BUT IN COMMON IS THE FACT THAT MEX-
        ICAN AMERICANS OFTEN DO NOT HAVE THE
        TIME SENSE THAT IS EXPECTED OF THEM.
        TEACHERS CAN DO MUCH TO HELP THESE
        STUDENTS IF THEY DECIDE THEIR MAIN JOB IS
        TO TEACH THEM THE SUBJECTS THEY CAME
        TO COLLEGE TO LEARN, AND NOT TO WASTE
        TIME ATTEMPTING TO MAKE THEIR TIME
        SCHEDULING AND STUDY HABITS CONFORM
        TO STANDARDS OTHER THAN THEIR OWN.
        THESE STUDENTS NEED FRIENDSHIP FROM
        BOTH FACULTY AND STUDENTS. COUNSELING,
        TUTORING, AND REMEDIAL READING AND
        WRITING MEASURES MUST ALSO BE EM-
        PLOYED.
ACCN   001500

1734 AUTH **SPECIAL POPULATIONS SUB-TASK PANEL ON
        MENTAL HEALTH OF HISPANIC AMERICANS.**
TITL   HISPANIC MENTAL HEALTH: REPORT TO THE
        PRESIDENT'S COMMISSION ON MENTAL HEALTH.
SRCE   *LOS ANGELES: SPANISH SPEAKING MENTAL
        HEALTH RESEARCH CENTER, 1978.*
INDX   POLICY, HEALTH DELIVERY SYSTEMS, MENTAL
        HEALTH, HEALTH, SPANISH SURNAMED, MEXI-
        CAN AMERICAN, PUERTO RICAN-M, PRIMARY
        PREVENTION, MENTAL HEALTH PROFESSION,
        CULTURAL FACTORS, PROGRAM EVALUATION,
        BILINGUAL-BICULTURAL PERSONNEL, FINANC-
        ING, CROSS CULTURAL, REVIEW
ABST   BEGINNING WITH A SUMMARY OF THE MENTAL
        HEALTH STATUS OF HISPANIC AMERICANS, THIS
        REPORT PRESENTS 28 RECOMMENDATIONS
        FOR THE IMPROVEMENT OF RESEARCH, DELIV-
        ERY OF MENTAL HEALTH SERVICES, AND PRE-
        VENTION PROGRAMS. THE RAPIDLY GROWING
        HISPANIC POPULATION IS HETEROGENEOUS,
        AS IT VARIES WIDELY IN NATIONAL ORIGIN,
        RACE, DEMOGRAPHIC DIMENSIONS, AND CUL-
        TURAL/LINGUISTIC CHARACTERISTICS. HIS-
        PANIC GROUPS HAVE MAINTAINED THEIR LAN-
        GUAGE, CULTURAL HERITAGE, AND ETHNIC
        IDENTITY; AND PERHAPS DUE TO THIS FAILURE
        TO "ASSIMILATE," THEY HAVE BEEN DENIED AN
        EQUITABLE SHARE OF THE NATION'S RE-

SOURCES AND OPPORTUNITIES, INCLUDING
ADEQUATE HEALTH AND MENTAL HEALTH CARE.
THE INCREASED PARTICIPATION OF THIS
POPULATION IN NATIONAL HEALTH POLICY DE-
SIGN IS THE SINGLE MOST IMPORTANT ELE-
MENT IN THE IMPROVEMENT OF HISPANIC
MENTAL HEALTH. 91 REFERENCES.
ACCN   002211

1735 AUTH **SPEISS, J. M., & SPEISS, M. L.**
TITL   REINFORCED READINESS REQUISITES: A CUL-
        TURALLY RELEVANT BEHAVIOR MODIFICATION
        PROGRAM FOR MEXICAN AMERICAN, INDIAN,
        AND BLACK CHILDREN.
SRCE   *PROCEEDINGS OF THE 81ST ANNUAL CONVEN-
        TION, AMERICAN PSYCHOLOGICAL ASSOCIA-
        TION, 1973. 8(2), 639-640.*
INDX   BEHAVIOR MODIFICATION, MEXICAN AMERI-
        CAN, CROSS CULTURAL, INSTRUCTIONAL
        TECHNIQUES, ATTITUDES, SCHOLASTIC
        ACHIEVEMENT, CHILDREN, SEX COMPARISON,
        READING, PROCEEDINGS
ABST   THE "REINFORCED READINESS REQUISITES"
        PROGRAM WAS DESIGNED AS A CULTURALLY
        RELEVANT MEANS OF INSTILLING MOTIVATION
        IN MINORITY SCHOOL CHILDREN. IT EMPLOYS
        BEHAVIOR MODIFICATION STRATEGIES DI-
        RECTED TOWARD THE ACQUISITION OF SKILLS
        NECESSARY FOR OPTIMAL LEARNING. TWO 36-
        WEEK FIELD TESTS WERE CONDUCTED ON
        2,963 CHILDREN IN RURAL AND URBAN AREAS
        IN THE SOUTHWEST. SUBJECTS WERE 3 TO 7
        YEARS-OLD, AND THE PREPONDERANT MA-
        JORITY WERE MEXICAN AMERICAN, NATIVE
        AMERICAN, AND BLACK. AN EXPERIMENTAL
        GROUP OF 1,242 SUBJECTS WAS ADMINIS-
        TERED THE PROGRAM, WHILE THE REMAINING
        787 SUBJECTS DID NOT RECEIVE THE PRO-
        GRAM AND SERVED AS A CONTROL GROUP.
        LESSONS WERE PRESENTED ON VISUAL DIS-
        CRIMINATION, ASSOCIATIVE VOCABULARY,
        AURAL DISCRIMINATION, LISTENING, AND NU-
        MERICAL CONCEPTS. CULTURALLY UNFAMIL-
        IAR MATERIAL WAS DELETED. REWARDS—GIVEN
        ON THE BASIS OF GROUP RATHER THAN INDI-
        VIDUAL ACHIEVEMENT—WERE INITIALLY PRO-
        VIDED ON A CONTINUOUS REINFORCEMENT
        SCHEDULE. THIS WAS FOLLOWED BY INTER-
        MITTENT REWARDS, TOKEN REINFORCEMENT,
        AND THEN A GRADUAL TAPERING OFF UNTIL
        DESIRED PERFORMANCE WAS MAINTAINED
        THROUGH SUBJECTS' OWN MOTIVATION AND
        TEACHER PRAISE. RESULTS WERE THAT: (1)
        THE EXPERIMENTAL GROUP SHOWED A SUB-
        STANTIALLY HIGHER GAIN THAN THE CONTROL
        GROUP IN READING READINESS AND RELATED
        ENTRY LEVEL SKILL BEHAVIORS; (2) THE EX-
        PERIMENTAL GROUP MAINTAINED THEIR PER-
        FORMANCE IN THE ABSENCE OF TANGIBLE RE-
        WARDS; (3) THE PROGRAM WAS EQUALLY
        EFFECTIVE FOR BOYS AND GIRLS AND FOR ALL
        THREE ETHNIC GROUPS; AND (4) TEACHERS
        FELT POSITIVELY ABOUT THE PROGRAM, SEEING
        IT AS A SYSTEMATIC WAY OF ACCOMPLISHING
        DESIRED TEACHING GOALS. 4 REFERENCES.
ACCN   001508

1736 AUTH **SPENCE, A. G., MISHRA, S. P., & GHOZEIL, S.**

TITL HOME LANGUAGE AND PERFORMANCE ON STANDARDIZED TESTS.

SRCE *ELEMENTARY SCHOOL JOURNAL, 1971, 71(6), 309-313.*

INDX LANGUAGE ACQUISITION, EMPIRICAL, MEXICAN AMERICAN, CHILDREN, SCHOLASTIC ACHIEVEMENT, BILINGUAL, ABILITY TESTING, METROPOLITAN READINESS TEST, STANFORD-BINET INTELLIGENCE TEST, WISC, ARIZONA, SOUTHWEST

ABST A SAMPLE OF 146 SIX YEAR-OLD MEXICAN AMERICAN CHILDREN FROM TWELVE ELEMENTARY SCHOOLS IN TUCSON, ARIZONA, WERE EVALUATED TO ASCERTAIN THE RELATIONSHIP BETWEEN HOME LANGUAGE PATTERNS OF PARENTS AND THE CHILDREN'S PERFORMANCE ON A BATTERY OF STANDARDIZED TESTS OF INTELLECTUAL ABILITIES. BASED ON INTERVIEWS WITH BOTH PARENTS OF EACH CHILD, THE FAMILIES WERE DIVIDED INTO TWO GROUPS—99 FAMILIES WHO SPOKE ONLY SPANISH AT HOME AND 47 FAMILIES WHO SPOKE ENGLISH AND SPANISH. THEN THE CHILDREN WERE ADMINISTERED THE METROPOLITAN READINESS TESTS, THE VAN ALSTYNE PICTURE VOCABULARY TEST, AND VOCABULARY SUBTESTS FROM THE STANFORD-BINET AND THE WECHSLER INTELLIGENCE SCALES. FROM THE DATA IT APPEARS THAT THE CHILDREN IN BILINGUAL HOMES HAVE SOME MEASURABLY SIGNIFICANT INTELLECTUAL ADVANTAGES OVER THOSE CHILDREN WHO WERE INSTRUCTED AT HOME IN SPANISH ONLY. NEVERTHELESS, THE TWO GROUPS OF CHILDREN SEEMED INSUFFICIENTLY PREPARED FOR ACADEMIC ACHIEVEMENT AS THEY WERE EQUALLY DISADVANTAGED ON ALL OF THE FOLLOWING ITEMS: (1) KNOWLEDGE OF ENGLISH WORDS; (2) LISTENING ABILITY IN ENGLISH; (3) ABILITY TO MATCH ENGLISH WORDS AND CONCEPTS; (4) USE OF THE ALPHABET; (5) ABILITY TO COPY; AND (6) KNOWLEDGE OF NUMBERS. 7 REFERENCES.

ACCN 001509

1737 AUTH **SPIELBERGER, C. D., GONZALEZ-REIGOSA, F., MARTINEZ-URRUTIA, A, NATALICIO, L. F. S., & NATALICIO, D. S.**

TITL DEVELOPMENT OF THE SPANISH EDITION OF THE STATE-TRAIT ANXIETY INVENTORY.

SRCE *INTERAMERICAN JOURNAL OF PSYCHOLOGY, 1971, 5(3-4), 145-158.*

INDX ANXIETY, TEST RELIABILITY, CROSS CULTURAL, EMPIRICAL, TEST VALIDITY, PUERTO RICAN-I, TEXAS, SOUTHWEST, BILINGUAL, CULTURE-FAIR TESTS

ABST TO CONSTRUCT A-STATE AND A-TRAIT ANXIETY SCALES SUITABLE FOR USE IN INTERAMERICAN CROSS-CULTURAL RESEARCH, THE STATE-TRAIT ANXIETY INVENTORY (STAI) WAS TRANSLATED INTO SPANISH WITH THE ASSISTANCE OF PSYCHOLOGISTS FROM 10 LATIN AMERICAN COUNTRIES. TO EVALUATE TEST RELIABILITY AND EQUIVALENCE OF THE SPANISH AND ENGLISH FORMS, THESE SCALES WERE GIVEN IN COUNTERBALANCED ORDER TO BILINGUAL SUBJECTS IN TEXAS AND PUERTO RICO. IN BOTH SAMPLES, HIGH ITEM-REMAIN-

DER CORRELATIONS AND ALPHA COEFFICIENTS RANGING FROM .82 TO .95 ESTABLISHED THE INTERNAL CONSISTENCY OF THE SPANISH A-STATE AND A-TRAIT SCALES. HIGH RELIABILITY WAS ALSO FOUND FOR THE SPANISH A-TRAIT SCALE BUT NOT THE A-STATE SCALE, WHICH WAS INFLUENCED, AS EXPECTED, BY TRANSITORY SITUATIONAL STRESS. IT IS CONCLUDED THAT THE SPANISH STAI PROVIDES INTERNALLY CONSISTENT AND RELIABLE SCALES FOR MEASURING STATE AND TRAIT ANXIETY, ESSENTIALLY EQUIVALENT TO THE ENGLISH STAI A-STATE AND A-TRAIT SCALES. 17 REFERENCES. (JOURNAL ABSTRACT MODIFIED)

ACCN 002212

1738 AUTH **STANG, D. J.**

TITL HISPANIC PROFESSIONALS DECRY LOW NUMBERS.

SRCE *APA MONITOR, JANUARY 1977, PP. 16.*

INDX REPRESENTATION, MENTAL HEALTH PROFESSION, PROFESSIONAL TRAINING, SPANISH SURNAMED, ESSAY, PROCEEDINGS

ABST REPORTS PRESENTED AT A MEETING AT THE SPANISH SPEAKING MENTAL HEALTH RESEARCH CENTER, UCLA, DOCUMENTED A CONTINUING PATTERN OF SEVERE HISPANIC UNDERREPRESENTATION AT ALL LEVELS OF THE MENTAL HEALTH PROFESSIONS. THIS CRITICAL SHORTAGE IS CONSIDERED TO BE A SIGNIFICANT FACTOR RESPONSIBLE FOR THE LOW QUANTITY AND QUALITY OF MENTAL HEALTH CARE DELIVERED TO HISPANICS. ANALYSES OF CURRENT REPRESENTATION AT TRAINING INSTITUTIONS SUGGEST AN ABSENCE OF SYSTEMATIC EFFORTS TO INCREASE OR EVEN MAINTAIN GRADUATE TRAINING OPPORTUNITIES FOR HISPANICS. A SIZABLE POOL OF QUALIFIED BUT UNFUNDED MINORITY APPLICANTS EXISTS, AND PROFESSIONAL AND GOVERNMENT AGENCIES SHOULD TAKE THE LEAD IN (1) STUDYING THE NEEDS IN HISPANIC MENTAL HEALTH, AND (2) PROMOTING TRAINING OPPORTUNITIES.

ACCN 001510

1739 AUTH **STANG, D. J., & PEELE, D.**

TITL THE STATUS OF MINORITIES IN PSYCHOLOGY.

SRCE *IN E. L. OLMEDO & S. LOPEZ (EDS.), HISPANIC MENTAL HEALTH PROFESSIONALS (MONOGRAPH NO. 5). LOS ANGELES: UNIVERSITY OF CALIFORNIA, SPANISH SPEAKING MENTAL HEALTH RESEARCH CENTER, 1977, PP. 31-42.*

INDX MENTAL HEALTH PROFESSION, REPRESENTATION, PROFESSIONAL TRAINING, EDUCATION, HIGHER EDUCATION, EMPIRICAL, SPANISH SURNAMED, CROSS CULTURAL, COLLEGE STUDENTS, EQUAL OPPORTUNITY

ABST A SPECIAL TASK FORCE OF THE AMERICAN PSYCHOLOGICAL ASSOCIATION (APA) PRESENTS DATA ON MINORITY REPRESENTATION IN GRADUATE PSYCHOLOGY PROGRAMS, FACULTY IN SELECTED PSYCHOLOGY DEPARTMENTS, THE APA MEMBERSHIP, AND THE APA GOVERNANCE STRUCTURE. (1) PROPORTIONATELY, NEARLY TWICE AS MANY BLACKS AND HISPANICS AS ANGLOS DROP OUT OF THE

EDUCATIONAL SYSTEM BEFORE ENTERING COLLEGE. (2) MINORITY REPRESENTATION IN POST-GRADUATE PSYCHOLOGY PROGRAMS INCREASED SUBSTANTIALLY FROM 1955 TO 1972, AND THE COMPLETION OF DOCTORATES BY MINORITIES ALSO INCREASED DURING THIS PERIOD. (3) FROM 1970 TO 1973, MINORITY ENROLLMENT IN GRADUATE PROGRAMS HAS REMAINED STABLE AT APPROXIMATELY 7%. HISPANICS HAVE ACCOUNTED FOR 1.4% OF THE GRADUATE ENROLLMENT IN THIS PERIOD. (4) AMONG SELECTED FIELDS OF STUDY IN PSYCHOLOGY, BLACKS AND HISPANICS HAVE BEEN CONCENTRATED IN COUNSELING PROGRAMS. (5) DATA FROM 1972-1976 REVEAL THAT 95% OF PSYCHOLOGY FACULTY WERE ANGLO. (6) FROM 1969 TO 1976, THE MINORITY REPRESENTATION IN APA TASK FORCES AND COMMITTEES INCREASED FROM 1% TO APPROXIMATELY 10%. (7) IN 1976, THE MINORITY PERCENTAGE OF APA MEMBERSHIP WAS 3%. IN CONCLUSION, IT IS RECOMMENDED THAT TO IMPROVE MINORITY REPRESENTATION IN PSYCHOLOGY THERE SHOULD BE MORE FINANCIAL ASSISTANCE FOR MINORITIES (THROUGH NIMH AND APA CO-SPONSORED MINORITY FELLOWSHIPS) AND THE FORMATION OF APA TASK FORCES AND COMMITTEES SPECIFICALLY CONCERNED WITH MINORITY REPRESENTATION. 9 REFERENCES.

ACCN   001511

1740 AUTH   **STAPLES, R.**
TITL   THE MEXICAN AMERICAN FAMILY: ITS MODIFICATIONS OVER TIME AND SPACE.
SRCE   *PHYLON, 1971, 32(3), 179-192.*
INDX   MEXICAN AMERICAN, FAMILY STRUCTURE, ACCULTURATION, MIGRATION, ESSAY, VALUES
ABST   AN ANALYSIS OF THE HISTORICAL AND CONTEMPORARY MEXICAN AMERICAN (MA) FAMILY IS PROVIDED FOR A BETTER UNDERSTANDING OF THEIR CULTURAL MANIFESTATIONS. THE MA FAMILY UNIT DIFFERS FROM THE AMERICAN FAMILY IN THAT IT IS EXTENDED TO INCLUDE SUCH RELATIVES AS GRANDPARENTS, GRANDCHILDREN, UNCLES, AUNTS, AND COUSINS. SUCH A UNIT PROVIDES SECURITY IN A HOSTILE AND ALIEN SOCIETY. IN ADDITION, IT PLAYS A PART IN THE CARE OF THE AGED OR UNMARRIED MOTHERS INSTEAD OF PLACING THEM IN COMMUNITY FACILITIES. THE ROLES FOR EACH FAMILY MEMBER ARE SHARPLY DEFINED. THE FATHER IS CONSIDERED THE AUTHORITARIAN FIGURE WHO IS HIGHLY RESPECTED. THE MOTHER IS SUBMISSIVE, FAITHFUL, DEVOTED, AND RESPECTFUL TO HER HUSBAND. THE MOTHER'S MAJOR RESPONSIBILITY IS THE REARING OF CHILDREN. IN MEXICAN HOMES, BOYS AND GIRLS ARE GIVEN A DIFFERENTIAL UPBRINGING, THE BOYS BEING TRAINED FOR THE WORLD, AND THE GIRLS FOR THE HOME. MEXICAN CHILDREN ARE BROUGHT UP WITH AN EMPHASIS ON RESPECT AND AUTHORITY. UNLIKE THE RURAL MA'S WHO ARE CLOSEST TO THE EXTENDED FAMILY PATTERN, THE URBAN MA'S HAVE TAKEN ON THE VALUES OF THE ANGLO-AMERICAN

CULTURE OF A NUCLEAR FAMILY PATTERN. INTEGRATION INTO THE BROADER SOCIETY FREQUENTLY RESULTS IN WEAKENING OF THE MA FAMILY. THE TASK OF MA PARENTS IS TO INCULCATE CULTURAL PRIDE IN THE MEXICAN CHILD. AT THE SAME TIME, THEY MUST ENCOURAGE HIS ACCEPTANCE OF THE SKILLS AND PATTERNS NEEDED TO ADJUST AND TO SURVIVE IN THE LARGER SOCIETY. 16 REFERENCES.

ACCN   001512

1741 AUTH   **STATE UNIVERSITY OF NEW YORK.**
TITL   MINORITY GROUP ENROLLMENT, HOUSING AND FINANCIAL AID STATISTICS: FALL 1969 THROUGH FALL 1971. (REPORT NO. 34)
SRCE   *NEW YORK: CENTRAL STAFF OFFICE OF INSTITUTIONAL RESEARCH, STATE UNIVERSITY OF NEW YORK, 1972.*
INDX   SPANISH SURNAMED, COLLEGE STUDENTS, EQUAL OPPORTUNITY, HIGHER EDUCATION, REPRESENTATION, EMPIRICAL, NEW YORK, EAST
ABST   FIFTEEN TABLES PRESENT STATISTICAL DATA FROM 1969 TO 1971 ON MINORITY STUDENT ENROLLMENT, HOUSING, AND FINANCIAL AID AT 68 INSTITUTIONS UNDER THE PROGRAM OF THE STATE UNIVERSITY OF NEW YORK—UNIVERSITY CENTERS; UNIVERSITY COLLEGES; HEALTH SCIENCE CENTERS; AND SPECIAL, STATUTORY, AGRICULTURAL, TECHNICAL, AND COMMUNITY COLLEGES. DATA FROM 1968 ARE ALSO INCLUDED IN A SUMMARY TABLE. FOUR MINORITY GROUPS ARE REPRESENTED—BLACKS, ORIENTALS, AMERICAN INDIANS, AND SPANISH-SURNAMED AMERICANS. RESULTS SHOW THAT, WITH FEW EXCEPTIONS, THE PERCENTAGE OF MINORITY GROUP ENROLLMENT HAS INCREASED EACH YEAR IN ALL INSTITUTIONS, FROM AN OVERALL ENROLLMENT OF 6.5% IN 1968 TO 12.6% IN 1971. THE NUMBER OF FINANCIAL AWARDS TO MINORITIES INCREASED EACH YEAR, AS DID THE PERCENTAGE OF AWARDS GRANTED THEM. UNIVERSITY-OWNED AND UNIVERSITY-SUPPORTED HOUSING STATISTICS ALSO SHOW SIMILAR OVERALL GAINS. INCLUDED IN AN APPENDIX ARE 33 UNIVERSITY PUBLICATIONS ON STUDENT POPULATION CHARACTERISTICS, ENROLLMENT TRENDS, AND RELATED TOPICS.

ACCN   001513

1742 AUTH   **STATON, R. D.**
TITL   A COMPARISON OF MEXICAN AND MEXICAN-AMERICAN FAMILIES.
SRCE   *THE FAMILY COORDINATOR, 1972, 21(3), 325-330.*
INDX   ACCULTURATION, ATTITUDES, AUTHORITARIANISM, CULTURAL CHANGE, CULTURAL FACTORS, CULTURE, FEMALE, MALE, FAMILY STRUCTURE, FAMILY ROLES, FICTIVE KINSHIP, MEXICAN, MEXICAN AMERICAN, MEXICO, REVIEW, SEX COMPARISON, SEX ROLES
ABST   AN ATTEMPT WAS MADE TO ASCERTAIN SOME OF THE MAJOR FEATURES OF THE MEXICAN FAMILY WHICH HAVE BEEN RETAINED BY THE MEXICAN AMERICAN FAMILY WITHIN THE UNITED STATES. AVAILABLE LITERATURE WHICH COMMENTS ON THE FAMILY SYSTEMS WAS SUR-

VEYED. SUFFICIENT INFORMATION FOR COMPARISONS WAS FOUND CONCERNING MALE-FEMALE RELATIONSHIPS, FAMILY ORGANIZATION, COURTSHIP AND MARRIAGE, HUSBAND-WIFE RELATIONSHIPS, AND PARENT-CHILD RELATIONSHIPS. PRESENT LITERATURE LARGELY PRESENTS ONLY A GENERALIZED VIEW OF BOTH FAMILIES. MANY VARIABLES SUCH AS RELIGION, SOCIAL CLASS, LANGUAGE, EDUCATION, PHYSICAL AND SOCIAL MOBILITY, ACCULTURATION, AND ASSIMILATION ARE NOT APPROPRIATELY CONSIDERED IN THE CASE OF THE MEXICAN AMERICAN FAMILY. 13 REFERENCES. (JOURNAL ABSTRACT)

ACCN 002523

1743 AUTH **STATON, R. D.**
TITL A COMPARISON OF MEXICAN AND MEXICAN-AMERICAN FAMILIES.
SRCE *FAMILY COORDINATOR, 1972, 21(3), 325-330.*
INDX MEXICAN, MEXICAN AMERICAN, FAMILY STRUCTURE, ACCULTURATION, SEX ROLES, FATHER-CHILD INTERACTION, FAMILY ROLES, REVIEW, MARRIAGE, EXTENDED FAMILY, ROLE EXPECTATIONS, MALE
ABST SOME OF THE MAJOR FEATURES OF THE MEXICAN FAMILY WHICH HAVE BEEN RETAINED BY THE MEXICAN AMERICAN FAMILY WITHIN THE UNITED STATES ARE DISCUSSED. AVAILABLE LITERATURE WHICH COMMENTED ON THESE FAMILY SYSTEMS WAS SURVEYED. SUFFICIENT INFORMATION FOR COMPARISONS WAS FOUND CONCERNING MALE-FEMALE RELATIONSHIPS, FAMILY ORGANIZATION, COURTSHIP AND MARRIAGE, HUSBAND-WIFE RELATIONSHIPS, AND PARENT-CHILD RELATIONSHIPS. IN BOTH FAMILIES, MALE AND FEMALE RELATIONSHIPS ARE FOUNDED ON THE CULTURAL BELIEF OF THE BIOLOGICAL, INTELLECTUAL, AND SOCIAL SUPERIORITY OF THE MALE AND INFERIORITY OF THE FEMALE. BOTH MEXICAN AND MEXICAN AMERICAN FAMILIES ARE PATRIARCHAL, THE BASIC FAMILY UNIT IS THE NUCLEAR FAMILY, AND THE FAMILY IS MORE IMPORTANT THAN THE INDIVIDUAL. EMPHASIS IN BOTH FAMILIES IS ON SUBMISSION AND OBEDIENCE TO THE FATHER. ATTITUDES ON COURTSHIP AND MARRIAGE AND TOWARD THE SEXUAL RELATIONSHIP BETWEEN HUSBAND AND WIFE ARE SLIGHTLY MORE LIBERAL IN THE MEXICAN AMERICAN FAMILY, BUT THE PATTERNS ARE ESSENTIALLY THE SAME. THE FATHER IN MEXICAN AMERICAN FAMILIES EXPRESSES AFFECTION FOR HIS CHILDREN MUCH MORE THAN MEXICAN FAMILIES. MANY VARIABLES (SUCH AS RELIGION, SOCIAL CLASS, LANGUAGE, EDUCATION, PHYSICAL AND SOCIAL MOBILITY, ACCULTURATION, AND ASSIMILATION) ARE NOT APPROPRIATELY CONSIDERED IN THE LITERATURE PRESENTLY AVAILABLE. 32 REFERENCES. (NCMHI ABSTRACT)

ACCN 001514

1744 AUTH **STAVENHAGEN, R.**
TITL LA APLICACION DE UNA CEDULA DE ENTREVISTA PARA EL ESTUDIO DE LA FAMILIA URBANA EN MEXICO. (THE USE OF AN INTERVIEW SCHEDULE FOR THE STUDY OF THE URBAN FAMILY IN MEXICO.)
SRCE *REVISTA MEXICANA DE CIENCIAS POLITICAS Y SOCIALES, 1957, 3, 209-225. (SPANISH)*
INDX RESEARCH METHODOLOGY, SURVEY, MEXICAN, URBAN, SES
ABST WITH THE GOAL OF ASSESSING THE ADEQUACY OF SURVEY INTERVIEW METHODOLOGY IN MEXICO, A LARGE (BUT UNSPECIFIED) NUMBER OF HOUSEHOLD HEADS IN THE POOR SECTIONS OF MEXICO CITY WERE INTERVIEWED IN 1957. QUESTIONS ENCOMPASSED ELEVEN AREAS: DEMOGRAPHICS, ECONOMIC CONDITIONS, MATERIAL LEVEL OF THE HOME, RELIGION, HEALTH, LEISURE ACTIVITIES, GOVERNMENTAL ATTITUDES, UNION AND POLITICAL ATTITUDES, AUTHORITY WITHIN THE FAMILY, INTERPERSONAL RELATIONSHIPS OUTSIDE THE FAMILY, AND PERSONAL ASPIRATIONS. ALL QUESTIONS IN THE INTERVIEW WERE "OBJECTIVE"—I.E., OF THE "YES/NO" AND MULTIPLE CHOICE VARIETY. THE EXCLUSIVE USE OF SUCH OBJECTIVE QUESTIONS WAS BASED UPON THE STUDY'S CONCERN WITH THE ESTABLISHMENT OF NORMS AND FREQUENCIES RATHER THAN WITH THE INTERPRETATION OF INDIVIDUAL CASES. THE AUTHOR CONCLUDES THAT THE SURVEY QUESTIONNAIRE IS A PARTICULARLY EFFECTIVE METHODOLOGY WHEN (1) IT PERMITS IMPRESSIONS OF A WELL-TRAINED INTERVIEWER AND (2) PROVIDES QUANTITATIVE DATA WHICH HAVE SOCIALLY IMPORTANT RESULTS FROM A QUALITATIVE POINT OF VIEW. THE AUTHOR ADDS THAT THE RESULTS OF THE SURVEY WILL BE PRESENTED IN A FUTURE ARTICLE. 7 REFERENCES.

ACCN 000621

1745 AUTH **STEDMAN, J. M., & ADAMS, R. L.**
TITL ACHIEVEMENT AS A FUNCTION OF LANGUAGE COMPETENCE. BEHAVIOR ADJUSTMENT, AND SEX IN YOUNG. DISADVANTAGED MEXICAN AMERICAN CHILDREN.
SRCE *JOURNAL OF EDUCATIONAL PSYCHOLOGY, 1972, 63(5), 411-417.*
INDX LANGUAGE COMPREHENSION, BILINGUALISM, SEX COMPARISON. CONFLICT RESOLUTION, MEXICAN AMERICAN, CHILDREN, SCHOLASTIC ACHIEVEMENT. EMPIRICAL, SES, TEXAS, SOUTHWEST
ABST LANGUAGE COMPETENCE IN BOTH ENGLISH AND SPANISH AND NONLINGUISTIC BEHAVIOR MEASURES WERE OBTAINED FROM 122 MEXICAN AMERICAN HEAD START ENROLLEES. SEVENTY-SIX AVAILABLE SUBJECTS WERE LATER RETESTED FOR ACHIEVEMENT AT THE END OF THE FIRST GRADE. RESULTS INDICATE THAT THE TEACHER BEHAVIOR RATING OF INTROVERSION-EXTROVERSION CONSTITUTED THE STRONGEST PREDICTOR OF LANGUAGE ACHIEVEMENT. WHEREAS ENGLISH-LANGUAGE COMPETENCE PROVED TO BE THE STRONGEST PREDICTOR OF MATH. SPANISH-LANGUAGE COMPETENCE FAILED TO PREDICT ANY LANGUAGE VARIABLE. SEX PROVED NOT TO BE A STRONG PREDICTOR OF ANY ACHIEVEMENT CRITERIA AND FAILED TO COR-

RELATE SIGNIFICANTLY WITH ANY ACHIEVE-MENT VARIABLE. THE BEHAVIOR PATTERNS OF THE MORE EXTROVERTED MEXICAN AMERI-CAN CHILD, WHICH POSSIBLY MAKE HIM MORE RECEPTIVE TO THE TEACHER-STUDENT INTER-ACTION, ARE DISCUSSED. 14 REFERENCES.

ACCN   001515

1746 AUTH   **STEDMAN, J. M., & ADAMS, R. L.**
TITL   TEACHER PERCEPTION OF BEHAVIORAL AD-JUSTMENT AS A FUNCTION OF LINGUISTIC ABILITY IN MEXICAN AMERICAN HEADSTART CHILDREN.
SRCE   *PSYCHOLOGY IN THE SCHOOLS, 1973, 10(2), 221-225.*
INDX   TEACHERS, ATTITUDES, LINGUISTIC COMPE-TENCE, MEXICAN AMERICAN, CHILDREN, BI-LINGUAL, SCHOLASTIC ACHIEVEMENT, DIS-CRIMINATION, EMPIRICAL, SEX COMPARISON, TEXAS, SOUTHWEST
ABST   THE RELATIONSHIP BETWEEN THE LINGUISTIC ABILITY OF MEXICAN AMERICAN HEADSTART CHILDREN AND TEACHER PERCEPTION OF AD-JUSTMENT AS EXPRESSED IN TEACHER RAT-ING SCALES WAS INVESTIGATED. IT WAS HY-POTHESIZED THAT ENGLISH LANGUAGE ABILITY WOULD REPRESENT A POSITIVE CLASSROOM COPING SKILL AND WOULD BE RELATED POSI-TIVELY TO TEACHER RATINGS OF ADJUSTMENT, WHILE SPANISH LANGUAGE ABILITY WOULD BE RELATED NEGATIVELY OR UNRELATED TO TEACHER PERCEPTION OF ADJUSTMENT. THE SAMPLE CONSISTED OF MEXICAN AMERICAN CHILDREN (ALL 5 YEARS-OLD) ENROLLED IN A HEADSTART PROGRAM. BEHAVIOR MEASURES AND OVERALL ADJUSTMENT SCORES WERE OBTAINED BY MEANS OF THE CLASSROOM BE-HAVIOR INVENTORY, PRESCHOOL TO PRIMARY (CBI) INSTRUMENT. LANGUAGE ABILITY IN EN-GLISH AND SPANISH WAS ASSESSED BY MEANS OF TESTS OF BASIC LANGUAGE COMPETENCE IN ENGLISH AND SPANISH, LEVEL I: CHILDREN, AGES 3-6 (TBLC). RESULTS SUPPORT THE MA-JOR HYPOTHESES. DATA INDICATED THAT STU-DENTS HIGH IN ENGLISH LANGUAGE PROFI-CIENCY ALSO TEND TO RECEIVE HIGH BEHAVIORAL RATINGS FROM THEIR TEACH-ERS. THE OPPOSITE WAS TRUE FOR THOSE LOW IN ENGLISH LANGUAGE PROFICIENCY. THESE FINDINGS HELD FOR BOYS SEPARATELY, FOR GIRLS SEPARATELY, AND FOR CHILDREN TAUGHT BY MEXICAN AMERICAN TEACHERS AND CHILDREN TAUGHT BY NONMEXICAN AMERICAN TEACHERS. IT SEEMS ESPECIALLY IMPORTANT TO ISOLATE TEACHER BIAS IN OR-DER TO DETERMINE WHETHER THIS FACTOR HAS UNDUE INFLUENCE ON TEACHERS' BE-HAVIORAL RATINGS OF YOUNG MEXICAN AMERICAN CHILDREN. 17 REFERENCES. (NCMHI ABSTRACT)
ACCN   001516

1747 AUTH   **STEDMAN, J. M., & MCKENZIE, R. E.**
TITL   FAMILY FACTORS RELATED TO COMPETENCE IN YOUNG DISADVANTAGED MEXICAN AMERI-CAN CHILDREN.
SRCE   *CHILD DEVELOPMENT, 1971, 42(5), 1602-1607.*
INDX   EARLY CHILDHOOD EDUCATION, MEXICAN

AMERICAN, CHILDREN, CLASSROOM BEHAV-IOR, LINGUISTIC COMPETENCE, FAMILY STRUCTURE, FAMILY ROLES, EDUCATION, AT-TITUDES, SES, DEMOGRAPHIC, POVERTY, EM-PIRICAL, BILINGUALISM, TEACHERS, ABILITY TESTING, LANGUAGE ASSESSMENT, TEXAS, SOUTHWEST
ABST   134 MEXICAN AMERICAN 5 YEAR-OLD HEAD-START ENROLLEES IN SAN ANTONIO, TEXAS, WERE EVALUATED TO IDENTIFY HIGH AND LOW COMPETENCE GROUPS BASED ON LINGUISTIC ABILITY AND BEHAVIORAL ADJUSTMENT. THE TOTAL POPULATION WAS SCREENED AND GROUPS OF 20 HIGH COMPETENCE (HIGH LANGUAGE/ADJUSTMENT) AND 20 LOW COM-PETENCE (LOW LANGUAGE/ADJUSTMENT) CHILDREN WERE SELECTED FOR MORE DE-TAILED EVALUATION. ADEQUATE FAMILY DATA WERE OBTAINED, FOCUSING ON THREE VARI-ABLES: (1) SCHOOL-RELATED ATTITUDES; (2) ROLES WITHIN THE FAMILY; AND (3) SOCIAL DATA REGARDING THE OVERALL FAMILY CON-STELLATION. THE SEMANTIC DIFFERENTIAL TECHNIQUE MEASURED PARENTS' SELF-CON-CEPT, ROLES WITHIN THE FAMILY, AND CON-CEPTS RELATED TO THE CHILD'S SCHOOL AD-JUSTMENT. IN ADDITION, THE RELATIONSHIP BETWEEN LINGUISTIC ABILITY IN BOTH EN-GLISH AND SPANISH AND TEACHER BEHAVIOR RATINGS WAS EVALUATED. BOTH HIGH AND LOW COMPETENCE FAMILIES WERE FOUND TO BE NONMOBILE AND URBAN-BORN. HIGH COMPETENCE GROUPS HAD HIGHER RATES OF REMARRYING, HIGHER LEVELS OF MATER-NAL EDUCATION, AND LOWER RATES OF PRI-MARY SUPPORT THROUGH PUBLIC WELFARE. HIGH COMPETENCE FAMILIES ARE REPORTED TO SHOW SIGNS OF MORE ADEQUATE AD-JUSTMENT AND MORE FAVORABLE "SEMANTIC STRUCTURE" REGARDING SCHOOL RELATED CONCEPTS. TWO-WAY MEDIAN TESTS FOR EACH FACTOR ON THE CONCEPT "HOW THE TEACHER SEES THE MEXICAN AMERICAN CHILD" RE-VEALED SIGNIFICANT BETWEEN-GROUP DIF-FERENCES. HIGH COMPETENCE PARENTS SEE ANGLO TEACHERS AS VIEWING THEIR CHIL-DREN IN A MORE POSITIVE LIGHT. RESULTS IN-DICATE DIFFERENCES ON A NUMBER OF IM-PORTANT VARIABLES ASSOCIATED WITH PRESCHOOL CHILD ADJUSTMENT AND LIN-GUISTIC ABILITY. 6 REFERENCES.
ACCN   001517

1748 AUTH   **STEINMAN, M.**
TITL   LOW INCOME AND MINORITY GROUP PARTICI-PATION IN ADMINISTRATIVE PROCESSES: MEX-ICAN AMERICAN ORIENTATIONS TO HEALTH CARE SERVICES.
SRCE   *URBAN AFFAIRS QUARTERLY, 1976, 11(4), 523-544.*
INDX   ADULTS, ATTITUDES, COMMUNITY INVOLVE-MENT, CULTURAL FACTORS, ECONOMIC FAC-TORS, SOCIAL SERVICES, EDUCATION, EMPIRI-CAL, ENVIRONMENTAL FACTORS, HEALTH DELIVERY SYSTEMS, MEXICAN AMERICAN, POLITICS, SES, NEBRASKA, MIDWEST, URBAN, SURVEY
ABST   A COMPARISON IS MADE OF THE PARTICIPA-

TION OF LOW-INCOME MEXICAN AMERICANS (N = 149) IN TWO AREAS OF COMMUNITY INVOLVEMENT: (1) PARTICIPATION IN THE ADMINISTRATIVE PROCESSES OF PUBLIC HEALTH CARE SERVICES; AND (2) POLITICAL PARTICIPATION. PUBLIC SERVICE INVOLVEMENT IS DIFFERENTIATED FROM POLITICAL PARTICIPATION BY ITS CONCERN WITH IMMEDIATE PROBLEMS PERTINENT TO THE CONSUMER (E.G., HEALTH POLICY, WELFARE RIGHTS), WHILE POLITICAL PARTICIPATION IS CHARACTERIZED BY AN IDEOLOGICAL AND FUTURE ORIENTATION. IT IS ARGUED IN THE LITERATURE ON POLITICAL PARTICIPATION THAT LOW-INCOME AND MINORITY INDIVIDUALS TEND TO TAKE LITTLE ADVANTAGE OF PARTICIPATORY OPPORTUNITIES BECAUSE THEY LACK NECESSARY SKILLS AND EFFICACIOUS SELF-IMAGES. BUT THE EXTRAPOLATION FROM THIS LITERATURE TO EXPLAIN LOW RATES OF PARTICIPATION IN MORE ADMINISTRATIVE PROCESSES IS CHALLENGED. IT IS HYPOTHESIZED, INSTEAD, THAT CORRELATES OF ADMINISTRATIVE PARTICIPATION DIFFER FROM FACTORS EXPLAINING POLITICAL INVOLVEMENTS. IN THE STUDY'S SURVEY QUESTIONNAIRE, RESPONSES TO TWO QUESTIONS PROVIDED A DISTRIBUTION OF RESPONDENTS' INCLINATION TO PARTICIPATE IN HEALTH CARE; RATES OF POLITICAL PARTICIPATION WERE DETERMINED BY RATING RESPONDENTS ON TEN FORMS OF POLITICAL BEHAVIOR (VOTER REGISTRATION, DONATION OF MONEY TO A POLITICAL CAMPAIGN, ETC.). THE CORRELATES OF POLITICAL AND ADMINISTRATIVE PARTICIPATION WERE FOUND TO BE DISSIMILAR, SUGGESTING THE UTILITY OF EMPLOYING A DIFFERENT EXPLANATORY FRAME OF REFERENCE FOR EACH. 29 REFERENCES.

ACCN   002213

1749 AUTH   **STENGER, E. M.**
TITL   MAKING PSYCHIATRY MEANINGFUL: IMPLICATIONS FOR CHICANOS.
SRCE   *IN A. M. PADILLA & E. R. PADILLA (EDS.), IMPROVING MENTAL HEALTH AND HUMAN SERVICES FOR HISPANIC COMMUNITIES: SELECTED PRESENTATIONS FROM REGIONAL CONFERENCES. WASHINGTON, D.C.: NATIONAL COALITION OF HISPANIC MENTAL HEALTH AND HUMAN SERVICES ORGANIZATIONS (COSSMHO), 1977, PP. 19-22.*
INDX   MENTAL HEALTH PROFESSION, ESSAY, PSYCHOTHERAPY, CURANDERISMO, MENTAL HEALTH, COMMUNITY, CULTURAL FACTORS, TEXAS, SOUTHWEST, CULTURAL PLURALISM, MEXICAN AMERICAN
ABST   IN THIS ADDRESS DELIVERED AT A CONFERENCE IN SAN ANTONIO, TEXAS, CONSIDERATION OF THE CHICANO CLIENT'S CULTURE AND INDIVIDUAL NEEDS IS URGED. TOO OFTEN TRADITIONAL NORMS OF BEHAVIOR ARE RIGIDLY APPLIED TO THIS POPULATION IN AN EFFORT TO MOLD PRESENTING SYMPTOMS TO ESTABLISHED THEORY. HENCE, CHICANOS OFTEN RECEIVE THE SUBTLE MESSAGE FROM PSYCHOTHERAPISTS TO "CEASE TO BE AN INDIVIDUAL, FORGET YOUR CULTURAL DIFFERENCES AND FIT IN." THE OPPOSITE AP-

PROACH—ONE IN WHICH THE INDIVIDUAL'S NEEDS COME FIRST, PSYCHIATRIC THEORY SECOND—IS PRESENTED FOR CONSIDERATION. IN THE SAN ANTONIO CLINIC DESCRIBED, THE "HUMANNESS" OF THE CLIENTS IS THE ONLY VALID MEANS OF DIAGNOSIS. MOST OF THE STAFF ARE PARAPROFESSIONALS FROM THE BARRIO WHO SHARE A COMMON CULTURE AND LANGUAGE WITH THE PATIENTS. THE THERAPISTS ARE URGED TO RELATE TO THE CLIENTS AS FELLOW HUMAN BEINGS, "COMPADRES," NOT AS PSYCHOTHERAPISTS TALKING DOWN TO PATIENTS. AS A WAY OF INCORPORATING CLIENT CULTURE INTO THE TREATMENT PATTERN, THERE IS FREQUENT USE OF CHICANO "CURANDEROS" WHO ARE OFTEN MORE EFFECTIVE THAN TRAINED PROFESSIONALS OR EVEN PARAPROFESSIONALS. MOREOVER, BEYOND CONSIDERATION OF THE CULTURAL HERITAGE OF THE CLIENT, GREAT EFFORT IS MADE TO DISCERN THE COMPLEXITY AND DIVERSITY OF HIS OR HER INDIVIDUAL NEEDS. THE SUCCESS OF SUCH AN APPROACH TO CHICANO MENTAL HEALTH SUGGESTS THAT WHEN WE INSIST ON UTILIZING A TOTALLY HUMAN PERSPECTIVE IN RELATING TO A PERSON, WE ARE RESPONDING TO THAT PERSON'S DEEPEST NEEDS.

ACCN   001518

1750 AUTH   **STEPHAN, W. G.**
TITL   COGNITIVE DIFFERENTIATION IN INTERGROUP PERCEPTION.
SRCE   *SOCIOMETRY, 1977, 40(1), 50-58.*
INDX   CHILDREN, MEXICAN AMERICAN, CROSS CULTURAL, SOUTHWEST, URBAN, EMPIRICAL, INTERPERSONAL ATTRACTION, PREJUDICE
ABST   ON THE BASIS OF PREVIOUS RESEARCH INDICATING THAT THE PERCEPTIONS OF DISLIKED OTHERS ARE MORE DIFFERENTIATED THAN THE PERCEPTIONS OF LIKED OTHERS, IT WAS PREDICTED THAT IN-GROUP MEMBERS WOULD PERCEIVE THEIR OWN GROUP AS LESS DIFFERENTIATED THAN OUT-GROUPS. IT WAS ALSO PREDICTED THAT STUDENTS IN INTEGRATED SCHOOLS WOULD PERCEIVE OUT-GROUPS AS LESS DIFFERENTIATED THAN WOULD STUDENTS IN SEGREGATED SCHOOLS. IN A SOUTHWESTERN CITY, 750 FIFTH- AND SIXTH-GRADE BLACK, CHICANO, AND ANGLO CHILDREN FROM THREE SEGREGATED AND FIVE INTEGRATED SCHOOLS WERE STUDIED TO TEST THESE HYPOTHESES. THE SUBJECTS COMPLETED A QUESTIONNAIRE WHICH INCLUDED A MEASURE OF LIKING AND A MEASURE OF DIFFERENTIATION. THE RESULTS PROVIDED STRONG SUPPORT FOR THE FIRST PREDICTION AND WEAK SUPPORT FOR THE SECOND. THE FINDINGS FOR THE FIRST HYPOTHESIS ARE DISCUSSED IN TERMS OF THE NEED TO UNDERSTAND THE BEHAVIOR OF DISLIKED OTHERS AND THE OPERATION OF THE "HALO EFFECT" WHICH OCCURS WHEN AN INDIVIDUAL'S GENERAL IMPRESSION OF ANOTHER INFLUENCES HIS ASSESSMENT OF THE SPECIFIC TRAITS THAT PERSON POSSESSES. REGARDING THE SECOND HYPOTHESIS, IT WAS FOUND THAT INTERGROUP CONTACT, EXCEPT

BETWEEN HIGHLY DISSIMILAR GROUPS, WAS NOT AN IMPORTANT DETERMINANT OF THE DEGREE OF DIFFERENTIATION PERCEIVED IN OUTGROUPS. 36 REFERENCES. (JOURNAL ABSTRACT MODIFIED)

ACCN   002214

1751 AUTH **STEPHAN, W. G.**
TITL   STEREOTYPING: THE ROLE OF INGROUP-OUTGROUP DIFFERENCES IN CAUSAL ATTRIBUTION FOR BEHAVIOR.
SRCE   *JOURNAL OF SOCIAL PSYCHOLOGY, 1977, 101, 255-266.*
INDX   STEREOTYPES, EMPIRICAL, CHILDREN, CROSS CULTURAL, MEXICAN AMERICAN, SOUTHWEST, ATTITUDES, LOCUS OF CONTROL, ATTRIBUTION THEORY
ABST   A STUDY WAS DESIGNED TO TEST THE IDEA THAT INGROUP-OUTGROUP DIFFERENCES IN ATTRIBUTIONAL PROCESSES PLAY AN IMPORTANT PART IN THE ORIGIN OF STEREOTYPES. SPECIFICALLY, IT WAS HYPOTHESIZED THAT INGROUP MEMBERS WOULD MAKE MORE DISPOSITIONAL ATTRIBUTIONS TO POSITIVE BEHAVIORS AND FEWER DISPOSITIONAL ATTRIBUTIONS TO NEGATIVE BEHAVIORS THAN OUTGROUP MEMBERS WOULD. A QUESTIONNAIRE INCLUDING ITEMS ON ATTRIBUTIONS TO POSITIVE AND NEGATIVE BEHAVIOR AND INTER-ETHNIC ATTITUDES WAS GIVEN TO A TRIETHNIC SAMPLE OF 750 FIFTH- AND SIXTH-GRADE STUDENTS IN A SOUTHWESTERN CITY. THE HYPOTHESIS WAS WELL SUPPORTED FOR THE EVALUATION OF THE CHICANOS' BEHAVIOR, PARTIALLY SUPPORTED FOR THE EVALUATION OF ANGLOS' BEHAVIOR, AND UNSUPPORTED FOR THE EVALUATION OF BLACKS' BEHAVIOR. OTHER RESULTS INDICATING THAT ALL THREE GROUPS ATTRIBUTE POSITIVE BEHAVIOR TO THE ACTOR AND NEGATIVE BEHAVIOR TO THE SITUATION AND THAT ANGLOS MAKE MORE DISPOSITIONAL ATTRIBUTIONS THAN THE OTHER GROUPS ARE ALSO DISCUSSED. 22 REFERENCES. (JOURNAL ABSTRACT MODIFIED)

ACCN   002215

1752 AUTH **STEPHENS, M. I.**
TITL   ELICITED IMITATION OF SELECTED FEATURES OF TWO AMERICAN ENGLISH DIALECTS IN HEADSTART CHILDREN.
SRCE   *JOURNAL OF SPEECH AND HEARING RESEARCH, 1976, 19(3), 493-507.*
INDX   CHILDREN, SPANISH SURNAMED, MIDWEST, EMPIRICAL, CROSS CULTURAL, LANGUAGE ACQUISITION, LANGUAGE ASSESSMENT, LANGUAGE LEARNING, LINGUISTIC COMPETENCE
ABST   THREE MEASURES WERE USED TO CHECK THE BIDIALECTAL IMITATIVE FACILITY OF 100 BLACK, WHITE, AND SPANISH-SPEAKING MIDWESTERN HEADSTART CHILDREN. IN GENERAL, BLACKS AND SPANISH-SPEAKING SUBJECTS PERFORMED MORE ACCURATELY ON BLACK ENGLISH MARKERS THAN ON STANDARD ENGLISH MARKERS AND WHITES, THE REVERSE. WHEN THE CHILDREN DID MAKE AN ERROR ON THE FEATURE MARKER THEY USUALLY SUBSTITUTED THE OPPOSING DIALECTAL MARKER.

BLACKS AND SPANISH-SPEAKING SUBJECTS WERE MORE APT TO BE ACCURATE ON THE TOTAL SENTENCE WHEN IT WAS GIVEN IN BLACK ENGLISH. THE FACT THAT THE WHITES' STANDARD ENGLISH/BLACK ENGLISH GAP WAS CONSIDERABLY NARROWER THAN THE BLACKS ON THE MARKERS MAY BE DUE TO THEIR EXPOSURE TO BLACK ENGLISH IN THEIR VERBAL ENVIRONMENTS OR SIMPLY THEIR UNFAMILIARITY WITH STANDARD ENGLISH. SOME OF THE BLACK ENGLISH MARKERS ARE FEATURES CHARACTERISTIC OF STAGES IN THE ACQUISITION OF STANDARD ENGLISH. IN OMITTING MORPHOLOGICAL SUFFIXES AND RELYING ON CONTENTIVES, SPANISH-SPEAKING CHILDREN MAY HAVE BEEN EXHIBITING ASPECTS OF SECOND-LANGUAGE LEARNING RATHER THAN DISPLAYING A FAMILIARITY WITH BLACK ENGLISH. 24 REFERENCES. (JOURNAL ABSTRACT MODIFIED)

ACCN   002216

1753 AUTH **STERN, C., & BRYSON, J.**
TITL   COMPETENCE VERSUS PERFORMANCE IN YOUNG CHILDREN'S USE OF ADJECTIVAL COMPARATIVES.
SRCE   *CHILD DEVELOPMENT, 1970, 41(4), 1197-1201.*
INDX   CHILDREN, COGNITIVE DEVELOPMENT, PEABODY PICTURE-VOCABULARY TEST, CULTURAL FACTORS, CURRICULUM, EDUCATION, LINGUISTICS, LINGUISTIC COMPETENCE, LANGUAGE COMPREHENSION, BILINGUAL, LANGUAGE ACQUISITION, EMPIRICAL, MEXICAN AMERICAN, CALIFORNIA, SOUTHWEST
ABST   LINGUISTIC RESEARCH HAS REVEALED THAT GHETTO CHILDREN LACK FACILITY IN THE USE OF CERTAIN LANGUAGE STRUCTURES. THIS STUDY POSES TWO QUESTIONS: (1) CAN DISADVANTAGED CHILDREN BE TAUGHT TO PRODUCE THE STANDARD COMPARATIVE FORM OF THE ADJECTIVE—CONSIDERED A BASIC LACK IN THEIR LANGUAGE STRUCTURING ABILITY— AND (2) WHICH OF TWO METHODS OF INSTRUCTION WOULD BE MORE EFFECTIVE IN FACILITATING THIS PROCESS? SIXTEEN MEXICAN AMERICAN CHILDREN (50-60 MONTHS OLD) IN THE LOS ANGELES CHILDREN'S CENTERS WERE RANDOMLY ASSIGNED TO ONE OF TWO INSTRUCTIONAL TREATMENTS. THE STIMULI CONSISTED OF 10 PAIRED PICTURES PRESENTING AN ADJECTIVE (E.G., FAT PIG) AND ITS COMPARATIVE (E.G., FATTER PIG). IN THE FIRST INSTRUCTIONAL PROCEDURE THE CHILDREN WERE TOLD THE APPROPRIATE WORD AND ASKED TO ECHO IT. IN THE SECOND, THE RULE FOR FORMING THE COMPARATIVE WAS PROVIDED AND EMPHASIZED. TWO GROUPS RECEIVED THE ECHOIC REPETITION TRAINING AND TWO THE RULE TRAINING. AFTER TRAINING, BOTH TREATMENTS MADE SIGNIFICANT GAINS (.01 LEVEL), SCORING 85% OR BETTER ON THE LABELING POSTTEST. THIS GAIN WAS RETAINED OVER A 6-MONTH PERIOD. THIS STUDY INDICATES THAT IT IS POSSIBLE TO DEMONSTRATE COMPREHENSION OF THE CONCEPT OF COMPARISON WITHOUT POSSESSING THE LABELS WHICH CONVEY THIS CONCEPT IN THE PREFERRED TERMINOLOGY

OF A PARTICULAR LANGUAGE COMMUNITY. IT ALSO DEMONSTRATES THAT IF A CHILD HAS AN INTERNALIZED UNDERSTANDING OF COMPARISON, HE CAN, WITH A FEW LESSONS, LEARN TO PRODUCE THE APPROPRIATE LABELS, INDEPENDENT OF THE TYPE OF INSTRUCTION. 10 REFERENCES.

ACCN   001519

1754 AUTH   **STERN, C., & RUBLE, D.**
TITL   TEACHING NEW CONCEPTS TO NON-ENGLISH SPEAKING PRESCHOOL CHILDREN.
SRCE   *TESOL QUARTERLY, 1973, 7(3), 309-317.*
INDX   EARLY CHILDHOOD EDUCATION, INSTRUCTIONAL TECHNIQUES, MEXICAN AMERICAN, BILINGUALISM, EMPIRICAL, LANGUAGE COMPREHENSION, COGNITIVE DEVELOPMENT
ABST   PRESCHOOL SPANISH-SPEAKING MEXICAN AMERICAN CHILDREN WERE TESTED TO DETERMINE IF THEY WOULD LEARN A NEW CONCEPT (E.G., TALL-SHORT) MOST QUICKLY WHEN TAUGHT IN SPANISH, ENGLISH, OR BILINGUALLY. FIFTEEN CHILDREN FROM 4 HEADSTART CLASSES PARTICIPATED IN THE STUDY. THE PROCEDURE, AS RECORDED, INCLUDED: (1) PRETESTING WITH THE GOODENOUGH DRAW-A-MAN TEST AND THE EXPRESSIVE VOCABULARY INVENTORY IN BOTH ENGLISH AND SPANISH; (2) AN INSTRUCTIONAL PROGRAM IN SPANISH OR ENGLISH ONLY, OR BILINGUALLY; (3) A CRITERION TEST IN THE APPROPRIATE LANGUAGE USING A SERIES OF BOOKLETS DEVELOPED TO TEACH THE CONCEPTUAL TASK; AND (4) A POSTTEST. STUDY RESULTS DETERMINED, FIRST, THAT SPANISH-SPEAKING CHILDREN DID NOT DO BETTER WHEN THEY WERE TAUGHT A NEW CONCEPT IN SPANISH RATHER THAN IN ENGLISH OR BILINGUALLY, AND SECOND, THAT THERE WAS NO EVIDENCE THAT THE CHILDREN WHO HAD BEEN TAUGHT THE NEW CONCEPT IN ENGLISH WOULD BE ABLE TO ACQUIRE A SIMILAR CONCEPT PRESENTED IN ENGLISH MORE READILY THAN THE GROUP WHICH WAS TAUGHT THE FIRST CONCEPT IN SPANISH. THIRD, ON A SPANISH LANGUAGE CRITERION TEST, THE CHILDREN WHO WERE TAUGHT THE CONCEPTS IN ENGLISH DID AS WELL AS THE CHILDREN WHO WERE TAUGHT THE CONCEPTS IN SPANISH OR BILINGUALLY. IT IS SUGGESTED THAT AN EFFECTIVE WAY TO TEACH NEW CONCEPTS TO NON-ENGLISH SPEAKING CHILDREN IS BY SIMULTANEOUS OR ALTERNATING PRESENTATION IN BOTH THE FAMILIAR AND THE NEW LANGUAGE. 4 REFERENCES.

ACCN   001520

1755 AUTH   **STEVENS, E. P.**
TITL   MACHISMO AND MARIANISMO.
SRCE   *TRANSACTION-SOCIETY, 1973, 10(6), 57-63.*
INDX   CULTURAL FACTORS, SEX ROLES, ESSAY, SPANISH SURNAMED, STEREOTYPES, MACHISMO
ABST   ON THE ASSUMPTION THAT LATIN AMERICAN MEN AND WOMEN HAVE UNEQUIVOCAL CONCEPTIONS OF THEIR ROLES, THIS ESSAY ARGUES THAT THE INTERPERSONAL DYNAMICS OF THE EXISTING SOCIAL STRUCTURE AFFORD EACH SEX A COMPLIMENTARY SPHERE OF INFLUENCE THAT SATISFIES BASIC PERSONAL AND SOCIAL NEEDS. AFTER A DISCUSSION OF THE CHARACTERISTICS AND MANIFESTATIONS OF MACHISMO AND THE PARALLEL FEMALE ATTITUDES AND BEHAVIOR PATTERNS TERMED "MARIANISMO," IT IS CONCLUDED THAT PRESSURES TO CONFORM TO THE MACHO STEREOTYPE COME AS STRONGLY FROM THE WOMEN AS FROM THE MEN. THIS SECULAR CULT OF FEMININITY DRAWN FROM THE ADORATION OF THE VIRGIN MARY PICTURES ITS SUBJECTS AS SEMI-DIVINE, MORALLY SUPERIOR, AND SPIRITUALLY STRONGER THAN MEN. FEMALE CHILDREN ARE SOCIALIZED IN ATTITUDES OF SELF-ABNEGATION TOWARDS MALES, YET EVENTUALLY ATTAIN STATUS AS THEY MARRY, ENDURE A LIFE OF SUFFERING, AND BEAR CHILDREN WHO WILL PERPETUATE THE CULT OF MOTHER-WORSHIP. BASED ON THEIR ACKNOWLEDGED SPIRITUAL SUPERIORITY, WOMEN ENJOY STATUS AND POWER IN A CULTURE WHERE SPIRITUALITY IS HIGHLY VALUED. THE MACHISMO-MARIANISMO PATTERNS OF ATTITUDES AND BEHAVIOR PROVIDE CLEAR-CUT SEX-ROLE DEFINITIONS AND A STABLE SYMBIOSIS IN LATIN AMERICAN CULTURE. 5 REFERENCES.

ACCN   001521

1756 AUTH   **STEVENS, E. P.**
TITL   MEXICAN MACHISMO: POLITICS AND VALUE ORIENTATIONS.
SRCE   *THE WESTERN POLITICAL QUARTERLY, 1965, 18(4), 848-857.*
INDX   POLITICS, MEXICAN, CULTURAL FACTORS, ESSAY, MEXICO, HISTORY, MALE, SEX ROLES, POLITICAL POWER, MACHISMO, VALUES
ABST   TAKING THE HYPOTHESIS THAT POLITICS REFLECT THE DOMINANT VALUE PATTERNS OF A SOCIAL SYSTEM, THE AUTHOR EXAMINES THE CONNECTION BETWEEN THE MEXICAN POLITICAL SYSTEM AND THE CULT OF MACHISMO. THE "MAN'S WORLD" OF POLITICS WOULD BE EXPECTED TO BE CHARACTERIZED BY VIOLENCE, INTRANSIGENCE, AND CONFORMANCE TO MODELS OF ABSOLUTE AUTHORITARIANISM, ANARCHY, OR TOTALITARIANISM. A REVIEW OF MEXICAN HISTORY REVEALS PERIODS OF ABSOLUTE AUTHORITARIANISM AND NEAR-ANARCHY, BUT THE SCOPE OF DEVELOPMENT FROM 1925 TO THE PRESENT DOES NOT FALL INTO ANY OF THE ABOVE CATEGORIES. THE PRESENT POLITICAL SYSTEM CONTAINS MUCH OF A "RECONCILIATION" SYSTEM, CHARACTERIZED BY BEHIND-THE-SCENES COMPROMISES BETWEEN GROUPS. THE CURRENT PRACTICES OF PETITIONING AND MANEUVERING DISPLAY CHARACTERISTICS THAT MAY BE REGARDED AS FEMININE BEHAVIOR, DIRECTLY AT VARIANCE WITH THE PREDICTED VALUE ORIENTATION OF MACHISMO. IT HAS BEEN SUGGESTED THAT THROUGH IDENTIFICATION WITH THE DOMINANT PARTY, INDIVIDUALS AND GROUPS CAN EXPRESS THEIR NEED-DISPOSITIONS OF AGGRESSIVENESS AND THEREBY BE REASSURED THAT POLITICAL AFFAIRS ARE BEING CONDUCTED IN A MANLY WAY. THE PRESIDENT BEHAVES IN A MANNER REMINIS-

CENT OF THE POWERFUL AND INTRANSIGENT MACHO, WITH POLITICIANS PLAYING THE ROLE OF "FEMININE" MANEUVERERS. HOWEVER, SINCE PRESENT POLITICAL BEHAVIOR DOES NOT CORRELATE WITH THE DOMINANT VALUE ORIENTATION OF MACHISMO, IT IS CONCLUDED THAT THE POLITICAL SYSTEM OF A COUNTRY IS NEITHER A PRODUCT OF NOR EXPLICABLE BY THE "CULTURE" OF A COUNTRY AS SEEN IN ITS PERSONALITY SYSTEMS AND SOCIAL SYSTEM. 30 REFERENCES.

ACCN   001522

1757 AUTH   **STEWARD, D., & STEWARD, M.**
TITL   EARLY LEARNING IN THE FAMILY: A REPORT OF RESEARCH IN PROGRESS.
SRCE   *CHARACTER POTENTIAL, 1974, 6(4), 171-176.*
INDX   SOUTHWEST, FEMALE, CALIFORNIA, CHILDREN, CROSS CULTURAL, DYADIC INTERACTION, EARLY CHILDHOOD EDUCATION, MALE, MOTHER-CHILD INTERACTION, RELIGION, SES, COGNITIVE DEVELOPMENT, LEARNING, FAMILY ROLES, MEXICAN AMERICAN, EMPIRICAL
ABST   TEACHER-LEARNER DYADS OF THREE ETHNIC GROUPS (CHINESE, ANGLO, AND MEXICAN AMERICAN) WERE STUDIED TO ASSESS THE NATURE OF EARLY LEARNING IN THE HOME. A STUDY OF MOTHERS (BAY AREA, CALIFORNIA RESIDENTS) TEACHING THEIR 3 YEAR-OLD SONS WAS COMPARED TO A STUDY OF MOTHERS TEACHING A CHILD OF THE SAME OR DIFFERENT ETHNIC AND SOCIAL CLASS. MOTHERS WERE VIDEOTAPED WHILE TEACHING CHILDREN TWO GAMES (A SORTING TASK AND A MOTOR TASK). A PARENT INTERACTION CODE WAS DEVELOPED AS AN OBSERVATIONAL INSTRUMENT IN THE HOME. THE CODE CONCEPTUALIZED A DYADIC TEACHER-LEARNING INTERACTION LOOP COMPOSED OF FOUR INTERACTIONS: (1) ALERTING (THE WAY A PARENT GAINS THE ATTENTION OF THE CHILD); (2) FORMAT (THE PROCESS BY WHICH THE PARENT GIVES INSTRUCTIONS TO THE CHILD); (3) CHILD RESPONSE; AND (4) PARENT FEEDBACK. RESULTS SHOW THAT TEACHING STRATEGIES AND CHILD RESPONSES DIFFERED BY ETHNIC GROUP AND BY MOTHER TEACHING OWN OR ANOTHER'S SON. YOUNG CHILDREN FROM THE THREE ETHNIC GROUPS, WHEN PAIRED WITH THEIR MOTHERS, EXPERIENCED DIFFERENT LEARNING ENVIRONMENTS (E.G., ANGLO MOTHERS PACED THEIR CHILDREN TWICE AS FAST AS MEXICAN AMERICAN MOTHERS). SECOND, NON-MOTHER TEACHERS ELICITED A RANGE OF CHILD RESPONSES (E.G., THE MEXICAN AMERICAN CHILDREN WORKING WITH TEACHERS OTHER THAN THEIR MOTHER SHOWED A BROADENED RESPONSE REPERTOIRE). THIRD, MOTHERS TEACHING CHILDREN OF DIFFERING ETHNIC BACKGROUNDS WERE UNIFORMLY NICER TO CHILDREN, INCREASING POSITIVE FEEDBACK AND DECREASING NEGATIVE FEEDBACK. IT IS CONCLUDED THAT FURTHER INVESTIGATIONS OF EARLY LEARNING EXPERIENCES AND THEIR PREDICTIVE VALUE IN LATER CROSS-ETHNIC LEARNING EXPERIENCES ARE NEEDED. IMPLICATIONS OF RESEARCH FINDINGS FOR RELI-

GIOUS EDUCATORS ARE DISCUSSED. 21 REFERENCES.
ACCN   001523

1758 AUTH   **STEWARD, M., & STEWARD, D.**
TITL   EFFECT OF SOCIAL DISTANCE ON TEACHING STRATEGIES OF ANGLO AMERICAN AND MEXICAN MOTHERS.
SRCE   *DEVELOPMENTAL PSYCHOLOGY, 1974, 10(6), 797-807.*
INDX   ENVIRONMENTAL FACTORS, MEXICAN AMERICAN, CROSS CULTURAL, MOTHER-CHILD INTERACTION, SES
ABST   THE VARIABLE OF SOCIAL DISTANCE BETWEEN TEACHER AND LEARNER WAS EXAMINED BY OBSERVING THE PATTERN OF INTERACTION BETWEEN MOTHERS AND THEIR OWN PRESCHOOL SONS—BOYS FROM A SIMILAR BACKGROUND, AND BOYS FROM A DIFFERENT ETHNIC AND SOCIAL CLASS BACKGROUND. ANGLO AMERICAN AND MEXICAN AMERICAN MOTHERS FROM MIDDLE AND LOWER CLASSES WERE VIDEOTAPED AS THEY TAUGHT A COGNITIVE AND A MOTOR TASK TO EACH OF THREE CHILDREN. THE PARENT INTERACTION CODE WAS EMPLOYED TO ANALYZE THE TEACHING LOOP BEHAVIOR. PROGRAMMATIC AND INSTRUCTIONAL VARIABLES WERE DIFFERENT BUT STABLE FOR EACH ETHNIC GROUP ACROSS SOCIAL DISTANCE, AND PATTERNS OF FEEDBACK AND CHILD RESPONSE SHIFTED SIGNIFICANTLY ACROSS SOCIAL DISTANCE. 30 REFERENCES. (NCMHI ABSTRACT)
ACCN   001524

1759 AUTH   **STEWARD, M., & STEWARD, D.**
TITL   THE OBSERVATION OF ANGLO-, MEXICAN-, AND CHINESE-AMERICAN MOTHERS TEACHING THEIR YOUNG SONS.
SRCE   *CHILD DEVELOPMENT, 1973, 44(2), 329-337.*
INDX   MEXICAN AMERICAN, CROSS CULTURAL, MOTHER-CHILD INTERACTION, CHILDREARING PRACTICES, SOCIALIZATION, EMPIRICAL, LEARNING
ABST   PARENTS WERE OBSERVED TEACHING PRESCHOOL CHILDREN A SORTING AND A MOTOR SKILL GAME. MOTHERS AND THEIR 3 YEAR-OLD SONS FROM SEVEN ETHNIC GROUPS PARTICIPATED. INTERACTION WAS VIDEOTAPED. CODERS WERE SELECTED FROM EACH ETHNIC GROUP. DATA WERE CODED USING A PARENT INTERACTION CODE WHICH ANALYZED PROGRAMMATIC VARIABLES (TOTAL TIME, INPUT, AND PACING) AND TEACHING LOOP VARIABLES (ALERT, FORMAT, CHILD RESPONSE, AND FEEDBACK). THE SINGLE BEST PREDICTOR OF MATERNAL TEACHING OR CHILD RESPONSE WAS ETHNICITY. CHILDREN EXPERIENCED DIFFERENT LEARNING ENVIRONMENTS WHICH MAY RESULT IN DIFFERENT SKILLS AND EXPECTATIONS BROUGHT BY THEM INTO THE CLASSROOM. 23 REFERENCES. (JOURNAL ABSTRACT MODIFIED)
ACCN   001525

1760 AUTH   **STEWART, D. N.**
TITL   EFFECTS OF SEX AND ETHNIC VARIABLES ON THE PROFILES OF THE ILLINOIS TEST OF PSY-

CHOLINGUISTICS AND WECHSLER INTELLI-GENCE SCALE OF CHILDREN.

SRCE   *PSYCHOLOGICAL REPORTS, 1976, 38, 53-54.*

INDX   ITPA, WISC, INTELLIGENCE TESTING, MENTAL RETARDATION, SEX COMPARISON, CROSS CULTURAL, MEXICAN AMERICAN, CHILDREN, LEARNING DISABILITIES, LANGUAGE LEARN-ING, IMPAIRMENT

ABST   A STUDY OF THE EFFECTS OF SEX AND ETHNI-CITY (BLACK, MEXICAN AMERICAN, OR ANGLO AMERICAN) VARIABLES ON THE ILLINOIS TEST OF PSYCHOLINGUISTIC ABILITIES AND WISC PROFILES OF 42 MENTALLY RETARDED, 42 NORMAL, AND 41 CHILDREN WITH DIAGNOSED LEARNING OR LANGUAGE PROBLEMS AGED 6-10 YEARS INDICATED THAT WHILE SUCH EF-FECTS MAY ATTAIN STATISTICAL SIGNIFI-CANCE, THE AMOUNT OF VARIANCE AC-COUNTED FOR BY THE VARIABLES IS SMALL. FINDINGS QUESTION THE PRACTICAL SIGNIFI-CANCE OF SUCH EFFECTS. 2 REFERENCES. (AUTHOR SUMMARY MODIFIED)

ACCN   001526

1761 AUTH   **STEWART, I. S.**

TITL   CULTURAL DIFFERENCES IN THE ATTRIBU-TIONS AND INTENTIONS OF ANGLOS AND CHI-CANOS IN AN ELEMENTARY SCHOOL (DOC-TORAL DISSERTATION, UNIVERSITY OF ILLINOIS AT URBANA-CHAMPAIGN, 1972).

SRCE   *DISSERTATION ABSTRACTS INTERNATIONAL, 1973, 34(2), 520A. (UNIVERSITY MICROFILMS NO. 73-17439.)*

INDX   CULTURAL FACTORS, CLASSROOM BEHAVIOR, ATTRIBUTION THEORY, MEXICAN AMERICAN, CROSS CULTURAL

ABST   TO IDENTIFY CULTURAL DIFFERENCES IN PER-CEPTIONS OF CLASSROOM BEHAVIOR, AN EX-PLORATORY INVESTIGATION WAS MADE OF THE RESPONSES OF ANGLO TEACHERS, PAR-ENTS, AND CHILDREN (N=32) AND CHICANO PARENTS AND CHILDREN (N=20) FROM ONE SCHOOL IN A SMALL ILLINOIS TOWN. USING THE FRAMEWORK OF ATTRIBUTION THEORY, CRITICAL INCIDENTS OF CULTURAL CONFLICT INVOLVING CHICANO CHILDREN IN THE CLASSROOM WERE IDENTIFIED AND USED TO ELICIT ATTRIBUTES AND INTENTIONS FROM EACH RESPONDENT. ALTHOUGH DIFFERENCES BETWEEN ANGLOS AND CHICANOS IN THEIR RESPONSES WERE DEMONSTRATED, THESE DIFFERENCES WERE NEITHER CLEAR NOR UN-COMPLICATED. ANGLOS AND CHICANOS WERE MORE SIMILAR IN THEIR DESCRIPTIONS OF IN-CIDENTS THAN IN THEIR SUGGESTIONS AS TO WHAT TO DO ABOUT THEM. ALL GROUPS HAD SIMILAR PERCEPTIONS OF ANGLO SUBJECTS, BUT THEY DIFFERED IN THEIR PERCEPTIONS OF CHICANOS. THE GREATER TENDENCY OF CHICANO PARENTS TO DESCRIBE THE STIMU-LUS PERSON AS NONCOMPETITIVE SET THEM APART FROM THE ANGLOS AND, TO A LESSER EXTENT, FROM THE CHICANO CHILDREN. A BROADER AND MORE COMPLEX VIEW OF THE EDUCATIONAL NEEDS OF CHICANO CHILDREN IS RECOMMENDED. THEY SHOULD BE PRO-VIDED WITH GUIDANCE IN DEFINING THEIR CLASSROOM ROLES AND IN DEVELOPING A

MORE POSITIVE SELF-IMAGE. EDUCATORS ARE ENCOURAGED TO FIND WAYS OF INCREASING COMMUNICATION BETWEEN HOME AND SCHOOL. 73 REFERENCES.

ACCN   001527

1762 AUTH   **STILWELL, W. E., & THORESEN, C. E.**

TITL   SOCIAL MODELING AND VOCATIONAL BEHAV-IORS OF MEXICAN-AMERICAN AND NON-MEXI-CAN-AMERICAN ADOLESCENTS.

SRCE   *VOCATIONAL GUIDANCE QUARTERLY, 1972, 21, 279-286.*

INDX   ADOLESCENTS, CROSS CULTURAL, EMPIRI-CAL, MALE, MEXICAN AMERICAN, MODELING, SOUTHWEST, VOCATIONAL COUNSELING, CALIFORNIA, SES

ABST   AN EXPLORATORY STUDY IS REPORTED WHICH EXAMINED VARIOUS SOCIAL MODELING TECH-NIQUES DESIGNED TO ENCOURAGE STUDENT INTEREST IN VOCATIONAL PROGRAMS. THE EFFECTS OF PARTICIPANT-OBSERVATION AND ETHNIC GROUP MEMBERSHIP WERE ALSO IN-VESTIGATED. A SAMPLE OF 68 MEXICAN AMERICAN AND 179 NON-MEXICAN AMERICAN 10TH GRADE BOYS AT TWO HIGH SCHOOLS IN NORTHERN CALIFORNIA WERE RANDOMLY AS-SIGNED TO ONE OF FOUR TREATMENT CONDI-TIONS. THE SCHOOLS VARIED IN TERMS OF HIGH OR LOW PROPORTION OF MEXICAN AMERICANS AND IN TERMS OF LOW OR MIDDLE CLASS STATUS. THE 2 EXPERIMENTAL CONDI-TIONS INCLUDED A VIDEOTAPE WITH A MEXI-CAN AMERICAN OR NON-MEXICAN MODEL. THE 2 ACTIVE CONTROLS WERE AUDIOTAPE ALONE OR SCRIPT ALONE. THE CRITERION MEASURES WERE A STUDENT REACTION SHEET (SRS) GIVEN IMMEDIATELY AFTER TREATMENT, A VOCATIONAL EDUCATION ATTITUDE QUES-TIONNAIRE (VEAQ), A PROJECT TALENT INTER-EST INVENTORY (PTII) GIVEN 2 DAYS AFTER TREATMENT, AND AN EDUCATION INFORMA-TION-SEEKING INVENTORY (EISI) GIVEN 3 WEEKS AFTER TREATMENT. A 3-WAY 2X2X2 ANALYSIS OF COVARIANCE WAS USED TO TEST THE HYPOTHESES. IN GENERAL, SUBJECTS AS-SIGNED TO VIDEO-MEDIA DID NOT SCORE HIGHER ON THE CRITERION MEASURES, AND SUBJECTS DID NOT PERFORM BETTER IF THE VIDEO MODEL WAS OF THE SAME ETHNICITY AS THE OBSERVER. THE EXCEPTION TO THE LATTER FINDING WAS A SIGNIFICANT INTER-ACTION BETWEEN ETHNICITY OF OBSERVER AND MODEL ON THE PTII. THAT IS, MEXICAN AMERICAN SUBJECTS TENDED TO INCREASE INTERESTS WHEN A MEXICAN AMERICAN VIDEO MODEL WAS USED WHILE NON-MEXICAN AMERICANS DID BETTER WITH A NON-MEXI-CAN MODEL. THE STUDY DEMONSTRATES THE FEASIBILITY OF ADMINISTERING VIDEO PRE-SENTED TRAINING IN FIELD SETTINGS, AND SUGGESTS THAT MEXICAN AMERICAN STU-DENTS ARE POSITIVE AND RESPONSIVE TO CA-REER PLANNING INTERVENTIONS. 25 REFER-ENCES.

ACCN   002414

1763 AUTH   **STODDARD, E. R.**

TITL   THE ADJUSTMENT OF MEXICAN AMERICAN

BARRIO FAMILIES TO FORCED HOUSING RE-
LOCATION.

SRCE   *SOCIAL SCIENCE QUARTERLY, 1973, 53(4), 749-
759.*

INDX   PSYCHOSOCIAL ADJUSTMENT, MEXICAN
AMERICAN, HOUSING, STRESS, SOCIAL
STRUCTURE, COMMUNITY, TEXAS, SOUTH-
WEST

ABST   TO TEST SPECIFIC HYPOTHESES RELATING
SEVERAL OBJECTIVE VARIABLES TO SELF-
EVALUATED SUCCESSFUL READJUSTMENT, 58
LOWER-CLASS MEXICAN AMERICAN FAMILIES
RELOCATED FROM AN EL PASO, TEXAS, BAR-
RIO WERE INTERVIEWED. THE DIRECTION AND
ASSOCIATION OF SUCCESSFUL READJUST-
MENT WITH SUCH FACTORS AS DISTANCE FROM
SCHOOLS, RESIDENCE LENGTH, HOME OWN-
ERSHIP, AND PARENTS' EDUCATION WERE STA-
TISTICALLY ANALYZED. SUCCESSFUL OR SAT-
ISFACTORY ADJUSTMENT WAS REPORTED BY
86.5% OF THE FAMILIES. AS PREDICTED, THE
MOST WELL-ADJUSTED FAMILIES INCLUDED
THOSE WHO WERE CLOSE TO AN ELEMENTARY
SCHOOL, OWNED THEIR OWN HOMES OR WERE
RENTING A HOUSE, WERE CITIZENS, HAD A
HIGHER EDUCATIONAL LEVEL, AND WHOSE
RELOCATION DID NOT FORCE THE PURCHASE
OF AN AUTOMOBILE. SUCCESSFULLY READ-
JUSTED FAMILIES TENDED TO RELY ON OFFI-
CIAL INFORMATION SOURCES AND GOVERN-
MENTAL ASSISTANCE OR SELF-HELP IN THEIR
MOVE, RATHER THAN ON ASSISTANCE FROM
FRIENDS OR RELATIVES. OF MAJOR CONCERN
TO THE MAJORITY WAS THE PRESERVATION OF
THOSE SOCIAL RELATIONSHIPS WHICH EX-
ISTED WITHIN THE BARRIO. IT WAS THE LOSS
OF THE "MINI-NEIGHBORHOOD" (I.E., A NET-
WORK OF SEVERAL FAMILIES LOCKED TO-
GETHER IN AN INTEGRATED PATTERN OF RE-
CIPROCAL VISITING) WHICH WAS MOST
LAMENTED. MORE IMPORTANT THAN KINSHIP
LOYALTIES, THE "MINI-NEIGHBORHOOD"
EMERGED AS THE CRITICAL SOCIAL UNIT TO
BE CONSIDERED IN RELOCATION PLANNING.
ITS THEORETICAL IMPLICATIONS SHOULD BE
PURSUED, WITH FURTHER RESEARCH NEEDED
TO CLARIFY THIS CONCEPT. 23 REFERENCES.

ACCN   001528

1764 AUTH   **STODDARD, E. R.**

TITL   MEXICAN AMERICANS.

SRCE   *NEW YORK: RANDOM HOUSE, 1973.*

INDX   MEXICAN AMERICAN, ACCULTURATION, VAL-
UES, HISTORY, REVIEW, STEREOTYPES, ECO-
NOMIC FACTORS, ETHNIC IDENTITY, EDUCA-
TION, CULTURE, MIGRANTS, POLITICS, CHICANO
MOVEMENT, POVERTY, SES, ADOLESCENTS,
PREJUDICE, RELIGION, TEXAS, CALIFORNIA,
SOUTHWEST, FAMILY STRUCTURE, SEX COM-
PARISON, LABOR FORCE, BOOK, SOCIAL
STRUCTURE, BIBLIOGRAPHY

ABST   FIFTH IN THE RANDOM HOUSE "ETHNIC GROUPS
IN COMPARATIVE PERSPECTIVE" SERIES, THIS
VOLUME ATTEMPTS TO OFFER THE MOST AC-
CURATE PICTURE POSSIBLE OF THE HETERO-
GENEITY WITHIN MEXICAN AMERICAN SOCIAL
STRUCTURE. THE BOOK FOCUSES ON CHICA-
NOS': (1) SOCIAL HISTORY; (2) SOCIAL ORGA-

NIZATIONS; (3) CULTURAL CONFLICTS; (4) EDU-
CATIONAL DEVELOPMENT; (5) RELIGION; (6)
ECONOMIC STATUS; AND (7) POLITICAL ACTIV-
ISM. EACH CHAPTER PROVIDES A GENERAL
HISTORICAL BACKGROUND ON THE TOPIC
AND THEN OFFERS THE AUTHOR'S PERSONAL
VIEWPOINT—WHICH GENERALLY TENDS TO BE
PESSIMISTIC. ON THE SUBJECT OF IDENTITY,
FOR EXAMPLE, IT IS ARGUED THAT THE CHI-
CANO, TO RID HIMSELF OF HIS INFERIOR STA-
TUS, MUST EITHER REJECT HIS ETHNIC ANCES-
TRY OR REJECT THE DOMINANT SOCIETY, THUS
REPUDIATING HIS RIGHT TO DETERMINE HIS
OWN IDENTITY. IN PARTICULAR, THE CHI-
CANO'S STRONG IDENTIFICATION WITH HIS
ETHNIC GROUP—RESULTING IN "CHICAN-
ISMO—HAS GENERATED SERIOUS CLASHES
WITH A RIGIDLY REPRESSIVE, DOMINANT SO-
CIETY. IF ECONOMIC AND POLITICAL PARITY
ARE TO BE ACHIEVED, AN UNUSUAL AMOUNT
OF COOPERATION BETWEEN ANGLOS AND
CHICANOS WILL BE NECESSARY. HOWEVER,
SOLUTIONS BASED ON SUCH COOPERATION
ARE GENERALLY UNAVAILABLE AT THE PRES-
ENT TIME. A BIBLIOGRAPHY OF SECONDARY
SOURCES FROM 1926 TO 1972 COMPLETES
THE VOLUME. 255 REFERENCES.

ACCN   001845

1765 AUTH   **STOKER, D. H.**

TITL   MEXICANS IN THE UNITED STATES.

SRCE   *PENNSYLVANIA PSYCHIATRIC QUARTERLY, 1966,
6(3), 30-37.*

INDX   MEXICAN AMERICAN, CULTURAL FACTORS,
PSYCHOTHERAPY, ESSAY

ABST   THE TREATMENT OF PSYCHOLOGICAL DISOR-
DERS OF MEXICAN AMERICAN PSYCHIATRIC
PATIENTS HAS BEEN INFLUENCED VERY LITTLE
BY INVESTIGATIONS OF THE CULTURAL BASES
OF PERSONALITY. AFTER REVIEWING SOME OF
THE LITERATURE, IT IS CONCLUDED THAT (1)
MEXICAN AMERICAN PSYCHIATRIC PATIENTS
SHOW CLEAR AND CONSISTENT DIFFERENCES
IN PSYCHOPATHOLOGY AND PERSONALITY
STRUCTURE, (2) AN ALTERNATIVE METHODO-
LOGICAL APPROACH TO THE STUDY OF CUL-
TURE AND PERSONALITY MAY BE THAT OF
VIEWING THE DISTURBED MEMBERS OF A SO-
CIETY, (3) IT IS UNREALISTIC TO EXPECT PEOPLE
WITH WIDELY DIFFERING NEED AND VALUE
SYSTEMS TO RESPOND FAVORABLY TO SOCIAL
INSTITUTIONS (SUCH AS THE SCHOOLS) WHICH
ARE HEAVILY WEIGHTED BY ANGLO NEEDS
AND VALUES, AND (4) IT WOULD SEEM THAT A
REORIENTATION OF THE TREATMENT OF SO-
CIAL PROBLEMS IS NEEDED—WHETHER IT BE
IN PSYCHOTHERAPY, EDUCATION, OR THE RE-
DUCTION OF POVERTY. 27 REFERENCES. (ERIC
ABSTRACT MODIFIED)

ACCN   001530

1766 AUTH   **STOKER, D. H., ZURCHER, L. A., & FOX, W.**

TITL   WOMEN IN PSYCHOTHERAPY: A CROSS CUL-
TURAL COMPARISON.

SRCE   *THE INTERNATIONAL JOURNAL OF SOCIAL
PSYCHIATRY, 1968-69, 15(1), 5-22.*

INDX   FEMALE, VALUES, CROSS CULTURAL, PSY-
CHOTHERAPY, CULTURAL FACTORS, INTER-

PERSONAL RELATIONS, MEXICAN AMERICAN, SEX ROLES, SYMPTOMATOLOGY, PSYCHOPATHOLOGY, ARIZONA, SOUTHWEST

ABST PSYCHOPATHOLOGICAL MANIFESTATIONS FOUND IN 25 ANGLO AND 25 MEXICAN AMERICAN FEMALE PATIENTS MATCHED FOR AGE, INCOME, AND EDUCATION AT AN ARIZONA MENTAL HEALTH CENTER WERE COMPARED AND SET IN THE CONTEXT OF OTHER RELEVANT CASE DATA. SIGNIFICANT DIFFERENCES WERE FOUND: MEXICAN AMERICANS HAD A HIGHER FREQUENCY OF NEUROTIC DISORDERS CENTERING AROUND DEPENDENCY CONFLICTS AND FRUSTRATIONS, WHILE ANGLOS MORE OFTEN EXHIBITED CHARACTER DISORDERS RELATING TO GUILT FEELINGS AND DOUBTS ABOUT SELF-WORTH. ANGLOS MANIFESTED A CONSISTENT PATTERN OF DISRUPTION OF INTERPERSONAL RELATIONSHIPS REFLECTING CULTURAL VALUES FOR ACHIEVEMENT AND COMPETITION. THIS WAS NOT FOUND IN MEXICAN AMERICANS, AS THEIR PSYCHOPATHOLOGY REFLECTED CULTURAL VALUES FOR PARTICULARISM, THE FEMALE "MARTYR" ROLE, AND MALE MACHISMO. THE MEXICAN AMERICAN FAMILY ACCEPTS AND SUPPORTS THE AFFLICTED, HESITATING TO REFER KIN TO A CENTER FOR TREATMENT. ANGLO FAMILIES FEEL NEITHER EQUIPPED NOR WILLING TO COPE, AND THEY TEND TO SEEK OUTSIDE ASSISTANCE. ALTHOUGH MEXICAN AMERICAN PATHOLOGY IS GENERALLY DIAGNOSED AS LESS CHRONIC AND SEVERE, CASE OUTCOMES ARE TERMED LESS SUCCESSFUL BECAUSE A LARGE NUMBER DROP OUT OF THERAPY. QUESTIONS ARE RAISED, THEREFORE, REGARDING THE APPROPRIATENESS OF TREATMENT AVAILABLE. 38 REFERENCES.

ACCN 001531

1767 AUTH **STOKER, D. H., & MEADOW, A.**
TITL CULTURAL DIFFERENCES IN CHILD GUIDANCE CLINIC PATIENTS.
SRCE *INTERNATIONAL JOURNAL OF SOCIAL PSYCHIATRY, 1974, 20(3-4), 186-202.*
INDX CULTURAL FACTORS, CHILDREN, HEALTH DELIVERY SYSTEMS, CROSS CULTURAL, MEXICAN AMERICAN, FAMILY STRUCTURE, EMPIRICAL, SEX COMPARISON, PSYCHOPATHOLOGY, SES, SYMPTOMATOLOGY
ABST THE PSYCHOPATHOLOGICAL, PSYCHOLOGICAL, AND FAMILIAL PROCESSES AND THERAPEUTIC TREATMENT OF MEXICAN AMERICAN AND ANGLO AMERICAN CHILDREN ARE DISCUSSED. CASE FILES OF 152 MEXICAN AMERICAN AND 152 ANGLO AMERICAN CHILDREN WERE RANDOMLY SELECTED FROM THE FILES OF THREE CHILD GUIDANCE CLINICS IN THE SOUTHWESTERN PART OF THE COUNTRY. EACH CASE WAS MATCHED ROUGHLY FOR GROSS YEARLY FAMILY INCOME. A LIST OF 74 SYMPTOMATIC BEHAVIORS WAS CONSTRUCTED THROUGH READING A NUMBER OF CASE HISTORIES. RESULTS OF THE ANALYSIS INDICATE WHICH SYMPTOMS WERE FOUND SIGNIFICANTLY MORE FREQUENTLY IN EACH GROUP, COMPARED SEPARATELY WITH EACH OTHER GROUP. FINDINGS INDICATE SIGNIFICANT AND CONSISTENT DIFFERENCES IN PSYCHOPATHOLOGY BETWEEN THE FOUR DIFFERENT SEX-CULTURE SAMPLES. FINDINGS ARE RELATED TO CULTURALLY DETERMINED ASPECTS OF FAMILY STRUCTURE, FAMILY INTERACTION, ROLE CONFLICTS, AND PERSONALITY STRUCTURE. 3 REFERENCES. (NCMHI ABSTRACT)

ACCN 001532

1768 AUTH **STONES, M. E.**
TITL SCHOOL ADMINISTRATOR ATTITUDES AND RACISM.
SRCE *INTEGRATED EDUCATION: A REPORT ON RACE AND SCHOOLS, 1973, 11(2), 54-59.*
INDX ADMINISTRATORS, ATTITUDES, PREJUDICE, EDUCATION, SURVEY, EMPIRICAL, TEXAS, SOUTHWEST
ABST TO ASSESS RACIAL ATTITUDES TOWARDS BLACK STUDENTS, QUESTIONNAIRES WERE MAILED TO 142 RANDOMLY SELECTED SCHOOL PRINCIPALS IN THREE MAJOR TEXAS CITIES. 66 QUESTIONNAIRES WERE RETURNED BY 44 WHITE, 17 BLACK, AND 9 CHICANO PRINCIPALS. THE FINDINGS REVEAL A WIDE VARIETY OF ATTITUDES AMONG ADMINISTRATORS ON SOCIAL DISTANCE, KNOWLEDGE OF DISCRIMINATION, RACIAL STEREOTYPING, SCHOOL SEGREGATION, BUSING, AND THE ADMINISTRATORS' OWN ROLE IN RACIAL ISSUES. A SIZABLE NUMBER OF ADMINISTRATORS DISPLAYED PERSONAL BARRIERS AGAINST OTHER ETHNIC GROUPS. ALTHOUGH MOST WERE AWARE OF PRACTICES OF DISCRIMINATION, SOME HELD STEREOTYPES OF BLACK PEOPLE AS LESS AMBITIOUS AND LAW-ABIDING. MOST WERE OPPOSED TO BUSING AND FELT THAT INTEGRATION WOULD BE MORE HARMFUL TO BLACK EDUCATION THAN TO WHITE. RACIAL PROBLEMS WERE FELT TO BE THE MOST COMMON SERIOUS PROBLEM THE PRINCIPALS FACED. ALMOST ALL FELT TEACHERS AND ADMINISTRATORS NEEDED MORE TRAINING IN DEALING WITH MINORITY GROUPS. MORE EXTENSIVE TRAINING FOR SCHOOL PERSONNEL ON RACIAL ISSUES, BETTER COMMUNITY RELATIONS PROGRAMS, AND FURTHER RESEARCH IN THIS FIELD ARE RECOMMENDED.

ACCN 001533

1769 AUTH **STRAUS, M. A.**
TITL COMMUNICATION, CREATIVITY, AND PROBLEM SOLVING ABILITY OF MIDDLE- AND WORKING-CLASS FAMILIES IN THREE SOCIETIES.
SRCE *AMERICAN JOURNAL OF SOCIOLOGY, 1968, 73(4), 417-430.*
INDX SES, CROSS CULTURAL, EMPIRICAL, PUERTO RICAN-I, GROUP DYNAMICS, ACHIEVEMENT MOTIVATION, MINNESOTA, MIDWEST
ABST DATA ON ABILITY TO SOLVE A LABORATORY PROBLEM ARE REPORTED FOR SAMPLES OF MIDDLE- AND WORKING-CLASS FAMILIES IN BOMBAY, INDIA, MINNEAPOLIS, MINNESOTA, AND SAN JUAN, PUERTO RICO. IN ALL THREE SAMPLES, WORKING-CLASS FAMILY GROUPS WERE LESS SUCCESSFUL IN SOLVING THE PROBLEM THAN MIDDLE-CLASS FAMILIES. THREE FACTORS WHICH COULD ACCOUNT FOR THE POORER PROBLEM-SOLVING ABILITY

OF THE WORKING-CLASS SAMPLES WERE IN-VESTIGATED. A "DIFFERENTIAL MOTIVATION" THEORY WAS TESTED BY MEANS OF AN INDEX OF THE EFFORT EXPENDED IN THE TASK. THE RESULTS SHOWED NO SOCIAL CLASS DIFFER-ENCE. TESTS OF A "COMMUNICATION BLOCK" AND A "COGNITIVE STYLE" THEORY REVEALED LARGE SOCIAL CLASS DIFFERENCES IN VOL-UME OF INTRAFAMILY COMMUNICATION AND IN CREATIVITY. IT IS CONCLUDED THAT THE DIFFERENCES IN PROBLEM-SOLVING ABILITY, AS WELL AS RESTRICTED WORKING-CLASS COMMUNICATION AND CREATIVITY (WHICH AP-PEAR PARTLY TO EXPLAIN THE DIFFERENCES IN PROBLEM-SOLVING ABILITY) ARE SIMILAR IN ALL THREE SOCIETIES, IN SPITE OF VAST DIF-FERENCES IN CULTURE. HOWEVER, THE MORE URBANIZED AND INDUSTRIALIZED THE SOCI-ETY, THE SMALLER THE SOCIAL CLASS DIFFER-ENCE. 37 REFERENCES. (JOURNAL ABSTRACT MODIFIED)

ACCN   001534

1770 AUTH   **STRAYER, R., & ELLENHORN, L.**
TITL   VIETNAM VETERANS: A STUDY EXPLORING AD-JUSTMENT PATTERNS AND ATTITUDES.
SRCE   *JOURNAL OF SOCIAL ISSUES, 1975, 31(4), 81-93.*
INDX   PSYCHOSOCIAL ADJUSTMENT, AUTHORITARI-ANISM, ROTTER INTERNAL-EXTERNAL SCALE, EMPIRICAL, MEXICAN AMERICAN, CROSS CUL-TURAL, ADULTS, DEPRESSION, VETERANS, CALIFORNIA, SOUTHWEST, URBAN
ABST   TO IDENTIFY DIFFERENCES BETWEEN VETER-ANS WHO EXPERIENCED ADJUSTMENT PROB-LEMS AND THOSE ABLE TO COPE WITH WAR EXPERIENCES AND INTEGRATE THEMSELVES INTO CIVILIAN LIFE, 40 VIETNAM VETERANS (25 WHITE, 7 BLACK, AND 8 MEXICAN AMERICAN) LIVING IN SOUTHERN CALIFORNIA WERE IN-TERVIEWED AND TESTED. THE DATA WERE COLLECTED THROUGH IN-DEPTH STRUC-TURED INTERVIEWS AND THE ADMINISTERING OF A BALANCED VERSION OF THE CALIFORNIA F SCALE, THE INTERNAL-EXTERNAL (I-E) CON-TROL SCALE, AND A SENTENCE COMPLETION TEST SPECIFICALLY DESIGNED FOR THIS STUDY. THESE VETERANS INDICATED THAT THE AD-JUSTMENT PROCESSES THEY FACED UPON RE-TURN TO CIVILIAN LIFE WERE UNUSUALLY DIF-FICULT AND COMPLEX. SEVERE DEPRESSION, HOSTILITY, AND GUILT FEELINGS CHARACTER-IZED MANY OF THEM. THE VETERAN'S PERCEP-TION OF THE EXTENT AND INTENSITY OF HIS COMBAT INVOLVEMENT AS WELL AS HIS PAR-TICIPATION IN ATROCITIES IS CLOSELY RE-LATED TO HIS OVERALL ADJUSTMENT TO CIVILIAN LIFE. INTRACEPTION VERSUS AU-THORITARIANISM ON THE PART OF THESE VETERANS TENDS TO DIFFERENTIATE BETWEEN THOSE WHO WITHDRAW AND ARE APATHETIC UPON RETURN AND THOSE WHO FIND EM-PLOYMENT OR SCHOOLING AND ARE IN FAVOR OF THE WAR EFFORT. RACE IS ALSO A DIS-CRIMINATING FACTOR, WITH BLACK AND MEX-ICAN AMERICAN VETERANS BEING FAR MORE OFTEN UNEMPLOYED, OPPOSED TO THE WAR, AND PERCEIVING THEMSELVES AS LESS ABLE

TO CONTROL THEIR OWN PERSONAL WORLD. 5 REFERENCES. (JOURNAL ABSTRACT MODI-FIED)

ACCN   001535

1771 AUTH   **STREVENS, P.**
TITL   SECOND LANGUAGE LEARNING.
SRCE   *JOURNAL OF THE AMERICAN ACADEMY OF ARTS AND SCIENCES, 1973(SUMMER), 149-160.*
INDX   LANGUAGE LEARNING, ESSAY, INSTRUC-TIONAL TECHNIQUES, HISTORY
ABST   THE SEARCH FOR A SINGLE MOST EFFECTIVE METHOD OF LANGUAGE INSTRUCTION OVER THE PAST FIFTY YEARS BEGAN WITH THE CLAS-SICAL GRAMMAR-TRANSLATION METHOD BEING REPLACED IN THE 1920'S BY THE DI-RECT METHOD OF HEARING THE LANGUAGE SPOKEN. IN THE 30'S AND 40'S, THIS WAS RE-PLACED BY THE AUDIO-LINGUAL AND AUDIO-VISUAL METHODS. SINCE 1950 THE FIELD HAS BEEN GREATLY AFFECTED BY NEW DEVELOP-MENTS IN LINGUISTICS. NO ONE METHOD, HOWEVER, HAS BEEN FOUND TO WORK WELL IN ALL SITUATIONS, AND NO ONE THEORY HAS INTEGRATED ALL FACTORS INVOLVED IN TEACHING AND LEARNING A SECOND LAN-GUAGE. EXPERIMENTATION INVOLVING LAN-GUAGE LABS, STATISTICAL SURVEYS, ETC., HAS PRODUCED RESULTS WHICH ARE EITHER AMBIGUOUS OR TOO SPECIFIC TO BE OF VALUE IN GENERAL APPLICATION. LANGUAGE LEARNING CANNOT BE ASSUMED TO BE SUF-FICIENTLY HOMOGENEOUS FOR A SINGLE METHOD TO FIT ALL CIRCUMSTANCES, AND SUCCESS OR FAILURE CANNOT BE ATTRIB-UTED TO METHOD ALONE. AN ADEQUATE AP-PROACH MUST TAKE INTO ACCOUNT SUCH VARIABLES AS (1) THE LEARNER'S AGE, VOL-UNTARY PARTICIPATION, AND LEVEL OF PRO-FICIENCY, (2) THE ORGANIZATIONAL ASPECTS OF HIS LEARNING ENVIRONMENT, AND (3) THE LANGUAGE IN WHICH THE INSTRUCTION IS GIVEN. THE AIMS OF LANGUAGE LEARNING MUST BE ADEQUATELY STATED, REALISTIC, AND RELEVANT TO THE LEARNER. THE QUES-TION OF OPTIMUM QUANTITY AND INTENSITY OF INSTRUCTION, IMPEDIMENTS TO LEARNING SUCH AS DISTRACTION AND OVERCROWDING, AND OTHER NEGATIVE FACTORS NEED TO BE CONSIDERED. INDIVIDUALS DIFFER IN WILL-INGNESS TO LEARN AND IN THEIR OWN EX-PECTATIONS OF SUCCESS AND FAILURE, WHILE TEACHERS VARY IN THEIR POSSESSION OF EF-FECTIVE SKILLS. METHODS AND MATERIALS CHOSEN MUST BE RELEVANT AND OF INTER-EST TO THE LEARNER. THE FUTURE OF SEC-OND LANGUAGE LEARNING EMERGES AS A TASK REQUIRING A MORE COMPLEX BUT RE-ALISTIC APPROACH TO IDENTIFICATION OF THOSE FACTORS MAXIMIZING SUCCESS AND MINIMIZING FAILURE FOR EACH SET OF LEARNERS. 17 REFERENCES.

ACCN   001536

1772 AUTH   **STROM, R., & JOHNSON, A.**
TITL   THE PARENT AS A TEACHER.
SRCE   *EDUCATION, 1974, 95(1), 40-43.*
INDX   PARENTAL INVOLVEMENT, EARLY CHILDHOOD

EDUCATION, CHILDREARING PRACTICES, LEARNING, MEXICAN, ATTITUDES

ABST TO TEST AND THEREBY IMPROVE "FAMILY IN-FLUENCE" POTENTIAL IN PRESCHOOL PARENT-INVOLVEMENT PROGRAMS, AN EIGHT-WEEK TRAINING PROGRAM WAS INSTITUTED WITH 70 ANGLO, BLACK, AND MEXICAN AMERICAN MOTHERS. AN INSTRUMENT FOR PARENTAL SELF-ASSESSMENT WAS DEVISED—THE PARENT AS A TEACHER INVENTORY (PAAT). THIS INVENTORY WAS ACCOMPANIED BY A QUESTIONNAIRE MEASURING THE CHILD'S PERCEPTIONS OF PARENTAL BEHAVIOR ALONG FIVE DIMENSIONS: CONTROL; CREATIVITY; FRUSTRATION; PLAY; AND TEACHING-LEARNING. ANALYSIS OF EACH DIMENSION IDENTIFIED STRENGTHS AND WEAKNESSES OF PARENTS' CHILDREARING PRACTICES. THE TRAINING PROGRAM FOCUSED ON THE USE OF TOYS AS AN INSTRUCTIONAL MEDIUM FOR HOME CURRICULUM, AND THE PAAT WAS USED AS A PREMEASURE, POSTMEASURE, AND DIAGNOSTIC MEASURE DURING THE TRAINING. THE RESULTS DEMONSTRATED SIGNIFICANT GAINS IN SELF-CONCEPT AMONG MOTHERS AS WELL AS CHILDREN. THE MOTHERS' KNOWLEDGE OF THE TEACHING-LEARNING PROCESS AND THE CHILDREN'S VERBAL SKILLS ALSO SHOWED SIGNIFICANT IMPROVEMENT. 11 REFERENCES. (ERIC ABSTRACT MODIFIED)

ACCN 001537

1773 AUTH STUMPHAUZER, J. S., AIKEN, T. W., & VELOZ, E. V.

TITL EAST SIDE STORY: BEHAVIORAL ANALYSIS OF A HIGH JUVENILE CRIME COMMUNITY.

SRCE BEHAVIORAL DISORDERS, 1977, 2, 76-84.

INDX CALIFORNIA, SOUTHWEST, ADOLESCENTS, URBAN, EMPIRICAL, BEHAVIOR MODIFICATION, POLICE-COMMUNITY RELATIONS, GANGS, RESEARCH METHODOLOGY, COMMUNITY, PEER GROUP, DELINQUENCY, ENVIRONMENTAL FACTORS, ECONOMIC FACTORS, SURVEY, MALE, FEMALE

ABST SINCE THE SEVERE GANG PROBLEMS IN LOS ANGELES ARE NOT BEING IMPROVED BY TRADITIONAL PSYCHOTHERAPEUTIC OR LAW ENFORCEMENT TECHNIQUES, THE AUTHORS PROPOSE AN ALTERNATIVE APPROACH. AN EXPANDED BEHAVIORAL ANALYSIS MODEL IS OFFERED, BY WHICH AN ENTIRE EAST LOS ANGELES (ELA) COMMUNITY AND A SPECIFIC GANG (EASTSIDE LOMA) CAN BE STUDIED FOR WAYS CRIME BEHAVIOR IS LEARNED AND WAYS NON-DELINQUENT BEHAVIOR CAN BE REINFORCED. SPECIFICALLY, THE MODEL PROBES ASSETS, DEFICITS, EXCESSES, AND CONTROLLING VARIABLES. A QUESTIONNAIRE ADMINISTERED TO POLICE OFFICERS REVEALED THEIR ATTITUDE THAT FIREARMS AND TRUANCY ARE MAJOR EXCESSES IN THE COMMUNITY AND THAT LACK OF CRIME PREVENTION PROGRAMS IS THE CHIEF DEFICIT. HOWEVER, BASED ON A PRELIMANARY ANALYSIS OF THE EASTSIDE LOMA GANG, THE AUTHORS ALSO CONCLUDE THAT DELINQUENT BEHAVIOR IS OFTEN INDIRECTLY REINFORCED BY MANY PARENTS, POLICE OFFICERS, COMMUNITY MEMBERS, AND

AGENCIES IN THE AREA. FINALLY, A BEHAVIORAL ANALYSIS OF NON-DELINQUENTS REVEALED THAT REINFORCEMENT FOR SUCH BEHAVIOR USUALLY COMES FROM A STRONG FAMILY, FROM PEERS NOT IN GANG LIFE, AND FROM OTHER INFLUENTIAL ADULTS IN THE COMMUNITY. IN CONCLUSION, FURTHER BEHAVIORAL ANALYSIS OF NON-DELINQUENTS IS RECOMMENDED. 13 REFERENCES.

ACCN 002217

1774 AUTH STYBEL, L. J.

TITL PSYCHOTHERAPEUTIC OPTIONS IN THE TREATMENT OF CHILD AND ADOLESCENT HYDROCARBON INHALERS.

SRCE AMERICAN JOURNAL OF PSYCHOTHERAPY, 1977, 31(4), 525-532.

INDX ADOLESCENTS, CASE STUDY, CROSS CULTURAL, INHALANT ABUSE, MEXICAN AMERICAN, PSYCHOTHERAPY, SOUTHWEST, TEXAS, CHILDREN, POLICY

ABST HYDROCARBON INHALATION, OR SNIFFING, BY PREADOLESCENTS AND ADOLESCENTS IS CONSIDERED A MAJOR PUBLIC HEALTH PROBLEM IN LOW SES AREAS WITH LARGE CONCENTRATIONS OF MEXICAN AMERICANS. SNIFFERS ARE CATAGORIZED INTO THREE TYPES: A SOCIAL SNIFFER, A MODERATE SNIFFER, AND A CHRONIC SNIFFER. SURVEY DATA SUGGEST THAT THESE CATAGORIES DESCRIBE 75%, 15%, AND 11% OF ALL ADOLESCENT SNIFFERS, RESPECTIVELY. SOCIAL SNIFFING APPEARS TO REFLECT A SOCIOLOGICAL PROBLEM, MODERATE SNIFFING REFLECTS A NEUROTIC OR SITUATIONAL CONFLICT, AND CHRONIC SNIFFING REFLECTS A PSYCHOTIC COMPONENT. ACCORDINGLY, DIFFERENT TREATMENT APPROACHES ARE WARRANTED AND SOME GUIDELINES ARE SUGGESTED. CASE STUDIES ARE PRESENTED TO ILLUSTRATE THE TYPES OF SNIFFERS. 7 REFERENCES.

ACCN 002654

1775 AUTH SUAREZ, C.

TITL SEXUAL STEREOTYPES—PSYCHOLOGICAL AND CULTURAL SURVIVAL.

SRCE REGENERACION, 1973, 2(3), 17-21.

INDX STEREOTYPES, SEX ROLES, ACCULTURATION, MEXICAN AMERICAN, FAMILY ROLES, MENTAL HEALTH, CHILDREARING PRACTICES, DISCRIMINATION, EDUCATION, FEMALE, ATTITUDES

ABST THE CHICANA HAS BEEN A DOUBLE VICTIM OF SEXUAL AND ETHNIC STEREOTYPES, BEING PARTICULARLY BLAMED FOR CHILD REARING PRACTICES WHICH BLOCK HER CHILD'S ADVANCEMENT INTO ANGLO SOCIETY. THE DOMINANT SOCIAL SCIENCE THEORIES THAT THE CHICANO CHILD IS CULTURALLY DISADVANTAGED DUE TO THE DISORGANIZATION, LOW EXPECTATIONS, AND LACK OF INTELLECTUAL STIMULATION IN HIS FAMILY, THAT THE CHICANO FAMILY IS THE MAIN OBSTACLE TO THE CHILD'S ADVANCEMENT, AND THAT CHICANO CULTURE IS COMPOSED OF VALUES DETRIMENTAL TO THE CHILD ARE ALL BASED ON THE PREMISE THAT THE ANGLO CULTURE IS SUPERIOR TO OTHERS. APPRECIATION FOR THE

RICHNESS OF MEXICAN AMERICAN CULTURE AND AN ACCEPTANCE OF CULTURAL PLURALISM ARE ESSENTIAL IN THE EDUCATION OF THE CHICANO CHILD. RATHER THAN BEING SUITED ONLY FOR MENIAL JOBS OR VOCATIONAL EDUCATION, CHICANAS HAVE MANY STRENGTHS AND TALENTS THAT HAVE BEEN OVERLOOKED AND SHOULD BE DEVELOPED. THEY HAVE EMERGED IN POSITIONS OF POLITICAL AND INTELLECTUAL LEADERSHIP, AND SOCIETY MUST APPRECIATE AND ACCEPT THE CULTURAL DIFFERENCES WHICH MAKE THE CHICANA WHAT SHE IS. 6 REFERENCES.

ACCN   001538

1776 AUTH   **SUE, S.**
TITL   COMMUNITY MENTAL HEALTH SERVICES TO MINORITY GROUPS: SOME OPTIMISM, SOME PESSIMISM.
SRCE   *AMERICAN PSYCHOLOGIST, 1977, 32, 616-624.*
INDX   PSYCHOTHERAPY, HEALTH DELIVERY SYSTEMS, DISCRIMINATION, CROSS CULTURAL, MEXICAN AMERICAN, MENTAL HEALTH, RESOURCE UTILIZATION, DEMOGRAPHIC, COMMUNITY, EMPIRICAL
ABST   TO DETERMINE WHETHER MINORITY GROUPS, BY VIRTUE OF THEIR CULTURAL BACKGROUND, REQUIRE DIFFERENTIAL MENTAL HEALTH SERVICES FOR EFFECTIVE TREATMENT, DATA WERE COLLECTED ON 13,198 CLIENTS AT 17 SEATTLE COMMUNITY MENTAL HEALTH CENTERS OVER A THREE-YEAR PERIOD (83 MEXICAN AMERICAN, 100 ASIAN AMERICAN, 152 NATIVE AMERICAN, 959 BLACK, AND 11,904 WHITE CLIENTS). ANALYSIS OF SERVICES RECEIVED SUGGESTS THAT THE TREATMENT OF BLACKS DIFFERED FROM WHITES IN ALL THE VARIABLES EXAMINED (E.G., BLACKS MORE OFTEN RECEIVED INTAKE AND THERAPY FROM PARAPROFESSIONAL RATHER THAN PROFESSIONAL PERSONNEL), AND OVER 50% OF THE BLACKS FAILED TO RETURN AFTER ONE CONTACT, COMPARED TO 30% OF THE WHITES. ALTHOUGH MEXICAN AMERICAN, ASIAN AMERICAN, AND NATIVE AMERICAN CLIENTS TENDED TO RECEIVE THE SAME SERVICE MODALITIES AS WHITES, OVER 40% OF THE CLIENTS IN EACH OF THESE MINORITY GROUPS DROPPED OUT AFTER ONE CONTACT. IF DROPOUT RATES ARE SEEN AS INDICATORS OF UNRESPONSIVE SERVICES, THEN SOME MINORITY GROUP CLIENTS MAY BE RECEIVING NON-DISCRIMINATORY BUT CULTURALLY UNRESPONSIVE SERVICES AT MENTAL HEALTH FACILITIES. THE ADEQUACY OF SERVICES MUST THEREFORE BE EXAMINED ON AN INTERPERSONAL AS WELL AS INSTITUTIONAL LEVEL (I.E., TYPES OF SERVICES RENDERED). ATTENTION NEEDS TO BE FOCUSED ON THE DELIVERY OF APPROPRIATE TREATMENT IN THE CONTEXT OF THE CLIENT'S ETHNIC BACKGROUND AS WELL AS ON THE DEVELOPMENT OF BETTER INDICES OF "ADEQUACY" OF SERVICES. INSTEAD OF OFFERING IDENTICAL SERVICES TO ALL CLIENTS, IRRESPECTIVE OF ETHNICITY, IT IS RECOMMENDED THAT MORE RESPONSIVE SERVICES BE IMPLEMENTED BY MEANS OF (1) TRAINING MENTAL HEALTH CARE PROVIDERS FOR MINORITY GROUPS, (2) HIRING ETHNIC SPECIALISTS AS HEALTH CARE CONSULTANTS WITHIN EXISTING INSTITUTIONS, (3) ESTABLISHING INDEPENDENT BUT PARALLEL SERVICES WITHIN MINORITY COMMUNITIES, AND (4) DEVELOPING NEW MENTAL HEALTH DELIVERY SYSTEMS WHICH ARE APPROPRIATE FOR MINORITY GROUPS' CULTURAL TRADITIONS. 19 REFERENCES.

ACCN   001540

1777 AUTH   **SUE, S.**
TITL   TRAINING OF "THIRD WORLD" STUDENTS TO FUNCTION AS COUNSELORS.
SRCE   *JOURNAL OF COUNSELING PSYCHOLOGY, 1973, 20(1), 73-78.*
INDX   PARAPROFESSIONALS, COLLEGE STUDENTS, PSYCHOTHERAPY, ATTITUDES, HEALTH DELIVERY SYSTEMS, CALIFORNIA, SOUTHWEST
ABST   TO PROVIDE MORE RESPONSIVE COUNSELING SERVICES TO MINORITY STUDENTS, STAFF MEMBERS AT A LOS ANGELES STUDENT HEALTH PSYCHIATRIC CLINIC INITIATED A PROGRAM TO TRAIN MINORITY STUDENTS AS COUNSELORS FOR OTHER MINORITY STUDENTS. THE PROBLEM WAS THAT FEW MINORITY STUDENTS WERE SEEKING THE CLINIC'S SERVICES, AND ETHNIC STUDIES PROGRAM DIRECTORS WHO WERE CONSULTED EXPLAINED THAT MANY MINORITY STUDENTS AVOIDED TRADITIONAL MENTAL HEALTH SERVICES BECAUSE (1) THERE WERE FEW MINORITY THERAPISTS, (2) THE STUDENTS FELT THAT THE PSYCHOTHERAPEUTIC PROCESS WAS DESIGNED FOR THE WHITE MIDDLE CLASS, AND (3) THE CLINIC WAS IDENTIFIED WITH AN "ESTABLISHMENT" INSTITUTION. MINORITY STUDENTS WERE RECRUITED AND 70 STUDENTS REPRESENTING ASIAN-AMERICAN, AMERICAN INDIAN, BLACK, CHICANO, AND WHITE ETHNIC GROUPS WERE ENROLLED. INITIAL PROBLEMS AROSE IN DEFINING GOALS AND DEVELOPING TRUST BETWEEN STUDENTS AND STAFF, BUT AREAS OF COMPROMISE WERE FOUND. TRAINING CONSISTED OF (1) LECTURES ON THE CULTURAL BACKGROUND OF MINORITY GROUPS, COUNSELING TECHNIQUES, BEHAVIOR PATHOLOGY, ETC., AND (2) WEEKLY SMALL GROUP INTERACTION SESSIONS, CONSISTING OF ROLE PLAYING AND GROUP-ENCOUNTER EXPERIENCES. AFTER TRAINING, 20 OF THE 70 STUDENTS WERE SELECTED TO BE EMPLOYED AS PEER COUNSELORS. ALTHOUGH NO FORMAL PRE- OR POST-TRAINING LEVELS OF FUNCTIONING WERE OBTAINED, THE STUDENTS WERE JUDGED TO BE FUNCTIONING WELL IN THE THERAPEUTIC ROLE, AND PLANS WERE BEING MADE TO CONTINUE THE TRAINING OF MINORITY-GROUP PARAPROFESSIONALS. 13 REFERENCES.

ACCN   001541

1778 AUTH   **SUE, S., ALLEN, D. B., & CONAWAY, L.**
TITL   THE RESPONSIVENESS AND EQUALITY OF MENTAL HEALTH CARE TO CHICANOS AND NATIVE AMERICANS.
SRCE   *AMERICAN JOURNAL OF COMMUNITY PSYCHOLOGY, 1978, 6(2), 137-146.*

INDX   MENTAL HEALTH, MEXICAN AMERICAN, CROSS CULTURAL, HEALTH DELIVERY SYSTEMS, RESOURCE UTILIZATION, DEMOGRAPHIC, PSYCHOTHERAPY, CULTURAL FACTORS, EMPIRICAL, DISCRIMINATION, ADULTS, SES, PERSONNEL, COMMUNITY

ABST   A COMPARISON WAS MADE BETWEEN THE EFFECTIVENESS AND EQUALITY OF MENTAL HEALTH SERVICES RECEIVED BY MINORITY CLIENTS (83 CHICANO AND 152 NATIVE AMERICANS) AND SERVICES RECEIVED BY A RANDOM SAMPLE OF 1,190 ANGLO CLIENTS AT 17 SEATTLE COMMUNITY MENTAL HEALTH FACILITIES. FOUR TABLES DESCRIBE DEMOGRAPHIC CHARACTERISTICS OF CLIENTS, DIAGNOSES BY GROUP, PROGRAM ASSIGNMENT AND TREATMENT BY GROUP, AND TYPE OF PERSONNEL AT INTAKE AND DURING THERAPY. IT WAS FOUND THAT CHICANOS WERE UNDERREPRESENTED AND NATIVE AMERICANS OVERREPRESENTED AT THESE CENTERS. SECONDLY, EVEN THOUGH THESE MINORITY CLIENTS TENDED TO HAVE LOWER INCOME AND EDUCATIONAL LEVELS, THERE WAS NO EVIDENCE THAT THEY WERE RENDERED INFERIOR OR DISCRIMINATORY SERVICES. NEVERTHELESS, 42% OF THE CHICANOS AND 55% OF THE NATIVE AMERICANS FAILED TO RETURN TO THE CENTERS FOR TREATMENT, AS COMPARED TO 30% OF THE ANGLOS; AND THIS SUGGESTS THAT FOR ETHNIC GROUP CLIENTS, "EQUALITY" OF SERVICES MAY NOT MEAN "RESPONSIVE" SERVICES. EMPHASIS SHOULD THEREFORE BE PLACED UPON THE DEVELOPMENT OF SERVICES APPROPRIATE TO ETHNIC DIFFERENCES IN CULTURE, LIFE STYLES, AND EXPERIENCES. 16 REFERENCES.

ACCN   001542

1779 AUTH   **SWADESH, F. L.**
TITL   PROPERTY AND KINSHIP IN NORTHERN NEW MEXICO.
SRCE   *ROCKY MOUNTAIN SOCIAL SCIENCE JOURNAL, 1965, 2, 209-214.*
INDX   MEXICAN AMERICAN, FAMILY STRUCTURE, EXTENDED FAMILY, COMMUNITY, HISTORY, ENVIRONMENTAL FACTORS, COOPERATION, ECONOMIC FACTORS, MARRIAGE, SOCIAL STRUCTURE, NEW MEXICO, SOUTHWEST
ABST   DOCUMENTATION IS PRESENTED WHICH SUPPORTS THE HYPOTHESIS THAT THE RIO ARRIBA SECTION OF NORTHERN NEW MEXICO MAINTAINS A DISTINCTIVE SOCIAL STRUCTURE AS WELL AS PATTERNS OF EXISTENCE WHICH ARE DIFFERENT FROM OTHER REGIONS IN NEW MEXICO. THE HISTORY OF PROPERTY OWNERSHIP AND RULES OF KINSHIP IN THIS AREA REVEAL THE DEVELOPMENT OF COOPERATIVE PATTERNS OF BEHAVIOR IN LABOR AND RESIDENCE DUE TO LIMITED MANPOWER AND THE NEED FOR MUTUAL PROTECTION. SECONDLY, THE REGULATION OF MARRIAGE AND PROPERTY INHERITANCE REDUCED THE FRACTIONING OF PROPERTY AND, CONCOMITANTLY, INTRAFAMILY FEUDING. THIS LEADS TO THE INTENSIFICATION OF FRATERNAL RELATIONS. SUCH FRATERNAL BONDS OF KINSHIP HAVE BECOME THE PRIMARY BASE OF THE ECO-

NOMIC ORGANIZATION AND SOCIAL CONTROL WHICH DISTINGUISH THIS REGION FROM THE MORE PATRON-DOMINATED REGIONS OF SOUTHERN AND EASTERN NEW MEXICO. 7 REFERENCES.

ACCN   001544

1780 AUTH   **SWANSON, E., & DEBLASSIE, R.**
TITL   INTERPRETER EFFECTS ON THE WISC PERFORMANCE OF FIRST GRADE MEXICAN AMERICAN CHILDREN.
SRCE   *MEASUREMENT AND EVALUATION IN GUIDANCE, 1971, 4(3), 172-175.*
INDX   EXAMINER EFFECTS, WISC, PERFORMANCE EXPECTATIONS, MEXICAN AMERICAN, CHILDREN, BILINGUAL, BILINGUAL-BICULTURAL PERSONNEL
ABST   BASED ON THE PREMISE THAT LINGUISTIC BACKGROUND IS THE MOST IMPORTANT CONTAMINATING VARIABLE IN ASSESSING THE INTELLIGENCE OF THE MEXICAN AMERICAN CHILD, THIS STUDY EXPLORES THE SPECIFIC CONCEPTS THAT (1) IN TESTING SITUATIONS, WHITE ANGLO AMERICAN EXAMINERS CAN AROUSE ANXIETY IN MINORITY GROUP CHILDREN AND (2) THAT SPANISH-SPEAKING CHILDREN SHOULD BE TESTED IN SPANISH AS WELL AS ENGLISH FOR MORE ACCURATE DETERMINATION OF THEIR POTENTIAL. SUBJECTS WERE 41 MEXICAN AMERICAN FIRST GRADERS FROM TWO RURAL SCHOOLS IN CENTRAL NEW MEXICO WHO ENTERED FIRST GRADE IN SEPTEMBER, 1969 AND ATTENDED HEADSTART THE PREVIOUS SUMMER. CHILDREN WERE RANKED ACCORDING TO TOTAL IQ AND ASSIGNED TO TWO GROUPS. EXPERIMENTAL GROUP A (N=21) WAS ADMINISTERED THE WISC BY THE SENIOR AUTHOR AND AN INTERPRETER WELL KNOWN TO THE CHILDREN, WHO ENCOURAGED THEM TO RESPOND IN SPANISH IF THEY WISHED. CONTROL GROUP B (N=20) WAS ADMINISTERED THE TEST IN ENGLISH BY THE AUTHOR ALONE. RESULTS WERE THAT NONE OF THE MEAN DIFFERENCES BETWEEN VERBAL, PERFORMANCE AND FULL SCALE WISC IQ'S WAS STATISTICALLY SIGNIFICANT. THIS RAISES SOME QUESTIONS CONCERNING THE EFFECTS OF AN INTERPRETER IN INFLUENCING THE PERFORMANCE OF MEXICAN AMERICAN CHILDREN ON AN INTELLIGENCE TEST. HOWEVER, THE AUTHORS NOTE THAT THE FINDINGS BE APPLIED WITH CAUTION IN LIGHT OF THE SMALL N'S. MOREOVER, IT IS HOPED THAT THERE WILL BE FURTHER PROBES INTO THE EFFECTS OF A NON-ENGLISH MONOLINGUISTIC ORIENTATION PERFORMANCE IN TESTING AND LEARNING SITUATIONS AND ON COUNTER MEASURES TO REDUCE THEIR INHIBITING FACTORS. 10 REFERENCES.

ACCN   001545

1781 AUTH   **SWARTZ, J. D., TAPIA, L. L., & THORPE, J. S.**
TITL   PERCEPTUAL DEVELOPMENT OF MEXICAN SCHOOL CHILDREN AS MEASURED BY RESPONSES TO THE HOLTZMAN INKBLOT TECHNIQUE.

SRCE *REVISTA INTERAMERICANA DE PSICOLOGIA, 1967, 1(4), 289-295.*

INDX PERCEPTION, MEXICAN, CHILDREN, PROJECTIVE TESTING, EMPIRICAL

ABST THE CROSS CULTURAL GENERALITY OF THE RELATIONSHIP BETWEEN LEVEL OF PERCEPTUAL DEVELOPMENT AND SCORES ON VARIABLES FROM THE HOLTZMAN INKBLOT TECHNIQUE (HIT) IS INVESTIGATED. STUDIES OF U.S. CHILDREN SHOW CONSISTENT AGE TRENDS IN FIVE HIT SCORES, CONFIRMING SCORES AS INDICES OF LEVEL OF PERCEPTUAL DEVELOPMENT. THREE HUNDRED NORMAL MEXICAN SCHOOL CHILDREN (150 MALES, 150 FEMALES) RESIDING IN MEXICO CITY WERE ADMINISTERED THE HIT TO TEST THE APPLICABILITY OF THESE INDICES. SUBJECTS WERE SAMPLED FROM 22 DIFFERENT SCHOOL DISTRICTS WITHIN BOTH GOVERNMENT AND PRIVATE SCHOOL SYSTEMS AND ARE CONSIDERED REPRESENTATIVE OF THE SOCIOECONOMIC STRATA OF MEXICO CITY. FORM A OF HIT WAS ADMINISTERED INDIVIDUALLY TO SUBJECTS IN THE OLDEST (12 YEARS, 8 MONTHS) AND YOUNGEST (6 YEARS, 8 MONTHS) AGE GROUPS, WHILE FORM B WAS GIVEN TO MIDDLE AGE SUBJECTS (9 YEARS, 8 MONTHS). TWO-WAY CLASSIFICATION (SEX-BY-AGE) ANALYSES OF VARIANCE OF 11 SELECTED HIT VARIABLES REVEALED AGE-GROUP DIFFERENCES FOR EIGHT OF THE ELEVEN VARIABLES STUDIED, WITH SEVEN SHOWING CONSISTENT MONOTONIC INCREASES WITH AGE. FIVE OF THESE SEVEN VARIABLES (FORM APPROPRIATENESS, FORM DEFINITENESS, MOVEMENT, INTEGRATION, AND HUMAN) ARE THOSE WHICH PROVED TO BE RELIABLE AND MEANINGFUL INDICES OF PERCEPTUAL DEVELOPMENT IN PREVIOUS STUDIES IN THE UNITED STATES. HIT SCORES ARE CONFIRMED AS INDICES OF PERCEPTUAL DEVELOPMENT IN MEXICAN CHILDREN. 4 REFERENCES.

ACCN 001546

1782 AUTH **SWEET, J. A.**

TITL DIFFERENTIALS IN THE RATE OF FERTILITY DECLINE: 1960-1970.

SRCE *FAMILY PLANNING PERSPECTIVES, 1974, 6(2), 103-107.*

INDX FERTILITY, CROSS CULTURAL, MEXICAN AMERICAN, MEXICAN

ABST DECLINING FERTILITY RATES OF AMERICAN ETHNIC, ECONOMIC, AND SOCIAL SUBGROUPS ARE DOCUMENTED BASED ON DATA FROM THE 1960 AND 1970 U.S. CENSUS. FERTILITY IS INFERRED FROM THE AVERAGE NUMBER OF CHILDREN UNDER AGE THREE LIVING IN THE SAME HOUSEHOLD WITH THEIR OWN MOTHER (MARRIED AND UNDER 40). SHORTCOMINGS OF THE FERTILITY MEASURE ARE ACKNOWLEDGED AND INCLUDE MISCOUNTS DUE TO (1) INFANT AND CHILD MORTALITY BETWEEN BIRTH AND ENUMERATION, (2) CHILDREN LIVING OUT OF MOTHER'S HOME, AND (3) CHILDREN ACQUIRED BY MARRIAGE OR ADOPTION. STANDARDIZED AND CRUDE MARITAL FERTILITY RATES ARE PRESENTED FOR NINE GROUPS: BLACK, AMERICAN INDIANS, JAPANESE AMERI-CANS, CHINESE AMERICANS, PUERTO RICAN AMERICANS, MEXICAN AMERICANS, AMERICANS WITH SPANISH SURNAMES, AND RURAL AND URBAN WHITES. DIFFERENTIAL RATES OF FERTILITY AMONG URBAN WHITES BY EDUCATION, REGION OF RESIDENCE, HUSBAND'S INCOME, PARITY, AND DURATION SINCE FIRST MARRIAGE ARE ALSO GIVEN. DECLINING FERTILITY IN THE U.S. HAS BEEN MOST PRONOUNCED AMONG THREE GROUPS WHICH PREVIOUSLY HAD THE HIGHEST FERTILITY— BLACKS, AMERICAN INDIANS, AND MEXICAN AMERICANS. AMONG URBAN WHITES, FERTILITY DECLINE HAS BEEN HEAVILY CONCENTRATED AMONG THOSE OF LOW INCOME. CAUSES OF FERTILITY DECLINE INCLUDE (1) LATER MARRIAGE AND DELAY OF FIRST BIRTH, (2) POSTPONEMENT OF CHILDBEARING AFTER MARRIAGE, (3) INCREASED INTERVALS BETWEEN BIRTHS, AND (4) REDUCED COHORT SIZE. IMPLICATIONS OF THESE FERTILITY DECLINES MAY INCLUDE (1) CHANGES IN THE DYNAMICS OF LOCAL AREA GROWTH, (2) REDUCTION OF POVERTY, (3) IMPROVING INVESTMENTS PER CHILD IN THE EDUCATIONAL SYSTEM, AND (4) GREATER OPPORTUNITY FOR ECONOMIC ADVANCEMENT BY WOMEN. 8 REFERENCES.

ACCN 001547

1783 AUTH **SWIKARD, D. L., & SPILKA, K.**

TITL HOSTILITY EXPRESSION OF MINORITY AND MAJORITY GROUPS.

SRCE *JOURNAL OF CONSULTING PSYCHOLOGY, 1961, 25(3), 216-220.*

INDX DELINQUENCY, ADOLESCENTS, EMPIRICAL, AGGRESSION, CROSS CULTURAL, SPANISH SURNAMED, SEX COMPARISON, MALE, FEMALE, SES, COLORADO, SOUTHWEST, MMPI

ABST TO INVESTIGATE WHETHER MINORITY GROUP MEMBERSHIP AND LOW SES COMBINE TO PRODUCE A GREATER MANIFESTATION OF HOSTILITY THAN WOULD RESULT FROM THE FRUSTRATION OF POVERTY ALONE, 81 SPANISH AMERICAN AND NON-SPANISH WHITE MALE AND FEMALE DELINQUENTS ON PROBATION IN DENVER WERE ADMINISTERED THE SIEGEL MANIFEST HOSTILITY SCALE, THE ROSENWEIG PICTURE FRUSTRATION STUDY, THE SOCIAL DESIRABILITY SCALE EXTRACTED FROM THE MMPI BY EDWARDS, AND THE MMPI LIE SCALE. BECAUSE OF TENDENCIES ON THE PART OF DELINQUENTS TO GIVE A "GOOD IMPRESSION" ON PERSONALITY MEASURES, IT WAS NECESSARY TO CORRECT HOSTILITY MEASURES FOR SOCIAL DESIRABILITY. SOCIAL DESIRABILITY WAS FOUND TO RELATE NEGATIVELY TO MANIFEST AND EXTRAPUNITIVE MEASURES OF HOSTILITY, BUT POSITIVELY TO INTROPUNITIVE AND IMPUNITIVE MEASURES OF HOSTILITY. ONCE THE HOSTILITY MEANS WERE ADJUSTED TO REMOVE THE EFFECTS OF SOCIAL DESIRABILITY, SIGNIFICANCE WAS OBTAINED BETWEEN THE GROUPS ON THE MANIFEST HOSTILITY SCALE. THE SPANISH AMERICAN MALE GROUP WAS SHOWN TO MANIFEST SIGNIFICANTLY GREATER HOSTILITY ON THIS MEASURE THAN ANY OTHER GROUP. THE SPANISH AMERICAN FEMALES, HOWEVER, DID NOT REVEAL MORE

EVIDENCE OF HOSTILITY THAN EITHER OF THE NON-SPANISH WHITE GROUPS. 16 REFERENCES.

ACCN 001548

1784 AUTH **SZALAY, L. B., WILLIAMS, R. E., BRYSON, J. A., & WEST, G.**

TITL PRIORITIES, MEANINGS AND PSYCHOCULTURAL DISTANCE OF BLACK, WHITE AND SPANISH AMERICAN GROUPS.

SRCE *WASHINGTON, D. C.: AMERICAN INSTITUTES FOR RESEARCH, 1976.*

INDX CULTURE, PERSONALITY, FAMILY ROLES, FAMILY STRUCTURE, INTERPERSONAL RELATIONS, INTERPERSONAL ATTRACTION, ACCULTURATION, SEX ROLES, MARRIAGE, ECONOMIC FACTORS, SOCIAL MOBILITY, OCCUPATIONAL ASPIRATIONS, SCHOLASTIC ASPIRATIONS, EDUCATION, HEALTH, RELIGION, COPING MECHANISMS, STRESS, SPANISH SURNAMED, EMPIRICAL

ABST TO ASSESS PSYCHOCULTURAL SIMILARITIES AND DIFFERENCES IN ATTITUDES, PERCEPTIONS, AND PRIORITIES, A COMPARATIVE STUDY OF SPANISH AMERICANS, BLACKS, AND WHITES (N = 156) WAS CONDUCTED IN THE WASHINGTON, D.C. AREA. DATA ANALYSIS COMPARED AND CONTRASTED ETHNIC-RACIAL GROUPS, SEX, AGE GROUPS (YOUNG, MIDDLE-AGED, ELDERLY), AND SOCIOECONOMIC STRATA (HIGH, MIDDLE, AND LOW INCOME). THE RESEARCH METHOD WAS ASSOCIATE GROUP ANALYSIS WHICH DRAWS INFERENCES FROM SPONTANEOUS WORD ASSOCIATIONS. REACTIONS WERE ELICITED TO 160 KEY COMMUNICATION THEMES REPRESENTING TEN PROBLEM AREAS: (A) FAMILY; (B) FRIENDS; (C) SOCIETY, PEOPLE; (D) SEX, LOVE; (E) MONEY, ECONOMY; (F) PROFESSION, WORK; (G) EDUCATION; (H) HEALTH; (I) RELIGION; AND (J) PROBLEMS. SIGNIFICANT DIFFERENCES WERE OBTAINED FOR CERTAIN CONCEPTS (MENTAL HEALTH; DRUGS; PSYCHIATRISTS) RELEVANT TO THE PLANNING AND DELIVERY OF MENTAL HEALTH SERVICES, WHILE OTHER CONCEPTS (SELF, COMMUNITY, FEAR, SOCIETY) INDICATED HOW VARIOUS GROUPS PERCEIVE THEMSELVES AND THEIR SOCIAL ENVIRONMENT. INDEPENDENT MEASURES ALONG THE DIMENSIONS OF PERCEPTIONS, PRIORITIES, AND ATTITUDES REVEALED (1) THAT CULTURAL DIFFERENCES APPEARED TO BE THE MOST INFLUENTIAL VARIABLE, FOLLOWED BY SES, AGE, AND SEX, (2) INTRACULTURAL DIFFERENCES WERE SUBSTANTIALLY LESS THAN INTERCULTURAL DIFFERENCES, AND (3) THE OVERALL PSYCHOCULTURAL DISTANCE BETWEEN BLACKS AND WHITES WAS MUCH LESS THAN THAT BETWEEN SPANISH AMERICANS AND THE BLACKS AND WHITES. IN CONCLUSION, THREE EMPIRICAL CRITERIA FOR AN OPERATIONAL DEFINITION OF CULTURE ARE PRESENTED; AND IT IS SUGGESTED THAT IT IS POSSIBLE TO EVALUATE SUCH PROCESSES AS SOCIALIZATION, ACCULTURATION, AND CULTURAL INFLUENCE BY MEASURING THE CHANGES IN RELATIVE PSYCHOCULTURAL DIFFERENCE OVER TIME. 19 REFERENCES.

ACCN 001550

1785 AUTH **SZALAY, L. B., & BRYSON, J. A.**

TITL SUBJECTIVE CULTURE AND COMMUNICATION: A PUERTO RICAN-U.S. COMPARISON.

SRCE *JSAS CATALOG OF SELECTED DOCUMENTS IN PSYCHOLOGY, 1976, 6, 68. (MS. NO. 1288).*

INDX RESEARCH METHODOLOGY, CULTURE, PUERTO RICAN-I, CROSS CULTURAL, EMPIRICAL

ABST IN THESE TWO STUDIES A COMPARATIVE ANALYSIS OF U.S. AND PUERTO RICAN STUDENT GROUP REACTIONS TO SELECTED VERBAL AND PICTORIAL STIMULI ARE PRESENTED. IN THE FIRST STUDY, INFERENCES DRAWN FROM WORD-STIMULATED AND PICTURE-STIMULATED ASSOCIATIONS WERE COMPARED AT 3 LEVELS. AT THE LEVEL OF SINGLE SELECTED STIMULI, INFERENCES REVEALED GROUP-CHARACTERISTIC MEANINGS, PERCEPTIONS, AND EVALUATIONS OF SPECIFIC WORDS AND PICTURES. AT THE LEVEL OF MULTIPLE STIMULI (16-20) THE ANALYSIS INFORMED ON BROADER PROBLEM AREAS SUCH AS FAMILY AND EDUCATION. AT THE THIRD LEVEL, DESIGNED TO REFLECT SUBJECTIVE CULTURE, HUNDREDS OF THOUSANDS OF RESPONSES TO 160 STIMULUS WORDS AND 80 PICTURES PRODUCED INFORMATION ON CULTURAL PRIORITIES AND ON PERCEPTUAL AND ATTITUDINAL DISPOSITIONS. THE SECOND STUDY EXPLORED THE UTILITY OF WORD AND PICTURE STIMULATED ASSOCIATIONS IN ASSESSING THE EFFECTS OF COMMUNICATIONS ON U.S. AND PUERTO RICAN GROUPS. ASSOCIATIONS TO KEY THEMES AND PICTURES STRATEGICALLY CHOSEN FROM THE SELECTED PIECE OF COMMUNICATION WERE OBTAINED BOTH BEFORE AND AFTER THE PRESENTATION OF A SELECTED EDITORIAL OR FILM. RESULTS INDICATE THAT WORD ASSOCIATIONS PROVIDE A SOLID BASE FOR ASSESSING SPONTANEOUSLY OCCURRING PERCEPTUAL AND ATTITUDINAL EFFECTS BETWEEN CULTURE GROUPS. THIS COMPARISON OF THE UNITED STATES AND PUERTO RICAN CULTURE GROUPS HAS SHOWN THAT THE DIFFERENCES OBSERVED WERE GENERALLY IN LINE WITH CULTURAL DISPOSITIONS IDENTIFIED IN THE FIRST STUDY. THE HIGH DEGREE OF CONSISTENCY IN THE 2 STUDIES' FINDINGS SUGGESTS THAT WORD ASSOCIATIONS ARE EXTREMELY USEFUL IN REVEALING CULTURAL DISPOSITIONS, DESPITE MODE OF ELICITATION. MOREOVER, WORD ASSOCIATIONS CAN REVEAL GROUP SPECIFIC PERCEPTUAL AND ATTITUDINAL PRIORITIES WHICH LIE BELOW THE LEVEL OF AWARENESS—PRIORITIES SUPPRESSED BY RATIONALIZATIONS AND DESIRE FOR SOCIAL DESIRABILITY IN CONVENTIONAL METHODS OF QUESTIONING OR SCALING.

ACCN 001551

1786 AUTH **SZAPOCZNIK, J. (ED.)**

TITL MENTAL HEALTH, DRUG AND ALCOHOL ABUSE: AN HISPANIC ASSESSMENT OF PRESENT AND FUTURE CHALLENGES.

SRCE *WASHINGTON, D.C.: NATIONAL COALITION OF*

HISPANIC MENTAL HEALTH AND HUMAN SERVICES ORGANIZATIONS (COSSMHO), 1979.

INDX   ALCOHOLISM, DRUG ABUSE, MENTAL HEALTH, POLICY, EMPIRICAL, ESSAY, HEALTH DELIVERY SYSTEMS, RESOURCE UTILIZATION, PRIMARY PREVENTION, SOCIAL SERVICES, PARA-PROFESSIONALS, BILINGUAL-BICULTURAL PERSONNEL, PROFESSIONAL TRAINING, CULTURAL FACTORS, BOOK

ABST   THE FIVE PAPERS PRESENTED IN THIS VOLUME ARE AUTHORED BY HISPANIC RESEARCHERS AND SERVICE PROVIDERS IN THE FIELDS OF MENTAL HEALTH, ALCOHOLISM, AND DRUG ABUSE. THE THEMES WHICH, AT A GENERAL LEVEL, UNIFY THE VOLUME INCLUDE: (1) THE NEED FOR INCREASED HISPANIC INVOLVEMENT IN POLICY DEVELOPMENT; (2) AN EMPHASIS ON PREVENTION AND EARLY INTERVENTION; (3) THE INADEQUCY OF DATA ON THE INCIDENCE AND PREVALENCE OF PSYCHOSOCIAL DISORDERS AMONG HISPANICS; (4) THE PAUCITY OF HISPANIC MENTAL HEALTH PROFESSIONALS; AND (5) THE DEARTH OF RESEARCH ON HISPANIC MENTAL HEALTH PROBLEMS. SPECIFICALLY, THE FIRST PAPER ADDRESSES HISPANIC PRIORITIES FOR THE 1980'S, BASED ON THE RECOMMENDATIONS OF COSSMHO'S NATIONAL HISPANIC COMMITTEE REGARDING THE REPORTS FROM THE PRESIDENT'S COMMISSION ON MENTAL HEALTH. THE SECOND PAPER, BY FOCUSING ON MENTAL HEALTH POLICIES IN THE HISPANIC COMMUNITY, IDENTIFIES KEY FACTORS ACCOUNTING FOR HISPANIC UNDERUTILIZATION OF MENTAL HEALTH SERVICES. THE THIRD DISCUSSES THE INADEQUACY OF DATA FOR ESTIMATING THE INCIDENCE AND PREVALENCE OF DRUG ABUSE AMONG HISPANICS, AND IT THEN OFFERS RECOMMENDATIONS FOR PERSONNEL TRAINING AND MORE EFFECTIVE SERVICE DELIVERY PERTAINING TO THE DRUG ABUSE PROBLEM. IN THE FOURTH, THE FOCUS IS ON CULTURAL FACTORS WHICH IMPEDE HISPANICS' UTILIZATION OF ALCOHOLISM TREATMENT PROGRAMS ACROSS THE UNITED STATES. THE FINAL PAPER TRACES THE DEVELOPMENT OF THE STUDY OF "OCCUPATIOAL ALCOHOLISM," EMPHASIZING THE EFFECTIVENESS OF EARLY INTERVENTION STRATEGIES AS WELL AS THE NEED FOR A NEW, BROADER DEFINITION OF ALCOHOLISM, ITS ETIOLOGY, AND ITS TREATMENT. 85 REFERENCES.

ACCN   001779

1787 AUTH   **SZAPOCZNIK, J., DARUNA, P., SCOPETTA, M. A., & ARANALDE, M.**

TITL   THE CHARACTERISTICS OF CUBAN IMMIGRANT INHALANT ABUSERS.

SRCE   *AMERICAN JOURNAL DRUG ALCOHOL ABUSE, 1977, 4(3), 377-389.*

INDX   ADOLESCENTS, INHALANT ABUSE, DRUG ABUSE, SES, MALE, FLORIDA, CUBAN, SOUTH, EMPIRICAL

ABST   THE CHARACTERISTICS OF 13 CUBAN IMMIGRANT INHALANT ABUSERS ADMITTED TO THE MIAMI SPANISH FAMILY GUIDANCE CLINIC DURING A 1-YEAR PERIOD WERE STUDIED. THIS GROUP WAS FOUND TO BE SIMILAR TOIN-

HALANT ABUSERS IN THE NATIONAL PICTURE. THE INHALERS WERE ALL MALES, 12 TO 26 YEARS-OLD, FROM VERY LOW SOCIOECONOMIC LEVELS, LARGELY FROM DISRUPTED FAMILY BACKGROUNDS AND DISRUPTED NEIGHBORHOODS. THEY SHOWED POOR SCHOOL AND/OR EMPLOYMENT PERFORMANCE, SERIOUS ANTISOCIAL BEHAVIOR, AND OCCASIONAL HALLUCINATORY EXPERIENCES. THIS GROUP OF INHALERS WAS FOUND TO BE MULTIPLE SUBSTANCE ABUSERS AND MORE LIKELY TO BE CHARACTERIZED BY A PATTERN OF POLYDRUG ABUSE THAN BY THEIR ABUSE OF INHALANTS PER SE. THIS FINDING CONFIRMS A GENERAL NATIONAL TREND TOWARD THE ABUSE OF MULTIPLE RATHER THAN SINGLE SUBSTANCES. A COMPARISON OF INHALERS WITH A CAREFULLY CHOSEN CONTROL GROUP OF 16 CLIENTS (MATCHED BY NATIONALITY, SEX, AND AGE) INDICATES THAT THE TWO GROUPS ARE SIMILAR IN IMPORTANT WAYS. BOTH GROUPS PRESENT GENERAL PROFILES OF ACTING OUT ADOLESCENTS, AND TEND TO COME FROM LOW SOCIOECONOMIC LEVELS, DISRUPTED FAMILIES, AND POOR NEIGHBORHOODS. 31 REFERENCES. (JOURNAL ABSTRACT MODIFIED)

ACCN   002219

1788 AUTH   **SZAPOCZNIK, J., LASAGA, J., PERRY, P., & SOLOMON, J. R.**

TITL   OUTREACH IN THE DELIVERY OF MENTAL HEALTH SERVICES TO HISPANIC ELDERS.

SRCE   *HISPANIC JOURNAL OF BEHAVIORAL SCIENCES, 1979, 1(1), 21-40.*

INDX   GERONTOLOGY, CUBAN, FLORIDA, SOUTH, RESOURCE UTILIZATION, MASS MEDIA, EMPIRICAL, MENTAL HEALTH, COMMUNITY, HEALTH DELIVERY SYSTEMS

ABST   AN ASSESSMENT WAS MADE OF THE RELATIVE EFFECTIVENESS OF TWO OUTREACH EFFORTS DESIGNED TO INCREASE HISPANIC ELDERS' UTILIZATION OF SERVICES AT A MIAMI MENTAL HEALTH CLINIC. THE TWO MODALITIES COMPRISED (1) CONTACTING VARIOUS REFERRAL SOURCES, SUCH AS AGING AND SOCIAL SERVICE AGENCIES, PHYSICIANS, AND PRIESTS, AND (2) A MASS MEDIA CAMPAIGN AIMED DIRECTLY AT ELDERLY PERSONS POTENTIALLY IN NEED OF MENTAL HEALTH SERVICES. A VARIETY OF METHODS WITHIN EACH MODALITY WERE EXPLORED. THE DATA REVEALED THAT THE USE OF SPANISH-LANGUAGE MEDIA WAS HIGHLY EFFECTIVE, AND THAT PUBLIC SERVICE ANNOUNCEMENTS ON TELEVISION WERE BY FAR THE SINGLE MOST EFFECTIVE MEANS OF REACHING AND ATTRACTING HISPANIC ELDERS. THIS SUCCESS WAS MEASURED BY THE NUMBER OF HISPANIC ELDERS (1) CONTACTING THE MENTAL HEALTH CLINIC TO INQUIRE ABOUT SERVICES, OR (2) BECOMING CLIENTS AT THE CLINIC AS A RESULT OF THE OUTREACH EFFORT. FURTHERMORE, IT WAS FOUND THAT THESE OUTREACH EFFORTS WERE SUCCESSFUL IN ATTRACTING CLIENTS WHO WERE AT AN EARLY STAGE IN THE DEVELOPMENT OF PSYCHOSOCIAL PROBLEMS. IT IS CONCLUDED THAT HISPANIC ELDERS IN NEED OF MENTAL

HEALTH SERVICES CAN BE IDENTIFIED AND REACHED IF THERE IS SUFFICIENT COMMITMENT TO ESTABLISH THE NECESSARY OUTREACH COMPONENT THAT BRIDGES SERVICES TO THESE ELDERS. 9 REFERENCES. (JOURNAL ABSTRACT MODIFIED)

ACCN   001776

1789 AUTH   **SZAPOCZNIK, J., SCOPETTA, M. A., KURTINES, W., & ARANALDE, M.**

TITL   THEORY AND MEASUREMENT OF ACCULTURATION.

SRCE   *INTERAMERICAN JOURNAL OF PSYCHOLOGY, 1978, 12(2), 113-130.*

INDX   ACCULTURATION, CROSS GENERATIONAL, CUBAN, CULTURAL CHANGE, CULTURAL FACTORS, CULTURE, EMPIRICAL, SES, SPANISH SURNAMED, FLORIDA, SOUTH, TEST RELIABILITY, IMMIGRATION, TEST VALIDITY

ABST   IN AN ATTEMPT TO ACCOUNT FOR THE PHENOMENON OF INTERGENERATIONAL/ ACCULTURATIONAL DIFFERENCES IN IMMIGRANT FAMILIES, A PSYCHOSOCIAL MODEL OF ACCULTURATION WAS DEVELOPED. A SET OF BEHAVIORAL AND VALUE ITEMS WERE CONSTRUCTED AS ACCULTURATION SCALES AND THEN ADMINISTERED TO 265 CUBAN IMMIGRANTS LIVING IN MIAMI AND TO A CULTURAL REFERENCE GROUP OF 201 ANGLO AMERICANS. THE RESEARCH REVEALED THAT THE BEHAVIORAL SCALE PROVIDED A HIGHLY RELIABLE AND VALID MEASURE OF ACCULTURATION AND PROVED SUPERIOR TO THE VALUE SCALE IN ALMOST EVERY RESPECT. CONCLUSIONS WERE THAT BEHAVIORAL AND VALUE ACCULTURATION IN IMMIGRANTS ARE LINEAR FUNCTIONS OF THE AMOUNT OF TIME THE PERSON IS EXPOSED TO THE HOST CULTURE, AND THAT THE RATE AT WHICH THE BEHAVIORAL ACCULTURATION PROCESS TAKES PLACE IS A FUNCTION OF THE AGE AND SEX OF THE INDIVIDUAL. THE FINDINGS SUGGEST THAT INTERGENERATIONAL/ACCULTURATIONAL DIFFERENCES DEVELOP BECAUSE YOUNGER MEMBERS OF THE FAMILY ACCULTURATE MORE RAPIDLY THAN OLDER FAMILY MEMBERS. SAMPLE BEHAVIORAL SCALE ITEMS AND RELATIONAL VALUE SCALE ITEMS QUESTIONNAIRES ARE APPENDED. 15 REFERENCES.

ACCN   002220

1790 AUTH   **SZAPOCZNIK, J., SCOPETTA, M. A., & KING, O. E.**

TITL   THEORY AND PRACTICE IN MATCHING TREATMENT TO THE SPECIAL CHARACTERISTICS AND PROBLEMS OF CUBAN IMMIGRANTS.

SRCE   *JOURNAL OF COMMUNITY PSYCHOLOGY, 1978, 6, 112-122.*

INDX   ACCULTURATION, ADULTS, ADOLESCENTS, COPING MECHANISMS, CROSS GENERATIONAL, CUBAN, CULTURAL FACTORS, EMPIRICAL, ESSAY, EXTENDED FAMILY, FAMILY THERAPY, FAMILY STRUCTURE, IMMIGRATION, MENTAL HEALTH, PREJUDICE, RESOURCE UTILIZATION, FLORIDA, URBAN, DRUG ABUSE, SOUTH, POLICY, COMMUNITY, PROGRAM EVALUATION, PARAPROFESSIONALS, PSYCHOTHERAPY

ABST   WIDESPREAD MENTAL HEALTH PROBLEMS IN THE CUBAN IMMIGRANT POPULATION OF MIAMI PRESENT PROBLEMS FOR THE PROVIDERS OF MENTAL HEALTH SERVICES IN THE AREA, BECAUSE THE CUBANS HAVE SERIOUSLY UNDERUTILIZED THE ESTABLISHED ANGLO AMERICAN-ORIENTED TREATMENT PROGRAMS. BASED ON RESEARCH AND EXPERIENCE AT ENCUENTRO-SPANISH FAMILY GUIDANCE CLINIC IN MIAMI, THE AUTHORS SUGGEST TREATMENT PROCEDURES WHICH MATCH THE SPECIAL CHARACTERISTICS, PROBLEMS, VALUES, AND CLIENT EXPECTATIONS OF THIS POPULATION. A REVIEW OF THE LITERATURE SUPPORTS THIS RECOMMENDATION. STUDIES BY THE CLINIC'S STAFF WITH 50 DRUG ABUSERS, AND BY ONE OF THE AUTHORS WITH THE CLINIC'S LATIN PARAPROFESSIONAL COUNSELORS REVEALED CULTURAL VARIABLES IN THE MIAMI LATIN POPULATION WHICH WOULD BE RELEVANT FOR A CULTURALLY SENSITIVE TREATMENT MODEL. THESE INCLUDE: (1) A PREFERENCE FOR LINEAL RELATIONSHIPS BASED ON HIERARCHICAL OR VERTICAL STRUCTURES; (2) A STRONG FAMILY INFLUENCE; (3) AN ORIENTATION FOR AVOIDING THE COMPLEX NETWORK OF SOCIAL SYSTEMS IN THE HOST ENVIRONMENT; (4) A CRISIS-ORIENTED (PRESENT-TIME ORIENTATION) APPROACH TO TREATMENT AND REHABILITATION. ACCULTURATION PROBLEMS FACING CUBAN IMMIGRANT FAMILIES AND THEIR IMPLICATIONS FOR TREATMENT ARE DISCUSSED. THE AUTHORS CONCLUDE THAT ECOLOGICAL STRUCTURAL FAMILY THERAPY IS A TREATMENT OF CHOICE FOR DYSFUNCTIONS OF CUBAN IMMIGRANT FAMILIES. 44 REFERENCES. (JOURNAL ABSTRACT MODIFIED)

ACCN   002221

1791 AUTH   **TAKESIAN, S. A.**

TITL   A COMPARATIVE STUDY OF THE MEXICAN AMERICAN GRADUATE AND DROP OUT.

SRCE   *SAN FRANCISCO: R AND E RESEARCH ASSOCIATES, 1971. (REPRINTED FROM AN UNPUBLISHED DOCTORAL DISSERTATION, UNIVERSITY OF SOUTHERN CALIFORNIA, 1967.)*

INDX   MEXICAN AMERICAN, SCHOLASTIC ACHIEVEMENT, EDUCATION, ATTITUDES, TEACHERS, INTERPERSONAL RELATIONS, CLASSROOM BEHAVIOR, EMPIRICAL, ADOLESCENTS, REVIEW, CALIFORNIA, SOUTHWEST

ABST   BASED ON THE HYPOTHESIS THAT PUBLIC SCHOOL PROGRAMS DO NOT PROVIDE A POSITIVE EDUCATIONAL EXPERIENCE FOR THE MEXICAN AMERICAN POTENTIAL DROPOUT, 64 MEXICAN AMERICAN HIGH SCHOOL GRADUATES WERE COMPARED WITH 38 DROPOUTS FROM THE SAME HIGH SCHOOL DISTRICT IN SOUTHERN CALIFORNIA. DATA WERE OBTAINED FROM CUMULATIVE SCHOOL RECORDS AS WELL AS 58 PERSONAL INTERVIEWS. PERSONAL BACKGROUND, EDUCATIONAL VALUES, RELATIONSHIP TO THE COMMUNITY, ELEMENTARY AND SECONDARY SCHOOL EXPERIENCES, SCHOLASTIC ACHIEVEMENT, AND PARTICIPATION IN SCHOOL ACTIVITIES WERE EXAMINED TO DISCOVER ANY SIGNIFICANT

DIFFERENCES BETWEEN THE TWO GROUPS. SOCIAL EXPERIENCE AND SCHOLASTIC ACHIEVEMENT WERE FOUND TO BE SIGNIFICANT FACTORS, WITH ELEMENTARY SCHOOL EXPERIENCES BEING MORE IMPORTANT THAN SECONDARY. PERSONAL DATA, EDUCATIONAL VALUES, AND COMMUNITY RELATIONSHIPS DIFFERED SIGNIFICANTLY, WHILE PARTICIPATION IN SCHOOL ACTIVITIES WAS FOUND NOT TO BE AN IMPORTANT VARIABLE. THE FINDINGS WERE INTERPRETED IN TERMS OF THEIR IMPLICATIONS FOR THE EDUCATION OF MEXICAN AMERICAN STUDENTS, AND RECOMMENDATIONS TO BOTH ELEMENTARY AND SECONDARY SCHOOLS ARE MADE IN THE HOPE OF REDUCING THE RATE OF MEXICAN AMERICAN DROPOUTS. 157 REFERENCES.

ACCN   001552

1792 AUTH   **TALLMER, M.**
TITL   SOME FACTORS IN THE EDUCATION OF OLDER MEMBERS OF MINORITY GROUPS.
SRCE   *JOURNAL OF GERIATRIC PSYCHIATRY, 1977, 10(1), 89-98.*
INDX   GERONTOLOGY, PUERTO RICAN-M, SPANISH SURNAMED, ESSAY, REVIEW, ADULTS, ADULT EDUCATION, MEXICAN AMERICAN, POLICY
ABST   TO IMPLEMENT ADULT EDUCATION AS ONE SOLUTION TO THE PSYCHOLOGICAL AND BIOMEDICAL HAZARDS OF AGING, THE IMPLICATIONS OF MINORITY ETHNIC AFFILIATION IN THE EDUCATION OF THE ELDERLY ARE CONSIDERED. THE AGED AND ETHNIC MINORITIES HAVE MANY CHARACTERISTICS IN COMMON— LOW INCOME, LOW PRESTIGE, ALIENATION FROM SOCIETY, AND SIZE (BOTH GROUPS NUMBER ABOUT 20 MILLION). THE DISADVANTAGES OF MINORITY GROUP MEMBERSHIP, HOWEVER, ARE EXACERBATED IN OLD AGE. ALTHOUGH MINORITY GROUP ELDERLY INTERACT MORE FREQUENTLY WITH THEIR CHILDREN AND LIVE MORE OFTEN IN AN EXTENDED FAMILY SITUATION, THE EXTENT OF POVERTY, ILL HEALTH, AND THE LACK OF EDUCATIONAL AND MEDICAL RESOURCES RESULT IN SERIOUS CONCERNS FOR DAILY SURVIVAL. THE DIRECTION OF EDUCATION FOR OLDER MINORITY GROUP MEMBERS THEREFORE MUST DIFFER: (1) AS A RESULT OF FORCED RETIREMENT AT AN EARLIER AGE, MINORITY ELDERLY CAN AND SHOULD BE REACHED SOONER; (2) COURSES SHOULD FOCUS ON TOPICS OF IMMEDIATE AND UTILITARIAN SIGNIFICANCE— PRACTICAL ASPECTS OF MEDICAL SERVICES, DEALING WITH FAMILY TENSIONS, ETC.; AND (3) FLEXIBILITY AND INNOVATION SHOULD BE THE PRIME COMPONENTS IN TEACHING THE ELDERLY. THE FOCUS MUST BE ON EMPIRICALLY DOCUMENTED NEEDS, PROVIDING REASONABLE RESOURCES, AND OFFERING AS MUCH DIRECTIONAL ASSISTANCE AS POSSIBLE. 12 REFERENCES.

ACCN   002222

1793 AUTH   **TARDY, W.**
TITL   THE LANGUAGE HANDICAPPED PSYCHIATRIST AND PATIENT: THE BILINGUAL SITUATION. A SUMMARY OF A PANEL DISCUSSION.
SRCE   *IN E. R. PADILLA & A. M. PADILLA (EDS.), TRANSCULTURAL PSYCHIATRY: AN HISPANIC PERSPECTIVE (MONOGRAPH NO. 4). LOS ANGELES: UNIVERSITY OF CALIFORNIA, SPANISH SPEAKING MENTAL HEALTH RESEARCH CENTER, 1977, PP. 89-91.*
INDX   PSYCHOTHERAPY, MENTAL HEALTH PROFESSION, BILINGUAL-BICULTURAL PERSONNEL, ESSAY
ABST   IN THE TREATMENT OF A PATIENT WHO SPEAKS ANOTHER LANGUAGE, THE THERAPIST MUST USE HIS ABILITY TO EMPATHIZE BECAUSE NONVERBAL COMMUNICATION PLAYS A SIGNIFICANT ROLE IN ESTABLISHING RAPPORT. ON THE COGNITIVE LEVEL, THE THERAPIST CANNOT BE DEPENDENT ON A TRANSLATOR AND VERBAL CONTENT ALONE. AS HE GAINS INSIGHT INTO THE PATIENT'S INNER WORLD, HE MUST BE AWARE OF WHERE CULTURE ENDS AND PSYCHOPATHOLOGY BEGINS. IT IS SUGGESTED THAT BILINGUAL HOSPITAL STAFF, TRANSLATORS, AND VOLUNTEERS BE EMPLOYED IN THE SOLUTION OF THIS PROBLEM, AS WELL AS TELEPHONE TRANSLATION NETWORKS AND LOCAL SERVICES TO REFER PATIENTS TO PSYCHIATRISTS WHO SPEAK THEIR OWN LANGUAGE. MEDICAL PROGRAMS OFFERING COURSES EMPHASIZING LEARNING OF THE CULTURE AS WELL AS A SECOND LANGUAGE ARE RECOMMENDED. THERAPISTS SHOULD BE EXPECTED TO TAKE A MORE ACTIVE ROLE IN LEARNING THE LANGUAGE OF THE PATIENTS.

ACCN   001553

1794 AUTH   **TAVARES, J.**
TITL   THE MEXICAN AMERICAN CULTURE.
SRCE   *CALIFORNIA YOUTH QUARTERLY, 1969, 22(2), 3-11.*
INDX   MEXICAN AMERICAN, CULTURAL FACTORS, ADOLESCENTS, CHICANO MOVEMENT, PEER GROUP, DELINQUENCY, ESSAY, MACHISMO
ABST   REHABILITATION OF THE MEXICAN AMERICAN DELINQUENT BEGINS WITH RECOGNITION OF HIS PSYCHOLOGICAL AND CULTURAL SITUATION. ALTHOUGH THE MEXICAN AMERICAN COMMUNITY IS PROUD OF ITS CULTURAL HERITAGE, YOUNG PEOPLE HAVE FREQUENTLY DEVELOPED THEIR OWN ANGLO-MEXICAN SUBCULTURE WITH A "GANG" STYLE OF SOCIAL ORGANIZATION AND DIALECT BASED ON THE MEXICAN DIALECT OF "CALO." CERTAIN ASPECTS OF MEXICAN AMERICAN FAMILY LIFE CONTRIBUTE TO DISTRUST AND FEAR OF AUTHORITY FIGURES AND AN ATTITUDE OF ISOLATION FROM OTHER GROUPS. PEER GROUP ASSOCIATIONS PROVIDE A YOUTH WITH BOTH A SENSE OF IDENTITY AND A MEANS OF STREET JUSTICE. THE CULTURE EMPHASIZES MACHISMO, AND BECOMING A MAN MEANS ALCOHOL, SEX, AND POSSIBLY SOME VIOLENCE. MEXICAN AMERICANS IN CORRECTIONAL INSTITUTIONS CARRY OVER THEIR GROUP-ORIENTED SOCIAL PATTERN OF STRONG GROUP LOYALTIES, LITTLE SHOW OF EMOTION, AND VIOLENT BEHAVIOR IN DEFENSE OF ONE'S HONOR. THE "FIRMA DE LA RAZA CHICANO" WAS FORMED WITHIN THE INSTITUTIONS TO

ENABLE MEXICAN AMERICANS TO PROTECT THEMSELVES FROM OTHER ETHNIC GROUPS AND INSTITUTION STAFF MEMBERS. MEXICAN AMERICANS FEEL THAT THE "FIRMA" STRENGTHENS THEM CULTURALLY—I.E., THEY RESENT BEING DEPRIVED OF THE RIGHT TO SPEAK SPANISH OR BEING FORCED TO SOCIALIZE WITH OTHER ETHNIC GROUPS. THE CHICANO MOVEMENT ENCOURAGES MEXICAN AMERICANS WITHIN INSTITUTIONS TO SEEK EDUCATION AND VOCATIONAL TRAINING IN ORDER TO IMPROVE THEIR POLITICAL AND ECONOMIC SITUATION. IT IS SUGGESTED THAT MORE MINORITY STAFF BE EMPLOYED AND PROGRAMS WITHIN CORRECTIONAL INSTITUTIONS BE GEARED TO MEXICAN AMERICAN CULTURE AND THINKING. THESE SHOULD STRESS A HEALTHY APPROACH TO AUTHORITY, SMALL GROUP RELATIONS, AND THE PHYSICAL MANAGEMENT ASPECTS OF LIFE. THERE SHOULD BE GREATER OPPORTUNITY FOR LEARNING BY DOING AND A MORE CONSTRUCTIVE USE OF PEER GROUP INFLUENCE.

ACCN   001554

1795 AUTH   **TAVERA, H.**
TITL   AN ASSESSMENT OF CHICANO STUDENTS ON THE EDUCATIONAL OPPORTUNITY PROGRAM AT THE UNIVERSITY OF CALIFORNIA AT SANTA BARBARA. PART I: PROFILE OF THE EOP GRADUATE.
SRCE   *UNPUBLISHED MANUSCRIPT, UNIVERSITY OF CALIFORNIA, SANTA BARBARA, 1974. (AVAILABLE FROM DR. AMADO PADILLA, DEPARTMENT OF PSYCHOLOGY, UNIVERSITY OF CALIFORNIA, LOS ANGELES, CA 90024.)*
INDX   EDUCATIONAL ASSESSMENT, MEXICAN AMERICAN, COLLEGE STUDENTS, PROGRAM EVALUATION, SCHOLASTIC ACHIEVEMENT, EMPIRICAL, CALIFORNIA, SOUTHWEST
ABST   THIS STUDY ASKS: "ARE THERE MEASURABLE FACTORS WHICH ACCOUNT FOR UNIVERSITY OF CALIFORNIA EOP CHICANO STUDENTS' SUCCESS IN COLLEGE (I.E., GRADUATION VS. DROPPING-OUT)?" THE SAMPLE OF 119 SUBJECTS REPRESENTED HALF OF THE TOTAL CHICANO STUDENTS ENROLLED IN THE UNIVERSITY OF CALIFORNIA AT SANTA BARBARA UNDER THE EOP PROGRAM FROM 1967 TO 1974. SPECIFICALLY, THE SAMPLING PROCESS BEGAN WITH THE GROUPING OF THE ENTIRE EOP CHICANO POPULATION INTO FOUR CATEGORIES (DROP-OUT VS. GRADUATE; REGULAR VS. SPECIAL ACTION; FRESHMAN VS. TRANSFER STUDENT; MALE VS. FEMALE), AND THEN EVERY OTHER NAME WAS SELECTED. A "CHECKLIST" OF 72 VARIABLES WAS USED TO ACCUMULATE PERSONAL, FINANCIAL, AND ACADEMIC INFORMATION ON EACH STUDENT. THOUGH NO ONE FACTOR ACCOUNTED FOR SUCCESS IN COLLEGE, FINDINGS REVEALED THE FOLLOWING VARIABLES AS CHARACTERIZING THE CHICANO EOP GRADUATE: (1) A STRONG "C" AVERAGE IN HIGH SCHOOL OR COLLEGE PREP COURSES; (2) FIRST POSITION IN SIBLING ORDER; (3) A SPANISH-SPEAKING HOME; (4) INVOLVEMENT IN EXTRACURRICULAR ACTIVITIES IN HIGH SCHOOL; (5) 21 YEARS-

OLD UPON ADMISSION AND USUALLY A TRANSFER; (6) A "B-" AVERAGE WHILE IN COLLEGE; (7) DID NOT RECEIVE OVER 6 "INCOMPLETE" UNITS OR GET ON PROBATION; (8) HAS A SENSE OF CHICANO IDENTITY; AND (9) IS A MEMBER OF A CHICANO STUDENT ORGANIZATION. THE REPORT CONCLUDES THAT THERE IS A DIRE NEED FOR BETTER RECORD KEEPING FOR FURTHER RESEARCH INTO THIS QUESTION.
ACCN   001555

1796 AUTH   **TAYLOR, D.**
TITL   ETHNICITY AND BICULTURAL CONSIDERATIONS IN PSYCHOLOGY: MEETING THE NEEDS OF ETHNIC MINORITIES.
SRCE   *WASHINGTON, D.C.: AMERICAN PSYCHOLOGICAL ASSOCIATION, 1977.*
INDX   PROFESSIONAL TRAINING, MENTAL HEALTH, REPRESENTATION, EQUAL OPPORTUNITY, SPANISH SURNAMED, HIGHER EDUCATION, PROGRAM EVALUATION, POLICY, MENTAL HEALTH PROFESSION, COLLEGE STUDENTS, ESSAY
ABST   DURING THE COURSE OF A THREE YEAR APA MINORITY FELLOWSHIP PROGRAM (1974-1977) TO INCREASE THE NUMBER OF ETHNIC MINORITIES IN THE PROFESSION OF PSYCHOLOGY, FELLOWSHIP STIPENDS WERE AWARDED TO 115 SELECTED MINORITY STUDENTS PURSUING THE DOCTORATE AT 44 INSTITUTIONS. THIS PUBLICATION SUMMARIZES THE PROGRAM'S HISTORY, PHILOSOPHY, POLICIES, AND PROCEDURES, INCLUDING DESCRIPTIONS OF ANCILLARY PROGRAMS AND A LIST OF THE FELLOWS, 33 OF WHOM WERE SPANISH-SPEAKING OR SPANISH SURNAMED. SELECTION CRITERIA EMPHASIZED LEADERSHIP POTENTIAL AND SENSITIVITY TO ETHNIC MINORITY CONCERNS. THE PROBLEMS ENCOUNTERED BY MINORITIES IN TRADITIONAL ACADEMIC SETTINGS ARE REFLECTED IN THE ABSENCE OF RELEVANT ETHNIC ISSUES WITHIN THE CURRICULUM AND THE DIFFICULTY IN FINDING FACULTY MEMBERS WILLING TO ENDORSE OR PARTICIPATE IN THE STUDENTS' RESEARCH INTERESTS. IT IS SUGGESTED THAT SUPPORT PRACTICES (SUCH AS TUTORING, RELAXATION OF DEADLINES, AND FLEXIBILITY IN RESEARCH CONTENT AND METHODOLOGY) CAN BE INSTRUMENTAL IN PREVENTING FAILURE AMONG MINORITY STUDENTS. 5 REFERENCES.
ACCN   002223

1797 AUTH   **TAYLOR, M. E.**
TITL   EDUCATIONAL AND CULTURAL VALUES OF MEXICAN-AMERICAN PARENTS: HOW THEY INFLUENCE THE SCHOOL ACHIEVEMENT OF THEIR CHILDREN.
SRCE   *WASHINGTON, D.C.: OFFICE OF EDUCATION, DEPARTMENT OF HEALTH, EDUCATION, AND WELFARE, 1970. (ERIC DOCUMENT REPRODUCTION SERVICE NO. ED 050 842)*
INDX   CULTURAL FACTORS, EDUCATION, ATTITUDES, MEXICAN AMERICAN, SCHOLASTIC ACHIEVEMENT, SES, EMPIRICAL, CHILDREN, CALIFORNIA, SOUTHWEST, VALUES

ABST   TO DETERMINE THE EFFECTS OF RURAL PAR-ENTS' VALUES AND ATTITUDES UPON THE SCHOOL ACHIEVEMENT OF THEIR 3RD- AND 4TH-GRADE CHILDREN, 20 WORKING-CLASS MEXICAN AMERICAN FAMILIES, 21 ANGLO WORKING-CLASS FAMILIES, AND 24 ANGLO MIDDLE-CLASS FAMILIES IN THE SAN JOAQUIN VALLEY, CALIFORNIA, WERE SAMPLED. AC-CORDING TO RESULTS OF THE VALUE ORIEN-TATION SCHEDULE, ALL THREE GROUPS WERE ORIENTED TO THE PRESENT, WERE MORE "DOING" THAN "BEING" TYPES OF PEOPLE, AND WERE IN HARMONY WITH NATURE IN THEIR LIFE ACTIVITIES. RESULTS OF THE MIN-NESOTA SURVEY OF OPINIONS-EDUCATION SCALE INDICATED THAT ALTHOUGH THERE WERE SIGNIFICANT DIFFERENCES AMONG THE THREE GROUPS IN THEIR ATTITUDES TOWARD THE VALUE OF EDUCATION, ALL GROUPS WERE ON THE STRONG-POSITIVE SIDE OF THE ATTI-TUDE SCALE, WITH THE ANGLO MIDDLE-CLASS GROUP BEING THE STRONGEST. PUPIL ACHIEVEMENT SCORES COUPLED WITH IN-FORMATION ON PARENT'S ATTITUDES TOWARD EDUCATION REVEALED THAT PARENTAL ATTI-TUDES DID AFFECT THE CHILD'S SCHOOL ACHIEVEMENT, PARTICULARLY IN READING. AMONG THE MEXICAN AMERICAN FAMILIES AND THE ANGLO MIDDLE-CLASS FAMILIES, THE GREATER THE VALUE OF EDUCATION, THE HIGHER THE ACHIEVEMENT OF THEIR CHIL-DREN IN SCHOOL. AMONG THE ANGLO WORK-ING-CLASS GROUP, HOWEVER, THE PATTERN WAS ENTIRELY REVERSED. THE RESULTS TEND TO INDICATE THAT: (1) THE MEXICAN AMERI-CAN WORKING-CLASS CHILD IS ACHIEVING AT A HIGHER LEVEL THAN THE ANGLO LOWER-CLASS CHILD WHEN IQ IS HELD CONSTANT, AND IS PERHAPS MORE LIKE THE ANGLO MIDDLE-CLASS CHILD IN HIS ACHIEVEMENT MOTIVATION; (2) THE MEXICAN AMERICAN PAR-ENT DOES VALUE EDUCATION AND HIS ATTI-TUDE HAS A POSITIVE INFLUENCE UPON THE ACHIEVEMENT OF THE CHILD; AND (3) THE VALUE ORIENTATION FOR THE MEXICAN AMERICAN GROUP IS IDENTICAL TO THAT OF THE OTHER TWO ANGLO GROUPS. 60 REFER-ENCES. (ERIC ABSTRACT MODIFIED)

ACCN   001556

1798 AUTH   **TAYLOR, M. E.**

TITL   INVESTIGATION OF PARENT FACTORS AFFECT-ING THE ACHIEVEMENT OF MEXICAN-AMERI-CAN CHILDREN (DOCTORAL DISSERTATION, UNIVERSITY OF SOUTHERN CALIFORNIA, 1970).

SRCE   *DISSERTATION ABSTRACTS INTERNATIONAL, 1970, 31(2), 569A. (UNIVERSITY MICROFILMS NO. 70-13,673.)*

INDX   SCHOLASTIC ACHIEVEMENT, MEXICAN AMERI-CAN, ATTITUDES, SES, EMPIRICAL, CHILDREN, CULTURAL FACTORS, EDUCATION, CALIFOR-NIA, SOUTHWEST

ABST   THIS DISSERTATION PROVIDES A MORE COM-PLETE ACCOUNT OF THE METHODOLOGY AND RESULTS OF THE STUDY CITED ABOVE (TAY-LOR, 1970, ERIC DOCUMENT NO. ED 050 842). THE STUDENT SAMPLE WAS ADMINISTERED THE COMPREHENSIVE TEST OF BASIC SKILLS

AS A MEASURE OF SCHOOL ACHIEVEMENT. ADDITIONAL MATERIALS INCLUDE (1) REVIEW OF RELATED LITERATURE, (2) PLANNING AND CONDUCTING OF THE FIELD STUDY, (3) 45 TABLES, (4) 6 FIGURES, (5) SUMMARY OF DE-SCRIPTIVE DATA AND METHODS OF ANALYSIS, AND (6) SUMMARY OF FINDINGS. 61 REFER-ENCES.

ACCN   001557

1799 AUTH   **TEICHER, J. D., SINAY, R. D., & STUMPHAUZER, J. S.**

TITL   TRAINING COMMUNITY-BASED PARAPROFES-SIONALS AS BEHAVIOR THERAPISTS WITH FAMILIES OF ALCOHOL ABUSING ADOLES-CENTS.

SRCE   *AMERICAN JOURNAL OF PSYCHIATRY, 1976, 133(7), 847-850.*

INDX   PARAPROFESSIONALS, COMMUNITY INVOLVE-MENT, ALCOHOLISM, ADOLESCENTS, FAMILY STRUCTURE, REHABILITATION, PROFESSIONAL TRAINING, MEXICAN AMERICAN, CROSS CUL-TURAL, CASE STUDY

ABST   IN THIS PILOT PROGRAM AT THE UNIVERSITY OF SOUTHERN CALIFORNIA MEDICAL CENTER ADOLESCENT CRISIS WARD, PARAPROFES-SIONALS WERE TRAINED TO CONDUCT BEHAV-IORAL FAMILY THERAPY IN THEIR OWN COM-MUNITIES, DIRECTLY IN THE HOMES OF ALCOHOL-ABUSING ADOLESCENTS. TEN PAR-APROFESSIONALS (5 MEN AND 5 WOMEN; 8 MEXICAN AMERICANS AND 2 BLACKS) WERE SELECTED. TRAINED AS A GROUP FOR 6 MONTHS, THEY ATTENDED WEEKLY SESSIONS IN WHICH PRINCIPLES OF LEARNING AND FAMILY CONTRACTING WERE PRESENTED. IN ADDITION, THEY OBSERVED BEHAVIOR THER-APY WITH FAMILIES CONDUCTED BY PROFES-SIONALS, VIEWED FILMS ON SOCIAL LEARN-ING THEORY AND PRACTICES, COMPLETED A PROGRAMMED TRAINING MANUAL, AND READ RELATED MATERIALS. EACH TRAINEE WAS THEN REQUIRED TO GUIDE THREE FAMILIES THROUGH A TREATMENT PERIOD CONSISTING OF FOUR PHASES: (1) INITIAL CONTACT, (2) AS-SESSMENT, (3) NEGOTIATION OF CONTRACTS, (4) TERMINATION. TO DATE, 12 FAMILIES HAVE BEEN TREATED (8 MEXICAN AMERICAN, 4 BLACK) AND ALL 12 ADOLESCENTS PRE-SENTED SEVERE PROBLEMS RELATED TO AL-COHOL ABUSE, SCHOOL, THE LAW AND THEIR FAMILIES. A SERIES OF CONTRACTS HAVE BEEN NEGOTIATED BETWEEN THE PARA-PROFESSIONALS AND THE ADOLESCENT, HIS FAMILY, AND SOMETIMES HIS SCHOOL AND PROBATION OFFICIALS. ATTRITION OF PARA-PROFESSIONALS PRESENTED A PROBLEM IN IMPLEMENTATION OF THE PROGRAM (OF THE 10 SELECTED ONLY 4 COMPLETED THE TRAIN-ING). BUT THOSE WHO COMPLETED IT DEM-ONSTRATED THAT THE SPECIFICITY OF BEHAV-IORAL CONTRACTING METHODS PROVIDED USEFUL TOOLS THAT COULD BE LEARNED AND APPLIED ON A CONTINUAL BASIS IN THEIR COMMUNITY CENTERS. RESEARCHERS CON-CLUDE THAT THIS PILOT PROGRAM OFFERS A FRUITFUL MODEL FOR THE CONTINUED TRAIN-ING OF COMMUNITY-BASED PARAPROFES-

SIONALS IN FAMILY BEHAVIOR THERAPY WITH ALCOHOL-ABUSING ADOLESCENTS. 26 REFERENCES.

ACCN 001558

1800 AUTH **TELACU (THE EAST LOS ANGELES COMMUNITY UNION).**

TITL UNINCORPORATED EAST LOS ANGELES SOCIAL AND COMMUNITY ENVIRONMENTAL ASSESSMENT PROGRAM: PREFERENCES AND ISSUES SURVEY SUBPROGRAM (VOL. 2).

SRCE *LOS ANGELES: TELACU (THE EAST LOS ANGELES COMMUNITY UNION), 1976.*

INDX SURVEY, ATTITUDES, DELINQUENCY, AGGRESSION, GANGS, ENVIRONMENTAL FACTORS, HOUSING, JUDICIAL PROCESS, ECONOMIC FACTORS, EDUCATION, BILINGUAL-BICULTURAL EDUCATION, SCHOLASTIC ACHIEVEMENT, HEALTH DELIVERY SYSTEMS, SES, POVERTY, URBAN, MEXICAN AMERICAN, STEREOTYPES, CALIFORNIA, SOUTHWEST

ABST THIS 1976 SURVEY OF 1,200 HOUSEHOLD HEADS AND 150 NON-RESIDENT PROPERTY OWNERS AND BUSINESS PERSONS OF EAST LOS ANGELES WAS DESIGNED TO IDENTIFY THEIR PREFERENCES AND COMMUNITY PERCEPTIONS. AS ONE OF THREE SUB-PROGRAMS OF THE EAST LOS ANGELES SOCIO-ECONOMIC ASSESSMENT PROGRAM, THE SURVEY'S OBJECTIVE WAS TO OBTAIN INFORMATION ON ASSESSMENT OF COMMUNITY HUMAN RESOURCES, CHARACTERISTICS OF CONSUMERS, AND OPINIONS ON MAJOR ISSUES FACING THE COMMUNITY. RESPONSES REVEALED THAT RESIDENTS HAVE A GENERALLY POSITIVE OPINION OF THEIR COMMUNITY—AS OPPOSED TO THE STEREOTYPICAL OUTSIDERS' VIEW THAT EAST L.A. IS UNSAFE, UNATTRACTIVE, AND UNDESIRABLE. POSITIVE, UNALIENATED ATTITUDES EXTENDED TO MOST SOCIAL SERVICES AND PROGRAMS. 91% HAVE "SOME" OR A "GREAT DEAL" OF RESPECT FOR THE POLICE—CONTRAPOSED TO HOSTILITY TOWARD POLICE DISPLAYED IN THE MASS MEDIA. MOST ARE HOPEFUL CONCERNING THE SCHOOLS AND ESPECIALLY SUPPORTIVE OF INNOVATIVE BILINGUAL PROGRAMS. THIS LARGELY NON-TRANSIENT POPULATION INDICATED A DESIRE FOR COMMUNITY INVOLVEMENT AND A WILLINGNESS TO STRENGTHEN THEIR NEIGHBORHOOD THROUGH SOCIAL, ECONOMIC, AND PHYSICAL IMPROVEMENTS. ALL INDICATED STRONG CONCERN ABOUT JUVENILE DELINQUENTS—A SMALL BUT TROUBLESOME PART OF THE ADOLESCENT POPULATION. MOST SUGGESTED THE PROBLEM CAN BE CONFRONTED THROUGH IMPROVED JOB PROGRAMS, PARENTAL INVOLVEMENT, AND EDUCATIONAL EFFORTS. THE SURVEY CONCLUDES THAT INCREASED OPPORTUNITIES FOR RESIDENT AND BUSINESSPERSON INVOLVEMENT IN ALL AREAS OF COMMUNITY PLANNING CAN ONLY IMPROVE THE QUALITY OF LIFE IN THE AREA.

ACCN 001560

1801 AUTH **TELLER, C. H.**

TITL PHYSICAL HEALTH STATUS AND HEALTH CARE UTILIZATION IN THE TEXAS BORDERLANDS.

SRCE *IN S. R. ROSS, (ED.), VIEWS ACROSS THE BORDER: THE UNITED STATES AND MEXICO. ALBUQUERQUE: UNIVERSITY OF NEW MEXICO PRESS, 1978, PP. 256-279.*

INDX CULTURAL FACTORS, CURANDERISMO, DEMOGRAPHIC, DISEASE, ECONOMIC FACTORS, ESSAY, HEALTH, SES, HEALTH DELIVERY SYSTEMS, MEXICAN, MEXICO, MEXICAN AMERICAN, PHYSICIANS, NURSING, POVERTY, TEXAS, ENVIRONMENTAL FACTORS, NUTRITION, PERSONNEL, FERTILITY, RESOURCE UTILIZATION, SOUTHWEST

ABST THE PHYSICAL HEALTH NEEDS OF THE TEXAS BORDERLAND HISPANIC POPULATION WERE ANALYZED FROM THE PERSPECTIVE OF A LATIN AMERICAN DEMOGRAPHER-SOCIOLOGIST. THE METHODOLOGY INVOLVED 3 YEARS OF PARTICIPANT-OBSERVATION, PLUS INTERVIEWS AND QUESTIONNAIRE DISTRIBUTION. FIVE HEALTH STATUS INDICATORS (DISEASE SPECIFIC DEATH RATES; INFANT MORTALITY RATE; INFECTIOUS DISEASE RATES; MEDICAL HISTORIES; NUTRITIONAL STATUS) DESCRIBE HIGHER RATES OF INFECTIOUS DISEASE AND POOR NUTRITIONAL STATUS. DATA ANALYSIS REVEALS INADEQUATE HEALTH RESOURCES, PARTICULARLY IN THE AREA OF HEALTH PERSONNEL. REGARDING UTILIZATION, LEVELS OF DENTAL AND PRENATAL CARE AND CHILD IMMUNIZATION WERE FOUND TO BE QUITE LOW AND CORRESPOND TO THE DEFICIENCIES IN TYPES OF HEALTH PERSONNEL. TO MAKE UP FOR THESE DEFICIENCIES, TEXAS BORDER RESIDENTS CROSS OVER TO MEXICO TO OBTAIN NEEDED PRIMARY CARE SERVICES. RECOMMENDED IS THE COLLECTION OF BASIC DESCRIPTIVE DATA ON HEALTH STATUS AND THE INITIATION AND EVALUATION OF EXPERIMENTAL CHICANO-ORGANIZED AND ADMINISTERED CONSUMER HEALTH CORPORATIONS. 35 REFERENCES.

ACCN 002225

1802 AUTH **TEMPLE-TRUJILLO, R. E.**

TITL CONCEPTIONS OF THE CHICANO FAMILY.

SRCE *SMITH COLLEGE STUDIES IN SOCIAL WORK, 1974, 45(1), 1-2.*

INDX MEXICAN AMERICAN, CULTURAL FACTORS, ESSAY, FAMILY STRUCTURE, STEREOTYPES, REVIEW

ABST AN ANALYSIS OF THE LITERATURE ABOUT THE CHICANO FAMILY BECOMES AN ANALYSIS OF THE IDEOLOGICAL BIASES OF SOME AMERICAN SOCIAL SCIENTISTS. CONSPICUOUS IN THIS LITERATURE IS THE VIEW THAT PROBLEMS ABOUND IN THE CHICANO POPULATION—PROBLEMS SUCH AS LACK OF AUTONOMY AND INITIATIVE, LOW TOLERANCE TO FRUSTRATION, POOR DELAYED GRATIFICATION, ECONOMIC STAGNATION, AND INADEQUATE CONTROL OVER IMPULSES. BUT NO MATTER WHAT EXPLANATIONS ARE OFFERED, THESE STUDIES CONCLUDE THAT THE MAJOR PROBLEM LIES WITHIN THE STRUCTURE OF THE CHICANO FAMILY. MOST REVEALING OF ANALYSTS' BIASES HAVE BEEN THE STANDARDS AGAINST

WHICH THE CHICANO IS JUDGED AND FOUND TO BE DEFICIENT—E.G., "ANGLO CULTURE," "CONVENTIONAL CULTURE," AND THE "MIDDLE-CLASS AMERICAN FAMILY." THE IMPLICATION IS THAT ASSIMILATION AND/OR ACCEPTANCE OF THE DOMINANT SOCIETY'S VALUES IS THE CHICANO'S ONLY RECOURSE AGAINST PERSONAL DISINTEGRATION. HOWEVER, A MORE SYMPATHETIC ANALYSIS OF CHICANO FAMILY STRUCTURE—FOCUSING ON CHICANOS' EMPHASIS ON HUMAN RELATIONSHIPS AND SENSE OF COMMUNITY—WILL REVEAL STRENGTHS AND SUPPORTS WHICH THE FAMILY PROVIDES THE INDIVIDUAL, CONTRAPOSED TO A DOMINANT SOCIETY WHICH IS LARGELY INSENSITIVE TO HIS NEEDS. IN CONCLUSION, CONCEPTS COMMONLY USED TO CHARACTERIZE THE CHICANO FAMILY OFTEN OVERSIMPLIFY AND DISTORT A RICH AND COMPLEX SOCIAL REALITY; AND UNTIL SUCH CONCEPTS ARE QUESTIONED AND MADE MORE EXPLICIT, AN UNDERSTANDING OF THE CHICANO FAMILY CANNOT GO BEYOND THE PRESENT SELECTIVE AND DESCRIPTIVE LITERATURE. WHAT IS NEEDED IS A NEW FRAMEWORK BY WHICH TO VIEW THE CHICANO FAMILY—ONE THAT INCLUDES LARGER ECONOMIC AND POLITICAL REALITIES AND DOES NOT PLACE RESPONSIBILITY FOR PROBLEMS ON THE CHICANO "PSYCHE" ALONE. 21 REFERENCES.

ACCN   001561

1803 AUTH   **TENHOUTEN, W. D., LEI, T., KENDALL, F., & GORDON, W. C.**

TITL   SCHOOL ETHNIC COMPOSITION, SOCIAL CONTEXTS, AND EDUCATIONAL PLANS OF MEXICAN AMERICAN AND ANGLO HIGH SCHOOL STUDENTS.

SRCE   *AMERICAN JOURNAL OF SOCIOLOGY, 1971, 77(1), 89-107.*

INDX   MEXICAN AMERICAN, CROSS CULTURAL, EDUCATIONAL ASSESSMENT, ADOLESCENTS, EMPIRICAL, SCHOLASTIC ASPIRATIONS, CALIFORNIA

ABST   THIS STUDY IS A COMPARATIVE ANALYSIS OF THE PROCESS BY WHICH MEXICAN AMERICAN AND ANGLO HIGH SCHOOL STUDENTS IN THE LOS ANGELES SCHOOL DISTRICT DEVELOP CONCRETE PLANS TO GO TO COLLEGE. THE SAMPLE CONSISTED OF 1,404 HIGH SCHOOL SENIORS (315 MEXICAN AMERICAN BOYS, 309 MEXICAN AMERICAN GIRLS, 226 ANGLO BOYS, AND 229 ANGLO GIRLS) FROM SOCIAL STUDIES CLASSES IN FIVE URBAN SECONDARY SCHOOLS. THEIR COLLEGE PLANS WERE RELATED TO THE VARIABLES OF FAMILY SOCIOECONOMIC STATUS, SCHOOL ETHNIC COMPOSITION, MEASURED INTELLIGENCE, PARENTS' ASPIRATIONS, AND PEERS' ASPIRATIONS. PATH ANALYSES WERE DEVELOPED SEPARATELY FOR MEXICAN AMERICAN AND ANGLO BOYS AND GIRLS. FAMILY SOCIOECONOMIC STATUS WAS FOUND TO BE A WEAK PREDICTOR OF COLLEGE PLANS FOR ALL GROUPS BUT SERVES AS AN INDIRECT PREDICTOR FOR ANGLOS. BOTH ETHNIC GROUPS WERE FOUND TO BE MORE APT TO DEVELOP COLLEGE PLANS IN SCHOOLS DOMINATED BY THEIR OWN ETHNIC GROUP.

ALL OTHER VARIABLES DIRECTLY AFFECT COLLEGE PLANS. PEERS' ASPIRATIONS IS THE MOST PREDICTIVE VARIABLE FOR MEXICAN AMERICAN BOYS, WHILE PARENTS' ASPIRATIONS IS THE MOST PREDICTIVE FOR THE OTHER THREE GROUPS. 38 REFERENCES.

ACCN   001562

1804 AUTH   **TEPLIN, L. A.**

TITL   A COMPARISON OF RACIAL/ETHNIC PREFERENCES AMONG ANGLOS, BLACK AND LATINO CHILDREN.

SRCE   *AMERICAN JOURNAL OF ORTHOPSYCHIATRY, 1976, 46(4), 702-709.*

INDX   ACCULTURATION, ATTITUDES, CHILDREN, CROSS CULTURAL, CULTURAL FACTORS, SELF CONCEPT, EMPIRICAL, ETHNIC IDENTITY, SPANISH SURNAMED, SOUTHWEST, MIDWEST, URBAN, SEX COMPARISON, EXAMINER EFFECTS

ABST   WITH A FOCUS ON LATINO CHILDREN, A PHOTOCHOICE METHOD WAS USED TO COMPARE RACIAL/ETHNIC GROUP PREFERENCES OF BLACK, ANGLO, AND LATINO CHILDREN. ALL 398 SUBJECTS WERE THIRD- AND FOURTH-GRADE ELEMENTARY SCHOOL STUDENTS FROM 12 CLASSROOMS IN THE PUBLIC SCHOOL SYSTEM OF A LARGE MIDWESTERN CITY. THE SAMPLE INCLUDED APPROXIMATELY ONE-THIRD ANGLO, ONE-THIRD BLACK, AND ONE-THIRD LATINO STUDENTS. ALL SCHOOLS WERE RACIALLY/ETHNICALLY INTEGRATED. THE CHILDREN WERE PRESENTED WITH A GROUP OF 24 PRETESTED PHOTOGRAPHS OF CHILDREN UNKNOWN TO THEM, WHICH INCLUDED FOUR MALE AND FOUR FEMALE CHILDREN OF EACH RACIAL/ETHNIC "TYPE." CHILDREN WERE ASKED BY ONE OF TWO EXAMINERS (A BLACK FEMALE AND AN ANGLO FEMALE): "WHO WOULD YOU MOST LIKE TO HAVE AS A FRIEND HERE?" AND "WHO WOULD YOU MOST LIKE TO WORK WITH?" THE CHILDREN WERE ASKED TO MAKE SIX CHOICES. WHILE BOTH BLACK AND ANGLO CHILDREN CHOSE INGROUP PHOTOS, LATINOS PREFERRED PICTURES OF ANGLO CHILDREN. EXPLANATIONS OF THIS OUTCOME ARE EXPLORED, AND A COMPARISON BETWEEN THE SITUATION OF TODAY'S LATINO CHILD AND THE BLACK CHILD OF TEN YEARS AGO IS SUGGESTED. IT IS CONCLUDED THAT THE PARTICULAR WAYS IN WHICH THESE DIFFERENCES ARISE PROVIDE A BASE FOR FUTURE RESEARCH. 35 REFERENCES. (JOURNAL ABSTRACT MODIFIED)

ACCN   002226

1805 AUTH   **TERRY, C. E., & COOPER, R. L.**

TITL   A NOTE ON THE PERCEPTION AND PRODUCTION OF PHONOLOGICAL VARIATION.

SRCE   *MODERN LANGUAGE JOURNAL, 1969, 53(4), 254-255.*

INDX   PHONOLOGY, PUERTO RICAN-M, EMPIRICAL, BILINGUAL, BILINGUALISM, NEW YORK, EAST

ABST   THIS REPORT DESCRIBES THE PERCEPTION OF PHONOLOGICAL VARIATIONS BY MEMBERS OF THE SAME SPEECH COMMUNITY, RELATING ABILITY TO PERCEIVE THIS VARIATION TO SEVERAL CRITERION VARIABLES. AS PART OF AN INTENSIVE STUDY OF BILINGUALISM WITHIN A

PUERTO RICAN URBAN NEIGHBORHOOD NEAR NEW YORK CITY, THE SPEECH OF 45 BILINGUAL RESPONDENTS WAS SUBJECTED TO EXTENDED PHONETIC ANALYSIS. SELECTED ENGLISH AND SPANISH VARIABLES WERE STUDIED WITH RESPECT TO RESPONDENTS' ABILITY TO PERCEIVE DIFFERENCES BETWEEN ALTERNATIVE PHONETIC REALIZATIONS, I.E., 3 REALIZATIONS OF A GIVEN WORD. SIXTEEN ITEMS WERE PRESENTED IN ALL, THE FIRST HALF OF WHICH REPRESENTED SPANISH VARIABLES AND THE SECOND HALF ENGLISH VARIABLES. THE ABILITY TO PERCEIVE THE DISTINCTION IN EACH ITEM WAS ANALYZED ACCORDING TO THE RELATIVE FREQUENCIES WITH WHICH THE ALTERNATIVE REALIZATIONS WERE PRODUCED IN 5 ELICITATION CONTEXTS. PERFORMANCE WAS ALSO STUDIED ACCORDING TO RATINGS ON CRITERION SCALES OF: (1) ENGLISH REPERTOIRE RANGE; (2) ACCENTEDNESS—DEGREE TO WHICH THE PHONOLOGICAL AND SYNTACTIC STRUCTURE OF ONE LANGUAGE APPEARS TO INFLUENCE THE OTHER; AND (3) READING—THE DEGREE TO WHICH THE RESPONDENT WAS ABLE TO READ IN ONE LANGUAGE ONLY. CONCLUSIONS WERE THAT PUERTO RICAN BILINGUALS' PERCEPTION OF PHONOLOGICAL VARIATION IN SPANISH AND ENGLISH WAS NOT GENERALLY FOUND TO BE RELATED TO THE RELATIVE FREQUENCY OF THEIR PRODUCTION. PERCEPTION OF SOME ITEMS, HOWEVER, WAS RELATED TO PERFORMANCE ON THREE CRITERION VARIABLES. THIS SUGGESTS THAT THE USE OF SELECTED PERCEPTION ITEMS, WHICH ARE RELATIVELY EASY TO ADMINISTER, MIGHT BE USEFUL IN LANGUAGE SURVEYS WHERE THE VALIDITY OF MORE DIRECT QUESTIONING IS IN DOUBT. 3 REFERENCES.

ACCN   001563

1806 AUTH   **TESKE, R. H. C., JR., & NELSON, B. H.**
TITL   AN ANALYSIS OF DIFFERENTIAL ASSIMILATION RATES AMONG MIDDLE-CLASS MEXICAN AMERICANS.
SRCE   *SOCIOLOGICAL QUARTERLY, 1976, 17(2), 218-235.*
INDX   ACCULTURATION, MEXICAN AMERICAN, TEXAS, SOUTHWEST, ADULTS, MALE, ETHNIC IDENTITY, SOCIALIZATION, ATTITUDES, EMPIRICAL, SES
ABST   TO IDENTIFY VARIABLES EXPLAINING DIFFERENTIAL ASSIMILATION RATES, DATA WERE COLLECTED FROM A RANDOM SAMPLE OF 151 MIDDLE-CLASS MEXICAN AMERICANS RESIDING IN WACO, AUSTIN, MCALLEN, AND LUBBOCK, TEXAS. THREE LIKERT-TYPE SCALES DESIGNED TO MEASURE VARIOUS COMPONENTS OF THE ASSIMILATION PROCESS WERE DEVELOPED OUT OF ITEMS EXTRACTED FROM THREE STANDARDIZED INTERVIEW SCHEDULES: THE MEXICAN AMERICAN IDENTITY SCALE; THE MEXICAN AMERICAN INTERACTION SCALE; AND THE ANGLO INTERACTION SCALE. FINDINGS SUGGEST THAT EARLY SOCIALIZATION PATTERNS WHICH INCORPORATE A DISCONTINUOUS STATUS SEQUENCE AND A LACK OF REINFORCEMENT AS A MEXICAN AMERICAN INCREASE THE PROBABILITY THAT THE INDI-

VIDUAL WILL ASSIMILATE INTO THE BROADER AMERICAN CULTURAL SYSTEM. 46 REFERENCES. (AUTHOR ABSTRACT MODIFIED)
ACCN   002227

1807 AUTH   **TESKE, R. H. C., JR., & NELSON, B. H.**
TITL   MIDDLE CLASS MEXICAN AMERICANS AND POLITICAL POWER POTENTIAL: A DILEMMA.
SRCE   *JOURNAL OF POLITICAL AND MILITARY SOCIOLOGY, 1976, 4(1), 107-119.*
INDX   POLITICS, MEXICAN AMERICAN, URBAN, TEXAS, SOUTHWEST, POLITICAL POWER, SURVEY, EMPIRICAL, ACCULTURATION, SES, CHICANO MOVEMENT
ABST   THIS PAPER REPORTS FINDINGS CONCERNING THE POLITICAL ORIENTATIONS OF A SAMPLE OF MIDDLE-CLASS MEXICAN AMERICANS AND THEIR MEMBERSHIP IN POLITICAL ORGANIZATIONS. THE DATA WERE COLLECTED FROM A RANDOM PROBABILITY SAMPLE OF MIDDLE-CLASS MEXICAN AMERICANS IN FOUR URBAN COMMUNITIES IN TEXAS. IN BRIEF, THE INVESTIGATION FOUND LIMITED EVIDENCE OF MEMBERSHIP IN, OR MORAL SUPPORT FOR, MEXICAN AMERICAN POLITICAL ORGANIZATIONS. SUBSEQUENTLY, THE DILEMMA WHICH THESE FINDINGS SUGGEST FOR MEXICAN AMERICAN POLITICAL POWER IS DISCUSSED. 26 REFERENCES. (AUTHOR ABSTRACT)
ACCN   002228

1808 AUTH   **TESKE, R. H. C., JR., & NELSON, B. H.**
TITL   TWO SCALES FOR THE MEASUREMENT OF MEXICAN-AMERICAN IDENTITY.
SRCE   *INTERNATIONAL REVIEW OF MODERN SOCIOLOGY, 1973, 3(2), 192-203.*
INDX   ADULTS, CULTURAL FACTORS, ECONOMIC FACTORS, EMPIRICAL, MEXICAN AMERICAN, SES, SELF CONCEPT, TEST RELIABILITY, TEST VALIDITY TEXAS, SOUTHWEST, RURAL, ETHNIC IDENTITY, PEER GROUP, URBAN
ABST   TWO SCALES DESIGNED TO MEASURE MEXICAN AMERICAN IDENTITY AMONG MEXICAN AMERICAN MIDDLE CLASS MEMBERS OF THE POPULATION ARE PRESENTED. FOUR COMMUNITIES VARYING IN DISTANCE FROM THE BORDER WERE SELECTED FOR SAMPLING: MCALLEN, AUSTIN, LUBBOCK, AND WACO, TEXAS. THE CITY DIRECTORY FOR EACH COMMUNITY WAS USED TO ACQUIRE THE NAMES AND SPECIFIC OCCUPATION OF ALL SPANISH SURNAMED MALES EMPLOYED IN THE AREA. RANDOMLY ORDERED NAMES OF THE CHOSEN INDIVIDUALS WERE PRESENTED TO TRAINED INTERVIEWERS FOR CONTACT AND INTERVIEWING. THE TWO SCALES, THE IDENTITY SCALE, CONSISTING OF 16 ATTITUDINAL-TYPE ITEMS, AND THE INTERACTION SCALE, CONSISTING OF 19 BEHAVIORAL-TYPE ITEMS, WERE THEN ADMINISTERED TO AN UNSPECIFIED NUMBER OF RESPONDENTS. ITEM ANALYSIS AND ITEM CORRELATION WERE COMPUTED VIA THE KUDER-RICHARDSON FORMULA. IN ADDITION, A PANEL OF JUDGES WAS USED TO SUBJECTIVELY EVALUATE MEXICAN AMERICAN IDENTITY OF THE RESPONDENTS IN ONE OF THE COMMUNITIES. SPECIFICALLY, A HIGH CORRELATION BETWEEN SCORES ON THE TWO

SCALES WAS OBSERVED, REINFORCING THE SCALES' VALIDITY. ALTHOUGH IT WAS NOT INTENDED THAT CONCLUSIONS CONCERNING THE MEXICAN AMERICAN POPULATION BE DRAWN, SEVERAL OBSERVATIONS SEEM NOTEWORTHY: DISTANCE FROM THE BORDER DOES NOT APPEAR TO BE A VARIABLE WHICH AFFECTS SCORES IN THIS POPULATION; ON THE OTHER HAND, THE EVIDENCE DOES SUGGEST THAT THERE ARE SIGNIFICANT DIFFERENCES BETWEEN COMMUNITIES. FUTURE INVESTIGATION SHOULD INCLUDE IDENTIFICATION OF VARIABLES WHICH MAY ACCOUNT FOR THESE DIFFERENCES. 12 REFERENCES.

ACCN   002229

1809 AUTH   **THARP, R. G., MEADOW, A., LENNHOFF, S. G., & SATTERFIELD, D.**

TITL   CHANGES IN MARRIAGE ROLES ACCOMPANYING THE ACCULTURATION OF THE MEXICAN AMERICAN WIFE.

SRCE   *JOURNAL OF MARRIAGE AND THE FAMILY, 1968, 30(3), 404-412.*

INDX   MARRIAGE, SEX ROLES, FAMILY ROLES, MEXICAN AMERICAN, FEMALE, ACCULTURATION, EMPIRICAL, ARIZONA, SOUTHWEST, FEMALE

ABST   THE EFFECT OF ACCULTURATION ON MARRIAGE ROLES WAS EXAMINED AMONG 84 MEXICAN AMERICAN WIVES IN TUCSON, ARIZONA. A COMBINATION OF AREA AND CLUSTER SAMPLING TECHNIQUES WERE EMPLOYED TO SELECT TWO GROUPS OF 42 WIVES FOR HOME INTERVIEWS. BOTH GROUPS WERE EQUIVALENT IN AGE (AGE RANGE FROM 26 TO 70). ONE GROUP WAS ENGLISH-SPEAKING (HIGH ACCULTURATION) AND THE OTHER WAS SPANISH-SPEAKING (LOW ACCULTURATION). ITEM RESPONSES WERE ANALYZED FOR GROUP DIFFERENCES, AND HYPOTHESES WERE GENERALLY CONFIRMED: THE MORE ACCULTURATED THE GROUP, THE GREATER THE MARRIAGE ROLE CHANGE TOWARD AN EGALITARIAN-COMPANIONATE MARRIAGE PATTERN, OR IN RAINWATER'S TERMS, FROM A SEGREGATED TO A JOINT CONJUGAL ROLE PATTERN. THE OBSERVED MARRIAGE ROLE DIFFERENCE WAS FOUND TO BE TRUE ACROSS LEVELS OF EDUCATION AND LENGTH OF U.S. RESIDENCY BUT NOT NECESSARILY INCOME AND OCCUPATION LEVEL. IT IS RECOMMENDED THAT FUTURE RESEARCH ON MARRIAGE ROLES FOCUS ON CULTURAL VS. SES DIFFERENCES. 7 REFERENCES.

ACCN   001564

1810 AUTH   **THARP, R. G., & MEADOW, A.**

TITL   DIFFERENTIAL CHANGE IN FOLK DISEASE CONCEPTS.

SRCE   *REVISTA INTERAMERICANA DE PSICOLOGIA, 1973, 7(1-2), 55-63.*

INDX   CURANDERISMO, FOLK MEDICINE, ATTITUDES, MEXICAN AMERICAN, CROSS CULTURAL, CULTURAL FACTORS, COMMUNITY, EMPIRICAL, DISEASE, HEALTH, SURVEY, ACCULTURATION, ARIZONA, SOUTHWEST

ABST   TO DETERMINE HOW BELIEF IN FOLK DISEASES CHANGES IN THE PROCESS OF ACCULTURATION, 250 MEXICAN AMERICAN MALE AND FEMALE HOUSEHOLD HEADS WERE INTERVIEWED IN TUCSON, ARIZONA. TRADITIONAL MEXICAN DISEASES WERE CATEGORIZED BY ETIOLOGY INTO THREE TYPES—THOSE OF NATURALISTIC ORIGIN, EMOTIONAL ORIGIN, OR MAGICAL ORIGIN. THEN INFORMANTS WERE ASKED, ON A FIVE-POINT SCALE, THE DEGREE TO WHICH THEY AND HOUSEHOLD MEMBERS ADHERED TO THESE FOLK DISEASES. A "HOUSEHOLD ADHERENCE SCORE" WAS ASSIGNED, REFLECTING THE DEGREE OF BELIEF OF THE LEAST ACCULTURATED HOUSEHOLD MEMBER. A CHI SQUARE ANALYSIS REVEALED THAT FOLK DISEASES OF NATURALISTIC ORIGIN PERSIST LONGER THAN THOSE OF EMOTIONAL ORIGIN, WHICH, IN TURN, PERSIST LONGER THAN THOSE OF MAGICAL ORIGIN. IT IS CONCLUDED THAT IN THE PROCESS OF ACCULTURATION AND URBANIZATION, FOLK CONCEPTS ARE ABANDONED IN AN ORDERLY AND PREDICTABLE MANNER. IT IS NOT THE CONTENT OF A BELIEF WHICH DETERMINES ITS RATE OF CHANGE, BUT RATHER THE DEGREE OF CONGRUENCE OF THE BELIEF TO THE BELIEF SYSTEM OF THE NEW SUPERORDINATE CULTURE—SPECIFICALLY IN THIS CASE, THE DISEASE ETIOLOGY BELIEF SYSTEM IN THE UNITED STATES. 8 REFERENCES.

ACCN   001565

1811 AUTH   **THOMAS, A., CHESS, S., SILLEN, J., & MENDEZ, O.**

TITL   CROSS-CULTURAL STUDY OF BEHAVIOR IN CHILDREN WITH SPECIAL VULNERABILITIES TO STRESS.

SRCE   *IN D. F. RICKS, A. THOMAS & M. ROFF (EDS.), LIFE HISTORY RESEARCH IN PSYCHOPATHOLOGY. MINNEAPOLIS: UNIVERSITY OF MINNESOTA PRESS, 1974, PP. 53-67.*

INDX   CROSS CULTURAL, CHILDREN, STRESS, ANXIETY, ETHNIC IDENTITY, FAMILY STRUCTURE, PUERTO RICAN-M, SES, PSYCHOPATHOLOGY, MENTAL HEALTH, CULTURAL FACTORS, ENVIRONMENTAL FACTORS, EMPIRICAL, DEVIANCE, NEW YORK, EAST, URBAN

ABST   TWO SAMPLES OF CHILDREN, 31 PUERTO RICAN FROM WORKING-CLASS FAMILIES IN SPANISH HARLEM AND 42 ANGLO FROM MIDDLE- AND UPPER-MIDDLE-CLASS FAMILIES IN OTHER AREAS OF NEW YORK CITY, WHO PRESENTED BEHAVIOR DISORDERS BEFORE THE AGE OF 9 WERE STUDIED. BY MEANS OF PERIODIC PARENTAL INTERVIEWS AND PSYCHOLOGICAL TESTING OF THE CHILDREN DURING THE LONGITUDINAL STUDY, THE AGE OF ONSET AND TYPES OF BEHAVIORAL SYMPTOMS WERE DETERMINED TO BE DIFFERENT FOR THE TWO ETHNIC-SES GROUPS. THESE DIFFERENCES ARE DISCUSSED IN TERMS OF VARIATIONS IN ENVIRONMENTAL INFLUENCES, AS WELL AS DEMANDS AND STRESSES EXPERIENCED BY THE PUERTO RICAN AND ANGLO CHILDREN AND THEIR PARENTS. DIFFERENCES BETWEEN THE GROUPS, BOTH IN TERMS OF THE CHILD'S BEHAVIOR AND THE PARENTS' METHOD OF MANAGEMENT, WERE FOUND IN THESE SYMPTOM AREAS: SLEEP, MOTOR ACTIVITY, DISCIPLINE, LEARNING, AND SELF-IN-

FLICTED INJURIES. (1) ALMOST HALF THE PUERTO RICAN CHILDREN PRESENTED SLEEP PROBLEMS BETWEEN THE AGES OF 5 AND 9, WHEREAS COMPLAINTS ABOUT SLEEP PROBLEMS IN THE ANGLO MIDDLE-CLASS GROUP OCCURRED MORE FREQUENTLY IN THE PRESCHOOL PERIOD AND DECLINED SHARPLY AFTER SCHOOL AGE. (2) OVER 50% OF THE PUERTO RICAN PARENTS COMPLAINED ABOUT THEIR CHILD'S MOTOR ACTIVITY, WHILE ONLY ONE BRAIN DAMAGED ANGLO CHILD PRESENTED WITH THE SAME COMPLAINT—A SIGNIFICANT DIFFERENCE. (3) ALSO STATISTICALLY SIGNIFICANT WAS THE TWO TIMES HIGHER INCIDENCE OF DISCIPLINARY PROBLEMS IN THE PUERTO RICAN SAMPLE THAN THE MIDDLE-CLASS SAMPLE. (4) LEARNING PROBLEMS WERE MORE COMMON IN THE SCHOOL AGE, MIDDLE-CLASS CHILDREN. (5) ABOUT 25% OF THE PUERTO RICAN CHILDREN HAD INFLICTED INJURY ON THEMSELVES BY BODY OR HEAD BANGING OR BY SUSTAINING BURN OR RAZOR CUTS. SEVERAL HAD ALSO THREATENED SUICIDE WHEN DISCIPLINED OR FRUSTRATED. NO ANGLO, MIDDLE-CLASS PARENT REPORTED THIS SYMPTOM. THE STUDY EMPHASIZES THE NEED FOR UNDERSTANDING A CHILD'S SOCIAL AND CULTURAL BACKGROUND IN EVALUATING WHAT CONSTITUTES EXCESSIVE STRESS AND ADAPTIVE BEHAVIOR FOR THAT CHILD. IN DIAGNOSING AND TREATING BEHAVIOR DISORDERS IN MINORITY OR LOWER-CLASS CHILDREN, IT IS NEITHER APPROPRIATE NOR ACCURATE TO USE CRITERIA BASED ONLY ON DEVELOPMENTAL DATA FOR ANGLO, NATIVE-BORN, MIDDLE-CLASS CHILDREN. 5 REFERENCES. (AUTHOR SUMMARY MODIFIED)

ACCN 001566

1812 AUTH **THOMAS, A., HERTZIG, M. E., DRYMAN, I., & FERNANDEZ, P.**

TITL EXAMINER EFFECT IN IQ TESTING OF PUERTO RICAN WORKING-CLASS CHILDREN.

SRCE *AMERICAN JOURNAL OF ORTHOPSYCHIATRY, 1971, 41(5), 809-821.*

INDX EXAMINER EFFECTS, PUERTO RICAN-M, SES, CHILDREN, INTELLIGENCE TESTING, EMPIRICAL, WISC, NEW YORK, EAST

ABST THE WISC SCORES OF 116 NEW YORK CITY PUERTO RICAN WORKING-CLASS CHILDREN, 6 TO 15 YEARS-OLD, WERE MARKEDLY AFFECTED BY DIFFERENCES IN EXAMINER STYLE, ALTHOUGH THE TWO EXAMINERS WERE EQUIVALENT IN SEX, ETHNICITY, FLUENCY IN SPANISH AND ENGLISH, AND CLINICAL EXPERIENCE. SIGNIFICANTLY HIGHER PERFORMANCE LEVEL OCCURRED WITH THE EXAMINER WHO HAD KNOWN THE CHILDREN FOR MANY YEARS AND WHOSE BEHAVIOR ENCOURAGED ACTIVE PARTICIPATION, VERBALIZATION, AND REPEATED EFFORT ON THE CHILD'S PART. RESULTS INDICATE THAN THE PERFORMANCE LEVEL OF DISADVANTAGED CHILDREN ON STANDARDIZED TESTS OF INTELLECTUAL FUNCTIONING CAN BE RAISED BY EMPLOYING EXAMINATION PROCEDURES THAT ARE CONGRUENT WITH THEIR SPONTANEOUS COGNI-

TIVE STYLE. THIS SUGGESTS THAT THE ACADEMIC ACHIEVEMENT OF SUCH CHILDREN MAY ALSO BE IMPROVED BY THE USE OF SIMILAR TECHNIQUES OF INSTRUCTION IN SCHOOLS. 17 REFERENCES. (JOURNAL ABSTRACT MODIFIED)

ACCN 001567

1813 AUTH **THOMAS, C. S., & GARRISON, V.**

TITL A CASE OF THE DOMINICAN MIGRANT.

SRCE *IN R. S. BRYCE-LAPORTE & C. S. THOMAS (EDS.), ALIENATION IN CONTEMPORARY SOCIETY: A MULTIDISCIPLINARY EXAMINATION. NEW YORK: PRAEGER PRESS, 1976, PP. 216-260.*

INDX SPANISH SURNAMED, ANOMIE, CASE STUDY, MENTAL HEALTH, STRESS, ENVIRONMENTAL FACTORS, CULTURAL FACTORS, PSYCHOPATHOLOGY, FOLK MEDICINE, ESPIRITISMO, CULTURAL PLURALISM, ACCULTURATION, URBAN, ANXIETY, HEALTH, PSYCHOSOCIAL ADJUSTMENT, PSYCHOTHERAPY OUTCOME

ABST A DETAILED CASE STUDY IS PRESENTED WHICH DISCUSSES JUAN'S RECENT ATTACKS (ATAQUES). ATAQUE IS DEFINED AS A FOLK CONCEPT OF DISEASE AND IS EXAMINED FROM BOTH A MEDICAL AND FOLK PERSPECTIVE. JUAN'S FEELINGS OF ALIENATION IS SIMILAR TO THOSE WHO HAVE MIGRATED FROM THE RURAL DOMINICAN REPUBLIC TO A LARGE URBAN COMPLEX SUCH AS NEW YORK CITY. JUAN IS LIKE MANY RECENT MIGRANTS—HE IS MARRIED WITH THREE CHILDREN AND CANNOT SPEAK, WRITE, OR READ ENGLISH. JUAN HAD PREVIOUSLY SOUGHT HELP FROM MENTAL HEALTH CLINICS BUT NOW HAS TURNED TO A FOLK HEALER FOR TREATMENT OF HIS ATAQUES. IT IS FELT THAT THESE HEALTH AGENCIES BY TREATING JUAN FOR VARIOUS POSSIBLE ORGANIC ETIOLOGICAL BASES IGNORED THE REALITY THAT JUAN'S CONDITION WAS PROBABLY PRECIPITATED BY SOCIOCULTURAL STRESS FACTORS RESULTING FROM HIS INABILITY TO ADJUST TO HIS NEW ENVIRONMENT. THE CULTURAL VALUES THAT JUAN IDENTIFIES REGARDING THE FAMILY, COMPADRES, VARIOUS CULTS SUCH AS SANTERIA, KINSHIP, AND CONFIANZA ARE EXAMINED. JUAN'S ADJUSTMENT IS DESCRIBED IN FOUR STAGES: ENTHUSIASM AND EXPECTATIONS; DISILLUSIONMENT, LONELINESS, AND FRUSTRATION; ACCOMODATION; AND RETRIBALIZATION. EVEN THOUGH JUAN IS BEING TREATED BY AN ESPIRITIST, HE IS STILL SUFFERING FROM ATAQUES. IT IS CONCLUDED THAT THE NATIONAL HEALTH CARE SYSTEM NEEDS TO RECOGNIZE, ACCEPT, AND LEGITIMIZE OTHER CULTURAL METHODS AS VIABLE MEANS IN THE TREATMENT OF MENTAL HEALTH PROBLEMS. 73 REFERENCES.

ACCN 001568

1814 AUTH **THOMAS, C. S., & GARRISON, V.**

TITL A GENERAL SYSTEMS VIEW OF COMMUNITY MENTAL HEALTH.

SRCE *IN L. BELLAK & H. BARTEN (EDS.), PROGRESS IN COMMUNITY MENTAL HEALTH (VOL. 3). NEW YORK: BRUNNER/MAZEL, 1975, PP. 265-332.*

INDX CASE STUDY, NEW YORK, EAST, MENTAL HEALTH,

COMMUNITY, HEALTH DELIVERY SYSTEMS, CARIBBEAN

ABST IT IS NOT ENOUGH FOR COMMUNITY MENTAL HEALTH CENTER (CMHC) STAFF TO KNOW ONLY THE BROAD, GENERAL TRAITS SHARED BY THE SPANISH SPEAKING/SURNAME POPULATION. THIS ASSERTION IS BASED UPON AN IN-DEPTH CASE STUDY OF THE EPISODIC MENTAL ILLNESS OF "JUAN," A MIGRANT NEW YORK "JEFE DE FAMILIA" (FAMILY PATRIARCH) FROM A PEASANT SUBCULTURE IN THE DOMINICAN REPUBLIC. AN ANALYSIS OF THE INTRIGUES AND PRESSURES WHICH THAT SUBCULTURE CAN IMPOSE ON A "JEFE" POISED BETWEEN TWO WORLDS, TRACES JUAN'S "ATAQUE DE NERVIOS" TO AN INTERNECINE PLOT BY HIS BROTHER TO USURP JUAN'S DOMINANT ROLE IN THE DOMINICAN REPUBLIC. IT ALSO REVEALS THAT JUAN'S STATUS OF "JEFE" WOULD BE FURTHER IMPERILED BY ANY IMPLICATION OF "LOCURA" (MENTAL ILLNESS) WHICH SPELLS TOTAL INCOMPETENCE IN HIS CULTURE. IN VIEW OF THIS, IT IS ASKED: WHAT, IF ANYTHING, COULD CMHC STAFF DO TO HELP IF THEY POSSESSED ONLY THE USUAL MEDICAL AND PSYCHIATRIC HISTORY AND THE DEMOGRAPHIC AND SOCIAL STUDIES DATA OF THE CATCHMENT AREA? OBVIOUSLY THE OLD PARADIGM OF REFERRING TO GENERAL INDEXED TRAITS WOULD YIELD LITTLE ACCURATE INFORMATION ABOUT THE SUBTLE PRESSURES IMPERILING THE PATIENT'S MENTAL HEALTH. INSTEAD, A BETTER, MORE MANAGEABLE UNIT OF ANALYSIS IS NEEDED—SPECIFICALLY, THE "EGOCENTRIC SOCIAL NETWORK" SHOULD BE EXAMINED, INCLUDING A SYSTEMIC THEORY OF "COMMUNITY," "MENTAL HEALTH," AND "INTEGRATION." THIS CAN BE DONE BY OBSERVING THE HABITUAL PATTERNS OF INTERACTION AND THE ROLES AND STATUSES RECOGNIZED BY ACTORS IN THESE INTERACTIONS. WHERE SUCH DETAILED ETHNOGRAPHIES ARE NOT AVAILABLE, THE DATA CAN BE OBTAINED FROM STATEMENTS OF PARAPROFESSIONAL CULTURE-CARRIERS (LIKE "ESPIRITISTAS"). THIS GENERAL SYSTEMS THEORY APPROACH CAN REDUCE THIS COMPLEX PROBLEM TO A LESS INEFFICIENT AND MORE MANAGEABLE SCALE. 60 REFERENCES.

ACCN 001569

1815 AUTH **THOMAS, E. C., & YAMAMOTO, K.**

TITL MINORITY CHILDREN AND THEIR SCHOOL RELATED PERCEPTIONS.

SRCE *JOURNAL OF EXPERIMENTAL EDUCATION, 1971, 40(1), 89-96.*

INDX CROSS CULTURAL, MEXICAN AMERICAN, ADOLESCENTS, SEMANTICS, EMPIRICAL, EDUCATION, ATTITUDES

ABST A SEMANTIC DIFFERENTIAL WAS ADMINISTERED TO 300 BLACK, 300 MEXICAN AMERICAN, AND 300 AMERICAN INDIAN CHILDREN IN SIXTH THROUGH EIGHTH GRADES TO STUDY THEIR ATTITUDES TO FOUR CURRICULUM CONCEPTS (SOCIAL STUDIES, LANGUAGE, SCIENCE, MATHEMATICS) AND FOUR PEOPLE (PARENT, TEACHER, CLASSMATES, MYSELF). NO OVERALL SEX OR GRADE DIFFERENCES

WERE FOUND, BUT ETHNICITY AND CONCEPT DIFFERENCES WERE SIGNIFICANT ON ALL THREE "PEOPLE FACTORS" (MOVEMENT, SECURITY, MERIT) AND ON BOTH "CURRICULUM FACTORS" (VIGOR, CERTAINTY). IN ADDITION, THERE WERE COMPLEX INTERACTIONS AMONG ETHNICITY, GRADE, AND SEX CONCEPTS. PARENT ENJOYED THE MOST FAVORABLE RATING FOR EACH ETHNIC GROUP, WHILE TEACHER WAS RANKED IN FOURTH POSITION ON TWO OF THE THREE FACTORS. GENERALLY, BLACK CHILDREN PROVIDED THE MOST FAVORABLE RATINGS ON PEOPLE AND INDIAN CHILDREN THE LEAST. OF THE CURRICULUM AREAS, LANGUAGE WAS RATED MOST VIGOROUS AND CERTAIN BY ALL ETHNIC GROUPS, WHILE SOCIAL STUDIES GENERALLY RANKED IN FOURTH POSITION. WHEN COMPARED WITH WHITE MIDDLE SCHOOL CHILDREN, THESE MINORITY CHILDREN IN RATHER FAVORABLE SCHOOL ENVIRONMENTS INDICATED GOOD SCHOOL-RELATED ATTITUDES. 18 REFERENCES.

ACCN 001570

1816 AUTH **THOMAS, P. H., CHINSKY, J. M., & ANDERSON, C. F.**

TITL A PRESCHOOL EDUCATIONAL PROGRAM WITH PUERTO RICAN CHILDREN: IMPLICATIONS AS A COMMUNITY INTERVENTION.

SRCE *JOURNAL OF COMMUNITY PSYCHOLOGY, 1973, 1(1), 18-22.*

INDX EARLY CHILDHOOD EDUCATION, PUERTO RICAN-M, PEABODY PICTURE-VOCABULARY TEST, EMPIRICAL, INTELLIGENCE TESTING, COMMUNITY INVOLVEMENT, PARAPROFESSIONALS, TEACHERS, SCHOLASTIC ACHIEVEMENT, BILINGUAL, EAST

ABST TO ASSESS THE VALUE OF HOME TUTORING, 57 PUERTO RICAN CHILDREN (AGES 21 TO 47 MONTHS) WERE STUDIED IN AN EASTERN U.S. COMMUNITY. THE CHILDREN WERE DIVIDED INTO TWO GROUPS: AN EXPERIMENTAL GROUP OF 36 CHILDREN WHO RECEIVED 1 HOUR OF TUTORING DAILY FOR 7 MONTHS; AND A MATCHED CONTROL GROUP OF 21 CHILDREN WHO DID NOT RECEIVE TUTORING. TUTORING WAS CONDUCTED BY 24 FEMALE, SPANISH-SPEAKING UNDERGRADUATES. THE TUTORING PROGRAM STRESSED BOTH INTELLECTUAL GROWTH (I.E., LANGUAGE AND COGNITIVE DEVELOPMENT) AND AFFECTIVE GROWTH (I.E., TUTORS WERE WARM, FRIENDLY, AND SOUGHT TO INSTILL A POSITIVE SELF-IMAGE). FOR THE PURPOSE OF COMPARISON, BOTH GROUPS OF CHILDREN WERE TESTED ON INTELLECTUAL AND BEHAVIORAL MEASURES, INCLUDING A SPANISH VERSION OF THE PEABODY PICTURE-VOCABULARY TEST AND THREE MERRILL PALMER SUBTESTS. RESULTS DETERMINED THAT THE EXPERIMENTAL GROUP SHOWED SIGNIFICANT INCREASES IN VOCABULARY, COLOR RECOGNITION AND LABELING, AS WELL AS MARGINAL GAINS IN IQ SCORES. MOREOVER, HOME INTERVENTION PROVED VALUABLE FOR REACHING OTHERWISE INACCESSIBLE CHILDREN AND FOR EXPOSING TUTORS TO CHILDREN'S TOTAL ENVIRONMENT. HOWEVER, DESPITE THE PROGRAM'S MANY STRENGTHS,

SOME SHORTCOMINGS EMERGED—E.G., MORE CULTURALLY SENSITIVE INTELLIGENCE TESTS NEED TO BE DEVELOPED; THE PROGRAM SHOULD HAVE HAD MORE INTERACTION WITH LOCAL SCHOOLS; AND THE COMMUNITY SHOULD HAVE BEEN MORE ACTIVELY ENCOURAGED TO CONTINUE THE PROGRAM BY ITSELF. 9 REFERENCES.

ACCN   001571

1817 AUTH   **THOMAS, P. J.**
TITL   ADMINISTRATION OF A DIALECTICAL SPANISH VERSION AND STANDARD ENGLISH VERSION OF THE PEABODY PICTURE VOCABULARY TEST.
SRCE   *PSYCHOLOGICAL REPORTS, 1977, 40, 747-750.*
INDX   BILINGUAL, CHILDREN, CULTURE-FAIR TESTS, EMPIRICAL, INTELLIGENCE TESTING, MEXICAN AMERICAN, PEABODY PICTURE-VOCABULARY TEST, SPANISH SURNAMED, TEXAS, SOUTHWEST, TEST RELIABILITY
ABST   THIS STUDY INVESTIGATED WHETHER SIGNIFICANT DIFFERENCES EXIST IN THE SCORES OBTAINED BY A SAMPLE OF CHILDREN OF MEXICAN DESCENT WHEN ADMINISTERED A SPANISH VERSION AND THE STANDARD ENGLISH VERSION OF THE PEABODY PICTURE VOCABULARY TEST. SUBJECTS WERE 78 SPANISH SURNAMED CHILDREN FROM THREE SMALL, RURAL SCHOOL DISTRICTS IN SOUTH CENTRAL TEXAS. THEY WERE DIVIDED INTO TWO GROUPS, ONE OF WHICH RECEIVED FORM A SPANISH VERSION FOLLOWED BY FORM B STANDARD ENGLISH VERSION AND THE OTHER, FORM A STANDARD ENGLISH VERSION FOLLOWED BY FORM B SPANISH VERSION. A GROUPS-BY-TRIALS ANALYSIS OF VARIANCE SHOWED THAT SUBJECTS SCORED SIGNIFICANTLY HIGHER ON THE STANDARD ENGLISH VERSION OF THE PEABODY. IN LIGHT OF THESE RESULTS IT WAS SUGGESTED THAT IT IS NOT NECESSARY TO TEST A CHILD IN THE SPANISH LANGUAGE UNLESS IT HAS FIRST BEEN DETERMINED THAT HIS ONLY LANGUAGE IS SPANISH. 6 REFERENCES. (JOURNAL ABSTRACT)

ACCN   002230

1818 AUTH   **THORNBURG, H. D.**
TITL   AN INVESTIGATION OF A DROPOUT PROGRAM AMONG ARIZONA'S MINORITY YOUTH.
SRCE   *EDUCATION, 1974, 94(3), 249-265.*
INDX   SCHOLASTIC ACHIEVEMENT, MEXICAN AMERICAN, DELINQUENCY, EMPIRICAL, SES, ATTITUDES, SELF CONCEPT, INTELLIGENCE, ARIZONA, SOUTHWEST
ABST   IN 1970-71 A SPECIAL ACADEMIC PROGRAM WAS DESIGNED TO ELEVATE ATTITUDES TOWARD SELF AND SCHOOL AND THEREBY STEM HIGH DROPOUT RATES AMONG MINORITY YOUTHS AT A RURAL ARIZONA HIGH SCHOOL. 265 9TH GRADE STUDENTS WERE DIVIDED INTO AN EXPERIMENTAL GROUP OF 126 SUBJECTS (LARGELY MEXICAN AMERICAN) AND A CONTROL GROUP OF 139 (MOSTLY ANGLO). EXPERIMENTAL STUDENTS WERE FURTHER RANDOMLY DIVIDED INTO A VOCATIONAL PROGRAM (AGRICULTURE AND HOME ECONOMICS) AND A SPECIAL ACADEMIC PROGRAM, TAUGHT VIA TEAM-TEACHING AND STRESSING

CORE ENGLISH AND MATH SUBJECTS. CONTROL STUDENTS RECEIVED REGULAR CLASSROOM ASSIGNMENTS. TESTS WERE ADMINISTERED IN THE FALL AND SPRING TO MONITOR CHANGES THAT COULD AFFECT DROPOUT BEHAVIORS. INITIALLY, ALL WERE ADMINISTERED A GENERAL INFORMATION SURVEY, THE LORGE-THORNDYKE INTELLIGENCE TEST, AND THE PUBLIC OPINION QUESTIONNAIRE (A TEST FOR MEASURING ATTITUDES TOWARD SCHOOL). ALSO, EXPERIMENTAL STUDENTS WERE ADMINISTERED THE TENNESSEE SELF-CONCEPT SCALE. THE PROJECT INDICATED THAT A SPECIAL ACADEMIC ENVIRONMENT WAS INSTRUMENTAL IN PRODUCING A MORE POSITIVE ATTITUDE TOWARD SELF AND SCHOOL. A GROWTH IN SELF-CONCEPT AND POSITIVE ATTITUDES TOWARD SCHOOL WAS EVIDENT AMONG HIGH-RISK DROPOUTS IN THE SPECIAL ACADEMIC PROGRAM, WHILE VOCATIONALLY PLACED AND REGULAR STUDENTS SHOWED A DROP. THE SPECIAL ACADEMIC PROGRAM ALSO SEEMED EFFECTIVE IN STEMMING OVERALL DROPOUT RATES: 9.3% OF THE STUDENTS IN THE SPECIAL ACADEMIC GROUP DROPPED OUT OF SCHOOL, COMPARED TO 18% IN THE VOCATIONAL GROUP AND 8.1% IN THE REGULAR CLASSROOMS. THESE FINDINGS SUGGEST THAT A SPECIAL ACADEMIC PROGRAM IN WHICH POSITIVE REINFORCEMENT TECHNIQUES ARE USED IS AN EFFECTIVE APPROACH TO THE PROBLEM OF CHRONIC DROPOUT TRENDS. THEY SUGGEST THAT THE SCHOOLS MIGHT CONSIDER WAYS OF DEVELOPING SPECIAL VOCATIONAL PROGRAMS THAT MEET THE SAME PRIMARY OBJECTIVES AS THE SPECIAL ACADEMIC PROGRAMS, WHILE TEACHING USABLE MANUAL SKILLS FOR POTENTIAL DROPOUTS. 39 REFERENCES.

ACCN   001572

1819 AUTH   **THORSELL, B. A.**
TITL   SELF-ESTEEM AND ETHNIC STATUS.
SRCE   *PAPER PRESENTED AT THE ANNUAL MEETING OF THE WESTERN PSYCHOLOGICAL ASSOCIATION, SACRAMENTO, CALIFORNIA, APRIL 24-26, 1975. (ABSTRACT)*
INDX   CROSS CULTURAL, ADOLESCENTS, ETHNIC IDENTITY, EMPIRICAL, SELF CONCEPT, MEXICAN AMERICAN, CALIFORNIA, SOUTHWEST
ABST   A SAMPLE OF 162 MALE SUBJECTS BETWEEN THE AGES OF 11 AND 17 WAS CHOSEN AT RANDOM FROM THREE LOS ANGELES PUBLIC SCHOOLS. THE SUBJECTS INCLUDED 75 WHITE, 63 CHICANO, AND 24 BLACK ADOLESCENTS. EACH WAS ASKED TO WRITE TWENTY STATEMENTS WHICH HE THOUGHT BEST ANSWERED THE QUESTION "WHO ARE YOU?" THE RESPONSES WERE FOUND TO BE CLASSIFIABLE INTO FOUR CATEGORIES: PHYSICAL CHARACTERISTICS, SOCIAL ROLES, LIKES-DISLIKES, AND SELF-EVALUATIONS. ALL SELF-EVALUATION RESPONSES WERE FURTHER CLASSIFIED AS EITHER "POSITIVE," "NEGATIVE," OR "NEUTRAL," AND AN ANALYSIS OF THE RELATIONSHIP BETWEEN THE SUBJECT'S ETHNIC STATUS AND SELF-ESTEEM, AS INDICATED BY HIS SELF-EVALUATIONS, WAS CARRIED OUT. AL-

THOUGH TWO-THIRDS OF ALL SUBJECTS' SELF-EVALUATIONS WERE CLASSIFIABLE AS POSITIVE, SIGNIFICANT DIFFERENCES WERE NOTED BETWEEN POSITIVE TO NEGATIVE OR NEUTRAL RESPONSES FOR EACH ETHNIC GROUP. BLACKS YIELDED THE GREATEST PROPORTION OF POSITIVE EVALUATIONS, WHITES THE NEXT LARGEST, CHICANOS THE SMALLEST. THESE RESULTS CONTRADICT THE BELIEF, SUPPORTED BY SOME STUDIES, THAT LOW SELF-ESTEEM AND A NEGATIVE SELF-CONCEPT ARE CHARACTERISTIC OF BLACKS AND OTHER OPPRESSED MINORITIES. IN THIS STUDY, BOTH BLACKS AND CHICANOS EXHIBIT RELATIVELY HIGH SELF-ESTEEM AND POSITIVE SELF-CONCEPTS, AND BLACKS EXCEED WHITES SUBSTANTIALLY IN THIS REGARD. THE REASONS FOR THIS MAY LIE IN HEIGHTENED ETHNIC PRIDE OVER THE PAST SEVERAL YEARS WHICH MAY HAVE AFFECTED THE SUBJECTS IN THIS RESEARCH WHILE THEY WERE QUITE YOUNG. FURTHER RESEARCH IS NEEDED TO FULLY ASSESS THE IMPACT OF THESE FACTORS IN MINORITY COMMUNITIES ON SELF-ESTEEM AND SELF-CONCEPT.

ACCN   001573

1820 AUTH   **THORSELL, B. A., & CHAMBERS, R.**
TITL   THE ADJUDICATION PROCESS AND SELF-CONCEPT.
SRCE   *PERSONALITY AND SOCIAL PSYCHOLOGY BULLETIN, 1974, 1(1), 327-329.*
INDX   ADOLESCENTS, MEXICAN AMERICAN, CULTURAL FACTORS, CROSS CULTURAL, SELF CONCEPT, EMPIRICAL, DELINQUENCY, MALE, CALIFORNIA, SOUTHWEST, VALUES
ABST   QUESTIONNAIRES ADMINISTERED IN SOUTHERN CALIFORNIA TO 82 MALE JUVENILE DELINQUENTS (16 BLACK, 19 CHICANO, AND 47 WHITE) AND 75 WHITE JUNIOR HIGH SCHOOL NONDELINQUENTS REVEALED THAT (1) THE JUVENILE OFFENDERS EXHIBITED SIGNIFICANTLY MORE NEGATIVE SELF-CONCEPTIONS AS MEASURED BY THE TWENTY STATEMENTS TEST, AND (2) THE DEGREE OF THE OFFENDERS' SELF-CONCEPTION WAS SIGNIFICANTLY RELATED TO ETHNICITY. WHITE DELINQUENTS HAD THE HIGHEST DEGREE OF NEGATIVENESS IN SELF-CONCEPT (58.2%), CHICANOS RANKED SECOND (52.8%), WHILE BLACKS RANKED THE LOWEST, AS ONLY 22.5% HAD NEGATIVE SELF-CONCEPTS. THE FINDING FOR BLACKS CONTRADICTS THE COMMON ARGUMENT THAT ALL JUVENILE OFFENDERS HAVE A NEGATIVE SELF-CONCEPT. IT IS SUGGESTED THAT THE NEGATIVE SELF-CONCEPTIONS DISPLAYED BY WHITES AND CHICANOS IN THIS STUDY INVOLVE A QUESTIONING OF PERSONAL WORTH AND AN INTERNALIZATION OF THE REJECTION OF SOCIETY. BUT AT THE SAME TIME, THE PHENOMENON OF "MACHISMO" MAY ENABLE THE CHICANO OFFENDER TO EFFECT A SELF-CONCEPT THAT REFLECTS THE VALUES OF MANLINESS AND HONOR, DESPITE HIS OWN DIMINISHED SENSE OF SELF-WORTH. 12 REFERENCES. (PASAR ABSTRACT MODIFIED)
ACCN   001574

1821 AUTH   **TILLY, C.**
TITL   MIGRATION TO AMERICAN CITIES.
SRCE   *IN D. MOYNIHAN (ED.), TOWARD A NATIONAL URBAN POLICY. NEW YORK: BASIC BOOKS, 1970, PP. 152-168.*
INDX   MIGRATION, RURAL, URBAN, SOCIAL MOBILITY, OCCUPATIONAL ASPIRATIONS, SES, PUERTO RICAN-M, ESSAY
ABST   PATTERNS OF URBAN MIGRATION WITHIN THE U.S. CAN BE ATTRIBUTED TO FACTORS OF OCCUPATIONAL INFORMATION, JOB OPPORTUNITIES, AND COST. WHILE SOME ANALYSTS FEEL THAT EVERY GROUP OF MIGRANTS TO AMERICAN CITIES UNDERGOES THE SAME GENERAL PROCESS OF INTEGRATION INTO THE CITY'S LIFE, OTHERS THINK THAT ALTHOUGH THIS WAS TRUE OF EUROPEAN IMMIGRANTS OF THE PAST, DECREASING DEMANDS FOR UNSKILLED LABOR AND SOLIDIFICATION OF RACIAL DISCRIMINATION HAVE CHANGED THE SITUATION ENTIRELY. THREE RECENT GROUPS OF MIGRANTS ARE EXAMINED: PUERTO RICANS AND APPALACHIANS BRIEFLY, AND NEGROES IN MORE DETAIL. THE POLITICAL STATUS OF PUERTO RICO, INEXPENSIVE AIR TRANSPORTATION BETWEEN SAN JUAN AND NEW YORK, AND A STRONG DEMAND FOR WORKERS COMBINED TO ATTRACT 30-40,000 PUERTO RICAN MIGRANTS PER YEAR UNTIL THE 1960'S, THEN THE RATE DROPPED TO ONE-HALF. PUERTO RICANS STARTED ON THE BOTTOM, YET IN TERMS OF THE TRADITIONAL SIGNS OF A GROUP'S SUCCESS IN AMERICA, IT APPEARS THAT THIS GROUP MAY BE FOLLOWING THE PATH OF THEIR EUROPEAN PREDECESSORS. COMPARISON AMONG PUERTOS, RICANS, APPALACHIANS, AND NEGROES LEAVES IT UNCLEAR AS TO WHETHER NEGROES WOULD BE EXPECTED TO FOLLOW THE SAME PATTERN, BUT IT IS CLEAR THAT (1) FOR THE NEGRO THE PRESENCE OF RACIAL DISCRIMINATION MAKES THE EXIT FROM THE GHETTO SLOW AND PAINFUL, AND (2) MANY OF THE CIRCUMSTANCES THOUGHT TO BE CONSEQUENCES OF MIGRATION ARE ACTUALLY EFFECTS OF THE ORGANIZATION OF CITY LIFE ITSELF. FUTURE ALTERNATIVES TO URBAN MIGRATION ARE MENTIONED.
ACCN   001575

1822 AUTH   **TODER, F. A.**
TITL   AN ALTERNATE METHOD OF FUNCTIONING FOR THE SCHOOL PSYCHOLOGIST.
SRCE   *PSYCHOLOGY IN THE SCHOOLS, 1975, 12(4), 404-408.*
INDX   CHILDREN, ATTITUDES, CONFLICT RESOLUTION, CULTURAL FACTORS, EDUCATIONAL COUNSELING, ESSAY, BEHAVIOR MODIFICATION, EDUCATION, MEXICAN AMERICAN, PROFESSIONAL TRAINING, PROGRAM EVALUATION, RURAL, CALIFORNIA, SOUTHWEST, SPANISH SURNAMED
ABST   REMEDIATION HAS LONG BEEN THE PRIMARY EMPHASIS OF THE APPLIED PSYCHOLOGIST; AND IN THE SCHOOLS THE FOCUS HAS TRADITIONALLY BEEN ON IDENTIFICATION AND TREATMENT OF LEARNING AND BEHAVIOR PROBLEMS. HOWEVER, RECENTLY A SHIFT TO-

WARD PREVENTION AND MENTAL HEALTH HAS TAKEN PLACE. THIS PAPER PRESENTS AN APPROACH TO IN-SERVICE TRAINING FOR TEACHERS AS CHANGE AGENTS, ATTEMPTING TO BE RELEVANT TO STUDENTS' NEEDS. THE APPROACH PROVIDES THEM WITH ADDITIONAL SENSITIVITY AND SKILLS IN RECOGNIZING AND REMEDIATING LEARNING AND/OR BEHAVIOR PROBLEMS WHILE ENHANCING THE LEARNER'S ENVIRONMENT. THE RESULTS IN A SEMIRURAL MEXICAN AMERICAN COMMUNITY ARE DESCRIBED. A COURSE DESCRIPTION, WHICH INCLUDES BOTH OUTLINE AND EXCERPTS FROM TEACHER PROJECTS, IS APPENDED. 14 REFERENCES. (AUTHOR ABSTRACT MODIFIED)

ACCN   002231

1823 AUTH   **TORO-CALDER, J.**
TITL   ENFOQUES MEDICO, LEGAL Y SOCIOLOGICO EN LA CATEGORIZACION DEL ADICTO A DROGAS: LA BUSQUEDA DE ALTERNATIVAS. (FOCUS ON THE MEDICAL, LEGAL AND SOCIOLOGICAL ASPECTS IN THE CATEGORIZATION OF THE DRUG ADDICT: THE SEARCH FOR ALTERNATIVES.)
SRCE   *REVISTA DE CIENCIAS SOCIALES, 1975, 4(19), 425-455. (SPANISH)*
INDX   ESSAY, PUERTO RICAN-I, DRUG ADDICTION, DRUG ABUSE, LEGISLATION, SOCIAL SCIENCES
ABST   IN PUERTO RICO, SCIENTIFIC KNOWLEDGE OF DRUG ABUSE IS IMPEDED BY THE NEGATIVE ATTITUDES OF SOCIETY AND BY LIMITATIONS IN MEDICAL, LEGAL, AND SOCIOLOGICAL APPROACHES TO THE PROBLEM. THE MEDICAL APPROACH IS LIMITED IN SCOPE, CONSIDERING DRUG USE ONLY AS AN ILLNESS TO THE EXCLUSION OF SOCIAL-PSYCHOLOGICAL FACTORS. THE LEGAL ORIENTATION CONSIDERS THE ADDICT AN OFFENDER AND CONFINES ITS ACTIVITIES TO THAT OF LEGAL PUNISHMENT. THE SOCIOLOGICAL APPROACH, ALTHOUGH WIDENING ITS SCOPE TO INCLUDE EXAMINATION OF SOCIOCULTURAL FACTORS, SEEMS TO LACK A PROFOUND UNDERSTANDING OF THE ADDICT. IN VIEW OF THESE LIMITATIONS, AN ALTERNATIVE ORIENTATION IS RECOMMENDED—ONE WHICH CONSIDERS THE ADDICT AS A HUMAN BEING WITH HIS OWN SPECIAL PROBLEMS AND WHICH FREES THE ADDICT FROM LIMITATIONS IMPOSED BY THE TRADITIONAL ALTERNATIVES OFFERED BY SOCIETY. THE PROPER ORIENTATION SHOULD ENCOMPASS MEDICAL, PSYCHOLOGICAL, AND SOCIOLOGICAL CONSIDERATIONS OF THE PROBLEM. IT IS CONCLUDED THAT IN ORDER TO CREATE A PUBLIC AWARENESS OF THE DRUG PROBLEM, INFORMATION FROM OTHER COUNTRIES SHOULD BE STUDIED AND THEIR SOLUTIONS ADOPTED WHEN APPLICABLE TO THE SOCIAL REALITIES OF PUERTO RICO. 19 REFERENCES. (JOURNAL ABSTRACT MODIFIED)

ACCN   002307

1824 AUTH   **TORO-CALDER, J., CAFERINA, C., & RECKLESS, W. C.**
TITL   A COMPARATIVE STUDY OF PUERTO RICAN ATTITUDES TOWARD THE LEGAL SYSTEM DEALING WITH CRIME.
SRCE   *JOURNAL OF CRIMINAL LAW, CRIMINOLOGY AND POLICE SCIENCE, 1968, 59(4), 536-541.*
INDX   PUERTO RICAN-I, ATTITUDES, CRIMINOLOGY, ADULTS, EMPIRICAL, CORRECTIONS, CROSS CULTURAL, CPI
ABST   A SAMPLE OF 612 MALE PUERTO RICAN PRISONERS, LABORERS, PRISON GUARDS, AND POLICE WERE ADMINISTERED A QUESTIONNAIRE CONSISTING OF THE SOCIALIZATION SCALE OF THE CALIFORNIA PSYCHOLOGICAL INVENTORY, 89 "LAW ITEMS" DEALING WITH ATTITUDES TOWARD CRIMINAL LAW, THE COURT SYSTEM, AND LAW ENFORCEMENT OFFICIALS, AND THE CRISSMAN MORAL JUDGMENT SCALE. RESULTS DEMONSTRATED THAT PRISONERS HAD THE MOST UNFAVORABLE ATTITUDES TOWARDS THE LAW, FOLLOWED BY LABORERS, WHILE PRISON GUARDS HAD FAVORABLE ATTITUDES AND POLICE OFFICIALS HAD THE MOST FAVORABLE ATTITUDES. THE SAME ATTITUDINAL GRADIENT WAS FOUND TO EXIST IN OHIO, ONTARIO, QUEBEC, ROME, ATHENS, WEST PAKISTAN, AND SOUTH KOREA. BY COMPARISON, THE PUERTO RICAN PRISONERS RANKED THIRD HIGHEST AMONG THE OTHER SEVEN NATIONAL GROUPS SAMPLED IN UNFAVORABLE ATTITUDES TOWARD THE LEGAL SYSTEM. IT IS FELT THAT THE FAVORABLE TO UNFAVORABLE DIRECTION OF ATTITUDES TOWARD THE LEGAL INSTITUTIONS ON THE PART OF VARIOUS ADULT GROUPS INDICATES AN INTERNALIZATION OF LIFE EXPERIENCES WHICH ARE RELATED TO INVOLVEMENT AND NONINVOLVEMENT IN DELINQUENCY AND CRIME. SUCH ATTITUDES MIGHT BE USED AS A CRIMINALITY INDEX, INDICATING DIRECTION TOWARD OR AWAY FROM INVOLVEMENT IN CRIME AS AN ADULT. 2 REFERENCES. (JOURNAL ABSTRACT MODIFIED)

ACCN   001576

1825 AUTH   **TORRES-MATRULLO, C.**
TITL   ACCULTURATION AND PSYCHOPATHOLOGY AMONG PUERTO RICAN WOMEN IN MAINLAND UNITED STATES.
SRCE   *AMERICAN JOURNAL OF ORTHOPSYCHIATRY, 1976, 46(4), 710-719.*
INDX   FEMALE, ADULTS, NEW JERSEY, EAST, PSYCHOPATHOLOGY, EMPIRICAL, ACCULTURATION, PUERTO RICAN-M
ABST   OF 72 PUERTO RICAN WOMEN LIVING IN NEW JERSEY INCLUDED IN THIS STUDY, THOSE WHO WERE LESS ACCULTURATED WERE FOUND TO BE MORE LIKELY TO EXHIBIT PSYCHOPATHOLOGY AS MEASURED ON THE WITTENBORN PSYCHIATRIC RATING SCALES. LEVEL OF ACCULTURATION WAS DETERMINED BY MEANS OF DEMOGRAPHIC DATA AND INTERVIEW QUESTIONS. SUBJECTS HIGH IN ACCULTURATION EXHIBITED HEALTHIER PERSONAL ADJUSTMENT AS SHOWN BY GOUGH'S ADJECTIVE CHECK LIST, WHILE THE LESS ACCULTURATED SUBJECTS INDICATED A POOR SELF-IMAGE AND NEGATIVE PERSONAL ADJUSTMENT. FAMILY AND SEX ROLE ATTITUDES AS MEASURED BY

AN ADAPTED AND TRANSLATED VERSION OF THE INCOMPLETE SENTENCE BLANK WERE NOT FOUND TO CHANGE SIGNIFICANTLY WITH ACCULTURATION, BUT THEY DID DIFFER ACCORDING TO SUBJECTS' LEVEL OF EDUCATION. EDUCATION WAS FOUND TO BE AN IMPORTANT VARIABLE INFLUENCING DIFFERENCES IN PERSONALITY ADJUSTMENT, PSYCHOPATHOLOGY, AND ATTITUDE CHANGE, WITH THE MORE HIGHLY EDUCATED SUBJECTS CONSISTENTLY SCORING LOWER ON ALL SCALES OF PSYCHOPATHOLOGY. RESULTS SUGGEST THAT RECENT ARRIVALS FROM PUERTO RICO, ESPECIALLY POOR AND UNEDUCATED WOMEN, ARE A HIGH RISK GROUP THAT WARRANTS CLINICAL ATTENTION AND EXTENDED SYSTEMS OF EMOTIONAL SUPPORT. THE IMPORTANCE OF THE DEVELOPMENT OF EDUCATIONAL OPPORTUNITIES IN ORDER TO COUNTERACT THE DEMORALIZATION AND HELPLESSNESS INHERENT IN BEING OF LIMITED EDUCATION AND CULTURALLY DIFFERENT IN THE U.S. IS EMPHASIZED. 38 REFERENCES.

ACCN   002455

1826 AUTH   **TORRES-MATRULLO, C.**
TITL   ACCULTURATION AND PSYCHOPATHOLOGY AMONG PUERTO RICAN WOMEN IN MAINLAND UNITED STATES (DOCTORAL DISSERTATION, RUTGERS UNIVERSITY, 1974.)
SRCE   *DISSERTATION ABSTRACTS INTERNATIONAL, 1974, 35, 3041A. (UNIVERSITY MICROFILMS NO. 74-27,664.)*
INDX   PUERTO RICAN-M, FEMALE, EMPIRICAL, ACCULTURATION, PSYCHOPATHOLOGY, FAMILY ROLES, SEX ROLES, ATTITUDES, SELF CONCEPT, PSYCHOSOCIAL ADJUSTMENT
ABST   THE DISSERTATION PROVIDES A MORE COMPLETELY DETAILED ACCOUNT OF THE STUDY CITED ABOVE (TORRES-MATRULLO, 1976). INCLUDED IN THE DISSERTATION BUT NOT IN THE ABOVE ARTICLE ARE: (1) A LENGTHIER REVIEW OF THE LITERATURE; (2) A DETAILED ACCOUNT OF THE METHODOLOGY AND RESULTS, INCLUDING 5 EXTENSIVE TABLES; (3) 3 APPENDICES WHICH CONSIST OF THE STUDY'S RESEARCH INSTRUMENTS; AND (4) 122 REFERENCES, COMPARED TO THE 38 REFERENCES CITED IN THE 1976 ARTICLE.
ACCN   001577

1827 AUTH   **TORREY, E. F.**
TITL   THE CASE FOR THE INDIGENOUS THERAPIST.
SRCE   *ARCHIVES OF GENERAL PSYCHIATRY, 1969, 20(3), 365-373.*
INDX   REVIEW, PSYCHOTHERAPY, FOLK MEDICINE, HEALTH DELIVERY SYSTEMS, ESSAY
ABST   PROLIFERATION OF MENTAL HEALTH CENTERS COMBINED WITH A PROFESSIONAL MANPOWER SHORTAGE NECESSITATE CONSIDERATION OF THE USE OF THE INDIGENOUS THERAPIST IN FORMAL PSYCHIATRIC SERVICES. THE ROLE OF PATIENT EXPECTATIONS AND THE EFFECT OF PERSONAL QUALITIES OF THE THERAPIST IN PRODUCING PSYCHOTHERAPEUTIC CHANGE HAVE BEEN RECOGNIZED IN TRADITIONAL MEDICINE. DIRECT OBSERVATION OF THE INDIGENOUS THERAPIST AT WORK GIVES EVIDENCE OF HIS EFFECTIVENESS IN PRODUCING POSITIVE RESULTS. EXAMPLES ARE CITED FROM OTHER CULTURES AND WITHIN THE U.S. WHERE HOSPITAL ATTENDANTS, MENTAL PATIENTS, COLLEGE STUDENTS, HOUSEWIVES, AND MEDICAL STUDENTS HAVE BEEN TRAINED TO CONDUCT THERAPY THAT COMPARES FAVORABLY TO THAT CONDUCTED BY PROFESSIONALS. MAJOR OBSTACLES TO THE ACCEPTANCE OF INDIGENOUS THERAPISTS ARE EXAMINED, AND SOLUTIONS UTILIZING SELECTIVE SANCTION OF THERAPISTS AND THERAPEUTIC TECHNIQUES ARE SUGGESTED. THE PROBLEM OF RESISTANCE ON THE PART OF THE MENTAL HEALTH PROFESSION IS ALSO DISCUSSED. 57 REFERENCES.
ACCN   001578

1828 AUTH   **TORREY, E. F.**
TITL   THE IRRELEVANCY OF TRADITIONAL MENTAL HEALTH SERVICES FOR URBAN MEXICAN AMERICANS.
SRCE   *PAPER PRESENTED AT THE MEETINGS OF THE AMERICAN ORTHOPSYCHIATRY ASSOCIATION, 1970.*
INDX   MENTAL HEALTH, HEALTH DELIVERY SYSTEMS, URBAN, MEXICAN AMERICAN, RESOURCE UTILIZATION, ESSAY, PSYCHOTHERAPY, CULTURAL FACTORS, CALIFORNIA, SOUTHWEST
ABST   AN ASSESSMENT OF MENTAL HEALTH SERVICES IN SAN JOSE AND SURROUNDING SANTA CLARA COUNTY POINTS OUT THE IRRELEVANCE FOR AND CONSEQUENT UNDERUTILIZATION BY MEXICAN AMERICANS OF SUCH SERVICES. THERE ARE NO PUBLIC OR PRIVATE FACILITIES LOCATED WITHIN THE DISTRICT WHICH HAS THE LARGEST CONCENTRATION OF MEXICAN AMERICANS. LESS THAN 5% OF THE COUNTY MENTAL HEALTH STAFF SPEAK ANY SPANISH. AND BECAUSE AMERICAN MENTAL HEALTH SERVICES ARE CLASS BOUND, THEY OFTEN DEGRADE ETHNIC MINORITIES AND, IN GENERAL, ARE UNRESPONSIVE TO THE LOWER SOCIOECONOMIC CLASS TO WHICH MOST MEXICAN AMERICANS BELONG. SINCE ANGLO AND MEXICAN AMERICAN CULTURES HAVE DIFFERENT CONCEPTUALIZATIONS OF MENTAL DISORDERS AND THERAPY (WITH MEXICAN AMERICANS HAVING THEIR OWN TRADITIONAL MENTAL HEALTH SERVICES, INVOLVING THE USE OF CURANDEROS), IT IS IMPERATIVE THAT THE CURRENT MODEL FOR MENTAL HEALTH SERVICES BE MODIFIED. THE CONTROL OF MENTAL HEALTH SERVICES SHOULD BE PLACED IN THE HANDS OF THE MEXICAN AMERICAN COMMUNITY, AND THE SERVICES SHOULD BE PROVIDED BY THOSE MOST CAPABLE WITHIN THE CONTEXT OF COMMUNITY NEEDS. 23 REFERENCES.
ACCN   001579

1829 AUTH   **TORREY, E. F.**
TITL   THE MIND GAME: WITCHDOCTORS AND PSYCHIATRISTS.
SRCE   *NEW YORK: EMERSON HALL PUBLISHERS, 1972.*
INDX   PSYCHOTHERAPISTS, CROSS CULTURAL, MEXICAN AMERICAN, REVIEW, CASE STUDY, ATTITUDES, INDIGENOUS POPULATIONS, ROLE EX-

PECTATIONS, CURANDERISMO, PSYCHO-THERAPY, RELIGION, CALIFORNIA, SOUTH-WEST, CULTURAL FACTORS, MENTAL HEALTH, CULTURAL PLURALISM, PSYCHOTHERAPY OUTCOME, BOOK

ABST EMPHASIZING CROSS-CULTURAL COMPARI-SON, THE AUTHOR (A PSYCHIATRIST) EXAM-INES THE ROLE OF "PSYCHOTHERAPIST" IN TERMS OF FOUR FACTORS: (1) PERSONALITY CHARACTERISTICS; (2) PATIENT EXPECTATIONS ABOUT GETTING WELL; (3) SHARING WITH THE PATIENT THE SAME WORLD VIEW; AND (4) SPE-CIFIC THERAPUTIC TECHNIQUES. THIS COM-PARATIVE ANALYSIS INCLUDES CASE STUDIES OF THERAPISTS IN THE U.S. AND OTHER COUNTRIES (E.G., A ZAR PRIEST IN ETHIOPIA, A "MANAG" IN BORNEO, AND A CALIFORNIA PSY-CHIATRIST), ALL OF WHOM ARE FOUND TO BE REMARKABLY SIMILAR. ONE CHAPTER IS DE-VOTED TO FOLK THERAPISTS IN MEXICAN AMERICAN CULTURE (I.E., CURANDEROS), DE-SCRIBING THEIR ENVIRONMENTAL MANIPULA-TIONS AND THEIR TECHNIQUES OF SUGGES-TION, CONFESSION, AND FAMILY THERAPY—ALL WITH STRONG RELIGIOUS OVERTONES. THE CONCLUDING CHAPTERS DISCUSS THE IMPLICATIONS OF THE "SAMENESS" OF PSY-CHOTHERAPISTS AROUND THE WORLD. THIS FINDING SUGGESTS THE NEED FOR EXPERI-MENTAL AND INNOVATIVE APPROACHES TO THE RECRUITMENT, TRAINING, AND ACCREDI-TATION OF PSYCHOTHERAPISTS IN ALL CUL-TURES. TO DEMONSTRATE THIS POINT, CASE ILLUSTRATIONS OF FUTURE MENTAL HEALTH SERVICES FOR ESKIMOS AND MEXICAN AMERI-CANS ARE OUTLINED. 433 REFERENCES.

ACCN 001749

1830 AUTH **TORREY, E. F.**

TITL PSYCHIATRIC SERVICES FOR MEXICAN AMERI-CANS.

SRCE *UNPUBLISHED MANUSCRIPT, AUGUST 26, 1968. (AVAILABLE FROM THE AUTHOR, DEPARTMENT OF PSYCHIATRY, STANFORD MEDICAL CENTER, STANFORD, CALIFORNIA.)*

INDX HEALTH DELIVERY SYSTEMS, MEXICAN AMERI-CAN, CULTURE, STRESS, ACCULTURATION, ES-SAY, PARAPROFESSIONALS, FOLK MEDICINE, PSYCHOTHERAPY

ABST IN AN EFFORT TO CONCEPTUALIZE PSYCHIAT-RIC SERVICES RELEVANT TO MEXICAN AMERI-CAN CULTURAL VALUES AND NEEDS, THIS PA-PER (1) DESCRIBES MAJOR POINTS OF CULTURAL STRESS, (2) EXAMINES INDIGE-NOUS PSYCHIATRIC BELIEFS, ILLNESSES, AND THERAPIES, (3) COMMENTS ON THE CLASS ORIENTATION OF AMERICAN PSYCHIATRY, AND (4) OFFERS SUGGESTIONS FOR MORE EFFEC-TIVE TREATMENT OF MENTAL ILLNESS AMONG MEXICAN AMERICANS. POINTS OF STRESS IN-CLUDE ACCULTURATION, SEX ROLE EXPECTA-TIONS, A HOSTILE WORLD-VIEW, MISTRUST OF EXTRA-FAMILIAL BONDS, AND THE FEAR AND SUPPRESSION OF EMOTIONS. MOST MENTAL ILLNESSES ARE CONCEPTUALIZED WITHIN THE CULTURE AS SUPERNATURAL OR EMOTION-ALLY CAUSED (E.G., MAL OJO, MAL PUESTO, AND SUSTO). ETIOLOGY, SYMPTOMS, OCCUR-RENCE, TREATMENT (INCLUDING A DESCRIP-TION OF TYPES OF INDIGENOUS THERAPISTS AND THERAPEUTIC TECHNIQUES), AND THE PSYCHOSOCIAL FUNCTION OF MENTAL ILL-NESS ARE DISCUSSED. THE PREVAILING MIDDLE-CLASS ORIENTATION OF AMERICAN PSYCHIATRY IS VIEWED AS INADEQUATE IN THE TREATMENT OF THE MAJORITY OF MEXI-CAN AMERICANS. IT IS RECOMMENDED THAT PSYCHIATRIC SERVICES INCLUDE THE SELEC-TION AND IN-SERVICE TRAINING OF INDIGE-NOUS THERAPISTS, AND THE SETTING OF THE GOALS AND TERMS OF THERAPY BY THE PA-TIENT AND HIS FAMILY. INDIGENOUS CON-CEPTS OF ILLNESS AND THERAPY SHOULD BE USED AND A BROAD RANGE OF SERVICES AP-PROPRIATE TO PATIENT EXPECTATIONS MADE AVAILABLE. 29 REFERENCES.

ACCN 001580

1831 AUTH **TOULIATOS, J., & LINDHOLM, B. W.**

TITL BEHAVIOR PROBLEMS OF ANGLO AND MEXI-CAN-AMERICAN CHILDREN.

SRCE *JOURNAL OF ABNORMAL CHILD PSYCHOLOGY, 1976, 4(3), 299-304.*

INDX CHILDREN, EMPIRICAL, CLASSROOM BEHAV-IOR, DELINQUENCY, PERSONALITY, MEXICAN AMERICAN, SES, SEX COMPARISON, CROSS CULTURAL, TEXAS, SOUTHWEST, MALE, FE-MALE

ABST IN TEXAS, 1,999 ANGLO AMERICAN AND 192 MEXICAN AMERICAN ELEMENTARY SCHOOL CHILDREN WERE COMPARED ON THE FOUR FACTORS OF THE BEHAVIOR PROBLEM CHECK LIST (BPCL). TEACHERS PROVIDED BACK-GROUND INFORMATION AND BPCL RATINGS. THE ANGLO CHILDREN WERE RATED AS HAV-ING MORE PROBLEMS THAN THE MEXICAN AMERICAN CHILDREN ON THE SCALES OF CONDUCT DISORDER, INADEQUACY-IMMATU-RITY, AND SOCIAL DELINQUENCY. SIGNIFICANT INTERACTIONS OF GRADE, SEX, AND SOCIAL CLASS WITH ETHNIC GROUP WERE REVEALED FOR TWO OF THE FACTORS: (1) HIGHER SES ANGLO MALES HAD MORE PERSONALITY DIS-ORDER PROBLEMS THAN MEXICAN AMERICAN MALES, WHILE LOWER SES BOYS EX-HIBITED FEWER; (2) ANGLO GIRLS OF HIGHER SES HAD EQUAL OR FEWER PROBLEMS THAN MEXICAN AMERICAN GIRLS, WHILE LOWER SES ANGLO GIRLS WERE RATED AS HAVING MORE. MEASURES OF SOCIALIZED DELIN-QUENCY REVEALED THAT THE NUMBER OF THESE PROBLEMS INCREASED FOR ANGLOS AND DECREASED FOR MEXICAN AMERICANS AS THEY PASSED FROM KINDERGARTEN THROUGH THE FIFTH GRADE, AND THAT AN-GLO MALES PRESENTED GREATER SOCIAL-IZED DELINQUENCY PROBLEMS THAN DID MEXICAN AMERICANS. 9 REFERENCES. (JOUR-NAL ABSTRACT MODIFIED)

ACCN 002234

1832 AUTH **TOULIATOS, J., & LINDHOLM, B. W.**

TITL A CANONICAL CORRELATION ANALYSIS OF DE-MOGRAPHIC INFORMATION AND THE BEHAV-IOR PROBLEM CHECKLIST.

SRCE   *PSYCHOLOGY IN THE SCHOOLS, 1976, 13(5), 15-18.*

INDX   DEMOGRAPHIC, CLASSROOM BEHAVIOR, PERSONALITY, SEX COMPARISON, EDUCATION, CHILDREN, DELINQUENCY, MEXICAN AMERICAN, CROSS CULTURAL, EMPIRICAL

ABST   A CANONICAL CORRELATIONAL ANALYSIS WAS CONDUCTED ON DEMOGRAPHIC INFORMATION AND THE BEHAVIOR PROBLEM CHECKLIST (BPCL) IN ORDER (1) TO EMPLOY THE DEMOGRAPHIC INFORMATION IN A MANNER THAT HAD NOT BEEN POSSIBLE USING OTHER METHODS, AND (2) TO EXAMINE THE FOUR FACTORS OF THE BPCL (CONDUCT DISORDER; PERSONALITY DISORDER; INADEQUACY-IMMATURITY; AND SOCIALIZED DELINQUENCY) AS A GENERAL MEASURE OF MENTAL HEALTH AND MENTAL ILLNESS. SUBJECTS INCLUDED 2005 WHITE AND 209 MEXICAN AMERICAN 1ST-5TH GRADERS OF BOTH SEXES, VARIOUS SOCIAL CLASSES, AND IN REGULAR OR SPECIAL EDUCATION PROGRAMS. THE CHILDREN'S TEACHERS RATED THEM ON THE BPCL AND ALSO PROVIDED THE DEMOGRAPHIC INFORMATION. IT WAS FOUND THAT THE FOUR FACTORS ON THE BPCL WERE SIGNIFICANTLY CORRELATED, AND ALSO THAT THERE WERE THREE SIGNIFICANT CANONICAL CORRELATIONS BETWEEN THE DEMOGRAPHIC INFORMATION AND THE BPCL RATINGS: (1) BEING FEMALE AND IN REGULAR CLASSES WAS RELATED TO NOT HAVING BEHAVIOR PROBLEMS; (2) BEING MALE, IN THE HIGHER SOCIAL CLASSES, AND IN REGULAR EDUCATION CLASSES WAS RELATED TO NOT HAVING BEHAVIOR PROBLEMS; AND (3) BEING IN THE HIGHER GRADES, IN THE LOWER SOCIAL CLASSES, AND IN REGULAR EDUCATION CLASSES WAS RELATED TO HAVING SOCIALIZED DELINQUENCY SYMPTOMS. 6 REFERENCES. (JOURNAL ABSTRACT MODIFIED)

ACCN   001581

1833 AUTH   **TOWNSEND, D. R., & ZAMORA, G. L.**

TITL   DIFFERING INTERACTION PATTERNS IN BILINGUAL CLASSROOMS.

SRCE   *CONTEMPORARY EDUCATION, 1975, 46(3), 196-202.*

INDX   BILINGUAL-BICULTURAL EDUCATION, MEXICAN AMERICAN, CHILDREN, CLASSROOM BEHAVIOR, TEACHERS, ATTITUDES, INSTRUCTIONAL TECHNIQUES, EMPIRICAL, BILINGUAL, BILINGUAL-BICULTURAL PERSONNEL, TEXAS, SOUTHWEST

ABST   FIFTY-SIX TEACHERS AND ASSISTANT TEACHERS IN A BILINGUAL EARLY CHILDHOOD EDUCATION CENTER IN TEXAS WERE COMPARED TO ASCERTAIN DIFFERENCES IN THEIR VERBAL (SPANISH VS. ENGLISH) AND NONVERBAL INTERACTIONS WITH CHILDREN. FIFTY-THREE OF THE TEACHERS WERE MEXICAN AMERICAN; THE CHILDREN WERE AGES 3 AND 4, 98% WERE MEXICAN AMERICAN, AND OVER 90% WERE MONOLINGUAL SPANISH. THE INSTRUMENT FOR RECORDING CLASSROOM INTERACTION WAS THE SYSTEM FOR CODING INTERACTION WITH MULTIPLE PHASES (SCIMP). THE FINDINGS REVEALED SIGNIFICANT DIFFERENCES IN TEACHER AND ASSISTANT TEACHER BEHAVIORS AS WELL AS IN THE BEHAVIORS OF ALL 56 SUBJECTS WHEN THEY TAUGHT IN THE TWO LANGUAGES: (1) IN THE VERBAL DIMENSION, TEACHERS USED MORE PRAISE, ACCEPTANCE, AND ENCOURAGEMENT; (2) IN THE NONVERBAL DIMENSION, ASSISTANT TEACHERS DEMONSTRATED MORE "NEGATIVE NODDING OF HEAD" AND "NEGATIVE USE OF EYES," WHILE TEACHERS SHOWED A MUCH HIGHER PERCENTAGE OF "COMBINED POSITIVE NONVERBAL BEHAVIORS;" AND (3) WITH RESPECT TO SPANISH VS. ENGLISH INSTRUCTION, THE SUBJECTS DEMONSTRATED MORE QUESTION-ASKING BEHAVIOR IN SPANISH BUT MORE DIRECTION-GIVING BEHAVIOR IN ENGLISH. ON THE BASIS OF THESE AND A NUMBER OF OTHER DIFFERENCES, IT IS RECOMMENDED THAT SCHOOL ADMINISTRATORS CONSIDER THE EFFECT UPON STUDENTS OF AN ASSISTANT TEACHER WHOSE INTERACTION PATTERN DIFFERS FROM THAT OF THE TEACHER. SECONDLY, IT APPEARS THAT SPECIFIC INTERACTION PATTERNS MAY BE FOUND WHICH ARE MORE EFFECTIVE IN ONE LANGUAGE THAN ANOTHER, AND THEREFORE FURTHER INVESTIGATIONS OF BILINGUAL EDUCATION ARE RECOMMENDED. 15 REFERENCES.

ACCN   001582

1834 AUTH   **TRAUTMAN, E. C.**

TITL   THE SUICIDAL FIT: A PSYCHOBIOLOGIC STUDY ON PUERTO RICAN IMMIGRANTS.

SRCE   *ARCHIVES OF GENERAL PSYCHIATRY, 1961, 5(1), 76-83.*

INDX   SUICIDE, ANXIETY, DEPRESSION, PUERTO RICAN-M, EAST, SEX COMPARISON, EMPIRICAL, NEW YORK

ABST   A CLINICAL AND PSYCHOLOGICAL STUDY ON THE SUICIDAL ATTEMPTS OF 93 PUERTO RICAN IMMIGRANTS—76 FEMALES AND 17 MALES—WHO WERE ADMITTED TO LINCOLN HOSPITAL IN NEW YORK CITY BETWEEN JUNE, 1957 AND DECEMBER, 1958 IS PRESENTED. THE BASIC EMOTIONAL ILLNESS, THE DEVELOPMENT OF THE SUICIDAL ATMOSPHERE, THE CONTRIBUTING AND PRECIPITATING CAUSES, AND THE BREAKDOWN OF THE ANTISUICIDAL BARRIER ARE DISCUSSED. ALSO, IT IS POINTED OUT THAT THERE IS A CORRELATION BETWEEN THE SUICIDAL FIT AND SEX, AGE, AND THE MENSES. THE RESULTS PROVIDE A FRAMEWORK FOR INVESTIGATING OTHER TYPES OF SUICIDE ATTEMPTS IN DIFFERENT DIAGNOSTIC CATEGORIES, SUCH AS ACUTE OR CHRONIC DEPRESSION, DELUSIONAL PSYCHOSIS, OR DELIRIOUS PANIC. IN EACH CASE THERE WAS AN EMOTIONAL TRAUMA, MOUNTING INNER TENSION AND STIMULATION, AND FINALLY THE SUICIDAL FIT, CHARACTERIZED BY A TRANCE-LIKE BEHAVIOR IN WHICH THERE WAS NO FEAR OF DEATH. THE QUICK IMPULSIVE WAY THAT THE AUTOMATIC FLIGHT REACTION FOLLOWED THE COLLAPSE OF LIFE-PERSERVING CONTROLLED BEHAVIOR (THE ANTISUICIDAL BARRIER) SUGGESTS THAT AN INCREASING STIMULATION OF THE DIENCEPHALON HAD ALREADY BEGUN BEFORE THE CRISIS WAS

REACHED, TRIGGERING THE FINAL BREAK-THROUGH OF THE AUTOMATIC REACTIONS. THE ACTION SPECIFICITY OF THE SUICIDE EPISODE CAN BE RELATED, THEN, TO THE DEPTH OF THE BREAK IN THE ANTISUICIDAL BARRIER. 12 REFERENCES.

ACCN   001583

1835 AUTH   **TRAUTMAN, E. C.**
TITL   SUICIDE ATTEMPTS OF PUERTO RICAN IMMIGRANTS.
SRCE   *PSYCHIATRIC QUARTERLY, 1961, 35(4), 544-554.*
INDX   SUICIDE, IMMIGRATION, EMPIRICAL, PSYCHOPATHOLOGY, PUERTO RICAN-M, STRESS, ANXIETY, ANOMIE, DEPRESSION
ABST   THE EMOTIONAL DISTURBANCE OF PUERTO RICAN IMMIGRANTS TO NEW YORK CITY WHO ATTEMPTED SUICIDE IS STUDIED AND THE RELATIONSHIP TO THE IMMIGRATION SITUATION IS EVALUATED. NINETY-THREE PUERTO RICAN ATTEMPTED SUICIDE CASES REVEAL THAT THE INTERRUPTION AND SUBSEQUENT DISTURBANCE OF THE INDIVIDUAL'S SOCIAL AND CULTURAL STABILITY THROUGH IMMIGRATION CAUSES PERSONALITY CONFLICTS AND EMOTIONAL ILLNESS, OUT OF WHICH AN ATMOSPHERE CONDUCIVE TO SUICIDE CAN DEVELOP. TWO PHASES OF THE IMMIGRATION SITUATION CAN BE SPECIFIED. THE FIRST IS THE SUDDEN DISRUPTION OF THE FAMILIAR LIFE SITUATION AND THE SOCIAL DISLOCATION THAT CAUSE A "HANGOVER DEPRESSION" AFTER EMIGRATION. THE SECOND IS THE TRANSITION PERIOD OF ADAPTING; THE CHANGE OF SOCIAL CONCEPTS AND CULTURAL VALUES CAUSES CONFLICTS AND DISINTEGRATION OF THE FAMILY, LEADING TO UNHAPPINESS AND TENSION WITH TRENDS TOWARD SUICIDE. THE TYPICAL FORM OF SUICIDE ATTEMPT IN ALL CASES IS THE "SUICIDAL FIT," WHICH IS A CONVERSION REACTION OF A NONPSYCHOTIC INDIVIDUAL IN AN ACUTE EMOTIONAL STATE. 10 REFERENCES.
ACCN   001584

1836 AUTH   **TREPPER, T. S., & ROBERTSON, D. J.**
TITL   THE EFFECTS OF I.T.A. ON THE READING ACHIEVEMENT OF MEXICAN-AMERICAN CHILDREN: A FOLLOW-UP.
SRCE   *READING IMPROVEMENT, 1975, 12(3), 177-183.*
INDX   CHILDREN, READING, INSTRUCTIONAL TECHNIQUES, EMPIRICAL, CALIFORNIA, SOUTHWEST, MEXICAN AMERICAN, BILINGUAL, PROGRAM EVALUATION, ATTITUDES, MATHEMATICS, URBAN, LEARNING
ABST   IN EAST LOS ANGELES, 37 MEXICAN AMERICAN BILINGUAL FIFTH-GRADE CHILDREN WERE RETESTED IN READING, MATH, AND ATTITUDES TOWARD SCHOOL TO SEE IF PREVIOUSLY REPORTED GAINS RELATED TO THE USE OF THE INITIAL TEACHING ALPHABET (ITA) OVER TRADITIONAL ORTHOGRAPHY (TO) HAD BEEN SUSTAINED. ANOTHER 255 SECOND-, THIRD-, AND FIFTH-GRADE CHILDREN WERE TESTED TO COMPARE THE EFFECTIVENESS OF 'ITA' AND 'TO'. RESULTS FOR THE RETEST GROUP INDICATED NO SIGNIFICANT DIFFERENCES BETWEEN 'ITA' AND 'TO'; HOWEVER, SIGNIFICANT

DIFFERENCES WERE FOUND BETWEEN THE 'ITA' AND THE 'TO' GROUPS FOR THE OTHERS. IT IS CONCLUDED THAT 'ITA' CAN BE AN EFFECTIVE TOOL IN THE TEACHING OF READING (AND POSSIBLY ALSO IN THE AREAS OF MATH AND ATTITUDES TOWARD SCHOOL) AMONG MEXICAN AMERICAN BILINGUAL CHILDREN. 10 REFERENCES. (NCMHI ABSTRACT MODIFIED)

ACCN   002235

1837 AUTH   **TREVINO, A. L., & LOPEZ, S.**
TITL   PROFESSIONAL HISPANIC PERSONNEL: AN ANNOTATED BIBLIOGRAPHY.
SRCE   *IN E. L. OLMEDO & S. LOPEZ (EDS.), HISPANIC MENTAL HEALTH PROFESSIONALS (MONOGRAPH NO. 5). LOS ANGELES: UNIVERSITY OF CALIFORNIA, SPANISH SPEAKING MENTAL HEALTH RESEARCH CENTER, 1977, PP. 85-98.*
INDX   BIBLIOGRAPHY, PROFESSIONAL TRAINING, REPRESENTATION, HIGHER EDUCATION, EDUCATION, EMPLOYMENT, MENTAL HEALTH PROFESSION, DISCRIMINATION, MEDICAL STUDENTS, CURRICULUM
ABST   FIFTY-THREE BOOKS AND JOURNAL ARTICLES ARE CITED, DATING FROM 1967 TO 1977, EACH PERTAINING TO THE DEGREE OF HISPANIC REPRESENTATION IN THE VARIOUS PROFESSIONS RELATED TO MENTAL HEALTH. AN INDICATIVE ABSTRACT, ROUGHLY 100 WORDS IN LENGTH, FOLLOWS EACH TITLE. SUBJECTS INCLUDE THE RELATIVE FREQUENCY OF SPANISH-SURNAME AMERICANS IN (1) PROFESSIONAL ASSOCIATIONS, (2) PH.D. AND OTHER GRADUATE STUDENT TRAINING PROGRAMS, (3) COLLEGE FACULTIES, AND (4) JOBS IN PRIVATE INDUSTRIES. THE MENTAL HEALTH FIELDS ENCOMPASSED WITHIN THIS BIBLIOGRAPHY ARE NURSING, SOCIAL WORK, SOCIOLOGY, PSYCHOLOGY, PSYCHIATRY, AND MEDICAL SCHOOLS.
ACCN   001585

1838 AUTH   **TREVINO, B. G.**
TITL   BILINGUAL INSTRUCTION IN THE PRIMARY GRADES.
SRCE   *MODERN LANGUAGE JOURNAL, 1970, 54(4), 255-256.*
INDX   BILINGUAL-BICULTURAL EDUCATION, MEXICAN AMERICAN, CHILDREN, SCHOLASTIC ACHIEVEMENT, CALIFORNIA ACHIEVEMENT TESTS, EMPIRICAL, TEXAS, SOUTHWEST
ABST   A PROGRAM IS DISCUSSED WHICH ATTEMPTED IN A TEXAS ELEMENTARY SCHOOL TO COMPENSATE FOR POOR SCHOLASTIC ACHIEVEMENT OF MEXICAN AMERICAN CHILDREN BY USING BILINGUAL INSTRUCTION FOR ALL STUDENTS IN THE THREE PRIMARY GRADES. THE PROJECT ENCOURAGED A SELF-HELP PROGRAM ON THE PART OF THE STUDENTS. RAW ARITHMETIC SCORES ON THE CALIFORNIA ACHIEVEMENT TEST FOR CHILDREN COMPLETING 3 YEARS OF BILINGUAL INSTRUCTION WERE CONVERTED INTO GRADE PLACEMENT EQUIVALENTS. RESULTS SHOW THAT ONLY ONE SPANISH-SPEAKING CHILD FELL BELOW THE NATIONAL NORM IN BASIC ARITHMETIC. IT IS SUGGESTED THAT THE SOLUTION TO LOW ACHIEVEMENT FOR SPANISH-

SPEAKING CHILDREN MAY BE FOUND THROUGH THE USE OF SPANISH IN THE PRIMARY GRADES. IT IS ALSO PROPOSED THAT A SECOND LANGUAGE MAY BE TAUGHT IN THE PRIMARY GRADES WITHOUT HAMPERING THE NORMAL ACHIEVEMENT OF ANY CHILD.

ACCN   001586

1839 AUTH   **TREVINO, F. M., & BRUHN, J. G.**
TITL   INCIDENCE OF MENTAL ILLNESS IN A MEXICAN-AMERICAN COMMUNITY.
SRCE   *PSYCHIATRIC ANNALS, 1977, 7(12), 33-51.*
INDX   MENTAL HEALTH, PSYCHOPATHOLOGY, MEXICAN AMERICAN, TEXAS, SOUTHWEST, SES, SEX COMPARISON, URBAN, RESOURCE UTILIZATION, EMPIRICAL, HEALTH DELIVERY SYSTEMS, SYMPTOMATOLOGY
ABST   TO ASSESS THE NEED FOR THERAPEUTIC AND PREVENTIVE PROGRAMS, THE SOCIAL AND GEOGRAPHIC CHARACTERISTICS OF 276 MEXICAN AMERICAN OUTPATIENTS AT A TEXAS COMMUNITY MENTAL HEALTH CENTER WERE ANALYZED. ETHNICITY, MARITAL STATUS, EDUCATION, SEX, AND AGE WERE CORRELATED WITH DIAGNOSTIC CATEGORIES AND CENSUS TRACTS. THE PATIENTS WERE MOST LIKELY TO BE SINGLE, UNEMPLOYED, RESIDING IN THE LESS AFFLUENT AREAS OF THE CITY, AND HAVING ONLY AN EIGHTH GRADE OR LESS EDUCATION. MOST MALE PATIENTS WERE DIAGNOSED AS EITHER SCHIZOPHRENIC, HAVING ALCOHOL OR DRUG PROBLEMS, OR TRANSIENT SITUATIONAL BEHAVIOR DISORDERS. MOST FEMALES WERE DIAGNOSED AS NEUROTIC. IT IS CONCLUDED THAT CULTURAL AND ECONOMIC FACTORS ENCOURAGE MEXICAN AMERICANS TO UTILIZE HEALTH CARE SYSTEMS SELECTIVELY. EXCEPT FOR PSYCHOSES, MOST OF THE PATIENTS HAD DIAGNOSES INDICATING PERSONAL, INTERPERSONAL, OR CULTURAL ADJUSTMENT DIFFICULTIES, AND IT IS HYPOTHESIZED THAT IT IS THESE PEOPLE WHO EITHER CHOOSE OR ARE FORCED TO SEEK HELP FROM OUTSIDE THE MEXICAN AMERICAN CULTURE. 16 REFERENCES.
ACCN   002236

1840 AUTH   **TROTTER, R. T., & CHAVIRA, J. A. (EDS.)**
TITL   EL USO DE ALCOHOL: A RESOURCE BOOK FOR SPANISH SPEAKING COMMUNITIES.
SRCE   *ATLANTA, GA.: SOUTHERN AREA ALCOHOL EDUCATION AND TRAINING PROGRAM, INC., 1977.*
INDX   BIBLIOGRAPHY, ALCOHOLISM, SPANISH SURNAMED, MEXICAN AMERICAN, PUERTO RICAN-M, PRIMARY PREVENTION, BOOK
ABST   DESIGNED AS A RESOURCE FOR INDIVIDUALS DOING ALCOHOL EDUCATION, PREVENTION, TREATMENT, OR RESEARCH IN U.S. SPANISH-SPEAKING COMMUNITIES, THIS BOOK DOCUMENTS AND ANALYZES PUBLISHED AND UNPUBLISHED WORKS ON ALCOHOL USE AND ABUSE IN SUCH COMMUNITIES. IT ALSO DOCUMENTS A CRITICAL NEED FOR ADDITIONAL RESEARCH, ADDITIONAL MODELS FOR PREVENTION AND TREATMENT, AND ADDITIONAL NATIONAL, REGIONAL, AND LOCAL CONCERN FOR ALCOHOL RELATED PROBLEMS IN SPANISH-SPEAKING COMMUNITIES. THE CHAPTERS HAVE BEEN DIVIDED INTO AREAS THAT ARE INTENDED TO MAKE IT A USEFUL RESOURCE DOCUMENT. CHAPTER II (THE FIRST SEGMENT OF THE CRITICAL ANNOTATED BIBLIOGRAPHY) IS DIVIDED INTO A SECTION COVERING GENERAL CROSS CULTURAL RESEARCH ON ALCOHOL USE AND ABUSE AND A SECTION SPECIFICALLY DEALING WITH LATIN AMERICAN RESEARCH. CHAPTER III (THE SECOND SECTION OF THE ANNOTATED BIBLIOGRAPHY) CONTAINS ARTICLES ON MEXICAN AMERICAN COMMUNITIES, PUERTO RICAN COMMUNITIES, AND OTHER SPANISH-SPEAKING COMMUNITIES IN THE UNITED STATES. CHAPTER IV IS A REVIEW OF AVAILABLE PREVENTION AND EDUCATION RESOURCES. CHAPTER V IS A COLLECTION OF ORIGINAL ARTICLES WRITTEN IN RESPONSE TO A GENERAL INVITATION TO MAKE UNPUBLISHED MATERIALS AVAILABLE TO THE AUTHORS FOR POSSIBLE INCLUSION IN THE MONOGRAPH. FINALLY, CHAPTER VI OFFERS A BRIEF SUMMARY OF FINDINGS AND RECOMMENDATIONS. 82 REFERENCES.
ACCN   002237

1841 AUTH   **TRUEX, G. F.**
TITL   MEASUREMENT OF INTERSUBJECT VARIATIONS IN CATEGORIZATIONS.
SRCE   *JOURNAL OF CROSS-CULTURAL PSYCHOLOGY, 1977, 8(1), 71-82.*
INDX   MEXICAN, BILINGUAL, LANGUAGE ASSESSMENT, LINGUISTICS, EMPIRICAL, ADULTS, MALE
ABST   VARIATIONS IN SORTS OF 13 RURAL MEXICAN SPANISH "HAVE" VERBS WERE ANALYZED USING TWO APPROACHES TO MEASURING INTERSUBJECT VARIATIONS: (1) MEASUREMENT OF SUBJECT DIFFERENCES FROM A STANDARD CATEGORIZATION; AND (2) DIRECT COMPARISON OF PAIRS OF INDIVIDUAL SUBJECT'S SORTS. TWENTY-FOUR LITERATE ADULT MALES, BILINGUAL IN SPANISH AND ZAPOTEC, PARTICIPATED IN THE RESEARCH. THE DIRECT COMPARISON OF PAIRS REVEALED A CONSISTENT STRUCTURE FOR A SUBSET OF THE SUBJECTS NOT REVEALED BY THE FIRST APPROACH. COMPARISON OF SUBJECT'S SORTS TO THE EMPIRICALLY DERIVED MODELS OF THE VERBS INDICATES THAT A SUBSET OF THE SUBJECTS HAVE SORTS ISOMORPHIC TO THE EMPIRICAL MODEL AT THE FIRST CUT LEVEL AND MUCH CLOSER TO THE EMPIRICAL MODEL AT THE SECOND CUT LEVEL. THUS, THE EMPIRICAL MODEL APPEARS TO REFLECT AGREEMENT FOR SOME SUBJECTS ABOUT THE STRUCTURAL RELATIONS AMONG THE VERBS. 10 REFERENCES. (JOURNAL ABSTRACT MODIFIED)
ACCN   002238

1842 AUTH   **TRUJILLO, C.**
TITL   COMPARATIVE USE OF MENTAL HEALTH RESOURCES BY MEXICAN AMERICANS AND ANGLO AMERICANS.
SRCE   *UNPUBLISHED MANUSCRIPT, DEPARTMENT OF*

PSYCHOLOGY, UNIVERSITY OF CALIFORNIA, LOS ANGELES, 1977.

INDX   MEXICAN AMERICAN, MENTAL HEALTH, HEALTH DELIVERY SYSTEMS, RESOURCE UTILIZATION, EMPIRICAL, SES, PSYCHOPATHOLOGY, STRESS, POVERTY, CROSS CULTURAL, COPING MECHANISMS, SURVEY, CALIFORNIA, SOUTHWEST

ABST   THIS STUDY OF MEXICAN AMERICAN UNDERUTILIZATION OF MENTAL HEALTH FACILITIES ASKS TWO CENTRAL QUESTIONS: (1) DO ANGLOS AND MEXICAN AMERICANS OF SIMILAR SES, NOW DISTINGUISHED ONLY BY DISTINCTIVE CULTURES, RESPOND DIFFERENTLY TO EMOTIONAL PROBLEMS?; AND (2) DO THE TWO GROUPS DIFFER IN THEIR RECOMMENDED SOURCES OF HELP TO PROBLEMS OF ANXIETY, DEPRESSION, ATTEMPTED SUICIDE, BEWITCHMENT, ALCOHOLISM, AND DRUG ADDICTION? THREE SOUTHERN CALIFORNIA TOWNS WERE RANDOMLY SAMPLED AND A TOTAL OF 666 MEXICAN AMERICANS AND 340 ANGLO AMERICANS WERE INTERVIEWED. RESULTS SHOWED THAT LOW SES MEMBERS OF BOTH ETHNIC GROUPS DID NOT MAKE MORE USE OF MENTAL HEALTH RESOURCES THAN MIDDLE AND HIGH GROUPS. IN FACT, WHEN SES IS CONTROLLED AND BOTH ETHNIC SAMPLES ARE COMPARED, THERE ARE MANY SIMILARITIES IN UTILIZATION AND REFERRAL PATTERNS. THE MAJOR DISCREPANCY THAT ARISES IS THE LOWER USE OF PSYCHOLOGISTS BY MEXICAN AMERICANS. THIS CAN BE ACCOUNTED FOR BY LINGUISTIC PROBLEMS, CULTURE-CLASS DIFFERENCES THAT RETARD COMMUNICATION, AND DISCOURAGING INSTITUTIONAL POLICIES. NO MAJOR DIFFERENCES ABOUT PERCEPTIONS OF MENTAL ILLNESS WERE FOUND BETWEEN THE TWO GROUPS. HOWEVER, FURTHER INVESTIGATION IS RECOMMENDED INTO THE AREAS OF MEXICAN AMERICANS' PERCEPTIONS AND ATTITUDES TOWARD MENTAL ILLNESS, THEIR RELIANCE ON FRIENDS AND RELATIVES IN TIMES OF CRISIS, SOURCES OF MENTAL STRESS, LEVELS OF ACCULTURATION, PATTERNS OF ASSESSMENT OF NEEDS, AND EVALUATIONS OF SATISFACTION WITH VARIOUS RESOURCES. 19 REFERENCES.

ACCN   001587

1843 AUTH   **TRUJILLO, R. G., & STEVENSON, R. M.**

TITL   THIRD WORLD STUDENTS AND COUNSELING: A SELECTED BIBLIOGRAPHY.

SRCE   *SANTA BARBARA: UNIVERSITY OF CALIFORNIA, UNIVERSITY LIBRARY, 1978.*

INDX   BIBLIOGRAPHY, MEXICAN AMERICAN, PUERTO RICAN-M, SPANISH SURNAMED, CROSS CULTURAL, EDUCATIONAL COUNSELING, SOCIAL SERVICES, CARIBBEAN

ABST   A BIBLIOGRAPHY FOCUSING ON COUNSELING MINORITY GROUPS WAS COMPLETED TO MEET THE INCREASING DEMAND FOR BIBLIOGRAPHIC TOOLS DEALING WITH ETHNIC STUDIES AND SERVICES. THE FOCUS IS ON COUNSELING IN EDUCATIONAL SETTINGS, BUT SOME WORKS DISCUSS COUNSELING IN A COMMUNITY SETTING. THE LITERATURE SEARCH WAS LIMITED TO THE PERIOD FROM 1965 TO DECEMBER OF 1977. THE BIBLIOGRAPHY IS DI-

VIDED INTO FIVE MAIN SECTIONS: (1) WORKS DEALING WITH COUNSELING THE CHICANO AND OTHER SPANISH-SPEAKING GROUPS (42 CITATIONS); (2) AMERICAN INDIANS (20 CITATIONS); (3) BLACKS (128 CITATIONS); (4) ASIAN AMERICANS (7 CITATIONS); AND (5) GENERAL WRITINGS DISCUSSING COUNSELING OF MINORITIES (175 CITATIONS). TWO CITATIONS RELATE TO ALASKANS AND HAITIANS. EACH SECTION IS ARRANGED ALPHABETICALLY BY AUTHOR.

ACCN   002239

1844 AUTH   **TUDDENHAM, R. D., BROOKS, J., & MILKOVICH, L.**

TITL   MOTHERS' REPORTS OF BEHAVIOR OF TEN-YEAR-OLDS: RELATIONSHIPS WITH SEX, ETHNICITY AND MOTHERS' EDUCATION.

SRCE   *DEVELOPMENTAL PSYCHOLOGY, 1974, 10(6), 959-995.*

INDX   MOTHER-CHILD INTERACTION, SEX ROLES, MEXICAN AMERICAN, EDUCATION, FAMILY STRUCTURE, ETHNIC IDENTITY, CROSS CULTURAL, CHILDREN, URBAN, TEST RELIABILITY, PERSONALITY, PERFORMANCE EXPECTATIONS

ABST   MOTHERS' DESCRIPTIONS OF THEIR 9 YEAR-OLD, 10 YEAR-OLD, AND 11 YEAR-OLD CHILDREN WERE SECURED BY MEANS OF A BEHAVIOR INVENTORY OF 100 ITEMS, TO BE SORTED INTO "TRUE," "NOT TRUE," AND "UNCERTAIN" CATEGORIES. FINDINGS ARE REPORTED FOR 2212 WHITES, 641 BLACKS, 117 ORIENTALS, AND 79 CHICANOS FROM AN URBAN, LARGELY MIDDLE-CLASS SAMPLE, BROKEN DOWN BY ETHNICITY, SEX OF CHILD, AND IN THE CASE OF WHITES AND BLACKS, BY EDUCATION OF THE MOTHER. COMPARISONS WITH SEVEN OTHER STUDIES, BOTH AMERICAN AND BRITISH, SHOW NOTEWORTHY AGREEMENT IN PROBLEM PREVALENCE, DESPITE MAJOR DIFFERENCES IN SAMPLES AND IN METHODS OF INVESTIGATION. 16 REFERENCES. (JOURNAL ABSTRACT)

ACCN   001588

1845 AUTH   **TURNER, P. R.**

TITL   ACADEMIC PERFORMANCE OF MEXICAN AMERICANS.

SRCE   *INTEGRATED EDUCATION, 1973, 11(3), 3-6.*

INDX   SCHOLASTIC ACHIEVEMENT, PERFORMANCE EXPECTATIONS, MEXICAN AMERICAN, SES, BILINGUALISM, EDUCATIONAL ASSESSMENT, TEACHERS, ATTITUDES, EMPIRICAL, ARIZONA, SOUTHWEST

ABST   A COGNITIVE ANTHROPOLOGICAL APPROACH WAS EMPLOYED TO DISCOVER DIFFERENCES BETWEEN ACADEMICALLY SUCCESSFUL MEXICAN AMERICAN (MA) HIGH SCHOOL STUDENTS WHO MIGHT GO ON TO COLLEGE AND UNSUCCESSFUL STUDENTS WHO PROBABLY WOULD NOT. SIX MA STUDENTS (3 SUCCESSFUL AND 3 UNSUCCESSFUL) IN ONE ARIZONA HIGH SCHOOL CLASS WERE INTERVIEWED IN-DEPTH, AS WERE THEIR PARENTS AND THEIR TEACHER. IT WAS FOUND THAT THE COGNITIVE MAPPING OF THE SCHOOL SITUATION DIFFERED SOMEWHAT BETWEEN THE STUDENTS, PARENTS, AND TEACHER; HOWEVER, VERY

FEW COGNITIVE DIFFERENCES WERE FOUND BETWEEN THE SUCCESSFUL AND UNSUCCESSFUL STUDENTS NOR BETWEEN THEIR RESPECTIVE PARENTS. IN ACCOUNTING FOR THIS LACK OF A DIFFERENCE IT WAS DISCOVERED THAT THE TEACHER WAS CONSISTENTLY ADJUSTING THE STUDENTS' GRADES UPWARDS TO ENCOURAGE THEM AND ALSO TO FIT IN WITH THE PATTERN OF GRADING PREVALENT AT THE SCHOOL. THE TEACHER WAS AWARE THAT THE STUDENTS WERE NOT DOING AS WELL AS THEIR GRADES INDICATED, BUT THE STUDENTS AND THEIR PARENTS WERE NOT AWARE OF THIS. IT IS SUGGESTED THAT MA PARENTS INSIST UPON FINDING OUT HOW THEIR CHILDREN'S ACHIEVEMENT COMPARES TO CITY-WIDE AND NATIONAL ACADEMIC STANDARDS, AND ALSO THAT AN INTEGRATED SCHOOL SYSTEM WOULD BETTER PREPARE MA STUDENTS TO COMPETE WITHIN AMERICAN SOCIETY. 2 REFERENCES.

ACCN   001589

1846 AUTH   **TURNER, R. G., & HORN, J. M.**
TITL   PERSONALITY CORRELATES OF HOLLAND'S OCCUPATIONAL TYPES: A CROSS CULTURAL STUDY.
SRCE   *JOURNAL OF VOCATIONAL BEHAVIOR, 1975, 6(3), 379-389.*
INDX   BILINGUAL, COLLEGE STUDENTS, EMPIRICAL, FEMALE, PERSONALITY ASSESSMENT, SPANISH SURNAMED, TEXAS, SOUTHWEST, MALE, MEXICAN AMERICAN
ABST   HOLLAND'S THEORY OF VOCATIONAL CHOICE POSITS THAT MOST PERSONS IN OUR CULTURE CAN BE CATEGORIZED AS ONE OF 6 PERSONALITY TYPES: REALISTIC; INVESTIGATIVE; ARTISTIC; SOCIAL; ENTERPRISING; OR CONVENTIONAL. THESE PERSONALITY TYPES, MOREOVER, ARE VERIFIABLE BY PERSONS' VOCATIONAL INTERESTS. IN THE PRESENT STUDY THIS THESIS WAS INVESTIGATED IN A GROUP OF 402 MEXICAN AMERICAN STUDENTS (234 MALES, 168 FEMALES) ENROLLED IN A DEVELOPMENTAL STUDIES PSYCHOLOGY CLASS AT SAN ANTONIO COLLEGE DURING 1970-1972. ETHNIC IDENTIFICATION WAS BASED UPON SUBJECTS HAVING A SPANISH SURNAME OR STATING ON AN ORIENTATION QUESTIONNAIRE THAT SPANISH WAS THE LANGUAGE PREDOMINATELY SPOKEN AT HOME. OCCUPATIONAL SCALE SCORES ON THE KUDER OCCUPATIONAL INTEREST SURVEY WERE USED TO CLASSIFY SUBJECTS INTO HOLLAND'S OCCUPATIONAL TYPES. MULTIPLE DISCRIMINANT ANALYSIS OF GROUPS' GUILFORD-ZIMMERMAN TEMPERAMENT SURVEY SCALE SCORES RESULTED IN SIGNIFICANT OVERALL GROUP DIFFERENTIATION AND TWO SIGNIFICANT DISCRIMINANT FUNCTIONS FOR MALES, BUT NO SIGNIFICANT RESULTS FOR FEMALES. ALTHOUGH THE PERSONALITY CHARACTERISTICS OF THE MALE GROUPS PROVIDE STRONG SUPPORT FOR THE GENERALIZABILITY OF HOLLAND'S CHARACTERIZATION TO MEXICAN AMERICAN MALES, THE SAME CAN NOT BE SAID FOR THE WOMEN. THE GENERALIZABILITY OF HOLLAND'S GROUP CHARACTERIZA-

TIONS TO WOMEN IN GENERAL—AND TO MEXICAN AMERICAN WOMEN IN PARTICULAR—REMAINS A MATTER FOR FUTURE INVESTIGATION. 13 REFERENCES. (JOURNAL ABSTRACT MODIFIED)

ACCN   002240

1847 AUTH   **TURNER, R. G., & HORN, J. M.**
TITL   STANDARD PSYCHOLOGICAL TEST RESPONSES OF A GROUP OF MEXICAN-AMERICANS.
SRCE   *JAS CATALOG OF SELECTED DOCUMENTS IN PSYCHOLOGY, 1975, 4, 210.*
INDX   CULTURAL FACTORS, COLLEGE STUDENTS, MEXICAN AMERICAN, PERSONALITY ASSESSMENT, EMPIRICAL, OCCUPATIONAL ASPIRATIONS, TEXAS, SOUTHWEST
ABST   TO INVESTIGATE WHETHER MEXICAN AMERICANS SHOW DISTINCTIVE PATTERNS OF RESPONSE ON TESTS COMMONLY USED IN GUIDANCE SITUATIONS, THE RESULTS OF THE AMERICAN COLLEGE TEST, THE GUILFORD-ZIMMERMAN TEMPERAMENT SURVEY, AND THE KUDER OCCUPATIONAL INTEREST SURVEY (FORM DD) WERE ADMINISTERED TO 456 MEXICAN AMERICAN MALE AND FEMALE COLLEGE STUDENTS IN TEXAS. THE STUDENTS SIGNIFICANTLY DIFFERED FROM THE GUILFORD-ZIMMERMAN NORMATIVE GROUP ON MORE THAN HALF OF THE SCALES, SCORING LOWER IN THE MEASURES OF ACTIVITY, RESTRAINT, SOCIABILITY, EMOTIONAL STABILITY, OBJECTIVENESS, PERSONAL RELATIONS, AND MASCULINITY. DISTINCTIVE PATTERNS OF RESPONSE TO THE KUDER WERE ALSO FOUND, AS THE MEXICAN AMERICANS SCORED HIGH ONLY ON CERTAIN SCALES. THE JOB INTERESTS THE WOMEN MOST FREQUENTLY LISTED WERE DENTAL ASSISTANT, NURSE, AND STENOGRAPHER, AS WELL AS THE COLLEGE MAJORS OF NURSING AND ELEMENTARY EDUCATION. FOR MEN, BRICKLAYER, PODIATRIST, PHYSICAL THERAPIST, AUTOMOBILE SALESMAN, AND THE COLLEGE MAJORS OF PHYSICAL AND ELEMENTARY EDUCATION WERE MOST COMMONLY LISTED. THE MOST STRIKING OMISSION OCCURRED FOR THOSE SUBSCALES DEALING WITH LAW OR POLITICAL SCIENCE. THESE DIFFERENCES SEEM MOST ATTRIBUTABLE TO ETHNIC BACKGROUND, AND THEY RAISE SERIOUS QUESTIONS ABOUT THE USE OF NORMATIVE DATA IN PROFILE INTERPRETATIONS FOR MEXICAN AMERICANS. IT IS RECOMMENDED THAT IN THE ABSENCE OF DATA INDICATING BEHAVIORAL DIFFERENCES, FURTHER VALIDATION OF PERSONALITY AND INTEREST TESTS IS NECESSARY FOR THE MEXICAN AMERICAN POPULATION. 10 REFERENCES.

ACCN   001590

1848 AUTH   **TURNER, R. G., & SURACE, S. J.**
TITL   ZOOT-SUITERS AND MEXICANS: SYMBOLS IN CROWD BEHAVIOR.
SRCE   *THE AMERICAN JOURNAL OF SOCIOLOGY, 1956, 62(1), 14-20.*
INDX   STEREOTYPES, MEXICAN AMERICAN, GROUP DYNAMICS, DISCRIMINATION, EMPIRICAL, MASS MEDIA, CALIFORNIA, SOUTHWEST

ABST   A CONTENT ANALYSIS OF 173 NEWSPAPER REFERENCES TO THE MEXICAN AMERICAN COMMUNITY OVER A TEN YEAR PERIOD PRIOR TO THE LOS ANGELES "ZOOT-SUIT RIOTS" OF 1943 WAS CONDUCTED TO TEST THE FOLLOWING HYPOTHESIS: OVERT HOSTILE CROWD BEHAVIOR IS USUALLY PRECEDED BY A PERIOD IN WHICH KEY SOCIAL SYMBOLS ARE STRIPPED OF FAVORABLE CONNOTATIONS AND INSTEAD BECOME UNAMBIGUOUSLY UNFAVORABLE. THE NEWSPAPER STORIES WERE ANALYZED IN TERMS OF FIVE TYPES OF PORTRAYAL OF MEXICAN AMERICANS: (1) FAVORABLE DEPICTIONS; (2) UNFAVORABLE; (3) NEUTRAL; (4) "NEGATIVE-FAVORABLE," DENYING ACCUSATIONS AGAINST MEXICAN AMERICANS; AND (5) THE "ZOOTER" THEME, IDENTIFIED WITH CRIME AND SEXUAL VIOLENCE. ALTHOUGH NO APPRECIABLE DECLINE IN THE PERCENTAGE OF FAVORABLE THEMES WAS FOUND OVERALL, THE THREE YEAR PERIOD PRIOR TO THE RIOTS SHOWED A 60% DECLINE IN TRADITIONAL REFERENCES AND A MARKED EMERGENCE OF THE "ZOOTER" THEME. DURING THE 30 DAYS IMMEDIATELY SURROUNDING THE RIOTS, TRADITIONAL THEMES DISAPPEARED COMPLETELY AND 74% OF ALL REFERENCES CENTERED AROUND THE "ZOOTER" THEME. THUS, TRADITIONAL AMBIVALENCE TOWARDS THE SYMBOL "MEXICAN" WAS REPLACED BY THE CLEARLY UNFAVORABLE CONNOTATIONS OF A NEW SYMBOL WHICH SANCTIONED OVERT CROWD HOSTILITY. 10 REFERENCES.

ACCN   001591

1849 AUTH   **U.S. BUREAU OF THE CENSUS.**

TITL   CENSUS OF POPULATION: 1970. PERSONS OF SPANISH ORIGIN (FINAL REPORT PC(2)-1C).

SRCE   *WASHINGTON, D.C.: U.S. GOVERNMENT PRINTING OFFICE, 1973.*

INDX   SPANISH SURNAMED, CENSUS, SEX COMPARISON, HOUSING, RURAL, URBAN, MARRIAGE, SCHOLASTIC ACHIEVEMENT, POVERTY, SES, BILINGUALISM, EMPIRICAL, DEMOGRAPHIC

ABST   A STATISTICAL REPORT BASED ON DATA FROM THE 1970 U.S. CENSUS OF POPULATION PRESENTS DEMOGRAPHIC DATA FOR PERSONS OF SPANISH ORIGIN, CROSS-CLASSIFIED BY VARIOUS SOCIAL AND ECONOMIC CHARACTERISTICS FOR THE U.S., REGIONS, SELECTED STATES, AND STANDARD METROPOLITAN STATISTICAL AREAS (SMSA'S). MORE THAN 9 MILLION PERSONS IDENTIFIED THEMSELVES AS BEING OF MEXICAN, PUERTO RICAN, CUBAN, CENTRAL OR SOUTH AMERICAN, OR "OTHER" SPANISH ORIGIN IN THE 1970 CENSUS QUESTIONNAIRE. DATA OBTAINED FROM A 5% SAMPLE, ADJUSTED TO REPRESENT THIS TOTAL POPULATION, PROVIDE THE BASIS FOR 17 STATISTICAL TABLES. TABLE 1 PRESENTS DATA FOR THE SPANISH ORIGIN POPULATION BY TYPE OF ORIGIN, CROSS-CLASSIFIED BY SEX AND URBAN-RURAL RESIDENCE FOR THE U.S., REGIONS, DIVISIONS, AND STATES. TABLE 2 SHOWS DATA BY RACE FOR THE TOTAL SPANISH ORIGIN POPULATION, EXCLUDING URBAN-RURAL RESIDENCE. TABLES 3-12 CONTAIN DATA ON CHARACTERISTICS SUCH AS AGE, RACE, HOUSEHOLD RELATIONSHIP, MARITAL STATUS, EDUCATION, EMPLOYMENT STATUS, OCCUPATION, INCOME IN 1969, AND HOUSING. MOST OF THESE TABLES INCLUDE DATA BY URBAN-RURAL RESIDENCE FOR THE UNITED STATES AND SELECTED STATES. IN TABLES 13-17, STATISTICS ON SOCIAL, ECONOMIC, AND HOUSING CHARACTERISTICS ARE GIVEN FOR 29 SMSA'S WITH 50,000 OR MORE PERSONS OF SPANISH ORIGIN AND 31 PLACES WITH 25,000 OR MORE PERSONS OF SPANISH ORIGIN. APPENDICES A THROUGH E INCLUDE INFORMATION ON (1) GENERAL INFORMATION CONCERNING THE DATA, (2) AREA CLASSIFICATIONS, (3) DEFINITIONS AND EXPLANATIONS OF SUBJECT CHARACTERISTICS, (4) ACCURACY OF THE DATA, AND (5) PUBLICATION AND COMPUTER SUMMARY TAPE PROGRAMS. MAPS INCLUDED SHOW STANDARD METROPOLITAN STATISTICAL AREAS OF THE U.S. IN 1970 AND REGIONS AND GEOGRAPHIC DIVISIONS OF THE U.S.

ACCN   001592

1850 AUTH   **U.S. BUREAU OF THE CENSUS.**

TITL   CENSUS OF POPULATION: 1970. PERSONS OF SPANISH SURNAME (FINAL REPORT PC(2)-1D).

SRCE   *WASHINGTON, D.C.: U.S. GOVERNMENT PRINTING OFFICE, 1973.*

INDX   SPANISH SURNAMED, CENSUS, SEX COMPARISON, HOUSING, RURAL, URBAN, MARRIAGE, SCHOLASTIC ASPIRATIONS, POVERTY, SES, EMPIRICAL, DEMOGRAPHIC, SOUTHWEST

ABST   A STATISTICAL REPORT BASED UPON DATA FROM THE 1970 U.S. CENSUS OF POPULATION PRESENTS DEMOGRAPHIC DATA ON THE APPROXIMATELY 4.7 MILLION PERSONS WITH SPANISH-SURNAMES IDENTIFIED IN THE FIVE SOUTHWESTERN STATES (ARIZONA, CALIFORNIA, COLORADO, NEW MEXICO, AND TEXAS). DATA OBTAINED FROM A 5% SAMPLE, ADJUSTED TO REPRESENT THIS TOTAL POPULATION, PROVIDE THE BASIS FOR 19 STATISTICAL TABLES. TABLES 1 AND 2 PRESENT DATA ON THE RACE, NATIVITY, PARENTAGE, AND COUNTRY OF ORIGIN OF PERSONS OF SPANISH-SURNAME BY SEX AND URBAN-RURAL RESIDENCE FOR U.S. REGIONS AND STATES. TABLES 3 AND 4 PROVIDE A BREAKDOWN ON MOTHER-TONGUE OF SPANISH-SURNAME PERSONS BY NATIVITY, PARENTAGE, COUNTRY OF ORIGIN, MARITAL STATUS, AND SEX. TABLES 6-18 CONTAIN DATA ON SUCH CHARACTERISTICS AS AGE, HOUSEHOLD RELATIONSHIP, MARITAL STATUS, EDUCATION, EMPLOYMENT STATUS, INCOME IN 1969, AND HOUSING. TABLE 19 PRESENTS DATA ON PERSONS OF SPANISH-SURNAME BY NATIVITY. APPENDICES A THROUGH E INCLUDE INFORMATION ON (1) GENERAL INFORMATION CONCERNING THE DATA, (2) AREA CLASSIFICATIONS, (3) DEFINITIONS AND EXPLANATIONS OF SUBJECT CHARACTERISTICS, (4) ACCURACY OF THE DATA, AND (5) PUBLICATION AND COMPUTER SUMMARY TAPE PROGRAMS. MAPS INCLUDED SHOW METROPOLITAN STATISTICAL AREAS OF THE U.S. IN 1970 AS WELL AS REGIONS AND GEOGRAPHIC DIVISIONS OF THE U.S.

ACCN   001593

1851 AUTH   **U.S. BUREAU OF THE CENSUS.**
     TITL   CENSUS OF THE POPULATION: 1970. LOW-IN-
            COME POPULATION (FINAL REPORT PC (2)-9A).
     SRCE   *WASHINGTON, D.C.: U.S. GOVERNMENT PRINT-
            ING OFFICE, 1973.*
     INDX   CENSUS, SPANISH SURNAMED, HOUSING, SEX
            COMPARISON, MARITAL STABILITY, MARRIAGE,
            FERTILITY, FAMILY STRUCTURE, EMPLOYMENT,
            SCHOLASTIC ACHIEVEMENT, SES, EMPIRICAL,
            DEMOGRAPHIC, ECONOMIC FACTORS, EDU-
            CATION, POVERTY, RURAL, URBAN
     ABST   A SUBJECT REPORT OF THE 1970 CENSUS OF
            POPULATION PRESENTS NATIONAL STATISTICS
            ON THE SOCIAL, ECONOMIC, AND HOUSING
            CHARACTERISTICS OF THOSE OF LOW-IN-
            COME (POVERTY) STATUS IN 1969. THE MA-
            JORITY OF THE TABLES ARE BASED ON A 5%
            SAMPLE ADJUSTED TO REPRESENT THE TOTAL
            POPULATION. 36 TABLES CONSIST OF DATA ON
            THE POVERTY STATUS OF THE POPULATION,
            CROSS-CLASSIFIED BY SUCH CHARACTERIS-
            TICS AS GEOGRAPHIC DISTRIBUTION, RACE,
            ETHNIC ORIGIN, MIGRATION, FERTILITY, SIZE
            OF FAMILY AND NUMBER OF CHILDREN, EDU-
            CATION, EMPLOYMENT STATUS, OCCUPATION,
            SOURCE OF INCOME, AMOUNT OF INCOME, IN-
            COME DEFICIT, AND SELECTED HOUSING
            CHARACTERISTICS. FOR ANALYTIC PURPOSES,
            MOST TABLES CONTAIN COMPARABLE DATA
            FOR THE TOTAL U.S. POPULATION. TWO ADDI-
            TIONAL TABLES PRESENT (1) THE COMPLETE
            MATRIX OF 1969 INCOME THRESHOLDS AT THE
            POVERTY LEVEL, AND (2) SELECTED CHARAC-
            TERISTICS OF FAMILIES AND UNRELATED INDI-
            VIDUALS WITH INCOME ALLOCATED. APPEND-
            ICES A THROUGH E CONTAIN GENERAL
            INFORMATION CONCERNING THE DATA, AREA
            CLASSIFICATIONS, DEFINITIONS AND EXPLA-
            NATIONS OF SUBJECT CHARACTERISTICS,
            QUALIFICATIONS OF ACCURACY OF THE DATA,
            AND INFORMATION ON THE PUBLICATION AND
            COMPUTER SUMMARY TAPE PROGRAM.
     ACCN   001594

1852 AUTH   **U.S. BUREAU OF THE CENSUS.**
     TITL   CHARACTERISTICS OF THE SPANISH SURNAME
            POPULATION BY CENSUS TRACT, FOR SMSA'S
            IN ARIZONA: 1970 (PC(S1)-57).
     SRCE   *WASHINGTON, D.C.: U.S. GOVERNMENT PRINT-
            ING OFFICE, 1974.*
     INDX   CENSUS, DEMOGRAPHIC, EDUCATION, EMPIR-
            ICAL, EMPLOYMENT, FAMILY STRUCTURE,
            HOUSING, SPANISH SURNAMED, SOUTHWEST,
            ARIZONA, POVERTY, SES, URBAN, MALE, FE-
            MALE
     ABST   THIS REPORT PRESENTS INFORMATION ON
            PERSONS OF SPANISH SURNAME LIVING IN
            CENSUS TRACTS OF 400 OR MORE PERSONS
            OF SPANISH SURNAME WITHIN STANDARD
            METROPOLITAN STATISTICAL AREAS (SMSA'S)
            IN THE STATE OF ARIZONA ON APRIL 1, 1970. AT
            THIS TIME, ARIZONA HAD A SPANISH SURNAME
            POPULATION OF 246,390, ABOUT 67% OF WHICH
            LIVED IN THE TWO SMSA'S IN THE STATE—
            PHOENIX AND TUCSON. THE CENSUS DATA
            ARE BASED ON A SAMPLE OF 15% OF THE

POPULATION. THIS SUPPLEMENTARY CENSUS
REPORT IS COMPRISED OF THREE MAIN TEXT
TABLES AND ONE APPENDIX TABLE. TABLE
ONE PRESENTS DATA ON AGE, SEX, RELATION-
SHIP TO HEAD OF HOUSEHOLD, TYPE OF
HOUSEHOLD, SCHOOL ENROLLMENT, YEARS
OF SCHOOL COMPLETED, AND RESIDENCE IN
1965. IN TABLE TWO, EMPLOYMENT STATUS,
FAMILY INCOME, AND POVERTY STATUS ARE
GIVEN. TABLE THREE PRESENTS HOUSING
CHARACTERISTICS FOR HOUSEHOLDS WITH A
SPANISH SURNAME HEAD. THE APPENDIX TABLE
DELINEATES PERSONS OF SPANISH SURNAME
BY RACE FOR URBAN AND RURAL RESIDENCE,
STANDARD METROPOLITAN STATISTICAL AREAS,
AND SELECTED PLACES IN ARIZONA.
     ACCN   002241

1853 AUTH   **U.S. BUREAU OF THE CENSUS.**
     TITL   CHARACTERISTICS OF THE SPANISH SURNAME
            POPULATION BY CENSUS TRACT, FOR SMSA'S
            IN NEW MEXICO: 1970 (PC(S1)-60).
     SRCE   *WASHINGTON, D.C.: U.S. GOVERNMENT PRINT-
            ING OFFICE, 1974.*
     INDX   CENSUS, DEMOGRAPHIC, EDUCATION, EMPIR-
            ICAL, EMPLOYMENT, FAMILY STRUCTURE,
            HOUSING, SPANISH SURNAMED, SOUTHWEST,
            NEW MEXICO, POVERTY, SES, URBAN, RURAL,
            MALE, FEMALE
     ABST   BASED ON A SAMPLE OF 15% OF THE POPU-
            LATION, THIS CENSUS REPORT PRESENTS IN-
            FORMATION ON PERSONS OF SPANISH SUR-
            NAME IN THE STATE OF NEW MEXICO ON APRIL
            1, 1970. AT THIS TIME, NEW MEXICO HAD A
            SPANISH SURNAME POPULATION OF 324,248
            PERSONS, OR ABOUT 32% OF THE TOTAL
            STATE POPULATION. THREE TABLES CONTAIN
            DATA ON THE SPANISH SURNAME POPULATION
            FOR THE ALBUQUERQUE SMSA (THE ONLY
            SMSA IN THE STATE), AND FOR EACH CENSUS
            TRACT WITH AT LEAST 400 PERSONS OF SPAN-
            ISH SURNAME WITHIN THE SMSA. TABLE ONE
            SHOWS DATA ON AGE, SEX, RELATIONSHIP TO
            HEAD OF HOUSEHOLD, TYPE OF HOUSEHOLD,
            SCHOOL ENROLLMENT, YEARS OF SCHOOL
            COMPLETED, AND RESIDENCE IN 1965. EM-
            PLOYMENT STATUS, FAMILY INCOME, AND POV-
            ERTY STATUS ARE GIVEN IN TABLE TWO. TABLE
            THREE PRESENTS HOUSING CHARACTERIS-
            TICS FOR HOUSEHOLDS WITH A SPANISH SUR-
            NAME HEAD. APPENDIX TABLE A PRESENTS
            RACE OF PERSONS OF SPANISH SURNAME FOR
            URBAN AND RURAL RESIDENCE, SMSA'S, AND
            SELECTED PLACES IN NEW MEXICO IN 1970.
     ACCN   002242

1854 AUTH   **U.S. BUREAU OF THE CENSUS.**
     TITL   CHARACTERISTICS OF THE SPANISH SURNAME
            POPULATION BY CENSUS TRACT, FOR SMSA'S
            IN TEXAS: 1970 (PC(S1)-61).
     SRCE   *WASHINGTON, D.C.: U.S. GOVERNMENT PRINT-
            ING OFFICE, 1974.*
     INDX   ADOLESCENTS, ADULTS, CHILDREN, CENSUS,
            DEMOGRAPHIC, ECONOMIC FACTORS, EDU-
            CATION, HOUSING, FEMALE, MALE, SES, SUR-
            VEY, SPANISH SURNAMED, EMPLOYMENT,
            TEXAS, SOUTHWEST
     ABST   THIS REPORT PRESENTS DATA ON PERSONS

OF SPANISH SURNAME LIVING IN CENSUS TRACTS OF 400 OR MORE PERSONS OF SPANISH SURNAME WITHIN SMSA'S IN THE STATE OF TEXAS ON APRIL 1, 1970—SUPPLEMENTING PREVIOUSLY PUBLISHED 1970 CENSUS REPORTS, SERIES PHC (1), IN WHICH DATA WERE PRESENTED FOR THE COMBINED GROUP, "PERSONS OF SPANISH LANGUAGE OR SPANISH SURNAME." IN THIS REPORT, TABLE 1 SHOWS DATA ON: AGE, SEX, RELATIONSHIP TO HEAD OF HOUSEHOLD, TYPE OF HOUSEHOLD, SCHOOL ENROLLMENT, YEARS OF SCHOOL COMPLETED, AND RESIDENCE IN 1965. EMPLOYMENT STATUS, FAMILY INCOME, AND POVERTY STATUS ARE GIVEN IN TABLE 2. TABLE 3 PRESENTS HOUSING CHARACTERISTICS FOR HOUSEHOLDS WITH A SPANISH SURNAME HEAD. A TABLE "RACE OF PERSONS OF SPANISH SURNAME FOR URBAN AND RURAL RESIDENCE, SELECTED STANDARD METROPOLITAN STATISTICAL AREAS, AND SELECTED PLACES, FOR TEXAS: 1970," IS APPENDED.

ACCN   002243

1855 AUTH   **U.S. BUREAU OF THE CENSUS.**
TITL   COMPARISON OF PERSONS OF SPANISH SURNAME AND PERSONS OF SPANISH ORIGIN IN THE UNITED STATES. (TECHNICAL PAPER NO. 38)
SRCE   *WASHINGTON, D.C.: U.S. GOVERNMENT PRINTING OFFICE, 1975.*
INDX   BILINGUAL, CENSUS, CENTRAL AMERICA, CUBAN, DEMOGRAPHIC, ECONOMIC FACTORS, EDUCATION, EMPIRICAL, MEXICAN AMERICAN, PUERTO RICAN-M, SES, SOUTH AMERICA, SPANISH SURNAMED, ETHNIC IDENTITY
ABST   COMPARATIVE DATA ARE PRESENTED ON THE CHARACTERISTICS OF THE SPANISH SURNAME POPULATION AND THE SPANISH ORIGIN POPULATION IN THE U.S., BASED ON THE MARCH 1971 CURRENT POPULATION SURVEY. THE PRIMARY PURPOSE OF THE REPORT IS TO ILLUSTRATE THE RELATIONSHIP BETWEEN THESE TWO IDENTIFIERS OF THE POPULATION OF SPANISH ANCESTRY AND TO DETERMINE THE EXTENT TO WHICH SPANISH SURNAME CAN BE USED AS A PROXY FOR IDENTIFYING PERSONS OF SPANISH ORIGIN. A HIGH CORRELATION WOULD ALLOW THE EXPANSION OF STATISTICAL DATA ON THE SPANISH ANCESTRY POPULATION THROUGH THE CODING OF SPANISH SURNAME IN THE EXISTING ADMINISTRATIVE AND VITAL RECORDS. PERSONS OF SPANISH ORIGIN ARE DEFINED AS THOSE PERSONS INDICATING THEIR ORIGIN AS MEXICAN, PUERTO RICAN, CUBAN, CENTRAL OR SOUTH AMERICAN, OR "OTHER SPANISH," WHILE PERSONS OF SPANISH SURNAME ARE IDENTIFIED BY MEANS OF A CODING OPERATION IN WHICH EACH SURNAME IN THE SURVEY IS COMPARED TO A LIST OF MORE THAN 8,000 SPANISH SURNAMES. THE FOLLOWING DEMOGRAPHIC AND SOCIOECONOMIC CHARACTERISTICS BY SPANISH ORIGIN AND SPANISH SURNAME ARE COMPARED: (1) AGE; (2) YEARS OF SCHOOL COMPLETED; (3) MARITAL STATUS; (4) INCOME; (5) CURRENT LANGUAGE; AND (6) SPECIFIC DEMOGRAPHIC MEASURES. IDENTIFICATION

BY SPANISH SURNAME WAS FOUND TO PROVIDE A FAIR APPROXIMATION OF THE SPANISH ORIGIN POPULATION IN THE FIVE SOUTHWESTERN STATES OF THE U.S., BUT NOT IN THE STATES OUTSIDE THIS AREA. TWENTY-SIX TABLES ILLUSTRATE CENSUS FINDINGS. 5 REFERENCES.

ACCN   002244

1856 AUTH   **U.S. BUREAU OF THE CENSUS.**
TITL   EMPLOYMENT PROFILES OF SELECTED LOW-INCOME AREAS: NEW YORK, N.Y.—PUERTO RICAN POPULATION OF SURVEY AREAS (PHC(3)-3).
SRCE   *WASHINGTON, D.C.: U.S. GOVERNMENT PRINTING OFFICE, 1972.*
INDX   ADULTS, CENSUS, DEMOGRAPHIC, ECONOMIC FACTORS, EDUCATION, EMPLOYMENT, FAMILY STRUCTURE, FERTILITY, HOUSING, JOB PERFORMANCE, LABOR FORCE, POVERTY, PUERTO RICAN-M, SES, NEW YORK, EAST, URBAN, MIGRATION, SPANISH SURNAMED, CROSS CULTURAL
ABST   FOCUSING ON PUERTO RICANS IN THE NEW YORK AREA, THIS REPORT PRESENTS STATISTICS FROM THE CENSUS EMPLOYMENT SURVEY (CES), CONDUCTED AS PART OF THE OVERALL PROGRAM OF THE 1970 CENSUS OF POPULATION AND HOUSING. DETAILED SOCIOECONOMIC INFORMATION ON EMPLOYMENT RELATED PROBLEMS FOR THIS AREA WAS COLLECTED THROUGH INTERVIEWS WITH PERSONS 16 YEARS OF AGE OR OLDER IN OVER 20,000 HOUSEHOLDS. TABLES A TO N PRESENT GENERAL DEMOGRAPHIC CHARACTERISTICS OF THE POPULATION BY THE MOST IMPORTANT LABOR FORCE AND SOCIOECONOMIC FACTORS. THESE TABLES INCLUDE DATA FOR EACH RACE AND SPANISH ORIGIN GROUP COMPRISING 5% OR MORE OF THE AREA'S POPULATION. TABLES 1 TO 18 PRESENT CURRENT LABOR FORCE AND EMPLOYMENT STATUS STATISTICS BY DEMOGRAPHIC CATEGORIES FOR THOSE RACIAL/ETHNIC GROUPS COMPRISING 20% OR MORE OF THE AREA'S POPULATION. TABLES 19 TO 31 PRESENT THE SAME DETAILED DEMOGRAPHIC CHARACTERISTICS BY THE WORK EXPERIENCE OF THE POPULATION IN THE LAST 12 MONTHS. INFORMATION ON JOB TRAINING AND WORK HISTORY OF THE POPULATION IS PRESENTED IN TABLES 32 TO 39. STATISTICS ON FAMILY INCOME AND THE MIGRATION PATTERN OF AREA RESIDENTS ARE PRESENTED IN TABLES 40 TO 54.

ACCN   002245

1857 AUTH   **U.S. BUREAU OF THE CENSUS.**
TITL   PERSONS OF SPANISH ORIGIN IN THE UNITED STATES: NOVEMBER 1969. (SERIES P-20, NO. 213).
SRCE   *WASHINGTON D.C.: U.S. GOVERNMENT PRINTING OFFICE, FEBRUARY, 1971.*
INDX   CENSUS, DEMOGRAPHIC, BILINGUALISM, EDUCATION, READING, MARRIAGE, MEXICAN AMERICAN, EMPIRICAL, SPANISH SURNAMED, PUERTO RICAN-I, EMPLOYMENT, SES
ABST   THIS STATISTICAL REPORT, BASED UPON A U.S.

CENSUS SAMPLE SURVEY OF 863 COUNTIES AND INDEPENDENT CITIES, FOCUSES ON THE SOCIAL AND ECONOMIC CHARACTERISTICS OF 9.2 MILLION PERSONS OF SPANISH ORIGIN LIVING IN THE UNITED STATES. 27 TABLES PRESENT DATA ON TYPES OF SPANISH ORIGIN, MOTHER TONGUE, LANGUAGE USUALLY SPO-KEN AT HOME, EDUCATIONAL ATTAINMENT, LIT-ERACY, EMPLOYMENT, OCCUPATIONAL LEVEL, AND INCOME. IN TABLES 1-5, PERSONS OF SPANISH ORIGIN ARE CLASSIFIED BY PLACE OF BIRTH, PLACE OF RESIDENCE, AGE, ORIGIN OF WIFE, AND ORIGIN OF HOUSEHOLD HEAD. THE INCIDENCE OF SPANISH AS THE MOTHER TONGUE AND/OR LANGUAGE SPOKEN IN THE HOME IS REPORTED IN TABLES 6-13 FOR DIF-FERENT TYPES OF SPANISH ORIGIN, PLACES OF BIRTH, AND RESIDENCE IN THE U.S. PER-SONS REPORTING ABILITY TO READ AND WRITE THEIR MOTHER TONGUE AND/OR LANGUAGE SPOKEN IN THE HOME ARE LISTED IN TABLES 14-20 BY AGE, SEX, AND EDUCATIONAL ATTAIN-MENT. TABLES 21-24 REPORT EMPLOYMENT STATUS AND OCCUPATIONS BY ORIGIN, AGE, SEX, AND LITERACY. FAMILY INCOME IS RE-PORTED BY ORIGIN, AGE, AND MOTHER TONGUE OF HOUSEHOLD HEAD IN TABLES 25-27. FINALLY, THE APPENDIX PROVIDES: (1) DEFI-NITIONS OF KEY TERMS; (2) RELIABILITY ESTI-MATES OF THE DATA; AND (3) A PORTION OF THE SURVEY QUESTIONNAIRE.

ACCN   001595

1858 AUTH   **U.S. BUREAU OF THE CENSUS.**
    TITL   PUERTO RICANS IN THE UNITED STATES (PC(2)1E).
    SRCE   *WASHINGTON, D.C.: U.S. GOVERNMENT PRINT-ING OFFICE, 1973.*
    INDX   CENSUS, DEMOGRAPHIC, ECONOMIC FAC-TORS, EDUCATION, EMPLOYMENT, FAMILY STRUCTURE, HOUSING, LABOR FORCE, MAR-RIAGE, POVERTY, PUERTO RICAN-M, SES, UR-BAN, RURAL, SEX COMPARISON, MALE, FE-MALE, EAST, SOUTH, WEST, MIDWEST, SOUTHWEST
    ABST   THIS REPORT PRESENTS 30 TABLES WITH DE-TAILED STATISTICS ON SELECTED SOCIAL, ECONOMIC, AND HOUSING CHARACTERISTICS OF PERSONS OF PUERTO RICAN BIRTH AND PERSONS OF PUERTO RICAN PARENTAGE FOR THE UNITED STATES, REGIONS, DIVISIONS, STATES, CITIES, AND SELECTED STANDARD METROPOLITAN STATISTICAL AREAS (SMSA'S). THE STATISTICS ARE BASED ON THE 1970 CEN-SUS OF POPULATION, WHICH USED A 15% SAMPLE TO REPRESENT THE TOTAL POPULA-TION. APPENDIX A PROVIDES GENERAL INFOR-MATION CONCERNING THE PRESENTATION OF DATA IN THIS SERIES OF REPORTS AND THE COLLECTION AND PROCESSING PROCEDURES OF THE 1970 CENSUS. APPENDIX B DESCRIBES THE VARIOUS AREA CLASSIFICATIONS AND ALSO EXPLAINS THE RESIDENCE RULES USED IN COUNTING THE POPULATION. APPENDIX C PROVIDES BRIEF DEFINITIONS AND EXPLANA-TIONS OF SUBJECTS COVERED IN CROSS-CLASSIFICATIONS IN THE REPORT. APPENDIX D PRESENTS INFORMATION ON SOURCES OF ER-

ROR IN THE DATA, SAMPLING VARIABILITY, RA-TIO ESTIMATION, AND EDITING PROCEDURES. APPENDIX E SUMMARIZES THE DATA DISSEMI-NATION PROGRAM.

ACCN   002246

1859 AUTH   **U.S. BUREAU OF THE CENSUS.**
    TITL   SELECTED CHARACTERISTICS OF PERSONS OF MEXICAN, PUERTO RICAN AND OTHER SPAN-ISH ORIGIN: MARCH 1971 (SERIES P-20, NO. 224).
    SRCE   *WASHINGTON, D.C.: U.S. GOVERNMENT PRINT-ING OFFICE, 1971.*
    INDX   CENSUS, SES, POVERTY, DEMOGRAPHIC, SEX COMPARISON, ECONOMIC FACTORS, MEXICAN AMERICAN, PUERTO RICAN-M, SPANISH SUR-NAMED, LABOR FORCE, EDUCATION, SCHO-LASTIC ACHIEVEMENT, MARRIAGE, EMPIRICAL
    ABST   A STATISTICAL REPORT BASED ON DATA FROM THE MARCH 1971 CURRENT POPULATION SUR-VEY PRESENTS SOCIAL AND ECONOMIC CHAR-ACTERISTICS FOR PERSONS AND FAMILIES OF MEXICAN, PUERTO RICAN, AND OTHER SPAN-ISH ORIGINS. TABLES INCLUDED ARE: (1) U.S. POPULATION BY RACE, ETHNIC ORIGIN, AND SEX; (2) AGE DISTRIBUTION BY ETHNIC ORIGIN; (3) MEDIAN FAMILY INCOME IN 1970 BY AGE OF HEAD OF HOUSEHOLD AND ETHNIC ORIGIN; (4) INCOME IN 1970 OF PERSONS 25 YEARS-OLD AND OVER BY SEX AND ETHNIC ORIGIN; (5) PERSONS BELOW THE LOW-INCOME LEVEL IN 1970, BY SEX AND BY ETHNIC ORIGIN OF HEAD OF HOUSEHOLD FOR THE U.S. AND FOR FIVE SOUTHWESTERN STATES; (6) LABOR FORCE PARTICIPATION AND UNEMPLOYMENT RATES OF PERSONS 16-64 YEARS-OLD BY AGE, SEX, AND ETHNIC ORIGIN; (7) EMPLOYED MEN 16 YEARS-OLD AND OVER BY MAJOR OCCUPA-TION GROUP AND ETHNIC ORIGIN; (8) LEVEL OF EDUCATION FOR THOSE 25 YEARS-OLD AND OVER BY ETHNIC ORIGIN AND FAMILY RE-LATIONSHIP; (9) FAMILIES BY NUMBER OF OWN CHILDREN UNDER 18, SEX OF HEAD OF HOUSEHOLD, AND ETHNIC ORIGIN; AND (10) MARITAL STATUS BY ETHNIC ORIGIN. COMPA-RABLE DATA ON THE TOTAL WHITE AND NE-GRO POPULATIONS ARE ALSO INCLUDED.

ACCN   001596

1860 AUTH   **U.S. BUREAU OF THE CENSUS.**
    TITL   SELECTED CHARACTERISTICS OF PERSONS OF MEXICAN, PUERTO RICAN AND OTHER SPAN-ISH ORIGIN: MARCH 1972.
    SRCE   *WASHINGTON, D.C.: U.S. GOVERNMENT PRINT-ING OFFICE, JULY 1972. (ERIC DOCUMENT RE-PRODUCTION SERVICE NO. ED 070 546)*
    INDX   SPANISH SURNAMED, CENSUS, SEX COMPARI-SON, HOUSING, RURAL, URBAN, MARRIAGE, SCHOLASTIC ACHIEVEMENT, POVERTY, SES, EMPIRICAL, DEMOGRAPHIC, PUERTO RICAN-M, SOUTHWEST
    ABST   DATA ON A VARIETY OF SOCIAL AND ECO-NOMIC CHARACTERISTICS FOR HISPANIC PER-SONS AND FAMILIES IN THE UNITED STATES (MEXICAN, PUERTO RICAN, CUBAN, AND OTHER SPANISH ORIGIN) AND COMPARATIVE DATA FOR THE REMAINING POPULATION WERE SE-LECTED FROM THE MARCH 1972 BUREAU OF

THE CENSUS CURRENT POPULATION SURVEY (CPS). REVISIONS IN THE MARCH 1972 CPS, AS COMPARED TO THE 1970 CPS, INCLUDE THE INTRODUCTION OF 1970 CENSUS-BASED POPULATION CONTROLS AND METROPOLITAN RESIDENCE DEFINITION, THE USE OF 1970 CENSUS SAMPLING MATERIALS FOR PART OF THE SAMPLE, A CHANGE IN THE AVERAGE SEGMENT SIZE FROM 6 TO 4 HOUSING UNITS FOR PART OF THE SAMPLE, AND A CHANGE IN THE FIRST STAGE RATIO ESTIMATION PROCEDURE. THE 10 TABLES CONTAIN INFORMATION CONCERNING: (1) U.S. POPULATION BY ETHNIC ORIGIN; (2) AGE DISTRIBUTION BY ETHNIC ORIGIN; (3) CHARACTERISTICS OF FAMILIES BY ETHNIC ORIGIN; (4) PERCENT OF THE POPULATION 25 YEARS OLD AND OVER WHO HAD COMPLETED LESS THAN 5 YEARS OF SCHOOL OR 4 YEARS OF HIGH SCHOOL OR MORE, BY ETHNIC ORIGIN; (5) LABOR FORCE PARTICIPATION OF PERSONS 16 TO 64 YEARS OLD, BY AGE, SEX, AND ETHNIC ORIGIN; (6) UNEMPLOYMENT RATES FOR PERSONS 16 TO 64 YEARS OLD, BY AGE, SEX, AND ETHNIC ORIGIN; (7) EMPLOYED MEN 16 YEARS OLD AND OVER, BY MAJOR OCCUPATION AND ETHNIC ORIGIN; (8) MEDIAN INCOME IN 1971 BY YEARS OF SCHOOL COMPLETED FOR MALES 25 YEARS OLD AND OVER BY ETHNIC ORIGIN; (9) FAMILY INCOME IN 1971 BY ETHNIC ORIGIN; AND (10) LOW-INCOME STATUS IN 1971 OF PERSONS OF SPANISH ORIGIN FOR THE U.S. AND 5 SOUTHWESTERN STATES. 5 REFERENCES. (ERIC ABSTRACT MODIFIED)

ACCN   001597

1861 AUTH   **U.S. BUREAU OF THE CENSUS.**
TITL   SUPPLEMENTARY REPORT. PERSONAS DE DESCENDENCIA HISPANA (PERSONS OF SPANISH ANCESTRY) (SERIES PC(SI)-30).
SRCE   *WASHINGTON, D.C.: U.S. GOVERNMENT PRINTING OFFICE, FEBRUARY, 1973. (SPANISH)*
INDX   SPANISH SURNAMED, MEXICAN AMERICAN, CENSUS, DEMOGRAPHIC, EMPIRICAL, CUBAN, PUERTO RICAN-M, SOUTH AMERICA, BILINGUAL, CENTRAL AMERICA
ABST   BASED UPON A 5% SAMPLE SURVEYED AS PART OF THE 1970 CENSUS OF POPULATION, THIS REPORT DELINEATES THE GEOGRAPHIC DISTRIBUTION OF THE MORE THAN 9 MILLION HISPANICS LIVING IN THE UNITED STATES. TEN TABLES ARE PRESENTED. TABLES A THROUGH D PROVIDE AN OVERVIEW, SUMMARIZING THE TOTAL NUMBER OF (A) HISPANICS IN THE U.S., (B) SPANISH SURNAMED IN THE FIVE SOUTHWESTERN STATES, (C) SPANISH-SPEAKING PERSONS IN THE U.S., AND (D) PERSONS BORN IN LATIN AMERICA NOW LIVING IN THE U.S. THE REMAINING 6 TABLES OFFER A MORE PRECISE BREAKDOWN BY EXAMINING THE POPULATION DISTRIBUTION IN U.S. REGIONS, DIVISIONS, 50 STATES, AND SELECTED SMSA'S IN EACH OF THE 50 STATES. IN TERMS OF THESE GEOGRAPHIC AREAS, TABLES 1 AND 2 REPORT ON THE NUMBER OF MEXICANS, PUERTO RICANS, CUBANS, AND "OTHER" HISPANICS. TABLES 3 AND 4 REPORT ON THE NUMBER OF SPANISH-

SPEAKING PERSONS IN THESE AREAS. AND TABLES 5 AND 6 DELINEATE THE NUMBER OF PERSONS BORN IN MEXICO, PUERTO RICO, CUBA, AND "ALL OTHER" LATIN AMERICAN COUNTRIES. 1 REFERENCE.

ACCN   001598

1862 AUTH   **U.S. BUREAU OF THE CENSUS.**
TITL   VOTER PARTICIPATION IN NOVEMBER 1972 (SERIES P-20, NO. 244).
SRCE   *WASHINGTON, D.C.: U.S. GOVERNMENT PRINTING OFFICE, DECEMBER, 1972.*
INDX   CENSUS, DEMOGRAPHIC, SEX COMPARISON, CROSS CULTURAL, · POLITICS, POLITICAL POWER, EMPIRICAL, ADULTS, SPANISH SURNAMED, SURVEY
ABST   VOTER PARTICIPATION DATA, BASED ON A SERIES OF QUESTIONS ADMINISTERED TO A SAMPLE OF PERSONS OF VOTING AGE TWO WEEKS AFTER THE ELECTIONS OF NOV. 7, 1972, ARE REPORTED IN THIS CURRENT POPULATION REPORT OF THE BUREAU OF THE CENSUS. QUESTIONS WERE DESIGNED TO PROVIDE INFORMATION ON VOTING BEHAVIOR BY AGE, REGION, RACE, AND SEX. ELECTION PARTICIPATION WAS FOUND TO VARY SIGNIFICANTLY (95% CONFIDENCE LIMIT) BY AGE, SEX, AND RACE. OF THE 11 MILLION PERSONS 18 TO 20 YEARS-OLD, 48% REPORTED VOTING, COMPARED TO 71% OF THE PERSONS 45 TO 64 YEARS-OLD. A SMALLER PROPORTION OF WOMEN (62%) THAN MEN (64%) REPORTED HAVING VOTED. APPROXIMATELY 65% OF WHITES, 52% OF NEGROES, AND 38% OF PERSONS OF SPANISH ORIGIN REPORTED THAT THEY VOTED. IN ADDITION TO THE NOVEMBER, 1972, ELECTION DATA, TWO TABLES REPORT VOTER PARTICIPATION RATES AND REGISTRATION FOR THE 1966, 1968, AND 1970 ELECTIONS.

ACCN   001599

1863 AUTH   **U.S. BUREAU OF THE CENSUS.**
TITL   1970 CENSUS OF POPULATION. SUPPLEMENTARY REPORT. CHARACTERISTICS OF THE SPANISH SURNAMED POPULATION BY CENSUS TRACT, FOR SMSA'S IN CALIFORNIA: 1970 (PC(S1)-58).
SRCE   *WASHINGTON, D.C.: U.S. GOVERNMENT PRINTING OFFICE, MAY 1974.*
INDX   CENSUS, DEMOGRAPHIC, SPANISH SURNAMED, FAMILY STRUCTURE, SCHOLASTIC ACHIEVEMENT, HOUSING, SES, POVERTY, ECONOMIC FACTORS, EDUCATION, EMPIRICAL, EMPLOYMENT, URBAN, CALIFORNIA, SOUTHWEST
ABST   FOCUSING EXCLUSIVELY ON CALIFORNIA, THIS SUPPLEMENTARY REPORT OF THE 1970 CENSUS OF POPULATION PRESENTS INFORMATION ON PERSONS OF SPANISH SURNAME LIVING IN CENSUS TRACTS OF 400 OR MORE PERSONS OF SPANISH SURNAME WITHIN STANDARD METROPOLITAN STATISTICAL AREAS (SMSA'S). THE FIRST OF THREE TABLES PRESENTS GENERAL AND SOCIAL CHARACTERISTICS OF PERSONS OF SPANISH SURNAME, INCLUDING AGE, SEX, RELATIONSHIP TO HEAD OF HOUSEHOLD, TYPE OF HOUSEHOLD, SCHOOL ENROLLMENT, YEARS OF SCHOOL COMPLETED, AND RESI-

DENCE IN 1965. THE SECOND TABLE REPORTS ECONOMIC CHARACTERISTICS, INCLUDING EMPLOYMENT STATUS, FAMILY INCOME, AND POVERTY STATUS. TABLE THREE PRESENTS HOUSING CHARACTERISTICS FOR HOUSE-HOLDS WITH A SPANISH-SURNAME HEAD. FI-NALLY, APPENDIX TABLE 'A' PRESENTS RACE OF PERSONS OF SPANISH SURNAME FOR UR-BAN AND RURAL RESIDENCE, SELECTED SMSA'S, AND SELECTED PLACES IN CALIFOR-NIA.

ACCN   001600

1864 AUTH   **U.S. COMMISSION ON CIVIL RIGHTS.**
      TITL   ETHNIC ISOLATION OF MEXICAN AMERICANS IN THE PUBLIC SCHOOLS OF THE SOUTHWEST (MEXICAN AMERICAN EDUCATIONAL STUDY, REPORT I).
      SRCE   *WASHINGTON, D.C.: U.S. GOVERNMENT PRINT-ING OFFICE, APRIL 1971.*
      INDX   MEXICAN AMERICAN, DISCRIMINATION, EDU-CATION, DEMOGRAPHIC, BILINGUAL-BICUL-TURAL PERSONNEL, EQUAL OPPORTUNITY, REPRESENTATION, ADMINISTRATORS, TEACH-ERS, SOUTHWEST
      ABST   FROM THIS COMMISSION'S STUDY OF THE DE-MOGRAPHIC CHARACTERISTICS AND ETHNIC ISOLATION OF MEXICAN AMERICAN STUDENTS AND STAFF IN THE SOUTHWEST, THREE BASIC FINDINGS EMERGE: (1) PUBLIC SCHOOL PU-PILS ARE SEVERELY ISOLATED BY SCHOOL DIS-TRICT; (2) MEXICAN AMERICANS ARE UNDER-REPRESENTED ON SCHOOL AND DISTRICT PROFESSIONAL STAFFS AND ON BOARDS OF EDUCATION; AND (3) THE MAJORITY OF MEXI-CAN AMERICAN STAFF SCHOOL BOARD MEM-BERS ARE FOUND IN PREDOMINANTLY MEXI-CAN AMERICAN SCHOOLS OR DISTRICTS. FOUR OF THE LARGEST SCHOOL DISTRICTS IN THE SOUTHWEST—LOS ANGELES, DENVER, ALBU-QUERQUE, AND TUCSON—ACCOUNT FOR A SIGNIFICANT PERCENTAGE OF THE DISPRO-PORTIONATELY HIGH MEXICAN AMERICAN SCHOOL ENROLLMENT. HOWEVER, CONSID-ERABLE IMBALANCE ALSO EXISTS IN SMALL OR MEDIUM DISTRICTS THROUGHOUT THE SOUTHWEST, AND CAN BE FOUND IN BOTH PREDOMINANTLY MEXICAN AMERICAN AND PREDOMINANTLY ANGLO DISTRICTS. CALIFOR-NIA, ALONE OF THE 5 SOUTHWESTERN STATES, HAS TAKEN ACTION AGAINST THE PROBLEM, ENACTING LEGISLATION THAT DECLARES A SCHOOL IMBALANCED "IF THE PERCENTAGE OF PUPILS OF ONE OR MORE RACIAL GROUP DIFFERS BY MORE THAN 15%," AND MANDATES SUCH DISTRICTS TO FIND MEASURES TO COR-RECT SUCH IMBALANCE. 61 REFERENCES.
      ACCN   001601

1865 AUTH   **U.S. COMMISSION ON CIVIL RIGHTS.**
      TITL   THE EXCLUDED STUDENT: EDUCATIONAL PRACTICES AFFECTING MEXICAN AMERICANS IN THE SOUTHWEST (MEXICAN AMERICAN EDUCATIONAL STUDY, REPORT III).
      SRCE   *WASHINGTON, D.C.: U.S. GOVERNMENT PRINT-ING OFFICE, MAY 1972. (STOCK NO. 0500-0074)*
      INDX   MEXICAN AMERICAN, BILINGUAL-BICULTURAL

EDUCATION, INSTRUCTIONAL TECHNIQUES, COMMUNITY INVOLVEMENT, EMPIRICAL
      ABST   THROUGH A COMMISSION HEARING IN SAN ANTONIO, TEXAS, AND A SURVEY OF SCHOOL DISTRICTS REPRESENTING 80% OF THE TOTAL CHICANO ENROLLMENT IN ARIZONA, CALI-FORNIA, COLORADO, NEW MEXICO, AND TEXAS (A TOTAL OF OVER ONE MILLION CHICANO STUDENTS), THIS STUDY ASCERTAINED THAT DEPRIVATION BY EXCLUSION IS BEING PRAC-TICED AGAINST MEXICAN AMERICAN STU-DENTS IN THE SCHOOL DISTRICTS OF THOSE STATES. THE DOMINANCE OF ANGLO VALUES IS APPARENT IN: (1) THE CURRICULA ON ALL EDUCATIONAL LEVELS; (2) THE CULTURAL CLI-MATE WHICH IGNORES OR DENIGRATES MEXI-CAN AMERICAN MORES AND THE USE OF THE SPANISH LANGUAGE; AND (3) THE EXCLUSION OF THE MEXICAN AMERICAN COMMUNITY FROM FULL PARTICIPATION IN MATTERS PERTAINING TO SCHOOL POLICIES AND PRACTICES. AL-THOUGH SOME INNOVATIONS ARE NOTED WHICH BEGIN TO CLOSE THE GAP BETWEEN THE TWO ETHNIC GROUPS (I.E., BILINGUAL PROGRAMS AND USE OF EDUCATIONAL CON-SULTANTS), THE COMMISSION SEES IMMEDI-ATE NEED FOR FURTHER PROCEDURES TO UNIFY THESE DISPARATE GROUPS. CORREC-TIVE ACTIONS WILL ENABLE ALL AMERICANS TO PARTICIPATE EQUALLY IN THE NATION'S IM-PRESSIVE EDUCATIONAL TRADITION. 76 REF-ERENCES.
      ACCN   001602

1866 AUTH   **U.S. COMMISSION ON CIVIL RIGHTS.**
      TITL   FULFILLING THE LETTER AND SPIRIT OF THE LAW: DESEGREGATION OF THE NATION'S PUB-LIC SCHOOLS.
      SRCE   *WASHINGTON, D.C.: U.S. GOVERNMENT PRINT-ING OFFICE, AUGUST 1976.*
      INDX   EDUCATION, CHILDREN, LEADERSHIP, PER-SONNEL, ATTITUDES, SPANISH SURNAMED, LEGISLATION, DISCRIMINATION, INTEGRATION, POLICY, EMPIRICAL, SURVEY, COMMUNITY IN-VOLVEMENT, PARENTAL INVOLVEMENT
      ABST   THE COMMISSION'S REPORT IS BASED UPON INFORMATION FROM FOUR FULL COMMISSION HEARINGS, FOUR STATE ADVISORY COMMIT-TEE OPEN MEETINGS, A MAIL SURVEY OF 1,291 SCHOOL DISTRICTS, AND 900 IN-DEPTH INTER-VIEWS WITH PERSONNEL IN 29 SCHOOL DIS-TRICTS THROUGHOUT THE COUNTRY. THOSE ASPECTS OF SCHOOL DESEGREGATION WHICH ARE DISCUSSED BY THE COMMISSION IN-CLUDE: (1) THE ROLE OF COMMUNITY AND SCHOOL LEADERSHIP; (2) PREPARATION OF THE COMMUNITY; (3) RESTRUCTURING OF SCHOOL DISTRICTS; (4) DESEGREGATION AND THE QUALITY OF EDUCATION; (5) MINORITY STAFF; (6) CLASSROOM DESEGREGATION; (7) EXTRACURRICULAR ACTIVITIES; (8) STUDENTS' ATTITUDES; AND (9) DISCIPLINE IN DESEGRE-GATED SCHOOLS. THE REPORT CONCLUDES THAT IN MOST COMMUNITIES DESEGREGA-TION HAS GONE PEACEFULLY AND SMOOTHLY. THE SUPPORT FOR DESEGREGATION BY LO-CAL LEADERS HAS GENERALLY RESULTED IN INSTITUTIONAL RENEWAL, BETTER COMMU-

NITY RACE RELATIONS, AND A HIGHER LEVEL OF PARENTAL INVOLVEMENT. NEVERTHELESS, MANY SCHOOL DISTRICTS (PARTICULARLY THE LARGER ONES) REMAIN SEGREGATED, AND WIDE REGIONAL VARIATIONS STILL EXIST. 445 REFERENCES.

ACCN   002249

1867 AUTH   **U.S. COMMISSION ON CIVIL RIGHTS.**
TITL   INEQUALITY IN SCHOOL FINANCING: THE ROLE OF THE LAW (CLEARINGHOUSE PUBLICATION NO. 39).
SRCE   *WASHINGTON, D.C.: U.S. GOVERNMENT PRINT-ING OFFICE, AUGUST 1972.*
INDX   ECONOMIC FACTORS, EDUCATIONAL ASSESS-MENT, DISCRIMINATION, EMPIRICAL, EQUAL OPPORTUNITY, TEXAS, SOUTHWEST
ABST   THIS STUDY WAS ORIGINALLY PREPARED AS A LEGAL APPENDIX TO "MEXICAN AMERICAN EDUCATION IN TEXAS: A FUNCTION OF WEALTH," A REPORT BY THE UNITED STATES COMMIS-SION ON CIVIL RIGHTS, ON THE IMPACT WHICH THE FINANCING OF EDUCATION IN TEXAS HAS HAD ON THE MEXICAN AMERICAN COMMU-NITY. HOWEVER, BECAUSE ITS SUBJECT MAT-TER HAS IMPLICATIONS FAR BEYOND THE MEX-ICAN AMERICAN CHILDREN IN TEXAS, THIS SURVEY OF THE LAW WAS PUBLISHED SEPA-RATELY. IT GIVES A BRIEF HISTORY OF THE MOVEMENT TOWARD EQUALITY OF EDUCA-TIONAL OPPORTUNITY IN THE UNITED STATES AND REVIEWS RECENT COURT DECISIONS MANDATING EQUALITY IN EDUCATIONAL EX-PENDITURES. FINALLY, IT RAISES SOME OF THE CRITICAL QUESTIONS THUS FAR UNAN-SWERED BY EITHER THE COURTS OR THE LEG-ISLATURE REGARDING THE RAMIFICATIONS OF THESE COURT DECISIONS: (1) THE RECENT COURT DECISIONS STRIKING DOWN STATE SYSTEMS OF SCHOOL FINANCE BECAUSE OF INTRASTATE INEQUALITY MAY NOT BE THE PANACEA FOR MINORITY GROUP SCHOOL CHILDREN; AND (2) MASS MIGRATIONS OF WHITE PERSONS OUT OF THE CENTRAL CITIES TO THE SUBURBS HAVE PLACED TREMENDOUS BURDENS ON CENTRAL CITY .SCHOOL DIS-TRICTS, AND SO A MEANS OF FINANCING MUST BE DEVELOPED WHICH TAKES THIS INTO CONSIDERATION. 302 REFERENCES.

ACCN   001603

1868 AUTH   **U.S. COMMISSION ON CIVIL RIGHTS.**
TITL   METHODOLOGICAL APPENDIX OF RESEARCH METHODS EMPLOYED IN THE MEXICAN AMERI-CAN EDUCATIONAL STUDY.
SRCE   *WASHINGTON, D.C.: U.S. GOVERNMENT PRINT-ING OFFICE, JANUARY 1972.*
INDX   MEXICAN AMERICAN, RESEARCH METHOD-OLOGY, BILINGUAL-BICULTURAL EDUCATION, SURVEY, EDUCATION, SOUTHWEST
ABST   (NOTE: THIS 156-PAGE MONOGRAPH DE-SCRIBES THE RESEARCH METHODOLOGY FOR THE U.S. COMMISSION ON CIVIL RIGHTS' RE-PORTS I THRU VI, ALL CITED IN THE PRESENT BIBLIOGRAPHY.) THE MEXICAN AMERICAN EDUCATION STUDY FOCUSED ON EDUCA-TIONAL CONDITIONS, PRACTICES, AND SCHO-LASTIC ACHIEVEMENT EXPERIENCED BY MEXI-

CAN AMERICANS IN THE SOUTHWEST UNITED STATES. THE FIRST PHASE INVOLVED ANALYSIS OF DATA FROM HEW'S 1968 ELEMENTARY AND SECONDARY SCHOOL SURVEY OF ETHNIC BACKGROUND OF STUDENTS AND STAFF IN ARIZONA, CALIFORNIA, COLORADO, NEW MEXICO, AND TEXAS. THE SECOND PHASE CONSISTED OF A MAIL SURVEY IN WHICH A QUESTIONNAIRE WAS SENT TO 538 SCHOOL DISTRICT SUPERINTENDENTS, REQUESTING INFORMATION ON ETHNICITY AND EDUCATION OF DISTRICT PERSONNEL AND BOARD MEM-BERS, POLICY CONCERNING THE USE OF SPANISH, AND THEIR SUPPORT OF IN-SERVICE TRAINING OF TEACHERS OF MEXICAN AMERI-CAN STUDENTS. 1,166 SCHOOL PRINCIPALS WERE ALSO SURVEYED REGARDING STAFFING PATTERNS, FACILITIES, ABILITY GROUPINGS, READING ACHIEVEMENT, AND MEXICAN AMERICAN PARTICIPATION IN SCHOOL AF-FAIRS. IN THE FINAL PHASE, PERSONAL INTER-VIEWS WERE CONDUCTED WITH PRINCIPALS AND COUNSELORS IN 52 URBAN, SUBURBAN, AND RURAL SCHOOLS IN THREE STATES. EX-TERNAL SCHOOL AND CLASSROOM CONDI-TIONS WERE OBSERVED AND PUPIL-TEACHER INTERACTION RECORDED IN 494 CLASS-ROOMS USING THE FLANDERS INTERACTION ANALYSIS AND THE OBSERVATION SCHEDULE AND RECORD. SUPPLEMENTARY DATA ON IN-COME AND EDUCATIONAL ATTAINMENT OF STUDENTS' FAMILIES WERE GATHERED. ALL QUESTIONNAIRES, RESEARCH INSTRUMENTS, AND AN ASSESSMENT OF THE QUALITY OF THE DATA ARE INCLUDED IN 10 APPENDICES.

ACCN   001604

1869 AUTH   **U.S. COMMISSION ON CIVIL RIGHTS.**
TITL   MEXICAN AMERICAN EDUCATION IN TEXAS: A FUNCTION OF WEALTH (MEXICAN AMERICAN EDUCATIONAL STUDY, REPORT IV).
SRCE   *WASHINGTON, D.C.: U.S. GOVERNMENT PRINT-ING OFFICE, AUGUST 1972.*
INDX   MEXICAN AMERICAN, ECONOMIC FACTORS, EDUCATION, DISCRIMINATION, EMPIRICAL, EQUAL OPPORTUNITY, EDUCATIONAL ASSESS-MENT, FINANCING, TEXAS, SOUTHWEST
ABST   IN THIS FOURTH REPORT ON MEXICAN AMERI-CAN EDUCATION IN THE SOUTHWEST, THE COMMISSION EXAMINED THE EFFECTS OF THE TEXAS SCHOOL FINANCING PLAN ON MEXI-CAN AMERICAN STUDENTS. SPECIFICALLY, THE REPORT EXAMINES DISPARITIES IN: (1) STATE AID TO LOCAL SCHOOL DISTRICTS, IN PAR-TICULAR THE MINIMUM FOUNDATION PRO-GRAM, WHICH PROVIDES 96% OF STATE EDU-CATION FUNDS; (2) PROPERTY VALUATION WITHIN DISTRICTS; (3) PROPERTY TAX EFFORT, OR THE RATE AT WHICH PROPERTY IS TAXED WITHIN SCHOOL DISTRICTS; AND (4) THE ECO-NOMIC BURDEN OF PROPERTY TAXES ON MEX-ICAN AMERICAN AND ANGLO CITIZENS. ON ALL FOUR COUNTS, PREDOMINANTLY MEXI-CAN AMERICAN DISTRICTS COME OUT SEC-OND BEST IN COMPARISON WITH PREDOMI-NANTLY ANGLO DISTRICTS. STATE AID DOES LITTLE TO EQUALIZE THE DISPARITIES IN REVE-NUE BETWEEN THESE SCHOOL DISTRICTS. AS

A CONSEQUENCE, THE AMOUNT OF MONEY SPENT FOR THE EDUCATION OF MANY CHICANO STUDENTS IS THREE-FIFTHS THAT SPENT TO EDUCATE ANGLO CHILDREN. 39 REFERENCES. (AUTHOR SUMMARY MODIFIED)

ACCN   001605

1870 AUTH   **U.S. COMMISSION ON CIVIL RIGHTS.**
TITL   MEXICAN AMERICANS AND THE ADMINISTRATION OF JUSTICE: BAIL.
SRCE   *IN N. R. YETMAN & C. H. STEELE (EDS.), MAJORITY AND MINORITY: THE DYNAMICS OF RACIAL AND ETHNIC RELATIONS. BOSTON: ALLYN AND BACON, 1975, PP. 422-426.*
INDX   CORRECTIONS, CRIMINOLOGY, CULTURAL FACTORS, DISCRIMINATION, ESSAY, FARM LABORERS, JUDICIAL PROCESS, MEXICAN AMERICAN, SOUTHWEST
ABST   THE SYSTEM OF BAIL IN THE SOUTHWEST FREQUENTLY IS USED MORE SEVERELY AGAINST MEXICAN AMERICANS THAN AGAINST ANGLOS AS A FORM OF DISCRIMINATION. IN CERTAIN CASES, MEXICAN AMERICAN DEFENDANTS ARE FACED WITH EXCESSIVELY HIGH BAIL. DEFENDANTS IN OTHER CASES ARE HELD WITHOUT ANY OPPORTUNITY TO PUT UP BAIL OR ARE PURPOSELY CONFUSED BY LOCAL OFFICIALS ABOUT THE BAIL HEARING SO THAT THEY UNKNOWINGLY FORFEIT THEIR BAIL. EVEN IN THE ABSENCE OF SUCH ABUSES, THE HIGH COST UNDER THE TRADITIONAL BAIL SYSTEM PREVENTS MANY MEXICAN AMERICANS FROM BEING RELEASED PRIOR TO THEIR TRIAL, WHILE OTHERS ACCUSED OF SIMILAR CRIMES GO FREE MERELY BECAUSE THEY CAN AFFORD TO PAY A BAIL BONDSMAN TO PUT UP THEIR BAIL. IN SOME JURISDICTIONS, ALTERNATIVES TO THE TRADITIONAL CASH BAIL SYSTEMS ARE BEING TRIED, INCLUDING THE RELEASE OF DEFENDANTS ON THEIR OWN RECOGNIZANCE. (AUTHOR ABSTRACT MODIFIED)
ACCN   002251

1871 AUTH   **U.S. COMMISSION ON CIVIL RIGHTS.**
TITL   STRANGER IN ONE'S LAND.
SRCE   *WASHINGTON, D.C.: U.S. GOVERNMENT PRINTING OFFICE, MAY 1970.*
INDX   COMMUNITY INVOLVEMENT, CULTURAL FACTORS, DISCRIMINATION, ECONOMIC FACTORS, EDUCATION, EMPLOYMENT, IMMIGRATION, JUDICIAL PROCESS, MEXICAN AMERICAN, MEXICAN, MIGRANTS, POVERTY, PROCEEDINGS, SOUTHWEST, POLITICS
ABST   AN ACCOUNT IS PRESENTED OF THE CIVIL RIGHTS COMMISSION'S 1968 HEARINGS IN SAN ANTONIO, TEXAS, ON THE PROBLEMS OF THE MEXICAN AMERICAN COMMUNITY. RUBEN SALAZAR, A CALIFORNIA JOURNALIST, EDITORIALLY REPORTS ON THE COMMISSION'S FINDINGS IN SIX AREAS: LANGUAGE; THE MEXICAN AMERICAN BORDER AND IMMIGRATION; POVERTY; EDUCATION; EMPLOYMENT; AND LEGAL JUSTICE. PRIOR TO THE HEARINGS, APPROXIMATELY 1,000 PERSONS WERE INTERVIEWED, AND VOLUMES OF DATA WERE COLLECTED AND ANALYZED BY COMMISSION STAFF. NEARLY 80 PERSONS WERE REQUESTED TO SPEAK UNDER SUBPOENA—INCLUDING BARRIO RESI-

DENTS, STATE OFFICIALS, BUSINESSMEN, FARM WORKERS, STUDENTS, AND SCHOOL SUPERINTENDENTS. THE REPORT, PUBLISHED FOR THE PURPOSE OF STIMULATING PUBLIC INTEREST AND CONCERN, DOCUMENTS ECONOMIC DEPRIVATION, RELEGATION TO MENIAL EMPLOYMENT, EDUCATIONAL SUPPRESSION, AND RESTRICTED OPPORTUNITY IN ALMOST EVERY PHASE OF LIFE. THE HEARING AIDED NATIONAL GOVERNMENT IN RECOGNIZING THE MEXICAN AMERICAN AS HAVING UNIQUE PROBLEMS REQUIRING SEPARATE CONSIDERATION. THE COMMITTEE WAS INSTITUTED AS A PERMANENT AGENCY UNDER PRESIDENT NIXON.

ACCN   002253

1872 AUTH   **U.S. COMMISSION ON CIVIL RIGHTS.**
TITL   TEACHERS AND STUDENTS: DIFFERENCES IN INTERACTION WITH MEXICAN AMERICAN AND ANGLO STUDENTS (MEXICAN AMERICAN EDUCATION STUDY, REPORT V).
SRCE   *WASHINGTON, D.C.: U.S. GOVERNMENT PRINTING OFFICE, 1973.*
INDX   MEXICAN AMERICAN, CHILDREN, ADOLESCENTS, TEACHERS, INSTRUCTIONAL TECHNIQUES, DISCRIMINATION, CLASSROOM BEHAVIOR, EMPIRICAL, SCHOLASTIC ACHIEVEMENT, SOUTHWEST
ABST   THIS IS THE FIFTH IN THE COMMISSION'S SERIES OF REPORTS INVESTIGATING BARRIERS TO EQUAL EDUCATIONAL OPPORTUNITIES FOR MEXICAN AMERICANS IN THE PUBLIC SCHOOLS OF THE SOUTHWEST. IT FOCUSES ON THE DENIAL OF THESE OPPORTUNITIES AS REFLECTED IN THE DIFFERENCES IN THE CLASSROOM VERBAL INTERACTIONS OF TEACHERS WITH MEXICAN AMERICAN AND ANGLO CHILDREN. FINDINGS ARE BASED UPON INFORMATION FROM OBSERVATIONS AND INTERVIEWS OBTAINED IN 429 CLASSROOMS OF SCHOOLS IN THREE GEOGRAPHICAL AREAS OF CALIFORNIA, NEW MEXICO, AND TEXAS. THE PICTURE OF VERBAL INTERACTION THAT EMERGES IS ONE IN WHICH MEXICAN AMERICAN STUDENTS ARE NEGLECTED IN COMPARISON TO ANGLO STUDENTS—E.G., TEACHERS WERE FOUND TO PRAISE OR ENCOURAGE ANGLO CHILDREN CONSIDERABLY MORE THAN MEXICAN AMERICANS, AND THEY DIRECTED QUESTIONS TO MEXICAN AMERICAN STUDENTS MUCH LESS OFTEN THAN THEY DID TO ANGLO STUDENTS. THUS, IT IS NOT SURPRISING TO FIND THAT MEXICAN AMERICAN CHILDREN SPEAK SIGNIFICANTLY LESS IN THE CLASSROOM THAN DO ANGLO CHILDREN. THIS PATTERN OF TEACHER-STUDENT INTERACTION IS SEEN TO MIRROR THE EDUCATIONAL NEGLECT OF MEXICAN AMERICAN STUDENTS THROUGHOUT THE EDUCATIONAL SYSTEM IN THE SOUTHWEST. IN THE COMMISSION'S VIEW, IT IS THE SCHOOLS AND TEACHERS, NOT THE CHILDREN, WHO ARE FAILING. THIS FAILURE WILL CONTINUE UNTIL FUNDAMENTAL CHANGES ARE MADE IN TEACHER TRAINING, CURRICULUMS, AND OTHER EDUCATIONAL PROGRAMS. 19 REFERENCES.

ACCN   001606

1873 AUTH **U.S. COMMISSION ON CIVIL RIGHTS.**

TITL TOWARD QUALITY EDUCATION FOR MEXICAN AMERICANS (MEXICAN AMERICAN EDUCATIONAL STUDY, REPORT VI).

SRCE *WASHINGTON, D.C.: U.S. GOVERNMENT PRINTING OFFICE, FEBRUARY 1974.*

INDX CURRICULUM, POLICY, EDUCATION, PROFESSIONAL TRAINING, LEGISLATION, CHILDREN, SOUTHWEST, SCHOLASTIC ACHIEVEMENT, TEACHERS, CULTURAL PLURALISM, MEXICAN AMERICAN, BILINGUAL-BICULTURAL EDUCATION, BILINGUAL-BICULTURAL PERSONNEL, EDUCATIONAL COUNSELING, EQUAL OPPORTUNITY

ABST BASED UPON EXAMINATION OF THOSE ASPECTS OF SCHOOLS' EDUCATIONAL PROGRAM AND STAFFING PATTERNS WHICH BEAR ON THEIR FAILURE TO PROVIDE EQUAL EDUCATIONAL OPPORTUNITY FOR MEXICAN AMERICAN CHILDREN, THE COMMISSION RECOMMENDS CORRECTIVE ACTION ON VARIOUS GOVERNMENTAL AND EDUCATIONAL LEVELS. INFORMATION WAS DERIVED FROM THE COMMISSION'S MAIL SURVEY AND FIELD STUDY, A REVIEW OF THE RESEARCH LITERATURE, AND CONSULTATION WITH EDUCATIONAL EXPERTS. FOUR AREAS OF STUDY WERE INVESTIGATED: (1) SCHOOL CURRICULUM AND ITS RELEVANCE TO THE MEXICAN AMERICAN CHILD; (2) THE PRACTICES OF GRADE RETENTION, ABILITY GROUPING, AND PLACEMENT IN CLASSES FOR THE EDUCABLE MENTALLY RETARDED; (3) THE ADEQUACY OF TEACHER EDUCATION IN RELATION TO THE NEEDS OF CHICANO STUDENTS; AND (4) THE KIND OF EDUCATIONAL COUNSELING AVAILABLE. A FINAL SECTION DEALS WITH THE EXTENT OF EFFORTS MADE UNDER TITLE VI OF THE CIVIL RIGHTS ACT OF 1964 TO ASSURE EQUAL EDUCATIONAL SERVICES. THE REPORT CONCLUDES WITH NUMEROUS, CAREFULLY DETAILED RECOMMENDATIONS WHICH CENTER AROUND THREE MAIN POINTS: (1) MEXICAN AMERICAN LANGUAGE, HISTORY, AND CULTURE MUST BE INCORPORATED INTO THE EDUCATIONAL CURRICULUM; (2) MEXICAN AMERICANS MUST BE FULLY REPRESENTED IN THE EDUCATIONAL DECISION-MAKING PROCESS; AND (3) ALL LEVELS OF GOVERNMENT SHOULD PROVIDE THE FUNDS NEEDED TO IMPLEMENT THESE RECOMMENDATIONS. APPENDICES INCLUDE THE METHOD OF DISTRICT SURVEY AND A REVIEW OF RESEARCH ON THE EFFECTS OF GRADE RETENTION. 159 REFERENCES.

ACCN 001607

1874 AUTH **U.S. COMMISSION ON CIVIL RIGHTS.**

TITL THE UNFINISHED EDUCATION: OUTCOMES FOR MINORITIES IN THE FIVE SOUTHWESTERN STATES (MEXICAN AMERICAN EDUCATIONAL STUDY, REPORT II).

SRCE *WASHINGTON, D.C.: U.S. GOVERNMENT PRINTING OFFICE, OCTOBER 1971.*

INDX SCHOLASTIC ACHIEVEMENT, MEXICAN AMERICAN, EMPIRICAL, READING, CURRICULUM, EDUCATION, CROSS CULTURAL, SOUTHWEST

ABST IN THIS SECOND IN ITS SERIES OF REPORTS INVESTIGATING THE NATURE OF EDUCATIONAL

OPPORTUNITIES FOR MEXICAN AMERICANS IN THE PUBLIC SCHOOLS OF ARIZONA, CALIFORNIA, COLORADO, NEW MEXICO, AND TEXAS, ATTENTION IS FOCUSED ON THE PERFORMANCE OF THE SCHOOLS AS REFLECTED IN THE ACHIEVEMENT OF THEIR PUPILS. INFORMATION WAS GATHERED PRIMARILY THROUGH A SURVEY OF SUPERINTENDENTS AND PRINCIPALS IN 538 SOUTHWESTERN SCHOOL DISTRICTS HAVING ENROLLMENT AT LEAST 10 PERCENT SPANISH SURNAMED. THE BASIC FINDING WAS THAT MEXICAN AMERICAN STUDENTS DO NOT OBTAIN THE SAME BENEFITS OF PUBLIC EDUCATION AS THEIR ANGLO PEERS. WITHOUT EXCEPTION, MEXICAN AMERICANS ACHIEVED AT A LOWER RATE THAN ANGLOS ON FIVE MEASURES: (1) THEIR SCHOOL HOLDING POWER IS LOWER; (2) THEIR READING ACHIEVEMENT IS POORER; (3) THEIR REPETITION OF GRADES IS MORE FREQUENT; (4) THEIR OVER-AGENESS IS MORE PREVALENT; AND (5) THEY PARTICIPATE IN EXTRACURRICULAR ACTIVITIES LESS THAN THEIR ANGLO COUNTERPARTS. THIS REPORT SOUGHT ONLY TO PRESENT OBJECTIVE FACTS, NOT TO REFLECT ON THEIR CAUSES. HOWEVER, IT IS URGED THAT THESE WIDE DIFFERENCES BETWEEN MEXICAN AMERICAN AND ANGLO STUDENTS IN THE SOUTHWEST BE CONSIDERED MATTERS OF CRUCIAL CONCERN TO THE NATION. 48 REFERENCES.

ACCN 001608

1875 AUTH **U.S. DEPARTMENT OF HEALTH, EDUCATION, AND WELFARE.**

TITL MINORITIES AND WOMEN IN THE HEALTH FIELDS: APPLICANTS, STUDENTS AND WORKERS (DHEW PUBLICATION NO. (HRA) 76-22).

SRCE *WASHINGTON, D.C.: U.S. GOVERNMENT PRINTING OFFICE, 1975.*

INDX PROFESSIONAL TRAINING, REPRESENTATION, HEALTH DELIVERY SYSTEMS, MEXICAN AMERICAN, FEMALE, EQUAL OPPORTUNITY, PUERTO RICAN-M, NURSING, MEDICAL STUDENTS, SPANISH SURNAMED, MALE

ABST THIS REPORT UPDATES AND EXPANDS A 1974 REPORT ON THE DEGREE OF REPRESENTATION OF FEMALES AND MINORITIES IN VARIOUS HEALTH FIELDS. OF THE 89 TABLES PRESENTED, 13 REPORT THE RACIAL-ETHNIC AND SEX REPRESENTATION AMONG STUDENTS AND PRACTITIONERS IN THE ENTIRE HEALTH FIELD. THE REMAINING 76 TABLES PRESENT DATA FOR EACH OF 19 HEALTH OCCUPATIONS. REGARDING RACIAL-ETHNIC REPRESENTATION, THE PROPORTION OF MINORITY PRACTITIONERS AND STUDENTS WAS FOUND TO VARY AMONG THE SEVERAL HEALTH OCCUPATIONS— E.G., FROM 27% OF NURSING AIDES, ORDERLIES, AND ATTENDANTS TO 9.6% OF REGISTERED NURSES, 6.9% OF PHYSICIANS, AND LESS THAN 1% OF VETERINARIANS. THE SUBSTANTIAL INCREASES IN FIRST-YEAR ENROLLMENT OF MINORITY STUDENTS, HOWEVER, INDICATES A MAJOR SHIFT IN THE FUTURE RACIAL-ETHNIC BALANCE IN HEALTH OCCUPATIONS. REGARDING FEMALE REPRESENTATION, THE PROPORTION OF FEMALES IN VARI-

OUS HEALTH OCCUPATIONS LIKEWISE VARIED—FROM 5% OF PHARMACISTS TO OVER 95% OF NURSES. HOWEVER, THE TRADITION OF PREDOMINANTLY MALE AND FEMALE OCCUPATIONS APPEARS TO BE CHANGING—EVIDENT IN THE FINDING THAT THE PROPORTION OF FEMALES ENTERING MEDICINE INCREASED TO 22% IN 1974-75, AND THAT THE PROPORTION OF MALES ADMITTED TO NURSING PROGRAMS INCREASED TO 6% IN 1971-72.

ACCN   001609

1876 AUTH   **U.S. DEPARTMENT OF HEALTH, EDUCATION, AND WELFARE.**

TITL   REPORT OF THE SOUTHWEST STATES CHICANO CONSUMER CONFERENCE ON HEALTH (DHEW PUBLICATION NO. HSM 73-6208).

SRCE   *ROCKVILLE, MD: U.S. DEPARTMENT OF HEALTH, EDUCATION, AND WELFARE, 1972.*

INDX   HEALTH, COMMUNITY, HEALTH DELIVERY SYSTEMS, MEXICAN AMERICAN, PROCEEDINGS, COMMUNITY INVOLVEMENT, TEXAS, SOUTHWEST

ABST   THIS 1972 CONFERENCE HELD IN SAN ANTONIO, TEXAS, SIGNALED A CONCERTED NATIONAL MOVEMENT ON THE PART OF CHICANO COMMUNITY AND HEALTH LEADERS AT LOCAL, STATE, AND HSMHA LEVELS, TO IDENTIFY HEALTH AS A MAJOR CHICANO PRIORITY AMONG MIGRANTS, RURAL POOR, AND BARRIO RESIDENTS. THE CONFERENCE ALSO EXPRESSED CONCERN WITH THE FRAGMENTED AND FREQUENTLY INSENSITIVE WAY THAT HEALTH SERVICES ARE DELIVERED IN SPANISH-SPEAKING COMMUNITIES. PRESENTATION OF A SERIES OF COMMUNITY HEALTH PROBLEMS (SUCH AS POOR PRIMARY CARE FACILITIES, INADEQUATE REPRESENTATION IN HEALTH CARE PLANNING, POOR TRAINING IN HYGIENE AND NUTRITION, ALCOHOLISM, DRUG ABUSE, AND UNSATISFACTORY CARE FOR THE AGED) WERE FOLLOWED BY DISCUSSIONS OF VARIOUS HSMHA PROGRAMS DESIGNED TO ALLEVIATE THESE PROBLEMS. SPECIFIC RECOMMENDATIONS APPROVED IN GENERAL SESSION REFLECTED BOTH THE FRUSTRATIONS AND ASPIRATIONS OF THE CHICANO CONSTITUENCY. SOME ADDRESSED THE PROBLEM OF ALLOCATION OF FUNDS FOR SERVICES WITH WHICH BARRIO RESIDENTS CANNOT IDENTIFY; OTHERS DISCUSSED THE ADMINISTRATION OF PROGRAMS THAT DISCRIMINATE AGAINST CHICANOS BY EXCLUDING THEM FROM PARTICIPATION AT ALL LEVELS. FOR CHICANO AND HSMHA GROUPS, THE CONFERENCE WAS SEEN AS A WORTHWHILE EVENT: COMMUNICATION LINKAGES WERE DEVELOPED; MODELS OF DELIVERY WERE IDENTIFIED; EXPERIENCES WERE SHARED; GAPS IN DELIVERY WERE IDENTIFIED; AND GAPS IN DELIVERY AND CONSUMER INVOLVEMENT WERE DEFINED.

ACCN   001610

1877 AUTH   **U.S. OFFICE OF CIVIL RIGHTS.**

TITL   RACIAL AND ETHNIC ENROLLMENT DATA FROM INSTITUTIONS OF HIGHER EDUCATION: FALL 1970.

SRCE   *WASHINGTON, D.C.: U.S. GOVERNMENT PRINTING OFFICE, 1972.*

INDX   COLLEGE STUDENTS, PROFESSIONAL TRAINING, SURVEY, EDUCATION, EQUAL OPPORTUNITY, HIGHER EDUCATION, CROSS CULTURAL, DEMOGRAPHIC, REPRESENTATION, EMPIRICAL, SPANISH SURNAMED

ABST   THE ENROLLMENT DATA FOR ETHNIC AND RACIAL GROUPS IN U.S. HIGHER EDUCATION INSTITUTIONS RECEIVING OR EXPECTING TO RECEIVE FEDERAL SUPPORT FOR 1972 ARE PRESENTED. THE DATA ARE LISTED BY INSTITUTION, STATE, AND REGION FOR UNDERGRADUATE, GRADUATE, AND PROFESSIONAL ENROLLMENTS OF FULL TIME STUDENTS. THE INSTITUTIONS OF THE 48 COTERMINOUS STATES AND THE DISTRICT OF COLUMBIA ARE PRESENTED IN THIS REPORT. IN ADDITION, AGGREGATE DATA FROM THE EARLIER 1968 AND 1970 SURVEYS ARE PRESENTED FOR COMPARISON PURPOSES.

ACCN   001611

1878 AUTH   **U.S. OFFICE OF EDUCATION.**

TITL   PROCEEDINGS OF THE NATIONAL CONFERENCE ON EDUCATIONAL OPPORTUNITIES FOR MEXICAN AMERICANS, APRIL 25-26, 1968.

SRCE   *AUSTIN, TEXAS: SOUTHWEST EDUCATIONAL DEVELOPMENT LABORATORY, 1968.*

INDX   EDUCATION, SCHOLASTIC ACHIEVEMENT, MEXICAN AMERICAN, BILINGUALISM, BILINGUAL-BICULTURAL EDUCATION, BILINGUAL-BICULTURAL PERSONNEL, URBAN, RURAL, LANGUAGE LEARNING, CURRICULUM, INSTRUCTIONAL TECHNIQUES

ABST   TO ESTABLISH PRIORITIES IN EDUCATION PROGRAM DEVELOPMENT AT THE LOCAL LEVEL, THIS 1968 CONFERENCE ADDRESSED THE SPECIAL NEEDS OF THE MEXICAN AMERICAN CHILD IN THREE AREAS: BILINGUAL EDUCATION, MIGRANT EDUCATION, AND URBAN EDUCATION. THE BILINGUAL EDUCATION SESSIONS DISCUSSED THE IMPLEMENTATION OF TITLE VII, AND ALSO FOCUSED ON IMPROVEMENT OF CURRICULUM, AND LANGUAGE AND READING SKILLS. THE CONCERN OF THE MIGRANT EDUCATION SESSIONS WAS (1) TRAINING OF PERSONNEL, (2) FUNDING, (3) LEGISLATION, (4) HEALTH AND NUTRITIONAL PROGRAMS, AND (5) CURRICULUM DEVELOPMENT FOR MIGRANTS. TWO MIGRANT DEMONSTRATION PROJECTS DESCRIBED A NEW COMPREHENSIVE EDUCATIONAL PROGRAM FOR ALL MEMBERS OF THE MIGRANT FAMILY, AND THE DEVELOPMENT OF A NEW CURRICULUM AND STAFF DEVELOPMENT PROGRAM. THE THEME OF THE URBAN EDUCATION DISCUSSION WAS THE MODEL CITIES PROGRAM WHICH PROVIDES GRANTS AND TECHNICAL ASSISTANCE FOR CITIES TO DEVELOP ALL-INCLUSIVE PROBLEM-SOLVING PROGRAMS, INCLUDING EDUCATIONAL PROJECTS. CONCURRENT DISCUSSION GROUPS INCLUDED PRESENTATIONS BY THE OFFICE OF CIVIL RIGHTS OF HEW, THE LIBRARY SERVICES DIVISION OF HEW, AND THE LATIN AMERICAN RESEARCH AND SERVICE AGENCY. AN EVALUATION OF THE CONFERENCE, CONDUCTED BY THE SOUTHWEST EDU-

CATIONAL DEVELOPMENT LABORATORY, IS IN-CLUDED IN THE APPENDIX.

ACCN 001612

1879 AUTH **UHLENBERG, P.**
TITL THE CHANGING FAMILY PATTERNS OF BLACKS, CHICANOS, AND WHITES: 1969-70.
SRCE *RESEARCH PREVIEWS, 1974, 21(1), 1-7.*
INDX FERTILITY, MEXICAN AMERICAN, FAMILY STRUCTURE, CROSS CULTURAL, DEMOGRAPHIC, FEMALE, ADULTS, MARITAL STABILITY, REVIEW, MARRIAGE
ABST BASED UPON AN EXAMINATION OF DATA FROM THE 1960 AND 1970 U.S. CENSUS OF POPULATION, THIS REPORT ADDRESSES THE QUESTION: "HAVE THE SIGNIFICANT CHANGES IN FAMILY STRUCTURE AND POPULATION GROWTH IN THE 1960'S AFFECTED BLACKS AND CHICANOS IN THE SAME WAY AS WHITES?" DURING THIS PERIOD THE U.S. DIVORCE RATE ROSE FROM 16 TO 26 PER 1,000; THE MEDIAN AGE AT FIRST MARRIAGE ROSE FROM 20.3 TO 20.8 YEARS; AND THE NUMBER OF TOTAL BIRTHS EXPECTED DROPPED FROM 3.1 TO 2.6. AMONG WHITE FEMALES THERE WAS A 28% INCREASE IN THE PERCENTAGE OF SINGLES, A 32% INCREASE IN THE PERCENT OF FIRST MARRIAGES DISSOLVED, AND A 27% DECREASE IN THE NUMBER OF CHILDREN. INCREASES IN EDUCATIONAL LEVEL PARTIALLY ACCOUNTED FOR THE INCREASE IN SINGLENESS AND THE DECLINE IN FERTILITY, BUT NOT FOR THE INCREASE IN DIVORCE. BLACK FEMALES EXHIBITED DISTINCTLY DIFFERENT FAMILY-BUILDING PATTERNS, YET CHANGES SEEN DURING THE 1960'S WERE IN THE SAME DIRECTION AND MAGNITUDE AS AMONG WHITES. DIFFERENCES COULD NOT BE ATTRIBUTED PRIMARILY TO DIFFERING EDUCATIONAL LEVELS. OF THE THREE ETHNIC GROUPS, CHICANAS HAD THE HIGHEST PERCENTAGE MARRIED, WERE INTERMEDIATE IN THE PERCENTAGE OF MARRIAGES INTACT, AND MOST SIMILAR TO BLACKS IN THEIR LEVEL OF REPRODUCTION. CHICANAS EXPERIENCED DECLINING FERTILITY AND INCREASED MARITAL INSTABILITY, BUT SHOWED LITTLE CHANGE IN THE INCIDENCE OF MARRIAGE. IT IS CONCLUDED THAT EACH ETHNIC GROUP IS CONTINUING A DISTINCTIVE LIFE-CYCLE PATTERN, AND DIFFERENCES BETWEEN THEM ARE NOT DECREASING. 8 REFERENCES.

ACCN 001613

1880 AUTH **UHLENBERG, P.**
TITL DEMOGRAPHIC CORRELATES OF GROUP ACHIEVEMENT: CONTRASTING PATTERNS OF MEXICAN AMERICANS AND JAPANESE AMERICANS.
SRCE *DEMOGRAPHY, 1972, 9(1), 119-128.*
INDX FERTILITY, MEXICAN AMERICAN, FAMILY STRUCTURE, CROSS CULTURAL, ACHIEVEMENT MOTIVATION, MARITAL STABILITY, SCHOLASTIC ACHIEVEMENT, SOCIAL MOBILITY, DEMOGRAPHIC, EMPIRICAL
ABST TO EXPLAIN WHY JAPANESE AMERICANS (JA) HAVE ACHIEVED MORE RAPID UPWARD SOCIAL MOBILITY THAN MEXICAN AMERICANS (MA), THIS STUDY CONTRASTED PATTERNS OF FAMILY SIZE, FAMILY STABILITY, AND TIMING OF FAMILY FORMATION CHARACTERISTIC OF THESE TWO GROUPS. DEMOGRAPHIC DATA REVEAL THAT MA'S COMMONLY ARE YOUNG WHEN THEY MARRY, YOUNG WHEN THEY BEGIN CHILDBEARING, HAVE HIGH RATES OF REPRODUCTION, AND HAVE HIGH RATES OF MARITAL INSTABILITY. JA'S, IN CONTRAST, DISPLAY JUST THE OPPOSITE PATTERN OF BEHAVIOR ON EACH OF THESE VARIABLES. IT IS THEREFORE CONCLUDED THAT THE DEMOGRAPHIC ENVIRONMENT EXPERIENCED BY JA YOUTHS MAY BE MORE CONDUCIVE TO EDUCATIONAL AND ECONOMIC ACHIEVEMENT THAN THAT ENCOUNTERED BY MA YOUTHS. THIS CONCLUSION IS SUPPORTED BY RESEARCH WHICH INDICATES THAT FAMILY SIZE AND STABILITY SIGNIFICANTLY INFLUENCE CHILDREN'S FUTURE ACHIEVEMENT. THUS AMONG JA'S, THEIR SMALL FAMILY SIZE GIVES THEIR CHILDREN A DECIDED ADVANTAGE. CONVERSELY, MA'S LARGE FAMILIES TEND TO RETARD THEIR CHILDREN'S PROGRESS BY (1) PRODUCING CROWDED HOME ENVIRONMENTS, AND (2) REDUCING THE AMOUNT OF PARENT-CHILD INTERACTION WHICH COULD PROMOTE ACHIEVEMENT MOTIVATION IN THE CHILDREN. SECONDLY, THE MA'S EARLY MARRIAGE, CHILDBEARING PATTERNS, AND MARITAL INSTABILITY ACT TO REDUCE EDUCATIONAL AND OCCUPATIONAL OPPORTUNITIES AND ALSO HINDER THE DEVELOPMENT OF APPROACHES TO CHILDREARING DIFFERENT FROM THOSE THE PARENTS THEMSELVES EXPERIENCED AS CHILDREN. 18 REFERENCES.

ACCN 001614

1881 AUTH **UHLENBERG, P.**
TITL FERTILITY PATTERNS WITHIN THE MEXICAN-AMERICAN POPULATION.
SRCE *SOCIAL BIOLOGY, 1973, 20(1), 30-39.*
INDX FERTILITY, MEXICAN AMERICAN, FAMILY STRUCTURE, DEMOGRAPHIC, CROSS GENERATIONAL, SEX ROLES, SES, IMMIGRATION, MIGRATION, BIRTH CONTROL
ABST THE HIGH FERTILITY RATE OF MEXICAN AMERICANS IN COMPARISON TO OTHER RACIAL OR ETHNIC GROUPS IN THE U.S. IS ANALYZED IN TERMS OF GENERATIONAL TRENDS IN FERTILITY, SOCIOECONOMIC DIFFERENTIALS, AND DEGREE OF URBANIZATION. DATA INDICATE THAT EVEN AFTER THREE GENERATIONS IN THE U.S., MEXICAN AMERICANS HAVE REPRODUCTIVE LEVELS MORE CHARACTERISTIC OF NONINDUSTRIAL THAN INDUSTRIAL POPULATIONS. DATA REVEAL EXTREME VARIATIONS WITHIN THE MEXICAN AMERICAN POPULATION, WITH THE MIDDLE CLASS HAVING THE SAME SIZE FAMILIES AS OTHER WHITES. FINDINGS SUGGEST THAT IT IS NOT PRESENCE IN, BUT RATHER INVOLVEMENT IN AN URBAN, INDUSTRIAL SOCIETY WHICH HAS GREATEST EFFECT IN FORCING MODIFICATION IN REPRODUCTIVE BEHAVIOR. ABSENCE OF INFORMATION ON DESIRED FAMILY SIZE PREVENTS DETERMINATION OF HOW MUCH THE

HIGH FERTILITY OF THE LOWER CLASS RESULTS FROM INABILITY TO PREVENT UNWANTED PREGNANCIES. 17 REFERENCES. (NCMHI ABSTRACT)

ACCN 001615

1882 AUTH **UHLENBERG, P.**

TITL MARITAL INSTABILITY AMONG MEXICAN AMERICANS: FOLLOWING THE PATTERNS OF BLACKS?

SRCE *SOCIAL PROBLEMS, 1972, 20(1), 49-56.*

INDX MARITAL STABILITY, MEXICAN AMERICAN, FAMILY STRUCTURE, DEMOGRAPHIC, CROSS CULTURAL, ENVIRONMENTAL FACTORS, CROSS GENERATIONAL, FAMILY ROLES, CULTURAL FACTORS, SEX ROLES, ECONOMIC FACTORS, MARRIAGE, CALIFORNIA, TEXAS, SOUTHWEST, MALE

ABST WHILE EXISTING LITERATURE REPEATEDLY STATES THAT RATES OF MARITAL INSTABILITY ARE LOW AMONG MEXICAN AMERICANS (MA), DATA FROM THE 1960 CENSUS SUGGEST OTHERWISE. A COMPARISON OF SUBGROUPS DEFINED BY GENERATION AND PLACE OF RESIDENCE (CALIFORNIA OR TEXAS) INDICATES A TREND TOWARD RAPIDLY INCREASING RATES OF MARITAL INSTABILITY FOR MA'S. THIRD GENERATION MA'S LIVING IN CALIFORNIA HAVE A LEVEL OF MARITAL INSTABILITY CLOSELY APPROACHING THAT OF BLACKS. AS AMONG BLACKS, THE INABILITY OF MANY MEXICAN AMERICAN MALES TO ADEQUATELY PROVIDE FOR THEIR FAMILIES AT THE LEVEL THEY DEEM NECESSARY, DUE TO LOW WAGES AND WIDESPREAD UNEMPLOYMENT, APPEARS TO BE AN IMPORTANT SOURCE OF MARITAL STRAIN. WHILE INCREASING MARITAL INSTABILITY MAY BE VIEWED AS AN ADAPTATION TO THEIR CURRENTLY DEPRIVED CIRCUMSTANCES, IT IS SUGGESTED THAT THIS INCREASING INSTABILITY MAY HINDER THE GROUP'S FUTURE ECONOMIC ADVANCEMENT. 12 REFERENCES. (JOURNAL ABSTRACT)

ACCN 001616

1883 AUTH **ULIBARRI, H.**

TITL THE BICULTURAL MYTH AND THE EDUCATION OF THE MEXICAN AMERICAN.

SRCE *IN A. CASTANEDA, M. RAMIREZ III, C. E. CORTES & M. BARRERA (EDS.), MEXICAN AMERICANS AND EDUCATIONAL CHANGE. NEW YORK: ARNO PRESS, 1974, PP. 285-313.*

INDX CULTURAL PLURALISM, CULTURE, MEXICAN AMERICAN, DISCRIMINATION, BILINGUAL-BICULTURAL PERSONNEL, EDUCATION, ACCULTURATION, SELF CONCEPT, URBAN, RURAL, BILINGUALISM, PSYCHOSOCIAL ADJUSTMENT, ESSAY, EDUCATION, ETHNIC IDENTITY, POLICY

ABST IN VIEW OF THEIR MINORITY STATUS AND LIMITED POWERS, MEXICAN AMERICANS MUST COLLECTIVELY AND INDEPENDENTLY UTILIZE THE EXISTING KNOWLEDGE BASE TO DEFINE PROBLEMS AND CARRY OUT SOLUTIONS, PARTICULARLY IN THE AREA OF EDUCATION. HISTORICALLY, EDUCATIONAL PROBLEMS OF THE MEXICAN AMERICAN HAVE BEEN ATTRIBUTED TO RACIAL INFERIORITY, LANGUAGE BARRIERS, CULTURAL DIFFERENCES, AND POV-

ERTY. CURRENTLY THERE IS CONFUSION ABOUT THE CORRELATION BETWEEN CULTURAL AND LANGUAGE FACTORS AND ACADEMIC SUCCESS. ONE POINT IS THAT THE CLASSROOM ENVIRONMENT HAS NOT BEEN SUITABLE FOR THE NEEDS OF THE MEXICAN AMERICAN STUDENT, EVIDENCED BY HIGH DROPOUT RATES AND LOW ACHIEVEMENT LEVELS. SECONDLY, THE PRESENT SCHOOL SYSTEM IS SAID TO (1) HAVE A MIDDLE CLASS BIAS, (2) HAVE SOCIOCULTURALLY INSENSITIVE TEACHERS, (3) EMPLOY TEACHING METHODS OUTSIDE THE CONTEXT OF THE MEXICAN AMERICAN SOCIOCULTURE, (4) STRESS ACCULTURATION AND ASSIMILATION, OMITTING SIGNIFICANT ASPECTS OF MEXICAN AMERICAN CULTURE, AND THEREBY CREATING NEGATIVE SELF CONCEPTS, AND (5) REFLECT SOCIETAL CONSTRAINTS WHICH LIMIT MEXICAN AMERICANS' OPPORTUNITIES TO PARTICIPATE AND ADVANCE IN THE AMERICAN SOCIAL MILIEU. FINALLY, ATTEMPTS AT FUSING BICULTURAL WITH BILINGUAL EDUCATION HAVE BEEN FRUSTRATED BY THE INABILITY TO FORM A CONSENSUS ON THE DEFINITION OF BICULTURALISM. IT IS CONCLUDED THAT PROGRAMS MUST BE DEVELOPED THAT ENHANCE CULTURAL PLURALITY AND FOSTER FEELINGS OF MUTUAL UNDERSTANDING AND RESPECT AMONG MEMBERS OF DIFFERENT ETHNIC AND CULTURAL BACKGROUNDS. 7 REFERENCES.

ACCN 001617

1884 AUTH **ULIBARRI, H.**

TITL BILINGUAL EDUCATION: A HANDBOOK FOR EDUCATORS.

SRCE *ALBUQUERQUE, NEW MEXICO: UNIVERSITY OF NEW MEXICO, 1970. (ERIC DOCUMENT REPRODUCTION SERVICE NO. ED 038 078)*

INDX BILINGUALISM, BILINGUAL-BICULTURAL EDUCATION, BILINGUAL-BICULTURAL PERSONNEL, BIBLIOGRAPHY, ACCULTURATION, CULTURAL PLURALISM, CURRICULUM, LANGUAGE LEARNING, EDUCATIONAL COUNSELING, CULTURAL FACTORS, INSTRUCTIONAL TECHNIQUES, EDUCATIONAL MATERIALS, TEACHERS, SPANISH SURNAMED

ABST DESIGNED PRIMARILY TO AID ADMINISTRATORS, THIS COMPREHENSIVE HANDBOOK ON BILINGUAL EDUCATION PRESENTS PROGRAM GUIDELINES, PROCEDURES FOR PROGRAM INITIATION, AND AN ANNOTATED BIBLIOGRAPHY SELECTED FROM REPORTS THAT WERE REVIEWED AND ANALYZED DURING THE COURSE OF THE PROJECT. BASED ON ANALYSES OF SOME 2,000 STUDIES AND REPORTS ON BILINGUAL AND BICULTURAL EDUCATION, THE WORK STRESSES SOCIAL, CULTURAL, AND PSYCHOLOGICAL CONSIDERATIONS IN SECTIONS TREATING: (1) OBJECTIVES OF BILINGUAL EDUCATION PROGRAMS; (2) PROGRAM DESCRIPTION; (3) TEACHER ROLE; (4) MATERIALS; (5) EVALUATION; (6) COUNSELING; AND (7) PROGRAM INITIATION AND IMPLEMENTATION. 212 ANNOTATED REFERENCES ARE PRESENTED IN THE APPENDIX. 690 REFERENCES. (ERIC ABSTRACT MODIFIED)

ACCN 001618

1885 AUTH **ULIBARRI, H.**

TITL THE EFFECTS OF CULTURAL DIFFERENCES IN THE EDUCATION OF SPANISH AMERICANS.

SRCE *UNPUBLISHED MANUSCRIPT, COLLEGE OF EDUCATION, NEW MEXICO UNIVERSITY, 1958. (ERIC DOCUMENT REPRODUCTION SERVICE NO. ED 019 156)*

INDX SPANISH SURNAMED, ACCULTURATION, CULTURAL FACTORS, EDUCATION, CAPITALISM, CULTURAL CHANGE, CULTURAL PLURALISM, CULTURE, CURANDERISMO, HISTORY, DISCRIMINATION, EQUAL OPPORTUNITY, ETHNIC IDENTITY, FAMILY STRUCTURE, FOLK MEDICINE, MARITAL STABILITY, POLITICAL POWER, RELIGION, SOCIAL MOBILITY, NEW MEXICO, SOUTHWEST, VALUES

ABST MANY SPANISH AMERICANS IN NEW MEXICO EXPERIENCE DIFFICULTIES TRACEABLE TO DIFFERING VALUES IN THE SPANISH AMERICAN AND AMERICAN CULTURES. THESE DIFFERENCES ARE EVIDENT IN THE AREAS OF POLITICAL ATTITUDES, EDUCATIONAL ATTAINMENT, RELIGIOUS ATTITUDES, HEALTH PRACTICES, RECREATIONAL ACTIVITIES, AND FAMILY LIFE. POLITICALLY, BECAUSE OF THE TRADITIONAL TWO-CLASS SYSTEM ("PEON" AND "PATRON") AND BECAUSE OF A PATTERN OF ACCOMODATION TO THE ANGLO, SPANISH AMERICANS HAVE NOT REALIZED OR EXERCISED THEIR VOTING POWERS. IN EDUCATION, SPANISH AMERICANS HAVE NOT ENJOYED EQUALIZED LEARNING ENVIRONMENTS BECAUSE THEIR CULTURAL ORIENTATION HAS BEEN IGNORED BY CURRICULA DEVELOPERS AND TEACHER TRAINING PROGRAMS. WITH RELIGION, THE TRADITIONAL SPANISH AMERICAN GOAL OF LIVING FOR A REWARD IN THE NEXT LIFE CLASHES WITH THE ANGLO CALVINISTIC ETHIC. IN HEALTH PRACTICES, REJECTION OF ANGLO MEDICAL CARE BY RURAL SPANISH AMERICANS CAN BE TRACED TO A TRADITION OF PHYSICAL AND MENTAL HEALTH CARE FOLK MEDICINE. AS IN ALL PHASES OF THE SPANISH AMERICAN CULTURE IN NEW MEXICO TODAY, THE FAMILY UNIT IS ON A VAST CONTINUUM OF ACCULTURATION IN WHICH THE TRADITIONAL EXTENDED FAMILY IS DISINTEGRATING. THE PHENOMENON OF THE WORKING WOMAN, AND THE ADVENT OF DIVORCE, PREVIOUSLY UNHEARD OF IN THIS CULTURE, ARE SEEN AS CAUSALLY RELATED. THIS MONOGRAPH BEGINS WITH AN HISTORICAL BACKGROUND OF NEW MEXICO AND CONCLUDES WITH AN EXTENSIVE BIBLIOGRAPHY. 42 REFERENCES.

ACCN 001619

1886 AUTH **ULIBARRI, H.**

TITL SOCIAL AND ATTITUDINAL CHARACTERISTICS OF MIGRANT AND EX-MIGRANT WORKERS— NEW MEXICO, COLORADO, ARIZONA AND TEXAS.

SRCE *UNPUBLISHED MANUSCRIPT, NEW MEXICO UNIVERSITY, 1965. (ERIC DOCUMENT REPRODUCTION SERVICE NO. ED 011 215)*

INDX SES, MIGRATION, ATTITUDES, CULTURAL FACTORS, SPANISH SURNAMED, FARM LABORERS, FAMILY STRUCTURE, SELF CONCEPT, TIME ORIENTATION

ABST THIS 79-PAGE MONOGRAPH IS A MORE DETAILED REPORT ON THE STUDY CITED BELOW (SEE ULIBARRI, 1971). ITEMS IN THIS REPORT WHICH ARE EXCLUDED FROM THE ABBREVIATED 1971 VERSION ARE: (1) 9 TABLES; (2) A LENGTHY DISCUSSION OF THE STUDY'S IMPLICATIONS FOR EDUCATION OF SPANISH-SPEAKING MIGRANT ADULTS; (3) THE STUDY'S QUESTIONNAIRE; AND (4) DETAILS OF THE STUDY'S 13 FACTOR SCALE OF SOCIAL AND ATTITUDINAL CHARACTERISTICS. 7 REFERENCES.

ACCN 001620

1887 AUTH **ULIBARRI, H.**

TITL SOCIAL AND ATTITUDINAL CHARACTERISTICS OF SPANISH-SPEAKING MIGRANT AND EX-MIGRANT WORKERS IN THE SOUTHWEST.

SRCE *IN N. N. WAGNER AND M. J. HAUG (EDS.), CHICANOS: SOCIAL AND PSYCHOLOGICAL PERSPECTIVES. SAINT LOUIS: C. V. MOSBY CO., 1971, PP. 164-170.*

INDX SPANISH SURNAMED, ACCULTURATION, SES, MEXICAN AMERICAN, MEXICAN, ATTITUDES, EMPIRICAL, MIGRATION, FARM LABORERS, SELF CONCEPT, RELIGION, TIME ORIENTATION, MIGRANTS

ABST THE PURPOSE OF THIS RESEARCH REPORT WAS TO COLLECT SOCIOLOGICAL DATA ON THE ATTITUDINAL ORIENTATIONS OF MIGRANT WORKERS. THE SAMPLE CONSISTED OF 65 PERSONS OF SPANISH AMERICAN HERITAGE. NO ATTEMPT AT RANDOMIZATION WAS MADE IN SELECTING THE SAMPLE. DATA WERE COLLECTED USING AN OPEN-ENDED TYPE INTERVIEW SCHEDULE. THOSE ATTITUDINAL CHARACTERISTICS SPECIFICALLY ISOLATED FOR STUDY WERE FAMILY, HEALTH, ECONOMICS, GOVERNMENT, CHILDREN, RELIGION, AND RECREATION. CONCLUSIONS WERE DRAWN THAT: (1) THE SAMPLE SHOWED PRESENT-TIME REWARD EXPECTATIONS IN ALL AREAS; (2) GREAT TIMIDITY AND PASSIVITY WAS SHOWN IN THE AREAS OF EDUCATION, HEALTH, AND ECONOMICS; (3) SATISFACTION WAS SHOWN IN FAMILY LIFE ALTHOUGH THE NUCLEAR FAMILY HAD IN MOST CASES REPLACED THE TRADITIONAL EXTENDED FAMILY; (4) THEY WERE FUTILITARIAN ABOUT THE EDUCATION OF THEIR CHILDREN; (5) THEY SHOWED TENDENCIES OF RESIGNATION TO THEIR ECONOMIC STATUS; AND (6) THE SAMPLE SHOWED DEFINITE ETHNOCENTRIC TENDENCIES. 5 REFERENCES. (ERIC ABSTRACT)

ACCN 001621

1888 AUTH **ULIBARRI, M.**

TITL AMBIENTE BILINGUE: PROFESSIONALS, PARENTS, AND CHILDREN.

SRCE *IN A. CASTANEDA, M. RAMIREZ III, C. E. CORTES & M. BARRERA (EDS.), MEXICAN AMERICANS AND EDUCATIONAL CHANGE. NEW YORK: ARNO PRESS, 1974, PP. 373-386.*

INDX BILINGUAL-BICULTURAL EDUCATION, BILINGUALISM, MEXICAN AMERICAN, EDUCATION, LANGUAGE LEARNING, CULTURAL PLURALISM, ACCULTURATION, BILINGUAL-BICULTURAL PERSONNEL, PARENTAL INVOLVEMENT, ESSAY, POLICY

ABST UNFORTUNATELY, BILINGUAL EDUCATION HAS OFTEN BEEN USED AS AN EXCUSE FOR NOT IMPLEMENTING BICULTURAL EDUCATION, EVEN THOUGH BOTH ARE ESSENTIAL COMPONENTS OF A TRULY BICULTURAL EDUCATIONAL SYSTEM. THE BASIC POINT IS THAT BICULTURALISM IMPLIES MUCH MORE THAN BILINGUALISM, AS IT INDICATES THE ABILITY TO OPERATE FULLY (NOT JUST VERBALLY) IN TWO CULTURES. MOREOVER, BICULTURAL EDUCATION CAN BE A STEPPING STONE, LEADING TO THE TRANSFORMATION OF THE PRESENT SOCIETY INTO A CULTURALLY PLURALISTIC SOCIETY. BILINGUAL EDUCATION ALONE CANNOT ACCOMPLISH THIS. WHAT IS REQUIRED IS A BASIC RESTRUCTURING OF THE EDUCATIONAL SYSTEM TO ENSURE THE COEXISTENCE OF TWO CULTURES; AND TO ACHIEVE THAT GOAL, THE TOTAL SCHOOL "AMBIENTE" (ENVIRONMENT) MUST BE TAKEN INTO ACCOUNT. 5 REFERENCES.

ACCN 001622

1889 AUTH **UPHAM, W. K., & WRIGHT, D. E.**
TITL POVERTY AMONG SPANISH AMERICANS IN TEXAS: LOW-INCOME FAMILIES IN A MINORITY GROUP (DEPARTMENTAL INFORMATION REPORT NO. 2).
SRCE *COLLEGE STATION, TEXAS: DEPARTMENT OF AGRICULTURAL ECONOMICS AND SOCIOLOGY, TEXAS A AND M UNIVERSITY, SEPTEMBER 1966. (ERIC DOCUMENT REPRODUCTION SERVICE NO. ED 024 520)*
INDX POVERTY, SES, MEXICAN AMERICAN, FAMILY STRUCTURE, ECONOMIC FACTORS, TEXAS, SOUTHWEST
ABST AN ANALYSIS OF 1960 CENSUS DATA IN TEXAS FOR PERSONS WITH SPANISH SURNAMES REVEALS A SIGNIFICANTLY HIGH RATE OF POVERTY (AS INDICATED BY AN ANNUAL FAMILY INCOME OF UNDER $3,000) WHEN COMPARED WITH OTHER ETHNIC GROUPS AND NATIONAL AVERAGES. IN PARTICULAR, A LARGE NUMBER OF MEXICAN AMERICAN FAMILIES WERE EXPERIENCING EXTREME POVERTY (INCOMES BELOW $2,000). AN ANALYSIS BY COUNTY SHOWS GREATER ECONOMIC DISADVANTAGE IN THE SOUTHERN PART OF THE STATE WHERE THE CONCENTRATION OF MEXICAN AMERICANS IS HIGHEST. THE POVERTY RATES OF MEXICAN AMERICANS AND THE REST OF THE POPULATION WERE SIMILAR IN THAT THE POVERTY RATES WERE MOST SEVERE FOR FAMILIES IN RURAL AREAS. IN ADDITION, THE PERCENTAGE OF MEXICAN AMERICAN FAMILIES WITH LOW INCOMES WAS HIGHER THE GREATER THE PROPORTION OF MEXICAN AMERICANS IN THE POPULATION. THE STUDY ALSO NOTES THAT MEXICAN AMERICANS IN TEXAS HAVE A LOWER LEVEL OF EDUCATIONAL ATTAINMENT AND GREATER FAMILY SIZE THAN BOTH ANGLO AMERICAN AND NON-WHITE GROUPS. ASSUMING A CAUSAL RELATIONSHIP BETWEEN POVERTY AND LOW EDUCATION, THE REPORT WARNS THAT NO REAL PROGRESS IS LIKELY TO BE MADE AGAINST THE PROBLEM UNLESS A WAY CAN BE FOUND TO RAISE GENERAL EDUCATIONAL LEVELS. 29 REFERENCES. (ERIC ABSTRACT MODIFIED)

ACCN 001624

1890 AUTH **URBAN ASSOCIATES INC.**
TITL A STUDY OF SELECTED SOCIO-ECONOMIC CHARACTERISTICS OF ETHNIC MINORITIES BASED ON THE 1970 CENSUS. VOLUME I: AMERICANS OF SPANISH ORIGIN (REPORT NO. HEW-PUB-(05)-75-120).
SRCE *WASHINGTON, D.C.: OFFICE OF THE ASSISTANT SECRETARY FOR PLANNING AND EVALUATION, 1974. (ERIC DOCUMENT REPRODUCTION SERVICE NO. ED 107 411)*
INDX SES, DEMOGRAPHIC, MEXICAN AMERICAN, CUBAN, PUERTO RICAN-M, SPANISH SURNAMED, ECONOMIC FACTORS, FERTILITY, FAMILY STRUCTURE, HOUSING, ENVIRONMENTAL FACTORS
ABST THIS REPORT IS THE FIRST IN A FOUR-VOLUME STUDY OF THE MAJOR BARRIERS TO THE DELIVERY OF CULTURALLY RELEVANT DHEW SERVICES TO PERSONS OF ETHNIC-MINORITY GROUP STATUS. IT FOCUSES ON AMERICANS OF SPANISH ORIGIN, AS DESIGNATED BY THE CENSUS BUREAU IN 1970—I.E., MEXICAN AMERICANS; PUERTO RICANS; CUBAN AMERICANS; CENTRAL AND SOUTH AMERICANS; AND "OTHER" SPANISH (THOSE PERSONS WHOSE FAMILIES ORIGINATED FROM SPAIN OR ELSE WHO WERE LIVING IN THE U.S. PRIOR TO 1848). DETAILED SOCIOECONOMIC DATA ON THE THREE LARGEST GROUPS (MEXICAN AMERICANS, PUERTO RICANS, AND CUBANS) WERE OBTAINED FROM CENSUS BUREAU PUBLICATIONS BASED UPON THE 1970 CENSUS. SECONDLY, NATIONAL AND LOCAL DATA ARE PRESENTED, FOCUSING ON SUCH CHARACTERISTICS AS IMMIGRATION AND IN-MIGRATION, GEOGRAPHIC AND AGE DISTRIBUTIONS, NATIVITY, FAMILY STRUCTURE, EDUCATION, EMPLOYMENT, INCOME, AND POVERTY. FINALLY, DATA FROM SELECTED LOCAL AREAS ARE PRESENTED TO HIGHLIGHT THOSE SITUATIONS WHEREIN LOCAL DATA DIFFER MARKEDLY FROM OR ARE OTHERWISE NOTABLE IN COMPARISON TO THE NATIONAL PICTURE. ALL DATA ARE SUMMARIZED IN TABULAR AND CHART FORM. 20 REFERENCES.

ACCN 001625

1891 AUTH **UZZELL, D.**
TITL SUSTO REVISTED: ILLNESS AS STRATEGIC ROLE.
SRCE *AMERICAN ETHNOLOGIST, 1974, 1(2), 369-378.*
INDX FOLK MEDICINE, SEX ROLES, SYMPTOMATOLOGY, HEALTH, CULTURAL FACTORS, ADULTS, DISEASE, MEXICAN, STRESS, FEMALE, MALE
ABST AS PART OF A GENERAL INQUIRY INTO ILLNESS BELIEFS IN THE MEXICAN VILLAGE OF SAN ANDRES ZAUTLA, OAXACA, THE NATURE AND OCCURRENCE OF SUSTO (I.E., "FRIGHT SICKNESS) WAS EXPLORED. IT WAS HYPOTHESIZED THAT THE SUSTO SYNDROME (CHARACTERIZED BY LISTLESSNESS, LOSS OF APPETITE, AND WITHDRAWAL FROM SOCIAL INTERACTION) WOULD HAVE A SOCIAL-PSYCHOLOGICAL BASIS, BEING THE CONSEQUENCE OF AN INDIVIDUAL'S INABILITY TO

MEET SOCIETAL EXPECTATIONS; SECONDLY, THE SEX WHICH EXPERIENCED MORE INTRA-CULTURAL STRESS WOULD EVIDENCE A GREATER SUSCEPTIBILITY TO SUSTO. DATA GATHERING BEGAN IN 1968 WITH FORMAL IN-TERVIEWS IN WHICH VILLAGERS LISTED THE NAMES, SYMPTOMS, CAUSES, AND CURES OF AS MANY ILLNESSES AS POSSIBLE. LISTS OF ILLNESSES THEREBY WERE GENERATED, AND THEN INFORMANTS WERE ASKED TO SORT THESE ACCORDING TO SUCH CRITERIA AS THE DANGEROUSNESS AND THE COST OF EACH ILLNESS. FINALLY, A LIST OF QUESTIONS ABOUT THESE ILLNESSES WAS PREPARED AND ADMIN-ISTERED TO A SAMPLE OF WOMEN (N=29) AND TO TWO GROUPS OF SCHOOL CHILDREN (N=18). DATA REVEAL THAT SUSTO IS MUCH MORE COMMON AMONG WOMEN THAN MEN (75% OF REPORTED SUSTO CASES WERE SUF-FERED BY WOMEN). CHILDREN WERE ALSO MORE LIKELY THAN MEN TO SUFFER SUSTO. THE GREATER SUSCEPTIBILITY OF WOMEN TO SUSTO APPEARS TO BE DUE TO TWO FAC-TORS: (1) THE PASSIVITY CHARACTERISTIC OF SUSTO IS A LESS EXTREME CHANGE OF IDEN-TITIES FOR WOMEN THAN MEN; AND (2) THE STRATEGIC ADVANTAGE FOR WOMEN TO AS-SUME THE SUSTO ROLE, ENABLING THEIR AC-QUISITION OF HOUSEHOLD DOMINANCE. SUSTO IS DESCRIBED AS A STRATEGIC "ILL-NESS ROLE" CHARACTERIZED BY FLEXIBLE CAUSAL FACTORS AND SYMPTOMS WHICH PROVIDE A PSYCHOLOGICAL EXPLANATION OF DEVIANT BEHAVIOR. THUS, AS WAS HY-POTHESIZED, SUSTO IS REPORTED TO IMPLY ROLE DISSATISFACTION RATHER THAN ROLE STRESS. 18 REFERENCES.

ACCN   001626

1892 AUTH   **VACA, N. C.**
TITL   THE MEXICAN AMERICAN IN THE SOCIAL SCI-ENCES 1912-1970. PART II: 1936-1970.
SRCE   *EL GRITO, 1970, 4(1), 17-51.*
INDX   MEXICAN AMERICAN, REVIEW, SOCIAL SCI-ENCES, CULTURAL PLURALISM, INTELLIGENCE TESTING, CULTURAL FACTORS, CULTURE, HIS-TORY
ABST   THE SOCIOLOGICAL, ANTHROPOLOGICAL, AND PSYCHOLOGICAL LITERATURE PERTAINING TO THE MEXICAN AMERICAN (MA) FROM 1932-1970 IS REVIEWED. THREE THEORETICAL THE-SES ARE EXAMINED AS CAUSAL EXPLANA-TIONS FOR THE SOCIAL ILLS THAT PLAGUE THE MA. FIRST, THE BIOLOGICAL DETERMINIST THEORY SUPPORTED THE NOTION OF THE IN-HERENT MENTAL INFERIORITY OF MA'S. SEC-OND, AFTER 1935 THE STRUCTURAL-ENVIRON-MENTAL DETERMINISM THEORY POSTULATED THAT THE CAUSES OF SOCIAL PROBLEMS OF THE MA COULD BE DIRECTLY TRACED TO THE ECONOMIC AND SOCIAL STRUCTURE OF AMERICAN SOCIETY. THIS POSTURE CALLED FOR A REEXAMINATION OF THE NATURE OF IN-TELLIGENCE TESTS (IQ), AND AN INQUIRY INTO THE POSSIBLE ENVIRONMENTAL INFLUENCES ON EDUCATION AND IQ TEST SCORES FOR THE MA CHILD. THIRD, ANOTHER THEORETICAL PERSPECTIVE TO GAIN POPULARITY AFTER

1935 WAS CULTURAL DETERMINISM. THIS VIEW POSTULATED THAT THE CULTURAL VALUES OF THE MA WERE THE MAIN CAUSE OF THE SO-CIAL ILLS ENCOUNTERED BY THIS ETHNIC GROUP. THE STRUGGLE FOR ASCENDANCY OCCURRED AMONG THESE THREE PERSPEC-TIVES WITH THE ULTIMATE TRIUMPH OF CUL-TURAL DETERMINISM PREVAILING AS THE DOMINANT ANALYTICAL APPROACH. WITH THIS THEORETICAL VIEW, SOCIAL WELFARE AGEN-CIES, THE POLICE, HOSPITALS, SCHOOLS, UNI-VERSITIES, AND NUMEROUS OTHER INSTITU-TIONS WHERE MA'S WERE FORCED INTO CONTACT, WERE COMPLETELY ABSOLVED OF ANY OPPRESSIVE POLICIES, LEAVING THE MA TO STAND IN RELIEF AS THE SOLE PERPETRA-TOR OF HIS ECONOMIC, SOCIAL, AND POLITI-CAL PLIGHT. 71 REFERENCES.
ACCN   001628

1893 AUTH   **VACA, N. C.**
TITL   THE MEXICAN AMERICAN IN THE SOCIAL SCI-ENCES 1912-1970. PART I: 1912-1935.
SRCE   *EL GRITO, 1969, 3(1), 3-24.*
INDX   MEXICAN AMERICAN, REVIEW, SOCIAL SCI-ENCES, IMMIGRATION, HISTORY
ABST   A REVIEW OF SOCIAL SCIENCE LITERATURE PERTAINING TO THE MEXICAN AMERICAN IS PRESENTED. IN PSYCHOLOGY THE FIRST YEARS OF CONCERN WERE CENTERED AROUND THE QUESTION OF THE PRESUMED INFERIORITY OF THE MEXICAN IMMIGRANT VERSUS THE DELE-TERIOUS EFFECTS OF THE SOCIAL CONDI-TIONS ON THE MEASUREMENT OF INTELLI-GENCE. SOCIOLOGY CONCERNED ITSELF WITH THE SOURCES OF THE SOCIAL ILLS THAT PLAGUED THE MEXICAN IMMIGRANTS, WITH ONE SEGMENT OF SOCIAL SCIENTISTS CLAIM-ING THE SOURCE TO BE THE CULTURAL HERI-TAGE OF THE MEXICAN WHILE ANOTHER SEG-MENT ACCUSED THE SOCIAL AND ECONOMIC CONDITION IN WHICH THE MEXICAN FOUND HIMSELF. THE DIVISIONS THAT OCCURRED IN THESE EARLY SOCIAL SCIENCE STUDIES ON THE MEXICAN AMERICAN, PARTICULARLY IN SOCIOLOGY, WERE TO BE MAINTAINED AND ENLARGED UPON THROUGH THE SUBSE-QUENT 35 YEARS BY SOCIAL SCIENTISTS. 24 REFERENCES.
ACCN   001627

1894 AUTH   **VALDES, T. M., & BAXTER, J. C.**
TITL   THE SOCIAL READJUSTMENT RATING QUES-TIONNAIRE: A STUDY OF CUBAN EXILES.
SRCE   *JOURNAL OF PSYCHOSOMATIC RESEARCH, 1976, 20(3), 231-236.*
INDX   ACCULTURATION, ADULTS, CROSS CULTURAL, CULTURAL FACTORS, EMPIRICAL, CUBAN, SES, SURVEY, TEXAS, SOUTHWEST, SOCIAL STRUC-TURE, STRESS, PSYCHOSOCIAL ADJUSTMENT
ABST   A REVISED FORM OF THE HOLMES AND RAHE SCALE WAS ADMINISTERED TO A GROUP OF 117 CUBAN EXILES. THE SUBJECTS PRE-SENTED SPECIAL CHARACTERISTICS AND LIFE EXPERIENCES FOR CROSS-CULTURAL COM-PARISON WITH 394 AMERICANS. THE CUBAN SAMPLE CONSISTED OF PERSONS WHO CAME TO THE U.S. AFTER 1958, AND WHO WERE 15

YEARS OR OLDER WHEN THEY EMIGRATED; 83% ARE IN THE PROFESSIONAL CATEGORY. THE DATA COLLECTION CONSISTED OF HOME INTERVIEWS CONDUCTED BY A SINGLE RESEARCHER, GENERALLY FAMILIAR WITH THE SAMPLE INTERVIEWEES. THE RESULTS OF ITEM RATINGS SUPPORT HOLMES AND RAHE'S HYPOTHESIS THAT PSYCHOSOCIAL PHENOMENA CAN BE EVALUATED ACROSS INDIVIDUALS AND ACROSS CULTURES. THE CUBAN AND AMERICAN ITEM RATINGS WERE REMARKABLY SIMILAR—A FACT POSSIBLY INFLUENCED BY THE EFFECTS OF SEVERAL YEARS OF ACCULTURATION AND BY THE PREDOMINANCE OF WELL-EDUCATED, MIDDLE-CLASS INDIVIDUALS IN THE CUBAN SAMPLE. IN GENERAL, FOR THE CUBANS, AREAS OF STRESS IN CULTURAL READJUSTMENT TO THE U.S. CENTER AROUND SEPARATION FROM THE HOMELAND AND FAMILY AS WELL AS CULTURAL DIFFERENCES IN FAMILY PATTERNS IN THE U.S. THE CUBANS DID NOT FEEL UNDULY REJECTED BY AMERICANS AND EXHIBITED A FAVORABLE EVALUATION OF THE SECOND CULTURE. REASONS FOR THIS PHENOMENON ARE DISCUSSED. 7 REFERENCES.

ACCN   002255

1895 AUTH   **VALDEZ, S. M.**
TITL   AN EXPLORATORY STUDY OF CHICANO PARENT PERCEPTIONS OF SCHOOL AND THE EDUCATION OF THEIR CHILDREN IN TWO OREGON COMMUNITY SETTINGS (DOCTORAL DISSERTATION, UNIVERSITY OF OREGON, 1974).
SRCE   *DISSERTATION ABSTRACTS INTERNATIONAL, 1974, 35(8), 4881A. (UNIVERSITY MICROFILMS NO. 75-3927.)*
INDX   MEXICAN AMERICAN, PARENTAL INVOLVEMENT, ATTITUDES, EDUCATIONAL ASSESSMENT, COMMUNITY, EDUCATION, ADULTS, DISCRIMINATION, OREGON
ABST   THIS STUDY CHALLENGES THE CLAIM THAT CHICANO PARENTS HAVE LITTLE TO OFFER THE SCHOOLS OR TO THE EDUCATION OF THEIR CHILDREN, AND INSTEAD CONTENDS THAT THESE PARENTS HAVE BEEN LARGELY IGNORED BY SCHOOLS ABOUT THEIR POTENTIAL ROLE IN THE EDUCATION PROCESS. 50 CHICANO PARENTS IN TWO RURAL OREGON COMMUNITIES WERE INTERVIEWED, AND ALL OF THEM EXPRESSED GREAT INTEREST AND CONCERN ABOUT THE EDUCATION OF THEIR CHILDREN. IN PARTICULAR, THE MAJORITY WERE ANXIOUS ABOUT THE HIGH RATE OF FAILURE OF THEIR CHILDREN IN THE UPPER GRADES. ALL PARENTS REPORTED HAVING RECEIVED SOME SORT OF COMMUNICATION INVITING THEIR SCHOOL PARTICIPATION, BUT MOST SPOKE OF BEING RELATIVELY UNINVOLVED AND UNINFORMED BECAUSE OF A LACK OF BILINGUAL SCHOOL PERSONNEL. PARENTS FROM BOTH COMMUNITIES COMPLAINED OF NEGATIVE PREJUDGMENTS BY SCHOOL OFFICIALS OF THEIR CHILDREN, ABUSES OF SUSPENSION POLICIES, AND OTHER BIASED APPLICATIONS OF SCHOOL RULES AND REGULATIONS. MOST REPORTED THAT THEIR EFFORTS TO CORRECT THESE ABUSES HAD RESULTED IN DISCOURAGEMENT. ALL PARENTS STATED THAT THEIR

OWN CULTURAL BACKGROUND AND EXPERIENCES WERE AN IMPORTANT ORIENTATION WHICH THEY WANTED THEIR CHILDREN TO RETAIN. THEY HOPED THAT MORE OF THE SCHOOL STAFF WOULD LEARN TO RESPECT THIS ORIENTATION. 90 REFERENCES.

ACCN   001629

1896 AUTH   **VALENCIA, A. A.**
TITL   BILINGUAL EDUCATION: A QUEST FOR BILINGUAL SURVIVAL.
SRCE   *IN A. CASTANEDA, M. RAMIREZ III, C. E. CORTES & M. BARRERA (EDS.), MEXICAN AMERICANS AND EDUCATIONAL CHANGE. NEW YORK: ARNO PRESS, 1974, PP. 345-362.*
INDX   BILINGUALISM, MEXICAN AMERICAN, BILINGUAL-BICULTURAL EDUCATION, LANGUAGE LEARNING, COGNITIVE DEVELOPMENT, ACCULTURATION, SES, CURRICULUM, INSTRUCTIONAL TECHNIQUES, TEACHERS, EDUCATION, ETHNIC IDENTITY, ESSAY
ABST   IF MEXICAN AMERICAN CULTURAL HERITAGE IS TO SURVIVE, BILINGUAL-BICULTURAL EDUCATION IS ESSENTIAL AND PUBLIC RESISTANCE TO IT MUST BE OVERCOME. COGNITIVE RESEARCH SUPPORTS THE PRACTICE OF INSTRUCTION IN A STUDENT'S FIRST LANGUAGE UNTIL HE IS FUNCTIONAL IN A SECOND. FURTHERMORE, BILINGUAL EDUCATION DEVELOPS COMMUNICATION SKILLS ACADEMICALLY AND ECONOMICALLY ADVANTAGEOUS TO BOTH ENGLISH AND SPANISH SPEAKERS. SEVERAL MODELS OF BILINGUAL EDUCATION ARE PRESENTED, AND THE SELECTION OF A MODEL CORRESPONDING TO THE PROFICIENCY LEVEL OF THE STUDENTS IS EMPHASIZED. THE TEACHING OF ENGLISH AS A SECOND LANGUAGE HAS BEEN USED IN THE PAST TO SHAPE IMMIGRANTS INTO THE ANGLO AMERICAN CULTURAL MOLD, ACCOMPANIED BY THE PHASING OUT OF THE NATIVE LANGUAGE. THE TIME HAS COME FOR THE RECOGNITION OF BILINGUALISM AS AN ADVANTAGE, NOT A HANDICAP. IN PARTICULAR, THE USE OF TWO LANGUAGES IS VERY APPROPRIATE IN THE MEXICAN AMERICAN AND NATIVE AMERICAN CULTURAL ENVIRONMENT OF THE SOUTHWEST. IN CONCLUSION, SINCE BILINGUALISM-BICULTURALISM SERVES TO PROMOTE GROUP IDENTITY, SELF-ESTEEM, AND CULTURAL PRIDE, DEMOCRACY MUST ALLOW FOR CULTURAL PLURALISM AND THE USE OF LANGUAGE AS A MEANS OF PERPETUATING AN ETHNIC GROUP'S CULTURE. 16 REFERENCES.

ACCN   001630

1897 AUTH   **VALENCIA-WEBER, G.**
TITL   A MODEL FOR PROVIDING PSYCHOLOGY GRADUATE TRAINING FOR HISPANICS.
SRCE   *PAPER PRESENTED AT THE NATIONAL HISPANIC CONFERENCE ON FAMILIES, SPONSORED BY THE NATIONAL COALITION OF HISPANIC MENTAL HEALTH AND HUMAN SERVICES ORGANIZATIONS, HOUSTON, OCTOBER 1978.*
INDX   HIGHER EDUCATION, COLLEGE STUDENTS, ESSAY, REPRESENTATION, PROGRAM EVALUATION, PROFESSIONAL TRAINING, CROSS CULTURAL, MENTAL HEALTH PROFESSION,

MIDWEST, OKLAHOMA, DEMOGRAPHIC, FINANCING, EDUCATIONAL COUNSELING

ABST A METHODOLOGY USED IN THE GRADUATE PSYCHOLOGY PROGRAM AT OKLAHOMA STATE UNIVERSITY (OSU) TO IDENTIFY, RECRUIT, AND RETAIN HISPANIC AND OTHER MINORITY STUDENTS IS PRESENTED. THE PROGRAM STRUCTURE—INCLUDING PROGRAM STAFF, RECRUITMENT PROCEDURES, ADMISSION PROCEDURES, AND POST-ADMISSION SERVICES—IS DESCRIBED IN DETAIL. OBSTACLES FOR THE PROGRAM INCLUDE THE TENDENCY FOR HISPANIC COLLEGE STUDENTS TO AVOID SCIENCE AND MATH CLASSES NECESSARY FOR ADMISSION TO GRADUATE PSYCHOLOGY PROGRAMS, THE LACK OF FINANCIAL AID FOR MINORITY GRADUATE STUDENTS, THE TENDENCY FOR EDUCATORS AND OTHER PLANNERS AT THE NATIONAL LEVEL TO FOCUS ON HISPANICS IN THE SOUTHWEST AND IGNORE THOSE IN THE MIDWEST, AND THE LACK OF MINORITY FACULTY. NEVERTHELESS, BY ITS STRONG COMMITMENT AND ATTENTION TO THE SPECIAL NEEDS OF MINORITY STUDENTS, OSU'S PSYCHOLOGY PROGRAM HAS SUCCEEDED IN RAISING MINORITY STUDENT ENROLLMENT TO 23% (20 STUDENTS). OF THESE, SEVEN STUDENTS ARE HISPANICS ENROLLED IN THE DOCTORATE PROGRAM. SUPPLEMENTING THE REPORT, PROVIDING SUPPORT FOR THE VALUE OF OSU'S PROGRAM, ARE NATIONAL STATISTICAL DATA WHICH DOCUMENT THE NEED FOR MORE HISPANIC GRADUATE STUDENTS AND PROFESSIONALS IN PSYCHOLOGY. 8 REFERENCES.

ACCN 002517

1898 AUTH **VALENCIA-WEBER, G.**

TITL TRANSRACIAL COMMUNICATION LITERATURE AS A GUIDE FOR OPERATING A MINORITY RECRUITMENT PROGRAM.

SRCE *PAPER PRESENTED AT THE ANNUAL MEETING OF THE WESTERN SPEECH COMMUNICATION ASSOCIATION, SAN FRANCISCO, NOVEMBER 1976.*

INDX DISCRIMINATION, EDUCATIONAL COUNSELING, INTERPERSONAL RELATIONS, CROSS CULTURAL, EQUAL OPPORTUNITY, PROFESSIONAL TRAINING, ESSAY, OKLAHOMA, MIDWEST, COLLEGE STUDENTS

ABST THE USE OF TRANSRACIAL COMMUNICATION SKILLS WAS EXAMINED IN A PROGRAM DESIGNED TO RECRUIT MINORITY PSYCHOLOGY STUDENTS TO OKLAHOMA STATE UNIVERSITY AND HELP THEM "SURVIVE" THE EXPERIENCE. IN THE PLANNING STAGES, TRANSRACIAL AND OTHER LITERATURE WHICH DISCUSSED ENVIRONMENTAL STRUCTURE, VERBAL BEHAVIOR, AND NONVERBAL BEHAVIOR WAS CONSULTED. ONCE THE PROGRAM WAS OPERATIONAL, DAILY INTAKE DATA WERE COLLECTED ON ALL INTERPERSONAL CONTACTS FOR THE FIRST 47 SERVICE DAYS OF THE PROGRAM—157 STUDENT VISITS. THE PROGRAM POPULATION INCLUDED AMERICAN INDIAN, BLACK, CHICANO, OTHER HISPANIC, AND ASIAN AMERICAN STUDENTS. COMBINING THE LITERATURE WITH EMPIRICAL OBSERVATION, THE FOLLOWING REMARKS

ABOUT TRANSRACIAL COMMUNICATION ARE MADE: (1) BEING HOSTED DURING ADMISSION INTERVIEWS BY A STUDENT WITH A SIMILAR MINORITY BACKGROUND FACILITATES INTERPERSONAL COMMUNICATION; (2) FREE ACCESS TO THE COORDINATOR—WITHOUT MONITORING BY A SECRETARY—HELPS CREATE AN ATMOSPHERE OF TRUST; (3) WHEN OFFICE HOURS ARE SET WITH TWO BASIC TYPES OF TIME AVAILABLE—DROP-IN AND APPOINTMENT TIME—ALL STUDENTS TEND TO BE MORE COMFORTABLE; (4) A PLEASANT, INFORMAL ATMOSPHERE GREATLY IMPROVES COMMUNICATION; (5) INFORMAL, ORDINARY LANGUAGE THAT ORIGINATES IN COMMUNICATOR SINCERITY, NOT A STRAINING AFTER IN-GROUP ETHNIC SLANG, IS ESSENTIAL FOR PROFESSIONAL/MINORITY STUDENT COMMUNICATION; AND (6) REGARDING NON-VERBAL BEHAVIORS (E.G., PHYSICAL CONTACT), NON-MINORITY PROFESSIONALS SHOULD NOT MODIFY THEIR BEHAVIORS BECAUSE MINORITY PEOPLE MAY INTERPRET SUCH BEHAVIORS AS INSINCERE. IN GENERAL, POSITIVE COMMUNICATION OUTCOMES IN THESE SETTINGS ARE THE RESULT OF DELIBERATE DESIGN, COMBINED WITH INDIVIDUAL COMMUNICATORS' WILLINGNESS TO RISK INTERACTIONS WHICH DIFFER FROM TRADITIONAL ACADEMIC PATTERNS. 15 REFERENCES.

ACCN 001631

1899 AUTH **VALENTINE, C. A.**

TITL THE INTERNATIONAL "CULTURE OF POVERTY," WITH IMPLICATIONS FOR SOCIAL SCIENCE AND SOCIAL POLICY.

SRCE *IN C. VALENTINE (ED.), CULTURE AND POVERTY: CRITIQUE AND COUNTER-PROPOSALS. CHICAGO: UNIVERSITY OF CHICAGO PRESS, 1968, PP. 48-77.*

INDX POVERTY, SOCIAL SCIENCES, MEXICO, MEXICAN, PUERTO RICAN, ESSAY, SES, CULTURE, PUERTO RICAN-I, PUERTO RICAN-M, REVIEW

ABST OSCAR LEWIS USES AN ANTHROPOLOGICAL APPROACH TOWARD THE "CULTURE OF POVERTY" AND HAS DONE WORK MAINLY WITH MEXICANS AND PUERTO RICANS. LEWIS'S FAILURE TO MAKE CLEAR CONNECTIONS AMONG HIS MAIN ELEMENTS OF ANALYSIS (I.E., THE INDIVIDUALS, THE FAMILY, THE COMMUNITY, LOWER-CLASS CULTURE, AND THE NATION) IS CLEARLY SEEN IN CONTRADICTIONS BETWEEN HIS CONCRETE EVIDENCE AND HIS THEORETICAL MODELS. FURTHER CRITICISM OF LEWIS'S THOUGHT IS PRESENTED, WITH EMPHASIS UPON THE "CULTURE OF POVERTY" AND HIS FORMULATIONS FOR CHANGE. LEWIS ULTIMATELY CHOOSES TO ELIMINATE THE "CULTURE OF POVERTY" RATHER THAN THE POVERTY ITSELF. 4 REFERENCES.

ACCN 001632

1900 AUTH **VALLE, J. R.**

TITL AMISTAD-COMPADRAZGO AS AN INDIGENOUS WEBWORK COMPARED WITH THE URBAN MENTAL HEALTH NETWORK (DOCTORAL DISSERTA-

TION, UNIVERSITY OF SOUTHERN CALIFORNIA, 1974).

SRCE   *DISSERTATION ABSTRACTS INTERNATIONAL, 1974, 35(5-6), 2486B-2487B. (UNIVERSITY MICROFILMS NO. 74-26,054.)*

INDX   FICTIVE KINSHIP, SOCIAL STRUCTURE, GROUP DYNAMICS, CALIFORNIA, EMPIRICAL, SOUTHWEST, EXTENDED FAMILY, URBAN, MENTAL HEALTH, CONFLICT RESOLUTION, MEXICAN AMERICAN, RESOURCE UTILIZATION, FOLK MEDICINE, PARAPROFESSIONALS

ABST   WHETHER OR NOT THE INSTITUTION OF AMISTAD-COMPADRAZGO—A SOCIAL GROUP WHOSE MEMBERS HELP EACH OTHER BY SHARING GOODS, SERVICES, OR PERSONAL SUPPORT—IS COMPATIBLE WITH FORMAL MENTAL HEALTH DELIVERY SYSTEMS TO URBAN CHICANOS IS EXAMINED. DATA WERE GATHERED VIA AN INTEGRATED FIELD RESEARCH METHODOLOGY COMBINING SURVEY AND PARTICIPANT-OBSERVATION TECHNIQUES. IN THE STATISTICALLY NON-GENERALIZABLE SAMPLE OF 187 CHICANO USERS OF MENTAL HEALTH SERVICES WHO WERE SURVEYED, WIDESPREAD AND CONCRETE EVIDENCE OF AMISTAD-COMPADRAZGO WEB RELATIONSHIPS WAS FOUND. THE AMISTAD WEBS WERE FOUND TO BE IN POSITIVE INTERACTION WITH THE MENTAL HEALTH SERVICES, WITH 84.2% OF THE 160 WEB-REPORTING RESPONDENTS INDICATING THAT THEIR WEBS AND THE SERVICE NETWORKS PERFORMED EITHER SIMILAR OR COMPLEMENTARY FUNCTIONS. MOREOVER, THERE WAS A STRONG TENDENCY AMONG RESPONDENTS TO COOPT THE SERVICE NETWORKS—I.E., 35% WERE FOUND TO BE ACTIVELY ENGAGED IN SOME FORM OF SERVICE DELIVERY BEYOND THEIR WEB-WORK RELATIONSHIPS. IT IS CONCLUDED THAT (1) AMISTAD-COMPADRAZGOS WILL BE FOUND AMONG CHICANOS IN URBAN AREAS WHERE CHICANOS FORM A MINIMUM OF 10% OF THE TOTAL POPULATION, AND (2) THESE AMISTAD-COMPADRAZGO CONNECTIONS WILL BE IN POSITIVE SUPPORTIVE RELATIONSHIP WITH LOCAL NETWORKS OF MENTAL HEALTH AND OTHER SERVICES. IT IS ALSO NOTED THAT THE INTEGRATED FIELD RESEARCH METHODOLOGY PROVED A HIGHLY APPROPRIATE VEHICLE FOR STUDYING CHICANO POPULATIONS, YIELDING HIGH QUALITY DATA. 114 REFERENCES.

ACCN   001633

1901 AUTH   **VALLE, J., & FIESTER, A. R.**
TITL   UTILIZATION PATTERNS OF MENTAL HEALTH SERVICES BY THE SPANISH SPEAKING-SPANISH SURNAMED POPULATION AND SERVICES RENDERED BY A COMMUNITY MENTAL HEALTH CENTER OF SOUTHEAST FLORIDA.

SRCE   *PRESENTED AT THE FIRST ANNUAL SOUTHEAST HISPANIC CONFERENCE ON HUMAN SERVICES, FEBRUARY 6, 1976.*

INDX   RESOURCE UTILIZATION, MENTAL HEALTH, HEALTH DELIVERY SYSTEMS, SPANISH SURNAMED, SES, CROSS CULTURAL, PSYCHOTHERAPY, REHABILITATION, EMPIRICAL, DIS-

CRIMINATION, PROGRAM EVALUATION, FLORIDA, SOUTH, POLICY

ABST   AN ANALYSIS OF SOCIODEMOGRAPHIC DATA AND UTILIZATION PATTERNS OF SPANISH-SPEAKING/SPANISH-SURNAME (SS/SS) CLIENTS OF THE PALM BEACH COUNTY COMMUNITY MENTAL HEALTH CENTER (CMHC) WAS CONDUCTED TO ASSESS THE STRENGTHS AND DEFICITS OF THE HEALTH CARE DELIVERY SYSTEM. CASE OPENING VARIABLES, DEMOGRAPHIC CHARACTERISTICS, AND TREATMENT VARIABLES OF 122 SS/SS CONSUMERS WERE EXAMINED TO ANSWER FOUR QUESTIONS: (1) WHAT ARE THE DIFFERENCES BETWEEN BLACK, SS/SS, AND ANGLO CLIENTS IN TERMS OF UTILIZATION PATTERNS AND SERVICES RECEIVED?; (2) WHAT ARE OTHER HUMAN SERVICE NEEDS OF SS/SS CONSUMERS?; (3) IS THE CARE SYSTEM PROVIDED THE SS/SS CONSUMER COMPARABLE AND EQUITABLE TO SERVICES RECEIVED BY ANGLO AND BLACK CLIENTELE?; AND (4) WHAT IS THE OUTCOME OF THE SS/SS EXPERIENCE AT THE MENTAL HEALTH CENTER? DATA REVEAL THAT THERE WAS NO DIFFERENCE IN USAGE OF OUTPATIENT SERVICES GIVEN TO THE THREE GROUPS, BUT PROPORTIONATELY TWICE AS MANY LATINO CLIENTS AS ANGLO OR BLACK CLIENTS WERE PLACED IN THE CMHC AFTERCARE PROGRAM. THE SS/SS WERE ALSO TWICE AS LIKELY TO BE PRESCRIBED A MAJOR TRANQUILIZER AND/OR ANTIDEPRESSANTS. THE DATA STRONGLY INDICATE THAT THERE IS AN UNDERUTILIZATION OF SERVICES BY SS/SS INDIVIDUALS AND THAT DIFFERENTIAL TREATMENT EXISTS FOR THIS GROUP. RECOMMENDED ARE (1) INCREASES IN THE NUMBER OF SS/SS THERAPISTS AND MENTAL HEALTH TECHNICIANS, (2) PROVISION OF NON-TRADITIONAL THERAPY, (3) ONGOING SYSTEM EVALUATION, AND (4) IMPROVEMENT OF PUBLIC RELATIONS AND/OR EDUCATION. 10 REFERENCES.

ACCN   001634

1902 AUTH   **VALLE, M.**
TITL   WHAT HOLDS SAMI BACK? A STUDY OF SERVICE DELIVERY IN A PUERTO RICAN COMMUNITY.

SRCE   *NEW YORK: VALLE CONSULTANTS, LTD., 1973.*

INDX   COMMUNITY, SOCIAL SERVICES, DEMOGRAPHIC, HEALTH DELIVERY SYSTEMS, SURVEY, EMPIRICAL, EXTENDED FAMILY, MENTAL HEALTH, FAMILY ROLES, CHILDREN, CHILDREARING PRACTICES, RESOURCE UTILIZATION, PUERTO RICAN-M, NEW YORK, EAST

ABST   TO OBTAIN FIRST-HAND INFORMATION REGARDING CHILD CARE PATTERNS, COMMUNITY CHILD CARE FACILITIES, AND OTHER NEEDS AMONG POVERTY-AREA PUERTO RICAN FAMILIES IN NEW YORK CITY, 213 PARENTS OR PARENT-SURROGATES WERE INTERVIEWED. THE SURVEY COVERED FAMILY AND HOUSEHOLD COMPOSITION, FAMILY MOBILITY AND ECONOMIC LEVEL, FACTORS INFLUENCING MIGRATION, PARENTAL ABSENCE, USE OF FOSTER CARE AND DAY-CARE SERVICE, USE OF PUBLIC AND PRIVATE AGENCIES IN NEW YORK AND IN PUERTO RICO, KNOWLEDGE OF

COMMUNITY FACILITIES, AND LANGUAGE USAGE. FINDINGS ARE LISTED IN 70 TABLES AND DISCUSSED. THE FOLLOWING RECOMMENDATIONS ARE MADE: (1) ESTABLISHMENT OF A FOSTER CARE AGENCY SPECIFICALLY TO SERVE PUERTO RICAN FAMILIES; (2) EXPANSION OF BILINGUAL-BICULTURAL DAY-CARE CENTERS; (3) A SHIFT FROM INSTITUTIONAL TO FOSTER HOME CARE WITH SHORT TERM PLACEMENT MADE WITHIN THE NEIGHBORHOOD; (4) SPECIAL EFFORTS TO IDENTIFY AND ASSIST MENTALLY ILL AND RETARDED CHILDREN; (5) MORE AGGRESSIVE RECRUITMENT OF SPANISH-SPEAKING STAFF TO ASSIST IN ALL PUBLIC AGENCIES AND INSTITUTIONS; (6) INFORMATION ON SOCIAL SERVICES PREPARED IN SPANISH AND DISTRIBUTED WITHIN POVERTY AREAS; AND (7) BILINGUAL JOB DEVELOPMENT PROGRAMS PUBLICIZED WITHIN POVERTY AREAS. GREATEST OF ALL IS THE NEED FOR AN INFORMED ADVOCATE TO FOCUS ATTENTION ON THE NEEDS OF THE PUERTO RICAN COMMUNITY.

ACCN   001635

1903 AUTH   **VALLE, R.**
   TITL   LOS BARRIOS DE EASTLOS: EAST LOS ANGELES AND COMPREHENSIVE MENTAL HEALTH PLANNING PERSPECTIVES.
   SRCE   *REPORT TO NATIONAL INSTITUTE OF MENTAL HEALTH (CONTRACT NO. 71-910), AUGUST 29, 1971.*
   INDX   COMMUNITY, MEXICAN AMERICAN, MENTAL HEALTH, HEALTH DELIVERY SYSTEMS, PROGRAM EVALUATION, EMPIRICAL, CALIFORNIA, SOUTHWEST
   ABST   PERSPECTIVES ARE PRESENTED OF THE CHICANO COMPREHENSIVE MENTAL HEALTH PLANNING PROJECT WHICH DESCRIBE THE HETEROGENEOUS NATURE OF THE CHICANO PEOPLE, THEIR MENTAL HEALTH NEEDS, AND MENTAL HEALTH PLANNING MODELS. THE VIEWS PRESENTED ARE FROM THE PROVIDER ORGANIZATIONS OF MENTAL HEALTH AS THEY REFLECT THE FERMENT IN EAST LOS ANGELES. IT IS POINTED OUT THAT THE CURRENT MENTAL HEALTH SYSTEMS OPERATING IN EAST LOS ANGELES ARE FRAGMENTED, UNDERMANNED, AND UNDERFINANCED. THE FEW EXISTING RESOURCES ARE EITHER STRAINED BEYOND THEIR CAPACITIES WITH REQUESTS FOR SERVICES OR ARE UNAVAILABLE TO THE SPANISH-SPEAKING CONSUMER. NECESSARY COMPONENTS FOR REVERSING THE SITUATION IN THE BARRIO ARE: (1) BUILDING A SATELLITE NETWORK WHICH WILL PLACE TEAMS OF SKILLED MENTAL HEALTH PROFESSIONALS AT ACCESSIBLE SPOTS THROUGHOUT THE COMMUNITY; (2) USING CHICANO CULTURAL STRENGTHS IN BUILDING A NEW SYSTEM OF SERVICE; (3) USING THE CHICANO COMMUNITY'S MANPOWER RESOURCES; (4) LAUNCHING A MASSIVE EDUCATION EFFORT; (5) TAILORING MENTAL HEALTH SERVICES TO THE DIFFERENT BARRIOS; (6) ENLARGING THE CONCEPT OF MENTAL HEALTH TO INCLUDE THE DYNAMICS OF ENVIRONMENTAL AND SOCIOECONOMIC PRESSURES; AND (7) INCREAS-

ING BILINGUAL-BICULTURAL PERSONNEL THROUGHOUT THE WHOLE MENTAL HEALTH SERVICE SYSTEM IN EAST LOS ANGELES. FURTHER RECOMMENDATIONS FOR STEPS TO IMPLEMENTATION ARE OFFERED IN THE AREA OF SERVICES, PLANNING, RESEARCH, AND TRAINING. THE FUNDING ROLE OF NIMH IS ALSO DISCUSSED.

ACCN   001636

1904 AUTH   **VALLEJO, E. M.**
   TITL   CHICANO COMPREHENSIVE MENTAL HEALTH PLANNING: FINAL REPORT.
   SRCE   *REPORT TO THE NATIONAL INSTITUTE OF HEALTH (CONTRACT NO. 71-979), SEPTEMBER 10, 1971.*
   INDX   MEXICAN AMERICAN, MENTAL HEALTH, PROGRAM EVALUATION, EMPIRICAL, COMMUNITY, CULTURAL PLURALISM, ATTITUDES, HEALTH DELIVERY SYSTEMS, CALIFORNIA, SOUTHWEST
   ABST   THE CHICANO COMPREHENSIVE MENTAL HEALTH PLANNING PROJECT (CCMHP) CONDUCTED IN LOS ANGELES IS CONCERNED WITH THE MENTAL HEALTH NEEDS OF THE COMMUNITY AS PERCEIVED BY THE RESIDENTS. APPROXIMATELY 200 CONSUMER GROUPS (BARRIO RESIDENTS) WERE IDENTIFIED AND CLUSTERED ON THE BASIS OF THEIR MAJOR AREAS OF CONCERN. THIS RESULTED IN THE EMERGENCE OF 11 TYPES OF CONSUMER GROUPS IDENTIFIED WITH RELIGION, EDUCATION, YOUTH, HEALTH, SOCIAL ACTION, SENIOR CITIZENS, CHICANO PROFESSIONALS, CIVIC POLITICS, LABOR, AND SOCIAL EVENTS. DATA WERE OBTAINED BY INTERVIEWING THE LEADERS OF THE CONSUMER GROUPS. IT WAS SHOWN THAT IN ORDER TO MEET THE MENTAL HEALTH NEEDS OF THE CHICANO: (1) THE CHICANO SHOULD BE ALLOWED TO REINFORCE HIS CULTURAL IDENTITY THROUGHOUT HIS LIFE; (2) INSTITUTIONS WHICH AFFECT THE FAMILY MUST AID IN THE CONTINUATION OF THE COHESIVENESS AND UNITY OF THE FAMILY; (3) THE INDIVIDUAL AND HIS FAMILY MUST FEEL THAT THEY HAVE THE CAPACITY TO ESTABLISH A SOLID ECONOMIC FOUNDATION; AND (4) EXPANSION AND REINFORCEMENT OF EXISTING CHANNELS TO INCREASE COMMUNITY PARTICIPATION AMONG THE RESIDENTS MUST CONTINUE. A DISCUSSION ON OTHER NEEDS FOR BARRIO-ORIENTED SERVICES IS FOLLOWED BY A NUMBER OF RECOMMENDATIONS. 5 REFERENCES.

ACCN   001637

1905 AUTH   **VALVERDE, G.**
   TITL   MEMORANDUM: ADMISSIONS DATA BY ETHNIC IDENTITY.
   SRCE   *UNPUBLISHED MANUSCRIPT, JUNE 30, 1976. (AVAILABLE FROM THE DEPARTMENT OF HEALTH, CENTER FOR HEALTH STATISTICS, SACRAMENTO, CALIF.)*
   INDX   RESOURCE UTILIZATION, MENTAL HEALTH, HEALTH DELIVERY SYSTEMS, SPANISH SURNAMED, SURVEY, EMPIRICAL, CROSS CULTURAL, CALIFORNIA, SOUTHWEST
   ABST   THE RESULTS OF A SURVEY OF TWELVE CALI-

FORNIA COUNTIES REGARDING MINORITY ADMISSIONS TO MENTAL HEALTH FACILITIES ARE REPORTED IN THIS MEMORANDUM FROM THE STATE OF CALIFORNIA CENTER FOR HEALTH STATISTICS. THE TWELVE COUNTIES COMPRISED 52% OF THE STATE'S TOTAL POPULATION AND 65% OF THE STATE'S MINORITY POPULATION. THE ETHNIC IDENTITY AND LANGUAGE PREFERENCES OF BOTH THE STAFF OF THE LOCAL MENTAL HEALTH CENTER AND THE RECIPIENTS OF SERVICES WERE ASCERTAINED IN THE ONE-MONTH SURVEY. SIX OF THE 12 COUNTIES WERE ABLE TO PROVIDE ADMISSIONS DATA WHILE 7 PROVIDED INFORMATION ON MENTAL HEALTH STAFF. TWO TABLES DELINEATE ADMISSIONS PER 1000 POPULATION AND UTILIZATION RATES BY ETHNIC GROUP FOR THE RESPONDING COUNTIES. BLACKS AND WHITES ARE REPORTED TO OVERUTILIZE SERVICES WHILE ASIANS AND THE SPANISH-SURNAMED UNDERUTILIZE SERVICES. UNDERUTILIZATION MAY INDICATE THAT SPANISH-SURNAMED AND ASIANS: (1) DO NOT NEED THE SERVICE PROVIDED; (2) REPRESENT A SUBCULTURE THAT IS NOT ADDRESSED BY THESE SERVICES; (3) LACK A COMMAND OF THE PREDOMINANT LANGUAGE; OR (4) DO NOT HAVE ACCESS TO SERVICES. AS PARTICIPATING COUNTIES HAD DISPARATE DATA COLLECTION, IT IS RECOMMENDED THAT UNIFORM METHODS BE INSTITUTED ACROSS THE STATE. 3 REFERENCES.

ACCN   001638

1906 AUTH   **VAN ARSDOL, M. D., JR., & SCHUERMAN, L. A.**
TITL   REDISTRIBUTION AND ASSIMILATION OF ETHNIC POPULATIONS: THE LOS ANGELES CASE.
SRCE   *DEMOGRAPHY, 1971, 8(4), 459-480.*
INDX   DEMOGRAPHIC, HOUSING, MEXICAN AMERICAN, DISCRIMINATION, MIGRATION, URBAN, REVIEW, COMMUNITY, CALIFORNIA, SOUTHWEST
ABST   REDISTRIBUTION RELATIVE TO METROPOLITAN GROWTH OF NEGRO, OTHER NON-WHITE, AND SPANISH-SURNAME POPULATIONS IS EXAMINED IN LOS ANGELES COUNTY FROM 1940 TO 1960 FOR A COMPARABLE GRID OF SUBAREAS. THE SUBAREAS ARE DEFINED RELATIVE TO THEIR MATURITY AT DIFFERENT TIME POINTS IN ORDER TO PARTIALLY CONTROL FOR POPULATION REDISTRIBUTION EFFECTS OF NEIGHBORHOOD LIFE HISTORIES, THE SPREAD OF OLDER SUBAREAS, AND THE PERSISTENCE OF NEIGHBORHOOD PATTERNS. SHIFTS IN ETHNIC CONCENTRATION ARE SHOWN FOR BOTH OLDER AND NEWER SUBAREAS. CONCURRENT CHANGES IN NEIGHBORHOOD SOCIAL STRUCTURES AND ETHNIC POPULATIONS ARE DESCRIBED. FINDINGS ARE CATEGORIZED UNDER THREE THEMES. FIRST, ETHNIC POPULATION INCREMENTS AND REDISTRIBUTION WERE GENERALLY RESTRICTED TO EXPANDING OLDER SUBAREAS. ETHNIC POPULATIONS DID NOT SPATIALLY EXPAND AT A RATE EQUAL TO THE SPREAD OF THE METROPOLIS OR OF OLDER SUBAREAS. SECOND, SEGREGATION IS GREATER IN BOTH OLDER AND NEWER NEIGHBORHOODS FOR NEGROES THAN

FOR OTHER ETHNIC POPULATIONS. NEGROES EXPERIENCED THE LARGEST PROPORTIONAL INCREMENTS IN BOTH OLDER AND NEWER SUBAREAS, AS WELL AS THE GREATEST STABILITY IN SUBAREA OCCUPANCY. FINALLY, THE SPATIAL SEPARATION OF ETHNIC POPULATIONS IMPEDES ASSIMILATION IN THAT UNIQUE PATTERNS OF NEIGHBORHOOD STRUCTURE COME TO CHARACTERIZE DIFFERENT ETHNIC POPULATIONS, AND CHANGES IN ETHNIC COMPOSITION ARE REFLECTED IN CHANGES IN NEIGHBORHOOD SOCIAL STRUCTURES. 39 REFERENCES. (AUTHOR ABSTRACT)

ACCN   001639

1907 AUTH   **VAN DUYNE, J. H., & GUTIERREZ, G.**
TITL   THE REGULATORY FUNCTION OF LANGUAGE IN BILINGUAL CHILDREN.
SRCE   *JOURNAL OF EDUCATIONAL RESEARCH, 1972, 66(3), 122-124.*
INDX   CHILDREN, BILINGUAL, EMPIRICAL, MEXICAN AMERICAN, PERFORMANCE EXPECTATIONS, LANGUAGE COMPREHENSION, BILINGUALISM, LANGUAGE ACQUISITION, ILLINOIS, MIDWEST, MIGRANTS
ABST   24 BILINGUAL, MEXICAN AMERICAN MIGRANT WORKERS' CHILDREN OF DEKALB COUNTY, ILLINOIS, WERE EVALUATED TO ASSESS PERFORMANCE ON A TWO-ASSOCIATION PERCEPTUAL MOTOR TASK WHEN GIVEN VERBAL INSTRUCTIONS IN EITHER SPANISH OR ENGLISH. SIX CHILDREN EACH WERE RANDOMLY SELECTED FROM THE DEKALB SCHOOL SYSTEM'S 4, 5, 6, AND 7 YEAR-OLD STUDENT POPULATION. ALL CHILDREN WERE GIVEN OPERANT CONDITIONING OF COLOR AND FORM DISCRIMINATION AND LABELING IN BOTH LANGUAGES PRIOR TO TASK PERFORMANCE. CANDY AND BALLOONS WERE OFFERED AS REINFORCEMENTS. SCORES REFLECTED THE NUMBER OF CORRECT RESPONSES TO 38 TEST STIMULI. A TWO-WAY ANALYSIS OF VARIANCE REVEALED A SIGNIFICANT DIFFERENCE BETWEEN LANGUAGE TREATMENTS: THE CHILDREN PERFORMED BETTER WITH SPANISH RATHER THAN ENGLISH INSTRUCTION. A SIGNIFICANT DIFFERENCE WAS ALSO OBSERVED BETWEEN AGE LEVELS: PERFORMANCE INCREASED WITH AGE. A SUBANALYSIS REVEALED THAT 5 YEAR-OLDS SCORED SIGNIFICANTLY HIGHER UNDER SPANISH TREATMENT. IT IS SUGGESTED THAT THE PERIOD FROM 5 TO 6 YEARS MAY BE THE TRANSITIONAL STAGE WHEN THE REGULATORY FUNCTION IS TRANSFERRED FROM THE "NONSPECIFIC IMPULSIVE ASPECTS" TO THE "SPECIFIC ELECTIVE SIGNIFICATIVE ASPECTS" OF LANGUAGE. THIS TRANSITIONAL PERIOD IN MONOLINGUAL CHILDREN OCCURS BETWEEN AGE 4 AND 5, INDICATING THAT BILINGUAL CHILDREN IN THE SAMPLE ARE APPROXIMATELY 1 YEAR RETARDED IN THIS LANGUAGE DEVELOPMENT. FINALLY, RESULTS ALSO INDICATE THAT THE MEXICAN AMERICAN CHILDREN IN THE STUDY WERE APPROXIMATELY 1 YEAR DELAYED IN SPANISH AND 2 YEARS DELAYED IN ENGLISH IN THEIR DEVELOPMENT OF THE "SPECIFIC ELECTIVE SIGNIFICATIVE ASPECTS" OF LANGUAGE.

CONCLUSIONS ARE CONFIRMED BY FINDINGS OF EARLIER INVESTIGATORS. 5 REFERENCES.

ACCN   001640

1908 AUTH   **VANKEEP, P. A., & RICE-WRAY, E. R.**
TITL   ATTITUDES TOWARD FAMILY PLANNING AND CONTRACEPTION IN MEXICO CITY.
SRCE   *STUDIES IN FAMILY PLANNING, 1973, 11(4), 305-309.*
INDX   ATTITUDES, BIRTH CONTROL, MEXICO, ADULTS, DEMOGRAPHIC, EMPIRICAL, FEMALE, FERTILITY, MEXICAN, FAMILY PLANNING, VALUES
ABST   IN MEXICO CITY, THE ATTITUDES OF CLIENTS AT A FAMILY PLANNING CLINIC (N = 250) TOWARD BASIC CONCEPTS OF FAMILY PLANNING AND CONTRACEPTION WERE COMPARED TO THOSE OF A RANDOMLY SELECTED SAMPLE OF THE CITY'S FEMALE POPULATION (N = 500). WOMEN AGES 16 TO 50, MARRIED AND LIVING WITH THEIR HUSBANDS, WERE GIVEN A QUESTIONNAIRE CONSISTING OF 18 STATEMENTS REVEALING THE RESPONDENT'S ATTITUDE TOWARD (1) THE IMPORTANCE OF A LARGE FAMILY, (2) THE EFFECT OF CONTRACEPTIVE PRACTICE ON INTERCOURSE AND THE MARITAL RELATIONSHIP, (3) THE INFLUENCE OF CONTRACEPTION ON ATTITUDES, (4) MACRO- AND MICRO-ECONOMIC CONSIDERATIONS IN DETERMINING FAMILY SIZE, AND (5) THE EFFECT OF CONTRACEPTIVES ON FUTURE OFFSPRING. RESPONDENTS ALSO INDICATED AGE, SOCIOECONOMIC STATUS, EDUCATIONAL ATTAINMENT, NUMBER OF LIVING CHILDREN, IDEAL FAMILY SIZE, AND CURRENT CONTRACEPTIVE PRACTICE. THE CLINIC SAMPLE WAS MORE INCLINED THAN THE CITY SAMPLE TO APPROVE OF FAMILY PLANNING. APPROVAL WAS GREATEST AMONG WOMEN AGES 21 TO 30, THOSE WITH A HIGHER SCHOOL-LEAVING AGE, AND THOSE FROM THE HIGHER SOCIO-ECONOMIC GROUPS. DATA INDICATE THAT THE CLINIC ATTENDER TYPICALLY HAS ACHIEVED DESIRED FAMILY SIZE WHILE THE AVERAGE WOMAN IN THE CITY SAMPLE HAS NOT. THE CITY SAMPLE WAS COMPARATIVELY IGNORANT ABOUT THE VARIOUS CONTRACEPTIVE METHODS AVAILABLE, AND ITS GREATER OPPOSITION TO CONTRACEPTIVE PRACTICE WAS EVIDENT IN ITS BELIEF THAT CONTRACEPTIVES CAN HAVE HARMFUL EFFECTS ON FUTURE OFFSPRING. WITH MEXICO'S EXPANDING, GOVERNMENT-SANCTIONED FAMILY PLANNING PROGRAM, KNOWLEDGE ABOUT SAFE, RELIABLE BIRTH CONTROL METHODS SHOULD FAVORABLY AFFECT ATTITUDES AND PRACTICES TOWARD FAMILY PLANNING.
ACCN   001641

1909 AUTH   **VARGAS, P.**
TITL   A PRELIMINARY ASSESSMENT OF NIDA PROGRAMS AND ACTIVITIES REGARDING THE INHALATION OF TOXIC SUSBSTANCES AS A DRUG ABUSE PROBLEM (SPECIAL REPORT TO THE DIRECTOR OF NIDA, DR. ROBERT L. DUPONT).
SRCE   *ROCKVILLE, MD.: NATIONAL INSTITUTE OF DRUG ABUSE, DECEMBER 1975.*
INDX   INHALANT ABUSE, DEMOGRAPHIC, GROUP DYNAMICS, SES, CULTURAL FACTORS, FAMILY ROLES, DRUG ABUSE, ESSAY, ADOLESCENTS, CHILDREN, BIBLIOGRAPHY, POLICY
ABST   AEROSOL INHALATION, ESTIMATED TO KILL ABOUT 125 AMERICANS EACH YEAR, IS CONSIDERED TO BE POTENTIALLY THE MOST DANGEROUS EXISTING DRUG PROBLEM. INHALANT ABUSE IS NOT CONFINED TO GLUE SNIFFING, BUT INCLUDES THE INGESTION OF TOXIC CHEMICALS AND HEAVY METALS (COPPER, ZINC, LEAD) CONTAINED IN SUCH COMMON AEROSOL DISPENSERS AS SPRAY PAINTS, DEODORANTS, AND HAIRSPRAYS. INHALANT ABUSE IS PREVALENT AMONG ALL SOCIOECONOMIC GROUPS, BUT BETWEEN-GROUP DIFFERENCES DO EXIST IN THE EXTENT OF ABUSE AND THE TYPE OF PRODUCTS USED TO ACHIEVE INTOXICATION. CURRENTLY, INHALANT ABUSE HAS RECEIVED LOW NATIONAL PRIORITY, WITH LESS THAN 0.2% OF THE FY1976 BUDGET ALLOCATED FOR RESEARCH AND PREVENTION. ATTENTION TO AEROSOL INHALATION IS OF SPECIAL URGENCY FOR MANY REASONS: (1) TOXIC SUBSTANCES IN AEROSOL PRODUCTS CAN BE MORE PHYSIOLOGICALLY DAMAGING THAN MOST HARD DRUGS; (2) INHALANT ABUSE IS ENGAGED IN BY THE VERY YOUNG; (3) IT INVOLVES UNCONTROLLED LEGAL AND INEXPENSIVE PRODUCTS READILY AVAILABLE TO YOUTHS; (4) LITTLE ATTENTION HAS BEEN PAID TO PREVENTION, TREATMENT, AND RESEARCH; (5) AEROSOL INHALATION SERVES AS A DRUG OF INITIATION, LEADING TO PROGRESSIVE INVOLVEMENT WITH ALCOHOL AND HARD DRUGS; (6) VIOLENT, AGGRESSIVE, AND DESTRUCTIVE BEHAVIORS ARE DIRECTLY ASSOCIATED WITH THE INHALATION OF AEROSOL SUBSTANCES; AND (7) INADEQUATE DATA ARE AVAILABLE TO DEFINE THE SCOPE AND NATURE OF THE DRUG ABUSE PROBLEM. IT IS ONLY THROUGH EARLY IMPLEMENTATION OF PREVENTIVE MEASURES THAT THERE CAN BE A REDUCTION OF THE IMMEDIATE AND LONG TERM SOCIAL AND INDIVIDUAL COSTS OF INHALANT ABUSE. AS AN APPENDIX TO THIS REPORT IS "BIBLIOGRAPHY ON THE INHALATION OF TOXIC SUBSTANCES," DATED THROUGH 1975 AND COMPRISED OF 590 REFERENCES. THERE ARE ALSO SIX OTHER APPENDICES CONSISTING OF JOURNAL-LENGTH ARTICLES DEALING WITH VARIOUS ASPECTS OF INHALANT ABUSE. 22 REFERENCES.
ACCN   001642

1910 AUTH   **VASQUEZ, A. G., & UHLIG, G. E.**
TITL   THE SPANISH-SPEAKING OF CHICAGO: EDUCATIONAL ISSUES.
SRCE   *JOURNAL OF INSTRUCTIONAL PSYCHOLOGY, 1975, 2(3), 2-8.*
INDX   SPANISH SURNAMED, EDUCATION, EDUCATIONAL COUNSELING, BILINGUAL-BICULTURAL EDUCATION, COMMUNITY, CULTURAL FACTORS, MEXICAN AMERICAN, CUBAN, CROSS CULTURAL, EMPIRICAL, EQUAL OPPORTUNITY, VOCATIONAL COUNSELING, PUERTO RICAN-M, BILINGUAL-BICULTURAL PERSONNEL, ADULTS, ILLINOIS, MIDWEST
ABST   DURING 1973 AND 1974 AN EXTENSIVE NEEDS ASSESSMENT OF THE SPANISH-SPEAKING

DIFFERENCES IN PRESCHOOL CHILDREN IS PRESENTED. FOURTEEN 5 YEAR-OLDS, FIVE BOYS AND NINE GIRLS, WERE DIVIDED INTO TWO GROUPS OF SEVEN, ONE MEXICAN AMERICAN (MA) AND THE OTHER ANGLO AMERICAN (AA). THE LEWINIAN CONCEPT OF LEVEL OF ASPIRATION AS DERIVED FROM ATKINSON'S MOTIVATIONAL THEORY FORMED THE BASIS FOR THIS STUDY. ESSENTIALLY, THE THEORY PREDICTS THAT HIGH N-ACHIEVERS ARE LESS LIKELY TO ALTER THEIR LEVEL OF ASPIRATION THAN ARE LOW N-ACHIEVERS. THE MATERIALS USED FOR THE EXPERIMENT CONSISTED OF A GLASS CONTAINER 25 CM. IN DIAMETER AND 10 PENNIES WHICH WERE USED AS TOSSING OBJECTS. THE S WAS ASKED TO GIVE AN ESTIMATE OF THE NUMBER HE THOUGHT HE WOULD GET IN THE CONTAINER. THE ESTIMATE WAS TERMED AS THE S'S LEVEL OF ASPIRATION (LA), AND THE ACTUAL NUMBER THROWN INTO THE CONTAINER WAS REFERRED TO AS THE ACHIEVEMENT LEVEL (AL). DATA REVEAL THAT THE DIFFERENCE WITH REGARD TO SOCIOCULTURAL BACKGROUND IS HIGHLY SIGNIFICANT. (1) THE MA GROUP IS MORE ADEPT AT SETTING REALISTIC GOALS WITH REGARD TO THE RISK TAKING IN THIS SITUATION. THE AA GROUP IS MUCH LESS ADEPT AT SETTING REALISTIC GOALS IN THIS RISK TAKING SITUATION. (2) BOTH THE MA AND AA GROUPS ARE SIGNIFICANTLY HIGHER IN LA AS COMPARED TO AL, BUT THE MA'S AL IS CONSIDERABLY NEARER TO THEIR LA. THE GENERAL ASSERTION THAT THERE ARE SIGNIFICANT MOTIVATIONAL AND BEHAVIOR DIFFERENCES IN DIFFERING SOCIOCULTURAL BACKGROUNDS IS SUPPORTED. 16 REFERENCES.

ACCN   001648

1917 AUTH   **VETTER, B. M., & BABCO, E. L.**
TITL   PROFESSIONAL WOMEN AND MINORITIES: A MANPOWER RESOURCE SERVICE.
SRCE   *WASHINGTON, D.C.: SCIENTIFIC MANPOWER COMMISSION, 1975.*
INDX   FEMALE, SEX COMPARISON, PROFESSIONAL TRAINING, EQUAL OPPORTUNITY, SPANISH SURNAMED, SCHOLASTIC ACHIEVEMENT, REPRESENTATION, EMPIRICAL, STEREOTYPES, FAMILY PLANNING
ABST   TO DATE, THE LITERATURE HAS FAILED TO PLACE THE ISSUE OF HIGHER BIRTH AND FERTILITY RATES AMONG MEXICAN AMERICANS THAN ANGLOS IN ITS PROPER CULTURAL CONTEXT. ASSUMPTIONS HAVE BEEN THAT BECAUSE OF (1) CATHOLIC BANS ON BIRTH CONTROL, (2) TRADITIONAL SUBMISSIVE, CHILDBEARING ROLES FOR WOMEN, AND (3) AUTHORITARIAN CHILD-PRODUCING ROLES FOR MALES, BIRTH RATES WILL CONTINUE TO SOAR. HOWEVER, THESE CONDITIONS ARE NOT UNIVERSAL TO ALL MEXICAN AMERICANS. THERE ARE CULTURAL VARIABLES WHICH INFLUENCE IDEAL FAMILY SIZE, THE DECISION TO LIMIT OR NOT LIMIT BIRTHS, AND THE ACTUAL PRACTICE OF ARTIFICIAL BIRTH CONTROL. IN GENERAL, GREATER DEGREES OF DEPENDENCE BEHAVIORS IN THE MEXICAN AMERICAN WIFE WILL INDICATE A GREATER DESIRE FOR A LARGER FAMILY AND WILL INDICATE A REJECTION OF THE CONCEPT OF ARTIFICIAL BIRTH CONTROL. CONVERSELY, A GREATER DEGREE OF EGALITARIANISM AND GREATER COMMUNICATION BETWEEN THE MEXICAN AMERICAN HUSBAND AND WIFE MAY INDICATE A GREATER LIKELIHOOD THAT THE WIFE WILL DESIRE A SMALLER FAMILY, AND WILL SEEK MEANS OF BIRTH CONTROL TO ACHIEVE THIS END. IT IS HOPED THAT THROUGH FURTHER RESEARCH NEW LIGHT CAN BE SHED ON THIS SUBJECT. WHEN A MORE REALISTIC PICTURE OF MEXICAN AMERICAN FAMILY STRUCTURE AND ATTITUDES TOWARD FAMILY PLANNING ARE OBTAINED THROUGH SOUND RESEARCH WITHIN A CULTURAL CONTEXT, MISLEADING ASSERTIONS ABOUT MEXICAN AMERICAN WOMEN AND BIRTH CONTROL ARE LESS LIKELY TO PREVAIL. 27 REFERENCES.

ACCN   001649

1918 AUTH   **VIGIL, D.**
TITL   ADAPTATION STRATEGIES AND CULTURAL LIFE STYLES OF MEXICAN AMERICAN ADOLESCENTS.
SRCE   *HISPANIC JOURNAL OF BEHAVIORAL SCIENCES, 1979, 1(4), 375-392.*
INDX   ADOLESCENTS, MEXICAN AMERICAN, ETHNIC IDENTITY, CALIFORNIA, SOUTHWEST, URBAN, CASE STUDY, EMPIRICAL, SEX COMPARISON, CROSS GENERATIONAL, STRESS, ACCULTURATION, SCHOLASTIC ACHIEVEMENT, ENVIRONMENTAL FACTORS, MEXICAN, SCHOLASTIC ASPIRATIONS
ABST   TO DETERMINE THE EFFECT OF DIFFERENT ENVIRONMENTS ON THE ACCULTURATION OF MEXICAN AMERICAN (MA) ADOLESCENTS, AN INVESTIGATION WAS CONDUCTED ON THE ADAPTATION STRATEGIES UTILIZED BY MA HIGH SCHOOL STUDENTS IN LOS ANGELES. A QUESTIONNAIRE WAS ADMINISTERED TO 80 SUBJECTS (39 IN AN URBAN SCHOOL, 41 IN A SUBURBAN SCHOOL) TO ASCERTAIN THEIR DEGREE OF ACCULTURATION ON A LIKERT-TYPE SCALE. SIX STUDENTS FROM EACH SCHOOL WERE THEN SELECTED FOR FURTHER STUDY—SPECIFICALLY, THE TWO MOST NATIVIST (MEXICAN-ORIENTED), THE TWO MOST INTERMEDIATE (CHICANO-ORIENTED), AND THE TWO MOST ACCULTURATED (ANGLO-ORIENTED). IN-DEPTH CASE STUDIES FOCUSING ON DIFFERENCES IN LIFESTYLES WERE COMPLETED ON THESE 12 STUDENTS. RESULTS INDICATE THAT THE URBAN STUDENTS EXPERIENCED MORE STRESS IN ACCULTURATION, ALTHOUGH THE MEXICAN-ORIENTED STUDENTS EXHIBITED MORE CONFIDENCE IN THEIR ETHNIC IDENTIFICATION AND PERFORMED BETTER ACADEMICALLY. THE SUBURBAN MEXICAN-ORIENTED STUDENTS OFTEN HAD DIFFICULTY IN PRACTICING THEIR CHOSEN CULTURAL LIFESTYLES. SUBURBAN CHICANO- AND ANGLO-ORIENTED STUDENTS LEANED MORE TOWARDS THE ANGLO SIDE OF THE ACCULTURATION CONTINUUM, BUT THEY STILL PARTICIPATED IN SUBCULTURAL (I.E., GANG-RELATED) ACTIVITIES.

21 REFERENCES. (JOURNAL ABSTRACT MODIFIED)

ACCN   001778

1919 AUTH   **VIGIL, J.**
TITL   ADOLESCENT CHICANO ACCULTURATION AND SCHOOL PERFORMANCE: THE ROLE OF SOCIAL ECONOMIC CONDITIONS AND URBAN-SUBURBAN ENVIRONMENTAL DIFFERENCES.
SRCE   *UNPUBLISHED DOCTORAL DISSERTATION, UNIVERSITY OF CALIFORNIA, LOS ANGELES, 1976.*
INDX   ACCULTURATION, BILINGUALISM, IMMIGRATION, MIGRATION, ECONOMIC FACTORS, SES, SOCIAL MOBILITY, OCCUPATIONAL ASPIRATIONS, SCHOLASTIC ASPIRATIONS, SCHOLASTIC ACHIEVEMENT, FAMILY ROLES, GANGS, PSYCHOSOCIAL ADJUSTMENT, LINGUISTIC COMPETENCE, ANXIETY, URBAN, EDUCATION, EMPIRICAL, MEXICAN AMERICAN, ADOLESCENTS, CALIFORNIA, SOUTHWEST
ABST   THIS STUDY INVESTIGATED THE RELATIONSHIP BETWEEN LEVEL OF ACCULTURATION, ENVIRONMENT (URBAN VS. SUBURBAN), AND ACADEMIC PERFORMANCE OF HIGH SCHOOL ADOLESCENT CHICANOS. A QUESTIONNAIRE COVERING PERSONAL, SOCIOCULTURAL, SOCIOECONOMIC, AND SUBCULTURAL ATTITUDES AND PRACTICES WAS DEVELOPED TO MEASURE DEGREE OF ACCULTURATION. IT WAS ADMINISTERED TO A RANDOM SAMPLE OF 80 CHICANOS (39 URBAN, 41 SUBURBAN) FROM TWO HIGH SCHOOLS. TWO METHODOLOGICAL STAGES WERE UTILIZED—THE FIRST A QUANTITATIVE, STATISTICAL ANALYSIS OF ALL 80 PARTICIPANTS; THE SECOND A COLLECTION OF ETHNOGRAPHIC DATA ON 12 SELECTED INFORMANTS WHO REPRESENTED MEXICAN, CHICANO, AND ANGLO CULTURAL TYPES. THIS SECOND STAGE WAS BASED ON AN ACCULTURATION TYPOLOGY DERIVED FROM QUANTITATIVE DATA. ALL TWELVE SUBJECTS IN THE SECOND STAGE WERE INTENSIVELY INTERVIEWED AND OBSERVED IN THE SCHOOL, HOME, AND COMMUNITY SETTING, AND LIFE HISTORIES WERE COMPILED ON EACH. CONCLUSIONS DRAWN FROM THESE DATA WERE THAT LEVEL OF ACCULTURATION IS NOT INDICATIVE OF SUCCESSFUL SCHOOL PERFORMANCE. MANY SPANISH-SPEAKERS FARED WELL IN SCHOOL. CONVERSELY, ENGLISH-SPEAKERS DID POORLY. MOREOVER, SUPERIOR BILINGUAL ABILITY WAS A GOOD OVERALL PREDICTOR OF SCHOOL SUCCESS. WITHIN THE SOCIAL/ECONOMIC REALM IT WAS DISCOVERED THAT SOCIAL MOBILITY ASPIRATIONS, REGARDLESS OF LEVEL OF ACCULTURATION, CORRELATED WITH A STRONGER SCHOOL RECORD. WHILE SUBURBAN CHICANOS WERE MORE ACCULTURATED, OF A HIGHER SOCIAL CLASS, AND GENERALLY MORE POSITIVE IN THEIR ATTITUDE TOWARD SCHOOL AS COMPARED WITH THE URBAN GROUP, THE LATTER WERE MORE SOCIALLY MOBILE AND POSSESSED A SLIGHTLY HIGHER GRADE POINT AVERAGE. FUTURE RESEARCH EFFORTS SHOULD WIDEN THE SCOPE OF THIS INQUIRY OF ACCULTURATION BY INCLUDING MORE DIVERSE SOCIAL CLASSES AND CONTRASTING ENVIRONMENTS THAN WERE EXAMINED IN THIS STUDY.

ACCN   001650

1920 AUTH   **VILLA, W.**
TITL   AN ASSESSMENT OF THE CHICANO STUDENTS ON THE EDUCATIONAL OPPORTUNITY PROGRAM AT THE UNIVERSITY OF CALIFORNIA AT SANTA BARBARA. PART II: PROFILE OF THE CHICANO EOP DROP-OUT AS COMPARED WITH THE CHICANO EOP GRADUATE.
SRCE   *UNPUBLISHED MANUSCRIPT, UNIVERSITY OF CALIFORNIA, SANTA BARBARA, 1974. (AVAILABLE FROM DR. AMADO PADILLA, DEPARTMENT OF PSYCHOLOGY, UNIVERSITY OF CALIFORNIA, LOS ANGELES, CA 90024.)*
INDX   COLLEGE STUDENTS, PROGRAM EVALUATION, EDUCATIONAL ASSESSMENT, SCHOLASTIC ACHIEVEMENT, CALIFORNIA, SOUTHWEST, EDUCATION, HIGHER EDUCATION, MALE, ETHNIC IDENTITY, PSYCHOSOCIAL ADJUSTMENT
ABST   THIS STUDY OF THE ATTRITION OF CHICANO EOP STUDENTS AT UCSB ASKS: "WHAT ARE THE INDICATORS THAT A STUDENT WILL EXPERIENCE DIFFICULTIES WHICH WILL LEAD TO DROPPING OUT?" OF THE SAMPLE OF 46 CHICANO DROPOUTS, 31 WERE MALE AND 15 FEMALE; 29 ENTERED UCSB FROM HIGH SCHOOL AND WERE CLASSIFIED AS SPECIAL-ACTION STUDENTS, WHILE 17 WERE COMMUNITY COLLEGE TRANSFERS. THIRTY OF THE 46 DID NOT MEET THE UNIVERSITY'S CRITERIA FOR ADMISSION. PERSONAL AND ACADEMIC INFORMATION ON EACH STUDENT WAS GATHERED AND EXAMINED. CONCLUSIONS WERE THAT: (1) SPECIAL-ACTION FRESHMAN MALES FROM AN URBAN AREA ARE PARTICULARLY VULNERABLE; (2) THE MAJOR FACTOR FOR DROPPING OUT IS PERSONAL REASONS; (3) THE DEGREE OF CULTURAL IDENTITY FELT BY THE STUDENT AND HIS/HER ABILITY TO PURSUE IT THROUGH CHICANO STUDENT ORGANIZATIONS AND THE CHICANO STUDIES CLASSES TEND TO HELP THE STUDENT COPE WITH THE CULTURAL IMPACT OF THE UNIVERSITY; AND (4) THERE IS A DIRECT CORRELATION BETWEEN GETTING INVOLVED IN EXTRACURRICULAR ACTIVITIES AT UCSB AND BEING A SUCCESSFUL EOP GRADUATE. FOR FUTURE RESEARCH, IT IS INDICATED THAT THE FOLLOWING QUESTIONS BE EXPLORED: (1) DO WOMEN DO BETTER THAN MEN?; AND (2) DO RURAL CHICANO EOP STUDENTS COPE WITH THE UNIVERSITY ENVIRONMENT MORE EASILY THAN URBAN CHICANO STUDENTS? 5 REFERENCES.

ACCN   002452

1921 AUTH   **VONTRESS, C. E.**
TITL   COUNSELING MIDDLE-AGED AND AGING CULTURAL MINORITIES.
SRCE   *PERSONNEL AND GUIDANCE JOURNAL, 1976, 55(1),132-135.*
INDX   ADULTS, BILINGUAL, CROSS CULTURAL, CULTURAL FACTORS, EMPLOYMENT, SPANISH SURNAMED, ESSAY, GERONTOLOGY, HEALTH, ANOMIE, PSYCHOSOCIAL ADJUSTMENT, DEPRESSION, PSYCHOTHERAPY, POVERTY

ABST COUNSELING PROBLEMS CONCERNING COMMUNICATION, EMPLOYMENT, HEALTH, AND LONELINESS ENCOUNTERED IN WORKING WITH MIDDLE-AGED AND AGED AMERICANS OF INDIAN, AFRICAN, HISPANIC, AND ASIAN DECENT ARE CONSIDERED. IN THE AREA OF COMMUNICATION, BILINGUAL-BICULTURAL BARRIERS MAY NECESSITATE THE USE OF INTERPRETERS, AND THIS CAN IMPEDE THE DEVELOPMENT OF COUNSELING RAPPORT. SECOND, TRANSFERENCE AND COUNTER TRANSFERENCE MAY BE INAPPROPRIATELY APPLIED, PARTICULARLY IN THE CASE OF A YOUNG COUNSELOR OF DIFFERENT RACIAL/ETHNIC BACKGROUND WORKING WITH AN ELDERLY MINORITY PERSON. EMPLOYMENT PROBLEMS ARE WIDESPREAD AMONG ELDERLY MINORITIES, PARTICULARLY FOR HISPANICS IN THE SOUTHWEST, WHO ARE UNEMPLOYED LARGELY DUE TO THE EXCESS OF UNSKILLED YOUNG PERSONS IN COMPETITION FOR THE SAME JOBS. A THIRD MAJOR AREA OF CONCERN IS HEALTH PROBLEMS OFTEN EXACERBATED BY POOR PERSONAL HEALTH HABITS, INACCESSABLE HEALTH FACILITIES, AND THE HIGH STRESS OF GHETTO LIFE. LONELINESS ACCOMPANYING DISENGAGEMENT FROM CENTRAL LIFE ROLES IS ANOTHER PROBLEM AREA FOR LOWER-CLASS MINORITIES, BEGINNING AS EARLY AS AGE 35 OR 40 AS OPPOSED TO 65 FOR NON-MINORITY MEMBERS. COUNSELORS MUST BE SENSITIVE TO THE UNIQUE PROBLEMS FACING THESE INDIVIDUALS WHO CONSTITUTE A MINORITY WITHIN THE MINORITIES. 25 REFERENCES.

ACCN 002256

1922 AUTH **WADDELL, J. O.**
TITL FROM DISSONANCE TO CONSONANCE AND BACK AGAIN: MEXICAN AMERICANS AND CORRECTIONAL PROCESSES IN A SOUTHWEST CITY.
SRCE *IN J. HELM (ED.), SPANISH SPEAKING PEOPLE IN THE UNITED STATES: PROCEEDINGS OF THE 1968 ANNUAL SPRING MEETING OF THE AMERICAN ANTHROPOLOGICAL SOCIETY. SEATTLE: UNIVERSITY OF WASHINGTON PRESS, 1968, PP. 134-144.*
INDX MEXICAN AMERICAN, CORRECTIONS, COGNITIVE DISSONANCE, JUDICIAL PROCESS, CONFLICT RESOLUTION, CULTURAL FACTORS, ESSAY, SOUTHWEST
ABST THE STRUCTURE OF PROBATION AND ITS AFFECT ON MEXICAN AMERICANS (MA) LIVING IN A SOUTHWESTERN CITY WHO ARE UNDER THE INFLUENCE OF THE COURT'S AUTHORITY ARE DISCUSSED. FESTINGER'S THEORY OF COGNITIVE DISSONANCE IS EMPLOYED TO EXPLORE THE VARIOUS ALTERNATIVES FOR REDUCING COGNITIVE STRAIN EXPERIENCED BY MA'S. THE CORRECTIONAL PROCESS IS SEEN AS A FORM OF DIRECTED, DEVELOPMENTAL CHANGE WITH A SUPERIOR PLANNING SEGMENT (THE COURT) AND A PLANNED-FOR SEGMENT (THE OFFENDERS). HOWEVER, INDIVIDUALS FROM THE PREDOMINANTLY LOWER-CLASS MA COMMUNITY AND INDIVIDUALS REPRESENTING THE PREDOMINANTLY MIDDLE-CLASS ANGLO AUTHORITY STRUCTURE OF THE COURT CONSTITUTE TWO ASSYMETRICAL SEGMENTS IN THE

CITY. THUS, STRUCTURED FEATURES OF A PROBATION SENTENCE THAT ARE PARTICULARLY INCONSISTENT WITH MA CORE VALUES (I.E., DRINKING RESTRICTIONS AND AVOIDING "HARMFUL OR DISREPUTABLE CHARACTERS) ALONG WITH DIFFICULTIES IN SEEKING AND MAINTAINING EMPLOYMENT AND COURT-CONTROLLED RESOURCE DISTRIBUTION, INTENSIFY THE DISSONANCE IN VALUES BY KEEPING THE AWARENESS AT A CONSCIOUS LEVEL. THE MOST FREQUENTLY EMPLOYED ALTERNATIVE FOR MA'S WAS THAT OF TAKING A CHANCE WITH PROBATION, TRYING TO LEARN THE RULES IN ORDER TO SATISFY THE PROBATION OFFICER, BUT KEEPING THIS ATTITUDE COGNITIVELY COMPARTMENTALIZED FOR USE IN MAKING OFFICE REPORTS WITHOUT INTERFERING WITH THE EXISTING REFERENCE GROUP PATTERNS. FINALLY, IT IS BELIEVED THAT PROBATIONS FAIL BECAUSE INDIVIDUALS CANNOT HANDLE THE DISSONANCE THAT IS PROMOTED, AND COGNITIVE CONSONANCE IS MORE READILY AVAILABLE IN POTENTIALLY HARMFUL REFERENCE GROUPS EVEN IF THOSE IDENTITIES INCREASE THE LIKELIHOOD OF A PRISON SENTENCE. 7 REFERENCES.

ACCN 001651

1923 AUTH **WAGNER, B.**
TITL PARENT AND CHILD—WHAT'S THE SCORE? PARENTAL PREPARATION OF LEARNING ENVIRONMENTS FOR DELAYED AND NON-DELAYED INFANTS.
SRCE *PAPER PRESENTED AT THE ANNUAL MEETING OF THE SOUTHERN ASSOCIATION ON CHILDREN UNDER SIX, BAL HARBOR, FLORIDA, APRIL 1975. (ERIC DOCUMENT REPRODUCTION SERVICE NO. ED 114 211)*
INDX INFANCY, PARENTAL INVOLVEMENT, ENVIRONMENTAL FACTORS, LEARNING, SPANISH SURNAMED, SOCIALIZATION, TEXAS, SOUTHWEST
ABST THIS STUDY WAS DESIGNED TO ASSESS THE NEEDS OF PARENTS IN PREPARING HOME LEARNING ENVIRONMENTS FOR THEIR YOUNG CHILDREN. SUBJECTS INCLUDED 30 FAMILIES (10 ANGLO, 10 BLACK, AND 10 CHICANO) WITH CHILDREN FROM BIRTH TO 3 YEARS OF AGE. DATA ON APPROXIMATELY HALF OF THE FAMILIES HAS BEEN ANALYZED AND IS DISCUSSED. HALF OF THE SUBJECT POPULATION HAVE CHILDREN IDENTIFIED AS DEVELOPMENTALLY DELAYED/HIGH RISK. THESE CHILDREN WERE MATCHED WITH NORMAL (NONDELAYED) CHILDREN IN THE SAME ETHNIC GROUP. DATA WERE COLLECTED THROUGH VIDEOTAPES OF THE CHILD'S DAILY ACTIVITIES, OF THE PARENT AND CHILD HANDLING NEW MATERIALS, AND OF SEQUENCED ACTIVITIES BASED ON PIAGETIAN DEVELOPMENTAL TASKS DESIGNED TO EVALUATE THE CHILD'S DEVELOPMENTAL LEVEL. AFTER THE COMPLETION OF THE VIDEOTAPE SERIES, PARENTS' KNOWLEDGE OF CHILD DEVELOPMENT AND OF HOW HOME ENVIRONMENTS MAY BE PREPARED FOR THE OPTIMAL DEVELOPMENT OF CHILDREN WAS ASSESSED BY USE OF A PARENT QUESTIONNAIRE. AN OBSERVATION INSTRUMENT WAS THEN USED TO DETERMINE THE PARENTS' PER-

FORMANCE IN ACTUALLY PREPARING APPRO-PRIATE LEARNING ENVIRONMENTS FOR THEIR CHILDREN. PRELIMINARY RESULTS INDICATED THAT PARENTS OF ALL THREE ETHNIC GROUPS HAD SIGNIFICANTLY HIGHER KNOWLEDGE SCORES THAN PERFORMANCE SCORES IN THE PREPARATION OF THEIR CHILDREN'S LEARN-ING ENVIRONMENTS. 7 REFERENCES. (ERIC ABSTRACT)

ACCN   001652

1924 AUTH   **WALKER, J. R., & HAMILTON, L. S.**
TITL   A CHICANO/BLACK/WHITE ENCOUNTER.
SRCE   *PERSONNEL AND GUIDANCE JOURNAL, 1973, 51(7), 471-477.*
INDX   ATTITUDES, COLLEGE STUDENTS, CROSS CUL-TURAL, CULTURAL FACTORS, EMPIRICAL, MEN-TAL HEALTH, MEXICAN AMERICAN, PREJUDICE, PSYCHOTHERAPY, SEX COMPARISON, SPANISH SURNAMED, STEREOTYPES, SOUTHWEST, GROUP DYNAMICS
ABST   THIS STUDY EXAMINES WHAT HAPPENS WHEN MEMBERS OF THREE ETHNIC GROUPS SPEND EIGHTEEN HOURS TOGETHER IN AN "ENCOUN-TER WEEKEND." THE PARTICIPANTS WERE 14 SOUTHWESTERN UNIVERSITY STUDENTS—6 BLACKS, 4 CHICANOS, AND 4 WHITES—WITH 2 WHITE STUDENT PERSONNEL DEANS ACTING AS FACILITATORS. THERE WERE 2 FEMALES AND 2 MALES FROM EACH ETHNIC SUBGROUP PLUS 2 ADDITIONAL BLACK FEMALES. REA-SONABLE MATURITY AND EMOTIONAL STABIL-ITY, A RECORD OF "ACTIVISM," AND LACK OF PREVIOUS ENCOUNTER GROUP EXPERIENCE WERE THE SELECTION CRITERIA. THE GROUP MET FOR 18 HOURS, BEGINNING ON FRIDAY EVENING AND CULMINATING ON SUNDAY AFTERNOON. A VIDEOTAPE WAS MADE OF THE ENTIRE PROCEEDINGS AND WAS SUBSE-QUENTLY USED TO ANALYZE CHANGES IN GROUP BEHAVIOR. THE STAGES THE GROUP UNDERWENT ARE DESCRIBED IN TERMS OF ROGERS' FIFTEEN CLUSTERS OF OBSERVABLE EVENTS. IN GENERAL, IT WAS OBSERVED THAT THIS FACILITATION STYLE THAT PLACES THE MAJOR RESPONSIBILITY FOR GROUP PROG-RESS ON THE GROUP ITSELF BROUGHT ABOUT MARKED BEHAVIORAL CHANGES AS THE GROUP PROGRESSED FROM DISTRUST, SUSPI-CION, AND VIOLENT RHETORIC TO EFFECTIVE COMMUNICATION AND UNDERSTANDING. IT IS SUGGESTED THAT THE ENCOUNTER GROUP CAN BE A PROMISING SOCIAL TOOL FOR HELPING PEOPLE LEARN TO BE MORE HUMAN WITH ONE ANOTHER. 11 REFERENCES. (JOUR-NAL ABSTRACT MODIFIED)

ACCN   001653

1925 AUTH   **WALSH, J. F., & D'ANGELO, R.**
TITL   IQ'S OF PUERTO RICAN HEADSTART CHILDREN ON THE VANE KINDERGARTEN TEST.
SRCE   *JOURNAL OF SCHOOL PSYCHOLOGY, 1971, 9(2), 173-176.*
INDX   PUERTO RICAN-M, EARLY CHILDHOOD EDU-CATION, INTELLIGENCE TESTING, EMPIRICAL, NEW YORK, EAST, CHILDREN
ABST   THE USE OF THE VANE KINDERGARTEN INTEL-LIGENCE TEST WITH PUERTO RICAN CHILDREN

IN NEW YORK CITY IS EVALUATED. SUBJECTS INCLUDED 225 PUERTO RICAN CHILDREN BE-TWEEN 4 1/2 AND 6 YEARS OF AGE ENROLLED IN HEADSTART CENTERS IN THE BOROUGHS OF THE BRONX AND MANHATTAN. NO SIGNIFI-CANT DIFFERENCE FOR FULL SCALE SCORES WAS FOUND BETWEEN VANE'S STANDARDIZA-TION SAMPLE AND THE PUERTO RICAN GROUP ON THE VOCABULARY SUBTEST, PUERTO RI-CAN SUBJECTS EARNED LOWER MEAN SCORES; ON THE PERCEPTUAL-MOTOR SUBTESTS, THEY SCORED HIGHER THAN THE NORMATIVE GROUP. THE PUERTO RICAN LOWER VOCABULARY SCORES CONFIRM STUDIES SHOWING POORER LANGUAGE PERFORMANCE IN BILINGUAL CHILDREN FROM LOWER SOCIO-ECONOMIC GROUPS. THE HIGHER PUERTO RICAN PER-CEPTUAL-MOTOR SCORES ARE ATTRIBUTED TO THE INCLUSION OF ALL BILINGUAL CHIL-DREN IN THE SAMPLE. BILINGUAL PUERTO RI-CAN PRE-SCHOOLERS ARE REPORTED TO FUNCTION AT A GENERALLY HIGHER INTEL-LECTUAL LEVEL THAN MONOLINGUAL PRE-SCHOOLERS. THE INCLUSION OF SUBGROUP SAMPLES OF PUERTO RICAN SUBJECTS TESTED WITH ENGLISH LANGUAGE MATERIAL IN NOR-MATIVE TEST DATA IS QUESTIONED. 2 REFER-ENCES. (JOURNAL ABSTRACT MODIFIED)

ACCN   001654

1926 AUTH   **WALSH, M. A.**
TITL   THE DEVELOPMENT OF A RATIONALE FOR A PROGRAM TO PREPARE TEACHERS FOR SPAN-ISH-SPEAKING CHILDREN IN THE BILINGUAL-BICULTURAL ELEMENTARY SCHOOL.
SRCE   *SAN FRANCISCO: R AND E RESEARCH ASSOCI-ATES, 1976.*
INDX   MEXICAN AMERICAN, SCHOLASTIC ACHIEVE-MENT, BILINGUAL-BICULTURAL EDUCATION, EDUCATION, PROFESSIONAL TRAINING, BILIN-GUALISM, COMMUNITY INVOLVEMENT, TEACH-ERS, CURRICULUM, BILINGUAL-BICULTURAL PERSONNEL, ESSAY, INSTRUCTIONAL TECH-NIQUES, TEXAS, SOUTHWEST
ABST   THE DEVELOPMENT OF A PROGRAM FOR THE PREPARATION OF TEACHERS OF SPANISH-SPEAKING CHILDREN IN A BILINGUAL-BICUL-TURAL ELEMENTARY SCHOOL IN TEXAS IS DOCUMENTED. THE PLANNING PROCESS BE-GAN WITH A REVIEW OF THE LITERATURE RE-GARDING BILINGUAL EDUCATION PLUS A QUESTIONNAIRE SURVEY OF 50 CHIEF STATE SCHOOL OFFICERS. NEXT, TWELVE EDUCA-TORS—IDENTIFIED THROUGH THE QUESTION-NAIRE AS KNOWLEDGEABLE IN THE FIELD OF BILINGUAL EDUCATION—WERE SELECTED TO ATTEND A CONFERENCE ON BILINGUAL EDU-CATION SPONSORED BY ST. EDWARDS UNIVER-SITY, JANUARY, 1971. LINGUISTIC AND CUL-TURAL COMPETENCIES NEEDED BY BILINGUAL EDUCATORS WERE IDENTIFIED THROUGH IN-TERVIEWS WITH, AND A QUESTIONNAIRE AD-MINISTERED TO, THE 12 EDUCATORS. IDENTI-FIED COMPETENCIES INCLUDED A KNOWLEDGE OF (1) PHONOLOGY, MORPHOLOGY, AND SYN-TAX OF ENGLISH AND SPANISH, (2) PSY-CHOLOGY OF LANGUAGE LEARNING, (3) PSY-CHOSOCIAL ASPECTS OF BILINGUALISM, (4)

THE NATURE OF CULTURE AND ITS IMPACT ON PERSONALITY, (5) HISTORICAL AND GEOGRAPHIC CIRCUMSTANCES THAT HAVE SHAPED MEXICAN AMERICAN CULTURE IN THE SOUTHWEST, AND (6) THE RELATIONSHIP BETWEEN LANGUAGE AND CULTURE. THE RESULTING PRODUCT WAS RATIONALE FOR THE DEVELOPMENT OF A BILINGUAL EDUCATION TRAINING PROGRAM, CONSISTING OF (1) A DISCUSSION OF THE UNDERLYING PHILOSOPHY OF THE PROGRAM, (2) CONCEPTUALIZATION OF PROFESSIONAL NEEDS IN THE BILINGUAL SCHOOL, AND (3) A DEFINITION OF PROGRAM OBJECTIVES. FOLLOWING THE DOCUMENTATION OF PROGRAM DEVELOPMENT, AN APPROVED CURRICULUM FOR TEACHERS OF SPANISH-SPEAKING CHILDREN IN BILINGUAL-BICULTURAL ELEMENTARY SCHOOLS IN THE SOUTHWEST IS OUTLINED. 88 REFERENCES.

ACCN   001655

1927 AUTH   **WASSERMAN, N., PLUTCHIK, R., DEUTSCH, R., & TAKETOMO, Y.**

TITL   A MUSIC THERAPY EVALUATION SCALE AND ITS CLINICAL APPLICATION TO MENTALLY RETARDED ADULT PATIENTS.

SRCE   *JOURNAL OF MUSIC THERAPY, 1973, 10(2), 64-77.*

INDX   MUSIC, THERAPEUTIC COMMUNITY, MENTAL RETARDATION, ADULTS, BEHAVIOR THERAPY, PUERTO RICAN-M, EMPIRICAL

ABST   THREE EVALUATION SCALES DEVELOPED TO ASSESS MUSICAL APTITUDES AND SOCIAL BEHAVIOR IN HOSPITALIZED MENTALLY RETARDED PATIENTS WERE USED TO QUANTITATIVELY IDENTIFY CHANGES DURING THE COURSE OF A 3-MONTH MUSIC THERAPY PROGRAM. SIXTEEN ADULT PATIENTS (4 WOMEN, 12 MEN) PARTICIPATED IN THE PROGRAM. THREE PATIENTS WERE PUERTO RICAN, FOUR BLACK, AND NINE WERE WHITE. ELEVEN PATIENTS WERE EPILEPTIC, TWO WERE CLASSIFIED AS IDIOT SAVANTS, ONE HAD DOWN'S SYNDROME, AND ONE WAS CATATONIC. THE DEGREE OF RETARDATION RANGED FROM MODERATE TO PROFOUND AS DETERMINED BY THE STANFORD-BINET OR CATTELL INFANT INTELLIGENCE SCALE. MENTAL AGE RANGED FROM 1.5 TO 6.9 YEARS. SOCIAL BEHAVIOR AND MUSICAL APTITUDE WERE EVALUATED TWICE (AT A 1-MONTH INTERVAL) IN THREE MUSICAL GROUPS—RHYTHM, SINGING, AND VOCAL DYNAMICS. INVESTIGATORS ATTEMPTED TO ANSWER THREE QUESTIONS: (1) WAS THERE AGREEMENT BETWEEN INDEPENDENT OBSERVERS ON EVALUATIONS OF MUSICAL APTITUDE AND SOCIAL BEHAVIOR?; (2) WAS THERE A CHANGE IN APTITUDE AND BEHAVIOR DURING EXPOSURE TO MUSIC THERAPY?; AND (3) WAS THERE A RELATIONSHIP BETWEEN THE LEVEL OF MUSICAL APTITUDE AND THAT OF SOCIAL BEHAVIOR, AS EVALUATED BY RATING SCALES AND IQ SCORES?; RESULTS SHOW (1) THERE WAS INTER-RATER RELIABILITY IN EVALUATING MUSIC APTITUDE AND SOCIAL BEHAVIOR, (2) THERE WERE NO SIGNIFICANT CHANGES IN MUSICAL APTITUDE AND SOCIAL BEHAVIOR DURING THE EVALUATION PERIOD,

AND (3) PATIENTS WITH HIGHER IQS FUNCTION BETTER, BOTH MUSICALLY AND SOCIALLY, THAN THOSE WITH LOWER IQS. ALTHOUGH THERE WERE NO SIGNIFICANT CHANGES AS MEASURED BY THE EVALUATION SCALES, THERE WERE PATIENTS WHO SHOWED IMPROVEMENT IN THEIR SOCIAL BEHAVIOR IN THE MUSIC THERAPY SETTING. 7 REFERENCES.

ACCN   001656

1928 AUTH   **WASSERMAN, S. A.**

TITL   EXPRESSED 'HUMANITARIAN' AND 'SUCCESS' VALUES OF FOUR-YEAR-OLD MEXICAN-AMERICAN, NEGRO AND ANGLO BLUE-COLLAR AND WHITE-COLLAR CHILDREN (DOCTORAL DISSERTATION, UNIVERSITY OF CALIFORNIA, LOS ANGELES, 1969).

SRCE   *DISSERTATION ABSTRACTS INTERNATIONAL, 1969, 30(11), 5091A. (UNIVERSITY MICROFILMS NO. 70-08238.)*

INDX   COOPERATION, COMPETITION, CHILDREN, MEXICAN AMERICAN, CROSS CULTURAL, SES, ATTITUDES, EMPIRICAL, SEX COMPARISON, VALUES

ABST   THE DISSERTATION PROVIDES A MORE DETAILED ACCOUNT OF THE STUDY CITED BELOW (WASSERMAN, 1971). INCLUDED ARE: (1) A REVIEW OF THE LITERATURE ON VALUES AND CONTRASTING VALUE-ORIENTATIONS AND SYSTEMS; (2) A DETAILED ACCOUNT OF THE RESEARCH METHOD AND ANALYSIS OF THE DATA; (3) IMPLICATIONS FOR EARLY CHILDHOOD EDUCATION; AND (4) RECOMMENDATIONS FOR FURTHER RESEARCH. THE RESEARCH INSTRUMENT, ENTITLED VALUE PREFERENCE INVENTORY, IS APPENDED. 84 REFERENCES.

ACCN   001657

1929 AUTH   **WASSERMAN, S. A.**

TITL   VALUES OF MEXICAN AMERICAN, NEGRO, AND ANGLO BLUE-COLLAR AND WHITE-COLLAR CHILDREN.

SRCE   *CHILD DEVELOPMENT, 1971, 42(5), 1625-1628.*

INDX   ATTITUDES, MEXICAN AMERICAN, CROSS CULTURAL, CHILDREN, SES, SEX COMPARISON, EMPIRICAL, COOPERATION, COMPETITION, VALUES

ABST   THE RELATIONSHIP BETWEEN 4 YEAR-OLD CHILDREN'S EXPRESSED HUMANITARIAN AND SUCCESS VALUE PREFERENCES AND THEIR RELATED ETHNICITY, SOCIOECONOMIC STATUS, AND SEX IS INVESTIGATED. A SAMPLE OF 180 CHILDREN INCLUDED AN EQUAL NUMBER OF MEXICAN AMERICAN (MA), NEGRO (N), AND ANGLO (A) CHILDREN FROM BLUE- AND WHITE-COLLAR BACKGROUNDS. THE HUMANITARIAN VALUES EXAMINED ARE HELPFULNESS, COOPERATION, CONCERN FOR OTHERS, AND SHARING; THE SUCCESS VALUES ARE COMPETITION, STATUS, EXPERTISE SEEKING, AND COMPLETION OF TASK. THE INSTRUMENTS (16 PICTURES) DEPICTED VALUE CONFLICT SITUATIONS, WITH EIGHT VALUES ILLUSTRATED BY TWO SITUATIONS EACH. FINDINGS INDICATE THAT THE SCORES OF A CHILDREN ARE HIGHER THAN THOSE OF MA AND N CHILDREN. FOR THE HUMANITARIAN VALUE COMPLEX THE DIF-

FERENCES ARE SIGNIFICANT FOR THE A AND N CHILDREN, BUT NOT FOR MA CHILDREN WHEN COMPARED EITHER WITH A OR N CHILDREN. FOR THE SUCCESS VALUE COMPLEX, HOWEVER, SIGNIFICANT DIFFERENCES ARE FOUND BETWEEN SCORES OF A AND MA, AND BETWEEN A AND N CHILDREN. CHILDREN OF DIFFERENT ETHNIC GROUPS MAY HAVE INTERNALIZED CERTAIN SUCCESS AND HUMANITARIAN VALUES IN DIFFERING DEGREES. FOUR YEAR-OLD A CHILDREN APPEAR TO HAVE INTERNALIZED SUCCESS VALUES TO A GREATER DEGREE PRIOR TO THEIR ENTRANCE INTO KINDERGARTEN OR FIRSTGRADE. THESE VALUES MAY BE PARTICULARLY SIGNIFICANT TO A CHILD'S SUCCESS IN SCHOOL AS IT IS PRESENTLY CONSTITUTED, AND TO LATER SUCCESS IN THE OCCUPATIONAL HIERARCHY OF SOCIETY. IT IS SUGGESTED THAT MINORITY CHILDREN EXPERIENCE VALUE CONFLICT IN SCHOOL. 13 REFERENCES.

ACCN   001658

1930 AUTH   **WATSON, J. B., & SAMORA, J.**
TITL   SUBORDINATE LEADERSHIP IN A BICULTURAL COMMUNITY: AN ANALYSIS.
SRCE   *AMERICAN SOCIOLOGICAL REVIEW, 1954, 19(4), 413-421.*
INDX   COLORADO, SOUTHWEST, LEADERSHIP, MEXICAN AMERICAN, COMMUNITY INVOLVEMENT, STEREOTYPES, POLITICAL POWER, POLITICS, ATTITUDES, CULTURAL FACTORS, FARM LABORERS, EMPIRICAL, SES
ABST   DEFICIENCIES IN COMMUNITY LEADERSHIP AMONG MEXICAN AMERICANS ARE REVEALED IN THIS STUDY OF A SOUTHERN COLORADO MOUNTAIN TOWN (POPULATION 2,500; 58% SPANISH-SPEAKING). THE DATA WERE GATHERED IN 1949-50 BY SOCIOLOGY GRADUATE STUDENTS (UNIVERSITY OF WASHINGTON), HOWEVER THE METHODOLOGY IS NOT DESCRIBED. THE MEXICAN AMERICAN RESIDENTS—PREDOMINANTLY LOW PAID AGRICULTURAL WORKERS—SHARE IN COMMON A NUMBER OF GRIEVANCES CONCERNING SCHOOLING, HOUSING, AND POLITICS. YET, THEY SHOW A STRONG TENDENCY TO SHRINK FROM LEADERSHIP ROLES BOTH IN INTER- AND INTRA-ETHNIC ORGANIZATIONS. THREE REASONS ARE POSITED TO ACCOUNT FOR THIS: (1) TRADITIONAL PATTERNS OF LEADERSHIP, AS THE "PATRON" OR "JEFE DE FAMILIA" SYSTEMS ARE INADEQUATE FOR PROMOTING COMMUNITY LEADERSHIP; (2) A GENERAL SUSPICION OF FELLOW MEXICAN AMERICANS WHO ARE "SUCCESSFUL" IN THE EYES OF ANGLOS; AND (3) INSUFFICIENT LEADERSHIP SKILLS—SUCH AS POOR LITERACY, LACK OF COMMAND OF ENGLISH, AND INADEQUATE KNOWLEDGE OF THE SOCIAL, POLITICAL, AND LEGAL PRACTICES OF THE DOMINANT SOCIETY. AN EXTENSIVE DISCUSSION OF THE "PATRON" SYSTEM IN THE SOUTHWEST IS PRESENTED; AND THE PHENOMENON OF ANGLO STEREOTYPING OF THE SPANISH-SPEAKING AS EITHER "REAL SPANISH" (HENCE, "GOOD") OR MERE "MEXICANS" IS DESCRIBED. IT IS CONCLUDED THAT THE COMBINATION OF ANGLO STEREOTYPING AND MEXICAN AMERICAN ATTITUDES ABOUT LEADERSHIP CAUSE MEXICAN AMERICANS' LEADERSHIP DEFICIENCIES IN THIS COMMUNITY. 10 REFERENCES.

ACCN   001659

1931 AUTH   **WEAVER, C. N.**
TITL   ACCIDENTS AS A MEASURE OF THE CULTURAL ADJUSTMENT OF MEXICAN AMERICANS.
SRCE   *THE SOCIOLOGICAL QUARTERLY, 1970, 11, 119-125.*
INDX   SES, MEXICAN AMERICAN, JOB PERFORMANCE, ACCULTURATION, CULTURAL FACTORS, PERFORMANCE EXPECTATIONS, ADULTS, CROSS CULTURAL, LABOR FORCE, TEXAS, SOUTHWEST
ABST   TO TEST THE HYPOTHESIS THAT THE STRESSES OF ACCULTURATION CAN CAUSE GREATER ON-THE-JOB ACCIDENTS AMONG MEXICAN AMERICANS, ACCIDENT RATES AMONG MEXICAN AMERICAN AND ANGLO WORKERS AT THE SAN ANTONIO HOUSING AUTHORITY AND AT THE POLICE AND FIRE DEPARTMENTS WERE EXAMINED. AT THE HOUSING AUTHORITY (TOTAL STAFF 191 = 82 MEXICAN AMERICANS, 109 ANGLOS AND OTHERS) THE ACTUAL NUMBER OF ACCIDENTS INVOLVING MEXICAN AMERICANS, ANGLOS, AND OTHERS WERE COMPARED WITH THE EXPECTED NUMBER OF ACCIDENTS BASED UPON THEIR REPRESENTATION ON THE STAFF. THE RESULTS SHOW THAT THE MEXICAN AMERICAN MAINTENANCE EMPLOYEES CONTRIBUTED LESS TO THE TOTAL NUMBER OF ON-THE-JOB ACCIDENTS THAN WOULD BE EXPECTED. SECONDLY, THERE WAS NO STATISTICALLY SIGNIFICANT DIFFERENCE BETWEEN MEXICAN AMERICANS AND OTHER EMPLOYEES IN TERMS OF ACCIDENTS WHICH INVOLVED A COST IN EMPLOYEE HOURS OFF THE JOB. BECAUSE A SIMILAR PICTURE EMERGES FROM THE ACCIDENT RECORDS OF BOTH THE POLICE AND FIRE DEPARTMENTS, IT IS CONCLUDED THAT THE RESULTS DO NOT SUPPORT THE HYPOTHESIS. 14 REFERENCES.

ACCN   001660

1932 AUTH   **WEAVER, C. N.**
TITL   A COMPARATIVE STUDY OF THE MEXICAN-AMERICAN MAINTENANCE EMPLOYEES AT THE SAN ANTONIO HOUSING AUTHORITY.
SRCE   *BUSINESS STUDIES, NORTH TEXAS STATE UNIVERSITY, FALL 1968.*
INDX   CULTURAL FACTORS, JOB PERFORMANCE, STEREOTYPES, EMPIRICAL, CROSS CULTURAL, MEXICAN AMERICAN, EMPLOYMENT, ADULTS, MALE, TEXAS, SOUTHWEST
ABST   IN THIS COMPARISON OF THE JOB PERFORMANCE OF SPANISH-SURNAME EMPLOYEES WITH THE PERFORMANCE OF THEIR NON-SPANISH-SURNAMED FELLOW WORKERS, IT WAS HYPOTHESIZED THAT THERE SHOULD BE NO DIFFERENCES BETWEEN THE JOB PERFORMANCES OF THE TWO GROUPS. THE DATA WERE DERIVED FROM THE PERSONNEL RECORDS OF THE HOUSING AUTHORITY OF SAN ANTONIO, TEXAS—RECORDS WHICH PROVIDED INFORMATION ON ACCIDENT RATES AND THE AMOUNT

OF SICK LEAVE AND ANNUAL LEAVE TAKEN. REGARDING SICK LEAVE, THE STUDY REVEALED THAT WHAT DIFFERENCE EXISTED BETWEEN THE TWO GROUPS INDICATED BETTER PERFORMANCE BY THE SPANISH-SURNAME EMPLOYEES. SIMILAR FINDINGS WERE REPORTED WITH RESPECT TO PERCENT OF ANNUAL LEAVE. MOREOVER, NO EVIDENCE WAS FOUND TO SUPPORT THE CONTENTION THAT THERE IS A DIFFERENCE IN ACCIDENT RATES BETWEEN THE MEXICAN AMERICANS AND ANGLOS. IN SUM, THE FINDINGS OF THIS STUDY CAST DOUBT ON THE ASSUMPTION THAT THE ORGANIZATIONAL BEHAVIOR OF MEXICAN AMERICANS IS LESS ADEQUATE THAN THAT OF ANGLO AMERICANS. LITTLE EVIDENCE WAS FOUND TO SUPPORT THE BELIEF THAT THERE ARE INNATE, PSYCHOLOGICAL, OR CULTURAL FACTORS WHICH LIMIT THE EFFECTIVENESS OF THE MEXICAN AMERICAN EMPLOYEE IN THE JOB SITUATION. 4 REFERENCES.

ACCN 001661

1933 AUTH **WEAVER, C. N.**
TITL A COMPARISON OF THE JOB PERFORMANCE OF MEXICAN AMERICAN AND ANGLO AMERICAN EMPLOYEES WITH SIMILAR LEVELS OF EDUCATION.
SRCE *JOURNAL OF EDUCATIONAL RESEARCH, 1971, 22(1), 26-33.*
INDX JOB PERFORMANCE, MEXICAN AMERICAN, CROSS CULTURAL, SCHOLASTIC ACHIEVEMENT, EMPIRICAL, LABOR FORCE, STEREOTYPES
ABST AS A WHOLE, THE MEXICAN AMERICAN POPULATION HAS NOT SHARED IN THE BENEFITS OF THE HIGH-LEVEL U.S. ECONOMY. THE MEXICAN AMERICANS ARE NOT PROPORTIONATELY REPRESENTED IN THE BETTER-PAID, HIGHER-STATUS OCCUPATIONAL CATEGORIES. THIS STUDY, CONDUCTED IN SEVERAL ORGANIZATIONS IN SAN ANTONIO, TEXAS, REVEALS THAT THE JOB PERFORMANCE OF MEXICAN AMERICANS IS COMPARABLE TO THAT OF ANGLOS, PROVIDED THEIR LEVELS OF EDUCATION ARE SIMILAR. IT APPEARS, THEREFORE, THAT THE CURRENT WIDESPREAD EFFORTS TO INCREASE THE LEVEL OF EDUCATION OF MEXICAN AMERICANS IS A WORTHWHILE APPROACH TO SOLVING THE PROBLEMS ASSOCIATED WITH THEIR DISADVANTAGED STATUS. 8 REFERENCES. (JOURNAL ABSTRACT)
ACCN 001662

1934 AUTH **WEAVER, C. N., & GLENN, N. D.**
TITL THE JOB PERFORMANCE OF MEXICAN-AMERICANS.
SRCE *SOCIOLOGY AND SOCIAL RESEARCH, 1970, 54(4), 477-494.*
INDX JOB PERFORMANCE, MEXICAN AMERICAN, CROSS CULTURAL, EMPIRICAL, LABOR FORCE, STEREOTYPES, TEXAS, SOUTHWEST
ABST MEXICAN AMERICAN AND ANGLO AMERICAN WORKERS IN THE SAME JOBS AND ORGANIZATIONS IN SAN ANTONIO, TEXAS, WERE COMPARED IN EFFICIENCY RATINGS AND SEVERAL OBJECTIVE INDICATORS OF JOB PERFORMANCE. MEXICAN AMERICAN POLICEMEN AND

FIREMEN AND YOUNG MEXICAN AMERICAN POSTAL CLERKS TOOK SOMEWHAT MORE SICK LEAVE THAN THEIR ANGLO CO-WORKERS, BUT OTHERWISE THE MEXICAN AMERICANS EXCEEDED OR ABOUT EQUALLED THE ANGLOS IN THE RATINGS AND INDICATORS. THESE FINDINGS ARE NOT CONCLUSIVE EVIDENCE AGAINST THE WIDESPREAD BELIEF THAT TRADITIONAL MEXICAN CULTURE IS DETRIMENTAL TO JOB PERFORMANCE AND ECONOMIC ADVANCEMENT, BUT THEY INDICATE THAT ANY SUCH INFLUENCE IS NOT VERY GREAT AMONG MODERATELY ACCULTURATED WORKERS UNDER THE CONDITIONS THAT EXIST IN SAN ANTONIO. 9 REFERENCES. (JOURNAL ABSTRACT)

ACCN 001663

1935 AUTH **WEAVER, J. L.**
TITL HEALTH CARE COSTS AS A POLITICAL ISSUE: COMPARATIVE RESPONSES OF CHICANOS AND ANGLOS.
SRCE *SOCIAL SCIENCE QUARTERLY, 1973, 53(4), 846-854.*
INDX HEALTH, URBAN, CROSS CULTURAL, MEXICAN AMERICAN, SURVEY, SES, COMMUNITY INVOLVEMENT, CHICANO MOVEMENT
ABST URBAN CHICANOS AND ANGLOS WERE SURVEYED TO ASSESS (1) EXPERIENCE WITH THE HEALTH CARE INDUSTRY, (2) OPINION OF PREVAILING PRICE STRUCTURE, AND (3) SUPPORT OF FIVE HEALTH COST REDUCTION SCHEMES. SURVEY RESPONDENTS WERE SELECTED AT RANDOM FROM CENSUS TRACTS TO OBTAIN EQUAL SAMPLES BY MEDIAN ANNUAL INCOME ($8,000-$14,000, AND UNDER $8,000). BILINGUAL COLLEGE COEDS AND ANGLO INTERVIEWERS COMPLETED 484 INTERVIEWS (79% ANGLO, 15% CHICANO, 6% OTHER). DETAILED MEDICAL HISTORIES OF EACH FAMILY DURING THE 6 MONTHS PRIOR TO THE INTERVIEW INCLUDED NAMES AND ADDRESSES OF CARE PROVIDERS AND PRESCRIBED TREATMENTS UNDERTAKEN. RESPONDENTS' VIEWS ON THE GOVERNMENT'S ROLE IN REDUCING HEALTH CARE COSTS WERE ASSESSED BY THEIR (1) OPINION OF COSTLINESS (TOO HIGH, REASONABLE, A BARGAIN) OF HOSPITALIZED CARE, PHYSICIANS' AND DENTISTS' SERVICES, AND PRESCRIBED DRUGS, AND (2) APPROVAL OR DISAPPROVAL OF FIVE HEALTH COST REDUCING PROPOSALS. WHILE BOTH POPULATIONS REGARD HEALTH CARE COSTS AS TOO HIGH, THE CHICANO COMMUNITY EXPRESSED SUPPORT FOR COST CUTTING PROPOSALS TO A MUCH GREATER DEGREE THAN THE ANGLOS. THE CONCERN ABOUT RISING HEALTH CARE COSTS MAY OFFER A FOCUS FOR WIDESPREAD POLITICAL MOBILIZATION WITHIN THE CHICANO COMMUNITY. 9 REFERENCES.
ACCN 001665

1936 AUTH **WEAVER, J. L.**
TITL MEXICAN AMERICAN HEALTH CARE BEHAVIOR: A CRITICAL REVIEW OF THE LITERATURE.
SRCE *SOCIAL SCIENCE QUARTERLY, 1973, 54(1), 85-102.*

INDX   MEXICAN AMERICAN, HEALTH, REVIEW, CULTURE, CURANDERISMO, MENTAL HEALTH, STEREOTYPES, FOLK MEDICINE, HEALTH DELIVERY SYSTEMS, CULTURAL FACTORS, CULTURE, RESOURCE UTILIZATION

ABST   THE METHODOLOGY, CONTENT, AND RELIABILITY OF THREE DECADES OF SOCIAL SCIENCE LITERATURE CONCERNING THE HEALTH BEHAVIOR OF MEXICAN AMERICANS IS REVIEWED. IN THE LATE 1940'S, ETHNOGRAPHIC STUDIES PLACED MEXICAN AMERICAN HEALTH CARE BEHAVIOR IN A CULTURAL PERSPECTIVE, WITH FOLK MEDICINE AT ITS CORE. MID- AND LATE-1950'S STUDIES, CONSISTING OF ETHNOGRAPHIES OF WORKING-CLASS RURAL AND VILLAGE POPULATIONS, DESCRIBED AN UNDIFFERENTIATED, HOMOGENEOUS POPULATION DISTRUSTFUL OF SCIENTIFIC MEDICINE AND RELIANT UPON FOLK PRACTICES. WORK OF THE 1960'S UTILIZED SURVEY RESEARCH METHODS AND ETHNOGRAPHIC DATA TO INVESTIGATE SUBSECTIONS OF THE MEXICAN AMERICAN POPULATION. OF THE LITERATURE REVIEWED, THERE ARE NO SYSTEMATIC WIDE-RANGING STUDIES OF HEALTH BEHAVIOR. IT IS RECOMMENDED THAT THREE QUESTIONS BE ADDRESSED IN NEW RESEARCH: (1) IS THERE A MEXICAN AMERICAN HEALTH CARE SUBCULTURE?; (2) IS UTILIZATION OF PUBLIC AND PRIVATE PROVIDERS A FUNCTION OF ETHNICITY?; AND (3) DO SPANISH-SPEAKING HEALTH PROVIDERS AND STAFF INCREASE UTILIZATION OF A HEALTH PROGRAM? 52 REFERENCES.

ACCN   001666

1937 AUTH   **WEAVER, T.**
TITL   SAMPLING AND GENERALIZATION IN ANTHROPOLOGICAL RESEARCH ON SPANISH SPEAKING GROUPS.

SRCE   *IN J. HELM (ED.), SPANISH SPEAKING PEOPLE IN THE UNITED STATES: PROCEEDINGS OF THE 1968 ANNUAL SPRING MEETING OF THE AMERICAN ETHNOLOGICAL SOCIETY. SEATTLE: UNIVERSITY OF WASHINGTON PRESS, 1968, PP. 1-18.*

INDX   SOCIAL SCIENCES, RESEARCH METHODOLOGY, SPANISH SURNAMED, DEMOGRAPHIC, CULTURAL FACTORS, ESSAY

ABST   THE USE OF MORE RIGOROUS AND SOPHISTICATED SAMPLING TECHNIQUES IN ANTHROPOLOGICAL STUDIES AND THE NEED FOR REPRESENTING THE TOTAL RANGE OF CULTURAL VARIATION PRESENT IN SUCH A COMPLEX GROUP AS THE SPANISH-SPEAKING (SS) POPULATION OF NEW MEXICO IS THE FOCUS OF THIS ARTICLE. AT PRESENT, GENERALIZATIONS FAIL TO ACCOUNT FOR STATUS, STRATIFICATION, SUBCULTURAL, ECONOMIC, AND OTHER DIFFERENCES IN THIS POPULATION AS A WHOLE. FURTHERMORE, ANTHROPOLOGISTS ARE NOT OVERLY CONCERNED WITH SAMPLING BECAUSE: (1) THE SMALL COMMUNITY SIZE ALLOWS FOR TOTAL ENCOMPASSING; (2) THERE IS A BIAS AGAINST QUANTITATIVE TECHNIQUES; (3) SOCIETIES UNDER STUDY HAVE NOT HAD WIDE CLASS AND STATUS DIFFERENTIATION; AND (4) SMALL CLOSED SYSTEMS ARE NOT SEEN AS PARTS OF LARGER

SOCIETIES. INDICATORS FROM POPULATION STATISTICS OF THE SS OF NEW MEXICO (I.E., RURAL-URBAN, NATIVITY OR PARENTAGE, MEDIAN AGE, YEARS OF EDUCATION, SCHOOL ENROLLMENT, OCCUPATION, AND INCOME) REVEAL WIDE VARIATIONS AMONG NATIVE BORN, MIXED PARENTAGE AND MEXICAN BORN. CONCLUSIONS ARE THAT: (1) SUBCULTURAL AREAS OF SS PERSONS CAN BE IDENTIFIED IN NEW MEXICO BASED ON DEMOGRAPHIC DATA; (2) DATA SUPPORT A DISTINCTION BASED ON SUBCULTURAL FACTORS; AND (3) LITTLE CAN BE ASCERTAINED FROM AVAILABLE DATA AS TO THE TOTAL SS POPULATION OR OTHER SEGMENTS OTHER THAN THE RURAL-FARMING-PASTORAL SUBCULTURE. IN ADDITION, THERE IS EVIDENCE FOR DISTINGUISHING A SPANISH AMERICAN FROM A MEXICAN AMERICAN SUBCULTURE. CURRENT ANTHROPOLOGICAL SAMPLING TECHNIQUES ARE OUTLINED AND SUGGESTED STEPS IN FIELD WORK ON COMPLEX GROUPS ARE PRESENTED. 46 REFERENCES.

ACCN   001667

1938 AUTH   **WEAVER, T.**
TITL   USE OF HYPOTHETICAL SITUATIONS IN A STUDY OF SPANISH-AMERICAN ILLNESS REFERRAL SYSTEMS.

SRCE   *HUMAN ORGANIZATION, 1970, 29(2), 140-152.*

INDX   HEALTH DELIVERY SYSTEMS, RESEARCH METHODOLOGY, SPANISH SURNAMED, EMPIRICAL, HEALTH, FOLK MEDICINE, COPING MECHANISMS, NEW MEXICO, SOUTHWEST

ABST   THE "HYPOTHETICAL SITUATION" TECHNIQUE AS AN ETHNOGRAPHIC TOOL CONSISTS OF DEVISING HYPOTHETICAL SITUATIONS IN THE LIFE OF A PEOPLE TO DIRECT THE DISCUSSIONS OF INFORMANTS. THIS TECHNIQUE WAS USED IN A STUDY OF THE INDIGENOUS REFERRAL SYSTEM FOR ILLNESS IN NORTHERN NEW MEXICO VILLAGES. INTERVIEWS WERE CONDUCTED WITH (1) SINGLE INFORMANTS (CURANDEROS, THEIR PATIENTS, AND PATIENTS' RELATIVES), AND (2) GROUPS OF INFORMANTS (ACCULTURATED SPANISH AMERICANS FROM LARGER TOWNS AND CITIES). THE RESULTS FROM 17 MONTHS OF INTERVIEWS, FROM 1959 TO 1962, REVEALED THAT THERE ARE FOUR SUCCESSIVE STAGES OF HEALTH CONSULTATION. IN STAGE ONE, INVOLVING MINOR ILLNESSES AND THE BEGINNINGS OF MAJOR ILLNESSES, CONSULTATION AND MEDICATION COME FROM KIN GROUP PROVIDERS. IN STAGE TWO, FRIENDS, NEIGHBORS, AND OTHER KNOWLEDGEABLE COMMUNITY MEMBERS ARE CONSULTED. IN STAGE THREE, LOCALLY AND CULTURALLY DEFINED EXPERTS IN CURING COMMON ILLNESSES (I.E., CURANDEROS) ARE CONSULTED. FINALLY, IT IS IN STAGE FOUR WHEREIN URBAN PROFESSIONALS—SCIENTIFICALLY TRAINED AND OF A DIFFERENT CULTURE THAN THE PATIENT—ARE CONSULTED. THERE IS SUFFICIENT EVIDENCE TO INDICATE THAT THE STRUCTURAL AND FUNCTIONAL ASPECTS OF THIS ILLNESS REFERRAL SYSTEM ARE SIMILAR ACROSS CULTURES. 27 REFERENCES.

ACCN   001668

1939 AUTH   **WEBER, R. E.**
TITL   NEUROLOGICAL IMPAIRMENT.
SRCE   *SAN FERNANDO, CALIF.: MONTAL EDUCA-TIONAL ASSOCIATES, FEBRUARY 1972.*
INDX   MENTAL RETARDATION, MEXICAN AMERICAN, CHILDREN, ESSAY, LEARNING DISABILITIES, SPECIAL EDUCATION, SYMPTOMATOLOGY
ABST   THE NEEDS OF THE NEUROLOGICALLY HANDI-CAPPED BILINGUAL/BICULTURAL CHICANITO ARE CONSIDERED IN A DISCUSSION OF THE DEFINITION, ETIOLOGY, INCIDENCE, SYMP-TOMATOLOGY, TREATMENT, AND CONSE-QUENCES OF NEUROLOGIC IMPAIRMENT. THE NEUROLOGICALLY IMPAIRED, ACCOUNTING FOR 8-10% OF THE SCHOOL-AGE POPULA-TION, EXHIBIT ABERRANT PHYSICAL, INTEL-LECTUAL, EMOTIONAL AND SOCIAL DEVELOP-MENT. THE ETIOLOGY OF NEUROLOGICAL IMPAIRMENT MAY BE TRACED TO (1) GENETIC ABERRATION, (2) DISEASE, (3) BIRTH COMPLI-CATION/TRAUMA, (4) ENVIRONMENTAL TRAUMA, AND (5) POOR NUTRITION DURING THE PRE-NATAL, PERINATAL, OR POSTNATAL COURSE. DIAGNOSTIC EVALUATIONS (I.E., MEDICAL EX-AMINATION, PSYCHOLOGICAL TESTING, TEACHER EVALUATION, AND SELF-EVALUA-TION) REVEAL SYMPTOMATOLOGY INCLUDING VISUAL AND AUDITORY PERCEPTUAL DISOR-DERS, MOTOR DYSFUNCTION, AND TEMPORAL DISORIENTATION. THE AVERAGE NEUROLOGI-CALLY IMPAIRED CHILD IS CHARACTERIZED BY A POOR SELF-IMAGE, MANIFESTED ANXIETY, OVER-REACTIVENESS, OVER-SENSITIVITY, LOW FRUSTRATION THRESHOLDS, POOR STRESS TOLERANCE, AND DIFFICULTY IN ADAPTING TO CHANGE. THE BASIC SOCIAL DRIVES, CURIOS-ITY, NEED FOR STATUS, AND COMPANIONSHIP ARE OFTEN BLUNTED AND FRUSTRATED. THE ADAPTATION PROBLEMS OF THE CHICANITO ARE GREATLY EXACERBATED BY A NEURO-LOGIC IMPAIRMENT, PARTICULARLY WHERE LANGUAGE IS CONCERNED. RECOMMENDA-TIONS WHICH WOULD IMPROVE SERVICES TO THE BILINGUAL/BICULTURAL, NEUROLOGI-CALLY IMPAIRED CHICANO CHILD INCLUDE: (1) RECRUIT AND TRAIN BILINGUAL/BICULTURAL SPECIAL EDUCATION PERSONNEL; (2) DE-VELOP PROGRAMS FOR EARLY DIAGNOSIS AND INTERVENTION; (3) PROMOTE COMPREHEN-SIVE PRE-SCHOOL PROGRAMS; (4) INCREASE PARENTAL UNDERSTANDING OF THEIR CHILD'S EDUCATIONAL RIGHTS THROUGH PARENT GROUP ORGANIZATION; (5) CORRECT THE MISLABELING OF BILINGUAL MINORITY CHIL-DREN AS MENTALLY RETARDED; (6) PROVIDE SENSITIVITY TRAINING FOR NORMAL CHIL-DREN AND EDUCATIONAL PROFESSIONALS; AND (7) ENCOURAGE NORMALIZATION THROUGH INTEGRATION OF SPECIAL EDUCA-TION WITH THE REGULAR EDUCATIONAL SYS-TEM. 39 REFERENCES.
ACCN   001669

1940 AUTH   **WECLEW, R. V.**
TITL   THE NATURE, PREVALENCE, AND LEVEL OF AWARENESS OF "CURANDERISMO" AND SOME OF ITS IMPLICATIONS FOR COMMUNITY MEN-TAL HEALTH.
SRCE   *COMMUNITY MENTAL HEALTH JOURNAL, 1975, 11(2), 145-154.*
INDX   MEXICAN AMERICAN, FOLK MEDICINE, CUR-ANDERISMO, MENTAL HEALTH, HEALTH DELIV-ERY SYSTEMS, MENTAL HEALTH PROFESSION, PARAPROFESSIONALS, EMPIRICAL, COMMU-NITY, CROSS CULTURAL, RESOURCE UTILIZA-TION, ADULTS, URBAN, BILINGUAL-BICUL-TURAL PERSONNEL, ILLINOIS, MIDWEST
ABST   A STUDY ON EXPLORATORY RESEARCH INTO THE NATURE, PREVALENCE, AND LEVEL OF AWARENESS OF CURANDERISMO (MEXICAN FOLK PSYCHIATRY) IS PRESENTED; ALSO, SOME OF ITS RAMIFICATIONS FOR COMMUNITY MEN-TAL HEALTH, AS PERCEIVED BY THE STAFF OF TWO COMMUNITY MENTAL HEALTH CENTERS SERVING LARGELY MEXICAN AMERICAN POPU-LATIONS ON CHICAGO'S SOUTH SIDE, ARE DIS-CUSSED. THE SAMPLE INTERVIEWED CON-SISTED OF VIRTUALLY THE ENTIRE STAFF—29 PERSONS IN ALL, 14 FROM ONE COMMUNITY MENTAL HEALTH CENTER AND 15 FROM THE OTHER. DATA COLLECTION WAS DONE INDI-VIDUALLY WITH A 4 PAGE, 31 QUESTION INTER-VIEW, MADE UP OF PERSONAL DATA QUES-TIONS, MULTIPLE CHOICE QUESTIONS, AND OPEN ENDED ONES. THESE FINDINGS SHOW THAT THERE IS NO ONE UNIVERSAL DEFINI-TION OF CURANDERO, THAT THE PREVALENCE OF CURANDERISMO IS NOT DETERMINED, AND THAT ALTHOUGH THE CURANDERO AND MEN-TAL HEALTH WORKER SEE THE CLIENT SEPA-RATELY, A COOPERATION IN TREATMENT AND AN AGREEMENT ON THERAPEUTIC GOALS ARE DEVELOPING. 7 REFERENCES. (NCMHI AB-STRACT)
ACCN   001670

1941 AUTH   **WEIGEL, R. H., WISER, P. L., & COOK, S. W.**
TITL   THE IMPACT OF COOPERATIVE LEARNING EX-PERIENCES ON CROSS-ETHNIC RELATIONS AND ATTITUDES.
SRCE   *JOURNAL OF SOCIAL ISSUES, 1975, 31(1), 219-244.*
INDX   ATTITUDES, CROSS CULTURAL, MEXICAN AMERICAN, ETHNIC IDENTITY, GROUP DYNAM-ICS, INTEGRATION, ADOLESCENTS, INTERPER-SONAL RELATIONS, CULTURAL FACTORS, EM-PIRICAL, EDUCATION, DISCRIMINATION, CLASSROOM BEHAVIOR, COOPERATION, IN-STRUCTIONAL TECHNIQUES, INTERPERSONAL ATTRACTION, TEACHERS
ABST   A FIELD EXPERIMENT EXAMINED THE EFFECTS OF COOPERATIVE INTERETHNIC CONTACT ON ETHNIC RELATIONS AND ATTITUDES IN THE SETTING OF NEWLY DESEGREGATED JUNIOR AND SENIOR HIGH SCHOOLS. COOPERATIVE INTERETHNIC CONTACT WAS INDUCED IN THE EXPERIMENTAL CLASSROOMS BY MEANS OF A TEACHING METHOD WHICH EMPHASIZED THE USE OF SMALL INTERDEPENDENT STUDENT WORK GROUPS COMPOSED OF WHITE, BLACK, AND MEXICAN AMERICAN STUDENTS. RESULTS INDICATED THAT THE INTERETHNIC GROUP METHOD RECEIVED A FAVORABLE ENDORSE-MENT FROM THE TEACHERS, PRODUCED SUB-

STANTIALLY MORE CROSS-ETHNIC HELPING BEHAVIOR, AND PROMOTED GREATER RELATIVE RESPECT AND LIKING FOR MEXICAN AMERICAN CLASSMATES AMONG WHITE STUDENTS. 38 REFERENCES. (JOURNAL ABSTRACT)

ACCN   001671

1942 AUTH   **WEIGEL, R. H., & QUINN, T. E.**
TITL   ETHNIC DIFFERENCES IN COOPERATIVE BEHAVIOR: A NON-CONFIRMATION.
SRCE   *PSYCHOLOGICAL REPORTS, 1977, 40, 666.*
INDX   ADOLESCENTS, COMPETITION, COOPERATION, CROSS CULTURAL, CULTURAL FACTORS, DYADIC INTERACTION, EMPIRICAL, MALE, URBAN, PERSONALITY, PUERTO RICAN-M, EAST, MASSACHUSETTS
ABST   TO TEST PREVIOUS RESEARCH FINDINGS WHICH INDICATE THAT SUBCULTURAL VARIATIONS EXIST IN CHILDREN'S DISPOSITIONS FOR COOPERATION, 148 13 YEAR-OLD URBAN BOYS WERE ASSIGNED TO ONE OF 6 EXPERIMENTAL CONDITIONS (WHITE-WHITE, BLACK-BLACK, PUERTO RICAN-PUERTO RICAN, WHITE-BLACK, WHITE-PUERTO RICAN, AND BLACK-PUERTO RICAN). THE BOYS WERE ASKED TO COMPLETE A VERSION OF MADSEN'S COOPERATION BOARD GAME, A GAME IN WHICH PRIZE WINNINGS CAN BE MAXIMIZED ONLY IF THE PAIRED SUBJECTS COOPERATIVELY ASSIST ONE ANOTHER. COOPERATION WAS MEASURED IN TERMS OF LENGTH OF TIME TAKEN TO COMPLETE THE GAME AND NUMBER OF PRIZES WON. NO SIGNIFICANT DIFFERENCES WERE FOUND AMONG THE SIX CONDITIONS WITH RESPECT TO EITHER TIME TO SOLUTION SCORES OR NUMBER OF PRIZES WON. RESULTS SUGGEST THAT AT LEAST BY THE TIME URBAN YOUTH HAVE REACHED THEIR TEENAGE YEARS, ETHNIC DIFFERENCES IN DISPOSITIONS TO COOPERATE OR COMPETE HAVE BECOME NEGLIGIBLE. 4 REFERENCES.

ACCN   002260

1943 AUTH   **WEIGERT, A. J., & THOMAS, D. L.**
TITL   SOCIALIZATION AND RELIGIOSITY: A CROSS-NATIONAL ANALYSIS OF CATHOLIC ADOLESCENTS.
SRCE   *SOCIOMETRY, 1970, 33(3), 305-325.*
INDX   SOCIALIZATION, RELIGION, ADOLESCENTS, CROSS CULTURAL, EMPIRICAL, PUERTO RICAN-I, MEXICAN, ATTITUDES, NEW YORK, MINNESOTA, MIDWEST, EAST, MALE
ABST   A CROSS-NATIONAL INVESTIGATION RELATING DIMENSIONS OF RELIGIOSITY (BELIEF, EXPERIENCING, KNOWLEDGE, AND PRACTICE) TO ADOLESCENTS' PERCEPTIONS OF THE CONTROL AND SUPPORT RECEIVED FROM PARENTS, IS REPORTED. SUBJECTS WERE CHOSEN FROM MIDDLE-CLASS, CATHOLIC BOYS' HIGH SCHOOLS IN FOUR CITIES—NEW YORK; ST. PAUL; SAN JUAN, PUERTO RICO; AND MERIDA, YUCATAN. THE CITIES SELECTED WERE CONCEIVED AS LYING ON TWO CONTINUA: A LATIN TO ANGLO CULTURE CONTINUUM, AND AN URBAN CONTINUUM. THESE CONTINUA ARE TAKEN AS REPRESENTING DIFFERENCES IN FAMILY STRUCTURE FROM AUTHORITARIAN AND PA-

TRIARCHAL (MERIDA) TO EGALITARIAN AND BILATERAL (NEW YORK). A SHORT FORM OF THE CORNELL PARENT BEHAVIOR DESCRIPTION AND A RELIGIOSITY QUESTIONNAIRE WERE ADMINISTERED TO SUBJECTS. EXCEPT FOR THE MERIDA SAMPLE AND THE KNOWLEDGE DIMENSION, THE A PRIORI HYPOTHESIS THAT ADOLESCENTS PERCEIVING A HIGH (LOW) DEGREE OF CONTROL AND SUPPORT SCORE HIGHEST (LOWEST) ON RELIGIOSITY IS MODERATELY VERIFIED, DUE MAINLY TO A POSITIVE RELATIONSHIP BETWEEN SUPPORT AND RELIGIOSITY. REASONS GIVEN FOR CHURCH ATTENDANCE REVEAL DIFFERENT PATTERNS FOR THE LATIN AND ANGLO SAMPLES. ANGLOS ATTEND CHURCH BECAUSE OF PARENTAL EXPECTATIONS, WHEREAS LATINS GIVE SELF-EXPECTATIONS. FOR THE ANGLO SAMPLES, THE FINDINGS DEMONSTRATE THE USEFULNESS OF SOCIALIZATION VARIABLES IN UNDERSTANDING RELIGIOSITY, AND THE DIFFERENCES ACROSS SAMPLES POINT TO THE IMPORTANCE OF REASONS FOR RELIGIOUS BEHAVIOR. 39 REFERENCES.

ACCN   001672

1944 AUTH   **WEILAND, A., & COUGHLIN, R.**
TITL   SELF-IDENTIFICATION AND PREFERENCES: A COMPARISON OF WHITE AND MEXICAN AMERICAN FIRST AND THIRD GRADERS.
SRCE   *JOURNAL OF CROSS-CULTURAL PSYCHOLOGY, 1979, 10(3), 356-365.*
INDX   MEXICAN AMERICAN, CROSS CULTURAL, EMPIRICAL, CHILDREN, MIDWEST, INTERPERSONAL ATTRACTION, SELF CONCEPT, ETHNIC IDENTITY
ABST   THE ETHNIC IDENTIFICATION SKILLS AND ETHNIC PREFERENCES OF 66 WHITE AND MEXICAN AMERICAN (MA) CHILDREN IN A MIDWESTERN SCHOOL SCHOOL WERE INVESTIGATED. THE SUBJECTS INCLUDED 19 WHITE AND 14 MA FIRST GRADERS AND 17 WHITE AND 16 MA THIRD GRADERS. THE TWO-PART TESTS CONSISTED OF A SELF- AND PICTURE-IDENTIFICATION SECTION AND A CLASSMATE PREFERENCE SECTION. ETHNIC IDENTIFICATION WAS MEASURED BY SUBJECTS' SELECTING A PHOTO OF A MALE OR FEMALE WHITE, MA, OR BLACK CHILD. PREFERENCES FOR ETHNIC GROUPS WERE INDICATED BY THE SELECTION OF A CLASSMATE IN RESPONSE TO EACH OF A SERIES OF PREFERENCE QUESTIONS. ALL SUBJECTS WERE ABLE TO IDENTIFY OTHER PERSONS ALONG AN ETHNIC DIMENSION. ALL WHITE SUBJECTS INDICATED STRONG PREFERENCES FOR WHITE CLASSMATES. WITH ONE EXCEPTION, MA'S PREFERENCES FOR WHITE VS. MA CLASSMATES DID NOT SIGNIFICANTLY DIFFER FROM CHANCE. 22 REFERENCES. (JOURNAL ABSTRACT MODIFIED)

ACCN   001729

1945 AUTH   **WEINBERG, M. (ED.)**
TITL   MEXICAN AMERICANS, PUERTO RICANS.
SRCE   *RESEARCH REVIEW OF EQUAL EDUCATION, 1977, 1(WHOLE ISSUE NO. 2).*
INDX   EDUCATION, MEXICAN AMERICAN, PUERTO RICAN-M, HISTORY, SOCIAL MOBILITY, ACCUL-

TURATION, POLITICAL POWER, READING, HIGHER EDUCATION, INTEGRATION, REVIEW, CHILDREN, ADOLESCENTS, COLLEGE STUDENTS

ABST NINETEEN RESEARCH STUDIES ON MEXICAN AMERICAN AND PUERTO RICAN CHILDREN ARE CITED, SUMMARIZED, AND DISCUSSED. SEVEN SEPARATE AREAS CONCERNING MEXICAN AMERICANS ARE REVIEWED: (1) HISTORY; (2) SOCIAL MOBILITY AND ASSIMILATION; (3) COMMUNITY POWER; (4) READING PROBLEMS; (5) MEXICAN AMERICAN LITERATURE; (6) HIGHER EDUCATION; AND (7) DESEGREGATION. IT IS OBSERVED THAT EDUCATIONAL PROBLEMS OF MEXICAN AMERICANS MUST BE PLACED IN AN HISTORICAL PERSPECTIVE AND SHOULD ADDRESS SUCH ISSUES AS ECONOMIC STATUS, THE LANGUAGE PROBLEM, THE EDUCATIONAL ROLE OF THE CATHOLIC CHURCH, AND ETHNIC IDENTITY. ALTHOUGH LITTLE RESEARCH HAS BEEN PUBLISHED ON THE PROBLEMS OF PUERTO RICAN EDUCATION, AN OVERVIEW OF THE RESEARCH IS PRESENTED. VIRTUALLY ALL THE STUDIES FOR BOTH GROUPS ARE CONTAINED IN DOCTORAL DISSERTATIONS AND HAVE NOT BEEN DISSEMINATED WIDELY. 19 REFERENCES.

ACCN 002261

1946 AUTH **WEINER, N. L.**
TITL THE EFFECT OF EDUCATION ON POLICE ATTITUDES.
SRCE *JOURNAL OF CRIMINAL JUSTICE, 1974, 2(4), 317-328.*
INDX POLICE-COMMUNITY RELATIONS, ATTITUDES, DEMOGRAPHIC, PREJUDICE, PUERTO RICAN-M, HIGHER EDUCATION, EMPIRICAL, MINNESOTA, MIDWEST
ABST TO DETERMINE IF COLLEGE-EDUCATED POLICEMEN ARE MORE TOLERANT THAN THEIR NON-COLLEGE COUNTERPARTS, 396 MINNESOTA POLICEMEN COMPLETED A DEMOGRAPHIC AND ATTITUDE QUESTIONNAIRE. THE INSTRUMENT COMPRISED THE SHEATSLY PRO-INTEGRATION SCALE, NIEDERHOFFER'S POLICE CYNICISM SCALE, THE MINNESOTA SURVEY OF OPINION LAW SCALE, AND THE BOGARDUS SOCIAL DISTANCE SCALE. RESULTS SHOW SIGNIFICANT DIRECT RELATIONSHIPS BETWEEN ONLY FIVE OF THE FIFTEEN ATTITUDE FACTORS AND POLICEMEN'S LEVEL OF EDUCATION: (1) ATTITUDES TOWARD BLACKS AND PUERTO RICANS AS FAMILY, FRIENDS, OR NEIGHBORS; (2) ATTITUDES TOWARD ITALIANS; (3) ATTITUDES TOWARD BLACKS AND PUERTO RICANS AS CO-WORKERS, U.S. CITIZENS, OR U.S. VISITORS; (4) ATTITUDES TOWARD BLACK PROTEST; AND (5) ATTITUDES TOWARD BLACK RIGHTS. THIS INDICATES THAT THERE IS A TENDENCY FOR MORE EDUCATED POLICEMEN TO BE MORE ACCEPTING OF ETHNIC GROUPS. HOWEVER, IT IS CONCLUDED THAT, IN GENERAL, THE EDUCATIONAL LEVEL OF THE POLICE DOES NOT SIGNIFICANTLY AFFECT THEIR ATTITUDES. THIS IS DUE, IN PART, TO THE VOCATIONAL ORIENTATION OF MANY POLICE COLLEGE STUDENTS AND TO THE PERVASIVE EFFECT OF THE POLICE ROLE. AS IT NOW EX-

ISTS, POLICE EDUCATION IS TOO VOCATIONAL, AND INSTEAD IT SHOULD BE CENTERED IN THE LIBERAL ARTS—NOT AS A CURE-ALL, BUT AS A BROADENING EXPERIENCE. 40 REFERENCES.

ACCN 001673

1947 AUTH **WEISENBERG, M., KREINDLER, M. L., SCHACHAT, R., & WERBOFF, J.**
TITL PAIN: ANXIETY AND ATTITUDES IN BLACK, WHITE AND PUERTO RICAN PATIENTS.
SRCE *PSYCHOSOMATIC MEDICINE, 1975, 37(2), 123-135.*
INDX PUERTO RICAN-M, ADULTS, ANXIETY, ATTITUDES, HEALTH, STRESS, PERCEPTION, CROSS CULTURAL, EAST
ABST REACTIONS TO PAIN AND THE CONCOMITANT ANXIETY OF 25 BLACK, 24 WHITE, AND 26 PUERTO RICAN PATIENTS IN AN OUTPATIENT DENTAL EMERGENCY CLINIC WERE STUDIED. MEASURES USED INCLUDED: (1) THE STATE-TRAIT ANXIETY INVENTORY; (2) PALMAR SWEAT PRINTS; (3) AN INTERVIEW TO OBTAIN PATIENT CHARACTERISTICS AND ATTITUDES TOWARD PAIN; (4) THE DENTAL ANXIETY SCALE; AND (5) A POSTTREATMENT DENTIST RATING. NO PHYSIOLOGICAL DIFFERENCES WERE OBTAINED WITH PALMAR SWEAT PRINTS; AND NO DIFFERENCES BETWEEN ETHNIC AND RACIAL GROUPS IN AMOUNT OF PAIN, TYPE, OR NUMBER OF SYMPTOMS WERE OBTAINED. BUT, SIGNIFICANT TRAIT ANXIETY DIFFERENCES DID EMERGE—PUERTO RICANS HAD THE HIGHEST LEVEL OF TRAIT ANXIETY, WHITES THE LOWEST, WITH BLACKS IN THE MIDDLE. THE DENTAL ANXIETY SCALE ALSO YIELDED DIFFERENCES, WITH PUERTO RICANS SCORING HIGHEST, BLACKS LOWEST, AND WHITES IN BETWEEN. ATTITUDE DIFFERENCES REFLECTED A RELATIVE WILLINGNESS TO DENY, GET RID OF, OR AVOID DEALING WITH THE PAIN. ON THIS SCALE, PUERTO RICAN SUBJECTS SCORED HIGHEST, WHITES LOWEST, AND BLACKS WERE IN BETWEEN. 46 REFERENCES.

ACCN 001674

1948 AUTH **WELCH, S., COMER, J., & STEINMAN, M.**
TITL INTERVIEWING IN A MEXICAN AMERICAN COMMUNITY: AN INVESTIGATION OF SOME POTENTIAL SOURCES OF RESPONSE BIAS.
SRCE *THE PUBLIC OPINION QUARTERLY, 1973, 37(1), 115-126.*
INDX MEXICAN AMERICAN, COMMUNITY, RESEARCH METHODOLOGY, EMPIRICAL, NEBRASKA, MIDWEST
ABST THIS SURVEY OF MEXICAN AMERICAN HOUSEHOLD HEADS IN TWO NEBRASKA COUNTIES ASKS: IF MEXICAN AMERICANS SUBJECT THEMSELVES TO INTERVIEWS, GIVEN LANGUAGE DIFFICULTIES, DIFFERENT ETHNIC STATUS OF THE INTERVIEWER, AND POSSIBLE ILLEGAL ENTRY, HOW CONSISTENT AND RELIABLE ARE THEIR RESPONSES? THERE WERE 178 PERSONS IN THE SAMPLE, 55% FEMALE. ALL RESPONDENTS WERE GIVEN THE OPTION OF TAKING THE INTERVIEW IN ENGLISH OR IN SPANISH, AND 22% CHOSE THE LATTER. INTERVIEWING WAS DONE IN THREE WAYS: BY A PROFESSIONAL ANGLO WORKING ALONE, BY

A SPECIALLY TRAINED MEXICAN AMERICAN WORKING ALONE, AND BY A PROFESSIONAL ANGLO AND A MEXICAN AMERICAN ASSOCIATE WORKING TOGETHER. FINDINGS WERE THAT IF EDUCATION AND AGE ARE CONTROLLED, INITIAL DIFFERENCES DISAPPEAR BETWEEN THOSE INTERVIEWED IN ENGLISH AND SPANISH, AND AMONG THOSE INTERVIEWED BY AN ANGLO, A MEXICAN AMERICAN, OR A COMBINATION OF THE TWO. IN SUM, THE FINDINGS SUPPORT THE CONCEPT THAT INTERVIEW DATA CAN BE OBTAINED FROM MEXICAN AMERICANS WITH ABOUT THE SAME DEGREE OF RELIABILITY AS FROM ANY OTHER GROUP. 7 REFERENCES.

ACCN   001675

1949 AUTH   **WELFARE PLANNING COUNCIL, LOS ANGELES REGION.**

TITL   EAST LOS ANGELES HEALTH: A COMMUNITY REPORT FROM A PROJECT AND CONFERENCES ON HEALTH PROBLEMS AND PRIORITIES IN EAST LOS ANGELES.

SRCE   *LOS ANGELES: LOS ANGELES WELFARE PLANNING COUNCIL, FEBRUARY 1970.*

INDX   MEXICAN AMERICAN, HEALTH, HEALTH DELIVERY SYSTEMS, EMPIRICAL, ALCOHOLISM, GERONTOLOGY, EMPLOYMENT, REPRESENTATION, EQUAL OPPORTUNITY, MENTAL HEALTH, MENTAL RETARDATION, ADOLESCENTS, DRUG ABUSE, ADULTS, ECONOMIC FACTORS, CALIFORNIA, SOUTHWEST, SURVEY, PROGRAM EVALUATION, RESOURCE UTILIZATION, COMMUNITY

ABST   IN ORDER TO DELINEATE THE MAJOR PROBLEMS AND PRIORITIES FOR ITS HEALTH SYSTEM AS PERCEIVED BY THE EAST LOS ANGELES (ELA) COMMUNITY, THE LOS ANGELES WELFARE PLANNING COUNCIL COLLECTED INFORMATION FROM AND ABOUT THE ELA COMMUNITY RESIDENTS AND HEALTH SERVICES IN THREE DISTINCT WAYS: (1) THROUGH BILINGUAL MEXICAN AMERICAN INTERVIEWERS WHO SURVEYED THE ELA RESIDENTS; (2) THROUGH A COMBINED COMMUNITY RESIDENTS' AND SERVICE WORKERS' CONFERENCE; AND (3) THROUGH STATISTICS OF THE AGENCIES OPERATING IN THE ELA AREA. THE REPORT COVERS THIRTEEN PROBLEM AREAS IDENTIFIED AS HEALTH CARE PRIORITIES BY THE COMMUNITY. AMONG THESE ARE: ALCOHOLISM, SENIOR CITIZENS, DENTAL CARE, HOSPITAL AND EMERGENCY CARE, HEALTH PROBLEMS OF THE YOUTH, SERVICES FOR THE MENTALLY RETARDED, NARCOTIC AND OTHER DRUG USAGE, AND HEALTH MANPOWER NEEDS. EACH PROBLEM AREA IS PRESENTED BY (1) ITS MAJOR ISSUES, (2) GENERAL AND SPECIFIC RECOMMENDATIONS, AND (3) FACTUAL ANALYSIS USING THE INFORMATION GATHERED FROM THE COMMUNITY INTERVIEWS, CONFERENCE, AND AGENCY STATISTICS. A SEPARATE SECTION PRESENTS THE PLANNING COUNCIL'S RECOMMENDATIONS AND COMMENTS. TWENTY-NINE TABLES AND FIVE APPENDICES PROVIDE STATISTICAL AND METHODOLOGICAL DATA RELATED TO THE STUDY. THE REPORT PROVIDES A USEFUL OVERVIEW OF THE HEALTH NEEDS OF THE EAST LOS ANGELES COMMUNITY AS PERCEIVED BY ITS RESIDENTS AND ITS SERVICE PROVIDERS.

ACCN   001676

1950 AUTH   **WELLISCH, D., & HAYS, J. R.**

TITL   A CROSS CULTURAL STUDY OF THE PREVALENCE AND CORRELATES OF STUDENT DRUG USE IN THE UNITED STATES AND MEXICO.

SRCE   *BULLETIN ON NARCOTICS, 1974, 26(1), 31-42.*

INDX   DRUG ABUSE, SES, ADOLESCENTS, ALCOHOLISM, INHALANT ABUSE, SEX COMPARISON, CROSS CULTURAL, MEXICAN, ATTITUDES, EMPIRICAL, DRUG ADDICTION

ABST   BASELINE SURVEY DATA CONCERNING DRUG USE AND ABUSE WERE COLLECTED ON 229 STUDENTS (172 MALES, 57 FEMALES), AGES 15 TO 18, IN MONTERREY, MEXICO. THE RESULTS WERE COMPARED TO SIMILAR DATA FROM THE HOUSTON INDEPENDENT SCHOOL DISTRICT (HISD). AN 87-ITEM MULTIPLE-CHOICE QUESTIONNAIRE WAS DESIGNED TO SHOW THE FREQUENCY OF USE OF NINE SUBSTANCES (TOBACCO; ALCOHOL; MARIJUANA; COUGH SYRUP; SOLVENTS; STIMULANTS; HALLUCINOGENS; BARBITUATES; AND OPIATES OR COCAINE) OVER THREE TIME PERIODS (EVER USED; USED IN PAST 6 MONTHS; USED IN PAST 7 DAYS). ANALYSIS REVEALED THAT THE MEXICAN YOUTHS HAD A MUCH LOWER PREVALENCE OF DRUG USE THAN THE HOUSTON GROUP; IN PARTICULAR, THE MONTERREY STUDENTS' USE OF OPIATES OR COCAINE WAS ONE-FIFTH THAT OF THE HOUSTON STUDENTS. SIMILARITIES BETWEEN THE TWO GROUPS WERE ALSO FOUND: (1) ALCOHOL AND TOBACCO WERE THE MOST USED SUBSTANCES, AND (2) MALE USE OF THE NINE SUBSTANCES WAS SIGNIFICANTLY GREATER THAN FEMALE USE IN BOTH CULTURES. CROSS-TABULATIONS REVEALED DIFFERENCES BETWEEN USERS AND NON-USERS IN BELIEFS, ATTITUDES, AND ACTIVITIES: (1) GRADE AVERAGE AND FUTURE EXPECTATIONS ABOUT GRADE AVERAGE WERE INVERSELY RELATED TO DRUG USE; (2) LACK OF LIFE DIRECTION FIGURED SIGNIFICANTLY IN THE LIVES OF DRUG USERS; AND (3) INCREASING AGE WAS POSITIVELY CORRELATED TO DRUG USE. ALTHOUGH A POSITIVE CORRELATION WAS FOUND IN THE HOUSTON SAMPLE BETWEEN DRUG USE AND THE PARENTS' EDUCATION LEVEL AND INCOME, NO SUCH RELATIONSHIP WAS FOUND IN THE MONTERREY SAMPLE. STUDENTS IN BOTH CULTURES SAW THE BEST MEANS OF DRUG EDUCATION TO BE LIVE PANELS OF PROFESSIONALS AND FORMER USERS. THE LEAST EFFECTIVE PROGRAM WAS BOOKS OR READINGS ON THE ISSUE. CROSS-CULTURALLY, THE ORIGINAL SOURCE OF DRUGS FOR DRUG USERS WAS ALMOST ALWAYS A FRIEND OF THE SAME AGE. SOURCES OF HELP FOR DRUG-RELATED PROBLEMS DIFFERED BETWEEN THE TWO SAMPLES, AS TWICE AS MANY MONTERREY STUDENTS (52%) AS HOUSTON STUDENTS (26%) SAID THEY WOULD GO TO THEIR PARENTS FOR HELP. FUTURE COMPARATIVE STUDIES ARE RECOMMENDED TO DETERMINE HOW PAT-

TERNS OF DRUG USE BEHAVIOR DEVELOP FROM CULTURE TO CULTURE. 12 REFERENCES.

ACCN   001677

1951 AUTH   **WENGER, D. A., BARTH, G., & GITHENS, J. H.**
TITL   NINE CASES OF SPHINGOMYELIN LIPIDOSIS, A NEW VARIANT IN SPANISH-AMERICAN CHILDREN: JUVENILE VARIANT OF NIEMANN-PICK DISEASE WITH FOAMY AND SEA-BLUE HISTIOCYTES.
SRCE   *AMERICAN JOURNAL OF DISEASES OF CHILDREN, 1977, 131, 955-961.*
INDX   CASE STUDY, DISEASE, MENTAL RETARDATION, MEXICAN AMERICAN, PHYSICAL DEVELOPMENT, COLORADO, SOUTHWEST, SYMPTOMATOLOGY, HEALTH, CHILDREN
ABST   DESCRIBED ARE NINE SPANISH AMERICAN CHILDREN FROM FIVE FAMILIES WITH AN UNUSUAL HEREDITARY LIPID STORAGE DISEASE. THE FAMILY ORIGINS WERE IN TWO SMALL SOUTHERN COLORADO TOWNS. THE CLINICAL COURSE VARIED, BUT ALL OF THE CHILDREN WERE FOUND TO BRUISE EASILY AND TO HAVE SPLENOMEGALY, AND MOST HAD HEPATOMEGALY. POSTNATAL JAUNDICE AND HEPATITIS OCCURRED IN FOUR. IMPAIRMENT OF VERTICAL GAZE AND INTELLECTUAL AND NEUROLOGIC DETERIORATION OCCURRED IN MOST OF THE PATIENTS WITH THE ONSET OF THE DISEASE—USUALLY IN CHILDHOOD. THE BONE MARROW IN ALL PATIENTS EXAMINED CONTAINED BOTH FOAMY AND SEA-BLUE HISTIOCYTES. SPHINGOMYELINASE LEVELS IN SKIN FIBROBLAST CULTURES WERE GREATLY DECREASED IN SEVEN OF THE EIGHT CASES EVALUATED. IT IS BELIEVED THAT THESE PATIENTS HAVE A SPHINGOMYELIN LIPIDOSIS AND REPRESENT A VARIANT OF THE NIEMANN-PICK DISEASE. CLINICAL AND ENZYMATIC FINDINGS ARE COMPARED WITH THOSE OF OTHER CASES IN THE LITERATURE. 27 REFERENCES. (AUTHOR ABSTRACT)
ACCN   002306

1952 AUTH   **WENK, M. G.**
TITL   ADJUSTMENT AND ASSIMILATION: THE CUBAN REFUGEE EXPERIENCE.
SRCE   *INTERNATIONAL MIGRATION REVIEW, 1968, 3(1), 38-49.*
INDX   IMMIGRATION, MIGRATION, SPANISH SURNAMED, PSYCHOSOCIAL ADJUSTMENT, SES, SOCIAL MOBILITY, SCHOLASTIC ACHIEVEMENT, SEX COMPARISON, ACCULTURATION, EMPIRICAL, CUBAN
ABST   THE BACKGROUND, EDUCATION, FAMILY COMPOSITION, ADAPTATION, AND ASSIMILATION OF CUBAN REFUGEES LIVING IN THE UNITED STATES ARE INVESTIGATED. TWO HUNDRED CUBAN FAMILIES (534 ADULTS, 593 CHILDREN) WERE SELECTED AT RANDOM FROM U.S. IMMIGRATION DEPARTMENT FILES TO OBTAIN A NATIONWIDE, RESPRESENTATIVE SAMPLE. DATA WERE OBTAINED FROM DEPARTMENT FILES, AND THE 1127 RESPONDENTS WERE INTERVIEWED WITH AN 85-ITEM QUESTIONNAIRE. COMPLETION OF EDUCATION BEYOND ELEMENTARY SCHOOL WAS FOUND IN 80% OF THE RESPONDENTS. APPROXIMATELY 60% HAD PROFESSIONAL, BUSINESS, SKILLED, OR SEMI-SKILLED WORK BACKGROUNDS IN CUBA, AND 40% MAINTAINED THEIR OCCUPATIONAL STANDING WHEN EMPLOYED IN THE U.S. THE CUBAN REFUGEE UNEMPLOYMENT RATE (0.9%) IS SIGNIFICANTLY BELOW THE NATIONAL AVERAGE (3.5%). ONCE RESETTLEMENT HAS OCCURRED, THE TREND IS TOWARD PROFESSIONAL UPWARD MOBILITY AND OCCUPATIONAL IMPROVEMENT, INDICATING THAT THE REFUGEE IS A PRODUCTIVE ASSET TO HIS COMMUNITY. AVERAGE FAMILY INCOME WAS BETWEEN $6,000 AND $8,000 PER YEAR, AND ESPECIALLY AMONG YOUNG FAMILIES THERE WAS A TENDENCY FOR WIVES TO WORK TO IMPROVE FAMILY ECONOMIC STABILITY. RESPONDENTS WERE FOUND TO HAVE RELATIVELY GOOD LIVING CONDITIONS, AS THE MAJORITY (50%) HAD ACCOMODATIONS RENTING OVER $100 PER MONTH. IT IS CONCLUDED THAT THE MAJORITY OF CUBAN REFUGEES HAVE ASSIMILATED AND ADJUSTED QUICKLY (1 TO 3 YEARS), AND THE MAJORITY FELT THAT THEIR EXPECTATIONS OF THE U.S. HAVE BEEN FULFILLED. THE CUBAN IS FOUND TO BE A PRODUCTIVE, SELF-SUFFICIENT, PROGRESSIVE, AND GRATEFUL MEMBER OF THE COMMUNITY, WITH A DESIRE TO ADAPT TO U.S. LIFE. 2 REFERENCES.
ACCN   001678

1953 AUTH   **WERNER, N. E., & EVANS, I. M.**
TITL   PERCEPTION OF PREJUDICE IN MEXICAN AMERICAN PRESCHOOL CHILDREN.
SRCE   *PERCEPTUAL AND MOTOR SKILLS, 1968, 27(3), 1039-1046.*
INDX   PREJUDICE, MEXICAN AMERICAN, CHILDREN, DISCRIMINATION, EMPIRICAL
ABST   STRUCTURED DOLL PLAY INTERVIEWS WITH 40 MEXICAN AMERICAN 4 AND 5 YEAR-OLDS WERE CONDUCTED TO DETERMINE (1) WHEN AND WHERE DISCRIMINATION OF SKIN COLOR DIFFERENCE OCCURS, (2) WHEN AND WHERE EVALUATIONS ARE MADE ON THE BASIS OF SKIN COLOR, AND (3) THE RELATIONSHIP BETWEEN CHILD'S AGE, SEX, AND SCHOOL EXPOSURE TO RACIAL DISCRIMINATION AND EVALUATION. SUBJECTS WERE GROUPED BY SEX, AGE (4 AND 5 YEARS-OLD), AND WHETHER THEY WERE IN OR NOT IN SCHOOL. THERE WERE 5 SUBJECTS IN EACH OF THE 8 CELLS. THE IN-SCHOOL GROUP WAS SELECTED FROM 2 RACIALLY INTEGRATED DAY-CARE CENTERS SERVING A LOW-INCOME COMMUNITY. THE OUT OF SCHOOL GROUP WAS SELECTED FROM A LIST OF THE ECONOMIC OPPORTUNITY CENTER SERVING THE SAME COMMUNITY. SUBJECTS WERE GIVEN 8 MALE AND FEMALE DOLLS (4 WHITE, 4 BLACK) TO PLAY WITH FOR 5-12 MINUTES AND THEN ASKED 15 QUESTIONS TO ELICIT REACTIONS TO THE DOLLS. SIGNIFICANT DIFFERENCES OF AWARENESS OF SKIN COLOR WERE FOUND BETWEEN THE IN-SCHOOL AND OUT OF SCHOOL GROUPS, BUT NOT BY SEX OR AGE. WHEN DISCRIMINATION OCCURS, IT IS ASSOCIATED WITH AN EVALUATION OF LIGHT SKIN AS GOOD AND

DARK SKIN AS BAD. A QUALITATIVE ANALYSIS WAS BASED UPON THE SPONTANEOUS SORTINGS OF DOLLS, AND RESPONSES TO QUESTIONS CONCERNING THE GOOD AND BAD FATHER, MOTHER, BOY, AND GIRL. DOLL SORTING OCCURRED BASED ON SEX-ROLE DIFFERENCES RATHER THAN ON SKIN COLOR DISCRIMINATIONS. CHARACTERISTICS OF GOOD BEHAVIOR ON THE PART OF THE CHILDREN INCLUDED (1) INDEPENDENCE OR SELF-CARE, (2) AMENABILITY TO DISCIPLINE, AND (3) SHARING WITH OTHERS. CHARACTERISTICS OF GOOD OR BAD BEHAVIOR IN PARENTS DEPEND ON (1) PHYSICAL CARE FOR CHILD, (2) EMOTIONAL AVAILABILITY, AND (3) DISCIPLINE BEHAVIORS. SOME PROBLEMS OF IDENTIFICATION ARISE FOR THE MEXICAN AMERICAN CHILD WHOSE PERSONAL CHARACTERISTICS DIFFER FROM THOSE OF THE MAJORITY. RESULTS ARE RELATED TO COMPARABLE STUDIES WITH BLACK AND ORIENTAL CHILDREN. 11 REFERENCES.

ACCN   001679

1954 AUTH   **WEST, G. A.**
TITL   RACE ATTITUDES AMONG TEACHERS IN THE SOUTHWEST.
SRCE   *JOURNAL OF ABNORMAL AND SOCIAL PSYCHOLOGY, 1936, 31(3), 331-337.*
INDX   ATTITUDES, PREJUDICE, TEACHERS, PERSONALITY, MEXICAN AMERICAN, CHILDREN, EMPIRICAL, DISCRIMINATION, NEW MEXICO, SOUTHWEST
ABST   SURVEY DATA WAS OBTAINED FROM 72 ANGLO TEACHERS AND 60 SPANISH AMERICAN TEACHERS EMPLOYED IN INTEGRATED, RURAL PUBLIC SCHOOLS OF NEW MEXICO TO DETERMINE THE EXISTENCE OF RACIAL PREJUDICE AMONG TEACHERS, AND DIFFERENCES OF RACIAL ATTITUDE IN THE TWO GROUPS OF TEACHERS. THE PROPORTION OF PUPILS OF EACH RACE TAUGHT BY THE TEACHERS COULD NOT BE CONTROLLED. TEACHERS RESPONDED TO A LIST OF 21 PUPIL-TRAITS BY (1) CHOOSING THE RACE OF PUPIL THEY THOUGHT EXCELLED (SLIGHTLY SUPERIOR OR DECIDEDLY SUPERIOR) IN EACH OF THE TRAITS OR (2) INDICATING A "NO DIFFERENCE" RESPONSE. RESULTS INDICATE A TENDENCY FOR SPANISH AMERICAN TEACHERS TO RESPOND "NO DIFFERENCE" FOR THE 21 TRAITS ALMOST TWICE AS OFTEN AS ANGLOS (50% SPANISH AMERICAN, 27.5% ANGLO). A LARGE MAJORITY OF SPANISH AMERICAN AS COMPARED TO ANGLO TEACHERS INDICATED A "NO DIFFERENCE" RESPONSE IN THE FOLLOWING TRAITS: HONESTY; COOPERATION; SULLENNESS; ABILITY TO TAKE CRITICISM; EASE OF MOTIVATION; INTELLIGENCE; SPORTSMANSHIP; EASE OF DISCIPLINE; CONSIDERATENESS; AMBITION; COURTESY; EMOTIONAL STABILITY; TRUSTWORTHINESS; MORALITY; AND DISINCLINATION TO HOLD GRUDGES. THE ANGLO TEACHERS CLAIMED SUPERIORITY FOR PUPILS OF THEIR OWN RACE TO A GREATER EXTENT THAN THE SPANISH AMERICAN TEACHERS. WHILE THE SPANISH AMERICAN TEACHERS EXPRESS AN ATTITUDE OF RACIAL EQUALITY, ANGLO TEACHERS INDICATE AN ATTITUDE OF SUPERIORITY IN THEIR RESPONSES. 1 REFERENCE.

ACCN   001680

1955 AUTH   **WIGNALL C. M., & KOPPIN, L. L.**
TITL   MEXICAN AMERICAN USAGE OF STATE MENTAL HOSPITAL FACILITIES.
SRCE   *COMMUNITY MENTAL HEALTH JOURNAL, 1967, 3(2), 137-148.*
INDX   MEXICAN AMERICAN, RESOURCE UTILIZATION, MENTAL HEALTH, ADULTS, EMPIRICAL, HEALTH, CULTURAL FACTORS, CROSS CULTURAL, DISCRIMINATION, FEMALE, MALE, COLORADO, SOUTHWEST
ABST   A COMPARISON BETWEEN MEXICAN AMERICANS (MA) AND NON-MEXICAN AMERICANS IN THE USE OF STATE MENTAL HOSPITAL FACILITIES OF COLORADO IS PROVIDED. INFORMATION WAS OBTAINED BY ANALYZING PUBLIC MENTAL HOSPITAL ADMISSION RATES FOR ONE YEAR. THE FINDINGS SHOW THAT: (1) THE ADMISSION RATE FOR MA MALES IS HIGHER THAN THAT FOR NON-MA MALES; (2) THE CHANCES FOR BEING ADMITTED TO THE STATE HOSPITAL INCREASE WITH AGE FOR NON-MA MALES, WHILE THE CHANCES FOR ADMISSION ARE GREATER IN THE AGE RANGE 20 TO 64 YEARS FOR MA MALES; (3) THE MA FEMALE ALCOHOLIC ADMISSION RATE IS SIGNIFICANTLY HIGHER THAN THAT FOR NON-MA FEMALES FOR THE DENVER-COLORADO SPRINGS METROPOLITAN AREA; AND (4) A LOWER OVERALL ADMISSION RATE IS FOUND IN THE NORTHEASTERN AREA OF COLORADO THAN FOR THE OTHER FOUR REGIONS OF THE STATE. IT IS SUGGESTED THAT A FACTOR WHICH PARTIALLY ACCOUNTS FOR THE EARLIER ADMISSION OF MA MALES TO THE STATE MENTAL HOSPITAL IS THAT THEY ARE FORCED INTO INDEPENDENCE SEVERAL YEARS EARLIER THAN MOST NON-MA CHILDREN. CULTURAL DIFFERENCE AS IT OPERATES IN THE SOCIAL BREAKDOWN SYNDROME IS ANOTHER FACTOR THAT MAY ACCOUNT FOR HIGHER ADMISSION RATES FOR MA MALES AND FOR MA ALCOHOLIC FEMALES. FINALLY, THE PATIENTS' DISTANCE FROM THE HOSPITAL MAY BE YET ANOTHER FACTOR THAT ACCOUNTS FOR THE LOW ADMISSION RATES FROM NORTHEASTERN COLORADO. THE DIFFERENCES IN MA USAGE OF STATE MENTAL HOSPITAL FACILITIES MUST BE THE END PRODUCTS OF ECONOMIC AND SOCIAL DISCRIMINATION. 7 REFERENCES.

ACCN   001685

1956 AUTH   **WILLIAMS, C. H.**
TITL   UTILIZATION OF PERSISTING CULTURAL VALUES OF MEXICAN-AMERICANS BY WESTERN PRACTITIONERS.
SRCE   *IN P. SINGER (ED.), TRADITIONAL HEALING: NEW SCIENCE OR NEW COLONIALISM? NEW YORK: CONCH MAGAZINE LIMITED, 1977, PP. 108-122.*
INDX   CURANDERISMO, FOLK MEDICINE, MEXICAN AMERICAN, ESSAY, HISTORY, CULTURAL FACTORS, HEALTH, MENTAL HEALTH

ABST   THIS ESSAY EXAMINES THE HISTORICAL BACK-GROUND OF MEXICAN AMERICAN DISEASE CONCEPTS, THE PERSISTENCE OF CURANDER-ISMO, AND ETHNICAL PROBLEMS IN UTILIZA-TION OF CURANDEROS BY WESTERN THERA-PISTS. THE MAIN THEMES OF MEXICAN AMERICAN CULTURE ARE FAMILY AND RELI-GION. THE CURANDERO RECOGNIZES THIS SOCIOCULTURAL CONTEXT OF DISEASE BY FOCUSING ON THE REINTEGRATION OF THE PATIENT WITH HIS FAMILY AND COMMUNITY. THREE CASE STUDIES ARE PRESENTED TO DEMONSTRATE HOW FOLK CONCEPTS, WHEN RECOGNIZED BY WESTERN THERAPISTS, CAN RESULT IN INCREASED PATIENT RAPPORT AND AN ENHANCED THERAPEUTIC SETTING. IT IS SUGGESTED THAT CURANDEROS MAY BE CON-SULTED IN SOMEWHAT THE SAME WAY AS OTHER NON-MEDICAL PROFESSIONALS (E.G., CLERGYMEN, MARRIAGE COUNSELORS), OR THEY MAY BE HIRED AS THERAPEUTIC ASSIS-TANTS UNDER PROFESSIONAL SUPERVISION. 7 REFERENCES.

ACCN   002263

1957 AUTH   **WILLIAMS, F., WHITEHEAD, J. L., & MILLER, L. M.**

TITL   ETHNIC STEREOTYPING AND JUDGMENTS OF CHILDREN'S SPEECH.

SRCE   *SPEECH MONOGRAPHS, 1971, 38(3), 168-170.*

INDX   STEREOTYPES, CHILDREN, ATTITUDES, LAN-GUAGE ASSESSMENT, EMPIRICAL, MEXICAN AMERICAN, TEXAS, SOUTHWEST

ABST   TO ASSESS THE EFFECT OF ETHNIC STEREO-TYPING ON LANGUAGE CHARACTERIZATION, 44 UNIVERSITY OF TEXAS UNDERGRADUATE ELEMENTARY EDUCATION MAJORS (2 MALE, 42 FEMALE) RATED THE LANGUAGE CHARACTER-ISTICS OF STANDARD AND NONSTANDARD EN-GLISH-SPEAKING WHITE, BLACK, AND MEXI-CAN AMERICAN CHILDREN. RATINGS WERE BASED ON OBSERVATIONS OF 90-SECOND VID-EOTAPE IMAGES OF CHILDREN, MATCHED WITH STANDARD AND NONSTANDARD ENGLISH AU-DIO TRACKS. TWO WEEKS PRIOR TO THE VID-EOTAPE SESSIONS, SUBJECTS COMPLETED FORMS REQUESTING RATINGS OF BLACK, WHITE, AND MEXICAN AMERICAN CHILDREN BASED ON SUBJECTS' EXPERIENCES WITH EACH ETHNIC GROUP. THESE RATINGS INDICATED SUBJECTS' STEREOTYPED ATTITUDES. IN THE VIDEOTAPE SESSIONS, GROUPS OF 5 OR 6 SUBJECTS VIEWED (1) A BLACK OR MEXICAN AMERICAN CHILD WHOSE NONSTANDARD SPEECH HAD BEEN DUBBED BY ENGLISH STANDARD SPEECH, (2) A BLACK OR MEXICAN AMERICAN CHILD SPEAKING NONSTANDARD ENGLISH, AND (3) A WHITE CHILD SPEAKING STANDARD ENGLISH. THE RATING INSTRU-MENT OF CHILDREN'S SPEECH CONSISTED OF TWO DIMENSIONS DERIVED FROM THE DE-TROIT DIALECT STUDY (I.E., CONFIDENCE-EA-GERNESS AND ETHNICITY-NONSTANDARD-NESS), WITH EACH DIMENSION COMPRISED OF FIVE BIPOLAR, SEMANTIC DIFFERENTIAL CON-CEPTS. RESULTS DEMONSTRATED THAT ETH-NICITY AFFECTED THE RATINGS OF CHIL-DREN'S LANGUAGE. FOR BLACK CHILDREN,

THE BIAS WAS IN THE DIRECTION OF EXPECT-ING THEM TO SOUND MORE NONSTANDARD AND ETHNIC THAN THEIR WHITE PEERS. FOR MEXICAN AMERICAN CHILDREN, THE BIAS WAS TOWARD EXPECTING MORE ETHNIC-NON-STANDARDNESS AS WELL AS MORE RETI-CENCE AND NONCONFIDENCE IN SPEAKING. TWO LINES OF RESEARCH ARE RECOM-MENDED: (1) IDENTIFICATION OF THE PERCEP-TUAL BEHAVIOR AT THE "MOMENT OF STER-EOTYPING;" AND (2) DETERMINATION OF WHAT CONTRIBUTES TO AN INDIVIDUAL'S TENDENCY TO STEREOTYPE. 11 REFERENCES.

ACCN   001681

1958 AUTH   **WILLIAMS, F., & NAREMORE, R. C.**

TITL   LANGUAGE ATTITUDES: AN ANALYSIS OF TEACHER DIFERENCES.

SRCE   *SPEECH MONOGRAPHS, 1974, 41(4), 391-396.*

INDX   TEACHERS, ATTITUDES, STEREOTYPES, SCHO-LASTIC ACHIEVEMENT, LANGUAGE ASSESS-MENT, PHONOLOGY, MEXICAN AMERICAN, CROSS CULTURAL, CULTURAL FACTORS, BILIN-GUALISM, EDUCATION, TEXAS, SOUTHWEST

ABST   TEACHERS FROM RURAL AND URBAN SCHOOLS (N = 130) IN CENTRAL TEXAS RATED VIDEO-TAPED SPEECH SAMPLES OF BLACK, ANGLO, AND MEXICAN AMERICAN CHILDREN ON TWO GLOBAL DIMENSIONS—CONFIDENCE/EAGER-NESS AND ETHNICITY/NONSTANDARDNESS. THE TEACHERS THEMSELVES WERE CLASSIFIED INTO FIVE CATEGORIES. TYPE I, II, AND III TEACHERS WERE PREDOMINANTLY ANGLO, WHILE TYPE IV AND V TEACHERS WERE BLACK OR MEXICAN AMERICAN. TYPE II TEACHERS MAINLY TAUGHT ANGLO CHILDREN, TYPE III AND IV MAINLY TAUGHT MEXICAN AMERICAN CHILDREN, WHILE TYPE I AND V TAUGHT RA-CIALLY MIXED GROUPS OF STUDENTS. THE RE-SULTS REVEALED THAT TYPE I TEACHERS (NEARLY ONE-HALF OF THE SAMPLE) HAD A BIAS IN FAVOR OF ANGLO CHILDREN, RATING THEM HIGH ON CONFIDENCE AND STANDARD-NESS. THE OTHER FOUR TEACHER TYPES, IN CONTRAST, HAD SOME BIASES IN FAVOR OF MINORITY CHILDREN. IN GENERAL, THE TEACHERS' RATINGS CORRESPONDED TO THEIR ACADEMIC EXPECTATIONS OF THE THREE ETH-NIC GROUPS OF CHILDREN. ALTHOUGH THE SAMPLE WAS SMALL, THE FINDINGS STRONGLY CHALLENGE THE ASSUMPTION THAT TEACH-ERS ARE RELATIVELY HOMOGENEOUS. GIVEN SIMILAR SETS OF VIDEOTAPED CONVERSA-TIONS, THERE WERE MEASURABLE DIFFER-ENCES IN THE TEACHERS' RATINGS; AND THIS POINTS TO THE NEED FOR FURTHER RE-SEARCH INTO THE WAYS TEACHERS PERCEIVE CHILDREN. IN PARTICULAR, THEIR STEREO-TYPED BIASES MAY PROVE TO BE AN IMPOR-TANT FACTOR NOT ONLY IN RESEARCH, BUT IN TEACHER RECRUITMENT, TRAINING, AND JOB ASSIGNMENT. 13 REFERENCES.

ACCN   001682

1959 AUTH   **WILLIAMS, J. A., JR., BABCHUK, N., & JOHN-SON, D. R.**

TITL   VOLUNTARY ASSOCIATIONS AND MINORITY

STATUS: A COMPARATIVE ANALYSIS OF ANGLO, BLACK, AND MEXICAN AMERICANS.

SRCE *AMERICAN SOCIOLOGICAL REVIEW, 1973, 38(5), 637-646.*

INDX MEXICAN AMERICAN, CROSS CULTURAL, EMPIRICAL, COMMUNITY INVOLVEMENT, ETHNIC IDENTITY, URBAN, ADULTS, SEX COMPARISON, SES, TEXAS, SOUTHWEST

ABST THE VOLUNTARY ASSOCIATIONS OF 380 ANGLOS, BLACKS, AND MEXICAN AMERICANS WERE EXAMINED IN AUSTIN, TEXAS. ETHNICITY PROVED TO BE AN IMPORTANT VARIABLE IN PREDICTING SOCIAL PARTICIPATION, WITH BLACKS HAVING THE HIGHEST AND MEXICAN AMERICANS HAVING THE LOWEST PARTICIPATION RATE. USING MULTIPLE CLASSIFICATION ANALYSIS, A NUMBER OF STRUCTURAL VARIABLES WERE INTRODUCED AS CONTROLS AND THESE VARIABLES, PARTICULARLY EDUCATION, WERE FOUND TO BE RESPONSIBLE FOR THE DIFFERENCE BETWEEN ANGLOS AND MEXICAN AMERICANS. BLACKS CONTINUED TO HAVE SIGNIFICANTLY HIGHER RATES OF PARTICIPATION IN VOLUNTARY ASSOCIATIONS AFTER CONTROLLING FOR OTHER VARIABLES. THE FINDINGS TEND TO CAST DOUBT ON ISOLATION AND CULTURAL INHIBITION THEORIES AND TO SUPPORT COMPENSATORY AND ETHNIC COMMUNITY THEORIES FOR PARTICIPATION RATES. 33 REFERENCES. (JOURNAL ABSTRACT)

ACCN 001683

1960 AUTH **WILLIAMS, M. A.**

TITL A COMPARATIVE STUDY OF POSTSURGICAL CONVALESCENCE AMONG WOMEN OF TWO ETHNIC GROUPS: ANGLO AND MEXICAN-AMERICAN.

SRCE *COMMUNICATING NURSING RESEARCH, 1972, 5, 59-73.*

INDX CULTURAL FACTORS, FEMALE, MEXICAN AMERICAN, URBAN, CROSS CULTURAL, EMPIRICAL, SELF CONCEPT, HEALTH, SES, SEX ROLES, CALIFORNIA, SOUTHWEST, ATTITUDES, SYMPTOMATOLOGY, ADULTS, STRESS

ABST A COMPARATIVE INVESTIGATION OF 32 MEXICAN AMERICAN AND 32 ANGLO WOMEN WHO HAD UNDERGONE HYSTERECTOMIES, FOCUSED ON THE RELATIONSHIP OF LENGTH OF CONVALESCENCE TO STRESS EXPERIENCED AND ETHNICITY. THE STUDY WAS CONDUCTED IN A PRIVATE CATHOLIC HOSPITAL IN EAST SAN FRANCISCO. RESPONDENTS WERE SEEN BY AN INTERVIEWER AT AN AVERAGE OF 19 WEEKS AFTER DISCHARGE. THE INTERVIEWS, GENERALLY ABOUT 50 MINUTES IN LENGTH, WERE CONDUCTED VERBALLY AND TRANSCRIBED VERBATIM. BOTH GROUPS WERE SIMILAR IN MARITAL STATUS, IN THE NUMBER EMPLOYED OUTSIDE THE HOME, IN THE TYPE OF SURGICAL PROCEDURE, AND IN NUMBER OF DAYS OF HOSPITALIZATION. STATISTICALLY, THE MAIN HYPOTHESES OF THE STUDY WERE NOT UPHELD—THAT IS, ANGLO WOMEN DID NOT REPORT A HIGHER DEGREE OF PERCEIVED STRESS NOR HAVE A LONGER CONVALESCENT PERIOD THAN MEXICAN AMERICAN WOMEN. IN THE CONVALESCENT PERIOD, MEXICAN AMERICAN WOMEN TENDED TO CITE SOMEWHAT MORE PHYSICAL AND EMOTIONAL SYMPTOMS AND TO RESUME HOUSEHOLD DUTIES MORE SLOWLY. IMPLICATIONS OF THESE DIFFERENCES ARE DISCUSSED. HOWEVER, IT IS EMPHASIZED THAT, IN GENERAL, MANY MORE SIMILARITIES THAN DIFFERENCES CHARACTERIZED THE TWO GROUPS. ALSO, WIDE VARIATION WITHIN THE MEXICAN AMERICAN GROUP WAS DISCOVERED. THEIR RESPONSES RANGED FROM THOSE WHICH WERE INDISTINGUISHABLE FROM THE "TYPICAL ANGLO" RESPONSES TO THOSE WHICH WERE "TRADITIONALISTIC" IN NATURE. THE NEED FOR AN AWARENESS BY HEALTH PROFESSIONALS OF THIS TYPE OF DIVERSITY IS UNDERSCORED. 19 REFERENCES.

ACCN 002233

1961 AUTH **WIMBERLEY, A. S.**

TITL MUSIC IN PUERTO RICAN CULTURE.

SRCE *JOURNAL OF EDUCATION, 1967, 150(2), 43-54.*

INDX MUSIC, PUERTO RICAN-I, CULTURE, ACCULTURATION, ESSAY

ABST TO IDENTIFY THE EXPRESSION OF PUERTO RICAN CULTURE AND PERSONALITY THROUGH ITS MUSIC SINCE THE 1950'S, INTERVIEWS WERE CONDUCTED WITH MUSIC SCHOOL AND GENERAL EDUCATION ADMINISTRATORS, TEACHERS, AND STUDENTS AS WELL AS PRIVATE CITIZENS IN PUERTO RICO. THE RESULTS ARE DISCUSSED WITHIN THE FRAMEWORK OF THREE CONCEPTS. (1) A NATIVISTIC CONCERN TO PRESERVE AND RESTORE THE ISLAND'S MUSICAL HERITAGE HAS DEVELOPED IN RESPONSE TO AMERICAN INFLUENCES. (2) INFLUENCES MOLDING THE PUERTO RICAN PERSONALITY ARE REVEALED IN THE VARIOUS STYLES OF MUSIC—INFLUENCES SUCH AS THE MINGLING OF RACES AND ETHNIC GROUPS; PERSISTING AND CHANGING SENTIMENTAL STYLES AND MORES; RELIGIOUS BELIEFS; AND THE MOBILITY OF PUERTO RICANS TO AND FROM THE U.S. (3) MUSIC AS AN ENCULTURATIVE AGENT IN PUERTO RICAN CULTURE IS VIEWED IN TERMS OF (A) MUSIC IN EVERYDAY LIFE, AND (B) MUSIC IN THE PUBLIC SCHOOLS. IN EVERYDAY LIFE, MUSIC IS HANDED DOWN FROM ONE GENERATION TO THE NEXT, AND THE YOUNG LEARN OF RELIGIOUS BELIEFS, PATRIOTISM, AND THE MORES OF THE PUERTO RICAN PEOPLE. PUBLIC SCHOOLS OFFER CHORAL, INSTRUMENTAL, AND LISTENING ACTIVITIES, AND THE ESCUELAS LIBRES DE MUSICA (FREE SCHOOLS OF MUSIC) PREPARE TALENTED STUDENTS FOR THE CONSERVATORY OF MUSIC. THERE IS, HOWEVER, A LACK OF QUALIFIED MUSIC TEACHERS, AND THERE ALSO EXISTS A NEGATIVE ATTITUDE TOWARD HIGHER EDUCATION WHICH INHIBITS STUDENTS FROM ATTENDING MUSIC SCHOOLS. NEVERTHELESS, IT IS CONCLUDED THAT PUERTO RICAN MUSIC WILL CONTINUE TO BE A VITAL PART OF EVERYDAY LIFE. 14 REFERENCES.

ACCN 001684

1962 AUTH **WITKIN, H. A., PRICE-WILLIAMS, D., BERTINI,**

M., CHRISTIANSEN, B., OLTMAN, P. K., RAMIREZ, M., & VAN MEEL, J.

TITL SOCIAL CONFORMITY AND PSYCHOLOGICAL DIFFERENTIATION.

SRCE *INTERNATIONAL JOURNAL OF PSYCHOLOGY, 1974, 9(1), 11-29.*

INDX CONFORMITY, SOCIALIZATION, MEXICAN, COGNITIVE STYLE, RELIGION, ATTITUDES, AUTHORITARIANISM, CROSS CULTURAL, EMPIRICAL, CHILDREN, FIELD DEPENDENCE-INDEPENDENCE, REVIEW

ABST THIS STUDY EXAMINED THE ROLE OF SOCIALIZATION EXPERIENCES IN THE DEVELOPMENT OF PSYCHOLOGICAL DIFFERENTIATION. IN EACH OF THREE COUNTRIES (HOLLAND, ITALY, MEXICO) TWO VILLAGES WERE SELECTED AS PRESENTING A CONTRASTING PICTURE WITH REGARD TO DEGREE OF EMPHASIS ON CONFORMITY TO FAMILY, AND RELIGIOUS AND POLITICAL AUTHORITY. IT WAS HYPOTHESIZED THAT WITHIN THE PAIR OF VILLAGES IN EACH COUNTRY, CHILDREN FROM THE VILLAGE WHICH STRESSED SOCIAL CONFORMITY WOULD TEND TO BE MORE FIELD DEPENDENT AND SHOW OTHER SIGNS OF LESS DEVELOPED DIFFERENTIATION THAN CHILDREN FROM THE VILLAGE IN WHICH SOCIAL CONFORMITY WAS LESS EMPHASIZED. IN EACH OF THE SIX VILLAGES APPROXIMATELY 100 CHILDREN (BOYS AND GIRLS, AGED 9-11 AND 13-15) WERE STUDIED. DIFFERENTIATION WAS ASSESSED BY A BATTERY OF TESTS OF FIELD-DEPENDENCE-INDEPENDENCE AND THE FIGURE-DRAWING TEST. IN EVERY COMPARISON OF MEAN TEST SCORES BETWEEN PAIRS OF VILLAGES, IN EACH OF THE THREE COUNTRIES, CHILDREN FROM THE VILLAGE IN WHICH SOCIAL CONFORMITY WAS STRESSED OBTAINED SCORES REFLECTING LESS DIFFERENTIATED FUNCTIONING. VILLAGE DIFFERENCES WERE SIGNIFICANT FOR EVERY MEASURE OF DIFFERENTIATION IN ALL THREE COUNTRIES. ADDITIONAL ANALYSES OF THE DATA FROM THE TESTS OF DIFFERENTIATION AND OTHER TESTS USED YIELDED RESULTS ESSENTIALLY CONSISTENT WITH FINDINGS FROM PREVIOUS STUDIES. 56 REFERENCES. (JOURNAL ABSTRACT)

ACCN 001686

1963 AUTH **WOLF K. L.**

TITL GROWING UP AND ITS PRICE IN THREE PUERTO RICAN SUBCULTURES.

SRCE *PSYCHIATRY, 1952, 15(4), 401-433.*

INDX PUERTO RICAN-I, PERSONALITY, CULTURAL FACTORS, CHILDREN, EMPIRICAL, CHILDREARING PRACTICES, SOCIALIZATION, ADULTS, RURAL

ABST A COMPARISON OF THREE PUERTO RICAN SUBCULTURES IN TERMS OF THEIR MEMBERS' PERSONALITY CHARACTERISTICS SHOWS THAT THERE IS NO SUCH THING AS ONE UNIFORM PUERTO RICAN PERSONALITY TYPE, IN SPITE OF THE FAIRLY UNIFORM CULTURAL TRADITION. THE THREE CLASSES STUDIED WERE SMALL RURAL FARMERS, SUGAR WORKERS, AND THE MIDDLE CLASS OF A SMALL RURAL TOWN. IT IS POINTED OUT THAT EACH CLASS ATTEMPTS TO INSTILL NORMS ASSOCIATED WITH ITS "IDEAL PERSONALITY" IN ITS CHILDREN. THIS INVESTIGATION OF CHILD TRAINING AND ADULT BEHAVIOR PATTERNS EXAMINES THE PSYCHOLOGICAL REACTIONS TO THE CULTURE'S CONDITIONING ATTEMPTS; AND IT PLACES SPECIAL EMPHASIS ON POTENTIALLY STRESSFUL CONFLICTS ARISING FROM IDEAL AND REAL BEHAVIOR (I.E., FAMILY STRUCTURES; CONCEPTS OF AUTHORITY; MALE AND FEMALE ROLES; CHILDREARING PRACTICES; PSYCHOLOGICAL IMPLICATIONS OF AGGRESSION; ADOLESCENT BEHAVIOR; AND CULTURAL FACTORS). IT IS CONCLUDED THAT THE CONTRADICTORY NORMS OF IDEAL AND REAL BEHAVIOR AFFECT CHILDREN AT EVERY STAGE OF DEVELOPMENT.

ACCN 001687

1964 AUTH **WOLFRAM, W.**

TITL SOCIOLINGUISTIC ASPECTS OF ASSIMILATION: PUERTO RICAN ENGLISH IN NEW YORK CITY.

SRCE *ARLINGTON, VIRGINIA: CENTER FOR APPLIED LINGUISTICS, 1974.*

INDX ACCULTURATION, ADOLESCENTS, EMPIRICAL, LANGUAGE ACQUISITION, LANGUAGE ASSESSMENT, LINGUISTICS, MALE, PUERTO RICAN-M, URBAN, SEMANTICS, SYNTAX, SES, NEW YORK, EAST, CROSS CULTURAL, LINGUISTIC COMPETENCE

ABST TO EXPAND THE DESCRIPTIVE KNOWLEDGE OF AMERICAN SOCIAL DIALECTS, THE SPEECH OF 29 PUERTO RICAN AND 15 BLACK TEENAGE MALES FROM EAST HARLEM AND THE BRONX WAS ANALYZED USING SOCIOLINGUISTIC METHODS. WITH AN INTEREST IN THE NATURE OF LANGUAGE VARIATION AS IT RELATES TO LANGUAGES IN CONTACT, THE INVESTIGATOR WISHED TO DETERMINE THE RELATIVE INFLUENCE OF BLACK ENGLISH ON PUERTO RICAN ENGLISH (PRE). PRE IS DEFINED AS THE ENGLISH SPOKEN BY SECOND GENERATION TEENAGE MALES LIVING PREDOMINANTLY IN EAST HARLEM, NEW YORK. A DESCRIPTION OF THE RESIDENTIAL BACKGROUND OF INFORMANTS, DEGREE OF PUERTO RICAN AND BLACK CONTACT, SOCIOECONOMIC FACTORS, AND USE OF SPANISH AND BLACK ENGLISH IS PROVIDED. THE LINGUISTIC ANALYSIS IS BASED ON ONE-HOUR INTERVIEWS DIVIDED INTO THREE MAIN AREAS—FREE CONVERSATION, RESPONSE TO CERTAIN SENTENCE STIMULI, AND READINGS FROM PROSE AND WORD LISTS. THE FOLLOWING LINGUISTIC PHENOMENA ARE DESCRIBED BASED ON INTERVIEW DATA: (1) LINGUISTIC VARIABILITY; (2) THE VARIABLE; (3) SYLLABLE-FINAL ALVEOLAR STOPS; AND (4) NEGATION. SOCIOLINGUISTIC PRINCIPLES THAT EMERGED FROM THIS STUDY OF LANGUAGE CONTACT INCLUDE VESTIGIAL INTERFERENCE, CONVERGENT PROCESSES, ASSIMILATION VARIANTS, GRAMMATICAL AND PHONOLOGICAL ASSIMILATION, THE EMERGENCE OF NEW RULES, AND LINGUISTIC VARIABILITY. THE PRINCIPLES ELUCIDATED BY THIS RESEARCH ARE CORROBORATED BY OTHER VARIABLE STUDIES CONDUCTED ON OTHER POPULATIONS. 84 REFERENCES.

ACCN 001688

1965 AUTH **WOLKON, G. H., MORIWAKI, S., MANDEL, D. M., ARCHULETA, J., BUNJE, P., & ZIMMERMANN, S.**

TITL ETHNICITY AND SOCIAL CLASS IN THE DELIVERY OF SERVICES: ANALYSIS OF A CHILD GUIDANCE CLINIC.

SRCE *AMERICAN JOURNAL OF PUBLIC HEALTH, 1974, 64(7), 709-712.*

INDX SES, HEALTH DELIVERY SYSTEMS, CHILDREN, MENTAL HEALTH, RESOURCE UTILIZATION, EMPIRICAL, MEXICAN AMERICAN, DISCRIMINATION, CROSS CULTURAL, CALIFORNIA, SOUTHWEST

ABST A SOUTHERN CALIFORNIA, FEDERALLY FUNDED CHILD GUIDANCE CLINIC WAS EXAMINED TO DETERMINE IF LOWER CLASS AND MINORITY CLIENTS WERE MORE OFTEN PLACED ON WAITING LISTS AND HAD A HIGHER DROPOUT RATE THAN MAJORITY GROUP CLIENTS. DATA CONSISTED OF 325 REQUESTS FOR SERVICES IN A SIX-MONTH PERIOD (79% FROM CAUCASIAN FAMILIES; 11% FROM BLACK FAMILIES; AND 10% FROM MEXICAN AMERICAN FAMILIES). CLIENTS WERE ALSO GROUPED ACCORDING TO OCCUPATIONAL AND EDUCATIONAL STATUS. IT WAS FOUND THAT IN EACH EDUCATIONAL, OCCUPATIONAL, AND ETHNIC GROUP, A GREATER PROPORTION OF CLIENTS WAS PLACED ON WAITING LISTS THAN WAS ASSIGNED IMMEDIATE TREATMENT. MOREOVER, ALL THREE ETHNIC GROUPS HAD A VERY HIGH DROPOUT RATE, WITH NO SIGNIFICANT DIFFERENCES BETWEEN THEM. THE RESULTS ARE CONTRARY TO OTHER STUDIES WHICH HAVE DISCOVERED DISCRIMINATION IN SUCH CLINICS. HOWEVER, THE CLINIC'S NONDISCRIMINATORY POLICY IS UNDERMINED BY (1) THE HIGH PROPORTION OF CLIENTS (49%) WHO REQUEST SERVICE BUT ULTIMATELY NEVER SEE A THERAPIST, AND (2) THE LONG WAITING TIME BEFORE INTAKE (A MEDIAN OF 28 WEEKS). IT IS RECOMMENDED THAT THE CLINIC'S DELIVERY SYSTEM BE REAPPRAISED TO SHORTEN WAITING TIME, EMPLOY OTHER TREATMENT MODALITIES, AND RECEIVE INPUT FROM THE TARGET POPULATION. 9 REFERENCES.

ACCN 001689

1966 AUTH **WOOD, C. H., & BEAN, F. D.**

TITL OFFSPRING GENDER AND FAMILY SIZE: IMPLICATIONS FOR A COMPARISON OF MEXICAN AMERICANS AND ANGLO AMERICANS.

SRCE *JOURNAL OF MARRIAGE AND THE FAMILY, 1977, 39(1), 129-139.*

INDX ATTITUDES, BIRTH CONTROL, CROSS CULTURAL, CULTURAL FACTORS, DEMOGRAPHIC, EMPIRICAL, FAMILY STRUCTURE, FERTILITY, MEXICAN AMERICAN, SOUTHWEST, SES, ADULTS, FAMILY PLANNING

ABST THE QUESTIONS OF WHETHER AND HOW OFFSPRING GENDER PREFERENCES AFFECT EVENTUAL FAMILY SIZE ASSUME GREATER PROPORTIONS GIVEN RECENT TECHNOLOGICAL DEVELOPMENTS IN REPRODUCTIVE GENDER CONTROL AND GIVEN THE TREND IN THE UNITED STATES TOWARD PREFERENCES FOR SMALLER FAMILIES. USING 1970 U.S. CENSUS PUBLIC USE SAMPLE DATA FOR ANGLOS AND MEXICAN AMERICANS, THIS STUDY EXAMINES THE RELATIONSHIP BETWEEN THE GENDER OF CHILDREN ALREADY BORN AND THE LIKELIHOOD OF HAVING SUBSEQUENT CHILDREN. THE RESULTS INDICATE THAT COUPLES WITH PREVIOUS CHILDREN OF THE SAME GENDER ARE CONSISTENTLY MORE LIKELY TO BEAR AN ADDITIONAL CHILD COMPARED TO THOSE WITH A GENDER MIX. THOUGH PRESENT AMONG MEMBERS OF BOTH GROUPS, THIS RELATIONSHIP IS MORE PRONOUNCED AMONG ANGLOS THAN MEXICAN AMERICANS. THE EFFECTS OF WIFE'S EDUCATION ON THE LIKELIHOOD OF ANOTHER BIRTH WERE ALSO EXAMINED AND FOUND TO BE GREATER AMONG COUPLES WITH A GENDER MIX THAN AMONG THOSE WITH CHILDREN OF THE SAME GENDER. THE RELEVANCE OF THESE FINDINGS TO THE ISSUE OF WHAT KINDS OF WIVES OPT TO HAVE FEWER CHILDREN ARE DISCUSSED, AND THE REASONS WHY THE TREND TOWARD FAMILIES OF SMALLER SIZES MAY HEIGHTEN PARENTAL INTEREST IN THE GENDER OF EARLY-BORN CHILDREN ARE NOTED. 36 REFERENCES. (JOURNAL ABSTRACT)

ACCN 002168

1967 AUTH **WOODEN, S. L., & PETTIBONE, T. J.**

TITL A COMPARATIVE STUDY OF THREE BEGINNING READING PROGRAMS FOR THE SPANISH SPEAKING CHILD.

SRCE *JOURNAL OF READING BEHAVIOR, 1972-73, 5(3), 192-199.*

INDX EDUCATION, READING, CHILDREN, BILINGUALISM, LINGUISTICS, COGNITIVE DEVELOPMENT, PERCEPTION, SPANISH SURNAMED, EMPIRICAL, LANGUAGE LEARNING, EDUCATIONAL MATERIALS

ABST SINCE LANGUAGE SKILLS IN ENGLISH ARE UNDERDEVELOPED IN THE SPANISH-SPEAKING CHILD, A BEGINNING READING PROGRAM THAT EMPHASIZES LANGUAGE SKILL DEVELOPMENT IS CRUCIAL. TO EXAMINE THIS HYPOTHESIS, THREE APPROACHES TO BEGINNING READING WERE STUDIED: HOUGHTON MIFFLIN, A BASAL TEXT APPROACH; THE MIAMI LINGUISTIC READER SERIES; AND TREATMENT III, A LINGUISTIC AND PERCEPTO-COGNITIVE APPROACH UTILIZING THE MIAMI MATERIALS AND THE KINDERGARTEN EVALUATION OF LEARNING POTENTIAL (KELP). THE THREE PROGRAMS WERE ADMINISTERED TO 522 CHILDREN IN 24 RANDOMLY SELECTED FIRST GRADE CLASSROOMS FROM 4 SOUTHWESTERN SCHOOLS SERVING PREDOMINANTLY SPANISH-SPEAKING CHILDREN. IN ALL THREE CONDITIONS THE DURATION OF THE PROGRAM WAS APPROXIMATELY 7 MONTHS. THE RESULTS OF THE STUDY WERE THAT NONE OF THESE THREE READING APPROACHES WAS UNIQUELY EFFECTIVE IN BRINGING ABOUT HIGHER READING ACHIEVEMENT. THESE FINDINGS THEREFORE STRESS THE IMPORTANCE OF CAREFUL DIAGNOSIS FOR EACH SPANISH-SPEAKING CHILD WHO IS BEGINNING TO READ IN ENGLISH. IDEALLY, A BEGINNING READING PROGRAM THAT EMPHASIZES LANGUAGE AND RELATED SKILLS (SUCH AS LISTENING COM-

PREHENSION, SPATIAL RELATIONS, AND AUDITORY ASSOCIATIONS) WOULD MOST NEARLY MATCH THE ENTRY LEVEL NEEDS OF THIS POPULATION. 10 REFERENCES.

ACCN   001690

1968 AUTH **WRIGHT, C. R., MOTLEY, M. T., & PHELAN, J. G.**
TITL   DISCRIMINATION OF DIALECT FROM TEMPORAL PATTERNS OF THE SPEECH SIGNAL.
SRCE   *PSYCHOLOGICAL REPORTS, 1976, 38(3, PT. 2), 1059-1067.*
INDX   LINGUISTICS, CROSS CULTURAL, CULTURAL FACTORS, MEXICAN AMERICAN, COGNITIVE DEVELOPMENT, LANGUAGE ASSESSMENT, PHONOLOGY, EMPIRICAL
ABST   TO DETERMINE WHETHER DIALECT DISCRIMINATION COULD BE MADE ON THE BASIS OF TEMPORAL SEQUENCING (OR RHYTHM) OF THE SPEECH SIGNAL, SPEECH SAMPLES WERE COLLECTED FROM 90 S'S, IDENTIFIED AS BLACK, WHITE, AND MEXICAN AMERICAN. SAMPLES WERE MATCHED ON THE BASIS OF SIMILARITY OF CONTEXT. SIMILAR SAMPLES WERE RECORDED, USING A TRIAD TEST FORMAT. TWO RACIALLY SIMILAR AND ONE DIFFERENT SPEAKER (E.G., BLACK, BLACK, AND WHITE) FORMED A TRIAD. TWENTY-FOUR TRIADS WERE PUT TOGETHER AND RECORDED. AN ELECTRONIC LOGIC SYSTEM (SCHMITT TRIGGER DESIGN) GENERATED A NOISE ANALOGY (TEMPORAL PATTERN) FOR THE SPEECH SIGNAL. TWENTY-FOUR NOISE-ANALOGY TRIADS AND 24 SPEAKER TRIADS WERE PRESENTED TO GROUPS OF BLACK, WHITE, AND MEXICAN AMERICAN LISTENERS TO DETERMINE WHETHER ETHNICALLY IDENTIFIED LISTENER GROUPS COULD DISTINGUISH SPEAKERS' PATTERNS. OUR ETHNICALLY DISTINCT S'S WERE UNABLE TO DISTINGUISH BETWEEN DIALECTS ON THE BASIS OF TEMPORAL PATTERNS ALONE. THERE WAS A TENDENCY FOR ALL LISTENERS TO DETECT THE MEXICAN AMERICAN SPEECH AT THE CHANCE LEVEL. 2 REFERENCES. (AUTHOR SUMMARY)
ACCN   001691

1969 AUTH **WRIGHT, S.**
TITL   WORK RESPONSE TO INCOME MAINTENANCE: ECONOMIC, SOCIOLOGICAL, AND CULTURAL PERSPECTIVES.
SRCE   *SOCIAL FORCES, 1975, 53(4), 552-562.*
INDX   EMPLOYMENT, SES, ECONOMIC FACTORS, JOB PERFORMANCE, CULTURAL FACTORS, HEALTH, MENTAL HEALTH, PERSONALITY, SOCIAL SCIENCES, NEW JERSEY, PENNSYLVANIA, ADULTS, SURVEY, PUERTO RICAN-M, LABOR FORCE, CROSS CULTURAL, EMPIRICAL, EAST
ABST   DATA WERE DERIVED FROM THE NEW JERSEY-PENNSYLVANIA NEGATIVE INCOME TAX (NIT) EXPERIMENT TO EXAMINE THE ASSUMPTION THAT UNEARNED INCOME CREATES DISINCENTIVES TO WORK. THE BASE WAS A RANDOM SAMPLE OF POVERTY TRACTS IN TRENTON, PATERSON-PASSAIC, AND JERSEY CITY, NEW JERSEY, AND SCRANTON, PENNSYLVANIA. THE SAMPLE WAS LIMITED TO HOUSEHOLDS WITH INCOMES LESS THAN 1.5 TIMES THE POVERTY THRESHOLDS WHICH INCLUDED AT LEAST ONE 18-58 YEAR-OLD MALE ELIGIBLE FOR WORK. TOTAL N EQUALED 1,357, REPRESENTING COMPARABLE PROPORTIONS OF BLACK, WHITE, AND PUERTO RICAN FAMILIES. THE EXPERIMENT, LASTING THREE YEARS, INCLUDED PRE-ENROLLMENT AND QUARTERLY INTERVIEWS WITH THE ENTIRE SAMPLE. CONTRARY TO PREDICTIONS DERIVED FROM ECONOMIC THEORY AND CULTURE OF POVERTY SPECULATIONS, DATA FROM BLACK, WHITE, AND PUERTO RICAN MALE HEADS OF HOUSEHOLDS REVEALED: (1) NO SUCH DISINCENTIVE EFFECTS AMONG MALE HEADS OF HOUSEHOLDS; (2) CONSISTENT AND SIGNIFICANT EFFECTS ON WORK ACTIVITY OF PRIOR LABOR FORCE HISTORY, AGE, HEALTH, FAMILY STRUCTURE, EDUCATION, AND WELFARE STATUS; AND (3) THAT EVEN THOSE WHO EXHIBITED A VARIETY OF ALLEGEDLY DETRIMENTAL PERSONALITY TRAITS, AS DESCRIBED BY THE CULTURE OF POVERTY THESIS, AND THOSE LEAST INTEGRATED INTO THE WORK ETHIC STILL SHOWED NO WORK REDUCTION AS A RESULT OF NIT. 47 REFERENCES.

ACCN   001692

1970 AUTH **WRIGHT, S. J.**
TITL   REDRESSING THE IMBALANCE OF MINORITY GROUPS IN THE PROFESSIONS.
SRCE   *JOURNAL OF HIGHER EDUCATION, 1972, 43(3), 239-248.*
INDX   HIGHER EDUCATION, COLLEGE STUDENTS, PROFESSIONAL TRAINING, SCHOLASTIC ACHIEVEMENT, EDUCATIONAL COUNSELING, ECONOMIC FACTORS, EDUCATION, MEXICAN AMERICAN, PUERTO RICAN-M, CROSS CULTURAL, ESSAY
ABST   ALTHOUGH BLACKS, CHICANOS, PUERTO RICANS AND AMERICAN INDIANS CONSTITUTE 15% OF THE NATION'S POPULATION, THEY ARE SERIOUSLY UNDERREPRESENTED IN HIGHER EDUCATION, MAJOR VOCATIONS, AND PROFESSIONS. TO IMPROVE THIS SITUATION THE FOLLOWING INTERRELATED FACTORS ARE SUGGESTED: (1) IMPROVEMENT IN COUNSELING AND TEACHING IN THE PUBLIC SCHOOLS; (2) REDUCTION IN THE SECONDARY LEVEL DROPOUT RATE; AND THEREBY (3) INCREASING THE NUMBER ENROLLED IN UNDERGRADUATE EDUCATION. ADEQUATE FINANCIAL AID FOR HIGHER EDUCATION MUST BE PROVIDED AND MINORITY GROUPS MUST ACQUIRE MORE POLITICAL PRESSURE. INCLUDED AMONG NINE SHORT-RANGE EFFORTS ARE OPEN ADMISSIONS IN PUBLIC INSTITUTIONS AND BILINGUAL TEACHERS IN ELEMENTARY SCHOOLS FOR MINORITY GROUP PUPILS. LONG-RANGE EFFORTS SUGGESTED ARE: PREPARATION AND EMPLOYMENT OF HIGH SCHOOL COUNSELORS FOR DISADVANTAGED MINORITY STUDENTS; TEACHERS TO BE HELD ACCOUNTABLE FOR STUDENT ACHIEVEMENT; AND THE ESTABLISHMENT OF TWO NATIONAL COMMISSIONS TO STUDY TEACHING METHODS AND CURRICULUM OF INNER-CITY SCHOOLS. 7 REFERENCES. (PASAR ABSTRACT MODIFIED)
ACCN   001693

1971 AUTH **YAMAMOTO, J., JAMES, Q. C., BLOOMBAUM, M., & HATTAM, J.**
TITL RACIAL FACTORS IN PATIENT SELECTION.
SRCE *AMERICAN JOURNAL OF PSYCHIATRY, 1967, 124, 630-636.*
INDX PSYCHOTHERAPY, PSYCHOTHERAPISTS, MEXICAN AMERICAN, RESOURCE UTILIZATION, HEALTH DELIVERY SYSTEMS, SEX COMPARISON, DISCRIMINATION, PREJUDICE, MENTAL HEALTH, PSYCHOPATHOLOGY, EMPIRICAL, CALIFORNIA, SOUTHWEST
ABST A PREVIOUS STUDY OF 594 CONSECUTIVE ADMISSIONS (60% WHITE, 25% BLACK, 14% MEXICAN AMERICAN) TO THE PSYCHIATRIC OUTPATIENT CLINIC OF A SOUTHERN CALIFORNIA HOSPITAL INDICATED THAT PATIENTS WERE BEING TREATED DIFFERENTLY DEPENDING UPON FACTORS OF RACE. INVESTIGATING THIS POSSIBILITY OF PREJUDICE, THE PRESENT STUDY ADMINISTERED THE BOGARDUS SOCIAL DISTANCE SCALE AS WELL AS QUESTIONS ABOUT VARIOUS ETHNIC GROUPS (MEXICAN AMERICANS, BLACKS, AND ORIENTALS) TO 15 STAFF THERAPISTS. ALL THERAPISTS WERE CAUCASIAN AND EITHER PSYCHIATRISTS OR PSYCHIATRIC SOCIAL WORKERS. RESULTS REVEALED THAT DIFFERENCES IN THE BOGARDUS SCALE PREDICTED THE PROPORTION OF ETHNIC PATIENTS SEEN IN TREATMENT: (1) THE THERAPISTS WITH LOW ETHNOCENTRICITY MUCH MORE OFTEN TREATED ETHNIC MINORITY PATIENTS IN PROPORTIONS COMPARABLE WITH THE CAUCASIAN GROUPS; WHILE (2) THOSE THERAPISTS WITH GREATER FEELINGS OF ETHNOCENTRICITY LESS OFTEN SAW THEIR MINORITY GROUP PATIENTS IN TREATMENT LASTING 6 OR MORE WEEKS. IT IS CONCLUDED THAT MORE SYSTEMATIC STUDIES ARE REQUIRED OF THERAPISTS' ATTITUDES SO THAT THERAPISTS MAY BE TRAINED TO BE MORE EFFECTIVE IN TREATING ETHNIC MINORITY GROUPS. 13 REFERENCES. (JOURNAL ABSTRACT MODIFIED)
ACCN 001694

1972 AUTH **YAMAMOTO, J., JAMES, Q. C., & PALLEY, N.**
TITL CULTURAL PROBLEMS IN PSYCHIATRIC THERAPY.
SRCE *ARCHIVES OF GENERAL PSYCHIATRY, 1968, 19(1), 45-49.*
INDX PSYCHOTHERAPY, MEXICAN AMERICAN, ADULTS, EMPIRICAL, CULTURAL FACTORS, CROSS CULTURAL, DISCRIMINATION, PSYCHOTHERAPISTS, ATTITUDES, PREJUDICE, CALIFORNIA, SOUTHWEST
ABST THE TREATMENT OF 594 PATIENTS IN THE PSYCHIATRIC OUTPATIENT CLINIC AT THE LOS ANGELES COUNTY GENERAL HOSPITAL REVEALS CERTAIN CULTURAL PROBLEMS IN PSYCHIATRIC THERAPY. A COMPARISON OF TREATMENT EXPERIENCE AND THE RESPONSES OF THE PATIENTS AND THEIR THERAPISTS TO SIMILAR QUESTIONS CONCERNING IMPROVEMENT, FEELINGS OF LIKING OR DISLIKING, WHETHER ADDITIONAL VISITS WOULD BE OF BENEFIT, AND WHETHER THE PATIENTS RECEIVED SATISFACTORY TREATMENT WERE ANALYZED WITH

PATIENT EVALUATIONS OF THE THERAPIST AND THERAPIST PROGNOSIS OF THE PATIENT. THE RESULTS AMONG THE PATIENTS (65% OF WHOM WERE CAUCASIAN, 25% NEGRO, 9% MEXICAN AMERICAN, AND 1% ORIENTAL) WERE COMPARED. DATA FROM 301 PATIENTS ANALYZED INDICATE THAT NON-CAUCASIANS SELDOM CRITICIZE THEIR THERAPISTS. WHILE 61% OF THE NEGRO PATIENTS THOUGHT THE THERAPIST WAS PREJUDICED, ONLY 4.3% OF MEXICAN AMERICANS AND 4.3% OF CAUCASIANS FELT THE THERAPIST WAS PREJUDICED. A COMPARISON OF THE TREATMENT EXPERIENCES OF THE PATIENTS IN GROUP OR INDIVIDUAL PSYCHOTHERAPY REVEALED THAT ETHNIC PATIENTS WERE MORE OFTEN DISCHARGED OR SEEN FOR MINIMAL SUPPORTIVE PSYCHOTHERAPY. AFTER 9 MONTHS OF ACTIVE TREATMENT, THE ETHNIC GROUP PATIENTS WERE VIRTUALLY ABSENT. THERAPISTS FELT THEY DISLIKED 10.7% OF THE PATIENTS WHILE 10.5% OF THE PATIENTS DISLIKED THEIR THERAPISTS. IT IS CONCLUDED THAT PATIENTS FROM DIFFERENT CULTURAL BACKGROUNDS ARE LESS OFTEN OFFERED OR RECEIVE INTENSIVE THERAPY. IMPROVEMENT OF TREATMENT TECHNIQUES REQUIRES FURTHER STUDY OF THE ETHNOCENTRICITY OF THE THERAPIST AND THE LIFE EXPERIENCES OF NEGRO MEN. 11 REFERENCES.
ACCN 001695

1973 AUTH **YANOCHIK-OWEN, A., & WHITE, M.**
TITL NUTRITION SURVEILLANCE IN ARIZONA: SELECTED ANTHROPOMETRIC AND LABORATORY OBSERVATIONS AMONG MEXICAN AMERICAN CHILDREN.
SRCE *AMERICAN JOURNAL OF PUBLIC HEALTH, 1977, 67(2), 151-154.*
INDX HEALTH, NUTRITION, CHILDREN, MEXICAN AMERICAN, HEALTH DELIVERY SYSTEMS, CROSS CULTURAL, EMPIRICAL, PHYSICAL DEVELOPMENT, ARIZONA, SOUTHWEST
ABST A NUTRITION SURVEILLANCE SYSTEM IN PUBLIC HEALTH CLINICS IS PROVIDING DATA FOR PATIENT CARE AND PROGRAM PLANNING. THROUGH THIS SYSTEM, ARIZONA'S MEXICAN AMERICAN POPULATION HAS BEEN SHOWN TO DIFFER FROM OTHER ETHNIC GROUPS SEEN IN CLINIC. ANEMIA AND LOW HEIGHT-FOR-AGE ARE SIGNIFICANT PROBLEMS IN THE MEXICAN AMERICAN POPULATION. OVER-NUTRITION, IN THE FORM OF OVERWEIGHT AND HIGH CHOLESTEROL, IS ALSO A PROBLEM AMONG THE MEXICAN AMERICAN CLINIC POPULATION. 8 REFERENCES. (JOURNAL ABSTRACT)
ACCN 001696

1974 AUTH **YARBROUGH, C. L.**
TITL AGE-GRADE STATUS OF TEXAS CHILDREN OF LATIN AMERICAN DESCENT.
SRCE *JOURNAL OF EDUCATIONAL RESEARCH, 1946, 40(1), 14-27.*
INDX EDUCATIONAL ASSESSMENT, MEXICAN AMERICAN, ADOLESCENTS, EMPIRICAL, SCHOLASTIC ACHIEVEMENT, TEXAS
ABST THE AGE-GRADE STATUS OF SPANISH AMERICAN (SA) AND ANGLO AMERICAN (AA) SCHOOL

CHILDREN IN TEXAS IS EXAMINED. A COMPARISON OF THE CENSUS AND ENROLLMENT BY AGES ON A PERCENTAGE BASIS WAS OBTAINED. DATA REVEAL THAT THE DIFFERENCE IN PERCENTAGE OF ENROLLMENT BETWEEN SA AND AA IS MORE THAN 20%. IN PROPORTION TO THEIR NUMBERS, THERE ARE 2.7 TIMES AS MANY SA CHILDREN NOT ENROLLED IN SCHOOL AS THERE ARE AA PUPILS. SEVENTY-EIGHT PERCENT OF SA CHILDREN DO NOT REACH THE TWELFTH GRADE, COMPARED WITH 41.89% OF AA CHILDREN. APPROXIMATELY 34% OF SA CHILDREN ARE NOT ENROLLED IN SCHOOL, COMPARED WITH 14% OF AA STUDENTS. THERE IS A WIDE RANGE OF AGE FOR EACH GRADE, WITH LARGE NUMBERS OF OVERAGE CHILDREN IN BOTH GROUPS. THE PERCENT OF CHILDREN IN THE AA GROUP WHO ARE UNDERAGE, NORMAL, OR OVERAGE IS 34.6%, 40.77%, AND 24.56%, RESPECTIVELY, COMPARED WITH 8.1%, 23.58%, AND 68.26% FOR THE SA GROUP. THE MEAN AGE-GRADE STATUS OF SA CHILDREN ENROLLED IN SCHOOL IS 1.55 YEARS MORE THAN THE AA CHILDREN. THE WIDEST DISPARITY IN AGES BETWEEN THE TWO GROUPS OCCURS IN THE ELEMENTARY GRADES. GREAT NUMBERS OF SA CHILDREN ARE ENROLLED IN GRADES ONE TO EIGHT FROM 1 TO 11 YEARS OVERAGE. SPECIFIC CAUSES OF INADEQUACIES IN THE EDUCATION OF CHILDREN OF LATIN DESCENT ARE: POOR SOCIAL ATMOSPHERE; SEGREGATED BUILDINGS WITH POOR FACILITIES; POORLY TRAINED TEACHERS; AND IMPROPER ATTENTION TO THE NEEDS AND INTERESTS OF THE CHILDREN INVOLVED. RECOMMENDATIONS INCLUDE SCHOOL PROGRAMS TO MEET THE NEEDS AND INTERESTS OF SA CHILDREN.

ACCN   001697

1975 AUTH **YAWKEY, T. D., ARONIN, E. L., STREETT, M. A., & HINOJOSA, O. M.**

TITL   TEACHING ORAL LANGUAGE TO YOUNG MEXICAN AMERICANS.

SRCE   *ELEMENTARY ENGLISH, 1974, 51(2), 198-202; 238.*

INDX   MEXICAN AMERICAN, CHILDREN, BILINGUALISM, LANGUAGE LEARNING, EDUCATION, ESSAY, INSTRUCTIONAL TECHNIQUES, POLICY, CURRICULUM

ABST   IMPROVED EDUCATIONAL TECHNIQUES AND CURRICULUM DEVELOPMENT ARE NEEDED TO REMEDY THE PROBLEMS ASSOCIATED WITH TEACHING ENGLISH TO YOUNG MEXICAN AMERICANS. UPON ENTERING U.S. SCHOOLS, MEXICAN AMERICAN CHILDREN FACE PRESSURES OF AN ORAL ENGLISH ENVIRONMENT WHICH LEAD TO SETBACKS IN SELF-ESTEEM AND CONTRIBUTE TO HIGH RATES OF FAILURE, ABSENTEEISM, AND DROPOUTS. THE MAJOR DIFFICULTIES IN ACQUIRING PROFICIENCY IN ENGLISH AS A SECOND LANGUAGE ARE (1) THAT PERCEPTIONS OF SOUNDS OF ENGLISH ARE MADE IN TERMS OF STRUCTURES AND SOUNDS OF SPANISH, AND (2) THAT BASIC PHONETIC DIFFERENCES LEAD TO ENUNCIATION PROBLEMS. TO SOLVE SUCH PROBLEMS, ORAL LANGUAGE METHODS FOR BUILDING

PROFICIENCY IN ENGLISH SHOULD INCLUDE TEACHING IN SPANISH, BILINGUALISM, AND THE BILINGUAL AND BICULTURAL APPROACH. IN PARTICULAR, THE LATTER APPROACH—BASED UPON TEACHER MODELING, PATTERNING, CUING, AND TEACHER RESPONSE—HAS PROVEN TO BE EFFECTIVE IN DEVELOPING FACILITY IN ORAL ENGLISH. SUGGESTIONS FOR THE IMPROVEMENT OF CURRICULA FOR TEACHING ORAL ENGLISH TO MEXICAN AMERICANS INCLUDE: (1) STRESSING FUNCTIONAL VOCABULARY DEVELOPMENT; (2) INCORPORATING MEXICAN AMERICAN CULTURE INTO PROGRAMS; (3) LEARNING ORAL ENGLISH THROUGH SOCIAL INTERACTIONS; (4) RAPID ORAL DRILLING; AND (5) USE OF BILINGUAL PERSONNEL. 18 REFERENCES.

ACCN   001698

1976 AUTH **YODER, R. D., & MOORE, R. A.**

TITL   CHARACTERISTICS OF CONVICTED DRUNKEN DRIVERS.

SRCE   *QUARTERLY JOURNAL OF STUDIES ON ALCOHOL, 1973, 34(3), 927-936.*

INDX   ALCOHOLISM, ADULTS, EMPIRICAL, MEXICAN AMERICAN, SOCIAL SERVICES, CORRECTIONS, CALIFORNIA, SOUTHWEST, CROSS CULTURAL

ABST   PERSONS CONVICTED OF DRIVING WHILE UNDER THE INFLUENCE OF ALCOHOL (DWI) AND ENROLLED IN A MANDATED UNIVERSITY OF CALIFORNIA AT SAN DIEGO EXTENSION SERVICE PROGRAM FOR DWI'S WERE EXAMINED. PERSONAL DATA FORMS WERE SUBMITTED BY 206 FIRST OFFENDERS AND 104 REPEAT OFFENDERS, OF WHOM 18% WERE WOMEN, 86% WERE ANGLOS, 10% MEXICAN AMERICANS, AND 3% AMERICAN INDIANS. PRIOR TO ARREST, 52% OF THE 140 PROBATIONERS WHO SUBMITTED NARRATIVES HAD BEEN DRINKING AT BARS OR POOL HALLS, AND 22% AT PARTIES, PICNICS, AND AT FRIENDS' HOMES. FATIGUE, STRESS, AND CONCURRENT USE OF OTHER DRUGS WERE ALSO INVOLVED. DENIAL OR PROJECTION OF GUILT WERE NOTED IN 31% OF THE NARRATIVES. ADDITIONALLY, THE MICHIGAN ALCOHOLISM SCREENING TEST (MAST) WAS GIVEN TO 201 FIRST OFFENDERS AND TO 68 REPEAT OFFENDERS. REPEAT OFFENDERS HAD SIGNIFICANTLY HIGHER MAST SCORES—INDICATING ALCOHOLISM—THAN FIRST OFFENDERS. MEAN BLOOD ALCOHOL CONCENTRATIONS WHEN ARRESTED AND PREVIOUS ARRESTS FOR ANY CAUSE WERE ALSO SIGNIFICANTLY HIGHER AMONG REPEAT OFFENDERS THAN AMONG THOSE CONVICTED OF DRUNK DRIVING FOR THE FIRST TIME. MANY OF THESE REPEAT OFFENDERS WERE AWARE THAT THEY HAD A DRINKING PROBLEM AND ASSERTED THAT THEY HAD TRIED TO SEEK HELP. ACCORDING TO PREARREST NARRATIVES, 92% OF THE DRINKING WAS DONE WITH FRIENDS, FAMILY, OR COWORKERS IN PLACES ACCESSIBLE ONLY BY AUTOMOBILE; YET 92% COULD RECOLLECT NO EFFORT MADE TO PREVENT THEM FROM DRIVING. 11 REFERENCES.

ACCN   001699

1977 AUTH **YOUNG, F. W., & YOUNG, R. C.**
TITL THE DIFFERENTIATION OF FAMILY STRUCTURE IN RURAL MEXICO.
SRCE *JOURNAL OF MARRIAGE AND THE FAMILY, 1968, 30, 154-161.*
INDX SCHOLASTIC ASPIRATIONS, OCCUPATIONAL ASPIRATIONS, EDUCATION, HOUSING, NUTRITION, HEALTH, MEXICO, MEXICAN, RURAL, FAMILY STRUCTURE, EMPIRICAL, RESEARCH METHODOLOGY, ECONOMIC FACTORS, FAMILY ROLES
ABST THE CONCEPT OF "STRUCTURAL DIFFERENTIATION" IS DEFINED AS THE CAPACITY OF A SOCIAL SYSTEM TO PROCESS A DIVERSITY OF INFORMATION—AND USUALLY, THIS TERM IS SYNONYMOUS WITH "SOCIAL DIVISION OF LABOR" IN A WHOLE SOCIETY. IN THE PRESENT STUDY, IT IS CONCEPTUALLY APPLIED TO RURAL MEXICAN FAMILIES AND IS EMPIRICALLY EXPLORED THROUGH 13 DEMOGRAPHIC AND SOCIOLOGICAL MEASURES. A SAMPLE OF 215 FAMILIES FROM THREE SMALL COMMUNITIES NORTHEAST OF MEXICO CITY WERE GIVEN MEASURES RANGING FROM CONVENTIONAL LEVEL-OF-LIVING INDICES TO SCALES OF FOOD CONSUMPTION AND PARTICIPATION IN FIESTAS. A PRINCIPAL COMPONENTS ANALYSIS WAS PERFORMED AND RESULTED IN TWO MAIN FACTORS, ACCOUNTING FOR 52% AND 38%, RESPECTIVELY, OF THE VARIANCE AFTER ROTATION. THE FIRST FACTOR SUPPORTS THE SINGULARITY OF THE DIFFERENTIATION DIMENSION, WHILE THE SECOND REFLECTS A FARM CONTINUITY DIMENSION. CONSTRUCTION OF A FAMILY DIFFERENTIATION SCALE WHICH IS SYSTEMATIC AND UNIFORMALLY SENSITIVE IN DIVERSE CONTEXTS AND CULTURES IS ADVOCATED IN ORDER TO DEVELOP A CROSS-CULTURALLY VALID MEASURE. FINALLY, THE DIFFERENTIATION CONCEPT IS CONTRASTED TO COGNATE TERMS, AND A REINTERPRETATION OF THE CLASSICAL INDUSTRIALIZATION-CONJUGAL FAMILY ASSOCIATION IS OFFERED. 11 REFERENCES. (JOURNAL ABSTRACT MODIFIED)
ACCN 001700

1978 AUTH **YOUNG, R. K.**
TITL TRANSFERENCIA E INHIBICION RETROACTIVA CON BILINGUES. (TRANSFER AND RETROACTIVE INHIBITION WITH BILINGUALS.)
SRCE *REVISTA INTERAMERICANA DE PSICOLOGIA, 1967, 1(13), 223-230.*
INDX BILINGUAL, COLLEGE STUDENTS, EMPIRICAL, LANGUAGE ASSESSMENT, ADOLESCENTS, BILINGUALISM
ABST THE RESULTS OF THREE EXPERIMENTS ON THE LEARNING AND RETENTION OF WORD LISTS PRESENTED IN THE TWO LANGUAGES (SPANISH AND ENGLISH) OF BILINGUALS ARE PRESENTED. THE METHOD OF INVESTIGATION INVOLVED PRESENTING THE SUBJECTS WITH TWO LISTS OF ISOLATED WORDS OF PAIRS OF NOUNS, FIRST IN ENGLISH AND THEN IN SPANISH, AND VICE VERSA. THE SUBJECTS OF THE FIRST EXPERIMENT WERE 48 HIGH SCHOOL STUDENTS WHO COULD SPEAK AND READ IN ENGLISH BUT COULD ONLY SPEAK AND UNDERSTAND SPANISH. THE SECOND EXPERIMENT INCLUDED 40 SPANISH-ENGLISH BILINGUAL COLLEGE STUDENTS WHOSE DOMINANT LANGUAGE WAS ENGLISH BUT WHO COULD ALSO READ AND SPEAK SPANISH. THE SUBJECTS IN THE THIRD EXPERIMENT WERE 40 COLLEGE STUDENTS, ALL OF THEM BILINGUALS BUT HALF OF THEM HAD ENGLISH AS THEIR DOMINANT LANGUAGE AND THE OTHER HALF HAD SPANISH. RESULTS INDICATE THAT THE LANGUAGES OF A BILINGUAL ARE NOT TWO INDEPENDENT SETS OF RESPONSES AND THAT THE ASSOCIATIONS FORMED IN ONE LANGUAGE ARE STRONGLY INFLUENCED BY THE ASSOCIATIONS FORMED IN THE OTHER. IMPLICATIONS FOR BILINGUAL SCHOOL CHILDREN ARE DISCUSSED.
ACCN 001701

1979 AUTH **YOUNG, R. K., & NAVAR, M. I.**
TITL RETROACTIVE INHIBITION WITH BILINGUALS.
SRCE *JOURNAL OF EXPERIMENTAL PSYCHOLOGY, 1968, 77(1), 109-115.*
INDX BILINGUAL, MEXICAN AMERICAN, EMPIRICAL, LANGUAGE ASSESSMENT, ADULTS
ABST A GROUP OF 40 BILINGUALS LEARNED TWO PAIRED-ASSOCIATE LISTS, AN ENGLISH LIST AND A SPANISH LIST, AND THEN RELEARNED THE FIRST LIST. THE TRANSFER PARADIGM EMPLOYED WAS A-B, A'-B'R, WHERE THE ITEMS OF THE SECOND LIST ARE TRANSLATIONS OF THE FIRST BUT WITH THE TRANSLATED STIMULI BEING REPAIRED WITH DIFFERENT TRANSLATED RESPONSES. IN CONTRAST TO EXPECTATIONS FROM PREVIOUS RESEARCH, THE RETROACTIVE INHIBITION (RI) OBTAINED WAS RELATED NEITHER TO THE DOMINANT LANGUAGE OF THE SUBJECT NOR TO THE ORDER OF THE LISTS LEARNED. THE RI OBTAINED WAS CONSIDERED IN LIGHT OF THE HYPOTHESIS THAT NONREINFORCED EVOCATION OF THE FIRST LIST RESPONSES DURING THE SECOND LIST LEARNING IS RELATED TO RI. FORGETTING IN ONE LANGUAGE OCCURS AS A FUNCTION OF ASSOCIATIONS FORMED IN ANOTHER LANGUAGE. IN ADDITION, LANGUAGE DOMINANCE DOES NOT APPEAR TO BE RELATED TO THE AMOUNT OF FORGETTING. IT IS CONCLUDED THAT THE TWO LANGUAGES OF A BILINGUAL ARE INTERDEPENDENT AND NOT INDEPENDENT. 9 REFERENCES.
ACCN 001702

1980 AUTH **YOUNG, R. K., & SAEGERT, J.**
TITL TRANSFER WITH BILINGUALS.
SRCE *PSYCHONOMIC SCIENCE, 1966, 6(4), 161-162.*
INDX BILINGUAL, MEXICAN AMERICAN, ADOLESCENTS, EMPIRICAL, LANGUAGE ASSESSMENT, COGNITIVE STYLE, LANGUAGE LEARNING
ABST TRANSFER WAS INVESTIGATED IN A GROUP OF 48 BILINGUAL HIGH SCHOOL JUNIORS. EACH SUBJECT LEARNED TWO SERIAL LISTS COMPOSED OF 12 COMMON NOUNS, ONE IN ENGLISH AND THE OTHER IN SPANISH. HALF OF THE SUBJECTS LEARNED THE ENGLISH LIST FIRST AND THE SPANISH LIST SECOND; AND FOR THE SECOND HALF, THE ORDER OF LEARNING WAS REVERSED. THREE TRANSFER

CONDITIONS WERE EMPLOYED: (1) SAME ORDER (THE SECOND LIST CONTAINED ITEMS TRANSLATED FROM THE FIRST IN THE SAME ORDER); (2) RANDOM ORDER (THE ITEMS TRANSLATED FROM THE FIRST LIST WERE RANDOMLY REARRANGED); AND (3) CONTROL (THE SECOND LIST ITEMS WERE UNRELATED TO THE FIRST). THE BASIC DESIGN WAS A 2 BY 3 FACTORIAL, WITH ORDER OF LANGUAGE LEARNING AND CONDITION OF TRANSFER BEING THE MAJOR VARIABLES. IN ADDITION, TWO SAMPLES OF ITEMS AND EQUAL NUMBERS OF MALES AND FEMALES WERE USED IN EACH CONDITION TO BRING THE FULL DESIGN TO A 2 BY 3 BY 2 BY 2 FACTORIAL. TWO SUBJECTS WERE CONTAINED IN EACH OF THE 24 EXPERIMENTAL CELLS. RESULTS INDICATE THAT THE AMOUNT OF TRANSFER WAS THE SAME FROM ENGLISH TO SPANISH AS FROM SPANISH TO ENGLISH. ABOUT 50% POSITIVE TRANSFER WAS OBTAINED IN THE SAME ORDER CONDITION AND ABOUT 13% NEGATIVE TRANSFER WAS OBTAINED IN THE RANDOM ORDER CONDITION. THUS, THE ASSOCIATIONS FORMED WITHIN THE CONTEXT OF ONE LANGUAGE CAN BOTH FACILITATE OR INTERFERE WITH THE FORMATION OF NEW ASSOCIATIONS IN A SECOND LANGUAGE. 3 REFERENCES. (JOURNAL ABSTRACT MODIFIED)

ACCN   001703

1981 AUTH   **YOUNG, R. K., & WEBBER, A.**
TITL   POSITIVE AND NEGATIVE TRANSFER WITH BILINGUALS.
SRCE   *JOURNAL OF VERBAL LEARNING AND VERBAL BEHAVIOR, 1967, 6(6), 874-877.*
INDX   BILINGUAL, MEXICAN AMERICAN, EMPIRICAL, LANGUAGE ASSESSMENT, ADULTS
ABST   AN INVESTIGATION OF THE TRANSFER EFFECTS OF LEARNING A PAIRED-ASSOCIATE LIST IN ONE LANGUAGE THEN TRANSFERRING TO A PAIRED-ASSOCIATE LIST IN A SECOND LANGUAGE WAS CONDUCTED. TWENTY BILINGUALS LEARNED A SPANISH LIST AND THEN AN ENGLISH LIST, AND 20 OTHER BILINGUALS LEARNED AN ENGLISH LIST AND THEN A SPANISH LIST. TWO TRANSFER SUBGROUPS WERE EMPLOYED WITHIN EACH GROUP. IN THE EQUIVALENT GROUP, THE SECOND LIST WAS A DIRECT TRANSLATION OF THE FIRST, WITH THE ARRANGEMENT OF THE ITEMS IN EACH PAIR BEING HELD CONSTANT FROM THE FIRST TO THE SECOND LISTS (A-B, A'-B'). IN THE REPAIRED GROUP, THE SECOND LIST CONSISTED OF ITEMS WHICH WERE TRANSLATED FROM THE FIRST, BUT WHICH HAD THE RESPONSES REPAIRED WITH OTHER STIMULI (A-B, A'-B'R). IT WAS FOUND THAT POSITIVE TRANSFER OCCURRED FOR THE EQUIVALENT GROUPS BOTH FROM ENGLISH TO SPANISH AND FROM SPANISH TO ENGLISH. FOR THE REPAIRED GROUPS, NEGATIVE TRANSFER OCCURRED FROM SPANISH TO ENGLISH BUT NO TRANSFER OCCURRED FROM ENGLISH TO SPANISH. 5 REFERENCES.
ACCN   001704

1982 AUTH   **YOUNG, R. K., & WEBBER, A.**

TITL   STANDARDIZATION OF MEXICAN TRIGRAMS.
SRCE   *PSYCHONOMIC SCIENCE, 1968, 11(10), 354.*
INDX   BILINGUAL, COLLEGE STUDENTS, EMPIRICAL, LANGUAGE ASSESSMENT, MEXICAN AMERICAN, LANGUAGE COMPREHENSION
ABST   THE PRESENT PAPER REPORTS AN ATTEMPT TO STANDARDIZE A LARGE NUMBER OF CONSONANT-VOWEL-CONSONANT TRIGRAMS ON A SAMPLE OF SPANISH SPEAKERS. A TOTAL OF 92 NATIONAL UNIVERSITY OF MEXICO STUDENTS GAVE "YES" OR "NO" RESPONSES TO EACH OF 987 TRIGRAMS IN RESPONSE TO QUESTIONS ABOUT WHETHER OR NOT THE TRIGRAM LOOKED OR SOUNDED LIKE A WORD. THE NUMBER OF "YES" RESPONSES FOR EACH TRIGRAM WAS USED TO DEFINE ITS MEANINGFULNESS AND THIS NUMBER VARIED FROM A LOW OF 3 TO A HIGH OF 90. INTERNAL CONSISTENCY AND COMPARISONS WITH OTHER STUDIES SUGGEST THAT THE RELIABILITY OF THE RATINGS WAS HIGH. 3 REFERENCES. (JOURNAL ABSTRACT)
ACCN   001705

1983 AUTH   **YZAGUIRRE, R.**
TITL   ACCESSIBILITY OF THE HISPANIC AMERICAN POPULATION TO THE DECISION AND POLICY-MAKING PROCESS IN THE PRIVATE AND PUBLIC INSTITUTIONS OF THE U.S.
SRCE   *PAPER PRESENTED AT THE NATIONAL COUNCIL OF LA RAZA AWARDS BANQUET FOR NATIONAL HISPANIC LEADERS, HOUSTON, NOVEMBER 1976.*
INDX   POLITICAL POWER, ADMINISTRATORS, POLITICS, EDUCATION, ECONOMIC FACTORS, CULTURAL FACTORS, REPRESENTATION, RELIGION, ESSAY, PROCEEDINGS, MEXICAN AMERICAN, LEADERSHIP, DISCRIMINATION, EMPLOYMENT, EQUAL OPPORTUNITY
ABST   OVER THE PAST DECADE, THE HISPANIC COMMUNITY HAS MOVED FROM BEING THE INVISIBLE MINORITY TO BEING A GROUP WITH KNOWLEDGE THAT BY 1990 IT WILL CONSTITUTE THE NATION'S LARGEST MINORITY. HOWEVER, THE LATINO'S LACK OF ACCESS AND REPRESENTATION TO THE INSTITUTIONS WHICH CONTROL HIS OR HER LIFE GREATLY DIMINISHES THE ABILITY TO SENSITIZE THESE INSTITUTIONS TO THE HISPANICS' BASIC NEEDS. HISPANICS ARE SYSTEMATICALLY DENIED ACCESS TO MOST OF THE MAJOR PRIVATE AND PUBLIC INSTITUTIONS OF THE UNITED STATES—THE FEDERAL EMPLOYMENT SYSTEM; FEDERAL ADVISORY BODIES; ELECTED AND APPOINTED OFFICES; SCHOOL BOARDS; THE JUDICIAL SYSTEM; BOARDS AND STAFFS OF PHILANTHROPIC FOUNDATIONS; CORPORATE DECISION-MAKING BOARDS; AND DECISION-MAKING BODIES WITHIN THE CATHOLIC CHURCH. THE PROBLEM CENTERS AROUND A LACK OF CONSCIOUSNESS ON THE PART OF LATINOS AND A BASIC LACK OF POWER. IT IS THIS POWERLESSNESS WHICH DENIES HISPANICS ON ALL LEVELS ACCESS TO EQUAL OPPORTUNITY IN EDUCATION, INCOME, JOBS, AND JUSTICE. WHEN HISPANICS BEGIN TO GRASP AND ACT ON THIS REALITY, PARTICIPA-

TION IN A TRULY PLURALISTIC SOCIETY WILL BECOME A REALITY. 8 REFERENCES.

ACCN   001706

1984 AUTH   **YZAGUIRRE, R.**
      TITL   A NEW ADMINISTRATION. . . UNFULFILLED PROMISES?
      SRCE   *AGENDA, JANUARY/FEBRUARY 1977, P. 2.*
      INDX   POLITICAL POWER, POLITICS, REPRESENTATION, ESSAY, MEXICAN AMERICAN, TEXAS, NEW YORK, ILLINOIS, MIDWEST, EAST, SOUTHWEST
      ABST   THE CHANGE IN PRESIDENTIAL ADMINISTRATIONS (FORD/CARTER) DID NOT BRING ABOUT THE PROMISED INCREASED CHICANO/LATINO GOVERNMENTAL INPUT AND INCREASED PUBLICITY REGARDING CHICANO/LATINO CONCERNS. EXPECTATIONS FOR CHANGE HAD BEEN NOURISHED BY CAMPAIGN RHETORIC. IN RESPONSE, A LARGE TURNOUT OF LATINO VOTERS GAVE THE CARTER/MONDALE TICKET THE MARGIN OF VICTORY IN SEVERAL STATES (TEXAS, NEW YORK, ILLINOIS). LATINO DEMANDS FOR GOVERNMENTAL INVOLVEMENT CAN BE FOLLOWED-UP THROUGH LETTER WRITING, CALLING CONGRESSIONAL REPRESENTATIVES, REQUESTING POSITIONS AND APPOINTMENTS IN THE ADMINISTRATION, AND EXPRESSING CONCERNS THROUGH THE MEDIA. ADDITIONALLY, THE CHICANO/LATINO MUST IDENTIFY AND HOLD ACCOUNTABLE COMMUNITY "BROKERS" OR AGENTS NEGOTIATING ON BEHALF OF THE HISPANIC POPULATION. TO AVOID HISPANICS AS "WINDOW DRESSINGS" IN THE ADMINISTRATION, THOSE APPOINTED SHOULD HAVE A RECORD OF COMPETENCY AND COMMITMENT AND MUST REPRESENT A COMMUNITY CONSTITUENCY. POLITICIANS, FOUNDATIONS, CORPORATIONS, AND OTHER CENTERS OF POWER ARE REPORTEDLY GUILTY OF ENGAGING LATINO ADMINISTRATORS WITH NO CONSTITUENCIES TO ENSURE "BOSS" LOYALTY. DIRECT CONFRONTATION IS FELT TO BE THE ONLY SOLUTION TO THE LONGSTANDING PROBLEM OF LATINO UNDERREPRESENTATION IN GOVERNMENT.

ACCN   001707

1985 AUTH   **ZAHN, M. A., & BALL, J. C.**
      TITL   FACTORS RELATED TO CURE OF OPIATE ADDICTION AMONG PUERTO RICAN ADDICTS.
      SRCE   *THE INTERNATIONAL JOURNAL OF THE ADDICTIONS, 1972, 7(2), 237-245.*
      INDX   DRUG ADDICTION, REHABILITATION, DRUG ABUSE, EMPIRICAL, CRIMINOLOGY, ADULTS, PUERTO RICAN-M
      ABST   STUDIES OF NARCOTIC ADDICTS INDICATE THAT CHANCES OF RELAPSE FOLLOWING TREATMENT ARE HIGH. STILL, A SIZEABLE PROPORTION OF NARCOTIC ADDICTS DO NOT RETURN TO CHRONIC USE OF OPIATES, AND THIS STUDY DELINEATES FACTORS ASSOCIATED WITH SUCH CURES. A FIELD, FOLLOW-UP STUDY WAS CONDUCTED OF 108 MALE PUERTO RICANS WHO PREVIOUSLY WERE ADDICTS. INTERVIEWS, RECORDS, AND URINALYSIS IDENTIFIED 21 CURED SUBJECTS (20%) WHO HAD BEEN DRUG-FREE FOR THREE YEARS. COMPARISONS BETWEEN THE CURED AND THE 87

NONCURED SUBJECTS ON SOCIAL BACKGROUND FACTORS REVEALED THAT THE CURED SUBJECTS HAD FEWER ARRESTS PRIOR TO TREATMENT, AND FEWER OF THESE WERE FOR NARCOTIC VIOLATIONS. THEY WERE LESS LIKELY TO HAVE BEEN HEROIN ADDICTS, AND THEY TENDED TO BEGIN DRUG USE AT A LATER AGE THAN THE NONCURED SUBJECTS. AMONG THE TREATMENT-RELATED VARIABLES, CURES CORRELATED WITH SHORTER LENGTH OF HOSPITAL STAY AND WITH A SINGLE ADMISSION. WITH REGARD TO OUTCOME VARIABLES, THE CURED SUBJECTS WERE MORE LIKELY TO BE LIVING WITH THEIR SPOUSES. ALMOST 50% WERE STEADILY EMPLOYED, AND 90% WERE ARREST-FREE FOR THE PREVIOUS THREE YEARS. 18 REFERENCES.

ACCN   001708

1986 AUTH   **ZAKS, V. C.**
      TITL   THE CHICANO IDENTITY QUESTIONNAIRE.
      SRCE   *PAPER PRESENTED AT THE ANNUAL CONVENTION OF THE WESTERN PSYCHOLOGICAL ASSOCIATION, SACRAMENTO, CALIFORNIA, APRIL 26, 1975.*
      INDX   SELF CONCEPT, ETHNIC IDENTITY, CULTURE, MEXICAN AMERICAN, EMPIRICAL, ADULTS, RESEARCH METHODOLOGY, CROSS CULTURAL, COLLEGE STUDENTS
      ABST   TO DE-EMPHASIZE TRADITIONAL BEHAVIOR AS A MEASURE OF CHICANO ETHNIC IDENTITY AND TO BEGIN LOOKING AT THE SUBJECTIVE SIDE OF ETHNICITY, A 50-ITEM LIKERT INSTRUMENT QUESTIONNAIRE WAS DEVISED. THE QUESTIONNAIRE FOCUSES ON THREE AREAS (RECOGNITION OF ONE'S ETHNIC BACKGROUND, ACCEPTANCE OF SELF AS A MEMBER OF THAT GROUP, AND ATTRIBUTION OF POSITIVE VALUE TO THAT GROUP) AND WAS ADMINISTERED TO THREE GROUPS OF CHICANO JUNIOR COLLEGE STUDENTS—41 CHICANO MEMBERS OF CAMPUS ETHNIC ORGANIZATIONS; 60 CHICANO NON-MEMBERS; AND 35 STUDENTS OF VARIOUS OTHER ETHNIC BACKGROUNDS, 10 OF WHOM WERE LATINO BUT NOT CHICANO. FINALLY CONDENSED TO 19 ITEMS, THE QUESTIONNAIRE SIGNIFICANTLY DIFFERENTIATED BETWEEN THE ETHNIC CLUB MEMBERS AND NON-MEMBERS. MEAN TOTAL SCORES CONTRADICT THE PASSIVE STEREOTYPE OF "TRADITIONAL" MEXICAN AMERICANS. THE SCORES OF LATINOS CLOSELY RESEMBLED THOSE OF CHICANOS, WHILE THE NON-LATINOS SCORED SIGNIFICANTLY LOWER IN ETHNIC IDENTIFICATION THAN CHICANOS AND OTHER LATINOS. IN TERMS OF SELF-DESCRIPTION, CLUB MEMBERS WERE MORE ASSERTIVE ABOUT THEIR ETHNIC IDENTITY AND LESS LIKELY TO ACCEPT LABELS IMPOSED BY THE DOMINANT CULTURE. THREE TIMES AS MANY CHICANO ETHNIC IDENTIFIERS AS NONIDENTIFIERS CLAIMED SPANISH AS THEIR PRIMARY LANGUAGE. HOWEVER, COUNTER TO THE VIEW OF ETHNIC IDENTIFIERS AS PASSIVE INDIVIDUALS, THE SPANISH SPEAKING IDENTIFIERS WERE "UNTRADITIONAL" WITH RESPECT TO SELF-DESCRIPTION AND ACTIVE PARTICIPATION IN AN ETHNIC, SOCIO-POLITICAL

GROUP. FINALLY, INTRA-GROUP DIFFERENCES WERE FOUND TO BE IMPORTANT ETHNIC INDICATORS, ALTHOUGH THEY ARE OFTEN OVERLOOKED IN THE LITERATURE. 5 REFERENCES.

ACCN   001709

1987 AUTH   **ZAMM, M.**
TITL   READING DISABILITIES: A THEORY OF COGNITIVE INTEGRATION.
SRCE   *JOURNAL OF LEARNING DISABILITIES, 1973, 6(2), 95-101.*
INDX   COGNITIVE DEVELOPMENT, READING, CHILDREN, MEMORY, LINGUISTIC COMPETENCE, SCHOLASTIC ACHIEVEMENT, SES, PUERTO RICAN-M, REVIEW, LEARNING DISABILITIES, LANGUAGE ACQUISITION, LANGUAGE LEARNING
ABST   THE DIFFICULTY OF TEACHING BLACK AND PUERTO RICAN CHILDREN IN POVERTY AREAS TO READ IS EXAMINED IN TERMS OF A THEORY OF COGNITIVE INTEGRATION. IT IS SUGGESTED THAT MANY BLACK AND PUERTO RICAN CHILDREN HAVE DIFFICULTY MAKING TOTALLY INTEGRATED RESPONSES TO WORDS BECAUSE OF COGNITIVE DISINTEGRATION WHICH BLOCKS NOT ONLY THE READING OF WORDS BUT ALSO COMPREHENSION. THE DEVELOPMENTAL BASIS OF SUCH DIFFICULTIES— WHEN THE WRITINGS OF PIAGET, J. HUNT, AND D. HEBB ARE CONSIDERED—LIE IN A POVERTY OF KEY TACTUAL AND EMOTIONAL EXPERIENCES AT CRUCIAL STAGES IN DEVELOPMENT. THIS CAUSES DIFFICULTIES IN COORDINATED NEURAL FUNCTIONING AND CAN FORM THE BASIS OF COGNITIVE DYSFUNCTION. POSSIBLE REMEDIES FOR SUCH PROBLEMS MIGHT BE FOUND IN THE USE OF READING AND COGNITIVE DEVELOPMENT DESIGN WHICH STIMULATE DIAGNOSIS AT EVERY STAGE, LEARNING AT AN INDIVIDUAL PACE, REJECTION OF UNIDIMENSIONAL PROGRAMS, AND SUPPORT FOR A MULTIMETHOD TREATMENT APPROACH. 10 REFERENCES.

ACCN   001710

1988 AUTH   **ZEINER, A. R., PAREDES, A., & COWDEN, L.**
TITL   PHYSIOLOGIC RESPONSES TO ETHANOL AMONG THE TARAHUMARA INDIANS.
SRCE   *ANNALS OF THE NEW YORK ACADEMY OF SCIENCES, 1976, 273, 151-158.*
INDX   ALCOHOLISM, INDIGENOUS POPULATIONS, MEXICO, CULTURAL FACTORS, EMPIRICAL, CROSS CULTURAL, ADULTS, MALE
ABST   TO TEST THE HYPOTHESIS THAT BIOLOGICAL DIFFERENCES IN SENSITIVITY TO ETHANOL ACCOUNT FOR DIFFERENCES IN THE INCIDENCE OF ALCOHOL ABUSE AMONG DIFFERENT ETHNIC GROUPS, 28 ADULT MALE TARAHUMARA INDIANS OF MEXICO WERE ASSIGNED TO EITHER AN EXPERIMENTAL ETHANOL CONDITION OR A PLACEBO CONTROL GROUP. BASELINE BLOOD PRESSURE, HEART RATE, SKIN POTENTIAL RESPONSE, EAR LOBE TEMPERATURE, AND DIGITAL PULSE WAVE AMPLITUDE WERE RECORDED; NEXT, THE ETHANOL SUBJECTS WERE GIVEN A DRINK CONTAINING 0.66 CC OF ETHANOL/KG OF BODY WEIGHT; AND FINALLY, PHYSIOLOGICAL MEASURES WERE TAKEN AGAIN. BOTH EXPERIMENTAL AND

CONTROL GROUPS EXHIBITED A STRONG VASODILATION EFFECT, BUT IN CONTRAST TO A PREVIOUS EXPERIMENT WITH CAUCASIAN SUBJECTS, ONLY THE ETHANOL GROUP SHOWED A HEART RATE INCREASE. ALTHOUGH TEMPERATURE CHANGES FROM THE EAR LOBE WERE NOT FOUND TO BE SENSITIVE TO ETHANOL IN THE DOSE ADMINISTERED, FREQUENCY OF SPONTANEOUS SKIN POTENTIAL RESPONSES PROVED TO BE A SENSITIVE INDEX OF ETHANOL INGESTION. IN THREE OF THE FOUR RELIABLE PHYSIOLOGICAL MEASURES RECORDED WITH THE TARAHUMARANS, THE CHANGES WERE NOT OF THE MAGNITUDE RECORDED IN THE EARLIER EXPERIMENT WITH CAUCASIANS. SINCE THE TARAHUMARANS WERE FOUND TO REACH A LOWER PEAK BLOOD ALCOHOL CONCENTRATION AND TO METABOLIZE ETHANOL FASTER THAN CAUCASIANS, IT IS SUGGESTED THAT THE DIFFERENTIAL BIOLOGICAL SENSITIVITY HYPOTHESIS MAY BE MORE LIMITED THAN PREVIOUSLY SUSPECTED AND IS IN NEED OF REVISION. 21 REFERENCES.

ACCN   001711

1989 AUTH   **ZIMMERING, P., TOOLAN, J., SAFRIN, R., & WORTIS, S. B.**
TITL   HEROIN ADDICTION IN ADOLESCENT BOYS.
SRCE   *JOURNAL OF NERVOUS AND MENTAL DISEASES, 1951, 114(1), 19-34.*
INDX   DRUG ADDICTION, PUERTO RICAN-M, ADOLESCENTS, EMPIRICAL, PERSONALITY, RORSCHACH TEST, WAIS, NEW YORK, EAST
ABST   A REPORT OF MEDICAL AND PSYCHIATRIC ASPECTS OF ADOLESCENT HEROIN ADDICTION IS BASED ON THE STUDY OF 22 CONSECUTIVE ADMISSIONS FOR ADDICTION AT THE BOYS' WARD OF BELLEVUE HOSPITAL, NEW YORK, IN 1951. SUBJECTS, AGES 14 TO 17 YEARS, WERE REFERRED FROM CHILDREN'S COURT, SOCIAL AGENCIES, AND PARENTS. COMPLETE MEDICAL AND PSYCHIATRIC EVALUATION (INCLUDING THE WECHSLER ADULT INTELLIGENCE SCALE AND RORSCHACH TEST) WAS CARRIED OUT DURING THE THREE- TO FIVE-WEEK HOSPITAL STAY. SOCIAL FACTORS BELIEVED TO BE IMPORTANT COMPONENTS OF THE ADDICTION PROBLEM INCLUDE (1) RACE, AS 21/22 PATIENTS WERE BLACK OR OF PUERTO RICAN DESCENT, AND (2) LIVING CONDITIONS, AS ALL ADDICTS CAME FROM AREAS CHARACTERIZED BY POVERTY, CONGESTION, SLUM-LIKE CONDITIONS, AND HIGH DELINQUENCY. INCREASED DRUG USE MAY BE ASSOCIATED WITH DRASTIC PERSONALITY CHANGES, ANTISOCIAL BEHAVIOR, AND SERIOUS AND OCCASIONALLY FATAL HEPATITIS. THE ORIGIN OF THE ADDICTION IS DETERMINED NOT BY THE CHEMICAL EFFECTS OF THE DRUG BUT BY THE PSYCHOLOGICAL STRUCTURE OF THE PATIENT. COMMON CHARACTER TRAITS OF THE ADOLESCENT ADDICT GROUP INCLUDE: (1) LACK OF AGGRESSION; (2) STRONG ATTACHMENT TO MOTHER; (3) POOR OBJECT RELATIONSHIP; (4) OMNIPOTENT STRIVING; AND (5) A TENDENCY TO REGRESS. THE MANAGEMENT OF THE GROWING ADOLESCENT DRUG PROB-

LEM IS FELT TO BE A SOCIAL-PSYCHOLOGICAL AND POLICE PROBLEM. SUGGESTED IS THE REMOVAL OF THE YOUTHFUL ADDICT TO IN-STITUTIONS FOR NORMAL BOYS FOR PERIODS UP TO 2 OR 3 YEARS, WITH PERIODIC TRIALS AT HOME. 19 REFERENCES.

ACCN   001712

1990 AUTH   **ZIMMERING, P., & TOOLAN, J.**
TITL   DRUG ADDICTION IN ADOLESCENTS.
SRCE   *JOURNAL OF NERVOUS AND MENTAL DISEASE, 1952, 116(3), 262-265.*
INDX   DRUG ADDICTION, SELF CONCEPT, PUERTO RI-CAN-M, ADOLESCENTS, EMPIRICAL, NEW YORK, EAST
ABST   COMMON CHARACTERISTICS OF ADOLES-CENT DRUG ADDICTS ADMITTED TO THE PSY-CHIATRIC DIVISION OF BELLEVUE HOSPITAL FROM 1949-1951 ARE REVIEWED. ADMISSION RATES OF NARCOTIC ADDICTS UNDER 21 IN-CREASED FROM 1 CASE IN 1949, TO 11 CASES IN 1950, AND TO 301 CASES IN 1951. ADOLES-CENT HEROIN ADDICTION IS DESCRIBED AS A PROGRESSION FROM "SNORTING" TO "SKIN POPPING," AND FINALLY TO "MAINLINING" WITH ASSOCIATED TRUANCY, RENUNCIATION OF SO-CIAL TIES, AND CRIMINAL ACTIVITY. COMMON CHARACTERISTICS SHARED BY THE ADDICT GROUP INCLUDE (1) NEGRO OR PUERTO RI-CAN DESCENT, (2) ATYPICAL DELINQUENT BE-HAVIOR (NONAGGRESSIVENESS, VERBAL AD-EPTNESS, SOCIAL GRACEFULLNESS), (3) SUSTAINED RELATIONSHIP WITH MOTHER AND ABSENT FATHERS, (4) WEAK OBJECT RELA-TIONSHIPS, (5) INHIBITIONS OF WORK AND SCHOOL, AND (6) SIMILAR DRUG INDUCED EX-PERIENCES (EUPHORIA, HEIGHTENED SELF-ESTEEM, FANTASIES OF OMNIPOTENCE, AND WITHDRAWAL FROM SOCIAL EXPERIENCE). A DYNAMIC COMPLEX OF ECONOMIC AND SO-CIAL FACTORS—IN PARTICULAR, THE IN-ABILITY TO HANDLE AGGRESSIVE DRIVES—DE-TERMINE ADOLESCENT ADDICTION. DISCUSSANTS BRIEFLY NOTE (1) THE CHANGE IN AGE (OLD TO YOUNG) AND RACIAL (WHITE TO NON-WHITE) COMPOSITION OF ADDICTS SINCE THE 1920'S, (2) THE ABSENCE OF ADO-LESCENT DRUG WITHDRAWAL REACTIONS, (3) THE ABSENCE OF MIXED ADDICTIONS, AND (4) THE PROBLEM OF THE DRUG PEDDLER IN THE COMMUNITY. 2 REFERENCES.

ACCN   001713

1991 AUTH   **ZIMMERMAN, B. J., & PIKE, E. O.**
TITL   EFFECTS OF MODELING AND REINFORCEMENT ON THE ACQUISITION AND GENERALIZATION OF QUESTION-ASKING BEHAVIOR.
SRCE   *CHILD DEVELOPMENT, 1973, 43(3), 892-907.*
INDX   MODELING, LINGUISTIC COMPETENCE, LEARNING, BEHAVIOR MODIFICATION, INTER-PERSONAL RELATIONS, POVERTY, CULTURAL FACTORS, MEXICAN AMERICAN, CHILDREN, CROSS CULTURAL, EMPIRICAL
ABST   THE QUESTION-ASKING BEHAVIOR OF DISAD-VANTAGED MEXICAN AMERICAN SECOND-GRADE CHILDREN WAS FOUND READILY MOD-IFIABLE USING AN ADULT MODEL OFFERING CONTINGENT PRAISE. LOWER LEVELS OF RE-SPONSE WERE PRODUCED WHEN ONLY PRAISE WAS PRESENTED. BOTH CONDITIONS NUMER-ICALLY SURPASSED AN UNTREATED CONTROL GROUP'S QUESTION-ASKING LEVELS. CAUSAL RELATIONSHIPS WERE ESTABLISHED BETWEEN THE TREATMENT VARIATIONS AND CHILD QUESTION PRODUCTION THROUGH A MUL-TIPLE BASELINE PROCEDURE WHICH PRO-DUCED STAGGERED INCREASES AND DE-CREASES WHEN TREATMENT WAS EITHER REINSTATED OR WITHDRAWN, RESPECTIVELY. SOME GENERALIZATION OF QUESTION-ASK-ING BEHAVIOR WAS OBSERVED WHEN A NEW TEACHER WHO DID NOT MODEL OR PRAISE WAS INTRODUCED. AFTER TRAINING, INDI-VIDUAL POSTTESTING REVEALED THAT ONLY THE CHILDREN WHO OBSERVED THE MODEL AND WERE PRAISED FOR THEIR QUESTIONS PRODUCED SIGNIFICANTLY MORE QUESTIONS THAN THE CONTROL GROUP WHEN PRE-SENTED WITH UNFAMILIAR STIMULUS CARDS. 20 REFERENCES. (JOURNAL ABSTRACT)

ACCN   001714

1992 AUTH   **ZIMMERMAN, B. J., & ROSENTHAL, T. L.**
TITL   OBSERVATION, REPETITION, AND ETHNIC BACKGROUND IN CONCEPT ATTAINMENT AND GENERALIZATION.
SRCE   *CHILD DEVELOPMENT, 1972, 43(2), 605-613.*
INDX   COGNITIVE STYLE, MEXICAN AMERICAN, CHIL-DREN, EMPIRICAL, CROSS CULTURAL, CUL-TURAL FACTORS
ABST   AN INVESTIGATION OF OBSERVATION, REPETI-TION IN CONCEPT ATTAINMENT, AND GENER-ALIZATION AMONG 64 MEXICAN AMERICAN (MA) AND 64 ANGLO AMERICAN (AA) FIFTH-GRADE PUPILS IS PRESENTED. SUBJECTS RANGED IN AGE FROM 10-0 TO 12-7, WITH A MEAN OF 10-7 YEARS. TWO SETS OF 12 STIMU-LUS CARDS WERE PREPARED. THE CONCEPT INVOLVED LEARNING TO PICK THE FORM BOTH ADJACENT TO A LARGE DOTTED FORM AND IN THE DIRECTION OF THE SMALLER BOTTOM NUMBER. ALL CHILDREN RECEIVED FEEDBACK ON CORRECT RESPONSES DURING PERFORM-ANCE-PHASE TRIALS. THE DESIGN FACTORI-ALLY COMPARED ETHNICITY X MODELING OR NONMODELING TRAINING X REPETITION OR NON-REPETITION OF A RULE SUMMARY. DATA INDICATE THAT BOTH MODELING AND REPETI-TION IMPROVE PERFORMANCE. PRIOR MOD-ELING GROUPS REDUCE ERRORS FASTER THAN NONMODELING GROUPS. CONCEPT GENER-ALIZATION IS AIDED BY MODELING AND BY REPETITION WHICH MAINLY DETERMINE LATER VERBALIZATION OF THE ROLE. ALTHOUGH AA SURPASS MA PUPILS, THE PATTERN OF RE-SULTS IS SIMILAR FOR BOTH SAMPLES. ETHNIC BACKGROUND DID NOT INTERFERE WITH ANY TREATMENT VARIATION AND THE MA CHIL-DREN SIGNIFICANTLY EXCEEDED THEIR OWN BASELINE SCORES BY TRANSFERRING THE CONCEPT TO THE NEW, GENERALIZED ITEMS. 9 REFERENCES.

ACCN   001715

1993 AUTH   **ZIMMERMAN, I. L., STEINER, V. G., & POND, R. I.**

TITL LANGUAGE STATUS OF PRESCHOOL MEXICAN-AMERICAN CHILDREN—IS THERE A CASE AGAINST EARLY BILINGUAL EDUCATION?

SRCE *PERCEPTUAL AND MOTOR SKILLS, 1974, 38(1), 227-230.*

INDX LINGUISTIC COMPETENCE, LANGUAGE ASSESSMENT, CHILDREN, MEXICAN AMERICAN, BILINGUAL-BICULTURAL EDUCATION, EMPIRICAL, LANGUAGE ACQUISITION, EARLY CHILDHOOD EDUCATION, BILINGUAL

ABST THE ACTUAL ENGLISH AND SPANISH LANGUAGE SKILLS OF YOUNG CHILDREN OF MEXICAN AMERICAN HERITAGE AS THEY RELATE TO PROGRESS MADE IN ENGLISH-LANGUAGE PRESCHOOL PROGRAMS WERE STUDIED. WHEN 253 SUBJECTS FROM A PREDOMINANTLY MEXICAN AMERICAN COMMUNITY WERE EXAMINED FOR LANGUAGE COMPETENCE IN BOTH ENGLISH AND SPANISH UPON ENTERING PRESCHOOL PROGRAMS, A SIGNIFICANT PERCENTAGE PROVED MARKEDLY DEFICIENT IN BOTH LANGUAGES. FURTHER, LESS THAN 20% WERE FLUENT IN SPANISH ONLY. NEVERTHELESS, SUCH CHILDREN WERE ABLE TO PROGRESS IN ENGLISH-LANGUAGE PRESCHOOL PROGRAMS. THIS SUGGESTS THAT AN ARBITRARY PLACEMENT OF YOUNG CHILDREN IN BILINGUAL PROGRAMS WITHOUT ADEQUATE PRIOR ASSESSMENT TO DETECT ACTUAL LANGUAGE NEEDS AND COMPETENCIES MAY BE LESS PRODUCTIVE THAN IMMEDIATE ENGLISH INSTRUCTION. 4 REFERENCES. (NCMHI ABSTRACT)

ACCN 001716

1994 AUTH **ZINN, M. B.**

TITL POLITICAL FAMILISM: TOWARD SEX ROLE EQUALITY IN CHICANO FAMILIES.

SRCE *AZTLAN, 1975, 6(1), 13-26.*

INDX SEX ROLES, MEXICAN AMERICAN, FAMILY ROLES, ACCULTURATION, ESSAY, POLITICAL POWER, FAMILY STRUCTURE, CHICANO MOVEMENT, FEMALE

ABST FAMILISM—I.E., CULTURAL AND POLITICAL ACTIVISM INVOLVING THE TOTAL FAMILY UNIT—HAS BEEN A DEFINING FEATURE OF "EL MOVIMIENTO" FOR CHICANO LIBERATION, AND IT HAS ALSO PLAYED AN IMPORTANT ROLE IN TRANSFORMING TRADITIONAL FAMILY AND SEX ROLES IN MEXICAN AMERICAN (MA) CULTURE. THUS, SOME CHANGES IN THE MA FAMILY WHICH WERE ATTRIBUTED TO MODERNIZATION OR ACCULTURATION PROVE, INSTEAD, TO BE A PRODUCT OF FAMILY ACTIVISM. SPECIFICALLY, FAMILISM HAS OPERATED AS A MECHANISM OF CULTURAL RESISTANCE DURING PERIODS WHEN POLITICAL RESISTANCE WAS NOT POSSIBLE. IN THIS WAY, "EL MOVIMIENTO" HAS HAD AN INTEGRATING EFFECT BY GUARDING FAMILY MEMBERS FROM THE OPPRESSION AND HOSTILITIES OF ANGLO SOCIETY. SECONDLY, "EL MOVIMIENTO" HAS HAD A ROLE-EQUALIZING EFFECT WITHIN THE FAMILY BY CHANGING THE STATUS OF MA WOMEN. AS CHICANAS HAVE BECOME INVOLVED IN POLITICAL ACTIVISM WHICH HAS SOUGHT RACIAL EQUALITY, THEY HAVE SIMULTANEOUSLY BECOME MORE AWARE OF THEIR OWN SUBORDINATION TO MEN. THUS, THE WOMEN'S INVOLVEMENT IN "EL MOVIMIENTO" HAS BEGUN TO TRANSFORM PATTERNS OF MALE EXCLUSIVENESS WHILE ALSO FORGING NEW DIRECTIONS FOR ACHIEVING THE GOALS OF "LA RAZA." 37 REFERENCES.

ACCN 001717

1995 AUTH **ZIRKEL, P. A.**

TITL SELF-CONCEPT AND THE "DISADVANTAGE" OF ETHNIC GROUP MEMBERSHIP AND MIXTURE.

SRCE *REVIEW OF EDUCATIONAL RESEARCH, 1971, 41(3), 211-225.*

INDX SELF CONCEPT, PROGRAM EVALUATION, EDUCATION, CULTURAL FACTORS, MEXICAN AMERICAN, CHILDREN, REVIEW, RESEARCH METHODOLOGY, ESSAY

ABST ALTHOUGH THE FINDINGS CONCERNING THE RELATIONSHIP OF SELF-CONCEPT TO ETHNIC GROUP MEMBERSHIP AND MIXTURE MAY SEEM EQUIVOCAL AND INCONCLUSIVE, IT IS SAFE TO SAY AT LEAST THAT ETHNIC GROUP MEMBERSHIP AND MIXTURE MAY EITHER ENHANCE OR DEPRESS THE SELF-CONCEPT OF A DISADVANTAGED CHILD. WHETHER SELF-CONCEPT IS SIGNIFICANTLY AFFECTED DEPENDS TO A LARGE EXTENT ON THE EFFORTS THAT SOCIETY AND THE SCHOOLS EXPEND ON DESEGREGATION AND THE DISADVANTAGED. MEANWHILE, THE "BLACK PRIDE" MOVEMENT AND THE NASCENT MOVEMENTS OF CHICANO, INDIAN, AND PUERTO RICAN POWER INDICATE THAT THE SUPPOSED DISADVANTAGE OF SUCH STUDENTS CAN BE TURNED INTO AN ADVANTAGE—THAT IS, AN ENHANCED SELF-CONCEPT. MOREOVER, WHETHER SUCH PROGRAMS AS BILINGUAL AND BICULTURAL EDUCATION AND BLACK STUDIES CAN USE THE SO-CALLED DISADVANTAGES OF ETHNIC MINORITY PUPILS FOR THEIR SCHOLASTIC SELF-REALIZATION MERITS THE ATTENTION OF SCHOOLMEN AND SCHOLARS ALIKE. 116 REFERENCES.

ACCN 001718

1996 AUTH **ZIRKEL, P. A., & GABLE, R. K.**

TITL THE RELIABILITY AND VALIDITY OF VARIOUS MEASURES OF SELF-CONCEPT AMONG ETHNICALLY DIFFERENT ADOLESCENTS.

SRCE *MEASUREMENT AND EVALUATION IN GUIDANCE, 1977, 10(1), 48-54.*

INDX ADOLESCENTS, CROSS CULTURAL, SELF CONCEPT, CULTURE-FAIR TESTS, EMPIRICAL, TEST RELIABILITY, TEST VALIDITY, PUERTO RICAN-M, POLICY

ABST AN EXAMINATION OF THE TEST-RETEST RELIABILITY AND CONSTRUCT VALIDITY OF FIVE SELF-CONCEPT MEASURES WAS CONDUCTED AMONG 218 7TH AND 8TH GRADE STUDENTS (45 BLACK, 41 WHITE, 132 PUERTO RICAN) FROM INNER-CITY SCHOOLS. THE MEASURES (NONVERBAL, VERBAL, PICTORIAL, AND OBSERVER-RATINGS) WERE ADMINISTERED ON A TEST-RETEST BASIS OVER A 3-WEEK PERIOD. STABILITY RELIABILITIES AND INTERCORRELATION MEASURES WERE COMPUTED TO TEST RELIABILITY AND CONSTRUCT VALIDITY. THE RESULTS INDICATE THAT EVALUATIONS OF SELF-

CONCEPT ENHANCEMENT PROGRAMS FOR DIFFERENT ETHNIC GROUPS SHOULD GIVE CONSIDERABLE ATTENTION TO THE SELECTION OF EVALUATION MEASURES. IN PARTICULAR, THE COMPLEX NATURE OF THE SELF-CONCEPT CONSTRUCT AS WELL AS THE MODERATE CONVERGENCE OF CURRENT MEASURING INSTRUMENTS SUGGEST THE USE OF MULTIPLE EVALUATION MEASURES. STUDENT RESPONSE OR OBSERVER-RATING MEASURES OF SELF-CONCEPT SHOULD NOT BE EMPLOYED WITHOUT EXAMINATION OF CONTENT VALIDITY WITH RESPECT TO IMPORTANT CULTURAL VARIABLES. LANGUAGE OF THE EXAMINER AND EXAMINEE AS WELL AS THE TYPE OF ITEM AND RESPONSE FORMAT SHOULD ALSO BE INVESTIGATED MORE THOROUGHLY. 29 REFERENCES. (JOURNAL ABSTRACT MODIFIED)

ACCN   002596

1997 AUTH   **ZIRKEL, P. A., & GREENE, J. F.**

TITL   THE VALIDATION OF PARALLEL TESTING OF AURAL ABILITY AS AN INDICATOR OF BILINGUAL DOMINANCE.

SRCE   *PSYCHOLOGY IN THE SCHOOLS, 1974, 21(2), 153-157.*

INDX   BILINGUALISM, EDUCATION, LANGUAGE ASSESSMENT, CHILDREN, ABILITY TESTING, EARLY CHILDHOOD EDUCATION, EMPIRICAL, PUERTO RICAN-M, CONNECTICUT

ABST   THE VALIDITY OF THE PICTURE-TYPE PARALLEL TEST OF AURAL ABILITY WAS EVALUATED AS A PRACTICAL CLASSROOM INSTRUMENT TO DETERMINE DEGREE OF STUDENT BILINGUALISM. THE ORAL VOCABULARY SUBTEST (OV) OF THE INTER-AMERICAN TEST OF GENERAL ABILITIES (LEVEL I, ALTERNATE FORMS AG-1-DES AND GA-1-CE) COMPOSED OF 25 MULTIPLE CHOICE PICTORIAL ITEMS WAS ADMINISTERED IN SPANISH AND ENGLISH TO 62 BILINGUAL, 1ST GRADE PUPILS IN A LARGE CONNECTICUT CITY. RESULTS OF OV TESTS WERE COMPARED TO LENGTH OF RESIDENCE IN THE U.S. AND TO THREE CRITERION MEASURES—TEACHER RATINGS, BILINGUAL BACKGROUND SCHEDULE (BBS), AND PARENT RATINGS. THE RELATIONSHIP BETWEEN OV SCORES AND THOSE OF CRITERION INSTRUMENTS WERE EVALUATED USING (1) SIMPLE CORRELATIONS, (2) CANONICAL CORRELATIONS, AND (3) DISCRIMINANT ANALYSIS. OV SCORES CORRELATED SIGNIFICANTLY WITH THE RESULTS OF ALL THREE CRITERION MEASURES. ADDITIONALLY, THE INSTRUMENT WAS ABLE TO DISCRIMINATE SUCCESSFULLY BETWEEN THOSE PUPILS WHO HAD BEEN ON THE MAINLAND MORE OR LESS THAN 4 YEARS. IT IS CONCLUDED THAT PARALLEL TESTING OF AURAL ABILITY IS A PROMISING PRACTICAL TECHNIQUE FOR THE ASSESSMENT OF LANGUAGE DOMINANCE OF SPANISH-SPEAKING STUDENTS IN THE EARLY GRADES. 30 REFERENCES.

ACCN   001720

1998 AUTH   **ZIRKEL, P. A., & MOSES, E. G.**

TITL   SELF-CONCEPT AND ETHNIC GROUP MEMBERSHIP AMONG PUBLIC SCHOOL STUDENTS.

SRCE   *AMERICAN EDUCATIONAL RESEARCH JOURNAL, 1971, 8(2), 253-265.*

INDX   SELF CONCEPT, PUERTO RICAN-M, CHILDREN, EMPIRICAL, CROSS CULTURAL

ABST   ONE HUNDRED TWENTY 5TH AND 6TH GRADERS (61 BOYS, 59 GIRLS) WERE EVALUATED TO DETERMINE: (1) IF DIFFERENCES EXISTED IN THE SELF-CONCEPT OF BLACK, PUERTO RICAN, AND WHITE STUDENTS, AND (2) THE EXTENT TO WHICH THESE DIFFERENCES WERE INFLUENCED BY THE MINORITY OR MAJORITY STATUS OF EACH GROUP WITHIN THE SCHOOL. SUBJECTS WERE DRAWN FROM THREE ELEMENTARY SCHOOLS IN SIMILAR SOCIOECONOMIC SECTIONS OF A LARGE CONNECTICUT CITY. EACH SCHOOL HAD BLACK, PUERTO RICAN, AND WHITE STUDENTS, BUT EACH HAD A DIFFERENT ONE OF THESE GROUPS AS A MAJORITY. 40 STUDENTS WERE SELECTED FROM EACH OF THE THREE SCHOOLS, 20 REPRESENTING THE MAJORITY AND 10 REPRESENTING THE MINORITY. GROUPS WERE MATCHED FOR SEX, SES, AND IQ. THE 42-ITEM COOPERSMITH SELF-ESTEEM INVENTORY WAS ADMINISTERED YIELDING SELF-ESTEEM SCORES AND SELF, SOCIAL-SELF, AND SCHOOL-SELF SUBSCORES. RESULTS SHOW THAT ETHNIC GROUP MEMBERSHIP IN PUBLIC SCHOOL SIGNIFICANTLY AFFECTS THE SELF-CONCEPT OF INDIVIDUAL STUDENTS. THE SIGNIFICANT ETHNIC GROUP DIFFERENCE IS ATTRIBUTABLE TO THE LOWER SELF-CONCEPT OF THE PUERTO RICAN STUDENTS IN THE STUDY. THE SELF-CONCEPT OF THE PUERTO RICAN CHILDREN WAS LOWEST WHEN THEY WERE IN A SCHOOL WITH A WHITE RATHER THAN A BLACK MAJORITY. IT IS THEREFORE CONCLUDED THAT LOWER SELF-CONCEPT IS DUE TO THE TYPES OF ETHNIC GROUPS PRESENT IN A SCHOOL AND NOT TO THE MINORITY-MAJORITY PROPORTION OF THE GROUPS. 55 REFERENCES.

ACCN   001719

1999 AUTH   **ZUNICH, M.**

TITL   PERCEPTIONS OF INDIAN, MEXICAN, NEGRO, AND WHITE CHILDREN CONCERNING THE DEVELOPMENT OF RESPONSIBILITY.

SRCE   *PERCEPTUAL AND MOTOR SKILLS, 1971, 32(3), 796-798.*

INDX   MEXICAN AMERICAN, CROSS CULTURAL, ADOLESCENTS, EMPIRICAL, ATTRIBUTION OF RESPONSIBILITY, SOCIALIZATION, COGNITIVE DEVELOPMENT, CHILDREN, SEX COMPARISON

ABST   FIVE HUNDRED SIXTY-FOUR 6TH GRADE BOYS AND GIRLS (102 AMERICAN INDIAN, 162 MEXICAN AMERICAN, 148 BLACK, AND 152 WHITE) WERE EVALUATED (1) TO TEST THE HYPOTHESIS THAT CHILDREN'S PERCEPTIONS CONCERNING THE DEVELOPMENT OF RESPONSIBILITY ARE INDEPENDENT OF ETHNICITY, AND (2) TO LEARN WHETHER OR NOT THEIR PERCEPTIONS DIFFER FROM THOSE OF MOTHERS. THE 25-ITEM CHILDREN'S RESPONSIBILITY INVENTORY WAS ADMINISTERED TO ELICIT THE AGE AT WHICH SIX TYPES OF RESPONSIBILITY COULD BE ASSUMED: (1) CARE OF CLOTHING; (2) CHILDREN'S RELATIONSHIPS; (3) CLEANLINESS; (4) HOUSEHOLD TASKS; (5) PERFORM-

ANCE OF ACTIVITIES ALONE; AND (6) PLAYING ALONE. FINDINGS INDICATE THAT BOYS BELIEVE THAT CHILDREN ARE ABLE TO ASSUME RESPONSIBILITY EARLIER THAN GIRLS BELIEVE THEY CAN. SUBSTANTIAL AGREEMENT EXISTED BETWEEN THE PERCEPTIONS OF MOTHERS AND THE CHILDREN CONCERNING THE AGES AT WHICH CHILDREN SHOULD ASSUME RESPONSIBILITY. CHI SQUARE ANALYSIS FAILED TO SUPPORT THE STUDY'S HYPOTHESIS, AS ETHNIC DIFFERENCES WERE FOUND TO EXIST IN FIVE OF THE SIX RESPONSIBILITY AREAS. FINDINGS ALSO SUGGEST THAT WITHIN ANY AGE GROUP THERE IS A RANGE OF LEVELS OF MATURITY, AND THESE LEVELS MUST BE TAKEN INTO ACCOUNT IN EVALUATING CHILDREN'S BEHAVIORS. 1 REFERENCE.

ACCN   001721

2000 AUTH   **ZURCHER, L. A.**
TITL   PARTICULARISM AND ORGANIZATIONAL POSITION: A CROSS-CULTURAL ANALYSIS.
SRCE   *JOURNAL OF APPLIED PSYCHOLOGY, 1968, 52(2), 139-144.*
INDX   CROSS CULTURAL, PEER GROUP, MEXICAN AMERICAN, ADULTS, EMPIRICAL, MEXICAN, JOB PERFORMANCE, VALUES, ROLE EXPECTATIONS
ABST   THE STOUFFER-TOBY ROLE CONFLICT SCALE, A MEASURE OF PARTICULARISM (THE VALUE FOR INSTITUTIONALIZED OBLIGATIONS OF FRIENDSHIP), WAS ADMINISTERED TO 230 EMPLOYEES IN 13 BANK BRANCHES IN MEXICO AND THE UNITED STATES. FINDINGS SUPPORT THE HYPOTHESIS THAT FOR BOTH BANK OFFICERS AND LINE EMPLOYEES, MEXICANS ARE SIGNIFICANTLY MORE PARTICULARISTIC THAN MEXICAN AMERICANS, WHO IN TURN ARE SIGNIFICANTLY MORE PARTICULARISTIC THAN ANGLO AMERICANS. THE HYPOTHESIS THAT, BY ETHNIC GROUP, OFFICERS ARE LESS PARTICULARISTIC THAN LINE EMPLOYEES WAS PARTIALLY SUPPORTED. THE CULTURAL DEVELOPMENT OF PARTICULARISM AND THE POTENTIAL IMPACT OF THAT VALUE UPON ORGANIZATIONAL BEHAVIOR ARE DISCUSSED. SOME SUGGESTIONS ARE OFFERED TO MANAGEMENT AND TO RESEARCHERS CONCERNING THE IMPORTANCE OF UNDERSTANDING THE INTERACTIONS AMONG SPECIFIC VALUE ORIENTATIONS AND SPECIFIC ORGANIZATIONAL BEHAVIORS, AND CONCERNING THE IMPLICATIONS OF SUCH INTERACTIONS FOR EMPLOYEE SATISFACTION AND ORGANIZATIONAL INTEGRITY. 24 REFERENCES. (JOURNAL ABSTRACT)

ACCN   001722

2001 AUTH   **ZURCHER, L. A., MEADOW, A., & ZURCHER, S.**
TITL   VALUE ORIENTATION, ROLE CONFLICT AND ALIENATION FROM WORK: A CROSS-CULTURAL STUDY.
SRCE   *AMERICAN SOCIOLOGICAL REVIEW, 1965, 30(4), 539-548.*
INDX   VALUES, ROLE EXPECTATIONS, JOB PERFORMANCE, CROSS CULTURAL, MEXICAN, ADULTS, EMPIRICAL, MEXICAN AMERICAN, ANOMIE, ARIZONA, SOUTHWEST, NEW MEXICO
ABST   ROLE CONFLICT AND ALIENATION SCALES WERE ADMINISTERED TO 38 MEXICAN, 43 MEXICAN AMERICAN, AND 149 ANGLO BANK EMPLOYEES IN ARIZONA AND NORTHERN MEXICO TO CROSS-CULTURALLY TEST THE RELATIONSHIP BETWEEN VALUE ORIENTATION AND JOB SATISFACTION. IT WAS HYPOTHESIZED THAT MEXICANS ARE MORE "PARTICULARISTIC" (I.E., VALUING OBLIGATIONS TO FRIENDS) WHILE ANGLOS ARE MORE "UNIVERSALISTIC" (I.E., VALUING OBLIGATIONS TO SOCIETY); AND SINCE THE BANK IS A UNIVERSALISTIC WORK ORGANIZATION, THEN MEXICANS WOULD BE MORE ALIENATED FROM WORK THAN ANGLOS, AND MEXICAN AMERICANS WOULD BE IN AN INTERMEDIATE POSITION. THE TEST INSTRUMENTS INCLUDED THE STOUFFER-TOBY ROLE CONFLICT SCALE (A MEASURE OF PARTICULARISM) AND THE PEARLIN ALIENATION FROM WORK SCALE. RESULTS PARTIALLY SUPPORTED THE HYPOTHESIZED CULTURAL DIFFERENCES. THE MEXICAN EMPLOYEES PROVED TO BE SIGNIFICANTLY MORE ALIENATED FROM WORK THAN THE OTHER TWO GROUPS, HOWEVER THERE WAS NO SIGNIFICANT DIFFERENCE IN JOB ALIENATION BETWEEN THE MEXICAN AMERICAN AND ANGLO EMPLOYEES. IT WAS ALSO DISCOVERED THAT PARTICULARISM AND JOB ALIENATION DECREASE AS (1) LENGTH OF EMPLOYMENT INCREASES, (2) LEVEL OF POSITION INCREASES, (3) JOB SATISFACTION INCREASES, AND (4) PLANS TO CONTINUE WITH THE BANK AS A CAREER INCREASE. 30 REFERENCES.

ACCN   001723

2002 AUTH   **ZUSMAN, M. E., & OLSON, A. O.**
TITL   GATHERING COMPLETE RESPONSE FROM MEXICAN-AMERICANS BY PERSONAL INTERVIEW.
SRCE   *JOURNAL OF SOCIAL ISSUES, 1977, 33(4), 46-55.*
INDX   MEXICAN AMERICAN, MIGRANTS, INDIANA, MIDWEST, FARM LABORERS, SEX COMPARISON, ADULTS, CHILDREN, RESEARCH METHODOLOGY, SURVEY, EMPIRICAL, RURAL, TEST RELIABILITY
ABST   A SURVEY QUESTIONNAIRE REGARDING INDIANA'S MIGRANT EDUCATION PROGRAM WAS ADMINISTERED TO MEXICAN AMERICAN MIGRANT FARM WORKER FAMILIES (95 PARENTS, 71 CHILDREN). AS PART OF THE LARGER STUDY, THIS REPORT EXAMINES THE SUBJECTS' COMPLETENESS OF RESPONSE IN TERMS OF (1) SAMPLE MORTALITY, (2) ITEM NONRESPONSE, AND (3) DEPTH OF DETAIL TO OPEN-ENDED QUESTIONS. COMPARISONS WERE MADE WITH RESPECT TO SUBJECTS' AGE AND SEX AND TO THE TYPE OF ITEM ADMINISTERED. REGARDING SAMPLE MORTALITY, NO INDIVIDUALS REFUSED TO BE INTERVIEWED. REGARDING ITEM NONRESPONSE, THE NONRESPONSE RATE WAS 3.2 FOR PARENTS AND 2.1 FOR CHILDREN OUT OF 40 ITEMS. OF PARTICULAR IMPORTANCE, YOUNG PARENTS (AGES 26-35) WERE LEAST LIKELY TO RESPOND TO TWO SENSITIVE, OPEN-ENDED QUESTIONS CONCERNING THE QUALITY OF THE MIGRANT EDUCATION PROGRAM. THIS SUGGESTS THAT OLDER RESPONDENTS ARE

MORE WILLING TO DISCUSS SENSITIVE IS-
SUES. WITH RESPECT TO THE DEPTH OF DE-
TAIL GIVEN TO OPEN-ENDED QUESTIONS, PAR-
ENTS WERE WILLING TO PROVIDE ONLY A
MODERATE DEGREE OF DETAIL, ESPECIALLY
FOR PERCEPTUAL/ATTITUDINAL ITEMS. IT IS
CONCLUDED, OVERALL, THAT THE PERSONAL
INTERVIEW WITH THIS POPULATION DOES NOT
GATHER COMPLETE RESPONSES. CONSE-
QUENTLY, SOCIAL ACTION STUDIES WILL BE
MOST SUCCESSFUL IN GENERALIZING ABOUT
MIGRANT FARM WORKERS IF THEY RELY EX-
CLUSIVELY ON DEMOGRAPHIC, FACTUAL DATA;
IF PERCEPTUAL/ATTITUDINAL ITEMS ARE IN-
CLUDED, THERE WILL BE A MUCH GREATER
RISK OF A HIGH RATE OF INCOMPLETE RE-
SPONSE. 13 REFERENCES.

ACCN   001807

NATIONAL UNIVERSITY
LIBRARY   SAN DIEGO
030520